highlights
drugs and
clinical considerations

2 atenolol

ENDO: Increased hypoglycemic response to insulin
GI: *Nausea, diarrhea,* vomiting, mesenteric arterial thrombosis, ischemic colitis
GU: Impotence, decreased libido
HEMA: Agranulocytosis, thrombocytopenia purpura
INTEG: Rash, fever, alopecia
RESP: Bronchospasm, dyspnea, wheezing, pulmonary edema

PHARMACOKINETICS

PO: Peak 2-4 hr; onset 1 hr; duration 24 hr; half-life 6-9 hr; excreted unchanged in urine, feces (50%); protein binding 5%-15%

INTERACTIONS

- Mutual inhibition: sympathomimetics (cough, cold preparations)

...ase: hypotension, bradycardia—...ne, hydrALAZINE, methyldopa, ...m, anticholinergics, digoxin, dilti... verapamil, cardiac glycosides, an...ertensives

...ase: hypoglycemia—insulins, oral ...diabetics

...crease: hypertension amphetamines, ...HEDrine, pseudoephedrine

Decrease: effect—insulin, oral antidiabetic agents, theophylline, DOPamine, MAOIs

Drug/Herb

Increase: atenolol effect—hawthorn

Decrease: atenolol effect—ephedra (ma huang)

Drug/Lab Test

Increase: blood glucose, BUN, K, triglycerides, uric acid, ANA titer

NURSING CONSIDERATIONS

Assess:

- I&O, weight daily; watch for CHF (rales/crackles, jugular vein distention, weight gain, edema)
- Hypertension: B/P, pulse q4hr; note rate, rhythm, quality; apical/radial pulse before administration; notify prescriber of any significant changes (<50 bpm); ECG
- Baselines in renal/hepatic studies before therapy begins

Perform/provide:

- Storage protected from light, moisture; place in cool environment

Evaluate:

- Therapeutic response: decreased B/P after 1-2 wk, increased activity tolerance, decreased anginal pain

Teach patient/family:

- **Not to discontinue product abruptly, taper over 2 wk (angina); to take at same time each day as directed**
- Not to use OTC products unless directed by prescriber
- To report bradycardia, dizziness, confusion, depression, fever
- To take pulse at home; advise when to notify prescriber
- To limit alcohol, smoking, sodium intake
- To comply with weight control, dietary adjustments, modified exercise program
- To carry emergency ID to identify product, allergies, conditions being treated
- To avoid hazardous activities if dizziness is present
- To change position slowly
- That product may mask symptoms of hypoglycemia in diabetic patients
- To use contraception while taking this product, pregnancy category (D)

TREATMENT OF OVERDOSE:

Lavage, IV atropine for bradycardia, IV theophylline for bronchospasm, dextrose for hypoglycemia, digoxin, O_2, diuretic for cardiac failure, hemodialysis

Nurse Alert

Genetic Implications

Life-threatening side effects are emphasized

Nursing considerations provide guidance throughout the nursing process

Mosby's 2013 NURSING DRUG REFERENCE

Mosby's 2013 NURSING DRUG REFERENCE

Linda Skidmore-Roth, RN, MSN, NP
Consultant
Littleton, Colorado

Formerly, Nursing Faculty
New Mexico State University
Las Cruces, New Mexico
El Paso Community College
El Paso, Texas

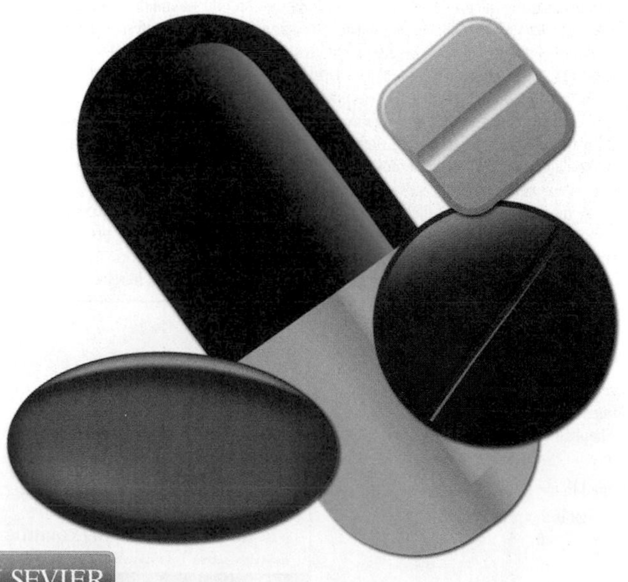

ELSEVIER

ELSEVIER
MOSBY

3251 Riverport Lane
St. Louis, Missouri 63043

MOSBY'S 2013 NURSING DRUG REFERENCE,
TWENTY-SIXTH EDITION

ISBN: 978-0-323-08642-4
ISSN: 1044-8470

Notices

Knowledge and best practice in this field are constantly changing. As new research and experience broaden our understanding, changes in research methods, professional practices, or medical treatment may become necessary.

Practitioners and researchers must always rely on their own experience and knowledge in evaluating and using any information, methods, compounds, or experiments described herein. In using such information or methods they should be mindful of their own safety and the safety of others, including parties for whom they have a professional responsibility.

With respect to any drug or pharmaceutical products identified, readers are advised to check the most current information provided (i) on procedures featured or (ii) by the manufacturer of each product to be administered, to verify the recommended dose or formula, the method and duration of administration, and contraindications. It is the responsibility of practitioners, relying on their own experience and knowledge of their patients, to make diagnoses, to determine dosages and the best treatment for each individual patient, and to take all appropriate safety precautions.

To the fullest extent of the law, neither the Publisher nor the authors, contributors, or editors, assume any liability for any injury and/or damage to persons or property as a matter of products liability, negligence or otherwise, or from any use or operation of any methods, products, instructions, or ideas contained in the material herein.

ISBN: 978-0-323-08642-4

Director, eContent Solutions: Robin Carter
Content Development Specialist:
Shephali Graf
Content Coordinator: Kevin Korinek

Publishing Services Manager:
Pat Joiner-Myers
Senior Project Manager: Joy Moore
Senior Book Designer: Amy Buxton

Printed in the United States of America
Last digit is the print number:
9 8 7 6 5 4 3 2 1

Consultants

Timothy Loren Brenner, PharmD, BCOP
Clinical Pharmacy Specialist
UPMC Cancer Centers
Pittsburgh, Pennsylvania

Claudia Chiesa, PhD, RPh
Staff Pharmacist
Catalina Pharmacy Management Services
Tucson, Arizona

David S. Chun, PharmD
Richmond Heights, Missouri

Shelley Fess, MS, RN, AOCN, CRNI
Assistant Professor of Nursing
Monroe Community College
Rochester, New York

Amanda Gross, RPh
Clinical Pharmacist
University of Colorado Hospital
Aurora, Colorado

Nicholas B. Hampton, PharmD
Clinical Decision Support Pharmacist
BJC HealthCare
St. Louis, Missouri

Joshua J. Neumiller, PharmD, CDE, CGP, FASCP
Assistant Professor
Washington State University
Spokane, Washington

Christopher T. Owens, PharmD, BCPS
Associate Professor and Chair
Department of Pharmacy Practice
Idaho State University College of Pharmacy
Pocatello, Idaho

Adam B. Pesaturo, PharmD, BCPS
Critical Care Pharmacist
Department of Pharmacy Services
Baystate Medical Center
Springfield, Massachusetts

Randolph E. Regal, PharmD, RPh, BS
Clinical Associate Professor
Adult Internal Medicine
University of Michigan Hospitals and College of Pharmacy
Ann Arbor, Michigan

Sheila Seed, PharmD, MPh, RPh
Associate Professor of Pharmacy Practice
Massachusetts College of Pharmacy and Health Sciences–Worcester/Manchester
Worcester, Massachusetts

Travis E. Sonnet, PharmD, FASCP
Clinical Assistant Professor
Washington State University
Spokane, Washington

Patricia Ann Talbert, RN, AAS
Horticulturist, Aromatherapist, Herbalist
Baxter Regional Medical Center
Mountain Home, Arkansas

Shamim Tejani, PharmD
Clinical Pharmacist
Adelante Healthcare
Phoenix, Arizona

Kristin A. Tuiskula, PharmD, RPh
Assistant Professor
Massachusetts College of Pharmacy and Health Sciences
Worcester, Massachusetts

Kristine C. Willett, PharmD
Associate Professor
Massachusetts College of Pharmacy and Health Sciences
Manchester, New Hampshire

Preface

Since the first publication of *Mosby's Nursing Drug Reference* in 1988, more than 100 U.S. and Canadian pharmacists and consultants have reviewed the book's content closely. Today, *Mosby's 2013 Nursing Drug Reference* is more up to date than ever—with features that make it easy to find critical information fast!

NEW FEATURES

- New full-color design to spotlight critical and safety-related information
- More than 20 recent FDA-approved drugs located throughout the book and in **Appendix A** (see Contents for a complete list). Included are monographs for:
  - belatacept (Nulojix)—for kidney transplant rejection
  - indacaterol (Arcapta)—for COPD
  - rilpivirine (Edurant)—for HIV
  - rivaroxaban (Xarelto)—for DVT
- Updated Evolve website

NEW FACTS

This edition features more than 2000 new drug facts, including:

- New drugs and dosage information
- Newly researched side effects and adverse reactions
- New and revised Black Box Warnings
- The latest precautions, interactions, and contraindications
- IV therapy updates
- Revised nursing considerations
- Updated patient/family teaching guidelines

ORGANIZATION

This reference is organized into three main sections:

- Drug categories
- Individual drug monographs (in alphabetical order by generic name)
- Appendixes (identified by the wide, blue thumb tabs on the edge)

The guiding principle behind this book is to provide fast, easy access to drug information and nursing considerations. Every detail—from the paper, typeface, cover, binding, use of color, and appendixes—has been carefully chosen with the user in mind.

INDIVIDUAL DRUG MONOGRAPHS

This book contains monographs for more than 1300 generic and 4500 trade medications. Common trade names are given for all drugs regularly used in the United States and Canada, with drugs available only in Canada identified by a maple leaf ✱.

The following information is provided, whenever possible, for safe, effective administration of each drug:

High-alert status: Identifies high-alert drugs with a label and icon. Visit the Institute for Safe Medication Practices (ISMP) at http://www.ismp.org/tools/highalertmedications.pdf for a list of medications and drug classes with the greatest potential for patient harm if they are used in error.

"Tall Man" lettering: Uses the capitalization of distinguishing letters to avoid medication errors and is required by the FDA for drug manufacturers.

Pronunciation: Helps the nurse master complex generic names.

Rx/OTC: Identifies prescription or over-the-counter drugs.

Functional and chemical classifications: Allows the nurse to see similarities and dissimilarities among drugs in the same functional but different chemical classes.

Do not confuse: Presents drug names that might easily be confused within each appropriate monograph.

Action: Describes pharmacologic properties concisely.

Uses: Lists the conditions the drug is used to treat.

Unlabeled uses: Describes drug uses that may be encountered in practice but are not yet FDA-approved.

Dosages and routes: Lists all available and approved dosages and routes for adult, pediatric, and geriatric patients.

Available forms: Includes tablets, capsules, extended-release, injectables (IV, IM, SUBCUT), solutions, creams, ointments, lotions, gels, shampoos, elixirs, suspensions, suppositories, sprays, aerosols, and lozenges.

Side effects: Groups these reactions by alphabetical body system, with common side effects *italicized* and life-threatening reactions (those that are potentially fatal and/or permanently disabling) in **bold, red type** for emphasis.

Contraindications: Lists conditions under which the drug absolutely should not be given, including FDA pregnancy safety categories D or X.

Precautions: Lists conditions that require special consideration when the drug is prescribed, including FDA pregnancy safety categories A, B, or C.

Black Box Warnings: Identifies FDA warnings that highlight serious and life-threatening adverse effects.

Pharmacokinetics: Outlines metabolism, distribution, and elimination.

Interactions: Includes confirmed drug interactions, followed by the drug or nutrient causing that interaction, when applicable.

Drug/herb: Highlights potential interactions between herbal products and prescription or OTC drugs.

Drug/food: Identifies many common drug interactions with foods.

Drug/lab test: Identifies how the drug may affect lab test results.

Nursing considerations: Identifies key nursing considerations for each step of the nursing process: Assess, Administer, Perform/Provide, Evaluate, and Teach Patient/Family. Instructions for giving drugs by various routes (e.g., PO, IM, IV) are included, with route subheadings in bold.

Compatibilities: Lists syringe, Y-site, and additive compatibilities and incompatibilities. If no compatibilities are listed for a drug, the necessary compatibility testing has not been done and that compatibility information is unknown. To ensure safety, assume that the drug may not be mixed with other drugs unless specifically stated.

"Nursing Alert" icon ⚠: Highlights a critical consideration.

Treatment of overdose: Provides drugs and treatment for overdoses where appropriate.

APPENDIXES

Selected new drugs: Includes comprehensive information on 26 key drugs approved by the FDA during the past 12 months.

Ophthalmic, otic, nasal, and topical products: Provides essential information for more than 140 ophthalmic, otic, nasal, and topical products commonly used today, grouped by chemical drug class.

Vaccines and toxoids: Features an easy-to-use table with generic and trade names, uses, dosages and routes, and contraindications for 39 key vaccines and toxoids.

I am indebted to the nursing and pharmacology consultants who reviewed the manuscript and thank them for their criticism and encouragement. I would also like to thank Robin Carter and Shephali Graf, my editors, whose active encouragement and enthusiasm have made this book better than it might otherwise have been. I am likewise grateful to Joy Moore and Graphic World Inc. for the coordination of the production process and assistance with the development of the new edition.

Linda Skidmore-Roth

FDA pregnancy categories

A	No risk demonstrated to the fetus in any trimester
B	No adverse effects in animals; no human studies available
C	Only given after risks to the fetus are considered; animal studies have shown adverse reactions; no human studies available
D	Definite fetal risks, may be given in spite of risks if needed in life-threatening conditions
X	Absolute fetal abnormalities; not to be used at any time during pregnancy

Note: **UK** = Unknown fetal risk (used in this text but not an official FDA pregnancy category)

Contents

DRUG CATEGORIES, 1

EVOLVE WEBSITE

α-ADRENERGIC BLOCKERS

ACTION: α-Adrenergic blockers act by binding to α-adrenergic receptors, causing dilation of peripheral blood vessels. Lowers peripheral resistance, resulting in decreased B/P.

USES: α-adrenergic blockers are used for benign prostatic hyperplasia, pheochromocytoma, prevention of tissue necrosis and sloughing associated with extravasation of IV vasopressors.

CONTRAINDICATIONS: Hypersensitive reactions may occur, and allergies should be identified before these products are given. Patients with MI, coronary insufficiency, angina, or other evidence of CAD should not use these products.

Administer:

- Starting with low dose, gradually increasing to prevent side effects
- With food or milk for GI symptoms

SIDE EFFECTS: The most common side effects are hypotension, tachycardia, nasal stuffiness, nausea, vomiting, and diarrhea.

PHARMACOKINETICS: Onset, peak, and duration vary among products.

INTERACTIONS: Vasoconstrictive and hypertensive effects of EPINEPHrine are antagonized by α-adrenergic blockers.

POSSIBLE NURSING DIAGNOSES:

- Risk for injury *[adverse reactions]*
- Insomnia *[adverse reactions]*
- Impaired urinary elimination *[uses]*

NURSING CONSIDERATIONS

Assess:

- Electrolytes: K, Na, Cl, CO_2
- Weight daily, I&O
- B/P lying, standing before starting treatment, q4hr thereafter
- Nausea, vomiting, diarrhea
- Skin turgor, dryness of mucous membranes for hydration status

Evaluate:

- Therapeutic response: decreased B/P, increased peripheral pulses

Teach patient/family:

- To avoid alcoholic beverages
- To report dizziness, palpitations, fainting
- To change position slowly or fainting may occur
- To take product exactly as prescribed
- To avoid all OTC products (cough, cold, allergy) unless directed by prescriber

SELECTED GENERIC NAMES

α 1 blockers

silodosin

tamsulosin

ANESTHETICS—GENERAL/LOCAL

ACTION: Anesthetics (general) act on the CNS to produce tranquilization and sleep before invasive procedures. Anesthetics (local) inhibit conduction of nerve impulses from sensory nerves.

USES: General anesthetics are used to premedicate for surgery, induction and maintenance in general anesthesia. For local anesthetics, refer to individual product listing for indications.

CONTRAINDICATIONS: Persons with cerebrovascular accident, increased intracranial pressure, severe hypertension, cardiac decompensation should not use these products since severe adverse reactions can occur.

Precautions: Anesthetics (general) should be used with caution in the geriatric, CVD (hypotension, bradydysrhythmias), renal/hepatic disease, Parkinson's disease, children <2 yr. The precaution for anesthetics (local) is pregnancy.

Administer:

- Anticholinergic preoperatively to decrease secretions
- Only with crash cart, resuscitative equipment nearby

SIDE EFFECTS: The most common side effects are dystonia, akathisia, flexion of arms, fine tremors, drowsiness, restlessness, and hypotension. Also common are chills, respiratory depression, and laryngospasm.

PHARMACOKINETICS: Onset, peak, and duration vary widely among products. Most products are metabolized in the liver and excreted in urine.

INTERACTIONS: MAOIs, tricyclics, phenothiazines may cause severe hypotension or hypertension when used with local anesthetics. CNS depressants will potentiate general and local anesthetics.

POSSIBLE NURSING DIAGNOSES:

General:

- Risk for injury *[adverse reactions]*
- Deficient knowledge *[teaching]*

Local:

- Deficient knowledge *[teaching]*
- Acute pain *[uses]*

NURSING CONSIDERATIONS

Assess:

- VS q10min during IV administration, q30min after IM dose

Perform/provide:

- Quiet environment for recovery to decrease psychotic symptoms

Evaluate:

- Therapeutic response: maintenance of anesthesia, decreased pain

SELECTED GENERIC NAMES (INJECTABLES ONLY)

General anesthetics

droperidol
etomidate
fentaNYL
fentaNYL/droperidol
fentaNYL transdermal
fospropofol
midazolam
propofol
thiopental

Local anesthetics

lidocaine
procaine
ropivacaine
tetracaine

ANTACIDS

ACTION: Antacids are basic compounds that neutralize gastric acidity and decrease the rate of gastric emptying. Products are divided into those containing aluminum, magnesium, calcium, or a combination of these.

USES: Antacids decrease hyperacidity in conditions such as peptic ulcer disease, reflux esophagitis, gastritis, and hiatal hernia.

CONTRAINDICATIONS: Sensitivity to aluminum or magnesium products may cause hypersensitive reactions. Aluminum products should not be used by persons sensitive to aluminum; magnesium products should not be used by persons sensitive to magnesium. Check for sensitivity before administering.

Precautions: Magnesium products should be given cautiously to patients with renal insufficiency and during pregnancy and breastfeeding. Sodium content of antacids may be significant; use with caution for patients with hypertension, congestive heart failure or for those on a low-sodium diet.

Administer:

- Not to take other products within 1-2 hr of antacid administration, since antacids may impair absorption of other products
- All products with an 8-oz glass of water to ensure absorption in the stomach
- Another antacid if constipation occurs with aluminum products

SIDE EFFECTS: The most common side effect caused by aluminum-containing antacids is constipation, which may lead to fecal impaction and bowel obstruction. Diarrhea occurs often when magnesium products are given. Alkalosis may occur when systemic products are used. Constipation occurs more frequently than laxation with calcium carbonate. The release of CO_2 from carbonate-containing antacids causes belching, abdominal distention, and flatulence. Sodium bicarbonate may act as a systemic antacid and produce systemic electrolyte disturbances and alkalosis. Calcium carbonate and sodium bicarbonate may cause rebound hyperacidity and milk-alkali syndrome. Alkaluria may occur when products are used on a long-term basis, particularly in persons with abnormal renal function.

PHARMACOKINETICS: Duration is 20-40 min. If ingested 1 hr after meals, acidity is reduced for at least 3 hr.

INTERACTIONS: Products whose effects may be increased by some antacids: quiNIDine, amphetamines, pseudoephedrine, levodopa, valproic acid, dicumarol. Products whose effects may be decreased by some antacids: cimetidine, corticosteroids, ranitidine, iron salts, phenothiazines, phenytoin, digoxin, tetracyclines, ketoconazole, salicylates, isoniazid.

POSSIBLE NURSING DIAGNOSES:

- Constipation *[adverse reactions]*
- Diarrhea *[adverse reactions]*
- Chronic pain *[uses]*

NURSING CONSIDERATIONS

Assess:

- Aggravating and alleviating factors of epigastric pain or hyperacidity; identify the location, duration, and characteristics of epigastric pain
- GI symptoms, including constipation, diarrhea, abdominal pain; if severe abdominal pain with fever occurs, these products should not be given
- Renal symptoms, including increasing urinary pH, electrolytes

Evaluate:

- Therapeutic response: absence of epigastric pain, and decreased acidity

SELECTED GENERIC NAMES

aluminum hydroxide
bismuth subsalicylate
calcium carbonate
magnesium oxide
sodium bicarbonate

ANTI-ALZHEIMER AGENTS

ACTION: Anti-Alzheimer agents improve cognitive functioning by increasing acetylcholine and inhibiting cholinesterase in the CNS. Do not cure condition, but improve symptoms.

USES: Anti-Alzheimer agents are used for the treatment of Alzheimer's symptoms.

CONTRAINDICATIONS: Persons with hypersensitivity reactions should not use these products.

Precautions: Anti-Alzheimer agents should be used cautiously in pregnancy (C), breastfeeding, sick sinus syndrome,

GI bleeding, bladder obstruction, and seizures.

Administer:

- Lowest possible dose for therapeutic result; adjust dose to response

SIDE EFFECTS:
The most common side effects are nausea, vomiting, diarrhea, dry mouth, insomnia, dizziness, as well as urinary frequency, incontinence, and rash. The most serious side effects are seizures and dysrhythmias.

PHARMACOKINETICS:
Onset, peak, and duration vary widely among products. Most products are metabolized in the liver and excreted by the kidneys.

INTERACTIONS:
Increased synergistic reactions may occur with succinylcholine, cholinesterase inhibitors, and cholinergic agonists. There may be a decrease in the action of anticholinergics, and there may be additive effects when used with cholinergic agents.

POSSIBLE NURSING DIAGNOSES:

- Chronic confusion *[uses]*
- Deficient knowledge *[teaching]*
- Noncompliance *[teaching]*

NURSING CONSIDERATIONS

Assess:

- B/P, hypotension, hypertension
- Mental status: affect, mood, behavioral changes, depression, confusion
- GI status: nausea, vomiting, anorexia, diarrhea
- GU status: urinary frequency, incontinence

Perform/provide:

- Assistance with ambulation during beginning therapy if dizziness, ataxia occur

Evaluate:

- Therapeutic response: decrease in confusion, improved mood

Teach patient/family:

- To report side effects, adverse reactions to health care provider
- To use exactly as prescribed, at regular intervals
- Not to increase or abruptly decrease dose; serious consequences may result
- That product is not a cure, but relieves symptoms

SELECTED GENERIC NAMES

donepezil
galantamine
memantine
rivastigmine

ANTIANGINALS

ACTION:
Antianginals are divided into the nitrates, calcium channel blockers, and β-adrenergic blockers. The nitrates dilate coronary arteries, causing decreased preload, and dilate systemic arteries, causing decreased afterload. Calcium channel blockers dilate coronary arteries and decrease SA/AV node conduction. β-Adrenergic blockers decrease heart rate so that myocardial O_2 use is decreased. Dipyridamole selectively dilates coronary arteries to increase coronary blood flow.

USES:
Antianginals are used in chronic stable angina pectoris, unstable angina, vasospastic angina. Some (i.e., calcium channel blockers and β-blockers) may be used for dysrhythmias and in hypertension.

CONTRAINDICATIONS:
Persons with known hypersensitivity, increased intracranial pressure, or cerebral hemorrhage should not use some of these products.

Precautions: Antianginals should be used with caution in postural hypotension, pregnancy, breastfeeding, children, renal disease, and hepatic injury.

SIDE EFFECTS:
The most common side effects are postural hypotension, headache, flushing, dizziness, nausea,

edema, and drowsiness. Also common are rash, dysrhythmias, and fatigue.

PHARMACOKINETICS: Onset, peak, and duration vary widely among coronary products. Most products are metabolized in the liver and excreted in urine.

INTERACTIONS: Interactions vary widely among products. Check individual monographs for specific information.

POSSIBLE NURSING DIAGNOSES:

- Decreased cardiac output *[adverse reactions]*
- Risk for injury *[uses]*
- Deficient knowledge *[teaching]*
- Acute pain *[uses]*
- Ineffective cardiac tissue perfusion *[uses]*

NURSING CONSIDERATIONS

Assess:

- Orthostatic B/P, pulse
- Pain: duration, time started, activity being performed, character
- Tolerance if taken over long period
- Headache, light-headedness, decreased B/P; may indicate a need for decreased dosage

Perform/provide:

- Storage protected from light, moisture; place in cool environment

Evaluate:

- Therapeutic response: decrease, prevention of anginal pain

Teach patient/family:

- To keep tabs in original container
- Not to use OTC products unless directed by prescriber
- To report bradycardia, dizziness, confusion, depression, fever
- To take pulse at home, advise when to notify prescriber
- To avoid alcohol, smoking, sodium intake
- To comply with weight control, dietary adjustments, modified exercise program
- To carry emergency ID to identify product that you are taking, allergies
- To make position changes slowly to prevent fainting

SELECTED GENERIC NAMES

Nitrates

isosorbide
nitroglycerin

β-Adrenergic blockers

atenolol
dipyridamole
metoprolol
nadolol
propranolol

Calcium channel blockers

amlodipine
diltiazem
niCARdipine
NIFEdipine
verapamil

Miscellaneous

ranolazine

ANTIANXIETY AGENTS

ACTION: Benzodiazepines potentiate the action of GABA, including any other inhibitory transmitters in the CNS resulting in decreased anxiety. Most agents cause a decrease in CNS excitability.

USES: Anxiety is relieved in conditions such as generalized anxiety disorder and phobic disorders. Benzodiazepines are also used for acute alcohol withdrawal to prevent delirium tremens, and some products are used for relaxation before surgery.

CONTRAINDICATIONS: These products are contraindicated in hypersensitivity, acute closed-angle glaucoma, children <6 mo, hepatic disease (clonazepam), and breastfeeding (diazepam). **Precautions:** Antianxiety agents should be used cautiously in geriatric or debilitated patients. Usually smaller doses are needed since metabolism is slowed. Persons with renal/hepatic disease may show delayed excretion. ClonazePAM may increase the incidence of seizures.

Administer:

- With food or milk for GI symptoms; may give crushed if patient is unable to swallow whole (tabs only, no controlled- or sustained-release products)

SIDE EFFECTS: The most common side effects are dizziness, drowsiness, blurred vision, and orthostatic hypotension. Most adverse reactions are mediated through the CNS. There is the potential for abuse and physical dependence with some products.

PHARMACOKINETICS: Most of these agents are metabolized by the liver and excreted via the kidneys.

INTERACTIONS: Increased CNS depression may occur when given with other CNS depressants. These products should be used together cautiously. Alcohol should not be used, as fatal reactions have occurred. The serum concentration and toxicity may be increased when used with benzodiazepines.

POSSIBLE NURSING DIAGNOSES:

- Anxiety *[uses]*
- Risk for injury *[adverse reactions]*
- Deficient knowledge *[teaching]*

NURSING CONSIDERATIONS

Assess:

- B/P (lying and standing), pulse; if systolic B/P drops 20 mm Hg, hold product and notify prescriber; orthostatic hypotension can be severe
- Hepatic/renal studies: AST, ALT, bilirubin, creatinine, LDH, alk phos
- Physical dependency and withdrawal with some products, including headache, nausea, vomiting, muscle pain, and weakness after long-term use

Evaluate:

- Therapeutic response: decreased anxiety, increased relaxation

Teach patient/family:

- That product should not be used for everyday stress or long-term use; not to take more than prescribed amount since product is habit forming
- To avoid driving and activities that require alertness since drowsiness and dizziness may occur
- To abstain from alcohol, other psychotropic medications unless directed by prescriber
- Not to discontinue abruptly; after extended periods, withdrawal symptoms may occur

SELECTED GENERIC NAMES

Benzodiazepines

ALPRAZolam
chlordiazePOXIDE
clonazePAM
diazepam
LORazepam
midazolam
oxazepam
temazepam
triazolam

Miscellaneous

busPIRone
doxepin
hydrOXYzine
PARoxetine
venlafaxine

ANTIASTHMATICS

ACTION: Bronchodilators are divided into anticholinergics, α/β-adrenergic agonists, β-adrenergic agonists, and phosphodiesterase inhibitors. Also included in antiasthmatic agents are corticosteroids, leukotriene antagonists, mast cell stabilizers, and monoclonal antibodies. Anticholinergics act by inhibiting interaction of acetylcholine at receptor sites on bronchial smooth muscle. α/β-Adrenergic agonists act by relaxing bronchial smooth muscle and increasing diameter of nasal passages. β-Adrenergic agonists act by action on β_2-receptors, which relaxes bronchial smooth muscle. Phosphodiesterase inhibitors act by blocking phosphodiesterase and increasing cAMP, which mediates smooth muscle relaxation in the respiratory system. Corticosteroids act by decreasing inflammation in the bronchial system. Leukotriene receptor antagonists decrease leukotrienes, and mast cell stabilizers decrease histamine; both act to decrease bronchospasm.

USES: Antiasthmatics are used for bronchial asthma; bronchospasm associated with bronchitis, emphysema, or other obstructive pulmonary diseases; Cheyne-Stokes respirations; and prevention of exercise-induced asthma. Some products are used for rhinitis and other allergic reactions.

CONTRAINDICATIONS: Persons with hypersensitivity, closed-angle glaucoma, tachydysrhythmias, and severe cardiac disease should not use some of these products.

Precautions: Antiasthmatics should be used with caution in breastfeeding, pregnancy, hyperthyroidism, hypertension, prostatic hypertrophy, and seizure disorders.

Administer:

- Inhaled product after shaking; exhale, place mouthpiece in mouth, inhale slowly, hold breath, remove, exhale slowly
- PO product with meals to decrease gastric irritation

SIDE EFFECTS: The most common side effects are tremors, anxiety, nausea, vomiting, and irritation in the throat. The most serious adverse reactions are bronchospasm and dyspnea.

PHARMACOKINETICS: Onset, peak, and duration vary widely among products. Most products are metabolized by the liver and excreted in urine.

INTERACTIONS: Interactions vary widely among products. Check individual monographs for specific information.

POSSIBLE NURSING DIAGNOSES:

- Activity intolerance *[uses]*
- Ineffective airway clearance *[uses]*
- Risk for injury *[adverse reactions]*
- Deficient knowledge *[teaching]*
- Noncompliance *[teaching]*

NURSING CONSIDERATIONS

Assess:

- Respiratory function: vital capacity, forced expiratory volume, ABGs, lung sounds, heart rate and rhythm, aggravating and alleviating factors

Perform/provide:

- Storage of inhaled product in light-resistant container; do not expose to temps over 86° F (30° C)
- Gum, small sips of water for dry mouth

Evaluate:

- Therapeutic response: decrease severity and number of asthma attacks; absence of dyspnea, wheezing

Teach patient/family:

- To avoid hazardous activities; drowsiness or dizziness may occur with some products
- To obtain blood work as required; some products require blood levels to be drawn
- Avoid all OTC medications unless approved by provider
- To report side effects, including insomnia, heart palpitations, light-headedness; these side effects may occur with some products

SELECTED GENERIC NAMES

Bronchodilators

albuterol
arformoterol
atropine
formoterol

ipratropium
levalbuterol
terbutaline
theophylline
tiotropium

Adrenergics

EPINEPHrine

Corticosteroids

beclomethasone
betamethasone
budesonide
cortisone
dexamethasone
flunisolide
fluticasone
hydrocortisone
methylPREDNISolone
predniSONE
triamcinolone

Leukotriene antagonists

zafirlukast

Mast cell stabilizers

cromolyn

Monoclonal antibodies

omalizumab

ANTICHOLINERGICS

ACTION: Anticholinergics inhibit the muscarinic actions of acetylcholine at receptor sites in the autonomic nervous system. Anticholinergics are also known as antimuscarinic products.

USES: Anticholinergics are used for a variety of conditions: decreasing involuntary movements in parkinsonism (benztropine, trihexyphenidyl); bradydysrhythmias (atropine); nausea and vomiting (scopolamine); and as cycloplegic mydriatics (atropine, homatropine, scopolamine, cyclopentolate, tropicamide). Gastrointestinal anticholinergics are used to decrease motility (smooth muscle tone) in the GI, biliary, and urinary tracts and for their ability to decrease gastric secretions (propantheline, glycopyrrolate).

CONTRAINDICATIONS: Persons with closed-angle glaucoma, myasthenia gravis, or GI/GU obstruction should not use some of these products.

Precautions: Anticholinergics should be used with caution in patients who are geriatric, pregnant, or breastfeeding or in those with prostatic hypertrophy, congestive heart failure, or hypertension; use with caution in presence of high environmental temperature.

Administer:

- Parenteral dose with patient recumbent to prevent postural hypotension
- With or after meals to prevent GI upset; may give with fluids other than water
- Parenteral dose slowly; keep in bed for at least 1 hr after dose; monitor vital signs
- After checking dose carefully; even slight overdose can lead to toxicity

SIDE EFFECTS: The most common side effects are dry mouth, constipation, urinary retention, urinary hesitancy, headache, and dizziness. Also common is paralytic ileus.

PHARMACOKINETICS: Onset, peak, and duration vary widely among products. Most products are metabolized in the liver and excreted in urine.

INTERACTIONS: Increased anticholinergic effects may occur when used with MAOIs and tricyclics and amantadine. Anticholinergics may cause a decreased effect of phenothiazines and levodopa.

POSSIBLE NURSING DIAGNOSES:

- Decreased cardiac output *[uses]*
- Constipation *[adverse reactions]*
- Deficient knowledge *[teaching]*

NURSING CONSIDERATIONS

Assess:

- I&O ratio; retention commonly causes decreased urinary output
- Urinary hesitancy, retention; palpate bladder if retention occurs
- Constipation; increase fluids, bulk, exercise if this occurs
- For tolerance over long-term therapy, dose may need to be increased or changed
- Mental status: affect, mood, CNS depression, worsening of mental symptoms during early therapy

Perform/provide:

- Storage at room temperature
- Hard candy, frequent drinks, sugarless gum to relieve dry mouth

Evaluate:

- Therapeutic response: decreased secretions, absence of nausea and vomiting

Teach patient/family:

- To avoid driving or other hazardous activities; drowsiness may occur
- To avoid OTC medication: cough, cold preparations with alcohol, antihistamines unless directed by prescriber

SELECTED GENERIC NAMES

atropine
benztropine
glycopyrrolate
hyoscyamine
scopolamine (transdermal)
solifenacin

ANTICOAGULANTS

ACTION: Anticoagulants interfere with blood clotting by preventing clot formation.

USES: Anticoagulants are used for deep venous thrombosis, PE, MI, open-heart surgery, disseminated intravascular clotting syndrome; atrial fibrillation with embolization, transfusion, and dialysis.

CONTRAINDICATIONS: Persons with hemophilia and related disorders, leukemia with bleeding, peptic ulcer disease, thrombocytopenic purpura, blood dyscrasias, acute nephritis, and subacute bacterial endocarditis should not use these products.

Precautions: Anticoagulants should be used with caution in alcoholism, geriatric patients, and pregnancy.

Administer:

- At same time each day to maintain steady blood levels
- In abdomen between pelvic bone, rotate sites; do not massage area or aspirate when giving SUBCUT injection; do not pull back on plunger, leave in for 10 sec, apply gentle pressure for 1 min
- Without changing needles
- Avoiding all IM inj that may cause bleeding

SIDE EFFECTS: The most serious adverse reactions are hemorrhage, agranulocytosis, leukopenia, eosinophilia, and thrombocytopenia, depending on the specific product. The most common side effects are diarrhea, rash, and fever.

PHARMACOKINETICS: Onset, peak, and duration vary widely among products. Most products are metabolized in the liver and excreted in urine.

INTERACTIONS: Salicylates, corticosteroids, and nonsteroidal antiinflammatories will potentiate the action of anticoagulants. Anticoagulants may cause serious effects; check individual monographs.

POSSIBLE NURSING DIAGNOSES:

- Risk for injury *[side effects]*
- Deficient knowledge *[teaching]*
- Ineffective cardiac tissue perfusion *[uses]*

NURSING CONSIDERATIONS

Assess:

- Blood studies (Hct, platelets, occult blood in stools) q3mo
- Partial PT, which should be $1^1/_2$-2 × control PPT daily, also APTT, ACT
- B/P; watch for increasing signs of hypertension
- Bleeding gums, petechiae, ecchymosis; black, tarry stools; hematuria
- Fever, skin rash, urticaria
- Needed dosage change q1-2wk

Perform/provide:

- Storage in tight container

Evaluate:

- Therapeutic response: decrease of DVT

Teach patient/family:

- To avoid OTC preparations that may cause serious product interactions unless directed by prescriber
- That product may be held during active bleeding (menstruation), depending on condition
- To use soft-bristle toothbrush to avoid bleeding gums; to avoid contact sports, use electric razor
- To carry emergency ID identifying product taken
- To report any signs of bleeding: gums, under skin, urine, stools

SELECTED GENERIC NAMES

argatroban
dabigatran
desirudin
enoxaparin
fondaparinux
heparin
lepirudin
tinzaparin
warfarin

ANTICONVULSANTS

ACTION: Anticonvulsants are divided into the barbiturates, benzodiazepines, hydantoins, succinimides, and miscellaneous products. Barbiturates and benzodiazepines are discussed in separate sections. Hydantoins act by inhibiting the spread of seizure activity in the motor cortex. Succinimides act by inhibiting spike and wave formation; they also decrease amplitude, frequency, duration, and spread of discharge in seizures.

USES: Hydantoins are used in generalized tonic-clonic seizures, status epilepticus, and psychomotor seizures. Succinimides are used for absence (petit mal) seizures. Barbiturates are used in generalized tonic-clonic and cortical focal seizures.

CONTRAINDICATIONS: Hypersensitive reactions may occur, and allergies should be identified before these products are given.

Precautions: Persons with renal/hepatic disease should be watched closely.

Administer:

- With food, milk to decrease GI symptoms

SIDE EFFECTS: Bone marrow depression is the most life-threatening adverse reaction associated with hydantoins or succinimides. The most common side effects are GI symptoms. Other common side effects for hydantoins are gingival hyperplasia and CNS effects such as nystagmus, ataxia, slurred speech, and mental confusion.

PHARMACOKINETICS: Onset, peak, and duration vary widely among products. Most products are metabolized in the liver and excreted in urine, bile, and feces.

INTERACTIONS: Decreased effects of estrogens, oral contraceptives (hydantoins).

POSSIBLE NURSING DIAGNOSES:

- Injury, risk for *[uses]*
- Noncompliance *[teaching]*

NURSING CONSIDERATIONS

Assess:

- Renal studies, including BUN, creatinine, serum uric acid, urine creatinine clearance before and during therapy
- Blood studies: RBC, Hct, Hgb, reticulocyte counts weekly for 4 wk then monthly
- Hepatic studies: AST, ALT, bilirubin, creatinine
- Mental status, including mood, sensorium, affect, behavorial changes; if mental status changes, notify prescriber
- Eye problems, including need for ophthalmic exam before, during, and after treatment (slit lamp, funduscopy, tonometry)
- Allergic reactions, including red, raised rash; if this occurs, product should be discontinued
- Blood dyscrasia, including fever, sore throat, bruising, rash, jaundice
- Toxicity, including bone marrow depression, nausea, vomiting, ataxia, diplopia, CV collapse, Stevens-Johnson syndrome

Perform/provide:

- Good oral hygiene as it is important for hydantoins

Evaluate:

- Therapeutic response: decreased seizure activity; document on patient's chart

Teach patient/family:

- To carry emergency ID stating products taken, condition, prescriber's name, phone number
- To avoid driving, other activities that require alertness

SELECTED GENERIC NAMES

Barbiturates

PHENobarbital
primidone
thiopental

Hydantoins

fosphenytoin
phenytoin

Miscellaneous

acetaZOLAMIDE
carBAMazepine
clonazePAM
diazepam
ezogabine
felbamate
gabapentin
lacosamide
lamoTRIgine
magnesium sulfate
rufinamide
tiagabine
topiramate
valproate/valproic acid, divalproex sodium
vigabatrin
zonisamide

ANTIDEPRESSANTS

ACTION: Antidepressants are divided into the tricyclics, MAOIs, and miscellaneous antidepressants (SSRIs). The tricyclics work by blocking reuptake of norepinephrine and serotonin into nerve endings and increasing action of norepinephrine and serotonin in nerve cells. MAOIs act by increasing concentrations of endogenous EPINEPHrine, norepinephrine, serotonin, and DOPamine in storage sites in CNS by inhibition of MAO; increased concentration reduces depression.

USES: Antidepressants are used for depression and, in some cases, enuresis in children.

CONTRAINDICATIONS: The contraindications to antidepressants are seizure disorders, prostatic hypertrophy and severe renal/hepatic/cardiac disease depending on the type of medication.

Precautions: Antidepressants should be used cautiously in suicidal patients, severe depression, schizophrenia, hyperactivity, diabetes mellitus, pregnancy, and geriatric patients.

Administer:

- Increased fluids if urinary retention occurs, bulk in diet, if constipation occurs
- With food or milk for GI symptoms

SIDE EFFECTS: The most serious adverse reactions are paralytic ileus, acute renal failure, hypertension, and hypertensive crisis, depending on the specific product. Common side effects are dizziness, drowsiness, diarrhea, dry mouth, urinary retention, and orthostatic hypotension.

PHARMACOKINETICS: Onset, peak, and duration vary widely among products. Most products are metabolized in the liver and excreted in urine.

INTERACTIONS: Interactions vary widely among products. Check individual monographs for specific information.

POSSIBLE NURSING DIAGNOSES:

- Ineffective coping *[uses]*
- Risk for injury *[uses/adverse reactions]*
- Deficient knowledge *[teaching]*

NURSING CONSIDERATIONS

Assess:

- B/P (lying, standing), pulse q4hr; if systolic B/P drops 20 mm Hg, hold product, notify prescriber; take VS q4hr in patients with cardiovascular disease
- Blood studies: CBC, leukocytes, differential, cardiac enzymes if patient is receiving long-term therapy
- Hepatic studies: AST, ALT, bilirubin, creatinine
- Weight q wk; appetite may increase with product
- EPS, primarily in geriatric patients: rigidity, dystonia, akathisia
- Mental status: mood, sensorium, affect, suicidal tendencies, increase in psychiatric symptoms: depression, panic
- Urinary retention, constipation; constipation is more likely to occur in children, geriatric patients
- Withdrawal symptoms: headache, nausea, vomiting, muscle pain, weakness; do not usually occur unless product was discontinued abruptly
- Alcohol consumption; if alcohol is consumed, hold dose until morning

Perform/provide:

- Storage in tight container at room temperature; do not freeze
- Assistance with ambulation during beginning therapy since drowsiness, dizziness occur
- Safety measures including side rails primarily in geriatric patients
- Checking to see PO medication swallowed
- Gum, hard candy, or frequent sips of water for dry mouth

Evaluate:

- Therapeutic response: decreased depression

Teach patient/family:

- That therapeutic effects may take 2-3 wk
- To use caution in driving, other activities requiring alertness because of drowsiness, dizziness, blurred vision
- To avoid alcohol ingestion, other CNS depressants
- Not to discontinue medication quickly after long-term use; may cause nausea, headache, malaise
- To wear sunscreen or wide-brimmed hat since photosensitivity may occur

SELECTED GENERIC NAMES

Tetracyclics
mirtazapine
Tricyclics
amitriptyline
clomiPRAMINE
desipramine
doxepin
imipramine
nortriptyline
Miscellaneous
buPROPion
DULoxetine
trazodone
venlafaxine
SSRIs
citalopram
escitalopram
FLUoxetine
fluvoxamine
PARoxetine
sertraline

ANTIDIABETICS

ACTION: Antidiabetics are divided into the insulins that decrease blood glucose, phosphate, and potassium and increase blood pyruvate and lactate; and oral antidiabetics that cause functioning β-cells in the pancreas to release insulin and improve the effect of endogenous and exogenous insulin.

USES: Insulins are used for ketoacidosis and diabetes mellitus types 1 and 2; oral antidiabetics are used for stable adult-onset diabetes mellitus type 2.

CONTRAINDICATIONS: Hypersensitive reactions may occur, and allergies should be identified before these products are given. Oral antidiabetics should not be used in juvenile or brittle diabetes, diabetic ketoacidosis, or severe renal/hepatic disease.

Precautions: Oral antidiabetics should be used with caution in the geriatric patient, in cardiac disease, pregnancy, breastfeeding, and in the presence of alcohol.

Administer:

- Insulin after warming to room temperature by rotating in palms to prevent lipodystrophy from injecting cold insulin
- Human insulin to those allergic to beef or pork
- Oral antidiabetic 30 min before meals

SIDE EFFECTS: The most common side effect of insulin and oral antidiabetics is hypoglycemia. Other adverse reactions to oral antidiabetics include blood dyscrasias; hepatotoxicity; and, rarely, cholestatic jaundice. Adverse reactions to insulin products include allergic responses and, more rarely, anaphylaxis.

PHARMACOKINETICS: Onset, peak, and duration vary widely among products. Oral antidiabetics are metabolized in the liver, with metabolites excreted in urine, bile, and feces.

INTERACTIONS: Interactions vary widely among products. Check individual monographs for specific information.

POSSIBLE NURSING DIAGNOSES:

- Imbalanced nutrition: more than body requirements *[uses]*

NURSING CONSIDERATIONS

Assess:

- Blood, urine glucose levels during treatment to determine diabetes control (oral products)
- Fasting blood glucose, 2 hr PP (60-100 mg/dl normal fasting level) (70-130 mg/dl normal 2-hr level)
- Hypoglycemic reaction that can occur during peak time

Perform/provide:
- Rotation of inj sites when giving insulin; use abdomen, upper back, thighs, upper arm, buttocks; rotate sites within one of these regions; keep a record of sites

Evaluate:
- Therapeutic response: decrease in polyuria, polydipsia, polyphagia, clear sensorium; absence of dizziness; stable gait

Teach patient/family:
- To avoid alcohol and salicylates except on advice of prescriber
- Symptoms of ketoacidosis: nausea, thirst, polyuria, dry mouth, decreased B/P; dry, flushed skin; acetone breath, drowsiness, Kussmaul respiration
- Symptoms of hypoglycemia: headache, tremors, fatigue, weakness; that candy or sugar should be carried to treat hypoglycemia
- To test urine for glucose/ketones tid if this product is replacing insulin
- To continue weight control, dietary restrictions, exercise, hygiene
- To obtain yearly eye exams

SELECTED GENERIC NAMES

glipiZIDE
glyBURIDE
insulin aspart
insulin detemir
insulin glargine
insulin glulisine
insulin lispro
insulin, regular
insulin, regular concentrated
linagliptin
liraglutide
metformin
miglitol
pioglitazone
repaglinide
rosiglitazone
saxagliptan
sitagliptin

ANTIDIARRHEALS

ACTION: Antidiarrheals work by various actions, including direct action on intestinal muscles to decrease GI peristalsis; by inhibiting prostaglandin synthesis responsible for GI hypermotility; by acting on mucosal receptors responsible for peristalsis; or by decreasing water content of stools.

USES: Antidiarrheals are used for diarrhea of undetermined causes.

CONTRAINDICATIONS: Persons with severe ulcerative colitis, pseudomembranous colitis with some products.

Precautions: Antidiarrheals should be used with caution in the geriatric patient, pregnancy, breastfeeding, children, dehydration.

Administer:
- For 48 hr only

SIDE EFFECTS: The most serious adverse reactions of some products are paralytic ileus, toxic megacolon, and angioneurotic edema. The most common side effects are constipation, nausea, dry mouth, and abdominal pain.

PHARMACOKINETICS: Onset, peak, and duration vary widely among products. Most products are metabolized in the liver and excreted in urine.

INTERACTIONS: Interactions vary widely among products. Check individual monographs for specific information.

POSSIBLE NURSING DIAGNOSES:

- Constipation *[adverse reactions]*
- Diarrhea *[uses]*
- Deficient fluid volume *[adverse reactions]*
- Deficient knowledge *[teaching]*

NURSING CONSIDERATIONS

Assess:

- Electrolytes (K, Na, Cl) if on long-term therapy
- Bowel pattern before; for rebound constipation after termination of medication
- Response after 48 hr; if no response, product should be discontinued
- Dehydration in children

Evaluate:

- Therapeutic response: decreased diarrhea

Teach patient/family:

- To avoid OTC products
- Not to exceed recommended dose

SELECTED GENERIC NAMES

bismuth subsalicylate
loperamide

ANTIDYSRHYTHMICS

ACTION: Antidysrhythmics are divided into four classes and miscellaneous antidysrhythmics:

- Class I increases the duration of action potential and effective refractory period and reduces disparity in the refractory period between a normal and infarcted myocardium; further subclasses include Ia, Ib, Ic
- Class II decreases the rate of SA node discharge, increases recovery time, slows conduction through the AV node, and decreases heart rate, which decreases O_2 consumption in the myocardium
- Class III increases the duration of action potential and the effective refractory period
- Class IV inhibits calcium ion influx across the cell membrane during cardiac depolarization; decreases SA node discharge; decreases conduction velocity through the AV node
- Miscellaneous antidysrhythmics include those such as adenosine, which slows conduction through the AV node, and digoxin, which decreases conduction velocity and prolongs the effective refractory period in the AV node

USES: Antidysrhythmics are used for PVCs, tachycardia, hypertension, atrial fibrillation, angina pectoris.

CONTRAINDICATIONS: Contraindications vary widely among products.

Precautions: Precautions vary widely among products.

SIDE EFFECTS: Side effects and adverse reactions vary widely among products.

PHARMACOKINETICS: Onset, peak, and duration vary widely among products.

INTERACTIONS: Interactions vary widely among products. Check individual monographs for specific information.

POSSIBLE NURSING DIAGNOSES:

- Decreased cardiac output *[uses]*
- Diarrhea *[adverse reactions]*
- Impaired gas exchange *[adverse reactions]*
- Ineffective cardiac tissue perfusion *[uses]*

NURSING CONSIDERATIONS

Assess:

- ECG continuously to determine product effectiveness, premature ventricular contractions, or other dysrhythmias
- IV inf rate to avoid causing nausea, vomiting
- For dehydration or hypovolemia

• B/P continuously for hypotension, hypertension
• I&O ratio
• Serum potassium
• Edema in feet and legs daily

Evaluate:
• Therapeutic response: decrease in B/P in hypertension; decreased B/P, edema, moist crackles in congestive heart failure

Teach patient/family:
• To comply with dosage schedule, even if patient is feeling better
• To report bradycardia, dizziness, confusion, depression, fever

SELECTED GENERIC NAMES

Class I
moricizine
Class Ia
disopyramide
procainamide
quiNIDine
Class Ib
lidocaine
phenytoin
Class Ic
flecainide
propafenone
Class II
acebutolol
esmolol
propranolol
sotalol
Class III
amiodarone
dronedarone
ibutilide
Class IV
verapamil
Miscellaneous
adenosine
atropine
digoxin

ANTIEMETICS

ACTION: The antiemetics are divided into the 5-HT3 receptor antagonists, the phenothiazines, and the miscellaneous products. The 5HT3 receptor antagonists work by blocking serotonin peripherally, centrally, and in the small intestine. The phenothiazines act by blocking the chemoreceptor trigger zone in the brain. The miscellaneous products work by either decreasing motion sickness or delaying gastric emptying.

USES: Antiemetics are used to prevent nausea and vomiting due to cancer chemotherapy, radiotherapy, and surgery (5-HT3 receptor antagonists); some of the miscellaneous products (antihistamines) work by decreasing motion sickness. Most other products are used for many types of nausea and vomiting.

CONTRAINDICATIONS: Persons developing hypersensitive reactions should not use these products.

Precautions: Antiemetics should be used cautiously in pregnancy, breastfeeding, hepatic disease, and some GI disorders.

Administer:
• Prophylactically, before nausea and vomiting occur, in cancer chemotherapy

SIDE EFFECTS: The most common side effects are headache, dizziness, fatigue, and diarrhea.

PHARMACOKINETICS: Onset, peak, and duration vary widely among products. Most products are metabolized by the liver and excreted by the kidneys.

INTERACTIONS: Interactions vary widely among products. Check individual monographs for specific information. Other CNS depressants increase CNS depression.

POSSIBLE NURSING DIAGNOSES:

- Deficient fluid volume *[uses]*
- Risk for injury *[uses, adverse reactions]*
- Deficient knowledge *[teaching]*
- Imbalanced nutrition: less than body requirements *[uses]*

NURSING CONSIDERATIONS

Assess:

- For reason for nausea, vomiting; absence of nausea and vomiting after giving product
- For hypersensitivity reactions: rash, bronchospasm with some products

Perform/provide:

- Storage at room temperature vial/ampules, oral products

Evaluate:

- Therapeutic response: absence or decreasing nausea and vomiting after use

Teach patient/family:

- To avoid hazardous activities if dizziness occurs; ask for assistance if hospitalized
- To rise slowly to prevent orthostatic hypotension
- To teach all aspects of product usage
- Conservative methods to control nausea and vomiting such as sips of water or other fluids and dry crackers

SELECTED GENERIC NAMES

5-HT3 antagonists

dolasetron
granisetron
ondansetron
palonosetron

Phenothiazines

chlorproMAZINE
prochlorperazine
promethazine

Miscellaneous

aprepitant
fosaprepitant
meclizine
metoclopramide
scopolamine
trimethobenzamide

ANTIFUNGALS (SYSTEMIC)

ACTION: Antifungals act by increasing cell membrane permeability in susceptible organisms by binding sterols and decreasing potassium, sodium, and nutrients in the cell.

USES: Antifungals are used for infections of histoplasmosis, blastomycosis, coccidioidomycosis, cryptococcosis, aspergillosis, phycomycosis, candidiasis, sporotrichosis causing severe meningitis, septicemia, and skin infections.

CONTRAINDICATIONS: Persons with severe bone depression or hypersensitivity should not use these products.

Precautions: Antifungals should be used with caution in renal/hepatic disease and pregnancy.

Administer:

- IV using in-line filter (mean pore diameter >1 μm) using distal veins; check for extravasation, necrosis q8hr
- Product only after C&S confirms organism; make sure product is used in life-threatening infections

SIDE EFFECTS: The most serious adverse reactions include renal tubular acidosis, permanent renal impairment, anuria, oliguria, hemorrhagic gastroenteritis, acute hepatic failure, and blood dyscrasias. Some common side effects include hypokalemia, nausea, vomiting, anorexia, headache, fever, and chills.

PHARMACOKINETICS: Onset, peak, and duration vary widely among products. Most products are metabolized in the liver and excreted in urine.

INTERACTIONS: Interactions vary widely among products. Check individual monographs for specific information.

POSSIBLE NURSING DIAGNOSES:

- Risk for infection *[uses]*
- Risk for injury *[adverse reactions]*
- Deficient knowledge *[teaching]*

NURSING CONSIDERATIONS

Assess:

- VS q15-30min during first infusion; note changes in pulse, B/P
- I&O ratio; watch for decreasing urinary output, change in specific gravity; discontinue product to prevent permanent damage to renal tubules
- Blood studies: CBC, K, Na, Ca, Mg q2wk
- Weight weekly; if weight increases over 2 lb/wk, edema is present; renal damage should be considered
- For renal toxicity: increasing BUN, if >40 mg/dl or if serum creatinine >3 mg/dl; product may be discontinued or dosage reduced
- For hepatotoxicity: increasing AST, ALT, alk phos, bilirubin
- For allergic reaction: dermatitis, rash; product should be discontinued, antihistamines (mild reaction) or EPINEPHrine (severe reaction) administered
- For hypokalemia: anorexia, drowsiness, weakness, decreased reflexes, dizziness, increased urinary output, increased thirst, paresthesias
- For ototoxicity: tinnitus (ringing, roaring in ears), vertigo, loss of hearing (rare)

Perform/provide:

- Protection from light during inf, cover with foil
- Symptomatic treatment as ordered for adverse reactions: aspirin, antihistamines, antiemetics, antispasmodics
- Storage protected from moisture and light; diluted sol is stable for 24 hr

Evaluate:

- Therapeutic response: decreased fever, malaise, rash, negative C&S for infecting organism

Teach patient/family:

- That long-term therapy may be needed to clear infection (2 wk-3 mo depending on type of infection)

SELECTED GENERIC NAMES

amphotericin B
anidulafungin
caspofungin
fluconazole
itraconazole
ketoconazole
micafungin
nystatin
posaconazole
voriconazole

ANTIHISTAMINES

ACTION: Antihistamines compete with histamines for H_1-receptor sites. They antagonize in varying degrees most of the pharmacologic effects of histamines.

USES: Antihistamines are used to control the symptoms of allergies, rhinitis, and pruritus.

CONTRAINDICATIONS: Hypersensitivity to H_1-receptor antagonists occurs rarely. Patients with acute asthma and lower respiratory tract disease should not use these products since thick secretions may result. Other contraindications include closed-angle glaucoma, bladder neck obstruction, stenosing peptic ulcer, symptomatic prostatic hypertrophy, newborns, and breastfeeding.

Precautions: Antihistamines must be used cautiously in conjunction with intraocular pressure since they increase intraocular pressure. Caution should also be used in geriatric patients, those with renal/cardiac disease, hypertension, seizure disorders, pregnancy, and those breastfeeding.

Administer:

• With food or milk to decrease GI symptoms; absorption may be decreased slightly

• Whole (sustained-release tabs)

SIDE EFFECTS: Most products cause drowsiness; however, fexofenadine and loratadine produce little, if any, drowsiness. Other common side effects are headache and thickening of bronchial secretions. Serious blood dyscrasias may occur but are rare. Urinary retention, GI effects occur with many of these products.

PHARMACOKINETICS: Onset varies from 20-60 min, with duration lasting 4-24 hr. In general, pharmacokinetics vary widely among products.

INTERACTIONS: Barbiturates, opioids, hypnotics, tricyclics, or alcohol can increase CNS depression when taken with antihistamines.

POSSIBLE NURSING DIAGNOSES:

• Ineffective airway clearance *[uses]*

NURSING CONSIDERATIONS

Assess:

• I&O ratio; be alert for urinary retention, frequency, dysuria; product should be discontinued if these occur

• CBC during long-term therapy since hemolytic anemia, although rare, may occur

• Blood dyscrasias: thrombocytopenia, agranulocytosis (rare)

• Respiratory status: rate, rhythm, increase in bronchial secretions, wheezing, chest tightness

• Cardiac status: palpitations, increased pulse, hypotension

Perform/provide:

• Hard candy, gum; frequent rinsing of mouth for dryness

Evaluate:

• Therapeutic response: absence of allergy symptoms, itching

Teach patient/family:

• To notify prescriber if confusion, sedation, hypotension occur

• To avoid driving, other hazardous activity if drowsiness occurs

• To avoid concurrent use of alcohol, other CNS depressants

• To discontinue a few days before skin testing

SELECTED GENERIC NAMES

brompheniramine
budesonide
cetirizine
chlorpheniramine
cyproheptadine
desloratadine
diphenhydrAMINE
fexofenadine
levocetirizine
loratadine
promethazine

ANTIHYPERTENSIVES

ACTION: Antihypertensives are divided into angiotensin-converting enzyme (ACE) inhibitors, β-adrenergic blockers, calcium channel blockers, centrally acting adrenergics, diuretics, peripherally acting antiadrenergics, and vasodilators. β-Blockers, calcium channel blockers, and diuretics are discussed in separate sections. Angiotensin-converting enzyme inhibitors act by selectively suppressing renin-angiotensin I to angiotensin II; dilation of arterial and venous vessels occurs. Centrally acting adrenergics act by inhibiting the sympathetic vasomotor center in the CNS that reduces impulses in the sympathetic nervous system; B/P, pulse rate, and cardiac output decrease. Peripherally acting antiadrenergics inhibit sympathetic vasoconstriction by inhibiting release of norepinephrine and/or depleting norepinephrine stores in adrenergic nerve endings. Vasodilators act on arteriolar smooth muscle by producing direct relaxation or vasodilation; a reduction in B/P, with concomitant increases in heart rate and cardiac output, occurs.

USES: Antihypertensives are used for hypertension. Some products are used for heart failure not responsive to conventional therapy. Some products are used in hypertensive crisis, angina, and for some cardiac dysrhythmias.

CONTRAINDICATIONS: Hypersensitive reactions may occur, and allergies should be identified before these products are given. Antihypertensives should not be used in children or in patients with heart block.

Precautions: Antihypertensives should be used with caution in geriatric and dialysis patients and in the presence of hypovolemia, leukemia, and electrolyte imbalances.

SIDE EFFECTS: The most common side effects are hypotension, bradycardia, tachycardia, headache, nausea, and vomiting. Side effects and adverse reactions may vary widely between classes and specific products.

PHARMACOKINETICS: Onset, peak, and duration vary widely among products. Most products are metabolized in the liver, with metabolites excreted in urine, bile, and feces.

INTERACTIONS: Interactions vary widely among products. Check individual monographs for specific information.

POSSIBLE NURSING DIAGNOSES:

- Decreased cardiac output *[uses]*
- Diarrhea *[adverse reactions]*
- Impaired gas exchange *[adverse reactions]*
- Ineffective cardiac tissue perfusion *[uses]*

NURSING CONSIDERATIONS

Assess:

- Blood studies: neutrophil; decreased platelets occur with many of the products
- Renal studies: protein, BUN, creatinine; watch for increased levels that may indicate nephrotic syndrome; obtain baselines in renal and hepatic function studies before beginning treatment
- Edema in feet and legs daily
- Allergic reaction, including rash, fever, pruritus, urticaria: product should be discontinued if antihistamines fail to help
- Symptoms of congestive heart failure: edema, dyspnea, wet crackles, B/P
- Renal symptoms: polyuria, oliguria, frequency

Perform/provide:

- Supine or Trendelenburg position for severe hypotension

Evaluate:

- Therapeutic response: decrease in B/P in hypotension; decreased B/P, edema, moist crackles in congestive heart failure

Teach patient/family:

- To comply with dosage schedule, even if feeling better
- To rise slowly to sitting or standing position to minimize orthostatic hypotension

SELECTED GENERIC NAMES

Aldosterone receptor antagonist

eplerenone

Angiotensin-converting enzyme inhibitors

benazepril
enalapril
fosinopril
quinapril
ramipril
trandolapril

Angiotensin II receptor blockers

azilsartan
candesartan
eprosartan
irbesartan
losartan

olmesartan
telmisartan
valsartan

Centrally acting adrenergics
cloNIDine
methyldopa

Peripherally acting antiadrenergics
doxazosin
prazosin
terazosin

Vasodilators
ambrisentan
fenoldopam
hydrALAZINE
minoxidil
nitroprusside

Antiadrenergic combined α-/β-blocker
labetalol

Direct renin inhibitors
aliskiren

ANTIINFECTIVES

ACTION: Antiinfectives are divided into several groups, which include but are not limited to penicillins, cephalosporins, aminoglycosides, sulfonamides, tetracyclines, monobactam, erythromycins, and quinolones. These products act by inhibiting the growth and replication of susceptible bacterial organisms.

USES: Antiinfectives are used for infections of susceptible organisms. These products are effective against bacterial, rickettsial, and spirochetal infections.

CONTRAINDICATIONS: Hypersensitivity reactions may occur. Allergies should be identified before these products are given. Cross-sensitivity can occur between products of different classes (penicillins and cephalosporins). Many persons allergic to penicillins are also allergic to cephalosporins.

Precautions: Antiinfectives should be used with caution in persons with renal/hepatic disease.

Administer:

- For 10-14 days to ensure organism death, prevention of superinfection
- Product after C&S completed; product may be taken as soon as C&S is drawn

SIDE EFFECTS: The most common side effects are nausea, vomiting, and diarrhea. Adverse reactions include bone marrow depression and anaphylaxis.

PHARMACOKINETICS: Onset, peak, and duration vary widely among products. Most products are metabolized in the liver. Metabolites are excreted in urine, bile, and feces.

INTERACTIONS: Interactions vary widely among products. Check individual monographs for specific information.

POSSIBLE NURSING DIAGNOSES:

- Diarrhea *[adverse reactions]*
- Risk for infection *[uses]*

NURSING CONSIDERATIONS

Assess:

- Nephrotoxicity: increased BUN, creatinine
- Blood studies: AST, ALT, CBC, Hct, bilirubin; test monthly if patient is on long-term therapy
- Bowel pattern daily; if severe diarrhea occurs, product should be discontinued
- Urine output; if decreasing, notify prescriber; may indicate nephrotoxicity
- Allergic reaction: rash, fever, pruritus, urticaria; product should be discontinued
- Bleeding: ecchymosis, bleeding gums, hematuria, stool guaiac daily
- Overgrowth of infection: perineal itching, fever, malaise, redness, pain, swelling, drainage, rash, diarrhea, change in cough, sputum

Evaluate:
• Therapeutic response, including absence of fever, fatigue, malaise, draining wounds

Teach patient/family:
• To comply with dosage schedule, even if feeling better
• To report sore throat, bruising, bleeding, joint pain; may indicate blood dyscrasias (rare)

SELECTED GENERIC NAMES

Aminoglycosides
amikacin
azithromycin
clarithromycin
gentamicin
neomycin
streptomycin
tobramycin

Cephalosporins
cefaclor
cefadroxil
ceFAZolin
cefdinir
cefditoren
cefepime
cefixime
cefotaxime
cefprozil
ceftaroline
ceftibuten
cefuroxime
cephalexin
cephradine

Fluoroquinolones
ciprofloxacin
gemifloxacin
levofloxacin
norfloxacin
ofloxacin

Miscellaneous
adefovir dipivoxil
DAPTOmycin
doripenem
ertapenem
fidaxomicin
meropenem
peginterferon alfa-2a
telavancin
vancomycin

Penicillins
amoxicillin/clavulanate
ampicillin/sulbactam
imipenem/cilastatin
nafcillin
oxacillin
penicillin G benzathine
penicillin G
penicillin G procaine
penicillin V
piperacillin
ticarcillin
ticarcillin/clavulanate

Sulfonamides
sulfasalazine

Tetracyclines
doxycycline
minocycline
tetracycline

ANTILIPIDEMICS

ACTION: Antilipidemics are divided into three categories or subclassifications; HMG-CoA reductase inhibitors (statins), bile acid sequestrants, and miscellaneous products. The HMG-CoA reductase inhibitors work by reduction of an enzyme that is responsible for the beginning step in cholesterol production. Bile acid sequestrants work by binding cholesterol in the GI system. The miscellaneous products work by various actions.

USES: Primary hypercholesterolemia in individuals as an adjunct with other lifestyle changes.

CONTRAINDICATIONS: Persons breastfeeding (some products) or those with hypersensitivity to any product or severe hepatic disease should not take these products. Antilipidemics are identified as pregnancy category X on some products.

Precautions: Some products are identified as pregnancy category C.

Administer:

- As directed by health care provider; times will vary with medication used

SIDE EFFECTS: The most common side effects are headache, dizziness, fatigue, insomnia, peripheral edema, dysrhythmias, sinusitis, pharyngitis, abdominal pain, diarrhea, constipation, flatulence, and back pain.

PHARMACOKINETICS: Pharmacokinetics and pharmacodynamics vary with each product.

INTERACTIONS: Interactions vary widely among products. Check individual monographs for specific information.

POSSIBLE NURSING DIAGNOSES:

- Constipation *[adverse reactions]*
- Diarrhea *[adverse reactions]*
- Deficient knowledge *[teaching]*
- Noncompliance *[teaching]*

NURSING CONSIDERATIONS

Assess:

- Obtain a diet and lifestyle history, including exercise, smoking, alcohol, and stress-related activities

Perform/provide:

- Protection from sunlight and heat

Evaluate:

- Therapeutic response: decrease in triglycerides and LDL cholesterol levels

Teach patient/family:

- All aspects of medication use
- To combine medication with lifestyle changes, including low-cholesterol diet, decreasing LDL in diet; avoid smoking, alcohol, and sedentary daily routine

SELECTED GENERIC NAMES

HMG-CoA reductase inhibitors

atorvastatin
fluvastatin
lovastatin
pitavastatin
pravastatin
simvastatin

Bile acid sequestrants

cholestyramine
colesevelam
colestipol

Miscellaneous

ezetimibe
fenofibrate
fenofibric acid
gemfibrozil
niacin
niacinamide

ANTINEOPLASTICS

ACTION: Antineoplastics are divided into alkylating agents, antimetabolites, antibiotic agents, hormonal agents, and miscellaneous agents. Alkylating agents act by cross-linking strands of DNA. Antimetabolites act by inhibiting DNA synthesis. Antibiotic agents act by inhibiting RNA synthesis and by delaying or inhibiting mitosis. Hormones alter the effects of androgens, luteinizing hormone, follicle-stimulating hormone, and estrogen by changing the hormonal environment.

USES: Antineoplastics uses vary widely among products and classes of products. They are used to treat leukemia, Hodgkin's disease, lymphomas, and other tumors throughout the body.

CONTRAINDICATIONS: Hypersensitive reactions may occur, and allergies should be identified before these products are given. Also, persons with severe hepatic/renal disease should not use these products unless the benefits outweigh the risks.

Precautions: Persons with bleeding, severe bone marrow depression, or renal/hepatic disease should be watched closely.

Administer:

- Checking IV site for irritation; phlebitis
- EPINEPHrine for hypersensitivity reaction
- Antibiotics for prophylaxis of infection

SIDE EFFECTS: Most products cause thrombocytopenia, leukopenia, and anemia. If these reactions occur, the product may have to be stopped until the problem is corrected. Other side effects include nausea, vomiting, glossitis, and hair loss. Some products also cause hepatotoxicity, nephrotoxicity, and cardiotoxicity.

PHARMACOKINETICS: Onset, peak, and duration vary widely among products. Most products cross the placenta and are excreted in breast milk and in urine.

INTERACTIONS: Toxicity may occur when used with other antineoplastics or radiation.

POSSIBLE NURSING DIAGNOSES:

- Risk for infection *[adverse reactions]*
- Imbalanced nutrition: less than body requirements *[adverse reactions]*
- Impaired oral mucous membrane *[adverse reactions]*

NURSING CONSIDERATIONS

Assess:

- CBC, differential, platelet count weekly; withhold product if WBC is $<4000/mm^3$ or platelet count is $<75{,}000/mm^3$; notify prescriber of results
- Renal function studies: BUN, creatinine, serum uric acid, and urine CCr before and during therapy
- I&O ratio; report fall in urine output of 30 ml/hr
- Monitor temp q4hr (may indicate beginning infection)
- LFTs before and during therapy (bilirubin, AST, ALT, LDH), monthly, or as needed
- Bleeding, including hematuria, guaiac, bruising or petechiae, mucosa, or orifices q8hr; obtain prescription for viscous Xylocaine (lidocaine)
- Yellowing of skin, sclera, dark urine, clay-colored stools, itchy skin, abdominal pain, fever, diarrhea
- Edema in feet, joint pain, stomach pain, shaking
- Inflammation of mucosa, breaks in skin

Perform/provide:

- Strict asepsis, protective isolation if WBC levels are low
- Comprehensive oral hygiene, using careful technique and soft-bristle brush

Evaluate:

- Therapeutic response: decreased tumor size

Teach patient/family:

- To report signs of infection, including increased temp, sore throat, malaise
- To report signs of anemia, including fatigue, headache, faintness, SOB, irritability
- To report bleeding; to avoid use of razors or commercial mouthwash

SELECTED GENERIC NAMES

Alkylating agents

bendamustine
busulfan
CARBOplatin
carmustine
chlorambucil
CISplatin
cyclophosphamide

dacarbazine
melphalan
oxaliplatin
Antimetabolites
capecitabine
cytarabine
decitabine
etoposide
fludarabine
fluorouracil
mercaptopurine
methotrexate
pemetrexed
Antibiotic agents
bleomycin
DACTINomycin
DAUNOrubicin
DOXOrubicin
epirubicin
mitomycin
mitoxantrone
Hormonal agents
estramustine
flutamide
fulvestrant
goserelin
irinotecan
leuprolide
megestrol
nilutamide
tamoxifen
topotecan
Miscellaneous
alemtuzumab
anastrozole
asparaginase
azacitidine
bortezomib
brentuximab
cabazitaxel
cetuximab
crizotinib
dasatinib
eribulin
erlotinib
gemcitabine
ibritumomab
imatinib
interferon alfa-2a
interferon alfa-2b
ipilimumab
irinotecan
ixabepilone
lapatinib
nilotinib
panitumumab
procarbazine
ranibizumab
riTUXimab
sipuleucel-T
sunitinib
vinBLAStine
vinCRIStine
vinorelbine

ANTIPARKINSON AGENTS

ACTION: Antiparkinson agents are divided into cholinergics, DOPamine, and monoamine oxidase type B agonists. Cholinergics work by blocking or competing at central acetylcholine receptors. DOPamine agonists work by decarboxylation to DOPamine or by activation of dopamine receptors. Monoamine oxidase type B inhibitors work by increasing dopamine activity by inhibiting MAO type B activity.

USES: Antiparkinson agents are used alone or in combination for patients with Parkinson's disease.

CONTRAINDICATIONS: Persons with hypersensitivity, closed-angle glaucoma, and undiagnosed skin lesions should not use these products.

Precautions: Antiparkinson agents should be used with caution in pregnancy, breastfeeding, children, renal/cardiac/hepatic disease, and affective disorder.

Administer:

- Product up until NPO before surgery
- Dosage adjustment depending on patient response
- With meals; limit protein taken with drug
- Only after MAOIs have been discontinued for 2 wk

SIDE EFFECTS: Side effects and adverse reactions vary widely among products. The most common side effects include involuntary movements, headache, numbness, insomnia, nightmares, nausea, vomiting, dry mouth, and orthostatic hypotension.

PHARMACOKINETICS: Onset, peak, and duration vary widely among products. Most products are metabolized in the liver and excreted in urine.

INTERACTIONS: Interactions vary widely among products. Check individual monographs for specific information.

POSSIBLE NURSING DIAGNOSES:

- Risk for injury *[uses]*
- Deficient knowledge *[teaching]*
- Impaired physical mobility *[uses]*

NURSING CONSIDERATIONS

Assess:

- B/P, respiration
- Mental status: affect, mood, behavioral changes, depression, complete suicide assessment

Perform/provide:

- Assistance with ambulation, during beginning therapy
- Testing for diabetes mellitus, acromegaly if on long-term therapy

Evaluate:

- Therapeutic response: decrease in akathisia, increased mood

Teach patient/family:

- To change positions slowly to prevent orthostatic hypotension
- To report side effects: twitching, eye spasm; indicate overdose
- To use product exactly as prescribed; if product is discontinued abruptly, parkinsonian crisis may occur

SELECTED GENERIC NAMES

amantadine
benztropine
bromocriptine
carbidopa-levodopa
pramipexole
rasagiline
selegiline
tolcapone

ANTIPLATELETS

ACTION: The antiplatelets are divided into the platelet aggregation inhibitors, platelet adhesion inhibitors, and the glycoprotein IIb, IIIa inhibitors. The platelet aggregation inhibitors work by action on thrombin; the platelet adhesion inhibitors work by inhibition of phosphodiesterase; and the glycoprotein IIb, IIIa inhibitors work by preventing fibrin from binding to glycoprotein IIb, IIIa receptors.

USES: Antiplatelets are used to prevent MI and stroke; other products are used for coronary syndromes.

CONTRAINDICATIONS: Persons developing hypersensitive reactions should not use these products.

Precautions: Antiplatelets should be used cautiously in pregnancy, breastfeeding, and bleeding disorders.

Administer:

• With heparin or other aspirin (some products)

SIDE EFFECTS:
The most common side effects are headache, dizziness, bleeding, and diarrhea.

PHARMACOKINETICS:
Onset, peak, and duration vary widely among products. Most products are metabolized by the liver and excreted by the kidneys.

INTERACTIONS:
Interactions vary widely among products. Check individual monographs for specific information.

POSSIBLE NURSING DIAGNOSES:

• Risk for injury *[uses, adverse reactions]*

• Deficient knowledge *[teaching]*

NURSING CONSIDERATIONS

Assess:

• For reason for use of these products

• For hypersensitivity reactions with some products

• For bleeding from orifices, in stool, urine

• Blood studies: platelets, Hgb, Hct, PT/APTT, and INR

Perform/provide:

• Storage at room temperature vial/ampules, oral products

Evaluate:

• Therapeutic response: absence of MI, stroke or other coronary syndromes

Teach patient/family:

• To avoid hazardous activities if drowsiness, dizziness occurs; to ask for assistance if hospitalized

• About all aspects of product usage

SELECTED GENERIC NAMES

Platelet aggregation inhibitors

cilostazol
clopidogrel
ticlopidine

Platelet adhesion inhibitors

dipyridamole

Glycoprotein IIb, IIIa inhibitors

eptifibatide
tirofiban

ANTIPSYCHOTICS

ACTION:
Antipsychotics/neuroleptics are divided into several subgroups: phenothiazines, thioxanthenes, butyrophenones, dibenzoxazepines, dibenzodiazepines, and indolones and other heterocyclic compounds. Although chemically different, these subgroups share many pharmacologic and clinical properties. All antipsychotics work to block postsynaptic dopamine receptors in the brain that are responsible for psychotic behavior, including hallucinations, delusions, and paranoia.

USES:
Antipsychotic behavior is decreased in conditions such as schizophrenia, paranoia, and mania. These agents are also effective for severe anxiety, intractable hiccups, nausea, vomiting, behavioral problems in children, and for relaxation before surgery.

CONTRAINDICATIONS:
Persons with hepatic damage, severe hypertension or coronary disease, cerebral arteriosclerosis, blood dyscrasias, bone marrow depression, parkinsonism, severe depression, closed-angle glaucoma, children <12 yr, or persons withdrawing from alcohol or barbiturates should not use antipsychotics until these conditions are corrected.

Precautions: Caution must be used when antipsychotics are given to geriatric patients since metabolism is slowed and adverse reactions can occur rapidly. Hepatic/renal disease may cause poor metabolism and excretion of the product. Seizure threshold is decreased with these products; increases in the dose of anticonvulsants may be required. Persons with diabetes mellitus, prostatic hypertrophy, chronic respiratory disease, and peptic ulcer disease should be monitored closely.

Administer:

- Antiparkinson agent if EPS occur
- Liquid concentrates mixed in glass of juice or cola since taste is unpleasant; avoid contact with skin when preparing liquid concentrate or parenteral medications
- Patient should remain lying down for at least 30 min after IM inj

SIDE EFFECTS:

The most common side effects include EPS such as pseudoparkinsonism, akathisia, dystonia, and tardive dyskinesia, which may be controlled by use of antiparkinson agents. Serious adverse reactions such as hypotension, agranulocytosis, cardiac arrest, and laryngospasm have occurred. Other common side effects include dry mouth and photosensitivity.

PHARMACOKINETICS:

Onset, peak, and duration vary widely with different products and routes. Products are metabolized by the liver, are excreted in urine as metabolites, are highly bound to plasma proteins, cross the placenta, and enter breast milk. Half-life can be extended over 3 days.

INTERACTIONS:

Because other CNS depressants can cause oversedation, these combinations should be used carefully. Anticholinergics may decrease the therapeutic actions of phenothiazines and also cause increased anticholinergic effects.

POSSIBLE NURSING DIAGNOSES:

- Chronic confusion *[uses]*

NURSING CONSIDERATIONS

Assess:

- Bilirubin, CBC, hepatic studies q mo since these products are metabolized in the liver and excreted in urine
- I&O ratio: palpate bladder if low urinary output occurs, since urinary retention occurs with many of these products
- Affect, orientation, LOC, reflexes, gait, coordination, sleep pattern disturbances
- Dizziness, faintness, palpitations, tachycardia on rising
- B/P (lying and standing); wide fluctuations between lying and standing B/P may require dosage or product change since orthostatic hypotension is occurring
- EPS, including akathisia, tardive dyskinesia, pseudoparkinsonism

Perform/provide:

- Supervised ambulation until stabilized on medication; do not involve in strenuous exercise program because fainting is possible; patient should not stand still for long periods
- Increased fluids to prevent constipation
- Sips of water, candy, gum for dry mouth

Evaluate:

- Therapeutic response: decrease in excitement, hallucinations, delusions, paranoia; reorganization of thought patterns, speech

Teach patient/family:

- To rise from sitting or lying position gradually since fainting may occur
- To avoid hot tubs, hot showers, or tub baths since hypotension may occur
- To wear a sunscreen or protective clothing to prevent burns
- To take extra precautions during hot weather to stay cool; heat stroke can occur
- To avoid driving, other activities requiring alertness until response to medication is known
- That drowsiness or impaired mental/motor activity is evident the first 2 wk, but tends to decrease over time

SELECTED GENERIC NAMES

Phenothiazines

chlorproMAZINE
fluphenazine

prochlorperazine
thioridazine
Butyrophenone
haloperidol
Miscellaneous
aripiprazole
asenapine
iloperidone
loxapine
lurasidone
olanzapine
paliperidone
quetiapine
risperidone
ziprasidone

ANTIPYRETICS

ACTION: Antipyretics act on the CNS to control fever and also inhibit prostaglandin production.

USES: Antipyretics are used to decrease fever.

CONTRAINDICATIONS: Persons developing hypersensitive reactions should not use these products.

Precautions: Antipyretics should be used cautiously in pregnancy, breastfeeding, hepatic disease, geriatric patients, and those with certain GI disorders.

Administer:
- Around the clock to keep fever reduced

SIDE EFFECTS: The most common side effects are nausea, vomiting, and rash.

PHARMACOKINETICS: Onset, peak, and duration vary widely among products. Most products are metabolized by the liver and excreted by the kidneys.

INTERACTIONS: Interactions vary widely among products. Check individual monographs for specific information.

POSSIBLE NURSING DIAGNOSES:
- Risk for injury *[uses, adverse reactions]*
- Deficient knowledge *[teaching]*

NURSING CONSIDERATIONS
Assess:
- Temperature frequently
- For reason for use and expected outcome
- For hypersensitivity reactions: rash, bronchospasm with some products

Perform/provide:
- Storage at room temperature

Evaluate:
- Therapeutic response: absence or decreasing fever after use

Teach patient/family:
- All aspects of product usage

SELECTED GENERIC NAMES
acetaminophen
aspirin
choline/magnesium salicylates
choline salicylate
ibuprofen
ketoprofen
magnesium salicylate
naproxen
salsalate

ANTIRETROVIRALS

ACTION: Antiretrovirals act by blocking DNA synthesis.

USES: Antiretrovirals are used for HIV infections and chronic hepatitis C to slow the progression of the disease.

CONTRAINDICATIONS: Persons with hypersensitivity should not use these products.

Precautions: Antiretrovirals should be used cautiously in renal/hepatic disease, pregnancy, and breastfeeding. Protease inhibitors should be used cautiously in diabetes.

Administer:

- In equal intervals around the clock

SIDE EFFECTS:

The most common side effects are nausea, vomiting, anorexia, headache, and diarrhea. The most serious adverse reactions are nephrotoxicity and blood dyscrasias.

PHARMACOKINETICS:

Onset, peak, and duration vary widely among products. Most products are metabolized by the liver and excreted by the kidneys.

INTERACTIONS:

Interactions vary widely among products. Check individual monographs for specific information.

POSSIBLE NURSING DIAGNOSES:

- Risk for infection *[uses]*
- Risk for injury *[adverse reactions]*
- Deficient knowledge *[teaching]*
- Noncompliance *[teaching]*

NURSING CONSIDERATIONS

Assess:

- For signs of HIV infection; increased CD4 counts, decreased viral load; signs of chronic hepatitis C
- Patients with compromised renal system; since product is excreted slowly in poor renal system function, toxicity may occur rapidly

Perform/provide:

- Storage at room temperature

Evaluate:

- Therapeutic response: decreased viral load, increased CD4 count, improvement in the symptoms of HIV/AIDS

Teach patient/family:

- To report sore throat, fever, fatigue; may indicate superinfection
- That medication does not cure condition or prevent infecting others but controls symptoms
- That product must be taken around the clock, in equal intervals, to maintain blood levels for duration of therapy
- To notify prescriber of side effects such as bruising, bleeding, fatigue, malaise; may indicate blood dyscrasias

SELECTED GENERIC NAMES

Nonnucleoside reverse transcriptase inhibitors

delavirdine
efavirenz
etravirine
nevirapine

Nucleoside reverse transcriptase inhibitors

abacavir
didanosine
emtricitabine
lamiVUDine
stavudine
tenofovir
zidovudine

Protease inhibitors

amprenavir
atazanavir
boceprevir
fosamprenavir
indinavir
nelfinavir
ritonavir
saquinavir
tipranavir

Fusion inhibitors

enfuvirtide

Miscellaneous

raltegravir

ANTITUBERCULARS

ACTION:

Antituberculars act by inhibiting RNA or DNA or by interfering with lipid and protein synthesis, thereby decreasing tubercle bacilli replication.

USES:

Antituberculars are used for pulmonary tuberculosis.

CONTRAINDICATIONS: Persons with severe renal disease or hypersensitivity should not use these products.

Precautions: Antituberculars should be used with caution with pregnancy, breastfeeding, and hepatic disease.

Administer:

- For some of these agents on empty stomach, 1 hr before meals (only for isoniazid and rifampin) or 2 hr after meals
- Antiemetic if vomiting occurs
- After C&S is completed; q mo to detect resistance

SIDE EFFECTS: They vary widely among products. Most products can cause nausea, vomiting, anorexia, and rash. Serious adverse reactions include renal failure, nephrotoxicity, ototoxicity, and hepatic necrosis.

PHARMACOKINETICS: Onset, peak, and duration vary widely among products. Most products are metabolized in the liver and excreted in urine.

INTERACTIONS: Interactions vary widely among products. Check individual monographs for specific information.

POSSIBLE NURSING DIAGNOSES:

- Risk for infection *[uses]*
- Risk for injury *[adverse reactions]*
- Deficient knowledge *[teaching]*
- Noncompliance *[teaching]*

NURSING CONSIDERATIONS

Assess:

- Signs of anemia: Hct, Hgb, fatigue
- Hepatic studies q wk: ALT, AST, bilirubin
- Renal status before, q mo: BUN, creatinine, output, specific gravity, urinalysis
- Hepatic status: decreased appetite, jaundice, dark urine, fatigue

Evaluate:

- Therapeutic response: decreased symptoms of TB, culture negative

Teach patient/family:

- That compliance with dosage schedule, duration is necessary
- That scheduled appointments must be kept; relapse may occur
- To avoid alcohol while taking product
- To report flulike symptoms: excessive fatigue, anorexia, vomiting, sore throat; unusual bleeding, yellowish discoloration of skin/eyes

SELECTED GENERIC NAMES

ethambutol
isoniazid
pyrazinamide
rifabutin
rifampin
streptomycin

ANTITUSSIVES/EXPECTORANTS

ACTION: Antitussives act by suppressing the cough reflex by direct action on the cough center in the medulla. Expectorants act by liquefying and reducing the viscosity of thick, tenacious secretions.

USES: Antitussives/expectorants are used to treat cough occurring in pneumonia, bronchitis, TB, cystic fibrosis, and emphysema; as an adjunct in atelectasis (expectorants); and nonproductive cough (antitussives).

CONTRAINDICATIONS: Some products are contraindicated in hypothyroidism, pregnancy, and breastfeeding.

Precautions: Some products should be used cautiously in asthmatic, geriatric, and debilitated patients.

Administer:

- Decreased dose to geriatric patients; their metabolism may be slowed

SIDE EFFECTS: The most common side effects are drowsiness, dizziness, and nausea.

PHARMACOKINETICS: Onset, peak, and duration vary widely among products. Some products are metabolized in the liver and excreted in urine.

INTERACTIONS: Interactions vary widely among products. Check individual monographs for specific information.

POSSIBLE NURSING DIAGNOSES:

- Ineffective airway clearance *[uses]*
- Deficient knowledge *[teaching]*

NURSING CONSIDERATIONS

Assess:

- Cough: type, frequency, character (including sputum)

Perform/provide:

- Increased fluids to liquefy secretions
- Humidification of patient's room

Evaluate:

- Therapeutic response: absence of cough

Teach patient/family:

- To avoid driving, other hazardous activities until patient is stabilized on this medication
- To avoid smoking, smoke-filled rooms, perfumes, dust, environmental pollutants, cleaners that increase cough

SELECTED GENERIC NAMES

acetylcysteine
benzonatate
codeine
dextromethorphan
diphenhydrAMINE
guaiFENesin
HYDROcodone

ANTIVIRALS

ACTION: Antivirals act by interfering with DNA synthesis that is needed for viral replication.

USES: Antivirals are used for mucocutaneous herpes simplex virus, herpes genitalis (HSV-1, HSV-2), varicella infections, herpes zoster, and herpes simplex encephalitis.

CONTRAINDICATIONS: Persons with hypersensitivity or immunosuppressed individuals should not use these products.

Precautions: Antivirals should be used cautiously in renal/hepatic disease, pregnancy, and breastfeeding.

Administer:

- Increased fluids to 3 L/day to decrease crystalluria when given IV

SIDE EFFECTS: The most common side effects are nausea, vomiting, anorexia, headache, and diarrhea. The most serious adverse reactions are nephrotoxicity and blood dyscrasias.

PHARMACOKINETICS: Onset, peak, and duration vary widely among products. Most products are metabolized by the liver and excreted by the kidneys.

INTERACTIONS: Interactions vary widely among products. Check individual monographs for specific information.

POSSIBLE NURSING DIAGNOSES:

- Risk for infection *[uses]*
- Risk for injury *[adverse reactions]*
- Deficient knowledge *[teaching]*

NURSING CONSIDERATIONS

Assess:

- For signs of infection, anemia
- Patients with a compromised renal system; since product is excreted slowly in poor renal system function, toxicity may occur rapidly
- Renal studies: urinalysis, BUN, serum creatinine or decreased CCr may indicate nephrotoxicity; I&O ratio; report hematuria, oliguria, fatigue, weakness; check for protein in the urine during treatment

- C&S before treatment, agent may be taken as soon as culture is taken; repeat C&S after treatment
- Bowel pattern before, during treatment; if severe abdominal pain with bleeding occurs, agent should be discontinued
- Skin reactions: rash, urticaria, itching
- Hepatic studies: AST, ALT
- Blood studies: WBC, RBC, Hct, Hgb, bleeding time; blood dyscrasias

Perform/provide:

- Storage at room temperature for up to 12 hr after reconstitution

Evaluate:

- Therapeutic response: absence or control of infection

Teach patient/family:

- To report sore throat, fever, fatigue; may indicate superinfection
- That medication does not prevent infecting others or cure condition but controls symptoms
- That product must be taken around the clock in equal intervals to maintain blood levels for duration of therapy
- To notify prescriber of side effects such as bruising, bleeding, fatigue, malaise; may indicate blood dyscrasias

SELECTED GENERIC NAMES

acyclovir
amantadine
cidofovir
docosanol
entecavir
famciclovir
foscarnet
ganciclovir
lamiVUDine
maraviroc
oseltamivir
penciclovir
valacyclovir
valganciclovir
zanamivir

β-ADRENERGIC BLOCKERS

ACTION: β-Blockers are divided into selective and nonselective blockers. Selective β-blockers competitively block stimulation of β_1-receptors in cardiac smooth muscle; these products produce chronotropic and inotropic effects. Nonselective blockers produce a fall in blood pressure without reflex tachycardia or reduction in heart rate through a mixture of β-blocking effects; elevated plasma renins are reduced.

USES: β-Blockers are used for hypertension, ventricular dysrhythmias, and prophylaxis of angina pectoris.

CONTRAINDICATIONS: Hypersensitive reactions may occur, and allergies should be identified before these products are given. β-Adrenergic blockers should not be used in heart block, congestive heart failure, or cardiogenic shock.

Precautions: β-Blockers should be used with caution in geriatric patients, or in renal/thyroid disease, COPD, coronary artery disease, diabetes mellitus, pregnancy, and asthma.

Administer:

- PO before meals and at bedtime; tabs may be crushed or swallowed whole
- Reduced dosage in renal dysfunction

SIDE EFFECTS: The most common side effects are orthostatic hypotension, bradycardia, diarrhea, nausea, and vomiting. Serious adverse reactions include blood dyscrasias, bronchospasm, and congestive heart failure.

PHARMACOKINETICS: Onset, peak, and duration vary widely among products. Most products are metabolized in the liver, with metabolites excreted in urine, bile, and feces.

INTERACTIONS: Interactions vary widely among products. Check individual monographs for specific information.

POSSIBLE NURSING DIAGNOSES:

- Decreased cardiac output *[uses]*
- Diarrhea *[adverse reactions]*
- Impaired gas exchange *[adverse reactions]*
- Ineffective cardiac tissue perfusion *[uses]*

NURSING CONSIDERATIONS

Assess:

- Renal studies: protein, BUN, creatinine; watch for increased levels that may indicate nephrotic syndrome; obtain baselines in renal/hepatic function studies before beginning treatment
- I&O, weight daily
- B/P during beginning treatment and periodically thereafter; pulse q4hr, note rate, rhythm, quality
- Apical/radial pulse before administration; notify prescriber of significant changes
- Edema in feet and legs daily

Evaluate:

- Therapeutic response: decrease in B/P in hypertension; decreased B/P, edema, moist crackles in congestive heart failure

Teach patient/family:

- To comply with dosage schedule even if feeling better
- To rise slowly to sitting or standing position to minimize orthostatic hypotension
- To report bradycardia, dizziness, confusion, depression, and fever
- To take pulse at home; advise when to notify prescriber
- To comply with weight control, dietary adjustment, modified exercise program
- To wear support hose to minimize effects of orthostatic hypotension
- Not to discontinue product abruptly; taper over 2 wk; may precipitate angina

SELECTED GENERIC NAMES

Selective β_1-receptor blockers

acebutolol
atenolol
esmolol
metoprolol
nebibolol
β2-receptor blockers
indacaterol

Combined α_1-, β_1-, and β_2-receptor blocker

labetalol

Nonselective β_1- and β_2-blockers

carteolol
nadolol
propranolol
timolol

BONE RESORPTION INHIBITORS

ACTION: Bone resorption inhibitors are divided into biphosphonates and selective estrogen receptor modulators. Biphosphonates act by absorbing calcium phosphate crystals in bone and may directly block dissolution of hydroxyapatite crystals of bone, inhibiting normal and abnormal bone resorption and mineralization. Selective estrogen receptor modulators act by reducing resorption of bone and decreasing bone turnover; medicated through estrogen receptor binding.

USES: Bone resorption inhibitors are used for prevention and treatment of osteoporosis in postmenopausal women, treatment of Paget's disease, and treatment of osteoporosis in men.

CONTRAINDICATIONS: Persons developing hypersensitive reactions or those with hypocalcemia should not use these products.

Precautions: Bone resorption inhibitors should be used cautiously in pregnancy, breastfeeding, hepatic/renal disease, geriatric patients, and some GI disorders.

Administer:

- For 6 months or more in Paget's disease

SIDE EFFECTS:
The most common side effects are nausea, vomiting, headache, bone pain, and rash.

PHARMACOKINETICS:
Onset, peak, and duration vary widely among products. Most products are taken up by the bones and excreted by the kidneys.

INTERACTIONS:
Interactions vary widely among products. Check individual monographs for specific information.

POSSIBLE NURSING DIAGNOSES:

- Risk for injury *[uses, adverse reactions]*
- Deficient knowledge *[teaching]*

NURSING CONSIDERATIONS

Assess:

- For reason for use and expected outcome
- For bone density test; hormonal status (women) before starting treatment and thereafter
- For hypercalcemia: paresthesia, twitching, laryngospasm; Chvostek's, Trousseau's signs

Perform/provide:

- Storage at room temperature

Evaluate:

- Therapeutic response: increase in bone mass, absence of fractures

Teach patient/family:

- To remain upright for at least 30 min after taking, to prevent esophageal irritation
- To teach all aspects of product usage
- To use weight-bearing exercise to increase bone density

SELECTED GENERIC NAMES

Bisphosphonates

alendronate
etidronate
ibandronate
pamidronate
risedronate

Selective estrogen receptor modulators

raloxifene

Monoclonal antibody

denosumab

CALCIUM CHANNEL BLOCKERS

ACTION:
Calcium channel blockers act by inhibiting calcium ion influx across the cell membrane in cardiac and vascular smooth muscle. This action produces relaxation of coronary vascular smooth muscle, dilates coronary arteries, slows SA/AV node conduction, and dilates peripheral arteries.

USES:
Calcium channel blockers are used for chronic stable angina pectoris, vasospastic angina, dysrhythmias, hypertension, and unstable angina.

CONTRAINDICATIONS:
Persons with 2nd-/3rd-degree heart block, sick sinus syndrome, hypotension of <90 mm Hg systolic, Wolff-Parkinson-White syndrome, or cardiogenic shock should not use these products since worsening of those conditions may occur.

Precautions: Congestive heart failure since edema may be increased. Hypotension may worsen since B/P is decreased. Patients with renal/hepatic disease should use these products cautiously since they are metabolized in the liver and excreted by the kidneys.

Administer:

- PO before meals and at bedtime

SIDE EFFECTS:
The most common side effects are dysrhythmias and edema. Also common are headache, fatigue, drowsiness, and flushing.

PHARMACOKINETICS: Onset, peak, and duration vary widely with route of administration. Products are metabolized by the liver and excreted in the urine primarily as metabolites.

INTERACTIONS: Increased levels of digoxin and theophylline may occur when used with these products. Increased effects of β-blockers and antihypertensives may occur with calcium channel blockers.

POSSIBLE NURSING DIAGNOSES:

- Decreased cardiac output *[adverse reactions]*
- Ineffective cardiac tissue perfusion *[uses]*

NURSING CONSIDERATIONS

Assess:

- Cardiac system: B/P, pulse, respirations, ECG intervals (PR, QRS, QT)

Evaluate:

- Therapeutic response: decreased anginal pain; decreased B/P, dysrhythmias

Teach patient/family:

- How to take pulse before taking product; patient should record or graph pulses to identify changes
- To avoid hazardous activities until stabilized on this product since dizziness commonly occurs
- The need for compliance in all areas of medical regimen, including diet, exercise, stress reduction, and product therapy

SELECTED GENERIC NAMES

amlodipine
clevidipine
diltiazem
felodipine
isradipine
niCARdipine
NIFEdipine
verapamil

CARDIAC GLYCOSIDES

ACTION: Cardiac glycosides act by inhibiting sodium and potassium ATPase and then making more calcium available to activate contracted proteins. Cardiac contractility and cardiac output are increased.

USES: Cardiac glycosides are used for congestive heart failure, atrial fibrillation, atrial flutter, atrial tachycardia, and rapid digitalization in these disorders.

CONTRAINDICATIONS: Hypersensitive reactions may occur, and allergies should be identified before these products are given. Also, persons with ventricular tachycardia, ventricular fibrillation, and carotid sinus syndrome should not use these products.

Precautions: Persons with acute MI and those who have or may develop serum potassium, calcium, or magnesium imbalances should use these products cautiously. Also, geriatric patients and those with AV block, severe respiratory disease, hypothyroidism, or renal/hepatic disease should exercise caution when these products are prescribed.

Administer:

- K supplements if ordered for K levels <3 mg/dl

SIDE EFFECTS: The most common side effects are cardiac disturbances, headache, hypotension, and GI symptoms. Also common are blurred vision and yellow-green halos.

PHARMACOKINETICS: Onset, peak, and duration vary widely with the route of administration. Digitoxin is inactivated by the liver, and inactive metabolites are excreted in urine. Digoxin is excreted in urine mainly as the parent product and metabolites.

INTERACTIONS: Toxicity may occur when used with diuretics, succinylcholine, quiNIDine, and thioamines. Increased blood levels may occur with propantheline bromide, spironolactone, quiNIDine, verapamil, aminoglycosides (PO), amiodarone, anticholinergics, and quiNINE. Diuretics may increase toxicity.

POSSIBLE NURSING DIAGNOSES:

- Decreased cardiac output *[adverse reactions]*
- Ineffective cardiac tissue perfusion *[uses]*

NURSING CONSIDERATIONS

Assess:

- Cardiac system: B/P, pulse, respirations, and increased urine output
- Apical pulse for 1 min before giving product; if pulse <60 bpm, take again in 1 hr; if still <60 bpm, notify prescriber
- Electrolytes: K, Na, Cl, Mg; renal function studies, including BUN and creatinine; and blood studies, including AST, ALT, bilirubin
- I&O ratio, daily weights
- Monitor therapeutic product levels

Evaluate:

- Therapeutic response: decreased weight, edema, pulse, respiration; increased urine output

Teach patient/family:

- How to take pulse before taking product; patient should record or graph pulse to identify changes
- To avoid hazardous activities until stabilized on this product, since dizziness commonly occurs
- About the need for compliance in all areas of medical regimen, including diet, exercise, stress reduction, product therapy

SELECTED GENERIC NAME

digoxin

CHOLINERGICS

ACTION: Cholinergics act by preventing destruction of acetylcholine, which increases concentration at sites where acetylcholine is released. This exaggerates the effects of acetylcholine and facilitates transmission of impulses across the myoneural junction. Cholinergics may also act by stimulating receptors for acetylcholine.

USES: Cholinergics are used for myasthenia gravis, as antagonists of nondepolarizing neuromuscular blockade, postoperative bladder distention and urinary distention, and postoperative ileus.

CONTRAINDICATIONS: Persons with obstruction of the intestine or renal system should not use these products.

Precautions: Caution should be used in patients with bradycardia, hypotension, seizure disorders, bronchial asthma, coronary occlusion, hyperthyroidism, breastfeeding, and in children.

Administer:

- Only with atropine sulfate available for cholinergic crisis
- Only after all other cholinergics have been discontinued
- Increased doses if tolerance occurs
- Larger doses after exercise or fatigue
- On empty stomach for better absorption

SIDE EFFECTS: The most serious adverse reactions are respiratory depression, bronchospasm, constriction, laryngospasm, respiratory arrest, seizures, and paralysis. The most common side effects are nausea, diarrhea, and vomiting.

PHARMACOKINETICS: Onset, peak, and duration vary widely among products. Most products are metabolized in the liver and excreted in urine.

INTERACTIONS: Interactions vary widely among products. Check individual monographs for specific information.

POSSIBLE NURSING DIAGNOSES:

- Deficient knowledge *[teaching]*
- Noncompliance *[teaching]*
- Impaired urinary elimination *[uses]*

NURSING CONSIDERATIONS

Assess:

- VS, respiration q8hr
- I&O ratio; check for urinary retention or incontinence
- Bradycardia, hypotension, bronchospasm, headache, dizziness, seizures, respiratory depression; product should be discontinued if toxicity occurs

Perform/provide:

- Storage at room temperature

Evaluate:

- Therapeutic response: increased muscle strength, hand grasp; improved muscle gait; absence of labored breathing (if severe)

Teach patient/family:

- That product is not a cure; it only relieves symptoms (myasthenia gravis)
- To carry emergency ID specifying myasthenia gravis, products taken

SELECTED GENERIC NAMES

bethanechol
neostigmine
physostigmine
pyridostigmine

CHOLINERGIC BLOCKERS

ACTION: Cholinergic blockers inhibit or block acetylcholine at receptor sites in the autonomic nervous system.

USES: Many cholinergic blockers are used to decrease secretions before surgery, to reverse neuromuscular blockade, and to decrease motility of GI, biliary, urinary tracts. Other products are used for parkinsonian symptoms, including dystonia associated with neuroleptic products.

CONTRAINDICATIONS: Hypersensitivity can occur, and allergies should be identified before administering these products. Persons with GI and GU obstruction should not use these products since constipation and urinary retention may occur. They are also contraindicated in closed-angle glaucoma and myasthenia gravis.

Precautions: Caution must be used when these products are given to geriatric patients since metabolism is slowed. Also, persons with tachycardia or prostatic hypertrophy should use these products with caution.

Administer:

- With food or milk to decrease GI symptoms
- Parenteral dose with patient recumbent to prevent postural hypotension; give parenteral dose slowly, monitoring vital signs

SIDE EFFECTS: The most common side effects are dryness of the mouth and constipation, which can be prevented by frequent rinsing of the mouth and by increasing water and bulk in the diet.

PHARMACOKINETICS: Onset, peak, and duration vary with route.

INTERACTIONS: Increase in anticholinergic effect occurs when used with opioids, barbiturates, antihistamines, MAOIs, phenothiazines, and amantadine.

POSSIBLE NURSING DIAGNOSES:

- Impaired physical mobility *[uses]*
- Chronic pain *[uses]*

NURSING CONSIDERATIONS

Assess:

• I&O ratio; be alert for urinary retention, frequency, dysuria; product should be discontinued if these occur
• Urinary hesitancy, retention; palpate bladder if retention occurs
• Constipation; increase fluids, bulk, exercise
• For tolerance over long-term therapy; dose may have to be increased or changed
• Mental status: affect, mood, CNS depression, worsening of mental symptoms during early therapy

Perform/provide:

• Hard candy, gum, frequent rinsing of mouth for dryness

Evaluate:

• Therapeutic response: absence of cramps and EPS

Teach patient/family:

• To avoid driving, other hazardous activities if drowsiness occurs
• To avoid concurrent use of cough, cold preparations with alcohol, antihistamines unless directed by prescriber
• To use with caution in hot weather since medication may increase susceptibility to heat stroke

SELECTED GENERIC NAMES

atropine
benztropine
glycopyrrolate
scopolamine

CORTICOSTEROIDS

ACTION: Corticosteroids are divided into glucocorticoids and mineralocorticoids. Glucocorticoids decrease inflammation by the suppression of migration of polymorphonuclear leukocytes, fibroblasts, increased capillary permeability, and lysosomal stabilization. They also have varied metabolic effects and modify the body's immune responses to many stimuli. Mineralocorticoids act by increasing resorption of sodium by increasing hydrogen and potassium excretion in the distal tubule.

USES: Glucocorticoids are used to decrease inflammation and for immunosuppression. In addition, some products may be given for allergy, adrenal insufficiency, or cerebral edema. Mineralocorticoids are given for adrenal insufficiency or adrenogenital syndrome.

CONTRAINDICATIONS: Hypersensitivity may occur and should be identified before administering. Since these products mask infection, they should not be used in systemic fungal infections or amebiasis. Mothers taking pharmacologic doses of corticosteroids should not breastfeed.

Precautions: Caution must be used when these products are prescribed for diabetic patients since hyperglycemia may occur. Also, patients with glaucoma, seizure disorders, peptic ulcer, impaired renal function, congestive heart failure, hypertension, ulcerative colitis, or myasthenia gravis should be monitored closely if corticosteroids are given. Use with caution in children, the geriatric patients, and during pregnancy.

Administer:

• With food or milk to decrease GI symptoms
• Take single daily or alternate-day doses in the morning before 9 AM (for replacement therapy)

SIDE EFFECTS: The most common side effects include change in behavior, including insomnia and euphoria; GI irritation, including peptic ulcer; metabolic reactions, including hypokalemia, hyperglycemia, and carbohydrate intolerance; and sodium and fluid retention. Most adverse reactions are dose dependent.

PHARMACOKINETICS: For oral preparations, the onset of action occurs between 1 and 2 hr, and duration can be up to 2 days, with a half-life of 2-4 days. Pharmacokinetics vary widely among products. These products cross the placenta and appear in breast milk.

INTERACTIONS: Decreased corticosteroid effect may occur with barbiturates, rifampin, and phenytoin; corticosteroid dose may have to be increased. There is a possibility of GI bleeding when used with salicylates and indomethacin. Corticosteroids may reduce salicylate levels. When using with digoxin, glycosides, potassium-depleting diuretics, and amphotericin, serum potassium levels should be monitored.

POSSIBLE NURSING DIAGNOSES:

- Disturbed body image *[adverse reactions]*
- Risk for infection *[adverse reactions]*
- Risk for suicide *[adverse reactions]*

NURSING CONSIDERATIONS

Assess:

- Potassium, blood glucose, urine glucose while on long-term therapy; hypokalemia and hyperglycemia are common
- Weight daily; notify prescriber of weekly gain >5 lb since these products alter fluid and electrolyte balance
- I&O ratio; be alert for decreasing urinary output and increasing edema
- Plasma cortisol levels during long-term therapy (normal level is 138-635 nmol/L SI units when drawn at 8 AM)
- Infection: increased temp, WBC, even after withdrawal of medication; product masks symptoms of infection
- Adrenal insufficiency: nausea, anorexia, fatigue, dizziness, dyspnea, weakness, joint pain
- Potassium depletion: paresthesias, fatigue, nausea, vomiting, depression, polyuria, dysrhythmias, weakness
- Mental status: affect, mood, behavioral changes, aggression; if severe personality changes occur, including depression, product may have to be tapered and then discontinued

Evaluate:

- Therapeutic response: decreased inflammation

Teach patient/family:

- That emergency ID as steroid user should be carried
- Not to discontinue this medication abruptly; adrenal crisis can result
- All aspects of product use, including cushingoid symptoms
- To take with meals or a snack
- To avoid exposure to chickenpox or measles if taking immunosuppressives

SELECTED GENERIC NAMES

Glucocorticoids

beclomethasone
betamethasone
cortisone
dexamethasone
hydrocortisone
methylPREDNISolone
prednisoLONE
predniSONE
triamcinolone

DIURETICS

ACTION: Diuretics are divided into subgroups: thiazides and thiazide-like diuretics, loop diuretics, carbonic anhydrase inhibitors, osmotic diuretics, and potassium-sparing diuretics. Each one of these subgroups has its own mechanism of action. Thiazides and thiazide-like diuretics increase excretion of water and sodium by inhibiting resorption in the early distal tubule. Loop diuretics inhibit resorption of sodium and chloride in the thick ascending limb of the loop of Henle. Carbonic anhydrase inhibitors increase sodium excretion by decreasing sodium-hydrogen ion exchange throughout the renal tubule. Carbonic anhydrase inhibitors also decrease secretion of aqueous humor in the eye and thus decrease intraocular pressure. Osmotic diuretics increase the osmotic pressure of glomerular filtrate, thus decreasing net absorption of sodium. The potassium-sparing diuretics interfere with sodium resorption at the distal tubule, thus decreasing potassium excretion.

USES:
B/P is reduced in hypertension; edema is reduced in congestive heart failure; intraocular pressure is decreased in glaucoma.

CONTRAINDICATIONS:
Persons with electrolyte imbalances (Na, Cl, K), dehydration, or anuria should not be given these products until the problem is corrected.

Precautions: Caution must be used when diuretics are given to geriatric patients since electrolyte disturbances and dehydration can occur rapidly. Hepatic/renal disease may cause poor metabolism and excretion of the product.

Administer:

- In AM to avoid interference with sleep if using product as a diuretic
- K replacement if K is <3 mg/dl

SIDE EFFECTS:
Hypokalemia, hyperuricemia, and hyperglycemia occur most frequently with thiazide diuretics. Aplastic anemia, blood dyscrasias, volume depletion, and dehydration may occur when thiazide-like diuretics, loop diuretics, or carbonic anhydrase inhibitors are given. Side effects and adverse reactions vary widely for the miscellaneous products.

PHARMACOKINETICS:
Onset, peak, and duration vary widely among the different subgroups of these products.

INTERACTIONS:
Cholestyramine and colestipol will decrease the absorption of thiazide diuretics. Concurrent use of thiazides with diazoxide may increase hyperuricemia, hyperglycemia, and antihypertensive effects of thiazides. Ototoxicity may occur when loop diuretics are used with aminoglycosides. Thiazide and loop diuretics may increase therapeutic and toxic effects of lithium.

POSSIBLE NURSING DIAGNOSES:

- Decreased cardiac output *[adverse reactions]*
- Excess fluid volume *[uses]*

NURSING CONSIDERATIONS

Assess:

- Weight, I&O daily to determine fluid loss; check skin turgor for dehydration
- Electrolytes: K, Na, Cl; include BUN, blood glucose, CBC, serum creatinine, blood pH, ABGs, uric acid, Ca; electrolyte imbalances may occur quickly
- B/P (lying and standing); postural hypotension may occur since fluid loss occurs first from intravascular spaces
- Signs of metabolic alkalosis, including drowsiness and restlessness
- Signs of hypokalemia with some products: postural hypotension, malaise, fatigue, tachycardia, leg cramps, weakness

Evaluate:

- Therapeutic response: improvement in edema of feet, legs, sacral area daily if medication is being used in congestive heart failure; improvement in B/P if medication is being used as a diuretic; improvement in intraocular pressure if medication is being used to decrease aqueous humor in the eye

Teach patient/family:

- To take product early in the day (diuretic) to prevent nocturia

DRUG CATEGORIES

SELECTED GENERIC NAMES

Thiazides
chlorothiazide
hydrochlorothiazide
Thiazide-like
chlorthalidone
indapamide
metolazone
Loop
bumetanide
furosemide
torsemide
Carbonic anhydrase inhibitor
acetaZOLAMIDE
Potassium-sparing
amiloride
spironolactone
Osmotics
mannitol

HISTAMINE H_2 ANTAGONISTS

ACTION: Histamine H_2 antagonists act by inhibiting histamine at the H_2-receptor site in parietal cells, which inhibits gastric acid secretion.

USES: Histamine H_2 antagonists are used for short-term treatment of duodenal and gastric ulcers and maintenance therapy for duodenal ulcer; gastroesophageal reflux disease.

CONTRAINDICATIONS: Persons with hypersensitivity should not use these products.

Precautions: Caution should be used in pregnancy, breastfeeding, child <16 yr, organic brain syndrome, hepatic/renal disease.

Administer:

- With meals for prolonged product effect
- Antacids 1 hr before or 1 hr after cimetidine
- IV slowly; bradycardia may occur; give over 30 min

SIDE EFFECTS: The most serious adverse reactions are agranulocytosis, thrombocytopenia, neutropenia, aplastic anemia, and exfoliative dermatitis. The most common side effects are confusion (not with ranitidine), headache, and diarrhea.

PHARMACOKINETICS: Onset, peak, and duration vary widely among products. Most products are metabolized in the liver and excreted in urine.

INTERACTIONS: Antacids interfere with absorption of histamine H_2 antagonists. Check individual monographs for specific information.

POSSIBLE NURSING DIAGNOSES:

- Risk for injury *[bleeding]*
- Deficient knowledge *[teaching]*
- Chronic pain *[uses]*

NURSING CONSIDERATIONS

Assess:

- Gastric pH (>5 should be maintained)
- I&O ratio, BUN, creatinine

Perform/provide:

- Storage of diluted sol at room temperature for up to 48 hr

Evaluate:

- Therapeutic response: decreased pain in abdomen

Teach patient/family:

- That gynecomastia, impotence may occur but are reversible
- To avoid driving, other hazardous activities until patient is stabilized on this medication
- To avoid black pepper, caffeine, alcohol, harsh spices, extremes in temperature of food
- To avoid OTC preparations: aspirin, cough, cold preparations
- That product must be continued for prescribed time to be effective
- To report bruising, fatigue, malaise; blood dyscrasias may occur

SELECTED GENERIC NAMES

cimetidine
famotidine
ranitidine

IMMUNOSUPPRESSANTS

ACTION: Immunosuppressants act by inhibiting lymphocytes (T).

USES: Most immunosuppressants are used for organ transplants to prevent rejection.

CONTRAINDICATIONS: Products are contraindicated in hypersensitivity.

Precautions: Caution should be used in severe renal/hepatic disease and pregnancy.

Administer:

- For several days before transplant surgery
- With meals for GI upset or product mixed with chocolate milk
- With oral antifungal for *Candida* infections

SIDE EFFECTS: The most serious adverse reactions are albuminuria, hematuria, proteinuria, renal failure, and hepatotoxicity. The most common side effects are overgrowth of oral *Candida,* gum hyperplasia, tremors, and headache. The most serious adverse reactions for azathioprine are hematologic (leukopenia and thrombocytopenia) and GI (nausea and vomiting). There is a risk of secondary infection.

PHARMACOKINETICS: Onset, peak, and duration vary widely among products. Most products are metabolized in the liver and excreted in urine.

INTERACTIONS: Interactions vary widely among products. Check individual monographs for specific information.

POSSIBLE NURSING DIAGNOSES:

- Risk for infection *[adverse reactions]*
- Risk for injury *[uses]*
- Deficient knowledge *[teaching]*

NURSING CONSIDERATIONS

Assess:

- Renal studies: BUN, creatinine at least q mo during treatment, 3 mo after treatment
- Hepatic studies: alk phos, AST (SGOT), ALT (SGPT), bilirubin
- Product blood levels during treatment
- Hepatotoxicity: dark urine, jaundice, itching, light-colored stools; product should be discontinued

Evaluate:

- Therapeutic response: absence of rejection

Teach patient/family:

- To report fever, chills, sore throat, fatigue since serious infections may occur
- To use contraceptive measures during treatment and for 12 wk after ending therapy

SELECTED GENERIC NAMES

azaTHIOprine
basiliximab
cycloSPORINE
everolimus
muromonab-CD3
sirolimus
tacrolimus

LAXATIVES

ACTION: Laxatives are divided into bulk products, lubricants, osmotics, saline laxative stimulants, and stool softeners. Bulk laxatives work by absorbing water and expanding to increase moisture content and bulk in the stool. Lubricants increase water retention in the stool causing reabsorption of water in the bowel. Osmotics increase distention and promote peristalsis. Saline draws water into the intestinal lumen. Stimulants act by increasing peristalsis by direct effect on the intestine. Stool softeners reduce surface tension of liquids of the bowel.

USES:
Laxatives are used as a preparation for bowel and rectal exam, constipation, and stool softener.

CONTRAINDICATIONS:
Persons with GI obstruction, perforation, gastric retention, toxic colitis, megacolon, abdominal pain, nausea, vomiting, or fecal impaction should not use these products.
Precautions: Caution should be used in rectal bleeding, large hemorrhoids, and anal excoriation.

Administer:
- Swallow tabs whole; do not break, crush, or chew
- Alone only with water for better absorption; do not take within 1 hr of antacids, milk, or cimetidine

SIDE EFFECTS:
The most common side effects are nausea, abdominal cramps, and diarrhea.

PHARMACOKINETICS:
Onset, peak, and duration vary among products.

INTERACTIONS:
Interactions vary widely among products. Check individual monographs for specific information.

POSSIBLE NURSING DIAGNOSES:
- Constipation *[uses]*
- Diarrhea *[adverse reactions]*
- Deficient knowledge *[teaching]*

NURSING CONSIDERATIONS
Assess:
- Blood, urine electrolytes if product is used often by patient
- I&O ratio to identify fluid loss
- Cause of constipation: identify whether fluids, bulk, or exercise missing from lifestyle
- Cramping, rectal bleeding, nausea, vomiting; if these symptoms occur, product should be discontinued

Evaluate:
- Therapeutic response: decrease in constipation

Teach patient/family:
- Not to use laxatives for long-term therapy; bowel tone will be lost
- That normal bowel movements do not always occur daily
- Not to use in presence of abdominal pain, nausea, vomiting
- To notify prescriber of abdominal pain, nausea, vomiting
- To notify prescriber if constipation is unrelieved or if symptoms of electrolyte imbalance: muscle cramps, pain, weakness, dizziness

SELECTED GENERIC NAMES
Bulk laxatives
methylcellulose
psyllium
Osmotic agents
glycerin
lactulose
Saline laxatives
magnesium salts
Stimulants
bisacodyl
Stool softener
docusate

NEUROMUSCULAR BLOCKING AGENTS

ACTION:
Neuromuscular blocking agents are divided into depolarizing and nondepolarizing blockers. They act by inhibiting transmission of nerve impulses by binding with cholinergic receptor sites.

USES: Neuromuscular blocking agents are used to facilitate endotracheal intubation and skeletal muscle relaxation during mechanical ventilation, surgery, or general anesthesia.

CONTRAINDICATIONS: Persons who are hypersensitive should not be given this product.

Precautions: Caution should be used in pregnancy, thyroid disease, collagen disease, cardiac disease, breastfeeding, children <2 yr, electrolyte imbalances, dehydration, neuromuscular disease (myasthenia gravis), and respiratory disease.

Administer:

- Using nerve stimulator by anesthesia provider to determine neuromuscular blockade
- Anticholinesterase to reverse neuromuscular blockade
- IV undiluted over 1-2 min (only by qualified person, usually an anesthesiologist)

SIDE EFFECTS: The most serious adverse reactions are prolonged apnea, bronchospasm, cyanosis, respiratory depression, and malignant hyperthermia. The most common side effects are bradycardia and decreased motility.

PHARMACOKINETICS: Onset, peak, and duration vary widely among products. Most products are metabolized in the liver and excreted in urine.

INTERACTIONS: Aminoglycosides potentiate neuromuscular blockade. Check individual monographs for specific information.

POSSIBLE NURSING DIAGNOSES:

- Risk for injury *[adverse reactions]*
- Deficient knowledge *[teaching]*

NURSING CONSIDERATIONS

Assess:

- For electrolyte imbalances (K, Mg); may lead to increased action of this product
- VS (B/P, pulse, respirations, airway) q15min until fully recovered; rate, depth, pattern of respirations, strength of hand grip
- I&O ratio; check for urinary retention, frequency, hesitancy
- Recovery: decreased paralysis of face, diaphragm, leg, arm, rest of body
- Allergic reactions: rash, fever, respiratory distress, pruritus; product should be discontinued

Perform/provide:

- Storage in light-resistant container, cool area
- Reassurance if communication is difficult during recovery from neuromuscular blockade

Evaluate:

- Therapeutic response: paralysis of jaw, eyelid, head, neck, rest of body

SELECTED GENERIC NAMES

atracurium
pancuronium
rocuronium
succinylcholine
vecuronium

NONSTEROIDAL ANTIINFLAMMATORIES

ACTION: Nonsteroidal antiinflammatories decrease prostaglandin synthesis by inhibiting an enzyme needed for biosynthesis.

USES: Nonsteroidal antiinflammatories are used to treat mild to moderate pain, osteoarthritis, rheumatoid arthritis, and dysmenorrhea.

DRUG CATEGORIES

CONTRAINDICATIONS:
Persons with hypersensitivity, asthma, or severe renal/hepatic disease should not use these products.

Precautions: Caution should be used in pregnancy, breastfeeding, children, geriatric patients, bleeding/GI/cardiac disorders, and hypersensitivity to other antiinflammatory agents.

Administer:

- With food to decrease GI symptoms; however, best to take on empty stomach to facilitate absorption

SIDE EFFECTS:
The most serious adverse reactions are nephrotoxicity (dysuria, hematuria, oliguria, azotemia), blood dyscrasias, and cholestatic hepatitis. The most common side effects are nausea, abdominal pain, anorexia, dizziness, and drowsiness.

PHARMACOKINETICS:
Onset, peak, and duration vary widely among products. Most products are metabolized in the liver and excreted in urine.

INTERACTIONS:
Interactions vary widely among products. Check individual monographs for specific information.

POSSIBLE NURSING DIAGNOSES:

- Deficient knowledge *[teaching]*
- Impaired physical mobility *[uses]*
- Noncompliance *[teaching]*
- Chronic pain *[uses]*

NURSING CONSIDERATIONS

Assess:

- Renal, hepatic, blood studies: BUN, creatinine, AST, ALT, Hgb, before treatment, periodically thereafter
- Audiometric, ophthalmic examination before, during, and after treatment
- For eye, ear problems: blurred vision, tinnitus; may indicate toxicity

Perform/provide:

- Storage at room temperature

Evaluate:

- Therapeutic response: decreased pain, stiffness in joints; decreased swelling in joints; ability to move more easily

Teach patient/family:

- To report blurred vision, ringing, roaring in ears; may indicate toxicity
- To avoid driving, other hazardous activities if dizziness, drowsiness occur, especially in geriatric patients
- To report change in urine pattern, increased weight, edema, increased pain in joints, fever, blood in urine; indicate nephrotoxicity
- That therapeutic effects may take up to 1 mo

SELECTED GENERIC NAMES

celecoxib
diclofenac
ibuprofen
indomethacin
ketoprofen
ketorolac
nabumetone
naproxen
piroxicam
sulindac

OPIOID ANALGESICS

ACTION:
Opioid analgesics act by depressing pain impulse transmission at the spinal cord level by interacting with opioid receptors. Products are divided into opiates and nonopiates.

USES:
Most opioid analgesics are used to control moderate to severe pain and are used before and after surgery.

CONTRAINDICATIONS:
Hypersensitive reactions occur frequently. Check for sensitivity before administering. These products should be used cautiously if opiate addiction is suspected.

Precautions: Caution must be used when these products are given to a person with an addictive personality since the possibility of addiction is so great. Also, they may worsen intracranial pressure. Persons with severe heart disease, hepatic/renal disease, respiratory conditions, or seizure disorders should be monitored closely for worsening condition.

Administer:

- With antiemetic if nausea or vomiting occurs
- When pain is beginning to return; determine dosage interval by response

SIDE EFFECTS: GI symptoms, including nausea, vomiting, anorexia, constipation, and cramps, are the most common side effects. Other common side effects include light-headedness, dizziness, and sedation. Serious adverse reactions such as respiratory depression, respiratory arrest, circulatory depression, and increased intracranial pressure may result but are less common and usually dose dependent.

PHARMACOKINETICS: Onset of action is immediate by IV route and rapid by IM and PO routes. Peak occurs from 1-2 hr, depending on route, with a duration of 2-8 hr. These agents cross the placenta and appear in breast milk.

INTERACTIONS: Barbiturates, other opioids, hypnotics, antipsychotics, or alcohol can increase CNS depression when taken with opioids.

POSSIBLE NURSING DIAGNOSES:

- Impaired gas exchange *[adverse reactions]*
- Acute pain *[uses]*

NURSING CONSIDERATIONS

Assess:

- I&O ratio; be alert for urinary retention, frequency, and dysuria; product should be discontinued if these occur
- Respiratory dysfunction: respiratory depression, rate, rhythm, character; notify prescriber if respirations are <12/min
- CNS changes: dizziness, drowsiness, hallucinations, euphoria, LOC, pupil reaction
- Allergic reactions: rash, urticaria
- Need for pain medication; use pain scoring

Perform/provide:

- Assistance with ambulation; patient should not be ambulating during product peak

Evaluate:

- Therapeutic response: decrease in pain

Teach patient/family:

- To report any symptoms of CNS changes, allergic reactions, or SOB
- That physical dependency may result when used for extended periods
- That withdrawal symptoms may occur, including nausea, vomiting, cramps, fever, faintness, anorexia
- To avoid alcohol and other CNS depressants

SELECTED GENERIC NAMES

buprenorphine
butorphanol
codeine
fentaNYL
fentaNYL transdermal
HYDROmorphone
meperidine
methadone
morphine
nalbuphine
oxyCODONE
oxymorphone
pentazocine
remifentanil

SALICYLATES

ACTION: Salicylates have analgesic, antipyretic, and antiinflammatory effects. The analgesic and antiinflammatory activities may be mediated through the inhibition of prostaglandin synthesis. Antipyretic action results from inhibition of the hypothalamic heat-regulating center.

USES: The primary uses of salicylates are relief of mild to moderate pain and fever and in inflammatory conditions such as arthritis, thromboembolic disorders, and rheumatic fever.

CONTRAINDICATIONS: Hypersensitivity to salicylates is common. Check for sensitivity before administering. Persons with bleeding disorders, GI bleeding, and vit K deficiency should not use these products since salicylates increase PT. Children should not use these products since salicylates have been associated with Reye's syndrome.

Precautions: Caution is needed when salicylates are given to patients with anemia, hepatic/renal disease, and Hodgkin's disease. Caution should also be exercised in pregnancy and breastfeeding.

Administer:

- With food or milk to decrease gastric irritation; give 30 min before or 1 hr after meals with a full glass of water

SIDE EFFECTS: The most common side effects are GI symptoms and rash. Serious blood dyscrasias and hepatotoxicity may result when used for long periods at high doses. Tinnitus or impaired hearing may indicate that blood salicylate levels are reaching or exceeding the upper limit of the therapeutic range.

PHARMACOKINETICS: Onset of action occurs in 15-30 min, with a peak of 1-2 hr and a duration up to 6 hr. These products are metabolized by the liver and excreted by the kidneys.

INTERACTIONS: Increased effects of anticoagulants, insulin, methotrexate, heparin, valproic acid, and oral sulfonylureas may occur when used with salicylates. Aspirin may decrease serum concentrations of nonsteroidal antiinflammatory agents.

POSSIBLE NURSING DIAGNOSES:

- Activity intolerance *[uses]*
- Impaired physical mobility *[uses]*
- Acute pain *[uses]*
- Chronic pain *[uses]*
- Ineffective thermoregulation *[uses]*

NURSING CONSIDERATIONS

Assess:

- Hepatic/renal studies: AST, ALT, bilirubin, creatinine, LDH, alk phos, BUN if patient is on long-term therapy since these products are metabolized and excreted by the liver and kidneys
- Blood studies: CBC, hematocrit, hemoglobin, and PT if patient is on long-term therapy since these products increase the possibility of bleeding and blood dyscrasias
- Hepatotoxicity: dark urine, clay-colored stools; yellowing of skin, sclera; itching, abdominal pain, fever, diarrhea, which may occur with long-term use
- Ototoxicity: tinnitus; ringing, roaring in ears; audiometric testing is needed before and after long-term therapy

Evaluate:

- Therapeutic response: decreased pain, fever

Teach patient/family:

- That blood glucose levels should be monitored closely if patient is diabetic
- Not to exceed recommended dosage; acute poisoning may result
- That therapeutic response takes 2 wk in arthritis
- To avoid use of alcohol since GI bleeding may result
- To notify prescriber of ringing in the ears or persistent GI pain

• To take with full glass of water to reduce risk of lodging in esophagus

SELECTED GENERIC NAMES

aspirin
choline salicylate
magnesium salicylate
salsalate

SEDATIVES/HYPNOTICS

ACTION: Sedatives/hypnotics depress the CNS; some products at the cerebral cortex, others inhibit transmitters in the CNS.

USES: Sedatives/hypnotics are used for the treatment of sleep disorders, seizures, muscle spasms, and alcohol withdrawal.

CONTRAINDICATIONS: Persons with hypersensitivity reactions should not use these products.

Precautions: Sedatives/hypnotics should be used cautiously in pregnancy (C) and breastfeeding.

Administer:

• Lowest possible dose for therapeutic result; adjust dose to response

SIDE EFFECTS: The most common side effects are nausea and drowsiness. The most serious side effects are Stevens-Johnson syndrome, blood dyscrasias, and risk of dependency.

PHARMACOKINETICS: Onset, peak, and duration vary widely among products. Most products are metabolized in the liver and excreted by the kidneys.

INTERACTIONS: Increased CNS depression may occur with other CNS depressants such as alcohol, opiates, antipsychotics, and antidepressants.

POSSIBLE NURSING DIAGNOSES:

• Deficient knowledge *[teaching]*
• Noncompliance *[teaching]*
• Insomnia *[uses]*

NURSING CONSIDERATIONS

Assess:

• Mental status: affect, mood, behavioral changes, depression, confusion; seizure activity

Perform/provide:

• Assistance with ambulation during beginning therapy if dizziness, ataxia occur

Evaluate:

• Therapeutic response: ability to sleep throughout the night; absence or decreasing seizure activity

Teach patient/family:

• That these products should only be used for short-term insomnia
• Not to drive or engage in other hazardous activities while taking these products
• To avoid breastfeeding while taking these products
• To avoid alcohol or other CNS depressants since drowsiness will increase
• That some of the products take 2 nights to be effective
• To report side effects, adverse reactions to health care provider
• To use exactly as prescribed, at regular intervals

SELECTED GENERIC NAMES

Barbiturates

PHENobarbital

Benzodiazepines

chlordiazePOXIDE
clorazepate
diazepam
flurazepam
LORazepam
midazolam
oxazepam
temazepam
triazolam

Miscellaneous products
chloral hydrate
dexmedetomidine
droperidol
eszopiclone
hydrOXYzine
promethazine
ramelteon
zaleplon
zolpidem

SKELETAL MUSCLE RELAXANTS

ACTION: Most skeletal muscle relaxants inhibit synaptic responses in the CNS by stimulating receptors and decreasing neurotransmission, decreasing pain and spasticity.

USES: Skeletal muscle relaxants are used for musculoskeletal disorders with pain or spasticity related to spinal cord injuries.

CONTRAINDICATIONS: Persons with hypersensitivity should not use these products.
Precautions: Skeletal muscle relaxants should be used cautiously in pregnancy (C), peptic ulcer, renal/hepatic disease, stroke, seizure disorder, diabetes, breastfeeding, and geriatric patients.
Administer:
- When pain is beginning to return, not after pain is severe

SIDE EFFECTS: The most common side effects are dizziness, weakness, fatigue, drowsiness, and headache. Some products can cause seizures, CV collapse, and severe CNS depression.

PHARMACOKINETICS: Pharmacokinetics varies widely among products. Check individual monographs for specific information.

INTERACTIONS: CNS depressants used with skeletal muscle relaxants may lead to increased CNS depression.

POSSIBLE NURSING DIAGNOSES:

- Risk for injury *[adverse reactions]*
- Deficient knowledge *[teaching]*
- Impaired physical mobility *[uses]*
- Acute pain *[uses]*
- Chronic pain *[uses]*

NURSING CONSIDERATIONS

Assess:
- Pain: character, location, duration, alleviating/aggravating factors

Perform/provide:
- Storage in dry area, away from heat and sunlight

Evaluate:
- Therapeutic response: decreased pain or spasticity

Teach patient/family:
- Not to use with other CNS depressant unless prescriber approved
- That many products require 1-2 mo of treatment for full effect
- To avoid hazardous activities until response to medication is known
- That most products should not be discontinued quickly, but tapered over 1-2 wk

SELECTED GENERIC NAMES

Centrally acting
baclofen
carisoprodol
cyclobenzaprine
diazepam
methocarbamol
Direct-acting
dantrolene

THROMBOLYTICS

ACTION: Thrombolytics act by activating conversion of plasminogen to plasmin (fibrinolysin). Plasmin is able to break down clots (fibrin).

USES: Thrombolytics are used to treat DVT, pulmonary embolism, arterial thrombosis, arterial embolism, arteriovenous cannula occlusion, lysis of coronary artery thrombi after MI, and acute, evolving transmural MI.

CONTRAINDICATIONS: Persons with hypersensitivity, active bleeding, intraspinal surgery, neoplasms of the CNS, ulcerative colitis/enteritis, severe hypertension, renal/hepatic disease, hypocoagulation, COPD, subacute bacterial endocarditis, rheumatic valvular disease, cerebral embolism/thrombosis/hemorrhage, recent intraarterial diagnostic procedure or surgery (10 days), and recent major surgery should not use these products.

Precautions: Caution should be used in arterial emboli from left side of heart and pregnancy.

Administer:

- As soon as thrombi identified; not useful for thrombi over 1 wk old
- Cryoprecipitate or fresh, frozen plasma if bleeding occurs
- Loading dose at beginning of therapy; may require increased loading doses
- Heparin after fibrinogen level is over 100 mg/dl; heparin inf to increase PTT to 1.5-2 × baseline for 3-7 days
- About 10% of patients have high streptococcal antibody titers requiring increased loading doses
- IV therapy using 0.8 μm filter

SIDE EFFECTS: Serious adverse reactions include GI, GU, intracranial retroperitoneal bleeding, and anaphylaxis. The most common side effects are decreased Hct, urticaria, headache, and nausea.

PHARMACOKINETICS: Onset, peak, and duration vary widely among products. Most products are metabolized in the liver and excreted in urine.

INTERACTIONS: Interactions vary widely among products. Check individual monographs for specific information.

POSSIBLE NURSING DIAGNOSES:

- Risk for injury *[uses]*

NURSING CONSIDERATIONS

Assess:

- VS, B/P, pulse, resp, neurologic signs, temp at least q4hr; temp >104° F (40° C) indicator of internal bleeding; cardiac rhythm following intracoronary administration; systolic pressure increase of >25 mm Hg should be reported to prescriber
- For neurologic changes that may indicate intracranial bleeding
- Retroperitoneal bleeding: back pain, leg weakness, diminished pulses
- Allergy: fever, rash, itching, chill; mild reaction may be treated with antihistamines
- For bleeding during 1st hr of treatment: hematuria, hematemesis, bleeding from mucous membranes, epistaxis, ecchymosis
- Blood studies (Hct, platelets, PTT, PT, TT, aPTT) before starting therapy; PT or APTT must be <2× control before starting therapy or PT q3-4hr during treatment

Perform/provide:

- Storage of reconstituted product in refrigerator; discard after 24 hr
- Bed rest during entire course of treatment

Evaluate:

- Therapeutic response: resolution of thrombosis, embolism

Teach patient/family:

- To avoid venous or arterial puncture, inj, rectal temp

• To treat fever with acetaminophen or aspirin
• To apply pressure for 30 sec to minor bleeding sites; to inform prescriber if this does not attain hemostasis; to apply pressure dressing

SELECTED GENERIC NAMES

alteplase
tenecteplase
urokinase

THYROID HORMONES

ACTION: Thyroid hormones act by increasing metabolic rates resulting in increased cardiac output, O_2 consumption, body temp, blood volume, growth, development at cellular level, respiratory rate, and enzyme system activity.

USES: Thyroid hormones are used for thyroid replacement.

CONTRAINDICATIONS: Persons with adrenal insufficiency, MI, or thyrotoxicosis should not use these products.
Precautions: Geriatric patients and those with angina pectoris, hypertension, ischemia, cardiac disease, diabetes mellitus or insipidus should be watched closely when using these products. Caution should be used in pregnancy (A) and breastfeeding.
Administer:
• At same time each day to maintain product level
• Only for hormone imbalances; not to be used for obesity, male infertility, menstrual conditions, lethargy

SIDE EFFECTS: The most common side effects include insomnia, tremors, tachycardia, palpitations, angina, dysrhythmias, weight loss, and changes in appetite. Serious adverse reactions include thyroid storm.

PHARMACOKINETICS: Pharmacokinetics vary widely among products. Check individual monographs for specific information.

INTERACTIONS:

• Impaired absorption of thyroid products may occur when administered with cholestyramine, iron products (separate by 4-5 hr)
• Increased effects of anticoagulants, sympathomimetics, tricyclics, catecholamines may occur
• Decreased effects of digoxin, glycosides, insulin, hypoglycemics may occur
• Decreased effects of thyroid products may occur with estrogens

POSSIBLE NURSING DIAGNOSES:

• Disturbed body image *[adverse reactions]*
• Deficient knowledge *[teaching]*
• Noncompliance *[teaching]*

NURSING CONSIDERATIONS

Assess:
• B/P, pulse before each dose
• I&O ratio
• Weight daily in same clothing, using same scale, at same time of day
• PT should be closely monitored, and dosage of anticoagulant therapy may need adjustment
• Height, growth rate if given to a child
• T_3, T_4, which are decreased; radioimmunoassay of TSH, which is increased; ratio uptake, which is decreased if patient is on too low a dosage of medication
• Increased nervousness, excitability, irritability; may indicate overdosage, usually after 1-3 wk of treatment
• Cardiac status: angina, palpitation, chest pain, change in VS
Perform/provide:
• Removal of medication 4 wk before RAIU test
Evaluate:
• Therapeutic response: absence of depression; increased weight loss; diuresis;

pulse; appetite; absence of constipation; peripheral edema; cold intolerance; pale, cool, dry skin; brittle nails; alopecia; coarse hair; menorrhagia; night blindness; paresthesias; syncope; stupor; coma; rosy cheeks

Teach patient/family:
- That hair loss will occur in child and is temporary
- To report excitability, irritability, anxiety, chest pain, palpitations, increased pulse, excessive sweating, heat intolerance; indicates overdose
- Not to switch brands unless directed by prescriber
- That hypothyroid child will show almost immediate behavior/personality change
- That treatment product is not to be taken to reduce weight
- To avoid OTC preparations with iodine; read labels
- To avoid iodine in food: iodinized salt, soybeans, tofu, turnips, some seafood, some bread

SELECTED GENERIC NAMES

levothyroxine (T_4)
liothyronine (T_3)
liotrix
thyroid USP

VASODILATORS

ACTION: Vasodilators have various modes of action. Check individual monographs for specific action.

USES: Vasodilators are used to treat intermittent claudication, arteriosclerosis obliterans, vasospasm and muscular ischemia, ischemic cerebrovascular disease, hypertension, and angina.

CONTRAINDICATIONS: Some products are contraindicated in acute MI, paroxysmal tachycardia, and thyrotoxicosis.

Precautions: Caution should be used in uncompensated heart disease or peptic ulcer disease.

Administer:
- With meals to reduce GI symptoms

SIDE EFFECTS: The most common side effects are headache, nausea, hypotension, hypertension, and ECG changes.

PHARMACOKINETICS: Onset, peak, and duration vary widely among products. Most products are metabolized in the liver and excreted in urine.

INTERACTIONS: Interactions vary widely among products. Check individual monographs for specific information.

POSSIBLE NURSING DIAGNOSES:

- Decreased cardiac output *[uses]*
- Deficient knowledge *[teaching]*
- Ineffective cardiac tissue perfusion *[uses]*

NURSING CONSIDERATIONS

Assess:
- Bleeding time in individuals with bleeding disorders
- Cardiac status: B/P, pulse, rate, rhythm, character; watch for increasing pulse

Perform/provide:
- Storage in tight container at room temperature

Evaluate:
- Therapeutic response: ability to walk without pain, increased temp in extremities, increased pulse volume

Teach patient/family:
- That medication is not a cure; may need to be taken continuously
- That it is necessary to quit smoking to prevent excessive vasoconstriction
- That improvement may be sudden, but usually occurs gradually over several weeks
- To report headache, weakness, increased pulse, as product may have to be decreased or discontinued

DRUG CATEGORIES

• To avoid hazardous activities until stabilized on medication; dizziness may occur

SELECTED GENERIC NAMES

bosentan
dipyridamole
hydrALAZINE
isoxsuprine
minoxidil
nesiritide

VITAMINS

ACTION: The action of vitamins varies widely among products and classes. Check individual monographs for specific information.

USES: Vitamins are used to correct and prevent vitamin deficiencies.

CONTRAINDICATIONS: Hypersensitive reactions may occur, and allergies should be identified before these products are given.

Administer:

• PO with food for better absorption

SIDE EFFECTS: There are no side effects or adverse reactions with the water-soluble vitamins (C, B). However, fat-soluble vitamins (A, D, E, K) may accumulate in the body and cause adverse reactions (see individual monographs).

PHARMACOKINETICS: Onset, peak, and duration vary widely among products. Check individual monographs for specific information.

POSSIBLE NURSING DIAGNOSES:

• Imbalanced nutrition: less than body requirements *[uses]*

NURSING CONSIDERATIONS

Perform/provide:

• Storage in tight, light-resistant container

Evaluate:

• Therapeutic response: no vitamin deficiency

Teach patient/family:

• Not to take more than prescribed amount

SELECTED GENERIC NAMES

Fat-soluble

phytonadione (vitamin K_1)
vitamin A
vitamin D
vitamin E

Water-soluble

ascorbic acid (C)
cyanocobalamin (B_{12})
pyridoxine (B_6)
riboflavin (B_2)
thiamine (B_1)

Miscellaneous

multivitamins

abacavir (Rx)

(ah-bak'ah-veer)

Ziagen

Func. class.: Antiretroviral

Chem. class.: Nucleoside reverse transcriptase inhibitor (NRTI)

Do not confuse:
abacavir/amprenavir

ACTION: A synthetic nucleoside analog with inhibitory action against HIV-1; inhibits replication of the virus by incorporating into cellular DNA by viral reverse transcriptase, thereby terminating the cellular DNA chain

USES: In combination with other antiretroviral agents for HIV-1 infection (not to be used with lamivudine or tenofovir)
Unlabeled uses: HIV prophylaxis following occupational exposure

CONTRAINDICATIONS

Black Box Warning: Hypersensitivity, moderate severe hepatic disease

Precautions: Pregnancy (C), breastfeeding, children <3 mo, granulocyte count <1000/mm^3 or Hgb <9.5 g/dl, severe renal disease, impaired hepatic function, HLA B5701

Black Box Warning: Lactic acidosis

DOSAGE AND ROUTES

- **Adult and adolescent ≥16 yr: PO** 300 mg bid or 600 mg/day with other antiretrovirals
- **Adolescent <16 yr and child ≥3 mo: PO** 8 mg/kg bid, max 300 mg bid with other antiretrovirals

Hepatic dose

- **Adult: PO** (Child-Pugh 5-6) (oral sol) 200 mg bid

HIV prophylaxis (unlabeled)

- **Adult: PO** 300 mg bid to be added to the basic 2-drug regimen ×4 wk

Available forms: Tabs 300 mg; oral sol 20 mg/ml

Administer:

- Give in combination with other antiretrovirals with or without food
- Reduce dose in hepatic disease, use oral sol
- Without regard to meals

SIDE EFFECTS

CNS: *Fever, headache, malaise, insomnia,* paresthesia
GI: *Nausea, vomiting, diarrhea, anorexia,* cramps, abdominal pain, increased AST, ALT, **hepatotoxicity, hepatomegaly with steatosis**
HEMA: **Granulocytopenia, anemia, lymphopenia**
INTEG: *Rash,* urticaria, hypersensitivity reactions
META: **Lactic acidosis**
OTHER: **Fatal hypersensitivity reactions, MI**
RESP: Dyspnea

PHARMACOKINETICS

Rapid/extensive absorption, distributed to extravascular space then erythrocytes; 50% plasma protein binding; extensively metabolized to inactive metabolites; half-life 1½ hr; excreted in urine, feces (unchanged)

INTERACTIONS

- Do not coadminister with abacavir-containing products

⚠ **Increase:** **possible lactic acidosis—ribavirin**
Increase: abacavir levels—alcohol
Decrease: abacavir levels—tipranavir
Decrease: levels of—methadone
Drug/Lab Test
Increase: glucose, triglycerides, GGT

NURSING CONSIDERATIONS

Assess:

- Symptoms of HIV and possible infections; increased temp

⚠ **Lactic acidosis (elevated lactate levels, increased LFTs), severe hepatomegaly with steatosis, discontinue treatment** and do not restart; may have large liver, elevated AST, ALT, lactate levels

Black Box Warning: Fatal hypersensitivity reactions: fever, rash, nausea, vomiting, fatigue, cough, dyspnea, diarrhea, abdominal discomfort; treatment should be discontinued and not restarted; those with HLA B5701 are at great risk for hypersensitivity; obtain genetic testing for HLA B5701 before starting treatment

⚠ **Blood dyscrasias** (anemia, granulocytopenia): bruising, fatigue, bleeding, poor healing

- Renal studies: BUN, serum uric acid, CCr before, during therapy; these may be elevated throughout treatment

Black Box Warning: Hepatic studies before and during therapy: bilirubin, AST, ALT, amylase, alk phos, creatine phosphokinase, creatinine, q mo

- Blood counts q2wk; monitor viral load and CD4 counts during treatment; watch for decreasing granulocytes, Hgb; if low, therapy may have to be discontinued and restarted after hematologic recovery; blood transfusions may be required

Perform/provide:

- Storage in cool environment; protect from light; oral sol stored at room temperature; do not freeze

Evaluate:

- Therapeutic response: increased CD4 count, decrease viral load

Teach patient/family:

- That product is not a cure but will control symptoms; patient is still infective, may pass AIDS virus on to others

⚠ To notify prescriber of sore throat, swollen lymph nodes, malaise, fever; other infections may occur; to stop product if skin rash, fever, cough, shortness of breath, GI symptoms, and to notify prescriber immediately; advise all health care providers that allergic reaction has occurred with abacavir

- That follow-up visits must be continued because serious toxicity may occur; blood counts must be done
- To use contraception during treatment; if patient is pregnant, register with the Antiretroviral Pregnancy Registry at 1-800-258-4263
- Give patient Medication Guide and Warning Card, discuss points on guide
- That other products may be necessary to prevent other infections and that drug is taken with other antiretrovirals
- Not to drink alcohol while taking this product

abatacept (Rx)

(ab-a-ta′sept)

Orencia

Func. class.: Antirheumatic agent (disease modifying); biologic response modifier

ACTION: A selective costimulation modulator, inhibits T-lymphocytes, inhibits production of tumor necrosis factor (TNF-α), interferon-γ, interleukin-2, which are involved in immune and inflammatory reactions

USES: Polyarticular juvenile rheumatoid arthritis; moderate to severe rheumatoid arthritis; acute, chronic rheumatoid arthritis that has not responded to other disease-modifying agents, may use in combination with DMARDs; do not use with TNF antagonists (adalimumab, etanercept, infliximab), anakinra

CONTRAINDICATIONS: Hypersensitivity, TB, viral hepatitis

Precautions: Pregnancy (C), breastfeeding, children, geriatric patients, recurrent infections, COPD

DOSAGE AND ROUTES

Rheumatoid arthritis

- **Adult:** Subcut 125 mg within a day after single IV loading dose, then 125 mg weekly; weekly subcut dose may be initiated without an IV loading dose for those unable to receive an infusion
- **Adult >100 kg: IV INF** 1 g over 30 min, give at 2, 4 wk after first inf, then q4wk

- **Adult 60-100 kg: IV INF** 750 mg over 30 min, give at 2, 4 wk after first inf, then q4wk
- **Adult <60 kg: IV INF** 500 mg over 30 min, give at 2, 4 wk after first inf, then q4wk

Juvenile rheumatoid arthritis (JRA)/juvenile idiopathic arthritis (JIA)

- **Adolescent and child ≥6 yr and >100 kg: IV INF** 1000 mg over 30 min q2wk × 2 doses, then 1000 mg over 30 min q4wk starting at wk 8
- **Adolescent and child ≥6 yr and 75-100 kg: IV INF** 750 mg over 30 min q2wk × 2 doses, then 750 mg over 30 min q4wk starting at wk 8
- **Adolescent and child ≥6 yr and <75 kg: IV INF** 10 mg/kg over 30 min q2wk × 2 doses then 10 mg/kg q4wk starting at wk 8

Available forms: Lyophilized powder, single-use vials 250 mg; sol for inj 125 mg/ml

Administer:

Intermittent IV INF route

- To reconstitute, remove plastic flip top from vial and wipe the top with alcohol wipe; insert syringe needle into vial and direct stream of sterile water for inj on the wall of vial; rotate vial until mixed; vent with needle to rid foam after reconstitution (25 mg/ml); further dilute in 100 ml NS from a 100-ml inf bag/bottle; withdraw the needed volume (2 vials remove 20 ml; 3 vials remove 30 ml, 4 vials remove 40 ml); slowly add the reconstituted Orencia sol from each vial into the inf bag/bottle using the same disposable syringe supplied; mix gently, discard unused portions of vials; do not use if particulate is present or discolored; give over 30 min; use non–protein-binding filter (0.2-1.2 microns), protect from light
- Do not admix with other sol or medications

SUBCUT route

- Use prefilled syringe for subcut only (do not use for IV); only those trained should use this system; allow syringe to warm to room temp (30-60 mins), do not speed up warming process in any way; the amount of liquid should be between the 2 lines on the barrel, do not use the syringe if there is more or less liquid; inject into fronts of thighs, outer area of upper arm, or abdomen except for 2-inch area around the navel; do not inject into tender, bruised area
- Gently pinch skin and hold firmly, insert needle at 45-degree angle, inject full amount in 125-mg syringe
- Rotate injection sites

SIDE EFFECTS

CNS: Headache, asthenia, dizziness
CV: *Hypo/hypertension*
GI: Abdominal pain, dyspepsia, nausea
INTEG: Rash, *inj site reaction,* flushing, urticaria, pruritus
RESP: *Pharyngitis, cough, URI,* non-URI, *rhinitis,* wheezing
SYST: **Anaphylaxis, malignancies,** angioedema, serious infections

PHARMACOKINETICS

Terminal half-life 14.3 days, steady state 60 days

INTERACTIONS

- Do not give concurrently with vaccines; immunizations should be brought up to date before treatment
- Do not use with TNF antagonists: adalimumab, etanercept, infliximab; anakinra
- Avoid use with corticosteroids, immunosuppressives, atropine, scopolamine, halothane

NURSING CONSIDERATIONS

Assess:

- **RA:** pain, stiffness, ROM, swelling of joints during treatment
- For latent/active TB, viral hepatitis before beginning treatment
- For inj site pain, swelling
- Patient's overall health at each visit; product should not be given with active infections

⚠ **Infection:** sinusitis, urinary tract infection, influenza, bronchitis; serious infections have occurred

Perform/provide:

• Storage in refrigerator; do not use expired vials, protect from light, do not freeze

Evaluate:

• Therapeutic response: decreased inflammation, pain in joints

Teach patient/family:

• That product must be continued for prescribed time to be effective
• To use caution when driving; dizziness may occur
• Not to have vaccinations while taking this product
• About patient information included in packaging

RARELY USED
⚠ HIGH ALERT

abciximab (Rx)

(ab-six′i-mab)

ReoPro

Func. class.: Platelet aggregation inhibitor

USES: Used with heparin and aspirin to prevent acute cardiac ischemia after percutaneous transluminal coronary angioplasty (PTCA) in patients at high risk for reclosure of affected arteries

Unlabeled uses: Acute MI, Kawasaki disease (child)

CONTRAINDICATIONS: Hypersensitivity to this product or murine protein; GI, GU bleeding; CVA within 2 yr, bleeding disorders, intracranial neoplasm, intracranial arteriovenous malformations, intracranial aneurysm, platelet count $<100,000/mm^3$, recent surgery, aneurysm, uncontrolled severe hypertension, vasculitis, coagulopathy

DOSAGE AND ROUTES

Percutaneous coronary intervention (PCI)

• **Adult: IV BOL** 250 mcg (0.25 mg)/kg 10-60 min before PCI followed by 0.125 mcg/kg/min **CONT INF** for 12 hr

MI (unlabeled)

• **Adult: IV BOL** 0.25 mg/kg over 5 min, then 0.125 mcg/kg/min (max 10 mcg/min); **IV INF** for 12 hr unless complications

abiraterone

See Appendix A—Selected new drugs

acarbose (Rx)

(ay-car′bose)

Precose

Func. class.: Oral antidiabetic

Chem. class.: α-Glucosidase inhibitor

Do not confuse:

Precose/preCare

ACTION: Delays digestion/absorption of ingested carbohydrates by inhibiting α-glucosidase, results in smaller rise in postprandial blood glucose after meals; does not increase insulin production

USES: Type 2 diabetes mellitus, alone or in combination with a sulfonylurea, metformin

Unlabeled uses: Adjunct in type 1 diabetes mellitus

CONTRAINDICATIONS: Breastfeeding, hypersensitivity, diabetic ketoacidosis, cirrhosis, inflammatory bowel disease, ileus, colonic ulceration, partial intestinal obstruction, chronic intestinal disease, serum creatinine >2 mg/dl, CCr <25 ml/min

Precautions: Pregnancy (B), children, renal/hepatic disease

DOSAGE AND ROUTES

- **Adult >60 kg: PO** 25 mg tid initially, with 1st bite of meal; maintenance dose may be increased to 50-100 mg tid; dosage adjustment at 4-8 wk intervals
- **Adult <60 kg: PO** max 50 mg tid

Type 1 diabetes mellitus (unlabeled)

- **Adult: PO** 50 mg tid with meals × 2 wk, then 100 mg tid with meals

Available forms: Tabs 25, 50, 100 mg

Administer:

PO route

- With 1st bite of each meal 3 ×/day

SIDE EFFECTS

GI: *Abdominal pain, diarrhea, flatulence,* increased serum transaminase level

PHARMACOKINETICS

Poor systemic absorption, peak 1 hr, metabolized in GI tract, excreted as intact product in urine, half-life 2 hr

INTERACTIONS

Increase: acetaminophen toxicity—acetaminophen combined with alcohol

Increase or decrease: glycemic control—androgens, lithium, bortezomib, quinolones

Decrease: effect of digoxin

- Do not use with gatifloxacin

Increase: hypoglycemia—sulfonylureas, insulin, MAOIs, salicylates, fibric acid derivatives, bile acid sequestrants, ACE inhibitors, angiotensin II receptor antagonists, beta blockers

Decrease: effect, increase hyperglycemia—digestive enzymes, intestinal absorbents, thiazide diuretics, loop diuretics, corticosteroids, estrogen, progestins, oral contraceptives, sympathomimetics, isoniazid, phenothiazines; protease inhibitors, atypical antipsychotics, carbonic anhydrase inhibitors, cyclosporine, tacrolimus, baclofen

Drug/Herb

Increase: hypoglycemia—chromium, garlic, horse chestnut

Drug/Lab Test

Increase: ALT, AST, bilirubin

Decrease: calcium, vit B_6, Hgb, Hct

NURSING CONSIDERATIONS

Assess:

- **Hypoglycemia** (weakness, hunger, dizziness, tremors, anxiety, tachycardia, sweating), hyperglycemia; even though product does not cause hypoglycemia, if patient is on sulfonylureas or insulin, hypoglycemia may be additive; if hypoglycemia occurs, treat with dextrose, or, if severe, with IV glucose or glucagon
- Monitor AST, ALT q3mo × 1 yr and periodically thereafter; if elevated, dose may need to be reduced or discontinued; A1c q3mo, monitor serum glucose
- For stress, surgery, or other trauma that may require change in dose
- GI side effects for tolerability/compliance

Perform/provide:

- Storage in tight container in cool environment

Evaluate:

- Therapeutic response: improved signs/symptoms of diabetes mellitus (decreased polyuria, polydipsia, polyphagia; clear sensorium, absence of dizziness, stable gait)

Teach patient/family:

- The symptoms of hypo/hyperglycemia, what to do about each
- That medication must be taken as prescribed; explain consequences of discontinuing medication abruptly; that insulin may need to be used for stress, including trauma, surgery, fever
- To avoid OTC medications, herbal supplements unless approved by health care provider
- That diabetes is a lifelong illness; that the diet and exercise regimen must be followed; that this product is not a cure
- To carry emergency ID and a glucose source; to avoid sugar, because sugar is blocked by acarbose
- That blood glucose monitoring is required to assess product effect

- Not to breastfeed
- That GI side effects may occur

acebutolol (Rx)

(a-se-byoo′toe-lole)

Apo-Acebutolol ✦, Gen-Acebutolol ✦, Nu-Acebutolol ✦, Sectral

Func. class.: Antihypertensive, antidysrhythmic (II)

Chem. class.: β_1-Blocker

ACTION: Competitively blocks stimulation of β-adrenergic receptors within vascular smooth muscle; decreases rate of SA node discharge, increases recovery time, slows conduction of AV node resulting in decreased heart rate (negative chronotropic effect), which decreases O_2 consumption in myocardium due to β_1-receptor antagonism; also decreases renin-angiotensin-aldosterone system at high doses, inhibits β_2-receptors in bronchial system (high doses)

USES: Mild to moderate hypertension, management of PVCs

Unlabeled uses: Chronic stable angina

CONTRAINDICATIONS: Hypersensitivity to this agent or β-blockers; cardiogenic shock, heart block (2nd, 3rd degree), sinus bradycardia, CHF, cardiac failure

Precautions: Pregnancy (B), breastfeeding, children, major surgery, peripheral vascular disease, diabetes mellitus, COPD, asthma, well-compensated heart failure, thyroid/renal/hepatic disease, psoriasis; abrupt discontinuation, myasthenia gravis, vasoplastic angina

DOSAGE AND ROUTES

Hypertension

- **Adult: PO** 400 mg/day or in 2 divided doses; may be increased to desired response; maintenance 200-1200 mg/day in 2 divided doses
- **Geriatric: PO** max 800 mg/day

Ventricular dysrhythmia

- **Adult: PO** 200 mg bid, may increase gradually; usual range 600-1200 mg/day; should be tapered over 2 wk before discontinuing
- **Geriatric:** Max 800 mg/day

Renal dose

- **Adult: PO** CCr 25-49 ml/min, reduce dose by 50%; CCr <25 ml/min, reduce dose by 75%

Available forms: Caps 200, 400 mg; tabs 100, 200, 400 mg ✦

Administer:

PO route

- Before meals, at bedtime; tab may be crushed or swallowed whole; give with food to prevent GI upset
- Avoid abrupt discontinuation; severe hypertension may occur

SIDE EFFECTS

CNS: *Insomnia, fatigue, dizziness, mental changes,* memory loss, hallucinations, depression, lethargy, drowsiness, strange dreams, catatonia, headache

CV: **Profound hypotension, bradycardia,** CHF, *cold extremities, postural hypotension,* **2nd-/3rd-degree heart block,** edema

EENT: Sore throat; dry, burning eyes

ENDO: Increased hyper/hypoglycemic response to insulin

GI: *Nausea, diarrhea,* vomiting, **mesenteric arterial thrombosis, ischemic colitis,** flatulence

GU: *Impotence,* decreased libido, dysuria, nocturia, polyuria

HEMA: **Agranulocytosis, thrombocytopenia, purpura**

INTEG: Rash, flushing, pruritus, sweating, alopecia, dry skin

MISC: Facial swelling, weight gain, decreased exercise tolerance

MS: Joint pain, cramping

RESP: **Bronchospasm,** dyspnea, wheezing, cough

PHARMACOKINETICS

Rapid absorption, onset 1-1½ hr, peak 2½-3½ hr, duration 10-12 hr, half-life 3-4 hr, metabolized in liver, 30%-40% excreted in urine, protcin binding 10%-26%, crosses placenta, enters breast milk (small amounts)

INTERACTIONS

- Attenuated effects: sulfonylureas

Increase: hypotension, bradycardia—hydrALAZINE, methyldopa, prazosin, anticholinergics, cardiac glycosides, verapamil, diuretics, calcium channel blockers, cimetidine, amiodarone, cloNIDine, haloperidol, MAOIs

Increase: hypoglycemic effect—insulin

Decrease: antihypertensive effects—NSAIDs, calcium, other antihypertensives

Decrease: bronchodilation—theophyllines, β_2-agonists

Decrease: effect of thyroid hormones, sympathomimetics

Drug/Herb

Decrease: antihypertensive effect of ephedra

Increase: acebutolol effect—hawthorn

Drug/Lab Test

Increase: serum lipoprotein levels, BUN, potassium, triglyceride, uric acid, LDH, AST, ALT, blood glucose, alk phos

Positive: ANA titer

NURSING CONSIDERATIONS

Assess:

- B/P during beginning treatment, periodically thereafter; note rate, rhythm, quality of heartbeat; apical/radial pulse before administration; notify prescriber of any significant changes (pulse <50 bpm); signs of CHF (dyspnea, crackles, weight gain, JVD)
- Baselines in renal, hepatic studies before therapy begins
- Edema in feet, legs daily: monitor I&O
- Skin turgor, dryness of mucous membranes for hydration status, especially in geriatric patients

Perform/provide:

- Storage protected from light, moisture; place in cool environment

Evaluate:

- Therapeutic response: decreased B/P after 1-2 wk; decreased dysrhythmias

Teach patient/family:

⚠ Not to discontinue product abruptly because severe cardiac reactions may occur, taper over 2 wk; do not double dose; if a dose is missed, take as soon as remembered up to 4 hr before next dose

- That drug may mask signs of hypoglycemia or alter blood glucose levels
- Not to use OTC products containing α-adrenergic stimulants (such as nasal decongestants, OTC cold preparations) unless directed by prescriber
- To report low pulse, dizziness, confusion, depression, fever
- To take pulse, B/P at home; advise when to notify prescriber
- To comply with weight control, dietary adjustments, modified exercise program
- To carry emergency ID to identify product, allergies
- To avoid hazardous activities if dizziness, drowsiness is present
- To report symptoms of CHF: difficult breathing, especially on exertion or when lying down, night cough, swelling of extremities
- To continue with required lifestyle changes (exercise, diet, weight loss, stress reduction)

TREATMENT OF OVERDOSE:

Lavage, IV atropine for bradycardia, IV theophylline for bronchospasm, O_2, diuretic for cardiac failure, glucagon for hypoglycemia, IV diazepam (or phenytoin) for seizures, calcium chloride, vasopressors

acetaminophen (otc)

(a-seat-a-mee′noe-fen)

Acephen, Aminofen, Apacet, APAP, Apo-Acetaminophen ♣, Apra, Children's Feverall, Equaline Children's Pain Relief, Equaline Infant's Pain Relief, Genapap, GoodSense Acetaminophen, GoodSense Children's Pain Relief, Infantaire, Leader Children's Pain Reliever, Mapap, Maranox, Meda, Neopap, Ofirmev, Oraphen-PD, Q-Pap, Q-Pap Children's, Redutemp, Ridenol, Silapap, Tapanol, Tempra, T-Painol, Tylenol, UniAce, Walgreen's Non-Aspirin, XS pain reliever, Walgreen's Acetaminophen

Func. class.: Nonopioid analgesic, antipyretic

Chem. class.: Nonsalicylate, paraaminophenol derivative

ACTION: May block pain impulses peripherally that occur in response to inhibition of prostaglandin synthesis; does not possess antiinflammatory properties; antipyretic action results from inhibition of prostaglandins in the CNS (hypothalamic heat-regulating center)

USES: Mild to moderate pain or fever, arthralgia, dental pain, dysmenorrhea, headache, myalgia, osteoarthritis

Unlabeled uses: Migraine

CONTRAINDICATIONS: Hypersensitivity

Precautions: Pregnancy (B), (C) IV; breastfeeding, geriatric patients, anemia, renal/hepatic disease, chronic alcoholism

DOSAGE AND ROUTES

- **Adult/child >12 yr: PO/RECT** 325-650 mg q4-6hr prn, max 4 g/day; weight ≥50 kg IV 1000 mg q6hr or 650 mg q4hr prn, max single dose 1000 mg, min dosing interval 4 hr; weight <50 kg IV 15 mg/kg/dose q6hr or 12.5 mg/kg/dose q4hr, max single dose 15 mg/kg, min dosing interval 4 hr, max 75 mg/kg/day from all sources
- **Child ≥2 yr and <50 kg: IV** 15 mg/kg/dose q6hr or 12.5 mg/kg/dose q4hr, max single dose 15 mg/kg, min dosing interval 4 hr, max 75 mg/kg/day from all sources
- **Child 1-12 yr: PO** 10-15 mg/kg q4-6hr, max 5 doses/24 hr
- **Child 1-12 yr: RECT** 10-20 mg/kg/dose q4-6hr
- **Neonate: RECT** 10-15 mg/kg/dose q6-8hr

Migraine (unlabeled)

- **Adult and adolescent: PO/RECT** 500-1000 mg, max 1 g/dose or max 4 g/day

Available forms: Rect supp 80, 120, 325, 650 mg; soft chew tabs 80, 160 mg; caps 500 mg; elix 120, 160, 325 mg/5 ml; oral disintegrating tab 80, 160 ml; oral drops 80 mg/0.8 ml, liquid 500 mg/5 ml, 80 mg/ml; tabs 325, 500, 650 mg; sol for inj 1000 mg/100 ml

Administer:

PO route

- Crushed or whole, do not crush EXT REL product; chewable tabs may be chewed; give with full glass of water
- With food or milk to decrease gastric symptoms if needed
- Susp after shaken well

Intermittent IV INF route

- No further dilution needed; do not add other medications to vial or inf device
- For doses equal to single vial, averted IV set may be used to deliver directly from vial; for doses less than a single vial, withdraw dose and place in an empty sterile syringe, plastic IV container, or glass bottle; infuse over 15 min

- Discard unused portion; if seal is broken, vial penetrated, or drug transferred to another container, give within 6 hr

SIDE EFFECTS

CNS: Stimulation, drowsiness
GI: Nausea, vomiting, abdominal pain; **hepatotoxicity, hepatic seizure (overdose), GI bleeding**
GU: Renal failure (high, prolonged doses)
HEMA: Leukopenia, neutropenia, hemolytic anemia (long-term use), thrombocytopenia, pancytopenia
INTEG: Rash, urticaria
SYST: Hypersensitivity
TOXICITY: Cyanosis, anemia, neutropenia, jaundice, pancytopenia, CNS stimulation, delirium followed by vascular collapse, seizures, coma, death

PHARMACOKINETICS

85%-90% metabolized by liver, excreted by kidneys; metabolites may be toxic if overdose occurs; widely distributed; crosses placenta in low concentrations; excreted in breast milk; half-life 1-4 hr
PO: Onset 10-30 min, peak ½-2 hr, duration 4-6 hr, well absorbed
RECT: Onset slow, peak 1-2 hr, duration 4-6 hr, absorption varies

INTERACTIONS

- Hypoprothrombinemia: warfarin, long-term use, high doses of acetaminophen
- Renal adverse reactions: NSAIDs, salicylates

Increase: hepatotoxicity—barbiturates, alcohol, carbamazepine, hydantoins, rifampin, rifabutin, isoniazid, diflunisal, zidovudine, lamotrigine, imatinib
Decrease: absorption—colestipol, cholestyramine

Drug/Herb
Decrease: acetaminophen effect—St. John's wort
Increase: hepatotoxicity—echinacea (rare)

Drug/Lab Test
Interference: chemstrip G, Dextrostix, Visidex II, 5-HIAA

NURSING CONSIDERATIONS

Assess:

- Hepatic studies: AST, ALT, bilirubin, creatinine before therapy if long-term therapy is anticipated; may cause hepatic toxicity at doses >4 g/day with chronic use
- Renal studies: BUN, urine creatinine, occult blood, albumin, if patient is on long-term therapy; presence of blood or albumin indicates nephritis
- Blood studies: CBC, PT if patient is on long-term therapy
- I&O ratio; decreasing output may indicate renal failure (long-term therapy)
- For fever and pain: type of pain, location, intensity, duration
- **Chronic poisoning: rapid, weak pulse; dyspnea; cold, clammy extremities; report immediately to prescriber**
- **Hepatotoxicity: dark urine; clay-colored stools; yellowing of skin, sclera; itching; abdominal pain; fever; diarrhea if patient is on long-term therapy**
- **Allergic reactions: rash, urticaria; if these occur, product may have to be discontinued**

Perform/provide:

- Storage of suppositories <80° F (27° C)

Evaluate:

- Therapeutic response: absence of pain using pain scoring; fever

Teach patient/family:

⚠ **Not to exceed recommended dosage; acute poisoning with liver damage may result; tell parents of children to check products carefully; that acute toxicity includes symptoms of nausea, vomiting, abdominal pain and that prescriber should be notified immediately; that toxicity may occur when used with other combination products**

- Not to use with alcohol, herbals without approval of prescriber

- To recognize signs of chronic overdose: bleeding, bruising, malaise, fever, sore throat
- That those with diabetes may notice blood glucose monitoring changes
- To notify prescriber of pain or fever lasting more than 3 days

TREATMENT OF OVERDOSE:
Product level, gastric lavage, activated charcoal; administer oral acetylcysteine to prevent hepatic damage *(see acetylcysteine monograph)*; monitor for bleeding

acetaZOLAMIDE (Rx)
(a-set-a-zole′a-mide)

Apo-Acetazolamide ♣, Diamox Sequels

Func. class.: Diuretic, carbonic anhydrase inhibitor, antiglaucoma agent, antiepileptic

Chem. class.: Sulfonamide derivative

Do not confuse:
acetaZOLAMIDE/acetoHEXAMIDE
Diamox/Trimox/Dobutrex

ACTION: Inhibits carbonic anhydrase activity in proximal renal tubules to decrease reabsorption of water, sodium, potassium, bicarbonate resulting in increased urine volume and alkalinization of urine; decreases carbonic anhydrase in CNS, increasing seizure threshold; able to decrease secretion of aqueous humor in eye, which lowers intraocular pressure

USES: Open-angle glaucoma, angle-closure glaucoma (preoperatively, if surgery delayed), seizures (petit mal, grand mal, mixed, absence), edema in CHF, product-induced edema, acute altitude sickness

Unlabeled uses: Urine alkalinization, metabolic alkalosis in mechanical ventilation, decrease CSF production in infants with hydrocephalus, familial periodic paralysis, nystagmus

CONTRAINDICATIONS: Hypersensitivity to sulfonamides, severe renal/hepatic disease, electrolyte imbalances (hyponatremia, hypokalemia), hyperchloremic acidosis, Addison's disease, long-term use for closed-angle glaucoma, adrenocortical insufficiency

Precautions: Pregnancy (C), breastfeeding, hypercalciuria, respiratory acidosis, pulmonary obstruction/emphysema, COPD

DOSAGE AND ROUTES

Angle-closure glaucoma
- **Adult: PO/IV** 250 mg q4hr or 250 mg bid for short-term therapy

Open-angle glaucoma
- **Adult: PO/IV** 250 mg/day in divided doses for amounts of more than 250 mg or 500 mg **SR** bid, max 1 g/day

Edema in CHF
- **Adult: PO/IV** 250-375 mg/day or 5 mg/kg in AM, give for 2 days, then 1-2 days drug free
- **Child: PO/IV** 5 mg/kg/day or 150 mg/m^2 in AM

Seizures
- **Adult: PO/IV** 8-30 mg/kg/day, in 1-4 divided doses, usual range 375-1000 mg/day; **ER** not recommended with seizures
- **Child: PO/IV** 8-30 mg/kg/day in divided doses tid or qid, or 300-900 mg/m^2/day, not to exceed 1 g/day

Altitude sickness
- **Adult: PO** 250 mg q6-12hr; **EXT REL** 500 mg q12-24hr, start therapy 24-48 hr before ascent and give for ≥48 hr after arrival at high altitude
- **Geriatric: PO** 250 mg bid, use lowest effective dose

Renal dose
- **Adult: PO/IV** CCr 10-50 ml/min give dose q12hr; CCr <10 ml/min, avoid use

Infants with hydrocephalus (unlabeled)
- **Infant: PO/IV** 5 mg/kg q6hr, may increase by 25 mg/kg/day; max 100 mg/kg/day

Urine alkalinization (unlabeled)
• **Adult: IV** 5 mg/kg/dose, repeat 2-3× over 24 hr
Familial periodic paralysis (unlabeled)
• **Adult: PO** 250-375 mg/day in divided doses
Metabolic alkalosis in mechanical ventilation (unlabeled)
• **Adult: IV** 500 mg as a single dose or 250 mg q6hr × 4 doses
Vestibular nystagmus (unlabeled)
• **Adult: PO** 250 mg, increase by 250 mg q3days; max 3 g/day in divided doses
Available forms: Tabs 125, 250 mg; ext rel caps 500 mg; inj 500 mg
Administer:
• In AM to avoid interference with sleep if using product as diuretic
• Potassium replacement if potassium level is <3 mg/dl
PO route
• Do not break, crush, or chew sus rel caps; this product should be used for altitude sickness, glaucoma
• With food if nausea occurs; absorption may be decreased slightly
IV route
• After diluting 500 mg in ≥5 ml sterile water for inj; **direct IV:** give at 100-500 mg/min; **intermittent INF:** may be diluted further in LR, D_5W, $D_{10}W$, 0.45% NaCl, 0.9% NaCl, or Ringer's sol and infused over 15-30 min; use within 24 hr of dilution

Additive compatibilities: cimetidine, ranitidine

SIDE EFFECTS

CNS: Anxiety, *confusion,* seizures, *depression,* dizziness, *drowsiness, fatigue,* headache, *paresthesia,* stimulation
EENT: Myopia, tinnitus
ENDO: *Hyperglycemia*
GI: *Nausea, vomiting, anorexia, diarrhea,* melena, *weight loss,* **hepatic insufficiency, cholestatic jaundice, fulminant hepatic necrosis,** *taste alterations,* **bleeding**
GU: *Frequency, polyuria,* uremia, glucosuria, hematuria, dysuria, crystalluria, renal calculi
HEMA: **Aplastic anemia, hemolytic anemia, leukopenia, thrombocytopenia, purpura, pancytopenia**
INTEG: *Rash,* pruritus, urticaria, fever, **Stevens-Johnson syndrome,** photosensitivity, flushing, **toxic epidermal necrolysis**
META: *Hypokalemia, hyperchloremic acidosis,* hyponatremia, sulfonamide-like reactions, metabolic acidosis

PHARMACOKINETICS

65% absorbed if fasting (oral), 75% absorbed if given with food; half-life 2½-5½ hr; excreted unchanged by kidneys (80% within 24 hr), crosses placenta
PO: Onset 1-1½ hr, peak 2-4 hr, duration 8-12 hr
PO-SUS REL: Onset 2 hr, peak 8-12 hr, duration 18-24 hr
IV: Onset 2 min, peak 15 min, duration 4-5 hr

INTERACTIONS

Increase: action of—amphetamines, flecainide, memantine, phenytoin, procainamide, quinidine, anticholinergics, methenamine, mecamylamine, ephedrine, memantine, mexiletene, quinidine, folic acid antagonists
Increase: excretion of lithium, primidone
Increase: osteomalacia—carbamazepine, ethotoin
Increase: toxicity—salicylates, cycloSPORINE
Increase: hypokalemia—corticosteroids, amphotericin B, corticotropin, ACTH
Increase: cardiac toxicity if hypokalemia develops—arsenic trioxide, cardiac glycosides, levomethadyl
Increase: renal stone formation, heat stroke—topiramate (avoid concurrent use)
Decrease: primidone levels

Drug/Lab Test
Increase: glucose, bilirubin, calcium, uric acid
Decrease: thyroid iodine uptake
False positive: urinary protein, 17 hydroxysteroid

NURSING CONSIDERATIONS

Assess:

- Edema: weight daily, I&O daily to determine fluid loss; effect of product may be decreased if used daily; monitor geriatric patients for dehydration
- Ocular status: intraocular pressure, ophthalmologic examination
- For cross-sensitivity with other sulfonamides and this product
- B/P lying, standing; postural hypotension may occur
- Electrolytes: K, Na, Cl; also BUN, blood glucose, CBC, serum creatinine, blood pH, ABGs, LFTs; I&O, platelet count, patient may need to be on a high-potassium diet; identify signs of hypokalemia (vomiting, fatigue, weakness)
- **Seizures:** neurologic status, provide seizure precaution

Perform/provide:

- Storage in dark, cool area; use reconstituted solution within 24 hr

Evaluate:

- Therapeutic response: improvement in edema of feet, legs, sacral area daily if medication is being used for CHF; decrease in aqueous humor if medication is being used for glaucoma; decreased frequency of seizures, prevention of altitude sickness

Teach patient/family:

- To take exactly as prescribed; if dose is missed, take as soon as remembered; do not double dose
- Altitude sickness: to avoid rapid ascent
- Diabetic: that drug may increase blood glucose and to monitor blood glucose
- To use sunscreen to prevent photosensitivity
- To avoid hazardous activities if drowsiness occurs
- To increase fluids to 2-3 L/day if not contraindicated

⚠ **To report nausea, vertigo, rapid weight gain, change in stools, weakness, numbness, rash, sore throat, bleeding/bruising; Stevens-Johnson syndrome, toxic epidermal necrolysis (blistering, red rash that spreads)**

TREATMENT OF OVERDOSE:

Lavage if taken orally; monitor electrolytes; administer dextrose in saline; monitor hydration, CV, renal status

acetylcholine ophthalmic

See Appendix B

acetylcysteine (Rx)

(a-se-teel-sis′tay-een)

Acetadote, Mucomyst ✱

Func. class.: Mucolytic; antidote—acetaminophen

Chem. class.: Amino acid L-cysteine

ACTION: Decreases viscosity of secretions by breaking disulfide links of mucoproteins; serves as a substrate in place of glutathione, which is necessary to inactivate toxic metabolites with acetaminophen overdose

USES: Acetaminophen toxicity; bronchitis; cystic fibrosis; COPD; atelectasis
Unlabeled uses: Prevention of contrast medium nephrotoxicity, distal intestinal obstruction, giant papillary conjunctivitis (GPC)

CONTRAINDICATIONS: Hypersensitivity, increased intracranial pressure, status asthmaticus
Precautions: Pregnancy (B), breastfeeding, hypothyroidism, Addison's disease, CNS depression, brain tumor, asthma, renal/hepatic disease, COPD, psychosis, alcoholism, seizure disorders,

bronchospasms, asthma, anaphylactoid reactions, fluid restriction, weight <40 kg

DOSAGE AND ROUTES

Acetaminophen toxicity

• **Adult and child: PO** 140 mg/kg, then 70 mg/kg q4hr × 17 doses to total of 1330 mg/kg; **IV** loading dose 150 mg/kg over 60 min (dilution 150 mg/kg in 200 ml of D_5); maintenance dose 1: 50 mg/kg over 4 hr (dilution 50 mg/kg in 500 ml D_5): maintenance dose 2: 100 mg/kg over 16 hr (dilution 100 mg/kg in 1000 ml D_5)

Mucolytic

• **Adult and child: INSTILL** 1-20 ml (10%-20% sol) q6-8hr prn or 3-5 ml (20% sol) or 6-10 ml (10% sol) tid or qid; nebulization (face mask, mouthpiece, tracheostomy) 1-10 ml of a 20% sol, or 2-20 ml of a 10% sol, q6-8hr; nebulization (tent, croupette) may require large dose, up to 300 ml/treatment

Nephrotoxicity prophylaxis (unlabeled)

• **Adult: PO** 600 mg bid, given day before and day of administration of contrast media or **IV** 150 mg/kg in 500 ml NS over 30 min before contrast, then 50 mg/kg in 500 ml NS over the next 4 hr; **IV BOL** 1200 mg before contrast medium and 1200 mg **PO** bid for 48 hr (MI undergoing angioplasty)

Giant papillary conjunctivitis (GPC) (unlabeled)

• **Adult: OPHTHALMIC** 1%-2% sol prepared by mixing in artificial tears, administer topically 4-6 ×/day

Meconium ileus (unlabeled)

• **Child: PO/RECT** 5-30 ml of 10% sol, 3-6 ×/day, usual dose 10 ml 4×/day

Available forms: Oral sol 10%, 20%; inj 20% (200 mg/ml)

Administer:

PO route

• **Antidotal use:** induce emesis or lavage; give within 24 hr; dilute 10% or 20% sol to a 5% sol with diet soda, may use water if giving via gastric tube; dilution of 10% sol 1:1, 20% sol 1:3

Direct intratracheal instill route

• By syringe: 1-2 ml of 10%-20% sol up to q1hr

• Decreased dose to geriatric patients; metabolism may be slowed

• Only if suction machine is available

• Before meals ½-1 hr for better absorption, to decrease nausea

• 20% sol diluted with NS or water for inj; may give 10% sol undiluted

• Only after patient clears airway by deep breathing, coughing

IV route

• **21-hr regimen:** loading dose: dilute 150 mg/kg in 200 ml D_5W; maintenance dose 1: dilute 50 mg/kg in 500 ml D_5W; maintenance dose 2: dilute 100 mg/kg in 1000 ml D_5W, give loading dose over 15 min, give maintenance dose 1 over 4 hr; give maintenance dose 2 over 16 hr, administer sequentially without time between doses

SIDE EFFECTS

CNS: *Dizziness, drowsiness,* headache, fever, chills

CV: Hypotension, flushing tachycardia

EENT: *Rhinorrhea,* tooth damage

GI: *Nausea,* stomatitis, constipation, vomiting, anorexia, **hepatotoxicity,** diarrhea

INTEG: Urticaria, rash, fever, clamminess, pruritus

RESP: **Bronchospasm,** burning, **hemoptysis,** chest tightness, cough

MISC: **Anaphylaxis, angioedema**

PHARMACOKINETICS

PO: (antidote), peak 1-2 hr, duration 4 hr

INH/INSTILL: Onset 5-10 min, peak 10 min, duration 1 hr

Excreted in urine, half-life 5.6 hr (adult), 11 hr (newborn)

IV: Protein binding 83%

INTERACTIONS

• Do not use with iron, copper, rubber, nickel

Increase: effect—nitrates

NURSING CONSIDERATIONS

Assess:

- Mucolytic use: cough—type, frequency, character, including sputum
- Rate, rhythm of respirations, increased dyspnea; sputum; discontinue if bronchospasm occurs
- VS, cardiac status including checking for dysrhythmias, increased rate, palpitations
- ABGs for increased CO_2 retention in asthma patients
- **Antidotal use:** LFTs, PT, BUN, creatinine, glucose, electrolytes, acetaminophen levels; inform prescriber if dose is vomited or vomiting is persistent
- Nausea, vomiting, rash; notify prescriber if these occur

Perform/provide:

- Storage in refrigerator; use within 96 hr of opening
- Assistance with inhaled dose: bronchodilator if bronchospasm occurs; mechanical suction if cough insufficient to remove excess bronchial secretions
- Gum, hard candy, frequent rinsing of mouth for dryness of oral cavity

Evaluate:

- Therapeutic response: absence of purulent secretions when coughing, clear lung sounds (mucolytic use); absence of hepatic damage with acetaminophen toxicity

Teach patient/family:

- About mucolytic use
- That unpleasant odor will decrease after repeated use
- That discoloration of sol after bottle is opened does not impair its effectiveness
- To report vomiting because dose may need to be repeated

acyclovir (Rx)

(ay-sye′kloe-veer)

Apo-Acyclovir ✱, Gen-Acyclovir ✱, Nu-Acyclovir ✱, ratio-Acyclovir ✱, Zovirax

Func. class.: Antiviral

Chem. class.: Purine nucleoside analog

ACTION: Interferes with DNA synthesis by conversion to acyclovir triphosphate, thereby causing decreased viral replication

USES: Mucocutaneous herpes simplex virus, herpes genitalis (HSV-1, HSV-2), varicella infections, herpes zoster, herpes simplex encephalitis

Unlabeled uses: Bell's palsy, prevention of CMV, Epstein-Barr virus, esophagitis, hairy leukoplakia, prevention of herpes labialis, herpes simplex, herpes simplex ocular prophylaxis, keratoconjunctivitis, pharyngitis, pneumonitis, prevention of postherpetic neuralgia, proctitis, stomatitis, tracheobronchitis, varicella prophylaxis

CONTRAINDICATIONS: Hypersensitivity to this product, valacyclovir

Precautions: Pregnancy (B), breastfeeding, renal/hepatic/neurologic disease, electrolyte imbalance, dehydration, hypersensitivity to famciclovir, ganciclovir, penciclovir, valganciclovir

DOSAGE AND ROUTES

Herpes simplex (recurrent)

- **Adult: PO** 400 mg 3 ×/day for 5 days or 200 mg 5 ×/day × 5 days
- **Adult and child >12 yr: IV INF** 5 mg/kg over 1 hr q8hr × 7 days, use ideal body weight for patients with obesity
- **Infant >3 mo/child <12 yr: IV INF** 10 mg/kg q8hr × 7 day; if HIV infected 5-10 mg/kg q8hr (moderate to severe)
- **Neonate: IV INF** 10 mg/kg q8hr × 10 days, may use higher dose

Genital herpes

• **Adult: PO** 200 mg q4hr (5 ×/day while awake) for 5 days to 6 mo depending on whether initial, recurrent, or chronic; **IV** 5 mg/kg q8hr × 5 days

Herpes simplex encephalitis

• **Adult: IV** 10 mg/kg over 1 hr q8hr × 10 days

• **Child 3 mo-12 yr: IV** 20 mg/kg q8hr × 10 days

• **Child birth-3 mo: IV** 10 mg/kg q8hr × 10 days

Herpes zoster

• **Adult: PO** 800 mg q4hr while awake × 7-10 days; **IV** 10 mg/kg q8hr × 7 days

Herpes zoster (shingles) immunocompromised patients

• **Adult/adolescent: PO** 800 mg q4hr 5×/day for 7-10 days; **IV** 10 mg/kg q8hr × 7 days

• **Child ≥12 yr: IV** 10 mg/kg/dose q8hr × 7 days

• **Infant/child <12 yr: IV** 20 mg/kg/dose q8hr × 7-10 days

Herpes zoster (shingles) immunocompetent

• **Adult: PO** 800 mg q4hr 5×/day × 7-10 days; start within 48-72 hr of rash onset

Varicella (chickenpox) immunocompetent

• **Adult/adolescent/child >40 kg: PO** 800 mg 4×/day × 5 days

• **Child ≥2 yr and ≤40 kg: PO** 20 mg/kg/dose (max 800 mg) 4×/day × 5 days

Mucosal/cutaneous herpes simplex infections in immunosuppressed patients

• **Adult and child >12 yr: IV** 5 mg/kg q8hr × 7 days

• **Infant >3 mo/child <12: IV** 10 mg/kg q8hr × 7 days

Renal dose

• **Adult and child: PO/IV** CCr >50 ml/min 100% dose q8hr, CCr 25-50 ml/min 100% dose q12hr, CCr 10-25 ml/min 100% dose q24hr, CCr 0-10 ml/min 50% dose q24hr

Bell's palsy (unlabeled)

• **Adult: PO** 400-800 mg 5 ×/day × 7 days, given with predniSONE

Hairy leukoplakia in HIV (unlabeled)

• **Adult: PO** 800 mg q6hr × 20 days

CMV prophylaxis (unlabeled)

• **Adult: IV** 500 mg/m^2 q8hr

Herpes simplex in pneumonitis/esophagitis/tracheobronchitis/proctitis/stomatitis/pharyngitis (unlabeled)

• **Adult and adolescent: IV** 5-10 mg/kg q8hr × 2-7 days or **PO** 200 mg q4hr 5×/day × 7-10 days or 400 mg 3-5 ×/day × 10 or more days

• **Child 6 mo-12 yr: IV** 1000 mg/day in 3-5 divided doses × 7-14 days

Herpes simplex prophylaxis for chronic suppression therapy (unlabeled)

• **Adult and adolescent: PO** 400 mg bid up to 12 mo

• **Child: PO** 800-1000 mg/day in 2-5 divided doses, max 80 mg/kg/day

Available forms: Caps 200 mg; tabs 400, 800 mg; powder for inj 500, 1000 mg; sol for inj 50 mg/ml; oral susp 200 mg/5 ml

Administer:

PO route

• Do not break, crush, or chew caps

• May give without regard to meals, with 8 oz of water

• Shake susp before use

Intermittent IV INF route

• Increase fluids to 3 L/day to decrease crystalluria; most critical during first 2 hr after IV

• Reconstitute with 10 ml compatible sol/500 mg or 20 mg/1 g of product, conc of 50 mg/ml, shake, further dilute in 50-125 ml compatible sol; use within 12 hr; give over at least 1 hr (constant rate) by inf pump to prevent nephrotoxicity; do not reconstitute with sol containing benzyl alcohol in neonates

Solution compatibilities: D_5W, LR, or NaCl (D_5 0.9% NaCl, 0.9% NaCl) sol

Y-site compatibilities: Alemtuzumab, alfentanil, allopurinol, amikacin, aminophylline, amphotericin B cholesteryl, amphotericin B liposome, ampicillin, anidulafungin, argatroban, atracurium, bivalirudin, buprenorphine, busulfan, butorphanol, calcium chloride/gluconate, CARBOplatin, cefazolin, cefonicid, cefoperazone, cefotaxime, cefoxitin, ceftazidime, ceftizoxime, cefTRIAXone, cefuroxime, cephapirin, chloramphenicol, cholesteryl sulfate complex, cimetidine, clindamycin, dexamethasone sodium phosphate, dimenhyDRINATE, DOXOrubicin, doxycycline, erythromycin, famotidine, filgrastim, fluconazole, gallium, gentamicin, granisetron, heparin, hydrocortisone sodium succinate, hydromorphone, imipenem/cilastatin, LORazepam, magnesium sulfate, melphalan, methylPREDNISolone sodium succinate, metoclopramide, metroNIDAZOLE, multivitamin, nafcillin, oxacillin, paclitaxel, penicillin G potassium, PENTobarbital, perphenazine, piperacillin, potassium chloride, propofol, ranitidine, remifentanil, sodium bicarbonate, tacrolimus, teniposide, theophylline, thiotepa, ticarcillin, tobramycin, trimethoprim-sulfamethoxazole, vancomycin, vasopressin, voriconazole, zidovudine

SIDE EFFECTS

CNS: Tremors, confusion, lethargy, hallucinations, **seizures**, dizziness, headache, encephalopathic changes

EENT: Gingival hyperplasia

GI: Nausea, vomiting, diarrhea, increased ALT/AST, abdominal pain, glossitis, colitis

GU: **Oliguria, proteinuria, hematuria,** vaginitis, moniliasis, **glomerulonephritis, acute renal failure,** changes in menses, polydipsia

HEMA: **Thrombotic thrombocytopenia purpura, hemolytic uremic syndrome** (immunocompromised patients)

INTEG: Rash, urticaria, pruritus, pain or phlebitis at IV site, unusual sweating, alopecia, **Stevens-Johnson syndrome**

MS: Joint pain, leg pain, muscle cramps

PHARMACOKINETICS

Distributed widely; crosses placenta; CSF concentrations are 50% plasma; protein binding 9%-33%

PO: Absorbed minimally, onset unknown, peak $1^1/_2$-2 hr, terminal half-life $3^1/_2$ hr

IV: Onset immediate, peak immediate, duration unknown, half-life 20 min-3 hr (terminal); metabolized by liver, excreted by kidneys as unchanged product (95%)

INTERACTIONS

Increase: CNS side effects; zidovudine

Increase: levels, toxicity—probenecid, mycophenolate

Increase: nephrotoxicity—aminoglycosides

Increase: concentrations of—entecavir, pemetrexed, tenofovir

Decrease: action of—hydantoins, valproic acid

- Zoster vaccine: avoid use

Drug/Lab Test

Increase: BUN, creatinine

NURSING CONSIDERATIONS

Assess:

- Signs of infection, anemia
- **Toxicity:** any patient with compromised renal system because product is excreted slowly with poor renal system function; toxicity may occur rapidly
- Hepatic, renal studies: AST, ALT; urinalysis, protein, BUN, creatinine, CCr, watch for increasing BUN and serum creatinine or decreased CCr; I&O ratio; report hematuria, oliguria, fatigue, weakness; may indicate **nephrotoxicity;** check for protein in urine during treatment
- Blood studies: WBC, RBC, Hct, Hgb, bleeding time; blood dyscrasias may occur; product should be discontinued
- C&S before product therapy; product may be taken as soon as culture is taken; repeat C&S after treatment; determine the presence of other infections
- Bowel pattern before, during treatment; if severe abdominal pain with

bleeding occurs, product should be discontinued
• Skin eruptions: rash, urticaria, itching
• Allergies before treatment, reaction of each medication; place allergies on chart in bright red letters
• Neurologic status with herpes encephalitis

Perform/provide:
• Storage at room temp for up to 12 hr after reconstitution; if refrigerated, sol may show a precipitate that clears at room temp; yellow discoloration does not affect potency
• Adequate intake of fluids (2 L) to prevent deposits in kidneys

Evaluate:
• Therapeutic response: absence of itching, painful lesions; crusting and healed lesions; decreased symptoms of chickenpox; healing, decreased pain with herpes zoster

Teach patient/family:
• To take as prescribed; if dose is missed, take as soon as remembered up to 1 hr before next dose; do not double dose
• That product may be taken orally before infection occurs; product should be taken when itching or pain occurs, usually before eruptions
• That sexual partners need to be told that patient has herpes because they can become infected; condoms must be worn to prevent reinfections
• Not to touch lesions to avoid spreading infection to new sites
• That product does not cure infection, just controls symptoms and does not prevent infecting others
• **Superinfection:** to report sore throat, fever, fatigue
• That product must be taken in equal intervals around the clock to maintain blood levels for duration of therapy
• **Blood dyscrasias:** to notify prescriber of side effects of bruising, bleeding, fatigue, malaise
• To seek dental care during treatment to prevent gingival hyperplasia
• That women with genital herpes are more likely to develop cervical cancer; to keep all gynecologic appointments

TREATMENT OF OVERDOSE:
Discontinue product, hemodialysis, resuscitate if needed

acyclovir topical
See Appendix B

adalimumab (Rx)
(add-a-lim′yu-mab)

Humira

Func. class.: Antirheumatic agent (disease modifying), immunomodulator, anti-TNF

Chem. class.: Recombinant human IgG1 monoclonal antibody, DMARD

Do not confuse:
Humira/Humulin/Humalog

ACTION: A form of human IgG1 monoclonal antibody specific for human tumor necrosis factor (TNF); elevated levels of TNF are found in patients with rheumatoid arthritis

USES: Reduction of signs and symptoms and inhibition of progression of structural damage in patients with moderate to severe active rheumatoid arthritis who are ≥18 years of age and who have not responded to other disease-modifying agents, juvenile rheumatoid arthritis (JRA), psoriatic arthritis, Crohn's disease, moderate to severe plaque psoriasis, ankylosing spondylitis

CONTRAINDICATIONS: Hypersensitivity

Precautions: Pregnancy (B), breastfeeding, children, geriatric patients, CNS demyelinating disease, lymphoma, CHF, hepatitis B carriers, manitol hypersensitivity, latex allergy, neoplastic disease

Black Box Warning: Active infections, risk of lymphomas/leukemias, TB

DOSAGE AND ROUTES

Rheumatoid arthritis/ankylosing spondylitis/psoriatic arthritis

• **Adult: SUBCUT** 40 mg every other wk or every wk if not combined with methotrexate; **IV** (unlabeled) 0.25-3 mg/kg q2-4wk

Juvenile rheumatoid arthritis

• **Child ≥4 yr/adolescent ≥30 kg: SUBCUT** 40 mg every other wk

• **Child ≥4 yr/adolescent ≥15 kg to <30 kg: SUBCUT** 20 mg every other wk

• **Child ≥4 yr/adolescent <15 kg: SUBCUT** 24 mg/m^2 BSA (up to 40 mg total) every other wk, then 20 mg every other wk

Crohn's disease

• **Adult: SUBCUT** 160 mg given as 4 inj on day 1 or 2 inj each on days 1 and 2, then 80 mg at wk 2 and 40 mg every other wk starting at wk 4

Plaque psoriasis

• **Adult: SUBCUT** 80 mg baseline as 2 inj then 40 mg every other wk starting 1 wk after initial dose × 16 wk

Available form: Inj 40 mg/0.8 ml; 20 mg/0.4 ml (pediatric)

Administer:

SUBCUT route

• Do not admix with other sol or medications; do not use filter; protect from light; give at 45-degree angle using abdomen, thighs; rotate inj sites; discard unused portions

SIDE EFFECTS

CNS: *Headache*
CV: *Hypertension*
EENT: *Sinusitis*
GI: Abdominal pain, nausea, hepatic damage
HEMA: Leukopenia pancytopenia, aplastic anemia, agranulocytopenia
INTEG: *Rash, inj site reaction*
MISC: Flulike symptoms, UTI, back pain, lupuslike syndrome, increased cancer risk, *antibody development to this drug;* risk of infection (TB, invasive fungal infections, other opportunistic infections), may be fatal, Stevens-Johnson syndrome
RESP: *URI,* pulmonary fibrosis

PHARMACOKINETICS

Absorption 65%, terminal half-life 2 wk, lower clearance with advancing age (40-75 yr), high RA factor

INTERACTIONS

Increase: serious infections—other TNF blockers, rilonacept

• Do not use with anakinra

• Do not give concurrently with vaccines; immunizations should be brought up to date before treatment

NURSING CONSIDERATIONS

Assess:

• **RA:** pain, stiffness, ROM, swelling of joints before, during treatment

• For inj site pain, swelling, redness; usually occur after 2 inj (4-5 days), use cold compress to relieve pain/swelling

Black Box Warning: For infections (fever, flulike symptoms, dyspnea, change in urination, redness/swelling around any wounds), stop treatment if present; some serious infections including sepsis may occur, may be fatal; patients with active infections should not be started on this product

• Latent TB before therapy, treat before starting this product

• **Anaphylaxis, latex allergy:** stop therapy if lupuslike syndrome develops

• **Blood dyscrasias:** CBC, differential periodically

Black Box Warning: For neoplastic disease (lymphomas/leukemia)

Evaluate:

• Therapeutic response: decreased inflammation, pain in joints, decreased joint destruction

Teach patient/family:

• About self-administration if appropriate: inj should be made in thigh, abdomen, upper arm; rotate sites at least 1 inch from old site; do not inject in areas that are bruised, red, hard

• That if medication is not taken when due, inject next dose as soon as remembered and inject next dose as scheduled

• Not to take any live virus vaccines during treatment
• To report signs of infection, allergic reaction, or lupuslike syndrome

adefovir (Rx)

(add-ee-foh′veer)

Hepsera

Func. class.: Antiviral

Chem. class.: Adenosine monophosphate analog

ACTION: Inhibits hepatitis B virus DNA polymerase by competing with natural substrates and by causing DNA termination after its incorporation into viral DNA; causes viral DNA death

USES: Chronic hepatitis B

CONTRAINDICATIONS: Hypersensitivity

Precautions: Pregnancy (C), labor, breastfeeding, children, geriatric patients, dialysis, females, obesity, organ transplant

Black Box Warning: Severe renal disease, impaired hepatic function, lactic acidosis, HIV

DOSAGE AND ROUTES

• **Adult/adolescent: PO** 10 mg/day, optimal duration unknown

Renal dose

• **Adult: PO** CCr ≥50 ml/min 10 mg q24hr; CCr 30-49 ml/min 10 mg q48hr; CCr 10-29 ml/min 10 mg q72hr; hemodialysis 10 mg q7days after dialysis

Available forms: Tabs 10 mg

Administer:

• By mouth without regard for food

SIDE EFFECTS

CNS: *Headache*

GI: *Dyspepsia,* abdominal pain, nausea, vomiting, diarrhea, hepatomegaly, flatulence, **pancreatitis**

GU: Hematuria, glycosuria, **nephrotoxicity, Fanconi syndrome, renal failure**

MISC: Fever, rash, weight loss, cough

PHARMACOKINETICS

PO: Rapidly absorbed from GI tract, peak 1¾ hr, excreted by kidneys 45%, terminal half-life 7.48 hr

INTERACTIONS

Increase: serum conc and possible toxicity—aminoglycosides, memantine, emtricitabine, efavirenz, dofetilide, digoxin, cyclosporine, amiloride, quiNINE, quiNIDine, procainamide, pemetrexed, midodrine, metformin, NSAIDs, vancomycin, trospium, triamterene, tenofovir, tacrolimus, ranitidine, cimetidine, morphine

Black Box Warning: Increase: NNRTIs, NRTIs, antiretroviral protease inhibitors

Drug/Lab Test

Increase: ALT, AST, amylase, creatine kinase

NURSING CONSIDERATIONS

Assess:

Black Box Warning: For nephrotoxicity: increasing CCr, BUN

Black Box Warning: For HIV before beginning treatment, because HIV resistance may occur in chronic hepatitis B patients

Black Box Warning: For lactic acidosis, severe hepatomegaly with stenosis; for use of NNRTIs, NRTIs, antiretroviral protease inhibitors (PIs), lactic acidosis with severe hepatomegaly is more common

• Geriatric patients more carefully; may develop renal, cardiac symptoms more rapidly

Black Box Warning: For exacerbations of hepatitis after discontinuing treatment, monitor LFTs, hepatitis B serology

Perform/provide:

• Storage in cool environment; protect from light

Evaluate:
- Therapeutic response: decreased symptoms of chronic hepatitis B, improving LFTs

Teach patient/family:
- That optimal duration of treatment is unknown, that product is not a cure, that transmission may still occur
- To avoid use with other medications unless approved by prescriber
- To notify prescriber of decreased urinary output
- To avoid breastfeeding

⚠ HIGH ALERT

adenosine (Rx)

(a-den′oh-seen)

Adenocard, Adenoscan

Func. class.: Antidysrhythmic

Chem. class.: Endogenous nucleoside

ACTION: Slows conduction through AV node, can interrupt reentry pathways through AV node, and can restore normal sinus rhythm in patients with paroxysmal supraventricular tachycardia (PSVT)

USES: PSVT, as a diagnostic aid to assess myocardial perfusion defects in CAD, Wolff-Parkinson-White (WPW) syndrome

Unlabeled uses: Wide-complex tachycardia diagnosis

CONTRAINDICATIONS: Hypersensitivity, 2nd- or 3rd-degree AV block, sick sinus syndrome, atrial flutter, atrial fibrillation, ventricular tachycardia, bronchospastic lung disease, symptomatic bradycardia, bundle branch block, heart transplant, unstable angina

Precautions: Pregnancy (C), breastfeeding, children, geriatric patients, asthma

DOSAGE AND ROUTES

Antidysrhythmic
- **Adult and child >50 kg: IV BOL** 6 mg; if conversion to normal sinus rhythm does not occur within 1-2 min, give 12 mg by rapid **IV BOL**; may repeat 12-mg dose again in 1-2 min
- **Infant and child <50 kg: IV BOL** 0.1 mg/kg; if not effective, increase dose by 0.05-0.1 mg/kg q2min to a max of 0.3 mg/kg/dose
- **Neonate: IV BOL** 0.05 mg/kg by rapid IV BOL, may increase by 0.05 mg/kg q2min, max 0.3 mg/kg/dose

Diagnostic use
- **Adult: IV INF** 140 mcg/kg/min × 6 min

Wolff-Parkinson-White (WPW) syndrome
- **Adult/adolescent/child ≥50 kg:** Rapid **IV BOL** 6 mg, follow with saline flush; then **IV BOL** 12 mg if needed

Wide-complex tachycardia diagnosis (unlabeled)
- **Adult/adolescent/child ≥50 kg:** Rapid **IV BOL** 6 mg, follow with saline flush; then **IV BOL** 12 mg if needed

Available forms: Adenocardi Inj 3 mg/ml in prefilled syringes; Adenoscani 3 mg/ml in vials

Administer:
- Warm to room temp; crystals will dissolve

IV, direct route
- **Adenocard:** undiluted; give 6 mg or less by rapid inj over 1-2 sec; if using an IV line, use port near insertion site, flush with NS (20 ml), then elevate arm

Intermittent INF (diagnostic testing)
- Use 30-ml vial, undiluted, by peripheral vein at a rate of 140 mcg/kg/min over 6 min for a total dose of 0.84 mg/kg, inject Thallium 201 as close to venous access as possible after 3 min of inf

Y-site compatibilities: abciximab

Solution compatibilities: D_5LR, D_5W, LR, 0.9% NaCl

A

SIDE EFFECTS

CNS: Lightheadedness, dizziness, arm tingling, numbness, apprehension, blurred vision, headache
CV: Chest pain, pressure, atrial tachydysrhythmias, sweating, palpitations, hypotension, *facial flushing,* AV block, **cardiac arrest, ventricular dysrhythmias**
GI: *Nausea,* metallic taste, throat tightness, groin pressure
RESP: *Dyspnea, chest pressure,* hyperventilation, **bronchospasm (asthmatics)**

PHARMACOKINETICS

Cleared from plasma in <30 sec, half-life 10 sec, converted to inosine/adenosine monophosphate

INTERACTIONS

Increase: risk for higher degree of heart block—carbamazepine
Increase: risk for ventricular fibrillation—digoxin, verapamil
• Smoking: increase tachycardia
Increase: effects of adenosine—dipyridamole
Decrease: activity of adenosine—theophylline or other methylxanthines (caffeine)
Drug/Herb
Increase: adenosine effect—ginger
Decrease: adenosine effect—guarana, green tea

NURSING CONSIDERATIONS

Assess:
• I&O ratio, electrolytes (K, Na, Cl)
• **Cardiopulmonary status:** B/P, pulse, respiration, rhythm, ECG intervals (PR, QRS, QT); check for transient dysrhythmias (PVCs, PACs, sinus tachycardia, AV block)
• Respiratory status: rate, rhythm, lung fields for crackles, watch for respiratory depression; bilateral crackles may occur in **CHF** patient; increased respiration, increased pulse, product should be discontinued
• CNS effects: dizziness, confusion, psychosis, paresthesias, seizures; product should be discontinued
Perform/provide:
• Storage at room temperature; sol should be clear; discard unused product
Evaluate:
• Therapeutic response: normal sinus rhythm or diagnosis of perfusion defect
Teach patient/family:
• To report facial flushing, dizziness, sweating, palpitations, chest pain; usually transient
• To rise from sitting or standing slowly to prevent orthostatic hypotension

TREATMENT OF OVERDOSE:

Defibrillation, vasopressor for hypotension, theophylline

aflibercept

See Appendix A—Selected new drugs

albumin, human 5%/25% (Rx)

(al-byoo′min)
Albuked, Albuminar, Albutein, Buminate, Flexbumin, Plasbumin
Func. class.: Plasma volume expander
Chem. class.: Placental human plasma

ACTION: Exerts oncotic pressure, which expands volume of circulating blood and maintains cardiac output

USES: Restores plasma volume after burns, hyperbilirubinemia, shock, hypoproteinemia, prevention of cerebral edema, cardiopulmonary bypass procedures, ARDS, nephrotic syndrome

CONTRAINDICATIONS: Hypersensitivity, CHF, severe anemia, renal insufficiency, pulmonary edema

Precautions: Pregnancy (C), decreased salt intake, decreased cardiac reserve, lack of albumin deficiency, renal/hepatic disease, chronic anemia

DOSAGE AND ROUTES

Burns

• **Adult: IV** dose to maintain plasma albumin at 3-4 mg/dl

Shock

• **Adult: IV** rapidly give 5% sol, when close to normal inf at ≤2-4 ml/min (25% sol ≤1 ml/min)

• **Child: IV** 0.5-1 g/kg/dose 5% sol, may repeat as needed, max 6 g/kg/day

Nephrotic Syndrome

• **Adult: IV** 100-200 ml of 25% and loop diuretic × 7-10 days

Hypoproteinemia

• **Adult: IV** 25 g, may repeat in 15-30 min, or 50-75 g of 25% albumin infused at ≤2 ml/min

• **Child and infant: IV** 0.5-1 g/kg/dose over 2-4 hr, may repeat q1-2days

Hyperbilirubinemia/erythroblastosis fetalis

• **Infant: IV** 1 g/kg 1-2 hr before transfusion

Available forms: Inj (5%) 50 mg/ml, (25%) 250 mg/ml

Administer:

IV route

• Slowly, to prevent fluid overload; dilute with NS for injection or D_5W; 5% is given undiluted; 25% may be given diluted or undiluted; give over 30-60 min, use inf pump, use large-gauge needle; inf must be completed within 4 hr

• 5% solution may be used with hypovolemic/intravascular depletion

• 25% solution may be used with sodium/fluid restrictions

Solution compatibilities: LR, NaCl, Ringer's, D_5W, $D_{10}W$, $D_{21/2}W$, NaCl 0.9%, dextrose/Ringer's, dextrose/LR

Y-site compatibilities: Diltiazem, LORazepam

SIDE EFFECTS

CNS: Fever, chills, flushing, headache

CV: Fluid overload, hypotension, erratic pulse, tachycardia

GI: Nausea, vomiting, increased salivation

INTEG: Rash, urticaria

RESP: Altered respirations, pulmonary edema

PHARMACOKINETICS

In hyponutrition states, metabolized as protein/energy source; terminal half-life 21 days

INTERACTIONS

Drug/Lab Test

Increase: sodium, serum albumin

Decrease: Hct, Hgb

False increase: alk phos

NURSING CONSIDERATIONS

Assess:

• Blood studies Hct, Hgb; if serum protein declines, dyspnea, hypoxemia can result

• Decreased B/P, erratic pulse, respiration

• I&O ratio: urinary output may decrease

⚠ **Circulatory/pulmonary overload:** CVP, pulmonary wedge pressure distended neck veins indicate circulatory overload; shortness of breath, anxiety, insomnia, expiratory crackles, frothy blood-tinged cough, cyanosis indicate pulmonary overload

• Allergy: fever, rash, itching, chills, flushing, urticaria, nausea, vomiting, hypotension, requires discontinuation of inf, use of new lot if therapy reinstituted; premedicate with diphenhydrAMINE

Perform/provide:

• Adequate hydration before, during administration

• Check type of albumin; some stored at room temp, some need to be refrigerated, use within 4 hr of opening

Evaluate:
- Therapeutic response: increased B/P, decreased edema, increased serum albumin levels, increased plasma protein

Teach patient/family:
- Reason for product; to report hypersensitivity

albuterol (Rx)

(al-byoo′ter-ole)

Accuneb, Gen-Salbutamol ♣, Novo-Salmol ♣, Proair HFA, Proventil, Proventil HFA, ReliOn, Ventolin HFA, VoSpire ER

Func. class.: Adrenergic β_2-agonist, sympathomimetic, bronchodilator

Do not confuse:
albuterol/atenolol
Ventolin/Vantin
Proventil/Prinivil
Salbutamol/salmeterol

ACTION: Causes bronchodilation by action on β_2 (pulmonary) receptors by increasing levels of cAMP, which relaxes smooth muscle; produces bronchodilation, CNS, cardiac stimulation as well as increased diuresis and gastric acid secretion; longer acting than isoproterenol

USES: Prevention of exercise-induced asthma, acute bronchospasm, bronchitis, emphysema, bronchiectasis, or other reversible airway obstruction

Unlabeled uses: Hyperkalemia in dialysis patients

CONTRAINDICATIONS: Hypersensitivity to sympathomimetics, tachydysrhythmias, severe cardiac disease, heart block

Precautions: Pregnancy (C), breastfeeding, cardiac/renal disease, hyperthyroidism, diabetes mellitus, hypertension, prostatic hypertrophy, angle-closure glaucoma, seizures, exercise-induced bronchospasm (aerosol) in children <12 yr, hypoglycemia

DOSAGE AND ROUTES

Bronchospasm prophylaxis
- **Adult and child ≥4 yr: INH** (metered-dose inhaler) 2 puffs q4-6hr as needed

Other respiratory conditions
- **Adult and child ≥12 yr: INH** (metered-dose inhaler) 1 puff q4-6hr; **PO** 2-4 mg tid-qid, max 32 mg; **NEB/IPPB** 2.5 mg tid-qid
- **Geriatric: PO** 2 mg tid-qid, may increase gradually to 8 mg tid-qid
- **Child 2-12 yr: INH** (metered-dose inhaler) 0.1 mg/kg tid (max 2.5 mg tid-qid); **NEB/IPPB** 0.1-0.15 mg/kg/dose tid-qid or 1.25 mg tid-qid for child 10-15 kg or 2.5 mg tid-qid for child >15 kg

Hyperkalemia (unlabeled)
- **Adult: ORAL INH** (albuterol nebulizer sol) 10-20 mg

Available forms: Aerosol 90 mcg/actuation; oral syr 2 mg/5 ml; tabs 2, 4 mg; ext rel 4, 8 mg; INH sol 0.5, 0.83, 1, 2, 5 mg/ml; powder for INH (Ventodisk) 200, 400 mcg; INH cap 200 mcg; 100 mcg/spray, 80 INH/canister, 200 INH/canister

Administer:

PO route
- Do not break, crush, or chew ext rel tabs; give with meals to decrease gastric irritation
- **Oral sol** to children (no alcohol, sugar)

Inhalation route
- For geriatric patients and children, a spacing device is advised
- After shaking metered-dose inhaler, exhale, place mouthpiece in mouth, inhale slowly while depressing inhaler, hold breath, remove, exhale slowly; give INH at least 1 min apart
- **NEB/IPPB** diluting 5 mg/ml sol/2.5 ml 0.9% NaCl for INH; other sol do not require dilution; for neb O_2 flow or compressed air 6-10 L/min
- Gum, sips of water for dry mouth

SIDE EFFECTS

CNS: *Tremors, anxiety,* insomnia, headache, dizziness, stimulation, *restlessness,* hallucinations, flushing, irritability

CV: Palpitations, tachycardia, angina, hypo/hypertension, dysrhythmias
EENT: Dry nose, irritation of nose and throat
GI: Heartburn, nausea, vomiting
MISC: Flushing, sweating, anorexia, bad taste/smell changes, hypokalemia
MS: Muscle cramps
RESP: Cough, wheezing, dyspnea, **paradoxical bronchospasm**, dry throat

PHARMACOKINETICS

Extensively metabolized in the liver and tissues, crosses placenta, breast milk, blood-brain barrier
PO: Onset ½ hr, peak 2-3 hr, duration 4-6 hr, half-life 2.7-6 hr, well absorbed
PO-ER: Onset ½ hr; peak 2-3 hr; duration 8-12 hr
INH: Onset 5-15 min, peak 1-1½ hr, duration 3-6 hr, half-life 4 hr

INTERACTIONS

Increase: ECG changes/hypokalemia—potassium-losing diuretics
Increase: severe hypotension—oxytocics
Increase: toxicity—theophylline
Increase: action of aerosol bronchodilators
Increase: action of albuterol—tricyclics, MAOIs, other adrenergics; do not use together
Increase: CV effects—atomoxetine, selegiline
Decrease: albuterol—other β-blockers
Drug/Herb
Increase: stimulation—caffeine (cola nut, green/black tea, guarana, yerba maté, coffee, chocolate)

NURSING CONSIDERATIONS

Assess:
- Respiratory function: vital capacity, forced expiratory volume, ABGs; lung sounds, heart rate and rhythm, B/P, sputum (baseline and peak); whether patient has not received theophylline therapy before giving dose
- Patient's ability to self-medicate
- For evidence of allergic reactions
- For paradoxical bronchospasm; hold medication, notify prescriber if bronchospasm occurs

Perform/provide:
- Storage in light-resistant container; do not expose to temperatures of more than 86° F (30° C)

Evaluate:
- Therapeutic response: absence of dyspnea, wheezing after 1 hr, improved airway exchange, improved ABGs

Teach patient/family:
- To use exactly as prescribed; to take missed dose when remembered, alter dosing schedule; not to use OTC medications; that excess stimulation may occur
- About use of inhaler: review package insert with patient; use demonstration; return demonstration; shake, prime before 1st use and when not used for >2 wk; release 4 test sprays into air, away from the face
- To avoid getting aerosol in eyes (blurring of vision may result) or using near flames or sources of heat
- To wash inhaler in warm water daily and dry; to track number of inhalations used and to discard product when labeled inhalations have been used
- To avoid smoking, smoke-filled rooms, persons with respiratory infections

⚠ That **paradoxical bronchospasm** may occur; to stop product immediately, call prescriber
- To limit caffeine products such as chocolate, coffee, tea, colas

TREATMENT OF OVERDOSE:

Administer β_1-adrenergic blocker, IV fluids

⚠ Nurse Alert

⚠ HIGH ALERT

aldesleukin, IL-2 (Rx)

(al-dess-loo′ken)

Proleukin

Func. class.: Antineoplastic—miscellaneous

Chem. class.: Interleukin-2, human recombinant (cytokine)

Do not confuse:
aldesleukin/oprelvekin
Proleukin/oprelvekin/Prokine

ACTION: Enhancement of lymphocyte mitogenesis and stimulation of IL-2–dependent cell lines; enhancement of lymphocyte cytotoxicity; induction of killer cell activity; induction of interferon-γ production; results in activation of cellular immunity, production of cytokines, and inhibition of tumor growth

USES: Metastatic renal cell carcinoma in adults; melanoma (metastatic)
Unlabeled uses: Acute myelogenous leukemia (AML), cutaneous T-cell lymphoma (CTCL), HIV, Hansen's disease (leprosy), mycosis fungoides, non-Hodgkin's lymphoma, phase II for HIV in combination with zidovudine

CONTRAINDICATIONS: Hypersensitivity, abnormal thallium stress test or pulmonary function tests, organ allografts, angina, cardiac tamponade, MI, GI bleeding/perforation, psychosis, renal failure, pulmonary insufficiency, seizures, ventricular tachycardia

Black Box Warning: Cardiac/pulmonary disease, coma

Precautions: Pregnancy (C), breastfeeding, children, CNS metastases, bacterial infections, renal/hepatic disease, anemia, thrombocytopenia, scleroderma, vasculitis

Black Box Warning: Capillary leak syndrome, infection

DOSAGE AND ROUTES

Renal cell cancer/malignant melanoma

• **Adult: IV INF without LAK cells** 600,000 international units/kg (0.037 mg/kg) over 15 min q8hr × 14 doses, off 9 days, repeat schedule for another 14 doses for a max of 28 doses/course; **SUBCUT (unlabeled)** 1800 international units/m² up to 18 million international units q day × 5 days then 2-day rest period, repeat q wk × 6-8 wk; **Cont IV INF (unlabeled)** 18 million international units/m² × 2 (5 day cycles), separate by 3-7 day rest period

Hansen's disease (leprosy) (unlabeled)

• **Adult: INTRADERMAL** 180,000 international units inj into each lesion bid × 8 days

Acute myelogenous leukemia (AML) (unlabeled)

• **Adult: IV** 9 million international units/m²/day over 1 hr on days 1-5 and 8-12 q6wk, max 4 cycles (for patients who have had 2nd remission after standard treatment)

Refractory non-Hodgkin's lymphoma/cutaneous T-cell lymphoma (CTCL) (mycosis fungoides) (unlabeled)

• **Adult: CONT IV INF** 20 million international units/m²/day for 3 courses of 5, 4, 3 days during weeks 1, 3, 5, respectively

HIV (unlabeled)

• **Adult: IV** 18 million international units/m²/day × 5 days q2mo × 6 cycles; **SUBCUT** 3-18 million international units/m²/day

Available forms: Powder for inj 22 million international units/vial

Administer:

SUBCUT route (unlabeled)

• Take care not to inject intradermally

Intermittent IV INF route

• Premedicate with antipyretic, H_2 blocker, antiemetics, antibiotic; use meperidine; dopamine drip for hypotention, IV fluids

• IV after diluting 22 million international units (1.3 mg)/1.2 ml sterile water for inj at site of vial and swirl, do not shake; dilute dose with 50 ml D_5W and give over 15 min; use plastic bag; do not use an in-line filter, give through Y-tube or 3-way stopcock; warm to room temperature before use

Continuous IV INF route

• Dilute appropriate reconstituted IV sol in a sufficient amount of D_5W inj containing 0.1% albumin human to 5-60 mcg/ml
• Do not use an in-line filter
• Hydrocortisone, dexamethasone, or sodium bicarbonate (1 mEq/1 ml) for extravasation, apply ice compresses
• Antiemetic 30-60 min before giving product to prevent vomiting
• DOPamine 1-5 kg/min before onset of hypotension; decreased dose preserves kidney output

Y-site compatibilities: Amikacin, amphotericin B, calcium gluconate, diphenhydrAMINE, DOPamine, fluconazole, foscarnet, gentamicin, heparin, IV fat emulsion, magnesium sulfate, metoclopramide, morphine, ondansetron, piperacillin, potassium chloride, ranitidine, ticarcillin, tobramycin, TPN #145, trimethoprim-sulfamethoxazole

SIDE EFFECTS

CNS: Mental status changes, dizziness, sensory dysfunction, syncope, motor dysfunction, *fever, chills,* headache, impaired memory, depression, sleep disturbances, hallucinations, rigors, neuropathy

CV: *Hypotension,* sinus tachycardia, dysrhythmias, bradycardia, PVCs, PACs, myocardial ischemia, **myocardial infarction, cardiac arrest, capillary leak syndrome, CVA**

EENT: Reversible visual changes

GI: *Nausea, vomiting, diarrhea, stomatitis, anorexia,* GI bleeding, dyspepsia, constipation, **intestinal perforation/ileus,** jaundice, ascites

GU: **Oliguria/anuria, proteinuria, hematuria, dysuria, renal failure**

HEMA: *Anemia,* **thrombocytopenia, leukopenia, coagulation disorders, leukocytosis, eosinophilia**

INTEG: *Pruritus, erythema, rash,* dry skin, **exfoliative dermatitis,** purpura, petechiae, urticaria

MS: Arthralgia, myalgia

RESP: Pulmonary congestion, *dyspnea,* **pulmonary edema, respiratory failure,** apnea, tachypnea, pleural effusion, wheezing

SYST: Infection

PHARMACOKINETICS

Half-life 85 min; onset, 4 wk; duration, variable

INTERACTIONS

Increase: hypotension—antihypertensives
• Reduced antitumor effectiveness: glucocorticoids
• Unpredictable reactions: psychotropics

Increase: toxicity—aminoglycosides, indomethacin, cytotoxic chemotherapy, methotrexate, asparaginase, DOXOrubicin

Decrease: immune response—live virus vaccines; do not use concurrently

Drug/Lab Test

Increase: bilirubin, BUN, serum creatinine, transaminase, alk phos; hypomagnesemia, acidosis hypocalcemia, hypophosphatemia, hypo/hyperkalemia, hyperuricemia, hypoalbuminemia, hypoproteinemia, hyponatremia, alkalosis (toxic effect of product)

NURSING CONSIDERATIONS

Assess:

• CBC, differential, platelet count weekly; may withhold product if WBC is <2000/mm^3 or platelet count is <75,000/mm^3; notify prescriber of these results

Black Box Warning: Capillary leak syndrome including a drop in mean arterial pressure (2-12 hr after initiating therapy); hypotension and hypoperfusion will occur; if B/P <90 mm Hg, use CVP, ECG, VS

- Renal studies: BUN, serum uric acid, urine CCr, electrolytes before, during therapy; I&O ratio; report fall in urine output to <30 ml/hr
- Monitor temp q4hr, chest x-ray, lipid profile, weight
- Hepatic studies before, during therapy: bilirubin, AST, ALT, alk phos, LDH as needed or monthly

⚠ ECG; ST-T wave changes, low QRS and T, possible dysrhythmias (sinus tachycardia, PVCs); ejection fraction

Black Box Warning: Baselines in pulmonary function; document FEV >2 L or ≥75% before therapy; monitor temp q4hr, pulse oximetry, dyspnea, crackles, ABGs; watch for respiratory failure, intubate if necessary

- Stress thallium study before therapy; document normal ejection fraction, unimpaired wall motion
- Bleeding: hematuria, guaiac, bruising petechiae
- Buccal cavity q8hr for dryness, sores, ulceration, white patches, oral pain, bleeding, dysphagia
- Local irritation, pain, burning at inj site
- GI symptoms: frequency of stools, cramping; acidosis, signs of dehydration: rapid respirations, poor skin turgor, decreased urine output, dry skin, restlessness, weakness

Perform/provide:

- Rinsing of mouth tid-qid with water, club soda; brushing of teeth bid-tid with soft brush or cotton-tipped applicators for stomatitis; use unwaxed dental floss
- Increased fluid when able to reduce renal problems
- Storage of diluted product in refrigerator; protect from light, do not freeze; administer within 48 hr; bring to room temp before infusing; discard unused portion

Evaluate:

- Therapeutic response: decreased tumor size, spread of malignancy

Teach patient/family:

- To use nonhormonal contraceptive method during therapy
- To report complaints, side effects to nurse, prescriber
- To avoid foods with citric acid, hot foods, foods with rough texture
- To avoid alcohol, salicylates, steroids, vaccinations; GI bleeding may occur
- To report bleeding, white spots, ulcerations in mouth to prescriber; tell patient to examine mouth daily
- To avoid crowds and persons with infections when granulocyte count is low
- That visual problems may occur but are reversible

alemtuzumab (Rx)

(a-lem-too′zoo-mab)

Campath

Func. class.: Antineoplastic—miscellaneous

Chem. class.: Monoclonal antibody

ACTION: Composed of recombinant DNA-derived humanized monoclonal antibody (campath-1H), binds to CD52 antigen present on surface of B and T lymphocytes, causes lysis of leukemic cells

USES: B-cell chronic lymphocytic leukemia that has been treated with alkylating agents and that has failed fludarabine therapy

Unlabeled uses: Cutaneous T-cell lymphoma (CTCL) (mycosis fungoides), prophylaxis/treatment of GVHD, non-Hodgkin's lymphoma (NHL), stem cell transplant, refractory T-cell prolymphocytic leukemia; subcut route

CONTRAINDICATIONS: Hypersensitivity

Precautions: Pregnancy (C), breastfeeding, children

Black Box Warning: Infusion-related reactions, bone marrow suppression, fungal/viral infection, active systemic infection, immunodeficiency

DOSAGE AND ROUTES

Chronic lymphocytic leukemia (CLL)

• **Adult:** **IV** 3 mg over 2 hr/day; when tolerated increase to 10 mg; when 10 mg tolerated increase to 30 mg/day, maintenance is 30 mg/day 3 ×/wk on alternate days for 12 wk, titration usually takes 3-7 days, max single dose 30 mg; max weekly dose 90 mg; **SUBCUT** (unlabeled) 3 mg on day 1, if tolerated give 10 mg on day 3, then target dose of 30 mg on day 5

Dose adjustments for neutropenia/ thrombocytopenia

• **Adult:** **IV** ANC ≤250/mol; platelets ≤25,000; 1st time hold dose; 2nd time hold dose, then resume at 10 mg; if delay is more than 7 days, start at 3 mg; 3rd time, stop completely; ANC 500/mol, platelets 50,000 if delay is more than 7 days, start at 3 mg and increase as tolerated

Available forms: Sol for inj 30 mg/ml

Administer:

Intermittent IV INF route

• Do not give IV push or bolus

• Withdraw amount needed, use 5-micron filter before dilution, check for particulate matter and discoloration; dilute with 100 ml sterile 0.9% NaCl or D_5W, gently invert to mix; do not add other products or infuse in same IV tubing, give over 2 hr

• Do not shake ampule

Black Box Warning: Give diphenhydrAMINE 50 mg and acetaminophen 650 mg ½ hr before inf; give hydrocortisone 200 mg to decrease severe inf reactions; give trimethoprim-sulfamethoxazole DS bid 3 ×/wk and famciclovir 250 mg bid; continue for 2 mo or until CD41 ≥200 cells/mm^3, whichever is later

SUBCUT route (unlabeled)

• Do not shake vial before use; each vial is for single use, discard any unused portion; inspect for particulate, sol should be clear and colorless; no dilution needed; withdraw needed amount, inject, take care not to inject intradermally

SIDE EFFECTS

CNS: *Dizziness, insomnia,* depression, headache, tremor, somnolence, fatigue, drowsiness, weakness, anxiety

CV: *Hypo/hypertension, tachycardia, edema, chest pain, supraventricular tachycardia,* CHF

GI: *Anorexia, diarrhea,* constipation, *nausea, stomatitis, vomiting, abdominal pain, dyspepsia*

HEMA: Anemia, neutropenia, thrombocytopenia, pancytopenia, purpura, epistaxis

INTEG: *Rash,* local reaction, pruritus

MISC: Rigors, *fever, infusion reactions,* sepsis, risk for fatal infection

MS: Back pain

RESP: Cough, pneumonia, rhinitis, bronchospasm, dyspnea, pharyngitis

PHARMACOKINETICS

Complete bioavailability, half-life 12 days, steady state 6 wk, binds to CD52 receptors

INTERACTIONS

Increase: bone marrow depression—radiation, other antineoplastics

Decrease: antibody reaction—live virus vaccines

Drug/Lab Test

Interference: diagnostic tests that involve antibodies

NURSING CONSIDERATIONS

Assess:

• CBC, platelets q wk or more often if myelosuppression occurs; CD4+ after therapy until recovery of >200 cells/μl; irradiate blood if transfusions are required to prevent GVHD

Black Box Warning: For symptoms of infection; chills, fever, headache, may be masked by product fever; do not administer product if infection is present

• CNS reaction: LOC, mental status, dizziness, confusion

• Cardiac status: lung sounds; ECG before and during treatment, especially with cardiac disease; monitor B/P hypotensive effect during administration

Black Box Warning: Bone marrow depression: bruising, bleeding, blood in stools, urine, sputum, emesis

Perform/provide:

- Storage of reconstituted sol for ≤8 hr at room temp, do not freeze; protect from light

Evaluate:

- Therapeutic response: decrease in production of malignant lymphocytes

Teach patient/family:

- To take acetaminophen for fever
- To avoid hazardous tasks because confusion, dizziness may occur
- To report signs of infection: sore throat, fever, diarrhea, vomiting
- To avoid breastfeeding; effects are unknown, do not resume for ≥3 mo after last dose
- To use contraception during treatment and for 6 mo after completion
- To avoid immunizations with live vaccines

alendronate (Rx)

(al-en-drone′ate)

Apo-Alendronate ✦, CO Alendronate ✦, Fosamax, Gen-Alendronate ✦, Novo-Alendronate ✦, PMS-Alendronate ✦

Func. class.: Bone-resorption inhibitor

Chem. class.: Bisphosphonate

Do not confuse:
Fosamax/Flomax

ACTION: Decreases rate of bone resorption and may directly block dissolution of hydroxyapatite crystals of bone, inhibits osteoclast activity

USES: Treatment and prevention of osteoporosis in postmenopausal women, treatment of osteoporosis in men, Paget's disease, treatment of corticosteroid-induced osteoporosis in postmenopausal women not receiving estrogen and in men who are on continuing corticosteroid treatment with low bone mass

CONTRAINDICATIONS: Hypersensitivity to bisphosphonates, delayed esophageal emptying, inability to sit or stand for 30 min, hypocalcemia

Precautions: Pregnancy (C), breastfeeding, children, CCr <35 ml/min, esophageal disease, ulcers, gastritis, poor dental health, increased esophageal cancer risk

DOSAGE AND ROUTES

Osteoporosis in postmenopausal women

- **Adult and geriatric: PO** 10 mg/day or 70 mg q wk

Osteoporosis in men

- **Adult: PO** 10 mg/day or 70 mg q wk

Paget's disease

- **Adult and geriatric: PO** 40 mg/day × 6 mo, consider retreatment for relapse

Prevention of osteoporosis

- **Adult/postmenopausal female: PO** 5 mg/day or 35 mg/wk

Corticosteroid-induced osteoporosis in postmenopausal women (not receiving estrogen)

- **Adult: PO** 10 mg/day

Corticosteroid-induced osteoporosis in men or premenopausal women

- **Adult: PO** 5 mg/day

Renal dose

- **Adult: PO** CCr ≤35 ml/min, not recommended

Available forms: Tabs 5, 10, 35, 40, 70 mg; oral sol 70 mg/75 ml

Administer:

- For 6 months to be effective for Paget's disease
- **Tablet:** take with 8 oz of water 30 min before 1st food, beverage, or medication of the day
- Do not lie down for ≥30 min after dose, do not take at bedtime or before rising
- **Liquid:** use oral syringe or calibrated device; give in AM with ≥2 oz of water

≥30 min before food, beverage, or medication

SIDE EFFECTS

CNS: Headache
CV: Atrial fibrillation
GI: Abdominal pain, constipation, nausea, vomiting, esophageal ulceration, acid reflux, dyspepsia, esophageal perforation, diarrhea, esophageal cancer
META: Hypophosphatemia, hypocalcemia
MS: Bone pain, osteonecrosis of the jaw, bone fractures
SYST: Angioedema, Stevens-Johnson syndrome, toxic epidermal necrolysis

PHARMACOKINETICS

Bioavailability 60%, protein binding 78%, rapidly cleared from circulation, taken up mainly by bones, eliminated primarily through kidneys; after bound to bone, half-life >10 yr

INTERACTIONS

Increase: GI adverse reactions—NSAIDs, salicylates, H_2 blockers, proton pump inhibitors (PPIs), gastric mucosal agents
Decrease: absorption—antacids, calcium supplements, aminoglycosides
Drug/Food
Decrease: absorption when used with caffeine, orange juice, food

NURSING CONSIDERATIONS

Assess:

⚠ Serious reactions: angioedema, Stevens-Johnson syndrome, toxic epidermal necrolysis, atrial fibrillation

• Hormonal status if a woman, before treatment

• **For osteoporosis:** bone density test before and during treatment

• **For Paget's disease:** increased skull size, bone pain, headache; decreased vision, hearing

• Electrolytes; BUN/creatinine; calcium, phosphorous, magnesium, potassium

• **For hypercalcemia:** paresthesia, twitching, laryngospasm; Chvostek's, Trousseau's signs

• Alk phos levels, baseline and periodically, 2 × upper limit of normal is indicative of Paget's disease

• Dental status: regular dental exams should be performed; dental extractions (cover with antiinfectives before procedure)

Perform/provide:

• Storage in cool environment, out of direct sunlight

Evaluate:

• Therapeutic response: increased bone mass, absence of fractures

Teach patient/family:

• To remain upright for 30 min after dose to prevent esophageal irritation; if dose is missed, skip dose, do not double doses or take later in day; to take in AM before food, other meds; to take with 6-8 oz of water only (no mineral water)

• To take calcium, vit D if instructed by health care provider

• To perform weight-bearing exercise to increase bone density

• To let health care provider know if pregnant or if pregnancy is planned or if breastfeeding; to inform dentist of the use of this product

• To maintain good oral hygiene

alfuzosin (Rx)

(al-fyoo'zoe-sin)

Apo-Alfuzosin ♣, Uroxatral

Func. class.: Urinary tract, antispasmodic, α_1-agonist

Chem. class.: Quinazolone

ACTION: Binds to α_{1A}-adrenoceptor subtype located mainly in the prostate, relaxing smooth muscles

USES: Symptoms of benign prostatic hyperplasia
Unlabeled uses: Lower urinary tract symptoms, erectile dysfunction with sildenafil

CONTRAINDICATIONS: Hypersensitivity, moderate to severe hepatic

impairment; not indicated for use in women or children, breastfeeding
Precautions: Pregnancy (B) but not used in females, geriatric patients; CAD, coronary insufficiency, mild hepatic disease, mild/moderate/severe renal disease, history of QT prolongation or coadministration with meds known to prolong QT interval, torsades de pointes, syncope, surgery, prostate cancer, orthostatic hypotension, ocular surgery, dysrhythmias, angina

DOSAGE AND ROUTES

• **Adult: PO EXT REL** 10 mg/day, taken after same meal each day
Available forms: Ext rel tabs 10 mg
Administer:
PO route
• Do not break, crush, chew tabs; give with food; take at same time each day

SIDE EFFECTS

CNS: *Dizziness, headache,* fatigue, flushing
CV: Postural hypotension (dizziness, lightheadedness, fainting) within a few hours of administration, chest pain, tachycardia, angina
GI: Nausea, abdominal pain, dyspepsia, constipation, diarrhea, liver injury, jaundice
INTEG: Rash, urticaria, **angioedema**, pruritus
GU: Impotence, priapism
MISC: Body pain in general, xerostomia, rhinitis
RESP: Upper respiratory infection, pharyngitis, bronchitis, sinusitis

PHARMACOKINETICS

Peak 8 hr, elimination half-life 10 hr, extensively metabolized in liver by CYP3A4 enzyme, excreted via urine (11% unchanged), moderately protein binding (82%-90%)

INTERACTIONS

• Not to be taken with prazosin, terazosin, doxazosin
Increase: QT prolongation (slight)—class IA/III antidysrhythmics
Increase: effects of alfuzosin—alcohol
Increase: effects—CYP3A4 inhibitors (ketoconazole, itraconazole, and ritonavir); do not use together
Increase: hypotension—β-blockers, phosphodiesterase 5 inhibitors, nitrates

NURSING CONSIDERATIONS

Assess:
• **Prostatic hyperplasia:** change in urinary patterns (hesitancy, dribbling, dysuria, urgency), baseline and throughout treatment
• **Serious skin reactions: angioedema**
Perform/provide:
• Storage in tight container in cool environment
Evaluate:
• Therapeutic response: decreased symptoms of benign prostatic hyperplasia
Teach patient/family:
• To take at same time each day with food; to not double doses
• Not to drive or operate machinery for 4 hr after 1st dose or after dosage increase, dizziness may occur
• About orthostatic hypotension; to rise slowly from sitting or lying
• To avoid all OTC products unless approved by prescriber
• To notify prescriber of fainting, dizziness
• That ED is a side effect and is temporary

aliskiren (Rx)

(a-lis′kir-en)

Tekturna

Func. class.: Antihypertensive
Chem. class.: Direct renin inhibitor

ACTION: Renin inhibitor that acts on the renin-angiotensin system (RAS)

USES: Hypertension, alone or in combination with other antihypertensives

CONTRAINDICATIONS:
Hypersensitivity

Black Box Warning: Pregnancy (D) 2nd, 3rd trimester

Precautions: Pregnancy (C) 1st trimester, breastfeeding, children, geriatric patients, angioedema, aortic/renal artery stenosis, cirrhosis, CAD, dialysis, hyper/hypokalemia, hyponatremia, hypotension, hypovolemia, renal/hepatic disease, surgery, diabetes, seizures

DOSAGE AND ROUTES

- **Adult: PO** 150 mg/day, may increase to 300 mg/day if needed, max 300 mg/day

Available forms: Tabs 150, 300 mg

Administer:

- PO; do not use with a high-fat meal
- Daily with a full glass of water, titrate up to achieve correct dose
- Do not discontinue abruptly, correct electrolyte/volume depletion before treatment

SIDE EFFECTS

CV: Orthostatic hypotension, hypotension

CNS: Headache, dizziness

GI: Diarrhea

GU: Renal stones, increased uric acid

INTEG: Rash

META: Hyperkalemia

MISC: Angioedema, cough

PHARMACOKINETICS

Poorly absorbed, bioavailability 2.3%, peak 1-3 hr, steady state 7-8 days, 91% excreted unchanged in the feces, half-life 24 hr

INTERACTIONS

Increase: potassium levels—ACE inhibitors, angiotensin receptor antagonists, potassium supplements, potassium-sparing diuretics

Increase: hypotension—other antihypertensives, diuretics

Increase: aliskiren levels—atorvastatin, itraconazole, ketoconazole, cyclosporine; concurrent use is not recommended

Decrease: levels of warfarin

Drug/Food

Decrease: absorption—high-fat meal

Drug/Lab Test

Increase: uric acid, CPK, BUN, serum creatinine, potassium

Decrease: Hct, Hgb

NURSING CONSIDERATIONS

Assess:

- Renal studies: uric acid, serum creatinine, BUN may be increased; potassium, hyperkalemia may occur

⚠ **Allergic reactions: angioedema** may occur (swelling of face; trouble breathing, swallowing)

- Daily dependent edema in feet, legs; weight, B/P, orthostatic hypotension; if there is a significant drop in B/P, place patient in supine position, give IV 0.9% NaCl

Perform/provide:

- Storage in tight container at room temp

Evaluate:

- Therapeutic response: decrease in B/P

Teach patient/family:

- About the importance of complying with dosage schedule even if feeling better; that if dose is missed, take as soon as possible; that if it is almost time for the next dose, take only that dose; do not double dose

Black Box Warning: To notify if pregnancy is planned or suspected; if pregnant, product will need to be discontinued

- How to take B/P and normal reading for age group
- Not to use OTC products including herbs, supplements unless approved by prescriber
- To report to prescriber immediately: dizziness, faintness, chest pain, palpitations, uneven or rapid heart beat, headache, severe diarrhea, swelling of tongue

or lips, trouble breathing, difficulty swallowing, tightening of the throat
• Not to operate machinery or perform hazardous tasks if dizziness occurs
• To avoid faintness; not to get up, stand up rapidly

allopurinol (Rx)
(al-oh-pure′i-nole)
Aloprim, Apo-Allopurinol ✱, Zyloprim
Func. class.: Antigout drug, antihyperuricemic
Chem. class.: Xanthene oxidase inhibitor

Do not confuse:
allopurinol/Apresoline
Zyloprim/Zovirax

ACTION: Inhibits the enzyme xanthine oxidase, reducing uric acid synthesis

USES: Chronic gout, hyperuricemia associated with malignancies, recurrent calcium oxalate calculi, uric acid calculi

CONTRAINDICATIONS: Hypersensitivity
Precautions: Pregnancy (C), breastfeeding, children, renal/hepatic disease

DOSAGE AND ROUTES
Increased uric acid levels in malignancies
• **Adult: PO** 600-800 mg/day in divided doses for 2-3 days; start up to 1-2 days before chemotherapy; **IV INF** 200-400 mg/m^2/day, max 600 mg/day 24-48 hr before chemotherapy, may be divided at 6-, 8-, 12-hr intervals
• **Child 6-10 yr: PO** 300 mg/day, adjust dose after 48 hr
• **Child <6 yr: PO** 150 mg/day, adjust dose after 48 hr
• **Child: IV INF** 200 mg/m^2/day, initially as a single dose or divided q6-12hr

Recurrent calculi
• **Adult: PO** 200-300 mg/day in a single dose or divided bid-tid, max 300 mg/dose, 800 mg/day
Uric acid nephropathy prevention
• **Adult and child >10 yr: PO** 600-800 mg/day × 2-3 days
Gout (mild)
• **Adult: PO** 100 mg/day, increase q wk based on uric acid levels, max 800 mg/day; maintenance dose 100-200 mg bid-tid
Gout (moderate-severe)
• **Adult: PO** 400-600 mg/day in a single dose or divided bid-tid, max 800 mg/day, doses >300 mg should be given in divided doses
Renal dose
• **Adult: PO/IV** CCr 81-100 ml/min 300 mg/day; CCr 61-80 ml/min 250 mg/day; CCr 41-60 ml/min 200 mg/day; 21-40 ml/min 150 mg/day; CCr 10-20 ml/min 100-200 mg/day; CCr 3-9 ml/min 100 mg/day or 100 mg every other day; CCr <3 ml/min 100 mg q24hr or longer or 100 mg every 3rd day
Available forms: Tabs, scored 100, 300 mg; powder for inj 500 mg/vial
Administer:
PO route
• With meals to prevent GI symptoms; may crush, add to foods or fluids
• A few days before antineoplastic therapy
Intermittent IV INF route
• Reconstitute 30-ml vial with 25 ml of sterile water for inj; dilute to desired conc (≤6 mg/ml) with 0.9% NaCl for inj or D_5 for inj; begin inf within 10 hr

Y-site compatibilities: Acyclovir, aminophylline, amphotericin B lipid complex, anidulafungin, argatroban, atenolol, aztreonam, bivalirudin, bleomycin, bumetanide, buprenorphine, butorphanol, calcium gluconate, CARBOplatin, caspofungin, ceFAZolin, cefoperazone, cefotetan, ceftazidime, ceftizoxime, cefTRIAXone, cefuroxime, CISplatin, cyclophosphamide, DACTINomycin, DAUNOrubicin citrate liposome, dexamethasone, dexmedetomidine, docetaxel, DOXOrubicin liposomal, enalaprilat, etoposide, famotidine, fenoldopam, filgrastim, fluconazole, fludarabine, fluorouracil, furosemide, gallium, ganciclovir, gatifloxacin, gemcitabine, gemtuzumab, granisetron hydrochloride, heparin, hydrocortisone phosphate, hydrocortisone succinate, HYDROmorphone, ifosfamide, linezolid injection, LORazepam, mannitol, mesna, methotrexate, metroNIDAZOLE, milrinone, mitoxantrone, morphine, nesiritide, octreotide, oxytocin, paclitaxel, pamidronate, pantoprazole, pemetrexed, piperacillin, piperacillin-tazobactam, plicamycin, potassium chloride, ranitidine, sodium acetate, sulfamethoxazole-trimethoprim, teniposide, thiotepa, ticarcillin, ticarcillin-clavulanate, tigecycline, tirofiban, vancomycin, vasopressin, vinBLAStine, vinCRIStine, voriconazole, zidovudine, zoledronic acid

SIDE EFFECTS

CNS: *Headache,* drowsiness, neuritis, paresthesia

EENT: Retinopathy, cataracts, epistaxis

GI: *Nausea, vomiting, anorexia, malaise,* metallic taste, cramps, peptic ulcer, diarrhea, stomatitis

HEMA: **Agranulocytosis, thrombocytopenia, aplastic anemia, pancytopenia, leukopenia, bone marrow suppression, eosinophilia**

INTEG: Fever, chills, dermatitis, pruritus, purpura, erythema, ecchymosis, alopecia, rash, **Stevens-Johnson syndrome**

MISC: Myopathy, arthralgia, hepatomegaly, **cholestatic jaundice, renal failure, exfoliative dermatitis**

PHARMACOKINETICS

Protein binding <1%, half-life 1-2 hr

PO: Peak 1.5 hr; excreted in feces, urine

IV: Peak up to 30 min

INTERACTIONS

Increase: kidney stone formation—ammonium chloride, vit C, potassium/sodium phosphate

Increase: rash—ampicillin, amoxicillin

Increase: action of oral anticoagulants, oral antidiabetics, theophylline

Increase: hypersensitivity—ACE inhibitors, thiazides

Increase: bone marrow depression—antineoplastics (mercaptopurine, azaTHIOprine)

Increase: xanthine nephropathy, calculi—rasburicase

NURSING CONSIDERATIONS

Assess:

- **For gout:** joint pain, swelling; may use with NSAIDs for acute gouty attacks; uric acid levels q2wk; uric acid levels should be ≤6 mg/dl
- CBC, AST, BUN, creatinine before starting treatment, periodically
- I&O ratio; increase fluids to 2 L/day to prevent stone formation and toxicity
- For rash, hypersensitivity reactions, discontinue allopurinol

Evaluate:

- Therapeutic response: decreased pain in joints, decreased stone formation in kidneys, decreased uric acid levels

Teach patient/family:

- To take as prescribed; if dose is missed, take as soon as remembered; do not double dose; that tabs may be crushed
- To increase fluid intake to 2 L/day
- To report skin rash, stomatitis, malaise, fever, aching; product should be discontinued
- To avoid hazardous activities if drowsiness or dizziness occurs
- To avoid alcohol, caffeine; will increase uric acid levels
- To avoid large doses of vit C; kidney stone formation may occur
- To reduce dairy products, refined sugars, sodium, meat if taking for calcium oxalate stones

almotriptan (Rx)

(al-moh-trip′tan)

Axert

Func. class.: Antimigraine agent, abortive

Chem. class.: 5-HT_1-receptor agonist, triptan

ACTION: Binds selectively to the vascular 5-$HT_{1B/1D/1F}$-receptors, exerts antimigraine effect

USES: Acute treatment of migraine with or without aura (adult/adolescent/child ≥12 yr)

CONTRAINDICATIONS: Hypersensitivity, acute MI, angina, CV disease, CAD, stroke, vasospastic angina, ischemic heart disease or risk for, peripheral vascular syndrome, uncontrolled hypertension, basilar or hemiplegic migraine

Precautions: Pregnancy (C), postmenopausal women, men >40 yr, breastfeeding, children <18 yr, geriatric patients, risk factors for CAD, MI; hypercholesterolemia, obesity, diabetes, impaired renal/hepatic function, sulfonamide hypersensitivity, cardiac dysrhythmias, Raynaud's disease, tobacco smoking, Wolff-Parkinson-White syndrome

DOSAGE AND ROUTES

- **Adult, adolescent, and child ≥12 yr: PO** 6.25-12.5 mg; may repeat dose after 2 hr; max 2 doses/24 hr, 25 mg/day or 4 treatment cycles within any 30-day period

Hepatic/renal dose CCr 10-30 ml/min

- **Adult: PO** 6.25 mg initially, max 12.5 mg

Available forms: Tabs 6.25, 12.5 mg

Administer:

- Avoid using more than 2 ×/wk; rebound headache may occur
- Swallow tabs whole; do not break, crush, chew

SIDE EFFECTS

CNS: *Tingling, hot sensation, burning, feeling of pressure, tightness, numbness, dizziness, sedation,* headache, anxiety, fatigue, cold sensation, **seizures**

CV: *Flushing,* palpitations, tachycardia, **coronary artery vasospasm, MI, ventricular fibrillation, ventricular tachycardia**

EENT: Throat, mouth, nasal discomfort; vision changes

GI: Nausea, xerostomia

INTEG: Sweating

MS: *Weakness, neck stiffness,* myalgia

RESP: Chest tightness, pressure

PHARMACOKINETICS

Onset of pain relief 2 hr; peak 1-3 hr; duration 3-4 hr; bioavailability 70%; protein binding 35%; metabolized in the liver (metabolite), metabolized by MAO-A, CYP2D6, CYP3A4; excreted in urine (40%), feces (13%); half-life 3-4 hr

INTERACTIONS

Increase: serotonin syndrome—SSRIs, SNRIs, serotonin-receptor agonists, sibutramine

Increase: vasospastic effects—ergot, ergot derivatives, other 5-HT_1 agonists; avoid concurrent use

⚠ **Increase: almotriptan effect—MAOIs, CYP2D6 inhibitors; do not use together**

Increase: plasma concentration of almotriptan—(CYP3A4 inhibitors) itraconazole, ritonavir, erythromycin, ketoconazole

Drug/Herb

- Avoid use with feverfew

Increase: serotonin syndrome—St. John's wort

NURSING CONSIDERATIONS

Assess:

- **Migraine:** pain location, aura, duration, intensity, nausea, vomiting
- **Serotonin syndrome: occurs in those taking SSRIs, SNRIs; agitation, confusion, hallucinations, diaphoresis, hypertension, diarrhea, fever, tremor**

• B/P; signs/symptoms of coronary vasospasms
• For stress level, activity, recreation, coping mechanisms
• Neurologic status: LOC, blurring vision, nausea, vomiting, tingling, hot sensation, burning, feeling of pressure, numbness, flushing preceding headache
• **Tyramine foods** (pickled products, beer, wine, aged cheese), food additives, preservatives, colorings, artificial sweeteners, chocolate, caffeine, which may precipitate these types of headaches

Perform/provide:
• Quiet, calm environment with decreased stimulation from noise, bright light, excessive talking

Evaluate:
• Therapeutic response: decrease in severity of migraine

Teach patient/family:
• To report chest pain, drowsiness, dizziness, tingling, flushing
• To use contraception while taking product, to notify prescriber if pregnancy is planned or suspected, to avoid breastfeeding
• That if one dose does not relieve migraine to take another after 2 hr
• That product does not prevent or reduce number of migraine attacks; use to relieve attack only

alprazolam (Rx)

(al-pray′zoe-lam)

Gen-Alprazolam ✱, Niravam, Xanax, Xanax XR

Func. class.: Antianxiety
Chem. class.: Benzodiazepine (short/intermediate acting)

Controlled Substance Schedule IV

Do not confuse:
alprazolam/lorazepam
Xanax/Lanoxin/Tylox/Zantac

ACTION: Depresses subcortical levels of CNS, including limbic system, reticular formation

USES: Anxiety, panic disorders with or without agoraphobia, anxiety with depressive symptoms

Unlabeled uses: Premenstrual dysphoric disorders, insomnia, PMS, alcohol withdrawal syndrome

CONTRAINDICATIONS: Pregnancy (D), breastfeeding, hypersensitivity to benzodiazepines, closed-angle glaucoma, psychosis, addiction

Precautions: Geriatric patients, debilitated patients, hepatic disease, obesity, severe pulmonary disease

DOSAGE AND ROUTES

Anxiety disorder
• **Adult: PO** 0.25-0.5 mg tid, may increase q3-4days if needed, max 4 mg/day in divided doses
• **Geriatric: PO** 0.125-0.25 mg bid; increase by 0.125 as needed

Panic disorder
• **Adult: PO** 0.5 mg tid, may increase up to 1 mg/day q3-4days, max 10 mg/day; **EXT REL** (Xanax XR) give daily in AM, 0.5-1 mg initially, maintenance 3-6 mg/day

Hepatic dose
• Reduce dose

Premenstrual dysphoric disorders/PMS (unlabeled)
• **Adult: PO** 0.25 mg bid-qid starting on day 16-18 of menses, taper over 2-3 days when menses occurs, max 4 mg/day

Insomnia (unlabeled)
• **Adult: PO** 0.25-0.5 mg at bedtime

Available forms: Tabs 0.25, 0.5, 1, 2 mg; ext rel tabs (Xanax XR) 0.5, 1, 2, 3 mg; orally disintegrating tabs 0.25, 0.5, 1, 2 mg; oral sol 1 mg/ml

Administer:
• Tabs may be crushed, mixed with food, fluids if patient is unable to swallow medication whole; do not break, crush, chew ext rel (XR), give ext rel tab in AM

• With food or milk for GI symptoms; high-fat meal will decrease absorption
• To discontinue, decrease by 0.5 mg q3days
• May divide total daily doses into more times/day if anxiety occurs between doses
• Orally disintegrating tabs on tongue to dissolve and swallow

SIDE EFFECTS

CNS: *Dizziness, drowsiness,* confusion, headache, anxiety, tremors, stimulation, fatigue, depression, insomnia, hallucinations, memory impairment, poor coordination
CV: *Orthostatic hypotension,* ECG changes, tachycardia, hypotension
EENT: *Blurred vision,* tinnitus, mydriasis
GI: Constipation, dry mouth, nausea, vomiting, anorexia, diarrhea, weight gain/loss, increased appetite
GU: Decreased libido
INTEG: Rash, dermatitis, itching, angioedema

PHARMACOKINETICS

PO: Well absorbed; widely distributed; onset 30 min; peak 1-2 hr; duration 4-6 hr; *oral disintegrating tab* peak 1.5-2 hr; therapeutic response 2-3 days; metabolized by liver (CYP3A4), excreted by kidneys; crosses placenta, breast milk; half-life 12-15 hr, protein binding 80%

INTERACTIONS

Increase: alprazolam action—CYP3A4 inhibitors (cimetidine, disulfiram, erythromycin, fluoxetine, isoniazid, itraconazole, ketoconazole, metoprolol, propoxyphene, propanolol, valproic acid)
Increase: CNS depression—anticonvulsants, alcohol, antihistamines, sedative/hypnotics, opioids
Decrease: sedation—xanthines
Decrease: alprazolam action—CYP3A4 inducers (barbiturates, rifampin)
Decrease: action of levodopa
Decrease: product level—cigarette smoking

Drug/Herb

Increase: CNS depression—kava, melatonin, St. John's wort, valerian

Drug/Food

Increase: product level—grapefruit juice

Drug/Lab Test

Increase: AST/ALT, alk phos
Decrease: Hct

NURSING CONSIDERATIONS

Assess:

• Mental status: anxiety, mood, sensorium, orientation, affect, sleeping pattern, drowsiness, dizziness, especially in geriatric patients both before and during treatment
• B/P lying, standing; pulse; if systolic B/P drops 20 mm Hg, hold product, notify prescriber
• Hepatic, blood studies: AST, ALT, bilirubin, creatinine, LDH, alk phos, CBC; may cause neutropenia, decreased Hct, increased LFTs
⚠ **Physical dependency, withdrawal symptoms:** anxiety, panic attacks, agitation, seizures, headache, nausea, vomiting, muscle pain, weakness; withdrawal seizures may occur after rapid decrease in dose or abrupt discontinuation; because duration of action is short, considered to be the product of choice for geriatric patients

Evaluate:

• Therapeutic response: decreased anxiety, restlessness, sleeplessness

Teach patient/family:

• Not to double doses; take exactly as prescribed; if dose is missed, take within 1 hr as scheduled; that product may be taken with food
• Not to use for everyday stress or for more than 4 mo unless directed by prescriber; not to take more than prescribed amount; that product may be habit forming; that memory impairment is a result of long-term use
• To avoid OTC preparations unless approved by prescriber

• Not to discontinue medication abruptly after long-term use
• To avoid driving, activities that require alertness because drowsiness may occur
• To avoid alcohol, other psychotropic medications unless directed by prescriber
• To rise slowly or fainting may occur, especially among geriatric patients
• That drowsiness may worsen at beginning of treatment

TREATMENT OF OVERDOSE:
Lavage, VS, supportive care, flumazenil

RARELY USED

alprostadil (Rx)
(al-pros′ta-dil)

Caverject, Caverject Impulse, Edex, Muse, Prostin VR Pediatric

Func. class.: Hormone

USES: To maintain patent ductus arteriosus (temporary treatment), erectile dysfunction

CONTRAINDICATIONS: Hypersensitivity, respiratory distress syndrome, those at risk for priapism

DOSAGE AND ROUTES
Patent ductus arteriosus
• **Infant: IV INF** 0.05-0.1 mcg/kg/min until desired response, then reduce to lowest effective amount, max 0.4 mcg/kg/min

Erectile dysfunction of vasculogenic or mixed etiology, psychogenic
• **Men: INTRACAVERNOSAL** 2.5 mcg, may increase by 2.5 mcg, may then increase by 5-10 mcg until adequate response occurs (max 60 mcg/dose); **INTRAURETHRAL** 125-250 mcg, max 2 doses/24 hr, max dose 1000 mcg; administer as needed to achieve erection

⚠ HIGH ALERT

alteplase (tissue plasminogen activator, t-PA) (Rx)
(al-ti-plaze′)

Activase, Cathflo

Func. class.: Thrombolytic enzyme
Chem. class.: Tissue plasminogen activator (TPA)

Do not confuse:
alteplase/Altace

ACTION: Produces fibrin conversion of plasminogen to plasmin; able to bind to fibrin, convert plasminogen in thrombus to plasmin, which leads to local fibrinolysis, limited systemic proteolysis

USES: Lysis of obstructing thrombi associated with acute MI, ischemic conditions that require thrombolysis (i.e., PE, unclotting arteriovenous shunts, acute ischemic CVA), central venous catheter occlusion (Cathflo)
Unlabeled uses: Arterial thromboembolism, deep vein thrombosis (DVT), occlusion prophylaxis, percutaneous coronary intervention (PCI), subarachnoid hemorrhage

CONTRAINDICATIONS: Active internal bleeding, history of CVA, severe uncontrolled hypertension, intracranial/intraspinal surgery/trauma (within 3 mo), aneurysm, brain tumor, platelets $<$100,000 mm^3, bleeding diathesis including INR $>$1.7 or PR $>$15 sec, arteriovenous malformation, subarachnoid hemorrhage, intracranial hemorrhage, uncontrolled hypertension, seizure at onset of stroke
Precautions: Pregnancy (C), breastfeeding, children, geriatric patients, neurologic deficits, mitral stenosis, recent GI/GU bleeding, diabetic retinopathy, subacute bacterial endocarditis, arrhythmias, diabetic hemorrhage retinopathy,

CVA, recent major surgery, hypertension, acute pericarditis, hemostatic defects, significant hepatic disease, septic thrombophlebitis, occluded AV cannula at seriously infected site

DOSAGE AND ROUTES

MI (standard infusion)

• **Adult >65 kg:** 100 mg total given over 3 hr as follows: 6- to 10-mg IV BOL over 1-2 min; remaining 50-54 mg given over the remainder of the hr; during 2nd, 3rd hr 20 mg given by **CONT IV INF** (20 mg/hr)

• **Adult <65 kg:** 1.25 mg/kg over 3 hr: 60% during 1st hr (6%-10% as bolus); remaining 50% given over remainder of hr; during 2nd hr, 20% of dose given by CONT IV INF; 20% given during 3rd hr by CONT IV INF

MI (accelerated infusion)

• **Adult >67 kg:** 100 mg total dose: give 15-mg IV bolus, then 50 mg over 30 min, then 35 mg over 60 min

• **Adult <67 kg:** 15-mg IV bolus, then 0.75 mg/kg (max 50 mg) over 30 min, then 0.5 mg/kg (max 35 mg) over next 60 min

Pulmonary embolism

• **Adult: IV** 100 mg over 2 hr, then heparin

Acute ischemic stroke

• **Adult: IV** 0.9 mg/kg, max 90 mg; give as **INF** over 1 hr, give 10% of dose **IV BOL** over 1st min

Occluded venous access devices

• **Adult/child ≥30 kg: IV** 2 mg/2 ml instilled in occluded catheter, may repeat if needed after 2 hr

• **Child 10-29 kg: IV** 110% of lumen volume, max 2 mg/2 ml instilled in occluded catheter, may repeat if needed after 2 hr

Arterial thromboembolism (unlabeled)

• **Adult: IV** 2 mg/hr for up to 5 hr

Deep venous thrombosis (DVT) (unlabeled)

• **Adult: IV** 4 mcg/kg/min as 2-hr inf, then 1 mcg/kg/min × 33 hr

Percutaneous coronary intervention (PCI) (unlabeled)

• **Adult: INTRACARDIAC** 20 mg over 5 min then 50 mg over the next 60 min

Occlusion prophylaxis (unlabeled)

• **Adult >30 kg:** Do not exceed 2 mg in 2 ml; may use up to 2 doses 120 min apart

Available forms: Powder for inj 50 mg (29 million international units/vial), 100 mg (58 million international units/vial); lyophilized powder for inj 2 mg

Administer:

Intermittent IV INF route

• After reconstituting with provided diluent, add appropriate amount of sterile water for inj (no preservatives) 20-mg vial/20 ml or 50-mg vial/50 ml to make 1 mg/ml, mix by slow inversion or dilute with NaCl, D_5W to a conc of 0.5 mg/ml; 1.5 to <0.5 mg/ml may result in precipitation of product; use 18G needle; flush line with NaCl after administration, give over 3 hr for MI, 2 hr for PE

• Heparin therapy after thrombolytic therapy is discontinued, TT, ACT, or APTT less than 2× control (about 3-4 hr); treatment can be initiated before coagulation study results obtained, inf should be discontinued if pretreatment INR >1.7, PT >15 sec, or elevated aPTT is identified

• Use reconstituted IV solution within 8 hr or discard

Y-site compatibilities: Eptifibatide, lidocaine, metoprolol, propranolol

• **Cathflo Actinase:** reconstitute by using 2.2 ml of sterile water provided and injecting in vial, direct flow into powder (1 mg/ml), foam will disappear after standing; swirl, do not shake, sol will be pale yellow or clear, use within 8 hr, instill 2 ml of reconstituted sol into occluded catheter, try to aspirate after ½ hr; if unable to remove, allow 2 hr, a 2nd dose may be used; aspirate 5 ml of blood to remove clot and product, irrigate with normal saline

SIDE EFFECTS

CV: Sinus bradycardia, cholesterol microembolization, ventricular tachycardia, accelerated idioventricular rhythm, bradycardia, recurrent ischemic stroke, hypotension
EENT: Orolingual angioedema
INTEG: Urticaria, rash
SYST: GI, GU, intracranial, retroperitoneal bleeding, *surface bleeding,* anaphylaxis, fever

PHARMACOKINETICS

Cleared by liver, 80% cleared within 10 min of product termination, onset immediate, peak 45 min, duration 4 hr, half-life 35 min

INTERACTIONS

Increase: bleeding—anticoagulants, salicylates, dipyridamole, other NSAIDs, abciximab, eptifibatide, tirofiban, clopidogrel, ticlopidine, some cephalosporins, plicamycin, valproic acid
Increase: orolingual angioedema—ACE inhibitors
Decrease: effect—nitroglycerin
Drug/Herb
Increase: risk for bleeding—feverfew, garlic, ginger, ginkgo, ginseng, green tea
Drug/Lab Test
Increase: PT, APTT, TT

NURSING CONSIDERATIONS

Assess:

• Treatment is not recommended for patients with acute ischemic stroke >3 hr after symptom onset or with minor neurologic deficits or rapidly improving symptoms

• VS, B/P, pulse, respirations, neurologic signs, temp at least q4hr; temp >104° F (40° C) indicates internal bleeding; monitor rhythm closely; ventricular dysrhythmias may occur with hyperfusion; monitor heart, breath sounds, neurologic status, peripheral pulses; assess neurologic status, neurologic change may indicate intracranial bleeding; those with severe neurologic deficit (NIH SS >22) at presentation have increased risk of hemorrhage

⚠ **For bleeding** during 1st hour of treatment and 24 hr after procedure: hematuria, hematemesis, bleeding from mucous membranes, epistaxis, ecchymosis; guaiac all body fluids, stools; do not use 150 mg or more total dose because intracranial bleeding may occur

⚠ **Hypersensitivity:** fever, rash, itching, chills, facial swelling, dyspnea, notify prescriber immediately; stop product, keep resuscitative equipment nearby; mild reaction may be treated with antihistamines

• Previous allergic reactions or streptococcal infection; alteplase may be less effective

• Blood studies (Hct, platelets, PTT, PT, TT, APTT) before starting therapy; PT or APTT must be less than 2× control before starting therapy TT or PT q3-4hr during treatment

• **MI:** ECG continuously, cardiac enzymes, radionuclide myocardial scanning/coronary angiography; chest pain intensity, character; monitor those with major early infarct signs on CT scan with substantial edema, mass effect, midline shift

• PE: pulse, B/P, ABGs, rate/rhythm of respirations

• **Occlusion:** have patient exhale then hold breath when connecting/disconnecting syringe to prevent air embolism

• **Cholesterol embolism:** purple toe syndrome, acute renal failure, gangrenous digits, hypertension, livedo reticularis, pancreatitis, MI, cerebral infarction, spinal cord infarction, retinal artery occlusion, bowel infarction, rhabdomyolysis

Perform/provide:

• Avoidance of invasive procedures, inj, rectal temp

• Pressure for 30 sec to minor bleeding sites; 30 min to sites of atrial puncture followed by pressure dressing; inform prescriber if this does not attain hemostasis; apply pressure dressing

• Storage of powder at room temperature or refrigerate; protect from excessive light

Evaluate:

• Therapeutic response: lysis of thrombi

Teach patient/family:

• The purpose and expected results of the treatment; to report adverse reactions

aluminum hydroxide (OTC)

Func. class.: Antacid, hypophosphatemic

Chem. class.: Aluminum product, phosphate binder

ACTION:
Neutralizes gastric acidity; binds phosphates in GI tract, these phosphates are then excreted

USES:
Antacid, hyperphosphatemia in chronic renal failure; adjunct in gastric, peptic, duodenal ulcers; hyperacidity, reflux esophagitis, heartburn, stress ulcer prevention in critically ill, GERD

Unlabeled uses: GI bleeding

CONTRAINDICATIONS:
Hypersensitivity to product or aluminum products

Precautions: Pregnancy (C), breastfeeding, geriatric patients, fluid restriction, decreased GI motility, GI obstruction, dehydration, renal disease, sodium-restricted diets

DOSAGE AND ROUTES

Antacid

• **Adult: PO** 600 mg 1 hr after meals, at bedtime, max 6 doses/day

Hyperphosphatemia

• **Adult: PO** 300-600 mg tid

• **Child: PO** 50-150 mg/kg/day in 4-6 divided doses

GI bleeding

• **Infant: PO** 2-5 ml/dose q1-2hr

• **Child: PO** 5-15 ml/dose q1-2hr

Available forms: Susp 320 mg/5 ml, 600 mg/5 ml

Administer:

• 2 tsp (10 ml) will neutralize 20 mEq of acid

PO route

• Hyperphosphatemia: give with 8 oz water, meals unless contraindicated

• Laxatives or stool softeners if constipation occurs, especially for geriatric patients

• After shaking susp

NG route

• By nasogastric tube if patient unable to swallow

SIDE EFFECTS

GI: *Constipation,* anorexia, **obstruction,** fecal impaction

META: *Hypophosphatemia,* hypercalciuria

PHARMACOKINETICS

PO: Onset 20-40 min, duration 1-3 hr, excreted in feces

INTERACTIONS

Decrease: effectiveness of—allopurinol, amprenavir, cephalosporins, corticosteroids, delavirdine, digoxin, gabapentin, gatifloxacin, H_2-antagonists, iron salts, isoniazid, ketoconazole, penicillamine, phenothiazines, phenytoin, quinidine, quinolones, tetracyclines, thyroid hormones, ticlopidine, anticholinergics; separate by at least 4-6 hr

Drug/Food

Decrease: product effect—high-protein meal

NURSING CONSIDERATIONS

Assess:

• Pain: location, intensity, duration, character, aggravating, alleviating factors

• Phosphate, calcium levels because product is bound in GI system

• Hypophosphatemia: anorexia, weakness, fatigue, bone pain, hyporeflexia

• Constipation; increase bulk in diet if needed

Evaluate:
- Therapeutic response: absence of pain, decreased acidity, healed ulcers, decreased phosphate levels

Teach patient/family:
- To increase fluids to 2 L/day unless contraindicated; measures to prevent constipation
- **Antacid:** not to use for prolonged periods for patients with low serum phosphate or patients on low-sodium diets
- That stools may appear white or speckled
- To check with prescriber after 2 wk of self-prescribed antacid use
- To separate from other medications by 2 hr
- **Hyperphosphatemia:** to avoid phosphate foods (most dairy products, eggs, fruits, carbonated beverages) during product therapy

amantadine (Rx)
(a-man′ta-deen)

Gen-Amantadine ✱

Func. class.: Antiviral, antiparkinsonian agent

Chem. class.: Tricyclic amine

Do not confuse:
amantadine/ranitidine/rimantidine

ACTION: Prevents uncoating of nucleic acid in viral cell, thereby preventing penetration of virus to host; causes release of DOPamine from neurons

USES: Prophylaxis or treatment of influenza type A, EPS, parkinsonism, Parkinson's disease

Unlabeled uses: Neuroleptic malignant syndrome, MS-associated fatigue

CONTRAINDICATIONS: Hypersensitivity, breastfeeding, children <1 eczematic rash

Precautions: Pregnancy (C), geriatric patients, epilepsy, CHF, orthostatic hypotension, psychiatric disorders, renal/hepatic disease, peripheral edema

DOSAGE AND ROUTES

Influenza type A
- **Adult and child >9 yr: PO** 200 mg/day in single dose or divided bid
- **Geriatric: PO** No more than 100 mg/day
- **Child 1-8 yr: PO** 4.4-8.8 mg/kg/day divided bid-tid, max 150 mg/day

Extrapyramidal reaction/parkinsonism
- **Adult: PO** 100 mg bid up to 400 mg/day in EPS; give for 1 wk then 100 mg as needed up to 400 mg for parkinsonism

Renal dose
- **Adult: PO** CCr 30-50 ml/min 200 mg 1st day then 100 mg/day; CCr 15-29 ml/min 100 mg 1st day then 100 mg on alternate days; CCr 15 ml/min reduce dose and interval to 200 mg q7days

MS-associated fatigue (unlabeled)
- **Adult: PO** 200 mg/day or 100 mg bid

Neuroleptic malignant syndrome (unlabeled)
- **Adult: PO** 100 mg bid × 3 wk

Available forms: Caps 100 mg; oral sol 50 mg/5 ml; tab 100 mg

Administer:
- **Prophylaxis:** before exposure to influenza; continue for 10 days after contact; **treatment:** initiate within 24-48 hr of onset of symptoms, continue for 24-48 hr after symptoms disappear
- After meals for better absorption to decrease GI symptoms; at least 4 hr before bedtime to prevent insomnia
- In divided doses to prevent CNS disturbances: headache, dizziness, fatigue, drowsiness

SIDE EFFECTS

CNS: *Headache, dizziness,* drowsiness, fatigue, *anxiety,* psychosis, *depression, hallucinations,* tremors, seizures, confusion, *insomnia*

CV: *Orthostatic hypotension,* CHF

EENT: Blurred vision

GI: *Nausea, vomiting,* constipation, dry mouth, anorexia

GU: *Frequency, retention*

HEMA: Leukopenia, agranulocytosis

A

INTEG: Photosensitivity, dermatitis, livedo reticularis

PHARMACOKINETICS

PO: Onset 48 hr, peak 1-4 hr, half-life 24 hr, not metabolized, excreted in urine (90%) unchanged, crosses placenta, excreted in breast milk

INTERACTIONS

Increase: anticholinergic response—atropine, other anticholinergics
Increase: CNS stimulation—CNS stimulants
Decrease: amantadine effect—metoclopramide, phenothiazines
Decrease: renal excretion of amantadine—triamterene, hydrochlorothiazide
Decrease: effect—intranasal influenza vaccine; avoid use 2 wk before or 48 hr after amantadine
Drug/Lab Test
Increase: BUN, creatinine, alk phos, CK, LDH, bilirubin, AST, ALT, GGT

NURSING CONSIDERATIONS

Assess:

- I&O ratio; report frequency, hesitancy; serum BUN, creatinine baseline
- Hematologic status for leukopenia, agranulocytosis
- **CHF** (weight gain, jugular venous distention, dyspnea, crackles)
- Bowel pattern before, during treatment
- Skin eruptions, photosensitivity after administration of product
- Respiratory status: rate, character, wheezing, tightness in chest
- Allergies before treatment, reaction to each medication
- Signs of infection
- **Livedo reticularis:** mottling of the skin, usually red; edema; itching in lower extremities
- **Parkinson's disease:** gait, tremors, akinesia, rigidity

⚠ **Toxicity:** confusion, behavioral changes, hypotension, seizures

Perform/provide:

- Storage in tight, dry container

Evaluate:

- Therapeutic response: absence of fever, malaise, cough, dyspnea with infection; tremors, shuffling gait with Parkinson's disease

Teach patient/family:

- To change body position slowly to prevent orthostatic hypotension
- About aspects of product therapy: to report dyspnea, weight gain, dizziness, poor concentration, dysuria, behavioral changes
- To avoid hazardous activities if dizziness, blurred vision occurs
- To take product exactly as prescribed; parkinsonian crisis may occur if product is discontinued abruptly; not to double dose; if a dose is missed, not to take within 4 hr of next dose; caps may be opened and mixed with food
- To avoid alcohol
- Not to breastfeed

TREATMENT OF OVERDOSE:

Withdraw product, maintain airway, administer EPINEPHrine, aminophylline, O_2, IV corticosteroids, physostigmine

ambrisentan (Rx)

(am-bri-sen′tan)

Letairis

Func. class.: Antihypertensive
Chem class.: Vasodilator/endothelin receptor antagonist

ACTION: Endothelin-1 receptor antagonist; endothelin-1 is vasoconstrictor

USES: Pulmonary arterial hypertension, alone or in combination with other antihypertensives

CONTRAINDICATIONS: Breastfeeding, hypersensitivity

Black Box Warning: Pregnancy (X)

Precautions: Children, females, geriatric patients, hepatitis, anemia, heart failure, jaundice, peripheral edema, hepatic disease

DOSAGE AND ROUTES

• **Adult: PO** 5 mg/day; may increase to 10 mg/day if needed

Hepatic dose

• **Adult: PO** Discontinue if AST/ALT >5× ULN, or if elevations are accompanied by bilirubin >2× ULN, or other signs of liver dysfunction

Available forms: Tabs 5, 10 mg

Administer:

• Do not break, crush, chew tabs
• Daily with a full glass of water without regard to food
• Do not discontinue abruptly
• Only those facilities enrolled in the LEAP program may administer this product

SIDE EFFECTS

CNS: *Headache,* fever, flushing, fatigue
CV: Orthostatic hypotension, hypotension, *peripheral edema,* palpitations
EENT: Sinusitis, rhinitis
GI: Abdominal pain, constipation, anorexia, hepatotoxicity
GU: Decreased sperm counts
HEMA: *Anemia*
INTEG: Rash, angioedema
RESP: Pharyngitis, dyspnea, pulmonary edema, veno-occlusive disease (VOD)

PHARMACOKINETICS

Rapidly absorbed, peak 2 hr, protein binding 99%, metabolized by CYP3A4, CYP2C19, terminal half-life 15 hr, effective half-life 9 hr

INTERACTIONS

• Possibly increase ambrisentan: cimetidine, clopidogrel, efavirenz, felbamate, fluoxetine, modafinil, oxcarbazepine, ticlopidine

Increase: hypotension—other antihypertensives, diuretics, MAOIs

Increase: ambrisentan—CYP3A4 inhibitors (amprenavir, aprepitant, atazanavir, clarithromycin, conivaptan, cycloSPORINE, dalfopristin, danazol, darunavir, erythromycin, estradiol, imatinib, itraconazole, ketoconazole, nefazodone, nelfinavir, propoxyphene, quinupristin, ritonavir, RU-486, saquinavir, tamoxifen, telithromycin, troleandomycin, zafirlukast); CYP2C19/CYP3A4 (chloramphenicol, delavirdine, fluconazole, fluvoxamine, isoniazid, voriconazole)

Decrease: ambrisentan—CYP3A4 inducers (carbamazepine, PHENobarbital, phenytoin, rifampin)

Decrease: ambrisentan absorption—mefloquine, niCARdipine, propafenone, quiNIDine, ranolazine, tacrolimus, testosterone

Drug/Herb

• Need for ambrisentan dosage change: St. John's wort, ephedra (ma huang)

Drug/Food

• Avoid use with grapefruit products

Drug/Lab Test

Increase: LFTs, bilirubin
Decrease: Hct, Hgb

NURSING CONSIDERATIONS

Assess:

• **Pulmonary status:** improvement in breathing, ability to exercise; pulmonary edema that may indicate veno-occlusive disease
• Blood studies: CBC with differential; Hct, Hgb may be decreased
• Liver function tests: AST, ALT, bilirubin

Black Box Warning: Assess pregnancy status before giving this product; pregnancy category X

Perform/provide:

• Storage in tight container at room temp

Evaluate:

• Therapeutic response: decrease in B/P; decreased shortness of breath

Teach patient/family:

• The importance of complying with dosage schedule even if feeling better

Black Box Warning: To notify if pregnancy is planned or suspected (if pregnant, product will need to be discontinued, pregnancy test done monthly); to use two contraception methods while taking this product

A

- Not to use OTC products including herbs, supplements unless approved by prescriber
- To report to prescriber immediately: dizziness, faintness, chest pain, palpitations, uneven or rapid heart rate, headache
- To report hepatic dysfunction: nausea/vomiting, anorexia, fatigue, jaundice, right upper quadrant abdominal pain, itching, fever, malaise

amifostine (Rx)

(a-mi-foss'teen)

Ethyol

Func. class.: Cytoprotective agent for cisplatin/radiation

ACTION: Binds and detoxifies damaging metabolites of cisplatin, alkylating agents, DNA-reactive agents, ionizing radiation by converting this product by alk phos in tissue to an active free thiol compound

USES: To reduce renal toxicity when cisplatin is given repeatedly for ovarian cancer; to reduce xerostomia (dry mouth) after radiation therapy for head, neck cancer

Unlabeled uses: To prevent or reduce cisplatin-induced neurotoxicity, cyclophosphamide-induced granulocytopenia; to prevent or reduce toxicity of radiation therapy; to reduce toxicity of paclitaxel, myelodysplastic syndrome (MDS)

CONTRAINDICATIONS: Breastfeeding, hypersensitivity to mannitol, aminothiol; hypotension, dehydration

Precautions: Pregnancy (C), children, geriatric patients, CV disease, hypocalcemia, MI, radiation therapy, stroke, dehydration, hypotension, chemotherapy, exfoliative dermatitis

DOSAGE AND ROUTES

Reduction of renal damage with cisplatin

- **Adult: IV** 910 mg/m^2/day within 1/2 hr before chemotherapy, give over 15 min; may reduce dose to 740 mg/m^2 if higher dose is poorly tolerated

Xerostomia prophylaxis

- **Adult: IV** 200 mg/m^2/day over 3 min as inf 15-30 min before radiation therapy

Bone marrow suppression prophylaxis/nephrotoxicity prophylaxis/neurotoxicity prophylasis (unlabeled)

- **Adult: IV** 100-340 mg/m^2/day over 15 min before each dose of chemotherapy/radiation

Myelodysplastic syndrome (MDS) (unlabeled)

- **Adult: IV** 100 mg/m^2 3×/wk, max 300 mg/m^2 3×/wk

Available forms: Powder for inj, lyophilized 500 mg/vial

Administer:

Intermittent IV INF route

- Intermittent inf after reconstituting 500 mg/9.7 ml of sterile 0.9% NaCl, further dilute with 0.9% NaCl to concentration of 5-40 mg/ml, give over 15 min within 1/2 hr of chemotherapy, place patient in supine position during inf
- **Xerostomia:** Give over 3 min 15-30 min before radiation

Y-site compatibilities: Amikacin, aminophylline, amphotericin B liposome, ampicillin, ampicillin/sulbactam, aztreonam, bivalirudin, bleomycin, bumetanide, buprenorphine, butorphanol, calcium gluconate, carboplatin, carmustine, caspofungin, cefazolin, cefotaxime, cefotetan, cefoxitin, ceftazidime, ceftizoxime, ceftriaxone, cefuroxime, cimetidine, ciprofloxacin, clindamycin, cyclophosphamide, cytarabine, dacarbazine, dactinomycin, daptomycin, DAUNOrubicin, dexamethasone, dexmedetomidine, diltiazem, diphenhydrAMINE, DOBUTamine, docetaxel, DOPamine, DOXOrubicin, doxycycline, droperidol, enalaprilat, epirubicin, ertapenem, etoposide, famotidine, fenoldopam, floxuridine, fluconazole, fludarabine, fluorouracil, furosemide, gallium, gentamicin, granisetron, haloperidol, heparin, hydrocortisone, HYDROmorphone, idarubicin, ifosfamide, imipenem-cilastatin, leucovorin, levofloxacin, linezolid, lorazepam, magnesium sulfate, mannitol, mechlorethamine, meperidine, mesna, methotrexate, methylPREDNISolone, metoclopramide, metronidazole, mezlocillin, milrinone, mitomycin, morphine, nalbuphine, nesiritide, netilmicin, octreotide, ondansetron, oxaliplatin, paclitaxel, palonosetron, pantoprazole, pemetrexed, piperacillin, plicamycin, potassium chloride, promethazine, ranitidine, sodium bicarbonate, streptozocin, tacrolimus, teniposide, thiotepa, ticarcillin, ticarcillin/clavulanate, tigecycline, tirofiban, tobramycin, trastuzumab, trimethoprim-sulfamethoxazole, trimetrexate, vancomycin, vinBLAStine, vinCRIStine, voriconazole, zidovudine

Solution compatibility: 0.9% NaCl

Additive incompatibilities: Do not mix with other products

SIDE EFFECTS

CNS: Dizziness, somnolence, loss of consciousness, seizures

CV: *Hypotension*

EENT: *Sneezing*

GI: *Nausea, vomiting,* hiccups, *diarrhea*

INTEG: Flushing, feeling of warmth

MISC: *Hypocalcemia,* rash, chills, anaphylaxis, toxic epidermal necrolysis, toxicoderma, Stevens-Johnson syndrome, exfoliative dermatitis, erythema multiforme

PHARMACOKINETICS

Metabolized to free thiol compound, half-life 8 min, onset 5-8 min

INTERACTIONS

Increase: hypotension—antihypertensives

Drug/Lab

Decrease: calcium

NURSING CONSIDERATIONS

Assess:

- B/P before and q5min during inf; antihypertensives should be discontinued 24 hr before inf if severe hypotension occurs, give IV 0.9% NaCl to expand fluid volume, place patient in modified Trendelenburg position
- Fluid status before administration; administer antiemetic before administration to prevent severe nausea and vomiting; may also give dexamethasone 20 mg IV and a serotonin antagonist such as ondansetron, dolasetron, granisetron
- Calcium levels before and during treatment; may cause hypocalcemia, calcium supplements may be needed
- **Xerostomia:** mouth lesions, dry mouth during therapy
- **Anaphylaxis:** Rash, pruritus, wheezing, laryngeal edema, discontinue; give antihistamines, EPINEPHrine depending on severity; reactions may be delayed, if severe product should be permanently discontinued; other serious skin disorders (Stevens-Johnson syndrome, toxic epidermal necrolysis, Toxicoderma, erythema multiforme, exfoliative dermatitis)

Evaluate:

- Therapeutic response: prevention of renal toxicity associated with cisplatin therapy; decreased xerostomia associated with radiation therapy of head, neck cancer

Teach patient/family:

- To stay supine during inf, B/P will be monitored often
- To drink fluids
- To report signs, symptoms, severe reactions
- The reason for the medication and expected results
- That side effects may include severe nausea, vomiting, decreased B/P, chills, dizziness, somnolence, hiccups, sneezing, skin reactions
- Not to breastfeed

A

amikacin (Rx)

(am-i-kay'sin)

Amikin

Func. class.: Antiinfective

Chem. class.: Aminoglycoside

Do not confuse:
Amikin/Amicar
Amikacin/anakinra

ACTION: Interferes with protein synthesis in bacterial cells by binding to ribosomal subunits, which causes misreading of genetic code; inaccurate peptide sequence forms in protein chain, thereby causing bacterial death

USES: Severe systemic infections of CNS, respiratory tract, GI tract, urinary tract, bone, skin, soft tissues caused by *Staphylococcus aureus (MSSA), Pseudomonas aeruginosa, Escherichia coli, Enterobacter, Acinetobacter, Providencia, Citrobacter, Serratia, Proteus, Klebsiella pneumoniae*
Unlabeled uses: *Mycobacterium avium* complex (intrathecal or intraventricular) in combination; aerosolization, actinomycotic mycetoma, febrile neutropenia

CONTRAINDICATIONS: Pregnancy (D), mild to moderate infections, hypersensitivity to aminoglycosides, sulfites
Precautions: Breastfeeding, neonates, geriatric patients, myasthenia gravis, Parkinson's disease

Black Box Warning: Hearing impairment, renal/neuromuscular disease

DOSAGE AND ROUTES

Severe systemic infections

• **Adult and child: IV INF** 10-15 mg/kg/day in 2-3 divided doses q8-12hr in 100-200 ml D_5W over 30-60 min, max 1.5 g; use for 7-10 days; decreased doses are needed with poor renal function as determined by blood levels, renal studies; **pulse dosing** (once-daily dosing) may be used with some infections; **IM** 10-15 mg/kg/day in divided doses q8-12hr; daily or extended-interval dosing as an alternative dosing regimen

• **Infant: IV/IM** 10 mg/kg initially then 7.5 mg/kg q12hr

• **Neonate: IV/IM** 10 mg/kg initially then 7.5 mg/kg q12hr

• **Premature neonate:** 10 mg/kg initially then 7.5 mg/kg q8-12hr

Severe urinary tract infections

• **Adult: IM** 10-15 mg/kg/day divided q8-12hr

Hemodialysis

• **Adult: IM/IV** 7.5 mg/kg followed by 5 mg/kg 3×/wk after each dialysis session (for TIW dialysis)

Renal dose (pulse dosing)

• **Adult: IV** CCr 40-59 ml/min 15 mg/kg q36hr; CCr 20-39 ml/min 15 mg/kg q48hr; <20 ml/min adjust based on serum concentrations and MIC

Mycobacterium avium complex (MAC) (unlabeled)

• **Adult and adolescent: IV** 7.5-15 mg/kg divided q12-24hr as part of multiple-drug regimen

• **Child: IV** 15-30 mg/kg/day divided q12-24hr as part of multiple-drug regimen, max 1.5 g/day

Actinomycotic mycetoma (unlabeled)

• **Adult: IM/IV** 15 mg/kg/day in 2 divided doses × 3 wk with co-trimoxazole for 5 wk; repeat cycle once, may be repeated 2×

Available forms: Inj 50, 250 mg/ml

Administer:

IM route

• Inj in large muscle mass; rotate inj sites

• Bicarbonate to alkalinize urine if ordered for UTI; product most active in alkaline environment

Intermittent IV INF route

- Dilute 500 mg of product/100-200 ml of D_5W, 0.9% NaCl and give over 1/2-1 hr; dilute in sufficient volume to allow for inf over 1-2 hr (infants); flush after administration with D_5W or 0.9% NaCl; sol clear or pale yellow; discard if precipitate or dark color develops
- In children, amount of fluid will depend on ordered dose; in infants, infuse over 1-2 hr
- In evenly spaced doses to maintain blood level, separate from penicillins by at least 1 hr

Y-site compatibilities: Acyclovir, aldesleukin, alfentanil, amifostine, aminophylline, amiodarone, amsacrine, anidulafungin, ascorbic acid, atracurium, atropine, aztreonam, benztropine, bivalirudin, bumetanide, buprenorphine, butorphanol, calcium chloride/gluconate, CARBOplatin, caspofungin, cefazolin, cefepime, cefonicid, cefotaxime, cefotetan, cefoxitin, ceftazidime, ceftizoxime, cefTRIAXone, cefuroxime, chloramphenicol, chlorproMAZINE, cimetidine, cisatracurium, CISplatin, clindamycin, codeine, cyanocobalamin, cyclophosphamide, cycloSPORINE, cytarabine, DACTINomycin, DAPTOmycin, dexamethasone, dexmedetomidine, digoxin, diltiazem, diphenhydrAMINE, DOBUTamine, docetaxel, DOPamine, doripenem, doxacurium, DOXOrubicin, doxycycline, eftifibatide, enalaprilat, ePHEDrine, EPINEPHrine, epirubicin, epoetin alfa, ertapenem, erythromycin, esmolol, etoposide, famotidine, fentaNYL, filgrastim, fluconazole, fludarabine, fluorouracil, foscarnet, furosemide, gemcitabine, gentamicin, glycopyrrolate, granisetron, hydrocortisone, HYDROmorphone, IDArubicin, ifosfamide, IL-2, imipenem/cilastin, isoproterenol, ketorolac, labetalol, levofloxacin, lidocaine, linezolid, lorazepam, magnesium sulfate, mannitol, mechlorethamine, melphalan, meperidine, metaraminol, methotrexate, methoxamine, methyldopate, methylPREDNISolone, metoclopramide, metoprolol, metronidazole, midazolam, milrinone, mitoxantrone, morphine, multivitamins, nafcillin, nalbuphine, naloxone, niCARdipine, nitroglycerin, nitroprusside, norepinephrine, octreotide, ondansetron, oxaliplatin, oxytocin, paclitaxel, palonosetron, pantoprazole, papaverine, pemetrexed, penicillin G, pentazocine, perphenazine, PHENobarbital, phenylephrine, phytonadione, piperacillin/tazobactam, potassium chloride, procainamide, prochlorperazine, promethazine, propranolol, protamine, pyridoxime, quinupristin/dalfopristin, rantidine, remifentanil, riTUXimab, rocuromium, sargramostim, sodium acetate, sodium bicarbonate, succinylcholine, sufentanil, tacrolimus, teniposide, theophylline, thiamine, thiotepa, ticarcillin/clavulanate, tigecycline, tirofiban, tobramycin, tolazoline, trimethaphan, urokinase, vancomycin, vasopressin, vecuronium, verapamil, vinCRIStine, vinorelbine, voriconazole, warfarin, zidovudine

SIDE EFFECTS

CNS: Confusion, depression, numbness, tremors, **seizures**, muscle twitching, **neurotoxicity**, dizziness, vertigo, tinnitus, **neuromuscular blockade with respiratory paralysis**

CV: Hypo/hypertension, palpitations

EENT: *Ototoxicity,* deafness, visual disturbances

GI: *Nausea, vomiting, anorexia;* increased ALT, AST, bilirubin; hepatomegaly, **hepatic necrosis**, splenomegaly

GU: **Oliguria, hematuria, renal damage, azotemia, renal failure, nephrotoxicity**

HEMA: **Agranulocytosis, thrombocytopenia, leukopenia, eosinophilia, anemia**

INTEG: *Rash,* burning, urticaria, dermatitis, alopecia

PHARMACOKINETICS

IM: Onset rapid, peak 1-2 hr, leads to unpredictable concentrations, IV preferred

IV: Onset immediate, peak 15-30 min; plasma half-life 2-3 hr, prolonged up to 7 hr in infants; not metabolized; excreted unchanged in urine; crosses placental barrier; poor penetration into CSF; removed by hemodialysis

INTERACTIONS

• Mask ototoxicity: dimenhyDRINATE, ethacrynic acid

Increase: serum trough and peak—NSAIDs

Increase: nephrotoxicity—cephalosporins, acyclovir, vancomycin, amphotericin B, cycloSPORINE, loop diuretics, cidofovir

Increase: neuromuscular blockade, respiratory depression—anesthetics, nondepolarizing neuromuscular blockers

Drug/Lab Test

Increase: BUN, ALT, AST, bilirubin, LDH, alk phos, creatinine

Decrease: Ca, Na, K, Mg

NURSING CONSIDERATIONS

Assess:

• C&S before starting treatment to identify organism

• Weight before treatment; calculation of dosage is usually based on ideal body weight but may be calculated on actual body weight

• I&O ratio; urinalysis daily for proteinuria, cells, casts; report sudden change in urine output

• VS during infusion; watch for hypotension, change in pulse

• IV site for thrombophlebitis including pain, redness, swelling q30min; change site if needed; apply warm compresses to discontinued site

• Serum aminoglycoside conc; serum peak, drawn at 30-60 min after IV infusion or 60 min after IM inj, trough level drawn just before next dose; peak 20-30 mcg/ml, trough 4-8 mcg/ml; adjust dosage per levels

• Urine pH if product used for UTI; urine should be kept alkaline

Black Box Warning: Renal impairment by securing urine for CCr, BUN, serum creatinine; lower dosage should be given with renal impairment; nephrotoxicity may be reversible if product stopped at 1st sign

Black Box Warning: Deafness: audiometric testing, ringing, roaring in ears, vertigo; assess hearing before, during, after treatment

• Dehydration: high specific gravity, decrease in skin turgor, dry mucous membranes, dark urine

• Overgrowth of infection: increased temp, malaise, redness, pain, swelling, perineal itching, diarrhea, stomatitis, change in cough, sputum

• Vestibular dysfunction: nausea, vomiting, dizziness, headache; product should be discontinued if severe

Black Box Warning: Neuromuscular blockade; respiratory paralysis may occur

Perform/provide:

• Adequate fluids of 2-3 L/day, unless contraindicated, to prevent irritation of tubules

Evaluate:

• Therapeutic response: absence of fever, draining wounds, negative C&S after treatment

Teach patient/family:

• If dose is missed to take as soon as possible and then space remaining doses for the day at regular intervals

• To report headache, dizziness, symptoms of overgrowth of infection, renal impairment; symptoms of neurotoxicity, hepatotoxicity

⚠ To report loss of hearing; ringing, roaring in ears; feeling of fullness in head

• To report hypersensitivity: rash, itching, trouble breathing, facial edema; notify health care provider

TREATMENT OF HYPERSENSITIVITY:

Hemodialysis, exchange transfusion in the newborn, monitor serum levels of product, may give ticarcillin or carbenicillin

amiloride (Rx)

(a-mill'oh-ride)

Apo-Amiloride ✱, Midamor

Func. class.: Potassium-sparing diuretic

Chem. class.: Pyrazine

Do not confuse:
amiloride/amlodipine

ACTION: Inhibits sodium, potassium ATPase in the distal tubule, cortical collecting duct resulting in inhibition of sodium reabsorption and decreasing potassium secretion

USES: Edema in CHF in combination with other diuretics, for hypertension, adjunct with other diuretics to maintain potassium, polyuria due to lithium administration

Unlabeled uses: Ascites

CONTRAINDICATIONS: Anuria, hypersensitivity, impaired renal function, diabetic nephropathy

Black Box Warning: Hyperkalemia

Precautions: Pregnancy (B), breastfeeding, children, geriatric patients, dehydration, diabetes, respiratory acidosis, hyponatremia

DOSAGE AND ROUTES

- **Adult: PO** 5-10 mg/day in 1-2 divided doses; may be increased to 10-20 mg/day if needed

Renal dose

- **Adult: PO** CCr 10-50 ml/min reduce dose by 50%; however, avoid if possible; CCr <10 ml/min contraindicated

Ascites (unlabeled)

- **Adult: PO** 10 mg/day, max 40 mg

Available forms: Tabs 5 mg

Administer:

- In AM to avoid interference with sleep if using as diuretic; if 2nd daily dose is needed, give in late afternoon
- With food; if nausea occurs, absorption may be decreased slightly

SIDE EFFECTS

CNS: *Headache,* dizziness, fatigue, weakness, paresthesias, tremor, depression, anxiety, encephalopathy

CV: *Orthostatic hypotension,* dysrhythmias, chest pain

EENT: Blurred vision, increased intraocular pressure

ELECT: Hyperkalemia, dehydration, hyponatremia, hypochloremia

GI: *Nausea, diarrhea,* dry mouth, *vomiting, anorexia,* cramps, constipation, abdominal pain, jaundice

GU: *Polyuria,* dysuria, urinary frequency, impotence

HEMA: Aplastic anemia, neutropenia

INTEG: *Rash, pruritus,* alopecia, urticaria

MS: Cramps

RESP: Cough, dyspnea, shortness of breath

PHARMACOKINETICS

15%-25% absorbed from GI tract; widely distributed; onset 2 hr; peak 3-4 hr; duration 24 hr; excreted in urine, feces; half-life 6-9 hr

INTERACTIONS

Black Box Warning: Hyperkalemia: other potassium-sparing diuretics, potassium products, ACE inhibitors, salt substitutes, cycloSPORINE, tacrolimus

- Lithium toxicity: lithium

Increase: action of antihypertensives

Decrease: effect of amiloride—NSAIDs

Drug/Herb

Increase: effect—hawthorn, horse chestnut

Drug/Food

- Possible hyperkalemia: foods high in potassium

Drug/Lab Test

Interference: GTT

NURSING CONSIDERATIONS

Assess:

- Weight, I&O daily to determine fluid loss; effect of product may be decreased if used daily
- Heart rate, B/P lying, standing; postural hypotension may occur
- Electrolytes: potassium, sodium, chloride; glucose (serum), BUN, CBC, serum creatinine, blood pH, ABGs, periodic ECG
- Discontinue potassium-sparing diuretics 3 days before GTT, hyperkalemia may occur
- **Hypokalemia:** weakness, polyuria, polydipsia, fatigue, ECG U wave

Black Box Warning: Hyperkalemia: fatigue, weakness, paresthesia, confusion, dyspnea, dysrhythmias, ECG changes

Evaluate:

- Therapeutic response: improvement in edema of feet, legs, sacral area daily if medication is being used for CHF; decreased B/P; prevention of hypokalemia (diuretics)

Teach patient/family:

- To take as prescribed; if dose is missed, to take when remembered within 1 hr of next dose; to take with food or milk for GI symptoms; to take early in day to prevent nocturia
- About adverse reactions: muscle cramps, weakness, nausea, dizziness, blurred vision
- To avoid potassium-rich foods: oranges, bananas; salt substitutes, dried fruits
- To rise slowly from sitting to standing to avoid orthostatic hypotension

TREATMENT OF OVERDOSE:

Lavage if taken orally, monitor electrolytes, administer sodium bicarbonate for potassium >6.5 mEq/L, IV glucose, kayoxalate as needed; monitor hydration, CV, renal status

amino acid injection (Rx)

(a-mee′noe)

FreAmine, HepatAmine

Func. class.: Nitrogen product

ACTION: Needed for anabolism to maintain structure, decrease catabolism, promote healing

USES: Hepatic encephalopathy, cirrhosis, hepatitis, nutritional support in cancer; burn or solid organ transplant patients; to prevent nitrogen loss when adequate nutrition by mouth, gastric, or duodenal tube cannot be obtained

CONTRAINDICATIONS: Hypersensitivity, severe electrolyte imbalances, anuria, severe liver damage, maple syrup urine disease, PKU, azotemia, genetic disease of amino acid metabolism

Precautions: Pregnancy (C), breastfeeding, children, renal disease, diabetes mellitus, CHF, sulfite sensitivity

DOSAGE AND ROUTES

- **Adult:** **IV** 80-120 g/day; 500 ml of amino acids/500 ml D_{50} given over 24 hr

Available forms: Inj; many strengths, types

Administer:

Continuous IV INF route

- Up to 40% protein and dextrose (up to 12.5%) via peripheral vein; stronger sol requires central IV administration
- TPN only mixed with dextrose to promote protein synthesis
- Immediately after mixing under strict aseptic technique, use inf pump, in-line filter (0.22 μm) unless mixed with fat emulsion and dextrose (3 in 1)

⚠ **Using careful monitoring technique; do not speed up inf; pulmonary edema, glucose overload will result**

SIDE EFFECTS

CNS: *Dizziness, headache,* confusion, loss of consciousness
CV: Hypertension, CHF, pulmonary edema
ENDO: *Hyperglycemia, rebound hypoglycemia, electrolyte imbalances, hyperosmolar syndrome, hyperosmolar hyperglycemic nonketotic syndrome,* alkalosis, acidosis, hypophosphatemia, hyperammonemia, dehydration, hypocalcemia
GI: Nausea, vomiting, liver fat deposits, abdominal pain
GU: Glycosuria, osmotic diuresis
INTEG: Chills, flushing, warm feeling, rash, urticaria, extravasation necrosis, phlebitis at inj site

INTERACTIONS

Decrease: protein-sparing effects—tetracycline

NURSING CONSIDERATIONS

Assess:

- Electrolytes (K, Na, Ca, Cl, Mg, Na HCO_3), blood glucose, ammonia, phosphate, ketones
- Renal, hepatic studies: BUN, creatinine, ALT, AST, bilirubin
- Weight changes, triglycerides before and after inf; vit A level with renal disease
- Inj site for extravasation: redness along vein, edema at site, necrosis, pain, hard, tender area; site should be changed immediately
- Respiratory function q4hr: auscultate lung fields bilaterally for crackles, respirations, quality, rate, rhythm
- Temp q4hr for increased fever, indicating infection; if infection suspected, discontinue inf, culture tubing and sol

⚠ For impending hepatic coma: asterixis, confusion, uremic fetor, lethargy

- **Hyperammonemia:** nausea, vomiting, malaise, tremors, anorexia, seizures

Perform/provide:

- Storage depending on type of sol; consult manufacturer
- Change of dressing and IV tubing to prevent infection q24-48hr if chills, fever, other signs of infection occur

Evaluate:

- Therapeutic response: weight gain, decrease in jaundice with liver disorders, increased LOC

Teach patient/family:

- The reason for use of TPN
- If chills, sweating are experienced to report at once
- About infusion pump and blood glucose monitoring

amino acid solution (Rx)

Clinimax, CliNimax E, NephrAmine

Func. class.: Nitrogen product

ACTION: Needed for anabolism to maintain structure, decrease catabolism, promote healing

USES: Nutritional support for cancer, trauma, intestinal obstruction, short bowel syndrome, severe malabsorption, burn or solid organ transplant patients

CONTRAINDICATIONS: Hypersensitivity, severe electrolyte imbalances, anuria, severe liver damage, maple syrup urine disease, PKU, azotemia, amino acid metabolism, genetic disorders
Precautions: Pregnancy (C), breastfeeding, children, renal disease, diabetes mellitus, CHF, sulfite sensitivity

DOSAGE AND ROUTES

- **Adult: IV** 1-1.5 g/kg/day titrated to patient's needs
- **Child: IV** 2-3 g/kg/day titrated to patient's needs

Available forms: Inj, many types, strengths

Administer:

Continuous IV INF route

- Up to 40% protein and dextrose (up to 12.5%) via peripheral vein; stronger sol requires central IV administration, use inf pump
- TPN only mixed with dextrose to promote protein synthesis
- Immediately after mixing in pharmacy under strict aseptic technique using laminar flow hood, use inf pump, in-line filter (0.22 μm) unless mixed with fat emulsion and dextrose (3 in 1)

⚠ Using careful monitoring technique; do not speed up inf; pulmonary edema, glucose overload will result

SIDE EFFECTS

CNS: Dizziness, headache, confusion, loss of consciousness

CV: Hypertension, CHF, pulmonary edema

ENDO: *Hyperglycemia, rebound hypoglycemia, electrolyte imbalances, hyperosmolar syndrome, hyperosmolar hyperglycemic nonketotic syndrome,* alkalosis, acidosis, hypophosphatemia, hyperammonemia, dehydration, hypocalcemia

GI: Nausea, vomiting, liver fat deposits, abdominal pain, jaundice

GU: Glycosuria, osmotic diuresis

INTEG: Chills, flushing, warm feeling, rash, urticaria, extravasation necrosis, phlebitis at inj site

NURSING CONSIDERATIONS

Assess:

- Electrolytes (K, Na, Ca, Cl, Mg, Na HCO_3), blood glucose, ammonia, phosphate
- Renal, hepatic studies: BUN, creatinine, ALT, AST, bilirubin
- Weight changes, triglycerides before, after inf; vit A level with renal disease
- Inj site for extravasation: redness along vein, edema at site, necrosis, pain, hard, tender area; site should be changed immediately
- Monitor respiratory function q4hr: auscultate lung fields bilaterally for crackles, respirations, quality, rate, rhythm
- Monitor temp q4hr for increased fever, indicating infection; if infection suspected, discontinue inf, culture tubing, bottle
- Urine glucose q6hr using Tes-Tape, Clinistix, which are not affected by inf substances; blood glucose is preferred testing method
- Hyperammonemia: nausea, vomiting, malaise, tremors, anorexia, seizures

Perform/provide:

- Storage depending on type of sol; consult label
- Change of dressing and IV tubing q24-48hr if chills, fever, other signs of infection occur

Evaluate:

- Therapeutic response: weight gain, decrease in jaundice with liver disorders, increased serum albumin

Teach patient/family:

- The reason for use of TPN
- That any chills, sweating should be reported at once
- About inf pump and blood glucose monitoring

aminophylline (theophylline ethylenediamine) (Rx)

(am-in-off'i-lin)

Phyllocontin ✦, Theochron, Theo-24, Uniphyl

Func. class.: Bronchodilator, spasmolytic

Chem. class.: Methylxanthine

ACTION: Exact mechanism unknown, relaxes smooth muscle of respiratory system by blocking phosphodiesterase, which increases cAMP; increased cAMP alters intracellular calcium ion movements; produces bronchodilation, increased pulmonary blood flow, relaxation of respiratory tract

USES:
Bronchial asthma, bronchospasm associated with chronic bronchitis, emphysema, apnea during infancy for respiratory/myocardial stimulation

Unlabeled uses: Methotrexate toxicity, sleep apnea, status asthmaticus

CONTRAINDICATIONS:
Hypersensitivity to xanthines, tachydysrhythmias

Precautions: Pregnancy (C), breastfeeding, children, geriatric patients, CHF, cor pulmonale, hepatic disease, diabetes mellitus, hyperthyroidism, hypertension, seizure disorder, irritation of the rectum/lower colon, alcoholism, active peptic ulcer disease

DOSAGE AND ROUTES

For updated dosages and routes, see Appendix A, pg 1246.

Available forms: Inj 250 mg/10 ml, 500 mg/20 ml, 100 mg/100 ml in 0.45% NaCl, 200 mg/100 ml in 0.45% NaCl; rect supp 250, 500 mg; tabs 100, 200 mg; ext rel tab 100, 200, 300, 400, 450, 600 mg; ext rel cap 100, 200, 300, 400; elixir 80 mg/15 ml

Administer:

- Avoid IM inj; pain and tissue damage may occur

PO route

- Avoid giving with food

Continuous IV INF route

- Only clear sol; flush IV line before dose
- May be **diluted** for IV inf in 100-200 ml in D_5W, $D_{10}W$, $D_{20}W$, 0.9% NaCl, 0.45% NaCl, LR
- **Give** loading dose over $^1/_2$ hr; max rate of inf 25 mg/min, use inf pump; after loading dose, give by cont inf

Syringe compatibilities: Heparin, metoclopramide, PENTobarbital, thiopental

Y-site compatibilities: Allopurinol, amifostine, amphotericin B, amrinone, aztreonam, ceftazidime, cholesteryl sulfate complex, cimetidine, cladribine, DOXOrubicin liposome, enalaprilat, esmolol, famotidine, filgrastim, fluconazole, fludarabine, foscarnet, gallium, granisetron, heparin sodium with hydrocortisone sodium succinate, labetalol, melphalan, meropenem, netilmicin, paclitaxel, pancuronium, piperacillin/tazobactam, potassium chloride, propofol, ranitidine, remifentanil, sargramostim, tacrolimus, teniposide, thiotepa, tolazoline, vecuronium

SIDE EFFECTS

CNS: Anxiety, restlessness, insomnia, *dizziness,* seizures, headache, lightheadedness, muscle twitching, tremors

CV: *Palpitations, sinus tachycardia,* hypotension, flushing, dysrhythmias, edema

GI: *Nausea, vomiting,* diarrhea, dyspepsia, anal irritation (suppositories), epigastric pain, reflux, anorexia

GU: Urinary frequency, SIADH

INTEG: Flushing, urticaria

MISC: Hyperglycemia

RESP: Tachypnea, increased respiratory rate

PHARMACOKINETICS

Metabolized by liver (caffeine); excreted in urine; crosses placenta; appears in breast milk; half-life 6.5-10.5 hr; half-life increased in geriatric patients, hepatic disease, CHF, neonates, premature infants; protein binding 40%

PO: Onset 1/4 hr, peak 1-2 hr, duration 6-8 hr, well absorbed
PO-ER: Onset unknown, peak 4-7 hr, duration 8-12 hr, well absorbed slowly
IV: Onset rapid, duration 6-8 hr
RECT: Onset erratic, peak 1-2 hr, duration 6-8 hr, supp absorbed erratically, sol absorbed quickly

INTERACTIONS

- Dose-dependent reversal of neuromuscular blockade
- Dysrhythmias: halothane
- May increase or decrease aminophylline levels: carbamazepine, loop diuretics, isoniazid

Increase: action of aminophylline, toxicity—cimetidine, nonselective β-blockers, erythromycin, clarithromycin, oral contraceptives, corticosteroids, interferons, fluoroquinolones, disulfiram, mexiletine, fluvoxamine, high doses of allopurinol, influenza vaccines, interferon, benzodiazepines
Increase: adverse reactions—tetracyclines
Increase: elimination—smoking
Decrease: effects of lithium
Decrease: effect of aminophylline—nicotine products, adrenergics, barbiturates, phenytoin, ketoconazole, rifampin

Drug/Herb

Increase: effects—cola tree, guarana, yerba maté, tea (black, green), horsetail, ginseng, Siberian ginseng
Decrease: effects—St. John's wort

Drug/Food

Increase: effect—xanthines
Increase: elimination by low-carbohydrate, high-protein diet; charcoal-broiled beef
Decrease: elimination by high-carbohydrate, low-protein diet

Drug/Lab Test

Increase: plasma-free fatty acids

NURSING CONSIDERATIONS

A

Assess:

- Theophylline blood levels (therapeutic level is 10-20 mcg/ml); toxicity may occur with small increase above 20 mcg/ml, especially in geriatric patients; whether theophylline was given recently (24 hr)
- Monitor I&O; diuresis occurs; dehydration may occur in geriatric patients or children
- Liver function tests: periodically, lower doses may be required in those with moderate to severe hepatic disease
- Respiratory rate, rhythm, depth; auscultate lung fields bilaterally; notify prescriber of abnormalities, monitor pulmonary function tests
- Allergic reactions: rash, urticaria; if these occur, product should be discontinued

Perform/provide:

- Storage of diluted sol for 24 hr if refrigerated

Evaluate:

- Therapeutic response: decreased dyspnea, respiratory stimulation for infants, clear lung fields bilaterally

Teach patient/family:

- To take doses as prescribed, not to skip dose, not to double dose
- To check OTC medications, current prescription medications for ePHEDrine; will increase CNS stimulation; not to drink alcohol or caffeine products (tea, coffee, chocolate, colas); to avoid large amounts of charcoal-grilled beef
- To avoid hazardous activities; dizziness may occur
- If GI upset occurs, to take product with 8 oz water; to avoid food because absorption may be decreased

⚠ To notify prescriber immediately about **toxicity:** insomnia, anxiety, nausea, vomiting, rapid pulse, seizures, flushing, headache, diarrhea

• To notify prescriber about changes in smoking habits because a change in dose may be required; to avoid smoking because it decreases drug blood levels and terminal half-life
• To increase fluids to 2 L/day to decrease secretion viscosity

⚠ ***HIGH ALERT***

amiodarone (Rx)

(a-mee-oh′da-rone)

Apo-Amiodarone ♣, Cordarone, Gen-Amiodarone ♣, Nexterone, Novo-Amiodarone ♣, Pacerone, PMS-Amiodarone ♣, ratio-Amiodarone ♣, Sandoz Amiodarone ♣

Func. class.: Antidysrhythmic (class III)

Chem. class.: Iodinated benzofuran derivative

Do not confuse:
amiodarone/Inamrinone
Cordarone/Inocor

ACTION: Prolongs duration of action potential and effective refractory period, noncompetitive α- and β-adrenergic inhibition; increases PR and QT intervals, decreases sinus rate, decreases peripheral vascular resistance

USES: Hemodynamically unstable ventricular tachycardia, supraventricular tachycardia, ventricular fibrillation not controlled by 1st-line agents
Unlabeled uses: Atrial fibrillation treatment/prophylaxis, atrial flutter, cardiac arrest, cardiac surgery, CPR, heart failure, PSVT, Wolff-Parkinson-White (WPW) syndrome

CONTRAINDICATIONS: Pregnancy (D), breastfeeding, neonates, infants, severe sinus node dysfunction, hypersensitivity, cardiogenic shock

Black Box Warning: 2nd-3rd degree AV block, bradycardia

Precautions: Children, goiter, Hashimoto's thyroiditis, electrolyte imbalances, CHF, respiratory disease

Black Box Warning: Severe hepatic disease, cardiac arrhythmias, pneumonitis, pulmonary fibrosis

DOSAGE AND ROUTES

Ventricular dysrhythmias
• **Adult: PO** Loading dose 800-1600 mg/day for 1-3 wk then 600-800 mg/day × 1 mo, maintenance 400 mg/day; **IV** loading dose (1st rapid) 150 mg over the first 10 min then slow 360 mg over the next 6 hr, maintenance 540 mg given over the remaining 18 hr, decrease rate of the slow inf to 0.5 mg/min
• **Child (unlabeled): PO** Loading dose 10-15 mg/kg/day in 1-2 divided doses for 4-14 days then 5 mg/kg/day
• **Child and infant: IV/INTRAOSSEOUS** (during CPR) 5 mg/kg as a bolus (PALS guidelines)

Perfusion tachycardia
• **Adult: IV** 5 mg/kg loading dose given over 20-60 min

Supraventricular dysrhythmias (atrial fibrillation, atrial flutter, PSVT, WPW syndrome) (unlabeled)
• **Adult: PO** 1.2-1.8 g/day divided until a total of 10 g has been given, then 200-400 mg/day (class IIa recommendation); **IV** 5-7 mg/kg over 30-60 min, then 1.2-1.8 g as **CONT IV INF** or in divided PO doses until 10 g, then 200-400 mg/day (class IIa recommendation)

• **Child and infant: PO** 10-20 mg/kg/day in divided doses for 7-10 days, then 5-10 mg/kg/day once daily

Available forms: Tabs 100, 200, 400 mg; inj 50 mg/ml

Administer:

PO route

• May be used with/without food but be consistent

IV, direct route

• **Peripheral:** max 2 mg/ml for more than 1 hr; preferred through central venous line with in-line filter; concentrations of more than 2 ml should be given by central line

• **Cardiac arrest:** give 300 bol; may repeat 150 mg after 3-5 min

Intermittent IV INF route

• **Rapid loading:** add 3 ml (150 mg), 100 ml D_5W (1.5 mg/ml), give over 10 min

• **Slow loading:** add 18 ml (900 mg), 500 ml D_5W (1.8 mg/ml), give over next 6 hr

Continuous IV INF route

• After 24 hr, dilute 50 ml to 1-6 mg/ml, give 1-6 mg/ml at 1 mg/min for the 1st 6 hr, then 0.5 mg/min

Y-site compatibilities: Amikacin, clindamycin, DOBUTamine, DOPamine, doxycycline, erythromycin, esmolol, gentamicin, insulin, isoproterenol, labetalol, lidocaine, metaraminol, metronidazole, midazolam, morphine, nitroglycerin, norepinephrine, penicillin G potassium, phenylephrine, potassium chloride, procainamide, tobramycin, vancomycin

Solution compatibility: D_5W, 0.9% NaCl

SIDE EFFECTS

CNS: *Headache, dizziness,* involuntary movement, *tremors, peripheral neuropathy,* malaise, *fatigue,* ataxia, *paresthesias,* insomnia

CV: *Hypotension, bradycardia,* sinus arrest, **CHF, dysrhythmias, SA node dysfunction, AV block,** increased defibrillation energy requirement

EENT: Blurred vision, halos, photophobia, *corneal microdeposits,* dry eyes

ENDO: *Hypo*/hyperthyroidism

GI: *Nausea, vomiting,* diarrhea, abdominal pain, *anorexia, constipation,* **hepatotoxicity**

GU: Epididymitis, ED

INTEG: Rash, photosensitivity, blue-gray skin discoloration, alopecia, spontaneous ecchymosis, **toxic epidermal necrolysis,** urticaria, **pancreatitis,** phlebitis (IV)

MISC: Flushing, abnormal taste or smell, edema, abnormal salivation, coagulation abnormalities

MS: Weakness, pain in extremities

RESP: **Pulmonary fibrosis/toxicity,** pulmonary inflammation, **ARDS; gasping syndrome if used with neonates**

PHARMACOKINETICS

PO: Onset 1-3 wk, peak 2-7 hr, half-life 26-107 days, metabolized by liver (CYP3A4, CYP2C8), excreted by kidneys, 99% protein binding

INTERACTIONS

Increase: QT prolongation—azoles, fluoroquinolones, macrolides

Increase: amiodarone concentrations, possible serious dysrhythmias-protease inhibitors

Increase: myopathy—HMG-CoA reductase inhibitors

Increase: bradycardia—β-blockers, calcium channel blockers

Increase: levels of cycloSPORINE, dextromethorphan, digoxin, disopyramide, flecainide, methotrexate, phenytoin, procainamide, quiNIDine, theophylline, class I antidysrhythmics

Increase: anticoagulant effects—warfarin

Drug/Food

• Toxicity: grapefruit juice

Drug/Lab Test

Increase: T_4, ALT, AST, GGT alk phos, cholesterol, lipids, PT, INR

Decrease: T_3

NURSING CONSIDERATIONS

Assess:

Black Box Warning: Pulmonary toxicity: dyspnea, fatigue, cough, fever, chest pain; product should be discontinued; for ARDS, pulmonary fibrosis, crackles, tachypnea

Black Box Warning: ECG continuously to determine product effectiveness; measure PR, QRS, QT intervals; check for PVCs, other dysrhythmias, B/P continuously for hypo/hypertension; report dysrhythmias, slowing heart rate; monitor amiodarone level: therapeutic 1-2.5 mcg/ml; toxic >2.5 mcg/ml

• I&O ratio; electrolytes (sodium, potassium, chloride); hepatic studies: AST, ALT, bilirubin, alk phos; for dehydration, hypovolemia

• Chest x-ray, thyroid function tests

• CNS symptoms: confusion, psychosis, numbness, depression, involuntary movements; product should be discontinued

• **Hypothyroidism:** lethargy; dizziness; constipation; enlarged thyroid gland; edema of extremities; cool, pale skin

• **Hyperthyroidism:** restlessness; tachycardia; eyelid puffiness; weight loss; frequent urination; menstrual irregularities; dyspnea; warm, moist skin

• Ophthalmic exams at baseline and periodically (PO)

• Cardiac rate, respirations: rate, rhythm, character, chest pain; start with patient hospitalized and monitored up to 1 wk; for rebound hypertension after 1-2 hr

Evaluate:

• Therapeutic response: decrease in ventricular tachycardia, supraventricular tachycardia, fibrillation

Teach patient/family:

• To take this product as directed; to avoid missed doses; not to use with grapefruit juice

• To use sunscreen or stay out of sun to prevent burns; that dark glasses may be needed for photophobia

• To report side effects immediately

• That skin discoloration is usually reversible

TREATMENT OF OVERDOSE:

O_2, artificial ventilation, ECG, administer DOPamine for circulatory depression, administer diazepam, thiopental for seizures, isoproterenol

amitriptyline (Rx)

(a-mee-trip′ti-leen)

Apo-Amitriptyline ✦

Func. class.: Antidepressant—tricyclic

Chem. class.: Tertiary amine

Do not confuse:

amitriptyline/nortriptyline/aminophylline

ACTION: Blocks reuptake of norepinephrine, serotonin into nerve endings, thereby increasing action of norepinephrine, serotonin in nerve cells

USES: Major depression

Unlabeled uses: Neuropathic pain, prevention of cluster/migraine headaches, fibromyalgia, ADHD, bulimia nervosa, diabetic neuropathy, enuresis, insomnia, panic disorder, postherpetic neuralgia, hiccups, social phobia

CONTRAINDICATIONS: Hypersensitivity to tricyclics, recovery phase of myocardial infarction

A

Precautions: Pregnancy (C), breastfeeding, geriatric patients, seizure disorders, prostatic hypertrophy, schizophrenia, psychosis, severe depression, increased intraocular pressure, closed-angle glaucoma, urinary retention, renal/hepatic/cardiac disease, hyperthyroidism, electroshock therapy, elective surgery

Black Box Warning: Children <12 yr, suicidal patients

DOSAGE AND ROUTES

Depression

- **Adult/adolescent: PO** 25-75 mg/day as single dose at bedtime or in divided doses, may increase to 200 mg/day; max 300 mg/day (if hospitalized)
- **Geriatric: PO** 10-25 mg at bedtime, may be increased to 150 mg/day

Cluster/migraine headache (unlabeled)

- **Adult: PO** 10-300 mg/day

Pain (unlabeled)

- **Adult: PO** 75-300 mg/day

Fibromyalgia/insomnia (unlabeled)

- **Adult: PO** 10-50 mg nightly

Enuresis (unlabeled)

- **Child 11-14 yr: PO** 50 mg at bedtime
- **Child 6-10 yr: PO** 25 mg at bedtime

ADHD/bulimia nervosa (unlabeled)

- **Adult: PO** 25 mg tid, titrate to 200 mg/day by 25-50 mg at weekly intervals
- **Child 6-12 yr: PO** 10-30 mg/day or 1-5 mg/kg/day in divided doses

Available forms: Tabs 10, 25, 50, 75, 100, 150 mg

Administer:

- Increase fluids, bulk in diet if constipation, urinary retention occur, especially in geriatric patients
- With food, milk for GI symptoms
- Crushed if patient unable to swallow medication whole
- Dosage at bedtime if oversedation occurs during day; may take entire dose at bedtime; geriatric patients may not tolerate once daily dosing

SIDE EFFECTS

CNS: *Dizziness, drowsiness,* confusion, headache, anxiety, tremors, stimulation, weakness, insomnia, nightmares, EPS (geriatric patients), increased psychiatric symptoms, **seizures, suicidal thoughts**

CV: *Orthostatic hypotension,* **ECG changes, tachycardia, hypertension, palpitations, dysrhythmias**

EENT: *Blurred vision,* tinnitus, mydriasis, ophthalmoplegia

GI: *Constipation, dry mouth,* weight gain, nausea, vomiting, **paralytic ileus,** increased appetite, cramps, epigastric distress, jaundice, **hepatitis,** stomatitis

GU: *Urinary retention*

HEMA: Agranulocytosis, thrombocytopenia, eosinophilia, leukopenia, aplastic anemia

INTEG: Rash, urticaria, sweating, pruritus, photosensitivity

PHARMACOKINETICS

Onset 45 min; peak 2-12 hr; therapeutic response 4-10 days; metabolized by liver to nortriptyline; excreted in urine, feces; crosses placenta; excreted in breast milk; half-life 10-46 hr

INTERACTIONS

⚠ **Hyperpyretic crisis, seizures, hypertensive episode: MAOIs**

Increase: risk for agranulocytosis—antithyroid agents

Increase: QT prolongation—procainamide, quinidine, amiodarone, tricyclics, class IA, III antidysrhythmics

Increase: amitriptyline levels, toxicity—cimetidine, fluoxetine, phenothiazines, oral contraceptives, antidepressants, carbamazepine, class IC antidysrhythmics

Increase: effects of direct-acting sympathomimetics (EPINEPHrine), alcohol, barbiturates, benzodiazepines, CNS depressants, opioids, sedative/hypnotics

Decrease: effects of guanethidine, clonidine, indirect-acting sympathomimetics (ePHEDrine)

Drug/Herb

Increase: serotonin syndrome—SAM-e, St. John's wort, yohimbe

Increase: CNS depression—kava, hops, chamomile, lavender, valerian

Drug/Lab Test

Increase: serum bilirubin, blood glucose, alk phos, LFTs

Decrease: WBCs, platelets, granulocytes

NURSING CONSIDERATIONS

Assess:

- B/P lying, standing; pulse q4hr; if systolic B/P drops 20 mm Hg, hold product, notify prescriber; take vital signs q4hr with CV disease; ECG for flattening of T wave, prolongation of QTc interval, bundle branch block, AV block, dysrhythmias in cardiac patients
- Blood studies: CBC, leukocytes, differential, cardiac enzymes if patient is receiving long-term therapy
- Hepatic studies: AST, ALT, bilirubin
- Weight q wk; appetite may increase with product
- EPS primarily in geriatric patients: rigidity, dystonia, akathisia

Black Box Warning: Mental status: mood, sensorium, affect, suicidal tendencies; increase in psychiatric symptoms: depression, panic; suicidal tendencies are higher in those ≤24 yr, restrict amount of product available

- Urinary retention, constipation; constipation is most likely to occur in children and geriatric patients
- **Withdrawal symptoms:** headache, nausea, vomiting, muscle pain, weakness; do not usually occur unless product was discontinued abruptly
- Alcohol consumption; if alcohol is consumed, hold dose until morning
- **Pain syndromes (unlabeled):** intensity, location, severity; use pain scale; product may be taken for 1-2 months before effective
- **Sexual dysfunction:** erectile dysfunction, decreased libido

Perform/provide:

- Storage at room temp; do not freeze
- Gum, hard sugarless candy, frequent sips of water for dry mouth

Evaluate:

- Therapeutic response: decrease in depression, absence of suicidal thoughts

Teach patient/family:

- To take medication as directed; not to double dose; that therapeutic effects may take 2-3 wk; not to discontinue medication quickly after long-term use: may cause nausea, headache, malaise
- To use caution when driving, performing other activities that require alertness because of drowsiness, dizziness, blurred vision; to avoid rising quickly from sitting to standing (especially geriatric patients); how to manage anticholinergic effects
- To avoid alcohol, other CNS depressants
- To wear sunscreen or large hat when outdoors, photosensitivity occurs
- That contraception is recommended during treatment; to avoid breastfeeding

TREATMENT OF OVERDOSE:

ECG monitoring, lavage; administer anticonvulsant, sodium bicarbonate

amLODIPine (Rx)

(am-loe′di-peen)

Norvasc

Func. class.: Antianginal, antihypertensive, calcium channel blocker

Chem. class.: Dihydropyridine

Do not confuse:

amLODIPine/amiloride

Norvasc/Navane/Norvir/Nascor

ACTION: Inhibits calcium ion influx across cell membrane during cardiac depolarization; produces relaxation of coronary vascular smooth muscle, peripheral vascular smooth muscle; dilates coronary vascular arteries; increases myocardial O_2 delivery in patients with vasospastic angina

USES: Chronic stable angina pectoris, hypertension, variant angina (Prinzmetal's angina); may coadminister with other antihypertensives, antianginals

Unlabeled uses: Hypertension (pediatric patients)

CONTRAINDICATIONS: Hypersensitivity to this product, severe aortic stenosis, severe obstructive CAD

Black Box Warning: Hypersensitivity to dihydropyridine

Precautions: Pregnancy (C), breastfeeding, children, geriatric patients, CHF, hypotension, hepatic injury

DOSAGE AND ROUTES

Coronary artery disease

- **Adult: PO** 5-10 mg/day
- **Geriatric: PO** 5 mg/day, max 10 mg/day

Hypertension

- **Adult: PO** 2.5-5 mg/day initially, max 10 mg/day
- **Geriatric: PO** 2.5 mg/day, may increase to 5 mg/day, max 10 mg/day
- **Child 6-16 yr (unlabeled): PO** 2.5-5 mg/day
- **Child <6 yr (unlabeled): PO** 0.05-0.2 mg/kg/day in 1-2 divided doses

Hepatic dose

- **Adult: PO** 2.5 mg/day; may increase to 10 mg/day (antihypertensive); 5 mg/day, may increase to 10 mg/day (antianginal)

Available forms: Tabs 2.5, 5, 10 mg

Administer:

- Once a day without regard to meals

SIDE EFFECTS

CNS: *Headache,* fatigue, dizziness, asthenia, anxiety, depression, insomnia, paresthesia, somnolence

CV: *Peripheral edema,* bradycardia, hypotension, palpitations, syncope, chest pain

GI: Nausea, vomiting, diarrhea, gastric upset, constipation, flatulence, anorexia, gingival hyperplasia, dyspepsia, dysphagia

GU: Nocturia, polyuria, sexual difficulties

INTEG: Rash, pruritus, urticaria, alopecia

OTHER: Flushing, muscle cramps, cough, weight gain, tinnitus, epistaxis

PHARMACOKINETICS

Peak 6-12 hr; half-life 30-50 hr; increased in geriatric patients, hepatic disease; metabolized by liver (CYP3A4); excreted in urine (90% as metabolites); protein binding >93%

INTERACTIONS

Increase: neurotoxicity—lithium

Increase: hypotension—alcohol, antihypertensives, nitrates, fentaNYL, quiNIDine

Increase: amLODIPine level—diltiazem

Decrease: antihypertensive effect—NSAIDs

Drug/Herb

Decrease: effect—yohimbe

Drug/Food

Increase: hypotensive effect—grapefruit juice

NURSING CONSIDERATIONS

Assess:

- Cardiac status: B/P, pulse, respirations, ECG; some patients have developed severe angina, acute MI after calcium channel blockers if obstructive CAD is severe
- I&O ratio, weight daily; CHF: peripheral edema, dyspnea, jugular vein distention, crackles
- Angina: intensity, location, duration of pain

Evaluate:

- Therapeutic response: decreased anginal pain, decreased B/P, increased exercise tolerance

Teach patient/family:

- To take product as prescribed, not to double or skip dose
- To avoid hazardous activities until stabilized on product, dizziness is no longer a problem
- To avoid OTC products unless directed by prescriber

- To comply in all areas of medical regimen: diet, exercise, stress reduction, product therapy, smoking cessation
- To notify prescriber of irregular heartbeat; shortness of breath; swelling of feet, face, hands; severe dizziness; constipation; nausea; hypotension; if chest pain does not improve
- To use correct technique when monitoring pulse; to contact prescriber if pulse <50 bpm
- To avoid large amounts of grapefruit juice, alcohol
- To change positions slowly to prevent orthostatic hypotension
- To continue with good oral hygiene to prevent gingival disease
- To use sunscreen, protective clothing to prevent photosensitivity
- To notify all health care providers of use of this product

TREATMENT OF OVERDOSE:

Defibrillation, β-agonists, IV calcium inotropic agents, diuretics, atropine for AV block, vasopressor for hypotension

amoxicillin (Rx)

(a-mox-i-sill'in)

Gen-Amoxicillin ✱, Moxatag

Func. class.: Antiinfective, antiulcer

Chem. class.: Aminopenicillin

Do not confuse:

amoxicillin/amoxapine/Amoxil

Trimox/Diamox/Tylox

Wymox/Tylox

ACTION: Interferes with cell wall replication of susceptible organisms; the cell wall, rendered osmotically unstable, swells and bursts from osmotic pressure; bactericidal: lysis mediated by bacterial cell wall autolysins

USES: Treatment of skin, respiratory, GI, GU infections, otitis media, gonorrhea; for gram-positive cocci *(Staphylococcus aureus, Streptococcus pyogenes, Streptococcus faecalis, Streptococcus pneumoniae)*, gram-negative cocci *(Neisseria gonorrhoeae, Neisseria meningitidis)*, gram-positive bacilli *(Corynebacterium diphtheriae, Listeria monocytogenes)*, gram-negative bacilli *(Haemophilus influenzae, Escherichia coli, Proteus mirabilis, Salmonella)*; β-lactase–negative organisms; prophylaxis of bacterial endocarditis; in combination with other products for treatment of *Helicobacter pylori*

Unlabeled uses: Lyme disease, anthrax treatment and prophylaxis, cervicitis, *Chlamydia trachomatis*, dental abscess/infection, dyspepsia, gastric ulcer, nongonococcal urethritis (NGU), periodontitis, typhoid fever

CONTRAINDICATIONS: Hypersensitivity to penicillins

Precautions: Pregnancy (B), breastfeeding, neonates, hypersensitivity to cephalosporins, severe renal disease, acute lymphocytic leukemia, mononucleosis, phenylketonuria

DOSAGE AND ROUTES

Systemic infections (severe)

- **Adult: PO** 750 mg-1.75 g/day in divided doses q8hr or q12hr
- **Child: PO** 20-50 mg/kg/day in divided doses q8hr or q12hr

Streptococcus pyogenes infection (pharyngitis/tonsillitis)

- **Adult/child >12 yr: PO EXT REL** 775 mg q day with meal × 10 days

Gonorrhea

- **Adult: PO** 3 g given with 1 g probenecid as a single dose followed by tetracycline or erythromycin therapy

Chlamydia trachomatis

- **Adult: PO** 500 mg/tid × 1 wk

Bacterial endocarditis prophylaxis (unlabeled)

- **Adult: PO** 2 g 1 hr before procedure
- **Child: PO** 50 mg/kg 1 hr before procedure; max 2 g

Renal disease

• **Adult: PO** CCr 10-30 ml/min 250-500 mg q12hr; CCr <10 ml/min 250-500 mg q24hr; do not use 775, 875 mg strength if CCr <30 ml/min

Lyme disease (unlabeled)

• **Adult: PO** 250-500 mg tid × 10-30 days

• **Child: PO** 20-50 mg/kg/day in divided doses q8hr × 10-30 days

Duodenal/gastric ulcer/dyspepsia from *H. pylori* infection (unlabeled)

• **Adult: PO** 1000 mg bid with lansoprazole or clarithromycin/omeprazole

Anthrax treatment/prophylaxis (unlabeled)

• **Adult and child >20 kg: PO** 500 mg q8hr × 10-14 days (prophylaxis), 60 days (treatment)

• **Child <20 kg: PO** 80 mg/kg divided in 3 doses q8hr × 60 days (treatment)

Available forms: Caps 250, 500 mg; chew tabs 125, 200, 250, 400 mg; tabs 250, 500, 875 mg; ext rel tab (Moxatag) 775 mg; susp 125, 200, 250, 400 mg/5 ml

Administer:

PO route

• **Susp:** shake well before each dose; may be used alone, mixed in drinks; use immediately; discard unused portion after 14 days

• Give around the clock; caps may be emptied, mixed with liquids if needed

• **Ext rel:** do not crush, chew, break

SIDE EFFECTS

CNS: Headache, **seizures**, agitation, confusion, dizziness, insomnia

GI: *Nausea, vomiting, diarrhea,* increased AST, ALT, abdominal pain, glossitis, colitis, **pseudomembranous colitis**, jaundice, cholestasis

HEMA: Anemia, increased bleeding time, **bone marrow depression, granulocytopenia, hemolytic anemia**

INTEG: *Urticaria, rash*

SYST: Anaphylaxis, respiratory distress, serum sickness, Stevens-Johnson syndrome, toxic epidermal necrolysis, exfoliative dermatitis

PHARMACOKINETICS

PO: Peak 2 hr, duration 6-8 hr, half-life 1-1⅓ hr, metabolized in liver, excreted in urine, crosses placenta, enters breast milk

INTERACTIONS

Increase: amoxicillin level—probenecid

Increase: anticoagulant action—warfarin

Increase: methotrexate levels—methotrexate

Decrease: effectiveness of oral contraceptives

Drug/Lab Test

Increase: AST/ALT, alk phos, LDH

False positive: direct Coombs' test

NURSING CONSIDERATIONS

Assess:

• I&O ratio; report hematuria, oliguria because penicillin in high doses is nephrotoxic

• Hepatic studies: AST, ALT

• Blood studies: WBC, RBC, Hgb, Hct, bleeding time

• Renal studies: urinalysis, protein, blood, BUN, creatinine

• C&S before product therapy; product may be given as soon as culture is taken

⚠ **Pseudomembranous colitis: bowel pattern before, during treatment; diarrhea, cramping, blood in stools; report to prescriber**

• Skin eruptions after administration of penicillin to 1 wk after discontinuing product

• Respiratory status: rate, character, wheezing, tightness in chest

⚠ **Anaphylaxis: rash, itching, dyspnea, facial/laryngeal edema**

Perform/provide:

• Adrenaline, suction, tracheostomy set, endotracheal intubation equipment on unit

• Adequate intake of fluids (2 L) during diarrhea episodes
• Scratch test to assess allergy after securing order from prescriber; usually done when penicillin is only product of choice
• Storage in tight container; after reconstituting, oral susp refrigerated for 14 days

Evaluate:
• Therapeutic response: absence of infection; prevention of endocarditis, resolution of ulcer symptoms

Teach patient/family:
• That caps may be opened, contents taken with fluids; that chewable form is available; to take as prescribed, not to double dose
• All aspects of product therapy: to complete entire course of medication to ensure organism death (10-14 days); that culture may be taken after completed course of medication
• To use nonhormonal form of contraception
⚠ To report sore throat, fever, fatigue, diarrhea **(superinfection or agranulocytopenia),** blood in stool, abdominal pain **(pseudomembranous colitis),** decreased urinary output
• That product must be taken in equal intervals around the clock to maintain blood levels; to take without regard to food
• To wear or carry emergency ID if allergic to penicillins

TREATMENT OF ANAPHYLAXIS: Withdraw product, maintain airway; administer EPINEPHrine, aminophylline, O_2, IV corticosteroids

amoxicillin/clavulanate (Rx)

(a-mox-i-sill'in)

Amoclan, Apo-Amoxi Clav ✤, Augmentin, Augmentin XR, Clavulin ✤

Func. class.: Broad-spectrum antiinfective

Chem. class.: Aminopenicillin β-lactamase inhibitor

Do not confuse:
Augmentin/amoxicillin

ACTION: Bacteriocidal, interferes with cell wall replication of susceptible organisms; the cell wall, rendered osmotically unstable, swells and bursts from osmotic pressure; lysis mediated by bacterial cell wall autolytic enzymes, combination increases spectrum of activity against β-lactamase–resistant organisms

USES: Lower respiratory tract infections, sinus infections, pneumonia, otitis media, skin infection, UTI; effective for strains of *Escherichia coli, Proteus mirabilis, Haemophilus influenzae, Streptococcus faecalis, Streptococcus pneumoniae,* and some β-lactamase–producing organisms
Unlabeled uses: Actinomycotic mycetoma, chancroid, dental infections, dentoalveolar infection, melioidosis, pericoronitis, SARS

CONTRAINDICATIONS: Hypersensitivity to penicillins, severe renal disease, dialysis, jaundice
Precautions: Pregnancy (B), breastfeeding, neonates, children, hypersensitivity to cephalosporins; renal/GI disease, asthma, colitis, diabetes, eczema, leukemia, mononucleosis, viral infections, phenylketonuria

DOSAGE AND ROUTES

- **Adult: PO** 250-500 mg q8hr or 500-875 mg q12hr, depending on severity of infection
- **Child ≤40 kg: PO** 20-90 mg/kg/day in divided doses q8-12hr

Renal disease

- **Adult: PO** CCr 10-30 ml/min dose q12hr; CCr <10 ml/min dose q24hr; do not use 875-mg strength or ext rel if CCr <30 ml/min; Augmentin XR is contraindicated with renal disease

Available forms: Tabs 250, 500, 875 mg/125 mg clavulanate; chew tabs 200/28.5, 400/57 mg; powder for oral susp 250/28.5, 200/28.5, 400/57, 600/42.9 mg/5 ml; ext rel tabs (XR) 1000 mg amoxicillin, 62.5 mg clavulanate; powder for oral susp (ES) 600 mg amoxicillin, 42.9 mg clavulanate

Administer:

PO route

- Do not break, crush, chew XR (ext rel) product

⚠ Only as directed; two 250-mg tabs not equivalent to one 500-mg tab due to strength of clavulanate

- Shake susp well before each dose; may be used alone, mixed in drinks; use immediately, discard unused portion of susp after 14 days
- Give around the clock
- Give with light meal for increased absorption

SIDE EFFECTS

CNS: Headache, fever, **seizures**, agitation, insomnia

GI: *Nausea, diarrhea, vomiting,* increased AST/ALT, abdominal pain, glossitis, colitis, black tongue, **pseudomembranous colitis**

GU: Oliguria, proteinuria, hematuria, *vaginitis, moniliasis,* **glomerulonephritis**

HEMA: Anemia, **bone marrow depression, granulocytopenia, leukopenia, eosinophilia,** thrombocytopenic purpura

INTEG: *Rash,* urticaria, dermatitis, **toxic epidermal necrolysis**

META: Hypo/hyperkalemia, alkalosis, hypernatremia

SYST: **Anaphylaxis, respiratory distress, serum sickness, superinfection, Stevens-Johnson syndrome,** candidiasis

PHARMACOKINETICS

PO: Peak 2 hr, duration 6-8 hr, half-life 1-$1\frac{1}{3}$ hr, metabolized in liver, excreted in urine, crosses placenta, excreted in breast milk, removed by hemodialysis

INTERACTIONS

Increase: amoxicillin levels—probenecid

Increase: anticoagulant effect—warfarin

Increase: skin rash—allopurinol

Decrease: action of oral contraceptives

Drug/Food

Decrease: absorption by a high-fat meal

Drug/Lab Test

Increase: AST/ALT, alk phos, LDH

False positive: direct Coombs' test

NURSING CONSIDERATIONS

Assess:

⚠ Nephrotoxicity at high doses: I&O ratio; report hematuria, oliguria

- Hepatic studies: AST, ALT
- Blood studies: WBC, RBC, Hgb, Hct, bleeding time
- Renal studies: urinalysis, protein, blood, BUN, creatinine; if urine output decreases, long-acting products should not be used
- C&S before product therapy; product may be given as soon as culture is taken

⚠ **Pseudomembranous colitis:** bowel pattern before, during treatment; diarrhea, cramping, blood in stools; report to prescriber

- Respiratory status: rate, character, wheezing, tightness in chest

⚠ **Anaphylaxis:** rash, itching, dyspnea, facial/laryngeal edema; skin eruptions after administration of penicillin to 1 wk after discontinuing product

Perform/provide:

• Adrenaline, suction, tracheostomy set, endotracheal intubation equipment on unit

• Adequate intake of fluids (2 L) during diarrhea episodes

• Scratch test to assess allergy after securing order from prescriber; usually done when penicillin is only product of choice

• Storage in refrigerator for 10 days

Evaluate:

• Therapeutic response: absence of infection

Teach patient/family:

• To take as prescribed, not to double dose

• All aspects of product therapy: to complete entire course of medication to ensure organism death (10-14 days); that culture may be taken after completed course of medication

⚠ To report sore throat, fever, fatigue **(superinfection or agranulocytosis);** diarrhea, cramping, blood in stools **(pseudomembranous colitis)**

• That product must be taken in equal intervals around the clock to maintain blood levels

• To wear or carry emergency ID if allergic to penicillins

• To use alternative contraceptive measures if using oral contraceptives; to use cautiously if breastfeeding (effects unknown)

TREATMENT OF HYPERSENSITIVITY:
Withdraw product, maintain airway, administer EPINEPHrine, aminophylline, O_2, IV corticosteroids for anaphylaxis

AMPHOTERICIN B

amphotericin B lipid based (Rx)

Abelcet

amphotericin B liposomal (Rx)

AmBisome

Func. class.: Antifungal

Chem. class.: Amphoteric polyene

ACTION:
Increases cell membrane permeability in susceptible fungi by binding sterols; alters cell membrane, thereby causing leakage of cell components, cell death

USES:
Histoplasmosis, blastomycosis, aspergillosis, coccidioidomycosis, cryptococcosis, aspergillosis, zygomycosis, candidiasis, sporotrichosis, cryptococcal meningitis; mucomycosis caused by mucormycosis, *Rhizopus, Absidia, Entomorphthora, Basidiobolus*

Unlabeled uses: Candiduria (bladder irrigation), funguria, *Acremonium* sp., coccidioidomycosis prophylaxis, histoplasmosis prophylaxis, *Fusarium* sp., sinusitis, febrile neutropenia

CONTRAINDICATIONS:
Hypersensitivity, severe bone marrow depression

Precautions: Pregnancy (B), breastfeeding, children, renal disease, anemia, hypokalemia, hypomagnesemia, infections

Black Box Warning: Fungal infections

DOSAGE AND ROUTES

Abelcet

• **Adult and child: IV** 5 mg/kg/day as a single inf given at 2.5 mg/kg/hr

AmBisome

Fungal infections

• **Adult and child: IV** 3-5 mg/kg q24hr

Visceral leishmaniasis
• **Adult:** IV 3-4 mg/kg q24hr days 1-5, and days 14, 21 (immunocompetent), and days 10, 17, 24, 31, 38 (immunocompromised)
Fungal/histoplasmosis (unlabeled)
• **Adult:** IV 3 mg/kg/day
Available forms: *Lipid complex:* susp for inj 100 mg/20-ml vial; *liposome:* powder for inj 50-mg vial
Administer:
• Do not confuse 4 different types; these are not interchangeable: conventional amphotericin B, amphotericin B cholesteryl, amphotericin B lipid complex, amphotericin B liposome
IV route
• Product only after C&S confirms organism, product needed to treat condition; make sure product used for life-threatening infections
Liposomal complex
IV route
• Reconstitute with 12 ml sterile water/50-ml vial (4 mg/ml), shake, use 5-micron filter, dilute in D_5W (1-2 mg/ml), flush IV line with D_5W inj prior to use or use separate IV line; use filter ≥1-micron, give over 2 hr

Y-site compatibilities: Acyclovir, amifostine, aminophylline, anidulafungin, atropine, azithromycin, bivalirudin, bumetanide, buprenorphine, busulfan, butorphanol, CARBOplatin, carmustine, cefazolin, cefoxitin, ceftizoxime, cefTRIAXone, cefuroxime, cimetidine, clindamycin, cyclophosphamide, cytarabine, DACTINomycin, DAPTOmycin, dexamethasone, dexmedetomidine, diphenhydrAMINE, doxacurium, enalaprilat, ePHEDrine, EPINEPHrine, eptifibatide, ertapenem, esmolol, etoposide, famotidine, fenoldopam, fentanyl, fludarabine, fluorouracil, fosphenytoin, furosemide, granisetron, haloperidol, heparin, hydrocortisone, HYDROmorphone, ifosfamide, isoproterenol, ketorolac, levorphanol, lidocaine, linezolid, mesna, methotrexate, methylPREDNISolone, metoprolol, milrinone, mitomycin, nesiritide, nitroglycerin, nitroprusside, octreotide, oxaliplatin, oxytocin, palonosetron, pancuronium, pantoprazole, pemetrexed, PENTobarbital, PHENObarbital, phenylephrine, piperacillin/tazobactam, potassium chloride, procainamide, ranitidine, SUFentanil, tacrolimus, theophylline, thiopental, thiotepa, ticarcillin/clavulanate, tigecycline, trimethoprim-sulfamethoxazole, vasopressin, vinCRIStine, voriconazole, zidovudine
Lipid complex
IV route
• Shake vial until dissolved, withdraw dose using 18G needle, replace needle from syringe with product using 5-micron filter needle (use needle for 4 vials or less), empty contents in IV of D_5W (1 mg/ml), give at 2.5 mg/kg/hr, use inf pump

Y-site compatibilities: anidulafungin, ertapenem, octreotide

SIDE EFFECTS

CNS: *Headache, fever, chills,* peripheral nerve pain, paresthesias, peripheral neuropathy, **seizures**, dizziness
CV: Bradycardia, hypotension, **cardiac arrest**
EENT: Tinnitus, deafness, diplopia, blurred vision
GI: *Nausea, vomiting, anorexia,* diarrhea, cramps, **hemorrhagic gastroenteritis, acute liver failure**
GU: *Hypokalemia,* azotemia, hyposthenuria, **renal tubular acidosis**, nephrocalcinosis, **permanent renal impairment, anuria, oliguria**
HEMA: Normochromic, normocytic anemia, **thrombocytopenia, agranulocytosis, leukopenia, eosinophilia,** hypokalemia, hyponatremia, hypomagnesemia
INTEG: *Burning, irritation,* pain, necrosis at inj site with extravasation, flushing, dermatitis, skin rash (topical route)
MS: Arthralgia, myalgia, generalized pain, weakness, weight loss
SYST: **Stevens-Johnson syndrome, toxic epidermal neurolysis, exfoliative dermatitis, anaphylaxis**

PHARMACOKINETICS

IV: Peak 1-2 hr; initial half-life (LAmB) mean 4-6 days; metabolized in liver; excreted in urine (metabolites), breast milk; protein binding 90%; penetrates poorly CSF, bronchial secretions, aqueous humor, muscle, bone; terminal half-life lipid complex mean 7 days, liposomal mean 4-6 days

INTERACTIONS

Increase: nephrotoxicity—other nephrotoxic antibiotics (aminoglycosides, CISplatin, vancomycin, cycloSPORINE, polymyxin B)

Increase: hypokalemia—corticosteroids, digoxin, skeletal muscle relaxants, thiazides

NURSING CONSIDERATIONS

Assess:

- VS q15-30min during first inf; note changes in pulse, B/P
- I&O ratio; watch for decreasing urinary output, change in specific gravity; discontinue product to prevent permanent damage to renal tubules
- Blood studies: CBC, K, Na, Ca, Mg q2wk, BUN, creatinine 2-3 ×/wk
- Weight weekly; if weight increases by more than 2 lb/wk, edema is present; renal damage should be considered

⚠ **For renal toxicity:** increasing BUN, serum creatinine; if BUN is >40 mg/dl or if serum creatinine is >3 mg/dl, product may be discontinued, dosage reduced

⚠ **For hepatotoxicity:** increasing AST, ALT, alk phos, bilirubin

- **For allergic reaction:** dermatitis, rash; product should be discontinued, antihistamines (mild reaction) or EPINEPHrine (severe reaction) administered
- **For hypokalemia:** anorexia, drowsiness, weakness, decreased reflexes, dizziness, increased urinary output, increased thirst, paresthesias
- **For ototoxicity:** tinnitus (ringing, roaring in ears), vertigo, loss of hearing (rare)

Perform/provide:

- Acetaminophen and diphenhydrAMINE 30 min before inf to reduce fever, chills, headache
- Storage protected from moisture and light; diluted solution stable for 24 hr at room temp

Evaluate:

- Therapeutic response: decreased fever, malaise, rash, negative C&S for infecting organism

Teach patient/family:

- That long-term therapy may be needed to clear infection (2 wk-3 mo, depending on type of infection)
- To notify prescriber of bleeding, bruising, or soft-tissue swelling

ampicillin (Rx)

(am-pi-sill'in)

NovoAmpicillin ♣

Func. class.: Antiinfective—broad-spectrum

Chem. class.: Aminopenicillin

Do not confuse:

Omnipen/imipenem

ACTION: Interferes with cell wall replication of susceptible organisms; the cell wall, rendered osmotically unstable, swells, bursts from osmotic pressure; lysis mediated by cell wall autolysins

USES: Effective for gram-positive cocci *(Staphylococcus aureus, Streptococcus pyogenes, Streptococcus faecalis, Streptococcus pneumoniae)*, gram-negative cocci *(Neisseria meningitidis)*, gram-negative bacilli *(Haemophilus influenzae, Proteus mirabilis, Salmonella, Shigella, Listeria monocytogenes)*, gram-positive bacilli; meningitis, GI/GU/respiratory infections, endocarditis, septicemia, otitis media

Unlabeled uses: Biliary tract infection, shigellosis, typhoid fever, PID, OB/GYN infections, leptospirosis

A

CONTRAINDICATIONS:

Hypersensitivity to penicillins, antimicrobial resistance

Precautions: Pregnancy (B), breastfeeding, neonates, hypersensitivity to cephalosporins, renal disease, mononucleosis

DOSAGE AND ROUTES

Systemic infections

- **Adult and child ≥40 kg: PO** 250-500 mg q6hr; **IV/IM** 2-8 g/day in divided doses q4-6hr
- **Child <40 kg: PO** 50-100 mg/kg/day in divided doses q6-8hr; **IV/IM** 100-200 mg/kg/day in divided doses q6-8hr

Bacterial meningitis

- **Adult and adolescent: IM/IV** 150-200 mg/kg/day in divided doses q3-4hr; IDSA dose IV 12 g in divided doses q4hr
- **Infant and child: IM/IV** 150-200 mg/kg/day in divided doses q3-4hr; IDSA dose IV 300 mg/kg/day in divided doses q6hr
- **Neonates >7 days and >2000 g: IM/IV** 200 mg/kg/day in divided doses q6hr; IDSA dose IV 200 mg/kg/day in divided doses q6-8hr

Gonorrhea (urethritis)

- **Adult and child ≥45 kg: PO** 3.5 g given with 1 g probenecid as a single dose (not recommended by CDC)

Prevention of bacterial endocarditis

- **Adult: IM/IV** 2 g 30 min before procedure
- **Child: IM/IV** 50 mg/kg 30 min before procedure, max 2 g

GI/GU infections other than *N. gonorrhoeae*

- **Adult and child >20 kg: PO** 250-500 mg q6hr, may use larger dose for more serious infections
- **Child ≤20 kg: PO** 50-100 mg/kg/day in divided doses q6hr

Renal disease

- **Adult and child:** CCr 10-50 ml/min extend to q6-12hr; CCr <10 ml/min extend to q12-16hr

Shigellosis in AIDS patients (unlabeled)

- **Adult: PO** 500 mg qid × 5 days (not recommended by CDC)

Typhoid fever (unlabeled)

- **Adult/adolescent/child: IV** 100 mg/kg/day in divided doses q6hr × 14 days or more

Available forms: Powder for inj 125, 250, 500 mg, 1, 2, 10 g; IV inj 500 mg, 1, 2 g; caps 250, 500 mg; powder for oral susp 125, 250/5 ml

Administer:

PO route

- On empty stomach with plenty of water for best absorption (1-2 hr before meals or 2-3 hr after meals)
- Shake susp well before each dose

IM route

- **Reconstitute** by adding 0.9-1.2 ml/125-mg vial; 0.9-1.9 ml/250-mg vial; 1.2-1.8 ml/500-mg vial; 2.4-7.4 ml/1-g vial; 6.8 ml/2-g vial

IV route

- **IV direct:** after diluting with sterile water 0.9-1.2 ml/125 mg product, administer over 3-5 min (up to 500 mg), 10-15 min (>500 mg)

Intermittent IV INF route

- May be diluted in 50 ml or more of D_5W, D_5 0.45% NaCl to a conc of 30 mg/ml or less; IV sol is stable for 1 hr; give at prescribed rate, do not give in same tubing as aminoglycosides, separate by ≥1 hr

Y-site compatibilities: Acyclovir, alprostadil, amifostine, aminocaproic acid, anidulafungin, atenolol, bivalirudin, bleomycin, CARBOplatin, CISplatin, clarithromycin, cyclophosphamide, DACTINomycin, DAPTOmycin, dexmedetomidine, docetaxel, doxacurium, DOXOrubicin liposome, eptifibatide, etoposide, filgrastim, fludarabine, fluorouracil, foscarnet, gatafloxacin, gemcitabine, granisetron, hetastarch, ifosfamide, irinotecan, levofloxacin, linezolid, mechlorethamine, methotrexate, metroNIDAZOLE, octreotide, ofloxacin, oxaliplatin, paclitaxel, palonosetron, pamidronate, pancuronium, pantoprazole, pemetrexed, perphenazine, propofol, remifentanil, riTUXimab, rocuronium, sodium acetate, teniposide, thiotepa, tigecycline, tirofiban, TNA, trastuzumab, vinCRIStine, vit B/C, voriconazole

SIDE EFFECTS

CNS: Lethargy, hallucinations, anxiety, depression, twitching, coma, seizures
GI: *Nausea, vomiting, diarrhea,* pseudomembranous colitis, stomatitis
GU: Oliguria, proteinuria, hematuria, *vaginitis, moniliasis,* glomerulonephritis
HEMA: Anemia, increased bleeding time, bone marrow depression, granulocytopenia, leukopenia, eosinophilia, hemolysis
INTEG: *Rash, urticaria,* erythema multiforme
MISC: Anaphylaxis, serum sickness, Stevens-Johnson syndrome, toxic epidermal necrolysis

PHARMACOKINETICS

Half-life 50-110 min; metabolized in liver; excreted in urine, bile, breast milk; crosses placenta; removed by dialysis
PO: Peak 2 hr, duration 6-8 hr
IM: Peak 1 hr
IV: Peak 5 min

INTERACTIONS

Increase: ampicillin concentrations—probenecid
Increase: ampicillin-induced skin rash—allopurinol
Decrease: effectiveness of oral contraceptives

Drug/Lab Test
Increase: AST, ALT
Decrease: conjugated estrone during pregnancy, conjugated estriol
False positive: urine glucose, direct Coombs' test

NURSING CONSIDERATIONS

Assess:

- Infection: characteristics of wound, sputum, WBC; baseline, periodically; C&S before product therapy, product may be taken as soon as culture is taken

⚠ **Nephrotoxicity:** I&O ratio; report hematuria, oliguria; renal studies: urinalysis, protein, blood, BUN, creatinine

- Hepatic studies: AST, ALT
- Blood studies: WBC, RBC, Hgb, Hct, bleeding time
- Bowel pattern before, during treatment
- Skin eruptions after administration of penicillin to 1 wk after discontinuing product
- Respiratory status: rate, character, wheezing, tightness in chest

⚠ **Anaphylaxis:** rash, itching, dyspnea, facial swelling; stop product, notify prescriber, have emergency equipment available

Perform/provide:

- Adequate intake of fluids (2 L) during diarrhea episodes
- Scratch test to assess allergy after securing order from prescriber; usually done when penicillin is only product of choice
- Storage in tight container; after reconstituting, oral suspension refrigerated for 2 wk or stored at room temp for 1 wk

Evaluate:

- Therapeutic response: absence of fever, draining wounds, other symptoms of infection

Teach patient/family:

- That tabs may be crushed; caps may be opened, mixed with water
- To take oral ampicillin on empty stomach with full glass of water
- All aspects of product therapy: to complete entire course of medication to ensure organism death (10-14 days); that culture may be taken after completed course of medication

⚠ To report sore throat, fever, fatigue, diarrhea (may indicate **superinfection**); to report rash, other signs of allergy

- That product must be taken in equal intervals around the clock to maintain blood levels

- To wear or carry emergency ID if allergic to penicillins
- To use nonhormonal contraception because effectiveness of hormonal contraceptives decreased
- **Pseudomembranous colitis:** diarrhea with blood or pus; notify prescriber

TREATMENT OF ANAPHYLAXIS: Withdraw product, maintain airway; administer EPINEPHrine, aminophylline, O_2, IV corticosteroids

ampicillin, sulbactam (Rx)

Unasyn

Func. class.: Antiinfective—broad-spectrum

Chem. class.: Aminopenicillin with β-lactamase inhibitor

ACTION: Interferes with cell wall replication of susceptible organisms; the cell wall, rendered osmotically unstable, swells, bursts from osmotic pressure; lysis due to cell wall autolytic enzymes; combination extends spectrum of activity by β-lactamase inhibition

USES: Skin infections, intraabdominal infections, pneumonia *(Staphylococcus aureus, Escherichia coli, Klebsiella, Proteus mirabilis, Bacteroides fragilis, Haemophilus influenzae, Enterobacter, Acinetobacter calcoaceticus)*, intraabdominal infections *(Enterobacter, Klebsiella, Bacteroides, E. coli)*, gynecologic infections *(E. coli, Bacteroides)*, meningitis, septicemia

Unlabeled uses: Aspiration pneumonia, bone/joint infections, gonorrhea, infectious arthritis, lower respiratory infections, osteomyelitis, PID, UTI

CONTRAINDICATIONS: Hypersensitivity to penicillins, ampicillin, sulbactam

Precautions: Pregnancy (B), breastfeeding, neonates, hypersensitivity to cephalosporins/carbapenems, renal disease, mononucleosis, viral infections, syphilis

DOSAGE AND ROUTES

- **Adult/adolescent/child ≥40 kg: IM/IV** 1.5-3 g q6hr, max 4 g/day sulbactam
- **Child ≤40 kg: IV** 150-300 mg/kg/day divided q6hr, max 4 g/day

Renal disease

- **Adult ≥40 kg: IM/IV** CCr 15-30 ml/min dose q12hr; CCr 5-15 ml/min dose q24hr

Available forms: Powder for inj 1.5 g (1 g ampicillin, 0.5 g sulbactam), 3 g (2 g ampicillin, 1 g sulbactam), 10 g (10 g ampicillin, 5 g sulbactam)

Administer:

IM route

- Reconstitute by adding 3.2 ml sterile water/1.5-g vial; 6.4 ml/3-g vial, give deep in large muscle, aspirate

IV, direct route

- After diluting 1.5 g/3.2 ml sterile water for inj or 3 g/6.4 ml (250 mg ampicillin/125 mg sulbactam), allow to stand until foaming stops; may give over 15 min

Intermittent IV INF route

- Dilute further in 50 ml or more of D_5W, NaCl; administer within 1 hr after reconstitution; give over 15-30 min, separate doses from aminoglycosides by ≥1 hr

Y-site compatibilities: Amifostine, aminocaproic acid, anidulafungin, atenolol, bivalirudin, bleomycin, CARBOplatin, cefepime, CISplatin, codeine, cyclophosphamide, cytarabine, DAPTOmycin, dexmedetomidine, docetaxel, doxacurium, eptifibatide, etoposide, fenoldopam, filgrastim, fludarabine, fluorouracil, gallium, gatifloxacin, gemcitabine, granisetron, hetastarch, irinotecan, levofloxacin, linezolid, methotrexate, metroNIDAZOLE, octreotide, oxaliplatin, paclitaxel, palonosetron, pamidronate, pancuronium, pantoprazole, pemetrexed, remifentanil, riTUXimab, rocuronium, tacrolimus, teniposide, thiotepa, tigecycline, tirofiban, TNA, TPN, trastuzumab, vencuronium, vinCRIStine, voriconazole

SIDE EFFECTS

CNS: Lethargy, hallucinations, anxiety, depression, twitching, coma, seizures

GI: *Nausea, vomiting, diarrhea,* increased AST/ALT, abdominal pain, glossitis, colitis, pseudomembranous colitis, hepatic necrosis/failure

GU: Oliguria, proteinuria, hematuria, *vaginitis, moniliasis,* glomerulonephritis, dysuria

HEMA: Anemia, increased bleeding time, bone marrow depression, granulocytopenia, leukopenia, eosinophilia, hemolysis

INTEG: Injection site reactions, rash, edema, urticaria

MISC: Anaphylaxis, serum sickness, toxic epidermal necrolysis, Stevens-Johnson syndrome

PHARMACOKINETICS

IV: Peak 5 min, half-life 50-110 min, little metabolized in liver, 75%-85% of both products excreted in urine, diffuses to breast milk, crosses placenta

INTERACTIONS

Increase: ampicillin-induced skin rash—allopurinol

Increase: ampicillin level—probenecid, disulfiram

Increase: methotrexate level—methotrexate

Decrease: effect of oral contraceptive

Drug/Lab Test

False positive: urine glucose, urine protein

NURSING CONSIDERATIONS

Assess:

- **Infection:** characteristics of wound, sputum; take temperature, WBC count; C&S before product therapy, product may be given as soon as culture is taken
- Bowel pattern before, during treatment
- Respiratory status: rate, character, wheezing, tightness in chest
- I&O ratio; report hematuria, oliguria because penicillin in high doses is nephrotoxic

⚠ Any patient with compromised renal system, because product excreted slowly with poor renal system function; toxicity may occur rapidly

- Hepatic studies: AST, ALT if on long-term therapy
- Blood studies: WBC, RBC, Hct, Hgb, bleeding time
- Renal studies: urinalysis, protein, blood, BUN, creatinine

⚠ **Anaphylaxis:** skin eruptions after administration of ampicillin to 1 wk after discontinuing product

- Allergies before treatment; reaction to each medication; report allergies

Perform/provide:

- Adrenaline, suction, tracheostomy set, endotracheal intubation equipment on unit for possible anaphylaxis
- Adequate intake of fluids (2 L) during diarrhea episodes
- Scratch test to assess allergy after securing order from prescriber; usually done when penicillin is only product choice
- Storage in tight container, out of light

Evaluate:

- Therapeutic response: absence of fever, draining wounds; negative C&S

Teach patient/family:

- That oral contraceptives may be reduced and a nonhormonal contraceptive should be used while taking this product if pregnancy is to be prevented
- To report superinfection: vaginal itching; loose, foul-smelling stools; black furry tongue

⚠ **Pseudomembranous colitis:** fever, diarrhea with pus, blood, mucus; may occur up to 4 wk after treatment; report immediately to health care provider

- To wear or carry emergency ID if allergic to penicillin products

A

TREATMENT OF ANAPHYLAXIS: Withdraw product, maintain airway; administer EPINEPHrine, aminophylline, O_2, IV corticosteroids

anagrelide (Rx)

(a-na′gre-lide)

Agrylin, Gen-Anagrelide ✱, PMS-Anagrelide ✱, Sandoz Anagrelide ✱

Func. class.: Antiplatelet

Chem. class.: Imidazo-quinazolinone

ACTION: Reduces platelet count and prevents early platelet shape changes in response to aggregating agents, thus inhibiting platelet aggregation

USES: Chronic myelogenous leukemia (CML), polycythemia vera, thrombocytosis

CONTRAINDICATIONS: Hypersensitivity

Precautions: Pregnancy (C), breastfeeding, children <16 yr, females, renal/hepatic/cardiac disease, hypotension, abrupt discontinuation

DOSAGE AND ROUTES

• **Adult: PO** 0.5 mg qid or 1 mg bid, may be adjusted after 1 wk, max 10 mg/day or 2.5 mg single dose; maintenance: titrate to lowest dose to maintain platelets <600,000/mcL; dosage range, 1.5-3 mg/day

Available forms: Caps 0.5, 1 mg

Administer:

• May give with food; monitor closely for dosage adjustment, better absorption on empty stomach

SIDE EFFECTS

CNS: *Headache, dizziness,* **seizures,** *paresthesia,* **CVA,** *fever*

CV: *Postural hypotension,* tachycardia, palpitations, **CHF, MI, cardiomyopathy, cardiomegaly, complete heart block, atrial fibrillation,** dysrhythmia, **chest pain**

EENT: Amblyopia, diplopia, tinnitus

GI: *Diarrhea, abdominal pain, nausea, flatulence, vomiting, anorexia,* constipation, pancreatitis

GU: Dysuria

HEMA: Anemia, thrombocytopenia, ecchymosis, lymphadenoma

INTEG: *Rash,* photosensitivity

MISC: *Edema, pain*

MS: Asthenia, back pain

RESP: *Dyspnea*

PHARMACOKINETICS

Peak 1 hr, duration >24 hr, metabolized in liver, excreted in feces/urine, terminal half-life 3-4 days

INTERACTIONS

Increase: bleeding risk—abciximab, anticoagulants, antineoplastics, antithymocyte globulin, aspirin, ciprofloxacin, cimetidine, eptifibatide, NSAIDs, thrombolytics, ticlopidine, tirofiban, SSRIs

Decrease: absorption—sucralfate

Drug/Herb

Increase: bleeding risk—green tea, feverfew, ginger, ginkgo, garlic, DHEA, horse chestnut, fish oils

NURSING CONSIDERATIONS

Assess:

⚠ **Blood dyscrasias: platelet counts q2day × 1 wk, q wk thereafter; response should begin after 1-2 wk; Hgb, WBC, LFTs, renal function studies (BUN, creatinine)**

• B/P, pulse during treatment until stable; B/P lying, standing; orthostatic hypotension common

• Cardiac status: chest pain, what aggravates, ameliorates condition

Perform/provide:

• Storage at room temp

Evaluate:

• Therapeutic response: decreased platelet count

Teach patient/family:
• That medication is not a cure: may have to be taken continuously in evenly spaced doses only as directed
• That it is necessary to quit smoking to prevent excessive vasoconstriction
• To avoid hazardous activities until stabilized on medication; dizziness may occur
• To rise slowly from sitting or lying to prevent orthostatic hypotension
• Not to use alcohol or OTC medications unless approved by prescriber; to use sunscreen, protective clothing to prevent burns; to avoid grapefruit, grapefruit juice
• To report cardiac reactions, increased bruising, bleeding
• To use contraception (if female, childbearing age) because fetal harm may occur
• To report product use if having any surgery
• Not to double dose; if dose is missed, to take as soon as remembered; if close to next dose, to omit dose

anakinra (Rx)

(an-ah-kin′rah)

Kineret

Func. class.: Antirheumatic (DMARD), immunomodulator

Chem. class.: Recombinant form of human interleukin-1 receptor antagonist (IL-1Ra)

ACTION: A form of human interleukin-1 receptor antagonist (IL-1Ra) produced by DNA technology; blocks activity of IL-1, thereby resulting in decreased inflammation, cartilage degradation, bone resorption

USES: Reduction in signs and symptoms of moderate to severe active rheumatoid arthritis in patients ≥18 yr who have not responded to other disease-modifying agents

Unlabeled uses: Cryopyrin-associated periodic syndromes (CAPS)

CONTRAINDICATIONS: Hypersensitivity to *Escherichia-coli*–derived proteins, product, latex; sepsis

Precautions: Pregnancy (B), breastfeeding, children, geriatric patients, renal impairment, active infections, immunosuppression, neoplastic disease, asthma

DOSAGE AND ROUTES

• **Adult: SUBCUT** 100 mg/day

Renal dose

• **Adult:** CCr <30 ml/min **SUBCUT** 100 mg every other day

Available form: Inj 100 mg/0.67 ml prefilled glass syringe

Administer:

SUBCUT route
• Do not use if cloudy, discolored, if particulate is present; protect from light
• Do not admix with other sol or medications; do not use filter; give at same time each day
• Apply cold compress before, after inj, allow sol to warm to room temp before use
• Use middle thigh, abdomen (outside 2 inches from navel), upper outer buttocks, upper outer area of arm; rotate sites, give inj at least 1 inch from old site; do not give in skin that is bruised, red, tender, hard; remove needle cover immediately before use, pull gently back on plunger, if no blood appears, inject entire contents of prefilled syringe; discard any unused portion

SIDE EFFECTS

CNS: *Headache*
CV: Cardiac arrest
EENT: *Sinusitis*
GI: *Abdominal pain, nausea, diarrhea*
HEMA: Neutropenia
INTEG: Rash, *inj site reaction,* allergic reaction
MISC: Flulike symptoms, infection

MS: *Worsening of RA, arthralgia*
RESP: *URI*

PHARMACOKINETICS

Terminal half-life 4-6 hr; eliminated renally

INTERACTIONS

• Do not give; use rilonacept
Increase: risk for severe infection—TNF-blocking agents
Decrease: antibody reactions—vaccines

NURSING CONSIDERATIONS

Assess:

• **Rheumatoid arthritis:** pain, stiffness, ROM, swelling of joints, baseline, periodically during treatment
• For inj site pain, swelling; usually occurs after 2 inj (4-5 days)
• For infections (increased WBC, fever, flulike symptoms); stop treatment if present
• CBC with differential, neutrophil counts before treatment, monthly × 3 mo, quarterly for up to 1 yr thereafter
• For allergic reactions (rash, dyspnea); discontinue if severe
• For urinary status: decreasing urinary output

Evaluate:

• Therapeutic response: decreased inflammation, pain in joints

Teach patient/family:

• Not to receive vaccines while taking this product; to update vaccines before treatment
• About self-administration, if appropriate: inj should be made in thigh, abdomen, upper arm; rotate sites at least 1 inch from old site; give at same time of day
• To notify prescriber if pregnancy is planned, suspected, to avoid breastfeeding; to notify prescriber of allergic reaction, decreasing urine output, signs/symptoms of infection

anastrozole (Rx)

(an-a-stroh′zole)

Arimidex

Func. class.: Antineoplastic
Chem. class.: Aromatase inhibitor

ACTION: Highly selective nonsteroidal aromatase inhibitor that lowers serum estradiol concentrations; many breast cancers have strong estrogen receptors

USES: Advanced breast carcinoma not responsive to other therapy in estrogen-receptor–positive patients (postmenopausal); patients with advanced disease taking tamoxifen, adjunct therapy for early breast cancer
Unlabeled uses: Uterine leiomyomata, breast cancer (in those who have received tamoxifen for 2-3 yr)

CONTRAINDICATIONS: Pregnancy (X), breastfeeding, hypersensitivity
Precautions: Children, geriatric patients, premenopausal women, osteoporosis, hepatic/cardiac disease

DOSAGE AND ROUTES

• **Adult: PO** 1 mg/day

Available forms: Tabs 1 mg

Administer:

• Give without regard to meals at same time of day

SIDE EFFECTS

CNS: *Hot flashes, headache, lightheadedness,* depression, dizziness, confusion, insomnia, anxiety, fatigue
CV: Chest pain, *hypertension,* thrombophlebitis, *edema,* angina, MI, cerebral infarct, CVA, vasodilation

GI: *Nausea, vomiting,* altered taste leading to anorexia, diarrhea, constipation, abdominal pain, dry mouth
GU: Vaginal bleeding, vaginal dryness, pelvic pain, pruritus vulvae, UTI
HEMA: Leukopenia
INTEG: *Rash,* Stevens-Johnson syndrome
MISC: Hypercholesterolemia
MS: Bone pain, myalgia, *asthenia,* bone loss/osteoporosis, arthralgia, fractures
RESP: Cough, sinusitis, dyspnea, pulmonary embolism

PHARMACOKINETICS

Peak 2 hr; half-life 50 hr; excreted in feces, urine, terminal half-life 50 hr

INTERACTIONS

• Do not use with oral contraceptives, estrogen, tamoxifen, androstenedione, DHEA

Drug/Lab Test
Increase: GGT, AST, ALT, alk phos, cholesterol, LDL

NURSING CONSIDERATIONS

Assess:
• Bone mineral density, cholesterol, lipid panel, periodically
⚠ **Serious skin reactions:** Stevens-Johnson syndrome

Perform/provide:
• Storage in light-resistant container at room temp

Evaluate:
• Therapeutic response: decreased tumor size, spread of malignancy

Teach patient/family:
• To report any complaints, side effects to prescriber
• That vaginal bleeding, pruritus, hot flashes reversible after discontinuing treatment
• To report continued vaginal bleeding immediately
• That **tumor flare**—increase in size of tumor, increased bone pain—may occur and will subside rapidly; may take analgesics for pain
• To take adequate calcium and vitamin D due to risk for bone loss/fractures

anidulafungin (Rx)

(a-nid-yoo-luh-fun′jin)

Eraxis

Func. class.: Antifungal, systemic
Chem. class.: Echinocandin

ACTION: Inhibits fungal enzyme synthesis; causes direct damage to fungal cell wall

USES: Esophageal candidiasis, *Candida albicans, C. glabrata, C. parapsilosis, C. tropicalis*
Unlabeled uses: Fungal prophylaxis, disseminated candidiasis, oropharyngeal candidiasis

CONTRAINDICATIONS: Hypersensitivity to product, other echinocandins
Precautions: Pregnancy (C), breastfeeding, children, severe hepatic disease

DOSAGE AND ROUTES

Candidemia and other Candida infections
• **Adult: IV** 200 mg loading dose on day 1 then 100 mg/day × 14 days or more until last positive culture

Esophageal candidiasis
• **Adult: IV** 100 mg loading dose on day 1 then 50 mg/day × 14 days, for at least 7 days after symptoms resolved

Fungal prophylaxis (unlabeled)
• **Adolescent and child 2-17 yr: IV** 1.5 mg/kg over 90 min then 0.75 mg/kg/day over 45 min × 5-28 days

Available forms: Powder for inj, lyophilized 50, 100 mg

Administer:

IV route

- ***Reconstitution:*** If dehydrated alcohol diluents supplied, use supplied diluent (dehydrated alcohol in water for inj); reconstitute each 50-mg vial/15 ml of diluents or 100-mg vial/30 ml (3.33 mg/ml); if diluents not supplied, reconstitute each 50-mg vial/15 ml sterile water for inj or 100-mg vial/30 ml of sterile water for inj (3.33 mg/ml)
- **Dilution: 200 mg loading dose inf with vials (dehydrated alcohol),** withdraw contents of 4 (50-mg reconstituted vials) or 2 (100-mg reconstituted vials)/500 ml of D_5W or NS (0.36 mg/ml); **200 mg loading dose inf with vials (sterile water for inj),** withdraw contents of 4 (50-mg reconstituted vials) or 2 (100-mg reconstituted vials)/200 ml of D_5W or NS, total volume 260 ml; **100 mg daily inf with vials (dehydrated alcohol),** withdraw contents of 1 (100-mg reconstituted vial) or 1 (50-mg reconstituted vial) and add to 250 ml D_5W or NS (0.36 mg/ml); **100 mg daily inf with vials (sterile water),** withdraw contents of 1 (100-mg reconstituted vial) or 2 (50-mg reconstituted vials)/100 ml D_5W or NS (total volume 130 ml); **50 mg daily inf (dehydrated alcohol),** withdraw 50-mg reconstituted vial/100 ml of D_5W or NS (0.43 mg/ml); **50 mg daily inf (dehydrated alcohol),** withdraw contents of 1 (50-mg reconstituted vial)/100 ml D_5W or NS final conc (0.43/ml)
- Inf rate max 1.1 mg/min (dehydrated alcohol); inf rate 1.4 mg/min (sterile water) or 84 ml/hr
- Give only as IV inf, not for IV bolus
- Do not use if cloudy or precipitated; do not admix

Y-site compatibilities: Acyclovir, alemtuzumab, alfentanil, allopurinol, amifostine, amikacin, aminocaproic acid, aminophylline, amiodarone, amphotericin B lipid complex, amphotericin B liposome, ampicillin, ampicillin sulbactam, argatroban, arsenic trioxide, atenolol, atracurium, azithromycin, aztreonam, bivalirudin, bleomycin, bumetanide, buprenorphine, busulfan, butorphanol, calcium chloride/gluconate, CARBOplatin, carmustine, caspofungin, ceFAZolin, cefepime, cefotaxime, cefotetan, cefoxitin, ceftazidime, ceftizoxime, cefTRIAXone, cefuroxime, chloramphenicol, chlorproMAZINE, cimetidine, ciprofloxacin, cisatracurium, CISplatin, clindamycin, cyclophosphamide, cycloSPORINE, cytarabine, dacarbazine, DACTINomycin, daunorubicin liposome, DAUNOrubicin hydrochloride, dexamethasone, dexmedetomidine, dexrazoxane, digoxin, diltiazem, diphenhydrAMINE, DOBUtamine, docetaxel, dolasetron, DOPamine, doripenem, doxacurium, DOXOrubicin, DOXOrubicin liposomal, doxycycline, droperidol, enalaprilat, ePHEDrine, EPINEPHrine, epirubicin, eptifibatide, erythromycin, esmolol, etoposide, etoposide phosphate, famotidine, fenoldopam, fentaNYL, fluconazole, fludarabine, fluorouracil, foscarnet, fosphenytoin, furosemide, gallium nitrate, ganciclovir, gatifloxacin, gemcitabine, gentamicin, glycopyrrolate, granisetron, haloperidol, heparin, hydrALAZINE, hydrocortisone, HYDROmorphone, hydrOXYzine, IDArubicin, ifosfamide, imipenem-cilastatin, inamrinone, insulin (regular), irinotecan, isoproterenol, ketorolac, labetalol, leucovorin, levofloxacin, lidocaine, linezolid injection, LORazepam, mannitol, mechlorethamine, melphalan, meperidine, meropenem, mesna, metaraminol, methotrexate, methyldopate, methylPREDNISolone, metoclopramide, metoprolol, metroNIDAZOLE, midazolam, milrinone, mitomycin, mitoxantrone, mivacurium, morphine, moxifloxacin, mycophenolate mofetil, nafcillin, naloxone, nesiritide, niCARdipine, nitroglycerin, nitroprusside, norepinephrine, octreotide, ondansetron, oxaliplatin, oxytocin, paclitaxel, palonosetron, pamidronate, pancuronium, pantoprazole, pemetrexed, pentamidine, pentazocine, PENTobarbital, PHENobarbital, phentolamine, phenylephrine, piperacillin-tazobactam, polymyxin B, potassium acetate/chloride, procainamide, prochlorperazine, promethazine, propranolol, quiNIDine, quinupristin-dalfopristin, ranitidine, remifentanil, rocuronium, sodium acetate, streptozocin, succinylcholine, SUFentanil, sulfamethoxazole-trimethoprim, tacrolimus, teniposide, theophylline, thiopental, thiotepa, ticarcillin, ticarcillin-clavulanate, tirofiban, tobramycin, topotecan, trimethobenzamide, vancomycin, vasopressin, vecuronium, verapamil, vinBLAStine, vinCRIStine, vinorelbine, voriconazole, zidovudine, zoledronic acid

SIDE EFFECTS

Candidemia/other *Candida* infections

CNS: Seizures, dizziness, *headache*

CV: DVT, atrial fibrillation, right bundle branch block, hypotension, sinus arrhythmia, thrombophlebitis superficial, ventricular extrasystoles, QT prolongation (rare)

GI: *Nausea, anorexia, vomiting, diarrhea, increased AST, ALT*

META: Hypokalemia

Esophageal candidiasis

CNS: *Headache*

GI: *Nausea, anorexia, vomiting, diarrhea,* hepatic necrosis

HEMA: Neutropenia, thrombocytopenia, leukopenia, coagulopathy

INTEG: *Rash,* urticaria, itching, flushing

META: Hypocalcemia, hyperglycemia, hyperkalemia, hypernatremia, hypomagnesium (rare)

MS: *Back pain, rigors*

PHARMACOKINETICS

Steady state after loading dose, distribution half-life 0.5-1 hr, terminal half-life 40-50 hr, protein binding 99%

INTERACTIONS

Increase: plasma concentrations—cycloSPORINE

Drug/Lab Test

Increase: amylase, bilirubin, CPK, creatinine, ECG, lipase

Decrease: platelets, magnesium, potassium, transferase, urea

NURSING CONSIDERATIONS

Assess:

• **Infection:** clearing of cultures during treatment; obtain culture at baseline and throughout treatment; product may be started as soon as culture is taken

⚠ **Blood dyscrasias (rare):** CBC (RBC, Hct, Hgb), differential, platelet count periodically; notify prescriber of results

• Hepatic studies before, during treatment: bilirubin, AST, ALT, alk phos, as needed; also uric acid

⚠ **Bleeding:** hematuria, heme-positive stools, bruising/petechiae of mucosa or orifices; blood dyscrasias can occur

• GI symptoms: frequency of stools, cramping; if severe diarrhea occurs, electrolytes may need to be given

Perform/provide:

• Store reconstituted vials at 59° F-86° F for up to 24 hr, do not freeze (dehydrated alcohol); store reconstituted vials at 36° F-46° F (sterile water) for up to 24 hr, do not freeze

Evaluate:

• Therapeutic response: decreased symptoms of *Candida* infection, negative culture

Teach patient/family:

• To notify prescriber if pregnancy is suspected, planned; use nonhormonal form of contraception while taking this product

• To avoid breastfeeding while taking this product

• To inform prescriber of renal/hepatic disease

• To report bleeding

• To report signs of infection: increased temp, sore throat, flulike symptoms

• To notify prescriber of nausea, vomiting, diarrhea, jaundice, anorexia, clay-colored stools, dark urine; hepatotoxicity may occur

⚠ HIGH ALERT

antihemophilic factor VIII (AHF) (Rx)

(an-tee-hee-moe-fill′ik)

Advate, Alphanate, Helixate FS, Hemofil M, Humate-P, Koate-DVI, Kogenate FS, Monarc-M, Monoclate-P, Recombinate, Xyntha

Func. class.: Hemostatic

Chem. class.: Factor VIII

Do not confuse:
Kogenate/Kogenate-2

ACTION: Necessary for clotting; activates factor X in conjunction with activated factor IX; transforms prothrombin to thrombin

USES: Prevention/treatment of hemophilia A, patients with acquired circulating factor VIII inhibitors, factor VIII deficiency; prevention of surgical bleeding, risk of thrombosis (von Willebrand disease)

CONTRAINDICATIONS: Hypersensitivity; mouse, hamster, bovine, porcine protein; lactation, HIV

Precautions: Pregnancy (C), neonates/infants, hepatic disease; blood types A, B, AB; factor VIII inhibitor, viral infection

DOSAGE AND ROUTES

Moderate hemorrhage

- **Adult and child:** IV 10-30 units/kg to achieve peak IVIII at 20%-60% of normal

Massive hemorrhage (general dosing)

- **Adult and child:** IV 30-50 units/kg to achieve peak FVIII at 60%-100% of normal

Minor hemorrhage

- **Adult and child:** IV 10-15 units/kg to achieve peak FVIII at 20%-30% of normal

Available forms: Inj 250, 500, 1000, 1500 units/vial (number of units noted on label)

Administer:

- Hepatitis A/B vaccination at birth, if diagnosed with hemophilia

IV route

- To prepare, administer factor VIII concentrates at 1st sign of danger
- After rotating gently to mix
- Warm to room temp using plastic syringe to reconstitute, administer; adheres to glass; use another needle as a vent when reconstituting
- After dilution with warm NS, D_5W, LR, give within 3 hr; complete dissolution may take up to 10 min

IV INF route

- Give at ≤2 ml/min if conc exceeds 34 units/ml or over 3 min if conc is <34 units/ml; filter before use

SIDE EFFECTS

CNS: Headache, *lethargy, chills, fever, flushing,* LOC

CV: *Hypotension,* tachycardia

GI: Nausea, vomiting, abdominal cramps, constipation, diarrhea, anorexia, jaundice, **viral hepatitis**

HEMA: **Thrombosis, hemolysis, risk of hepatitis B, risk of HIV, antibody formation**

INTEG: Rash, flushing, *urticaria,* stinging at inj site

MISC: **Anaphylaxis,** blurred vision, back pain

RESP: **Bronchospasm,** rhinitis, dyspnea, nosebleeds, wheezing, **pulmonary embolism**

PHARMACOKINETICS

IV: Half-life 4 hr, terminal 15 hr

NURSING CONSIDERATIONS

Assess:

- Blood studies (coagulation factors assay by % of normal: 5% prevents spontaneous hemorrhage, 30%-50% for surgery, 80%-100% for severe hemorrhage)
- I&O, urine color; notify prescriber if urine becomes orange, red

• Pulse: discontinue inf if significant increase
• Hct, Coombs' test with blood types A, B, AB
• Test for factor VIII inhibitors before starting treatment, may require concomitant antiinhibitor coagulant complex therapy
• **Allergy:** fever, rash, itching, jaundice; give diphenhydrAMINE HCl (Benadryl), continue therapy if reaction is mild
• Blood group of patient, donors (if applicable; most factor VIII not from specific blood group donors)

⚠ **Bleeding:** ankles, knees, elbows, other joints

Perform/provide:

• Storage in refrigerator; do not freeze; after reconstitution, do not refrigerate; give within 3 hr

Evaluate:

• Therapeutic response: absence of bleeding

Teach patient/family:

• To report any signs of bleeding: gums, under skin, urine, stools, emesis; review methods to prevent bleeding
• To avoid salicylates, NSAIDs (increase bleeding tendencies)
• To advise health professionals of treatment for hemophilia
• About the signs of viral hepatitis, AIDS
• That immunization for hepatitis B may be given first
• To report hives, urticaria, chest tightness, hypotension; may be monoclonal-antibody–derived factor VIII
• To be screened q2-3mo for HIV
• To carry emergency ID describing disease process
• To report suspected transmission of infection to respective manufacturers

⚠ HIGH ALERT

antithrombin III, human (Rx)

(an′tee-throm-bin)

ATryn, Thrombate III

Func. class.: Antithrombin

Chem. class.: Pooled human plasma

ACTION: Inactivates thrombin and the activated forms of factors IX, X, XI, XII, thereby resulting in the inhibition of coagulation

USES: During surgical or obstetric procedures, for thromboembolism in patients with known antithrombin III deficiency, deep venous thrombosis (DVT), pulmonary embolism

Unlabeled uses: Disseminated intravascular coagulation (DIC)

CONTRAINDICATIONS: Goat milk hypersensitivity

Precautions: Pregnancy (B), breastfeeding, children

DOSAGE AND ROUTES

• Dosage is individualized
• Expect a 1.4% rise from baseline for every 1 international unit/kg administered

Units required =

$$\frac{(\text{Desired level} - \text{Baseline}) \times \text{Weight in kg}}{1.4\%}$$

DIC (unlabeled)

• **Adult: IV** Target AT III at >100%-120%

Available forms: 500 units in 10 ml; 1000 units in 20 ml; powder for inj 1750 units

Administer:

• ATryn is not indicated for treatment of thromboembolic events with hereditary antithrombin deficiency

• Heparin after fibrinogen level is >100 mg/dl; heparin infusion to increase PTT to 1.5-2 × baseline for 3-7 days

IV route

• Only by IV route over 10-20 min (Thrombate III)

• After **reconstituting** 500 international units/10 ml of NS, D_5W; do not shake; rotate to dissolve; allow to warm to room temp; use within 3 hr of reconstitution; give 50 international units or less/min; max 100 international units/min using 0.22 or 0.45 microfilter

SIDE EFFECTS

CNS: Dizziness, chills, severe lightheadedness

GI: Nausea, cramps, bowel fullness

RESP: Shortness of breath

SYST: **Bleeding,** surface bleeding, **anaphylaxis,** vasodilatory effects

PHARMACOKINETICS

Biologic half-life 2.5 days, peak 15-30 min

INTERACTIONS

• Do not administer with other products in syringe, sol

Increase: bleeding risk—anticoagulants, thrombolytics, pentosan, NSAIDs, salicylates, low-molecular-weight heparins (LMWHs), platelet inhibitors, antineoplastics, antithymocyte globulin, strontium-89

Drug/Food

Increase: bleeding risk—fish oil, omega-3 fatty acids

Drug/Herb

Increase: bleeding risk—garlic, ginger, ginkgo, green tea, horse chestnut

NURSING CONSIDERATIONS

Assess:

• AT-III levels q12hr, maintain at >80% of normal activity until stabilized then daily before dose

• VS, B/P, pulse, respirations, neurologic signs, temp at least q4hr, temp of 104° F (40° C) (may indicate infection), platelet count, thromboplastin time, aPI, prothrombin time, fibrinogen levels, cardiac rhythm

⚠ **For child born of parents with hereditary AT-III deficiency, obtain AT-III levels immediately after birth**

⚠ **Retroperitoneal bleeding:** back pain, leg weakness, diminished pulses; for neurologic changes that may indicate intracranial bleeding

Perform/provide:

• Storage in refrigerator

Evaluate:

• Therapeutic response: absence of thrombi formation

Teach patient/family:

• About product use and expected results

• To report adverse reactions, bleeding, bruising

• That maintenance dosing not usually required

• That there are many drug, herb interactions; to obtain approval from health care provider before taking

antithymocyte

See lymphocyte immune globulin

apraclonidine ophthalmic

See Appendix B

aprepitant (Rx)

(ap-re′pi-tant)

Emend

fosaprepitant

Emend

Func. class.: Antiemetic

Chem. class.: Miscellaneous

ACTION: Selective antagonist of human substance P/neurokinin 1 (NK_1) receptors that decreases emetic reflex

USES:
Prevention of nausea/vomiting associated with cancer chemotherapy (highly emetogenic/moderately emetogenic), including high-dose cisplatin; used in combination with other antiemetics; postoperative nausea/vomiting

CONTRAINDICATIONS:
Hypersensitivity

Precautions: Pregnancy (B), breastfeeding, children, geriatric patients, hepatic disease

DOSAGE AND ROUTES

Highly emetogenic (aprepitant)

- **Adult: PO** Day 1 (1 hr before chemotherapy) aprepitant 125 mg with 12 mg dexamethasone **PO,** with 32 mg ondansetron IV; day 2 aprepitant 80 mg with 8 mg dexamethasone **PO;** day 3 aprepitant 80 mg with 8 mg dexamethasone **PO;** day 4 only dexamethasone 8 mg **PO; IV INF** 115 mg over 15 min, 30 min before chemotherapy as alternative to 1st dose of aprepitant on day 1 of regimen (fosaprepitant)

Moderately emetogenic

- **Adult: PO** Day 1 125 mg aprepitant with dexamethasone 12 mg **PO,** with ondansetron 8 mg **PO** × 2; days 2 and 3 80 mg aprepitant only (aprepitant); **IV INF** 115 mg over 15 min, 30 min before chemotherapy as alternative to 1st dose of aprepitant on day 1 of regimen (fosaprepitant)

Prevention of postoperative nausea/vomiting

- **Adult: PO** 40 mg within 3 hr of induction of anesthesia

Available forms: Caps 40, 80, 125 mg; powder for inj 115 mg; combo pack cap 80-125 mg

Administer:

PO route

- Do not break, crush, or chew
- PO on 3-day schedule, give with full glass of water 1 hr before chemotherapy, with or without food

Intermittent IV INF route

- Only approved as a substitute for the 1st dose of aprepitant in 3-day regimen
- **Reconstitution:** use aseptic technique; inject 5 ml 0.9% NaCl into the vial, directing stream to wall of vial to prevent foam; swirl (do not shake)
- Prepare inf bag with 110 ml NS; do not dilute, reconstitute with any divalent cations such as calcium, magnesium, including LR, Hartmann's sol
- Withdraw entire volume from vial, transfer to inf bag; total volume 115 ml (1 mg/1 ml)
- Gently invert bag 2-3 times; reconstituted sol stable for 24 hr at lower room temp or <25° C
- Visually inspect for particulates, discoloration
- Infuse over 15 min

SIDE EFFECTS

CNS: *Headache, dizziness,* insomnia, anxiety, depression, confusion, peripheral neuropathy

CV: Bradycardia, tachycardia, DVT, hypo/hypertension

GI: *Diarrhea, constipation,* abdominal pain, anorexia, gastritis, increased AST, ALT, *nausea,* vomiting, heartburn

GU: Increased BUN, serum creatine, proteinuria, dysuria

HEMA: Anemia, thrombocytopenia, neutropenia

INTEG: Pruritus, rash, urticaria

MISC: Asthenia, fatigue, dehydration, fever, hiccups, tinnitus, alopecia

SYST: Anaphylaxis

PHARMACOKINETICS

Absorption 60%-65%, peak 4 hr, metabolized in liver by CYP3A4 enzymes to active metabolite, half-life 9-12 hr, 95% protein bound, not excreted in kidneys, crosses blood-brain barrier

INTERACTIONS

Increase: aprepitant action—CYP3A4 inhibitors (ketoconazole, itraconazole, nefazodone, troleandomycin, clarithromycin, ritonavir, nelfinavir, diltiazem)

Increase: action of CYP3A4 substrates (pimozide, cisapride, dexamethasone, methylPREDNISolone, midazolam, alprazolam, triazolam, docetaxel, paclitaxel, etoposide, irinotecan, imatinib, ifosfamide, vinorelbine, vinBLAStine, vinCRIStine)
Decrease: aprepitant action—CYP3A4 inducers (rifampin, carbamazepine, phenytoin)
Decrease: action of CYP2C9 substrates (warfarin, TOLBUTamide, phenytoin), oral contraceptives
Decrease: action of both products—paroxetine
Drug/Food
Decrease: effect—grapefruit juice

NURSING CONSIDERATIONS

Assess:

⚠ **For hypersensitive reactions:** pruritus, rash, urticaria, anaphylaxis

- CV status: hypo/hypertension, bradycardia, tachycardia, DVT
- For absence of nausea, vomiting during chemotherapy

Perform/provide:

- Storage at room temp; keep in original bottles, blisters (PO)

Evaluate:

- Therapeutic response: absence of nausea, vomiting during cancer chemotherapy

Teach patient/family:

- To report diarrhea, constipation
- To take only as prescribed; to take 1st dose 1 hr before chemotherapy
- To report all medications and herbals to prescriber before taking this medication
- To use nonhormonal form of contraception while taking this agent and for 1 mo thereafter; oral contraceptive effect may be decreased
- That those patients also taking warfarin should have clotting monitored closely during 2-wk period after administration of aprepitant
- To avoid breastfeeding

arformoterol (Rx)

(ar-for-moe′ter-ole)

Brovana

Func. class.: Long-acting adrenergic β_2-agonist, sympathomimetic, bronchodilator

ACTION:
Causes bronchodilation by action on β_2 (pulmonary) receptors by increasing levels of cAMP, which relaxes smooth muscle; produces bronchodilation and CNS, cardiac stimulation as well as increased diuresis and gastric acid secretion; longer acting than isoproterenol

USES:
COPD, including chronic bronchitis, emphysema

CONTRAINDICATIONS:
Hypersensitivity to sympathomimetics, product, racemic formoterol; tachydysrhyhmias, severe cardiac disease, heart block, children, monotherapy in asthma

Black Box Warning: Actively deteriorating COPD

Precautions: Pregnancy (C), breastfeeding, cardiac disorders, hyperthyroidism, diabetes mellitus, hypertension, prostatic hypertrophy, angle-closure glaucoma, seizures, hypoglycemia

DOSAGE AND ROUTES

COPD

- **Adult: NEB** 15 mcg, bid, AM, PM

Available forms: Inh sol 15 mcg/2 ml
Administer:

- By nebulization only; no dilution needed, give over 10-15 min; sol should be colorless

SIDE EFFECTS

CNS: *Tremors, anxiety,* insomnia, headache, dizziness, stimulation, *restlessness,* hallucinations, flushing, irritability
CV: Palpitations, tachycardia, hypertension, angina, hypotension, dysrhythmias

EENT: Dry nose, irritation of nose, throat
GI: Heartburn, nausea, vomiting
MISC: Flushing, sweating, anorexia, bad taste/smell changes, hypokalemia, anaphylaxis
MS: Muscle cramps
RESP: Cough, wheezing, dyspnea, bronchospasm, dry throat

PHARMACOKINETICS

Onset 5 min; peak 1-1½ hr; duration 4-6 hr; terminal half-life (COPD) 26 hr; extensively metabolized by direct conjugation by CYP2D6, CYP2C19; crosses placenta; protein binding 52%-65%; excreted in urine 63%, feces 11%

INTERACTIONS

Increase: severe hypotension—oxytocics
Increase: toxicity—theophylline
Increase: ECG changes/hypokalemia—potassium-losing diuretics
Increase: action of nebulized bronchodilators
Increase: action of arformoterol—tricyclics, MAOIs, other adrenergics; do not use together
Decrease: arformoterol action, asthma-related death—other β-blockers
Drug/Herb
Increase: stimulation—caffeine (cola nut, green/black tea, guarana, yerba maté, coffee, chocolate)

NURSING CONSIDERATIONS

Assess:

Black Box Warning: Respiratory function: vital capacity, forced expiratory volume, ABGs; lung sounds, heart rate, rhythm, B/P, sputum (baseline, peak); actively deteriorating COPD may occur

- Whether patient has received theophylline therapy, other bronchodilators before giving dose
- Patient's ability to self-medicate
- For evidence of allergic reactions; anaphylaxis may occur
- For **paradoxical bronchospasm;** hold medication, notify prescriber if bronchospasm occurs

Perform/provide:
- Storage in refrigerator; if stored at room temp, discard after 6 wk or if past expiration date, whichever is sooner

Evaluate:
- Therapeutic response: absence of dyspnea, wheezing after 1 hr, improved airway exchange, improved ABGs

Teach patient/family:
- To use exactly as prescribed; that death has resulted from asthma with products similar to this one
- Not to use OTC medications because excess stimulation may occur

⚠ HIGH ALERT

argatroban (Rx)

(are-ga-troe′ban)
Func. class.: Anticoagulant
Chem. class.: Thrombin inhibitor

Do not confuse:
argatroban/Aggrastat

ACTION: Direct inhibitor of thrombin, it reversibly binds to thrombin active site

USES: Anticoagulation prevention/treatment of thrombosis in heparin-induced thrombocytopenia; adjunct to percutaneous coronary intervention (PCI) in those with history of HIT
Unlabeled uses: Acute MI, DIC, use in infants/children/adolescents

CONTRAINDICATIONS: Hypersensitivity, overt major bleeding
Precautions: Pregnancy (B), breastfeeding, children, intracranial bleeding, renal function impairment, hepatic disease, severe hypertension, after lumbar puncture, spinal anesthesia, major surgery, congenital/acquired bleeding, GI ulcers

A

DOSAGE AND ROUTES

DVT, Pulmonary Embolism

• **Adult: CONT IV INF** 2 mcg/kg/min; adjust dose until steady-state aPTT is 1.5-3× initial baseline, max 100 sec, max dose 10 mcg/kg/min

• **Infant/child/adolescent (unlabeled): CONT IV INF** 0.75 mcg/kg/min, monitor aPTT q2hr until stable then at least daily

Hepatic dose

• **Adult: CONT INF** 0.5 mcg/kg/min, adjust rate based on aPTT

Percutaneous coronary intervention (PCI) in HIT

• **Adult: IV INF** 25 mcg/kg/min and bolus of 350 mcg/kg given over 3-5 min, check ACT 5-10 min after bolus completed, proceed if ACT >300 sec; if ACT <300 sec, give another 150 mcg/kg **BOL,** increase inf rate to 30 mcg/kg/min, recheck ACT in 5-10 min; if ACT >450 sec, decrease inf rate to 15 mcg/kg/min, recheck ACT in 5-10 min; when ACT is therapeutic, continue for duration of procedure

Acute MI (unlabeled)

• **Adult: IV** 1-3 mcg/kg/min

DIC (unlabeled)

• **Adult: CONT IV** 0.7 mcg/kg/min

Available forms: Inj 100 mg/ml (2.5 ml; must dilute 100-fold)

Administer:

• Avoid all IM inj that may cause bleeding

IV, direct route

• **For PCI:** 350 mg/kg bol and continuous inf of 25 mcg/kg/min; check ACT 5-10 min after bolus

Intermittent IV INF route

• **Dilute** in 0.9% NaCl, D_5, LR to a final conc of 1 mg/ml; **dilute** each 2.5-ml vial 100-fold by mixing with 250 ml of diluent, mix by repeated inversion of the diluent bag for 1 min; may briefly be slightly hazy

• Dosage adjustment may be made after review of aPTT, max 10 mcg/kg/min

SIDE EFFECTS

CNS: *Fever,* intracranial bleeding, headache

CV: Atrial fibrillation, coronary thrombosis, MI, myocardial ischemia, coronary occlusion, ventricular tachycardia, bradycardia, *chest pain, hypotension*

GI: *Nausea, vomiting, abdominal pain, diarrhea,* GI bleeding

GU: Hematuria, abnormal kidney function, UTI

HEMA: Hemorrhage

MISC: *Back pain, headache,* infection

RESP: Pneumonia, dyspnea, coughing, hemoptysis

SYST: Sepsis

PHARMACOKINETICS

Metabolized in liver by P450 CYP3A 4/5, distributed to extracellular fluid, 54% plasma protein binding, half-life 39-51 min, excreted in feces, steady state 1-3 hr

INTERACTIONS

Increase: bleeding risk—antiplatelets, NSAIDs, salicylates, dipyridamole, clopidogrel, ticlopidine, heparin, warfarin, glycoprotein IIb/IIIa antagonists (abciximab, tirofiban, eptifibatide), thrombolytics (alteplase, reteplase, urokinase, tenecteplase), other anticoagulants

NURSING CONSIDERATIONS

Assess:

• Baseline aPTT before treatment; do not start treatment if aPTT ratio is ≥2.5, then check aPTT 2 hr after initiation of treatment and at least daily thereafter

• aPTT, which should be 1.5-3× control

⚠ **Bleeding** gums: petechiae; ecchymosis; black, tarry stools; hematuria/epistaxis; B/P; vaginal bleeding, possible hemorrhage

⚠ **Anaphylaxis:** dyspnea, rash during treatment

• Fever, skin rash, urticaria

Evaluate:

• Therapeutic response: absence or decrease of thrombosis

Teach patient/family:
- To use a soft-bristle toothbrush to avoid bleeding gums; avoid contact sports; use electric razor; avoid IM inj
- To report any signs of bleeding: gums, under skin, urine, stools
- To notify prescriber if planning to become pregnant, breastfeeding

aripiprazole (Rx)
(a-rip-ip-pra′zol)
Abilify, Abilify Discmelt
Func. class.: Antipsychotic
Chem. class.: Quinolinone

ACTION: Exact mechanism unknown; may be mediated through both DOPamine type 2 (D_2, D_3) and serotonin type 2 ($5\text{-}HT_{1A}$, $5\text{-}HT_{2A}$) antagonism

USES: Schizophrenia and bipolar disorder (adults and adolescents), agitation, mania, major depressive disorder, short-term mania or mixed episodes of bipolar disorder; irritability in patients with autism
Unlabeled uses: Psychosis in patients with dementia

CONTRAINDICATIONS: Breastfeeding, hypersensitivity, seizure disorders
Precautions: Pregnancy (C), geriatric patients, renal/hepatic/cardiac disease

Black Box Warning: Children, dementia, suicidal ideation

DOSAGE AND ROUTES

Major depressive disorder
- **Adult: PO** 2-5 mg/day as an adjunct to other antidepressant treatment; adjust by 5 mg at ≥1 wk (range, 2-15 mg/day)

Schizophrenia
- **Adult: PO** 10-15 mg/day; if needed, dosage may be increased to 30 mg/day after 2 wk; maintenance 15 mg/day; periodically reassess
- **Adolescent 13-17 yr: PO** 2 mg/day, may increase to 5 mg after 2 days, then 10 mg after 2 more days, max 30 mg/day

Bipolar disorder
- **Adult: PO** 15 mg/day, may increase to 30 mg if needed (monotherapy); adjunctive to lithium or valproate PO 10-15 mg qd, may increase to 30 mg if needed
- **Child >10 yr, adolescents: PO** 2 mg, titrate to 5 mg/day after 2 days to target of 10 mg/day after another 2 days

Agitation with bipolar disorder/schizophrenia
- **Adult: IM** 9.75 mg as a single dose, may start with a lower dose, max 30 mg/day

Irritability associated with autism
- **Child ≥6 yr, adolescents: PO** 2 mg/day, increase to 5 mg/day after 1 wk, may increase to 10-15 mg/day if needed; dose changes should not occur more frequently than q1wk

Potential CYP2D6 inhibitor, strong CYP3A4 inhibitors
- **Adult: PO** Reduce to 50% of usual dose, increase dose when CYP2D6, CYP3A4 inhibitor withdrawn

Combination of strong CYP3A4/CYP2D6 inhibitors
- **Adult: PO** reduce to 25% of usual dose

Acute psychosis (unlabeled)
- **Adults: PO** 15 mg/day, may increase to 20-30 mg/day after 3 wk

Available forms: Tabs 2, 5, 10, 15, 20, 30 mg; inj 9.75 mg/1.3 ml; orally disintegrating tab 10, 15 mg; oral sol 1 mg/ml

Administer:

PO route
- May be given without regard to meals
- Orally disintegrating tabs; do not open blister until ready to use, do not push tab through foil; place on tongue, allow to dissolve, swallow, do not divide
- Oral liquid: use calibrated measuring device

IM route
- Give IM only; inject slowly, deeply into muscle mass; discard unused portion

SIDE EFFECTS

CNS: *Drowsiness, insomnia, agitation, anxiety, headache,* seizures, neuroleptic malignant syndrome, *light-headedness,*

akathisia, asthenia, tremor, stroke, suicidal ideation, dystonia
CV: Orthostatic hypotension, tachycardia
EENT: *Blurred vision, rhinitis*
GI: *Constipation, nausea, vomiting,* jaundice, *weight gain*
INTEG: *Rash*
META: Hypoglycemia
RESP: *Cough*
SYST: Death among geriatric patients with dementia

PHARMACOKINETICS

PO: Absorption 87%; extensively metabolized by liver to a major active metabolite; plasma protein binding >99%; terminal half-life 75-146 hr; excretion via urine 25%, feces 55%; clearance decreased in geriatric patients

INTERACTIONS

Increase: effects of aripiprazole—CYP3A4 inhibitors (ketoconazole, erythromycin), CYP2D6 inhibitors (quiNIDine, FLUoxetine, PARoxetine); reduce dose of aripiprazole
Increase: sedation—other CNS depressants, alcohol
Increase: EPS—other antipsychotics, lithium
Decrease: aripiprazole level—famotidine, valproate
Decrease: effects of aripiprazole—CYP3A4 inducers (carbamazepine)
Drug/Herb
Decrease: aripiprazole effect—St. John's wort

NURSING CONSIDERATIONS

Assess:

Black Box Warning: Mental status before initial administration, children/young adults may exhibit suicidal thoughts/behaviors, therefore smallest amount of product should be given; do not use to treat elderly patients, dementia may occur

- Swallowing of PO medication; check for hoarding, giving of medication to other patients
- I&O ratio; palpate bladder if urinary output is low
- Bilirubin, CBC, LFTs q mo
- Affect, orientation, LOC, reflexes, gait, coordination, sleep pattern disturbances
- B/P standing and lying; also pulse, respirations; take q4hr during initial treatment; establish baseline before starting treatment; report drops of 30 mm Hg; watch for ECG changes
- Dizziness, faintness, palpitations, tachycardia on rising
- **EPS,** including akathisia (inability to sit still, no pattern to movements), tardive dyskinesia (bizarre movements of the jaw, mouth, tongue, extremities), pseudoparkinsonism (rigidity, tremors, pill rolling, shuffling gait)

⚠ **Neuroleptic malignant syndrome:** hyperthermia, increased CPK, altered mental status, muscle rigidity; notify prescriber immediately

- Constipation, urinary retention daily; if these occur, increase bulk, water in diet; stool softeners, laxatives may be needed

Perform/provide:

- Supervised ambulation until patient is stabilized on medication; do not involve patient in strenuous exercise program because fainting is possible; patient should not stand still for a long time
- Storage in tight, light-resistant container

Evaluate:

- Therapeutic response: decrease in emotional excitement, hallucinations, delusions, paranoia; reorganization of patterns of thought, speech

Teach patient/family:

- That orthostatic hypotension may occur; to rise from sitting or lying position gradually
- To avoid hot tubs, hot showers, tub baths; hypotension may occur
- To avoid abrupt withdrawal of this product; EPS may result; product should be withdrawn slowly
- To avoid OTC preparations (cough, hay fever, cold) unless approved by prescriber because serious product interactions may occur; to avoid use with alco-

hol, CNS depressants because increased drowsiness may occur

- To avoid hazardous activities if drowsy, dizzy
- About compliance with product regimen
- To report impaired vision, tremors, muscle twitching, urinary retention
- That heat stroke may occur in hot weather; to take extra precautions to stay cool
- To notify prescriber if pregnant or intending to become pregnant; not to breastfeed

Black Box Warning: To report suicidal thoughts/behaviors immediately

TREATMENT OF OVERDOSE:
Lavage if orally ingested; provide airway; *do not induce vomiting*

RARELY USED

armodafinil (Rx)
(ar-moe-daf'in-il)

Nuvigil

Controlled Substance Schedule IV

USES: Narcolepsy, obstructive sleep apnea/hypoapnea syndrome, circadian rhythm disruption (shift-work sleep problems)

CONTRAINDICATIONS: Hypersensitivity to this product or modafinil

DOSAGE AND ROUTES
Narcolepsy, obstructive sleep apnea/hypoapnea syndrome

- **Adult and adolescent ≥17 yr: PO** 150-250 mg in AM

Circadian rhythm disruption (shift work sleep problems)

- **Adult and adolescent ≥17 yr: PO** 150 mg at start of shift

ascorbic acid (vit C) (OTC, Rx)
(a-skor'bic)

Acerola C, Apo-C ✱, Ascor L-500, Cenolate, Equaline Vitamin C, Walgreens Gold Seal, and many more

Func. class.: Vit C—water-soluble vitamin

ACTION: Wound healing, collagen synthesis, antioxidant, carbohydrate metabolism

USES: Vit C deficiency, scurvy; delayed wound, bone healing; chronic disease; urine acidification; before gastrectomy; dietary supplement

Unlabeled uses: Common cold prevention

CONTRAINDICATIONS: Tartrazine, sulfite sensitivity; G6PD deficiency

Precautions: Pregnancy (C), gout, diabetes, renal calculi (large doses)

DOSAGE AND ROUTES
Dietary supplementation

- **Adult:** 50-500 mg/day
- **Child 14-18 yr: PO** 65 mg (female), 75 mg (male)
- **Child 9-13 yr: PO** 45 mg/day
- **Child 4-8 yr: PO** 25 mg/day
- **Child 1-3 yr: PO** 15 mg/day
- **Infant: PO** 40-50 mg/day

Scurvy

- **Adult: PO/SUBCUT/IM/IV** 100-250 mg/day × 2 wk then 50 mg or more daily
- **Child: PO/SUBCUT/IM/IV** 100-300 mg/day × 2 wk then 35 mg or more daily

Wound healing/chronic disease/fracture (may be given with zinc)

- **Adult: SUBCUT/IM/IV/PO** 200-500 mg/day for 1-2 mo
- **Child: SUBCUT/IM/IV/PO** 100-200 mg added doses for 1-2 mo

Urine acidification

- **Adult:** 4-12 g/day in divided doses
- **Child:** 500 mg q6-8hr

Available forms: Tabs 25, 50, 100, 250, 500, 1000, 1500 mg; effervescent tabs 1000 mg; chewable tabs 100, 250, 500 mg; timed-release tabs 500, 750, 1000, 1500 mg; timed-release caps 500 mg; crys 4 g/tsp; powder 4 g/tsp; liq 35 mg/0.6 ml; sol 100 mg/ml; syr 20 mg/ml, 500 mg/5 ml; inj SUBCUT, IM, IV 100, 250, 500 mg/ml

Administer:

PO route

- Do not crush or chew ext rel tab or caps
- Caps may be opened and contents mixed with jelly

IV, direct route

- 100 mg undiluted by direct IV over at least 1 min; rapid inf may cause fainting

Intermittent IV INF route

- Diluted with D_5W, D_5NaCl, NS, LR, Ringer's, sodium lactate and given over 15 min

Syringe compatibilities: Metoclopramide, aminophylline, theophylline

Y-site compatibilities: Warfarin

SIDE EFFECTS

CNS: Headache, insomnia, dizziness, fatigue, flushing

GI: Nausea, vomiting, diarrhea, anorexia, heartburn, cramps

GU: Polyuria, urine acidification, oxalate/urate renal stones, dysuria

HEMA: Hemolytic anemia in patients with G6PD

INTEG: Inflammation at inj site

PHARMACOKINETICS

PO/INJ: Readily absorbed PO, metabolized in liver; unused amounts excreted in urine (unchanged), metabolites; crosses placenta, breast milk

INTERACTIONS

Drug/Lab Test

False positive: negatives in glucose tests

False negative: occult blood, urine bilirubin, leukocyte determination

NURSING CONSIDERATIONS

Assess:

- I&O ratio; urine pH (acidification)
- Ascorbic acid levels throughout treatment if continued deficiency is suspected
- Nutritional status: citrus fruits, vegetables
- Inj sites for inflammation
- Thrombophlebitis if receiving large dose

Evaluate:

- Therapeutic response: absence of anorexia, irritability, pallor, joint pain, hyperkeratosis, petechiae, poor wound healing

Teach patient/family:

- Necessary foods to include in diet, such as citrus fruits
- That smoking decreases vit C levels; not to exceed prescribed dose; that excesses will be excreted in urine, except when taking timed-release forms

asenapine (Rx)

(a-sen′a-peen)

Saphris

Func. class.: Antipsychotic, atypical

Chem. class.: Benzisoxazole derivative

ACTION: Unknown; may be mediated through both DOPamine type 2 (D2) and serotonin type 2 (5-HT2A) antagonism

USES: Bipolar 1 disorder, schizophrenia

CONTRAINDICATIONS: Breastfeeding, hypersensitivity

Precautions: Pregnancy (C), children, geriatric patients, cardiac/renal/hepatic disease, breast cancer, Parkinson's disease, dementia, seizure disorder, CNS depression, agranulocytosis, QT prolongation, torsades de pointes, suicidal ideation, substance abuse

Black Box Warning: Dementia

DOSAGE AND ROUTES

Schizophrenia

• **Adult: SL** 5 mg bid, max 20 mg/day

Bipolar 1 disorder

• **Adult: SL** 10 mg bid, may decrease to 5 mg bid as needed, max 20 mg/day

Available forms: SL tab 5, 10 mg

Administer:

• Anticholinergic agent to be used for EPS

• ***SL tab:*** remove tab; place tab under tongue; after it dissolves, swallow; advise patient not to chew, crush, swallow tabs, not to eat, drink for 10 min

SIDE EFFECTS

CNS: *EPS, pseudoparkinsonism, akathisia, dystonia, tardive dyskinesia; drowsiness, insomnia, agitation, anxiety, headache,* **seizures, neuroleptic malignant syndrome,** dizziness

CV: Orthostatic hypotension, **sinus tachycardia; heart failure, QT prolongation, stroke, bundle branch block**

GI: *Nausea,* vomiting, *constipation,* weight gain, increased appetite; oral hypoesthesia/parasthesia (SL)

GU: Hyperprolactinemia, hyperglycemia, hyponatremia

HEMA: Thrombocytopenia

INTEG: Serious allergic reactions

PHARMACOKINETICS

Extensively metabolized by liver, protein binding 95%, peak 0.5-1.5 hr, terminal half-life 24 hr

INTERACTIONS

Increase: sedation—other CNS depressants, alcohol

Increase: EPS—CYP2D6 inhibitors/substrates (SSRIs)

Increase: EPS—other antipsychotics

Increase: asenapine excretion—carbamazepine

Increase: QT prolongation—class IA/III antidysrhythmics, some phenothiazines, β-agonists, local anesthetics, tricyclics, haloperidol, methadone, chloroquine, clarithromycin, droperidol, erythromycin, pentamidine

Decrease: asenapine action—CYP2D6 inducers (carbamazepine, barbiturates, phenytoins, rifampin)

Drug/Herb

Increase: CNS depression—kava

Increase: EPS—betel palm, kava

Drug/Lab Test

Increase: prolactin levels

NURSING CONSIDERATIONS

Assess:

⚠ **Mental status before initial administration; watch for suicidal thoughts and behaviors; dementia and death may occur among elderly patients**

• Affect, orientation, LOC, reflexes, gait, coordination, sleep pattern disturbances

• B/P standing and lying; also pulse, respirations; take these q4hr during initial treatment; establish baseline before starting treatment; report drops of 30 mm Hg; watch for ECG changes; QT prolongation may occur

• Dizziness, faintness, palpitations, tachycardia on rising

• **EPS,** including akathisia, tardive dyskinesia (bizarre movements of the jaw, mouth, tongue, extremities), pseudoparkinsonism (rigidity, tremors, pill rolling, shuffling gait)

• **Neuroleptic malignant syndrome:** hyperthermia, increased CPK, altered mental status, muscle rigidity

• Constipation daily; increase bulk, water in diet if needed

• Weight gain, hyperglycemia, metabolic changes with diabetes

Perform/provide:

• Supervised ambulation until patient stabilized on medication; do not involve patient in strenuous exercise program because fainting is possible; patient should not stand still for a long time

• Increased fluids to prevent constipation

• Storage in tight, light-resistant container

Evaluate:
• Therapeutic response: decrease in emotional excitement, hallucinations, delusions, paranoia; reorganization of patterns of thought, speech

Teach patient/family:
• That orthostatic hypotension may occur; to rise from sitting or lying position gradually
• To avoid hot tubs, hot showers, tub baths; hypotension may occur
• To avoid abrupt withdrawal of this product; EPS may result; product should be withdrawn slowly
• To avoid OTC preparations (cough, hay fever, cold) unless approved by prescriber; serious product interactions may occur; to avoid use of alcohol; increased drowsiness may occur
• To avoid hazardous activities if drowsy, dizzy
• About compliance with product regimen
• That heat stroke may occur in hot weather; to take extra precautions to stay cool
• To use contraception; to inform prescriber if pregnancy is planned, suspected

Black Box Warning: To report suicidal thoughts/behaviors immediately

TREATMENT OF OVERDOSE:
Lavage if orally ingested; provide airway; *do not induce vomiting*

asparaginase *Erwinia chrysanthemi*

See Appendix A—Selected new drugs

RARELY USED
⚠ HIGH ALERT

asparaginase (Rx)
(a-spare′a-gi-nase)

Elspar

Func. class.: Antineoplastic
Chem. class.: *Escherichia coli* enzyme

USES: Acute lymphocytic leukemia in combination with other antineoplastics

CONTRAINDICATIONS: Hypersensitivity to product or *E. coli* protein, thromboembolic disease, infants, breastfeeding, pancreatitis

DOSAGE AND ROUTES
In combination
• **Adult and child: IM/IV** 25,000 international units/m^2/wk × 2 wk or 6000 international units/m^2 every other day × 3-4 wk or 1000-20,000 international units/m^2 for 10-12 days

aspirin (OTC)
(as′pir-in)

APC-ASA Coated Aspirin ✦, A.S.A., Ascriptin Enteric, Aspergum, Aspirin ✦, Aspir-Low, Aspir-trin ✦, Bayer Aspirin, Bayer Children's Aspirin, Bufferin, Ecotrin, Equaline, Good Sense Aspirin, Halfprin, PMS-ASA ✦, St. Joseph Children's, St. Joseph's Adult, Walgreens Aspirin Adult

Func. class.: Nonopioid analgesic, nonsteroidal antiinflammatory, antipyretic, antiplatelet
Chem. class.: Salicylate

ACTION: Blocks pain impulses in CNS, reduces inflammation by inhibition of prostaglandin synthesis; antipyretic action results from vasodilation of peripheral vessels; decreases platelet aggregation

USES:
Mild to moderate pain or fever including RA, osteoarthritis, thromboembolic disorders; TIAs, rheumatic fever, post MI, prophylaxis of MI, ischemic stroke, angina, acute MI

Unlabeled uses: Prevention of cataracts (long-term use), prevention of pregnancy loss in women with clotting disorders, bone pain, claudication, colorectal cancer prophylaxis, Kawasaki disease, PCI, preeclampsia/thrombosis prophylaxis, vernal keratoconjunctivitis, pericarditis

CONTRAINDICATIONS:
Pregnancy (D) 3rd trimester, breastfeeding, children <12 yr, children with flulike symptoms, hypersensitivity to salicylates, tartrazine (FDC yellow dye #5), GI bleeding, bleeding disorders, vit K deficiency, peptic ulcer, acute bronchospasm, agranulocytosis, increased intracranial pressure, intracranial bleeding, nasal polyps, urticaria

Precautions: Abrupt discontinuation, acetaminophen/NSAIDs hypersensitivity, acid/base imbalance, alcoholism, ascites, asthma, bone marrow suppression in elderly patients, dehydration, G6PD deficiency, gout, heart failure, anemia, renal/hepatic disease, pre/postoperatively, gastritis

DOSAGE AND ROUTES

Arthritis

- **Adult: PO** 3 g/day in divided doses q4-6hr
- **Child >25 kg (55 lb): PO/RECT** 90-130 mg/kg/day in divided doses

Pain/fever

- **Adult: PO/RECT** 325-650 mg q4hr prn, max 4 g/day
- **Child 2-11 yr: PO** 10-15 mg/kg/dose q4hr, max 4 g/day

Thromboembolic disorders

- **Adult: PO** 325-650 mg/day or bid

Transient ischemic attacks (risk)

- **Adult: PO** 50-325 mg/day (grade 1A)

Evolving MI with ST segment elevation (STEMI)

- **Adult: PO** 160-325 mg nonenteric, chewed and swallowed immediately, maintenance 75-162 mg daily

MI, stroke prophylaxis

- **Adult: PO** 50-325 mg/day

Prevention of recurrent MI

- **Adult: PO** 75-162 mg/day

CABG

- **Adult: PO** 75-325 mg/day starting 6 hr postprocedure, continue for 1 yr

PTCA

- **Adult: PO** 325 mg 2 hr before surgery

Thrombosis prophylaxis in ACS (unlabeled)

- **Adult: PO** 160-325 mg nonenteric, chewed and swallowed immediately

Idiopathic/viral pericarditis (unlabeled)

- **Adult: PO** 800 mg tid-qid × 7-10 days with gradual tapering to 800 mg/day q wk for an additional 2-3 wk

Colorectal cancer prophylaxis (unlabeled)

- **Adult: PO** 325 mg every other day

Kawasaki disease (unlabeled)

- **Child: PO** 80-100 mg/kg/day in 4 divided doses, maintenance 3-5 mg/kg/day

Available forms: Tabs 81, 325, 500, 650, 800 mg; chewable tabs 81 mg; supp 300, 600 mg; gum 227 mg; enteric-coated tabs 81, 325, 500, 975 mg; ext rel tabs 800 mg; del rel tabs 325, 500 mg

Administer:

PO route

- Do not break, crush, or chew enteric product
- Crushed or whole; chewable tablets may be chewed
- ½ hr before planned exercise
- With food or milk to decrease gastric symptoms; separate by 2 hr from enteric products
- With 8 oz of water; sit upright for ½ hr after dose to facilitate product passing into stomach

SIDE EFFECTS

CNS: Stimulation, drowsiness, dizziness, confusion, **seizures**, headache, flushing, hallucinations, **coma**
CV: Rapid pulse, pulmonary edema
EENT: Tinnitus, hearing loss
ENDO: Hypoglycemia, hyponatremia, hypokalemia
GI: *Nausea, vomiting,* **GI bleeding,** diarrhea, heartburn, anorexia, **hepatitis**
HEMA: **Thrombocytopenia, agranulocytosis, leukopenia, neutropenia, hemolytic anemia,** increased PT, aPTT, bleeding time
INTEG: *Rash,* urticaria, bruising
RESP: Wheezing, hyperpnea
SYST: **Reye's syndrome (children), anaphylaxis, laryngeal edema**

PHARMACOKINETICS

Enteric metabolized by liver; inactive metabolites excreted by kidneys; crosses placenta; excreted in breast milk; half-life 15-20 min, up to 9 hr in large dose; rectal products may be erratic, protein binding 90%
PO: Onset 15-30 min, peak 1-2 hr, duration 4-6 hr, well absorbed
RECT: Onset slow, duration 4-6 hr

INTERACTIONS

Increase: Gastric ulcer risk—corticosteroids, antiinflammatories, NSAIDs, alcohol
Increase: bleeding—alcohol, plicamycin, cefamandole, thrombolytics, ticlopidine, clopidogrel, tirofiban, eptifibatide, anticoagulants
Increase: effects of warfarin, insulin, methotrexate, thrombolytic agents, penicillins, phenytoin, valproic acid, oral hypoglycemics, sulfonamides
Increase: salicylate levels—urinary acidifiers, ammonium chloride, nizatidine
Increase: hypotension—nitroglycerin
Decrease: effects of aspirin—antacids (high doses), urinary alkalizers, corticosteroids
Decrease: antihypertensive effect—ACE inhibitors
Decrease: effects of probenecid, spironolactone, sulfinpyrazone, sulfonylamides, NSAIDs, β-blockers, loop diuretics

Drug/Herb
Increase: risk of bleeding—feverfew, garlic, ginger, ginkgo, ginseng *(Panax),* horse chestnut

Drug/Food
Increase: risk of bleeding—fish oil (omega-3 fatty acids)
• Foods that acidify urine may increase aspirin level

Drug/Lab Test
Increase: coagulation studies, LFTs, serum uric acid, amylase, CO_2, urinary protein
Decrease: serum potassium, cholesterol
Interference: VMA, 5-HIAA, xylose tolerance test, TSH, pregnancy test

NURSING CONSIDERATIONS

Assess:
• **Pain:** character, location, intensity; ROM before and 1 hr after administration
• **Fever:** temp before and 1 hr after administration
• Hepatic studies: AST, ALT, bilirubin, creatinine if patient is receiving long-term therapy
• Renal studies: BUN, urine creatinine; I&O ratio; decreasing output may indicate renal failure (long-term therapy)
• Blood studies: CBC, Hct, Hgb, PT if patient is receiving long-term therapy
⚠ **Hepatotoxicity: dark urine, clay-colored stools, yellowing of skin, sclera, itching, abdominal pain, fever, diarrhea if patient is receiving long-term therapy**
• **Allergic reactions:** rash, urticaria; if these occur, product may have to be discontinued; patients with asthma, nasal polyps, allergies: severe allergic reaction may occur
• **Ototoxicity:** tinnitus, ringing, roaring in ears; audiometric testing needed before, after long-term therapy

• **Salicylate level:** therapeutic level 150-300 mcg/ml for chronic inflammation
• Edema in feet, ankles, legs
• Product history; many product interactions

Evaluate:
• Therapeutic response: decreased pain, inflammation, fever

Teach patient/family:
• To report any symptoms of hepatotoxicity, renal toxicity, visual changes, ototoxicity, allergic reactions, bleeding (long-term therapy)
• To avoid if allergic to tartrazine
• Not to exceed recommended dosage; acute poisoning may result
• To read labels on other OTC products because many contain aspirin, salicylates
• That the therapeutic response takes 2 wk (arthritis)
• To report tinnitus, confusion, diarrhea, sweating, hyperventilation
• To avoid alcohol ingestion; GI bleeding may occur
• That patients who have allergies, nasal polyps, asthma may develop allergic reactions
• To discard tabs if vinegar-like smell is detected
• That medication is not to be given to children or teens with flulike symptoms or chickenpox because Reye's syndrome may develop

TREATMENT OF OVERDOSE:
Lavage, activated charcoal, monitor electrolytes, VS

atazanavir (Rx)
(at-a-za-na'veer)

Reyataz

Func. class.: Antiretroviral
Chem. class.: Protease inhibitor

ACTION: Inhibits human immunodeficiency virus (HIV-1) protease, which prevents maturation of the infectious virus

USES: HIV-1 infection in combination with other antiretroviral agents

CONTRAINDICATIONS: Hypersensitivity

Precautions: Pregnancy (B), breastfeeding, children, geriatric patients, hepatic disease, alcoholism, drug resistance, AV block, diabetes, dialysis, elderly, females, hemophilia, hypercholesterolemia, immune reconstitution syndrome, lactic acidosis, pancreatitis

DOSAGE AND ROUTES
Antiretroviral-naive patients
• **Adult: PO** 400 mg/day (unable to take ritonavir); 300 mg with ritonavir 100 mg/day
• **Child ≥6 yr/adolescent ≥40 kg: PO** 300 mg with ritonavir 100 mg daily
• **Child ≥6 yr/adolescent 20 to <40 kg: PO** 200 mg with ritonavir 100 mg daily
• **Child ≥6 yr/adolescent 15 to <20 kg: PO** 150 mg with ritonavir 80 mg daily

Antiretroviral-experienced patients
• **Adult: PO** 300 mg with ritonavir 100 mg daily
• **Pregnant adults/adolescents (2nd/3rd trimester) with H2 blocker or tenofovir: PO** 400 mg with ritonavir 100 mg daily
• **Child ≥6 yr/adolescent ≥40 kg: PO** 300 mg with ritonavir 100 mg daily
• **Child ≥6 yr/adolescent 20 to <40 kg: PO** 200 mg with ritonavir 100 mg daily

Hepatic dose
• **Adult: PO** Child-Pugh B: 300 mg/day; Child-Pugh C: do not use

Available forms: Caps 100, 150, 200, 300 mg

Administer:
• With food; 2 hr before or 1 hr after antacid or didanosine, swallow cap whole

SIDE EFFECTS
CNS: Headache, depression, dizziness, insomnia, peripheral neurologic symptoms

GI: Vomiting, *diarrhea, abdominal pain, nausea,* hepatotoxicity

INTEG: *Rash,* Stevens-Johnson syndrome, *photosensitivity*
MISC: Fatigue, fever, arthralgia, back pain, cough, lipodystrophy, pain, gynecomastia, nephrolithiasis; **lactic acidosis, hyperbilirubinemia (pregnancy, females, obesity)**

PHARMACOKINETICS

Rapidly absorbed, absorption increased with food, peak 2½ hr, 86% protein bound, extensively metabolized in liver by CYP3A4, 27% excreted unchanged in urine/feces (minimal), half-life 7 hr

INTERACTIONS

⚠ **Increase: levels, toxicity of immunosuppressants (cycloSPORINE, sirolimus, tacrolimus, sildenafil), tricylic antidepressants, warfarin, calcium channel blockers, clarithromycin, chlorazepate, diazepam, irinotecan, HMG-CoA reductase inhibitors, antidysrhythmics, midazolam, triazolam, ergots, pimozide, other protease inhibitors**
Increase: effects of estrogens, oral contraceptives
Increase: atazanavir levels—CYP3A4 substrates, CYP3A4 inhibitors
Increase: hyperbilirubinemia—indinavir
Decrease: atazanavir levels—CYP3A4 inducers, rifampin, antacids, didanosine, efavirenz, proton pump inhibitors, H_2-receptor antagonists
Drug/Herb
Decrease: atazanavir levels—St. John's wort
Increase: myopathy, rhabdomyolysis—red yeast rice
Drug/Lab Test
Increase: AST, ALT, total bilirubin, amylase, lipase, CK
Decrease: Hgb, neurophils, platelets

NURSING CONSIDERATIONS

Assess:
⚠ **For hepatic failure; hepatic studies: ALT, AST, bilirubin**
- **For lactic acidosis, hyperbilirubinemia (females, pregnancy, obesity)**
- For signs of infection, anemia
- Bowel pattern before, during treatment; if severe abdominal pain with bleeding occurs, product should be discontinued; monitor hydration
- Viral load, CD4 count throughout treatment
- Skin eruptions, rash, urticaria, itching
- Allergies before treatment, reaction to each medication; place allergies on chart

Evaluate:
- Therapeutic response: increasing CD4 counts; decreased viral load, resolution of symptoms of HIV-1 infection

Teach patient/family:
- To take as prescribed with other antiretrovirals as prescribed; if dose is missed, to take as soon as remembered up to 1 hr before next dose; not to double dose, share with others
- That product must be taken daily to maintain blood levels for duration of therapy
- That product may cause photosensitivity; to use protective clothing, stay out of the sun
- To notify prescriber if diarrhea, nausea, vomiting, rash occurs; dizziness, lightheadedness may occur; ECG may be altered
- That product interacts with many products; St. John's wort; to advise prescriber of all products, herbal products used
- That redistribution of body fat may occur, the effect is not known
- That product does not cure HIV-1 infection, prevent transmission to others; only controls symptoms
- That, if taking phosphodiesterase type 5 inhibitor with atazanavir, there may be increased risk of phosphodiesterase type 5 inhibitor–associated adverse events (hypotension, prolonged penile erection); to notify physician promptly of these symptoms

atenolol (Rx)

(a-ten'oh-lole)

CO Atenolol ♣, Gen-Atenolol ♣, PMS-Atenolol ♣, RAN-Atenolol ♣, ratio-Atenolol ♣, Sandoz Atenolol ♣, Tenormin

Func. class.: Antihypertensive, antianginal

Chem. class.: β-Blocker, β_1-, β_2-blocker (high doses)

Do not confuse:
atenolol/albuterol
Tenormin/thiamine/Imuran

ACTION: Competitively blocks stimulation of β-adrenergic receptor within vascular smooth muscle; produces negative chronotropic activity (decreases rate of SA node discharge, increases recovery time), slows conduction of AV node, decreases heart rate, negative inotropic activity decreases O_2 consumption in myocardium; decreases action of renin-aldosterone-angiotensin system at high doses, inhibits β_2 receptors in bronchial system at higher doses

USES: Mild to moderate hypertension, prophylaxis of angina pectoris; suspected or known MI (IV use); MI prophylaxis

Unlabeled uses: Migraine prophylaxis, supraventricular tachycardia prophylaxis (PSVT), unstable angina, alcohol withdrawal, lithium-induced tremor

CONTRAINDICATIONS: Pregnancy (D), hypersensitivity to β-blockers, cardiogenic shock, 2nd- or 3rd-degree heart block, sinus bradycardia, cardiac failure, Raynaud's disease, pulmonary edema

Precautions: Breastfeeding, major surgery, diabetes mellitus, thyroid/renal disease, CHF, COPD, asthma, well-compensated heart failure, dialysis, myasthenia gravis

Black Box Warning: Abrupt discontinuation

DOSAGE AND ROUTES

- **Adult: PO** 25-50 mg/day, increasing q1-2wk to 100 mg/day; may increase to 200 mg/day for angina, up to 100 mg/day for hypertension
- **Child: PO** 0.8-1 mg/kg/dose initially; range, 0.8-1.5 mg/kg/day; max 2 mg/kg/day
- **Geriatric: PO** 25 mg/day initially

Chronic stable angina

- **Adult: PO** 50 mg/day, then 100 mg/day as needed after 7 days, max 200 mg/day

Post MI, MI prophylaxis

- **Adult: PO** 100 mg/day in 1-2 divided doses; may need for 1-3 yr after MI

Renal disease

- **Adult: PO** CCr 15-35 ml/min, max 50 mg/day; CCr <15 ml/min, max 25 mg/day; hemodialysis 25-50 mg after dialysis

PSVT prophylaxis (unlabeled)

- **Child: PO** 0.3-1.3 mg/kg/day

Ethanol withdrawal prevention (unlabeled)

- **Adult: PO** 50-100 mg/day

Migraine prophylaxis (unlabeled)

- **Adult: PO** 50-150 mg/day, titrate to response

Lithium-induced tremor (unlabeled)

- **Adult: PO** 50 mg/day

Available forms: Tabs 25, 50, 100 mg

Administer:

PO route

- Product before meals, at bedtime; tab may be crushed, swallowed whole
- Reduced dosage with renal dysfunction

SIDE EFFECTS

CNS: *Insomnia, fatigue, dizziness, mental changes,* memory loss, hallucinations, depression, lethargy, drowsiness, strange dreams, catatonia

CV: **Profound hypotension, bradycardia,** CHF, *cold extremities, postural hypotension, 2nd- or 3rd-degree heart block*

EENT: Sore throat; dry, burning eyes; blurred vision; stuffy nose

ENDO: Increased hypoglycemic response to insulin
GI: *Nausea, diarrhea,* vomiting, **mesenteric arterial thrombosis, ischemic colitis**
GU: Impotence, decreased libido
HEMA: **Agranulocytosis, thrombocytopenia purpura**
INTEG: Rash, fever, alopecia
RESP: **Bronchospasm,** dyspnea, wheezing, pulmonary edema

PHARMACOKINETICS

PO: Peak 2-4 hr; onset 1 hr; duration 24 hr; half-life 6-9 hr; excreted unchanged in urine, feces (50%); protein binding 5%-15%

INTERACTIONS

- Mutual inhibition: sympathomimetics (cough, cold preparations)

Increase: hypotension, bradycardia—reserpine, hydrALAZINE, methyldopa, prazosin, anticholinergics, digoxin, diltiazem, verapamil, cardiac glycosides, antihypertensives

Increase: hypoglycemia—insulins, oral antidiabetics

Increase: hypertension amphetamines, ePHEDrine, pseudoephedrine

Decrease: effect—insulin, oral antidiabetic agents, theophylline, DOPamine, MAOIs

Drug/Herb

Increase: atenolol effect—hawthorn

Decrease: atenolol effect—ephedra (ma huang)

Drug/Lab Test

Increase: blood glucose, BUN, K, triglycerides, uric acid, ANA titer

NURSING CONSIDERATIONS

Assess:

- I&O, weight daily; watch for CHF (rales/crackles, jugular vein distention, weight gain, edema)
- Hypertension: B/P, pulse q4hr; note rate, rhythm, quality; apical/radial pulse before administration; notify prescriber of any significant changes (<50 bpm); ECG
- Baselines in renal/hepatic studies before therapy begins

Perform/provide:

- Storage protected from light, moisture; place in cool environment

Evaluate:

- Therapeutic response: decreased B/P after 1-2 wk, increased activity tolerance, decreased anginal pain

Teach patient/family:

- ⚠ **Not to discontinue product abruptly, taper over 2 wk (angina); to take at same time each day as directed**
- Not to use OTC products unless directed by prescriber
- To report bradycardia, dizziness, confusion, depression, fever
- To take pulse at home; advise when to notify prescriber
- To limit alcohol, smoking, sodium intake
- To comply with weight control, dietary adjustments, modified exercise program
- To carry emergency ID to identify product, allergies, conditions being treated
- To avoid hazardous activities if dizziness is present
- To change position slowly
- That product may mask symptoms of hypoglycemia in diabetic patients
- To use contraception while taking this product, pregnancy category (D)

TREATMENT OF OVERDOSE:

Lavage, IV atropine for bradycardia, IV theophylline for bronchospasm, dextrose for hypoglycemia, digoxin, O_2, diuretic for cardiac failure, hemodialysis

atomoxetine (Rx)

(at-o-mox′eh-teen)

Strattera

Func. class.: Psychotherapeutic—miscellaneous

Chem. class.: Selective norepinephrine reuptake inhibitor

ACTION: Selective norepinephrine reuptake inhibitor; may inhibit the presynaptic norepinephrine transporter

USES: Attention deficit hyperactivity disorder

CONTRAINDICATIONS: Hypersensitivity, angle-closure glaucoma, arteriosclerosis, cardiac disease, cardiomyopathy, heart failure, jaundice, MAOI therapy, history of pleochromocytoma

Precautions: Pregnancy (C), breastfeeding, hepatic disease, angioedema, bipolar disorder, dysrhythmias, CAD, hypo/hypertension

Black Box Warning: Children <6 yr, suicidal ideation

DOSAGE AND ROUTES

- **Child ≤70 kg >6 yrs: PO** 0.5 mg/kg/day, increase after 3 days to target daily dose of 1.2 mg/kg in AM or evenly divided doses AM, late afternoon; max 1.4 mg/kg/day or 100 mg/day, whichever is less
- **Adult and child >70 kg: PO** 40 mg/day, increase after 3 days to target daily dose of 80 mg in AM or evenly divided doses AM, late afternoon; max 100 mg/day

Maintenance

- **Adolescent ≤15 yr and child ≥6 yr: PO** 1.2-1.8 mg/kg/day

Initial dose titration with strong CYP2D6 inhibitors

- **Adult and child >6 yr weighing >70 kg: PO** 40 mg/day each AM or 2 evenly divided doses, titrate to target of 80 mg/day if symptoms do not improve after 4 wk and dose is well tolerated

Hepatic dose

- Child-Pugh B: reduce dose by 50%; Child-Pugh C: reduce dose by 75%

Available forms: Caps 10, 18, 25, 40, 60, 80, 100 mg

Administer:

- Whole; do not break, crush, chew
- Gum, hard candy, frequent sips of water for dry mouth
- Without regard to food

SIDE EFFECTS

CNS: *Insomnia,* dizziness, headache, irritability, crying, mood swings, fatigue, hypoesthesia, lethargy, paresthesia

CV: *Palpitations,* hot flushes, tachycardia, increased B/P

ENDO: Growth retardation

GI: Dyspepsia, nausea, anorexia, dry mouth, weight loss, vomiting, diarrhea, constipation, hepatic injury

GU: Urinary hesitancy, retention, dysmenorrhea, erectile disturbance, ejaculation failure, impotence, prostatitis, abnormal orgasm, male pelvic pain

INTEG: Exfoliative dermatitis, sweating, rash

MISC: Cough, rhinorrhea, dermatitis, ear infection

PHARMACOKINETICS

Peak 1-2 hr, metabolized by liver, excreted by kidneys, 98% protein binding

INTERACTIONS

Increase: hypertensive crisis—MAOIs or within 14 days of MAOIs, vasopressors

Increase: cardiovascular effects of albuterol, pressor agents

Increase: effects of atomoxetine—CYP2D6 inhibitors (amiodarone, cimetidine [weak], clomipramine, delavirdine, gefitinib, imatinib, propafenone, quinidine [potent], ritonavir, citalopram, escitalopram, FLUoxetine, sertraline, PARoxetine, thioridazine, venlafaxine)

NURSING CONSIDERATIONS

Assess:

- VS, B/P; check patients with cardiac disease more often for increased B/P
- Height, growth rate q3mo in children; growth rate may be decreased

⚠ Mental status: mood, sensorium, affect, stimulation, insomnia, aggressiveness, suicidal ideation in children/young adults

- Appetite, sleep, speech patterns
- For increased attention span, decreased hyperactivity with ADHD

Evaluate:

- Therapeutic response: decreased hyperactivity (ADHD)

Teach patient/family:

- To avoid OTC preparations unless approved by prescriber
- To avoid alcohol ingestion
- To avoid hazardous activities until stabilized on medication
- To get needed rest; patients will feel more tired at end of day; not to take dose late in day, insomnia may occur

Black Box Warning: To report suicidal ideation

atorvastatin (Rx)

(a-tore′va-stat-in)

Lipitor

Func. class.: Antilipidemic

Chem. class.: HMG-CoA reductase inhibitor (statin)

Do not confuse:

Lipitor/Levatol

ACTION: Inhibits HMG-CoA reductase enzyme, which reduces cholesterol synthesis; high doses lead to plaque regression

USES: As adjunct for primary hypercholesterolemia (types Ia, Ib), dysbetalipoproteinemia, elevated triglyceride levels, prevention of CV disease by reduction of heart risk in those with mildly elevated cholesterol

Unlabeled uses: Atherosclerosis

CONTRAINDICATIONS: Pregnancy (X), breastfeeding, hypersensitivity, active hepatic disease

Precautions: Previous hepatic disease, alcoholism, severe acute infections, trauma, severe metabolic disorders, electrolyte imbalance

DOSAGE AND ROUTES

- **Adult: PO** 10-20 mg/day, usual range 10-80 mg/day, dosage adjustments may be made in 2-4 wk intervals, max 80 mg/day; patients who require >45% reduction in LDL may be started at 40 mg/day

Atherosclerosis (unlabeled)

- **Adult: PO** 80 mg/day

Available forms: Tabs 10, 20, 40, 80 mg

Administer:

- Total daily dose at any time of day without regard to meals

SIDE EFFECTS

CNS: Headache, asthenia

EENT: Lens opacities

GI: *Abdominal cramps, constipation, diarrhea, flatus, heartburn,* dyspepsia, **liver dysfunction, pancreatitis,** nausea, increased serum transaminase

GU: Impotence

INTEG: Rash, pruritus, alopecia; photosensitivity (rare)

MISC: Hypersensitivity

MS: Arthralgia, myalgia, **rhabdomyolysis**

RESP: Pharyngitis, sinusitis

PHARMACOKINETICS

Peak 1-2 hr, metabolized in liver, highly protein bound, excreted primarily in urine, half-life 14 hr, protein binding 98%

INTERACTIONS

Increase: rhabdomyolysis—azole antifungals, cycloSPORINE, erythromycin, niacin, gemfibrozil, clofibrate

Increase: serum level of digoxin

Increase: levels of oral contraceptives

Increase: levels of atorvastatin—erythromycin
Increase: effects of warfarin
Decrease: atorvastatin levels—colestipol
Drug/Herb
Decrease: effect—St. John's wort
Drug/Food
• Possible toxicity when used with grapefruit juice; oat bran may reduce effectiveness
Drug/Lab Test
Increase: bilirubin, alk phos, ALT, AST, CK
Interference: thyroid function tests

NURSING CONSIDERATIONS

Assess:
• **Hypercholesterolemia:** diet, obtain diet history including fat, cholesterol in diet; cholesterol triglyceride levels periodically during treatment; check lipid panel 6-12 wk after changing dose
• Hepatic studies q1-2mo, at initiation, 6, 12 wk after initiation or change in dose, periodically thereafter; AST, ALT, LFTs may be increased
• Renal studies in patients with compromised renal system: BUN, I&O ratio, creatinine
• Bowel status: constipation, stool softeners may be needed; if severe, add fiber, water to diet
⚠ **Rhabdomyolysis:** for muscle pain, tenderness, obtain CPK baseline; if markedly increased, product may need to be discontinued
Perform/provide:
• Storage in cool environment in tight container protected from light
Evaluate:
• Therapeutic response: decrease in LDL, total cholesterol, triglycerides, CAD; increase in HDL
Teach patient/family:
• That blood work and eye exam will be necessary during treatment
• To report blurred vision, severe GI symptoms, headache, muscle pain, weakness
• That previously prescribed regimen will continue: low-cholesterol diet, exercise program, smoking cessation
• **Not to take product if pregnant (X), breastfeeding; to avoid alcohol**
• To stay out of the sun; to use sunscreen, protective clothing to prevent photosensitivity (rare)

atovaquone (Rx)

(a-toe′va-kwon)
Mepron
Func. class.: Antiprotozoal
Chem. class.: Aromatic diamide derivative, analog of ubiquinone

ACTION: Interferes with DNA/RNA synthesis in protozoa

USES: *Pneumocystis jiroveci* infections in patients intolerant of trimethoprim-sulfamethoxazole, prophylaxis, *Toxoplasma gondii,* toxoplasmosis
Unlabeled uses: Babesiosis, malaria treatment/prophylaxis, toxoplasmosis prophylaxis, *Plasmodium* sp.

CONTRAINDICATIONS: Hypersensitivity or history of developing life-threatening allergic reactions to any component of the formulation, benzyl alcohol sensitivity
Precautions: Pregnancy (C), breastfeeding, neonates, hepatic disease, GI disease, respiratory insufficiency

DOSAGE AND ROUTES

Acute, mild, moderate *Pneumocystis jiroveci* pneumonia
• **Adult and adolescent 13-16 yr: PO** 750 mg with food bid for 21 days
***Pneumocystis jiroveci* pneumonia, prophylaxis**
• **Adult and adolescent: PO** 1500 mg/day with meal

Babesiosis (unlabeled)
- **Adult: PO** 750 mg q12hr with azithromycin (500-1000 mg on day 1 then 250 mg/day × 7-14 days)

Toxoplasmosis prophylaxis in AIDS (unlabeled)
- **Adult: PO** 1500 mg alone or in combination

Plasmodium falciparum **(unlabeled)**
- **Adult: PO** 250 mg with proguanil daily
- **Child: PO** 17 mg/kg with proguanil daily

Available forms: Susp 750 mg/5 ml
Administer:
- With high-fat food to increase absorption of product and higher plasma concentrations
- Oral susp, shake before using
- All contents of foil pouch

SIDE EFFECTS

CNS: *Dizziness, headache, anxiety, insomnia,* asthenia, fever
CV: Hypotension
GI: *Nausea, vomiting, diarrhea,* anorexia, increased AST/ALT, acute pancreatitis, constipation, abdominal pain
HEMA: Anemia, neutropenia
INTEG: Pruritus, urticaria, *rash*
META: Hyperkalemia, hypoglycemia, hyponatremia
OTHER: Cough, dyspnea

PHARMACOKINETICS

Excreted unchanged in feces (94%), highly protein bound (99%), half-life 2-3 days

INTERACTIONS

Increase: level of—zidovudine
Decrease: effect of atovaquone—rifampin, rifabutin, tetracycline
Drug/Lab Test
Increase: AST, ALT, alk phos
Decrease: glucose, neutrophils, Hgb, sodium

NURSING CONSIDERATIONS

Assess:
Infection: WBC, vital signs; sputum baseline, periodically; obtain specimens needed before giving 1st dose
- Bowel pattern before, during treatment
- Respiratory status: rate, character, wheezing, dyspnea; risk for respiratory infection
- Allergies before treatment, reaction to each medication

Evaluate:
- Therapeutic response: decreased temp, ability to breathe

Teach patient/family:
- To take with food to increase plasma concentrations

RARELY USED

atracurium (Rx)

(a-tra-kyoor′ee-um)
Func. class.: Neuromuscular blocker (nondepolarizing)

USES: Facilitation of endotracheal intubation, skeletal muscle relaxation during mechanical ventilation, surgery, or general anesthesia

CONTRAINDICATIONS: Hypersensitivity

Black Box Warning: Respiratory insufficiency

DOSAGE AND ROUTES

- **Adult and child >2 yr: IV BOL** 0.4-0.5 mg/kg then 0.08-0.1 mg/kg 20-45 min after 1st dose if needed for prolonged procedures; give smaller doses with halothane
- **Child 1 mo-2 yr: IV BOL** 0.3-0.4 mg/kg

⚠ HIGH ALERT

atropine (Rx)

(a'troe-peen)

Atreza, AtroPen, Sal-Tropine

Func. class.: Antidysrhythmic, anticholinergic parasympatholytic, antimuscarinic

Chem. class.: Belladonna alkaloid

Do not confuse:
atropine/Akarpine

ACTION: Blocks acetylcholine at parasympathetic neuroeffector sites; increases cardiac output, heart rate by blocking vagal stimulation in heart; dries secretions by blocking vagus

USES: Bradycardia <40-50 bpm, bradydysrhythmia, reversal of anticholinesterase agents, insecticide poisoning, blocking cardiac vagal reflexes, decreasing secretions before surgery, antispasmodic with GU, biliary surgery, bronchodilator, AV heart block

Unlabeled uses: Cardiac arrest, CPR, diarrhea, pulseless electrical activity, ventricular asystole, asthma

CONTRAINDICATIONS: Hypersensitivity to belladonna alkaloids, closed-angle glaucoma, GI obstructions, myasthenia gravis, thyrotoxicosis, ulcerative colitis, prostatic hypertrophy, tachycardia/tachydysrhythmias, asthma, acute hemorrhage, severe hepatic disease, myocardial ischemia, paralytic ileus

Precautions: Pregnancy (C), breastfeeding, children <6 yr, geriatric patients, renal disease, CHF, hyperthyroidism, COPD, hypertension, intraabdominal infection, Down syndrome, spastic paralysis, gastric ulcer

DOSAGE AND ROUTES

Bradycardia/bradydysrhythmia

- **Adult: IV BOL** 0.5-1 mg given q3-5min, max 3 mg
- **Child: IV BOL** 0.01 mg/kg up to 0.4 mg or 0.3 mg/m^2; may repeat q4-6hr; min dose 0.1 mg to avoid paradoxical reaction, max single dose 0.5 mg

Organophosphate poisoning

- **Adult and child: IM/IV** 1-2 mg hourly until muscarinic symptoms disappear; may need 6 mg q hr
- **Adult and child >90 lb, usually >10 yr: AtroPen** 2 mg
- **Child 40-90 lb, usually 4-10 yr: AtroPen** 1 mg
- **Child 15-40 lb: AtroPen** 0.5 mg
- **Infant <15 lb: IM/IV** 0.05 mg/kg q5-20min as needed

Presurgery

- **Adult and child >20 kg: SUBCUT/IM/IV** 0.4-0.6 mg 30-60 min before anesthesia
- **Child <20 kg: IM/SUBCUT** 0.01 mg/kg up to 0.4 mg ½-1 hr preop, max 0.6 mg/dose

Available forms: Inj 0.05, 0.1, 0.4, 0.5, 0.8, 1 mg/ml; tabs 0.4 mg; AtroPen 0.5, 1, 2 mg inj prefilled autoinjectors

Administer:

PO route

- Increased bulk, water in diet if constipation occurs
- ½ hr before meals

IM route

- Atropine flush may occur in children and is not harmful

AtroPen

- Use no more than 3 AtroPen inj unless under the supervision of trained medical provider
- Use as soon as symptoms appear (tearing, wheezing, muscle fasciculations, excessive oral secretions)

IV route

- Undiluted or diluted with 10 ml sterile water; give at 0.6 mg/min through Y-tube or 3-way stopcock; do not add to IV sol; may cause paradoxical bradycardia for 2 min

Y-site compatibilities: Amrinone, etomidate, famotidine, heparin, hydrocortisone, meropenem, nafcillin, potassium chloride, sufentanil, vit B/C

SIDE EFFECTS

CNS: Headache, dizziness, involuntary movement, confusion, psychosis, anxiety, coma, flushing, drowsiness, insomnia, weakness; delirium (geriatric patients)
CV: Hypo/hypertension, paradoxical bradycardia, angina, PVCs, tachycardia, ectopic ventricular beats
EENT: Blurred vision, photophobia, glaucoma, eye pain, pupil dilation, nasal congestion
GI: Dry mouth, nausea, vomiting, abdominal pain, anorexia, constipation, paralytic ileus, abdominal distention, altered taste
GU: Retention, hesitancy, impotence, dysuria
INTEG: Rash, urticaria, contact dermatitis, dry skin, flushing
MISC: Suppression of lactation, decreased sweating

PHARMACOKINETICS

Half-life 2-3 hr, terminal 12.5 hr, excreted by kidneys unchanged (70%-90% in 24 hr), metabolized in liver, 40%-50% crosses placenta, excreted in breast milk
PO: Onset ½ hr, peak ½-1 hr, duration 4-6 hr, well absorbed
IM/SUBCUT: Onset 15-50 min, peak 30 min, duration 4-6 hr, well absorbed
IV: Peak 2-4 min, duration 4-6 hr

INTERACTIONS

Increase: Mucosal lesions—potassium chloride tab
Increase: anticholinergic effects—tricyclics, amantadine, antiparkinson agents
Decrease: absorption—ketoconazole, levodopa
Decrease: effect of atropine—antacids

NURSING CONSIDERATIONS

Assess:
- I&O ratio; check for urinary retention, daily output
- **ECG** for ectopic ventricular beats, PVC, tachycardia in cardiac patients
- For bowel sounds, constipation
- Respiratory status: rate, rhythm, cyanosis, wheezing, dyspnea, engorged neck veins
- **Increased intraocular pressure:** eye pain, nausea, vomiting, blurred vision, increased tearing
- Cardiac rate: rhythm, character, B/P continuously
- Allergic reaction: rash, urticaria

Perform/provide:
- Sugarless hard candy, gum, frequent rinsing of mouth for dryness

Evaluate:
- Therapeutic response: decreased dysrhythmias, increased heart rate, secretions; GI, GU spasms; bronchodilation

Teach patient/family:
- To report blurred vision, chest pain, allergic reactions, constipation, urinary retention
- Not to perform strenuous activity in high temperatures; heat stroke may result
- To take as prescribed; not to skip or double doses
- Not to operate machinery if drowsiness occurs
- Not to take OTC products without approval of prescriber

TREATMENT OF OVERDOSE:

O_2, artificial ventilation, ECG; administer DOPamine for circulatory depression; administer diazepam or thiopental for seizures; assess need for antidysrhythmics

atropine ophthalmic

See Appendix B

RARELY USED

auranofin (Rx)

(au-rane′oh-fin)

Ridaura

Func. class.: Antiinflammatory, gold compound

Do not confuse:
Ridaura/Cardura

USES: RA; not for 1st-line therapy
Unlabeled uses: SLE, psoriatic arthritis, pemphigus

CONTRAINDICATIONS: Breastfeeding, children <6 yr, hypersensitivity to gold, necrotizing enterocolitis, pulmonary fibrosis, exfoliative dermatitis, recent radiation therapy, renal/hepatic disease, marked hypertension, uncontrolled CHF

Black Box Warning: Bone marrow suppression, blood dyscrasias, hematuria, anemia, diarrhea

DOSAGE AND ROUTES

• **Adult: PO** 6 mg/day or 3 mg bid; may increase to 9 mg/day after 3 mo

axitinib

See Appendix A—Selected new drugs

⚠ HIGH ALERT

azacitidine (Rx)

(a-za-sie-ti′deen)

Vidaza

Func. class.: Antineoplastic-nucleoside analogue

Chem. class.: DNA demethylation agent

Do not confuse:
azacitidine/azaTHIOprine

ACTION: Cytotoxic by producing damage to double-strand DNA during DNA synthesis

USES: Myelodysplastic syndrome (MDS)
Unlabeled uses: Acute myelogenous leukemia (AML), chronic myelogenous leukemia (CML)

CONTRAINDICATIONS: Pregnancy (D), hypersensitivity to product or mannitol, advanced malignant hepatic tumors
Precautions: Breastfeeding, children, geriatric patients, renal/hepatic disease, baseline albumin <30 g/L; a man should not father a child while taking product

DOSAGE AND ROUTES

• **Adult: SUBCUT/IV** 75 mg/m^2/day × 7 days q4wk, dose may be increased to 100 mg/m^2 if no response seen after 2 treatment cycles; minimum treatment, 4 cycles

Available forms: Powder for inj 100 mg

Administer:

• Use cytotoxic handling procedures

SUBCUT route

• **Reconstitute** with 4 ml sterile water for inj (25 mg/ml), inject diluents slowly into vial, invert vial 2-3 times, gently rotate; sol will be cloudy, use immediately; divide doses >4 ml into 2 syringes; invert contents 2-3 times, gently roll syringe between the palms for 30 sec immediately before administration, rotate inj site

Intermittent IV INF route

• **Reconstitute** each vial with 10 ml sterile water for inj, shake well until all solids are dissolved, withdraw sol (10 mg/ml), inject in 50-100 NS or LR inf run over 10-40 min

SIDE EFFECTS

CNS: Anxiety, depression, dizziness, fatigue, headache, fever, insomnia
CV: Cardiac murmur, hypotension, tachycardia, peripheral edema, chest pain
GI: Diarrhea, nausea, vomiting, anorexia, constipation, abdominal pain, distention, tenderness, hemorrhoids, mouth hemorrhage, tongue ulceration, stomatitis, dyspepsia, **hepatotoxicity, hepatic coma**
GU: **Renal failure, renal tubular acidosis,** dysuria, UTI
HEMA: **Leukopenia, anemia, thrombocytopenia, neutropenia, febrile neutropenia,** ecchymosis, petechiae
INTEG: Irritation at site, rash, sweating, pyrexia, pruritus
META: Hypokalemia
MS: Weakness, arthralgia, muscle cramps, myalgia, back pain
RESP: Cough, dyspnea, pharyngitis, **pleural effusion**

PHARMACOKINETICS

Rapidly absorbed, peak ½ hr, metabolized in the liver, half-life 4 hr, excreted in urine

INTERACTIONS

Increase: bone marrow depression—other antineoplastics

NURSING CONSIDERATIONS

Assess:
- For CNS symptoms: fever, headache, chills, dizziness
- Bone marrow suppression/hematologic response: CBC with differential, baseline WBC $\geq$3000/mm^3, absolute neutrophil count (ANC) $\geq$1500/mm^3, platelets $>$7500/mm^3, adjust dose based on nadir; ANC $<$500/mm^3, platelets $<$25,000/mm^3, give 50% dose next course; ANC 500-1500/mm^3, platelets 25,000-50,000/mm^3, give 67% next course; bruising, bleeding, blood in stools, urine, sputum, emesis; myelodysplastic syndrome (MDS), splenomegaly
- Buccal cavity q8hr for dryness, sores, or ulceration, white patches, oral pain, bleeding, dysphagia
- Myelodysplastic syndrome (MDS): severe anemia, cytopenias, splenomegaly
- Blood studies: BUN, bicarbonate, creatine, LFTs

Perform/provide:
- Increased fluid intake to 2-3 L/day to prevent dehydration unless contraindicated
- Rinsing of mouth tid-qid with water, club soda; brushing of teeth bid-tid with soft brush or cotton-tipped applicator for stomatitis; use unwaxed dental floss
- Nutritious diet with iron, vitamin supplement, low fiber, few dairy products

Evaluate:
- Therapeutic response: improvement in blood counts with refractory anemia or refractory anemia with excess blasts

Teach patient/family:
- To avoid crowds, persons with known infections; not to receive immunizations
- To avoid foods with citric acid or hot or rough texture if stomatitis is present; to drink adequate fluids
- To report stomatitis; any bleeding, white spots, ulcerations in mouth; to examine mouth daily, report symptoms, infection site reactions, pruritus, fever
- To use contraception during and for several months after therapy (pregnancy [D]); not to breastfeed; not to father a child while receiving product

azaTHIOprine (Rx)

(ay-za-thye′oh-preen)

Apo-Azathioprine ✤, Azasan, Gen-Azathioprine ✤, Imuran

Func. class.: Immunosuppressant
Chem. class.: Purine antagonist

Do not confuse:
Imuran/Imferon/Elmiron/IMDUR/Enduron/Tenormin
azaTHIOprine/azacitidine

ACTION:
Produces immunosuppression by inhibiting purine synthesis in cells

USES:
Renal transplants to prevent graft rejection, refractory rheumatoid arthritis

Unlabeled uses: Myasthenia gravis, chronic ulcerative colitis, Crohn's disease, Behçet's disease, autoimmune hepatitis, dermatomyositis, thrombocytopenic purpura, lupus nephritis, polymyositis, pulmonary fibrosis, systemic lupus erythematosus (SLE), Wegener's granulomatosis, vasculitis, atopic dermatitis

CONTRAINDICATIONS:
Pregnancy (D), hypersensitivity, breastfeeding

Precautions: Severe renal/hepatic disease, geriatric patients, thiopurine methyltransferase deficiency, infection

Black Box Warning: Bone marrow suppression, neoplastic disease, must be used by experienced clinician

DOSAGE AND ROUTES

Prevention of rejection

- **Adult and child: IV** 3-5 mg/kg/day then maintenance **(PO)** of ≥ 1-3 mg/kg/day

Refractory rheumatoid arthritis

- **Adult: PO** 1 mg/kg/day, may increase dose after 2 mo by 0.5 mg/kg/day and then q4wk, max 2.5 mg/kg/day

Lupus nephritis/SLE/Wegener's granulomatosis/idiopathic pulmonary fibrosis (unlabeled)

- **Adult: PO** 2-3 mg/kg/day

Atopic dermatitis (unlabeled)

- **Adult/adolescent ≥16 yr: PO** 2.5 mg/kg/day

Available forms: Tabs 50, 75, 100 mg; inj 100 mg

Administer:

- For several days before transplant surgery
- All medications PO if possible; avoid IM inj because bleeding may occur

PO route

- With meals to reduce GI upset

IV route

- Prepare in biologic cabinet with gown, gloves, mask

Direct IV

- **Dilute** to 10 mg/ml with 0.9% NaCl, 0.45% NaCl, D_5W, **give** over 5 min

Intermittent IV INF route

- **Reconstitute** 100 mg/10 ml of sterile water for inj; rotate to dissolve; **further dilute** with 50 ml or more saline or glucose in saline, **give** over ½-1 hr

Y-site compatibilities: Alfentanil, atracurium, atropine, benztropine, calcium gluconate, cycloSPORINE, enalaprilat, epoetin alfa, erythromycin, fentaNYL, fluconazole, folic acid, furosemide, glycopyrrolate, heparin, insulin, mannitol, mechlorethamine, metoprolol, naloxone, nitroglycerin, oxytocin, penicillin G, potassium chloride, propranolol, protamine, SUFentanil, trimetaphan, vasopressin

Solution compatibilities: D_5W, NaCl 0.9%, NaCl 0.45%

SIDE EFFECTS

GI: *Nausea, vomiting,* stomatitis, esophagitis, pancreatitis, hepatotoxicity, jaundice

HEMA: Leukopenia, thrombocytopenia, anemia, pancytopenia, bleeding

INTEG: Rash, alopecia

MISC: Serum sickness, Raynaud's symptoms, secondary malignancy, infection

MS: Arthralgia, muscle wasting

PHARMACOKINETICS

Metabolized in liver, excreted in urine (active metabolite), crosses placenta, half-life 3 hr

INTERACTIONS

Increase: leukopenia—ACE inhibitors, sulfamethoxazole-trimethoprim

Increase: myelosuppression—cycloSPORINE, mercaptopurine

Increase: action of azaTHIOprine—allopurinol

Decrease: immune response—vaccines, toxoids

Decrease: action of warfarin—warfarin
• Do not admix with other products

Drug/Lab Test
Increase: LFTs
Decrease: uric acid
Interference: CBC, differential count

NURSING CONSIDERATIONS

Assess:

• **For infection:** increased temp, WBC; sputum, urine
• I&O, weight daily, report decreasing urine output; toxicity may occur

Black Box Warning: Bone marrow suppression: severe leukopenia, pancytopenia, thrombocytopenia; Hgb, WBC, platelets during treatment monthly; if leukocytes are <3000/mm³ or platelets <100,000/mm³, product should be discontinued

⚠ **Hepatotoxicity:** if dark urine, jaundice, itching, light-colored stools, increased LFTs, product should be discontinued; hepatic studies: alk phos, AST, ALT, bilirubin
• **Arthritis:** pain, ROM, swelling, mobility before, during treatment

Evaluate:

• Therapeutic response: absence of graft rejection, immunosuppression in autoimmune disorders

Teach patient/family:

• To take as prescribed; not to miss doses; if dose is missed on daily regimen, to skip dose; if taking multiple doses/day, to take as soon as remembered
• That therapeutic response may take 3-4 mo with RA; to continue with prescribed exercise, rest, other medications
• To report fever, rash, severe diarrhea, chills, sore throat, fatigue because **serious infections** may occur; report unusual bleeding, bruising; signs/symptoms of **renal/hepatic toxicity**
• To use contraceptive measures during treatment, for 16 wk after ending therapy (pregnancy [D]); to avoid vaccinations
• To avoid crowds to reduce risk for infection
• To use soft-bristled toothbrush to prevent bleeding
• That treatment is ongoing to prevent transplant rejection

azelaic acid topical

See Appendix B

azelastine nasal agent

See Appendix B

azelastine ophthalmic

See Appendix B

azilsartan

See Appendix A—Selected new drugs

azithromycin (Rx)

(ay-zi-thro-my′sin)

CO Azithromycin ✤, ratio-Azithromycin ✤, Sandoz Azithromycin ✤, Zithromax, Zmax, Zithromax Tri Pak, Zithromax Z Pak

Func. class.: Antiinfective
Chem. class.: Macrolide (azalide)

Do not confuse:
azithromycin/erythromycin
Zithromax/Zinacef

ACTION: Binds to 50S ribosomal subunits of susceptible bacteria and suppresses protein synthesis; much greater spectrum of activity than erythromycin; more effective against gram-negative organisms

USES: Mild to moderate infections of the upper respiratory tract, lower respiratory tract; uncomplicated skin and skin structure infections caused by *Moraxella catarrhalis, Streptococcus pneumoniae, Streptococcus pyogenes, Staphylococcus aureus, Streptococcus agalactiae, Mycoplasma pneumoniae, Haemophilus influenzae, Clostridium, Legionella pneumophila;* NGU or cervicitis due to *Chlamydia trachomatis;* in children: acute otitis media *(H. influenzae, M. catarrhalis, S. pneumoniae)* **PO;** acute pharyngitis/tonsillitis (group A streptococcal) **PO;** acute skin/soft tissue infections **PO;** community-acquired pneumonia *(Chlamydia pneumoniae, H. influenzae, M. pneumoniae, S. pneumoniae)* **PO;** pharyngitis/tonsillitis *(S. pyogenes);* prophylaxis of disseminated *Mycobacterium avium* complex (MAC)

Unlabeled uses: Babesiosis, cholera, cystic fibrosis, dental abscess/infection, endocarditis prophylaxis, granuloma inguinale, *Helicobacter pylori, Klebsiella granulomatis,* Legionnaire's disease, Lyme disease, lymphogranuloma venereum, MAC, *Mycoplasma hominis,* periodontitis, pertussis, prostatitis, *Rickettsia tsutsugamushi, Salmonella typhi,* shigellosis, syphilis, toxoplasmosis, typhoid fever

CONTRAINDICATIONS:

Hypersensitivity to azithromycin, erythromycin, any macrolide

Precautions: Pregnancy (B), breastfeeding; geriatric patients; renal/hepatic/cardiac disease; <6 mo for otitis media; <2 yr for pharyngitis, tonsillitis

DOSAGE AND ROUTES

Most infections

• **Adult: PO** 500 mg on day 1 then 250 mg/day on days 2-5 for a total dose of 1.5 g

• **Child 2-15 yr: PO** 10 mg/kg on day 1 then 5 mg/kg × 4 days

Disseminated MAC infections

• **Adult: PO** 600 mg/day with ethambutol 15 mg/kg/day

Pelvic inflammatory disease

• **Adult: PO/IV** 500 mg **IV** q24hr × 2 doses then 500 mg **PO** q24hr × 7-10 days

Cervicitis, chlamydia, chancroid, nongonococcal urethritis, syphilis

• **Adult: PO** 1 g single dose

Gonorrhea

• **Adult: PO** 2 g single dose

Lower respiratory tract infections

• **Adult: PO** 500 mg day 1, then 250 mg × 4 days

• **Child: PO** 5-12 mg/kg/day × 5 days

Acute otitis media

• **Child >6 mo: PO** 30 mg/kg as a single dose or 10 mg/kg/day × 3 days or 10 mg/kg as a single dose on day 1 (max 500 mg/day) then 5 mg/kg on days 2-5 (max 250 mg/day)

Prevention of acute otitis media

• **Child: PO** 10 mg/kg q wk × 6 mo

Legionnaire's disease/early Lyme disease (unlabeled)

• **Adult: PO** 500 mg/day

Pertussis (unlabeled)

• **Adult: PO** 500 mg on day 1 then 250 mg/day for 2-5 days

• **Infant <6 mo: PO** 10 mg/kg/day × 5 days

Available forms: Tabs 250, 500, 600 mg; powder for inj 500 mg; susp 100, 200 mg/5 ml 1 g single-dose powder for susp; ext rel powder for susp 2 g

Administer:

PO route

• **Susp** 1 hr before meal or 2 hr after meal; reconstitute 1 g packet for susp with 60 ml water, mix, rinse glass with more water and have patient drink to consume all medication; packets not for pediatric use

Intermittent IV INF route

• **Reconstitute** 500 mg of product with 4.8 ml sterile water for inj (100 mg/ml); shake, **dilute** with 250 or 500 ml 0.9% NaCl, 0.45% NaCl, or LR to 1-2 mg/ml; diluted sol stable for 24 hr or 7 days if refrigerated

• **Give** 1 mg/ml sol over 3 hr or 2 mg/ml sol over 1 hr; never give IM or as bolus

Y-site compatibilities: Aminocaproic acid, amphotericin B liposome, anidulafungin, atenolol, bivalirudin, bleomycin, CARBOplatin, CISplatin, cytarabine, DAPTOmycin, dexmedetomidine, diphenhydrAMINE, docetaxcl, dolasetron, doripenem, doxacurium, droperidol, epirubicin, eptifibatide, ertapenem, fenoldopam, fluorouracil, IDArubicin, irinotecan, methochlorethamine, meperidine, nesiritide, octreotide, ondansetron, oxaliplatin, palonosetron, pamidronate, pantoprazole, pemetrexed, rocuronium, sodium acetate, tigecycline, tirofiban, TPN, vasopressin, vinCRIStine, voriconazole

SIDE EFFECTS

CNS: Dizziness, headache, vertigo, somnolence, myasthenia gravis
CV: Palpitations, chest pain
EENT: Hearing loss, tinnitus, loss of smell (anosmia)
GI: *Nausea, vomiting, diarrhea,* **hepatotoxicity,** abdominal pain, stomatitis, heartburn, dyspepsia, flatulence, melena, **cholestatic jaundice, pseudomembranous colitis,** tongue discoloration
GU: Vaginitis, moniliasis, nephritis
HEMA: Anemia
INTEG: Rash, urticaria, pruritus, photosensitivity
SYST: **Angioedema, Stevens-Johnson syndrome, toxic epidermal necrolysis**

PHARMACOKINETICS

PO: Peak 2-4 hr, duration 24 hr
IV: Peak end of inf; duration 24 hr; half-life 11-57 hr; excreted in bile, feces, urine primarily as unchanged product; may be inhibitor of P-glycoprotein

INTERACTIONS

Increase: toxicity—ergotamine
⚠ **Increase: Dysrhythmias—pimozide: fatal reaction**
Increase: effects of oral anticoagulants, digoxin, theophylline, methylPREDNISolone, cycloSPORINE, bromocriptine, disopyramide, triazolam, carBAMazepine, phenytoin, tacrolimus, nelfinavir
Decrease: clearance of triazolam
Decrease: absorption of azithromycin—aluminum, magnesium antacids

Drug/Lab Test
Increase: CPK, ALT, AST, bilirubin, BUN, creatinine, alk phos

NURSING CONSIDERATIONS

Assess:

- I&O ratio; report hematuria, oliguria with renal disease
- Hepatic studies: AST, ALT, CBC with differential
- Renal studies: urinalysis, protein, blood
- C&S before product therapy; product may be taken as soon as culture is taken; C&S may be repeated after treatment
- **Serious skin reactions: Stevens-Johnson syndrome, toxic epidermal necrolysis, angioedema; discontinue if rash develops, treat symptomatically**
- **Superinfection: sore throat, mouth, tongue; fever, fatigue, diarrhea, anogenital pruritus**
- **Pseudomembranous colitis: diarrhea, abdominal pain, fever, fatigue, anorexia; obtain CBC, serum albumin**
- Bowel pattern before, during treatment
- Respiratory status: rate, character; wheezing, tightness in chest: discontinue product

Perform/provide:

- Storage at room temperature

Evaluate:

- Therapeutic response: C&S negative for infection; decreased signs of infection

Teach patient/family:

⚠ **To report sore throat, fever, fatigue, severe diarrhea, anal/genital itching (may indicate superinfection)**

- Not to take aluminum-magnesium–containing antacids simultaneously with this product (PO)

⚠ To notify nurse of diarrhea, dark urine, pale stools; yellow discoloration of eyes, skin; severe abdominal pain
- To complete dosage regimen

TREATMENT OF HYPERSENSITIVITY: Withdraw product, maintain airway; administer EPINEPHrine, aminophylline, O_2, IV corticoster oids

azithromycin ophthalmic

See Appendix B

RARELY USED

aztreonam (Rx)

(az-tree′oh-nam)

Azactam, Cayston

Func. class.: Antibiotic—miscellaneous

USES: Urinary tract infection; septicemia; skin, muscle, bone infection; lower respiratory tract, intraabdominal infections; other infections caused by gram-negative organisms

CONTRAINDICATIONS: Hypersensitivity to product, penicillins, cephalosporins, severe renal disease

DOSAGE AND ROUTES

Urinary tract infections
- **Adult: IM/IV** 500 mg-1 g q8-12hr

Systemic infections
- **Adult: IM/IV** 1-2 g q8-12hr
- **Child: IM/IV** 90-120 mg/kg/day in divided doses q6-8hr; max 8 g/day **IV**

Severe systemic infections
- **Adult: IM/IV** 2 g q6-8hr; max 8 g/day; continue treatment for 48 hr after negative culture or until patient is asymptomatic

Cystic fibrosis with *Pseudomonas aeruginosa*
- **Adult, adolescent, child ≥7 yr: NEB** 75 mg tid × 28 days, then 28 days off; give q4hr or more; give bronchodilator before aztreonam

bacitracin topical

See Appendix B

baclofen (Rx)

(bak′loe-fen)

Apo-Baclofen ✤, Gen-Baclofen ✤, Lioresal, PMS-Baclofen ✤, ratio-Baclofen ✤

Func. class.: Skeletal muscle relaxant, central acting

Chem. class.: GABA chlorophenyl derivative

Do not confuse:
Lioresal/Lotensin

ACTION: Inhibits synaptic responses in CNS by stimulating GABAb receptor subtype, which decreases neurotransmitter function; decreases frequency, severity of muscle spasms

USES: Spasticity with spinal cord injury, multiple sclerosis

Unlabeled uses: Neuropathic pain, hiccups, trigeminal neuralgia/nystagmus, recurrent priapism

CONTRAINDICATIONS: Hypersensitivity

Precautions: Pregnancy (C), breastfeeding, geriatric patients, peptic ulcer disease, renal/hepatic disease, stroke, seizure disorder, diabetes mellitus

Black Box Warning: Abrupt discontinuation

DOSAGE AND ROUTES

- **Adult: PO** 5 mg tid × 3 days, then 10 mg tid × 3 days, then 15 mg tid × 3 days, then 20 mg tid × 3 days, then titrated to response, max 80 mg/day; **INTRATHECAL** use implantable intrathecal inf pump, use screening trial of 3 separate bol doses if needed 24 hr apart (50 mcg, 75 mcg, 100 mcg); patients who do not respond to 100 mcg should not be considered for chronic IT therapy; initial: double screening dose that produced result, give over 24 hr, increase by 10%-30% q24hr only; maintenance: 1200-1500 mcg/day

- **Child >2-7 yr: PO** 10-15 mg/day divided q8hr; titrate q3days by 5-15 mg/day to max 40 mg/day
- **Child ≥8 yr:** As above; max 60 mg/day
- **Child: INTRATHECAL** initial test dose same as adult; for small children, initial dose of 25 mcg/dose may be used; 25-1200 mcg/day inf titrated to response in screening phase
- **Geriatric: PO** 5 mg bid-tid

Neuropathic pain including trigeminal neuralgia (unlabeled)

- **Adult: PO** 10 mg tid, may increase by 10 mg every other day; max 80 mg/day

Hiccups (unlabeled)

- **Adult: PO** 10 mg qid

Recurrent priapism (unlabeled)

- **Adult: PO** 40 mg at bedtime

Available forms: Tabs 10, 20 mg; intrathecal inj 10 mg/20 ml (500 mcg/ml), 10 mg/5 ml (2000 mcg/ml); pharmacy can prepare extemperaneous liquid preparations

Administer:

PO route

- With meals for GI symptoms

IT route

- **For screening,** dilute to a concentration of 50 mcg/ml with NaCl for inj (preservative free), give test dose over 1 min; watch for decreasing muscle tone, frequency of spasm; if inadequate, use 2 more test doses q24hr; **maintenance inf** via implantable pump of 500-2000 mcg/ml because individual titration is required
- Do not give IT dose by inj, IV, IM, SUBCUT, epidural

Additive compatibilities: Clonidine, morphine, ziconotide

SIDE EFFECTS

CNS: *Dizziness, weakness, fatigue, drowsiness,* headache, *disorientation,* insomnia, paresthesias, tremors; **seizures, life-threatening CNS depression, coma; CNS infection** (IT)

CV: Hypotension, chest pain, palpitations, edema; **cardiovascular collapse (IT)**

EENT: Nasal congestion, blurred vision, mydriasis, tinnitus

GI: *Nausea,* constipation, *vomiting,* increased AST, alk phos, abdominal pain, dry mouth, anorexia

GU: Urinary frequency, hematuria

INTEG: Rash, pruritus

RESP: Dyspnea; respiratory failure (IT)

PHARMACOKINETICS

PO: Onset 3-4 days, peak 2-3 hr, duration >8 hr, half-life $2^1/_2$-4 hr, partially metabolized in liver, excreted in urine (unchanged)

INTRATHECAL: CSF levels with plasma levels 100 times that of the oral route, peak 4 hr, duration 4-8 hr

BOLUS: Onset $^1/_2$-1 hr

CONT INF: Onset 6-8 hr, peak 24-48 hr

INTERACTIONS

Increase: CNS depression—alcohol, tricyclics, opiates, barbiturates, sedatives, hypnotics, MAOIs

Increase: hypotension—antihypertensives

Drug/Herb

Increase: CNS depression—kava, valerian

Drug/Lab Test

Increase: AST, alk phos, blood glucose

NURSING CONSIDERATIONS

Assess:

- **Multiple sclerosis:** spasms, spasticity, ataxia; improvement should occur with product
- B/P, weight, blood glucose, hepatic function periodically

⚠ **Seizures:** for increased seizure activity with seizure disorders; product decreases seizure threshold; EEG in epileptic patients

- I&O ratio; check for urinary frequency
- Allergic reactions: rash, fever, respiratory distress
- Severe weakness, numbness in extremities
- Tolerance: increased need for medication, more frequent requests for medication, increased pain
- **Withdrawal symptoms:** CNS depression, dizziness, drowsiness, psychiatric symptoms
- **Intrathecal:** have emergency equipment nearby; assess test dose and titration; if no response, check pump, catheter for proper functioning

Perform/provide:

- Storage in tight container at room temperature
- Assistance with ambulation if dizziness, drowsiness occurs

Evaluate:

- Therapeutic response: decreased pain, spasticity

Teach patient/family:

- Not to discontinue medication quickly; hallucinations, spasticity, tachycardia will occur; product should be tapered off over 1-2 wk
- Not to take with alcohol, other CNS depressants
- To avoid hazardous activities if drowsiness, dizziness occurs; to rise slowly to prevent orthostatic hypotension
- To avoid using OTC medications; not to take cough preparations, antihistamines unless directed by prescriber
- To notify prescriber if nausea; headache; tinnitus; insomnia; confusion; constipation; inadequate, painful urination continues
- **MS:** may require 1-2 mo for full response

TREATMENT OF OVERDOSE:

Induce emesis of conscious patient, activated charcoal, dialysis, physostigmine to reduce life-threatening CNS side effects

balsalazide (Rx)

(ball-sal′a-zide)

Colazal

Func. class.: GI antiinflammatory
Chem. class.: Salicylate derivative

Do not confuse:
Colazal/Clozaril

ACTION:

Delivered intact to the colon, bioconverted to 5-ASA, may block production of arachidonic acid metabolites in the colon, topical rather than systemic action

USES:

Active, mild to moderate ulcerative colitis in adults and children

CONTRAINDICATIONS:

Hypersensitivity to salicylates/5-aminosalicylates

Precautions: Pregnancy (B), breastfeeding, children <5 yr, pyloric stenosis, renal disease, colitis, hepatitis

DOSAGE AND ROUTES

- **Adult: PO** 2250 mg (three 750-mg caps) tid × 8-12 wk, max 6.75 g/day
- **Adolescent/child 5-12 yr: PO** 2250 mg (three 750-mg caps) tid × 8 wk

Available forms: Caps 750 mg

Administer:

- Whole; do not crush, chew tabs; cap can be opened, contents sprinkled on applesauce
- With food in evenly divided doses
- With resuscitative equipment available; severe allergic reactions may occur
- Total daily dose evenly spaced throughout the day to minimize GI intolerance

SIDE EFFECTS

CNS: Headache, insomnia, fatigue, fever, dizziness

EENT: Dry eyes, rhinitis, sinusitis, blurred vision

GI: Nausea, vomiting, abdominal pain, diarrhea, anorexia, constipation, dyspep-

sia, flatulence, **GI bleeding, hepatic failure/necrosis, hepatitis**
MS: Arthralgia, back pain, myalgia
RESP: Cough, pharyngitis
SYST: Anaphylaxis

PHARMACOKINETICS

Low and variably absorbed, peak $1^1/_2$ hr, excreted in feces as metabolites, protein binding 99%, metabolized to mesalamine

INTERACTIONS

Increase: myelosuppression—mercaptopurine
Increase: effect—warfarin, azathioprine
Decrease: effect—thioguanine
• Avoid use of live varicella virus vaccine
Drug/Lab Test
Increase: AST, ALT, GGT, LDH, bilirubin, alk phos
False positive: urinary glucose test

NURSING CONSIDERATIONS

Assess:
• Renal studies: BUN, creatinine, urinalysis (long-term therapy)
• Allergic reaction: rash, dermatitis, urticaria, pruritus, dyspnea, bronchospasm
• Myelosuppression: CBC
Perform/provide:
• Storage in tight, light-resistant container at room temp
Evaluate:
• Therapeutic response: absence of fever, mucus in stools; resolution of symptoms of ulcerative colitis
Teach patient/family:
• To notify prescriber if symptoms do not improve; if colitis symptoms worsen; if rash, hives, respiratory problems occur

⚠ HIGH ALERT

basiliximab (Rx)

(bas-ih-liks′ih-mab)
Simulect
Func. class.: Immunosuppressant
Chem. class.: Murine/human monoclonal antibody (interleukin-2) receptor antagonist

ACTION: Binds to and blocks the IL-2 receptor, which is selectively expressed on the surface of activated T lymphocytes; impairs the immune system to antigenic challenges

USES: Acute allograft rejection in renal transplant patients when used with cycloSPORINE and corticosteroids
Unlabeled uses: Liver transplant rejection prophylaxis, graft-versus-host disease

CONTRAINDICATIONS: Breastfeeding, hypersensitivity to mannitol/murine, exposure to viral infections
Precautions: Pregnancy (B), children, geriatric patients, human anti-murine antibody

Black Box Warning: Infections

DOSAGE AND ROUTES

• **Adult/child ≥35 kg: IV** 20 mg × 2 doses; 1st dose within 2 hr before transplant surgery; 2nd dose 4 days after transplantation
• **Child/adolescent <35 kg: IV** 10 mg × 2 doses; 1st dose within 2 hr before transplant surgery; 2nd dose 4 days after transplantation
Available forms: Powder for inj 10, 20 mg
Administer:
Intermittent IV INF route
• **Reconstitute** 10 mg vial/2.5 ml or 20-mg vial in 5 ml sterile water for inj; shake gently to dissolve, **dilute** reconstituted sol in 25 ml (10 mg vial) or 50 ml

(20-mg vial) with 0.9% NaCl or D_5, gently invert bag, do not shake; **give** over ½ hr, do not admix

SIDE EFFECTS

CNS: *Pyrexia, chills, tremors, headache, insomnia, weakness, dizziness*
CV: *Chest pain,* angina, cardiac failure, hypotension, *hypertension, edema*
GI: *Vomiting, nausea, diarrhea, constipation, abdominal pain,* GI bleeding, *gingival hyperplasia, stomatitis*
INTEG: *Acne,* pruritus, impaired wound healing
META: *Acidosis, hypercholesterolemia, hyperuricemia, hypo/hyperkalemia, hypocalcemia, hypophosphatemia*
MISC: *Infection, moniliasis,* anaphylaxis, anemia, allergic reaction, dysuria, CMV infection, candidiasis
MS: *Arthralgia, myalgia*
RESP: *Dyspnea, wheezing,* pulmonary edema, *cough*

PHARMACOKINETICS

Peak ½ hr (adults); terminal half-life 7 days (adult), 9½ days (children)

INTERACTIONS

Increase: immunosuppression—other immunosuppressants
Drug/Herb
Decrease: St. John's wort, turmeric
Drug/Lab Test
Increase: cholesterol, BUN, uric acid, creatinine, K, Ca, blood glucose, Hgb, Hct
Decrease: Hgb, Hct, platelets, magnesium, phosphate

NURSING CONSIDERATIONS

Assess:

Black Box Warning: For infection: increased temp, WBC, sputum, urine; may be fatal (bacterial, protozoal, fungal)

- Blood studies: Hgb, WBC, platelets during treatment q mo; if leukocytes are <3000/mm³, product should be discontinued; electrolytes, B/P, edema assessment
- Hepatic studies: alk phos, AST, ALT, bilirubin

⚠ **Anaphylaxis, hypersensitivity:** dyspnea, wheezing, rash, pruritus, hypotension, tachycardia; if severe hypersensitivity reactions occur, product should not be used again

Perform/provide:
- Storage of reconstituted sol refrigerated for up to 24 hr or at room temp for 4 hr

Evaluate:
- Therapeutic response: absence of graft rejection

Teach patient/family:

Black Box Warning: To report fever, chills, sore throat, fatigue, serious infection may occur

- To avoid crowds, persons with known upper respiratory tract infections
- To use contraception during treatment
- To report GI symptoms, bleeding, allergic reactions

beclomethasone (Rx)

(be-kloe-meth′a-sone)

Apo-Beclomethasone ✦, QVAR

Func. class.: Corticosteroid, synthetic
Chem. class.: Glucocorticoid

Do not confuse:
beclomethasone/betamethasone

ACTION: Prevents inflammation by suppression of the migration of polymorphonuclear leukocytes, fibroblasts and the reversal of increased capillary permeability and lysosomal stabilization; does not suppress hypothalamus and pituitary function

USES: Chronic asthma, allergic/vasomotor rhinitis, nasal polyps

CONTRAINDICATIONS: Hypersensitivity, status asthmaticus (primary treatment)
Precautions: Pregnancy (C), breastfeeding, children <12 yr, nasal disease/

surgery, nonasthmatic bronchial disease; bacterial, fungal, viral infections of mouth, throat, lungs; HPA suppression, osteoporosis, Cushing's syndrome, diabetes mellitus, measles, cataracts, corticosteroid hypersensitivity, glaucoma, herpes infection

DOSAGE AND ROUTES

- **Adult and child >12 yr: ORAL INH** 40-80 mcg bid (alone) or 40-160 mcg bid (previous inhaled corticosteroids); max 320 mcg bid
- **Child 5-12 yr: ORAL INH** 40 mcg bid; max 80 mcg bid

Available forms: Oral inh 40, 80, 250 ♣mcg/metered spray

Administer:

- Bronchodilator spray; if used, should be used 1st, then wait a few minutes, then use this product
- Prime before 1st use or if not used for 7-10 days; prime by spraying 2 actuations into the air, away from the face; do not share inhaler
- **Oral inhalation** (metered-dose non-CFC aerosol) (QVAR); shake well, use spacer; after using, rinse mouth, gargle if possible; clean weekly with dry cloth/tissue, do not wash inhaler
- Titrated dose, use lowest effective dose

SIDE EFFECTS

CNS: *Headache*

EENT: *Hoarseness, candidal infection of oral cavity, sore throat,* loss of taste/smell, dysgeusia

ENDO: Hypothalmic-pituitary (HPA) suppression

GI: Dry mouth, dyspepsia

MISC: Angioedema, adrenal insufficiency, facial edema, Churg-Strauss syndrome (rare)

RESP: Bronchospasm, wheezing, cough

PHARMACOKINETICS

INH: Onset 1-4 wk; excreted in feces, urine (metabolites); half-life 2.8 hr; crosses placenta; metabolized in lungs, liver (by CYP3A)

NURSING CONSIDERATIONS

Assess:

- For fungal infection in mucous membranes
- Adrenal function periodically for HPA axis suppression during prolonged therapy, monitor growth/development

Perform/provide:

- Gum, rinsing of mouth for dry mouth

Evaluate:

- Therapeutic response: decreased dyspnea, wheezing, dry crackles

Teach patient/family:

- To gargle/rinse mouth after each use to prevent oral fungal infections
- That, during times of stress, systemic corticosteroids may be needed to prevent adrenal insufficiency; not to discontinue oral product abruptly, to taper slowly
- To notify prescriber if therapeutic response decreases; dosage adjustment may be needed
- Proper administration technique and cleaning technique
- About all aspects of product usage, including cushingoid symptoms
- About **adrenal insufficiency symptoms:** nausea, anorexia, fatigue, dizziness, dyspnea, weakness, joint pain, depression

beclomethasone nasal agent

See Appendix B

belatacept

(bel-a-ta′sept)

Nulojix

Func. class.: Biologic response modifier

Chem. class.: Fusion protein

ACTION:

Activated T lymphocytes are the mediators of immunologic rejection, this product is a selective T-cell costimulation blocker; blocks the CD28 mediated costimulation of T lymphocytes by binding to CD80 and CD86 on antigen-presenting cells; inhibits T lymphocyte proliferation and the production of the cytokines interleukin-2, interferon-gamma, interleukin-4, and TNF-alpha.

USES:
Kidney transplant rejection prophylaxis given with basiliximab induction, mycophenolate mofetil, corticosteroids

CONTRAINDICATIONS:
Hypersensitivity

Precautions: Breastfeeding, child/infant/neonate, pregnancy (C), diabetes mellitus, progressive multifocal leukoencephalopathy, immunosuppression, sunlight exposure, TB

Black Box Warning: Infection, organ transplant, requires an experienced clinician, secondary malignancy, post-transplant lymphoproliferation disorder (PTLD)

DOSAGE AND ROUTES

• **Adult: IV** 10 mg/kg rounded to the nearest 12.5 mg increment; give over 30 min the day of transplantation (day 1) but before transplantation, on day 5 approximately 96 hours after the day 1 dose 1, at the end of wk 2, at the end of wk 4, at the end of wk 8, and at the end of wk 12; maintenance dosage is 5 mg/kg rounded to the nearest 12.5 mg increment; give over 30 min at the end of wk 16 and every 4 wk +/- 3 days thereafter; doses should be calculated on actual body weight on the transplantation day unless the patient's weight varies by >10%

Available forms: Powder for inj 250 mg

Administer:

Black Box Warning: Only providers skilled in the use of immunosuppressant and management of transplant should use these products

IV route

• Visually inspect product for particulate matter, discoloration whenever sol/container permit, discard if present

• Calculate the number of drug vials required to provide total inf dose

• Reconstitute each vial/10.5 ml of sterile water for injection, 0.9% sodium chloride, D_5W, using the silicone-free disposable syringe provided with each vial and an 18 to 21G needle. If silicone-free disposable syringe is dropped or becomes contaminated, use a new silicone-free disposable syringe from inventory. If you need additional silicone-free disposable syringes, call 1-888-685-6549. If the powder is accidentally reconstituted using a different syringe than the one provided, the sol may develop a few translucent particles. Discard any sol prepared using siliconized syringes.

• Using aseptic technique, inject the diluent into the vial and direct the stream of diluent to the glass wall of the vial; to minimize foaming, rotate the vial and invert with gentle swirling until the contents are dissolved; do not shake when reconstituted (25 mg/ml), should be clear to slightly opalescent and colorless to pale yellow; do not use if opaque particles, discoloration, or other foreign particles are present.

• Calculate the total volume of the reconstituted 25 mg/ml sol required to provide the total inf dose; further dilute this volume with a volume of inf fluid equal to the volume of the reconstituted drug sol required to provide the prescribed dose. Use either NS or D_5W if drug was reconstituted with SWFI; use NS if drug was reconstituted with NS; use D_5W if drug was reconstituted with D_5W. With the same silicone-free disposable syringe used for reconstitution, withdraw the required amount of belatacept sol from the vial, inject it into the inf container, gently rotate the inf container to ensure mixing; final conc in inf container should range (2-10 mg/ml). Volume of 100 ml will be appropriate for most patients and doses, but total inf volumes ranging from 50-250 ml may be used. Discard any unused drug sol remaining in the vials; after reconstitution, immediately transfer the reconstituted sol from the vial to the inf bag or bottle; complete within 24 hr.

IV INF route

• Give over 30 min, use an inf set and a sterile, nonpyrogenic, low-protein-binding filter (0.2-1.2 mm), use a separate line

SIDE EFFECTS

CNS: Guillain-Barré syndrome, anxiety, dizziness, headache, fever, insomnia, tremor

EENT: Pharyngitis, stomatitis

GI: Abdominal pain, constipation, diarrhea, nausea, vomiting

GU: **Renal tubular necrosis, renal failure,** proteinuria, urinary incontinence

HEMA: Anemia, neutropenia, leucopenia, leukoencephalopathy

INTEG: Acne, alopecia

META: Hypercholesterolemia, hyperglycemia, hyper/hypokalemia, hypocalcemia, hypophosphatemia, hypomagnesemia

MS: Arthralgia

SYST: **Secondary malignancy, post-transplant lymphoproliferation disorder (PTLD), wound dehiscence, BK-virus associated neuropathy**

PHARMACOKINETICS

Half-life, 6.1-15.1 days during receipt of 10 mg/kg IV doses; during receipt of 5 mg/kg IV doses, terminal half-life 3.1-11.9; steady-state by wk 8 after transplantation and by month 6 during maintenance phase

INTERACTIONS

Increase: Basiliximab induction, mycophenolate mofetil

NURSING CONSIDERATIONS

Assess:

Black Box Warning: Transplant rejection: flu-like symptoms, decreasing urinary output, malaise; some may experience pain in area (rare; monitor BUN/creatinine)

Black Box Warning: Infection: monitor for fever, chills, increased WBC, **wound dehiscences**

Black Box Warning: Post-transplant lymphoproliferation disorder (PTLD): may lead to secondary malignancy (lymphoma) or infectious mononucleosis-like lesions; may be treated with antivirals or immunosuppressant; product may need to be discontinued

• Hyperlipidemia: monitor cholesterol, triglycerides; an anti-lipidemic may be needed

Perform/provide:

• Storage: refrigerated, protected from light ≤24 hr; max 4 hr of the total 24 hr can be at room temp and room light

Evaluate:

• Therapeutic response: Absence of renal transplant rejection

Teach patient/family:

• Reason for product and expected result

• To avoid exposure to sunlight, tanning beds, risk of secondary malignancy

• To avoid crowds, persons with known infections

• That repeated lab test will be needed

• To avoid with vaccines

• That immunosuppressants will be needed for life to prevent rejection; teach symptoms of rejection and to call provider immediately

belimumab

(be-lim′ue-mab)

Benlysta

Func. class.: Monoclonal antibody

Chem. class.: Disease-Modifying Antirheumatic Drugs (DMARDs)

ACTION:

Inhibits B lymphocyte stimulator (BLyS), which is needed for B-cell survival; normally, soluble BLyS binds to its receptors on B cells and allows B cell survival; binds BLyS and prevents binding to its receptors on B cells

USES:
Active, autoantibody-positive, systemic lupus erythematosus (SLE) in combination with standard therapy

CONTRAINDICATIONS:
Hypersensitivity

Precautions: Pregnancy (C), breastfeeding, children/infants, geriatric patients, African decent patients, depression, immunosuppression, infection, suicidal ideation, vaccination, secondary malignancy, cardiac disease; requires experienced clinician

DOSAGE AND ROUTES

- **Adult: IV** 10 mg/kg over 1 hr q2wk for the first 3 doses then q4wk

Available forms: Powder for injection 120, 400 mg

Administer:

- Only healthcare providers prepared to manage anaphylaxis should administer this product; may give premedication for prophylaxis against infusion and hypersensitivity reactions

Intermittent IV INF route

- Visually inspect particulate matter and discoloration whenever sol and container permits
- Give as IV inf only, do not give IV bolus or push; give over 1 hr and slow or stop if inf reactions occur
- Do not give with any other agents in the same IV line
- Allow to stand at room temp for 10-15 min before using
- Reconstitute with the appropriate amount of sterile water for injection to a final conc 80 mg/ml; add 1.5 ml of sterile water per 120 mg vial or 4.8 ml of sterile water per 400 mg vial
- When reconstituting, direct the stream of sterile water toward the side of the vial to minimize foaming; gently swirl the vial for 60 sec, allow to sit at room temp during reconstitution, gently swirling the vial for 60 sec q5min until the powder is dissolved; do not shake; reconstitution is complete in 10 to 30 min
- If a mechanical reconstitution device (swirler) is used to reconstitute, max 500 rpm swirled for ≤30 min.
- Sol should be opalescent and colorless to pale yellow and without particles; small air bubbles are expected; protect from sunlight
- Dilution: only dilute in 0.9% sodium chloride injection; dilute reconstituted sol with enough 0.9% sodium chloride injection (normal saline) to a total volume of 250 ml. From a 250-ml inf bag or bottle of normal saline, withdraw and discard a volume equal to the volume of the reconstituted sol required for the patient's dose; add the required volume of the reconstituted sol the infusion bag/bottle; gently invert to mix the sol
- Discard any unused sol that remains in the vials

SIDE EFFECTS

CNS: Headache, dizziness, anxiety, depression, fever, insomnia, migraine, **suicidal ideation**

CV: Bradycardia, hypotension

GI: Nausea, diarrhea

MISC: Rash, dyspnea, cystitis, leukopenia, myalgia, rash, bronchitis, nasopharyngitis, pharyngitis

SYST: **Anaphylaxis, angioedema, antibody formation, secondary malignancy, infection, influenza**

PHARMACOKINETICS

Terminal half-life 19.4 days; distribution half-life 1.75 days

NURSING CONSIDERATIONS

Assess:

- **SLE:** monitor for decreasing fever, malaise, fatigue, joint pain, myalgias
- **Suicidal ideation:** more common in those with pre-existing depression
- **Infection:** determine if a chronic or acute infection is present, may be fatal when used with this product; do not begin therapy if any products are being used for a chronic infection; leucopenia

may occur with this product and susceptibility to infections increased
• **Anaphylaxis,** infusion site reactions: if these occur, stop infusion
• **African descent patients:** use cautiously in these patients, may not respond to this product
• Cardiac disease: monitor closely for cardiovascular side effects, bradycardia, hypotension
• Pregnancy: determine if pregnant or if pregnancy is planned or suspected

Perform/provide:
• Storage in refrigerator or at room temp; total time from reconstitution to completion of inf max 8 hr

Evaluate:
• Positive response: Decreasing symptoms of SLE: decreasing fatigue, fever, malaise

Teach patient/family:
• To notify prescriber if pregnancy is planned or suspected, to use reliable contraception during and for 4 months after final treatment; to avoid breastfeeding
• To seek treatment immediately for serious hypersensitive reactions
• Not to receive vaccinations during treatment

benazepril (Rx)

(ben-aze′uh-pril)

Lotensin

Func. class.: Antihypertensive

Chem. class.: Angiotensin-converting enzyme (ACE) inhibitor

ACTION:
Selectively suppresses renin-angiotensin-aldosterone system; inhibits ACE, thus preventing conversion of angiotensin I to angiotensin II

USES:
Hypertension, alone or in combination with thiazide diuretics

Unlabeled uses: CHF, diabetic nephropathy, proteinuria, renal impairment

CONTRAINDICATIONS:
Breastfeeding, children, hypersensitivity to ACE inhibitors, angioedema

Black Box Warning: Pregnancy (D)

Precautions: Geriatric patients, impaired renal/hepatic function, dialysis patients, hypovolemia, blood dyscrasias, CHF, COPD, asthma, bilateral renal artery stenosis

DOSAGE AND ROUTES
• **Adult: PO** 10 mg/day initially, then 20-40 mg/day divided bid or daily (without a diuretic); reduce initial dose to 5 mg **PO** daily (with a diuretic); max 80 mg/day
• **Geriatric: PO** used on the basis of the clinical response
• **Child ≥6 yrs: PO** 0.2 mg/kg/day max 5 mg/day

Renal dose
• **Adult: PO** CCr <30 ml/min 5 mg **PO** daily, max 40 mg/day

Renal impairment due to diabetic nephropathy (unlabeled)
• **Adult: PO** 10 mg/day

Heart failure (unlabeled)
• **Adult: PO** 2-20 mg/day

Available forms: Tabs 5, 10, 20, 40 mg

Administer:
• May give without regard to food
• Do not discontinue product abruptly

SIDE EFFECTS
CNS: Anxiety, hypertonia, insomnia, paresthesia, headache, dizziness, fatigue
CV: Hypotension, postural hypotension, syncope, palpitations, angina
GI: Nausea, constipation, vomiting, gastritis, melena, diarrhea
GU: Increased BUN, creatinine, decreased libido, impotence, UTI
HEMA: Agranulocytosis, neutropenia
INTEG: Rash, flushing, sweating
META: Hyperkalemia, hyponatremia
MISC: Angioedema
MS: Arthralgia, arthritis, myalgia
RESP: Cough, asthma, bronchitis, dyspnea, sinusitis

PHARMACOKINETICS

Peak 1-2 hr fasting, 2-4 hr after food; protein binding 89%-95%; half-life 10-11 hr; metabolized by liver (metabolites); excreted in urine 33%

INTERACTIONS

Increase: hypotension—phenothiazines, nitrates, acute alcohol ingestion, diuretics, other antihypertensives
Increase: hyperkalemia—potassium-sparing diuretics, potassium supplements
Increase: myelosuppression—azathioprine
Increase: serum levels of lithium, digoxin
Decrease: hypotensive effects—NSAIDs

Drug/Herb
Increase: antihypertensive effect—hawthorn

Drug/Lab Test
Increase: AST, ALT, alk phos, bilirubin, uric acid, blood glucose
Positive: ANA titer
False positive: ANA titer

NURSING CONSIDERATIONS

Assess:

- **Hypertension:** B/P, pulse at baseline, periodically; B/P at peak/trough level of product; orthostatic hypotension, syncope when used with diuretic; notify prescriber of changes; monitor compliance
- **Blood dyscrasias:** neutrophils, decreased platelets; WBC with differential at baseline, q3mo; if neutrophils <1000/mm³, discontinue treatment; recommended with collagen-vascular disease
- Renal studies: protein, BUN, creatinine; increased levels may indicate nephrotic syndrome; monitor urine for protein; LFTs, uric acid, glucose may be increased
- Potassium levels, although hyperkalemia rarely occurs
- Allergic reactions: rash, fever, pruritus, urticaria; product should be discontinued if antihistamines fail to help
- Renal symptoms: polyuria, oliguria, frequency, dysuria
- **CHF (unlabeled):** edema in feet, legs daily; weight daily

Perform/provide:

- Storage in tight container at 86° F (30° C) or less

Evaluate:

- Therapeutic response: decrease in B/P

Teach patient/family:

- Not to use OTC products (cough, cold, allergy) unless directed by prescriber; not to use salt substitutes that contain potassium without consulting prescriber
- The importance of complying with dosage schedule, even if feeling better

Black Box Warning: To notify prescriber of pregnancy (D); product will need to be discontinued

- To rise slowly to sitting or standing position to minimize orthostatic hypotension
- To notify prescriber of mouth sores, sore throat, fever, swelling of hands or feet, irregular heartbeat, chest pain
- To report excessive perspiration, dehydration, vomiting, diarrhea; may lead to fall in B/P
- That product may cause dizziness, fainting, lightheadedness; that this may occur during first few days of therapy
- That product may cause skin rash or impaired perspiration
- How to take B/P, and normal readings for age-group

TREATMENT OF OVERDOSE:

0.9% NaCl IV INF, hemodialysis

HIGH ALERT

bendamustine (Rx)

(ben-da-muss′teen)

Treanda

Func. class.: Antineoplastic alkylating agent
Chem. class.: Mechlorethamine derivative

ACTION: Cross-linking DNA that causes single strand and double strand breaks, inhibits several mitotic checkpoints, combines alkylating and antimetabolite properties

USES:
Chronic lymphocytic leukemia, non-Hodgkin's lymphoma

Unlabeled uses: Mantle cell lymphoma (MCL)

CONTRAINDICATIONS:
Pregnancy (D), fetal harm may occur; breastfeeding, children, hepatic disease, renal impairment, hypersensitivity to product or mannitol

Precautions: Hyperuricemia, infusion-related reactions, myelosuppression, infection, skin reactions

DOSAGE AND ROUTES

Chronic lymphocytic leukemia

- **Adult: IV INF** 100 mg/m^2 over 30 min on days 1, 2 q28days up to 6 cycles

Non-Hodgkin's lymphoma

- *Adult:* **IV INF** 120 mg/m^2 over 60 min on days 1, 2 q21days up to 8 cycles

Mantle cell lymphoma (unlabeled)

- **Adult: IV INF** 90 mg/m^2 on days 1, 2 with rituximab on day 1 q28days for 6 cycles

Renal/hepatic dose

- **Adult: IV INF** CCr <40 ml/min, do not use; AST or ALT 2.5-10 × upper limit normal (ULN) or bilirubin 1.5-3 × ULN, do not use

Available forms: Powder for inj 25, 100 mg

Administer:

- Allopurinol to those at high risk for tumor lysis syndrome
- Blood transfusions, RBC colony-stimulating factors to counter anemia
- Antiemetic 30-60 min before giving product to prevent vomiting
- All medications PO; if possible, avoid IM inj if platelets are <100,000/mm^3

Intermittent IV INF route

- Prepare in biologic cabinet wearing gown, gloves, mask; avoid contact with skin, can cause burning, stain the skin brown; use cytotoxic handling procedures
- After **reconstituting** 100 mg product/20 ml or 25 mg/5 ml sterile water for inj (5 mg/ml), sol should be clear, colorless to pale yellow, completely dissolve in 5 min; if particulate is present, do not use
- Within 30 min of reconstitution, withdraw volume needed and **further dilute** in 500 ml NS or $D_{2.5}/_{0.45}$%NS to a final conc of 0.2-0.6 mg/ml; doses of ≤100 mg/m^2, **give** over 30 min; doses of >100 mg/m^2, **give** over 60 min
- Monitor for inf reactions; may use antihistamines or corticosteroids for grade 1, 2 reactions; if grade 3 or 4 occurs, discontinue if needed

SIDE EFFECTS

CNS: Asthenia, *fatigue,* fever, *headache,* chills, hypertension

CV: **Hypertension, hypertensive crisis**

GI: *Nausea, vomiting, diarrhea,* hyperbilirubinemia, *constipation,* stomatitis, *anorexia*

GU: **Renal failure**

HEMA: **Thrombocytopenia, leukopenia, anemia, lymphocytopenia, neutropenia, secondary malignancy, toxic epidermal necrolysis, tumor lysis syndrome**

INTEG: *Bulbous rash, pruritus,* extravasation

META: Hyperuricemia

SYST: **Anaphylaxis, infection, dehydration, severe skin toxicities, tumor lysis syndrome, Stevens-Johnson syndrome**

PHARMACOKINETICS

95% protein binding, metabolized by hydrolysis via CYP450 1A2, two metabolites are produced, half-life 40 min, 90% excreted unchanged (feces)

INTERACTIONS

Increase: agranulocytosis risk—clozapine (do not use concurrently)

Increase: bleeding risk—aspirin, anticoagulants, NSAIDs, platelet inhibitors, thrombolytics

Increase: myelosuppression—myelosuppressive agents

Increase: toxicity—other antineoplastics, radiation
Increase: adverse reactions, decreased antibody reaction—live vaccines
Increase: bendamustine—CYP1A2 inhibitors (atazanavir, cimetidine, ciprofloxacin, enoxacin, ethyl estradiol, fluvoxamine, mexiletine, norfloxacin, tacrine, thiabendazole, zileuton)
Decrease: bendamustine—CYP1A2 inducers (barbiturates, carbamazepine, rifampin)
Drug/Lab Test
Increase: LFTs

NURSING CONSIDERATIONS

Assess:

- **Blood dyscrasias:** CBC, differential, platelet count weekly; withhold product if WBC is <1000 or if platelet count is <75,000; notify prescriber of results
- Hepatic studies: AST, ALT, bilirubin
- Renal studies: BUN, serum uric acid, urine CCr before, during therapy; I&O ratio; report fall in urine output of 30 or 40 ml/hr; electrolytes
- Monitor for cold, cough, fever (may indicate beginning infection)
- For malignancy regression
- Bleeding: hematuria, guaiac, bruising, petechiae, mucosa, orifices q8hr
- **Serious skin toxicities:** toxic epidermal necrolysis, Stevens-Johnson syndrome; product should be discontinued
- **Tumor lysis syndrome:** monitor uric acid, potassium; may occur during 1st treatment cycle; use allopurinol for patients at high risk for this condition, usually during the 1st 2 wk; provide adequate hydration

Perform/provide:

- Storage of reconstituted sol in refrigerator for 24 hr or at room temp for 3 hr; protect from light; store vials at room temp

Evaluate:

- Therapeutic response: improvement in blood counts, morphology

Teach patient/family:

- To avoid hazardous activity that requires mental alertness
- To use contraception during therapy and for 3 mo after pregnancy (D)
- To avoid use of aspirin, ibuprofen, razors, commercial mouthwash
- To report signs of anemia (fatigue, irritability, SOB, faintness)
- To report signs of infection, myelosuppression, skin toxicities

benzocaine topical

See Appendix B

RARELY USED

benzonatate (Rx)

(ben-zoe′na-tate)

Tessalon Perles, Zonatuss

Func. class.: Antitussive, nonopioid

USES: Nonproductive cough

CONTRAINDICATIONS: Hypersensitivity

DOSAGE AND ROUTES

- **Adult and child: PO** 100 mg up to tid; max 600 mg/day

benztropine (Rx)

(benz′troe-peen)

Apo-Benztropine ♣, Cogentin

Func. class.: Cholinergic blocker, antiparkinson's agent
Chem. class.: Tertiary amine

ACTION: Blockade of central acetylcholine receptors

USES: Parkinson's symptoms, EPS associated with neuroleptic products, acute dystonic reactions, hypersalivation

B

CONTRAINDICATIONS:

Children <3 yr, hypersensitivity, closed-angle glaucoma, myasthenia gravis, GI/GU obstruction, peptic ulcer, megacolon, prostate hypertrophy, dementia, tardive dyskinesia

Precautions: Pregnancy (C), breastfeeding, children, geriatric patients, tachycardia, renal/hepatic disease, substance abuse history, dysrhythmias, hypo/hypertension, psychiatric patients

DOSAGE AND ROUTES

Drug-induced EPS

- **Adult: IM/IV/PO** 1-4 mg daily/bid; give **PO** dose as soon as possible
- **Child >3 yr: IM/IV/PO** 0.02-0.05 mg/kg/dose 1-2×/day
- **Geriatric: PO** 0.5 mg daily-bid, increase by 0.5 mg q5-6days; max 4 mg/day

Parkinson's symptoms

- **Adult: PO/IM** 0.5-1 mg at bedtime; increase by 0.5 mg q5-6days titrated to patient response, max 6 mg/day

Acute dystonic reactions

- **Adult: IM/IV** 1-2 mg, may increase to 1-2 mg bid **(PO)**

Available forms: Tabs 0.5, 1, 2 mg; inj 1 mg/ml

Administer:

PO route

- With or after meals to prevent GI upset; may give with fluids other than water
- At bedtime to avoid daytime drowsiness with parkinsonism

IM route

- Inject deeply in muscle

IV, direct route

- **Undiluted** IV (1 mg 5 1 ml): **give** 1 mg/1 min (rarely used)

Syringe compatibilities: Metoclopramide, perphenazine

Y-site compatibilities: Fluconazole, tacrolimus

SIDE EFFECTS

CNS: Anxiety, restlessness, irritability, delusions, hallucinations, headache, sedation, depression, incoherence, dizziness, memory loss; *confusion*, delirium (geriatric patients)

CV: Palpitations, tachycardia, hypotension, bradycardia

EENT: Blurred vision, photophobia, dilated pupils, difficulty swallowing, dry eyes, mydriasis, increased intraocular tension, closed-angle glaucoma

GI: *Dryness of mouth, constipation,* nausea, vomiting, abdominal distress, **paralytic ileus**, epigastric distress, xerostomia

GU: Urinary hesitancy/retention, dysuria

INTEG: Rash, urticaria, dermatoses

MISC: Increased temperature, flushing, decreased sweating, **hyperthermia, heat stroke**, numbness of fingers

MS: Muscular weakness, cramping

PHARMACOKINETICS

PO: Onset 1 hr, duration 6-10 hr

IM/IV: Onset 15 min, duration 6-10 hr

INTERACTIONS

Increase: anticholinergic effect—antihistamines, phenothiazines, tricyclics, disopyramide, quinidine

Decrease: absorption—antidiarrheals, antacids

Decrease: cholinergic effect of—bethanechol

NURSING CONSIDERATIONS

Assess:

- **Parkinsonism:** EPS, shuffling gait, muscle rigidity, involuntary movements, loss of balance
- I&O ratio; commonly causes decreased urinary output; urinary hesitancy, retention; palpate bladder if retention occurs
- Constipation: increase fluids, bulk, exercise if this occurs
- Mental status: affect, mood, CNS depression, worsening of mental symptoms during early therapy
- Use caution during hot weather; product may increase susceptibility to stroke by decreasing sweating

• With benztropine "buzz" or "high," patients may imitate EPS

Perform/provide:

• Storage at room temp

• Hard candy, gum, frequent drinks to relieve dry mouth

Evaluate:

• Therapeutic response: absence of involuntary movements after 2 days of treatment

Teach patient/family:

• That tabs may be crushed, mixed with food

• Not to discontinue product abruptly; to taper off over 1 wk or withdrawal symptoms may occur (EPS, tremors, insomnia, tachycardia, restlessness); to take as directed; not to double dose

• To avoid driving, other hazardous activities; drowsiness/dizziness may occur

• To avoid OTC medications: cough, cold preparations with alcohol, antihistamines, antacids, antidiarrheals within 2 hr unless directed by prescriber

• To change positions slowly to prevent orthostatic hypotension

• To use good oral hygiene, frequent sips of water, sugarless gum for dry mouth

RARELY USED

beractant (Rx)

(ber-ak'tant)

Survanta

Func. class.: Natural lung surfactant

USES: Prevention and treatment (rescue) of respiratory distress syndrome in premature infants

DOSAGE AND ROUTES

• **Newborn: INTRATRACHEAL INSTILL** 4 doses can be administered during the 1st 48 hr of life; give doses no more frequently than q6hr; each dose is 100 mg of phospholipids/kg birth weight

betamethasone (Rx)

(bay-ta-meth'a-sone)

Celestone

Func. class.: Corticosteroid, synthetic, long-acting

Do not confuse:

betamethasone/beclomethasone

ACTION: Decreases inflammation by suppressing the migration of polymorphonuclear leukocytes, fibroblasts and reversing increased capillary permeability, lysosomal stabilization

USES: Immunosuppression, severe inflammation

Unlabeled uses: Churg-Strauss syndrome, multiple myeloma, polyarteritis nodosa, polychondritis, pulmonary edema, temporal arteritis, Wegener's granulomatosis, prevention of hyaline membrane disease

CONTRAINDICATIONS: Children <2 yr, psychosis, hypersensitivity, idiopathic thrombocytopenia, acute glomerulonephritis, amebiasis, fungal infections, nonasthmatic bronchial disease, AIDS, TB, threadworm, high doses with traumatic brain injury

Precautions: Pregnancy (C), breastfeeding, diabetes mellitus, glaucoma, osteoporosis, seizure disorders, ulcerative colitis, CHF, myasthenia gravis, renal disease, esophagitis, peptic ulcer

DOSAGE AND ROUTES

• **Adult: PO** 0.6-7.2 mg/day; **IM** 0.6-9 mg/day in joint or soft tissue (sodium phosphate)

• **Child: PO** 62.5-250 mcg/kg/day in 3 divided doses; **IM** 17.5-250 mcg/kg/day in 3 divided doses every 3rd day or 5.8-8.75 mcg/kg/day as a single dose (adrenal insufficiency)

Acute graft-versus-host disease (GVHD)

• **Adult/adolescent/child: IM** (sodium phosphate and acetate combination) 0.5-9 mg/day; range, 1/3-1/2 of normal corticosteroid dose q12hr

Nonsuppurative thyroiditis

• **Adult/adolescent: PO** 0.6-7.2 mg/day as a single or divided dose; **IM** 0.5-9 mg/day in divided doses

• **Child: PO** 62.5-250 mcg/kg/day or 1.875-7.5 mg/m^2/day in 3-4 divided doses; **IM** 0.5-9 mg/day in divided doses

Other uses

• **Child: PO** 62.5-250 mcg/kg/day in 3 divided doses; **IM** 20.8-125 mcg/kg/day of the base q12-24hr

Maintenance with acute rheumatic carditis/polymyositis/SLE/temperol arteritis/Churg-Strauss syndrome/mixed connective-tissue disease/polyarteritis nodosa/relapsing polychondritis/polymyalgia rheumatica/vasculitis/Wegener's granulomatosis (unlabeled)

• **Adult: PO** 0.6-7.2 mg/day as a single or divided dose

• **Child: PO** 62.5-250 mcg/kg/day

Available forms: Effervescent tabs 500 mcg ♣; syr 600 mcg/5 ml; ext rel tab 1 mg; susp for inj (phosphate/acetate) 6 mg/ml

Administer:

PO route

• With food, milk to decrease GI symptoms

IM route

• Inj deeply in large muscle mass, rotate sites, avoid deltoid, use 21G needle

• In single dose in AM to prevent adrenal suppression; avoid SUBCUT administration, may damage tissue

SIDE EFFECTS

CNS: *Depression, flushing, sweating,* headache, bruising, mood changes

CV: *Hypertension,* **circulatory collapse, thromboembolism, embolism,** tachycardia, **necrotizing angiitis, CHF**

EENT: Fungal infections, increased intraocular pressure, blurred vision

GI: *Diarrhea, nausea, abdominal distention,* **GI hemorrhage,** *increased appetite,* **pancreatitis**

HEMA: **Thrombocytopenia**

INTEG: *Acne, poor wound healing, ecchymosis, bruising,* petechiae

MS: Fractures, osteoporosis, weakness, myopathy

PHARMACOKINETICS

Metabolized in liver, excreted in urine as metabolites, crosses placenta

PO: Onset 1-2 hr, peak 1 hr, duration 3 days

IM: Onset 10 min, peak 4-8 hr, duration 1-1½ days

INTERACTIONS

Increase: GI bleeding—NSAIDs, alcohol, salicylates, indomethacin

Increase: effects of betamethasone—CYP3A4 inhibitors (erythromycin, ketoconazole, itraconazole, ritonavir, saquinavir, indinavir)

Increase: hypokalemia—thiazides, loop diuretics, ticarcillin, amphotericin B, piperacillin

Increase: tendon rupture—fluoroquinolones

Decrease: action of betamethasone—barbiturates, rifampin, phenytoin

Decrease: effects of anticoagulants, antidiabetics, insulin, isoniazid, toxoids, vaccines, salicylates, oral contraceptives, somatrem, somatropin

Drug/Food

• Grapefruit juice should be avoided

Drug/Lab Test

Increase: cholesterol, sodium, blood glucose, uric acid, calcium, urine glucose

Decrease: calcium, potassium, T_4, T_3, thyroid ^{131}I uptake test, urine 17-OHCS, 17-KS, PBI

False negative: skin allergy tests

NURSING CONSIDERATIONS

Assess:

• **Infection:** increased temp, WBC even after withdrawal of medication; product masks infection symptoms

• **Adrenal insufficiency/crisis:** decreased B/P, nausea, vomiting, anorexia, weakness, weight loss, confusion, lethargy

• Potassium depletion: paresthesias, fatigue, nausea, vomiting, depression, polyuria, dysrhythmias, weakness

• Edema, hypo/hypertension, cardiac symptoms

• Mental status: affect, mood, behavioral changes, aggression

• Potassium, blood glucose, urine glucose while on long-term therapy; hypokalemia, hyperglycemia

• Weight daily; notify prescriber of weekly gain of >5 lb

• B/P, pulse; notify prescriber if chest pain occurs

• I&O ratio; be alert for decreasing urinary output, increasing edema

• Plasma cortisol levels during long-term therapy (normal level: 138-635 nmol/L SI units when drawn at 8 AM)

Perform/provide:

• Assistance with ambulation for patient with bone-tissue disease to prevent fractures

Evaluate:

• Therapeutic response: ease of respirations, decreased inflammation

Teach patient/family:

• That ID as corticosteroid user should be carried

• To notify prescriber if therapeutic response decreases; dosage adjustment may be needed

⚠ **Adrenal crisis:** not to discontinue abruptly

• To avoid all OTC products unless directed by prescriber; to avoid vaccines without prescriber approval

• All aspects of product usage, including cushingoid symptoms; to report black, tarry stools, abdominal pain to prescriber immediately

• **Adrenal insufficiency symptoms:** nausea, anorexia, fatigue, dizziness, dyspnea, weakness, joint pain

betamethasone topical

See Appendix B

betamethasone (augmented) topical

See Appendix B

betaxolol ophthalmic

See Appendix B

bethanechol (Rx)

(be-than′e-kole)

Urecholine

Func. class.: Urinary tract stimulant, cholinergic

Chem. class.: Synthetic choline ester

ACTION: Stimulates muscarinic ACH receptors directly; mimics effects of parasympathetic nervous system stimulation; stimulates gastric motility, micturition; increases lower esophageal sphincter pressure

USES: Urinary retention (postoperative, postpartum), neurogenic atony of bladder with retention

Unlabeled uses: Ileus, GERD, anticholinergic syndrome

CONTRAINDICATIONS: Hypersensitivity, severe bradycardia, asthma, severe hypotension, hyperthyroidism, peptic ulcer, parkinsonism, seizure disorders, CAD, COPD, coronary occlusion, mechanical obstruction, peritonitis, recent urinary/GI surgery, GI/GU obstruction

Precautions: Pregnancy (C), breastfeeding, children <8 yr, hypertension

DOSAGE AND ROUTES

- **Adult: PO** 10-50 mg bid-qid
- **Child (unlabeled): PO** 0.6 mg/kg/day in 3-4 divided doses

Ileus (unlabeled)

- **Adult: PO** 10-20 mg tid-qid before meals

Available forms: Tabs 5, 10, 25, 50 mg

Administer:

- To avoid nausea, vomiting, take on an empty stomach
- Only after all other cholinergics have been discontinued

SIDE EFFECTS

CNS: Dizziness, headache, malaise

CV: Hypotension, bradycardia, reflex tachycardia, **cardiac arrest, circulatory collapse**

EENT: Miosis, increased salivation, lacrimation, blurred vision

GI: *Nausea, bloody diarrhea, belching, vomiting, cramps, fecal incontinence*

GU: Urgency

INTEG: Rash, urticaria, flushing, increased sweating

RESP: **Acute asthma, dyspnea, bronchoconstriction**

PHARMACOKINETICS

PO: Onset 30-90 min, duration 6 hr

INTERACTIONS

Increase: severe hypotension—ganglionic blockers

Increase: action or toxicity—cholinergic agonists, anticholinesterase agents

Decrease: action of anticholinergics, procainamide, quiNIDine

Drug/Lab Test

Increase: AST, lipase/amylase, bilirubin

NURSING CONSIDERATIONS

Assess:

- **Urinary patterns:** retention, urgency
- B/P, pulse: observe after parenteral dose for 1 hr
- I&O ratio: check for urinary retention, urge incontinence
- **Toxicity:** bradycardia, hypotension, bronchospasm, headache, dizziness, seizures, respiratory depression; product should be discontinued if toxicity occurs

Perform/provide:

- Storage at room temp

Evaluate:

- Therapeutic response: absence of urinary retention, abdominal distention

Teach patient/family:

- To take product exactly as prescribed; 1 hr before meals or 2 hr after meals
- To make position changes slowly; orthostatic hypotension may occur
- To avoid driving, hazardous activities until effects are known

TREATMENT OF OVERDOSE:

Administer atropine 0.6-1.2 mg IV or IM (adult)

⚠ HIGH ALERT

bevacizumab (Rx)

(beh-va-kiz′you-mab)

Avastin

Func. class.: Antineoplastic—miscellaneous

Chem. class.: Monoclonal antibody

Do not confuse:

Avastin/Astelin

ACTION: DNA-derived monoclonal antibody selectively binds to and inhibits activity of human vascular endothelial growth factor (VEGF) to reduce microvascular growth and metastatic disease progression

USES: Non–small-cell lung cancer (NSCLC), metastatic carcinoma of the colon or rectum in combination with 5-FU IV; renal cell carcinoma, glioblastoma

Unlabeled uses: Adjunctive for pancreatic/neovascular/ovarian cancer; (wet) macular degeneration

CONTRAINDICATIONS:
Hypersensitivity

Precautions: Pregnancy (C), breastfeeding, children, geriatric patients, CHF, blood dyscrasias, CV disease, hypertension, surgery, thromboembolic disease, hamster protein/murine hypersensitivity

Black Box Warning: GI perforation, wound dehiscence

DOSAGE AND ROUTES

Non–small-cell lung cancer

• **Adult: IV** 15 mg/kg over 60-90 min with CARBOplatin and paclitaxel q3wk

Colorectal cancer

• **Adult: IV INF** 5-10 mg/kg q14days given over 90 min; if well tolerated, next inf may be given over 60 min; if 60-min infs well tolerated, subsequent infs may be given over 30 min

Metastatic renal cell carcinoma

• **Adult: IV** 10 mg/kg q2wk with interferon alfa 9 million units SUBCUT 3×/wk up to 52 wk

Glioblastoma single agent

• **Adult: IV** 10 mg/kg q2wk given over 60-90 min; 28 day cycle

Advanced pancreatic cancer (unlabeled)

• **Adult: IV** 10 mg/kg on days 1, 15 with gemcitabine 1000 mg/m^2 on days 1, 8, 15 in 28-day cycle

Metastatic Breast Cancer (unlabeled)

• **Adult: IV** 15 mg/kg on day 1 with docetaxel 100 mg/m^2 q3wk, up to 9 cycles (those who have not received previous chemotherapy)

Metastatic renal cell cancer (unlabeled)

• **Adult (single agent): IV** 10 mg/kg over 60-90 min q2wk; may be given in combination with other products

Ovarian cancer (unlabeled)

• **Adult: IV** 15 mg/kg q21days until unacceptable toxicity, disease progression

Neovascular (wet) macular degeneration (unlabeled)

• **Adult: INTRAVITREOUS INJ** 1.25 mg q mo

Available forms: Inj 25 mg/ml

Administer:

Intermittent IV INF route

• Do not give by IV bolus, IV push; do not shake vial

• Withdraw amount of product to be given, dilute in 100 ml 0.9% NaCl, discard any unused portion

Black Box Warning: Wound dehiscence: do not give for ≥28 days after surgery; make sure wound is healed before giving product

• Give as IV inf over 90 min for 1st dose and 60 min thereafter if well tolerated; subsequent inf may be given over 30 min; do not admix with dextrose

• **Rapid infusion rate (unlabeled):** give at rate of 0.5 mg/kg/min for all doses including initial inf (5 mg/kg over 10 min; 10 mg/kg over 20 min; 15 mg/kg over 30 min)

SIDE EFFECTS

CNS: *Asthenia, dizziness,* intracranial hemorrhage (malignant glioma), headache, fatigue, confusion

CV: Deep vein thrombosis, hypo/hypertension, hypertensive crisis

GI: Nausea, vomiting, *anorexia, diarrhea,* constipation, *abdominal pain,* colitis, stomatitis, GI hemorrhage/perforation

GU: Proteinuria, urinary frequency/urgency, nephrotic syndrome, ovarian failure

HEMA: Leukopenia, neutropenia, thrombocytopenia, microangiopathic hemolytic anemia, thromboembolism, bleeding

META: Bilirubinemia, hypokalemia

MISC: Exfoliative dermatitis, hemorrhage, non-GI fistula formation, alopecia, *impaired wound healing,* osteonecrosis of the jaw

RESP: Dyspnea, upper respiratory tract infection

PHARMACOKINETICS

Half-life 20 days, steady state 100 days

INTERACTIONS

• Avoid concurrent use with sunitab; microangiopathic hemolytic anemia may occur

NURSING CONSIDERATIONS

Assess:

- B/P; take frequently if hypertension develops
- For symptoms of infection; may be masked by product
- **CNS reaction:** dizziness, confusion
- **CHF:** crackles, jugular venous distention, dyspnea during treatment

⚠ **GU status** (proteinuria): nephrotic syndrome may occur; monitor urinalysis for increasing protein level; product should be held if protein ≥2 g/24 hr; resume when <2 g/24 hr

Black Box Warning: **GI perforation, serious bleeding, nephrotic syndrome, hypertensive crisis;** product should be discontinued permanently, surgery should be postponed

Evaluate:

- Therapeutic response: decrease in size of tumors

Teach patient/family:

- To avoid hazardous tasks because confusion, dizziness may occur
- To report signs of infection: sore throat, fever, diarrhea, vomiting
- Not to become pregnant while taking this product or for several months after discontinuing treatment
- To report bleeding, changes in urinary patterns, edema, abdominal pain
- To avoid immunizations

bicalutamide (Rx)

(bye-kal-u′ta-mide)

Casodex, CO Bicalutamide ✤, PMS-Bicalutamide ✤, ratio-Bicalutamide ✤, Sandoz Bicalutamide ✤

Func. class.: Antineoplastic hormone

Chem. class.: Nonsteroidal antiandrogen

Do not confuse:

Casodex/Kapidex

ACTION: Binds to cytosolic androgen in target tissue, which competitively inhibits the action to androgens

USES: Stage D-2 metastatic prostate cancer in combination with luteinizing-hormone–releasing hormone (LHRH) analog

Unlabeled uses: Recurrent priapism

CONTRAINDICATIONS: Pregnancy (X), women, hypersensitivity

Precautions: Breastfeeding, geriatric patients, renal/hepatic disease, diabetes mellitus

DOSAGE AND ROUTES

- **Adult: PO** 50 mg/day with LHRH analog

Recurrent priapism (unlabeled)

- **Adult: PO** 50 mg every other day

Available forms: Tabs 50 mg

Administer:

- At same time each day, either AM or PM, with/without food
- With LHRH treatment; start both products at same time

SIDE EFFECTS

CNS: Dizziness, paresthesia, insomnia, anxiety, neuropathy, headache

CV: CHF, *edema, hot flashes,* hypertension, chest pain, MI

GI: *Diarrhea, constipation, nausea,* vomiting, increased hepatic enzymes, anorexia, dry mouth, melena, *abdominal pain,* hepatitis

GU: *Nocturia, hematuria,* UTI, impotence, gynecomastia; urinary incontinence, frequency, dysuria, retention, urgency; breast tenderness, decreased libido

INTEG: Rash, sweating, dry skin, pruritus, alopecia

MISC: *Infection,* anemia, dyspnea, bone pain, headache, *asthenia, back pain,* flulike symptoms

PHARMACOKINETICS

Well absorbed; peak 31½ hr; metabolized by liver; excreted in urine, feces; half-life 5.8 days; 96% protein binding

INTERACTIONS

Increase: anticoagulation—anticoagulants

Increase: bicalutamide effects—CYP3A4 inhibitors (amiodarone, antiretrovirals, protease inhibitors, clarithromycin, dalfopristin, quinupristin, delavirdine, efavirenz, erythromycin, fluoxetine, fluvoxamine, imatinib, mifepristone, RU-486, nefazodone, some azole antifungals)

Decrease: bicalutamide effects—CYP3A4 inducers (barbiturates, bosentan, carBAMazepine, dexamethasone, nevirapine, oxcarbazepine, phenytoins, rifabutin, rifampin, rifapentine)

Drug/Herb

• May require dosage change when used with St. John's wort

Drug/Food

• Do not use with grapefruit juice

Drug/Lab Test

Increase: AST, ALT, bilirubin, BUN, creatinine

Decrease: Hgb, WBC

NURSING CONSIDERATIONS

Assess:

• For diarrhea, constipation, nausea, vomiting

• For hot flashes, gynecomastia; assure patient that these are common side effects

• Prostate-specific antigen, LFTs

Evaluate:

• Therapeutic response: decreased tumor size, decreased spread of malignancy

Teach patient/family:

• To recognize, report signs of anemia, hepatoxicity, renal toxicity

• That hair may be lost but that this is reversible after therapy is completed

• Not to use other products unless approved by prescriber

• To report severe diarrhea

• To use contraception while taking this product

bimatoprost ophthalmic

See Appendix B

bisacodyl (Rx, OTC)

(bis-a-koe′dill)

Alophen, APC-Bisacodyl ✱, Apo-Bisacodyl ✱, Bisac-Evac, Corrective, Correctol, Dacodyl, Dulcolax, Ex-Lax Ultra Tab, Femilax, Feminine, Femitrol, Good Sense Women's, Leader Laxative, ratio-Bisacodyl ✱, Top Care Laxative, Veracolate, Walgreens Gentle, Walgreens Women's

Func. class.: Laxative, stimulant

Chem. class.: Diphenylmethane

ACTION: Acts directly on intestine by increasing motor activity; thought to irritate colonic intramural plexus

USES: Short-term treatment of constipation; bowel or rectal preparation for surgery, examination

CONTRAINDICATIONS: Hypersensitivity, rectal fissures, abdominal pain, nausea, vomiting, appendicitis, acute surgical abdomen, ulcerated hemorrhoids, acute hepatitis, fecal impaction, intestinal/biliary tract obstruction

Precautions: Pregnancy (C), breastfeeding

DOSAGE AND ROUTES

• **Adult and child ≥12 yr: PO** 10-15 mg in PM or AM; may use up to 30 mg for bowel or rectal preparation; **RECT** 10 mg as a single dose; 30-ml enema

• **Child 3-11 yr: PO** 5-10 mg as a single dose; **RECT** 5-10 mg as a single dose

Available forms: Tabs 5 mg; enteric-coated tabs 5 mg; supp 5, 10 mg; enema 10 mg/30 ml

Administer:

PO route

- Swallow tabs whole with full glass of water; do not break, crush, chew tabs
- Alone only with water for better absorption; do not take within 1 hr of other products or within 1 hr of antacids, milk, H_2 antagonists; do not take enteric product with proton pump inhibitors
- In AM or PM

SIDE EFFECTS

CNS: Muscle weakness

GI: *Nausea, vomiting, anorexia, cramps,* diarrhea, rectal burning (suppositories)

META: Protein-losing enteropathy, alkalosis, hypokalemia, tetany; electrolyte, fluid imbalances

PHARMACOKINETICS

Small amounts metabolized by liver; excreted in urine, bile, feces, breast milk

PO: Onset 6-10 hr

RECT: Onset 15-60 min

INTERACTIONS

Increase: gastric irritation—antacids, milk, H_2-blockers, gastric acid pump inhibitors

NURSING CONSIDERATIONS

Assess:

- Blood, urine electrolytes if product is used often by patient
- I&O ratio to identify fluid loss
- Cause of constipation; identify whether fluids, bulk, exercise missing from lifestyle; determine use of constipating products
- **GI symptoms:** cramping, rectal bleeding, nausea, vomiting; if these symptoms occur, product should be discontinued

Evaluate:

- Therapeutic response: decrease in constipation

Teach patient/family:

- Not to use laxatives for long-term therapy because bowel tone will be lost
- That normal bowel movements do not always occur daily
- Not to use in presence of abdominal pain, nausea, vomiting
- To notify prescriber if constipation is unrelieved or if symptoms of electrolyte imbalance occur: muscle cramps, pain, weakness, dizziness

bismuth subsalicylate (OTC)

(bis′muth sub-sal-iss′uh-late)

Bismatrol, Equaline Stomach Relief, Good Sense Stomach Relief, GNP Pink Bismuth, Kao-Tin, Leader Pink Bismuth, Peptic Relief, Pepto-Bismol, Pink Bismuth, Top Care Stomach Relief, Walgreens Soothe

Func. class.: Antidiarrheal, weak antacid

Chem. class.: Salicylate

Do not confuse:
Kaopectate/Kayoxalate

ACTION: Inhibits the prostaglandin synthesis responsible for GI hypermotility, intestinal inflammation; stimulates absorption of fluid and electrolytes; binds toxins produced by *Escherichia coli*

USES: Diarrhea (cause undetermined), prevention of diarrhea when traveling; may be included to treat *Helicobacter pylori,* heartburn, indigestion, nausea

CONTRAINDICATIONS: Children <3 yr, children with chickenpox, history of GI bleeding, renal disease, flulike symptoms, hypersensitivity to product or salicylates

Precautions: Pregnancy (C), breastfeeding, geriatric patients, anticoagulant therapy, immobility, gout, diabetes mellitus, bleeding disorders, previous hypersensitivity to NSAIDs, *Clostridium-difficile*–associated diarrhea when used with antiinfectives for *H. pylori*

DOSAGE AND ROUTES

Antidiarrheal/Gastric Distress

• **Adult: PO** 2 tabs or 30 ml (15 ml extra/max strength) q30min or 2 tabs q60min, max 4.2 g/24 hr

Antiulcer (unlabeled)

• **Adult/adolescent: PO** 525 mg qid, max 4.2 g/24 hr; given with metronidazole or tetracycline

Available forms: Tabs 262 mg; chewable tabs 262 mg; susp 87 mg/5 ml, 130 mg/15 ml, 262 mg/15 ml, 525 mg/15 ml

Administer:

PO route

• Increased fluids to rehydrate patient
• **Susp:** shake liquid before using
• Tabs can be chewed, dissolved in mouth; caplets to be swallowed whole with water

SIDE EFFECTS

CNS: Confusion, twitching, neurotoxicity (high doses)

EENT: Hearing loss, tinnitus, metallic taste, blue gums, black tongue

GI: Increased fecal impaction (high doses), dark stools, constipation, diarrhea, nausea

HEMA: Increased bleeding time

PHARMACOKINETICS

PO: Onset 1 hr, peak 2 hr, duration 4 hr

INTERACTIONS

Increase: toxicity—salicylates, methotrexate

Increase: effects of oral anticoagulants, oral antidiabetics

Decrease: absorption of tetracycline, quinolones

Drug/Lab Test

Interference: radiographic studies of GI system

NURSING CONSIDERATIONS

Assess:

• **Diarrhea:** bowel pattern before product therapy, after treatment
• Electrolytes (K, Na, Cl) if diarrhea is severe or continues long term; assess skin turgor, other signs of dehydration

Evaluate:

• Therapeutic response: decreased diarrhea, absence of diarrhea when traveling; resolution of ulcers

Teach patient/family:

• To chew, dissolve medication in mouth; not to swallow whole; to shake liquid before using
• To avoid other salicylates unless directed by prescriber; not to give to children, possibility of Reye's syndrome
• That stools may turn black; that tongue may darken; that impaction may occur in debilitated patients
• To stop use if symptoms do not improve within 2 days or become worse or if diarrhea is accompanied by high fever

bisoprolol (Rx)

(bis-oh′pro-lole)

Apo-Bisoprolol ♣, PMS-Bisoprolol ♣, Sandoz Bisoprolol ♣, Zebeta

Func. class.: Antihypertensive

Chem. class.: β_1-Blocker

Do not confuse:

Zebeta/DiaBeta/Zetia

ACTION: Preferentially and competitively blocks stimulation of β_1-adrenergic receptors within cardiac muscle (decreases rate of SA node discharge, increases recovery time), slows conduction of AV node, decreases heart rate, which decreases O_2 consumption in myocardium; decreases renin-angiotensin-aldosterone system; inhibits β_2-receptors in bronchial and vascular smooth muscle at high doses

USES:
Mild to moderate hypertension
Unlabeled uses: Stable angina, stable CHF

CONTRAINDICATIONS:
Hypersensitivity to β-blockers, cardiogenic shock, heart block (2nd, 3rd degree), sinus bradycardia, CHF, cardiac failure
Precautions: Pregnancy (C), breastfeeding, children, major surgery, diabetes mellitus, thyroid/renal/hepatic disease, COPD, asthma, well-compensated heart failure, aortic or mitral valve disease, peripheral vascular disease, myasthenia gravis

Black Box Warning: Abrupt discontinuation

DOSAGE AND ROUTES
Hypertension
- **Adult: PO** 2.5-5 mg/day; may increase to 20 mg/day if necessary; max 20 mg/day

Renal/hepatic dose
- **Adult: PO** CCr <40 ml/min 2.5 mg, titrate upward

Angina (unlabeled)
- **Adult: PO** 5-20 mg/day

Heart failure (unlabeled)
- **Adult: PO** 1.25 mg/day × 48 hr, then 2.5 mg/day for 1st mo, then 5 mg/day; max 10 mg/day

Available forms: Tabs 5, 10 mg
Administer:
- Product before meals, bedtime; tab may be crushed, swallowed whole; may give without regard to meals
- Reduced dosage with renal/hepatic dysfunction

SIDE EFFECTS
CNS: Vertigo, headache, insomnia, fatigue, dizziness, mental changes, memory loss, hallucinations, depression, lethargy, drowsiness, strange dreams, catatonia, peripheral neuropathy
CV: **Ventricular dysrhythmias, profound hypotension, bradycardia, CHF,** cold extremities, postural hypotension, 2nd- or **3rd-degree heart block**
EENT: Sore throat; dry, burning eyes
ENDO: Increased hypoglycemic response to insulin
GI: Nausea, diarrhea, vomiting, **mesenteric arterial thrombosis, ischemic colitis,** flatulence, gastritis, gastric pain
GU: Impotence, decreased libido
HEMA: **Agranulocytosis, thrombocytopenia,** purpura, eosinophilia
INTEG: Rash, flushing, alopecia, pruritus, sweating
MISC: Facial swelling, weight gain, decreased exercise tolerance
MS: Joint pain, arthralgia
RESP: **Bronchospasm,** dyspnea, wheezing, cough, nasal stuffiness

PHARMACOKINETICS
Peak 2-4 hr, half-life 9-12 hr, 50% excreted unchanged in urine, protein binding 30%-36%, metabolized in liver to inactive metabolites

INTERACTIONS
Increase: hypotension—reserpine, guanethidine
Increase: myocardial depression—calcium channel blockers
Increase: antihypertensive effect—ACE inhibitors, α-blockers, calcium channel blockers, diuretics
Increase: bradycardia—digoxin, amiodarone
Increase: peripheral ischemia—ergots
Increase: antidiabetic effect—antidiabetics
Decrease: antihypertensive effect—NSAIDs, salicylates
Drug/Herb
Increase: β-blocking effect—hawthorn
Decrease: β-blocking effect—ephedra
Drug/Lab Test
Increase: AST, ALT, ANA titer, blood glucose, BUN, uric acid, K, lipoprotein
Interference: glucose/insulin tolerance tests

NURSING CONSIDERATIONS

Assess:

• **Hypertension:** B/P during beginning treatment, periodically thereafter; pulse q4hr: note rate, rhythm, quality; apical/radial pulse before administration; notify prescriber of any significant changes (pulse <50 bpm)

• Baselines of renal, hepatic studies before therapy begins

• **CHF:** I&O, weight daily; increased weight, jugular venous distention, dyspnea, crackles, edema in feet, legs daily

• Skin turgor, dryness of mucous membranes for hydration status, especially for geriatric patients

Perform/provide:

• Storage protected from light, moisture; place in cool environment

Evaluate:

• Therapeutic response: decreased B/P after 1-2 wk

Teach patient/family:

Black Box Warning: Not to discontinue product abruptly; may cause precipitate angina, rebound hypertension; evaluate noncompliance

• Not to use OTC products that contain α-adrenergic stimulants (e.g., nasal decongestants, OTC cold preparations) unless directed by prescriber

• To report bradycardia, dizziness, confusion, depression, fever, cold extremities

• To take pulse at home; advise when to notify prescriber

• To avoid alcohol, smoking, sodium intake

• To comply with weight control, dietary adjustments, modified exercise program

• To carry emergency ID to identify product, allergies

• To avoid hazardous activities if dizziness is present

⚠ To report symptoms of CHF: difficulty breathing, especially on exertion or when lying down, night cough, swelling of extremities

• That, if diabetic, product may mask signs of hypoglycemia or alter blood glucose levels

TREATMENT OF OVERDOSE:

Lavage, IV atropine for bradycardia; IV theophylline for bronchospasm; digoxin, O_2, diuretic for cardiac failure; hemodialysis, IV glucose for hypoglycemia; IV diazepam or phenytoin for seizures

⚠ HIGH ALERT

bivalirudin (Rx)

(bye-val-i-rue′din)

Angiomax

Func. class.: Anticoagulant

Chem. class.: Thrombin inhibitor

ACTION: Direct inhibitor of thrombin that is highly specific; able to inhibit free and clot-bound thrombin

USES: Unstable angina in patients undergoing percutaneous transluminal coronary angioplasty (PTCA), used with aspirin; heparin-induced thrombocytopenia, with/without thrombosis syndrome

Unlabeled uses: Acute MI, DVT prophylaxis

CONTRAINDICATIONS: Hypersensitivity, active bleeding, cerebral aneurysm, intracranial hemorrhage, recent surgery, CVA

Precautions: Pregnancy (B), breastfeeding, children, geriatric patients, renal function impairment, hepatic disease, asthma, blood dyscrasias, thrombocytopenia, GI ulcers, hypertension

DOSAGE AND ROUTES

• **Adult: IV BOL** 0.75 mg/kg then **IV INF** 1.75 mg/kg/hr for 4 hr; another **IV INF** may be used at 0.2 mg/kg/hr for ≤20 hr; this product is intended to be used with aspirin (325 mg/day) adjusted to body weight

Renal dose

• **Adult: IV** GFR 30-59 ml/min, give 1.75 mg/kg/hr; GFR 10-29 ml/min, give 1 mg/kg/hr; give dialysis-dependent patients 0.25 mg/kg/hr

Acute MI (unlabeled)

• **Adult: IV BOL** 0.25 mg/kg then **CONT IV INF** 0.5 mg/kg/hr × 12 hr

DVT prophylaxis (unlabeled)

• **Adult: SUBCUT** 1 mg/kg q8hr for those undergoing orthopedic surgery

Available forms: Inj, lyophilized 250 mg/vial

Administer:

• Before PTCA; give with aspirin (325 mg)

IV, direct route

• Dilute by adding 5 ml of sterile water for inj/250 mg bivalirudin, swirl until dissolved, further dilute in 50 ml of D_5W or 0.9% NaCl (5 mg/ml), give by bolus inj 0.75 mg/kg, then intermittent inf

Continuous IV INF route

• To each 250-mg vial add 5 ml of sterile water for inj, swirl until dissolved, further dilute in 500 ml D_5W or 0.9% NaCl (0.5 mg/ml); give inf after bolus dose at a rate of 1.75 mg/kg/hr; may give an additional inf at 0.2 mg/kg/hr

• Do not mix other IV medications with bivalirudin or provide via the same IV line as bivalirudin

Y-site compatibilities: Abciximab, acyclovir, alfentanil, allopurinol, amifostine, amikacin, aminocaproic acid, aminophylline, amphotericin B liposome, ampicillin, ampicillin-sulbactam, anidulafungin, argatroban, arsenic trioxide, atenolol, atracurium, atropine, azithromycin, aztreonam, bleomycin, bumetanide, buprenorphine, busulfan, butorphanol, calcium chloride/gluconate, capreomycin, CARBOplatin, carmustine, ceFAZolin, cefepime, cefoperazone, cefotaxime, cefotetan, cefoxitin, ceftazidime, ceftizoxime, cefTRIAXone, cefuroxime, chloramphenicol, cimetidine, ciprofloxacin, cisatracurium, CISplatin, clindamycin, cyclophosphamide, cycloSPORINE, cytarabine, dacarbazine, DACTINomycin, DAPTOmycin, DAUNOrubicin, DAUNOrubicin liposome, dexamethasone, dexmedetomidine, dexrazoxane, digoxin, diltiazem, diphenhydrAMINE, docetaxel, dolasetron, DOPamine, DOXOrubicin, DOXOrubicin liposomal, doxycycline, droperidol, enalaprilat, ePHEDrine, EPINEPHrine, epirubicin, epoprostenol, eptifibatide, ertapenem, erythromycin, esmolol, etoposide, etoposide phosphate, famotidine, fenoldopam, fentaNYL, fluconazole, fludarabine, fluorouracil, foscarnet, fosphenytoin, furosemide, gallium, ganciclovir, gatifloxacin, gemcitabine, gentamicin, glycopyrrolate, granisetron, haloperidol, heparin, hydrALAZINE, hydrocortisone, HYDROmorphone, hydrOXYzine, IDArubicin, ifosfamide, imipenem-cilastatin, inamrinone, insulin (regular), irinotecan, isoproterenol, ketorolac, labetalol, leucovorin, levofloxacin, lidocaine, linezolid, LORazepam, magnesium, mannitol, mechlorethamine, melphalan, meperidine, meropenem, mesna, methohexital, methotrexate, methyldopate, methylPREDNISolone, metoclopramide, metoprolol, metroNIDAZOLE, midazolam, milrinone, mitomycin, mitoxantrone, mivacurium, morphine, moxifloxacin, mycophenolate mofetil, nafcillin, nalbuphine, naloxone, nesiritide, niCARdipine, nitroglycerin, nitroprusside, norepinephrine, octreotide, ofloxacin, ondansetron, oxaliplatin, oxytocin, paclitaxel, palonosetron, pamidronate, pancuronium, pemetrexed, PENTobarbital, PHENobarbital, phenylephrine, piperacillin, piperacillin-tazobactam, polymyxin B, potassium acetate/chloride/phosphates, procainamide, promethazine, propranolol, ranitidine, remifentanil, rocuronium, sodium acetate/bicarbonate/phosphates, streptozocin, succinylcholine, SUFentanil, sulfamethoxazole-trimethoprim, tacrolimus, teniposide, theophylline, thiopental, thiotepa, ticarcillin, ticarcillin-clavulanate, tigecycline, tirofiban, tobramycin, topotecan, vasopressin, vecuronium, verapamil, vinBLAStine, vinCRIStine, vinorelbine, voriconazole, warfarin, zidovudine, zoledronic acid

SUBCUT injection (unlabeled)

• May be used for DVT prophylaxis

SIDE EFFECTS

CNS: *Headache, insomnia, anxiety, nervousness*

CV: *Hypo/hypertension, bradycardia*

GI: *Nausea, vomiting, abdominal pain, dyspepsia*

HEMA: Hemorrhage, thrombocytopenia

MISC: Pain at inj site, pelvic pain, urinary retention, fever

MS: *Back pain*

PHARMACOKINETICS

Excreted in urine, half-life 25 min, duration 1 hr, no protein binding

INTERACTIONS

Increase: bleeding risk—anticoagulants, aspirin, treprostinil, thrombolytics

Drug/Herb

Increase: bleeding risk—agrimony, alfalfa, angelica, anise, bilberry, black haw, bogbean, buchu, cat's claw, chamomile, chondroitin, devil's claw, dong quai, evening primrose, fenugreek, feverfew, fish oil, garlic, ginger, ginkgo, ginseng, horse chestnut, Irish moss, kava, kelp, kelpware, khella, licorice, lovage, lungwort, meadowsweet, motherwort, mugwort, nettle, papaya, parsley (large amts), pau d'arco, pineapple, poplar, prickly ash, red clover, safflower, saw palmetto, senega, skullcap, tonka bean, turmeric, wintergreen, yarrow

Decrease: anticoagulant effect—coenzyme Q10, flax, glucomannan, goldenseal, guar gum

NURSING CONSIDERATIONS

Assess:

• Baseline and periodic ACT, APTT, PT, INR, TT, platelets, Hgb, Hct

⚠ **Bleeding:** check arterial and venous sites, IM inj sites, catheters; all punctures should be minimized; fall in B/P or Hct may indicate hemorrhage

• Fever, skin rash, urticaria

• CV status: B/P, watch for hypo/hypertension, bradycardia

• Neurologic status: any focal or generalized deficits should be reported immediately

Perform/provide:

• Storage of reconstituted vials in refrigerator for up to 24 hr; store diluted conc at room temp for 24 hr

Evaluate:

• Therapeutic response: anticoagulation with PTCA; resolution of heparin-induced thrombocytopenia, thrombosis syndrome

Teach patient/family:

• About the reason for the product and expected results

• To report black, tarry stools; blood in urine; difficulty breathing

⚠ HIGH ALERT

bleomycin (Rx)

(blee-oh-mye′sin)

Bleoxane ✦

Func. class.: Antineoplastic, antibiotic

Chem. class.: Glycopeptide

ACTION: Inhibits synthesis of DNA, RNA, protein; derived from *Streptomyces verticillus;* phase specific to the G_2 and M phases; a nonvesicant, sclerosing agent

USES: Cancer of head, neck, penis, cervix, vulva of squamous cell origin; Hodgkin's/non-Hodgkin's disease; testicular carcinoma; as a sclerosing agent for malignant pleural effusion

Unlabeled uses: Cutaneous T-cell lymphoma (CTCL), hemangioma, Kaposi's sarcoma, malignant ascites, verruca plantaris/vulgaris, osteogenic sarcoma

CONTRAINDICATIONS:

Pregnancy (D), breastfeeding, hypersensitivity, prior idiosyncratic reaction

Precautions: Patients >70 yr old, renal/hepatic disease, respiratory disease

Black Box Warning: Idiosyncratic reaction, pulmonary fibrosis

DOSAGE AND ROUTES

Test dose

- **Adult and child (unlabeled): IM/IV/SUBCUT** ≤2 units for first 2 doses followed by 24 hr of observation
- **Adult and child: SUBCUT/IV/IM** 0.25-0.5 units/kg 1-2 ×/wk or 10-20 units/m^2, then 1 unit/day or 5 units/wk; may also be given by **CONT INF;** do not exceed total dose of 400 units during lifetime

Malignant pleural effusion

- **Adult:** 60 units diluted in 100 ml of 0.9% NaCl; intrapleural inj given through a thoracostomy tube after drainage of excess pleural fluid and complete lung expansion; remove after 4 hr

Renal dose

- **Adult/child:** CCr 40-50 ml/min reduce dose by 30%; CCr 30-39 ml/min reduce dose by 40%; CCr 20-29 ml/min reduce dose by 45%; CCr 10-19 ml/min reduce dose by 55%; CCr 5-10 ml/min reduce dose by 60%

Cutaneous T-cell lymphoma (CTCL) (unlabeled)

- **Adult: IV** 15 units twice weekly with vinBLAStine and predniSONE

Kaposi's sarcoma (unlabeled)

- **Adult: IV** 15 units q2wk with DOXOrubicin and vinCRIStine

Malignant ascites (unlabeled)

- **Adult: INTRACAVITARY** 60 units mixed in 50-100 ml 0.9% NaCl, injected into pleural space

Available forms: Powder for inj, 15, 30 units/vial

Administer:

- Antiemetic 30-60 min before giving product to prevent vomiting; continue antiemetics 6-10 hr after treatment
- Topical or systemic analgesics for pain of stomatitis as ordered; antihistamines and antipyretics for fever, chills
- May be given IM, subcut, IV, intrapleurally, intralesionally, intraarterially

IM/SUBCUT route

- After reconstituting 15 units/1-5 ml or 30 mg/2-10 ml of 0.9% NaCl or bacteriostatic water for inj, rotate inj sites; do not use products that contain benzyl alcohol when giving to neonates or that contain dextrose because of loss of potency

Intrapleural route

- 60 units/100 ml of 0.9% NaCl administered by MD through thoracostomy tube

IV route

- Use cytotoxic handling procedures
- After reconstituting 15- or 30-unit vial with 5 or 10 ml of NS, respectively, inj slowly over 10 min or after further dilution with 50-100 ml D_5W or 0.9% NaCl; give 15 units or less over 10 min through Y-tube or 3-way stopcock
- For patients with lymphoma, give 2 test doses of 2-5 units before initial dose; monitor for anaphylaxis

Y-site compatibilities: Acyclovir, alfentanil, allopurinol, amifostine, amikacin, aminocaproic acid, aminophylline, amiodarone, ampicillin, ampicillin-sulbactam, anidulafungin, atenolol, atracurium, azithromycin, aztreonam, bivalirudin, bumetanide, buprenorphine, busulfan, butorphanol, calcium chloride/gluconate, CARBOplatin, carmustine, caspofungin, cefazolin, cefepime, cefotaxime, cefotetan, cefoxitin, ceftazidime, ceftizoxime, cefTRIAXone, cefuroxime, chloramphenicol, chlorproMAZINE, cimetidine, ciprofloxacin, cisatracurium, CISplatin, clindamycin, codeine, cyclophosphamide, cycloSPORINE, cytarabine, dacarbazine, DACTINomycin, DAPTOmycin, DAUNOrubicin, dexamethasone, dexmedetomidine, dexrazoxane, digoxin, diltiazem, diphenhydrAMINE,

DOBUTamine, docetaxel, DOPamine, doxacurium, DOXOrubicin, DOXOrubicin liposomal, doxycycline, droperidol, enalaprilat, ePHEDrine, EPINEPHrine, epirubicin, ertapenem, erythromycin, esmolol, etoposide, famotidine, fenoldopam, fentaNYL, filgrastim, fluconazole, fludarabine, fluorouracil, foscarnet, fosphenytoin, furosemide, ganciclovir, gatifloxacin, gemcitabine, gentamicin, glycopyrrolate, granisetron, haloperidol, heparin, hydrALAZINE, hydrocortisone sodium succinate, HYDROmorphone, hydrOXYzine, IDArubicin, ifosfamide, imipenem-cilastatin, inamrinone, insulin (regular), irinotecan, isoproterenol, ketorolac, labetalol, leucovorin, levofloxacin, levorphanol, lidocaine, linezolid, lorazepam, magnesium sulfate, mannitol, mechlorethamine, melphalan, meperidine, meropenem, mesna, metaraminol, methohexital, methotrexate, methyldopate, methylPREDNISolone, metoclopramide, metoprolol, metroNIDAZOLE, midazolam, milrinone, minocycline, mitomycin, mitoxantrone, mivacurium, morphine, nafcillin, nalbuphine, naloxone, nesiritide, niCARdipine, nitroglycerin, nitroprusside, norepinephrine, octreotide, ondansetron, oxaliplatin, palonosetron, pamidronate, pancuronium, pantoprazole, pemetrexed, pentamidine, pentazocine, PENTobarbital, PHENobarbital, phenylephrine, piperacillin, piperacillin-tazobactam, polymyxin B, potassium chloride, potassium phosphates, procainamide, prochlorperazine, promethazine, propranolol, quiNIDine, ranitidine, remifentanil, riTUXimab, rocuronium, sargramostim, sodium acetate, sodium bicarbonate, sodium phosphates, succinylcholine, SUFentanil, sulfamethoxazole-trimethoprim, tacrolimus, teniposide, theophylline, thiopental, thiotepa, ticarcillin, ticarcillin-clavulanate, tirofiban, tobramycin, tolazoline, trastuzumab, trimethobenzamide, vancomycin, vasopressin, vecuronium, verapamil, vinBLAStine, vinCRIStine, vinorelbine, voriconazole, zidovudine

SIDE EFFECTS

CNS: Pain at tumor site, headache, confusion

CV: MI, stroke

GI: *Nausea, vomiting, anorexia, stomatitis, weight loss,* ulceration of mouth, lips

GU: Hemolytic-uremic syndrome

IDIOSYNCRATIC REACTION: Hypotension, *confusion, fever,* chills, wheezing

INTEG: *Rash, hyperkeratosis, nail changes, alopecia,* pruritus, acne, striae, peeling, hyperpigmentation

RESP: Fibrosis, pneumonitis, wheezing, pulmonary toxicity

SYST: Anaphylaxis, radiation recall, Raynaud's phenomenon

PHARMACOKINETICS

Half-life 2 hr; when CCr is >35 ml/min, half-life is increased with lower clearance; metabolized in liver; 50% excreted in urine (unchanged)

INTERACTIONS

- Avoid live virus vaccines concurrently

Increase: toxicity—other antineoplastics, radiation therapy, general anesthesia, filgrastim, sargramostim

Decrease: serum phenytoin levels—phenytoin, fosphenytoin

Drug/Lab Test

Increase: uric acid

NURSING CONSIDERATIONS

Assess:

- IM test dose in patients with lymphoma of 1-2 units before 1st 2 doses
- **Pulmonary toxicity/fibrosis:** pulmonary function tests; chest x-ray before, during therapy, should be obtained q2wk during treatment; pulmonary diffusion capacity for carbon monoxide (DLCO) monthly, if <40% of pretreatment value, stop treatment; treat pulmonary infection before treatment; dyspnea, crackles, unproductive cough, chest pain, tachypnea, fatigue, increased pulse, pallor, lethargy

- Temp q4hr; fever may indicate beginning infection
- Renal status: serum creatinine
- Effects of alopecia, skin color alterations on body image; discuss feelings about body changes
- Buccal cavity q8hr for dryness, sores, ulceration, white patches, oral pain, bleeding, dysphagia
- Local irritation, pain, burning, discoloration at inj site

Anaphylaxis: rash, pruritus, urticaria, purpuric skin lesions, itching, flushing, wheezing, hypotension; have emergency equipment available

Black Box Warning: Idiosyncratic reaction: hypotension, mental confusion, fever, chills, wheezing

Perform/provide:
- Storage for 2 wk after reconstituting if refrigerated or for 24 hr at room temp; discard unused portions
- Deep-breathing exercises with patient tid-qid; place patient in semi-Fowler's position
- Liquid diet: carbonated beverages; gelatin may be added if patient is not nauseated, vomiting
- Rinsing of mouth tid-qid with water, club soda; brushing of teeth with baking soda bid-tid with soft brush or cotton-tipped applicators for stomatitis; use unwaxed dental floss
- HOB raised to facilitate breathing

Evaluate:
- Therapeutic response: decrease in size of tumor

Teach patient/family:
- To report any complaints, side effects to nurse, prescriber
- To report any changes in breathing, coughing, fever
- That hair may be lost during treatment and that wig or hairpiece may make patient feel better; that new hair may be different in color, texture
- To avoid foods with citric acid, hot or rough texture
- To report any bleeding, white spots, ulcerations in mouth; to examine mouth daily and report symptoms
- To use contraception during treatment (pregnancy D), avoid breastfeeding
- Not to receive vaccines during treatment

boceprevir

(boe-se′pre-vir)

Victrelis

Func. class.: Antiviral, anti-hepatitis agents

ACTION: Prevents hepatitis C viral (HCV) replication by blocking the activity of HCV NS3/4A serine protease. Hepatitis C virus NS3/4A serine protease is an enzyme responsible for the conversion of HCV encoded polyproteins to mature/functioning viral proteins. These mature proteins, NS4A, NS4B, NS5A, and NS5B, are needed for viral replication.

USES: Hepatitis C infection

CONTRAINDICATIONS: Pregnancy (X), male partners of women who are pregnant

Precautions: Breastfeeding, neonates, infants, children, adolescents <18 years of age, anemia, neutropenia, thrombocytopenia, HIV, hepatitis B, decompensated hepatic disease, in liver or other organ transplants

DOSAGE AND ROUTES

Chronic hepatitis C infection (genotype 1) compensated liver disease (in those without cirrhosis, previously untreated with interferon and ribavirin therapy)

- **Adults: PO** Before starting therapy with boceprevir, peginterferon alfa and ribavirin must be given for 4 wk, then add boceprevir 800 mg (four 200 mg caps) PO TID (every 7-9 hours). Treatment length is determined by HCV RNA conc at treatment wk 4, 8, 12, and 24. If patient has undetectable HCV RNA conc at wk 8 and 24, discontinue all 3 medications at wk 28. If HCV RNA is detectable at wk 8 but undetectable at wk 24, continue the 3-drug regimen through wk 36, then give only peginterferon alfa and ribavirin through treatment wk 48. If the patient has a poor response to peginterferon alfa and ribavirin during the initial 4 wk, continue treatment with all 3 medications for a total of 48 wks. Discontinue the 3-drug regimen if the HCV RNA conc >100 international units/ml at treatment wk 12 or a detectable HCA RNA conc at treatment wk 24.

Chronic hepatitis C infection (genotype 1) compensated liver disease (in those without cirrhosis, previous partial responders/ relapsers to interferon and ribavirin therapy)

• **Adults: PO** Before starting therapy with boceprevir, peginterferon alfa and ribavirin must be given for 4 wk; then add boceprevir 800 mg (four 200 mg caps) PO TID (every 7-9 hours). Treatment length is determined by HCV RNA concentrations at treatment wk 8, 12, and 24. If patient has undetectable HCV RNA concentrations at wks 8 and 24, discontinue all 3 medications at wk 36. If HCV RNA is detectable at wk 8 but undetectable at wk 24, continue the 3-drug regimen through wk 36 and then administer only peginterferon alfa and ribavirin through treatment wk 48. Discontinue the 3-drug regimen if the patient has an HCV RNA concentration >100 international units/ml at treatment wk 12 or a detectable HCA RNA concentration at treatment wk 24. It is recommended to continue all 3 medications through wk 48 if the response prior to treatment with peginterferon alfa and ribavirin was <2-log reduction in HCV RNA at wk 12.

Chronic hepatitis C infection (genotype 1) compensated liver disease with cirrhosis

• **Adults: PO** Before starting therapy with boceprevir; peginterferon alfa and ribavirin must be given for 4 wk; then add boceprevir 800 mg (four 200 mg caps) PO TID (every 7-9 hours) to peginterferon alfa and ribavirin for an additional 44 wk (48 wk total)

Available forms: Caps 200 mg

Administer:

• Only use in combination with peginterferon alfa and ribavirin; never give as monotherapy.

• Discontinue in hepatitis C virus (HCV) if RNA concentrations ≥100 international units/ml at wk 12 or a confirmed detectable HCV RNA concentrations at wk 24

• Any contraindication to peginterferon alfa or ribavirin also applies to boceprevir. See ribavirin or peginterferon alfa monographs for additional information regarding contraindications and warnings associated with these products

• Give with food

SIDE EFFECTS

When used in combination with peginterferon/ribavarin

CNS: *Fatigue, chills, asthenia*, insomnia, irritability, dizziness

GI: Nausea, vomiting, diarrhea, dysgeusia, decreased appetite, xerostomia

HEMA: Anemia (Hgb <10 g/dL), neutropenia, thrombocytopenia

INTEG: *Alopecia, rash*, xerosis

MISC: *Arthralgia, exertional dyspnea*

INTERACTIONS

⚠ **Increase:** life-threatening reactions of each product: alfuzosin, ergots (dihydroergotamine, ergotamine, ergonovine, methylergonovine), cisapride, pimozide, lovastatin, simvastatin, ezetimibe, niacin with simvastatin and boceprevir; triazolam, oral midazolam; sildenafil, tadalafil (pulmonary arterial hypertension); do not use concurrently

Increase: adverse reactions of each product—phosphodiesterase type 5 (PDE5) inhibitors (for erectile dysfunction), acetaminophen, alfentanil, aliskiren, almotriptan, alosetron, alprazolam, aminophylline, amiodarone, amitriptyline, amlodipine, aripiprazole, astemizole, atorvastatin, atorvastin, bepridil, boceprevir, bosentan, budesonide, bupivacaine, buprenorphine, buspirone, carvedilol, cevimeline, chloroquine, cilostazol, cinacalcet, citalopram, clarithromycin, clomipramine, clonazepam, clopidogrel, clozapine, colchicine, cyclobenzaprine, cyclosporine, dapsone, daunorubicin, desipramine, desloratadine, dexamethasone, dexlansoprazole, dextromethorphan, diazepam, diclofenac, digoxin, diltiazem, disopyramide, disulfiram, docetaxel, dolasetron, donepezil, doxorubicin, droperidol, dutasteride, ebastine, eletriptan, eplerenone, erlotinib, erythromycin, estazolam, eszopiclone, ethosuximide, etoposide, exemestane, felodipine, fentaNYL, fexofenadine, finasteride, flecainide, flunitrazepam, flurazepam, galantamine, gefitinib, glyburide, granisetron, halofantrine, haloperidol, hydrocodone, ifosfamide, imipramine, indiplon, irinotecan, isradipine, itraconazole, ivermectin, ixabepilone, ketoconazole, lansoprazole, lidocaine, loperamide, loratadine, losartan, maraviroc, mefloquine, meloxicam, mirtazapine, mitomycin, montelukast, morphine, nateglinide, niCARdipine, NIFEdipine, nisoldipine, nortriptyline, omeprazole, ondansetron, oxybutynin, oxycodone, paclitaxel, palonosetron, paricalcitol, plicamycin, posaconazole, prasugrel, praziquantel, propafenone, quazepam, quetiapine, quinacrine, quinidine, ramelteon, repaglinide, rifabutin, risperidone, ropivacaine, salmeterol, selegiline, sertraline, sibutramine, silodosin, sirolimus, sitaxsentan, solifenacin, SUFentanil, sunitinib, systemic corticosteroids, tacrolimus, telithromycin, teniposide, terfenadine, testosterone, theophylline, tiagabine, tinidazole, tolterodine, tolvaptan, tramadol, trazodone, vardenafil, venlafaxine, verapamil, vinBLAStine, vinCRIStine, voriconazole, warfarin, and others; use cautiously, may need to reduce dose

Increase: hyperkalemia—drospirenone

Decrease: estrogen levels—ethinyl estradiol

Decrease: boceprevir effect—CYP3A4 inhibitors (phenytoin, carBAMazepine, phenobarbital, rifampin)

Decrease: effect of—methadone

Possible treatment failure: efavirenz, ritonavir, atazanavir, lopinavir with ritonavir

Drug/Herb

- Do not use with St. John's wort

NURSING CONSIDERATIONS

Assess:

⚠ **Pregnancy: obtain a pregnancy test prior to, monthly during, and for 6 mo after treatment is completed; those who are not willing to practice strict contraception should not receive treatment with these products; report any cases of prenatal ribavirin exposure to the Ribavirin Pregnancy registry at (800) 593-2214**

- **Anemia:** monitor hemoglobin prior to, at treatment wk 4, 8, 12, and as needed. If Hgb is <10 g/dL, decrease ribavirin dosage; if Hgb is <8.5 g/dL, discontinuation of therapy is recommended; boceprevir dosage should not be altered based on adverse reactions; anemia may be managed through ribavirin dose modifications; never alter the dose of boceprevir. If anemia persists despite a reduction in ribavirin dose, consider discontinuing boceprevir. If management of anemia requires permanent discontinuation of ribavirin, treatment with boceprevir MUST also be permanently discontinued. Once boceprevir has been discontinued, it must not be restarted; monitor CBC with differential at treatment wk 4, 8, 12, and at other treatment points as needed

Teach patient/family:

- To use 2 forms of effective contraception (intrauterine devices and barrier methods) during treatment and for 6 mo after treatment (pregnancy X), to avoid breastfeeding

boric acid otic

See Appendix B

bortezomib (Rx)

(bor-tez′oh-mib)

Velcade

Func. class.: Antineoplastic—miscellaneous

Chem. class.: Proteasome inhibitor

ACTION:

Reversible inhibitor of chymotrypsin-like activity in mammalian cells; causes delay in tumor growth by disrupting normal homeostatic mechanisms

USES:

Multiple myeloma previously untreated or when at least 2 other treatments have failed; mantle cell lymphoma who have received ≥1 prior therapy

Unlabeled uses: Non-Hodgkin's lymphoma (NHL)

CONTRAINDICATIONS:

Pregnancy (D), breastfeeding; hypersensitivity to product, boron, mannitol

Precautions: Children, geriatric patients, peripheral neuropathy, renal/hepatic disease, hypotension, tumor lysis syndrome, thrombocytopenia, infection, diabetes mellitus, bone marrow suppression

DOSAGE AND ROUTES

Multiple myeloma (previously untreated)

• **Adult: IV BOL** Give for nine 6-wk cycles; cycles 1-4, 1.3 mg/m²/dose given on days 1, 4, 8, 11, then a 10-day rest period (days 12-21), then give again on days 22, 25, 29, 32, then a 10-day rest period (days 33-42); given with melphalan (9 mg/m²/day on days 1-4) and predniSONE (60 mg/m²/day on days 1-4); during cycles 5-9, give bortezomib 1.3 mg/m²/dose on days 1, 8, 22, 29 with melphalan (9 mg/m²/day on days 1-4) and predniSONE (60 mg/m²/day on days 1-4); this 6-wk cycle is considered 1 course; at least 72 hr should elapse between consecutive doses

Mantle cell lymphoma

• **Adult: IV BOL** 1.3 mg/m²/dose on days 1, 4, 8, 11 followed by a 10-day rest period (days 12 to 21); max 8 cycles

Hepatic dose

• **Adult: IV** bilirubin >1.5 × ULN, reduce to 0.7 mg/m² during cycle 1; consider dose escalation to 1 mg/m² or further reduction to 0.5 mg/m² during next cycles based on tolerability

Non-Hodgkin's Lymphoma (unlabeled)

• **Adult: IV BOL** 1.3 mg/m² on days 1, 4, 8, 11 repeated q21 days

Available forms: Lyophilized powder for inj 3.5 mg

Administer:

IV bolus route:

• **Reconstitute** each vial with 3.5 ml of 0.9% NaCl (1 mg/ml); sol should be clear/colorless; **inj** as bolus over 3-5 sec

• Wear protective clothing during handling, preparation; avoid contact with skin

SIDE EFFECTS

CNS: Anxiety, insomnia, dizziness, headache, *peripheral neuropathy,* rigors, paresthesia

CV: *Hypotension,* edema, CHF

GI: Abdominal pain, *constipation, diarrhea,* dyspepsia, nausea, *vomiting,* anorexia

HEMA: *Anemia,* neutropenia, thrombocytopenia
MISC: Dehydration, weight loss, herpes zoster, rash, pruritus, blurred vision
MS: *Fatigue, malaise, weakness,* arthralgia, bone pain, muscle cramps, myalgia, back pain, tumor lysis syndrome
RESP: Cough, pneumonia, dyspnea, URI

PHARMACOKINETICS

Half-life 9-15 hr, protein binding 83%, metabolized by CYP450 enzymes (3A4, 2D6, 2C19, 2C9, 1A2)

INTERACTIONS

- Do not use hematopoietic progenitor cells (sargramostim, GM-CSF, filgrastim, G-CSF) within 24 hr of chemotherapy
- Oral hypoglycemics: may result in hypo/hyperglycemia

Increase: risk for bleeding—anticoagulants, NSAIDs, platelet inhibitors, salicylates, thrombolytics
Increase: hypotension—antihypertensives
Increase: peripheral neuropathy—amiodarone, antivirals (amprenavir; atazanavir; didanosine, lamiVUDine, 3TC; ritonavir; stavudine, zidovudine), chloramphenicol, CISplatin, colchicine, cycloSPORINE, dapsone, disulfiram, docetaxel, gold salts, HMG-CoA reductase inhibitors, iodoquinol, INH, metroNIDAZOLE, nitrofurantoin, oxaliplatin, paclitaxel, penicillamine, phenytoin, sulfasalazine, thalidomide, vinBLAStine, vinCRIStine, zalcitabine ddc, isoniazid, statins, others
Increase: toxicity or decrease efficacy when administered with products that induce or inhibit CYP3A4
Drug/Herb
Increase: toxicity or decrease efficacy—St. John's wort

NURSING CONSIDERATIONS

Assess:
- Hematologic status: platelets, CBC throughout treatment; platelets $\geq 70 \times 10^9$/L and ANC $\geq 1.0 \times 10^9$/L before any cycle; nonhematologic toxicities should be grade 1 or baseline before any cycle
- For extravasation at inj site
- B/P, fluid status, peripheral neuropathy symptoms

Evaluate:
- Therapeutic response: improvement of multiple myeloma symptoms

Teach patient/family:
- To use contraception while taking this product (pregnancy [D]); to avoid breastfeeding
- To monitor blood glucose levels if diabetic
- To contact prescriber about new or worsening peripheral neuropathy, severe vomiting, diarrhea, easy bruising, bleeding, infection
- To avoid driving, operating machinery until effect is known
- To avoid using other medications unless approved by prescriber

bosentan (Rx)

(boh′sen-tan)

Tracleer

Func. class.: Vasodilator
Chem. class.: Endothelin receptor antagonist

ACTION:
Peripheral vasodilation occurs via the antagonism of the effect of endothelin on endothelium and vascular smooth muscle

USES:
Pulmonary arterial hypertension with WHO class III, IV symptoms
Unlabeled uses: Septic shock to improve microcirculatory blood flow, functional class II pulmonary arterial hypertension

CONTRAINDICATIONS:
Pregnancy (X), hypersensitivity, CVA, CAD
Precautions: Breastfeeding, children, geriatric patients, mitral stenosis
Black Box Warning: Hepatic disease

DOSAGE AND ROUTES

- **Adult and adolescent >40 kg: PO** 62.5 mg bid × 4 wk then 125 mg bid
- **Adult and adolescent <40 kg: PO** 62.5 mg bid

Available forms: Tabs 62.5, 125 mg

Administer:

- Give without regard to meals
- Only available through the TAP program
- Do not stop product abruptly; taper

SIDE EFFECTS

CNS: Headache, flushing, fatigue, fever
CV: *Hypo/hypertension,* palpitations, edema of lower limbs
GI: Abnormal hepatic function, diarrhea, dyspepsia, **hepatotoxicity**
HEMA: Anemia, leukopenia, neutropenia, lymphopenia, thrombocytopenia
INTEG: Pruritus, **anaphylaxis,** rash, **Stevens-Johnson syndrome, toxic epidermal necrolysis**
MISC: Oligospermia, tumor lysis syndrome
SYST: Secondary malignancy

PHARMACOKINETICS

Metabolized by and an inducer of CYP2C9, CYP3A4, possibly CYP2C19; metabolized by the liver; terminal half-life 5 hr; steady state 3-5 days

INTERACTIONS

- Do not coadminister cycloSPORINE with bosentan; bosentan is increased, cycloSPORINE is decreased
- Do not coadminister glyBURIDE with bosentan; glyBURIDE is decreased significantly, bosentan is also decreased, hepatic enzymes may be increased

Increase: bosentan effects—CYP2C9, CYP3A4 inhibitors
Increase: bosentan level—ketoconazole
Decrease: effects of warfarin, hormonal contraceptives, statins

Drug/Lab Test
Increase: ALT, AST
Decrease: Hgb, Hct

NURSING CONSIDERATIONS

Assess:

- **Serious skin toxicities:** Stevens-Johnson syndrome, toxic epidermal necrolysis
- B/P, pulse during treatment until stable
- Blood studies: Hct, Hgb may be decreased
- **Hepatic toxicity:** vomiting, jaundice; product should be discontinued; hepatic studies: AST, ALT, bilirubin; hepatic enzymes may increase; if ALT/AST >3× and ≤5× ULN, decrease dose or interrupt treatment and monitor AST/ALT q2wk; if bilirubin >2× ULN or signs of hepatitis or hepatic disease are present, stop treatment

Perform/provide:

- Storage at room temp

Evaluate:

- Therapeutic response: decrease in pulmonary hypertension

Teach patient/family:

- To report jaundice, dark urine, joint pain, fatigue, malaise, bruising, easy bleeding; may indicate blood dyscrasias
- To avoid pregnancy; to use nonhormonal form of contraception
- That lab work will be required periodically

brentuximab

(bren-tuk′see-mab)

Adcetris

Func. class.: Monoclonal antibody; antineoplastic

ACTION: The anticancer activity is due to the binding of the ADC to CD30-expressing cells, followed by the internalization and transportation of the ADC-CD30 complex to lysosomes and the release of MMAE via selective proteolytic cleavage. MMAE binds to tubulin and disrupts the microtubule network within the cell, inducing cell cycle arrest and apoptotic death of the cells

USES:
For the treatment of Hodgkin's disease after failure of autologous stem cell transplant (ASCT) or after failure of at least 2 prior multi-agent chemotherapy regimens in patients who are not ASCT candidates; for the treatment of non-Hodgkin's lymphoma (NHL); for the treatment of systemic anaplastic large cell lymphoma (sALCL) after failure of at least 1 prior multi-agent chemotherapy regimen

CONTRAINDICATIONS
Hypersensitivity, pregnancy (category D)

Precautions: Breastfeeding, children, infants, neonates, neutropenia, peripheral neuropathy, tumor lysis syndrome (TLS)

Black Box Warning: Progressive multifocal leukoencephalopathy (PML)

DOSAGE AND ROUTES

- **Adult:** **IV** 1.8 mg/kg over 30 min every 3 wk until a maximum of 16 cycles, disease progression, or unacceptable toxicity. For patients >100 kg, max weight used for dosage calculation should be 100 kg, which translates to no more than 180 mg/dose

Dose adjustments for toxicity due to peripheral neuropathy:

- For grade <3: no dosage adjustments are recommended; for new or worsening grade 2-3: interrupt treatment until toxicity resolves to grade ≤1; when resuming treatment, reduce dosage to 1.2 mg/kg IV q3wk; for grade 4: discontinue treatment

Dose adjustments for toxicity due to neutropenia:

- For neutropenia grade <3: no dosage adjustments; for grade 3-4 neutropenia: interrupt treatment until toxicity resolves to baseline or grade ≤2; consider the use of growth factors (CSFs) for subsequent cycles of therapy; for grade 4 neutropenia despite the use of growth factors: discontinue treatment or reduce the dose to 1.2 mg/kg IV q3wk

Available forms: Powder for inj 50 mg

Administer:

Intermittent IV INF route

- Visually inspect for particulate matter and discoloration whenever sol and container permit
- Only as an IV inf, do not give as an IV push or bolus
- Use cytotoxic handling procedures
- Do not mix, or administer as an infusion, with other IV products
- Calculate the dose (mg) and the number of vials required. For patients weighing >100 kg, use 100 kg to calculate the dose; reconstitute each 50-mg vial per 10.5 ml of sterile water for inj (5 mg/ml)
- Direct the stream of sterile water toward the wall of the vial and not directly at the cake or powder; gently swirl the vial to aid in dissolution, do not shake
- Discard any unused portion left in the vial
- After reconstitution, dilute immediately with ≥100 ml of 0.9% sodium chloride, 5% dextrose, or lactated ringers solution to a final concentration (0.4 mg/ml-1.8 mg/ml)
- Infuse over 30 min

SIDE EFFECTS

CNS: Headache, dizziness, fever, peripheral neuropathy, anxiety, chills, confusion, fatigue, paresthesias, insomnia, night sweats

CV: Peripheral edema, supraventricular arrhythmia

GI: Abdominal pain, nausea, vomiting, constipation, diarrhea, weight loss

INTEG: Rash, pruritus, alopecia, xerosis

RESP: **Pneumothorax, pneumonitis, pulmonary embolism,** dyspnea, cough

SYST: **Anaphylaxis, tumor lysis syndrome,** antibody formation, **Stevens-Johnson Syndrome**

PHARMACOKINETICS

Protein binding is 68%-82%, only a small amount is metabolized; potent inhibitors or inducers of CYP3A4 may alter action; ADC peak at end of infusion; MME peak 1-3 days; terminal half-life is 4–6 days; 3 components are released: MMAE (monomethyl auristatin E), ADC, and the total antibody; the half-life of MMAE a component is 3.43-3.6 days

INTERACTIONS

Increase: brentuximab component action: ketoconazole, boceprevir, delavirdine, isoniazid, indinavir, itraconazole, dalfopristin; quinupristin, telithromycin, tipranavir, rifampin, ritonavir
Increase non-infectious pulmonary toxicity: bleomycin, do not use together
Drug/Herb
• Increased brentuximab component action: St. John's Wort

NURSING CONSIDERATIONS

Assess:
• Tumor lysis syndrome (TLS): assess for hyperkalemia, hypophosphatemia, hypocalcemia; may develop renal failure may use allopurinol or rasburicase to prevent TLS; monitor serum BUN/creatinine
• Pregnancy: determine if pregnancy is planned or suspected, pregnancy category D
• Peripheral neuropathy: Progressive multifocal leukoencephalopathy (PML): Assess for weakness, or paralysis, vision loss, impaired speech, and cognitive deterioration; often fatal
• Monitor CBC, serum
Perform/provide:
• Use the diluted sol immediately or store in refrigerator for ≤24 hr after reconstitution; do not freeze
Evaluate:
• Decreasing symptoms of Hodgkin's disease (increased lymph nodes, night sweats, weight loss, splenomegaly, hepatomegaly)
Teach patient/family:
• To report immediately weakness, change in vision, impaired speech
• To use reliable contraception (pregnancy D); to avoid breastfeeding

brimonidine ophthalmic

See Appendix B

brinzolamide ophthalmic

See Appendix B

bromfenac ophthalmic

See Appendix B

bromocriptine (Rx)

(broe-moe-krip′teen)

Apo-Bromocriptine ♣, Cycloset, Parlodel, PMS-Bromocriptine ♣

Func. class.: Dopamine receptor agonist, antiparkinson agent

Chem. class.: Ergot alkaloid derivative

Do not confuse:
Parlodel/pindolol/Provera

ACTION: Inhibits prolactin release by activating postsynaptic dopamine receptors; activation of striatal dopamine receptors may be reason for improvement in Parkinson's disease

USES: Parkinson's disease, amenorrhea/galactorrhea caused by hyperprolactinemia, infertility, acromegaly, pituitary adenomas, adjunct for type 2 diabetes
Unlabeled uses: Neuroleptic malignant syndrome, alcoholism, premenstrual syndrome, mastalgia, cocaine withdrawal, premenstrual breast symptoms

CONTRAINDICATIONS:

Severe ischemic disease, uncontrolled hypertension, severe peripheral vascular disease; hypersensitivity to ergot, bromocriptine; migraine, preeclampsia

Precautions: Pregnancy (B), breastfeeding, children, renal/hepatic disease, pituitary tumors, peptic ulcer disease, sulfite hypersensitivity, pulmonary fibrosis, dementia, GI bleeding, bipolar disorder

DOSAGE AND ROUTES

Hyperprolactinemia

- **Adult: PO** 1.25-2.5 mg with meals; may increase by 2.5 mg q3-7days, usual range 2.5-15 mg/day

Acromegaly

- **Adult: PO** 1.25-2.5 mg × 3 days at bedtime; may increase by 1.25-2.5 mg q3-7days; usual range 20-30 mg/day, max 100 mg/day

Parkinson's disease

- **Adult: PO** 1.25 mg bid with meals; may increase q2-4wk by 2.5 mg/day, max 100 mg/day; levodopa should be continued while bromocriptine is being instituted

Pituitary adenoma

- **Adult: PO** 1.25 mg bid-tid; may increase over several wk to 10-20 mg/day

Type 2 diabetes (Cycloset only)

- **Adult: PO** (initially) 0.8 mg daily in AM within 2 hr of waking; titrate by 0.8 mg/day no more than q wk to max 1.6-4.8 mg/day

Neuroleptic malignant syndrome (unlabeled)

- **Adult: PO** 2.5-10 mg tid

Cocaine withdrawal (unlabeled)

- **Adult: PO** 0.625 mg qid × 42 days

Alcoholism (unlabeled)

- **Adult: PO** 7.5 mg/day

Mastalgia (unlabeled)

- **Adult: PO** 2.5-7.5 bid starting 10-14 days before menses; discontinue when menses begins

Available forms: Caps 5 mg; tabs 2.5 mg; Cycloset tabs 0.8 mg

Administer:

- With meal to prevent GI symptoms
- At bedtime so that dizziness, orthostatic hypotension do not occur

SIDE EFFECTS

CNS: *Headache,* depression, restlessness, anxiety, nervousness, confusion, **seizures,** *hallucinations,* dizziness, fatigue, drowsiness, abnormal involuntary movements, psychosis

CV: Orthostatic hypotension, decreased B/P, palpitations, extrasystole, **shock,** dysrhythmias, bradycardia, **MI**

EENT: Blurred vision, diplopia, burning eyes, nasal congestion

GI: *Nausea, vomiting, anorexia,* cramps, constipation, diarrhea, dry mouth, GI hemorrhage

GU: Frequency, retention, incontinence, diuresis

INTEG: *Rash on face, arms;* alopecia; coolness, pallor of fingers, toes; peripheral edema

PHARMACOKINETICS

Peak 1-3 hr, duration 4-8 hr, 90%-96% protein bound, half-life 3 hr, metabolized by liver (inactive metabolites), 85%-98% of dose excreted in feces, >90% of absorbed dose undergoes 1st-pass metabolism

INTERACTIONS

- Disulfiram-like reaction: alcohol

Increase: action of antihypertensives, levodopa

Decrease: action of bromocriptine—phenothiazines, oral contraceptives, progestins, estrogens, haloperidol, loxapine, methyldopa, metoclopramide, MAOIs, reserpine

Drug/Lab Test

Increase: growth hormone, AST, ALT, CK, BUN, uric acid, alk phos

NURSING CONSIDERATIONS

Assess:

- B/P; establish baseline, compare with other readings; this product decreases B/P
- **Parkinson's symptoms:** pill rolling, shuffling gait, restlessness, tremors, postural instability before and during treatment
- **Neuroleptic malignant syndrome:** decreased temp, seizures, sweating, pulse indicates resolution of symptoms
- Change in size of soft-tissue volume with acromegaly

Perform/provide:

- Storage at room temp in tight, light-resistant container

Evaluate:

- Therapeutic response (Parkinson's disease): decreased dyskinesia, slow movements, drooling

Teach patient/family:

- That tabs may be crushed, mixed with food
- To change position slowly to prevent orthostatic hypotension
- To use contraceptives during treatment with this product; that pregnancy may occur; to use methods other than oral contraceptives
- That therapeutic effect for Parkinson's disease may take 2 mo
- To avoid hazardous activity if dizziness occurs
- To report symptoms of MI immediately

brompheniramine (Rx)

(brome-fen-ir'a-meen)

Bidhist, BPM, J-Tan PD, Lodrane 24, LoHist-12, Respa-BR, TanaCof-XR, VaZol

Func. class.: Antihistamine

Chem. class.: Alkylamine, H_1-receptor antagonist

ACTION: Acts on blood vessels, GI, respiratory system by competing with histamine for H_1-receptor site; decreases allergic response by blocking histamine

USES: Allergy symptoms, rhinitis, urticaria

CONTRAINDICATIONS: Children <2 yr, hypersensitivity to H_1-receptor antagonists, acute asthma attack, lower respiratory tract disease

Precautions: Pregnancy (C), breastfeeding, increased intraocular pressure, renal/cardiac disease, hypertension, bronchial asthma, seizure disorder, stenosed peptic ulcers, hyperthyroidism, prostatic hypertrophy, bladder neck obstruction, closed-angle glaucoma

DOSAGE AND ROUTES

- **Adult and child >12 yr: PO** 4-8 mg q6-8hr, max 24 mg/day; **EXT-REL** 6-12 mg bid-tid, max 24 mg/day
- **Child 6-11 yr: PO** 2 mg q6-8hr, max 12 mg/day; **EXT REL** 6-12 mg/day
- **Child 2-5 yr:** 1 mg q6-8hr, max 6 mg/day

Available forms: Tabs 4 mg; elix 2 mg/5 ml; caps 4 mg; chew tabs 12 mg; ext rel tabs 6 mg; ext rel caps 12 mg; liquid 8 mg, 12 mg/5 ml

Administer:

PO route

- Do not break, crush, chew ext rel forms
- With meals if GI symptoms occur; absorption may slightly decrease

SIDE EFFECTS

CNS: *Dizziness, drowsiness,* poor coordination, fatigue, anxiety, euphoria, confusion, paresthesia, neuritis, paradoxical excitation (children, elderly)

CV: Hypotension, palpitations, tachycardia

EENT: Blurred vision, dilated pupils, tinnitus, nasal stuffiness; dry nose, throat, mouth

GI: Nausea, vomiting, anorexia, constipation, diarrhea

GU: Retention, dysuria, frequency, impotence
HEMA: Thrombocytopenia, agranulocytosis, hemolytic anemia (rare)
INTEG: Photosensitivity
RESP: Thick secretions, wheezing, chest tightness

PHARMACOKINETICS

PO: Peak 2-5 hr, duration 48 hr; metabolized by liver, excreted by kidneys, excreted in breast milk, half-life 12-34 hr

INTERACTIONS

- Incompatible with aminophylline, insulins, PENTobarbital

Increase: CNS depression—barbiturates, opiates, hypnotics, tricyclics, alcohol
Increase: anticholinergic effect—MAOIs
Drug/Lab Test
Interference: skin allergy tests

NURSING CONSIDERATIONS

Assess:

- Urinary retention, frequency, dysuria; product should be discontinued if these occur
- CBC during long-term therapy
- **Blood dyscrasias:** thrombocytopenia, agranulocytosis (rare) during long-term therapy
- Respiratory status: rate, rhythm, increase in bronchial secretions, wheezing, chest tightness

Perform/provide:

- Hard candy, gum, frequent rinsing of mouth for dryness
- Storage in tight container at room temp

Evaluate:

- Therapeutic response: absence of running, congested nose, rashes

Teach patient/family:

- About all aspects of product use; to notify prescriber if confusion, sedation, hypotension occurs
- To avoid driving, other hazardous activities if drowsiness occurs
- To avoid alcohol, other CNS depressants while taking product

budesonide (Rx)

(byoo-des′oh-nide)

Entocort EC, Gen-Budesonide AQ ✦, Pulmicort, Pulmicort Flexhaler, Rhinocort Aqua

Func. class.: Glucocorticoid
Chem. class.: Nonhalogenated

ACTION: Prevents inflammation by depressing migration of polymorphonuclear leukocytes and fibroblasts, reversal of increased capillary permeability, and lysosomal stabilization; does not suppress hypothalamus or pituitary function

USES: Rhinitis; prophylaxis for asthma; Crohn's disease
Unlabeled uses: Microscopic colitis

CONTRAINDICATIONS: Hypersensitivity, status asthmaticus
Precautions: Pregnancy (C), inhaled form (B); breastfeeding; children; TB; fungal, bacterial, systemic viral infections; ocular herpes simplex; nasal septal ulcers; hepatic disease (caps)

DOSAGE AND ROUTES

Rhinitis (Rhinocort Aqua)

- **Adult and child >12 yr: SPRAY/INH** 256 mcg/day (2 sprays in each nostril AM, PM or 4 sprays in each nostril AM)

Asthma

- **Adult: INH** 360 mcg bid, max 720 mcg bid

Crohn's disease

- **Adult: PO** 9 mg/day AM × 8 wk

Available forms: Dry powder for INH 90, 180, 200 mcg/actuation (Pulmicort Flexhaler); 32 mcg/actuation (Rhinocort Aqua)

Administer:

PO route (Crohn's disease)

- Swallow caps whole; do not break, crush, chew

• May repeat 8-wk course if needed; may taper to 6 mg/day for 2 wk before cessation

Inhalation route (asthma)

• Use scissors to open pouch

SIDE EFFECTS

CNS: *Headache,* insomnia, hypertonia, syncope, dizziness, drowsiness

CV: Chest pain, hypertension, sinus tachycardia, palpitation

EENT: *Sinusitis, pharyngitis,* rhinitis, oral candidiasis

ENDO: Adrenal insufficiency, growth suppression in children

GI: Dry mouth, dyspepsia, nausea, vomiting, abdominal pain

MISC: Ecchymosis, fever, *hypersensitivity,* flulike symptoms, epistaxis, dysuria

MS: Back pain, myalgias, fractures

RESP: Nasal irritation, cough, nasal bleeding, *respiratory infections,* bronchospasm

PHARMACOKINETICS

Peak: Respules 4-6 wk, Rhinocort Aqua 2 wk, half-life 2-3.6 hr

Onset: Respules 2-8 days, Rhinocort Aqua 10 hr

Enters breast milk

INTERACTIONS

• Avoid using with products metabolized by CYP3A4 inhibition

• Avoid concurrent use of varicella live vaccine in pediatric patients

Decrease: budesonide metabolism—ketoconazole, cimetidine

NURSING CONSIDERATIONS

Assess:

• Respiratory status: rate, rhythm, increase in bronchial secretions, wheezing, chest tightness; provide fluids to 2 L/day to decrease thickness of secretions; check for oral candidiasis

• **Bronchospasm:** stop treatment, give bronchodilator

• Viral infections: corticosteroid use can mask infections

• Increased intraocular pressure: discontinue use if this occurs

Perform/provide:

• Storage at 59° F-86° F (15° C-30° C); keep away from heat, open flame

Evaluate:

• Therapeutic response: absence of asthma, rhinitis

Teach patient/family:

• To notify prescriber of pharyngitis, nasal bleeding, oral candidiasis

• Not to exceed recommended dose because adrenal suppression may occur

• To carry emergency ID that identifies steroid use

• To read and follow package directions

• To prevent exposure to infections (especially viral)

• To avoid taking with grapefruit juice (caps PO)

• To use good oral hygiene if using nebulizer or inhaler

• To avoid breastfeeding

• That burning or stinging may occur with first few doses of inhalation use

budesonide nasal agent

See Appendix B

bumetanide (Rx)

(byoo-met′a-nide)

Func. class.: Loop diuretic, antihypertensive

Chem. class.: Sulfonamide derivative

Do not confuse:

Bumex/Buprenex/Permax

ACTION: Acts on ascending loop of Henle by inhibiting reabsorption of chloride, sodium

USES: Edema in CHF, renal/hepatic disease, heart failure

Unlabeled uses: Hypercalcemia, hypertension, ascites

B

CONTRAINDICATIONS:
Hypersensitivity to sulfonamides, anuria, hepatic coma

Black Box Warning: Electrolyte imbalance

Precautions: Pregnancy (C), breastfeeding, neonates, ascites, severe renal disease, hepatic cirrhosis, blood dyscrasias, ototoxicity, hyperuricemia, hypokalemia, hyperglycemia, oliguria, hypomagnesemia, hypovolemia

Black Box Warning: Dehydration

DOSAGE AND ROUTES

- **Adult and adolescent: PO** 0.5-2.0 mg/day; may give 2nd or 3rd dose at 4-5 hr intervals, max 10 mg/day; may be given on alternate days or intermittently; **IV/IM** 0.5-1.0 mg; may give 2nd or 3rd dose at 2-3 hr intervals, not to exceed 10 mg/day
- **Child and infant (unlabeled): PO/IM/IV** 0.015-0.1 mg/kg daily or every other day, max 10 mg/day

Hypercalcemia (unlabeled)

- **Adult: IV** 1-2 mg q1-4hr to maintain urine output of 200-250 ml/hr; give saline before 1st dose of this product

Hypertension (unlabeled)

- **Adult and adolescent: PO** 0.5-2 mg/day, max 10 mg/day in 2 divided doses

Available forms: Tabs 0.5, 1, 2 mg; inj 0.25 mg/ml

Administer:

- In AM to avoid interference with sleep if using product as a diuretic; without regard to meals
- Potassium replacement if potassium is <3.0

PO route

- With food if nausea occurs; absorption may be decreased slightly

IV, direct route

- Direct IV undiluted slowly over 1-2 min through Y-tube, 3-way stopcock, or heplock

Intermittent IV INF route

- Dilute in LR, D_5W, 0.9% NaCl (rarely given by this method), give over 12 hr with renal disease

Syringe compatibilities: Doxapram

Y-site compatibilities: Acyclovir, alfentanil, allopurinol, amifostine, amikacin, aminocaproic acid, aminophylline, amiodarone, amoxicillin, amphotericin B lipid complex (Abelcet), amphotericin B liposome (AmBisome), anidulafungin, ascorbic acid injection, atenolol, atracurium, atropine, aztreonam, benztropine, bivalirudin, bleomycin, buprenorphine, butorphanol, calcium chloride/gluconate, CARBOplatin, caspofungin, cefamandole, cefazolin, cefepime, cefmetazole, cefonicid, cefoperazone, cefotaxime, cefotetan, cefoxitin, ceftazidime, ceftizoxime, ceftobiprole, cefTRIAXone, cefuroxime, cephalothin, cephapirin, chloramphenicol, cimetidine, cisatracurium, CISplatin, cladribine, clarithromycin, clindamycin, codeine, cyanocobalamin, cyclophosphamide, cycloSPORINE, cytarabine, DACTINomycin, DAPTOmycin, dexamethasone, dexmedetomidine, digoxin, diltiazem, diphenhydrAMINE, DOBUTamine, docetaxel, DOPamine, doripenem, doxacurium, DOXOrubicin, doxycycline, enalaprilat, ePHEDrine, EPINEPHrine, epirubicin, epoetin alfa, eptifibatide, ertapenem, erythromycin, esmolol, etoposide, famotidine, fentaNYL, filgrastim, fluconazole, fludarabine, fluorouracil, folic acid, furosemide, gatifloxacin, gemcitabine, gentamicin, glycopyrrolate, granisetron, heparin, hydrocortisone sodium succinate, HYDROmorphone, hydrOXYzine, IDArubicin, ifosfamide, imipenem-cilastatin, indomethacin, insulin (regular), irinotecan, isoproterenol, ketorolac, labetalol, levofloxacin, lidocaine, linezolid, LORazepam, magnesium sulfate, mannitol, mechlorethamine, melphalan, meperidine, metaraminol, methotrexate, methoxamine, methyldopate, methylPREDNISolone, metoclopramide, metoprolol, metroNIDAZOLE, mezlocillin, micafungin, miconazole, milrinone, mitoxantrone, morphine, moxalactam, multiple vitamins injection, mycophenolate, nafcillin, nalbuphine, naloxone, netilmicin, nitroglycerin, nitroprusside, norepinephrine, octreotide, ondansetron, oxacillin, oxaliplatin, oxytocin, palonosetron, pamidronate, pancuronium, pantoprazole, pemetrexed, penicillin G potassium/sodium, pentazocine, PENTobarbital, PHENobarbital, phenylephrine, phytonadione, piperacillin, piperacillin-tazobactam, polymyxin B, potassium chloride, procainamide, promethazine, propofol, propranolol, protamine, pyridoxine, quiNIDine, ranitidine, remifentanil, rifampin, ritodrine, riTUXimab, rocuronium, sodium acetate, sodium bicarbonate, succinylcholine, SUFentanil, tacrolimus, teniposide, theophylline, thiamine, thiotepa, ticarcillin, ticarcillin-clavulanate, tigecycline, tirofiban, TNA, tobramycin, tolazoline, TPN, tramadol, trastuzumab, trimetaphan, urokinase, vancomycin, vasopressin, vecuronium, verapamil, vinCRIStine, vinorelbine, voriconazole

SIDE EFFECTS

CNS: *Headache,* fatigue, weakness, *dizziness,* encephalopathy
CV: Chest pain, *hypotension,* circulatory collapse, ECG changes, dehydration
EENT: *Loss of hearing*
ELECT: *Hypokalemia, hypochloremic alkalosis, hypomagnesemia, hyperuricemia, hypocalcemia, hyponatremia*
ENDO: *Hyperglycemia*
GI: *Nausea,* diarrhea, dry mouth, vomiting, anorexia, cramps, upset stomach, abdominal pain, acute pancreatitis, jaundice
GU: *Polyuria,* renal failure, glycosuria, premature ejaculation, hypercholesterolemia
HEMA: Thrombocytopenia, leukopenia, granulocytopenia, hemoconcentration
INTEG: *Rash, pruritus,* purpura, Stevens-Johnson syndrome, sweating, photosensitivity
MS: Muscular cramps, arthritis, stiffness

PHARMACOKINETICS

Excreted by kidneys (50% unchanged), feces (20%); crosses placenta; excreted in breast milk; protein binding >96%; half-life 1-1½ hr, 6-15 hr in neonates
PO: Onset ½-1 hr, peak 1-2 hr, duration 3-6 hr
IM: Onset 40 min, peak 1-2 hr, duration 4-6 hr
IV: Onset 5 min, peak 15-30 min, duration 3-6 hr

INTERACTIONS

- Ototoxicity: aminoglycosides
- Hypokalemia: potassium-wasting products

Increase: toxicity—lithium, digoxin
Increase: diuresis, electrolyte loss—metolazone
Decrease: diuretic effect—indomethacin, NSAIDs, probenecid
Decrease: antidiabetic effects—antidiabetics
Drug/Herb
Increase: effect—hawthorn, horse chestnut
Decrease: effect of bumetanide—ginseng, ephedra

NURSING CONSIDERATIONS

Assess:

- For tinnitus; obtain audiometric testing for long-term IV treatment
- Weight, I&O daily to determine fluid loss; if urinary output decreases or azotemia occurs, product should be discontinued; safest dosage schedule is alternate days
- B/P lying, standing; postural hypotension may occur

Black Box Warning: Electrolyte imbalances: K, Na, Cl; include BUN, blood glucose, CBC, serum creatinine, blood pH, ABGs, uric acid, Ca, Mg; severe electrolyte imbalances should be corrected before starting treatment

- Blood glucose if patient is diabetic; blood uric acid levels in those with gout
- Improvement in edema of feet, legs, sacral area daily if medication is being used for CHF
- Signs of metabolic alkalosis: drowsiness, restlessness

• Signs of hypokalemia: postural hypotension, malaise, fatigue, tachycardia, leg cramps, weakness
• Rashes, temp elevation daily
• Confusion, especially in geriatric patients; take safety precautions if needed
• **Digoxin toxicity** in patients taking digoxin products: anorexia, nausea, vomiting, confusion, paresthesia, muscle cramps; **lithium toxicity** in those taking lithium

Evaluate:
• Therapeutic response: decreased edema, B/P

Teach patient/family:
• To increase fluid intake to 2-3 L/day unless contraindicated; to take potassium supplement; to rise slowly from lying or sitting position
• To recognize adverse reactions: muscle cramps, weakness, nausea, dizziness
• To take with food, milk for GI symptoms; to avoid alcohol
• To take early in day to prevent nocturia
• To use sunscreen to prevent photosensitivity

TREATMENT OF OVERDOSE:
Lavage if taken orally; monitor electrolytes; administer dextrose in saline; monitor hydration, CV, renal status

buprenorphine (Rx)
(byoo-pre-nor′feen)

Buprenex, Butrans

Func. class.: Opioid analgesic, partial agonist

Chem. class.: Thebaine derivative

Controlled Substance Schedule V (Parenteral); Schedule III (Tablet, TD)

Do not confuse:
Buprenex/Bumex

ACTION: Depresses pain impulse transmission at the spinal cord level by interacting with opioid receptors

USES: Moderate to severe pain, opiate agonist withdrawal

Unlabeled uses: Cocaine withdrawal

CONTRAINDICATIONS: Hypersensitivity, ileus

Precautions: Pregnancy (C), breastfeeding, substance abuse/alcoholism, increased intracranial pressure, MI (acute), severe heart disease, respiratory depression, renal/hepatic/pulmonary disease, hypothyroidism, Addison's disease

Black Box Warning: QT prolongation, use of heating pad

DOSAGE AND ROUTES
• **Adult: IM/IV** 0.3 mg q6hr prn, reduce dosage in geriatric patients, may repeat after 30-60 min; **EPIDURAL** (unlabeled) 4 mcg/kg or 2 mcg/kg (epidural inj); **TD** each patch is worn for 7 days (moderate-severe pain); **opioid-naive patients** (those taking <30 mg of oral morphine or equivalent before beginning treatment with TD buprenorphine), 5 mcg/hr q7days, overestimating dose can be fatal; **conversion from other opiate agonist therapy,** titrate from other opioids for up to 7 days to no more than 30 mg oral morphine or equivalent before beginning TD therapy, begin with 5 mcg/hr q7days; for those with daily dose of 30-80 mg oral morphine or equivalent, start with 10 mcg/hr q7days; for those taking >80 mg oral morphine or equivalent, start with 20 mcg/hr q7days
• **Child 2-12 yr: IM/IV** 2-6 mcg/kg q4-6hr

Available forms: Inj 0.3 mg/ml (1-ml vials); SL tab 2, 8 mg as base; TD system 5, 10, 20 mcg/hr (weekly)

Administer:
• Long-term use not recommended

Transdermal route

- Apply to clean, dry, intact skin; each patch should be worn for 7 days; do not apply direct heat source to patch, will increase absorption of product
- Apply to upper outer arm, upper chest/back, or side of chest

IM route

- In deep muscle mass

IV, direct route

- **Give** undiluted over 2 min, titrate to patient response
- With antiemetic if nausea, vomiting occur
- When pain is beginning to return; determine dosage interval by patient response

Additive compatibilities: Bupivacaine, glycopyrrolate, haloperidol

Syringe compatibilities: Glycopyrrolate, haloperidol, heparin, midazolam

Y-site compatibilities: Acyclovir, alfentanil, allopurinol, amifostine, amikacin, aminocaproic acid, amphotericin B liposome (AmBisone), anidulafungin, ascorbic acid injection, atenolol, atracurium, atropine, aztreonam, benztropine, bivalirudin, bleomycin, bumetanide, butorphanol, calcium chloride/gluconate, CARBOplatin, cefamandole, cefazolin, cefepime, cefmetazole, cefonicid, cefoperazone, cefotaxime, cefotetan, cefoxitin, ceftazidime, ceftizoxime, cefTRIAXone, cefuroxime, cephalothin, cephapirin, chloramphenicol, chlorproMAZINE, cimetidine, cisatracurium, CISplatin, cladribine, clindamycin, cyanocobalamin, cyclophosphamide, cycloSPORINE, cytarabine, D_5W-dextrose 5%, DACTINomycin, DAPTOmycin, dexamethasone, dexmedetomidine, digoxin, diltiazem, diphenhydrAMINE, DOBUTamine, docetaxel, DOPamine, doxacurium, DOXOrubicin HCl, doxycycline, enalaprilat, ePHEDrine, EPINEPHrine, epirubicin, epoetin alfa, eptifibatide, ertapenem, erythromycin, esmolol, etoposide, famotidine, fenoldopam, fentaNYL, filgrastim, fluconazole, fludarabine, gatifloxacin, gemcitabine, gentamicin, glycopyrrolate, granisetron, heparin, hydrocortisone, hydrOXYzine, IDArubicin, ifosfamide, imipenem-cilastatin, inamrinone, insulin (regular), irinotecan, isoproterenol, ketorolac, labetalol, lactated Ringer's injection, levofloxacin, lidocaine, linezolid, LORazepam, magnesium sulfate, mannitol, mechlorethamine, melphalan, meperidine, metaraminol, methicillin, methotrexate, methoxamine, methyldopate, methylPREDNISolone, metoclopramide, metoprolol, metroNIDAZOLE, mezlocillin, miconazole, midazolam, milrinone, minocycline, mitoxantrone, morphine, moxalactam, multiple vitamins injection, mycophenolate mofetil, nafcillin, nalbuphine, naloxone, nesiritide, netilmicin, nitroglycerin, nitroprusside, norepinephrine, octreotide, ondansetron, oxacillin, oxaliplatin, oxytocin, palonosetron, pamidronate, pancuronium, papaverine, pemetrexed, penicillin G potassium/sodium, pentamidine, pentazocine, phenylephrine, phytonadione, piperacillin, piperacillin-tazobactam, polymyxin B, potassium chloride, procainamide, prochlorperazine, promethazine, propofol, propranolol, protamine, pyridoxine, quiNIDine, ranitidine, remifentanil, Ringer's injection, ritodrine, riTUXimab, rocuronium, sodium acetate, succinylcholine, SUFentanil, tacrolimus, teniposide, theophylline, thiamine, thiotepa, ticarcillin, ticarcillin-clavulanate, tigecycline, tirofiban, TNA (3-in-1), tobramycin, tolazoline, TPN, trastuzumab, trimetaphan, urokinase, vancomycin, vasopressin, vecuronium, verapamil, vinCRIStine, vinorelbine, voriconazole

SIDE EFFECTS

CNS: *Drowsiness, dizziness, confusion, headache, sedation, euphoria,* increased intracranial pressure, amnesia

CV: Palpitations, bradycardia, change in B/P, tachycardia

EENT: Tinnitus, blurred vision, *miosis,* diplopia

GI: *Nausea,* vomiting, anorexia, constipation, cramps, dry mouth
GU: Dysuria, urinary retention
INTEG: *Rash,* urticaria, bruising, flushing, diaphoresis, pruritus
RESP: **Respiratory depression,** dyspnea, hypo/hyperventilation

PHARMACOKINETICS

Metabolized in liver by CYP3A4, excreted by kidneys and in feces, crosses placenta, excreted in breast milk, half-life $2^1/_2$-$3^1/_2$ hr, 96% bound to plasma proteins
IM: Onset 15 min, peak ½ hr, duration 6 hr
SL: Onset, peak, duration unknown, half-life 37 hr
IV: Onset 1 min, peak 5 min, duration 6 hr, half-life 2.2 hr

INTERACTIONS

Increase: effect with other CNS depressants—alcohol, opioids, sedative/hypnotics, antipsychotics, skeletal muscle relaxants, MAOIs
Increase: buprenorphine effect—CYP3A4 inhibitors (erythromycin, indinavir, ketoconazole, ritonavir, saquinavir)
Increase: QT prolongation—class IA, III antidysrhythmics
Decrease: buprenorphine effect—CYP3A4 inducers (carbamazepine, PHENobarbital, phenytoin, rifampin)
Drug/Herb
Increase: CNS depression—St. John's wort

NURSING CONSIDERATIONS

Assess:
- **Pain:** intensity, location, type before treatment, after 5 min (IV); need for pain medication, tolerance
- I&O ratio; check for decreasing output; may indicate urinary retention
- Bowel pattern; severe constipation can occur
- CNS changes, dizziness, drowsiness, hallucinations, euphoria, LOC, pupil reaction; withdrawal in opioid-dependent persons; if dependence occurs, within 2 wk of discontinuing product **withdrawal symptoms** will occur
- Allergic reactions: rash, urticaria
- Respiratory dysfunction: respiratory depression, character, rate, rhythm; notify prescriber if respirations are <12/min

Black Box Warning: QT prolongation: in those taking class Ia, III antidysrhythmics; patients with hypokalemia, cardiac instability (TD)

Evaluate:
- Therapeutic response: decrease in pain, absence of grimacing

Teach patient/family:
- To report any symptoms of CNS changes, allergic reactions
- That tolerance may result when used for extended periods; that long-term use not recommended
- To avoid hazardous activities such as driving unless reaction known

TREATMENT OF OVERDOSE:

Naloxone 0.4 mg ampule diluted in 10 ml 0.9% NaCl given by direct IV push 0.02 mg q2min (adult)

buPROPion (Rx)

(byoo-proe′pee-on)

Aplenzin, Budeprion SR, Budeprion XL, Buproban, Sandoz Bupropion ♣, Wellbutrin, Wellbutrin SR, Wellbutrin XL, Zyban

Func. class.: Antidepressant—miscellaneous smoking deterrent
Chem. class.: Aminoketone

Do not confuse:
buPROPion/busPIRone
Zyban/Diovan/Zagam

ACTION: Inhibits reuptake of DOPamine

USES: Depression (Wellbutrin), smoking cessation (Zyban); seasonal affective disorder

Unlabeled uses: Neuropathic pain, enhancement of weight loss, ADHD (attention-deficit/hyperactivity disorder)

CONTRAINDICATIONS:
Hypersensitivity, eating disorders, seizure disorders

Precautions: Pregnancy (C), breastfeeding, geriatric patients, renal/hepatic disease, recent MI, cranial trauma, seizure disorder

Black Box Warning: Children <18 yr, suicidal thinking/behavior (young adults)

DOSAGE AND ROUTES

Depression

• **Adult: PO** 100 mg bid initially then increase after 3 days to 100 mg tid if needed; may increase after 1 mo to 150 mg tid; **ER/SR** initially 150 mg AM, increase to 300 mg/day if initial dose is tolerated; Aplenzin 174 mg q AM, may increase to 348 mg q AM on day 4, may increase to 522 mg after several weeks if needed

• **Geriatric: PO** 50-100 mg/day, may increase by 50-100 mg q3-4days

Smoking cessation (Zyban)

• **Adult: SR** 150 mg q day × 3 days then 150 mg bid for remainder of treatment, initiate 1-2 wk before targeted "quit day," continue for 7-12 wk; in combination with nicotine TD, 150 mg q day × 3 days then 150 mg bid for remainder of treatment, give ≥8 hr apart, max 300 mg/day, initiate 1-2 wk before targeted "quit day," continue for 7-12 wk, may be continued for 8-20 wk

ADHD (unlabeled) (Wellbutrin)

• **Adult: PO** 100 mg bid, after ≥3 days titrate to 100 mg tid; SR 300 mg/day, 200 mg 8 AM, 100 mg 4 PM

Diabetic neuropathy/postherpetic neuralgia (unlabeled)(Wellbutrin SR)

• **Adult: PO** SR 150-300 mg/day

Available forms: Tabs 75, 100 mg; sus rel tabs (SR) 150; ext rel tab (XL) 100, 150, 300 mg; (SR-12 hr, XL-24 hr); tab ext rel (Aplenzin) 174, 348, 522 mg

Administer:

PO route

⚠ When switching to Aplenzin from Wellbutrin, Wellbutrin SR or XL, use these equivalents: 174 mg buPROPion HBr = 150 mg buPROPion HCl; 348 mg buPROPion HBr = 300 mg buPROPion HCl; 522 mg buPROPion HBr = 450 mg buPROPion HCl

• **Wellbutrin immediate rel,** separate by ≥6 hr, give in 3 divided doses; **Wellbutrin SR,** if multiple doses are used, separate by ≥8 hr; **Wellbutrin XL,** give daily in AM; **Zyban SR,** give in 2 divided doses, ≥8 hr apart; **Aplenzin ER,** give daily in AM, a larger dose of Aplenzin is needed because these products are not equivalent

• Do not break, crush, chew sus rel, ext rel tab

• At evenly spaced times to prevent seizures; seizure risk increases with high doses

• Increased fluids, bulk in diet if constipation occurs

• With food, milk for GI symptoms

• Sugarless gum, hard candy, frequent sips of water for dry mouth

• Avoid giving at night to prevent insomnia

SIDE EFFECTS

CNS: *Headache, agitation, dizziness, akinesia, bradykinesia, confusion,* seizures, delusions, *insomnia, sedation, tremors,* suicidal ideation

CV: *Dysrhythmias, hypertension,* palpitations, *tachycardia,* hypotension, complete AV block; QRS prolongation (overdose)

EENT: *Blurred vision, auditory disturbance*

GI: *Nausea, vomiting,* anorexia, diarrhea, *dry mouth,* increased appetite, *constipation,* altered taste

GU: Impotence, urinary frequency, retention, *menstrual irregularities*

INTEG: *Rash,* pruritus, *sweating,* Stevens-Johnson syndrome

MISC: *Weight loss or gain*

PHARMACOKINETICS

Onset 2-4 wk, half-life 14 hr, extensively metabolized by liver, some conversion to active metabolites, steady state 5-8 days, protein binding 84%, excreted in urine and feces

INTERACTIONS

⚠ **Increase:** **adverse reactions, seizures—levodopa, MAOIs, phenothiazines, antidepressants, benzodiazepines, alcohol, theophylline, systemic steroids**
Increase: buPROPion toxicity—ritonavir
Increase: buPROPion level—cimetidine
Increase: buPROPion effect—CYP2D6/CYP2B6 inhibitors
Decrease: effect of tamoxifen
Decrease: buPROPion effect—carBAMazepine, cimetidine, PHENobarbital, phenytoin or other products (CYP2D6); CYP2B6 inducers

Drug/Herb

Increase: CNS depression—kava, valerian

NURSING CONSIDERATIONS

Assess:

- Hepatic/renal function in patients with hepatic, kidney impairment
- For increased risk of seizures; if patient has excessively used CNS depressants and OTC stimulants, dosage of buPROPion should not be exceeded
- For smoking cessation after 7-12 wk; if progress has not been made, product should be discontinued

Black Box Warning: Mental status: mood, sensorium, affect, suicidal tendencies, increase in psychiatric symptoms

Perform/provide:

- Assistance with ambulation during beginning therapy because sedation occurs
- Safety measures, primarily for geriatric patients

Evaluate:

- Therapeutic response: decreased depression, ability to perform daily activities, ability to sleep throughout the night, smoking cessation

Teach patient/family:

- That therapeutic effects may take 2-4 wk; not to increase dose without prescriber's approval; that treatment for smoking cessation lasts 7-12 wk
- To use caution when driving, performing other activities that require alertness; sedation, blurred vision may occur
- To avoid alcohol, other CNS depressants; alcohol may increase risk of seizures
- Not to use with nicotine patches unless directed by prescriber; may increase B/P
- To notify prescriber immediately if urinary retention occurs
- That risk of seizures increased when dose exceeded, if patient has seizure disorder

⚠ **That suicidal ideas, behaviors, hostility, depression may occur in children or young adults**

- To notify prescriber if pregnancy is suspected, planned

TREATMENT OF OVERDOSE:

ECG monitoring; lavage, activated charcoal; administer anticonvulsant

busPIRone (Rx)

(byoo-spye′rone)

Apo-Buspirone ♣, BuSpar, BuSpar Dividose, CO Buspirone ♣, Gen-Buspirone ♣, PMS-Buspirone ♣

Func. class.: Antianxiety, sedative
Chem. class.: Azaspirodecanedione

Do not confuse:
busPIRone/buPROPion

ACTION: Acts by inhibiting the action of serotonin (5-HT); has shown little potential for abuse; a good choice with substance abuse

USES: Management and short-term relief of generalized anxiety disorders
Unlabeled uses: Autism

CONTRAINDICATIONS:

Children <18 yr, hypersensitivity

Precautions: Pregnancy (B), breastfeeding, geriatric patients, impaired hepatic/renal function

DOSAGE AND ROUTES

- **Adult: PO** 7.5 mg bid; may increase by 5 mg/day q2-3days, max 60 mg/day

Autism with anxiety (unlabeled)

- **Adult: PO** 5-15 mg tid after titration, max 60 mg/day
- **Child ≥5 yr: PO** 0.2-0.6 mg/kg/day, max 60 mg/day; titrate to higher dose

Hepatic/renal dose

- **Adult: PO** reduce by 25%-50% for mild-moderate hepatic disease; do not use for severe hepatic disease; CCr 11-70 ml/min reduce by 25%-50%, CCr <10 ml/min do not use

Available forms: Tabs 5, 7.5, 10, 15, 30 mg

Administer:

- With food, milk for GI symptoms; avoid grapefruit juice; give drug at same time of day, with/without food consistently
- Crushed if patient unable to swallow medication whole
- Sugarless gum, hard candy, frequent sips of water for dry mouth

SIDE EFFECTS

CNS: *Dizziness, headache, depression, stimulation, insomnia, nervousness, lightheadedness, numbness, paresthesia, incoordination,* nightmares, *tremors,* excitement, involuntary movements, confusion, akathisia, hostility

CV: *Tachycardia, palpitations,* hypo/hypertension, CVA, CHF, MI

EENT: *Sore throat, tinnitus, blurred vision, nasal congestion;* red, itching eyes; change in taste, smell

GI: *Nausea, dry mouth, diarrhea, constipation,* flatulence, increased appetite, rectal bleeding

GU: Frequency, hesitancy, menstrual irregularity, change in libido

INTEG: *Rash,* edema, pruritus, alopecia, dry skin

MISC: *Sweating,* fatigue, weight gain, fever

MS: *Pain, weakness,* muscle cramps, spasms

RESP: Hyperventilation, chest congestion, shortness of breath

PHARMACOKINETICS

Peak 40-90 min, half-life 2-3 hr, rapidly absorbed, metabolized by liver (CYP3A4), excreted in feces, protein binding 86%

INTERACTIONS

Increase: busPIRone—product metabolized by CYP3A4 (erythromycin, itraconazole, nefazodone, ketoconazole, ritonavir, several other protease inhibitors)

Increase: B/P—procarbazine, MAOIs; do not use together

Increase: CNS depression—psychotropic products, alcohol (avoid use)

Increase: serotonin syndrome—SSRIs, SNRIs, serotonin receptor agonists

Decrease: busPIRone effects—rifampin

Decrease: busPIRone action—products induced by CYP3A4 (rifampin, phenytoin, PHENobarbital, carBAMazepine, dexamethasone)

Drug/Food

Increase: peak concentration of busPIRone—grapefruit juice

NURSING CONSIDERATIONS

Assess:

- B/P lying, standing; pulse; if systolic B/P drops 20 mm Hg, hold product, notify prescriber
- CNS reactions because some may be unpredictable
- Mental status: mood, sensorium, affect, sleeping pattern, drowsiness, dizziness; withdrawal symptoms when dose reduced, product discontinued

Perform/provide:

- Safety measures if drowsiness, dizziness occurs
- Check to confirm PO medication swallowed

Evaluate:
- Therapeutic response: decreased anxiety, restlessness, sleeplessness

Teach patient/family:
- That product may be taken consistently with/without food
- To avoid OTC preparations, alcohol ingestion, other psychotropic medications unless approved by prescriber; to avoid large amounts of grapefruit juice
- To avoid activities that require alertness because drowsiness may occur
- Not to discontinue medication abruptly after long-term use; if dose missed, do not double
- To rise slowly because fainting may occur, especially among geriatric patients
- That drowsiness may worsen at beginning of treatment; that 1-2 wk of therapy may be required before therapeutic effects occur

⚠ HIGH ALERT

busulfan (Rx)

(byoo-sul′fan)

Busulfex, Myleran

Func. class.: Antineoplastic alkylating agent

Chem. class.: Bifunctional alkylating agent

Do not confuse:
Myleran/Leukeran

ACTION: Changes essential cellular ions to covalent bonding with resultant alkylation; this interferes with the normal biological function of DNA; activity is not phase specific; action is due to myelosuppression

USES: Chronic myelocytic leukemia, bone marrow ablation, stem cell transplant preparation with CML

CONTRAINDICATIONS: Pregnancy (D) 3rd trimester, breastfeeding, radiation, chemotherapy, blastic phase of chronic myelocytic leukemia, hypersensitivity

Precautions: Women of childbearing age and men, leukopenia, anemia, hepatotoxicity, renal toxicity, seizures, tumor lysis syndrome, hyperkalemia, hyperphosphatemia, hypocalcemia, hyperuricemia

Black Box Warning: Thrombocytopenia, neutropenia, secondary malignancy

DOSAGE AND ROUTES

Chronic myelocytic leukemia
- **Adult: PO** 4-8 mg/day or 1.8-4 mg/m²/day initially, reduce dose if WBC reaches 30,000-40,000/mm³, discontinue if WBC ≤20,000/mm³, maintenance 1-3 mg/day
- **Child: PO** 0.06-0.12 mg/kg/day or 1.8-4.6 mg/m²/day; reduce if WBC reaches 30,000-40,000/mm³, discontinue if WBC ≤20,000/mm³

Allogenic hemopoietic stem cell transplantation with chronic myelogenous leukemia
- **Adult: IV** 0.8 mg/kg over 2 hr, q6hr × 4 days (total 16 doses); give cyclophosphamide **IV** 60 mg/kg over 1 hr daily for 2 days starting after 16th dose of busulfan; **PO** (unlabeled) 1 mg/kg q6hr × 16 doses
- **Adolescent and child (unlabeled) >12 kg: IV** 0.8 mg/kg over 2 hr q6hr × 16 doses (4 days) then high-dose cyclophosphamide 50 mg/kg/day × 4 days
- **Infant/child ≤12 kg (unlabeled): IV** 1.1 mg/kg over 2 hr q6hr × 16 doses (4 days) then high-dose cyclophosphamide 50 mg/kg/day × 4 days

Available forms: Tabs 2 mg; inj 6 mg/ml

Administer:

PO route
- Give at same time daily on empty stomach

Intermittent IV INF route
- Prepare in biologic cabinet while wearing gloves, gown, mask; **dilute** with 10 times volume of product with D_5W, 0.9% NaCl, (0.5 mg/ml); when withdraw-

ing product, use needle with 5-micron filter provided, remove amount needed, remove filter, and **inject** product into diluent; always add product to diluent (not vice versa); stable for 8 hr at room temp (using D_5W) or 12 hr refrigerated; **give** by central venous catheter over 2 hr q6hr × 4 days, use inf pump, do not admix

- Give antiemetics before IV route on schedule
- In those with history of seizures, give phenytoin before IV drug to prevent seizures (using 0.9% NaCl)

Y-site compatibilities: Acyclovir, amphotericin B lipid complex, amphotericin B liposome, anidulafungin, atenolol, bivalirudin, bleomycin, caspofungin, codeine, DAPTOmycin, dexmedetomidine, diltiazem, docetaxel, ertapenem, fenoldopam, gatifloxacin, granisetron, HYDROmorphone, levofloxacin, linezolid, LORazepam, meperidine, metroNIDAZOLE, milrinone, nesiritide, octreotide acetate, ondansetron, palonosetron, pancuronium, piperacillin-tazobactam, riTUXimab, sodium acetate, tacrolimus, tigecycline, tirofiban, trastuzumab, vasopressin

SIDE EFFECTS

PO route

CV: *Hypotension,* thrombosis, *chest pain,* tachycardia, atrial fibrillation, heart block, pericardial effusion, cardiac tamponade (high dose with cyclophosphamide)

GI: *Anorexia, constipation, diarrhea, dry mouth, nausea, vomiting*

RESP: Alveolar hemorrhage, atelectasis, cough, hemoptysis, hypoxia, pleural effusion, pneumonia, sinusitis, pulmonary fibrosis

IV route

CNS: Cerebral hemorrhage, coma, seizures, *anxiety, depression, dizziness, headache,* encephalopathy, *weakness,* mental changes

EENT: *Pharyngitis, epistaxis,* cataracts

GI: Nausea, vomiting, *diarrhea, weight loss*

GU: Impotence, sterility, amenorrhea, gynecomastia, renal toxicity, hyperuremia, adrenal-insufficiency–like syndrome

HEMA: Thrombocytopenia, leukopenia, pancytopenia, severe bone marrow depression

INTEG: Dermatitis, hyperpigmentation, alopecia

OTHER: Chromosomal aberrations

RESP: Irreversible pulmonary fibrosis, pneumonitis

PHARMACOKINETICS

Well absorbed orally, excreted in urine, crosses placenta, excreted in breast milk, half-life 2.5 hr

INTERACTIONS

Increase: hepatotoxicity—thioguanine

Increase: cardiac tamponade—cyclophosphamide

Increase: toxicity—other antineoplastics, radiation

Increase: risk for bleeding—anticoagulants, salicylates

Increase: antibody response—live virus vaccines

Decrease: busulfan level—phenytoin

Decrease: busulfan clearance—acetaminophen, itraconazole

Drug/Lab Test

False positive: breast, bladder, cervix, lung cytology tests

NURSING CONSIDERATIONS

Assess:

Black Box Warning: CBC, differential, platelet count weekly; withhold product if WBC is $<15,000/mm^3$ or platelet count is $<150,000/mm^3$; notify prescriber of results; institute thrombocytopenia precautions; levels for withholding product will be different for children

Black Box Warning: Bone marrow status before chemotherapy; seizure history; bone marrow suppression may be prolonged (up to 2 mo)

• **Pulmonary fibrosis:** pulmonary function tests, chest x-ray films before, during therapy; chest film should be obtained q2wk during treatment; pulmonary fibrosis may occur up to 10 yr after treatment with busulfan
• Renal studies: BUN, serum uric acid, urine CCr before, during therapy; monitor ALT, alk phos, bilirubin, uric acid before and during treatment; I&O ratio; report fall in urine output of <30 ml/hr; hyperuricemia

Black Box Warning: For secondary malignancy within 5-8 yr of chronic oral therapy, long-term follow-up may be required

• Monitor for cold, fever, sore throat (may indicate beginning infection)
• Bleeding: hematuria, guaiac, bruising, petechiae; mucosa, orifices q8hr; no rectal temps
• Dyspnea, crackles, nonproductive cough, chest pain, tachypnea
• Inflammation of mucosa, breaks in skin; use viscous xylocaine for oral pain

Perform/provide:
• Comprehensive oral hygiene
• Strict medical asepsis, protective isolation if WBC levels low
• Increased fluid intake to 2-3 L/day to prevent urate deposits, calculi formation
• Storage in tight container

Evaluate:
• Therapeutic response: decreased exacerbations of chronic myelocytic leukemia

Teach patient/family:
• To avoid use of products that contain aspirin, ibuprofen; razors; commercial mouthwash
• To use effective contraception during and for at least 3 mo after treatment; to avoid breastfeeding
• To report signs of **anemia** (fatigue, headache, irritability, faintness, shortness of breath); symptoms of **infection;** jaundice; persistent cough, congestion, skin pigmentation, darkening of skin; sudden weakness, weight loss (may resemble adrenal insufficiency)
• To report symptoms of bleeding (hematuria, tarry stools)
• To avoid vaccinations, crowds, persons with known infections
• That impotence, amenorrhea can occur; that these are reversible after discontinuing treatment

butoconazole vaginal antifungal

See Appendix B

butorphanol (Rx)

(byoo-tor'fa-nole)

Apo-Butorphanol ♣, PMS-Butorphanol ♣

Func. class.: Opioid analgesic
Chem. class.: Mixed opioid antagonist, partial agonist

Controlled Substance Schedule IV

Do not confuse:
Stadol/Haldol/sotalol

ACTION: Depresses pain impulse transmission at the spinal cord level by interacting with opioid receptors

USES: Moderate to severe pain, general anesthesia induction/maintenance, headache, migraine, preanesthesia
Unlabeled uses: Pruritus

CONTRAINDICATIONS: Hypersensitivity to product, preservative; addiction (opioid)
Precautions: Pregnancy (C), breastfeeding, children <18 yr, addictive personality, increased intracranial pressure, respiratory depression, renal/hepatic disease, bowel impaction, CHF, MI

DOSAGE AND ROUTES

Moderate-severe pain

- **Adult: IM** 1-4 mg q3-4hr prn; **IV** 0.5-2 mg q3-4hr prn; **INTRANASAL** 1 spray in 1 nostril, may give another dose 1-1½ hr later; repeat if needed 3-4hr after last dose
- **Geriatric: IV** ½ adult dose at 2× the interval; **INTRANASAL** if no relief after 90-120 min, may repeat with 1 spray

Renal dose

- **Adult: INTRANASAL** max 1 mg followed by 1 mg after 90-120 min; **IM/IV** give 50% of dose (0.5 mg **IV**, 1 mg **IM**), do not repeat within 6 hr

Opioid-induced pruritus (unlabeled)

- **Adult: INTRANASAL** 1 mg (1 spray) in each nostril q4-6hr

Intractable pruritus with inflammatory skin or systemic disease (unlabeled)

- **Adult: INTRANASAL** 1-4 mg/day

Available forms: Inj 1, 2 mg/ml; nasal spray 10 mg/ml

Administer:

- With antiemetic if nausea, vomiting occur
- When pain beginning to return; determine dosage interval according to patient response

IM route

- Deeply in large muscle mass

IV direct route

- Undiluted at a rate of <2 mg/>3-5 min, titrate to patient response; inject directly in vein or tubing of free-flowing compatible IV inf

Syringe compatibilities: Atropine, chlorproMAZINE, cimetidine, diphenhydrAMINE, droperidol, fentaNYL, hydrOXYzine, meperidine, methotrimeprazine, metoclopramide, midazolam, morphine, pentazocine, perphenazine, prochlorperazine, promethazine, scopolamine, thiethylperazine

Y-site compatibilities: Acyclovir, alfentanil, allopurinol, amifostine, amikacin, aminocaproic acid, aminophylline, amphotericin B liposome (AmBisome), anidulafungin, ascorbic acid injection, atenolol, atracurium, atropine, aztreonam, benztropine, bivalirudin, bleomycin, bumetanide, buprenorphine, calcium chloride/gluconate, CARBOplatin, caspofungin, cefamandole, cefazolin, cefepime, cefmetazole, cefonicid, cefoperazone, cefotaxime, cefotetan, cefoxitin, ceftazidime, ceftizoxime, cefTRIAXone, cefuroxime, cephalothin, chlorproMAZINE, cimetidine, cisatracurium, CISplatin, cladribine, clindamycin, cyanocobalamin, cyclophosphamide, cycloSPORINE, cytarabine, DACTINomycin, DAPTOmycin, dexamethasone phosphate, dexmedetomidine, digoxin, diltiazem, diphenhydrAMINE, DOBUTamine, docetaxel, DOPamine, doxacurium, DOXOrubicin, DOXOrubicin liposomal, doxycycline, enalaprilat, ePHEDrine, EPINEPHrine, epirubicin, epoetin alfa, eptifibatide, ertapenem, erythromycin, esmolol, etoposide, famotidine, fenoldopam, fentaNYL, filgrastim, fluconazole, fludarabine, fluorouracil, gatifloxacin, gemcitabine, gentamicin, glycopyrrolate, granisetron, heparin, hydrocortisone, hydrOXYzine, IDArubicin, ifosfamide, imipenem-cilastatin, irinotecan, isoproterenol, ketorolac, labetalol, lactated Ringer's injection, levofloxacin, lidocaine, linezolid injection, LORazepam, magnesium, mannitol, mechlorethamine, melphalan, meperidine, metaraminol, methicillin, methotrexate, methoxamine, methyldopate, methylPREDNISolone, metoclopramide, metoprolol, metroNIDAZOLE, mezlocillin, miconazole, milrinone, minocycline, mitoxantrone, morphine, moxalactam, multiple vitamins injection, mycophenolate mofetil, nafcillin, nalbuphine, naloxone, nesiritide, netilmicin, niCARdipine, nitroglycerin, nitroprusside, norepinephrine, octreotide, ondansetron, oxacillin, oxaliplatin, oxytocin, palonosetron, pamidronate, pancuronium, papaverine, pemetrexed, penicillin G potassium/sodium, pentazocine, PHENobarbital, phenylephrine, phytonadione, piperacillin, piperacillin-tazobactam, polymyxin B, potassium chloride, procainamide, prochlorperazine, promethazine, propofol, propranolol, protamine, pyridoxine, quiNIDine, ranitidine, remifentanil, Ringer's injection, ritodrine, riTUXimab, rocuronium, sargramostim, sodium acetate, succinylcholine, SUFentanil, tacrolimus, teniposide, theophylline, thiamine, thiotepa, ticarcillin, ticarcillin-clavulanate, tigecycline, tirofiban, TNA, tobramycin, tolazoline, TPN, trastuzumab, trimetaphan, urokinase, vancomycin, vasopressin, vecuronium, verapamil, vinCRIStine, vinorelbine, voriconazole

SIDE EFFECTS

CNS: *Drowsiness, dizziness, confusion, headache, sedation, euphoria, weakness, hallucinations,* insomnia (nasal)

CV: Palpitations, bradycardia, hypotension

EENT: Tinnitus, blurred vision, miosis, diplopia, nasal congestion, unpleasant taste

GI: *Nausea, vomiting, anorexia, constipation, cramps*

GU: Dysuria, urinary retention

INTEG: Rash, urticaria, bruising, flushing, diaphoresis, pruritus

RESP: **Respiratory depression**, URI, sinusitis

PHARMACOKINETICS

Metabolized by liver, excreted by kidneys, crosses placenta, excreted in breast milk, half-life 2-9 hr, protein binding 80%

IM: Onset 5-15 min, peak 30-60 min, duration 3-4 hr

INTRANASAL: Onset within 15 min, peak 1-2 hr, duration 4-5 hr

IV: Onset 1 min, peak 4-5 min, duration 2-4 hr

INTERACTIONS

⚠ **Severe, fatal reactions: MAOIs**

Increase: CNS effects—alcohol, opioids, sedative/hypnotics, antipsychotics, skeletal muscle relaxants, other CNS depressants

NURSING CONSIDERATIONS

Assess:

- For decreasing output; may indicate urinary retention
- ⚠ **For withdrawal symptoms in opioid-dependent patients; PE, vascular occlusion, abscesses, ulcerations**
- CNS changes: dizziness, drowsiness, hallucinations, euphoria, LOC, pupil reaction
- Allergic reactions: rash, urticaria
- Respiratory dysfunction: respiratory depression, character, rate, rhythm; notify prescriber if respirations are <10/min
- Need for pain medication, physical dependence

Perform/provide:

- Storage in light-resistant container at room temp
- Safety measures: night-light, call bell within easy reach, assistance with ambulation, especially for geriatric patients

Evaluate:

- Therapeutic response: decrease in pain

Teach patient/family:

- To report any symptoms of CNS changes, allergic reactions
- That physical dependency may result when used for extended periods
- That withdrawal symptoms may occur: nausea, vomiting, cramps, fever, faintness, anorexia

TREATMENT OF OVERDOSE:

Naloxone HCl (Narcan) 0.2-0.8 mg IV, O_2, IV fluids, vasopressors

cabazitaxel
(ka-baz′i-tax′el)

Jevtana

Func class: Antineoplastic—miscellaneous

Chem class: Taxane

ACTION: Taxane that binds to tubulin, inhibits microtubule depolymerization, cell division, cell cycle arrest (G2/M) phase, cell proliferation; unlike other taxanes, this product may be useful for treating multidrug-resistant tumors

USES: Hormone-refractory prostate cancer in combination with prednisone in patients who have been previously treated who a docetaxel-containing regimen

CONTRAINDICATIONS: Pregnancy (D), hypersensitivity to this product

Black Box Warning: Hypersensitivity to polysorbate 80, neutropenia (ANC ≤1500/mm^3)

Precautions: Breastfeeding, children, elderly, diarrhea, hepatic disease, renal disease, sepsis, vomiting

DOSAGE AND ROUTES

- **Adult: IV INF** 25 mg/m^2 over 1 hr on day 1 with predniSONE 10 mg q day continuously; give q3wk cycles, for up to 10 cycles

Hepatic dose

- **Adult: IV INF** do not use if total bilirubin ULN ≥ or AST and/or ALT >1.5 times ULN

Available forms: Sol for inj 60 mg/1.5 ml

Administer:

- Use cytotoxic handling procedures
- Obtain neutrophil counts prior to administration; count should be >1500/mm^3
- Do not use PVC inf containers or polyurethane inf sets for preparation or administration
- **Premedicate** with diphenhydramine 25 mg IV or equivalent, dexamethasone 8 mg or equivalent, ranitidine 50 mg or equivalent, and antiemetics
- Do not use sol that is discolored or if particulate is present; sol should be clear, yellow to brownish; discard if first or second dilution is not clear; remove immediately if sol comes in contact with skin

Intermittent IV Inf:

- Two dilutions are required, both product and dilution are overfilled; ***first dilution:*** mix each vial of product (60 mg/1.5 ml) with the entire contents of supplied diluent (10 mg/ml); when transferring diluent, direct needle on side of vial, inject slowly to limit foaming; remove syringe and needle, gently mix with several inversions, do not shake; let stand for a few min; ***second dilution:*** withdraw required dose, further dilute withdrawn product with 0.9% NaCl or D_5 in a PVC-free container, remove syringe and needle, mix by gently inverting the bag/bottle (final concentration 0.1-0.26 mg/ml); if a dose of ≥65 mg is needed, use a larger volume of inf solution so the concentration is max 0.26 mg/ml; do not mix with other drugs; sol may crystallize over time, discard if this occurs, use sol within 8 hr (room temp), 24 hr (refrigerated); **give** over 1 hr, use 0.22 micrometer in-line filter

SIDE EFFECTS

CNS: *Peripheral neuropathy, dysgeusia, dizziness, headache, fatigue, fever*

CV: Dysrhythmia, peripheral edema, hypotension

GI: *Diarrhea, nausea, vomiting, constipation, abdominal pain, dyspepsia, anorexia, mucosal inflammation*

GU: Renal failure, dehydration, hematuria, urinary tract infection, dysuria, obstructive uropathy, infertility

HEMA: Neutropenia, febrile neutropenia, anemia, leucopenia, thrombocytopenia

MS: Back pain, arthralgia, muscle spasms
RESP: Cough, dyspnea
SYST: **Fatal infections, sepsis, anaphylaxis**

PHARMACOKINETICS

89%-92% protein binding, primarily bound to albumin and lipoproteins; equally distributed between blood and plasma; extensively metabolized by CYP3A4/5 in the liver and by CYP2C8 to a lesser extent; 80% eliminated within 2 wk, mainly in feces; half-life alpha, beta, gamma of 4 min, 2 hr, 95 hr, respectively

INTERACTIONS

Increase: bone marrow depression—other antineoplastics, radiation
Increase: cabazitaxel concentrations—strong CYP3A4 inhibitors (conivaptan, chloramphenicol, danazol, dalfopristin, delavirdine, ethinyl estradiol, fluvoxamine, imatinib, isoniazid, tipranavir, troleandomycin, zafirlukast, ketoconazole, itraconazole, clarithromycin, atazanavir, indinavir, nefazodone, nelfinavir, ritonavir, saquinavir, telithromycin, voriconazole); mild or moderate CYP3A4 inhibitors (basiliximab, fluoxetine, nicardipine, ranolazine, amiodarone, darunavir, diltiazem, miconazole, mifepristone [RU-486], posaconazole, propoxyphene, tamoxifen, erythromycin, verapamil, fluconazole)
Decrease: cabazitaxel concentrations—CYP3A4 inducers (rifampin, phenytoin, cabBAMazepine, rifabutin, rifapentine, PHENobarbital)
Decrease: immune response—vaccines

NURSING CONSIDERATIONS

Assess:

- **Anaphylaxis:** hypotension, dyspnea, generalized urticaria, bronchospasm, discontinue immediately; keep emergency equipment near; usually occurs during the first or second infusion; do not use this product again after severe hypersensitivity reactions
- **Infusion site reactions:** if given by regular IV rather than port (redness, inflammation, warmth)

Black Box Warning: Bone marrow depression: monitor CBC with differential prior to and after 1 wk, withhold if WBC <1500/mm^3 or platelets <100,000/mm^3; may not be a concern if erythropoietin agent given

- **Neurological side effects:** peripheral neuropathy, dizziness, headache; during infusion of product, ice on extremities periodically may prevent peripheral neuropathy
- **Musculoskeletal reactions:** back pain, arthralgia, muscle spasms
- **Renal failure:** has been fatal; monitor BUN, creatinine, serum electrolytes; usually associated with sepsis, dehydration, obstructive uropathy
- **Bleeding:** bruising, petechiae, hematuria, blood in emesis or stools; check mucosa orifices for stomatitis; obtain order for viscous Xylocaine if needed
- Monitor temp periodically; increased temp may indicate beginning infection
- Hepatic studies: AST, ALT, bilirubin, LDH, prior to and periodically during treatment; jaundice of skin, eyes; clay-colored stools, dark urine, itching skin, abdominal pain, fever, diarrhea
- Alopecia: effects on body image, discuss feelings about body changes

Teach patient/family:

- To use a nonhormonal form of contraception; to notify prescriber if pregnancy is planned or suspected (pregnancy category [D]); not to breastfeed
- That hair may be lost during treatment; a wig or hairpiece may make the patient feel better; new hair will be different in color, texture
- To avoid receiving vaccinations while using this product
- To report signs of infection: fever, sore throat, flulike symptoms; to avoid persons with known respiratory infections

calcitonin (rDNA) (Rx)

(kal-sih-toh′nin)

Apo-Calcitonin ✤, Fortical, Sandoz Calcitonin ✤

calcitonin (salmon) (Rx)

Miacalcin

Func. class.: Parathyroid agents (calcium regulator)

Chem. class.: Polypeptide hormone

ACTION: Decreases bone resorption, blood calcium levels; increases deposits of calcium in bones; opposes parathyroid hormone

USES: Paget's disease, postmenopausal osteoporosis, hypercalcemia

Unlabeled uses: Bone/neuropathic pain, diabetic neuropathy, osteolytic metastases, osteoporosis prophylaxis, phantom limb pain

CONTRAINDICATIONS: Hypersensitivity to this product, fish

Precautions: Pregnancy (C), breastfeeding, children, renal disease, osteogenic sarcoma, pernicious anemia

DOSAGE AND ROUTES

rDNA

Paget's disease

• **Adult: SUBCUT** 0.5 mg/day initially; may require 0.5 mg bid × 6 mo, then decrease until symptoms reappear

Salmon

Postmenopausal osteoporosis

• **Adult: SUBCUT/IM** 100 international units every other day; **INTRANASAL** 200 international units (1 spray) daily alternating nostrils daily, activate pump before 1st dose

Paget's disease

• **Adult: SUBCUT/IM** 100 international units/day, maintenance 50 international units daily, every other day or 3 × per wk

Hypercalcemia

• **Adult: SUBCUT/IM** 4 international units/kg q12hr, increase to 8 international units/kg q12hr if response is unsatisfactory

Neuropathic pain/phantom limb pain/diabetic neuropathy (unlabeled)

• **Adult: IV/SUBCUT** 100-200 international units/day for phantom limb pain **IV** 200 international units over 20 min and 2nd inf given

Bone pain due to osteoporosis, osteolytic metastases (unlabeled)

• **Adult: SUBCUT** 50-100 international units/day or **INTRANASAL** 200 international units in 1 nostril/day

Available forms: Inj 200 international units/ml; nasal spray 200 international units/actuation

Administer:

SUBCUT route (rDNA)

• By SUBCUT route only; rotate inj sites; use within 6 hr of reconstitution; **give** at bedtime to minimize nausea, vomiting

IM route (Salmon)

• After test dose of 10 international units/ml, 0.1 ml intradermally; watch for 15 min; **give** only with epinephrine, emergency meds available

• IM inj slowly into deep muscle mass; rotate sites; preferred route if volume is >2 ml

SIDE EFFECTS

CNS: Headache, tetany, chills, weakness, dizziness, fever

CV: Chest pressure

EENT: Nasal congestion, eye pain

GI: Nausea, diarrhea, vomiting, anorexia, abdominal pain, salty taste, epigastric pain

GU: Diuresis, nocturia, urine sediment, frequency

INTEG: Rash, flushing, pruritus of earlobes, edema of feet, reaction at inj site

MS: Swelling, tingling of hands, backache

RESP: Dyspnea

SYST: Anaphylaxis

PHARMACOKINETICS

IM/SUBCUT: Onset 15 min, peak 4 hr, duration 8-24 hr, metabolized by kidneys, excreted as inactive metabolites via kidneys

INTERACTIONS

Decrease: lithium effect

NURSING CONSIDERATIONS

Assess:

⚠ **Anaphylaxis, hypersensitivity reaction** (rash, fever, inability to breathe); emergency equipment should be nearby

• GI symptoms, polyuria, flushing, head swelling, tingling, headache; may indicate hypercalcemia

• Nutritional status; diet for sources of vit D (milk, some seafood), calcium (dairy products, dark green vegetables), phosphates

• Urinalysis (calcium should be kept at 9-10 mg/dl, vit D 50-135 international units/dl), alk phos baseline, q3-6mo; monitor urine hydroproline with Paget's disease, biochemical markers of bone formation/absorption, radiologic evidence of fracture; bone density (osteoporosis)

• **Toxicity (can occur rapidly),** increased drug level; have parenteral calcium on hand if calcium level drops too low; check for tetany (irritability, paresthesia, nervousness, muscle twitching, seizures, tetanic spasms)

• Urine for sediment

Perform/provide:

• Storage at <77° F (25° C); protect from light

Evaluate:

• Therapeutic response: calcium levels 9-10 mg/dl, decreasing symptoms of Paget's disease

Teach patient/family:

• About the method of inj if patient will be responsible for self-medication

• To report difficulty swallowing, any changes in side effects to prescriber immediately

Nasal

• To use alternating nostrils for nasal spray; use after allowing to warm to room temp; prime to get full spray

C

calcitriol vitamin D_3 (Rx)

(kal-sih-try′ole)

Calcijex, Rocaltrol

Func. class.: Parathyroid agent (calcium regulator)

Chem. class.: Vit D hormone

Do not confuse:

calcitriol/Calciferol

ACTION: Increases intestinal absorption of calcium, provides calcium for bones, increases renal tubular resorption of phosphate

USES: Hypocalcemia with chronic renal disease, hyperparathyroidism pseudohypoparathyroidism

Unlabeled uses: Osteopetrosis, osteoporosis, osteoporosis prophylaxis, rickets, familial hypophosphatemia

CONTRAINDICATIONS: Hypersensitivity, hyperphosphatemia, hypercalcemia, vit D toxicity

Precautions: Pregnancy (C), breastfeeding, renal calculi, CV disease

DOSAGE AND ROUTES

Hypocalcemia (stage 5 chronic kidney disease, on dialysis)

• **Adult and child ≥6 yr: PO** 0.25 mcg/day **IV** 0.5 mcg tid initially; may increase by 0.25 every other day q4-8wk

• **Child 1-5 yr: PO** 0.25-2 mcg/day

Renal osteodystrophy

• **Adult and child ≥3 yr: PO** 0.25 mcg/day, may increase to 0.5 mcg/day

• **Child <3 yr: PO** 0.01-0.015 mcg/kg/day

Hypoparathyroidism

• **Adult and child ≥6 yr: PO** 0.25 mcg/day, may increase q2-4wk, maintenance 0.5-2 mcg/day

- **Child 1-5 yr: PO** 0.25-0.75 mcg daily
- **Child <1 yr: PO** 0.04-0.08 mcg/kg/day

Rickets (unlabeled)

- **Adult and child: PO** 1 mcg/day

Familial hypophosphatemia (unlabeled)

- **Adult: PO** 2 mcg/day
- **Child: PO** 0.015-0.02 mcg/kg/day, maintenance 0.03-0.06 mcg/kg/day; max 2 mcg/day

Postmenopausal osteoporosis (unlabeled)

- **Adult: PO** 0.25 mcg bid, adjust to serum calcium levels

Osteopetrosis (unlabeled)

- **Child: PO** high-dose calcitriol 1-2 mcg/kg/day given in 4-6 divided doses

Osteoporosis prophylaxis in corticosteroid therapy (unlabeled)

- **Adult: PO** 0.5-1 mcg/day

Available forms: Caps 0.25, 0.5 mcg; inj 1 mcg/ml; oral sol 1 mcg/ml

Administer:

PO route

- Do not break, crush, chew caps
- Give without regard to meals

IV route

- Give by direct IV over 1 min

SIDE EFFECTS

CNS: Drowsiness, headache, vertigo, fever, lethargy, hallucinations
CV: Palpitations, hypertension
EENT: Blurred vision, photophobia
GI: Nausea, diarrhea, vomiting, jaundice, anorexia, dry mouth, constipation, cramps, metallic taste
GU: Polyuria, hypercalciuria, hyperphosphatemia, hematuria, thirst
MS: Myalgia, arthralgia, decreased bone development, weakness
SYST: Anaphylaxis

PHARMACOKINETICS

PO: Absorbed readily from GI tract, peak 10-12 hr, duration 3-5 days, half-life 3-6 hr, undergoes hepatic recycling, excreted in bile

INTERACTIONS

- Hypercalcemia: thiazide diuretics, calcium supplements
- Cardiac dysrhythmias: cardiac glycosides, verapamil
- Hypermagnesemia: magnesium antacids
- Toxicity: other vit D products

Increase: metabolism of vit D—phenytoin
Decrease: absorption of calcitriol—cholestyramine, mineral oil, fat-soluble vitamins

Drug/Food

- Large amounts of high-calcium foods may cause hypercalcemia

Drug/Lab Test

False increase: cholesterol
Interference: alk phos, electrolytes

NURSING CONSIDERATIONS

Assess:

- BUN, urinary calcium, PTH, creatinine, chloride, magnesium, electrolytes, phosphate; may increase calcium; should be kept at 9-10 mg/dl, vit D 50-135 international units/dl, phosphate 70 mg/dl; toxic reactions may occur rapidly
- **Hypercalcemia:** dry mouth, metallic taste, polyuria, bone pain, muscle weakness, headache, fatigue, change in LOC, dysrhythmias, increased respirations, anorexia, nausea, vomiting, cramps, diarrhea, constipation; paresthesia, twitching, dysrhythmias, Chvostek's sign, Trousseau's sign **(hypocalcemia)**
- Renal status: decreased urinary output (oliguria, anuria), edema in extremities, weight gain 5-7 lb, periorbital edema
- Nutritional status, diet for sources of vit D (milk, some seafood); calcium (dairy products, dark green vegetables), phosphates (dairy products) must be avoided

Perform/provide:

- Storage protected from light, heat, moisture
- Restriction of sodium, potassium if required; restriction of fluids if required for chronic renal failure

Evaluate:
- Therapeutic response: calcium 9-10 mg/dl; decreasing symptoms of hypocalcemia, hypoparathyroidism

Teach patient/family:
- About symptoms of hypercalcemia: renal stones, nausea, vomiting, anorexia, lethargy, thirst, bone or flank pain
- To avoid products with sodium: cured meats, dairy products, cold cuts, olives, beets, pickles, soups, meat tenderizers with chronic renal failure; products with potassium: oranges, bananas, dried fruit, peas, dark green leafy vegetables, milk, melons, beans
- To avoid OTC products that contain calcium, potassium, sodium with chronic renal failure
- To monitor weight weekly; to maintain fluid intake

calcium carbonate (PO-OTC)

AcidFree, Alka-Mints, Amitone, Apo-Cal ♣, Calcarb, Calci-Chew, Calci-Mix, Calcite ♣, Cal-Gest, Caltrate, Equaline Calcium, Leader Calcium, Maalox Antacid, Os-Cal 500, PMS-Calcium ♣, Rolaids Extra Strength Softchew, Tums, Tums E-X, Walgreens Calcium

calcium acetate (OTC)

(kal'see-um ass'e-tate)

Calphron, Eliphos, PhosLo

Func. class.: Antacid, calcium supplement

Chem. class.: Calcium product

Do not confuse:
Os-Cal/Asacol

ACTION: Neutralizes gastric acidity

USES: Antacid, calcium supplement; not suitable for chronic therapy, hyperphosphatemia, hypertension during pregnancy, osteoporosis, prevention, treatment of hypocalcemia, hypoparathyroidism

Unlabeled uses: Duodenal ulcer, PMS, stress gastritis

CONTRAINDICATIONS: Hypersensitivity, hypercalcemia, hyperparathyroidism, bone tumors

Precautions: Pregnancy (C), breastfeeding, geriatric patients, fluid restriction, decreased GI motility, GI obstruction, dehydration, renal disease

DOSAGE AND ROUTES

Nutritional supplement including osteoporosis prophylaxis
- **Adult ≥51 yr: PO** 1000-1500 mg/day elemental calcium (2500-3750 mg/day calcium carbonate)
- **Adult 19-50 yr: PO** 1000 mg/day elemental calcium (2500 mg/day calcium carbonate)

Chronic hypocalcemia
- **Adult: PO** 2-4 g/day elemental calcium (5-10 g/day calcium carbonate) in 3-4 divided doses
- **Child: PO** 45-65 mg/kg/day elemental calcium (112.5-162.5 mg/kg/day calcium carbonate) in 4 divided doses
- **Neonate: PO** 50-150 mg/kg/day elemental calcium (125-375 mg/kg/day in 4-6 divided doses, max 1 g/day)

Supplementation
- **Adolescent and child 9-18 yr: PO** 1300 mg elemental calcium (3250 mg calcium carbonate)
- **Child 4-8 yr: PO** 800 mg/day elemental calcium (2000 mg/day calcium carbonate)
- **Child 1-3 yr: PO** 500 mg/day elemental calcium (1250 mg/day calcium carbonate)
- **Infant 6-12 mo: PO** 270 mg/day elemental calcium based on total intake
- **Neonates and infants <6 mo: PO** 210 mg/day elemental calcium based on total intake

Hyperphosphatemia
• **Adult: PO** Individualized on response
Heartburn, dyspepsia, hyperacidity (OTC)
• **Adult: PO** 1-2 tabs q2hr, max 9 tabs/24 hr (Alka-mints); chew 2-4 tab q1hr prn, max 16 tabs (Tums regular strength); chew 2-4 tab q1hr prn, max 10 tabs (Tums E-X); chew 2-3 tabs q1hr prn, max 10 tabs/24 hr (Tums Ultra); chew 2 tabs q2-3hr, max 19 tabs/24 hr (Titralac Extra Strength)
Duodenal ulcer/stress gastritis (unlabeled)
• **Adult: PO** 80-140 mEq q1-3hr
PMS (unlabeled)
• **Adult: PO** (Tums EX, Tums Calcium for Life PMS) Chew 2 tabs bid
Available forms: calcium carbonate: chewable tabs 350, 420, 450, 500, 750, 1000, 1250 mg; tabs 500, 600, 650, 667, 1000, 1250, 1500 mg; gum 300, 450, 500 mg; susp 1250 mg/5 ml; caps 1250 mg; powder 6.5 g/packet; **calcium acetate:** tabs 250 mg (65 mg Ca), 667 mg (169 mg Ca), 668 mg (169 mg Ca), 1 g (250 mg Ca); caps 500 mg (125 mg Ca)
Administer:
PO route
• Do not give enteric-coated within 1 hr of calcium carbonate
• For ulcer treatment (adjunct): give 1 and 3 hr after meals and at bedtime
• For a phosphate binder: give 1 hr after each meal or snack and at bedtime
• For supplement: give 1-1½ hr after meals; avoid oxalic acid foods (spinach, rhubarb), phytic acid (brans, cereals) or phosphorus (milk, dairy), may decrease calcium absorption
• Suspension: shake well, use calibrated measuring device
• Laxatives or stool softeners if constipation occurs

SIDE EFFECTS

GI: *Constipation,* anorexia, nausea, vomiting, flatulence, diarrhea, rebound hyperacidity, eructation
GU: Calculi, hypercalciuria

PHARMACOKINETICS

⅓ of dose absorbed by small intestine, onset 20 min, duration 20-180 min, excreted in feces and urine, crosses placenta, must have adequate vit D for absorption

INTERACTIONS

Increase: digoxin toxicity—hypercalcemia
Increase: plasma levels of quiNIDine, amphetamines
Increase: hypercalcemia—thiazide diuretics
Decrease: levels of salicylates, calcium channel blockers, ketoconazole, iron salts, tetracyclines, fluoroquinolones, phenytoin, etidronate, risedronate, atenolol
Drug/Lab Test
False increase: chloride
False positive: benzodiazepines
False decrease: magnesium, oxylate, lipase

NURSING CONSIDERATIONS

Assess:
• Calcium (serum, urine), calcium should be 8.5-10.5 mg/dl, urine calcium should be 150 mg/day, monitor weekly; serum phosphate
⚠ **Milk-alkali syndrome:** nausea, vomiting, disorientation, headache
• Constipation; increase bulk in the diet if needed
• **Hypercalcemia:** headache, nausea, vomiting, confusion; hypocalcemia: paresthesia, twitching colic, dysrhythmias, Chvostek's sign, Trousseau's sign
• Those taking digoxin for toxicity
• Antacid—for abdominal pain, heartburn, indigestion before, after administration
Evaluate:
• Therapeutic response: absence of pain, decreased acidity; decreased hyperphosphatemia with renal failure
Teach patient/family:
• To increase fluids to 2 L unless contraindicated; to add bulk to diet for consti-

pation; to notify prescriber of constipation

- Not to switch antacids unless directed by prescriber; not to use as antacid for >2 wk without approval by prescriber
- That therapeutic dose recommendations are figured as elemental calcium
- To avoid excessive use of alcohol, caffeine, tobacco
- To avoid spinach, cereals, dairy products in large amounts

CALCIUM SALTS

calcium chloride (Rx)
calcium gluceptate (Rx)
calcium gluconate (Rx)
calcium lactate (Rx)

Func. class.: Electrolyte replacement—calcium product

ACTION: Caution needed for maintenance of nervous, muscular, skeletal function; enzyme reactions; normal cardiac contractility; coagulation of blood; affects secretory activity of endocrine, exocrine glands

USES: Prevention and treatment of hypocalcemia, hypermagnesemia, hypoparathyroidism, neonatal tetany, cardiac toxicity caused by hyperkalemia, lead colic, hyperphosphatemia, vit D deficiency, osteoporosis prophylaxis, calcium antagonist toxicity (calcium channel blocker toxicity)

Unlabeled uses: Electrolyte abnormalities in cardiac arrest, CPR

CONTRAINDICATIONS: Hypercalcemia, digoxin toxicity, ventricular fibrillation, renal calculi

Precautions: Pregnancy (C), breastfeeding, children, respiratory/renal disease, cor pulmonale, digitalized patient, respiratory failure, diarrhea, dehydration

DOSAGE AND ROUTES

Calcium chloride

- **Adult: IV** 500 mg-1 g q1-3days as indicated by serum calcium levels, give at <1 ml/min; **IV** 200 800 mg injected in ventricle of heart

Calcium gluceptate

- **Adult: IV** 5-20 ml; **IM** 2-5 ml

Calcium gluconate

- **Adult: PO** 0.5-2 g bid-qid; **IV** 0.5-2 g at 0.5 ml/min (10% solution); max **IV** dose 3 g
- **Child: PO/IV** 500 mg/kg/day in divided doses

Calcium lactate

- **Adult: PO** 325 mg-1.3 g tid with meals
- **Child: PO** 500 mg/kg/day in divided doses

Available forms: Many; check product listings

Administer:

PO route (only acetate, carbonate, citrate, glubionate, lactate, phosphate)

- Give in 3-4 divided doses with or 1 hr after meals, follow with full glass of water; if using as phosphate binder in renal dialysis, do not follow with water, do not give oral medications within 1 hr of oral calcium; *chew tab:* chew thoroughly; *effervescent tab:* dissolve in full glass of water; *oral powder:* mix and give with food; *oral solution:* give before meals; *oral suspension:* shake well

IM route

- Glycerophosphate, lactate may be given IM
- Do not give chloride, gluconate IM
- Use only if IV is not feasible
- Inject into gluteal region (adult), lateral thigh (child)
- Aspirate prior to inj
- Do not give chloride subcut

IV route

- Undiluted or diluted with equal amounts of NS to a 5% sol for inj, give 0.5-1 ml/min
- Through small-bore needle into large vein; if extravasation occurs, necrosis will result (IV)
- Remain recumbent 1/2 hr after IV dose

Calcium chloride

Additive compatibilities: Amikacin, amphotericin B, ampicillin, ascorbic acid, ceftriaxone, cephapirin, chloramphenicol, DOPamine, hydrocortisone, isoproterenol, lidocaine, methicillin, norepinephrine, penicillin G potassium, penicillin G sodium, pentobarbital, PHENobarbital, verapamil, vit B/C

Syringe compatibilities: Milrinone

Y-site compatibilities: Inamrinone, DOBUTamine, EPINEPHrine, esmolol, morphine, paclitaxel

Calcium gluceptate

Additive compatibilities: Ascorbic acid inj, isoproterenol, lidocaine, norepinephrine, phytonadione, sodium bicarbonate

Calcium gluconate

Additive compatibilities: Amikacin, aminophylline, ascorbic acid inj, cephapirin, chloramphenicol, cisatracurium, corticotropin, dimenhyDRINATE, DOXOrubicin liposome, erythromycin, furosemide, heparin, hydrocortisone, lidocaine, magnesium sulfate, methicillin, norepinephrine, penicillin G potassium, penicillin G sodium, PHENobarbital, potassium chloride, remifentanil, tobramycin, vancomycin, verapamil, vit B/C

Syringe compatibilities: Aldesleukin, allopurinol, amifostine, aztreonam, cefazolin, cefepime, ciprofloxacin, cladribine, DOBUTamine, enalaprilat, EPINEPHrine, famotidine, filgrastim, granisetron, heparin/hydrocortisone, labetalol, melphalan, midazolam, netilmicin, piperacillin/tazobactam, potassium chloride, prochlorperazine, propofol, sargramostim, tacrolimus, teniposide, thiotepa, tolazoline, vinorelbine, vit B/C

SIDE EFFECTS

CV: Shortened QT, heart block, hypotension, bradycardia, dysrhythmias; cardiac arrest (IV)

GI: Vomiting, nausea, constipation

HYPERCALCEMIA: Drowsiness, lethargy, muscle weakness, headache, constipation, coma, anorexia, nausea, vomiting, polyuria, thirst

INTEG: Pain, burning at IV site, severe venous thrombosis, necrosis, extravasation

PHARMACOKINETICS

Crosses placenta, enters breast milk, excreted via urine and feces, half-life unknown, protein binding 40%-50%

PO: Onset, peak, duration unknown, absorption from GI tract

IV: Onset immediate, duration 1/2-2 hr

INTERACTIONS

Increase: milk-alkali syndrome—antacids

Increase: dysrhythmias—digoxin glycosides

Increase: toxicity—verapamil

Increase: hypercalcemia—thiazide diuretics

Decrease: absorption of fluoroquinolones, tetracyclines, iron salts, phenytoin, thyroid hormones when calcium is taken PO

Decrease: effects of atenolol, verapamil

Drug/Herb

Increase: action/side effects—lily of the valley, pheasant's eye, shark cartilage, squill

Drug/Lab Test

Increase: 11-OHCS

Decrease: 17-OHCS

False decrease: magnesium

NURSING CONSIDERATIONS

Assess:

- **ECG for decreased QT and T wave inversion:** hypercalcemia, product should be reduced or discontinued, consider cardiac monitoring
- Calcium levels during treatment (8.5-11.5 g/dl is normal level); urine calcium if hypercaluria occurs
- Cardiac status: rate, rhythm, CVP (PWP, PAWP if being monitored directly)
- **Hypocalcemia:** muscle twitching, paresthesia, dysrhythmias, laryngospasm
- Digitalized patients frequently; an increase in calcium increases digoxin toxicity risk

Perform/provide:

- Seizure precautions: padded side rails, decreased stimuli (noise, light); place airway suction equipment, padded mouth gag if Ca levels are low
- Store at room temp

Evaluate:

- Therapeutic response: decreased twitching, paresthesias, muscle spasms; absence of tremors, seizures, dysrhythmias, dyspnea, laryngospasm; negative Chvostek's sign, negative Trousseau's sign

Teach patient/family:

- To add foods high in vit D
- To add calcium-rich foods to diet: dairy products, shellfish, dark green leafy vegetables; to decrease oxalate- and zinc-rich foods: nuts, legumes, chocolate, spinach, soy
- To prevent injuries; to avoid immobilization

RARELY USED

calfactant (Rx)

(cal-fak'tant)

Infasurf

Func. class.: Natural lung surfactant extract

USES: Prevention and treatment (rescue) of respiratory distress syndrome in premature infants

DOSAGE AND ROUTES

- **Newborn: INTRATRACHEAL INSTILL:** 3 ml/kg of birth weight given as 2 doses of 1.5 ml/kg; repeat doses of 3 ml/kg of birth wt until up to 3 doses 12 hr apart have been given

candesartan (Rx)

(can-deh-sar'tan)

Atacand

Func. class.: Antihypertensive

Chem. class.: Angiotensin II receptor (type AT_1) antagonist

ACTION: Blocks the vasoconstrictor and aldosterone-secreting effects of angiotensin II; selectively blocks the binding of angiotensin II to the AT_1 receptor found in tissues

USES: Hypertension, alone or in combination; CHF NYHA Class II-IV and ejection fraction ≤40%

CONTRAINDICATIONS: Hypersensitivity

Black Box Warning: Pregnancy (D) 2nd/3rd trimesters

Precautions: Pregnancy (C) 1st trimester, breastfeeding, children, geriatric patients, hypersensitivity to ACE inhibitors, volume depletion, renal/hepatic impairment

DOSAGE AND ROUTES

Hypertension

- **Adult: PO** single agent 16 mg/day initially in patients who are not volume depleted, range 8-32 mg/day; with diuretic or volume depletion 2-32 mg/day as single dose or divided bid
- **Adolescent and child ≥6 yr and weight >50 kg: PO** 8-16 mg q day or divided bid, adjust to B/P; usual range 4-32 mg/day, max 32 mg/day
- **Child ≥6 yr, weight <50 kg: PO** 4-8 mg/day or divided bid, adjust to B/P
- **Child ≥1 yr and <6 yr: PO** 0.2 mg/kg/day in 1 dose or in 2 divided doses, adjust to B/P, max 0.4 mg/kg/day

Heart failure

- **Adult: PO** 4 mg q day, may be doubled ≥2 wk, target dose 32 mg/day

Renal/hepatic disease
• **Adult: PO** ≤8 mg/day for severe renal disease/moderate hepatic disease, adjust dose as needed
Available forms: Tabs 4, 8, 16, 32 mg
Administer:
• Without regard to meals
• Oral liquid: shake well, do not freeze

SIDE EFFECTS

CNS: *Dizziness,* fatigue, headache
CV: Chest pain, peripheral edema, hypotension
EENT: Sinusitis, rhinitis, pharyngitis
GI: *Diarrhea,* nausea, abdominal pain, vomiting
GU: Renal failure
MS: Arthralgia, pain
RESP: *Cough, upper respiratory infection*
SYST: Angioedema

PHARMACOKINETICS

Peak 3-4 hr, protein binding 99%, half-life 9-12 hr, extensively metabolized, excreted in urine (33%) and feces (67%)

INTERACTIONS

Increase: lithium level—lithium
Increase: hyperkalemia—potassium, potassium-sparing diuretics
Increase: hypotension—ACE inhibitors, β-blockers, calcium channel blockers, α-blockers
Decrease: effect—salicylates, NSAIDs
Drug/Herb
Increase: antihypertensive effect—hawthorn
Decrease: antihypertensive effect—ephedra

NURSING CONSIDERATIONS

Assess:
⚠ **Serious hypersensitivity reaction:** angioedema, anaphylaxis: facial swelling, difficulty breathing (rare)

Black Box Warning: For pregnancy; this product can cause fetal death when given during pregnancy (D), 2nd/3rd trimester

• Response and adverse reactions, especially with renal disease
• B/P, pulse q4hr; note rate, rhythm, quality; electrolytes: K, Na, Cl; baselines of renal/hepatic studies before therapy begins
• **Heart failure:** jugular venous distention, weight, edema, dyspnea, crackles
Evaluate:
• Therapeutic response: decreased B/P
Teach patient/family:
• To comply with dosage schedule, even if feeling better
• To notify prescriber of mouth sores, fever, swelling of hands or feet, irregular heartbeat, chest pain
• That excessive perspiration, dehydration, vomiting, diarrhea may lead to fall in B/P; to consult prescriber if these occur
• To rise slowly to sitting or standing position to minimize orthostatic hypotension; that product may cause dizziness, fainting, lightheadedness

Black Box Warning: To notify prescriber immediately if pregnant; not to use if breastfeeding

• To avoid all OTC medications unless approved by prescriber; to inform all health care providers of medication use
• To use proper technique for obtaining B/P; to understand acceptable parameters

capecitabine (Rx)

(cap-eh-sit′ah-bean)
Xeloda
Func. class.: Antineoplastic, antimetabolite
Chem. class.: Fluoropyrimidine carbamate

Do not confuse:
Xeloda/Xenical

ACTION: Competes with physiologic substrate of DNA synthesis, thereby interfering with cell replication in the S phase of cell cycle (before mitosis); also interferes with RNA and protein synthesis; product is converted to 5-FU

USES:
Monotherapy for paclitaxel; anthracycline-resistant, metastatic breast, colorectal cancer when 5-FU monotherapy is preferred; treatment of colorectal cancer patients who have undergone complete resection of their primary tumors

Unlabeled uses: Biliary tract, ovarian cancer

CONTRAINDICATIONS:
Pregnancy (D), hypersensitivity to 5-FU, infants, severe renal impairment (CCr <30 ml/min), DPD deficiency

Precautions: Breastfeeding, children, geriatric patients, renal/hepatic disease

DOSAGE AND ROUTES

Metastatic breast cancer resistant to both paclitaxel and anthracycline or resistant to paclitaxel and when further anthracycline therapy is not indicated

• **Adult: PO** 2500 mg/m^2/day divided q12hr after a meal × 2 wk, repeat q3wk

Breast cancer (locally advanced/ metastatic) with docetaxel, previously treated with anthracycline

• **Adult: PO** 2500 mg/m^2/day divided q12hr after a meal on days 1-14, with docetaxel 75 mg/m^2 IV on day 1

Advanced/metastatic breast cancer (HER2 positive) previously treated with anthracycline, taxane, and trastuzumab

• **Adult: PO** 2000 mg/m^2/day divided q12hr after a meal on days 1-14 with lapatinib 1250 mg/day on days 1-21, repeat q21days

Metastatic/locally advanced breast cancer resistant to anthracycline, previously treated with a taxane or taxane resistant, and when further anthracycline is contraindicated

• **Adult: PO** 2000 mg/m^2/day divided q12hr on days 1-14 with ixabepilone 40 mg/m^2 IV over 3 hr, repeat q3wk

As an adjuvant for Dukes C colorectal cancer with a complete resection when fluoropyrimidine alone is preferred

• **Adult: PO** 2500 mg/m^2/day divided q12hr within 30 min of a meal × 2 wk, repeat q3wk for 8 cycles

First-line treatment of metastatic colorectal cancer when fluoropyrimidine alone is preferred

• **Adult: PO** 2500 mg/m^2/day divided q12hr after a meal × 2 wk, repeat q3wk

First-line treatment of metastatic colorectal cancer with oxaliplatin with or without bevacizumab (unlabeled)

• **Adult: PO** 2000 mg/m^2/day divided q12hr after a meal on days 1-14 with oxaliplatin on day 1, repeat q3wk

First-/second-line treatment of advanced colorectal cancer with oxaliplatin (unlabeled)

• **Adult: PO** 2000 mg/m^2/day divided q12hr on days 1-14 and oxaliplatin 130 mg/m^2 IV on day 1, repeat q3wk

Unresectable advanced/metastatic biliary tract cancer (unlabeled)

• **Adult: PO** 2500 mg/m^2 divided q12hr on days 1-14, then 7-day rest period; given with CISplatin 60 mg/m^2 IV over 1 hr on day 1, repeat q21days

Renal dose

• **Adult: PO** CCr 30-50 ml/min, decrease initial dose to 75% of usual dose; CCr <30 ml/min, contraindicated

Available forms: Tabs 150, 500 mg

Administer:

• **Dosage adjustments of capecitabine monotherapy based on most severe toxicity OR when used in combination with ixabepilone based on nonhematologic toxicity:** *Grade 1 toxicity:* maintain current dosage; *Grade 2 toxicity (1st appearance):* interrupt therapy until toxicity is resolved to grade 0–1; do not replace missed doses, begin the next cycle with 100% of the starting dose; *Grade 2 toxicity (2nd appearance):* interrupt therapy until toxicity is resolved to grade 0–1; do not replace missed doses, begin the next cycle with

75% of the starting dose; *Grade 2 toxicity (3rd appearance):* interrupt therapy until toxicity is resolved to grade 0–1; do not replace missed doses, begin the next cycle with 50% of the starting dose; *Grade 2 toxicity (4th appearance):* discontinue treatment permanently; *Grade 3 toxicity (1st appearance):* interrupt therapy until toxicity is resolved to grade 0–1

SIDE EFFECTS

CNS: Dizziness, *headache, paresthesia, fatigue,* insomnia

CV: Venous thrombosis

GI: *Nausea, vomiting, anorexia, diarrhea, stomatitis, abdominal pain, constipation, dyspepsia,* intestinal obstruction, necrotizing enterocolitis, hyperbilirubinemia, hepatic failure

HEMA: Neutropenia, lymphopenia, thrombocytopenia, anemia

INTEG: *Hand and foot syndrome, dermatitis,* nail disorders

OTHER: *Eye irritation, edema, myalgia,* limb pain, *pyrexia,* dehydration

RESP: *Cough, dyspnea,* pulmonary embolism

PHARMACOKINETICS

Readily absorbed, peak $1^1/_2$ hr, food decreases absorption, extensively metabolized in the liver, elimination half-life 45 min

INTERACTIONS

Increase: toxicity—leucovorin

Increase: capecitabine levels—antacids (aluminum, magnesium)

Increase: phenytoin level—phenytoin

Black Box Warning: Increase: bleeding risk—anticoagulants

Drug/Food

Increase: absorption; give within 30 min of a meal

NURSING CONSIDERATIONS

Assess:

- **Bone marrow suppression,** CBC (RBC, Hct, Hgb), differential, platelet count weekly; withhold product if WBC is <4000/mm^3, platelet count is <75,000/mm^3, or RBC, Hct, Hgb low; notify prescriber of these results; frequently monitor INR in those receiving warfarin concurrently
- Renal studies: BUN, serum uric acid, urine CCr, electrolytes before, during therapy
- Monitor temp q4hr; fever may indicate beginning infection; no rectal temps
- Hepatic studies before, during therapy: bilirubin, ALT, AST, alk phos as needed or monthly
- **Bleeding:** hematuria, heme-positive stools, bruising or petechiae of mucosa or orifices q8hr
- Dyspnea, crackles, unproductive cough, chest pain, tachypnea, fatigue, increased pulse, pallor, lethargy; personality changes with high doses
- **Hand and foot syndrome:** paresthesia, tingling, painful/painless swelling, blistering, erythema with severe pain of hands or feet
- **Toxicity:** severe diarrhea, nausea, vomiting, stomatitis, fever
- Buccal cavity q8hr for dryness, sores, ulceration, white patches, oral pain, bleeding, dysphagia
- **GI symptoms:** frequency of stools, cramping; if severe diarrhea occurs, fluid, electrolytes may need to be given

Perform/provide:

- Rinsing of mouth tid-qid with water, club soda; brushing of teeth bid-tid with soft brush or cotton-tipped applicators for stomatitis; use unwaxed dental floss

Evaluate:

- Therapeutic response: decreased tumor size, spread of malignancy

Teach patient/family:

- To avoid foods with citric acid, hot or rough texture if stomatitis is present; take with water within 30 min of end of meal

- To avoid pregnancy while taking this product; to avoid breastfeeding
- Not to double dose if dose is missed

⚠ To immediately report severe diarrhea, vomiting, stomatitis, fever of more than 100° F (37.8° C), hand and foot syndrome, anorexia

- To report signs of **infection:** increased temp, sore throat, flulike symptoms; signs of **anemia:** fatigue, headache, faintness, shortness of breath, irritability; **bleeding;** to avoid use of razors, commercial mouthwash
- OTC antidiarrheals for mild diarrhea (4-6 stools/day or diarrhea at night)

captopril (Rx)

(kap′toe-pril)

Apo-Capto ♣, Capoten, Gen-Captopril ♣, PMS-Captopril ♣

Func. class.: Antihypertensive

Chem. class.: Angiotensin-converting enzyme (ACE) inhibitor

Do not confuse:
captopril/Capitrol/carvedilol

ACTION: Selectively suppresses renin-angiotensin-aldosterone system; inhibits ACE; prevents conversion of angiotensin I to angiotensin II

USES: Hypertension, CHF, left ventricular dysfunction after MI, diabetic nephropathy

Unlabeled uses: Acute MI, hypertensive emergency/urgency, scleroderma renal crisis (SRC)

CONTRAINDICATIONS: Breastfeeding, children, hypersensitivity, heart block, potassium-sparing diuretics, bilateral renal artery stenosis, angioedema

Black Box Warning: Pregnancy (D)

Precautions: Dialysis patients, hypovolemia, leukemia, scleroderma, SLE, blood dyscrasias, CHF, diabetes mellitus, thyroid/renal/hepatic disease, COPD, asthma

DOSAGE AND ROUTES

Hypertension

- **Adult: PO** initial dose: 12.5-25 mg bid-tid; may increase to 50 mg bid-tid at 1-2 wk intervals; usual range: 25-150 mg bid-tid; max 450 mg/day
- **Child: PO** 0.3-0.5 mg/kg/dose, titrate up to 6 mg/kg/day in 2-4 divided doses
- **Neonate: PO** 0.05-0.1 mg/kg bid-tid, may increase as needed

CHF

- **Adult: PO** 25 mg bid; may increase to 50 mg tid; after 14 days, may increase to 150 mg tid if needed

Diabetic nephropathy

- **Adult: PO** 25 mg tid

Renal dose

- **Adult: PO** CCr >50 ml/min, no change; CCr 10-50 ml/min, decrease dose by 25%; CCr <10 ml/min, decrease dose by 50%

Acute MI (unlabeled) or post MI

- **Adult: PO** 6.25-12.5 mg tid, increase to 25 mg tid gradually

Hypertensive emergency/urgency (unlabeled)

- **Adult: PO** 25 mg, may repeat q30min

Available forms: Tabs 12.5, 25, 50, 100 mg

Administer:

- 1 hr before or 2 hr after meals
- **Oral sol:** may crush tab, dissolve in water; give within ½ hr; make sure tab completely dissolved

SIDE EFFECTS

CNS: Fever, chills

CV: *Hypotension,* postural hypotension, *tachycardia,* angina

GI: Loss of taste, increased LFTs

GU: Impotence, dysuria, nocturia, proteinuria, nephrotic syndrome, acute reversible renal failure, polyuria, oliguria, urinary frequency

HEMA: Neutropenia, agranulocytosis, pancytopenia, thrombocytopenia, anemia

INTEG: Rash, pruritus

MISC: Angioedema, hyperkalemia

RESP: Bronchospasm, *dyspnea, cough*

PHARMACOKINETICS

Peak 1 hr; duration 2-6 hr; half-life <2 hr, increased in renal disease; metabolized by liver (metabolites); excreted in urine; crosses placenta; excreted in breast milk, small amounts; protein binding 25%-30%

INTERACTIONS

- Do not use with potassium-sparing diuretics, sympathomimetics, potassium supplements

Increase: possible toxicity—lithium, digoxin

Increase: hypoglycemia—insulin, oral antidiabetics

Increase: hypotension—diuretics, other antihypertensives, phenothiazines, nitrates, acute alcohol ingestion

Decrease: captopril effect—antacids, NSAIDs, salicylates

Drug/Herb

Increase: antihypertensive effect—hawthorn

Decrease: antihypertensive effect—ephedra

Drug/Food

Decrease: absorption of captopril

Drug/Lab Test

Increase: AST, ALT, alk phos, bilirubin, uric acid, glucose

False positive: urine acetone, ANA titer

NURSING CONSIDERATIONS

Assess:

- **Blood dyscrasias:** blood studies: decreased platelets; WBC with differential at baseline and periodically q3mo; if neutrophils $<1000/mm^3$, discontinue treatment (recommended with collagen-vascular or renal disease)
- **Hypertension:** B/P, pulse rates at baseline, frequently
- Renal studies: protein, BUN, creatinine; watch for raised levels, may indicate nephrotic syndrome; increased LFTs, uric acid; glucose may be increased
- Allergic reaction: rash, fever, pruritus, urticaria; discontinue product if antihistamines fail to help
- **CHF:** edema, dyspnea, wet crackles, increased B/P, weight gain

Perform/provide:

- Storage in tight container at 86° F (30° C) or less

Evaluate:

- Therapeutic response: decrease in B/P with hypertension; edema, moist crackles (CHF)

Teach patient/family:

- To take 1 hr before or 2 hr after meals; not to discontinue product abruptly; if dose is missed, take as soon as remembered but not if almost time for next dose; not to double doses
- Not to use OTC products (cough, cold, or allergy) unless directed by prescriber; avoid salt substitutes, high-potassium or high-sodium foods
- To avoid sunlight or wear sunscreen if in sunlight because photosensitivity may occur
- To comply with dosage schedule, even if feeling better
- To rise slowly to sitting or standing position to minimize orthostatic hypotension
- To notify prescriber of mouth sores, sore throat, fever, swelling of hands or feet, irregular heartbeat, chest pain, signs of angioedema
- That excessive perspiration, dehydration, vomiting, diarrhea may lead to fall in B/P; to consult prescriber if these occur
- That dizziness, fainting, lightheadedness may occur during first few days of therapy
- That skin rash or impaired perspiration may occur
- How to take B/P and when to notify prescriber

Black Box Warning: To report if pregnancy is suspected or planned

TREATMENT OF OVERDOSE:

0.9% NaCl IV/INF; hemodialysis

carbachol ophthalmic

See Appendix B

carBAMazepine (Rx)

(kar-ba-maz′e-peen)

Apo-Carbamazepine ✦, Carbatrol, Epitol, Equetro, Gen-Carbamazepine CR ✦, PMS-Carbamazepine ✦, Sandoz-Carbamazepine ✦, Taro-Carbamazepine ✦, Tegretol, Tegretol-XR

Func. class.: Anticonvulsant

Chem. class.: Iminostilbene derivative

Do not confuse:
Tegretol/Toradol

ACTION: Exact mechanism unknown; appears to decrease polysynaptic responses and block posttetanic potentiation

USES: Tonic-clonic, complex-partial, mixed seizures; trigeminal neuralgia; bipolar disorder

Unlabeled uses: Neurogenic pain, psychotic behavior with dementia, diabetic neuropathy, agitation, hiccups

CONTRAINDICATIONS: Pregnancy (D), hypersensitivity to carBAMazepine or tricyclics, AV or bundle branch block

Black Box Warning: Bone marrow depression

Precautions: Breastfeeding, children <6 yr, glaucoma, cardiac/renal/hepatic disease, psychosis, alcoholism, hepatic porphyria

Black Box Warning: Hematologic disease, Asian patients, agranulocytosis, leukopenia, neutropenia, thrombocytopenia

DOSAGE AND ROUTES

Seizures

- **Adult and child >12 yr: PO** 200 mg bid, may be increased by 200 mg/day in weekly intervals, give in divided doses q6-8hr; maintenance 800-1200 mg/day, max 1600 mg/day (adult); max child 12-15 yr 1000 mg/day; max child >15 yr 1200 mg/day; adjust to minimum dose to control seizures; **EXT REL** give bid; rectal administration of **ORAL SUSP** 200 mg/10 ml or 6 mg/kg as a single dose
- **Child 6-12 yr: PO** tabs 100 mg bid or susp 50 mg qid; may increase by <100 mg q wk; max 1000 mg/day **EXT REL** tabs daily-bid
- **Child <6 yr: PO** 10-20 mg/kg/day in 2-3 divided doses, may increase every wk

Trigeminal neuralgia

- **Adult: PO** 100 mg bid with meals; may increase 100 mg q12hr until pain subsides, max 1200 mg/day; maintenance 200-400 mg bid

Diabetic neuropathy (unlabeled)

- **Adult: PO** 100 mg bid or 50 mg qid, titrate to 600-800 mg/day

Bipolar disorder

- **Adult: PO** (Equetro only) 200 mg bid, may adjust dose by 200 mg/day to desired response, max 1600 mg/day

Agitation due to dementia (unlabeled)

- **Adult: PO** 100 mg bid, may increase to 250-300 mg/day

Hiccups (unlabeled)

- **Adult: PO** 200 mg tid

Available forms: Chewable tabs 100, 200 mg; tabs 200 mg; ext rel tabs (XR) 100, 200, 400 mg; oral susp 100 mg/5 ml; ext rel caps 100, 200, 300 mg

Administer:

PO route

- Do not crush, chew ext rel tab; ext rel cap may be opened and beads sprinkled over food; patient should chew chewable tab, not swallow it whole
- With food, milk to decrease GI symptoms; shake oral susp before use
- Mix an equal amount of water, D_5W,

0.9% NaCl when giving by NG tube; flush tube with 100 ml of above sol

SIDE EFFECTS

CNS: *Drowsiness,* dizziness, unsteadiness, confusion, fatigue, paralysis, headache, hallucinations, worsening of seizures, speech disturbance, suicidal thoughts/behaviors

CV: Hypertension, CHF, dysrhythmias, AV block, hypotension, aggravation of cardiac artery disease

EENT: Tinnitus, dry mouth, blurred vision, diplopia, nystagmus, conjunctivitis

ENDO: SIADH (geriatric patients)

GI: *Nausea, constipation, diarrhea,* anorexia, vomiting, abdominal pain, stomatitis, glossitis, increased hepatic enzymes, hepatitis, hepatic porphyria

GU: Frequency, retention, albuminuria, glycosuria, impotence, increased BUN, renal failure

HEMA: Thrombocytopenia, leukopenia, agranulocytosis, leukocytosis, aplastic anemia, eosinophilia, increased PT

INTEG: *Rash,* Stevens-Johnson syndrome, urticaria, photosensitivity, toxic epidermal necrolysis

RESP: Pulmonary hypersensitivity (fever, dyspnea, pneumonitis)

PHARMACOKINETICS

Onset slow; peak 4-5 hr; metabolized by liver; excreted in urine, feces; crosses placenta, blood-brain barrier; excreted in breast milk; half-life 18-65 hr then 8-29 hr after 1st month; protein binding 76%; metabolized by CYP3A4

INTERACTIONS

- CNS toxicity: lithium

⚠ Fatal reaction: MAOIs

Increase: carBAMazepine levels—CYP3A inhibitors (cimetidine, clarithromycin, danazol, diltiazem, erythromycin, FLUoxetine, fluvoxamine, isoniazid, propoxyphene, valproic acid, verapamil, voriconazole)

Increase: effects of desmopressin, lithium, lypressin, vasopressin

Decrease: carBAMazepine effect—CYP1A2, CYP2C9 substrates

Decrease: effect of CYP3A inducers

Decrease: effects of benzodiazepines, doxycycline, felbamate, haloperidol, oral contraceptives, PHENobarbital, phenytoin, primidone, theophylline, thyroid hormones, warfarin

Decrease: carBAMazepine levels—CYP3A4 inducers (CISplatin, darunavir, delavirdine, DOXOrubicin, felbamate, nefazodone, oxcarbazepine, PHENobarbital, phenytoin, primidone, rifampin, theophylline)

Drug/Herb

Decrease: carBAMazepine metabolism, increased levels—echinacea

Decrease: anticonvulsant effect—St. John's wort

Drug/Food

Increase: peak concentration of carBAMazepine—grapefruit juice

NURSING CONSIDERATIONS

Assess:

Black Box Warning: Asian patients for serious skin reaction; genetic test before administration

- **Seizures:** character, location, duration, intensity, frequency, presence of aura
- **Trigeminal neuralgia:** facial pain including location, duration, intensity, character, activity that stimulates pain
- Renal studies: urinalysis, BUN, urine creatinine q3mo

Black Box Warning: Bone marrow depression: blood studies: RBC, Hct, Hgb, reticulocyte counts every wk for 4 wk then q3-6mo if on long-term therapy; if myelosuppression occurs, product should be discontinued; blood dyscrasias: fever, sore throat, bruising, rash, jaundice

- Hepatic studies: ALT, AST, bilirubin
- Product levels during initial treatment or when changing dose; should remain at 4-12 mcg/ml; anorexia may indicate increased blood levels

⚠ Mental status: mood, sensorium, affect, behavioral changes, **suicidal thoughts/behaviors;** if mental status changes, notify prescriber
- Eye problems: need for ophthalmic examinations before, during, after treatment (slit lamp, funduscopy, tonometry)
- Allergic reaction: purpura, red, raised rash; if these occur, product should be discontinued

⚠ Toxicity: bone marrow depression, nausea, vomiting, ataxia, diplopia, CV collapse, Stevens-Johnson syndrome

Perform/provide:
- Storage at room temp
- Hard candy, gum, frequent rinsing for dry mouth

Evaluate:
- Therapeutic response: decreased seizure activity; document on patient's chart

Teach patient/family:
- To carry emergency ID stating patient's name, products taken, condition, prescriber's name and phone number
- To avoid driving, other activities that require alertness usually for the first 3 days of treatment
- Not to discontinue medication quickly after long-term use
- To immediately report chills, rash, light-colored stools, dark urine, yellowing of skin and eyes, abdominal pain, sore throat, mouth ulcers, bruising, blurred vision, dizziness
- That urine may turn pink to brown

TREATMENT OF OVERDOSE:
Lavage, VS

carbidopa-levodopa (Rx)

(kar-bi-doe′pa)-(lee-voe-doe′pa)

Apo-Levocarb ✱, Atamet, Parcopa, Sinemet, Sinemet CR

Func. class.: Antiparkinson agent

Chem. class.: Catecholamine

ACTION:
Decarboxylation of levodopa in periphery is inhibited by carbidopa; more levodopa is made available for transport to the brain and for conversion to dopamine in the brain

USES:
Parkinson's disease, parkinsonism resulting from carbon monoxide, chronic manganese intoxication, cerebral arteriosclerosis

Unlabeled uses: Restless leg syndrome

CONTRAINDICATIONS:
Hypersensitivity, malignant melanoma, history of malignant melanoma or undiagnosed skin lesions resembling melanoma

Precautions: Pregnancy (C), breastfeeding, diabetes, closed-angle glaucoma, respiratory/cardiac/renal/hepatic disease, MI with dysrhythmias, seizures, peptic ulcer, depression

DOSAGE AND ROUTES

Beginning therapy for those not taking levodopa
- **Adult: PO** 25 mg carbidopa/100 mg levodopa tid, may increase daily or every other day by 1 tab to desired response (8 tabs/day); **EXT REL** tabs 50 mg carbidopa/200 mg levodopa bid

For those not taking levodopa ER
- 50 mg carbidopa/200 mg levodopa bid

For those taking levodopa ER
- Begin treatment with 10% more levodopa/day given q4-8hr, may increase or decrease dose q3days

For those taking levodopa <1.5 g/day
- **Adult: PO** 25 mg carbidopa/100 mg levodopa tid-qid, may increase daily to desired response

For those taking levodopa >1.5 g/day
- **Adult: PO** 25 mg carbidopa/250 mg levodopa tid-qid, may increase daily to desired response

Restless leg syndrome (RLS) (unlabeled)
- **Adult: PO** 25 mg carbidopa/100 mg levodopa, 1 tab at bedtime, may repeat if awakening within 2 hr or 50 mg

carbidopa/200 mg levodopa sus rel tab 1-2 tabs 1 hr before bedtime

Available forms: Tabs 10 mg carbidopa/100 mg levodopa, 25 mg carbidopa/100 mg levodopa, 25 mg carbidopa/250 mg levodopa; ext rel tab 25 mg/100 mg, 50 mg carbidopa/200 mg levodopa (Sinemet CR); oral disintegrating tab (Parcopa) 10 mg carbidopa/100 mg levodopa, 25 mg carbidopa/100 mg levodopa; 25 mg carbidopa/250 mg levodopa

Administer:

- Pyridoxine (B_6) not effective for reversing Sinemet or Sinemet CR

PO route

- Do not crush or chew **ext rel tabs;** they may be broken in half; adjust dosage to response
- **Oral disintegrating tab** by gently removing from bottle, placing on tongue and swallowing with saliva; after tab dissolves, liquid is not necessary
- With meals if GI symptoms occur; limit protein taken with product
- Only after nonselective MAOIs have been discontinued for 2 wk; if patient has been previously treated with levodopa, discontinue for at least 12 hr before change to carbidopa-levodopa

SIDE EFFECTS

CNS: *Involuntary choreiform movements, hand tremors, fatigue, headache, anxiety, twitching, numbness, weakness, confusion, agitation, insomnia, nightmares,* psychosis, hallucination, hypomania, severe depression, dizziness, impulsive behaviors, neuroleptic malignant syndrome

CV: *Orthostatic hypotension,* tachycardia, hypertension, palpitation

EENT: Blurred vision, diplopia, dilated pupils

GI: *Nausea, vomiting, anorexia, abdominal distress, dry mouth, flatulence, dysphagia,* bitter taste, diarrhea, constipation

HEMA: Hemolytic anemia, leukopenia, agranulocytosis

INTEG: Rash, sweating, alopecia

MISC: Urinary retention, incontinence, weight change, dark urine

PHARMACOKINETICS

PO: Onset 30 min, peak 1-3 hr, excreted in urine (metabolites)

EXT REL: Onset 4-6 hr

INTERACTIONS

- Hypertensive crisis: nonselective MAOIs

Increase: effects of levodopa—antacids, metoclopramide

Decrease: effects of levodopa—anticholinergics, hydantoins, papaverine, pyridoxine, benzodiazepines, antipsychotics

Drug/Lab Test

Increase: BUN, AST, ALT, bilirubin, alk phos, LDH, serum glucose

Decrease: BUN, creatinine, uric acid

False positive: urine ketones (dipstick), Coombs' test

False negative: urine glucose

False increase: urine protein

Drug/Food

Decrease: absorption of levodopa—protein

NURSING CONSIDERATIONS

Assess:

- **Parkinson's symptoms:** tremors, pill rolling, drooling, akinesia, rigidity, shuffling gait before, during treatment
- B/P, respiration; orthostatic B/P
- Mental status: affect, mood, behavioral changes, depression, complete suicide assessment
- **Toxicity:** muscle twitching, blepharospasm
- Renal, hepatic, hematopoietic tests; also for diabetes, acromegaly if on long-term therapy

Evaluate:

- Therapeutic response: decrease in akathisia/bradykinesis, tremor, rigidity, improved mood

Teach patient/family:
• To change positions slowly to prevent orthostatic hypotension
• To report side effects: twitching, eye spasms because these indicate overdose
• To use product as prescribed; if discontinued abruptly, parkinsonian crisis, neuroleptic malignant syndrome (NMS) may occur; to gradually taper
• That urine, sweat may darken
• To use physical activities to maintain mobility, lessen spasms
• That improvement may not occur for 2-4 mo; about "on-off phenomenon"

⚠ HIGH ALERT

CARBOplatin (Rx)

(kar-boe-pla′-tin)

Func. class.: Antineoplastic alkylating agent

Chem. class.: Platinum coordination compound

Do not confuse:
carboplatin/cisplatin

ACTION: Produces interstrand DNA cross-links and, to a lesser extent, DNA-protein cross-links; activity is not cell-cycle–phase specific

USES: Initial treatment of advanced ovarian cancer in combination with other agents; palliative treatment of ovarian carcinoma recurrent after treatment with other antineoplastic agents

Unlabeled uses: Acute lymphocytic leukemia (ALL), acute myelogenous leukemia (AML), bladder/breast/head/neck/lung/testicular cancer, bone marrow ablation, malignant glioma, neuroblastoma, non-Hodgkin's lymphoma, osteogenic sarcoma, soft-tissue sarcoma, stem-cell transplant preparation, Wilms' tumor, stage I seminoma

CONTRAINDICATIONS: Pregnancy (D), breastfeeding, hypersensitivity, significant bleeding, aluminum products used to prepare or administer CARBOplatin

Black Box Warning: Severe bone marrow depression, platinum compound hypersensitivity

Precautions: Geriatric patients, radiation therapy within 1 mo, other cancer chemotherapy within 1 mo, renal/hepatic disease

Black Box Warning: Anemia, infection

DOSAGE AND ROUTES

Advanced ovarian cancer
• **Adult (single agent): IV INF** initially 300 mg/m^2 on day 1 with cyclophosphamide, 600 mg/m^2 **IV** on day 1, repeat q4wk × 6 cycles; refractory tumors 360 mg/m^2 single dose, may repeat q4wk as needed, do not repeat until neutrophils >2000/mm^3 and platelets >100,000/mm^3

Renal dose
• **Adult (single agent): IV INF** CCr 41-59 ml/min, 250 mg/m^2, CCr 16-40 ml/min, 200 mg/m^2, do not use if CCr <15 ml/min

AML/ALL (unlabeled)
• **Adult: CONT IV INF** 315 mg/m^2/day × 5 days

Wilms' tumor (unlabeled)
• **Child: IV** 160 mg/m^2 × 5 days with etoposide 100 mg/m^2/day **IV**

Osteogenic sarcoma (unlabeled)
• **Adult/adolescent/child: IV** 560 mg/m^2 on day 1 with ifosfamide 2.65 g/m^2/day **IV** on days 1-3

Neuroblastoma/soft-tissue sarcoma (unlabeled)
• **Child: IV** 300-600 mg/m^2 q4wk or 400 mg/m^2/day for 2 days q4wk or 160 mg/m^2/day × 5 days q4wk

Available forms: Lyophilized powder for inj 50-, 150-, 450-mg vials; aqueous sol for inj 50 mg/5-ml vial, 150 mg/15-ml vial, 450 mg/45-ml vial, 600 mg/60-ml vial

Administer:
• Antiemetic 30-60 min before product and prn for vomiting

IV route

- Use cytotoxic handling procedures
- **Reconstitute** CARBOplatin 50, 150, or 450 mg with 5, 15, or 45 ml, respectively, of sterile water for inj, D_5W, or NaCl (10 mg/ml); then further **dilute** with the same sol to 0.5-4 mg/ml; **give** over 15 min or more (intermittent INF)
- **Continuous IV INF** over 24 hr; do not use needles or IV administration sets that contain aluminum; may cause precipitate or loss of potency

Solution compatibilities: D_5/0.2% NaCl, D_5/0.45% NaCl, D_5/0.9% NaCl, 0.9% NaCl, D_5W, sterile water for inj

Y-site compatibilities: Acyclovir, alfentanil, allopurinol, amifostine, amikacin, aminocaproic acid, aminophylline, amiodarone, amphotericin B lipid complex, amphotericin B liposome, ampicillin, ampicillin-sulbactam, anidulafungin, atenolol, atracurium, azithromycin, aztreonam, bivalirudin, bleomycin, bumetanide, buprenorphine, butorphanol, calcium chloride/gluconate, caspofungin, cefazolin, cefepime, cefoperazone, cefotaxime, cefotetan, cefoxitin, ceftazidime, ceftizoxime, ceftriaxone, cefuroxime, cimetidine, ciprofloxacin, cisatracurium, CISplatin, cladribine, clindamycin, codeine, cyclophosphamide, cycloSPORINE, cytarabine, DAPTOmycin, DAUNOrubicin, dexamethasone, dexmedetomidine, dexrazoxane, digoxin, diltiazem, diphenhydrAMINE, DOBUTamine, docetaxel, DOPamine, doripenem, doxacurium, DOXOrubicin, DOXOrubicin liposomal, doxycycline, droperidol, enalaprilat, ePHEDrine, EPINEPHrine, epirubicin, ertapenem, erythromycin, esmolol, etoposide, famotidine, fenoldopam, fentanyl, filgrastim, fluconazole, fludarabine, fluorouracil, foscarnet, fosphenytoin, furosemide, ganciclovir, gatifloxacin, gemcitabine, gentamicin, granisetron, haloperidol, heparin, hydrocortisone, HYDROmorphone, hydrOXYzine, IDArubicin, ifosfamide, imipenem-cilastatin, inamrinone, insulin (regular), irinotecan, isoproterenol, ketorolac, labetalol, levofloxacin, levorphanol, lidocaine, linezolid injection, lorazepam, magnesium sulfate, mannitol, melphalan, meperidine, meropenem, mesna, methohexital, methotrexate, methylPREDNISolone, metoclopramide, metoprolol, metroNIDAZOLE, micafungin, midazolam, milrinone, minocycline, mitoxantrone, mivacurium, morphine, nafcillin, nalbuphine, naloxone, nesiritide, niCARdipine, nitroglycerin, nitroprusside, norepinephrine, octreotide, ofloxacin, ondansetron, oxaliplatin, paclitaxel, palonosetron, pamidronate, pancuronium, pantoprazole, pemetrexed, pentamidine, PENTobarbital, PHENobarbital, phenylephrine, piperacillin, piperacillin-tazobactam, potassium chloride, potassium phosphates, prochlorperazine, promethazine, propofol, propranolol, ranitidine, remifentanil, riTUXimab, rocuronium, sargramostim, sodium acetate, sodium bicarbonate, sodium phosphates, succinylcholine, sufentanil, sulfamethoxazole-trimethoprim, tacrolimus, teniposide, theophylline, thiotepa, ticarcillin, ticarcillin-clavulanate, tigecycline, tirofiban, TNA, tobramycin, topotecan, TPN, trastuzumab, trimethobenzamide, vancomycin, vasopressin, vecuronium, verapamil, vinBLAStine, vinCRIStine, vinorelbine, voriconazole, zidovudine

SIDE EFFECTS

CNS: Seizures, central neurotoxicity, *peripheral neuropathy,* dizziness, confusion

CV: Cardiac abnormalities (fatal CV events), stroke

EENT: Tinnitus, hearing loss, *vestibular toxicity,* visual changes

GI: *Severe nausea, vomiting,* diarrhea, weight loss, mucositis, anorexia, constipation, taste change

HEMA: Thrombocytopenia, leukopenia, pancytopenia, neutropenia, anemia, bleeding

INTEG: *Alopecia,* dermatitis, rash, erythema, pruritus, urticaria

META: Hypomagnesemia, hypocalcemia, hypokalemia, hyponatremia, hyperuremia
SYST: Anaphylaxis

PHARMACOKINETICS

Initial half-life 1-2 hr, postdistribution half-life 2½-6 hr, not bound to plasma proteins, excreted by the kidneys

INTERACTIONS

Increase: nephrotoxicity or ototoxicity—aminoglycosides, amphotericin B
Increase: bleeding risk—aspirin, NSAIDs, thrombolytic agents
Increase: toxicity—radiation, bone marrow suppressants
Increase: myelosuppression—myelosuppressives
Decrease: phenytoin levels
Drug/Lab Test
Increase: AST, BUN, alk phos, bilirubin, creatinine

NURSING CONSIDERATIONS

Assess:

Black Box Warning: Bone marrow depression: CBC, differential, platelet count weekly; withhold product if neutrophil count is $<2000/mm^3$ or platelet count is $<100,000/mm^3$; notify prescriber of results; calcium, magnesium, phosphate, potassium, sodium, uric acid

- Renal studies: BUN, creatinine, serum uric acid; urine CCr before, during therapy; I&O ratio; report fall in urine output to <30 ml/hr
- Monitor temp q4hr (may indicate beginning infection)
- Hepatic studies before, during therapy (bilirubin, AST, ALT, LDH) as needed or monthly; jaundice of skin, sclera; dark urine, clay-colored stools, itchy skin, abdominal pain, fever, diarrhea

⚠ **Anaphylaxis:** hypotension, rash, pruritus, wheezing, tachycardia; notify prescriber after discontinuing product; resuscitation equipment should be available

- **Bleeding;** hematuria, stool guaiac, bruising, petechiae, mucosa or orifices q8hr
- Dyspnea, crackles, unproductive cough, chest pain, tachypnea
- Effects of alopecia on body image; discuss feelings about body changes

Perform/provide:

- Storage protected from light at room temp; reconstituted vials stable for 24 hr at room temp, Paraplatin multidose (10 mg/ml) vials stable for up to 14 days after entry into vial

Evaluate:

- Therapeutic response: decreasing size of tumor, spread of malignancy

Teach patient/family:

- To report ringing/roaring in the ears; numbness, tingling in face, extremities; weight gain
- That impotence or amenorrhea can occur; that this is reversible after treatment is discontinued; to notify prescriber if pregnancy is suspected or planned; that contraception should be used if patient is fertile
- Not to breastfeed during treatment
- To avoid OTC products with aspirin, NSAIDs, alcohol; not to receive vaccinations during treatment

⚠ To notify prescriber immediately of fever, fatigue, sore throat, bleeding, bruising, chills, back pain, blood in stools, dyspnea

- That hair may be lost during treatment; that a wig or hairpiece may make the patient feel better; that new hair may be different in color, texture
- To avoid crowds, persons with known infections; to avoid the use of razors, stiff-bristle toothbrushes

carboprost (Rx)

(kar′boe-prost)

Hemabate

Func. class.: Oxytocic, abortifacient

Chem. class.: Prostaglandin

ACTION: Stimulates uterine contractions, causes complete abortion in approximately 16 hr

USES: Abortion at 13-20 wk gestation, postpartum hemorrhage caused by uterine atony not controlled by other methods

Unlabeled uses: Hemorrhagic cystitis

CONTRAINDICATIONS: Hypersensitivity to this product or benzyl alcohol, severe CV/respiratory/renal/hepatic disease, PID

Precautions: Pregnancy (C), asthma, anemia, jaundice, diabetes mellitus, hypo/hypertension, seizure disorders, past uterine surgery

DOSAGE AND ROUTES

Pregnancy termination between 13-20 wk gestation

- **Adult: IM** 100 mcg (0.4 ml) test dose, then 250 mcg, then 250 mcg q1½-3½hr; may increase to 500 mcg if no response, max 12 mg total dose

Postpartum hemorrhage

- **Adult: IM** 250 mcg, repeat at 15-90-min intervals; max total dosage 2 mg

Hemorrhagic cystitis (unlabeled)

- **Adult: INTRAVESICULAR** 0.8 mg/dl in 50 ml of saline instilled into the bladder for 60 min, q6hr × 4 doses

Available forms: Inj 250 mcg/ml

Administer:

- In deep muscle mass; aspirate before inj, rotate inj sites if additional doses given

SIDE EFFECTS

CNS: *Fever, chills,* headache

GI: *Nausea, vomiting, diarrhea*

PHARMACOKINETICS

Peak 15-60 min, excreted in urine (major metabolites)

INTERACTIONS

Increase: action—other oxytocics

NURSING CONSIDERATIONS

Assess:

- B/P, pulse; watch for change that may indicate hemorrhage
- Respiratory rate, rhythm, depth; notify prescriber of abnormalities
- For length, duration of contractions; notify prescriber of contractions that last more than 1 min or absence of contractions; watch for signs of uterine rupture
- For incomplete abortion, pregnancy must be terminated by another method; product is teratogenic

Perform/provide:

- Storage in refrigerator

Evaluate:

- Therapeutic response: expulsion of fetus, control of bleeding

Teach patient/family:

- To report increased blood loss, abdominal cramps, increased temp, foul-smelling lochia

carisoprodol (Rx)

(kar-eye-soe-proe′dole)

Soma

Func. class.: Skeletal muscle relaxant, central acting

Chem. class.: Meprobamate congener

Do not confuse:

Soma/Soma Compound

ACTION: Depresses CNS by blocking interneuronal activity in descending reticular formation, spinal cord, thereby producing sedation

USES: Relieving pain, stiffness with musculoskeletal disorders

CONTRAINDICATIONS:
Hypersensitivity, intermittent porphyria

Precautions: Pregnancy (C), breastfeeding, geriatric patients, Asian patients, renal/hepatic disease, addictive personality

DOSAGE AND ROUTES

- **Adult/adolescent ≥16 yr: PO** 250-350 mg tid and at bedtime, max 3 wk of use

Available forms: Tabs 350 mg

Administer:

- With meals for GI symptoms
- For short term (2-3 wk), potential for habituation

SIDE EFFECTS

CNS: *Dizziness, weakness, drowsiness,* headache, tremor, depression, insomnia, ataxia, irritability, **seizures**

CV: Postural hypotension, tachycardia

EENT: Diplopia, temporary loss of vision

GI: *Nausea,* vomiting, hiccups, epigastric discomfort

HEMA: Eosinophilia

INTEG: Rash, pruritus, fever, facial flushing, **erythema multiforme**

RESP: Asthmatic attacks

SYST: **Angioedema, anaphylaxis**

PHARMACOKINETICS

PO: Onset 1/2 hr; peak 4 hr; duration 4-6 hr; extensively metabolized by liver, substrate of CYP2C19; excreted in urine; crosses placenta; excreted in breast milk (large amounts); half-life 8 hr

INTERACTIONS

- Do not use together with meprobamate

Increase: CNS depression—alcohol, tricyclics, opioids, barbiturates, sedatives, hypnotics

Drug/Herb

Increase: CNS depression—kava, valerian

Increase: metabolism of carisoprodol—St. John's wort

Drug/Lab Test

Increase: AST, alk phos, blood glucose

NURSING CONSIDERATIONS

Assess:

- **Pain,** stiffness, mobility, activities of daily living at baseline and throughout treatment
- **ECG in seizure patients;** poor seizure control has occurred among patients taking this product
- BUN, creatinine at baseline and periodically
- **Idiosyncratic reaction** (weakness, dizziness, blurred vision, confusion, euphoria), anaphylaxis within a few minutes or hours of 1st to 4th dose
- **Allergic reactions:** rash, fever, respiratory distress, anaphylaxis, angioedema
- **CNS depression:** dizziness, drowsiness, psychiatric symptoms, abuse potential

Perform/provide:

- Storage in tight container at room temp
- Assistance with ambulation if dizziness, drowsiness occurs, especially for geriatric patients

Evaluate:

- Therapeutic response: decreased pain, spasticity; increased ROM

Teach patient/family:

- To avoid hazardous activities if drowsiness, dizziness occur; not to drive while taking product
- To avoid using OTC medications (cough preparations, antihistamines) unless directed by prescriber; not to take with alcohol, other CNS depressants
- To report allergic reaction immediately: rash, swelling of tongue/lips, hives, dyspnea

TREATMENT OF OVERDOSE:
Activated charcoal, dialysis, lavage

⚠ HIGH ALERT

carmustine (Rx)

(kar-mus′teen)

BiCNU, Gliadel

Func. class.: Antineoplastic alkylating agent

Chem. class.: Nitrosourea

ACTION: Alkylates DNA, RNA; able to inhibit enzymes that allow for the synthesis of amino acids in proteins; activity is not cell-cycle–phase specific

USES: Brain tumors such as glioblastoma, medulloblastoma, brain stem glioma, astrocytoma, ependymoma, metastatic brain tumors; multiple myeloma (with predniSONE), non-Hodgkin's disease, Hodgkin's disease, other lymphomas; GI, breast, bronchogenic, renal carcinomas; wafer, as adjunct to surgery/radiation for patients newly diagnosed with high-grade malignant glioma

Unlabeled uses: Malignant melanoma, bone marrow ablation, mycosis fungoides, stem cell transplant preparation

CONTRAINDICATIONS: Pregnancy (D), breastfeeding, hypersensitivity, leukopenia, thrombocytopenia

Precautions: Dental disease, extravasation, females, infection, leukopenia, neutropenia, secondary malignancy, thrombocytopenia

Black Box Warning: Bone marrow suppression, pulmonary fibrosis

DOSAGE AND ROUTES

Carmustine should not be given until platelets >100,000/mm³ and WBC >4000/mm²

• **Adult: IV** 75-100 mg/m² over 1-2 hr × 2 days or 150-200 mg/m² × 1 dose q6-8wk or 40 mg/m²/day × 5 days q6wk

• **Adult: INTRACAVITARY** up to 8 wafers inserted into resection cavity

Malignant melanoma (unlabeled)

• **Adult: IV** 75-100 mg/m²/day for 2 days q6wk or 200 mg/m² as a slow inf q6-8wk

Stem cell transplant/bone marrow ablation (unlabeled)

• **Adult: IV** 450-600 mg/m² as a single dose or 2 divided doses q12hr at a rate of no more than 3 mg/m²/min

Available forms: Powder for inj 100 mg; wafer 7.7 mg (intracavitary)

Administer:

• Blood transfusions, RBC colony-stimulating factors to counter anemia

• Antiemetic 30-60 min before product to prevent vomiting

• All medications PO, if possible; avoid IM inj if platelets are <100,000/mm³

Wafer route

• If wafers are broken into several pieces, they should not be used

• Foil pouches may be kept at room temp for 6 hr if unopened

Intermittent IV INF route

• Prepare in biologic cabinet while wearing gown, gloves, mask; avoid contact with skin; can cause burning; stain the skin brown; use cytotoxic handling procedures; do not use if an oil film appears on vial (decomposition)

• After **diluting** 100 mg product/3 ml ethyl alcohol (provided), **further dilute** with 27 ml sterile water for inj; **then dilute** with 100-500 ml 0.9% NaCl or D_5W, **give** over 1 hr or more, reduce rate if discomfort is felt; use only glass containers, protect from light

• **Flush** IV line after carmustine with 10 ml 0.9% NaCl to prevent irritation at site

Y-site compatibilities: Amifostine, amphotericin B lipid complex, amphotericin B liposome, anidulafungin, aztreonam, bivalirudin, bleomycin, caspofungin, cefepime, codeine, DAPTOmycin, dexmedetomidine, docetaxel, ertapenem, etoposide, fenoldopam, filgrastim, fludarabine, gemcitabine, granisetron, levofloxacin, melphalan, meperidine, mitoxantrone, nesiritide, octreotide, ondansetron, paclitaxel, palonosetron, pamidronate, pantoprazole, pemetrexed, piperacillin-tazobactam, riTUXimab, sargramostim, sodium acetate, tacrolimus, teniposide, thiotepa, tigecycline, tirofiban, trastuzumab, vinCRIStine, vinorelbine, voriconazole

SIDE EFFECTS

GI: *Nausea, vomiting, anorexia, stomatitis,* hepatotoxicity
GU: *Azotemia,* renal failure
HEMA: Thrombocytopenia, leukopenia, myelosuppression, anemia
INTEG: Pain, burning, hyperpigmentation at inj site
RESP: Fibrosis, pulmonary infiltrate
SYST: Secondary malignant neoplastic disease

PHARMACOKINETICS

Degraded within 15 min; crosses blood-brain barrier; 70% excreted in urine within 96 hr; 10% excreted as CO_2, fate of 20% is unknown

INTERACTIONS

Increase: bleeding risk—aspirin, anticoagulants
Increase: myelosuppression—myelosuppressive agents
Increase: toxicity: other antineoplastics, radiation, cimetidine
Increase: adverse reactions, decreased antibody reaction—live vaccines
Decrease: effects of digoxin, phenytoins

NURSING CONSIDERATIONS

Assess:

- **Bone marrow suppression:** CBC, differential, platelet count weekly; withhold product if WBC is <4000 or platelet count is <100,000; notify prescriber of results
- Hepatic studies: AST, ALT, bilirubin
- **Pulmonary fibrosis/infiltrate:** pulmonary function tests, chest x-ray films before, during therapy; chest film should be obtained q2wk during treatment; monitor for dyspnea, cough, pulmonary fibrosis; infiltrate occurs after high doses or several low-dose courses
- Renal studies: BUN, serum uric acid, urine CCr before, during therapy; I&O ratio; report fall in urine output of 30 ml/hr
- Monitor for cold, cough, fever (may indicate beginning infection)
- **Bleeding:** hematuria, guaiac, bruising, petechiae, mucosa, orifices q8hr

Perform/provide:

- Storage of reconstituted sol in refrigerator for 24 hr or at room temp for 8 hr; protect from light
- Rinsing of mouth tid-qid with water or club soda; use of sponge brush for stomatitis
- Warm compresses at inj site for inflammation; reduce flow rate if patient complains of burning at inf site

Evaluate:

- Therapeutic response: decreasing size of tumor, spread of malignancy

Teach patient/family:

- To report any changes in breathing or coughing, to avoid smoking
- To avoid foods with citric acid, hot or rough texture if stomatitis is present; to report any bleeding, white spots, ulceration in mouth to prescriber; to examine mouth daily
- To avoid aspirin, ibuprofen, razors, commercial mouthwash
- To report signs of anemia (fatigue, irritability, shortness of breath, faintness); to report signs of infection (sore throat, fever); pulmonary toxicity can occur up to 15 yr after treatment
- To use contraception during treatment; to avoid breastfeeding, pregnancy (D)
- Not to receive live vaccines during treatment

carteolol ophthalmic

See Appendix B

C

carvedilol (Rx)

(kar-ved'i-lole)

Apo-Carvedilol ✤, Coreg, Coreg CR, PMS-Carvedilol ✤, RAN-Carvedilol ✤, ratio-Carvedilol ✤

Func. class.: Antihypertensive, α-/β-adrenergic blocker

Do not confuse:
carvedilol/captopril/carteolol

ACTION: A mixture of nonselective α-/β-adrenergic blocking activity; decreases cardiac output, exercise-induced tachycardia, reflex orthostatic tachycardia; causes vasodilation, reduction in peripheral vascular resistance

USES: Essential hypertension alone or in combination with other antihypertensives, CHF, LV dysfunction after MI, cardiomyopathy

Unlabeled uses: Angina, pediatric patients

CONTRAINDICATIONS: Hypersensitivity, asthma, class IV decompensated cardiac failure, 2nd- or 3rd-degree heart block, cardiogenic shock, severe bradycardia, pulmonary edema

Precautions: Pregnancy (C), breastfeeding, children, geriatric patients, cardiac failure, hepatic injury, peripheral vascular disease, anesthesia, major surgery, diabetes mellitus, thyrotoxicosis, emphysema, chronic bronchitis, renal disease

Black Box Warning: Abrupt discontinuation

DOSAGE AND ROUTES

Essential hypertension

• **Adult: PO** 6.25 mg bid × 7-14 days; if tolerated well, then increase to 12.5 mg bid × 7-14 days; if tolerated well, may be increased (if needed) to 25 mg bid; not to exceed 50 mg/day; **EXT REL** cap 20 mg/day, may increase after 7-14 days to 40 mg/day

Congestive heart failure

• **Adult: PO** 3.125 mg bid × 2 wk; if tolerated well, give 6.25 mg bid × 2 wk, then double q2wk to max dose of 25 mg bid <85 kg or 50 mg bid >85 kg; **EXT REL** caps (Coreg CR) 10 mg/day × 2 wk, increase to 20, 40, 80 mg/day over successive intervals of 2 wk

Postmyocardial infarction

• **Adult: PO** 6.25 mg bid with food × 3-10 days, lower starting dose may be used if indicated; titrate upward as tolerated; may increase to 12.5 mg bid then titrate to 25 mg bid; **PO EXT REL** 20 mg daily with food, lower starting dose of 10 mg/day may be used, titrate upward after 3-10 days, increase to 40 mg daily as required

Angina (unlabeled)

• **Adult: PO** 25-50 mg bid

Available forms: Tabs 3.125, 6.25, 12.5, 25 mg; ext rel cap 10, 20, 40, 80 mg

Administer:

• Product before meals, bedtime; tabs may be crushed or swallowed whole; give ext rel every AM with food; do not break, crush, chew ext rel cap; separate alcohol (including OTC products that contain ethanol) by ≥2 hr; caps may be opened and sprinkled over applesauce

Black Box Warning: Do not discontinue before surgery

SIDE EFFECTS

CNS: *Dizziness,* fatigue, weakness, somnolence, insomnia, ataxia, hyperesthesia, paresthesia, vertigo, depression, headache

CV: Bradycardia, *postural hypotension,* dependent edema, peripheral edema, AV block, extrasystoles, hypo/hypertension, palpitations, peripheral ischemia, CHF, pulmonary edema

GI: *Diarrhea,* abdominal pain, increased alk phos, ALT, AST

GU: Decreased libido, *impotence,* UTI

INTEG: Rash

MISC: Injury, back pain, viral infection, hypertriglyceridemia, thrombocytopenia, *hyperglycemia*
RESP: Rhinitis, pharyngitis, dyspnea, bronchospasm, cough

PHARMACOKINETICS

Peak 1-2 hr; readily and extensively absorbed PO; >98% protein binding; extensively metabolized by liver; excreted through bile into feces; terminal half-life 7-10 hr with increases in geriatric patients, hepatic disease

INTERACTIONS

Increase: conduction disturbances—calcium channel blockers
Increase: bradycardia, hypotension—levodopa, MAOIs, reserpine
Increase: hypoglycemia—antidiabetic agents
Increase: concentrations of digoxin
Increase: toxicity of carvedilol—cimetidine, other antihypertensives, nitrates, acute alcohol ingestion
Decrease: heart rate, B/P—clonidine
Decrease: carvedilol levels—rifampin, NSAIDs, thyroid medications
Drug/Herb
Increase: antihypertensive effect—hawthorn
Decrease: antihypertensive effect—ephedra (ma huang)
Drug/Lab Test
Increase: blood glucose, BUN, potassium, triglycerides, uric acid

NURSING CONSIDERATIONS

Assess:

- **Hypertension:** B/P when beginning treatment, periodically thereafter; pulse: note rate, rhythm, quality; apical/radial pulse before administration; notify prescriber of significant changes
- **CHF:** edema in feet, legs daily; fluid overload: dyspnea, weight gain, jugular venous distention, fatigue, crackles

Evaluate:

- Therapeutic response: decreased B/P with hypertension

Teach patient/family:

- To comply with dosage schedule even if feeling better; that improvement may take several weeks
- To rise slowly to sitting or standing position to minimize orthostatic hypotension
- To report bradycardia, dizziness, confusion, depression, fever, weight gain, SOB, cold extremities, rash, sore throat, bleeding, bruising
- To weigh, take pulse, B/P at home; to advise if weight gain of >2 lb/day or 5 lb/wk and when to notify prescriber

⚠ Not to discontinue product abruptly; to taper over 1-2 wk; life-threatening dysrhythmias may occur

- To avoid hazardous activities until stabilized on medication; dizziness may occur
- To avoid all OTC medications unless approved by prescriber
- To carry emergency ID with product name, prescriber information at all times
- To inform all health care providers of products, supplements taken

caspofungin (Rx)

(cas-po-fun′gin)

Cancidas

Func. class.: Antifungal, systemic
Chem. class.: Echinocandin

ACTION: Inhibits an essential component in fungal cell walls; causes direct damage to fungal cell wall

USES: Treatment of invasive aspergillosis and candidemia that has not responded to other treatment, including peritonitis, intraabdominal abscesses; susceptible species: *Aspergillus flavus, A. fumigatus, A. terreus, Candida albicans, C. glabrata, C. krusei, C. lusitaniae, C. parapsilosis, C. tropicalis,* esophageal candidiasis; empirical therapy for presumed fungal infection in febrile, neutropenic patients

Unlabeled uses: *Aspergillus niger,* fungal infections in premature neonates, neonates, infants, children <2 yr

CONTRAINDICATIONS:

Hypersensitivity to this product, other echinocandins, including mannitol

Precautions: Pregnancy (C), breastfeeding, children, geriatric patients, severe hepatic disease

DOSAGE AND ROUTES

- **Adult: IV** loading dose 50-70 mg on day 1 then 50 mg/day maintenance dose, depending on condition; max 70 mg/day
- **Adolescent/child/infant ≥3 mo: IV INF** 70 mg/m^2 loading dose then 50 mg/m^2/day; max 70 mg/day
- **Neonate and infant <3 mo (unlabeled): IV** 25 mg/m^2/day

Available forms: Powder for inj 50, 70 mg

Administer:

Intermittent IV INF route

- Allow to warm to room temp
- May administer loading dose on day 1
- Do not admix; do not use with dextrose, do not give as IV bolus
- **Reconstitute** 50-mg vial or 70-mg vial with 10.8 ml 0.9% NaCl, sterile water for inj or bacteriostatic water for inj (5 mg/ml or 7 mg/ml); **swirl** to dissolve, withdraw 10 ml reconstituted sol, and **further dilute** with 250 ml 0.9% NaCl, 0.45% NaCl, 0.225% NaCl, RL; **run** over 1 hr or more

Y-site compatibilities: Alfentanil, allopurinol, amifostine, amikacin, aminophylline, amiodarone, anidulafungin, atracurium, aztreonam, bleomycin, bumetanide, busulfan, butorphanol, calcium acetate, calcium chloride/gluconate, CARBOplatin, carmustine, ceftizoxime, chlorproMAZINE, cimetidine, ciprofloxacin, cisatracurium, CISplatin, cyclophosphamide, cycloSPORINE, dacarbazine, DACTINomycin, DAPTOmycin, DAUNOrubicin, dexmedetomidine, dexrazoxane, diltiazem, diphenhydrAMINE, DOBUTamine, docetaxel, dolasetron, DOPamine, doripenem, DOXOrubicin, doxycycline, droperidol, EPINEPHrine, epirubicin, erythromycin, esmolol, etoposide, famotidine, fenoldopam, fentanyl, fluconazole, fludarabine, ganciclovir, gatifloxacin, gemcitabine, gentamicin, glycopyrrolate, granisetron, haloperidol, hydrocortisone, HYDROmorphone, hydrOXYzine, IDArubicin, ifosfamide, imipenem-cilastatin, inamrinone, insulin (regular), irinotecan, isoproterenol, labetalol, leucovorin, levofloxacin, linezolid injection, magnesium, mannitol, mechlorethamine, melphalan, meperidine, meropenem, mesna, metaraminol, methyldopate, metoclopramide, metoprolol, midazolam, milrinone, minocycline, mitomycin, mitoxantrone, morphine, moxifloxacin, mycophenolate, nalbuphine, naloxone, niCARdipine, nitroglycerin, norepinephrine, octreotide, ondansetron, oxaliplatin, oxytocin, paclitaxel, palonosetron, pentamidine, pentazocine, phenylephrine, polymyxin B, potassium chloride, procainamide, prochlorperazine, promethazine, propranolol, quiNIDine, remifentanil, rocuronium, streptozocin, succinylcholine, sufentanil, tacrolimus, teniposide, theophylline, thiopental, thiotepa, tigecycline, tirofiban, tobramycin, topotecan, trimethobenzamide, vancomycin, vasopressin, vecuronium, verapamil, vinBLAStine, vinCRIStine, vinorelbine, voriconazole, zidovudine

SIDE EFFECTS

CNS: Dizziness, *headache*

CV: Sinus tachycardia

GI: Abdominal pain, *nausea, anorexia, vomiting, diarrhea, increased AST/ALT, alk phos*

HEMA: Thrombophlebitis, vasculitis, anemia

INTEG: *Rash, pruritus, inj site pain*

META: Hypokalemia

MS: Myalgia

RESP: Acute respiratory distress syndrome (ARDS)

SYST: Anaphylaxis

PHARMACOKINETICS

Metabolized in liver to inactive metabolites; excretion in feces, urine; phase II terminal half-life 9-11 hr; phase III terminal half-life 40-50 hr; protein binding 97%

INTERACTIONS

Increase: plasma concentrations—cycloSPORINE; may need dosage reduction
Decrease: levels of tacrolimus, sirolimus
Decrease: caspofungin levels—carBAMazepine, dexamethasone, efavirenz, nelfinavir, nevirapine, phenytoin, rifampin
Drug/Lab Test
Increase: AST, ALT, RBC, eosinophils
Decrease: HCT/Hgb, WBC, potassium

NURSING CONSIDERATIONS

Assess:

- **Infection;** clearing of cultures during treatment; obtain culture at baseline, throughout treatment; product may be started as soon as culture is taken (esophageal candidiasis); monitor cultures during HSCT for prevention of *Candida* infections
- Hepatic studies before, during treatment: bilirubin, AST, ALT, alk phos, as needed; obtain baseline renal studies
- **Hypersensitivity:** rash, pruritus, facial swelling; also for phlebitis
- GI symptoms: frequency of stools, cramping; if severe diarrhea occurs, electrolytes may need to be given

Perform/provide:

- Storage at room temp for up to 24 hr or refrigerated for 48 hr; store reconstituted sol at room temp for 1 hr prior to preparation of sol for administration

Evaluate:

- Therapeutic response: decreased symptoms of *Candida, Aspergillus* infections

Teach patient/family:

- To notify prescriber if pregnancy is suspected or planned; to use a nonhormonal form of contraception while taking this product; not to breastfeed while taking this product
- To inform prescriber of renal/hepatic disease
- To report bleeding, facial swelling, wheezing, difficulty breathing, itching, rash, hives, increasing warmth, flushing; anaphylaxis can occur

C

cefaclor

See cephalosporins—2nd generation

cefadroxil

cefazolin

See cephalosporins—1st generation

cefdinir

cefditoren pivoxil

cefepime

cefixime

cefotaxime

See cephalosporins—3rd generation

cefotetan

cefoxitin

See cephalosporins—2nd generation

cefpodoxime

See cephalosporins—3rd generation

cefprozil

See cephalosporins—2nd generation

ceftazidime

ceftibuten

ceftizoxime

ceftriaxone

See cephalosporins—3rd generation

cefuroxime

See cephalosporins—2nd generation

ceftaroline (Rx)

(sef-tar′oh-leen)

Teflaro

Func. class.: Cephalosporin action: Inhibits cell wall synthesis through binding to essential penicillin-binding protein (PBPs)

USES: Acute bacterial skin/skin structure infections (ABSSI), bacterial community-acquired pneumonia

CONTRAINDICATIONS: Cephalosporin hypersensitivity

Precautions: Child/infant/neonate, breastfeeding, elderly patients, antimicrobial resistance, carbapenem/penicillin hypersensitivity, coagulopathy, colitis, dialysis, diarrhea, GI disease, hypoprothrombinemia, IBS, pregnancy (B), pseudomembranous colitis, renal disease, ulcerative colitis, viral infection, vit K deficiency

DOSAGE AND ROUTES

- **Adult: IV** 600 mg q12hr × 5-14 days (skin/skin-structure infections) or × 5-7 days (bacterial community-acquired pneumonia)

Renal dose

- **Adult: IV** CCr >30-≤50 ml/min, 400 mg q12hr; CCr ≥15-≤30 ml/min, 300 mg q12hr, CCr ≤15 ml/min, 200 mg q12hr

Available forms: Powder for inj 400 mg, 600 mg

Administer:

Intermittent IV INF route

- Visually inspect for particulate matter, discoloration if sol or container permits
- **Reconstitute:** add 20 ml of sterile water to 400- or 600-mg vial (20 ml/ml for 400 mg; 30 mg/ml for 600 mg), mix gently until dissolved; **dilute** in 250 ml of 0.9% NaCl, 0.45% NaCl, LR, D_5, D2.5, **give** over 1 hr, do not admix, use within 6 hr at room temp or 24 hr refrigerated

SIDE EFFECTS

CV: Phlebitis

ENDO: Hypokalemia

GI: Diarrhea, nausea, vomiting, constipation, abdominal pain, pseudomembranous colitis (rare), elevated hepatic enzymes

INTEG: Rash, anaphylaxis

PHARMACOKINETICS

Protein binding 20%; excreted in urine 88%, feces 6%; half-life 2.66 hr; not hepatically metabolized

INTERACTIONS

Increase: prothrombin time risk—anticoagulants

NURSING CONSIDERATIONS

Assess:

- **Infection:** vital signs, sputum, WBC before, during therapy
- **Hypersensitivity:** before use, obtain a history of hypersensitivity reactions to cephalosporins, carbapenems, penicillins; cross-sensitivity may occur
- Obtain specimens for culture, sensitivity before beginning therapy
- **Anaphylaxis (rare):** rash, pruritus, laryngeal edema, dyspnea, wheezing; discontinue product, notify health care provider immediately, keep emergency equipment nearby
- **Pseudomembranous colitis:** diarrhea, abdominal pain, fever, bloody stools; report immediately if these occur; may occur several weeks after terminating therapy

Perform/provide:

- Store reconstituted sol in refrigerator

Evaluate:

- Therapeutic response: negative C&S, resolution of symptoms of infection

Teach patient/family:

- About the reason for treatment and expected result
- To immediately report rash, itching, difficulty breathing, bloody diarrhea, fever, abdominal pain

⚠ HIGH ALERT

celecoxib (Rx)

(sel-eh-cox′ib)

Celebrex

Func. class.: Nonsteroidal antiinflammatory, antirheumatic

Chem. class.: COX-2 inhibitor

Do not confuse:
Celebrex/Celexa/Cerebra/Cerebyx

ACTION: Inhibits prostaglandin synthesis by selectively inhibiting cyclooxygenase-2 (COX-2), an enzyme needed for biosynthesis

USES: Acute, chronic rheumatoid arthritis, osteoarthritis, acute pain, primary dysmenorrhea, ankylosing spondylitis, juvenile rheumatoid arthritis (JRA)

Unlabeled uses: Colorectal adenoma prophylaxis

CONTRAINDICATIONS: Pregnancy (D) 3rd trimester; hypersensitivity to salicylates, iodides, other NSAIDs, sulfonamides

Black Box Warning: CABG

Precautions: Pregnancy (C) 1st/2nd trimesters, breastfeeding, children <18 yr, geriatric patients, bleeding, GI/renal/hepatic/cardiac disorders, PVD, hypertension, severe dehydration, asthma

Black Box Warning: GI bleeding/perforation, peptic ulcer disease, MI, stroke

DOSAGE AND ROUTES

Do not exceed recommended dose; deaths have occurred

Acute pain/primary dysmenorrhea

• **Adult: PO** 400 mg initially, then 200 mg if needed on 1st day, then 200 mg bid prn on subsequent days; start with 1/2 dose for poor CYP2C9 metabolizers

Osteoarthritis

• **Adult: PO** 200 mg/day as a single dose or 100 mg bid; start with 1/2 dose for poor CYP2C9 metabolizers

• **Geriatric: PO** use lowest possible dose

Rheumatoid arthritis

• **Adult: PO** 100-200 mg bid; start with 1/2 dose for poor CYP2C9 metabolizers

Ankylosing spondylitis

• **Adult: PO** 200 mg/day or in divided doses (bid); start with 1/2 dose for poor CYP2C9 metabolizers

Juvenile rheumatoid arthritis (JRA)

• **Adolescent and child ≥2 yr (>25 kg): PO** 100 mg bid; start with 1/2 dose for poor CYP2C9 metabolizers

• **Child ≥2 yr (10-25 kg): PO** 50 mg bid; start with 1/2 dose for poor CYP2C9 metabolizers

Hepatic disease

• **Adult: PO** (Child-Pugh B) reduce dose by 50%

Colorectal adenoma prophylaxis (unlabeled)

• **Adult: PO** 400 mg bid × 6 mo

Available forms: Caps 50, 100, 200, 400 mg

Administer:

• Do not break, crush, chew, or dissolve caps with a full glass of water to enhance absorption; caps may be opened into applesauce or soft food, ingest immediately with water

• With food, milk to decrease gastric symptoms (with higher doses [400 mg bid]); do not increase dose

SIDE EFFECTS

CNS: *Fatigue, anxiety, depression, nervousness, paresthesia,* dizziness, insomnia

CV: Stroke, MI, tachycardia, CHF, angina, palpitations, dysrhythmias, hypertension, fluid retention

EENT: Tinnitus, hearing loss, blurred vision, glaucoma, cataract, conjunctivitis, eye pain

GI: Nausea, anorexia, vomiting, constipation, dry mouth, diverticulitis, gastritis,

gastroenteritis, hemorrhoids, hiatal hernia, stomatitis, **GI bleeding/ulceration**
GU: **Nephrotoxicity:** *dysuria,* **hematuria, oliguria, azotemia,** cystitis, UTI, **renal papillary necrosis**
HEMA: **Blood dyscrasias,** epistaxis, bruising, anemia, **platelet aggregation**
INTEG: **Serious (sometimes fatal) Stevens-Johnson syndrome, toxic epidermal necrolysis,** purpura, rash, pruritus, sweating, erythema, petechiae, photosensitivity, alopecia
RESP: Pharyngitis, SOB, pneumonia, coughing

PHARMACOKINETICS

Well absorbed, crosses placenta, bound to plasma proteins, metabolized by CYP2C9 in liver, very little excreted by kidneys/in feces, peak 3 hr, half-life 11 hr, protein binding ~97%

INTERACTIONS

Increase: bleeding risk—anticoagulants, SSRIs, antiplatelets, thrombolytics, salicylates, alcohol
Increase: adverse reactions—glucocorticoids, NSAIDs, aspirin
Increase: toxicity—lithium, antineoplastics, bisphosphonates
Increase: celecoxib blood level—fluconazole
Decrease: effect of aspirin, ACE inhibitors, thiazide diuretics, furosemide

Drug/Herb
Decrease: effect of feverfew
Increase: bleeding risk—garlic, ginger, ginkgo

Drug/Lab Test
Increase: ALT, AST, BUN

NURSING CONSIDERATIONS

Assess:
- **Pain** of rheumatoid arthritis, osteoarthritis; check ROM, inflammation of joints, characteristics of pain

Black Box Warning: For cardiac disease that may be worse after taking product; MI, stroke; do not use with coronary artery bypass graft (CABG)

- CBC during therapy; watch for decreasing platelets; if low, therapy may need to be discontinued, restarted after hematologic recovery; LFTs, serum creatinine/BUN, stool guaiac

Black Box Warning: For blood dyscrasias (thrombocytopenia): bruising, fatigue, bleeding, poor healing

- **GI toxicity:** black, tarry stools; abdominal pain

⚠ **Serious skin disorders:** Stevens-Johnson syndrome, toxic epidermal necrolysis; may be fatal

Evaluate:
- Therapeutic response: decreased pain, inflammation in arthritic conditions; decreased number of polyps

Teach patient/family:

⚠ Not to exceed recommended dose; to notify prescriber immediately of chest pain, skin eruptions; to stop product if these occur
- To check with prescriber to determine when product should be discontinued prior to surgery
- That product must be continued for prescribed time to be effective; to avoid other NSAIDs, aspirin, sulfonamides
- To notify prescriber if pregnancy is planned or suspected

⚠ To notify prescriber of GI symptoms: black, tarry stools; cramping or rash; edema of extremities; weight gain

⚠ To report bleeding, bruising, fatigue, malaise because blood abnormalities do occur
- To report possible respiratory infection: fever, SOB, coughing, painful swallowing

cephalexin

See cephalosporins—1st generation

CEPHALOSPORINS—1ST GENERATION

cefadroxil (Rx)
(sef-a-drox′ill)
Apo-Cefadroxil ✦
cefazolin (Rx)
(sef-a′zoe-lin)
cephalexin (Rx)
(sef-a-lex′in)
Keflex, Panixine
Func. class.: Antiinfective
Chem. class.: Cephalosporin (1st generation)

Do not confuse:
cephalexin/cefaclor

ACTION: Inhibits bacterial cell wall synthesis; renders cell wall osmotically unstable, leads to cell death; lysis mediated by cell wall autolytic enzymes

USES:

cefadroxil: Gram-negative bacilli: *Escherichia coli, Proteus mirabilis, Klebsiella* (UTI only); gram-positive organisms: *Streptococcus pneumoniae, Streptococcus pyogenes, Staphylococcus aureus;* upper, lower respiratory tract, urinary tract, skin infections; otitis media; tonsillitis; UTIs
cefazolin: Gram-negative bacilli: *Haemophilus influenzae, Escherichia coli, Proteus mirabilis, Klebsiella;* gram-positive organisms: *Staphylococcus aureus;* upper, lower respiratory tract, urinary tract, skin infections; bone, joint, biliary, genital infections; endocarditis, surgical prophylaxis, septicemia
cephalexin: Gram-negative bacilli: *Haemophilus influenzae, Escherichia coli, Proteus mirabilis, Klebsiella;* gram-positive organisms: *Streptococcus pneumoniae, Streptococcus pyogenes, Staphylococcus aureus;* upper, lower respiratory tract, urinary tract, skin, bone infections; otitis media

CONTRAINDICATIONS: Hypersensitivity to cephalosporins, infants <1 mo
Precautions: Pregnancy (B), breastfeeding, hypersensitivity to penicillins, renal disease

DOSAGE AND ROUTES

cefadroxil
• **Adult: PO** 1-2 g/day or q12hr in divided doses; loading dose of 1 g initially
• **Child: PO** 30 mg/kg/day in divided doses bid, max 2 g/day
Renal dose
• **Adult: PO** CCr 25-50 ml/min, 500 mg q12hr; CCr 10-24 ml/min, 500 mg q24hr; CCr <10 ml/min, 500 mg q36hr
Available forms: Caps 500 mg; tabs 1 g; oral susp 250, 500 mg/5 ml

cefazolin
Life-threatening infections
• **Adult: IM/IV** 1-2 g q6-8hr; max 12 g/day
• **Child >1 mo: IM/IV** 75-100 mg/kg in 3-4 divided doses; max 6 g/day
Mild/moderate infections
• **Adult: IM/IV** 250 mg-1 g q8hr, max 12 g/day
• **Child >1 mo: IM/IV** 25-50 mg/kg in 3-4 equal doses, max 6 g/day, or 2 g as a single dose
Renal dose
• **Adult: IM/IV** after loading dose, CCr 35-54 ml/min, dose q8hr; CCr 10-34 ml/min, 50% of dose q12hr; CCr <10 ml/min, 50% of dose q18-24hr
• **Child: IM/IV** CCr >70 ml/min, no dosage adjustment; CCr 40-70 ml/min after loading dose, reduce dose to 7.5-30 mg/kg q12hr; CCr 20-39 ml/min, give 3.125-12.5 mg/kg after loading dose q12hr; CCr 5-19 ml/min, 2.5-10 mg/kg after loading dose q24hr
Available forms: Inj 250, 500 mg, 1, 5, 10, 20 g; inf 500 mg, 1 g/50-ml vial

cephalexin
Moderate infections
• **Adult: PO** 250-500 mg q6hr, max 4 g/day

• **Child: PO** 25-50 mg/kg/day in 4 equal doses, max 4 g/day

Moderate skin infections

• **Adult: PO** 500 mg q12hr

Endocarditis prophylaxis

• 2 g 1 hr before procedure

Severe infections

• **Adult: PO** 500 mg-1 g q6hr
• **Child: PO** 50-100 mg/kg/day in 4 equal doses, max 4 g/day

Renal dose

• **Adult: PO** CCr 10-40 ml/min, 250-500 mg then 250-500 mg q8-12hr; CCr <10 ml/min, 250-500 mg then 250-500 mg q12-24hr

Available forms: Caps 250, 500 mg; tabs 250, 500 mg, 1 g; oral susp 125 mg, 250 mg/5 ml

Administer:

cefadroxil

• For 10-14 days to ensure organism death, prevent superinfection
• With food if needed for GI symptoms
• Shake susp, refrigerate, discard after 2 wk
• After C&S completed

cefazolin

IV route

• Check for irritation, extravasation often; dilute in 10 ml sterile water for inj, run over 3-5 min; may be further diluted with 50-100 ml of NS, D_5W sol, run over ½-1 hr by Y-tube or 3-way stopcock
• For 10-14 days to ensure organism death, prevent superinfection
• After C&S completed

Syringe compatibilities: DimenhyDRINATE, heparin, vit B complex

Y-site compatibilities: Acyclovir, alfentanil, allopurinol, alprostadil, amifostine, amikacin, aminocaproic acid, aminophylline, amphotericin B liposome, anidulafungin, ascorbic acid injection, atenolol, atracurium, atropine, aztreonam, benztropine, bivalirudin, bleomycin, bumetanide, buprenorphine, butorphanol, calcium gluconate, CARBOplatin, cefamandole, cefmetazole, cefonicid, cefoperazone, cefotetan, cefoxitin, cefpirome, ceftazidime, ceftizoxime, cefTRIAXone, cefuroxime, cephalothin, cephapirin, chloramphenicol, cimetidine, CISplatin, clindamycin, codeine, cyanocobalamin, cyclophosphamide, cycloSPORINE, cytarabine, DACTINomycin, DAPTOmycin, dexamethasone, dexmedetomidine, digoxin, diltiazem, docetaxel, doxacurium, doxapram, DOXOrubicin liposomal, enalaprilat, ePHEDrine, EPINEPHrine, epirubicin, epoetin alfa, eptifibatide, esmolol, etoposide, fenoldopam, fentaNYL, filgrastim, fluconazole, fludarabine, fluorouracil, folic acid (as sodium salt), foscarnet, furosemide, gallium, gatifloxacin, gemcitabine, gentamicin, glycopyrrolate, granisetron, heparin, hydrocortisone, hydrOXYzine, IDArubicin, ifosfamide, imipenem-cilastatin, indomethacin, insulin (regular), irinotecan, isoproterenol, ketorolac, lidocaine, linezolid, LORazepam, LR's injection, mannitol, mechlorethamine, melphalan, meperidine, metaraminol, methicillin, methotrexate, methoxamine, methyldopate, methylPREDNISolone, metoclopramide, metoprolol, metroNIDAZOLE, mezlocillin, miconazole, midazolam, milrinone, morphine, moxalactam, multiple vitamins injection, nafcillin, nalbuphine, naloxone, nesiritide, niCARdipine, nitroglycerin, nitroprusside, norepinephrine, octreotide, ondansetron, oxacillin, oxaliplatin, oxytocin, paclitaxel, palonosetron, pamidronate, pancuronium, pantoprazole, penicillin G potassium/sodium, peritoneal dialysis solution, perphenazine, PHENobarbital, phenylephrine, phytonadione, piperacillin, Plasma-Lyte M in dextrose 5%, polymyxin B, potassium chloride, procainamide, propofol, propranolol, ranitidine, remifentanil, Ringer's injection, ritodrine, riTUXimab, sargramostim, sodium acetate, sodium bicarbonate, succinylcholine, SUFentanil, tacrolimus, teniposide, tenoxicam, theophylline, thiamine, thiotepa, ticarcillin, ticarcillin-clavulanate, tigecycline, tirofiban, TNA, tolazoline, trastuzumab, trimetaphan, urokinase, vasopressin, vecuronium, verapamil, vinCRIStine, vitamin B complex with C, voriconazole, warfarin

cephalexin

- Shake susp, refrigerate, discard after 2 wk
- For 10-14 days to ensure organism death, prevent superinfection
- With food if needed for GI symptoms
- After C&S

SIDE EFFECTS

CNS: Headache, dizziness, weakness, paresthesia, fever, chills, seizures (with high doses)

GI: Nausea, vomiting, *diarrhea, anorexia,* pain, glossitis, bleeding; increased AST, ALT, bilirubin, LDH, alk phos; abdominal pain, **pseudomembranous colitis**

GU: Proteinuria, vaginitis, pruritus, candidiasis, increased BUN, **nephrotoxicity, renal failure**

HEMA: **Leukopenia, thrombocytopenia, agranulocytosis,** anemia, **neutropenia, lymphocytosis, eosinophilia, pancytopenia, hemolytic anemia**

INTEG: Rash, urticaria, dermatitis

RESP: Dyspnea

SYST: **Anaphylaxis, serum sickness,** superinfection, **Stevens-Johnson syndrome**

PHARMACOKINETICS

cefadroxil: Peak 1-1$^1/_2$ hr, duration 12-24 hr, half-life 1-2 hr, 20% bound by plasma proteins, crosses placenta, excreted in breast milk

cefazolin

IM: Peak $^1/_2$-2 hr, duration 6-12 hr, half-life 1$^1/_2$-2$^1/_4$ hr

IM: Peak 10 min, duration 6-12 hr, eliminated unchanged in urine, 75%-85% protein bound

cephalexin: Peak 1 hr, duration 6-12 hr, half-life 30-72 min, 5%-15% bound by plasma proteins, 80%-100% eliminated unchanged in urine, crosses placenta, excreted in breast milk

INTERACTIONS

Increase: prothrombin time—anticoagulants; use cautiously

Increase: toxicity—aminoglycosides, loop diuretics, probenecid

Drug/Lab Test

Increase: AST, ALT, alk phos, LDH, BUN, creatinine, bilirubin

False positive: urinary protein, direct Coombs' test, urine glucose

Interference: cross-matching

NURSING CONSIDERATIONS

Assess:

- Sensitivity to penicillin and other cephalosporins

⚠ **Nephrotoxicity: increased BUN, creatinine; urine output: if decreasing, notify prescriber**

- I&O daily
- Blood studies: AST, ALT, CBC, Hct, bilirubin, LDH, alk phos, Coombs' test monthly if patient is on long-term therapy
- Electrolytes: K, Na, Cl monthly if patient is on long-term therapy
- **Pseudomembranous colitis:** bowel pattern daily; if severe diarrhea occurs, product should be discontinued

⚠ **Anaphylaxis: rash, urticaria, pruritus, chills, fever, joint pain; angioedema; may occur a few days after therapy begins; discontinue product, notify prescriber immediately, keep emergency equipment nearby**

- Bleeding: ecchymosis, bleeding gums, hematuria, stool guaiac daily

⚠ **Overgrowth of infection: perineal itching, fever, malaise, redness, pain, swelling, drainage, rash, diarrhea, change in cough, sputum**

Evaluate:

- Therapeutic response: decreased symptoms of infection, negative C&S

Teach patient/family:

- To use yogurt or buttermilk to maintain intestinal flora, decrease diarrhea
- To take all medication prescribed for length of time ordered

⚠ To report sore throat, bruising, bleeding, joint pain (may indicate **blood dyscrasias** [rare]); diarrhea with mucus, blood (may indicate **pseudomembranous colitis**)

TREATMENT OF ANAPHYLAXIS: EPINEPHrine, antihistamines; resuscitate if needed

CEPHALOSPORINS—2ND GENERATION

cefaclor (Rx)
(sef′a-klor)
Ceclor, Raniclor

cefotetan (Rx)
(sef′oh-tee-tan)
Cefotan

cefoxitin (Rx)
(se-fox′i-tin)
Mefoxin

cefprozil (Rx)
(sef-proe′zill)
Cefzil

cefuroxime (Rx)
(sef-yoor-ox′eem)
Ceftin, cefuroxime, Zinacef

Func. class.: Antiinfective
Chem. class.: Cephalosporin (2nd generation)

Do not confuse:
cefaclor/cephalexin
Cefotan/Ceftin
cefprozil/cefazolin/cefuroxime
Cefzil/Ceftin

ACTION: Inhibits bacterial cell wall synthesis, renders cell wall osmotically unstable, leads to cell death by binding to cell wall membrane

USES:

cefaclor: Gram-negative bacilli: *Haemophilus influenzae, Escherichia coli, Proteus mirabilis, Klebsiella;* gram-positive organisms: *Streptococcus pneumoniae, Streptococcus pyogenes, Staphylococcus aureus;* respiratory tract, urinary tract, skin, bone, joint infections; otitis media

cefotetan: Gram-negative organisms: *Haemophilus influenzae, Escherichia coli, Enterobacter aerogenes, Proteus mirabilis, Klebsiella, Citrobacter, Salmonella, Shigella, Acinetobacter, Bacteroides fragilis, Neisseria, Serratia;* gram-positive organisms: *Streptococcus pneumoniae, Streptococcus pyogenes, Staphylococcus aureus;* upper and lower, serious respiratory tract, urinary tract, skin, bone, joint, gynecologic, gonococcal, intraabdominal infections

cefoxitin: Gram-negative bacilli: *Haemophilus influenzae, Escherichia coli, Proteus, Klebsiella, Bacteroides fragilis, Neisseria gonorrhoeae;* gram-positive organisms: *Streptococcus pneumoniae, Streptococcus pyogenes, Staphylococcus aureus;* anaerobes including *Clostridium;* lower respiratory tract, urinary tract, skin, bone, gynecologic, gonococcal infections; septicemia, peritonitis

cefprozil: Pharyngitis/tonsillitis; otitis media; secondary bacterial infection of acute bronchitis; acute bacterial exacerbation of chronic bronchitis; uncomplicated skin and skin-structure infections; acute sinusitis

cefuroxime: Gram-negative bacilli: *Haemophilus influenzae, Escherichia coli, Neisseria, Proteus mirabilis, Klebsiella;* gram-positive organisms: *Streptococcus pneumoniae, Streptococcus pyogenes, Staphylococcus aureus;* serious lower respiratory tract, urinary tract, skin, bone, joint, gonococcal infections; septicemia, meningitis

CONTRAINDICATIONS: Hypersensitivity to cephalosporins or related antibiotics; seizures

Precautions: Pregnancy (B), breastfeeding, children, GI/renal disease

DOSAGE AND ROUTES

cefaclor

- **Adult: PO** 250-500 mg q8hr, max 4 g/day
- **Child >1 mo: PO** 20-40 mg/kg/day in divided doses q8hr or total daily dose

may be divided and given q12hr, max 1 g/day

Available forms: Caps 250, 500 mg; oral susp 125, 187, 250, 375 mg/5 ml; chew tabs (Raniclor) 250, 375 mg

cefotetan

• **Adult: IM/IV** 1-2 g q12hr × 5-10 days

Renal dose

• **Adult: IM/IV** CCr 10-30 ml/min, give dose q24hr or ½ dose q12hr; CCr <10 ml/min, give dose q48hr or ½ dose q24hr

Perioperative prophylaxis

• **Adult: IV** 1-2 g ½-1 hr before surgery

Available forms: Inj 1, 2, 10 g

cefoxitin

• **Adult: IM/IV** 1-2 g q6-8hr

Renal dose

• **Adult: IM/IV** after loading dose, CCr 30-50 ml/min, 1-2 g q8-12hr; CCr 10-29 ml/min, 1-2 g q12-24hr; CCr <10 ml/min, 0.5-1 g q12-24hr

Uncomplicated gonorrhea (outpatient)

• **Adult/adolescent/child ≥45 kg: IM** 2 g as single dose with 1 g **PO** probenecid at same time

Severe infections

• **Adult: IM/IV** 2 g q4hr

• **Child ≥3 mo: IM/IV** 80-160 mg/kg/day divided q4-6hr; max 12 g/day

Available forms: Powder for inj 1, 2, 10 g

cefprozil

Renal dose

• CCr <30 ml/min, 50% of dose

Upper respiratory infections

• **Adult: PO** 500 mg q24hr × 10 days

Otitis media

• **Child 6 mo-12 yr: PO** 15 mg/kg q12hr × 10 days

Lower respiratory infections

• **Adult: PO** 500 mg q12hr × 10 days

Skin/skin-structure infections

• **Adult: PO** 250-500 mg q12hr × 10 days

Available forms: Tabs 250, 500 mg; susp 125, 250 mg/5 ml

cefuroxime

• **Adult and child: PO** 250 mg q12hr; may increase to 500 mg q12hr for serious infections

• **Adult: IM/IV** 750 mg-1.5 g q8hr for 5-10 days

Urinary tract infections

• **Adult: PO** 125 mg q12hr; may increase to 250 mg q12hr if needed

Otitis media

• **Child <2 yr: PO** 125 mg bid

• **Child >2 yr: PO** 250 mg bid

Surgical prophylaxis

• **Adult: IV** 1.5 g ½-1 hr prior to surgery

Severe infections

• **Adult: IM/IV** 1.5 g q6hr; may give up to 3 g q8hr for bacterial meningitis

• **Child >3 mo: IM/IV** 50-100 mg/kg/day or IM in divided doses q6-8hr

Uncomplicated gonorrhea

• **Adult:** 1.5 g **IM** as single dose with oral probenecid in 2 separate sites

Renal dose

• Dosage reduction indicated with severe renal impairment (CCr <20 ml/min)

Available forms: Tabs 125, 250, 500 mg; inj 150, 750 mg, 1.5, 7.5 g; inj 750 mg; 1.5 g powder; susp 125, 250 mg/5 ml

Administer:

• Do not break, crush, or chew ext rel tabs or caps

• On an empty stomach 1 hr before or 2 hr after a meal

cefaclor

• Shake susp, refrigerate, discard after 2 wk

• For 10-14 days to ensure organism death, prevent superinfection

• With food if needed for GI symptoms

• After C&S completed

cefotetan

• IV direct after diluting 1 g/10 ml sterile water for inj, give over 3-5 min; may be diluted further with 50-100 ml NS or D_5W; shake; run over ½-1 hr by Y-tube or 3-way stopcock; discontinue primary inf during administration

• May be stored 96 hr refrigerated or 24 hr at room temp

Y-site compatibilities: Allopurinol, amifostine, aztreonam, diltiazem, famotidine, filgrastim, fluconazole, fludarabine, heparin, insulin (regular), melphalan, meperidine, morphine, paclitaxel, remifentanil, sargramostim, tacrolimus, teniposide, theophylline, thiotepa

cefoxitin

IV route

• After diluting 1 g or less/10 ml or more D_5W, NS and give over 3-5 min; may be diluted further with 50-100 ml NS or D_5W; run over ½-1 hr by Y-tube or 3-way stopcock; discontinue primary inf during administration; give by cont inf at prescribed rate; may store 96 hr refrigerated or 24 hr at room temp
• For 10-14 days to ensure organism death, prevent superinfection
• After C&S completed

Syringe compatibilities: Heparin, insulin

Y-site compatibilities: Acyclovir, amifostine, amphotericin B cholesteryl sulfate complex, aztreonam, cyclophosphamide, diltiazem, DOXOrubicin liposome, famotidine, fluconazole, foscarnet, HYDROmorphone, magnesium sulfate, meperidine, morphine, ondansetron, perphenazine, remifentanil, teniposide, thiotepa

cefprozil

• For 10-14 days to ensure organism death, prevent superinfection
• After C&S
• Refrigerate/shake susp prior to use

cefuroxime

• For 10-14 days to ensure organism death, prevent superinfection
• With food if needed for GI symptoms
• After C&S obtained

Y-site compatibilities: Acyclovir, allopurinol, amifostine, atracurium, aztreonam, cyclophosphamide, diltiazem, famotidine, fludarabine, foscarnet, HYDROmorphone, melphalan, meperidine, morphine, ondansetron, pancuronium, perphenazine, remifentanil, sargramostim, tacrolimus, teniposide, thiotepa, vecuronium

SIDE EFFECTS

CNS: Dizziness, headache, fatigue, paresthesia, fever, chills, confusion

GI: *Diarrhea,* nausea, vomiting, anorexia, dysgeusia, glossitis, bleeding; increased AST, ALT, bilirubin, LDH, alk phos; abdominal pain, loose stools, flatulence, heartburn, stomach cramps, colitis, jaundice, pseudomembranous colitis

GU: Vaginitis, pruritus, candidiasis, increased BUN, nephrotoxicity, renal failure, pyuria, dysuria, reversible interstitial nephritis

HEMA: Leukopenia, thrombocytopenia, agranulocytosis, anemia, neutropenia, lymphocytosis, eosinophilia, pancytopenia, hemolytic anemia, leukocytosis, granulocytopenia

INTEG: Rash, urticaria, dermatitis, Stevens-Johnson syndrome

RESP: Dyspnea

SYST: Anaphylaxis, serum sickness, superinfection

PHARMACOKINETICS

cefaclor

PO: Peak ½-1 hr, half-life 36-54 min, 25% bound by plasma proteins, 60%-85% eliminated unchanged in urine in 8 hr, crosses placenta, excreted in breast milk (low concentrations)

cefotetan

IM/IV: Peak 1½-3 hr, half-life 3-5 hr, 75%-90% bound by plasma proteins, 50%-80% eliminated unchanged in urine, crosses placenta, excreted in breast milk

cefoxitin

Half-life 0.75-1 hr; 65%-80% bound by plasma proteins; 90%-100% eliminated unchanged in urine; crosses placenta, blood-brain barrier; eliminated in breast milk; not metabolized

IM: Peak 15-60 min

IV: Peak 3 min

cefprozil

PO: Peak 1.5 hr, protein binding 36%, elimination half-life 1.3 hr (normal renal function), 2 hr (hepatic disease), 5½-6 hr (end-stage renal disease), extensively metabolized to an active metabolite, eliminated in urine 60%

cefuroxime

Peak PO 2 hr, IM 45 min, IV 2-3 min, 66% excreted unchanged in urine, half-life 1-2 hr in normal renal function

INTERACTIONS

Increase: effect/toxicity—aminoglycosides, furosemide, probenecid

Increase: bleeding risk (cefotetan)—anticoagulants, thrombolytics, NSAIDs, antiplatelets, plicamycin, valproic acid

Decrease: absorption of cephalosporin—antacids

Decrease: effect of cephalosporin—H_2-blockers

Drug/Lab Test

False increase: creatinine (serum urine), urinary 17-KS

False positive: urinary protein, direct Coombs' test, urine glucose testing (Clinitest)

Interference: cross-matching

NURSING CONSIDERATIONS

Assess:

⚠ **Nephrotoxicity:** increased BUN, creatinine

- I&O ratio
- Blood studies: AST, ALT, CBC, Hct, bilirubin, LDH, alk phos, Coombs' test q monthly if patient is on long-term therapy
- Electrolytes: K, Na, Cl q mo if patient is on long-term therapy
- Bowel pattern daily; if severe diarrhea occurs, product should be discontinued; may indicate pseudomembranous colitis
- Urine output; if decreasing, notify prescriber (may indicate nephrotoxicity)

⚠ **Anaphylaxis:** rash, flushing, urticaria, pruritus, dyspnea; discontinue product, notify prescriber, have emergency equipment available

- **Bleeding:** ecchymosis, bleeding gums, hematuria, stool guaiac daily

⚠ **Overgrowth of infection:** perineal itching, fever, malaise, redness, pain, swelling, drainage, rash, diarrhea, change in cough, sputum

Evaluate:

- Therapeutic response: negative C&S

Teach patient/family:

- If diabetic, to use blood glucose testing
- To complete full course of product therapy; to report persistent diarrhea
- To use yogurt, buttermilk to maintain intestinal flora, decrease diarrhea
- To notify prescriber if breastfeeding or of any side effects

⚠ To report sore throat, bruising, bleeding, joint pain (may indicate blood dyscrasias [rare]); diarrhea with mucus, blood (pseudomembranous colitis)

TREATMENT OF ANAPHYLAXIS:
EPINEPHrine, antihistamines; resuscitate if needed

CEPHALOSPORINS—3RD/4TH GENERATION

cefdinir (Rx)
(sef′dih-ner)
Omnicef

cefditoren pivoxil (Rx)
(sef-dit′oh-ren pih-vox′il)
Spectracef

cefepime (Rx)
(sef′e-peem)
Maxipime (4th generation)

cefixime (Rx)
(sef-icks′ime)
Cefixime, Suprax

cefotaxime (Rx)
(sef-oh-taks′eem)
Claforan

cefpodoxime (Rx)
(sef-poe-docks′eem)
Vantin

ceftazidime (Rx)
(sef′tay-zi-deem)
Ceptaz, Fortaz, Tazicef, Tazidime

ceftibuten (Rx)
(sef-ti-byoo′tin)
Cedax

ceftizoxime (Rx)
(sef-ti-zox′eem)
Cefizox

ceftriaxone (Rx)
(sef-try-ax′one)
Rocephin

Func. class.: Broad-spectrum antibiotic
Chem. class.: Cephalosporin (3rd generation)

Do not confuse:
ceftazidime/ceftizoxime
Vantin/Ventolin

ACTION: Inhibits bacterial cell wall synthesis, renders cell wall osmotically unstable, leads to cell death

USES:

cefdinir: Community-acquired pneumonia, otitis media, sinusitis, pharyngitis, skin and skin-structure infections, acute exacerbations of chronic bronchitis, gram-negative bacilli: *Haemophilus influenzae, Haemophilus parainfluenzae, Moraxella catarrhalis;* gram-positive organisms: *Streptococcus pneumoniae, Streptococcus pyogenes, Staphylococcus aureus (MSSA)*
cefditoren pivoxil: Acute bacterial exacerbations of chronic bronchitis caused by *Haemophilus influenzae, Haemophilus parainfluenzae, Streptococcus pneumoniae, Moraxella catarrhalis*; pharyngitis/tonsillitis caused by *Streptococcus pyogenes*; uncomplicated skin and skin-structure infections caused by *Staphylococcus aureus, Streptococcus pyogenes;* community-acquired pneumonia
cefepime: Gram-negative bacilli: *Escherichia coli, Proteus, Klebsiella;* gram-positive organisms: *Streptococcus pneumoniae, Streptococcus pyogenes, Staphylococcus aureus;* lower respiratory tract, urinary tract, skin, bone infections; febrile neutropenia intraabdominal infection
cefixime: Uncomplicated UTI *(Escherichia coli, Proteus mirabilis)*, pharyngitis and tonsillitis *(Streptococcus pyogenes)*, otitis media *(Haemophilus influenzae)*, *Moraxella catarrhalis,* acute bronchitis and acute exacerbations of chronic bronchitis *(Streptococcus pneumoniae, H. influenzae)*, uncomplicated gonorrhea
cefotaxime: Gram-negative organisms: *Haemophilus influenzae, Haemophilus parainfluenzae, Escherichia coli, Enterococcus faecalis, Neisseria gonorrhoeae, Neisseria meningitidis, Proteus mirabilis, Klebsiella, Citrobacter, Serratia, Salmonella, Shigella Pseudo-*

monas; gram-positive organisms: *Streptococcus pneumoniae, Streptococcus pyogenes, Staphylococcus aureus;* serious lower respiratory tract, urinary tract, skin, bone, gonococcal infections; bacteremia, septicemia, meningitis, skin, skin-structure infections; CNS infections; perioperative prophylaxis

cefpodoxime: Gram-negative bacilli: *Neisseria gonorrhoeae, Haemophilus influenzae, Escherichia coli, Proteus mirabilis, Klebsiella;* gram-positive organisms: *Streptococcus pneumoniae, Streptococcus pyogenes, Staphylococcus aureus;* upper and lower respiratory tract, urinary tract, skin infections; otitis media; sexually transmitted diseases

ceftazidime: Gram-negative organisms: *Haemophilus influenzae, Escherichia coli, Enterobacter aerogenes, Pseudomonas aeruginosa, Proteus mirabilis, Klebsiella, Citrobacter, Enterobacter, Salmonella, Shigella, Acinetobacter, Bacteroides fragilis, Neisseria, Serratia;* gram-positive organisms: *Streptococcus pneumoniae, Streptococcus pyogenes, Staphylococcus aureus;* serious upper/lower respiratory tract, urinary tract, skin, gynecologic, bone, joint, intraabdominal infections; septicemia, meningitis, febrile neutropenia

ceftibuten: Pharyngitis/tonsillitis, otitis media, secondary bacterial infection of acute bronchitis

ceftizoxime: Gram-negative bacilli: *Haemophilus influenzae, Escherichia coli, Enterobacter aerogenes, Proteus mirabilis, Klebsiella, Enterobacter;* gram-positive organisms: *Streptococcus pneumoniae, Streptococcus pyogenes, Staphylococcus aureus;* serious lower respiratory tract, urinary tract, skin, intraabdominal infections; septicemia, meningitis, bone, joint infections; PID caused by *Neisseria gonorrhoeae*

ceftriaxone: Gram-negative bacilli: *Haemophilus influenzae, Escherichia coli, Enterobacter aerogenes, Proteus mirabilis, Klebsiella, Citrobacter, Enterobacter, Salmonella, Shigella, Acinetobacter, Bacteroides fragilis, Neisseria, Serratia;* gram-positive organisms: *Streptococcus pneumoniae, Streptococcus pyogenes, Staphylococcus aureus;* serious lower respiratory tract, urinary tract, skin, gonococcal, intraabdominal infections; septicemia, meningitis, bone, joint infections; otitis media; PID

CONTRAINDICATIONS:

Hypersensitivity to cephalosporins, infants <1 mo

Precautions: Pregnancy (B), breastfeeding, children, hypersensitivity to penicillins, GI/renal disease

DOSAGE AND ROUTES

cefdinir

Uncomplicated skin and skin-structure infections/community-acquired pneumonia

- **Adult and child ≥13 yr: PO** 300 mg q12hr × 10 days
- **Child 6 mo-12 yr: PO** 7 mg/kg q12hr or 14 mg/kg q24hr × 10 days

Acute exacerbations of chronic bronchitis/acute maxillary sinusitis

- **Adult and child ≥13 yr: PO** 300 mg q12hr or 600 mg q24hr × 10 days or 300 mg bid × 5 days for some infections

Pharyngitis/tonsillitis

- **Adult and child ≥13 yr: PO** 300 mg q12hr or 600 mg q24hr × 10 days
- **Child 6 mo-12 yr: PO** 7 mg/kg q12hr × 5-10 days or 14 mg/kg q24hr × 10 days

Renal dose

- CCr <30 ml/min, 300 mg/day (adult); 7 mg/kg/day (child)

Available forms: Caps 300 mg; susp 125 mg, 250 mg/5 ml

cefditoren pivoxil

- **Adult: PO** 200-400 mg bid × 10 days

Renal dose

- **Adult: PO** CCr 30-50 ml/min, max 200 mg bid; CCr <30 ml/min, max 200 mg daily

Available forms: Tabs 200 mg

cefepime

Febrile neutropenia

• **Adult/adolescent >16 yrs/child ≥ 40 kg: IV** 2 g q8hr × 7 days or until neutropenia resolves

• **Infant ≥2 mo/child/adolescent ≤16 yr and ≤40 kg: IV** 50 mg/kg/dose q8hr × 7-10 days or until neutropenia resolves

• **Neonate >14 days (unlabeled): IV** 50 mg/kg q12hr

• **Neonate ≤14 days (unlabeled): IV** 30 mg/kg q12hr

Urinary tract infections (mild to moderate)

• **Adult: IV/IM** 0.5-1 g q12hr × 7-10 days

Urinary tract infections (severe)

• **Adult/adolescent >16 yr/child ≥40 kg: IV** 2 g q12hr × 10 days

Pneumonia (moderate to severe)

• **Adult: IV** 1-2 g q12hr × 10 days

• Dosage reduction indicated with renal impairment (CCr <50 ml/min)

Uncomplicated gonorrhea

• **IM** 2 g as a single dose with 1 g **PO** probenecid at the same time

Available forms: Powder for inj 500 mg, 1, 2 g; 1 g/50 ml, 2 g/100 ml

cefixime

• **Adult: PO** 400 mg/day as a single dose or 200 mg q12hr

• **Child >50 kg or >12 yr: PO** use adult dosage

• **Child <50 kg or <12 yr: PO** 8 mg/kg/day as a single dose or 4 mg/kg q12hr

Renal dose

• CCr 21-60 ml/min, give 75% of dose; CCr <20 ml/min, give 50% of dose

Available forms: Tabs 400 mg; powder for oral susp 100 mg/5 ml

cefotaxime

• **Adult: IM/IV** 1-2 g q12hr

• **Child 1 mo-12 yr: IM/IV** 50-180 mg/kg/day divided q6hr

Severe infections

• **Adult: IM/IV** 2 g q4hr not to exceed 12 g/day

• **Child 1 mo-12 yr: IM/IV** 50-180 mg/kg/day in 4-6 divided doses

Uncomplicated gonorrhea

• **Adult: IM** 1 g

• Dosage reduction indicated for severe renal impairment (CCr <30 ml/min)

Available forms: Powder for inj 500 mg, 1, 2, 10 g; inj 1, 2 g premixed frozen

cefpodoxime

Pneumonia

• **Adult >13 yr: PO** 200 mg q12hr × 14 days

Uncomplicated gonorrhea

• **Adult >13 yr: PO** 200 mg as a single dose

Skin and skin structure

• **Adult >13 yr: PO** 400 mg q12hr × 7-14 days

Pharyngitis and tonsillitis

• **Adult >13 yr: PO** 100 mg q12hr × 10 days

• **Child 5 mo-12 yr: PO** 5 mg/kg q12hr (max 100 mg/dose or 200 mg/day) × 5-10 days

Uncomplicated UTI

• **Adult >13 yr: PO** 100 mg q12hr × 7 days; dosing interval increased with severe renal impairment

Acute otitis media

• **Child 5 mo-12 yr: PO** 5 mg/kg q12hr × 10 days

Available forms: Tabs 100, 200 mg; granules for susp 50 mg, 100 mg/5 ml

ceftazidime

• **Adult: IV/IM** 1-2 g q8-12hr × 5-10 days

• **Child: IV** 30-50 mg/kg q8hr, max 6 g/day

• **Neonate: IV** 30-50 mg/kg q12hr

Renal dose

• **Adult: IM/IV** CCr <50 ml/min, give q12hr; CCr 10-30 ml/min, give q24hr; CCr <10 ml/min, give q48-72hr

Available forms: Inj 250, 500 mg, 1, 2, 6 g

ceftibuten

• **Adult: PO** 400 mg/day × 10 days

• **Child 6 mo-12 yr: PO** 9 mg/kg/day × 10 days

Renal dose

• **Adult: PO** CCr 30-49 ml/min, give 200

mg q24hr; CCr 5-29 ml/min, give 100 mg q24hr

Available forms: Caps 400 mg; susp 90 mg, 180 mg/5 ml

ceftizoxime

- **Adult: IM/IV** 1-2 g q8-12hr, may give up to 4 g q8hr in life-threatening infections
- **Child >6 mo: IM/IV** 50 mg/kg q6-8hr

Renal dose

- **Adult: IM/IV** CCr <50-80 ml/min, give 500-1500 mg q8hr; CCr 5-49 ml/min, give 250-1000 mg q12hr

PID

- **Adult: IV** 2 g q8hr, may increase to 4 g q8hr in severe infections

Available forms: Powder for inj 500 mg, 1, 2, 10 g; premixed 1 g, 2 g/50 ml

ceftriaxone

- **Adult: IM/IV** 1-2 g/day, max 2 g q12-24hr
- **Child: IM/IV** 50-75 mg/kg/day in equal doses q12hr

Uncomplicated gonorrhea

- **Adult:** 250 mg **IM** as single dose
- Reduce dosage in severe renal impairment (CCr <10 ml/min)

Meningitis

- **Adult and child: IM/IV** 100 mg/kg/day in equal doses q12hr, max 4 g/day

Surgical prophylaxis

- **Adult: IV** 1 g $^1/_2$-2 hr before surgery

Available forms: Inj 250, 500 mg, 1, 2, 10 g

Administer:

- Change IV site q72hr

cefdinir

- Oral susp after adding 39 ml water to the 60-ml bottle or 65 ml water to the 120-ml bottle; discard unused portion after 10 days; give without regard to food, do not give within 2 hr of antacids, iron supplements
- After C&S completed

cefditoren pivoxil

- For 10 days to ensure organism death, prevent superinfection
- With food for GI symptoms, do not give with antacids
- After C&S completed

cefepime

Intermittent IV INF route

- IV after diluting in 50-100 ml or more D_5, NS; give over 30 min
- For 7-10 days to ensure organism death, prevent superinfection

Solution compatibilities: 0.9% NaCl, D_5, D_5W, 0.5%, 10% lidocaine, bacteriostatic water for inj with parabens/benzyl alcohol

Y-site compatibilities: DOXOrubicin liposome

cefixime

- For 10-14 days to ensure organism death, prevent superinfection
- Do not break, crush, or chew tab
- Without regard to food

cefotaxime

IV route

- IV after **diluting** 1 g/10 ml D_5W, NS, sterile water for inj, **give** over 3-5 min by Y-tube or 3-way stopcock; may be **diluted further** with 50-100 ml NS or D_5W; **run** over $^1/_2$-1 hr; discontinue primary inf during administration; may be **diluted** in larger vol of sol, given as a cont inf over 6-24 hr
- For 10-14 days to ensure organism death, prevent superinfection
- Thaw frozen container at room temp or refrigeration; do not force thaw by immersion or microwave; visually inspect container for leaks

Syringe compatibilities: Caffeine, diphenhyDRINATE, heparin, ofloxacin

Y-site compatibilities: Acyclovir, alfentanil, alprostadil, amifostine, amikacin, aminocaproic acid, aminophylline, anidulafungin, ascorbic acid injection, atenolol, atracurium, atropine, aztreonam, benztropine, bivalirudin, bleomycin, bumetanide, buprenorphine, butorphanol, caffeine, calcium chloride/gluconate, CARBOplatin, cefamandole, cefmetazole, cefonicid, cefoperazone, cefotetan, cefoxitin, ceftazidime (L-arginine), cefTRIAXone sodium, cefuroxime, cimetidine, CISplatin, clindamycin, codeine, cyanocobalamin, cyclophosphamide, cycloSPORINE, cytarabine, DACTINomycin,

DAPTOmycin, dexamethasone, dexmedetomidine, digoxin, diltiazem, docetaxel, DOPamine, doxacurium, doxycycline, enalaprilat, ePHEDrine, EPINEPHrine, epirubicin, epoetin alfa, eptifibatide, erythromycin, esmolol, etoposide, famotidine, fenoldopam, fentaNYL, fludarabine, fluorouracil, folic acid, furosemide, gatifloxacin, gentamicin, glycopyrrolate, granisetron, heparin, hydrocortisone, HYDROmorphone, ifosfamide, imipenem-cilastatin, insulin (regular), isoproterenol, ketorolac, lidocaine, linezolid, LORazepam, LR, magnesium sulfate, mannitol, mechlorethamine, melphalan, meperidine, metaraminol, methicillin, methotrexate, methoxamine, methyldopate, metoclopramide, metoprolol, metroNIDAZOLE, mezlocillin, miconazole, midazolam, milrinone, minocycline, mitoxantrone, morphine, moxalactam, multiple vitamins, mycophenolate, nafcillin, nalbuphine, naloxone, nesiritide, netilmicin, nitroglycerin, nitroprusside, norepinephrine, normal saline, octreotide, ofloxacin, ondansetron, ornidazole, oxacillin, oxaliplatin, oxytocin, paclitaxel, palonosetron, pamidronate, pancuronium, pantoprazole, papaverine, pefloxacin, pemetrexed, penicillin G potassium/sodium, pentamidine, pentazocine, PENTobarbital, peritoneal dialysis solution, perphenazine, PHENobarbital, phenylephrine, phenytoin, phytonadione, piperacillin, polymyxin B, potassium chloride, procainamide, prochlorperazine, promethazine, propofol, propranolol, protamine, pyridoxine, quiNIDine, quinupristin, ranitidine, remifentanil, Ringer's injection, ritodrine, riTUXimab, rocuronium, sargramostim, sodium acetate/bicarbonate, sodium fusidate, sodium lactate, succinylcholine, SUFentanil, sulfamethoxazole-trimethoprim, tacrolimus, teniposide, theophylline, thiamine, thiotepa, ticarcillin, ticarcillin-clavulanate, tigecycline, tirofiban, TNA, tobramycin, tolazoline, TPN, trastuzumab, trimetaphan, urokinase, vancomycin, vasopressin, vecuronium, verapamil, vinorelbine, voriconazole

cefpodoxime

- Do not break, crush, or chew tabs due to taste
- For 10-14 days to ensure organism death, prevent superinfection
- With food for better absorption; do not give within 2 hr of antacids, H_2-receptor antagonists

ceftazidime

IM route

- **Fortaz, Tazidime vials:** Reconstitute 500 mg or 1 g with 1.5 or 3 ml, respectively, of sterile or bacteriostatic water for inj or 0.5-1% lidocaine (approx 280 mg/ml)
- **Tazicef vials:** Reconstitute 1 g/3 ml sterile water for inj (approx 280 mg/ml)
- **Ceptaz vials:** Reconstitute 1 g/3 ml sterile or bacteriostatic water for inj or 0.5-1% lidocaine (approx 250 mg/ml)
- **Withdraw** dose while making sure needle remains in vial; **ensure** no CO_2 bubbles present; **inject** deeply in large muscle mass, **aspirate** before injection

IV route

- Visually inspect for particulate matter, discoloration, if possible
- **Fortaz, Tazicef, Tazidime packs: Reconstitute** 1 or 2 g/100 ml sterile water for inj or other compatible IV sol (10 or 20 mg/ml, respectively); reconstitution is done in two stages: first, **inject** 10 ml of the diluent into the pack and **shake** well to dissolve and become clear; CO_2 pressure inside container will occur, **insert** vent needle to release pressure; **add** remaining diluents, **remove** vent needle
- **Fortaz, Tazicef, Tazidime vials: Reconstitute** 500 mg, 1 g, 2 g with 5, 10, 10 ml, respectively, of sterile water for inj or other compatible IV solution (100, 95-100, or 170-180 mg/ml, respectively); **shake** well to dissolve
- **Fortaz, Tazidime ADD-Vantage vials (for IV only): Reconstitute** 1 or 2 g with NS, ½ NS, D_5W in either 50- or 100-ml flexible diluent container; to release CO_2 pressure, **insert** vent needle after dissolving, **remove** vent before using

• **Ceptaz packs: Reconstitute** 1 or 2 g/100 ml sterile water for inj or compatible IV sol (10 or 20 mg/ml, respectively); reconstitution is done in two stages: first, **inject** 10 ml of the diluent into the pack and **shake** well to dissolve, **add** the remaining diluent, **insert** vent needle before giving

• **Ceptaz vials: Reconstitute** 1 or 2 g/10 ml of sterile water for inj or compatible IV sol (90-95, or 170-180 mg/ml, respectively)

• **Ceptaz ADD-Vantage vials (for IV only): Reconstitute** 1 or 2 g with NS, ½ NS, or D_5W in either 50- or 100-ml diluent container

Direct Intermittent IV INF route

• **Vials: withdraw** dose while making sure needle remains in sol; make sure there are no CO_2 bubbles in syringe before inj; **inject** directly over 3-5 min or slowly into tubing of a free-flowing compatible IV solution

Intermittent IV INF route

• **Vials: withdraw** dose while making sure needle opening remains in sol; make sure there are no CO_2 bubbles in syringe before inj; infusion packs and ADD-Vantage systems ready for inf after reconstitution, **infuse** over 15-30 min

Syringe compatibilities: Cimetidine, dimenhyDRINATE, HYDROmorphone

Y-site compatibilities: Acyclovir, alfentanil, allopurinol, amifostine, amikacin, aminocaproic acid, aminophylline, amphotericin B lipid complex, anakinra, anidulafungin, atenolol, atropine sulfate, aztreonam, benzotropine, bivalirudin, bleomycin, bumetanide, buprenorphine, butorphanol, calcium gluconate, CARBOplatin, cefamandole, ceFAZolin, cefonicid, cefoperazone, cefotetan, cefoxitin, ceftazidime, ceftizoxime, cefTRIAXone, cefuroxime, cephalothin, cephapirin, cimetidine, ciprofloxacin, CISplatin, clindamycin, codeine, cyanocobalamin, cyclophosphamide, cycloSPORINE, cytarabine, DACTINomycin, DAPTOmycin, dexamethasone, dexmedetomidine, digoxin, diltiazem, docetaxel, DOPamine, doxacurium, doxapram, enalaprilat, ePHEDrine, EPINEPHrine, epoetin alfa, eptifibatide, esmolol, etoposide, famotidine, fenoldopam, fentaNYL, filgrastim, fludarabine, fluorouracil, folic acid, foscarnet, furosemide, gallium, gatifloxacin, gemcitabine, gentamicin, glycopyrrolate, granisetron, heparin, HYDROmorphone, ifosfamide, imipenem-cilastatin, indomethacin, insulin (regular), irinotecan, isepamicin, isoproterenol, isosorbide, ketamine, ketorolac, labetalol, levofloxacin, lidocaine, linezolid, LORazepam, LR, magnesium sulfate, mannitol, mechlorethamine, melphalan, meperidine, metaraminol, methicillin, methotrexate, methoxamine, methyldopate, methylPREDNISolone, metoclopramide, metoprolol, metroNIDAZOLE, miconazole, milrinone, morphine, moxalactam, multiple vitamin inj, nafcillin, nalbuphine, paclitaxel, ranitidine, remifentanil, tacrolimus, teniposide, theophylline, thiotepa, vinorelbine, zidovudine

ceftibuten

• For 10 days to ensure organism death, prevent superinfection

• Without regard to food

ceftizoxime

IV route

• IV after **diluting** 1 g/10 ml sterile water, shake and **give** over 3-5 min; may be **diluted further** with 50-100 ml NS or D_5W; give through Y-tube or 3-way stopcock; **run** over ½-1 hr

• For 10-14 days to ensure organism death, prevent superinfection

Y-site compatibilities: Acyclovir, alfentanil, allopurinol, amifostine, amikacin, aminocaproic acid, aminophylline, amiodarone, amphotericin B cholesteryl, amphotericin B liposome, anidulafungin, ascorbic acid injection, atenolol, atracurium, atropine, aztreonam, benztropine, bivalirudin, bleomycin, bumetanide, buprenorphine, butorphanol, calcium chloride/gluconate, CARBOplatin, caspofungin, cefamandole, ceFAZolin, cefmetazole, cefoperazone, cefotetan, ceftazidime, cefTRIAXone, cefuroxime, cephalothin, cephapirin, cimetidine, CISplatin, clindamycin, codeine, cyanocobalamin, cyclophosphamide, cycloSPORINE, cytarabine, DACTINomycin, DAPTOmycin, dexamethasone, dexmedetomidine, digoxin, diltiazem, diphenhydrAMINE, docetaxel, DOPamine, doxacurium, DOXOrubicin, DOXOrubicin liposomal, enalaprilat, ePHEDrine, EPINEPHrine, epirubicin, epoetin alfa, eptifibatide, esmolol, etoposide, fenoldopam, fentaNYL, fluconazole, fludarabine, fluorouracil, folic acid, foscarnet, furosemide, gatifloxacin, gemcitabine, gentamicin, glycopyrrolate, granisetron, heparin, hydrocortisone, HYDROmorphone, IDArubicin, ifosfamide, imipenem-cilastatin, insulin (regular), irinotecan, isoproterenol, ketorolac, labetalol, levofloxacin, lidocaine, linezolid, LORazepam, LR, magnesium sulfate, mannitol, mechlorethamine, melphalan, meperidine, methotrexate, methoxamine, methyldopate, metoclopramide, metoprolol, metroNIDAZOLE, mezlocillin, midazolam, milrinone, mitoxantrone, morphine, multiple vitamins injection, mycophenolate mofetil, nafcillin, naloxone, nesiritide, netilmicin, niCARdipine, nitroglycerin, nitroprusside, norepinephrine, octreotide, ondansetron, oxaliplatin, oxytocin, paclitaxel, palonosetron, pamidronate, pancuronium, pantoprazole, pemetrexed, penicillin G potassium/sodium, PHENobarbital, phenylephrine, phytonadione, piperacillin, polymyxin B, potassium chloride, propofol, propranolol, ranitidine, remifentanil, Ringer's, ritodrine, riTUXimab, rocuronium, sargramostim, sodium acetate/bicarbonate, succinylcholine, SUFentanil, tacrolimus, teniposide, theophylline, thiotepa, ticarcillin-clavulanate, tigecycline, tirofiban, TNA, tobramycin, TPN, trastuzumab, trimetaphan, vasopressin, verapamil, vinCRIStine, vinorelbine, voriconazole

ceftriaxone

- For 10-14 days to ensure organism death, prevent superinfection
- **IM** inj deeply in large muscle mass

IV route

- **IV** after **diluting** 250 mg/2.4 ml D_5W, water for inj, 0.9% NaCl; may be **further diluted** with 50-100 ml NS, D_5W, $D_{10}W$; shake; **run** over $^1/_2$-1 hr
- Do not mix with calcium salts

Y-site compatibilities: Acyclovir, alfentanil, allopurinol, amifostine, amikacin, aminocaproic acid, aminophylline, amiodarone, amphotericin B liposome, anidulafungin, atenolol, atracurium, atropine, aztreonam, benztropine, bivalirudin, bleomycin, bumetanide, buprenorphine, butorphanol, CARBOplatin, cefamandole, ceFAZolin, cefmetazole, cefonicid, cefoperazone, cefotaxime, cefotetan, cefoxitin, ceftazidime, ceftizoxime, cefuroxime, cephalothin, cephapirin, cimetidine, cisatracurium, CISplatin, codeine, cyanocobalamin, cyclophosphamide, cycloSPORINE, cytarabine, DACTINomycin, DAPTOmycin, dexamethasone, dexmedetomidine, digoxin, diltiazem, docetaxel, DOPamine, doxacurium, DOXOrubicin liposomal, doxycycline, drotrecogin alfa, enalaprilat, ePHEDrine, EPINEPHrine, epoetin alfa, eptifibatide, erythromycin, esmolol, etoposide, fenoldopam, fludarabine, fluorouracil, folic acid, foscarnet, furosemide, gallium, gatifloxacin, gemcitabine, gentamicin, glycopyrrolate, granisetron, heparin, hydrocortisone, HYDROmorphone, ifosfamide, indomethacin, insulin (regular), isoproterenol, ketorolac, lansoprazole, levofloxacin, lidocaine, linezolid, LORazepam, mannitol, mechlorethamine, melphalan, meperidine, metaraminol, methicillin, methotrexate, methoxamine, methyldopate, methylPREDNISolone, metoclopramide, metoprolol, metroNIDAZOLE, mezlocillin, miconazole, midazolam, milrinone, morphine, moxalactam, multiple vitamins injection, nafcillin, nalbuphine, naloxone, nesiritide, netilimicin, nitroglycerin, nitroprusside, norepinephrine, octreotide, oxacillin, oxaliplatin, oxytocin, paclitaxel, palonosetron, pamidronate, pancuronium, pantoprazole, pemetrexed, penicillin

G potassium/sodium, PHENobarbital, phenylephrine, phytonadione, piperacillin, polymyxin B, potassium chloride, procainamide, propofol, propranolol, pyridoxine, ranitidine, remifentanil, ritodrine, riTUXimab, rocuronium, sargramostim, sodium acetate/bicarbonate, succinylcholine, SUFentanil, tacrolimus, teniposide, theophylline, thiamine, thiotepa, ticarcillin, ticarcillin-clavulanate, tigecycline, tirofiban, tolazoline, trastuzumab, trimetaphan, urokinase, vasopressin, vecuronium, verapamil, vinCRIStine, voriconazole, warfarin, zidovudine

SIDE EFFECTS

CNS: Headache, dizziness, weakness, paresthesia, fever, chills, seizures, dyskinesia (cefdinir)
CV: Heart failure, syncope (cefdinir)
EENT: *Oral candidiasis*
GI: *Nausea, vomiting, diarrhea, anorexia,* pain, glossitis, **bleeding**; increased AST, ALT, bilirubin, LDH, alk phos; abdominal pain, **pseudomembranous colitis**; cholestasis (cefotaxime)
GU: **Proteinuria**, vaginitis, pruritus, *candidiasis,* increased BUN, **nephrotoxicity, renal failure**
HEMA: **Leukopenia, thrombocytopenia, agranulocytosis**, anemia, **neutropenia, lymphocytosis, eosinophilia, pancytopenia, hemolytic anemia**
INTEG: Rash, urticaria, dermatitis
RESP: Dyspnea
SYST: **Anaphylaxis, serum sickness, Stevens-Johnson syndrome, toxic epidermal necrolysis**

PHARMACOKINETICS

cefdinir
Unchanged in urine; crosses placenta, blood-brain barrier; eliminated in breast milk, not metabolized; 60%-70% protein binding, half-life 1.7 hr
cefditoren pivoxil
Well absorbed when broken down (prodrug), wide distribution, half-life 100 min, onset rapid, peak 0.5-3 hr, duration 12 hr, 88% protein binding
cefepime
Peak 79 min; half-life 2 hr; 20% bound by plasma proteins; 90% excreted unchanged in urine; crosses placenta, blood-brain barrier; excreted in breast milk, not metabolized
cefixime
PO: Peak 1-2 hr, half-life 3-4 hr, 65% bound by plasma proteins, 50% eliminated unchanged in urine, crosses placenta, excreted in breast milk
cefotaxime
Half-life 1 hr, 35%-65% is bound by plasma proteins, 40%-65% is eliminated unchanged in urine in 24 hr, 25% metabolized in the liver to active metabolites, excreted in breast milk (small amounts)
IM: Onset 30 min
IV: Onset 5 min
cefpodoxime
Half-life 3 hr, 21%-29% bound by plasma proteins, 30% eliminated unchanged in urine in 8 hr, crosses placenta, excreted in breast milk
ceftazidime
IM/IV:
Peak 1 hr, half-life 1-1$^1/_2$ hr, 90% bound by plasma proteins, 80% eliminated unchanged in urine, crosses placenta, excreted in breast milk
ceftibuten
PO: Peak 2-3 hr; plasma protein binding 65%, elimination half-life 2 hr, extensively metabolized to an active metabolite
ceftizoxime
Half-life 1.6 hr, 30% bound by plasma proteins, 36%-60% eliminated unchanged in urine, crosses placenta, excreted in breast milk
IM: Peak 1 hr
IV: Onset 5 min
ceftriaxone
Half-life 6-9 hr, 90% protein binding 58%-96%, eliminated unchanged in urine, crosses placenta, excreted in breast milk
IM: Peak 2-3 hr
IV: Onset 5 min

INTERACTIONS

Increase: bleeding—anticoagulants, thrombolytics, plicamycin, valproic acid, NSAIDs

Increase: toxicity—aminoglycosides, furosemide, probenecid

Decrease: absorption of cefdinir—iron

Drug/Food

Decrease: absorption—iron-rich cereal, infant formula

Drug/Lab Test

Increase: ALT, AST, alk phos, LDH, bilirubin, BUN, creatinine

False increase: creatinine (serum urine), urinary 17-KS

False positive: urinary protein, direct Coombs' test, urine glucose

Interference: cross-matching

NURSING CONSIDERATIONS

Assess:

- Sensitivity to penicillin, other cephalosporins

⚠ **Nephrotoxicity:** increased BUN, creatinine; urine output: if decreasing, notify prescriber

- Blood studies: AST, ALT, CBC, Hct, bilirubin, LDH, alk phos, Coombs' test monthly if patient is on long-term therapy
- Electrolytes: K, Na, Cl monthly if patient is on long-term therapy
- **Pseudomembranous colitis:** bowel pattern daily; if severe diarrhea occurs, product should be discontinued
- IV site for extravasation, phlebitis

⚠ **Anaphylaxis:** rash, urticaria, pruritus, chills, fever, joint pain, angioedema; may occur a few days after therapy begins

- Bleeding: ecchymosis, bleeding gums, hematuria, stool guaiac

⚠ **Overgrowth of infection:** perineal itching, fever, malaise, redness, pain, swelling, drainage, rash, diarrhea, change in cough, sputum

Evaluate:

- Therapeutic response: decreased symptoms of infection; negative C&S

Teach patient/family:

- If diabetic, to check blood glucose

⚠ To report sore throat, bruising, bleeding, joint pain, may indicate **blood dyscrasias (rare);** diarrhea with mucus, blood, may indicate **pseudomembranous colitis**

- To report persistent diarrhea
- That cefditoren can be taken with oral contraceptives

TREATMENT OF ANAPHYLAXIS:
EPINEPHrine, antihistamines; resuscitate if needed

cephradine

See cephalosporins—1st generation

certolizumab pegol (Rx)

(ser'tue-liz'oo-mab pegh'ol)

Cimzia

Func. class.: Biologic response modifier

Chem. class: Anti-tissue necrosis factor (anti-TNF) agent

ACTION:
Monoclonal antibody that neutralizes the activity of tumor necrosis factor α (TNF-α) found in Crohn's disease; decreases infiltration of inflammatory cells

USES:
Crohn's disease (moderate to severe) that has not responded to conventional therapy, rheumatoid arthritis (moderate to severe)

Unlabeled uses: Moderate to severe chronic plaque psoriasis, fistulizing Crohn's disease

CONTRAINDICATIONS:
Influenza, IV administration, sepsis, hypersensitivity

Black Box Warning: Infection

Precautions: Pregnancy (B), breastfeeding, children, geriatric patients, AIDS, coagulopathy, diabetes, fungal infection, heart failure, hepatitis, human antichimeric antibody, immunosuppression, leukopenia, MS, cancer, neurologic/renal disease, surgery, thrombocytopenia, TB, vaccinations

DOSAGE AND ROUTES

Crohn's disease (moderate to severe)

• **Adult: SUBCUT** 400 mg given as 2 inj at wk 0, 2, 4; if clinical response occurs, give 400 mg q4wk

Rheumatoid arthritis (moderate to severe)

• **Adult: SUBCUT** 400 mg q2wk × 3 doses then 200 mg q2wk; given with methotrexate

Crohn's disease (fistulizing)/ intolerant to infliximab (unlabeled)

• **Adult: SUBCUT** 400 mg wk 0, 2, 4 then 400 mg q4wk

Available forms: Powder for inj 400-mg kit

Administer:

SUBCUT route

• Give by subcut inj only

• Reconstitution: allow to warm to room temp; add 1 ml sterile water for inj to each vial; 2 vials will be needed for patients with Crohn's disease

• Gently swirl; do not shake; full reconstitution may take up to 30 min; reconstituted product may remain at room temp for up to 2 hr or refrigerated up to 24 hr

• If reconstituted product has been refrigerated, allow to warm to room temp

• Use 2 syringes and two 20G needles

• Withdraw reconstituted sol from each vial into separate syringes; each will contain 200 mg; switch 20G to 23G needle; inject into 2 separate sites in abdomen or thigh

SIDE EFFECTS

CNS: *Dizziness,* syncope, peripheral neuropathy, **fever, seizures, demyelinating disease of CNS**

CV: Hypotension, **heart failure, MI, cardiac dysrhythmia**

EENT: Optic neuritis, retinal hemorrhage, uveitis

GI: Increased LFTs, **hepatitis, bowel obstruction**

GU: UTI, renal disease

HEMA: Anemia, aplastic anemia, pancytopenia, thrombocytopenia

INTEG: *Rash, urticaria,* **angioedema**

MISC: Anaphylaxis, antibody formation, arthralgia, bleeding, infection, lupuslike symptoms, lymphadenopathy, **malignancies, serum sickness, suicidal ideation**

RESP: Dyspnea, upper respiratory tract infection

PHARMACOKINETICS

Peak 54-171 hr, terminal half-life 14 days

INTERACTIONS

• Do not administer live vaccines, toxoids concurrently

Increase: possible infections—abatacept, adalimumab, anakinra, etanercept, immunosuppressive agents, infliximab, rilonacept; do not use concurrently

Increase: possible malignancies—adalimumab, etanercept, infliximab

NURSING CONSIDERATIONS

Assess:

• Antinuclear antibody test (ANA), hepatitis B serology, CBC

• For rheumatoid arthritis, ROM, pain

• GI symptoms: nausea, vomiting, abdominal pain, hepatitis, increased LFTs

• Periodic blood counts (CBC)

• CV status: B/P, pulse, chest pain

⚠ **Allergic reaction, anaphylaxis:** rash, dermatitis, urticaria, dyspnea, hypotension, fever, chills; discontinue if severe; administer EPINEPHrine, corticosteroids, antihistamines; assess for allergies to murine proteins before starting therapy

Black Box Warning: Infection: discontinue if infection occurs; do not administer to patients with active infection

• Identify TB, risk for HBV before beginning treatment; TB test should be obtained; if present, TB should be treated prior to certolizumab treatment

Perform/provide:

• Storage in refrigerator; do not freeze

Evaluate:
- Therapeutic response: absence of fever, mucus in stools

Teach patient/family:
- Not to breastfeed while taking this product
- To notify prescriber of GI symptoms, hypersensitivity reactions, infections, fluid retention; redness, pain, swelling at inj site
- Not to operate machinery, drive if dizziness, vertigo occur

cetirizine (Rx, OTC)

(se-teer′i-zeen)

All Day Allergy, All Day Allergy Children's, Apo-Cetirizine ✷, GNP All Day Allergy, GNP Children's All Day Allergy, Good Sense All Day Allergy, Good Sense Children's All Day Allergy, Publix Allergy Children's, Reactine ✷, Top Care Children's All Day Allergy, Zyrtec, Zyrtec Children's

Func. class.: Antihistamine (2nd generation, peripherally selective)

Chem. class.: Piperazine, H_1-histamine antagonist

Do not confuse:
Zyrtec/Xanax/Zantac

ACTION: Acts on blood vessels, GI, respiratory system by competing with histamine for H_1-receptor site; decreases allergic response by blocking pharmacologic effects of histamine; minimal anticholinergic, sedative action

USES: Rhinitis, allergy symptoms, chronic idiopathic urticaria

Unlabeled uses: Asthma, atopic dermatitis

CONTRAINDICATIONS: Breastfeeding, newborn or premature infants, hypersensitivity to this product or hydrOXYzine, severe hepatic disease

Precautions: Pregnancy (B), children, geriatric patients, respiratory disease, angle-closure glaucoma, prostatic hypertrophy, bladder neck obstruction, asthma

DOSAGE AND ROUTES

Perennial/seasonal allergic rhinitis or idiopathic urticaria
- **Adult and child ≥6 yr: PO** 5-10 mg/day
- **Child 2-5 yr: PO** 2.5 mg/day, may increase to 5 mg/day or 2.5 mg bid
- **Child 1-2 yr: PO** 2.5 mg/day, may increase to 2.5 mg q12hr
- **Geriatric: PO** 5 mg/day, may increase to 10 mg/day

Self-treatment of hay fever/other respiratory allergies
- **Adult/adolescent/child ≥6 yr: PO** 10 mg/day; **ORAL SOL** 5-10 mg/day

Renal dose/hemodialysis/hepatic dose
- **Adult: PO** CCr 11-31 ml/min, 5 mg/day

Atopic dermatitis (unlabeled)
- **Child 6-12 yr: PO** 5-10 mg/day
- **Child 1-2 yr: PO** 0.25 mg/kg bid

Available forms: Tabs 5, 10 mg; syr 5 mg/5 ml, prefilled spoons 1 mg/ml; oral sol 5 mg/ml; liquid-filled caps 10 mg; chew tabs 5, 10 mg

Administer:
- Without regard to meals
- **Caps:** swallow whole, do not break, cut, chew, crush
- **Chew tabs:** chew before swallowing, may use with or without water
- **Oral liquid:** use calibrated measuring device

SIDE EFFECTS

CNS: *Headache,* stimulation, *drowsiness,* sedation, *fatigue,* confusion, blurred vision, tinnitus, restlessness, tremors; paradoxical excitation in children, geriatric patients

GI: *Dry mouth,* increased LFTs, constipation

INTEG: Rash, eczema, photosensitivity, urticaria

RESP: *Thickening of bronchial secretions,* dry nose, throat

PHARMACOKINETICS

Absorption rapid; onset ½ hr; peak 1-2 hr; duration 24 hr; protein binding 93%; half-life decreased in children, increased in renal/hepatic disease

INTERACTIONS

Increase: CNS depression—alcohol, opiates, sedative/hypnotics, other CNS depressants
Increase: anticholinergic/sedative effect—MAOIs
Increase: cetirizine effect—ritonavir
Drug/Food
- Food prolongs absorption by 1.7 hr

Drug/Lab Test
False negative: skin allergy tests

NURSING CONSIDERATIONS

Assess:
- **Allergy symptoms:** pruritus, urticaria, watering eyes at baseline and during treatment
- Respiratory status: rate, rhythm, increase in bronchial secretions, wheezing, chest tightness
- Blood studies: LFTs, BUN, creatinine at baseline, periodically

Perform/provide:
- Hard candy, gum, frequent rinsing of mouth for dryness
- Storage in tight, light-resistant container

Evaluate:
- Therapeutic response: absence of running or congested nose, rashes

Teach patient/family:
- About all aspects of product use; to notify prescriber if confusion, sedation, hypotension occur
- To avoid driving, other hazardous activity if drowsiness occurs
- To avoid alcohol, other CNS depressants, OTC antihistamines
- To avoid exposure to sunlight; burns may occur
- To use sugarless gum, candy, frequent sips of water to minimize dry mouth
- Not to breastfeed

TREATMENT OF OVERDOSE:

Administer diazepam, vasopressors, phenytoin IV

C

cetrorelix (Rx)

(set-roe-ree′lix)

Cetrotide

Func. class.: Gonadotropin-releasing hormone antagonist
Chem. class.: Synthetic decapeptide

ACTION:

Inhibitor of pituitary gonadotropin secretion; initially increases LH and FSH, induces a rapid suppression of gonadotropin secretion

USES:

For inhibition of premature LH surges in women undergoing controlled ovarian hyperstimulation
Unlabeled uses: Benign prostatic hyperplasia (BPH), endometriosis

CONTRAINDICATIONS:

Pregnancy (X), breastfeeding, hypersensitivity, latex allergy, renal disease
Precautions: Geriatric patients

DOSAGE AND ROUTES

Single-dose regimen
- **Adult: SUBCUT** 3 mg when serum estradiol level at appropriate stimulation response, usually on stimulation day 7; if hCG not given within 4 days after inj of 3 mg cetrorelix, give 0.25 mg daily until day of hCG administration

Multiple-dose regimen
- **Adult: SUBCUT** 0.25 mg given on stimulation day 5 (either morning or evening) or 6 (morning) and continued daily until day hCG is given

BPH (unlabeled)
- **Adult (male): SUBCUT** 5 mg bid × 2 days then 1 mg/day

Endometriosis (unlabeled)
- **Adult (female): SUBCUT** 3 mg q wk

Available forms: Inj 0.25, 3 mg

Administer:

SUBCUT route

• Attach yellow-marked needle to diluent syringe, dilute powder by injecting liquid from syringe into vial, leaving syringe on vial; gently swirl until clear, avoid bubbles; withdraw contents of vial back into syringe, replace yellow-marked needle with gray-marked needle

• SUBCUT using abdomen, 1 inch away from navel or upper thigh; swab inj area with disinfectant; clean a 2-inch circle and allow to dry; pinch up area between thumb and finger; insert needle 45-90 degrees to surface; if positioned correctly, no blood will be drawn back into syringe; reposition needle without removing it; rotate inj sites

SIDE EFFECTS

CNS: Headache
CV: Edema
ENDO: Ovarian hyperstimulation syndrome, abdominal pain (gyn)
GI: Nausea, vomiting, diarrhea
INTEG: Pain on inj; local site reactions, bruising, pruritus
Other: Rapid weight gain
RESP: Shortness of breath
SYST: Fetal death, anaphylaxis

PHARMACOKINETICS

Excreted in feces/urine, half-life depends on dosage, metabolized to metabolites, protein binding 86%

NURSING CONSIDERATIONS

Assess:

• Serum progesterone, LH; ovarian ultrasound day 7-14; pelvic exam, serum estradiol/gonadotropin; weight

• For suspected pregnancy; product should not be used, pregnancy (X)

• For latex allergy, product should not be used

⚠ For anaphylaxis during first inf

Perform/provide:

• Protection from light

Evaluate:

• Therapeutic response: pregnancy

Teach patient/family:

• To report abdominal pain, vaginal bleeding, nausea, vomiting, diarrhea, SOB, peripheral edema

• How to perform self-administration technique if needed

cetuximab (Rx)

(se-tux′i-mab)

Erbitux

Func. class.: Antineoplastic—miscellaneous, monoclonal antibody

Chem. class.: Epidermal growth factor receptor inhibitor

ACTION:

Not fully understood; binds to epidermal growth factor receptors (EGFRs); inhibits phosphorylation and activation of receptor-associated kinase, thereby resulting in inhibition of cell growth

USES:

Alone or in combination with irinotecan for EGFRs expressing metastatic colorectal carcinoma, head/neck cancer

Unlabeled uses: Front-line use for non–small-cell lung cancer in combination with CISplatin and vinorelbine

CONTRAINDICATIONS:

Hypersensitivity to this product, murine proteins

Precautions: Pregnancy (C), breastfeeding, children, geriatric patients; CV/renal/hepatic disease; ocular, pulmonary disorders

Black Box Warning: Arrhythmias, CAD, infusion-related reactions, radiation

DOSAGE AND ROUTES

• **Adult: IV INF** 400 mg/m^2 loading dose given over 120 min, max inf rate 5 ml/min; weekly maintenance dose (all other inf) is 250 mg/m^2 given over 60 min, max inf rate 5 ml/min (10 mg/min); premedicate with an H_1-antagonist (diphenhydrAMINE 50 mg IV); dosage adjustments made for inf reactions or dermatologic toxicity; other protocols used

Non–small-cell lung cancer (NSCLC) (unlabeled)

- **Adult: IV** 400 mg/m^2 over 120 min (max 5 ml/min) week 1 with weekly inf of 250 mg/m^2 over 60 min (max 5 ml/min) with cisplatin 80 mg/m^2 on day 1 and vinorelbine 25 mg/m^2 on days 1, 8

Available forms: Sol for inj 100 mg/50 ml, 200 mg/100 ml

Administer:

Intermittent IV INF route

- Use cytoxic handling procedures
- By IV inf only; do not give by IV push or bolus; do not shake or dilute
- **Inf pump:** draw up volume of vial using appropriate syringe/needle (vented spike or other appropriate transfer device); fill Erbitux into sterile evacuated container/bag, repeat until calculated volume put into the container; use new needle for each vial; give through in-line filter (low protein binding 0.22 micrometer); affix inf line and prime before starting inf, max rate 5 ml/min; flush line at end of inf with 0.9% NaCl, use a low protein binding 0.22-micrometer in-line filter
- **Syringe pump:** draw up volume of vial using appropriate syringe/needle (vented spike); place syringe into syringe driver of syringe pump and set rate; use in-line filter (low protein binding 0.22-micrometer); connect inf line, start inf after priming; repeat until calculated volume given
- Use new needle and filter for each vial, max 5 ml/min rate; use 0.9% NaCl to flush line after inf
- Do not piggyback to patient inf line
- Observe patient for adverse reactions for 1 hr after inf
- Inf reactions: if mild (grade 1 or 2), reduce all doses by 50%; if severe (grade 3 or 4), permanently discontinue

SIDE EFFECTS

CNS: *Headache, insomnia, depression,* aseptic meningitis

GI: *Nausea, diarrhea, vomiting, anorexia, mouth ulceration, dehydration, constipation, abdominal pain*

HEMA: Leukopenia, anemia

INTEG: Rash, pruritus, acne, dry skin, toxic epidermal necrolysis, angioedema, *blepharitis, cheilitis, cellulitis, cysts, alopecia, skin/nail disorder,* acute infusion reactions, other skin toxicities

MISC: *Conjunctivitis, asthma, malaise, fever,* renal failure, hypomagnesemia

MS: *Back pain*

RESP: Interstitial lung disease, *cough, dyspnea,* pulmonary embolus, *peripheral edema*

SYST: Anaphylaxis, sepsis, infection

PHARMACOKINETICS

Half-life 114 hr, steady state by 3rd wkly inf, peak 168-235 g/ml, trough 41-85 g/ml

INTERACTIONS

Drug/Lab:

Increase: LFTs

NURSING CONSIDERATIONS

Assess:

⚠ **Pulmonary changes:** lung sounds, cough, dyspnea; interstitial lung disease may occur, may be fatal; discontinue therapy if confirmed

⚠ **Serious hypersensitivity reactions:** toxic epidermal necrosis, angioedema, anaphylaxis

- GI symptoms: frequency of stools, dehydration, abdominal pain, stomatitis
- **K-RAS mutations** with metastatic colorectal carcinoma; if K-RAS mutation on codon 12 or 13 detected, patient should not receive anti-EGFR antibody therapy

Perform/provide:

- Storage refrigerated at 36° F-46° F, discard unused portions

Evaluate:

- Therapeutic response: decreased growth, spread of EGFR-expressing metastatic colorectal, head/neck carcinoma

Teach patient/family:
- To report adverse reactions immediately: shortness of breath, severe abdominal pain, skin eruptions
- About the reason for treatment, expected results
- To use contraception during treatment (pregnancy [C]), not to breastfeed
- To wear sunscreen and hats to limit sun exposure; sun exposure can exacerbate any skin reactions
- To avoid crowds, persons with known infections

charcoal, activated (OTC)

Actidose-Aqua, Actidose with Sorbitol, Charcoal Plus, Charcoal Plus DS, Charcocaps, EZ Char

Func. class.: Antiflatulent; antidote

ACTION: Binds poisons, toxins, irritants; increases adsorption in GI tract; inactivates toxins and binds until excreted

USES: Poisoning, overdose

Unlabeled uses: Diarrhea, flatulence

CONTRAINDICATIONS: Hypersensitivity to this product, unconsciousness, semiconsciousness, cyanide poisoning, mineral acids, alkalis, gag reflex depression, ethanol intoxication, intestinal obstruction, absent bowel sounds

Precautions: Pregnancy (C), hypersensitivity to quiNIDine, quiNINE

DOSAGE AND ROUTES

Children should not get more than 1 dose of products that contain sorbitol

Poisoning
- Tabs/caps should not be used for poisonings
- **Adult/adolescents: PO** (activated charcoal aqueous susp) 5-10 × estimated weight of drug/chemical ingested or 50-100 g dose, may repeat q4-6hr as needed; (activated charcoal with sorbitol susp) 50 g as a single dose, do not use multiple dosing
- **Child: PO** (activated charcoal aqueous susp) 1-2 g/kg/dose or 25-50 g dose, may repeat as needed q4-6hr
- **Infant: PO** (activated charcoal aqueous susp) 1 g/kg/dose, may repeat as needed q4-6hr

Diarrhea/flatulance (unlabeled)
- **Adult: PO** (CharcoCaps) 520 mg (2 caps) after meals or prn, max 4.16 g (16 cap)/day

Available forms: Powder 15, 25 ✱, 30, 40, 120, 240 g/container; oral susp 12.5 g/60 ml, 15 g/72 ml, 15 g/120 ml, 25 g/120 ml, 30 g/120 ml, 50 g/240 ml; 15 g/120 ml ✱, 25 g/125 ml, 50 g/225 ml, 50 g/250 ml

Administer:

PO route
- Give orally to those with intact gag reflexes, protected airways
- After inducing vomiting unless vomiting contraindicated (i.e., cyanide or alkalis)
- After mixing with water or fruit juice to form thick syrup; do not use dairy products, chocolate syrup to mix charcoal
- Repeat dose if vomiting occurs soon after dose; give with a laxative to promote elimination
- After spacing at least 2 hr before or after other products or absorption will be decreased
- Do not use tabs, caps to treat overdose

NG route
- Through nasogastric tube if patient unable to swallow

SIDE EFFECTS

GI: *Nausea, black stools,* vomiting, constipation, diarrhea, abdominal pain

OTHER: Pulmonary aspiration

PHARMACOKINETICS

PO: Excreted in feces, not absorbed, excreted unchanged in feces

INTERACTIONS

- Inactivation of acetylcysteine

Decrease: effects of acarbose, carBAMazepine, digoxin, ipecac, phenytoin

NURSING CONSIDERATIONS

Assess:

- Respiration, pulse, B/P to determine charcoal effectiveness if taken for barbiturate/opiate poisoning; intact gag reflex, serum electrolytes

Perform/provide:

- Storage in tightly closed container to prevent absorption of gases

Evaluate:

- Therapeutic response: LOC alert (poisoning)

Teach patient/family:

- That stools will be black
- How to prevent further poisonings

chloral hydrate (Rx)

(klor-al hye′drate)

Chloral Hydrate ODAN ✤, Somnote

Func. class.: Sedative/hypnotic, nonbarbiturate

Chem. class.: Chloral derivative

Controlled Substance Schedule IV (USA), Schedule F (Canada)

ACTION: Reduction product trichloroethanol produces mild cerebral depression, which causes sleep

USES: Sedation, short-term treatment of insomnia, anxiety, alcohol withdrawal

CONTRAINDICATIONS: Hypersensitivity to this product, triclofos; severe renal/hepatic disease, GI disorders (oral forms), gastritis

Precautions: Pregnancy (C), breastfeeding, geriatric patients, severe cardiac disease, depression, suicidal individuals, asthma, intermittent porphyria, esophagitis, gastric/duodenal ulcers, gastritis

DOSAGE AND ROUTES

Sedation

- **Adult: PO/RECT** 250 mg tid after meals; max 2 g/day
- **Child: PO** 25-50 mg/kg tid; max 500 mg tid

Insomnia

- **Adult: PO/RECT** 500 mg-1 g ½ hr before bedtime; max 2 g/day
- **Child: PO/RECT** 50 mg/kg (1 dose)

Alcohol withdrawal

- **Adult: PO/RECT** 500 mg-1 g q6hr; max 2 g/day

Postoperative pain/adjunct

- **Adult: PO** 250 mg tid after meals; max 2 g/day

Renal disease

- **Adult: PO/RECT** CCr <50 ml/min, avoid use

Available forms: Caps 500 mg; syr 250 mg, 500 mg/5 ml; supp 325, 650 mg

Administer:

- Do not break, crush, or chew caps
- On empty stomach with full glass of water or juice for best absorption and to decrease corrosion; dilute oral liquid with fluids; chilling syrup may mask unpleasant taste
- After meals to decrease GI symptoms if using for sedation
- ½-1 hr before bedtime for sleeplessness

SIDE EFFECTS

CNS: *Drowsiness,* dizziness, stimulation, nightmares, ataxia, hangover (rare), light-headedness, headache, paranoia, hallucinations

CV: Hypotension, dysrhythmias

GI: *Nausea, vomiting, flatulence, diarrhea,* unpleasant taste, **gastric necrosis,** abdominal pain

HEMA: **Eosinophilia, leukopenia**

INTEG: *Rash,* urticaria, **angioedema,** fever, purpura, eczema

RESP: **Depression**

PHARMACOKINETICS

PO: Onset 30 min-1 hr, duration 4-8 hr
RECT: Onset slow, duration 4-8 hr, metabolized by liver, excreted by kidneys (inactive metabolite) and in feces, crosses placenta, excreted in breast milk, metabolite highly protein bound

INTERACTIONS

Increase: action—oral anticoagulants, furosemide
Increase: action of both products—alcohol, CNS depressants
Decrease: effects of phenytoin
Drug/Lab Test
Interference: urine catecholamines, urinary 17-OHCS

NURSING CONSIDERATIONS

Assess:

- Mental status: mood, sensorium, affect, memory (long and short term)
- **Physical dependency:** more frequent requests for medication, tremors, anxiety, pinpoint pupils
- **Respiratory dysfunction:** respiratory depression, character, rate, rhythm; hold product if respirations <10/min or if pupils dilated (rare)
- History of substance abuse, cardiac disease, gastritis

Perform/provide:

- Assistance with ambulation after receiving dose, especially for geriatric patients
- Safety measures: night-light, call bell within easy reach
- Check to confirm PO medication swallowed
- Check dose of syrup carefully; fatal overdoses have occurred
- Storage in dark container, suppositories in refrigerator

Evaluate:

- Therapeutic response: ability to sleep at night, decreased amount of early morning awakening if taking product for insomnia

Teach patient/family:

- To avoid driving, other activities that require alertness
- To avoid alcohol ingestion, CNS depressants; serious CNS depression may result
- Not to discontinue medication quickly after long-term use; product should be tapered over 1-2 wk, delirium may occur
- That effects may take 2 nights to be noticed
- About alternative measures to improve sleep (reading, exercise several hours before bedtime, warm bath, warm milk, TV, self-hypnosis, deep breathing)
- To avoid breastfeeding

TREATMENT OF OVERDOSE:

Lavage, activated charcoal; monitor electrolytes, vital signs

chlorambucil (Rx)

(klor-am′byoo-sil)

Leukeran

Func. class.: Antineoplastic alkylating agent

Chem. class.: Nitrogen mustard

Do not confuse:

Leukeran/leucovorin/Leukine

ACTION: Alkylates DNA, RNA; inhibits enzymes that allow for the synthesis of amino acids in proteins; activity not cell-cycle–phase specific

USES: Chronic lymphocytic leukemia, non-Hodgkin's/Hodgkin's disease, other lymphomas

Unlabeled uses: Macroglobulinemia; ovarian, testicular carcinoma; Behçet's syndrome, Churg-Strauss syndrome; dermatomyositis, hydatidiform mole, thrombocytopenic purpura (ITP); lupus nephritis, nephrotic syndrome; pneumonitis; polyarteritis nodosa; polymyositis; rheumatoid arthritis, SLE; Wegener's granulomatosis; choriocarcinoma

CONTRAINDICATIONS:
Breastfeeding, radiation therapy within 1 mo, chemotherapy within 1 mo, thrombocytopenia, recent smallpox vaccination

Black Box Warning: Pregnancy (D)

Precautions: Children, *Pneumococcus* vaccination, tumor lysis syndrome

Black Box Warning: Bone marrow suppression, infertility, secondary malignancy

DOSAGE AND ROUTES

- **Adult: PO** 0.1-0.2 mg/kg/day × 3-6 wk initially then 4-10 mg/day maintenance
- **Geriatric: PO** initially ≤2-4 mg/day
- **Child: PO** 0.1-0.2 mg/kg/day (4.5 mg/m^2/day) in divided doses or 4.5 mg/m^2/day as 1 dose or in divided doses × 3-6 wk

Nephrotic syndrome (unlabeled)

- **Child: PO** 0.1-0.2 mg/kg/day with predniSONE × 8-12 wk

Macroglobulinemia (unlabeled)

- **Adult: PO** 2-10 mg/day × 9 days or 8 mg/m^2/day with predniSONE × 10 days, repeat q6-8wk as needed

Intractable idiopathic uveitis/Behçet's syndrome/Churg-Strauss syndrome/polyarteritis nodosa/Wegener's granulomatosis (unlabeled)

- **Adult: PO** 0.2 mg/kg/day

Dermatomyositis/pneumonitis/lupus nephritis/polymyositis related to SLE/rheumatoid arthritis (unlabeled)

- **Adult: PO** 0.1-0.2 mg/kg/day

Available forms: Tabs 2 mg

Administer:

- Give at bedtime with an antiemetic
- All products PO if possible, avoid IM inj when platelets <100,000/mm^3
- Allopurinol to maintain uric acid levels, alkalinization of urine; increase fluid intake to 2-3 L/day to prevent urate deposits, calculi formation

SIDE EFFECTS

CNS: Seizures, tremors, confusion, agitation, ataxia, hallucinations

GI: *Nausea, vomiting, diarrhea, weight loss,* hepatoxicity, *jaundice*

GU: Hyperuremia

HEMA: Thrombocytopenia, leukopenia, pancytopenia (prolonged use), permanent bone marrow depression

INTEG: Alopecia (rare), dermatitis, rash, Stevens-Johnson syndrome

RESP: Fibrosis, pneumonitis

PHARMACOKINETICS

Well absorbed orally, metabolized by liver, excreted in urine, half-life 2 hr

INTERACTIONS

- Filgrastim, sargramostim contraindicated 24 hr prior to or after chemotherapy
- Not to be used in combination with nalidixic acid
- Do not use with live virus vaccines

Increase: toxicity—other antineoplastics, radiation

Increase: bleeding risk—anticoagulants, salicylates

NURSING CONSIDERATIONS

Assess:

- Bleeding: hematuria, guaiac, bruising, petechiae of mucosa or orifices q8hr
- Jaundice of skin, sclera; dark urine, clay-colored stools; itchy skin, abdominal pain, fever, diarrhea
- Dyspnea, crackles, unproductive cough, chest pain, tachypnea
- Effects of alopecia on body image; discuss feelings about body changes (rare)

Black Box Warning: Bone marrow suppression: CBC, differential, platelet count weekly; withhold product if WBC is <2000 or granulocyte count is <1000/mm^3; notify prescriber of results

- **Pneumonitis/fibrosis:** pulmonary function tests, chest x-ray films before, during therapy; chest film should be obtained q2wk during treatment

• Renal studies: BUN, serum uric acid, urine CCr before, during therapy; I&O ratio; report urine output of <30 ml/hr

• Monitor temp q4hr (may indicate beginning infection)

• Hepatic studies before, during therapy (bilirubin, AST, ALT, LDH) as needed or monthly

Perform/provide:

• Storage in tight container, amber glass; store in refrigerator

Evaluate:

• Therapeutic response: decreased size of tumor, spread of malignancy

Teach patient/family:

• To report signs of infection: increased temp, sore throat, persistent cough, flu-like symptoms

• To report signs of anemia: fatigue, headache, faintness, SOB, irritability, seizures, jaundice, bruising

• To report bleeding; to avoid use of razors, commercial mouthwash

• To avoid use of aspirin products, ibuprofen

• To avoid vaccinations during treatment

Black Box Warning: To use contraception during and for several months after completion of therapy; may cause irreversible gonadal suppression; to avoid breastfeeding, pregnancy (D)

• To report any changes in breathing or coughing

• To drink 2-3 L of fluid daily unless contraindicated; to report drop in urine output

chloramphenicol (Rx)

(klor-am-fen′i-kole)

Pentamycetin ✱

Func. class.: Antiinfective—miscellaneous

Chem. class.: Dichloroacetic acid derivative

ACTION: Binds to 50S ribosomal subunit, which interferes with or inhibits protein synthesis

USES: Infections caused by *Haemophilus influenzae, Salmonella typhi, Rickettsia, Neisseria, Staphylococcus, Streptococcus, Escherichia coli,* mycoplasma, *Bacteroides;* meningitis, bacteremia; abdominal skin, soft-tissue infections; not to be used if less toxic products can be used

Unlabeled uses: *Bacillus anthracis,* glanders, melioidosis, plague, plague prophylaxis, psittacosis, *Stenotrophomonas maltophilia,* tularemia

CONTRAINDICATIONS: Hypersensitivity, severe renal/hepatic disease, minor infections, labor, influenza, tympanic membrane perforation

Precautions: Pregnancy (C), breastfeeding, infants, children, renal/hepatic disease, ulcerative colitis, pseudomembranous colitis

Black Box Warning: Bone marrow suppression

DOSAGE AND ROUTES

• **Adult and child: PO/IV** 50 mg/kg/day in divided doses q6hr, 100 mg/kg/day (for meningitis only), max 100 mg/kg/day

• **Premature infant and neonate: IV** 20 mg/kg loading dose, then 25 mg/kg/day in 4 divided doses q6hr 12 hr after loading dose

Available forms: Inj 1 g, caps 250 mg

C

Administer:

- Product must be taken in equal intervals around clock to maintain blood levels
- IM route not recommended

PO route

⚠ Do not break, crush, or chew caps

- Give oral form on empty stomach with full glass of water
- Store caps in airtight container at room temp

Intermittent IV INF route

- After **diluting** 1 g/10 ml sterile water for inj or D_5W (10% sol); **give** over >1 min; may be **further diluted** in 50-100 ml of D_5W; give through Y-tube, 3-way stopcock, or additive inf set; **run** over ½-1 hr

Syringe compatibilities: Ampicillin, cloxacillin, heparin, penicillin G sodium

Y-site compatibilities: Acyclovir, alfentanil, amikacin, aminophylline, anidulafungin, atenolol, atracurium, atropine, aztreonam, bivalirudin, bleomycin, bumetanide, buprenorphine, calcium chloride/gluconate, cefamandole, ceFAZolin, cefmetazole, cefonicid, cefoperazone, cefotetan, cefoxitin, cefuroxime, cephalothin, cephapirin, clindamycin, corticotropin, cyanocobalamin, cyclophosphamide, cycloSPORINE, DACTINomycin, DAPTOmycin, dexamethasone, digoxin, docetaxel, enalaprilat, ePHEDrine, EPINEPHrine, epoetin alfa, ertapenem, etoposide, fenoldopam, fentaNYL, fludarabine, folic acid, foscarnet, furosemide, glycopyrrolate, granisetron, heparin, hydrocortisone, HYDROmorphone, imipenem-cilastatin, indomethacin, insulin (regular), isoproterenol, ketorolac, lidocaine, linezolid, LORazepam, LR, magnesium sulfate, mannitol, methicillin, methylPREDNISolone, metoclopramide, metoprolol, metroNIDAZOLE, mezlocillin, miconazole, milrinone, mitoxantrone, morphine, moxalactam, multiple vitamins injection, naloxone, nesiritide, niCARdipine, nitroglycerin, nitroprusside, norepinephrine, octreotide, oxacillin, oxaliplatin, oxytocin, paclitaxel, palonosetron, pamidronate, pancuronium, penicillin G potassium/sodium, PENTobarbital, perphenazine, PHENobarbital, phenylephrine, phytonadione, piperacillin, piperacillin-tazobactam, potassium chloride, propranolol hydrochloride, ranitidine, Ringer's injection, ritodrine, sodium bicarbonate, succinylcholine, SUFentanil, tacrolimus, teniposide, theophylline, thiotepa, ticarcillin, ticarcillin-clavulanate, tirofiban, tobramycin, TPN, urokinase, vasopressin, voriconazole

SIDE EFFECTS

CNS: Headache, *depression,* confusion, peripheral neuritis

CV: **Gray baby syndrome in newborns: failure to feed, pallor, cyanosis, abdominal distention, irregular respiration, vasomotor collapse**

EENT: Optic neuritis, blindness

GI: *Nausea, vomiting, diarrhea,* abdominal pain, xerostomia, glossitis, colitis, pruritus ani

HEMA: **Anemia, thrombocytopenia, aplastic anemia, granulocytopenia, leukopenia, acute generalized exanthematous pustulosis (AGEP) (rare)**

INTEG: Itching, urticaria, contact dermatitis, rash

PHARMACOKINETICS

Absorbed well (PO), completely (IV); distributed widely, metabolized in liver; excreted in kidneys, unchanged; half-life 1½-4 hr

PO: Peak 1-2 hr, onset 15 min

IV: Peak inf end, onset rapid

INTERACTIONS

Increase: action of barbiturates, anticoagulants, hydantoins, iron products, antidiabetics, sulfonylureas

Decrease: action of vit B_{12}, folic acid, penicillins, rifampin

NURSING CONSIDERATIONS

Assess:

- Signs of infection, anemia

⚠ **Any patient with a compromised renal system; product is excreted slowly in poor renal system function; toxicity may occur rapidly**

- Hepatic studies: AST, ALT

Black Box Warning: Blood studies: WBC, RBC, Hct, Hgb, platelets, serum iron, reticulocytes; product should be discontinued if bone marrow depressed

- Renal studies: urinalysis, protein, blood, BUN, creatinine
- C&S before product therapy; may be given as soon as culture is taken
- Product level in impaired renal, hepatic systems; peak 10-25 mcg/ml, draw 90 min after IV dose, trough 5-15 mcg/ml prior to next dose
- Bowel pattern before, during treatment
- Skin eruptions, itching, dermatitis after administration
- Allergies before treatment, reaction to each medication

⚠ **Neonates for beginning gray baby syndrome: cyanosis, abdominal distention, irregular respiration, failure to feed; product should be discontinued immediately**

Perform/provide:

- Storage of reconstituted sol at room temp

Evaluate:

- Therapeutic response: decreased symptoms of infection

Teach patient/family:

- About all aspects of product therapy; that culture may be taken after complete course of medication
- To report sore throat, fever, fatigue, unusual bleeding, bruising; could indicate bone marrow depression (may occur weeks or months after termination of product)

TREATMENT OF HYPERSENSITIVITY: Withdraw product, maintain airway, administer EPINEPHrine, aminophylline, O_2, IV corticosteroids

chloramphenicol ophthalmic

See Appendix B

chloramphenicol otic

See Appendix B

chlordiazePOXIDE (Rx)

(klor-dye-az-e-pox′ide)

Apo-Chlordiazepoxide ♣, Librium

Func. class.: Antianxiety

Chem. class.: Benzodiazepine, long-acting

Controlled Substance Schedule IV

Do not confuse:
Librium/Librax

ACTION: Potentiates the actions of GABA, especially in the limbic system, reticular formation

USES: Short-term management of anxiety, acute alcohol withdrawal, preoperatively for relaxation

CONTRAINDICATIONS: Pregnancy (D), breastfeeding, children <6 yr, hypersensitivity to benzodiazepines, closed-angle glaucoma, psychosis

Precautions: Geriatric patients, debilitated, renal/hepatic disease, suicidal ideation, abrupt discontinuation

DOSAGE AND ROUTES

Mild anxiety

- **Adult: PO** 5-10 mg tid-qid
- **Geriatric: PO** 5 mg bid initially, increase as needed
- **Child >6 yr: PO** 5 mg bid-qid, max 10 mg bid-tid

Severe anxiety
• **Adult: PO** 25-50 mg tid-qid
Preoperatively
• **Adult: PO** 5-10 mg tid-qid on day before surgery
Alcohol withdrawal
• **Adult: PO** 50-100 mg q4-6hr prn, max 300 mg/day
Renal disease
• **Adult: PO** CCr <10 ml/min, give 50% dose
Available forms: Caps 5, 10, 25 mg
Administer:
PO route
• With food or milk for GI symptoms
• Crushed if patient is unable to swallow medication whole

SIDE EFFECTS

CNS: *Dizziness, drowsiness,* confusion, headache, anxiety, tremors, stimulation, fatigue, depression, insomnia, hallucinations
CV: *Orthostatic hypotension,* edema, ECG changes, tachycardia, hypotension
EENT: *Blurred vision,* tinnitus, mydriasis
GI: Constipation, dry mouth, nausea, vomiting, anorexia, diarrhea
GU: Irregular periods, decreased libido
HEMA: Agranulocytosis
INTEG: Rash, dermatitis, itching

PHARMACOKINETICS

PO: Onset 30 min, peak within 2 hr, duration 4-6 hr, metabolized by liver, excreted by kidneys, crosses placenta, excreted in breast milk, half-life 5-30 hr (increased in geriatric patients)

INTERACTIONS

Increase: CNS depression—CNS depressants, alcohol
Increase: chlordiazePOXIDE—cimetidine, disulfiram, FLUoxetine, isoniazid, ketoconazole, metoprolol, oral contraceptives, propranolol, valproic acid
Decrease: action of levodopa
Decrease: action of chlordiazePOXIDE—CYP3A4 inhibitors (protease inhibitors, barbiturates, rifamycins)

Drug/Lab Test
False increase: 17-OHCS
False positive: pregnancy test (some methods)

NURSING CONSIDERATIONS

Assess:
• B/P (lying, standing), pulse; if systolic B/P drops 20 mm Hg, hold product, notify prescriber
• Blood studies: CBC during long-term therapy; **blood dyscrasias** have occurred rarely
• Hepatic studies: AST, ALT, bilirubin, creatinine, LDH, alk phos during long-term therapy
• I&O; may indicate renal dysfunction
• For ataxia, oversedation of geriatric patients, debilitated patients
• Physical dependency, withdrawal symptoms: headache, nausea, vomiting, muscle pain, weakness after long-term use
• Mental status: mood, sensorium, affect, sleeping pattern, drowsiness, dizziness; suicidal tendencies; paradoxic reactions such as excitement, stimulation, acute rage
• For pregnancy; product should not be used during pregnancy (D)
Perform/provide:
• Assistance with ambulation during beginning therapy since drowsiness, dizziness occur
• Check to confirm that PO medication has been swallowed if patient is depressed, suicidal
• Sugarless gum, hard candy, frequent sips of water for dry mouth
Evaluate:
• Therapeutic response: decreased anxiety, restlessness, sleeplessness
Teach patient/family:
• That product may be taken with food
• Not to use product for everyday stress or use for more than 4 mo unless directed by prescriber
• Not to take more than prescribed amount; may be habit forming

- To avoid OTC preparations unless approved by prescriber
- To avoid driving, activities that require alertness because drowsiness may occur
- To avoid alcohol ingestion, other psychotropic medications unless directed by prescriber
- Not to discontinue medication abruptly after long-term use because this may precipitate seizures
- To rise slowly because fainting may occur, especially among geriatric patients
- That drowsiness may be worse at beginning of treatment
- To notify prescriber if pregnancy is suspected or planned
- To immediately report suicidal thoughts/behaviors

TREATMENT OF OVERDOSE:

Lavage, VS, supportive care, give flumazenil

chloroquine (Rx)

(klor′oh-kwin)

Aralen, Novo-Chloroquine ✱

Func. class.: Antimalarial

Chem. class.: Synthetic 4-aminoquinoline derivative

ACTION: Inhibits parasite replication, transcription of DNA to RNA by forming complexes with DNA of parasite

USES: Malaria of *Plasmodium vivax, P. malariae, P. ovale, P. falciparum* (some strains); amebiasis

Unlabeled uses: Discoid lupus erythematosus, polymorphous light eruption, rheumatoid arthritis, ulcerative colitis

CONTRAINDICATIONS: Hypersensitivity, retinal field changes

Precautions: Pregnancy (C), breastfeeding, children, blood dyscrasias, severe GI disease, neurologic disease, alcoholism, hepatic disease, G6PD deficiency, psoriasis, eczema, seizures, preexisting auditory damage, torsades de pointes

Black Box Warning: Infection

DOSAGE AND ROUTES

Acute malaria attacks

- **Adult: PO** 1000 mg (600-mg base), then 500 mg (300-mg base) in 6-8 hr, then 500 mg (300-mg base) q day × 2 days for a total of 2.5 g (1.5-g base) in 3 days
- **Adult/adolescent of low body weight, child/infant: PO** 16.5 mg (10-mg base)/kg, max 600-mg base; then 8.3 mg (5-mg base)/kg, max 300-mg base 6 hr after 1st dose; then 8.3 mg (5-mg base)/kg, max 300-mg base 24 hr after 1st dose; then 8.3 mg (5-mg base)/kg, max 300-mg base 36 hr after 1st dose

Malaria prophylaxis (in areas with chloroquine–sensitive P. falciparum)

- **Adult: PO** 500 mg (300-mg base) weekly on same day of each wk starting 2 wk before travel and for 8 wk after leaving

Extraintestinal amebiasis

- **Adult: PO** 1 g (600-mg base) daily × 2 days, then 500 mg (300-mg base) for ≥2-3 wk
- **Child (unlabeled): PO** 16.6 mg (10-mg base)/kg (max 300-mg base) daily × 2-3 wk

Rheumatoid arthritis/discoid lupus erythematosus (unlabeled)

- **Adult: PO** 250 mg (150-mg base) daily

Available forms: Tabs 250 mg (150-mg base), 500 mg (300-mg base) phosphate

Administer:

- Product in mg or base; they are different

PO route

- Before or after meals at same time each day to maintain product level

SIDE EFFECTS

CNS: Headache, stimulation, fatigue, **seizures**, psychosis, hallucinations, insomnia

CV: Hypotension, **heart block, asystole with syncope,** ECG changes, cardiomyopathy
EENT: *Blurred vision, corneal changes, retinal changes, difficulty focusing,* tinnitus, vertigo, deafness, photophobia, corneal edema
GI: *Nausea, vomiting, anorexia,* diarrhea, cramps
HEMA: **Thrombocytopenia, agranulocytosis, hemolytic anemia, leukopenia**
INTEG: Pruritus, pigmentary changes, skin eruptions, lichen-planus–like eruptions, eczema, **exfoliative dermatitis**

PHARMACOKINETICS

Metabolized in liver; excreted in urine, feces, breast milk; crosses placenta
PO: Peak 1-3 hr, half-life 3-5 days

INTERACTIONS

• Reduced oral clearance and metabolism of chloroquine: cimetidine
Increase: QT prolongation, torsades de pointes—class IA, III antidysrhythmics
Increase: effects—2D6 inhibitors (amiodarone, chlorpheniramine, FLUoxetine, haloperidol, ritonavir, paroxetine, terbinafine, ticlopidine); CYP3A4 inhibitors (diltiazem, verapamil, itraconazole, ketoconazole, erythromycin, doxycycline, clarithromycin)
Decrease: action of chloroquine—magnesium, aluminum compounds, kaolin; do not use concurrently
Decrease: effects of ampicillin, rabies vaccine (ID)

NURSING CONSIDERATIONS

Assess:

Black Box Warning: **Infection:** resistance is common, not to be used for *P. falciparum* acquired in areas of resistance or where prophylaxis has failed

• Ophthalmic test if long-term treatment or dosage of >150 mg/day
• Blood studies: CBC, since blood dyscrasias occur
• **ECG** during therapy; watch for depression of T waves, widening of QRS complex
• **Allergic reactions:** pruritus, rash, urticaria
• **Blood dyscrasias:** malaise, fever, bruising, bleeding (rare)
• **For ototoxicity** (tinnitus, vertigo, change in hearing); audiometric testing should be done before, after treatment
⚠ **For toxicity:** blurring vision; difficulty focusing; headache; dizziness; decreased knee, ankle reflexes; seizures, CV collapse; product should be discontinued immediately and IV fluids given
Perform/provide:
• Storage in tight, light-resistant container at room temp; keep inj in cool environment
Evaluate:
• Therapeutic response: decreased symptoms of infection
Teach patient/family:
• To take with meals or immediately after meals
• To use sunglasses in bright sunlight to decrease photophobia
• That urine may turn rust or brown color
• To report hearing, visual problems; fever, fatigue, bruising, bleeding; may indicate blood dyscrasias

TREATMENT OF OVERDOSE:

Administer barbiturate (ultrashort-acting), vasopressor; tracheostomy may be necessary

chlorothiazide (Rx)

(klor-oh-thye′a-zide)

Diuril

Func. class.: Diuretic
Chem. class.: Thiazide; sulfonamide derivative

Do not confuse:
chlorothiazide/chlorproMAZINE/chlorthalidone/chlorproPAMIDE

ACTION: Acts on distal tubule and thick ascending limb of the loop of Henle by increasing excretion of water, sodium, chloride, potassium, magnesium

USES:
Hypertension, diuresis, CHF, edema, nephrotic syndrome
Unlabeled uses: Hypercalciuria

CONTRAINDICATIONS:
Breastfeeding, hypersensitivity to thiazides or sulfonamides, hepatic coma, anuria, renal decompensation
Precautions: Pregnancy (C), geriatric patient, hypokalemia, renal/hepatic disease, gout, COPD, SLE, diabetes mellitus, hyperlipidemia

DOSAGE AND ROUTES

Hypertension

- **Adult: PO/IV** 500 mg-1 g/day may divide bid, max 2 g/day in divided doses

Edema

- **Adult: IV** 250 mg q6-12hr
- **Child >6 mo: PO** 10-20 mg/kg/day may divide bid
- **Child <6 mo: PO** 10-20 mg/kg/day in 2 doses

Renal dose

- **Adult: PO/IV** CCr <30 ml/min, do not use

Available forms: Tabs 250, 500 mg; powder for inj 500 mg; oral susp 250 mg/5 ml

Administer:

- In AM to avoid interference with sleep if using product as diuretic
- Potassium replacement if potassium <3 mg/dl
- With food if nausea occurs; absorption may be decreased slightly; dehydration may occur; tablets may be crushed
- **Susp:** shake well, measure with calibrated measuring device

IV direct/IV INF route

- May be given undiluted over 5 min or as inf
- Reconstitute: add 18 ml of sterile water for inj to vial (28 mg/ml)

Additive compatibilities: Cimetidine, lidocaine, ranitidine, sodium bicarbonate
Y-site compatibilities: Alprostadil

SIDE EFFECTS

CNS: Paresthesia, *headache, dizziness, fatigue*
CV: Irregular pulse, *orthostatic hypotension,* volume depletion
EENT: Blurred vision
ELECT: *Hypokalemia,* hypercalcemia, hyponatremia, hypomagnesemia, hyperuricemia, hypochloremia
GI: *Nausea, vomiting, anorexia, constipation, diarrhea,* pancreatitis, GI irritation, hepatitis
GU: *Urinary frequency,* polyuria, incontinence, ED
HEMA: Aplastic anemia, hemolytic anemia, leukopenia, agranulocytosis, thrombocytopenia, neutropenia
INTEG: *Rash, urticaria,* purpura, *photosensitivity,* fever, *alopecia,* exfoliative dermatitis
META: Hyperglycemia, *hyperuricemia,* increased creatinine, BUN
SYST: Anaphylaxis

PHARMACOKINETICS

PO: Onset 2 hr, peak 4 hr, duration 6-12 hr, crosses placenta, excreted in breast milk, excreted unchanged by kidneys, half-life 2 hr; not well absorbed

INTERACTIONS

- Hypokalemia: ticarcillin, glucocorticoids, amphotericin, mezlocillin, piperacillin

Increase: toxicity—lithium, nondepolarizing skeletal muscle relaxants, digoxin, allopurinol
Increase: hypotension—other antihypertensives, alcohol, nitrates
Decrease: absorption of thiazides—cholestyramine, colestipol
Decrease: diuretic action—NSAIDs

Drug/Herb

Increase: antihypertensive effect—hawthorn, horse chestnut
Decrease: antihypertensive effect—ephedra

Drug/Lab Test

Increase: calcium, amylase, parathyroid test, CPK

Decrease: PBI
False negative: tyramine tests
Interference: urine steroid tests

NURSING CONSIDERATIONS

Assess:

- Weight, I&O daily to determine fluid loss; effect of product may be decreased if used daily
- Rate, depth, rhythm of respirations; effect of exertion
- B/P lying, standing; postural hypotension may occur, especially in geriatric patients
- Electrolytes: sodium, potassium, chloride, calcium, magnesium; include BUN, blood glucose, CBC, serum creatinine, blood pH, ABGs, uric acid; glucose in urine if patient is diabetic
- Signs of metabolic alkalosis: drowsiness, restlessness
- Rashes, temp elevation daily
- Confusion, especially in geriatric patients; take safety precautions if needed

Evaluate:

- Therapeutic response: improvement in edema of feet, legs, sacral area daily if medication being used for CHF; decreased B/P; increased urinary output

Teach patient/family:

- To rise slowly from lying or sitting position because orthostatic hypotension may occur
- To notify prescriber of muscle weakness, cramps, nausea, dizziness
- That product may be taken with food or milk; to take at same time each day; not to double dose
- That blood glucose may be increased in diabetics
- To take early in day to avoid nocturia
- To use sunscreen; use protective clothing to prevent photosensitivity
- To weigh weekly and notify prescriber of change of >3 lb
- To eat diet high in potassium if recommended by prescriber; about high-potassium foods
- Not to take OTC medications without consulting prescriber, avoid alcohol, lithium

TREATMENT OF OVERDOSE:

Lavage if taken orally; monitor electrolytes; administer dextrose in saline; monitor hydration, CV, renal status

C

chlorpheniramine (OTC, Rx)

(klor-fen-ir′a-meen)

AHIST, Aller-Chlor, Allergy, Chlor-Pheniton, Chlor-Trimeton, Diabetic Tussin Allergy Relief, ED-Chlor-Tann, Equaline Allergy, Equate Chlortabs Allergy, Good Sense Allergy, Leader Allergy, P-Tann, Select Brand Chlorpheniramine, Tana Hist-PD, Teldrin, Top Care Allergy, Walfinate Allergy

Func. class.: Antihistamine (1st generation, nonselective)
Chem. class.: Alkylamine, H_1-receptor antagonist

Do not confuse:
Teldrin/Tedral

ACTION: Acts on blood vessels, GI system, respiratory system by competing with histamine for H_1-receptor site; decreases allergic response by blocking histamine

USES: Allergy symptoms, rhinitis, conjunctivitis (allergic)
Unlabeled uses: Nausea, vomiting due to motion sickness, pruritus, urticaria

CONTRAINDICATIONS: Newborns/neonates
Precautions: Pregnancy (B), breastfeeding, children, geriatric patients, increased intraocular pressure, cardiac/renal disease, hypertension, asthma, seizure disorder, hyperthyroidism, prostatic hypertrophy, GI obstruction, peptic ulcer disease, emphysema, hypersensitivity to H_1-receptor antagonists, lower respiratory tract disease, stenosed peptic ulcers,

bladder neck obstruction, closed-angle glaucoma

DOSAGE AND ROUTES

- **Adult and child ≥12 yr: PO** 4 mg tid-qid, max 24 mg/day; **EXT REL** 8-12 mg bid-tid, max 24 mg/day
- **Child 6-12 yr: PO** 2 mg q4-6hr, max 12 mg/day; **EXT REL** 8 mg bedtime or daily, **EXT REL** not recommended for child <6 yr
- **Child 2-5 yr: PO** (syrup) 1 mg q4-6hr, max 4 mg/day

For self-treatment of hay fever or other upper respiratory allergies

- **Adult/adolescent/child ≥12 yr: PO** 4 mg q4-6hr, max 24 mg/24 hr
- **Child 6-11 yr: PO** 2 mg q4-6hr, max 12 mg/24 hr

Motion sickness (unlabeled)

- **Adult: PO** 4-8 mg tid

Available forms: Chewable tabs 2 mg; tabs 4, 8, 12 mg; ext rel tabs 8, 12 mg; ext rel caps 8, 12 mg; syr 1 mg/5 ml, 2 mg/5 ml, 2.5 mg/5 ml

Administer:

- Avoid concurrent use with other CNS depressants
- Do not break, crush, or chew ext rel forms
- With meals for GI symptoms; absorption may slightly decrease
- Avoid use in children <2 yr

SIDE EFFECTS

CNS: *Dizziness, drowsiness,* poor coordination, fatigue, anxiety, euphoria, confusion, paresthesia, neuritis

EENT: Blurred vision; dilated pupils; tinnitus; nasal stuffiness; dry nose, throat, mouth

GI: Nausea, anorexia, diarrhea

GU: *Retention,* dysuria, urinary frequency

HEMA: **Thrombocytopenia, agranulocytosis, hemolytic anemia**

INTEG: Photosensitivity

RESP: Increased thick secretions, wheezing, chest tightness

PHARMACOKINETICS

Detoxified in liver, excreted by kidneys (metabolites/free drug), half-life 12-15 hr

PO: Onset ½ hr, duration 4-12 hr

PO-ER: Duration 8-24 hr

INTERACTIONS

Increase: CNS depression—barbiturates, opiates, hypnotics, tricyclics, alcohol

Increase: effect of chlorpheniramine—MAOIs

Increase: anticholinergic action—atropine, phenothiazines, quiNIDine, haloperidol

Drug/Lab Test

False negative: skin allergy tests

NURSING CONSIDERATIONS

Assess:

- Be alert for urinary retention, frequency, dysuria; product should be discontinued
- Respiratory status: rate, rhythm, increase in bronchial secretions, wheezing, chest tightness

Perform/provide:

- Hard candy, gum, frequent rinsing of mouth for dryness
- Storage in tight container at room temp

Evaluate:

- Therapeutic response: absence of running, congested nose, rashes, conjunctivitis

Teach patient/family:

- About all aspects of product use; to notify prescriber of confusion, sedation, hypotension, difficulty voiding
- To avoid driving, other hazardous activity if drowsiness occurs, especially geriatric patients
- To avoid concurrent use of alcohol

TREATMENT OF OVERDOSE:

Administer diazepam, vasopressors, phenytoin IV

chlorproMAZINE (Rx)

(klor-proe′ma-zeen)

Novo-ChlorproMAZINE ✤

Func. class.: Antipsychotic/antiemetic

Chem. class.: Phenothiazine-aliphatic

Do not confuse:
chlorproMAZINE/chlorproPAMIDE/prochlorperazine

ACTION:
Depresses cerebral cortex, hypothalamus, limbic system, which control activity aggression; blocks neurotransmission produced by dopamine at synapse; exhibits a strong α-adrenergic, anticholinergic blocking action; mechanism for antipsychotic effects is unclear

USES:
Psychotic disorders, mania, schizophrenia, anxiety, intractable hiccups in adults, nausea, vomiting; preoperatively for relaxation; acute intermittent porphyria, behavioral problems in children, nonpsychotic, demented patients, Tourette's syndrome

Unlabeled uses: Vascular headache, agitation, dementia, neonatal abstinence syndrome

CONTRAINDICATIONS:
Children <6 mo, hypersensitivity, circulatory collapse, liver damage, cerebral arteriosclerosis, coronary disease, severe hypo/hypertension, blood dyscrasias, coma, brain damage, bone marrow depression, alcohol/barbiturate withdrawal, closed-angle glaucoma

Precautions: Pregnancy (C), breastfeeding, geriatric patients, seizure disorders, hypertension, hepatic/cardiac disease, prostatic enlargement, Parkinson's disease, pulmonary disease

Black Box Warning: Dementia

DOSAGE AND ROUTES

Psychosis

- **Adult: PO** 10-50 mg q1-4hr initially then increase up to 2 g/day if necessary; **IM** 10-50 mg q1-4hr, usual dose 300-800 mg/day
- **Geriatric:** 10-25 mg daily-bid, increase by 10-25 mg/day q4-7days, max 800 mg/day
- **Child >6 mo: PO** 0.55 mg/kg q4-6hr; **IM** 0.5 mg/kg q6-8hr

Nausea and vomiting

- **Adult: PO** 10-25 mg q4-6hr prn; **IM** 25-50 mg q3hr prn; q6-8hr prn, max 400 mg/day; **IV** 25-50 mg daily-qid
- **Child ≥6 mo: PO** 0.55 mg/kg q4-6hr; **IM** q6-8hr; **IM** ≤5 yr or ≤22.7 kg, 40 mg; max **IM** 5-10 yr or 22.7-45.5 kg, 75 mg

Intractable hiccups

- **Adult: PO** 25-50 mg tid-qid; **IM** 25-50 mg (only if PO dose does not work); **IV** 25-50 mg in 500-1000 ml **NS** (only for severe hiccups)

Available forms: Tabs 10, 25, 50, 100, 200 mg; inj 25 mg/ml

Administer:

- Anticholinergic agent for EPS if ordered

PO route

- Do not break, crush, or chew ext rel caps
- With full glass of water, milk or with food to decrease GI upset
- Product in liquid form mixed in glass of juice or cola if hoarding is suspected
- Periodically attempt dosage reduction in those with behavioral problems

IM route

- IM, inject in deep muscle mass, do not give SUBCUT, no dilution needed; if irritation occurs, may dilute in NS or procaine 2%

IV route

Direct IV: After **diluting** 1 mg/1 ml with NS, **give** 1 mg or less/2 min or more, never give undiluted

Continuous IV INF: Dilute 25-50 mg/500-1000 NS or other compatible large IV sol, **give** slowly, protect from light

Syringe compatibilities: Atropine, benztropine, butorphanol, diphenhydrAMINE, doxapram, droperidol, fentaNYL, glycopyrrolate, hydromorphone, hydrOXYzine, meperidine, metoclopramide, midazolam, morphine, pentazocine, perphenazine, prochlorperazine, promazine, promethazine, scopolamine

Y-site compatibilities: Alfentanil, amikacin, amphotericin B lipid complex, amsacrine, anidulafungin, ascorbic acid injection, atenolol, atracurium, atropine, benztropine, bleomycin sulfate, buprenorphine, butorphanol, calcium chloride/gluconate, caspofungin, cimetidine, cisatracurium, CISplatin, cladribine, codeine, cyanocobalamin, cyclophosphamide, cycloSPORINE, cytarabine, DACTINomycin, DAPTOmycin, dexmedetomidine, digoxin, diltiazem, diphenhydrAMINE, DOBUTamine, docetaxel, DOPamine, doxacurium, DOXOrubicin, DOXOrubicin liposomal, doxycycline, enalaprilat, ePHEDrine, EPINEPHrine, epirubicin, erythromycin, esmolol, etoposide, famotidine, fenoldopam, fentaNYL, filgrastim, fluconazole, gatifloxacin, gemcitabine, gentamicin, glycopyrrolate, granisetron, hydrocortisone, HYDROmorphone, hydrOXYzine, IDArubicin, ifosfamide, isoproterenol, labetalol, levofloxacin, lidocaine, LORazepam, LR, magnesium sulfate, mannitol, mechlorethamine, meperidine, methicillin, methoxamine, methyldopate, methylPREDNISolone, metoclopramide, metoprolol, metroNIDAZOLE, miconazole, midazolam, milrinone, minocycline, mitoxantrone, morphine, multiple vitamins injection, mycophenolate mofetil, nafcillin, nalbuphine, naloxone, netilmicin, nitroglycerin, norepinephrine, octreotide, ondansetron, oxacillin, oxaliplatin, palonosetron, pamidronate, pancuronium, papaverine, penicillin G potassium, pentamidine, pentazocine, phytonadione, polymyxin B, potassium chloride, procainamide, prochlorperazine, promethazine, propofol, propranolol, protamine sulfate, pyridoxine, quiNIDine, quinupristin-dalfopristin, ranitidine, Ringer's injection, ritodrine, riTUXimab, rocuronium, sodium acetate, succinylcholine, SUFentanil, tacrolimus, teniposide, theophylline, thiamine, thiotepa, tirofiban, TNA, tolazoline, TPN, trimetaphan, vancomycin, vasopressin, vecuronium, verapamil, vinCRIStine, vinorelbine, vitamin B complex with C, voriconazole, zoledronic acid

SIDE EFFECTS

CNS: *EPS: pseudoparkinsonism, akathisia, dystonia, tardive dyskinesia,* seizures, *headache,* neuroleptic malignant syndrome, dizziness

CV: *Orthostatic hypotension,* hypertension, cardiac arrest, ECG changes, tachycardia

EENT: Blurred vision, glaucoma, dry eyes

ENDO: SIADH

GI: *Dry mouth, nausea, vomiting, anorexia, constipation,* diarrhea, cholestatic jaundice, weight gain

GU: Urinary retention, enuresis, impotence, amenorrhea, gynecomastia, breast engorgement

HEMA: Anemia, leukopenia, leukocytosis, agranulocytosis

INTEG: *Rash,* photosensitivity, dermatitis

RESP: Laryngospasm, dyspnea, respiratory depression

SYST: Death in geriatric patients with dementia

PHARMACOKINETICS

Metabolized by liver, excreted in urine (metabolites), crosses placenta, enters breast milk, 95% bound to plasma proteins, elimination half-life 10-30 hr

PO: Absorption variable, widely distributed, onset erratic 30-60 min, duration 4-6 hr

PO-ER: Onset 30-60 min, peak unknown, duration 10-12 hr

IM: Well absorbed, peak 15-20 min, duration 4-8 hr

RECT: Onset erratic, duration 3 hr

IV: Onset 5 min, peak 10 min, duration unknown

INTERACTIONS

Increase: CNS depression—other CNS depressants, alcohol, barbiturate anes-

thetics, antihistamines, sedatives/hypnotics, antidepressants
Increase: toxicity—EPINEPHrine
Increase: agranulocystosis—antithyroid agents
Increase: effects of both products—β-adrenergic blockers, alcohol
Increase: anticholinergic effects—anticholinergics, antidepressants, antiparkinsonian agents
Increase: valproic acid level
Decrease: lowered seizure threshold—anticonvulsants
Decrease: absorption—aluminum hydroxide, magnesium hydroxide antacids
Decrease: antiparkinson activity—levodopa, bromocriptine
Decrease: serum chlorproMAZINE—lithium, barbiturates
Decrease: anticoagulant effect—warfarin

Drug/Lab Test
Increase: hepatic studies, cardiac enzymes, cholesterol, blood glucose, prolactin, bilirubin, PBI, cholinesterase, ^{131}I, alk phos, leukocytes, granulocytes, platelets
Decrease: hormones (blood and urine)
False positive: pregnancy tests, PKU
False negative: urinary steroids, 17-OHCS

NURSING CONSIDERATIONS

Assess:
- Mental status: orientation, mood, behavior, presence and type of hallucinations before initial administration and monthly
- Any potentially reversible causes of behavior problems in geriatric patients before and during therapy
- Swallowing of PO medication; check for hoarding or giving of medication to other patients
- I&O ratio; palpate bladder if low urinary output occurs, especially in geriatric patients
- Bilirubin, CBC, LFTs, ocular exam; agranulocytosis, glaucoma, cholestatic jaundice may occur
- Urinalysis recommended before, during prolonged therapy
- Affect, orientation, LOC, reflexes, gait, coordination, sleep pattern disturbances
- B/P sitting, standing, lying; take pulse, respirations q4hr during initial treatment; establish baseline before starting treatment; report drops of 30 mm Hg; obtain baseline ECG; Q-wave and T-wave changes
- Dizziness, faintness, palpitations, tachycardia on rising

⚠ **Neuroleptic malignant syndrome:** hyperpyrexia, muscle rigidity, increased CPK, altered mental status, for acute dystonia (check chewing, swallowing, eyes, pill rolling)

- **EPS:** akathisia (inability to sit still, no pattern to movements), tardive dyskinesia (bizarre movements of the jaw, mouth, tongue, extremities), pseudoparkinsonism (rigidity, tremors, pill rolling, shuffling gait)
- Constipation, urinary retention daily; increase bulk, water in diet

Perform/provide:
- Supervised ambulation until stabilized on medication; do not involve in strenuous exercise program because fainting is possible; patient should not stand still for long periods
- Increased fluids, roughage to prevent constipation
- Candy, gum, sips of water for dry mouth
- Storage in tight, light-resistant container, oral sol in amber bottle

Evaluate:
- Therapeutic response: decrease in emotional excitement, hallucinations, delusions, paranoia; reorganization of patterns of thought, speech; increase in target behaviors

Teach patient/family:
- To use good oral hygiene; to use frequent rinsing of mouth, sugarless gum, candy, ice chips for dry mouth
- To avoid hazardous activities until product response is determined

• That orthostatic hypotension occurs often; to rise gradually from sitting or lying position
• To remain lying down for at least 30 min after IM inj
• To avoid hot tubs, hot showers, tub baths since hypotension may occur; that, during hot weather, heat stroke may occur; to take extra precautions to stay cool
• To avoid abrupt withdrawal of product or EPS may result; product should be withdrawn slowly
• To avoid OTC preparations (cough, hay fever, cold) unless approved by prescriber since serious product interactions may occur; avoid use with alcohol, increased drowsiness may occur
• To use a sunscreen and sunglasses to prevent burns
• To take antacids 2 hr before or after this product
• To report sore throat, malaise, fever, bleeding, mouth sores; CBC should be drawn and product discontinued
• To employ contraceptive measures
• That urine may turn pink or reddish brown

TREATMENT OF OVERDOSE:
Lavage if orally ingested; provide airway; *do not induce vomiting or use EPINEPHrine*

chlorthalidone (Rx)

(klor-thal′i-done)

Apo-Chlorthalidone ♣, Hygroton
Thalitone, Uridon ♣

Func. class.: Diuretic
Chem. class.: Thiazide-like phthalimidine derivative

Do not confuse:
Uridon/Vicodin
Hygroton/Regroton

ACTION: Acts on distal tubule and by blocking the reabsorption of sodium and chloride, thereby resulting in the increased excretion of water, sodium, chloride, potassium, magnesium, bicarbonate and possible arteriolar dilation

USES: Edema, hypertension, edema with CHF

CONTRAINDICATIONS: Hypersensitivity to thiazides or sulfonamides, anuria, renal decompensation, breastfeeding
Precautions: Pregnancy (B), geriatric patients, hypokalemia, renal/hepatic disease, gout, diabetes mellitus, hyperlipidemia, SLE, hypotension, CCr <25 ml/min

DOSAGE AND ROUTES
• **Adult: PO** 12.5-100 mg/day
Available forms: Tabs 25, 50, 100 mg
Administer:
• In AM to avoid interference with sleep if using product as a diuretic
• Potassium replacement if potassium <3 mg/dl
• With food if nausea occurs; absorption may be decreased slightly

SIDE EFFECTS
CNS: Paresthesia, headache, *dizziness, weakness,* fever
CV: Hypertension, orthostatic hypotension, palpitations, volume depletion
EENT: Blurred vision
ELECT: *Hypokalemia,* hypomagnesemia, hypercalcemia, hyponatremia, hypochloremia
GI: *Nausea, vomiting, anorexia,* constipation, diarrhea, pancreatitis, GI irritation, jaundice
GU: *Urinary frequency,* polyuria, uremia, glucosuria, impotence
HEMA: Aplastic anemia, hemolytic anemia, leukopenia, agranulocytosis, thrombocytopenia, neutropenia
INTEG: Rash, urticaria, purpura, photosensitivity
META: *Hyperglycemia, hyperuremia,* increased creatinine, BUN, gout

PHARMACOKINETICS

Onset 2 hr, peak 6 hr, duration 48-72 hr, excreted unchanged by kidneys, crosses placenta, enters breast milk, half-life 40-60 hr, protein binding 75%

INTERACTIONS

Increase: hyperglycemia, hypotension—diazoxide
Increase: hypokalemia—glucocorticoids, amphotericin B
Increase: toxicity of lithium, nondepolarizing skeletal muscle relaxants, allopurinol
Increase: hypotensive effect—alcohol
Decrease: absorption of thiazides—cholestyramine, colestipol

Drug/Herb
Increase: hypotension—hawthorn, horse chestnut
Decrease: antihypertensive effect—ephedra

Drug/Lab Test
Increase: Amylase, bilirubin, calcium, cholesterol, creatinine, low-density lipoproteins, serum/urine glucose (diabetics), triglycerides, uric acid
Decrease: PBI, parathyroid test, magnesium, potassium, sodium, urinary calcium

NURSING CONSIDERATIONS

Assess:
- **Hypertension:** B/P lying, standing; postural hypotension may occur
- Weight, I&O daily to determine fluid loss; effect of product may be decreased if used daily
- Electrolytes: K, Mg, Na, Cl; include BUN, blood glucose, CBC, serum creatinine, blood pH, ABGs, uric acid, Ca
- Blood glucose levels if patient is diabetic
- Signs of **metabolic alkalosis:** drowsiness, restlessness
- Signs of **hypokalemia:** postural hypotension, malaise, fatigue, tachycardia, leg cramps, weakness
- Rashes, temp elevation daily
- Confusion, especially among geriatric patients; take safety precautions if needed

Evaluate:
- Therapeutic response: improvement in edema of feet, legs, sacral area daily if medication used in CHF

Teach patient/family:
- To rise slowly from lying or sitting position
- To notify prescriber of muscle weakness, cramps, nausea, dizziness
- That product may be taken with food, milk
- To maintain adequate potassium intake
- That blood glucose may be increased in diabetics
- To use sunscreen to protect against photosensitivity
- To take early in day to avoid nocturia

TREATMENT OF OVERDOSE:

Lavage if taken orally, monitor electrolytes, administer dextrose in NS; monitor hydration, CV, renal status

cholestyramine (Rx)

(koe-less-tir′a-meen)

PMS-Cholestyramine ✦, Prevalite, Questran, Questran Light

Func. class.: Antilipemic
Chem. class.: Bile acid sequestrant

Do not confuse:
Questran/Quarzan

ACTION: Absorbs, combines with bile acids to form insoluble complex that is excreted through feces; loss of bile acids lowers LDL, cholesterol levels

USES: Primary hypercholesterolemia (esp. type IIa/IIb hyperlipoproteinemia), pruritus associated with biliary obstruction
Unlabeled uses: Diarrhea caused by excess bile acid

CONTRAINDICATIONS:
Hypersensitivity; biliary obstruction; hyperlipidemia III, IV, V

Precautions: Pregnancy (C), breastfeeding, children

DOSAGE AND ROUTES

- **Adult: PO** 4 g/day or bid, max 24 g/day
- **Child: PO** 240 mg/kg/day in 3 divided doses with food or drink, max 8 g/day titrated up over several weeks to decrease GI effects

Available forms: Powder for susp 4 g cholestyramine/packet or scoop; tab 1 g

Administer:

- Product daily or bid; give all other medications 1 hr before or 4-6 hr after cholestyramine to avoid poor absorption
- Product mixed with applesauce or stirred into beverage (2-6 oz), let stand for 2 min; do not take dry, avoid inhaling powder, avoid GI tube administration
- Supplemental doses of vit A, D, K if levels are low

SIDE EFFECTS

CNS: Headache, dizziness, drowsiness, vertigo, tinnitus, anxiety

GI: *Constipation, abdominal pain, nausea,* fecal impaction, hemorrhoids, flatulence, vomiting, steatorrhea, peptic ulcer

HEMA: **Bleeding,** increased PT

INTEG: Rash, irritation of perianal area, tongue, skin

META: Decreased vit A, D, K, red cell folate content; **hyperchloremic acidosis**

MS: Muscle, joint pain

PHARMACOKINETICS

PO: Excreted in feces, LDL lowered within 4-7 days, serum cholesterol lowered within 1 mo, duration 2-4 wk

INTERACTIONS

Decrease: absorption of warfarin; thiazides; cardiac glycosides; propranolol; corticosteroids; iron; thyroid hormones; acetaminophen; amiodarone; penicillin G; tetracyclines; clofibrate; gemfibrozil; glipiZIDE; vit A, D, E, K

Drug/Lab Test

Increase: AST, ALT, alk phos

Decrease: sodium, potassium

NURSING CONSIDERATIONS

Assess:

- Cardiac glycoside level if both products administered
- For signs of vit A, D, K deficiency
- **Hypercholesterolemia:** fasting LDL, HDL, total cholesterol, triglyceride levels, electrolytes if receiving extended therapy; diet history
- **Pruritus:** for signs of itching
- Bowel pattern daily; increase bulk, water in diet for constipation; diarrhea may also occur

Evaluate:

- Therapeutic response: decreased LDL, cholesterol level (hyperlipidemia); diarrhea, pruritus (excess bile acids)

Teach patient/family:

- ⚠ **About the symptoms of hypoprothrombinemia: bleeding mucous membranes, dark tarry stools, hematuria, petechiae; report immediately**
- That PKU patients should avoid Questran Light (contains aspartame and phenylalanine)
- About the importance of compliance
- That risk factors should be decreased: high-fat diet, smoking, alcohol consumption, absence of exercise
- That GI side effects will resolve with continued use

choline/magnesium salicylates (Rx)

Func. class.: Nonopioid analgesic

Chem. class.: Salicylate

ACTION:
Blocks pain impulses in CNS that occur in response to inhibition of prostaglandin synthesis; antipyretic action results from inhibition of hypothalamic heat-regulating center to produce vasodilation to allow heat dissipation

USES:
Mild to moderate pain or fever, including arthritis, juvenile rheumatoid arthritis

CONTRAINDICATIONS:
Children <3 yr, vit K deficiency, children with flulike symptoms, hypersensitivity to salicylates, GI bleeding, bleeding disorders, Reye's syndrome

Precautions: Pregnancy (C), breastfeeding, anemia, renal/hepatic disease, Hodgkin's disease

DOSAGE AND ROUTES
- **Adult: PO** 1500 mg bid
- **Child >37 kg: PO** 2.2 g of salicylate/day divided bid
- **Child <37 kg: PO** 50 mg of salicylate/kg/day divided bid

Available forms: Tabs 500, 750, 1000 mg; liquid 500 mg/5 ml

Administer:
- Mixed with fruit juice, carbonated beverage, water

SIDE EFFECTS
CNS: Stimulation, drowsiness, dizziness, confusion, **seizures**, headache, flushing, hallucinations, **coma**

CV: Rapid pulse, pulmonary edema

EENT: Tinnitus, hearing loss

ENDO: Hypoglycemia, hyponatremia, hypokalemia

GI: *Nausea, vomiting, GI bleeding, diarrhea, heartburn,* anorexia, **hepatitis, hepatotoxicity**

HEMA: **Thrombocytopenia, agranulocytosis, leukopenia, neutropenia, hemolytic anemia,** increased PT

INTEG: *Rash,* urticaria, bruising, sweating

RESP: Wheezing, hyperpnea, hyperventilation

PHARMACOKINETICS
Absorbed via GI tract; onset 15-30 min; metabolized by liver; crosses placenta; excreted in breast milk, by kidneys; half-life 2-3 hr; large doses 9-17 hr

INTERACTIONS
Increase: gastric ulcer—steroids, antiinflammatories, NSAIDs

Increase: bleeding—alcohol, aspirin, heparin, plicamycin

Increase: effects of anticoagulants, insulin, methotrexate, thrombolytic agents, penicillins, phenytoin, valproic acid, oral hypoglycemics, sulfonamides

Increase: salicylate levels—urinary acidifiers, ammonium chloride, nizatidine

Decrease: effects of choline salicylate: antacids (high doses), urinary alkalizers, corticosteroids

Decrease: effects of probenecid, spironolactone, sulfinpyrazone, sulfonamides, NSAIDs, β-blockers

Drug/Lab Test

Increase: coagulation studies, LFTs, serum uric acid, amylase, CO_2, urinary protein

Decrease: serum K, cholesterol

Interference: VMA, TSH, 5-HIAA

NURSING CONSIDERATIONS
Assess:
- **Pain:** location, intensity, character at baseline and 1-2 hr after dose
- Hepatic studies: AST, ALT, bilirubin, creatinine (long-term therapy)
- Renal studies: BUN, urine creatinine (long-term therapy); decreased urine output
- Blood studies: CBC, Hct, Hgb, PT (long-term therapy)
- I&O ratio; decreasing output may indicate renal failure (long-term therapy)

⚠ **Hepatotoxicity: dark urine; clay-colored stools; yellowing of skin, sclera; itching; abdominal pain; fever; diarrhea (long-term therapy)**
- Allergic reactions: rash, urticaria; product may have to be discontinued
- Ototoxicity: tinnitus, ringing, roaring in ears; audiometric testing needed before, after long-term therapy
- Edema in feet, ankles, legs
- Product history; many interactions

Evaluate:

• Therapeutic response: decreased pain, fever, stiffness of joints

Teach patient/family:

• To report any symptoms of **hepatotoxicity, renal toxicity,** visual changes, **ototoxicity,** allergic reactions, bleeding (long-term therapy)

• Not to exceed recommended dosage; acute poisoning may result

• To read label on other OTC products; many contain aspirin

• That therapeutic response takes 2 wk (arthritis)

• To avoid alcohol ingestion; GI bleeding may occur

• That if anticoagulants are given with product, product should be decreased 2 wk before surgery

TREATMENT OF OVERDOSE:

Lavage, activated charcoal, monitor electrolytes, VS

cidofovir (Rx)

(si-doh-foh′veer)

Vistide

Func. class.: Antiviral

Chem. class.: Nucleotide analog

ACTION:

Suppresses cytomegalovirus (CMV) replication by selective inhibition of viral DNA synthesis

USES:

CMV retinitis in patients with HIV; used with probenecid

Unlabeled uses: Adenovirus, condylomata acuminata, eczema vaccination, Epstein-Barr virus, generalized vaccinia, herpes genitalis/simplex, HPV, molluscum contagiosum, vaccinia necrosum, vaccinia, varicella-zoster, variola

CONTRAINDICATIONS:

Hypersensitivity to this product, probenecid, sulfa products; direct intraocular injection

Black Box Warning: Proteinuria, renal disease/failure

Precautions: Pregnancy (C), breastfeeding, children <6 mo, geriatric patients, preexisting cytopenias, renal function impairment, platelet count <25,000/mm^3

Black Box Warning: Neutropenia, infertility, secondary malignancy

DOSAGE AND ROUTES

• **Adult: IV** 5 mg/kg q wk × 2 wk then 3 mg/kg q2wk, give with probenecid

Renal dose

• **Adult: IV** CCr <55 ml/min, do not use; SCr increase of 0.3-0.4 mg/dl above baseline, decrease dose to 3 mg/kg; SCr increase of ≥0.5 mg/dl above baseline or ≥21 proteinuria, discontinue

Available forms: Inj 75 mg/ml

Administer:

• Use cytotoxic handling procedures

Intermittent IV INF route

• **Dilute** in 100 ml 0.9% saline sol before administration; probenecid must be given PO 2 g 3 hr prior to the cidofovir inf and 1 g at 2 and 8 hr after ending the cidofovir inf; **give** 1 L of 0.9% saline sol IV with each INF of cidofovir, give saline INF over 1-2 hr period immediately prior to cidofovir; patient should be given a 2nd L if the patient can tolerate the fluid load (2nd L given at time of cidofovir or immediately afterward, should be given over 1-3 hr)

• **Mix** under strict aseptic conditions using gloves, gown, and mask; use precautions for antineoplastic medications

• **Give** slowly; do not give by bolus IV, SUBCUT inj

• Use diluted sol within 24 hr, do not freeze; do not use sol with particulate matter or discoloration; allow to warm to room temp before using

SIDE EFFECTS

CNS: *Fever, chills,* coma, confusion, abnormal thoughts, *dizziness*, bizarre dreams, *headache*, psychosis, tremors, somnolence, paresthesia, *amnesia, anxiety, insomnia*, seizures

CV: Dysrhythmias, hypo/hypertension

EENT: Retinal detachment with CMV retinitis

GI: Abnormal LFTs, *nausea, vomiting, anorexia, diarrhea*, abdominal pain, hemorrhage

GU: Hematuria, increased creatinine, BUN, nephrotoxicity

HEMA: Granulocytopenia, thrombocytopenia, irreversible neutropenia, anemia, eosinophilia

INTEG: *Rash, alopecia, pruritus, acne*, urticaria, pain at inj site, phlebitis

RESP: Dyspnea

PHARMACOKINETICS

Terminal half-life 2.6 hr

INTERACTIONS

• **Nephrotoxicity:** amphotericin B, foscarnet, aminoglycosides, pentamidine IV, NSAIDs, salicylates; wait 7 days after use to begin cidofovir

NURSING CONSIDERATIONS

Assess:

• Culture before treatment is initiated; cultures of blood, urine, and throat may all be taken; CMV not confirmed by this method; diagnosis made by ophthalmic exam

Black Box Warning: Renal, hepatic, increased hemopoietic studies, BUN; serum creatinine, AST, ALT, creatinine, CCr, A-G ratio, baseline and drip treatment, blood counts should be done q2wk; watch for decreasing granulocytes, Hgb; if low, therapy may have to be discontinued and restarted after hematologic recovery; blood transfusions may be required

• For GI symptoms: severe nausea, vomiting, diarrhea; severe symptoms may necessitate discontinuing product

• Electrolytes and minerals: calcium, phosphorus, magnesium, sodium, potassium; watch closely for tetany during 1st administration

Black Box Warning: Blood dyscrasias (anemia, granulocytopenia); bruising, fatigue, bleeding, poor healing; leukopenia, neutropenia, thrombocytopenia: WBCs, platelets q2days during 2 ×/day dosing and every wk thereafter; check for leukopenias with daily WBC count in patients with prior leukopenia, with other nucleoside analogs, or for whom leukopenia counts are <1000 cells/mm^3 at start of treatment

• Allergic reactions: flushing, rash, urticaria, pruritus

• Monitor serum creatinine or CCr at least q2wk; give only to those with creatinine levels ≤1.5 mg/dl, CCr >55 ml/min, urine protein <100 mg/dl

Evaluate:

• Therapeutic response: decreased symptoms of CMV

Teach patient/family:

• To notify prescriber if sore throat, swollen lymph nodes, malaise, fever occur; may indicate other infections

• To report perioral tingling, numbness in extremities, paresthesias; report rash immediately

• That serious product interactions may occur if OTC products are ingested; check 1st with prescriber

• That product is not a cure but will control symptoms

• That regular ophthalmic exams must be continued

• That major toxicities may necessitate discontinuing product

• To use contraception during treatment; that infertility may occur; and that men should use barrier contraception for 90 days after treatment

TREATMENT OF OVERDOSE:

Discontinue product; use hemodialysis, increase hydration

cilostazol (Rx)

(sih-los′tah-zol)

Pletal

Func. class.: Platelet aggregation inhibitor

Chem. class.: Quinolinone derivative

Do not confuse:
Pletal/Plendil

ACTION:
Reversibly inhibits cellular phosphodiesterase; inhibits platelet aggregation induced by thrombin, ADP, collagen, arachidonic acid, EPINEPHrine, stress

USES:
Intermittent claudication

Unlabeled uses: Buerger's disease, percutaneous coronary intervention (PCI)

CONTRAINDICATIONS:
Hypersensitivity, acute MI, active bleeding conditions, hemostatic conditions

Black Box Warning: CHF

Precautions: Pregnancy (C), breastfeeding, children, geriatric patients, previous hepatic disease, cardiac/renal disease, increased bleeding risk, low platelet count, platelet dysfunction

DOSAGE AND ROUTES

• **Adult: PO** 100 mg bid taken ≥30 min before or 2 hr after breakfast and dinner or 50 mg bid if using products that inhibit CYP3A4 and CYP2C19; 12 wk of treatment may be needed for beneficial effect

PCI to prevent acute coronary thrombosis/Buerger's disease (unlabeled)

• **Adult: PO** 100 mg bid

Available forms: Tabs 50, 100 mg

Administer:

• Give bid 30 min before or 2 hr after meals; do not give with grapefruit juice

SIDE EFFECTS

CNS: *Dizziness,* headache

CV: *Palpitations, tachycardia,* nodal dysrhythmia, postural hypotension

EENT: Blindness, diplopia, ear pain, tinnitus, retinal hemorrhage

GI: *Nausea,* vomiting, *diarrhea,* GI discomfort, colitis, cholelithiasis, ulcer, esophagitis, gastritis, anorexia, *flatulence, dyspepsia*

GU: Cystitis, frequency, vaginitis, **vaginal hemorrhage,** hematuria

HEMA: Bleeding (epistaxis, hematuria, retinal hemorrhage, GI bleeding), thrombocytopenia, anemia, **polycythemia, aplastic anemia**

INTEG: *Rash,* urticaria, dry skin, **Stevens-Johnson syndrome**

MISC: *Back pain, headache, infection, myalgia, peripheral edema,* chills, fever, malaise, diabetes mellitus

RESP: *Cough, pharyngitis, rhinitis,* asthma, pneumonia

PHARMACOKINETICS

95%-98% protein binding; metabolism: hepatic extensively by CYP3A4, 2C19 enzymes; excreted in urine (74%), feces (20%); half-life 11-13 hr

INTERACTIONS

Increase: bleeding tendencies—anticoagulants, NSAIDs, thrombolytics, abciximab, eptifibatide, tirofiban, ticlopidine

Increase: cilostazol levels—CYP3A4, CYP2C19 inhibitors; diltiazem, erythromycin, clarithromycin, verapamil, protease inhibitors, omeprazole; exercise caution when coadministering with fluvoxamine, FLUoxetine, ketoconazole, isoniazid, gemfibrozil, omeprazole, itraconazole, voriconazole, fluconazole; reduce dose to 50 mg bid

Decrease: cilostazol levels—CYP3A4 inducers

Drug/Herb

Decrease: action—chamomile, coenzyme Q10, flax, goldenseal, St. John's wort

Drug/Food

- Do not use with grapefruit juice, toxicity may occur

NURSING CONSIDERATIONS

Assess:

- For underlying CV disease since CV risk is great; for CV lesions with repeated oral administration; do not administer to patients with CHF of any severity; for severe headache, signs of toxicity
- Blood studies: CBC q2wk, Hct, Hgb, PT

Evaluate:

- Therapeutic response: improved walking distance, duration; decreased pain

Teach patient/family:

- To report any unusual bleeding
- To report side effects such as diarrhea, skin rashes, subcutaneous bleeding
- That effects may take 2-4 wk; treatment of up to 12 wk may be required for necessary effect
- That reading the patient package insert is necessary
- That it is best to discontinue tobacco use
- That there are many drug and herb interactions; obtain approval from prescriber before use

cimetidine (OTC, Rx)

(sye-met′i-deen)

Acid Reducer, Apo-Cimetidine ✤, Equaline Acid Reducer, Gen-Cimetidine ✤, Good Sense Heartburn Relief, Leader Cimetidine, Nu-Cimet ✤, Select Brand Cimetidine, Tagamet, Tagamet HB, Top Care Heartburn Relief, Walgreens Cimetidine

Func. class.: H_2-histamine receptor antagonist

Chem. class.: Imidazole derivative

ACTION: Inhibits histamine at H_2-receptor site in the gastric parietal cells, which inhibits gastric acid secretion

USES: Short-term treatment of duodenal and gastric ulcers and maintenance; management of GERD (PO) and Zollinger-Ellison syndrome; prevention of upper GI bleeding; prevent, relieve heartburn, acid indigestion, upper GI bleeding

Unlabeled uses: Prevention of aspiration pneumonitis, stress ulcers, angioedema, molluscum contagiosum, NSAID-induced ulcer prophylaxis, verruca vulgaris

CONTRAINDICATIONS: Hypersensitivity

Precautions: Pregnancy (B), breastfeeding, children <16 yr, geriatric patients, organic brain syndrome, renal/hepatic disease

DOSAGE AND ROUTES

Short-term treatment of active ulcers

- **Adult: PO** 300 mg qid with meals, at bedtime × 8 wk or 400 mg bid, 800 mg at bedtime; after 8 wk, give bedtime dose only; **IV BOL** 300 mg/20 ml 0.9% NaCl over 1-2 min q6hr; **IV INF** 300 mg/50 ml D_5W over 15-20 min; **IM** 300 mg q6hr, max 2400 mg/day
- **Child: PO** 20-40 mg/kg/day; **IM/IV** 5-10 mg/kg q6-8hr

Prophylaxis of duodenal ulcer

- **Adult and child >16 yr:** 400 mg at bedtime or 300 mg bid

GERD

- **Adult: PO** 800-1600 mg/day in divided doses

Hypersecretory conditions (Zollinger-Ellison syndrome)

- **Adult: PO/IM/IV** 300-600 mg q6hr; may increase to 12 g/day if needed; OTC use ≤200 mg daily or bid, max 2×/wk

Upper GI bleeding prophylaxis

- **Adult: IV** 50 mg/hr; lowered in renal disease

Renal disease

- **Adult: PO/IV** CCr <30 ml/min, 300 mg q12hr

Aspiration pneumonitis prophylaxis (unlabeled)

• **Adult: IM/IV** 300 mg **IM** 1 hr before anesthesia then 300 mg **IV** q4hr until patient is alert, max 2400 mg/day

Severe urticaria/angioedema (unlabeled)

• **Adult: IV** 300 mg, diluted, appropriately, in combination with H_1-blocker

Molluscum contagiosum (unlabeled)

• **Child: PO** 40 mg/kg/day × 2 mo

Verruca vulgaris (unlabeled)

• **Child: PO** 30-40 mg/kg/day × 2 mo

Available forms: Tabs 100, 200, 300, 400, 800 mg; liq 200, 300 mg/5 ml; inj 300 mg/2 ml, 300 mg/50 ml 0.9% NaCl

Administer:

• With meals for prolonged product effect; antacids 1 hr before or 1 hr after cimetidine

IV route

• After **diluting** 300 mg/20 ml of 0.9% NaCl for inj; give by **direct IV over** ≥5 min; **Intermittent IV INF** may be **diluted** 300 mg/50 ml of D_5W; **run** over 15-20 min; or total daily dose (900 mg) diluted in 100-1000 ml D_5W given over 24 hr **Continuous IV INF**

Y-site compatibilities: Acyclovir, alfentanil, amifostine, amikacin, aminocaproic acid, aminophylline, amphotericin B lipid complex/liposome, anakinra, anidulafungin, ascorbic acid injection, atenolol, atracurium, atropine, aztreonam, benztropine, bivalirudin, bleomycin, bumetanide, buprenorphine, butorphanol, calcium chloride/gluconate, CARBOplatin, caspofungin, cefamandole, ceFAZolin, cefmetazole, cefonicid, cefotaxime, cefotetan, cefoxitin, ceftazidime, ceftizoxime, cefTRIAXone, cefuroxime, cephalothin, cephapirin, chlorpromazine, cisatracurium, CISplatin, cladribine, clarithromycin, clindamycin, codeine, cyanocobalamin, cyclophosphamide, cycloSPORINE, cytarabine, DACTINomycin, DAPTOmycin, dexamethasone, dexmedetomidine, digoxin, diltiazem, diphenhydrAMINE, DOBUTamine, docetaxel, DOPamine, doripenem, doxacurium, doxapram, DOXOrubicin, DOXOrubicin liposome, enalaprilat, ePHEDrine, EPINEPHrine, epirubicin, epoetin alfa, eptifibatide, ertapenem, erythromycin, esmolol, etoposide, famotidine, fenoldopam, fentaNYL, filgrastim, fluconazole, fludarabine, fluorouracil, folic acid, foscarnet, gallium, gatifloxacin, gemcitabine, gentamicin, gycopyrrolate, granisetron, heparin, hydrocortisone, HYDROmorphone, hydrOXYzine, IDArubicin, ifosfamide, imipenem-cilastatin, irinotecan, isoproterenol, ketorolac, labetalol, levofloxacin, lidocaine, linezolid, LORazepam, LR, magnesium sulfate, mannitol, mechlorethamine, melphalan, meperidine, metaraminol, meropenem, methicillin, methotrexate, methoxamine, methyldopate, methylPREDNIsolone, metoclopramide, metoprolol, metroNIDAZOLE, mezlocillin, miconazole, midazolam, milrinone, minocycline, mitoxantrone, morphine, moxalactum, multiple vitamin injection, mycophenolate, nafcillin, nalbuphine, naloxone, nesiritide, netilmicin, niCARdipine, nitroglycerin, nitroprusside, norepinephrine, octreotide, ondansetron, oxacillin, oxaliplatin, oxytocin, paclitaxel, palonosetron, pamidronate, pancuronium, pantoprazole, papaverine, pemetrexed, penicillin G sodium/potassium, pentamidine, pentazocine, phenylephrine, phytonadione, pipercillin, piperacillin/tazobactam, polymyxin B, potassium chloride, procainamide, prochlorperazine, promethazine, propofol, propranolol, protamine, pyridoxine, quiNIDine, quinupristin-dalfopristin, ranitidine, remifentanil, Ringers' ritodrine, riTUXimab, rocuronium, sargramostim, sodium acetate/bicarbonate, succinylcholine, SUFentanil, tacrolimus, teniposide, theophylline, thiamine, thiotepa, ticarcillin, ticarcillin-clavulanate, tigecycline, tirofiban, TNA, tobramycin, tolazoline, topotecan, TPN, trastuzumab, trimetaphan, urokinase, vancomycin, vasopressin, vecuronium, verapamil, vinCRIStine, vinorelbine, voriconazole, zidovudine, zoledronic acid

SIDE EFFECTS

CNS: *Confusion, headache,* depression, dizziness, anxiety, weakness, psychosis, tremors, **seizures**
CV: Bradycardia, tachycardia, **dysrhythmias**
GI: *Diarrhea,* abdominal cramps, **paralytic ileus, jaundice**
GU: Gynecomastia, galactorrhea, impotence, increase in BUN, creatinine
HEMA: **Agranulocytosis, thrombocytopenia, neutropenia, aplastic anemia, increase in PT**
INTEG: Urticaria, rash, alopecia, sweating, flushing, **exfoliative dermatitis**
RESP: **Pneumonia**

PHARMACOKINETICS

Half-life 1$^1/_2$-2 hr; 30%-40% metabolized by liver, excreted in urine (unchanged), crosses placenta, enters breast milk
PO: Onset 30 min, peak 45-90 min; duration 4-5 hr, well absorbed
IM/IV: Onset 10 min, peak $^1/_2$ hr, duration 4-5 hr, well absorbed (IM)

INTERACTIONS

Increase: toxicity due to CYP450 pathway—benzodiazepines, β-blockers, calcium channel blockers, carBAMazepine, chloroquine, lidocaine, metroNIDAZOLE, moricizine, phenytoin, quiNIDine, quiNINE, sulfonylureas, theophylline, tricyclics, valproic acid, warfarin
Decrease: absorption of cimetidine—antacids, sucralfate
Decrease: absorption—ketoconazole, itraconazole
Drug/Lab Test
Increase: alk phos, AST, creatinine, prolactin
False positive: gastroccult, hemoccult tests
False negative: TB skin tests

NURSING CONSIDERATIONS

Assess:
- Gastric pH (≥5 should be maintained); epigastric pain, duration, intensity; aggravating, ameliorating factors
- I&O ratio, BUN, creatinine, LFTs, CBC with differential periodically

Perform/provide:
- Storage of diluted sol at room temp up to 48 hr

Evaluate:
- Therapeutic response: decreased pain in abdomen; healing of ulcers; absence of gastroesophageal reflux, gastric pH of 5

Teach patient/family:
- That gynecomastia, impotence may occur, are reversible
- To avoid driving, other hazardous activities until stabilized on this medication; drowsiness or dizziness may occur
- To avoid black pepper, caffeine, alcohol, harsh spices, extremes in temp of food
- To avoid OTC preparations: aspirin; cough, cold preparations; condition may worsen
- That smoking decreases effectiveness of product
- That product must be taken exactly as prescribed and continued for prescribed time to be effective; not to double dose
- To report bruising, fatigue, malaise; blood dyscrasias may occur
- To report diarrhea, black tarry stools, sore throat, rash to prescriber

cinacalcet (Rx)

(sin-a-kal′set)

Sensipar

Func. class.: Calcium receptor agonist

Chem. class.: Polypeptide hormone

ACTION:
Directly lowers PTH levels by increasing sensitivity of calcium-sensing receptors to extracellular calcium

USES:
Hypercalcemia with parathyroid carcinoma, secondary hyperparathyroidism with chronic kidney disease for patient on dialysis, primary hyperparathyroidism

CONTRAINDICATIONS:
Hypersensitivity, hypocalcemia

Precautions: Pregnancy (C), breastfeeding, children, seizure disorders, hepatic disease

DOSAGE AND ROUTES

Parathyroid carcinoma

- **Adult: PO** 30 mg bid, titrate q2-4wk, with sequential doses of 30 mg bid, 60 mg bid, 90 mg bid, 90 mg tid-qid to normalize calcium levels

Secondary hyperparathyroidism

- **Adult: PO** 30 mg/day, titrate no more frequently than q2-4wk with sequential doses of 30, 60, 90, 120, 180 mg/day

Available forms: Tabs 30, 60, 90 mg

Administer:

- Swallow tabs whole; do not break, crush, or chew; use with food or right after a meal
- Can be used alone or in combination with vit D sterols, phosphate binders

Secondary hyperthyroidism

- Titrate q2-4wk to target iPTH consistent with National Kidney Foundation–Kidney Disease Outcomes Quality Initiative (NKF-K/DOQI) for chronic kidney disease patient on dialysis of 150-300 pg/ml; if iPTH <150-300 pg/ml, reduce dose of cinacalcet and/or vit D sterols or discontinue treatment

SIDE EFFECTS

CNS: Dizziness, asthenia, **seizures**, tetany, hallucinations, depression

CV: Hypertension, dysrhythmia exacerbation

GI: Nausea, diarrhea, vomiting, anorexia

MISC: Access infection, noncardiac chest pain, hypocalcemia

MS: Myalgia

PHARMACOKINETICS

93%-97% bound to plasma; proteins metabolized by CYP3A4, 2D6, 1A2; half-life 30-40 hr; renal excretion of metabolites (80% renal, 15% in feces)

INTERACTIONS

- Drugs metabolized by CYP3A4 (ketoconazole, erythromycin, itraconazole), CYP2D6 (flecainide, vinBLAStine, thioridazine, tricyclics): adjustments may be necessary

Drug/Food

Increase: action by high-fat meal

NURSING CONSIDERATIONS

Assess:

- **Hypocalcemia:** cramping, seizures, tetany, myalgia, paresthesia
- Calcium, phosphorous within 1 wk and iPTH 1-4 wk after initiation or dosage adjustment when maintenance established; measure calcium, phosphorus monthly; iPTH q1-3mo, target range 150-300 pg/ml for iPTH level; biochemical markers of bone formation/resorption; radiologic evidence of fracture; serum testosterone
- If calcium <8.4 mg/dl, do not start therapy

Perform/provide:

- Storage at <77° F (25° C)

Evaluate:

- Therapeutic response: calcium levels 9-10 mg/dl, decreasing symptoms of hypercalcemia

Teach patient/family:

- To take with food or shortly after a meal
- To report cramping, seizures, muscle pain, tingling, tetany immediately

ciprofloxacin (Rx)

(sip-ro-floks′a-sin)

Cipro, Cipro XR, CO Ciprofloxacin ♣, PMS-Ciprofloxacin ♣, ProQuin XR, RAN Ciprofloxacin ♣, ratio-Ciprofloxacin ♣, Sandoz Ciprofloxacin ♣, Taro-Ciprofloxacin ♣

Func. class.: Antiinfective—broad spectrum

Chem. class.: Fluoroquinolone

Do not confuse:
ciprofloxacin/cephalexin

ACTION: Interferes with conversion of intermediate DNA fragments into high-molecular-weight DNA in bacteria; DNA gyrase inhibitor

USES: Infection caused by susceptible *Escherichia coli, Enterobacter cloacae, Proteus mirabilis, Klebsiella pneumoniae, Proteus vulgaris, Citrobacter freundii, Serratia marcescens, Pseudomonas aeruginosa, Staphylococcus aureus, Staphylococcus epidermidis, Enterobacter, Campylobacter jejuni, Salmonella;* chronic bacterial prostatitis, acute sinusitis, postexposure inhalation anthrax, infectious diarrhea, typhoid fever, complicated intraabdominal infections, nosocomial pneumonia, urinary tract infections

Unlabeled uses: *Acinetobacter/woffii, Aeromonas hydrophila,* brucellosis, *Burkholderia, pseudomallei,* chancroid, cholera, dental infection, *Edwardsiella tarda,* endocarditis, *Enterobacter aerogenes,* granuloma inguinale, *Klebsiella oxytoca,* Legionnaire's disease, melioidosis, meningococcal infection prophylaxis, *Pasteurella multocida,* PID, periodontitis, pharyngitis, *Salmonella sp., Stenotrophomonas maltophilia,* tularemia, *Vibrio cholerae/parahaemolyticus/vulnificus, Yersinia enterocolitica*

CONTRAINDICATIONS: Hypersensitivity to quinolones

Precautions: Pregnancy (C), breastfeeding, children, geriatric patients, renal disease, epilepsy, QT prolongation, hypokalemia

Black Box Warning: Tendon pain/rupture, tendinitis

DOSAGE AND ROUTES

Uncomplicated urinary tract infections

- **Adult: PO** 250 mg q12hr × 3 days or 500 mg × q24hr × 3 days

Complicated/severe urinary tract infections

- **Adult: PO** 500 mg q12hr or 1000 mg q24hr × 7-14 days; **IV** 400 mg q12hr

Pyelonephritis, acute uncomplicated

- **Adult: PO** 1000 mg q24hr × 7-14 days q4-6wk

Respiratory, bone, skin, joint infections

- **Adult: PO** 500-750 mg q12hr × 7-14 days; **IV** 400 mg q12hr

Nosocomial pneumonia

- **Adult: IV** 400 mg q8hr × 10-14 days

Intraabdominal infections, complicated

- **Adult: PO** 500 mg q12hr × 7-14 days; **IV** 400 mg q12hr × 7-14 days, usually given with metroNIDAZOLE

Acute sinusitis, mild/moderate

- **Adult: PO** 500 mg q12hr × 10 days; **IV** 400 mg q12hr × 10 days

Inhalational anthrax (postexposure)

- **Adult: PO** 500 mg q12hr × 60 days; **IV** 400 mg q12hr × 60 days
- **Child: PO** 15 mg/kg/dose q12hr × 60 days, max 500 mg/dose; **IV** 10 mg/kg q12hr, max 400 mg/dose

Infectious diarrhea

- **Adult: PO** 500 mg q12hr × 5-7 days

Chronic bacterial prostatis

- **Adult: PO** 500 mg q12hr × 28 days; **IV** 400 mg q12hr × 28 days

Renal disease

• **Adult:** CCr 30-50 ml/min, **PO** 250-500 mg q12hr; CCr 5-29 ml/min, **PO** 250-500 mg q18hr; **IV** 200-400 mg q18-24hr

Available forms: Tabs 100, 250, 500, 750 mg; ext rel tabs (XR) 500, 1000 mg; inj 200 mg/20 ml, 400 mg/40 ml, 200 mg/100 ml D_5, 400 mg/200 ml D_5; oral susp 250 mg, 500 mg/5 ml

Administer:

• Do not use theophylline with this product, will cause toxicity

• Use caution when giving with antidysrhythmics IA, III

PO route

• Do not break, crush, chew XR (ext rel) product

• 2 hr before or 2 hr after antacids, zinc, iron, calcium

• Do not give oral susp by GI tube

IV route

• Over 1 hr as an inf, comes in premixed plastic inf container or diluted 20- or 40-ml vial to a final conc of 0.5-2 mg/ml of NS or D_5W; give through Y-tube or 3-way stopcock

• After clean-catch urine for C&S

Y-site compatibilities: Amifostine, anakinra, anidulafungin, atenolol, aztreonam, bivalirudin, bleomycin, calcium gluconate, CARBOplatin, caspofungin, ceftazidime, cisatracurium, CISplatin, clarithromycin, codeine, cytarabine, DACTINomycin, DAPTOmycin, dexmedetomidine, digoxin, diltiazem, diphenhydrAMINE, DOBUTamine, docetaxel, doripenem, DOPamine, doxacurium, DOXOrubicin, epirubicin, eptifibatide, ertapenem, etoposide, fenoldopam, fludarabine, gallium, gemcitabine, gentamicin, granisetron, HYDROmorphone, hydrOXYzine, IDArubicin, ifosfamide, irinotecan, lidocaine, linezolid, LORazepam, LR, mechlorethamine, meperidine, methotrexate, metoclopramide, metroNIDAZOLE, midazolam, midodrine, milrinone, mitoxantrone, mycophenolate, nesiritide, octreotide, ondansetron, oxaliplatin, oxytocin, paclitaxel, palonosetron, pamidronate, pancuronium, piperacillin, potassium acetate/chloride, promethazine, ranitidine, remifentanil, rocuronium, sodium chloride, tacrolimus, teniposide, thiotepa, tigecycline, tirofiban, TNA, tobramycin, trastuzumab, vasopressin, vecuronium, verapamil, vinCRIStine, vinorelbine, voriconazole

SIDE EFFECTS

CNS: *Headache*, dizziness, fatigue, insomnia, depression, ***restlessness,*** **seizures, confusion**

GI: *Nausea, diarrhea*, increased ALT/AST, dry mouth, flatulence, heartburn, *vomiting*, oral candidiasis, dysphagia, **pseudomembranous colitis**

HEMA: Bone marrow depression

INTEG: *Rash*, pruritus, urticaria, photosensitivity, flushing, fever, chills, **toxic epidermal necrolysis**

MISC: Anaphylaxis, Stevens-Johnson syndrome, visual impairment, QT prolongation

MS: Tremor, arthralgia, tendinitis, **tendon rupture**

PHARMACOKINETICS

PO: Peak 1 hr; half-life 3-4 hr; excreted in urine as active product, metabolites 35%-40%, 20%-40% protein binding

INTERACTIONS

Increase: nephrotoxicity—cycloSPORINE

Increase: ciprofloxacin levels—probenecid; monitor for toxicity

Increase: levels of theophylline, warfarin, monitor blood levels

Increase: QT prolongation—astemizole, droperidol, class IA/III antidysrhythmics, tricyclics, tetracyclines, local anesthetics, phenothiazines, haloperidol, risperidone, sertindole, ziprasidone, alfuzosin, arsenic trioxide, b-agonists, chloroquine, clozapine, cyclobenzapine, dasatinib, dolasetron, droperidol, flecainide, halogenated anesthetics, lapatinib, levomethadyl, macrolides, methadone, octreotide, ondansetron, paliperidone, palonosetron, pentamidine, propafenone, ranola-

zine, sunitinib, tacrolimus, terfenadine, vardenafil, vorinostat
Decrease: ciprofloxacin absorption—antacids that contain magnesium, aluminum; zinc, iron, sucralfate, enteral feedings, calcium
Drug/Food
Increase: effect of caffeine
Decrease: absorption—dairy products, food
Drug/Lab Test
Increase: AST, ALT, BUN, creatinine, LDH, bilirubin, alk phos, glucose, proteinuria, albuminuria
Decrease: WBC, glucose

NURSING CONSIDERATIONS

Assess:
- **Infection:** WBC, temperature before treatment, periodically
- **CNS symptoms:** headache, dizziness, fatigue, insomnia, depression
- Renal, hepatic studies: BUN, creatinine, AST, ALT
- I&O ratio, urine pH <5.5 is ideal

⚠ **Anaphylaxis:** fever, flushing, rash, urticaria, pruritus, dyspnea
- For tendon pain, especially in children

Perform/provide:
- Limited intake of alkaline foods, products: milk, dairy products, alkaline antacids, sodium bicarbonate; caffeine intake if excessive cardiac or CNS stimulation
- Increase in fluids to 3 L/day to avoid crystallization in kidneys

Evaluate:
- Therapeutic response: decreased pain, frequency, urgency, C&S; absence of infection

Teach patient/family:
- Not to take any products that contain magnesium, calcium (such as antacids), iron, aluminum with this product or within 2 hr of product
- To report tendon pain, chest pain, palpitations
- To ambulate, perform activities with assistance if dizziness occurs
- To complete full course of product therapy; not to double or miss doses
- To contact prescriber if adverse reaction occurs, if inflammation or pain in tendon occurs
- To frequently rinse mouth; use sugarless candy, gum for dry mouth
- To contact prescriber if taking theophylline

ciprofloxacin ophthalmic

See Appendix B

⚠ HIGH ALERT

CISplatin (Rx)

(sis′pla-tin)

Func. class.: Antineoplastic alkylating agent
Chem. class.: Platinum complex

Do not confuse:
CISplatin/CARBOplatin
Platinol/Paraplatin

ACTION: Alkylates DNA, RNA; inhibits enzymes that allow for the synthesis of amino acids in proteins; activity not cell-cycle–phase specific

USES: Advanced bladder cancer; adjunct in metastatic testicular cancer; osteosarcoma; soft-tissue sarcomas; adjunct in metastatic ovarian cancer; head, neck cancer; esophagus, prostate, lung, cervical cancer; lymphoma
Unlabeled uses: Astrocytoma; breast, gastric, head, neck, hepatocellular, lung, penile cancer; carcinoid, desmoid tumor; Hodgkin's disease, malignant glioma, malignant melanoma, neuroblastoma, non-Hodgkin's lymphoma (NHL), osteogenic sarcoma

CONTRAINDICATIONS: Pregnancy (D), breastfeeding; radiation or chemotherapy within 1 mo; thrombocytopenia; recent smallpox vaccination;

aluminum products used to prepare or administer CISplatin

Black Box Warning: Preexisting hearing impairment, bone marrow suppression, platinum compound hypersensitivity, renal disease/failure

Precautions: Geriatric patients, pneumococcus vaccination

DOSAGE AND ROUTES

Dosage protocols may vary

Metastatic testicular cancer

- **Adult: IV** 20 mg/m^2/day × 5 days, repeat q3wk for 2 cycles or more, depending on response

Advanced bladder cancer

- **Adult: IV** 50-70 mg/m^2 q3-4wk

Metastatic ovarian cancer

- **Adult: IV** 100 mg/m^2 q4wk or 75-100 mg/m^2 q3wk with cyclophosphamide; mix with 2 L NaCl and 37.5 g mannitol over 6 hr

Breast cancer (unlabeled)

- **Adult: IV** 60 mg as a single dose on days 23, 30 of a 60-day cycle with other antineoplastics

Hodgkin's/non-Hodgkin's lymphoma (unlabeled)

- **Adult and child: IV INF** 100 mg/m^2 24 hr continuous inf day 1 of 4-day regimen with cytarabine/dexamethasone q3-4wk

Gastric cancer (unlabeled)

- **Adult: IV** 75 mg/m^2 on day 1 with docetaxel 75 mg/m^2 and fluorouracil 750 mg/m^2 on days 1-5, q21days

Available forms: Inj 0.5 ✱, 1 mg/ml

Administer:

IV route

- Use cytotoxic handling procedures
- Do not use aluminum equipment during any preparation or administration, will form precipitate; do not refrigerate unopened powder or solution; protect from sunlight
- Prepare in biologic cabinet using gown, gloves, mask; do not allow product to come in contact with skin; use soap and water if contact occurs; use cytotoxic handling procedures
- Hydrate patient with 0.9% NaCl over 8-12 hr before treatment
- EPINEPHrine, antihistamines, corticosteroids for hypersensitivity reaction
- Antiemetic 30-60 min before product and prn; allopurinol to maintain uric acid levels, alkalinization of urine; diuretic (furosemide 40 mg IV) or mannitol after inf

Intermittent IV INF route

- **Dilute** 10 mg/10 ml or 50 mg/50 ml sterile water for inj, withdraw prescribed dose; **dilute** ½ dose with 1000 ml D_5 0.2 NaCl, D_5 0.45 NaCl with 37.5 g mannitol; IV INF is **given** over 3-4 hr; use a 0.45-μm filter; total dose 2 L over 6-8 hr; check site for irritation, phlebitis

Continuous IV INF route

- **Give** over 24 hr × 5 days

Additive compatibilities: CARBOplatin, cyclophosphamide, floxuridine, hydrOXYzine, ifosfamide, leucovorin, magnesium sulfate, mannitol, ondansetron

Solution compatibilities: D_5/0.225% NaCl, D_5/0.45% NaCl, D_5/0.9% NaCl, D_5/0.45% NaCl with mannitol 1.875%, D_5/0.33% NaCl with KCl 20 mEq and mannitol 1.875%, 0.9% NaCl, 0.45% NaCl, 0.3% NaCl, 0.225% NaCl

Syringe compatibilities: Bleomycin, cyclophosphamide, doxapram, droperidol, fluorouracil, furosemide, heparin, leucovorin, methotrexate, metoclopramide, vinBLAStine, vinCRIStine

Y-site compatibilities: Acyclovir, alfentanil, allopurinol, amikacin, aminophylline, amiodarone, ampicillin, ampicillin-sulbactam, anidulafungin, atenolol, atracurium, azithromycin, aztreonam, bivalirudin, bleomycin, bumetanide, buprenorphine, butorphanol, calcium chloride/gluconate, caspofungin, ceFAZolin, cefoperazone, cefotaxime, cefotetan, cefoxitin, ceftazidime, ceftizoxime, cefTRIAXone, cefuroxime, chlorproMAZINE, cimetidine, ciprofloxacin, cisatracurium, cladribine, clindamycin, codeine, cyclophosphamide, cycloSPORINE, cytarabine, DACTINomycin, DAPTOmycin, DAUNOrubicin, dexamethasone, dexmedetomidine, dexrazoxane, digoxin, diltiazem, diphenhydrAMINE, DOBUTamine, docetaxel, DOPamine, doripenem, doxacurium, DOXOrubicin, DOXOrubicin liposomal, doxycycline, droperidol, enalaprilat, ePHEDrine, EPINEPHrine, epirubicin, ertapenem, erythromycin, esmolol, etoposide, famotidine, fenoldopam, fentaNYL, filgrastim, fluconazole, fludarabine, fluorouracil, foscarnet, fosphenytoin, furosemide, ganciclovir, gatifloxacin, gemcitabine, gentamicin, glycopyrrolate, granisetron, haloperidol, heparin, hydrocortisone, HYDROmorphone, IDArubicin, ifosfamide, imipenem-cilastatin, inamrinone, indomethacin, irinotecan, isoproterenol, ketorolac, labetalol, leucovorin, levofloxacin, levorphanol, lidocaine, linezolid, LORazepam, magnesium sulfate, mannitol, melphalan, meperidine, meropenem, methohexital, methotrexate, methylPREDNISolone, metoclopramide, metoprolol, metroNIDAZOLE, midazolam, milrinone, minocycline, mitomycin, mitoxantrone, mivacurium, nafcillin, naloxone, nesiritide, niCARdipine, nitroglycerin, nitroprusside, norepinephrine, octreotide, ofloxacin, ondansetron, oxaliplatin, paclitaxel, palonosetron, pamidronate, pancuronium, pemetrexed, pentamidine, pentazocine, PENTobarbital, PHENobarbital, phenylephrine, phenytoin, piperacillin, polymyxin B, potassium chloride/phosphates, procainamide, prochlorperazine, promethazine, propofol, propranolol, quiNIDine, quinupristin-dalfopristin, ranitidine, remifentanil, riTUXimab, sargramostim, sodium acetate/bicarbonate/phosphates, succinylcholine, SUFentanil, sulfamethoxazole-trimethoprim, tacrolimus, teniposide, theophylline, thiopental, ticarcillin, ticarcillin-clavulanate, tigecycline, tirofiban, TNA, tobramycin, topotecan, trastuzumab, vancomycin, vasopressin, vecuronium, verapamil, vinBLAStine, vinCRIStine, vinorelbine, voriconazole, zidovudine, zoledronic acid

SIDE EFFECTS

CNS: **Seizures,** peripheral neuropathy
CV: Cardiac abnormalities
EENT: *Tinnitus, hearing loss, vestibular toxicity,* blurred vision, altered color perception
GI: *Severe nausea, vomiting, diarrhea, weight loss*
GU: **Renal tubular damage,** renal insufficiency, impotence, sterility, amenorrhea, gynecomastia, hyperuremia
HEMA: **Thrombocytopenia, leukopenia, pancytopenia**
INTEG: *Alopecia,* dermatitis
META: Hypomagnesemia, hypocalcemia, hypokalemia, hypophosphatemia
RESP: **Fibrosis**
SYST: **Anaphylaxis**

PHARMACOKINETICS

Absorption complete, metabolized in liver, excreted in urine, half-life 30-100 hr, accumulates in body tissues for several months, enters breast milk

INTERACTIONS

Increase: bleeding risk—aspirin, NSAIDs, alcohol
Increase: ototoxicity—bumetanide, ethacrynic acid, furosemide
Increase: myelosuppression—myelosuppressive agents, radiation
Increase: nephrotoxicity—aminoglycosides, loop diuretics, salicylates
Decrease: effects of phenytoin
Decrease: antibody response—live virus vaccines

Drug/Lab Test
Increase: uric acid, BUN, creatinine
Decrease: CCr, calcium, phosphate, potassium, magnesium
Positive: Coombs' test

NURSING CONSIDERATIONS

Assess:

Black Box Warning: Bone marrow depression: CBC, differential, platelet count weekly; withhold product if WBC is <4000 or platelet count is <100,000; notify prescriber of results

Black Box Warning: Renal studies: BUN, creatinine, serum uric acid, urine CCr before, electrolytes during therapy; dose should not be given if BUN <25 mg/dl; creatinine <1.5 mg/dl; I&O ratio; report fall in urine output of <30 ml/hr

⚠ **Anaphylaxis:** wheezing, tachycardia, facial swelling, fainting; discontinue product, report to prescriber; resuscitation equipment should be nearby

- Monitor temp q4hr; may indicate beginning infection
- Hepatic studies before, during therapy (bilirubin, AST, ALT, LDH) as needed or monthly

⚠ **Bleeding:** hematuria, guaiac, bruising, petechiae, mucosa or orifices q8hr; obtain prescription for viscous lidocaine (Xylocaine)

- Effects of alopecia on body image; discuss feelings about body changes
- Jaundice of skin, sclera; dark urine, clay-colored stools; itchy skin; abdominal pain; fever; diarrhea
- Edema in feet, joint pain, stomach pain, shaking, peripheral neuropathy

Perform/provide:

- Comprehensive oral hygiene
- All medications PO, if possible; avoid IM inj when platelets <100,000/mm^3
- Increase fluid intake to 2-3 L/day to prevent urate deposits, calculi formation; promote elimination of product

Evaluate:

- Therapeutic response: decreased tumor size, spread of malignancy

Teach patient/family:

- To report signs of infection: increased temp, sore throat, flulike symptoms
- To report signs of anemia: fatigue, headache, faintness, SOB, irritability
- To report bleeding, bruising, petechiae; to avoid use of razors, commercial mouthwash
- To avoid aspirin, ibuprofen, NSAIDs, alcohol; may cause GI bleeding
- To report any complaints or side effects to nurse or prescriber
- That impotence or amenorrhea can occur but is reversible after discontinuing treatment
- To report any changes in breathing, coughing
- To maintain adequate fluids; report decreased urine output, flank pain
- That hair may be lost during treatment; a wig or hairpiece may make patient feel better; new hair may be different in color, texture
- To report numbness, tingling in face or extremities; poor hearing; joint pain, swelling
- Not to receive vaccinations during treatment
- To use contraception during treatment and for 4 mo after (pregnancy D); product may cause infertility; to avoid breastfeeding

citalopram (Rx)

(sigh-tal′oh-pram)

Apo-Citalopram ✱, Celexa, CO Citalopram ✱, Gen-Citalopram ✱, PMS-Citalopram✱, RAN-Citalopram ✱, ratio-Citalopram ✱, Sandoz Citalopram ✱

Func. class.: Antidepressant

Chem. class.: Selective serotonin reuptake inhibitor (SSRI)

Do not confuse:

Celexa/Celebrex/Cerebyx/Cerebra

ACTION: Inhibits CNS neuron uptake of serotonin but not of norepinephrine; weak inhibitor of CYP450 enzyme system, thus making it more appealing than other products

USES: Major depressive disorder

Unlabeled uses: Premenstrual disorders, panic disorder, social phobia, impulsive aggression in children, obsessive-compulsive disorder in adolescents; treatment of psychotic symptoms in nondepressed demented patients; anxiety, hot flashes, menopause; adjunct in schizophrenia, PTSD

CONTRAINDICATIONS:

Hypersensitivity

Precautions: Pregnancy (C), breastfeeding, geriatric patients, renal/hepatic disease, seizure disorder, hypersensitivity to escitalopram

Black Box Warning: Children, suicidal ideation

DOSAGE AND ROUTES

Depression

- **Adult: PO** 20 mg/day AM or PM, may increase if needed to 40 mg/day after 1 wk; maintenance: after 6-8 wk of initial treatment, continue for 24 wk (32 wk total), reevaluate long-term usefulness (max 60 mg/day)

Hepatic dose/geriatric

- **Adult: PO** 20 mg/day, may increase to 40 mg/day if no response

Panic disorder (unlabeled)

- **Adult: PO** 20-60 mg/day

Premenstrual dysphoria/social phobia (unlabeled)

- **Adult: PO** 10-30 mg/day, used intermittently in premenstrual dysphoria

Available forms: Tabs 10, 20, 40 mg; oral sol 10 mg/5 ml

Administer:

- With food or milk for GI symptoms
- Crushed if patient is unable to swallow medication whole
- Dosages at bedtime if oversedation occurs during the day; may take entire dose at bedtime

SIDE EFFECTS

CNS: *Headache, nervousness, insomnia, drowsiness, anxiety, tremor, dizziness, fatigue, sedation, poor concentration, abnormal dreams, agitation,* **seizures,** apathy, euphoria, hallucinations, delusions, psychosis, **suicidal attempts, neuroleptic malignant-like syndrome reactions**

CV: *Hot flashes, palpitations,* angina pectoris, **hemorrhage,** hypertension, tachycardia, 1st-degree AV block, bradycardia, **MI,** thrombophlebitis

EENT: Visual changes, ear/eye pain, photophobia, tinnitus

GI: *Nausea, diarrhea, dry mouth, anorexia, dyspepsia, constipation, cramps, vomiting, taste changes, flatulence, decreased appetite*

GU: *Dysmenorrhea, decreased libido, urinary frequency, UTI,* amenorrhea, cystitis, impotence, urine retention

INTEG: *Sweating, rash, pruritus,* acne, alopecia, urticaria

MS: *Pain,* arthritis, twitching

RESP: *Infection, pharyngitis, nasal congestion, sinus headache, sinusitis, cough, dyspnea, bronchitis,* asthma, hyperventilation, pneumonia

SYST: *Asthenia, viral infection, fever, allergy, chills;* hyponatremia (geriatric patients), **serotonin syndrome**

PHARMACOKINETICS

Metabolized in liver by CYP3A4, CYP2C19; excreted in urine; steady state 1 wk; peak 4 hr; half-life 35 hr

INTERACTIONS

⚠ **Fatal reactions: do not use with MAOIs**

⚠ **Increase: QTc interval—pimoside, quinolones, ziprasidone; do not use together**

Increase: effect of tricyclics; use cautiously

Increase: serotonin syndrome—serotonin receptor agonists, SSRIs, tramadol, lithium, MAOIs, trazodone, SNRIs (venlafaxine, DULoxetine)

Increase: bleeding risk—NSAIDs, salicylates, thrombolytics, anticoagulants, antiplatelets

Increase: CNS effects—barbiturates, sedative/hypnotics, other CNS depressants

Increase: citalopram levels—macrolides, azole antifungals

Increase: plasma levels of β-blockers

Decrease: citalopram levels—carBAMazepine, cloNIDine

Drug/Herb

⚠ **Increase: serotonin syndrome—St. John's wort, SAM-e; fatal reaction may occur; do not use concurrently**

Increase: CNS stimulation—yohimbe

Drug/Lab Test

Increase: serum bilirubin, blood glucose, alk phos

Decrease: VMA, 5-HIAA

False increase: urinary catecholamines

NURSING CONSIDERATIONS

Assess:

⚠ **Mental status: mood, sensorium, affect, suicidal tendencies, increase in psychiatric symptoms, depression, panic**

⚠ **Serotonin syndrome: increased heart rate, sweating, dilated pupils, tremors, twitching, hyperthermia, agitation**

- B/P lying, standing, pulse q4hr; if systolic B/P drops 20 mm Hg, hold product, notify prescriber; take vital signs q4hr in patients with CV disease
- Weight weekly; appetite may decrease or increase with product
- ECG for flattening of T wave, bundle branch, AV block, dysrhythmias in cardiac patients
- Alcohol consumption; if alcohol is consumed, hold dose until AM
- Sexual dysfunction: erectile dysfunction, decreased libido

Perform/provide:

- Storage at room temp; do not freeze
- Assistance with ambulation during therapy, since drowsiness, dizziness occur
- Safety measures, primarily for geriatric patients
- Check to confirm PO medication swallowed
- Sugarless gum, hard candy, frequent sips of water for dry mouth

Evaluate:

- Therapeutic response: decreased depression

Teach patient/family:

- That therapeutic effect may take 4-6 wk, that patient may have increased anxiety 1st 5-7 days of therapy
- To use caution when driving, performing other activities that require alertness because of drowsiness, dizziness, blurred vision; to report signs, symptoms of bleeding
- To avoid alcohol, other CNS depressants

⚠ **That suicidal ideas, behavior may occur in children or young adults**

- To notify prescriber if pregnant, planning to become pregnant, or breastfeeding

⚠ **About the effects of serotonin syndrome: nausea/vomiting, tremors; if symptoms occur, to discontinue immediately, notify prescriber**

clarithromycin (Rx)

(klare-ith′row-my-sin)

Biaxin, Biaxin Filmtab, Biaxin XL

Func. class.: Antiinfective

Chem. class.: Macrolide

ACTION: Binds to 50S ribosomal subunits of susceptible bacteria and suppresses protein synthesis

USES: Mild to moderate infections of the upper and lower respiratory tract, uncomplicated skin and skin-structure infections caused by *Streptococcus pneumoniae, Mycoplasma pneumoniae, Legionella pneumophila, Moraxella catarrhalis, Neisseria gonorrhoeae, Corynebacterium diphtheriae, Listeria monocytogenes, Haemophilus influenzae, Streptococcus pyogenes, Staphylococcus aureus, Mycobacterium avium* complex (MAC); complex infection in AIDS patients; *Mycobacterium avium intracellulare, Helicobacter pylori* in combination with omeprazole, *H. parainfluenzae*

Unlabeled uses: Endocarditis prophylaxis, dyspepsia, gastric ulcer, Legionnaire's disease, pertussis, SARS

CONTRAINDICATIONS: Hypersensitivity to this product or macrolide antibiotics

Precautions: Pregnancy (C), breastfeeding, geriatric patients, renal/hepatic disease, QT prolongation

DOSAGE AND ROUTES

Acute exacerbation of chronic bronchitis

- **Adult: PO** 250-500 mg q12hr × 7-14 days or 1000 mg/day × 7 days (XL)

Pharyngitis/tonsillitis

- **Adult: PO** 250 mg q12hr × 10 days

Community-acquired pneumonia

- **Adult: PO** 250 mg q12hr × 7-14 days or 1000 mg/day × 7 days (XL)

MAC prophylaxis/treatment

- **Adult: PO** 500 mg bid; will require an additional antiinfective for active infection

***H. pylori* infection**

- **Adult: PO** 500 mg bid plus omeprazole 2 × 20 mg q AM (days 1-14), then omeprazole 20 mg q AM (days 15-28)

Acute maxillary sinusitis

- **Adult: PO** 500 mg q12hr × 14 days

Most infections

- **Child: PO** 7.5 mg/kg q12hr × 10 days, max 500 mg/dose for MAC

Renal dose

- **Adult and child: PO** CCr <30 ml/min, reduce dose by 50%

Legionnaire's disease/SARS/whooping cough/gastric ulcer/dyspepsia *(H. pylori)* (unlabeled)

- **Adult: PO** 500 mg q12hr; may be used in combination for some of these conditions

Endocarditis prophylaxis (unlabeled)

- **Adult: PO** 500 mg 1 hr before procedure

Available forms: Tabs 250, 500 mg; oral susp 125 mg/5 ml, 250 mg/5 ml; ext rel tab (XL) 500 mg

Administer:

- Do not break, crush, or chew tabs
- Adequate intake of fluids (2 L) during diarrhea episodes
- q12hr to maintain serum levels

SIDE EFFECTS

CV: Ventricular dysrhythmias, QT prolongation

GI: *Nausea, vomiting, diarrhea,* **hepatotoxicity,** *abdominal pain,* stomatitis, heartburn, anorexia, *abnormal taste,* **pseudomembranous colitis**

GU: Vaginitis, moniliasis

HEMA: Leukopenia, thrombocytopenia, increased INR

INTEG: Rash, urticaria, pruritus, **Stevens-Johnson syndrome, toxic epidermal necrolysis**

MISC: *Headache,* hearing loss

PHARMACOKINETICS

Peak 2-2.5 hr; duration 12 hr; half-life 3-4 hr; metabolized by liver; excreted in bile, feces; possible inhibition of P-glycoprotein

INTERACTIONS

Increase: dysrhythmias—cisapride, pimozide

Increase: levels, increase toxicity—ALPRAZolam, busPIRone, carBAMazepine, cycloSPORINE, digoxin, disopyramide, ergots, felodipine, fluconazole, omeprazole, tacrolimus, theophylline

Increase: oral anticoagulants effect—digoxin, theophylline, carBAMazepine

Increase: levels of HMG-CoA reductase inhibitors

Increase: action, risk for toxicity—all products metabolized by CYP3A enzyme system

Increase: effect of calcium channel blockers, midazolam, benzodiazepines, tacrolimus

Increase: QT prolongation—class IA, III antidysrhythmics

Increase or decrease action: zidovudine

Decrease: levels—rifampin, rifabutin

Drug/Lab Test

Increase: 17-OHCS/17-KS, AST, ALT, BUN, creatinine, LDH, total bilirubin

Decrease: folate assay, WBC

NURSING CONSIDERATIONS

Assess:

- **Infection:** wound characteristics, urine, stool, sputum, WBC, temp; C&S before product therapy; product may be given as soon as culture is taken; C&S may be repeated after treatment
- For ulcers: abdominal pain, bleeding in stools, emesis
- Renal, hepatic studies; report hematuria, oliguria
- Bowel pattern before, during treatment
- Respiratory status: rate, character, wheezing, tightness in chest; discontinue product
- Allergies before treatment, reaction to each medication
- **QT prolongation, ventricular dysrhythmias:** monitor ECG, cardiac status in those with underlying cardiac abnormalities
- **Serious skin reaction:** Stevens-Johnson syndrome, toxic epidermal necrolysis; product should be discontinued immediately

Perform/provide:

- Storage at room temp

Evaluate:

- Therapeutic response: C&S negative for infection

Teach patient/family:

- To take with full glass of water; may give with food to decrease GI symptoms
- ⚠ **To report sore throat, fever, fatigue; may indicate superinfection**
- ⚠ **To notify prescriber of diarrhea, dark urine, pale stools, yellow discoloration of eyes or skin, severe abdominal pain**
- To take at evenly spaced intervals; to complete dosage regimen
- To notify prescriber if pregnancy is suspected or planned

TREATMENT OF HYPERSENSITIVITY: Withdraw product, maintain airway, administer EPINEPHrine, aminophylline, O_2, IV corticosteroids

clevidipine (Rx)

(klev-id'i-peen)

Cleviprex

Func. class.: Calcium channel blocker (L-type)

Chem. class.: Dihydropyridine

ACTION: L-type calcium channels mediate the influx of calcium during depolarization in arterial smooth muscle; reduces mean arterial B/P by decreasing systemic vascular resistance

USES: Reduction of B/P when oral therapy not feasible

CONTRAINDICATIONS: Hypersensitivity to this product, eggs, soya lecithin; defective lipid metabolism; severe aortic stenosis, pancreatitis

Precautions: Pregnancy (C), labor, breastfeeding, children <18 yr, heart failure, hyperlipidemia, chronic hypertension, pheochromocytoma

DOSAGE AND ROUTES

- **Adult: CONT IV** 1-2 mg/hr; dose may be doubled q90sec initially; as B/P reaches goal, adjust dose less frequently (q5-10min) with smaller increases in dose; most patients require 4-6 mg/hr, max 32 mg/hr; no more than 1000 ml should be infused per 24-hr period due to lipid load restrictions

Available forms: Single-dose vial 50, 100 ml (0.5 mg/ml); IV emulsion

Administer:

Intermittent IV INF route

- Do not give through same line as other medications, do not dilute
- Gently invert several times before use; do not use if discolored or if particulate matter is present
- Give through central or peripheral line at 1-2 mg/hr, use infusion device

SIDE EFFECTS

CNS: Headache
CV: Hypotension, MI, sinus tachycardia, syncope, reflex tachycardia, atrial fibrillation
GI: Nausea, vomiting
GU: Renal failure

PHARMACOKINETICS

Onset 2-4 min; half-life initially 1 min, terminal 15 min; metabolized via esterases in blood, extravascular tissues; excreted in urine 63%-74%, feces 7%-22%; protein binding >99%

NURSING CONSIDERATIONS

Assess:
- Cardiac status: B/P, pulse, respiration, ECG; some patients have developed severe angina, acute MI after calcium channel blockers if obstructive CAD is severe; if not transitioned to other antihypertensive therapies after clevidipine inf, patients should be monitored ≥8 hr for rebound hypertension; monitor for rebound hypertension after product stoppage
- **Renal failure:** I&O ratio, weight daily; peripheral edema, dyspnea, jugular vein distention, crackles (perioperative hypertensive patients)

Perform/provide:
- Storage of vials in refrigerator, do not freeze; leave vials in carton until use; product is photosensitive but protection from light during administration is not required

Evaluate:
- Therapeutic response: decreased B/P

Teach patient/family:
- To notify prescriber immediately if neurological symptoms, visual changes, or symptoms of CHF occur
- To continue follow up for hypertension
- To notify prescriber if pregnancy is planned, suspected, or if breastfeeding

C

clindamycin HCl (Rx)

(klin-da-my′sin)

Cleocin HCl, Dalacin C ♣

clindamycin palmitate (Rx)

Cleocin Pediatric, Dalacin C Flavored Granules ♣

clindamycin phosphate (Rx)

Cleocin Phosphate, Dalacin C Phosphate Sterile Solution ♣

Func. class.: Antiinfective—miscellaneous
Chem. class.: Lincomycin derivative

ACTION: Binds to 50S subunit of bacterial ribosomes, suppresses protein synthesis

USES: Infections caused by staphylococci, streptococci, *Rickettsia, Fusobacterium, Actinomyces, Peptococcus, Bacteroides, Pneumocystis jiroveci*
Unlabeled uses: Acne rosacea, *Bacillus anthracis,* dental infections, folliculitis, malaria, pemphigus, periodontitis, *Pneumocystis jiroveci* pneumonia (PCP), toxoplasmosis

CONTRAINDICATIONS: Hypersensitivity to this product or lincomycin, tartrazine dye; ulcerative colitis/enteritis

Black Box Warning: Pseudomembranous colitis

Precautions: Pregnancy (B), breastfeeding, geriatric patients, GI/renal/hepatic disease, asthma, allergy

Black Box Warning: Diarrhea

DOSAGE AND ROUTES

- **Adult: PO** 150-450 mg q6-8hr, max 1.8 g/day; **IM/IV** 1.2-2.7 g/day in 2-4 divided doses, max 4800 mg/day
- **Child >1 mo: PO** 8-25 mg/kg/day in divided doses q6-8hr; **IM/IV** 20-40 mg/kg/day in 3-4 equal divided doses q6-8hr

• **Neonate: IM/IV** 15-20 mg/kg/day divided doses q6-8hr

PID

• **Adult: IV** 900 mg q8hr plus gentamicin

Bacterial endocarditis prophylaxis (unlabeled)

• **Adult:** 600 mg 1 hr before procedure

***P. jiroveci pneumonia* (unlabeled)**

• **Adult: PO** 1200-1800 mg/day in divided doses with 15-30 mg primaquine/day × 21 days

Available forms: *HCl:* caps 75, 150, 300 mg; *palmitate:* oral sol 75 mg/5 ml; *phosphate:* inj 150, 300, 600 mg base/4 ml; 900 mg base/ml; inj inf in D_5 300 mg, 600 mg, 900 mg

Administer:

• In equal intervals around the clock to maintain blood levels

PO route

• Do not break, crush, chew caps

• Orally with at least 8 oz of water

IM route

• IM deep inj; rotate sites; do not give >600 mg in single IM inj

Intermittent IV INF route

• By inf only; do not administer bolus dose; **dilute** 300-mg or 600-mg doses/50 ml of D_5W, NS; **give** over 10 or 20 min, respectively; 900-mg and 1200-mg doses/100 ml of compatible diluent and **give** over 30 or 40 min, respectively; final conc ≤12 mg/ml; if using ADD-Vantage vials, dilute containers with NS, D_5W, give over 10-60 min, rate max 30 mg/min, max 1.2 g/h

Rapid IV inj route

• Dilute as above, administer as rapid 1st dose only, then give at **cont inf** rate based on clindamycin levels

Syringe compatibilities: Amikacin, aztreonam, gentamicin, heparin

Y-site compatibilities: Acyclovir, alfentanil, amifostine, amikacin, aminocaproic acid, aminophylline, amiodarone, amphotericin B cholesteryl, amphotericin B lipid complex, amsacrine, anakinra, anidulafungin, ascorbic acid injection, atenolol, atracurium, atropine, aztreonam, benztropine, bivalirudin, bleomycin, bumetanide, buprenorphine, butorphanol, calcium chloride/gluconate, CARBOplatin, cefamandole, ceFAZolin, cefmetazole, cefonicid, cefoperazone, cefotaxime, cefotetan, cefoxitin, cefpirome, ceftazidime, ceftizoxime, ceftobiprole, cefuroxime, cephalothin, cephapirin, chloramphenicol, cimetidine, cisatracurium, CISplatin, codeine, cyanocobalamin, cyclophosphamide, cycloSPORINE, cytarabine, DACTINomycin, DAPTOmycin, dexamethasone, dexmedetomidine, digoxin, diltiazem, diphenhydrAMINE, docetaxel, DOPamine, doxacurium, DOXOrubicin, DOXOrubicin liposomal, doxycycline, enalaprilat, ePHEDrine, EPINEPHrine, epirubicin, epoetin alfa, eptifibatide, esmolol, etoposide, famotidine, fenoldopam, fentaNYL, fludarabine, fluorouracil, folic acid, foscarnet, furosemide, gatifloxacin, gemcitabine, gemtuzumab, gentamicin, glycopyrrolate, granisetron, heparin, hydrocortisone, HYDROmorphone, ifosfamide, imipenem-cilastatin, indomethacin, insulin (regular), irinotecan, isoproterenol, ketorolac, levofloxacin, lidocaine, linezolid, LORazepam, LR, magnesium sulfate, mannitol, mechlorethamine, melphalan, meperidine, metaraminol, methicillin, methotrexate, methoxamine, methyldopate, methylPREDNISolone, metoclopramide, metoprolol, metroNIDAZOLE, mezlocillin, miconazole, milrinone, morphine, moxalactam, multiple vitamins injection, nafcillin, nalbuphine, naloxone, nesiritide, netilmicin, niCARdipine, nitroglycerin, nitroprusside, norepinephrine, octreotide, ondansetron, oxacillin, oxaliplatin, oxytocin, paclitaxel, palonosetron, pamidronate, pancuronium, pantoprazole, pemetrexed, penicillin G potassium/sodium, pentazocine, perphenazine, PHENobarbital, phenylephrine, phytonadione, piperacillin, piperacillin-tazobactam, potassium chloride, procainamide, propofol, propranolol, protamine, pyridoxine, ranitidine, remifentanil, Ringer's, ritodrine, riTUXimab, rocuronium, sargramostim, sodium acetate/bicarbonate, succinylcholine, SUFentanil, tacrolimus, teniposide, theophylline, thiamine, thiotepa, ticarcillin, ticarcillin-clavulanate, tigecycline, tirofiban, TNA, tobramycin, tolazoline, TPN, trimetaphan, urokinase, vancomycin, vasopressin, vecuronium, verapamil, vinCRIStine, vinorelbine, vitamin B complex/C, voriconazole, zidovudine, zoledronic acid

SIDE EFFECTS

GI: *Nausea, vomiting, abdominal pain, diarrhea,* **pseudomembranous colitis,** anorexia, weight loss, increased AST/ALT, bilirubin, alk phos; jaundice
GU: *Vaginitis,* urinary frequency
INTEG: Rash, urticaria, pruritus, erythema, pain, abscess at inj site
SYST: **Stevens-Johnson syndrome, exfoliative dermatitis**

PHARMACOKINETICS

PO: Peak 45 min, duration 6 hr
IM: Peak 3 hr (adult), 1 hr (child); duration 8-12 hr; half-life $2^1/_2$ hr; metabolized in liver; excreted in urine, bile, feces as inactive metabolites; crosses placenta; excreted in breast milk

INTERACTIONS

• May block clindamycin effect: erythromycin, chloramphenicol
Increase: neuromuscular blockade—neuromuscular blockers
Decrease: absorption—kaolin
Drug/Lab Test
Increase: alk phos, bilirubin, CPK, AST, ALT

NURSING CONSIDERATIONS

Assess:
• **Infection:** C&S before product therapy; product may be given as soon as culture is taken
• VS, urine, stools, sputum
• Hepatic studies: AST, ALT if on long-term therapy
• B/P, pulse in patient receiving product parenterally
• **Pseudomembranous colitis:** bowel pattern before, during treatment; if severe diarrhea occurs, product should be discontinued
• Skin eruptions, itching, dermatitis after administration
• Respiratory status: rate, character, wheezing, tightness in chest
• **Serious skin reactions:** Stevens-Johnson syndrome, exfoliative dermatitis
• Allergies before treatment, reaction to each medication
Perform/provide:
• Storage at room temp (caps), up to 2 wk (reconstituted)
• EPINEPHrine, suction, tracheostomy set, endotracheal intubation equipment on unit
• Adequate intake of fluids (2 L) during diarrhea episodes
Evaluate:
• Therapeutic response: decreased temp, negative C&S
Teach patient/family:
• To take oral product with full glass of water; that antiperistaltic products may worsen diarrhea
• About all aspects of product therapy; to complete entire course of medication to ensure organism death (10-14 days); culture may be taken after medication course completed
⚠ To report sore throat, fever, fatigue; may indicate **superinfection**
• To take with food to reduce GI symptoms
• To notify nurse or prescriber of diarrhea with pus, mucous

TREATMENT OF HYPERSENSITIVITY:

• Withdraw product; maintain airway; administer EPINEPHrine, aminophylline, O_2, IV corticosteroids

clindamycin topical

See Appendix B

clobetasol topical

See Appendix B

clomiPHENE (Rx)

(kloe′mi-feen)

Clomid, Serophene

Func. class.: Ovulation stimulant

Chem. class.: Nonsteroidal antiestrogenic

Do not confuse:
clomiPHENE/clomiPRAMINE

ACTION: Increases LH, FSH release from the pituitary, which increases the maturation of the ovarian follicle, ovulation, and the development of the corpus luteum

USES: Female infertility (ovulatory failure)
Unlabeled uses: Oligospermia

CONTRAINDICATIONS: Pregnancy (X), hypersensitivity, hepatic disease, undiagnosed uterine bleeding, uncontrolled thyroid or adrenal dysfunction, intracranial lesion, ovarian cysts, endometrial carcinoma
Precautions: Hypertension, depression, seizures, diabetes mellitus, abnormal ovarian enlargement, ovarian hyperstimulation

DOSAGE AND ROUTES

- **Adult: PO** 50-100 mg/day × 5 days or 50-100 mg/day beginning on day 5 of menstrual cycle; may be repeated until conception occurs or 3 cycles of therapy completed

Oligospermia (unlabeled)

- **Adult (men): PO** 25 mg/day × 25 days then 5 days off cycle each mo

Available forms: Tabs 50 mg
Administer:

- After discontinuing estrogen therapy
- At same time daily to maintain product level

SIDE EFFECTS

CNS: *Headache, depression,* restlessness, anxiety, nervousness, fatigue, insomnia, dizziness, flushing
CV: Vasomotor flushing, phlebitis, **deep venous thrombosis**
EENT: Blurred vision, diplopia, photophobia
GI: *Nausea, vomiting, constipation,* abdominal pain, bloating
GU: Polyuria, urinary frequency, **birth defects, spontaneous abortions,** multiple ovulation, breast pain, oliguria, abnormal uterine bleeding, ovarian cyst, hypertrophy of ovary
INTEG: *Rash, dermatitis,* urticaria, alopecia

PHARMACOKINETICS

Metabolized in liver, excreted in feces

INTERACTIONS

Drug/Lab Test
Increase: FSH/LH, BSP, thyroxine, TBG

NURSING CONSIDERATIONS

Assess:

- LFTs before therapy: AST, ALT, alk phos
- Serum progesterone, urinary excretion of pregnanediol to identify occurrence of ovulation
- Ovarian size, cervical condition by pelvic examination
- For endometrial carcinoma in women >35 yr by endometrial biopsy

Evaluate:

- Therapeutic response: fertility

Teach patient/family:

- That multiple births are common
- To notify prescriber immediately if low abdominal pain occurs; may indicate ovarian cyst, cyst rupture
- To notify prescriber of photophobia, blurred vision, diplopia, abnormal bleeding, hot flashes, nausea, vomiting, headache
- That, if dose is missed, to double it next time; if more than one dose is missed, to call prescriber

• That response usually occurs 4-10 days after last day of treatment
• About the method for taking, recording basal body temp to determine whether ovulation has occurred
• If ovulation can be determined (there is a slight decrease in temp then a sharp increase with ovulation), to attempt coitus 3 days before and every other day until after ovulation
• If pregnancy is suspected, to notify prescriber immediately

clomiPRAMINE (Rx)

(kloe-mip′ra-meen)

Anafranil

Func. class.: Antidepressant, tricyclic
Chem. class.: Tertiary amine

Do not confuse:
clomiPRAMINE/clomiPHENE/chlorproMAZINE/desipramine/Norpramin

ACTION: Potentiates serotonin and norepinephrine; moderate anticholinergic effect

USES: Obsessive-compulsive disorder
Unlabeled uses: Panic disorder, autism, depression, premature ejaculation, dysphoria, phobias, anxiety, agoraphobia

CONTRAINDICATIONS: Hypersensitivity, immediate post-MI
Precautions: Pregnancy (C), breastfeeding, geriatric patients, seizures, cardiac disease, glaucoma, prostatic hypertrophy, urinary retention

Black Box Warning: Children, suicidal ideation

DOSAGE AND ROUTES

Obsessive-compulsive disorder
• **Adult: PO** 25 mg at bedtime, increase gradually over 4 wk to 75-250 mg/day in divided doses
• **Child 10-18 yr: PO** 25 mg/day gradually increased; max 3 mg/kg/day or 200 mg/day, whichever is smaller

Autism (unlabeled)
• **Adult: PO** 25 mg/day, may increase to 75-100 mg/day, max 250 mg/day
• **Child: PO** 25 mg/day, may increase if needed

Premature ejaculation (unlabeled)
• **Adult: PO** 25-50 mg/day

Depression (unlabeled)
• **Adult: PO** 25 mg at bedtime and increase gradually over 4 wk to 75-250 mg/day in divided doses
• **Child 10-18 yr: PO** 25-50 mg/day gradually increased; max 3 mg/kg/day or 200 mg/day, whichever is smaller

Available forms: Caps 25, 50, 75 mg
Administer:
• Do not break, crush, or chew caps
• Increased fluids, bulk in diet for constipation, especially for geriatric patients
• With food or milk for GI symptoms
• After titration, may be given as a single dose at bedtime to reduce daytime sedation

SIDE EFFECTS

CNS: *Dizziness, tremors, mania,* **seizures**, aggressiveness, EPS, drowsiness, headache, **neuroleptic malignant syndrome**, insomnia, agitation
CV: Hypotension, tachycardia, **cardiac arrest**
EENT: Blurred vision
ENDO: Galactorrhea, hyperprolactinemia
GI: *Constipation, dry mouth, nausea, dyspepsia,* weight gain, **hepatic toxicity**
GU: *Delayed ejaculation, anorgasmia,* urinary retention, decreased libido
HEMA: **Agranulocytosis, neutropenia, pancytopenia**
INTEG: Diaphoresis, photosensitivity
META: Hyponatremia
SYST: **Suicide in children, adolescents**

PHARMACOKINETICS

Onset ≥2 wk (depression), 4-10 wk (OCD); peak 2-6 hr; extensively bound to tissue and plasma proteins; demethylated in liver; active metabolites excreted in urine (50%-60%), feces (24%-32%); half-life 20-30 hr; steady state 1-2 wk

INTERACTIONS

Increase: hypertensive crisis, seizures, hypertensive episode—MAOIs
Increase: clomiPRAMINE levels—cimetidine, FLUoxetine, fluvoxamine, sertraline; do not use together
Increase: hypertensive effect—cloNIDine, EPINEPHrine, norepinephrine
Increase: clomiPRAMINE level—CYP1A2, CYP2D6
Increase: CNS depression—alcohol, CNS depressants, general anesthetics
Increase: QT prolongation—other tricyclics, phenothiazines, quinolones
Decrease: effect of cloNIDine, levodopa, skeletal muscle relaxants, haloperidol, opiates
Decrease: clomiPRAMINE levels—barbiturates, carBAMazepine, phenytoin

Drug/Herb

Increase: serotonin syndrome—St. John's wort; do not use concurrently
Increase: CNS depression—hops, kava, valerian

Drug/Lab Test

Increase: prolactin, TBG, AST, ALT, blood glucose
Decrease: serum thyroid hormone (T_3, T_4)

NURSING CONSIDERATIONS

Assess:

- B/P lying, standing; pulse q4hr; if systolic B/P drops 20 mm Hg, withhold product, notify prescriber; take VS q4hr in patients with CV disease
- **Neuroleptic malignant syndrome:** hyperpyrexia, rigidity, irregular pulse, diaphoresis
- **ECG** for flattening of T wave, QTc prolongation, bundle branch block, AV block, dysrhythmias in cardiac patients
- Blood studies: CBC, leukocytes, differential, cardiac enzymes if patient is receiving long-term therapy
- Hepatic studies: AST, ALT, bilirubin
- Mental status: mood, sensorium, affect, suicidal tendencies; increase in psychiatric symptoms: depression, panic, frequency of obsessive-compulsive behaviors; watch closely for evidence of suicidal thoughts in children, adolescents; seizure disorders
- Urinary retention, constipation; constipation more likely in children
- **Withdrawal symptoms:** headache, nausea, vomiting, muscle pain, weakness; not usual unless product discontinued abruptly
- Alcohol consumption; if alcohol consumed, withhold dose until AM

Perform/provide:

- Storage in tight container at room temp; do not freeze
- Assistance with ambulation during beginning therapy, since drowsiness, dizziness occurs
- Safety measures, primarily for geriatric patients
- Check to confirm PO medication swallowed
- Gum, hard candy, or frequent sips of water for dry mouth

Evaluate:

- Therapeutic response: decreased anxiety, depression

Teach patient/family:

- That the effects may take 4-6 wk to appear
- About risk for seizures
- To use caution when driving, performing other activities that require alertness because drowsiness, dizziness, blurred vision may occur
- To avoid alcohol, other CNS depressants
- Not to discontinue medication quickly after long-term use because this may cause nausea, headache, malaise
- That suicidal thoughts/behaviors may occur in children, young adults
- To wear sunscreen, protective clothing to prevent photosensitivity
- To notify prescriber if pregnancy is planned, suspected
- That men may experience a high incidence of sexual dysfunction

TREATMENT OF OVERDOSE:
ECG monitoring; induce emesis; lavage, activated charcoal; anticonvulsant; diazepam IV

clonazePAM (Rx)
(kloe-na′zi-pam)

Apo-Clonazepam ✱, CO Clonazepam ✱, Gen-Clonazepam ✱, Klonopin, PMS-Clonazepam ✱, ratio-Clonazepam ✱, Sandoz Clonazepam ✱

Func. class.: Anticonvulsant

Chem. class.: Benzodiazepine derivative

Controlled Substance Schedule IV

Do not confuse:
clonazePAM/LORazepam/clorazepate
Klonopin/cloNIDine

ACTION:
Inhibits spike, wave formation during absence seizures (petit mal); decreases amplitude, frequency, duration, spread of discharge during minor motor seizures

USES:
Absence, atypical absence, akinetic, myoclonic seizures; Lennox-Gastaut syndrome, panic disorder

Unlabeled uses: Anxiety, insomnia, nystagmus, restless leg syndrome

CONTRAINDICATIONS:
Pregnancy (D), hypersensitivity to benzodiazepines, acute closed-angle glaucoma, psychosis, severe hepatic disease

Precautions: Breastfeeding, geriatric patients, open-angle glaucoma, chronic respiratory disease, renal/hepatic disease

DOSAGE AND ROUTES
- **Adult: PO** up to 1.5 mg/day in 3 divided doses; may be increased 0.5-1 mg q3days until desired response, max 20 mg/day
- **Geriatric: PO** 0.25 daily-bid initially, increase by 0.25/day q7-14days as needed
- **Child <10 yr or <30 kg: PO** 0.01-0.03 mg/kg/day in divided doses q8hr, max 0.05 mg/kg/day; may be increased 0.25-0.5 mg q3days until desired response, max 0.1-0.2 mg/kg/day

Restless leg syndrome (RLS) (unlabeled)
- **Adult: PO** 0.5 mg tid or 0.5 mg in the evening and 30 min prior to bedtime

Insomnia/anxiety (unlabeled)
- **Adult: PO** 0.125-0.25 mg at bedtime, titrate up q3-4days as needed

Available forms: Tabs 0.5, 1, 2 mg; orally disintegrating tabs 0.125, 0.25, 0.5, 1, 2 mg

Administer:

PO route
- With food, milk for GI symptoms
- Orally disintegrating tablets: open pouch by peeling back foil on blister pack (do not push tab through foil), place on tongue, allow to dissolve; may be swallowed with/without water

SIDE EFFECTS
CNS: *Drowsiness,* dizziness, confusion, behavioral changes, tremors, insomnia, headache, **suicidal tendencies**, slurred speech, anterograde amnesia

CV: Palpitations, bradycardia, tachycardia

EENT: *Increased salivation, nystagmus, diplopia,* abnormal eye movements

GI: *Nausea, constipation,* polyphagia, anorexia, xerostomia, diarrhea, gastritis, sore gums

GU: Dysuria, enuresis, nocturia, retention, libido changes

HEMA: **Thrombocytopenia, leukocytosis, eosinophilia**

INTEG: Rash, alopecia, hirsutism

RESP: **Respiratory depression**, dyspnea, congestion

PHARMACOKINETICS

PO: Peak 1-2 hr, metabolized by liver, excreted in urine, half-life 18-50 hr, duration 6-12 hr, protein binding 85%

INTERACTIONS

Increase: clonazePAM effects—CYP3A4 inhibitors (azoles, cimetidine, clarithromycin, diltiazem, erythromycin, FLUoxetine), oral contraceptives

Increase: CNS depression—alcohol, barbiturates, opiates, antidepressants, other anticonvulsants, general anesthetics, hypnotics, sedatives

Decrease: clonazePAM effect—CYP3A4 inducers (carBAMazepine, PHENobarbital, phenytoin)

Drug/Herb

Increase: CNS depression—kava, chamomile, valerian

Increase: clonazePAM effect—ginkgo, melatonin

Decrease: clonazePAM effect—ginseng, St. John's wort

Drug/Lab Test

Increase: AST, alk phos, bilirubin

NURSING CONSIDERATIONS

Assess:

- **Seizures:** duration, type, intensity, with/without aura
- Blood studies: RBC, Hct, Hgb, reticulocyte counts q wk for 4 wk then monthly
- Hepatic studies: ALT, AST, bilirubin, creatinine
- Signs of physical withdrawal if medication suddenly discontinued

⚠ **Mental status:** mood, sensorium, affect, oversedation, behavioral changes, **suicidal thoughts/behaviors;** if mental status changes, notify prescriber

- Eye problems: need for ophthalmic exam before, during, after treatment (slit lamp, funduscopy, tonometry)
- Allergic reaction: red, raised rash; product should be discontinued

⚠ **Blood dyscrasias:** fever, sore throat, bruising, rash, jaundice

- **Toxicity:** bone marrow depression, nausea, vomiting, ataxia, diplopia, CV collapse; drug levels during initial treatment (therapeutic 20-80 ng/ml)

Perform/provide:

- Storage at room temp
- Assistance with ambulation during early part of treatment; dizziness occurs, especially among geriatric patients

Evaluate:

- Therapeutic response: decreased seizure activity; document on patient's chart

Teach patient/family:

- To carry emergency ID bracelet stating name, products taken, condition; prescriber's name, phone number
- To avoid driving, other activities that require alertness
- To avoid alcohol, other CNS depressants; increased sedation may occur
- Not to discontinue medication quickly after long-term use; to taper off over several wk
- To notify prescriber of yellowing of skin/eyes, clay-colored stools, bleeding, fever, extreme fatigue, sore throat, suicidal thoughts/behaviors

TREATMENT OF OVERDOSE:

Lavage, activated charcoal, flumazenil, monitor electrolytes, VS, administer vasopressors

cloNIDine (Rx)

(klon′i-deen)

Apo-Clonidine ✤, Catapres, Catapres-TTS, Duraclon, Kapvay

Func. class.: Antihypertensive

Chem. class.: Central α-adrenergic agonist

Do not confuse:

cloNIDine/KlonoPIN/clonazePAM
Catapres/Cataflam/Catarase

ACTION:

Inhibits sympathetic vasomotor center in CNS, which reduces impulses in sympathetic nervous system; blood pressure, pulse rate, cardiac output decrease, prevents pain signal transmission in CNS by α-adrenergic receptor stimulation of the spinal cord

USES:
Mild to moderate hypertension, used alone or in combination; severe pain in cancer patients (epidural)

Unlabeled uses: Opioid withdrawal, prevention of vascular headaches, treatment of menopausal symptoms, dysmenorrhea, attention-deficit/hyperactivity disorder (ADHD), autism, cycloSPORINE nephrotoxicity prophylaxis, diabetic neuropathy, ethanol withdrawal, Tourette's syndrome, hypertensive emergency

CONTRAINDICATIONS:
Hypersensitivity; (epidural) bleeding disorders, anticoagulants

Precautions: Pregnancy (C), breastfeeding, children <12 yr (transdermal), geriatric patients, noncompliant patients, MI (recent), diabetes mellitus, chronic renal failure, Raynaud's disease, thyroid disease, depression, COPD, asthma

Black Box Warning: Labor

DOSAGE AND ROUTES

Hypertension

- **Adult: PO/TRANSDERMAL** 0.1 mg bid then increase by 0.1-0.2 mg/day at weekly intervals until desired response; range 0.2-0.6 mg/day in divided doses
- **Geriatric: PO** 0.1 mg at bedtime, may increase gradually
- **Child: PO** 5-10 mcg/kg/day in divided doses q8-12hr, max 0.9 mg/day

Severe pain

- **Adult: CONT EPIDURAL INF** 30 mcg/hr
- **Child: CONT EPIDURAL INF** 0.5 mcg/kg/hr then titrate to response

Opioid withdrawal (unlabeled)

- **Adult: PO** 0.3-1.2 mg/day; may decrease by 50% × 3 days then decrease by 0.1-0.2 mg/day or discontinue

ADHD

- **Child: PO** 0.05 mg/kg/day in 3-4 divided doses × 8 wk, max 0.4 mg/day (unlabeled); Kapvay 0.1 mg at bedtime, increase dose by 0.1 mg/day up to 0.4 mg/day

Menopausal symptoms (unlabeled)

- **Adult: TRANSDERMAL** 0.1-mg patch q1wk; **PO** 0.05-0.4 mg/day

Tourette's syndrome (unlabeled)

- **Adult: PO** 0.15-0.2 mg/day

Hypertensive emergency (unlabeled)

- **Adult: PO** 0.1-0.2 mg q1hr to a total of 0.6 mg

Available forms: Tabs 0.025 ✱, 0.1, 0.2, 0.3 mg; transdermal 2.5, 5, 7.5 mg delivering 0.1, 0.2, 0.3 mg/24 hr, respectively; inj 100, 500 mcg/ml; ext rel tab 0.1 mg (Kapvay)

Administer:

PO route

- Give last dose at bedtime
- Do not crush, cut, chew, or break ext rel tabs

Transdermal route

- Once weekly; apply to site without hair; best absorption over chest or upper arm; rotate sites with each application; clean site before application; apply firmly, especially around edges

Epidural route

- Used for severe cancer pain
- May be used with opiates
- Use only if familiar with epidural inf devices

SIDE EFFECTS

CNS: *Drowsiness, sedation, headache, fatigue,* nightmares, insomnia, mental changes, anxiety, depression, hallucinations, delirium

CV: *Orthostatic hypotension, palpitations,* **CHF**, ECG abnormalities, sinus tachycardia

EENT: Taste change, parotid pain

ENDO: Hyperglycemia

GI: *Nausea, vomiting, malaise,* constipation, *dry mouth*

GU: Impotence, dysuria, nocturia, gynecomastia

INTEG: *Rash,* alopecia, facial pallor, pruritus, hives, edema, burning papules, excoriation (transdermal patches)

MISC: Withdrawal symptoms

MS: Muscle, joint pain; leg cramps

PHARMACOKINETICS

Absorbed well

PO: Onset ½ to 1 hr, peak 2-4 hr, duration 8-12 hr, half-life 6-12 hr

TRANSDERMAL: Onset 3 days; duration 1 wk; metabolized by liver (metabolites); excreted in urine (30% unchanged, inactive metabolites), feces; crosses blood-brain barrier; excreted in breast milk

INTERACTIONS

- AV block: verapamil

⚠ Life-threatening elevations of B/P: tricyclics, β-blockers

Increase: CNS depression—opiates, sedatives, hypnotics, anesthetics, alcohol

Increase: hypotensive effects—diuretics, other antihypertensive nitrates

Decrease: hypotensive effects—tricyclics, MAOIs, appetite suppressants, amphetamines, prazosin

Decrease: effect of levodopa

Drug/Herb

Increase: antihypertensive effect—hawthorn

Decrease: antihypertensive effect—ephedra, ginseng

Drug/Lab Test

Increase: blood glucose

Decrease: VMA, urinary catecholamines, aldosterone

NURSING CONSIDERATIONS

Assess:

- **Hypertension:** B/P, pulse; report significant changes
- **Opiate withdrawal (unlabeled):** fever, diarrhea, nausea, vomiting, cramps, insomnia, shivering, dilated pupils
- **Cancer pain:** location, intensity, character; alleviating, aggravating factors at baseline and frequently
- Edema in feet, legs daily; monitor I&O; check for falling output
- **Allergic reaction:** rash, fever, pruritus, urticaria; product should be discontinued if antihistamines fail to help
- **CHF:** edema, dyspnea, wet crackles, B/P
- Renal symptoms: polyuria, oliguria, frequency

Perform/provide:

- Storage of patches in cool environment, tablets in tight container

Evaluate:

- Therapeutic response: decrease in B/P with hypertension, decrease in withdrawal symptoms (opioid), decrease in pain

Teach patient/family:

- To avoid hazardous activities, since product may cause drowsiness
- To notify all health care providers of medication use
- Not to discontinue product abruptly or **withdrawal symptoms** may occur: anxiety, increased B/P, headache, insomnia, increased pulse, tremors, nausea, sweating; to comply with dosage schedule even if feeling better
- Not to use OTC (cough, cold, or allergy) products unless directed by prescriber
- To rise slowly to sitting or standing position to minimize orthostatic hypotension, especially among geriatric patients
- To notify prescriber of mouth sores, sore throat, fever, swelling of hands or feet, irregular heartbeat, chest pain, signs of **angioedema**
- About excessive perspiration, dehydration, vomiting; diarrhea may lead to fall in B/P; consult prescriber if these occur; that product may cause dizziness, fainting; that lightheadedness may occur during first few days of therapy
- That product may cause dry mouth; to use hard candy, saliva product, sugarless gum, or frequent rinsing of mouth
- That compliance is necessary; not to skip or stop product unless directed by prescriber; tolerance may develop with long-term use
- How to use patch; that patch comes in two parts: product patch and overlay to keep patch in place; not to trim or cut patch
- That response may take 2-3 days if product is given transdermally; on administration of patch, if switching from

tabs to patch, to taper tabs to avoid withdrawal

TREATMENT OF OVERDOSE:
Supportive treatment; administer tolazoline, atropine, DOPamine prn

clopidogrel (Rx)
(klo-pid′oh-grel)

Plavix

Func. class.: Platelet aggregation inhibitor

Chem. class.: Thienopyridine derivative

Do not confuse:
Plavix/Paxil/Elavil

ACTION:
Inhibits ADP-induced platelet aggregation

USES:
Reducing the risk of stroke, MI, vascular death, peripheral arterial disease in high-risk patients, acute coronary syndrome, transient ischemic attack (TIA), unstable angina

Unlabeled uses: Cardiac surgery (infant and child), Kawasaki disease

CONTRAINDICATIONS:
Hypersensitivity, active bleeding

Precautions: Pregnancy (B), breastfeeding, children, previous hepatic disease, increased bleeding risk, neutropenia, agranulocytosis, renal disease, Asian/Black/Caucasian patients

Black Box Warning: CYP2C19 allele (poor metabolizers)

DOSAGE AND ROUTES

Recent MI, stroke, peripheral arterial disease

- **Adult: PO** 75 mg/day with/without aspirin

Acute coronary syndrome

- **Adult: PO** loading dose 300 mg then 75 mg/day with aspirin

Cardiac surgery/other cardiac conditions (unlabeled)

- **Child ≤2 yr, infant, neonate: PO** 0.2 mg/kg/day for platelet inhibition

Available forms: Tabs 75, 300 mg

Administer:

- Without regard to food
- Should be discontinued 1 wk before surgery

SIDE EFFECTS

CNS: Headache, dizziness, depression, syncope, hypesthesia, neuralgia

CV: Edema, hypertension, chest pain

GI: Nausea, vomiting, diarrhea, constipation, GI discomfort, **GI bleeding, pancreatitis, hepatic failure**

GU: **Glomerulonephritis**

HEMA: Epistaxis, purpura, **bleeding, neutropenia, aplastic anemia, agranulocytosis, thrombotic thrombocytopenic purpura**

INTEG: Rash, pruritus, **anaphylaxis**

MISC: UTI, hypercholesterolemia, chest pain, fatigue, **intracranial hemorrhage, toxic epidermal necrolysis, Stevens-Johnson syndrome**, flulike syndrome

MS: Arthralgia, back pain

RESP: Upper respiratory tract infection, dyspnea, rhinitis, bronchitis, cough, **bronchospasm**

PHARMACOKINETICS
Rapidly absorbed; peak 1-3 hr; metabolized by liver (CYP3A4); excreted in urine, feces; half-life 8 hr; plasma protein binding 95%; effect on platelets after 3-7 days

INTERACTIONS

- Avoid use with CYP2C19 inhibitors (omeprazole, esomeprazole)

Increase: bleeding risk—anticoagulants, aspirin, NSAIDs, abciximab, eptifibatide, tirofiban, thrombolytics, ticlopidine, SSRIs, treprostinil, rifampin

Increase: action of some NSAIDs, phenytoin, TOLBUTamide, tamoxifen, torsemide, fluvastatin, warfarin

Decrease: clopidogrel effect—proton pump inhibitor (PPIs)
Decrease: CYP3A4 inhibitors/substrates—atorvastatin, simvastatin, cerivastatin
Drug/Herb
Increase: clopidogrel effect—feverfew, fish oil, omega-3 fatty acid, garlic, ginger, ginkgo biloba, green tea, horse chestnut
Decrease: clopidogrel effect—bilberry, saw palmetto
Drug/Lab Test
Increase: AST, ALT, bilirubin, uric acid, total cholesterol, nonprotein nitrogen (NPN)

NURSING CONSIDERATIONS

Assess:
⚠ **Thrombotic/thrombocytic purpura,** fever, thrombocytopenia, neurolytic anemia
• Symptoms of stroke, MI during treatment
• Hepatic studies: AST, ALT, bilirubin, creatinine (long-term therapy)
• Blood studies: CBC, differential, Hct, Hgb, PT, cholesterol (long-term therapy)
Evaluate:
• Therapeutic response: absence of stroke, MI
Teach patient/family:
• That blood work will be necessary during treatment
• To report any unusual bruising, bleeding to prescriber; that it may take longer to stop bleeding
• To take with food or just after eating to minimize GI discomfort
• To report diarrhea, skin rashes, subcutaneous bleeding, chills, fever, sore throat
• To tell all health care providers that clopidogrel is being used; may be held for 7 days before surgery

clorazepate (Rx)

(klor-az′e-pate)

Apo-Clorazepate ✱, Novo-Clopate ✱, Tranxene

Func. class.: Antianxiety, anticonvulsant, sedative/hypnotic
Chem. class.: Benzodiazepine, long-acting

Controlled Substance Schedule IV

Do not confuse:
clorazepate/clonazePAM

ACTION: Potentiates the actions of GABA, especially in the limbic system and the reticular formation

USES: Anxiety, acute alcohol withdrawal, adjunct for seizure disorders
Unlabeled uses: Insomnia

CONTRAINDICATIONS: Pregnancy (D), breastfeeding, children <9 yr, hypersensitivity to benzodiazepines, closed-angle glaucoma, psychosis
Precautions: Geriatric patients, debilitated, renal/hepatic disease, suicidal ideation, dependency problems

DOSAGE AND ROUTES

Anxiety
• **Adult: PO** 15-60 mg/day in divided doses or 7.5 mg tid
• **Geriatric: PO** 7.5 mg daily-bid
Alcohol withdrawal
• **Adult: PO** Day 1: 30 mg then 30-60 mg in divided doses; day 2, 45-90 mg in divided doses; day 3, 22.5-45 mg in divided doses; day 4, 15-30 mg in divided doses; then gradually reduce daily dose to 7.5-15 mg
Seizure disorders
• **Adult and child >12 yr: PO** 7.5 mg tid; may increase by 7.5 mg/wk or less, max 90 mg/day

• **Child 9-12 yr: PO** 3.75-7.5 mg bid; may increase by 3.75 mg/wk or less, max 60 mg/day

Insomnia (unlabeled)

• **Adult: PO** 7.5-15 mg at bedtime

• **Geriatric: PO** 3.75-7.5 mg at bedtime; max 15 mg at bedtime

Available forms: Tabs 3.75, 7.5, 15 mg

Administer:

• With food, milk for GI symptoms

• Crushed if patient cannot swallow whole

SIDE EFFECTS

CNS: *Dizziness, drowsiness,* confusion, headache, anxiety, tremors, stimulation, fatigue, depression, insomnia, hallucinations, lethargy

CV: *Orthostatic hypotension,* ECG changes, tachycardia, hypotension, chest pain

EENT: *Blurred vision,* tinnitus, mydriasis

GI: Constipation, dry mouth, nausea, vomiting, anorexia, diarrhea

INTEG: Rash, dermatitis, itching

PHARMACOKINETICS

PO: Onset 1 hr; peak 1-2 hr; duration up to 24 hr; metabolized by liver; excreted by kidneys; crosses placenta, breast milk; half-life 30-200 hr; 97% protein binding

INTERACTIONS

Increase: clorazepate effects—CNS depressants, alcohol, valproic acid, antidepressants, MAOIs, cimetidine, oral contraceptives, disulfiram, FLUoxetine, isoniazid, ketoconazole, propoxyphene, some β-blockers; CYP3A4 inhibitors

Decrease: clorazepate action—rifampin, barbiturates

Drug/Lab Test

Increase: AST, ALT

Decrease: Hct

NURSING CONSIDERATIONS

Assess:

• **Seizures:** location, duration, intensity, presence of aura

• B/P lying, standing; pulse; if systolic B/P drops 20 mm Hg, hold product, notify prescriber

• Blood studies: CBC during long-term therapy; blood dyscrasias have occurred rarely

• Hepatic studies: AST, ALT, bilirubin, creatinine, LDH, alk phos

• I&O; may indicate renal dysfunction

• **Mental status:** mood, sensorium, affect, sleeping pattern, drowsiness, dizziness; for delirium, tremors, hallucinations during alcohol withdrawal, suicidal thoughts/behaviors

• **Physical dependency, withdrawal symptoms:** headache, nausea, vomiting, muscle pain, weakness after long-term use

Perform/provide:

• Assistance with ambulation during beginning therapy because of drowsiness, dizziness, especially for geriatric patients

• Check to confirm that PO medication has been swallowed

• Sugarless gum, hard candy, frequent sips of water for dry mouth

Evaluate:

• Therapeutic response: decreased anxiety, restlessness, insomnia

Teach patient/family:

• That product may be taken with food

• That product is not to be used for everyday stress or used >4 mo unless directed by prescriber; not to take more than prescribed amount; that product may be habit forming

• To avoid OTC preparations unless approved by prescriber

• That those using product for seizure should carry ID with condition, medications used

• To notify prescriber if pregnancy is planned or suspected (pregnancy D)

• To notify all providers of medication use

• To avoid driving, activities that require alertness; that drowsiness may occur, especially among geriatric patients

• To avoid alcohol, other psychotropic medications unless directed by prescriber

• Not to discontinue medication abruptly after long-term use; that restlessness, insomnia, irritability may occur
• To rise slowly because fainting may occur
• That drowsiness may worsen at beginning of treatment

TREATMENT OF OVERDOSE:

Lavage, VS, supportive care, flumazenil

clotrimazole topical

See Appendix B

clotrimazole vaginal antifungal

See Appendix B

clozapine (Rx)

(kloz′a-peen)

Clozaril, FazaClo

Func. class.: Antipsychotic

Chem. class.: Tricyclic dibenzodiazepine derivative

Do not confuse:
Clozaril/Clinoril/Colazal

ACTION: Interferes with dopamine receptor binding with lack of EPS; also acts as an adrenergic, cholinergic, histaminergic, serotonergic antagonist

USES: Management of psychotic symptoms for schizophrenic patients for whom other antipsychotics have failed; recurrent suicidal behavior

Unlabeled uses: Agitation, bipolar disorder, psychosis in dementia, tremor in Parkinson's disease

CONTRAINDICATIONS: Hypersensitivity, severe granulocytopenia (WBC <3500 before therapy), coma

Black Box Warning: Myeloproliferative disorders, severe CNS depression, agranulocytosis, leukopenia, neutropenia, seizure disorder

Precautions: Pregnancy (B), breastfeeding, children <16 yr, geriatric patients; CV, pulmonary, cardiac, renal, hepatic disease; seizures, prostatic enlargement, closed-angle glaucoma, stroke

Black Box Warning: Bone marrow suppression, dementia, hypotension, myocarditis, orthostatic hypotension, seizures

DOSAGE AND ROUTES

• **Adult: PO** 12.5 mg daily or bid; may increase by 25-50 mg/day; normal range 300-450 mg/day after 2 wk; do not increase dose more than 2×/wk; max 900 mg/day; use lowest dose to control symptoms

Tremor in Parkinson's disease (unlabeled)

• **Adult: PO** 40 mg at bedtime

Dementia with multiple behavioral disturbances (unlabeled)

• **Geriatric: PO** 12.5 mg daily at bedtime, may increase by 12.5 mg every other day, max 50 mg/day

Available forms: Tabs 25, 50, 100, 200 mg; orally disintegrating tabs 25, 100 mg (Fazacio: 12.5, 150, 200 mg)

Administer:

• Patient-specific registration required before administration; if WBC <3500 cells/mm^3 or ANC <2000 cells/mm^3, therapy should not be started
• Check to confirm PO medication swallowed; monitor for hoarding or giving of medication to other patients, if hospitalized; avoid giving patient >7 days' worth of medication if outpatient
• **Orally disintegrating tab:** do not push through foil; leave in foil blister until ready to take, peel back foil, place tab in mouth; allow to dissolve, swallow; water is not needed

SIDE EFFECTS

CNS: Neuroleptic malignant syndrome, *sedation, salivation, dizziness, headache, tremors, sleep problems, akinesia, fever,* seizures, *sweating, akathisia, confusion, fatigue, insomnia,* depression, slurred speech, anxiety, *agitation,* dystonia, obsessive-compulsive symptoms

CV: *Tachycardia, hypo/hypertension,* chest pain, ECG changes, orthostatic hypotension

EENT: *Blurred vision*

GI: *Drooling or excessive salivation, constipation, nausea, abdominal discomfort, vomiting, diarrhea,* anorexia, *weight gain, dry mouth,* heartburn, *dyspepsia, gastroesophageal reflux*

GU: *Urinary abnormalities,* incontinence, ejaculation dysfunction; frequency, urgency, retention, dysuria

HEMA: Leukopenia, agranulocytosis, eosinophilia

MS: Weakness; pain in back, neck, legs; spasm, *rigidity*

OTHER: *Diaphoresis*

RESP: Dyspnea, nasal congestion, lower respiratory tract infection

SYST: Death among geriatric patients with dementia, aggravation of diabetes mellitus

PHARMACOKINETICS

Bioavailability 27%-47%; 97% protein bound; completely metabolized by liver enzymes involved in metabolism CYP1A2, 2D6, 3A4; excreted in urine (50%), feces (30%) (metabolites); half-life 8-12 hr

INTERACTIONS

Increase: CNS depression—CNS depressants, psychoactives, alcohol

Increase: clozapine level—caffeine, citalopram, FLUoxetine, sertraline, ritonavir, risperidone, CYP1A2 inhibitors (fluvoxamine), CYP3A4 inhibitors (ketoconazole, erythromycin)

Increase: plasma concentration—warfarin, digoxin, other highly protein-bound products

Increase: hypotension, respiratory, cardiac arrest, collapse—benzodiazepines

Decrease: clozapine level—CYP1A2 inducers (carBAMazepine, omeprazole, rifampin); PHENobarbital

Drug/Lab Test

Increase: LFTs, cardiac enzymes, cholesterol, blood glucose, bilirubin, PBI, cholinesterase, ^{131}I

False positive: pregnancy tests, PKU

False negative: urinary steroids, 17-OHCS

NURSING CONSIDERATIONS

Assess:

Black Box Warning: Myocarditis; if suspected, discontinue use; myocarditis usually occurs during 1st month of treatment

• Seizures; usually occur with higher doses

• I&O ratio; obtain baseline before treatment begins; palpate bladder if low urinary output occurs

Black Box Warning: Bone marrow depression: bilirubin, CBC, LFTs monthly; discontinue treatment if WBC <3000/mm^3 or ANC <1500/mm^3; test q wk; may resume when normal; if WBC <2000/mm^3 or ANC <1000/mm^3, discontinue

• Urinalysis recommended before, during prolonged therapy

• Affect, orientation, LOC, reflexes, gait, coordination, sleep pattern disturbances

Black Box Warning: Hypotension: B/P standing and lying; take pulse, respirations q4hr during initial treatment; establish baseline before starting treatment; report drops of 30 mm Hg

• Dizziness, faintness, palpitations, tachycardia on rising

• **EPS** including akathisia (inability to sit still, no pattern to movements), tardive dyskinesia (bizarre movements of the jaw, mouth, tongue, extremities), pseudoparkinsonism (rigidity, tremors, pill rolling, shuffling gait)

⚠ **Neuroleptic malignant syndrome:** tachycardia, seizures, fever, dyspnea, diaphoresis, increased/decreased B/P; notify prescriber immediately

• Constipation, urinary retention daily; if these occur, increase bulk, water in diet, especially for geriatric patients; stool softeners, laxatives may be needed

• If diabetic, check blood glucose levels

Perform/provide:

• Supervised ambulation until stabilized on medication; do not involve patient in strenuous exercise program because fainting is possible; patient should not stand still for long periods

• Storage in tight, light-resistant container

Evaluate:

• Therapeutic response: decrease in emotional excitement, hallucinations, delusions, paranoia, reorganization of patterns of thought, speech

Teach patient/family:

• About symptoms of agranulocytosis and need for blood tests weekly for 6 mo, then q2wk; to report flulike symptoms

• That orthostatic hypotension often occurs; to rise gradually from sitting or lying position; to avoid hot tubs, hot showers, tub baths; hypotension may occur

• To avoid abrupt withdrawal of this product because EPS may result; that product should be withdrawn over 1-2 wk

• To avoid OTC preparations (cough, hay fever, cold) unless approved by prescriber, since serious product interactions may occur; to avoid use with alcohol or CNS depressants, increased drowsiness may occur

• About compliance with product regimen

• About EPS and necessity for meticulous oral hygiene, since oral candidiasis may occur

Black Box Warning: To report sore throat, malaise, fever, bleeding, mouth sores; if these occur, CBC should be drawn and product discontinued

• That heat stroke may occur in hot weather; to take extra precautions to stay cool

• To avoid driving, other hazardous activities; seizures may occur

• To notify prescriber if pregnant or if pregnancy is intended; not to breastfeed

TREATMENT OF OVERDOSE:

Lavage, activated charcoal; provide an airway; do not induce vomiting

codeine (Rx)

(koe′deen)

Paveral ✱

Func. class.: Opiate analgesic, antitussive

Chem. class.: Opiate, phenathrene derivative

Controlled Substance Schedule II, III, IV, V (depends on content)

Do not confuse:
codeine/Lodine/iodine/Cardene

ACTION:

Depresses pain impulse transmission at the spinal cord level by interacting with opioid receptors; decreases cough reflex, GI motility

USES:

Moderate to severe pain

Unlabeled uses: Diarrhea, arthralgia, bone/dental pain, headache, migraine, myalgia, nonproductive cough

CONTRAINDICATIONS:

Breastfeeding, hypersensitivity to opiates, respiratory depression, increased intracranial pressure, seizure disorders, severe respiratory disorders

Precautions: Pregnancy (C), geriatric patients, cardiac dysrhythmias, prostatic hypertrophy, bowel impaction

DOSAGE AND ROUTES

Pain

- **Adult: PO/IM/SUBCUT** 15-60 mg q4hr prn
- **Child 6-17 yr: PO** 3 mg/kg/day in divided doses q4hr prn

Cough

- **Adult: PO** 10-20 mg q4-6hr, max 120 mg/day

Renal disease

- **Adult: PO** CCr 10-50 ml/min, 75% of dose; CCr <10 ml/min, 50% of dose

Diarrhea (unlabeled)

- **Adult: PO** 30 mg; may repeat qid prn

Arthralgia/bone pain/back pain/dental pain/headache/migraine/myalgia (unlabeled)

- **Adult: PO/IM/SUBCUT** 15-60 mg q4-6hr
- **Child ≥3 yr: IM/SUBCUT** 0.5-1 mg/kg or 15 mg/m^2 (max 60 mg/dose) q4-6hr

Available forms: Inj tab 30, 60 mg; tabs 15, 30, 60 mg; inj 15, 30 mg/ml

Administer:

Discontinue gradually after long-term use

IM/SUBCUT route

- Do not use if precipitate is present
- Usually given IM/SUBCUT
- With antiemetic for nausea, vomiting
- When pain is beginning to return; determine dosage interval by patient response

IV route

- **Direct IV:** Give slowly by direct inj

Syringe compatibilities: DimenhyDRINATE, glycopyrrolate, hydrOXYzine

Y-site compatibilities: Amifostine, amikacin, aminophylline, ammonium, ampicillin-sulbactam, aztreonam, bleomycin, bumetanide, busulfan, calcium gluconate, CARBOplatin, carmustine, ceFAZolin, cefotaxime, cefotetan, cefoxitin, ceftazidime, ceftizoxime, cefTRIAXone, cefuroxime, chlorproMAZINE, cimetidine, ciprofloxacin, CISplatin, clindamycin, cyclophosphamide, cycloSPORINE, cytarabine, DACTINomycin, DAUNOrubicin, dexamethasone, dexrazoxane, digoxin, diphenhydrAMINE, DOBUTamine, docetaxel, DOPamine, DOXOrubicin, doxycycline, droperidol, enalaprilat, etoposide, etoposide phosphate, famotidine, floxuridine, fluconazole, fludarabine, fluorouracil, gemcitabine, gentamicin, haloperidol, heparin, hydrocortisone phosphate, hydrocortisone succinate, hydrOXYzine, IDArubicin, ifosfamide, imipenem-cilastatin, leucovorin, levofloxacin, magnesium sulfate, mesna, metoclopramide, metroNIDAZOLE, mezlocillin, minocycline, mitomycin, mitoxantrone, netilmicin, ofloxacin, ondansetron, paclitaxel, plicamycin, potassium chloride, prochlorperazine, promethazine, ranitidine, sodium bicarbonate, streptozocin, teniposide, theophylline, thiotepa, ticarcillin, tobramycin, topotecan, trimethobenzamide, vancomycin, vinBLAStine, vinCRIStine, vinorelbine, zidovudine

SIDE EFFECTS

CNS: *Drowsiness, sedation,* dizziness, agitation, dependency, lethargy, restlessness, euphoria, **seizures**, hallucinations, headache, confusion

CV: Bradycardia, palpitations, orthostatic hypotension, tachycardia, **circulatory collapse**

GI: *Nausea, vomiting, anorexia, constipation,* dry mouth

GU: Urinary retention

INTEG: Flushing, rash, urticaria, pruritus

RESP: **Respiratory depression, respiratory paralysis,** dyspnea

SYST: **Anaphylaxis**

PHARMACOKINETICS

Bioavailability 60%-90%; peak ½-1 hr; duration 4-6 hr; metabolized by liver (CYP3A4); excreted by kidneys, in breast milk; crosses placenta; half-life 3 hr; protein binding 7%; altered codeine metabolism occurs in different ethnic groups

PO: Onset 30-60 min

IM: Onset 10-30 min

INTERACTIONS

Increase: CNS depression—CYP2D6, alcohol, opiates, sedative/hypnotics, antipsychotics, skeletal muscle relaxants

⚠ **Increase:** toxicity—MAOIs; use cautiously

Drug/Lab Test

Increase: lipase, amylase

NURSING CONSIDERATIONS

Assess:

- **Pain:** intensity, type, location, aggravating, alleviating factors; need for pain medication, tolerance; use pain scoring
- I&O ratio; check for decreasing output; may indicate urinary retention, especially among geriatric patients
- GI function: nausea, vomiting, constipation
- **Cough:** type, duration, ability to raise secretion for productive cough; do not use to suppress productive cough
- CNS changes, dizziness, drowsiness, hallucinations, euphoria, LOC, pupil reaction
- Allergic reactions: rash, urticaria

⚠ **Respiratory dysfunction:** respiratory depression, character, rate, rhythm; notify prescriber if respirations are <10/min, shallow

Perform/provide:

- Storage in light-resistant container at room temp
- Assistance with ambulation if needed
- Safety measures: top side rails, nightlight, call bell

Evaluate:

- Therapeutic response: decrease in pain, absence of grimacing, decreased cough, decreased diarrhea

Teach patient/family:

- Not to breastfeed
- To report any symptoms of CNS changes, allergic reactions
- That physical dependency may result after extended periods
- To decrease dry mouth use sugarless gum, rinse mouth often
- To change position slowly; orthostatic hypotension may occur
- To avoid hazardous activities if drowsiness, dizziness occurs
- To avoid alcohol, other CNS depressants unless directed by prescriber

TREATMENT OF OVERDOSE:

Naloxone 0.4-mg ampule diluted in 10 ml 0.9% NaCl and given by direct IV push, 0.02 mg q2min (adult)

colchicine (Rx)

(kol′chih-seen)

Colcrys

Func. class.: Antigout agent

Chem. class.: ***Colchicum autumnale*** alkaloid

ACTION:

Inhibits microtubule formation of lactic acid in leukocytes, which decreases phagocytosis and inflammation in joints

USES:

Gout, gouty arthritis (prevention, treatment); to arrest the progression of neurologic disability in those with MS

Unlabeled uses: Hepatic cirrhosis, Mediterranean fever, pericarditis, amyloidosis, Behçet's syndrome, biliary cirrhosis, dermatitis herpetiformis, idiopathic thrombocytopenic purpura, Paget's disease, pseudogout, pulmonary fibrosis

CONTRAINDICATIONS:

Pregnancy (D) (injectable), serious GI, severe cardiac/renal/hepatic disorders, hypersensitivity

Precautions: Pregnancy (C) (PO), breastfeeding, children, geriatric patients, blood dyscrasias, hepatic disease

DOSAGE AND ROUTES

Gout prevention

- **Adult: PO** 0.6-1.8 mg/day, depending on severity

Gout treatment
• **Adult: PO** 1.2 mg initially, then 0.6 mg 1 hr later (1.8 mg); for those on strong CYP3A4 inhibitor (during past 14 days), 0.6 mg initially, then 0.3 mg 1 hr later
Renal dose
• **Adult: PO** CCr <30 ml/min, for acute gout, do not repeat course for 2 wk; for familial Mediterranean fever, 0.3 mg daily, increase cautiously
Mediterranean fever (unlabeled)
• **Adult: PO** 0.6 mg qhr × 4 doses, then q2hr × 2 doses, then 1.2 mg q12hr × 2 days
Amyloidosis/biliary cirrhosis/dermatitis herpetiformis/Paget's disease/Behçet's syndrome/chronic idiopathic thrombocytopenic purpura/pulmonary fibrosis (unlabeled)
• **Adult: PO** 0.5-0.6 mg bid-tid
Available forms: Tabs 0.5, 0.6, 1 ✱ mg
Administer:
PO route
• With food for GI symptoms
• Cumulative doses ≤4 mg, renal patients ≤2 mg; when reached, administer only for 3 wk

SIDE EFFECTS

GI: *Nausea, vomiting, anorexia, malaise,* metallic taste, cramps, peptic ulcer, diarrhea
GU: **Hematuria, oliguria, renal damage**
HEMA: **Agranulocytosis, thrombocytopenia, aplastic anemia, pancytopenia**
INTEG: Chills, dermatitis, pruritus, purpura, erythema
MISC: Myopathy, alopecia, reversible azoospermia, peripheral neuritis

PHARMACOKINETICS

PO: Peak ½-2 hr, half-life 4.4 hr, deacetylates in liver, excreted in feces (metabolites/active product)

INTERACTIONS

Increase: toxicity—cycloSPORINE, clarithromycin, erythromycin
Increase: GI effects—NSAIDs, ethanol
Increase: bone marrow depression—radiation, bone marrow depressants, cycloSPORINE
Decrease: action of vit B_{12}; may cause reversible malabsorption
Drug/Lab Test
Increase: alk phos, AST
False positive: urine Hgb
Interference: urinary 17-hydroxycorticosteroids

NURSING CONSIDERATIONS

Assess:
• Relief of pain, uric acid levels returning to normal
• I&O ratio; observe for decrease in urinary output
⚠ **CBC, platelets, reticulocytes before, during therapy (q3mo); may cause aplastic anemia, agranulocytosis, decreased platelets**
• **Toxicity:** weakness, abdominal pain, nausea, vomiting, diarrhea; product should be discontinued, report symptoms immediately
Evaluate:
• Therapeutic response: decreased stone formation, decreased pain in kidney region, absence of hematuria, decreased pain in joints
Teach patient/family:
• To avoid alcohol, OTC preparations that contain alcohol
• To report any pain, redness, hard areas, usually in legs; rash, sore throat, fever, bleeding, bruising, weakness, numbness, tingling, nausea, vomiting, abdominal pain
• About the importance of complying with medical regimen (diet, weight loss, product therapy); about the possibility of bone marrow depression occurring
• Advise all providers of product use; surgery may increase possibility of acute gout symptoms

TREATMENT OF OVERDOSE:

D/C medication; may need opioids to treat diarrhea

colesevelam (Rx)

(koe-leh-seve′eh-lam)

WelChol

Func. class.: Antilipemic

Chem. class.: Bile acid sequestrant

ACTION: Absorbs, combines with bile acids to form insoluble complex excreted through feces; loss of bile acids lowers cholesterol levels

USES: Elevated LDL cholesterol, alone or in combination with HMG-COA reductase inhibitor; type 2 diabetes (adjunct)

CONTRAINDICATIONS: Hypersensitivity, biliary obstruction, dysphagia, bowel disease, primary biliary cirrhosis, triglycerides >300 mg/dl, fat-soluble vitamin deficiency

Precautions: Pregnancy (B), breastfeeding, children

DOSAGE AND ROUTES

Monotherapy

• **Adult: PO** 3 625-mg tabs bid with meals or 6 tabs daily with meal; may increase to 7 tabs if needed

Combination therapy

• **Adult: PO** 3 tabs bid with meals or 6 tabs daily with meal given with an HMG-CoA reductase inhibitor

Type 2 diabetes, adjunct (to improve glycemic control)

• **Adult and geriatric: PO** Approx 3.8 g (6 tabs)/day or approx 1.9 g (3 tabs) bid

Heterozygous familial hypercholesterolemia

• **Females (postmenarchal and >10 yr) and males ≥10 yr: PO** 1.875-g packet bid or 3.75-g packet daily dissolved in 4-8 oz of water with meal

Available forms: Tabs 625 mg; powder for oral susp 3.75 g

Administer:

• Swallow tabs whole; do not break, crush, or chew

• Drug daily or bid with meals; give all other medications 1 hr before or 4 hr after colesevelam; with liquid to avoid poor absorption

SIDE EFFECTS

CNS: Headache, dizziness, drowsiness, vertigo, tinnitus

GI: *Constipation, abdominal pain, nausea,* fecal impaction, hemorrhoids, flatulence, vomiting, GI obstruction

INTEG: Rash, irritation of perianal area, tongue, skin

MISC: Hypertriglycerides, hypoglycemia

MS: Muscle, joint pain

PHARMACOKINETICS

Excreted in feces, peak response 2 wk

INTERACTIONS

Decrease: absorption of diltiazem, gemfibrozil, mycophenolate, phenytoin, propranolol, warfarin, thiazides, digoxin, penicillin G, tetracyclines, corticosteroids, iron, thyroid, fat-soluble vitamins, glyburide

Decrease: action of—oral contraceptives

Drug/Lab Test

Increase: LFTs

NURSING CONSIDERATIONS

Assess:

• Cardiac glycoside level, if both products administered

• Fasting LDL, HDL, total cholesterol, triglyceride levels, electrolytes if on extended therapy

• Bowel pattern daily; increase bulk, water in diet for constipation

Evaluate:

• Therapeutic response: decreased total cholesterol level, LDL cholesterol, apolipoproteins

Teach patient/family:

• About the importance of compliance; toxicity may result if doses missed

• That risk factors should be decreased: high-fat diet, smoking, alcohol consumption, absence of exercise

colestipol (Rx)

(koe-les′ti-pole)

Colestid

Func. class.: Antilipemic

Chem. class.: Bile acid sequestrant

ACTION: Absorbs, combines with bile acids to form insoluble complex excreted through feces; loss of bile acids lowers cholesterol levels

USES: Primary hypercholesterolemia, xanthomas

Unlabeled uses: Digotoxin toxicity/overdose, pruritus, diarrhea due to increased bile acids after surgery

CONTRAINDICATIONS: Hypersensitivity, biliary obstruction

Precautions: Pregnancy (B), breastfeeding, children, bleeding disorders

DOSAGE AND ROUTES

- **Adult: PO** Tabs 2 g daily-bid, may increase q1mo, max 16 g/day; powder 5-30 g mixed with liquid daily or in divided doses

Digotoxin toxicity/overdose, digoxin overdose (unlabeled)

- Adult: **PO** 10 g then 5 g q6-8hr

Diarrhea/pruritus (unlabeled)

- **Adult: PO** granules 5 g daily-bid, may increase by 5 g/day at 1-2 mo intervals, max 30 g/day in 1-2 divided doses

Available forms: Powder/packet/scoop (granules) 5 g; tabs 1 g

Administer:

- Swallow tabs whole; do not break, crush, or chew; take tabs one at a time
- Product daily or bid; give all other medications 1 hr before or 4 hr after colestipol to avoid poor absorption; use of powdered products may not be bioequivalent with other products
- Product mixed in applesauce or stirred into beverage (2-6 oz); do not take dry; let stand for 2 min
- Supplemental doses of vit A, D, K if levels are low

SIDE EFFECTS

GI: *Constipation, abdominal pain, nausea,* fecal impaction, hemorrhoids, flatulence, vomiting, steatorrhea, peptic ulcer

HEMA: Bleeding, increased PT

INTEG: *Rash,* irritation of perianal area, tongue, skin

META: *Decreased vit A, D, K,* red folate content; **hyperchloremic acidosis**

PHARMACOKINETICS

PO: Onset 24-48 hr, peak/duration 30 days, excreted in feces after binding bile acids

INTERACTIONS

Decrease: action of atorvastatin, bexarotene, calcifediol, calcitriol, NSAIDs, ezetimibe, fenofibric acid, mycophenolate, phosphorous salts, vancomycin, thiazides, digoxin, warfarin, penicillin G, gemfibrozil, glipiZIDE, propranolol, phenytoin, TOLBUTamide, tetracycline, corticosteroids, iron, thyroid agents, fat-soluble vitamins

Drug/Lab Test

Increase: AST, ALT, alk phos, chloride, phosphorus, PT

Decrease: sodium, potassium, calcium

NURSING CONSIDERATIONS

Assess:

- Hypercholesterolemia: diet history: fat consumption in diet; serum cholesterol, triglyceride levels, electrolytes (extended therapy)
- Cardiac glycoside levels, if both products administered
- For signs of vit A, D, K deficiency
- **Diarrhea:** bowel pattern daily; increase bulk, water in diet if constipation develops

Evaluate:

- Therapeutic response: decreased LDL cholesterol; decreased pruritus, diarrhea

Teach patient/family:

⚠ About the **symptoms of hypoprothrombinemia:** bleeding mucous membranes; dark, tarry stools; hematuria, petechiae; report immediately

• That compliance is needed; not to miss or double doses

• That risk factors should be decreased: high-fat diet, smoking, alcohol consumption, absence of exercise

conivaptan (Rx)

(kon-ih-vap′tan)

Vaprisol

Func. class.: Vasopressin receptor antagonist

ACTION: Dual arginine vasopressin (AVP) antagonist with affinity for V_{1A}, V_2 receptors; level of AVP in circulating blood is critical for regulation of water, electrolyte balance and is usually elevated in euvolemic/hypervolemic hyponatremia

USES: Euvolemia hyponatremia in hospitalized patients; not indicated for CHF, hypervolemic hyponatremia

CONTRAINDICATIONS: Hypersensitivity, hypovolemia

Precautions: Pregnancy (C), breastfeeding, orthostatic disease, renal disease, heart failure, rapid correction of serum sodium

DOSAGE AND ROUTES

• **Adult: IV INF** loading dose 20 mg given over 30 min then **CONT IV** over 24 hr; after 1 day, give for an additional 1-3 days as a **CONT INF** of 20 mg/day total; can be titrated up to 40 mg/day if serum sodium is not rising at desired rate; max time 4 days

Hepatic/renal dose

• **Adult: IV**

• **Child-Pugh A-C or CCr 30-60 ml/min:** give IV loading dose over 10 min then **CONT IV INF** 10 mg over 24 hr × 2-4 days

Available forms: 5 mg/ml (20 mg/4 ml) in single-use ampule; 20 mg/100 ml in D_5 for inj

Administer:

IV route

• Withdraw 4 ml (20 mg), add to 100 ml D_5W, gently invert several times to mix, give over 30 min

Continuous IV INF route

• Withdraw 4 ml (20 mg), add to 250 ml D_5W, gently invert several times to mix, give over 24 hr; or give 40 mg in 250 ml D_5W, gently invert several times to mix, give over 24 hr

SIDE EFFECTS

CNS: Headache, confusion, insomnia

CV: Atrial fibrillation, hypo/hypertension, *orthostatic hypotension,* phlebitis

GI: Nausea, vomiting, constipation, dry mouth

GU: Hematuria, polyuria, UTI, pollakiuria

HEMA: Anemia

INTEG: Erythemia, inj site reaction

META: Dehydration, hypo/hyperglycemia, hypokalemia, hypomagnesia, hyponatremia

MISC: Oral candidiasis, pain, peripheral edema, pneumonia

PHARMACOKINETICS

Protein binding 99%, metabolized by CYP3A4, terminal half-life 5 hr

INTERACTIONS

Increase: effect of—CYP3A4 substrates (alfuzosin, aripiprazole, bexarolene, bortezomib, bosentan, bupivacaine, buprenorphine, carBAMazepine, cevimeline, cilostazol, cinacalcet, clopidogrel, colchicine, cyclobenzaprine, dapsone, darifenacin, disopyramide, docetaxel, donepezil, DOXOrubicin, dutasteride, eletriptan, eplerenone, ergots, erlotinib, eszopiclone, ethinyl estradiol, ethosuximide, etoposide, fentaNYL, galantamine, gefitinib, halofantrine, ifosfamide, irinotecan, levobupivacaine, levomethadyl, lidocaine, loperimide, loratadine, mefloquine, methadone, modafinil, paclitaxel, paricalcitrol, pimozide, praziquantel, quiNIDine, quiNINE, ramelteon, reboxetine, repaglinide, rifabutin, sibutramine, sildenafil, sirolimus, SUFentanil, sunitinib, tacrolimus, tamoxifen, teniposide, testosterone, tiagabine, tinidazole, trimetrexate, vardenafil, vinca alkaloids, ziprasidone, zolpidem, zonisamide); do not use concurrently

NURSING CONSIDERATIONS

Assess:

- Renal, hepatic function
- Frequent sodium volume status; overly rapid correction of sodium concentration (>12 mEq/L per 24 hr) may result in osmotic demyelination syndrome
- Neurologic status: confusion, headache
- CV status: atrial fibrillation, hypo/hypertension, orthostatic hypotension; monitor B/P, pulse
- Monitor other electrolytes (magnesium and potassium)

Evaluate:

- Therapeutic response: correction of serum sodium levels

Teach patient/family:

- To avoid pregnancy, breastfeeding while taking this product
- To report neurologic changes: headache, insomnia, confusion
- About administration procedure and expected results
- To report inj site pain, redness, swelling

CONTRACEPTIVES, HORMONAL

Monophasic, Oral

ethinyl estradiol/desogestrel (Rx)

Apri, Cesia, Desogen, Kariva, Mircette, Ortho-Cept, Reclipsen, Solia, Velivet

ethinyl estradiol/drospirenone (Rx)

Yasmin, Yaz 28

ethinyl estradiol/ethynodiol (Rx)

Kelnor 1/35, Zovia

ethinyl estradiol/levonorgestrel (Rx)

Alesse, Aviane-28, Enpresse, Jolessa, Lessina, Levlen, Levlite, Levora, Lutera, Nordette, Portia, Quasense, Seasonique, Sronyx

ethinyl estradiol/norethindrone (Rx)

Brevicon, Genora 0.5/35, Genora 1/35, Junel 21 1/20, Junel 21 1.5/20, Loestrin 21 1.5/30, Loestrin 21 1/20, Microgestin, Modicon, N.E.E 1/35, Nelova 0.5/35E, Nelova 1/35E, Norcept-E 1/35, Norethin 1/35E, Norinyl 1+35, Norlestrin 1/50, Norlestrin 2.5/50, Nortrel

ethinyl estradiol/norgestimate (Rx)

MonoNessa, Ortho-Cyclen, Previfem, Sprintec

ethinyl estradiol/norgestrel (Rx)

Cryselle, Lo/Ovral, Low-Ogestrel, Ogestrel, Ovral

mestranol/norethindrone (Rx)
Genora 1/50, Nelova 1/50m, Norethin 1/50m, Norinyl 1+50, Ortho-Novum 1/50

Biphasic, Oral

ethinyl estradiol/norethindrone (Rx)
Nelova 10/11, Ortho-Novum 10/11

Triphasic, Oral

ethinyl estradiol/desogestrel (Rx)
Cyclessa

ethinyl estradiol/norethindrone (Rx)
Necor 7/7/7, Nortrel 7/7/7, Ortho-Novum 7/7/7, Tri-Norinyl

ethinyl estradiol/norgestimate (Rx)
Ortho Tri-Cyclen, Ortho Tri-Cyclen Lo

ethinyl estradiol/levonorgestrel (Rx)
Enpresse, Tri-Levlen, Triphasil

Extended Cycle, Oral

ethinyl estradiol/levonorgestrel (Rx)
Seasonale

Progestin, Oral

norethindrone (Rx)
Errin, Ortho Micronor, Camila, Jolivette, Nor-Q D

Progressive Estrogen, Oral

ethinyl estradiol/norethindrone acetate (Rx)
Estrostep, Estrostep Fe

Emergency

levonorgestrel/ethinyl estradiol (Rx)
Preven

levonorgestrel (Rx)
Plan B

medroxyprogesterone (Rx)
Depo-Provera

Intrauterine

levonorgestrel (Rx)
Mirena

Implant

etonogestrel (Rx)
Implanon

Vaginal Ring

ethinyl estradiol/etonogestrel (Rx)
Nuva Ring

Transdermal

ethinyl estradiol/norelgestromin (Rx)
Ortho Evra

ACTION: Prevents ovulation by suppressing FSH and LH; *monophasic:* estrogen/progestin (fixed dose) used during a 21-day cycle; ovulation is inhibited by suppression of FSH and LH; thickness of cervical mucus and endometrial lining prevents pregnancy; *biphasic:* ovulation is inhibited by suppression of FSH and LH; alteration of cervical mucus, endometrial lining prevents pregnancy; *triphasic:* ovulation is inhibited by suppression of FSH and LH; change of cervical mucus, endometrial lining prevents pregnancy; variable doses of estrogen/progestin combinations may be similar to natural hormonal fluctuations; *extended cycle:* estrogen/progestin continuous for

84 days, off for 7 days, results in 4 menstrual periods/yr; *progressive estrogen:* constant progestin with 3 progressive doses of estrogen; *progestin-only pill, implant, intrauterine:* change of cervical mucus and endometrial lining prevents pregnancy; ovulation may be suppressed

USES:
To prevent pregnancy, regulation of menstrual cycle, treatment of acne in women >14 yr for whom other treatment has failed, emergency contraception; *injection:* inhibits gonadotropin secretion, ovulation, follicular maturation; *emergency:* inhibits ovulation and fertilization, decreases transport of sperm and egg from fallopian tube to uterus; *vaginal ring, transdermal:* inhibits ovulation, prevents sperm entry into uterus; *antiacne:* may decrease sex hormone binding globulin, results in decreased testosterone

CONTRAINDICATIONS:
Pregnancy (X), breastfeeding, women ≥40 yr, reproductive cancer, thrombophlebitis, MI, hepatic tumors, hepatic disease, CAD, CVA

Precautions: Depression, hypertension, renal disease, seizure disorders, lupus erythematosus, rheumatic disease, migraine headache, amenorrhea, irregular menses, breast cancer (fibrocystic), gallbladder disease, diabetes mellitus, heavy smoking, acute mononucleosis, sickle cell disease

DOSAGE AND ROUTES

Monophasic

- **Adult: PO** Take first tab on Sunday after start of menses × 21 days; skip 7 days, then repeat cycle; start on 1st day of menses × 21 days; skip 7 days, then repeat cycle; may contain 7 placebo tabs when 1 tab is taken daily

Biphasic

- **Adult: PO** Take 10 days of small progestin, then large progestin; estrogen is the same during cycle; skip 7 days, then repeat cycle; may contain 7 placebo tabs when 1 tab is taken daily

Triphasic

- **Adult: PO** Estrogen dose remains constant, progestin changes throughout 21-day cycle, some products contain 28 tabs per month

Extended cycle

- **Adult: PO** Start taking on 1st day of menses; continue for 84 days of active tab, then 7 days of placebo; repeat cycle

Progestin

- **Adult: PO** Start on 1st day of menses, then daily and continuously

Progressive estrogen

- **Adult: PO** Progestin dose remains constant, estrogen increases q7days throughout 21-day cycle, may include 7 placebo tabs for 28-day cycle

Emergency

- **Adult/adolescent:** Give within 72 hr of intercourse, repeat 12 hr later; **Plan B** 1 tab, then 1 tab 12 hr later; **Preven** 2 tab, then 2 tab 12 hr later; **Ovral (unlabeled)** 2 white tabs; **Lo/Ovral (unlabeled)** 4 white tabs; **Levlen (unlabeled), Nordette (unlabeled)** 4 orange tabs; **Triphasil (unlabeled), Tri-Levlen (unlabeled)** 4 yellow tabs

Injectable

- **Adult: IM (Depo-Provera)** 150 mg within 5 days of start of menses or within 5 days postpartum (must not be breastfeeding); if breastfeeding, give 6 wk postpartum, repeat q3mo

Intrauterine

- **Adult:** To be inserted using the levonorgestrel-releasing intrauterine system (LRIS) by those trained in procedure; inserted into uterine cavity within 7 days of the onset of menstruation; use should not exceed 5 yr per implant

Vaginal ring

- **Adult: VAG** Insert 1 ring on or prior to day 5 of cycle, leave in place 3 wk; remove for 1 wk, then repeat

Transdermal

- **Adult: TD** Apply patch within 7 days of menses, change weekly × 3 wk; no patch wk 4, repeat cycle

Implant

• **Adult: SUBDERMAL** In inner side of upper arm on days 1-5 of menses, replace q3yr

Acne

• **Adult: PO (Ortho Tri-Cyclen)** Take daily × 21 days, off 7 days

Administer:

• PO with food for GI symptoms; give at same time each day

• Subdermal implant of 6 caps effective for 5 yr, then should be removed

• IM inj deep in large muscle mass after shaking suspension; ensure patient not pregnant if inj are 2 wk or more apart

SIDE EFFECTS

CNS: Depression, fatigue, dizziness, nervousness, anxiety, headache

CV: Increased B/P, cerebral hemorrhage, thrombosis, pulmonary embolism, fluid retention, edema

EENT: Optic neuritis, retinal thrombosis, cataracts

ENDO: Decreased glucose tolerance, increased TBG, PBI, T_4, T_3

GI: *Nausea,* vomiting, cramps, diarrhea, bloating, constipation, change in appetite, cholestatic jaundice

GU: Breakthrough bleeding, amenorrhea, spotting, dysmenorrhea, galactorrhea, endocervical hyperplasia, vaginitis, cystitis-like syndrome, breast changes

HEMA: Increased fibrinogen, clotting factor

INTEG: *Chloasma, melasma,* acne, rash, urticaria, erythema, pruritus, hirsutism, alopecia, photosensitivity

PHARMACOKINETICS

Excreted in breast milk

INTERACTIONS

Decrease: oral contraceptives effectiveness—anticonvulsants, rifampin, analgesics, antibiotics, antihistamines, griseofulvin

Decrease: oral anticoagulants action

Drug/Herb

• Altered action: black cohosh

Decrease: oral contraceptives effect—saw palmetto, St. John's wort

Drug/Food

Increase: peak level—grapefruit juice

Drug/Lab Test

Increase: PT; clotting factors VII, VIII, IX, X; TBG, PBI, T_4, platelet aggregability, BSP, triglycerides, bilirubin, AST, ALT

Decrease: T_3, antithrombin III, folate, metyrapone test, GTT, 17-OHCS

NURSING CONSIDERATIONS

Assess:

• Glucose, thyroid function, LFTs

• Reproductive changes: changes in breasts, tumors; positive Pap smear; product should be discontinued

Evaluate:

• Therapeutic response: absence of pregnancy, endometriosis, hypermenorrhea

Teach patient/family:

• About detection of clots using Homan's sign

• To use sunscreen or avoid sunlight; photosensitivity can occur

• To take at same time each day to ensure equal product level

• To report GI symptoms that occur after 4 mo

• To use another birth control method during 1st week of oral contraceptive use

• To take another tablet as soon as possible if one is missed

• That, after product is discontinued, pregnancy may not occur for several months

• To report abdominal pain, change in vision, shortness of breath, change in menstrual flow, spotting, breakthrough bleeding, breast lumps, swelling, headache, severe leg pain

• That continuing medical care is needed: Pap smear and gynecologic examinations q6mo

• To notify health care providers and dentists of oral contraceptive use

RARELY USED

corticotropin (ACTH) (Rx)

(kor-ti-koe-troe′pin)

H.P. Acthar Gel

Func. class.: Pituitary hormone

USES: Testing of adrenocortical function, treatment of adrenal insufficiency caused by administration of corticosteroids (long term), MS, myasthenia gravis, infantile spasms in child <2 yr

CONTRAINDICATIONS: Hypersensitivity, scleroderma, osteoporosis, CHF, peptic ulcer disease, hypertension, systemic fungal infections, smallpox vaccination, recent surgery, ocular herpes simplex, primary adrenocortical insufficiency/hyperfunction

DOSAGE AND ROUTES

Acute exacerbations of multiple sclerosis

• **Adult: IM** 80-120 units/day × 14-21 days

Infantile spasms

• **Infant: IM GEL** 75 units/m^2 bid × 2 wk, increase if needed

cortisone (Rx)

(kor′ti-sone)

Cortone ♣

Func. class.: Corticosteroid, synthetic

Chem. class.: Glucocorticoid, short-acting

ACTION: Decreases inflammation by suppression of migration of polymorphonuclear leukocytes, fibroblasts, reversal of increased capillary permeability and lysosomal stabilization

USES: Inflammation, severe allergy, adrenal insufficiency, collagen disorders; respiratory, dermatologic, rheumatic disorders, CLL, ALL, Hodgkin's/non-Hodgkin's lymphoma, endocrine system disorders, eye disorders, Crohn's/ulcerative colitis, hypercalcemia of malignancy, mycosis fungoides, nephrotic syndrome, TB of meninges

Unlabeled uses: Temporal arteritis, Churg-Strauss syndrome, mixed connective-tissue disease, polyarteritis nodosa, relapsing polychondritis, polymyalgia rheumatica, vasculitis, Wegener's granulomatosis, multiple myeloma

CONTRAINDICATIONS: Pregnancy (D), children <2 yr, psychosis, hypersensitivity, idiopathic thrombocytopenia, acute glomerulonephritis, amebiasis, fungal infections, nonasthmatic bronchial disease, AIDS, TB, measles, varicella

Precautions: Breastfeeding, diabetes mellitus, glaucoma, osteoporosis, seizure disorders, ulcerative colitis, CHF, myasthenia gravis, renal/hepatic disease, esophagitis, peptic ulcer

DOSAGE AND ROUTES

• **Adult: PO** 25-300 mg/day or q2days, titrated to response

Multiple myeloma/temporal arteritis/Churg-Strauss syndrome/mixed connective-tissue disease/polyarteritis nodosa/relapsing polychondritis/polymyalgia rheumatica/vasculitis/Wegener's granulomatosis (unlabeled)

• **Adult: PO** 25-300 mg/day or alternate days

Available forms: Tabs 25 mg

Administer:

• Titrated dose; use lowest effective dose
• In 1 dose in AM to prevent adrenal suppression
• With food or milk to decrease GI symptoms

SIDE EFFECTS

CNS: *Depression, flushing, sweating,* headache, mood changes, insomnia

CV: *Hypertension,* circulatory collapse, thrombophlebitis, embolism, tachycardia, necrotizing angiitis, CHF, edema
EENT: Fungal infections, increased intraocular pressure, blurred vision, cataracts, glaucoma
GI: *Diarrhea, nausea, abdominal distention,* GI hemorrhage, increased appetite, pancreatitis, ulcerative esophagitis
HEMA: Thrombocytopenia
INTEG: Acne, poor wound healing, ecchymosis, bruising, petechiae, hirsutism
META: Sodium, fluid retention, potassium loss, diabetes
MS: Fractures, osteoporosis, weakness, loss of muscle mass

PHARMACOKINETICS

Peak 2 hr, duration $1^1/_2$ days, half-life 8-12 hr

INTERACTIONS

Increase: effect of—cyclosporine, tacrolimus
Increase: tendon rupture—fluoroquinolones
Increase: hypokalemia—thiazide/loop diuretics, amphotericin B
Increase: action of cortisone—salicylates, estrogens, indomethacin, hormonal contraceptives, ketoconazole, macrolide antiinfectives
Increase: side effects—alcohol, salicylates, NSAIDs
Decrease: effects of antidiabetics, toxoids, vaccines, salicylates, insulins
Decrease: cortisone action—barbiturates, rifampin, phenytoin, theophylline, acetylcholinesterases
Increase or decrease: effect of—anticoagulants

Drug/Lab Test
Increase: cholesterol, Na, blood glucose, uric acid, Ca, urine glucose
Decrease: Ca, K, T_4, T_3, thyroid ^{131}I uptake test, urine 17-OHCS, 17-KS
False negative: Skin allergy tests

NURSING CONSIDERATIONS

Assess:
- Potassium; blood glucose while receiving long-term therapy; hypokalemia, hyperglycemia may occur
- Weight daily; notify prescriber of weekly gain >5 lb
- B/P, pulse; notify prescriber if chest pain occurs
- I&O ratio; be alert for decreasing urinary output, increasing edema
- Plasma cortisol levels during long-term therapy (normal level: 138-635 nmol/L SI units if drawn at 8 AM)
- **Infection:** fever, WBC even after withdrawal of medication; product masks infection
- Potassium depletion: paresthesias, fatigue, nausea, vomiting, depression, polyuria, dysrhythmias, weakness
- Edema, hypertension, cardiac symptoms
- Mental status: affect, mood, behavioral changes, aggression
- Growth inhibition: monitor children receiving long-term therapy

Perform/provide:
- Assistance with ambulation for patient with bone-tissue disease to prevent fractures

Evaluate:
- Therapeutic response: decreased inflammation

Teach patient/family:
- That medical ID as corticosteroid user should be carried at all times
- To notify prescriber if therapeutic response decreases; that dosage adjustment may be needed

⚠ **Adrenal crisis:** not to discontinue abruptly or adrenal crisis can result
- To avoid all OTC products: salicylates, alcohol in cough products, cold preparations unless directed by prescriber; avoid high-sodium foods
- About all aspects of product usage, including cushingoid symptoms
- **About symptoms of adrenal insufficiency:** nausea, anorexia, fatigue, dizziness, dyspnea, weakness, joint pain

⚠ Nurse Alert

• To avoid exposure to chickenpox and measles
• To take PO dose in AM with food or fluid (milk)
• To report immediately black, tarry stools or abdominal pain; to report swelling, bruising, bone pain, visual changes, or mood changes

crizotinib

(kriz-oh′ti-nib)

XALKORI

Func. class.: Antineoplastic; biologic response modifiers

Chem. class.: Signal transduction inhibitors (STIs)

ACTION:

Inhibits receptor tyrosine kinases (anaplastic lymphoma kinase (ALK), Hepatocyte Growth Factor Receptor (HGFR, c-Met), Recepteur d'Origine Nantais (RON)

USES:

Locally advanced or metastatic non-small cell lung cancer (NSCLC) that is anaplastic lymphoma kinase (ALK)-positive as detected by an FDA-approved test

CONTRAINDICATIONS:

Pregnancy (D), breastfeeding

Precautions: Neonates, infants, children, adolescents, pneumonitis, severe hepatic disease, congenital long QT syndrome, severe renal impairment, end-stage renal disease, vision disorders

DOSAGE AND ROUTES

• **Adult: PO** 250 mg bid, continue as long beneficial

Dose adjustments for hematologic toxicities

• **For Grade 1-2:** no dosage adjustment needed; **Grade 3:** interrupt treatment until toxicity resolves to grade ≤2, then continue with the same dosage schedule. In case of recurrence after a grade 4 event with dose reduction, interrupt treatment until toxicity resolves to grade ≤2; when resuming treatment, reduce dosage to 250 mg PO daily; **Grade 4:** interrupt treatment until toxicity resolves to grade ≤2; when resuming treatment, reduce dosage to 200 mg PO bid. In case of grade 4 recurrence, permanently discontinue treatment

Dose adjustments for hepatic laboratory abnormalities

• **For Grade 1:** No dosage adjustment necessary; **Grade 2 ALT/AST elevations with grade ≤1 total bilirubin elevations:** no dosage adjustment necessary; **Grade 3-4 ALT/AST elevations with grade ≤1 total bilirubin elevations:** interrupt treatment until toxicity resolves to grade ≤1 or baseline; when resuming treatment, reduce dosage to 200 mg PO bid; in case of recurrence, interrupt treatment until toxicity resolves to grade ≤1, and when resuming treatment, reduce dosage to 250 mg PO daily; permanently discontinue treatment in case of further recurrence; **Grade 2-4 ALT/AST elevations with concurrent Grade 2-4 total bilirubin elevations (in the absence of cholestasis or hemolysis):** permanently discontinue treatment

Dose adjustments for pneumonitis not attributable to NSCLC progression, other pulmonary disease, infection, or radiation effect

• **For any grade pneumonitis:** permanently discontinue

Dose adjustment for QTc prolongation:

• **For Grade 1-2 QTc prolongation:** no dosage adjustment necessary; **For Grade 3 QTc prolongation:** interrupt treatment until toxicity resolves to grade ≤1; when resuming treatment, reduce dosage to 200 mg PO bid; in case of recurrence, interrupt treatment until toxicity resolves to grade ≤1 and when resuming treatment, reduce dosage to 250 mg PO daily; permanently discontinue in case of further recurrence; **For Grade 4 QTc prolongation:** permanently discontinue

Available forms: Cap 200, 250 mg
Administer:
- May be taken orally with or without food
- Have the patient swallow capsule whole; do not crush or chew
- If a dose is missed, it can be taken up to 6 hr before the next dose is due to maintain the twice daily regimen. Do not take both doses at the same time

SIDE EFFECTS

CNS: Dizziness, balance disorder, presyncope, neuropathy (motor and sensory), burning sensation, dysesthesia, hyperesthesia, hypoesthesia, neuralgia, paresthesias, peripheral neuropathy (motor and sensory), headache, insomnia
CV: QT prolongation, disseminated intravascular coagulation (DIC), septic shock, bradycardia
EENT: Diplopia, photopsia, photophobia, blurred vision, visual field defect, vitreous floaters, visual brightness, reduced visual acuity; esophageal disorders, dyspepsia, dysphagia, epigastric discomfort/pain, burning, esophagitis, esophageal obstruction/pain/spasm, esophageal ulceration, gastroesophageal reflux, odynophagia, and reflux esophagitis
GI: Nausea, diarrhea, vomiting, constipation, decreased appetite, dysgeusia, abdominal pain, abdominal discomfort/pain, stomatitis, oral ulceration, glossodynia, glossitis, cheilitis, mucosal inflammation, oropharyngeal pain/discomfort, oral pain, esophageal disorder, elevated hepatic enzymes and hyperbilirubinemia
HEMA: Grade 3/4 neutropenia, thrombocytopenia, lymphopenia
MISC: Fatigue, fever, edema, localized/peripheral edema, chest pain (unspecified), chest discomfort, musculoskeletal chest pain, arthralgia, back pain, *rash*
RESP: Severe, life-threatening pneumonitis, pneumonia, hypoxia, acute respiratory distress syndrome (ARDS), dyspnea, empyema, pulmonary hemorrhage, pulmonary embolism, upper respiratory tract infection (nasopharyngitis, pharyngitis, rhinitis), cough

PHARMACOKINETICS

Protein binding 91%; distribution into the tissues and plasma; metabolized by the CYP3A4/5; primary metabolic pathways are oxidation to metabolites; terminal half-life 42 hr; excreted 63% feces, 22% urine; unchanged drug 53% feces, 2.3% urine; absolute bioavailability is 43%; peak is 4-6 hr; steady state is reached within 15 days; dosage adjustments may need to be made in hepatic/renal disease and Asian Patients

INTERACTIONS

Increase: CYP3A4 inhibitors (ketoconazole, atazanavir, indinavir, itraconazole, nefazodone, nelfinavir, ritonavir, voriconazole, boceprevir, delavirdine, isoniazid, dalfopristin; quinupristin, tipranavir)
Decrease: CYP3A4 inducers (rifampin, carBAMazepine, PHENobarbital, phenytoin, rifabutin); antacids, H2-blockers, proton pump inhibitors (PPIs)
Increase: action of—midazolam
Avoid use with CYP3A4 substrates(alfentanil, cycloSPORINE, ergotamine, dihydroergotamine fentanyl, sirolimus, colchicine)
Increase: QT prolongation, torsades de pointes—arsenic trioxide, certain phenothiazines (chlorproMAZINE, mesoridazine, thioridazine), grepafloxacin, levomethadyl, pentamidine, probucol, sparfloxacin, troleandomycin, class IA antiarrhythmics (disopyramide, procainamide, quiNIDine), class III antiarrhythmics (amiodarone, dofetilide, ibutilide, sotalol), clarithromycin, ziprasidone, pimozide, haloperidol, halofantrine, quiNIDine, chloroquine, dronedarone, droperidol, erythromycin, methadone, posaconazole, propafenone, saquinavir, abarelix, amoxapine, apomorphine, asenapine, β-agonists, ofloxacin, eribulin, ezogabine, flecainide, gatifloxacin, gemifloxacin, halogenated anesthetics, ilo-

peridone, levofloxacin, local anesthetics, magnesium sulfate, potassium sulfate, sodium, maprotiline, moxifloxacin, nilotinib, norfloxacin, ciprofloxacin, olanzapine, paliperidone, some phenothiazines (fluphenazine, perphenazine, prochlorperazine, trifluoperazine), telavancin, tetrabenazine, tricyclic antidepressants, venlafaxine, vorinostat, citalopram, alfuzosin, clozapine, cyclobenzaprine, dolasetron, palonosetron, quetiapine, rilpivirine, sunitinib, tacrolimus, tacrolimus, vardenafil, indacaterol, dasatinib, fluconazole, lapatinib, lopinavir/ritonavir, mefloquine, octreotide, ondansetron, ranolazine, risperidone, telithromycin, vemurafenib

Drug/Herb

Do not use with St. John's Wort

Drug/Food

Do not use with grapefruit juice

NURSING CONSIDERATIONS

Assess:

- **Severe, life-threatening, or fatal treatment-related pneumonitis:** all cases occurred within 2 mo of treatment initiation; monitor for pulmonary symptoms that may indicate pneumonitis, other causes of pneumonitis should be excluded; permanently discontinue in patients with treatment-related pneumonitis l
- **Hepatic disease:** liver function test (LFT) abnormalities, altered bilirubin levels may occur during treatment; monitor LFTs and bilirubin levels prior to treatment, then monthly; more frequent testing is needed in those presenting with grade 2 or greater toxicities; laboratory alterations should be managed with dose reduction, treatment interruption, or discontinuation
- **QT prolongation** has been reported with use of product; therefore, avoid crizotinib use in those patients; monitor ECG and electrolytes in patients with congestive heart failure, bradycardia, electrolyte imbalance (hypokalemia, hypomagnesemia), or in patients taking concomitant medications known to prolong the QT interval; treatment interruption, dosage adjustment, treatment discontinuation may be needed in patients who develop QT prolongation
- **Vision disorders,** generally start within 2 wks of the start of therapy; ophthalmological evaluation should be considered, particularly if patients experience photopsia or new or increased vitreous floaters; caution should be used when driving or operating machinery by patients who experience vision disorders
- **Pregnancy/breastfeeding:** identify if pregnancy is planned or suspected (pregnancy category D), do not breastfeed

Perform/provide:

- Storage of capsules at room temperature

Evaluate:

- Decreasing spread of malignancy

Teach patient/family:

- That missed doses can be taken up to 6 hr before the next dose is due to maintain the twice daily regimen
- To use reliable contraception; both women and men of childbearing age should use adequate contraceptive methods during therapy and for at least 90 days after completing treatment, pregnancy category D
- To report immediately shortness of breath, cough, fatigue

cromolyn (OTC, Rx)

(kroe′moe-lin)

Gastrocrom Intal, Nasalcrom, Rynacrom ✥

Func. class.: Antiasthmatic

Chem. class.: Mast cell stabilizer

Do not confuse:

Nasalcrom/Nasalide

ACTION: Stabilizes the membrane of the sensitized mast cell, thus preventing the release of chemical mediators after an antigen-IgE interaction

USES:
Severe perennial bronchial asthma; prevention of exercise-induced bronchospasm; acute bronchospasm induced by environmental pollutants, mastocytosis, allergic rhinitis

Unlabeled uses: Food allergy, ulcerative colitis

CONTRAINDICATIONS:
Hypersensitivity to this product or lactose; status asthmaticus, acute asthma

Precautions: Pregnancy (B), breastfeeding, children <5 yr (aerosol); <2 yr (nebulizer); <2 yr (nasal sol); oral <2 yr; renal/hepatic disease, safety not established; cardiac dysrhythmias, CAD

DOSAGE AND ROUTES

Allergic rhinitis

- **Adult and child >2 yr: NASAL SOL** 1 spray in each nostril tid-qid, max 6 doses/day

To prevent exercise-induced bronchospasm

- **Adult and child >5 yr: INH** 2 metered sprays inhaled ≤1 hr prior to exercise

Bronchial asthma

- **Adult and child >5 yr: INH** 2 metered sprays using inhaler qid; **NEB** 20 mg qid by nebulization

Systemic mastocytosis

- **Adult and child >12 yr: PO** 200 mg qid ½ hr before meals and at bedtime
- **Child 2-12 yr: PO** 100 mg qid ½ before meals and at bedtime

Ulcerative colitis (unlabeled)

- **Adult: PO** (Gastrocrom) 200 mg qid 20 min before meals and at bedtime, may double dose after 2 wk
- **Child 2-14 yr: PO** (Gastrocrom) 100 mg qid 20 min before meals and at bedtime, may double dose after 2-3 wk

Available forms: Nasal sol 5.2 mg/metered spray (40 mg/ml); neb sol 20 mg/2 ml; aerosol 800 mcg/actuation; oral conc 100 mg/5 ml

Administer:

- For oral conc: break open ampule, squeeze contents into glass of water, stir, drink

SIDE EFFECTS

CNS: *Headache, dizziness,* neuritis, confusion, drowsiness

EENT: Throat irritation, cough, nasal congestion, burning eyes, nasal stinging/irritation, sneezing

GI: Nausea, vomiting, anorexia, dry mouth, bitter taste

GU: Urinary frequency, dysuria

INTEG: Rash, urticaria, angioedema

MS: Joint pain/swelling

Oral conc:

CNS: Dizziness, headache, paresthesia, migraine, seizures, psychosis, anxiety, depression, hallucinations, insomnia

CV: Tachycardia, PVCs, palpitations

GI: Diarrhea, nausea, abdominal pain, constipation, dyspepsia, stomatitis, vomiting

HEMA: Polycythemia, neutropenia, pancytopenia

INTEG: Pruritus, rash, flushing, photosensitivity

PHARMACOKINETICS

Excreted unchanged in feces, half-life 80 min, 63%-76% protein binding

NURSING CONSIDERATIONS

Assess:

- Eosinophil count during treatment
- Respiratory status: rate, rhythm, characteristics, cough, wheezing, dyspnea

Perform/provide:

- Gargle, sip of water to decrease irritation in throat (INH/Neb)

Evaluate:

- Therapeutic response: decrease in asthmatic symptoms; congested, runny nose

Teach patient/family:

Nasal sol

- Blow nose, hold pump between fingers; if 1st use, spray in air until fine mist occurs, insert nozzle in nostril, spray and breathe in through nose, repeat in other nostril

Aerosol (not for acute asthma)

- Take cover off mouthpiece, shake gently, breathe out slowly, place mouthpiece in mouth, close mouth around it, tilt head back, breathe in as the inhaler is depressed, remove, hold breath, then breathe out slowly

Inhalation

- Do not swallow sol
- Empty ampule into power-driven nebulizer as directed; do not combine different meds

Oral

- Take 1/2 hr before meals and at bedtime

cyanocobalamin (vit B_{12}) (OTC, Rx)

(sye-an-oh-koe-bal′a-min)

Alphamin, Anacobin ✱, Bedoz ✱, Cobex, Cobolin-M, Crystamine, Crysti-1000, Cyanabin ✱, Cyanoject, Cyomin, Ener-B, Hydrobexan, Hydro-Crysti-12

hydroxocobalamin (OTC, Rx)

Hydro Cobex, Hydroxycobal, LA-12, Nascobal, Neuroforte-R, Rubesol-1000, Rubramin PC, Shovite, Vibral LA, Vibral, Vitamin B_{12}

Func. class.: Vit B_{12}, water-soluble vitamin

ACTION: Needed for adequate nerve functioning, protein and carbohydrate metabolism, normal growth, RBC development, cell reproduction

USES: Vit B_{12} deficiency, pernicious anemia, vit B_{12} malabsorption syndrome, Schilling test, increased requirements with pregnancy, thyrotoxicosis, hemolytic anemia, hemorrhage, renal/hepatic disease, nutritional supplementation

CONTRAINDICATIONS: Hypersensitivity, optic nerve atrophy

Precautions: Pregnancy (A), breastfeeding, children

DOSAGE AND ROUTES

Cyanocobalamin

- **Adult: PO** Up to 1000 mcg/day **SUBCUT/IM** 30-100 mcg/day × 1 wk, then 100-200 mcg/mo

Schilling test

- **Adult and child: IM** 1000 mcg in 1 dose
- **Child: PO** Up to 1000 mcg/day **SUBCUT/IM** 30-50 mcg/day × 2 wk, then 100 mcg/mo; **NASAL** 500 mcg q wk

Hydroxocobalamin

- **Adult: SUBCUT/IM** 30-50 mcg/day × 5-10 days then 100-200 mcg/mo
- **Child: SUBCUT/IM** 30-50 mcg/day × 5-10 days then 30-50 mcg/mo

Available forms: *Cyanocobalamin:* tabs 25, 50, 100, 250, 500, 1000, 5000 mcg; ext rel tabs 100, 200, 500, 1000 mcg; lozenges 100, 250, 500 mcg; nasal jel 500 mcg/spray; inj 100, 1000 mcg/ml; *hydroxocobalamin:* inj 1000 mcg/ml

Administer:

PO route

- With fruit juice to disguise taste; immediately after mixing
- With meals if possible for better absorption; large doses should not be used because most is excreted

IM route

- By IM inj for pernicious anemia for life unless contraindicated

Intranasal route

- Avoid use within 1 hr of hot fluids, food

IV route

- IV route not recommended but may be admixed in TPN solution

Additive compatibilities: Ascorbic acid, chloramphenicol, hydrocortisone, metaraminol, vit B/C

Solution compatibilities: Dextrose/Ringer's or LR combinations, dextrose/saline combinations, D_5W, $D_{10}W$, 0.45% NaCl, Ringer's or LR sol

Y-site compatibilities: Alfentanil, amikacin, aminophylline, ascorbic acid, atracurium, atropine, azaTHIOprine, aztreonam, benztropine, bretylium, bumetanide, buprenorphine, butorphanol, calcium chloride/gluconate, cefamandole, ceFAZolin, cefmetazole, cefonicid, cefoperazone, cefotaxime, cefotetan, cefoxitin, ceftazidime, ceftizoxime, cefTRIAXone, cefuroxime, cephalothin, cephapirin, chloramphenicol, chlorproMAZINE, cimetidine, clindamycin, dexamethasone, digoxin, diphenhydrAMINE, DOBUTamine, DOPamine, doxycycline, enalaprilat, ePHEDrine, EPINEPHrine, epoetin alfa, erythromycin, esmolol, famotidine, fentaNYL, fluconazole, folic acid, furosemide, ganciclovir, gentamicin, glycopyrrolate, heparin, hydrocortisone, hydrOXYzine, imipenem-cilastatin, indomethacin, insulin (regular), isoproterenol hydrochloride, ketorolac, labetalol, lidocaine, magnesium, mannitol, meperidine, metaraminol, methicillin, methoxamine, methyldopate, methylPREDNISolone, metoclopramide, metoprolol, mezlocillin, miconazole, midazolam, minocycline, morphine, moxalactam, multiple vitamins injection, nafcillin, nalbuphine, naloxone, netilmicin, nitroglycerin, nitroprusside, norepinephrine, ondansetron, oxacillin, oxytocin, papaverine, penicillin G potassium/sodium, pentamidine, pentazocine, PENTobarbital, PHENobarbital, phentolamine, phenylephrine, phytonadione, piperacillin, polymyxin B, potassium chloride, procainamide, prochlorperazine, promethazine, propranolol, protamine, pyridoxine, quiNIDine, ranitidine, ritodrine, sodium bicarbonate, succinylcholine, SUFentanil, theophylline, thiamine, ticarcillin, ticarcillin-clavulanate, tobramycin, tolazoline, trimetaphan, urokinase, vancomycin, vasopressin, verapamil, vitamin B complex with C

SIDE EFFECTS

CNS: Flushing, optic nerve atrophy
CV: CHF, peripheral vascular thrombosis, pulmonary edema
GI: *Diarrhea*
INTEG: Itching, rash, pain at inj site
META: Hypokalemia
SYST: Anaphylactic shock

PHARMACOKINETICS

Gastric intrinsic factor must be present for absorption to occur; stored in liver, kidneys, stomach; 50%-90% excreted in urine; crosses placenta; excreted in breast milk

INTERACTIONS

Increase: absorption—predniSONE
Decrease: absorption—aminoglycosides, anticonvulsants, colchicine, chloramphenicol, aminosalicylic acid, potassium preparations, cimetidine

Drug/Herb

Decrease: vit B_{12} absorption—goldenseal

Drug/Lab Test

False positive: intrinsic factor

NURSING CONSIDERATIONS

Assess:

• For vit B_{12} deficiency: red, beefy tongue; psychosis; pallor; neuropathy
• GI function: diarrhea, constipation
• Potassium levels during beginning treatment in megaloblastic anemia; q6mo in pernicious anemia; folic acid, plasma vit B_{12} (after 1 wk), reticulocyte counts
• Nutritional status: egg yolks, fish, organ meats, dairy products, clams, oysters: good sources of vit B_{12}
• For pulmonary edema, worsening of CHF in cardiac patients

Perform/provide:

• Protection from light, heat

Evaluate:

• Therapeutic response: decreased anorexia, dyspnea on exertion, palpitations, paresthesias, psychosis, visual disturbances

Teach patient/family:

• That treatment must continue for life for pernicious anemia
• To eat a well-balanced diet

• To avoid contact with persons with infection; that infections are common

TREATMENT OF OVERDOSE:
Discontinue product

cyclobenzaprine (Rx)
(sye-kloe-ben′za-preen)

Amrix, Apo-Cyclobenzaprine ✦, Fexmid, Flexeril, Gen-Cyclobenzaprine ✦, PMS-Cyclobenzaprine ✦, ratio-Cyclobenzaprine ✦

Func. class.: Skeletal muscle relaxant, central acting

Chem. class.: Tricyclic amine salt

Do not confuse:
cyclobenzaprine/cyproheptadine

ACTION: Reduces tonic muscle activity at the brain stem; may be related to antidepressant effects

USES: Adjunct for relief of muscle spasm and pain in musculoskeletal conditions

Unlabeled uses: Fibromyalgia

CONTRAINDICATIONS: Children <12 yr, acute recovery phase of MI, dysrhythmias, heart block, CHF, hypersensitivity, intermittent porphyria, thyroid disease, QT prolongation

Precautions: Pregnancy (B), breastfeeding, geriatric patients, renal/hepatic disease, addictive personality

DOSAGE AND ROUTES

Muscloskeletal disorders
- **Adult/adolescent ≥15 yr: PO** 5 mg tid × 1 wk, max 30 mg/day × 3 wk
- **Adult: EXT REL** 15 mg/day, max 30 mg/day × 3 wk
- **Geriatric: PO** 5 mg tid

Fibromyalgia (unlabeled)
- **Adult: PO** 10 mg at bedtime, titrated up

Hepatic dose
- **Adult (mild hepatic disease): PO** 5 mg, titrate slowly

Available forms: Tabs 5, 10 mg; ext rel tab 15, 30 mg

Administer:
- Without regard to meals
- Do not crush, break, chew ext rel cap

SIDE EFFECTS

CNS: *Dizziness, weakness, drowsiness,* headache, tremor, depression, insomnia, confusion, paresthesia, nervousness

CV: Postural hypotension, tachycardia, dysrhythmias

EENT: Diplopia, temporary loss of vision

GI: *Nausea,* vomiting, hiccups, dry mouth, constipation, hepatitis

GU: Urinary retention, frequency, change in libido

INTEG: Rash, pruritus, fever, facial flushing, sweating

PHARMACOKINETICS

PO: Onset 1 hr, peak 3-8 hr, duration 12-24 hr, half-life 1-3 days, metabolized by liver, excreted in urine, crosses placenta, excreted in breast milk

INTERACTIONS

• Do not use within 14 days of MAOIs, tramadol

Increase: QT interval—erythromycin, levaquin

Increase: CNS depression—alcohol, tricyclics, opiates, barbiturates, sedatives, hypnotics

Drug/Herb

Increase: CNS depression—kava

NURSING CONSIDERATIONS

Assess:
- **Pain:** location, duration, mobility, stiffness at baseline, periodically
- **Allergic reactions:** rash, fever, respiratory distress
- Severe weakness, numbness in extremities

Perform/provide:
- Storage in tight container at room temp
- Assistance with ambulation if dizziness, drowsiness occur, especially for geriatric patients

Evaluate:
- Therapeutic response: decreased pain, spasticity; muscle spasms of acute, painful musculoskeletal conditions generally short term; long-term therapy seldom warranted

Teach patient/family:
- Not to discontinue medication abruptly; that insomnia, nausea, headache, spasticity, tachycardia will occur; that product should be tapered off over 1-2 wk
- Not to take with alcohol, other CNS depressants
- To avoid hazardous activities if drowsiness, dizziness occur
- To avoid using OTC medication (cough preparations, antihistamines) unless directed by prescriber
- To use gum, frequent sips of water for dry mouth

TREATMENT OF OVERDOSE:

Administer activated charcoal; use anticonvulsants if indicated; monitor cardiac function

cyclopentolate ophthalmic

See Appendix B

HIGH ALERT

cyclophosphamide (Rx)

(sye-kloe-foss′fa-mide)

Cytoxan, Procytox ♣

Func. class.: Antineoplastic alkylating agent

Chem. class.: Nitrogen mustard

Do not confuse:
cyclophosphamide/cycloSPORINE
Cytoxan/Cytosar/Cytotec/cytarabine

ACTION: Alkylates DNA is responsible for cross-linking DNA strands; activity is not cell-cycle–phase specific

USES: Hodgkin's disease; lymphomas; leukemia; cancer of female reproductive tract, breast, lung, prostate; multiple myeloma; neuroblastoma; retinoblastoma; Ewing's sarcoma; disseminated neuroblastoma, nephrotic syndrome

Unlabeled uses: Aplastic anemia, chronic idiopathic thrombocytopenic purpura, dermatomyositis, pneumonitis, polymyositis, SLE, scleroderma, RA, Behçet's syndrome, Churg-Strauss syndrome, polyarteritis nodosa, Wegener's granulomatosis, idiopathic pulmonary fibrosis, localized neuroblastoma, CLL

CONTRAINDICATIONS: Pregnancy (D), breastfeeding, severely depressed bone marrow function, hypersensitivity, prostatic hypertrophy, bladder neck obstruction

Precautions: Radiation therapy, cardiac disease

DOSAGE AND ROUTES

- **Adult: PO** Initially 1-5 mg/kg over 2-5 days, maintenance is 1-5 mg/kg; **IV** initially 40-50 mg/kg in divided doses over 2-5 days, maintenance 10-15 mg/kg q7-10 days or 3-5 mg/kg q3days
- **Child: PO/IV** 2-8 mg/kg or 60-250 mg/m^2 in divided doses for 6 or more days; maintenance 10-15 mg/kg q7-10 days or

30 mg/kg q3-4wk; dose should be reduced by half when bone marrow depression occurs

Neuroblastoma

• **Child and infant: PO** 150 mg/m^2/day, days 1-7 with DOXOrubicin (**IV** 35 mg/m^2 on day 8) q21days × 5 cycles

• **Child: IV** 70 mg/kg/day with hydration on days 1, 2 with DOXOrubicin and vinCRIStine q21days for courses 1, 2, 4, 6 alternating with CISplatin and etoposide q21days for courses 3, 5, 7

Breast cancer

• **Adult: PO** 100-200 mg/m^2/day or 2 mg/kg/day × 4-14 days; **IV** 500-1000 mg/m^2 on day 1 in combination with fluorouracil and methotrexate or DOXOrubicin or DOXOrubicin alone, also cyclophosphamide 600 mg/m^2; may be given dose-dense on day 1 of q14days with DOXOrubicin (60 mg/m^2) with growth-factor support

Operable node-positive breast cancer IV (TAC regimen)

• **Adult: IV** 500 mg/m^2 with DOXOrubicin (50 mg/m^2 **IV**) then docetaxel (75 mg/m^2) **IV** given 1 hr later q3wk × 6 cycles

Nephrotic syndrome

• **Adult: PO** 2-3 mg/kg/day for up to 12 wk when corticosteroids are unsuccessful

Aplastic anemia (unlabeled)

• **Adult: IV** 45-50 mg/kg divided over 4 days

Behçet's syndrome/Churg-Strauss syndrome/polyarteritis nodosa/uveitis/Wegener's granulomatosis (unlabeled)

• **Adult: PO** 1-2 mg/kg/day, **IV** 0.5-1 g/m^2

Rheumatoid arthritis (unlabeled)

• **Adult and child: PO** 1.5-2.5 mg/kg/day

CLL (unlabeled)

• **Adult: IV** 250 mg/m^2/day on days 1-3 with fludarabine 30 mg/m^2/day on days 1-3

Available forms: Inj 100, 200, 500 mg, 1, 2 g; tabs 25, 50 mg

Administer:

• In AM so product can be eliminated before bedtime

• Fluids IV or PO before chemotherapy to hydrate patient

• Antacid before oral agent; give after evening meal, before bedtime

• Antiemetic 30-60 min before product and prn

• Allopurinol or sodium bicarbonate to maintain uric acid levels, alkalinization of urine

PO route

• Take on empty stomach; do not crush, break, chew tabs

• May be taken as a single dose or divided doses

• Take in AM or afternoon, avoid evening

Intermittent IV INF route

• Use cytotoxic handling procedures

• IV after diluting 100 mg/5 ml of sterile water or bacteriostatic water; shake; let stand until clear; may be further diluted in ≤250 ml D_5 or NS; give 100 mg or less/min through 3-way stopcock of glucose or saline inf

• Use 21, 23, 25G needle; check site for irritation, phlebitis

Solution compatibilities: Amino acids 4.25%/D_{25}, D_5/0.9% NaCl, D_5W, 0.9% NaCl

Syringe compatibilities: Bleomycin, CISplatin, doxapram, DOXOrubicin, droperidol, fluorouracil, furosemide, heparin, leucovorin, methotrexate, metoclopramide, mitomycin, vinBLAStine, vinCRIStine

Y-site compatibilities: Acyclovir, alfentanil, allopurinol, amifostine, amikacin, aminocaproic acid, aminophylline, amiodarone, amphotericin B lipid complex, amphotericin B liposome, ampicillin, ampicillin-sulbactam, anidulafungin, atenolol, atracurium, azlocillin, aztreonam, bivalirudin, bleomycin, bumetanide, buprenorphine, butorphanol, calcium chloride/gluconate, CARBOplatin, caspofungin, cefamandole, ceFAZolin, cefepime, cefoperazone, cefotaxime, cefotetan, cefoxitin, ceftazidime, ceftizoxime, cefTRIAXone, cefuroxime, chloramphenicol, chlorproMAZINE, cimetidine, ciprofloxacin, cisatracurium, CISplatin, cladribine, clindamycin, codeine, cycloSPORINE, cytarabine, DACTINomycin, DAPTOmycin, DAUNOrubicin, dexamethasone, dexmedetomidine, dexrazoxane, digoxin, diltiazem, diphenhydrAMINE, DOBUTamine, docetaxel, dolasetron, DOPamine, doripenem, doxacurium, DOXOrubicin, DOXOrubicin liposomal, doxycycline, droperidol, enalaprilat, ePHEDrine, EPINEPHrine, epirubicin, ertapenem, erythromycin, esmolol, etoposide, famotidine, fenoldopam, fentaNYL, filgrastim, fluconazole, fludarabine, fluorouracil, foscarnet, fosphenytoin, furosemide, gallium, ganciclovir, gatifloxacin, gemcitabine, gentamicin, granisetron, haloperidol, heparin, hydrocortisone, HYDROmorphone, hydrOXYzine, IDArubicin, imipenem-cilastatin, inamrinone, insulin (regular), irinotecan, isoproterenol, kanamycin, ketorolac, labetalol, leucovorin, levofloxacin, levorphanol, lidocaine, linezolid, LORazepam, magnesium sulfate, mannitol, melphalan, meperidine, meropenem, mesna, methohexital, methotrexate, methylPREDNISolone, metoclopramide, metoprolol, metroNIDAZOLE, midazolam, milrinone, minocycline, mitomycin, mitoxantrone, mivacurium, morphine, nafcillin, nalbuphine, naloxone, nesiritide, nitroglycerin, nitroprusside, norepinephrine, octreotide, ondansetron, oxacillin, oxaliplatin, paclitaxel, palonosetron, pamidronate, pancuronium, pantoprazole, pemetrexed, penicillin G potassium, pentamidine, PENTobarbital, PHENObarbital, phenylephrine, piperacillin, piperacillin-tazobactam, potassium chloride/phosphates, procainamide, prochlorperazine, promethazine, propofol, propranolol, quinupristin-dalfopristin, ranitidine, rapacuronium, remifentanil, riTUXimab, rocuronium, sargramostim, sodium acetate/bicarbonate/phosphates, succinylcholine, SUFentanil, sulfamethoxazole-trimethoprim, tacrolimus, teniposide, theophylline, thiopental, thiotepa, ticarcillin, ticarcillin-clavulanate, tigecycline, tirofiban, TNA, tobramycin, topotecan, TPN, trastuzumab, vancomycin, vasopressin, vecuronium, verapamil, vinBLAStine, vinCRIStine, vinorelbine, voriconazole, zidovudine, zoledronic acid

SIDE EFFECTS

CNS: Headache, dizziness
CV: Cardiotoxicity (high doses), myocardial fibrosis
ENDO: SIADH, gonadal suppression
GI: *Nausea, vomiting, diarrhea, weight loss,* colitis, hepatotoxicity
GU: Hemorrhagic cystitis, *hematuria, neoplasms, amenorrhea, azoospermia, sterility, ovarian fibrosis*
HEMA: Thrombocytopenia, leukopenia, pancytopenia; myelosuppression
INTEG: *Alopecia,* dermatitis
META: Hyperuricemia
MISC: Secondary neoplasms, anaphylaxis
RESP: Pulmonary fibrosis, interstitial pneumonia

PHARMACOKINETICS

Metabolized by liver, excreted in urine, half-life 4-6½ hr, 50% bound to plasma proteins

INTERACTIONS

Increase: neuromuscular blockade—succinylcholine
Increase: cyclophosphamide toxicity—barbiturates
Increase: action of warfarin
Increase: bone marrow depression—allopurinol, thiazides
Increase: hypoglycemia—insulin
Decrease: digoxin levels—digoxin
Decrease: cyclophosphamide effect—chloramphenicol, corticosteroids
Decrease: antibody response—live virus vaccines

Drug/Herb

- Toxicity: St. John's wort

Drug/Lab Test

Increase: uric acid
Decrease: pseudocholinesterase

False positive: Pap smear
False negative: PPD, mumps, trichophytin, *Candida, Trichophyton,* Pap smear

NURSING CONSIDERATIONS

Assess:

• **Hemorrhagic cystitis;** renal studies: BUN, serum uric acid, urine CCr before, during therapy; I&O ratio; report fall in urine output <30 ml/hr

• **Bone marrow depression:** CBC, differential, platelet count baseline, weekly; withhold product if WBC is <2500 or platelet count is <75,000; notify prescriber of results

• Pulmonary function tests, chest x-ray films before, during therapy; chest film should be obtained q2wk during treatment

• Monitor temp q4hr; elevated temp may indicate beginning infection

• **Hepatotoxicity:** hepatic studies before, during therapy (bilirubin, AST, ALT, LDH), as needed; jaundice of skin, sclera; dark urine, clay-colored stools; itchy skin; abdominal pain; fever; diarrhea

• **Bleeding:** hematuria, guaiac, bruising or petechiae, mucosa or orifices q8hr

• Dyspnea, crackles, unproductive cough, chest pain, tachypnea

• Effects of alopecia on body image, discuss feelings about body changes

• Buccal cavity q8hr for dryness, sores or ulceration, white patches, oral pain, bleeding, dysphagia; obtain prescription for viscous lidocaine (Xylocaine)

⚠ Symptoms that indicate severe allergic reaction: rash, pruritus, urticaria, purpuric skin lesions, itching, flushing

Perform/provide:

• Storage in tight container at room temp

• Strict medical asepsis, protective isolation if WBC levels are low

• Increase fluid intake to 2-3 L/day to prevent urate deposits, calculi formation, reduce incidence of hemorrhagic cystitis

• Diet low in purines: organ meats (kidney, liver), dried beans, peas to maintain alkaline urine

• Rinsing of mouth tid-qid with water, club soda; brushing of teeth bid-tid with soft brush or cotton-tipped applicators for stomatitis; use unwaxed dental floss

• Warm compresses at inj site for inflammation

Evaluate:

• Therapeutic response: decreased tumor size, spread of malignancy

Teach patient/family:

• About protective isolation

• That amenorrhea can occur and may last up to 1 yr after therapy but is reversible after stopping treatment

• To report any changes in breathing or coughing

• That hair may be lost during treatment; a wig or hairpiece may make patient feel better; new hair may be different in color, texture

• To avoid foods with citric acid, hot or rough texture

• To report any bleeding, white spots, ulcerations in mouth to prescriber; to examine mouth daily

• To report signs of infection: increased temp, sore throat, flulike symptoms

• To report signs of anemia: fatigue, headache, faintness, SOB, irritability

• To report bleeding (bruising, hematuria, petechiae); to avoid use of razors, commercial mouthwash

• To use reliable contraception during and for 4 mo after treatment; not to breastfeed

• To avoid use of aspirin products, ibuprofen

• To avoid vaccinations during therapy

cycloSPORINE (Rx)

(sye′kloe-spor-een)

Gengraf, Neoral, Sandimmune, Pulminiq

Func. class.: Immunosuppressant
Chem. class.: Fungus-derived peptide

Do not confuse:
cycloSPORINE/cycloSERINE/cyclophosphamide

ACTION: Produces immunosuppression by inhibiting lymphocytes (T)

USES: Organ transplants (liver, kidney, heart) to prevent rejection, rheumatoid arthritis, psoriasis

Unlabeled uses: Recalcitrant ulcerative colitis, aplastic anemia, Crohn's disease, GVHD, thrombocytopenia purpura, lupus, nephritis, myasthenia gravis, psoriatic arthritis, atopic dermatitis

CONTRAINDICATIONS: Breastfeeding, hypersensitivity to polyxyethylated castor oil (inj only); psoriasis or RA in renal disease (Neoral/Gengraf); Gengraf/Neoral used with PUVA/UVB, methotrexate, coal tar; ocular infections

Black Box Warning: Uncontrolled, malignant hypertension; radiation in psoriasis, neoplastic disease, sunlight (UV) exposure, renal disease/failure

Precautions: Pregnancy (C), geriatric patients, severe hepatic disease

DOSAGE AND ROUTES

Prevention of transplant rejection (nonmodified)

- **Adult and child: PO** 15 mg/kg several hr before surgery, daily for 2 wk, reduce dosage by 2.5 mg/kg/wk to 5-10 mg/kg/day; **IV** 5-6 mg/kg several hr before surgery, daily, switch to PO form as soon as possible

Prevention of transplant rejection (modified)

- **Adult and child: PO** 4-12 mg/kg/day divided q12hr, depends on organ transplanted

Rheumatoid arthritis (Neoral/Gengraf)

- **Adult: PO** 2.5 mg/kg/day divided bid, may increase 0.5-0.75 mg/kg/day after 8-12 wk, max 4 mg/kg/day

Psoriasis (Neoral/Gengraf)

- **Adult: PO** 2.5 mg/kg/day divided bid, × 4 wk, then increase by 0.5 mg/kg/day q2wk, max 4 mg/kg/day

Idiopathic thrombocytopenia purpura (unlabeled)

- **Adult: PO** 1.25-2.5 mg/kg bid

Severe aplastic anemia (unlabeled)

- **Adult and child: PO** 12 mg/kg/day or 15 mg/kg/day (child) with antithymocyte globulin (ATG)

Atopic dermatitis (unlabeled)

- **Adult/adolescent/child ≥2 yr: PO** 5 mg/kg/day

Crohn's disease that is resistant to/intolerant of corticosteroids (unlabeled)

- **Adult: PO** 2.5-15 mg/kg/day (nonmodified)

Available forms: Oral sol 100 mg/ml; soft gel cap 25, 50, 100 mg; inj 50 mg/ml; sol for inh 300 mg/4.8 ml

Administer:

PO route

- Do not break, crush, or chew caps
- Use pipette provided to draw up oral sol; may mix with milk or juice; wipe pipette, do not wash
- For several days before transplant surgery; give at same time of day
- With corticosteroids
- With meals for GI upset or in chocolate milk, milk, or orange juice
- With oral antifungal for candida infections

Rheumatoid arthritis

- Give Neoral or Gengraf 2.5 mg/kg/day divided bid; may use with salicylates, NSAIDs, PO corticosteroids
- Always give the daily dose of Neoral/Gengraf in 2 divided doses on consistent schedule
- Give initial Sandimmune PO dose 4-12 hr prior to transplantation as a single dose of 15 mg/kg, continue the single daily dose for 1-2 wk, then taper 5%/wk to a maintenance dose of 5-10 mg/kg/day

Intermittent IV INF route

- After diluting each 50 mg/20-100 ml of 0.9% NaCl or D_5W; run over 2-6 hr, use an inf pump, glass inf bottles only

Continuous IV INF route

- May run over 24 hr
- **For Sandimmune parenteral**, give 1/3 of PO dose, initial dose 4-12 hr prior

to transplantation as a single IV dose 5-6 mg/kg/day, continue the single daily dose until PO can be used

Solution compatibilities: D_5W, NaCl 0.9%

Y-site compatibilities: Abciximab, alatrofloxacin, alfentanil, amikacin, aminocaproic acid, aminophylline, amphotericin B lipid complex, anidulafungin, argatroban, ascorbic acid injection, atenolol, atracurium, atropine, azaTHIOprine, aztreonam, benztropine, bivalirudin, bleomycin, bretylium, bumetanide, buprenorphine, butorphanol, calcium chloride/gluconate, CARBOplatin, carmustine, caspofungin, cefamandole, ceFAZolin, cefmetazole, cefonicid, cefoperazone, cefotaxime, cefotetan, cefoxitin, ceftaroline, ceftazidime, ceftizoxime, ceftobiprole, cefTRIAXone, cefuroxime, cephalothin, cephapirin, chloramphenicol, chlorproMAZINE, cimetidine, ciprofloxacin, CISplatin, clindamycin, codeine, cyanocobalamin, cyclophosphamide, cytarabine, DACTINomycin, DAPTOmycin, DAUNOrubicin, dexamethasone, dexmedetomidine, digoxin, diltiazem, diphenhydrAMINE, DOBUTamine, docetaxel, DOPamine, doripenem, doxacurium, DOXOrubicin, doxycycline, enalaprilat, ePHEDrine, EPINEPHrine, epirubicin, epoetin alfa, eptifibatide, ertapenem, erythromycin, esmolol, etoposide, famotidine, fenoldopam, fentaNYL, fluconazole, fludarabine, fluorouracil, folic acid, furosemide, gallium, ganciclovir, gatifloxacin, gemcitabine, gentamicin, glycopyrrolate, granisetron, heparin, hydrocortisone, HYDROmorphone, hydrOXYzine, ifosfamide, imipenem-cilastatin, indomethacin, irinotecan, isoproterenol, ketorolac, labetalol, lansoprazole, levofloxacin, lidocaine, linezolid, LORazepam, mannitol, mechlorethamine, meperidine, meropenem, methicillin, methotrexate, methoxamine, methyldopate, methylPREDNISolone, metoclopramide, metoprolol, metroNIDAZOLE, mezlocillin, micafungin, miconazole, midazolam, milrinone, minocycline, mitoxantrone, morphine, moxalactam, multiple vitamins injection, nafcillin, naloxone, nesiritide, netilmicin, nitroglycerin, nitroprusside, norepinephrine, octreotide, ondansetron, oxacillin, oxaliplatin, oxytocin, paclitaxel, palonosetron, pamidronate, pancuronium, pantoprazole, papaverine, pemetrexed, penicillin G potassium/sodium, pentamidine, pentazocine, phentolamine, phenylephrine, phytonadione, piperacillin, piperacillin-tazobactam, polymyxin B, potassium acetate/chloride, procainamide, prochlorperazine, promethazine, propofol, propranolol, protamine, pyridoxine, quiNIDine, quinupristin-dalfopristin, ranitidine, ritodrine, sargramostim, sodium acetate/bicarbonate, succinylcholine, SUFentanil, tacrolimus, teniposide, theophylline, thiamine, thiotepa, ticarcillin, ticarcillin-clavulanate, tigecycline, tirofiban, tobramycin, trimetaphan, urokinase, vancomycin, vasopressin, vecuronium, verapamil, vinCRIStine, vinorelbine, zoledronic acid

SIDE EFFECTS

CNS: *Tremors, headache,* **seizures, confusion**

GI: Nausea, vomiting, diarrhea, *oral candida, gum hyperplasia,* **hepatotoxicity,** pancreatitis

GU: **Albuminuria, hematuria, proteinuria, renal failure**

INTEG: Rash, acne, *hirsutism,* pruritus

META: Hyperkalemia, hypomagnesemia, hyperlipidemia, hyperuricemia

MISC: *Infection, hypertension*

PHARMACOKINETICS

Peak 4 hr; highly protein bound; half-life (biphasic) 1.2 hr, 25 hr; metabolized in liver; excreted in feces, 6% in urine; crosses placenta; excreted in breast milk

INTERACTIONS

Increase: action, toxicity of cycloSPORINE—allopurinol, amiodarone, amphotericin B, androgens, azole antifungals, β-blockers, bromocriptine, calcium channel blockers, carvedilol, cimetidine,

colchicine, corticosteroids, fluoroquinolones, foscarnet, imipenem-cilastatin, macrolides, metoclopramide, oral contraceptives, NSAIDs, melphalan, SSRIs
Increase: effects of digoxin, etoposide, HMG-CoA reductase inhibitors, methotrexate, potassium-sparing diuretics, sirolimus, tacrolimus
Decrease: cycloSPORINE action—anticonvulsants, nafcillin, orlistat, PHENObarbital, phenytoin, rifamycins, sulfamethoxazole-trimethoprim, terbinafine, ticlopidine
Decrease: antibody reaction—live virus vaccines

Drug/Food

- Slowed metabolism of product: grapefruit juice, food

NURSING CONSIDERATIONS

Assess:

- Renal studies: BUN, creatinine at least monthly during treatment, 3 mo after treatment
- Product blood level during treatment 12 hr after dose, toxic >400 ng/ml
- Hepatic studies: alk phos, AST, ALT, bilirubin; hepatotoxicity: dark urine, jaundice, itching, light-colored stools; product should be discontinued
- Serum lipids, magnesium, potassium, cycloSPORINE blood concentrations

⚠ **Encephalopathy:** impaired cognition, seizures, visual changes including blindness, loss of motor function, movement disorders and psychiatric changes; dosage reduction or discontinuation may be needed in severe cases

⚠ **Nephrotoxicity:** 6 wk after surgery, acute tubular necrosis, CyA trough level >200 ng/ml, gradual rise in creatinine (0.15 mg/dl/day), creatinine plateau <25% above baseline, intracapsular pressure <40 mm Hg

⚠ Signs/symptoms of encephalopathy, lymphoma

Evaluate:

- Therapeutic response: absence of rejection

Teach patient/family:

- To report fever, chills, sore throat, fatigue, since serious infections may occur; tremors, bleeding gums, increased B/P
- To use contraceptive measures during treatment, for 12 wk after ending therapy; to notify prescriber if pregnancy is planned or suspected
- To take at same time of day, every day; not to skip doses or double dose; not to use with grapefruit juice or receive vaccines; that there are many drug interactions; not to add new or discontinued products without approval of prescriber

Black Box Warning: To limit UV exposure

- That treatment is lifelong to prevent rejection; to identify signs of rejection
- To report severe diarrhea because drug loss may result
- About the signs of nephrotoxicity: increased B/P, tremors of the hands, changes in gums, increased hair on body, face
- To continue with all lab work and follow-up appointments
- That types of products are not interchangeable

cyproheptadine (Rx)

(si-proe-hep′ta-deen)

PMS-Cyproheptadine ✦

Func. class.: Antihistamine, H_1-receptor antagonist
Chem. class.: Piperidine

Do not confuse:
cyproheptadine/cyclobenzaprine

ACTION: Acts on blood vessels, GI, respiratory system by competing with histamine for H_1-receptor site; decreases allergic response by blocking histamine

USES: Allergy symptoms, rhinitis, pruritus, common cold, urticaria
Unlabeled uses: Appetite stimulant, management of vascular headache,

nightmares, posttraumatic stress disorder

CONTRAINDICATIONS:
Hypersensitivity to H_1-receptor antagonist, breastfeeding, closed-angle glaucoma, neonates/infants, peptic ulcers, bladder-neck obstruction, prostatic hypertrophy
Precautions: Pregnancy (B), geriatric patients, cardiac disease, asthma, ileus, urinary retention, COPD

DOSAGE AND ROUTES

- **Adult: PO** 4 mg tid-qid, not to exceed 0.5 mg/kg/day
- **Geriatric: PO** 4 mg bid, may increase if needed
- **Child 7-14 yr: PO** 4 mg bid-tid, not to exceed 16 mg/day
- **Child 2-6 yr: PO** 2 mg bid-tid, not to exceed 12 mg/day

Available forms: Tabs 4 mg; syr 2 mg/5 ml
Administer:
- With meals for GI symptoms; absorption may slightly decrease

SIDE EFFECTS

CNS: *Dizziness, drowsiness,* poor coordination, fatigue, anxiety, euphoria, confusion, paresthesia, neuritis
CV: Hypotension, palpitations, tachycardia
EENT: *Blurred vision,* dilated pupils; tinnitus; nasal stuffiness; dry nose, throat, mouth
GI: *Constipation, dry mouth,* nausea, vomiting, anorexia, diarrhea, weight gain, increased appetite
GU: *Retention,* dysuria, urinary frequency
HEMA: **Hemolytic anemia, leukopenia, thrombocytosis, agranulocytosis**
INTEG: Rash, urticaria, photosensitivity
RESP: Increased thick secretions, wheezing, chest tightness
SYST: **Anaphylactic shock**

PHARMACOKINETICS

PO: Duration 4-6 hr; metabolized in liver; excreted by kidneys (65%-75%), in feces (25%-35%); excreted in breast milk

INTERACTIONS

Increase: CNS depression—barbiturates, opiates, hypnotics, tricyclics, alcohol, other CNS depressants
Increase: anticholinergic effect—MAOIs
Drug/Lab Test
False negative: skin allergy tests

NURSING CONSIDERATIONS

Assess:
- I&O ratio; be alert for urinary retention, frequency, dysuria; product should be discontinued
- CBC during long-term therapy
- Respiratory status: rate, rhythm, increase in bronchial secretions, wheezing, chest tightness
- Cardiac status: palpitations, increased pulse, hypotension

Perform/provide:
- Hard candy, gum, frequent rinsing of mouth for dryness
- Storage in airtight container at room temperature

Evaluate:
- Therapeutic response: absence of running or congested nose, rashes

Teach patient/family:
- All aspects of product use; to notify prescriber of confusion, sedation, hypotension
- To avoid driving, other hazardous activity if drowsiness occurs, especially geriatric patients
- To avoid concurrent use of alcohol, other CNS depressants
- To avoid breastfeeding

TREATMENT OF OVERDOSE:
Ipecac syrup or lavage, diazepam, vasopressors, phenytoin IV

⚠ HIGH ALERT

cytarabine (Rx)

(sye-tare'a-been)

Ara-C, Cytosar ♣

cytarabine liposomal (Rx)

DepoCyt

Func. class.: Antineoplastic, antimetabolite

Chem. class.: Pyrimidine nucleoside analog

Do not confuse:
Cytosar/Cytoxan/Cytovene

ACTION: Competes with physiologic substrate of DNA synthesis, thus interfering with cell replication in the S phase of the cell cycle (before mitosis)

USES: Acute myelocytic leukemia, acute nonlymphocytic leukemia, chronic myelocytic leukemia; lymphomatous meningitis (intrathecal/intraventricular)
Unlabeled uses: Hodgkin's/non-Hodgkin's lymphoma, malignant meningitis, mantle cell lymphoma

CONTRAINDICATIONS: Pregnancy (D), hypersensitivity
Precautions: Breastfeeding, children, renal/hepatic disease, tumor lysis syndrome, infection, hyperkalemia, hyperphosphatemia, hyperuricemia, hypocalcemia

Black Box Warning: Bone marrow suppression

DOSAGE AND ROUTES

Acute myelogenous leukemia (AML)
• **Adult: CONT IV INF** 100 mg/m²/day × 7 days q2wk as single agent or 2-6 mg/kg/day (100-200 mg/m²/day) as a single dose or 2-3 divided doses for 5-10 days until remission, used in combination; maintenance 70-200 mg/m²/day for 2-5 days q mo; **SUBCUT/IM** maintenance 100 mg/m²/day × 5 days q28days

Meningeal leukemia
• **Adult/child: INTRATHECAL** 5-70 mg/m² variable daily × 4 days to q2-7days

Refractory acute Hodgkin's/ refractory non-Hodgkin's lymphoma (unlabeled)
• **Adult/child: IV** 2 g/m²/day; on day 5 q21days, with etoposide, methylPREDNISolone, and CISplatin

Carcinomatous meningitis (liposoma)
• **Adult: IT** 50 mg over 1-5 min q14days, during induction and consolidation wk 1, 3, 5, 7, 9, give another 50 mg **IT** wk 13; maintenance 50 mg q28days on wk 17, 21, 25, 29 use with dexamethasone 4 mg **PO/IV** × 5 day on each day of cytarabine

Renal dose
• **Adult CCr ≤60 ml/min, serum creatinine 1.5-1.9 mg/dl or increase of 0.5-1.2 mg/dl from baseline during treatment:** reduce to 1 g/m²/dose; **serum creatinine ≥2 mg/dl or change from baseline serum creatinine was 1.2 mg/dl:** reduce to 100 mg/m²/day

Available forms: Powder for inj 100, 500 mg, 1, 2 g; sus rel, (DepoCyt) liposomal for intrathecal use 10 mg/ml

Administer:
• Antiemetic 30-60 min before product and prn
• Allopurinol to maintain uric acid levels and alkalinization of the urine
• Topical or systemic analgesics for pain

IT route
• Use preservative-free NS, add 5 ml/100-mg vial or 10 ml/500-mg vial; use immediately, discard unused product
• Use dexamethasone with IT administration

IV route
• Use cytotoxic handling precautions

Direct IV route
• After diluting 100 mg/5 ml of sterile water for inj; given by direct IV over 1-3 min through free-flowing tubing (IV)

Intermittent IV INF route

- May be further diluted in 50-100 ml NS or D_5W, given over 30 min to 24 hr, depending on dose

Continuous IV INF route

- May also be given by continuous inf

Additive compatibilities: Corticotropin, DAUNOrubicin with etoposide, etoposide, hydrOXYzine, lincomycin, mitoxantrone, ondansetron, potassium chloride, prednisoLONE, sodium bicarbonate, vinCRIStine

Solution compatibilities: Amino acids, D_5/LR, D_5/0.2% NaCl, D_5/0.9% NaCl, D_{10}/0.9% NaCl, D_5W, invert sugar 10% in electrolyte #1, Ringer's, LR, 0.9% NaCl, sodium lactate 1/6 mol/L, TPN #57

Syringe compatibilities: Metoclopramide

Y-site compatibilities: Acyclovir, alfentanil, amifostine, amikacin, aminocaproic acid, aminophylline, amphotericin B lipid complex, amphotericin B liposome, ampicillin, ampicillin-sulbactam, amsacrine, anidulafungin, atenolol, atracurium, azithromycin, aztreonam, bivalirudin, bleomycin, bumetanide, buprenorphine, butorphanol, calcium chloride/gluconate, CARBOplatin, cefazolin, cefepime, cefoperazone, cefotaxime, cefotetan, cefoxitin, ceftazidime, ceftizoxime, cefTRIAXone, cefuroxime, chlorproMAZINE, cimetidine, ciprofloxacin, cisatracurium, CISplatin, cladribine, clindamycin, codeine, cyclophosphamide, cycloSPORINE, DAUNOrubicin, dexamethasone, dexmedetomidine, dexrazoxane, digoxin, diltiazem, diphenhydrAMINE, DOBUTamine, docetaxel, dolasetron, DOPamine, doxacurium, DOXOrubicin, DOXOrubicin liposomal, doxycycline, droperidol, enalaprilat, ePHEDrine, EPINEPHrine, ertapenem, erythromycin, esmolol, etoposide, famotidine, fenoldopam, fentaNYL, filgrastim, fluconazole, fludarabine, foscarnet, fosphenytoin, furosemide, gatifloxacin, gemcitabine, gemtuzumab, gentamicin, granisetron, haloperidol, heparin, hydrocortisone, HYDROmorphone, hydrOXYzine, IDArubicin, ifosfamide, imipenem-cilastatin, inamrinone, insulin (regular), irinotecan, isoproterenol, ketorolac, labetalol, leucovorin, levofloxacin, levorphanol, lidocaine, linezolid, LORazepam, magnesium sulfate, mannitol, melphalan, meperidine, meropenem, mesna, methohexital, methotrexate, methylPREDNISolone, metoclopramide, metoprolol, metroNIDAZOLE, midazolam, milrinone, minocycline, mitoxantrone, mivacurium, morphine, nalbuphine, naloxone, nesiritide, niCARdipine, nitroglycerin, nitroprusside, norepinephrine, octreotide, ofloxacin, ondansetron, oxaliplatin, paclitaxel, palonosetron, pamidronate, pancuronium, pantoprazole, pemetrexed, pentamidine, PENTobarbital, PHENobarbital, phenylephrine, piperacillin, piperacillin-tazobactam, potassium chloride/phosphates, procainamide, prochlorperazine, promethazine, propofol, propranolol, quinupristin-dalfopristin, ranitidine, rapacuronium, remifentanil, riTUXimab, rocuronium, sargramostim, sodium acetate/bicarbonate/phosphates, succinylcholine, SUFentanil, sulfamethoxazole-trimethoprim, tacrolimus, teniposide, theophylline, thiopental, thiotepa, ticarcillin, ticarcillin-clavulanate, tigecycline, tirofiban, TNA, tobramycin, trastuzumab, trimethobenzamide, vancomycin, vasopressin, vecuronium, verapamil, vinCRISTine, vinorelbine, voriconazole, zidovudine, zoledronic acid

SIDE EFFECTS

CNS: Neuritis, dizziness, headache, cerebellar syndrome, personality changes, ataxia, mechanical dysphasia, **coma; chemical arachnoiditis (IT)**

CV: Chest pain, **cardiopathy**

CYTARABINE SYNDROME: *Fever,* myalgia, bone pain, chest pain, *rash,* conjunctivitis, malaise (6-12 hr after administration)

EENT: Sore throat, conjunctivitis

GI: *Nausea, vomiting, anorexia, diarrhea, stomatitis,* **hepatotoxicity,** abdominal pain, hematemesis, **GI hemorrhage**

GU: Urinary retention, renal failure, hyperuricemia
HEMA: Thrombophlebitis, bleeding, thrombocytopenia, leukopenia, myelosuppression, anemia
INTEG: *Rash, fever,* freckling, cellulitis
META: Hyperuricemia
RESP: Pneumonia, dyspnea, pulmonary edema (high doses)
SYST: Anaphylaxis

PHARMACOKINETICS

INTRATHECAL: Half-life 100-236 hr; metabolized in liver; excreted in urine (primarily inactive metabolite); crosses blood-brain barrier, placenta
IV/SUBCUT: Distribution half-life 10 min, elimination half-life 1-3 hr

INTERACTIONS

- Do not use with live virus vaccines
- Do not use within 24 hr of chemotherapy—sargramostim, GM-CSF, filgrastim, G-CSF

Increase: toxicity—immunosuppressants, methotrexate, flucytosine, radiation, or other antineoplastics
Increase: bleeding risk—anticoagulants, platelet inhibitors, salicylates, thrombolytics, NSAIDs
Decrease: effects of oral digoxin, gentamicin

NURSING CONSIDERATIONS

Assess:

Black Box Warning: Bone marrow suppression: CBC (RBC, Hct, Hgb), differential, platelet count weekly; withhold product if WBC is <1000/mm³, platelet count is <50,000/mm³, or RBC, Hct, Hgb low; notify prescriber of these results

- Renal studies: BUN, serum uric acid, urine CCr, electrolytes before and during therapy
- I&O ratio; report fall in urine output to <30 ml/hr
- Monitor temp q4hr; fever may indicate beginning infection; no rectal temps
- **Hepatotoxicity:** hepatic studies before and during therapy: bilirubin, ALT, AST, alk phos, as needed or monthly; check for jaundice of skin, sclera; dark urine; clay-colored stools; pruritus; abdominal pain; fever; diarrhea
- Blood uric acid during therapy

⚠ For anaphylaxis: rash, pruritus, facial swelling, dyspnea; resuscitation equipment should be nearby

⚠ Chemical arachnoiditis (IT): headache, nausea, vomiting, fever; neck rigidity pain, meningism, CSF pleocytosis; may be decreased by dexamethasone

- Cytarabine syndrome 6-12 hr after inf: fever, myalgia, bone pain, chest pain, rash, conjunctivitis, malaise; corticosteroids may be ordered
- Bleeding: hematuria, heme-positive stools, bruising or petechiae, mucosa or orifices q8hr

⚠ Dyspnea, crackles, unproductive cough, chest pain, tachypnea, fatigue, increased pulse, pallor, lethargy; personality changes, with high doses; pulmonary edema may be fatal (rare)

- Buccal cavity q8hr for dryness, sores or ulceration, white patches, oral pain, bleeding, dysphagia
- Local irritation, pain, burning, discoloration at inj site
- GI symptoms: frequency of stools, cramping; antispasmodic may be used
- Acidosis, signs of dehydration: rapid respirations, poor skin turgor, decreased urine output, dry skin, restlessness, weakness

Perform/provide:

- Increased fluid intake to 2-3 L/day to prevent urate deposits and calculi formation unless contraindicated
- Diet low in purines: absence of organ meats (kidney, liver), dried beans, peas to prevent increased urate deposits
- Rinsing of mouth tid-qid with water, club soda; brushing of teeth bid-tid with soft brush or cotton-tipped applicators for stomatitis; use unwaxed dental floss

Evaluate:

- Therapeutic response: decreased tumor size, spread of malignancy

Teach patient/family:

- To report any coughing, chest pain, changes in breathing; may indicate beginning **pneumonia, pulmonary edema**
- To avoid foods with citric acid, spicy or rough texture if stomatitis is present, use sponge brush and rinse with water after each meal; to report stomatitis: any bleeding, white spots, ulcerations in mouth; to examine mouth daily, report any symptoms
- To report signs of **infection:** increased temp, sore throat, flulike symptoms; to avoid crowds, persons with infections
- To report signs of **anemia:** fatigue, headache, faintness, SOB, irritability
- To report bleeding; to avoid use of razors, commercial mouthwash, salicylates, NSAIDs, anticoagulants
- To use thrombocytopenia precautions
- To take fluids to 3 L/day to prevent renal damage
- To use reliable contraception during treatment and for 4 mo thereafter; not to breastfeed
- To avoid receiving vaccines during treatment
- That fever, headache, nausea, vomiting likely to occur

dabigatran

(da-bye-gat′ran)

Pradaxa

Func. class.: Anticoagulant-thrombin inhibitor

ACTION: Direct thrombin inhibitor that inhibits both free and clot-bound thrombin, prevents thrombin-induced platelet aggregation and thrombus formation by preventing conversion of fibrinogen to fibrin

USES: Stroke/systemic embolism prophylaxis with nonvalvular atrial fibrillation

Unlabeled uses: Deep venous thrombus (DVT), pulmonary embolism prophylaxis

CONTRAINDICATIONS: Hypersensitivity, bleeding

Precautions: Pregnancy (C), labor, obstetric delivery, breastfeeding, children, geriatric patients, abrupt discontinuation, anticoagulant therapy, renal disease, surgery

DOSAGE AND ROUTES

Stroke prophylaxis

- **Adult: PO** 150 mg bid

For conversion from an alternative anticoagulant to dabigatran

- When converting from warfarin to dabigatran, discontinue warfarin and initiate dabigatran therapy when the INR is <2.0; when converting from a parenteral anticoagulant to dabigatran, initiate dabigatran 0-2 hr before the time of the next scheduled anticoagulant dose or at the time of discontinuation of a continuously administered anticoagulant (e.g., intravenous unfractionated heparin)

For conversion from dabigatran to warfarin

- **Adult:** CCr >50 ml/min, start warfarin 3 days before discontinuing dabigatran; CCr 31-50 ml/min, start warfarin 2 days before discontinuing dabigatran; CCr 15-30 ml/min, start warfarin 1 day before discontinuing dabigatran

For conversion from dabigatran to parenteral anticoagulants

- **Adult: PO** discontinue dabigatran, start parenteral anticoagulant 12 hr (CCR ≥30 ml/min) or 24 hr (CCR <30 ml/min) after the last dabigatran dose

Renal dose

- **Adult: PO** CCr 15-30 ml/min, 75 mg bid

Deep venous thrombus (DVT)/ pulmonary embolism prophylaxis (unlabeled)

- **Adult: PO** 220 mg or 150 mg/day × 28-35 days, starting with ½ dose 1-4 hr after surgery

Administer
- Do not crush, break, chew, or empty contents of capsule
- If dose is missed, take as soon as remembered if on the same day; do not administer if <6 hr before next dose
- Without regard to food

SIDE EFFECTS

CNS: Intracranial bleeding
CV: Myocardial infarction
GI: Abdominal pain, dyspepsia, peptic ulcer, esophagitis, GERD, gastritis, GI bleeding
HEMA: Bleeding
INTEG: Rash, pruritus
SYST: Anaphylaxis (rare)

PHARMACOKINETICS

Protein binding 35%, half-life 12-17 hr (extended in renal disease), peak 1 hr, high-fat meal delays peak

INTERACTIONS

Increase: bleeding risk—amiodarone, other anticoagulants, clopidogrel, ketoconazole, quinidine, thrombolytics, verapamil
Decrease: dabigatran effect—rifampin

NURSING CONSIDERATIONS

Assess:
- **Bleeding:** blood in urine or emesis, dark tarry stools, lower back pain; caution with arterial/venous punctures, catheters, NG tubes; monitor vital signs frequently; elderly more prone to serious bleeding
- **Thrombosis/MI/emboli:** swelling, pain, redness, difficulty breathing, chest pain, tachypnea, cough, coughing up blood, cyanosis
- **Post-thrombotic syndrome:** pain, heaviness, itching/tingling, swelling, varicose veins, brownish/reddish skin discoloration, ulcers; use of ambulation, compression stockings, adequate anticoagulation can prevent this syndrome
- Serum creatinine

Perform/provide:
- Store in original package at room temp until time of use; discard after 30 days, protect from moisture

Evaluate:
- Therapeutic response: decreased thrombus formation/extension, absence of emboli, post-thrombotic effects

Teach patient/family:
- About the purpose and expected results of this product
- To report if bleeding is present

⚠ HIGH ALERT

dacarbazine (Rx)

(da-kar′ba-zeen)

DTIC ✦, DTIC-Dome

Func. class.: Antineoplastic alkylating agent

Chem. class.: Cytotoxic triazine

ACTION:

Alkylates DNA, RNA; inhibits DNA, RNA synthesis; also responsible for breakage, cross-linking of DNA strands; activity is not cell-cycle–phase specific

USES:

Hodgkin's disease, malignant melanoma

Unlabeled uses: Malignant pheochromocytoma in combination with cyclophosphamide and vinCRIStine, metastatic soft-tissue sarcoma in combination with other agents, carcinoma meningitis, neuroblastoma

CONTRAINDICATIONS:

Breastfeeding, hypersensitivity

Precautions: Renal disease

Black Box Warning: Pregnancy (C) 1st trimester, radiation therapy, hepatic disease, bone marrow suppression, secondary malignancy

DOSAGE AND ROUTES

Metastatic malignant melanoma

• **Adult:** IV 2-4.5 mg/kg/day × 10 days or 100-250 mg/m^2/day × 5 days; repeat q3-4wk depending on response

Hodgkin's disease

• **Adult:** IV 150 mg/m^2/day × 5 days with other agents, repeat q4wk; or 375 mg/m^2 on days 1 and 15 when given in combination, repeat q28 days

Osteogenic sarcoma (unlabeled)

• **Adult and child:** IV 250 mg/m^2/day as continuous inf × 4 days q28days

Soft-tissue sarcoma (unlabeled)

• **Adult and child:** IV 250-300 mg/m^2/day as continuous inf × 3 days q21-28 days

Carcinoma meningitis (unlabeled)

• **Adult:** INTRATHECAL 5-30 mg in a fixed dose 2-3 ×/wk until disease controlled

Available forms: Powder for inj 10, 100, 200 mg

Administer:

• Antiemetic 30-60 min before giving product to prevent vomiting, nausea; vomiting may subside after several doses

• Antibiotics for prophylaxis of infection

IV route

• Use cytotoxic handling precautions

Direct IV route

• After diluting 100 mg/9.9 ml of sterile water for inj (10 mg/ml), give by direct IV over 1 min through Y-tube or 3-way stopcock

Intermittent IV INF route

• May be further diluted in 50-250 ml D_5W or NS for inj, given as an inf over ½ hr

• Watch for extravasation; give 4 ml Na thiosulfate 10% plus 5 ml sterile water, 3-5 ml SUBCUT if needed

Y-site compatibilities: Amifostine, anidulafungin, atenolol, aztreonam, bivalirudin, bleomycin, caspofungin, DAPTOmycin, dexmedetomidine, docetaxel, DOXOrubicin, ertapenem, etoposide, fenoldopam, filgrastim, fludarabine, gemtuzumab, granisetron, levofloxacin, mechlorethamine, melphalan, nesiritide, octreotide, ondansetron, oxaliplatin, paclitaxel, palonosetron, pamidronate, quinupristin-dalfopristin, sargramostim, teniposide, thiotepa, tigecycline, tirofiban, vinorelbine, voriconazole, zoledronic acid

SIDE EFFECTS

CNS: Facial paresthesia, flushing, fever, malaise; confusion, headache, **seizures, cerebral hemorrhage,** blurred vision (high doses)

GI: *Nausea, anorexia, vomiting,* **hepatotoxicity** (rare)

HEMA: **Thrombocytopenia, leukopenia,** anemia

INTEG: *Alopecia,* dermatitis, pain at inj site, photosensitivity; severe sun reactions (high doses)

MISC: Flulike symptoms, malaise, fever, myalgia, hypotension

SYST: **Anaphylaxis**

PHARMACOKINETICS

Metabolized by liver; excreted in urine; half-life 35 min, terminal 5 hr, 5% protein bound

INTERACTIONS

• **Toxicity, bone marrow suppression:** bone marrow suppressants, radiation, other antineoplastics

• Bleeding: salicylates, anticoagulants

Increase: adverse reaction; decrease antibody reaction—live virus vaccines

Increase: nephrotoxicity—aminoglycosides

Increase: ototoxicity—loop diuretics

Decrease: dacarbazine effect—phenytoin, PHENobarbital

NURSING CONSIDERATIONS

Assess:

⚠ **Bone marrow suppression:** **CBC, differential, platelet count weekly; withhold product if WBC <4000 or platelet count <75,000; notify prescriber of results**

• Monitor temp q4hr; may indicate beginning infection

• Bleeding: hematuria, guaiac, bruising, petechiae of mucosa or orifices q8hr
• Effects of alopecia on body image, discuss feelings about body changes

Black Box Warning: Hepatic disease: jaundice of skin, sclera; dark urine; clay-colored stools; itchy skin; abdominal pain; fever; diarrhea; hepatic studies before, during therapy (bilirubin, AST, ALT, LDH) as needed or monthly

• Inflammation of mucosa, breaks in skin

⚠ **Hypersensitivity reactions, anaphylaxis,** discontinue product, administer meds for anaphylaxis

Perform/provide:

• Storage in light-resistant container in a dry area
• Increased fluid intake to 2-3 L/day to prevent urate deposits, calculi formation
• Warm compresses at inf site for inflammation

Evaluate:

• Therapeutic response: decreased tumor size, spread of malignancy

Teach patient/family:

• That patient should avoid prolonged exposure to sun, wear sunscreen
• That hair may be lost during treatment; that a wig or hairpiece may make the patient feel better; that new hair may be different in color, texture
• To report signs of **infection:** fever, sore throat, flulike symptoms
• To report signs of **anemia:** fatigue, headache, faintness, SOB, irritability
• To report bleeding; to avoid use of razors, commercial mouthwash
• To avoid aspirin products or ibuprofen

Black Box Warning: To use reliable contraceptives during and for several months after therapy; not to breastfeed

⚠ **HIGH ALERT**

DACTINomycin (Rx)

(dak-ti-noe-mye′sin)

Cosmegen

Func. class.: Antineoplastic, antibiotic

Do not confuse:
DACTINomycin/daptomycin

ACTION: Inhibits DNA, RNA, protein synthesis; derived from *Streptomyces parvullus;* replication is decreased by binding to DNA, which causes strand splitting; cell-cycle nonspecific; a vesicant

USES: Sarcomas, trophoblastic tumors in women, testicular cancer, Wilms' tumor, rhabdomyosarcoma

Unlabeled uses: Kaposi's sarcoma, malignant melanoma, osteogenic sarcoma, ovarian cancer, soft tissue sarcoma

CONTRAINDICATIONS: Children <6 mo, hypersensitivity, herpes infection

Black Box Warning: Pregnancy (D)

Precautions: Breastfeeding, renal/hepatic disease, bone marrow depression, tumor lysis syndrome, infection

Black Box Warning: Accidental exposure, extravasation, secondary malignancy

DOSAGE AND ROUTES

• **Adult: IV** 500 mcg/m²/day × 5 days; stop product for 2-4 wk then repeat cycle
• **Child: IV** 15 mcg/kg/day × 5 days not to exceed 500 mcg/day; stop product until bone marrow recovery, then repeat cycle

Choriocarcinoma/hydatidiform mole

• **Adult: IV** 1250 mcg/m² q14days × 4 cycles

Wilms' tumor/childhood rhabdomyosarcoma/Ewing's sarcoma
• **Adult and child:** IV 15 mcg/kg/day × 5 days
Germ cell testicular cancer
• **Adult and child:** IV 1000 mcg/m^2 as a single dose on day 1
Malignant melanoma (unlabeled)
• **Adult:** IV 1-1.5 mg/m^2
Soft tissue sarcoma/Kaposi's sarcoma (unlabeled)
• **Adult:** CONT IV INF 15 mcg/kg/day × 5 days q3mo
Germ testicular/ovarian cancer (unlabeled)
• **Adult and child:** IV 1000 mcg/m^2 as a single dose on day 1; used with VAB-6 regimen

Available forms: Inj 0.5 mg/vial

Administer:
• Antiemetic 30-60 min before product to prevent vomiting
• Increase fluids to 3 L/day

IV route
• Use cytotoxic handling precautions

Direct IV route
• After diluting 0.5-mg vial/1.1 ml sterile water for inj without preservative, give by direct IV at 0.5 mg over 1-3 min through Y-tube or 3-way stopcock if inf in progress

Intermittent IV INF route
• May be further diluted if required in 50 ml D_5W or NS for inf; run over 20-30 min; change needles between reconstitution and direct IV administration

Black Box Warning: Hydrocortisone, sodium thiosulfate to infiltration area, and ice compress after stopping inf

Y-site compatibilities: Acyclovir, alfentanil, allopurinol, amifostine, amikacin, aminophylline, amiodarone, amphotericin B colloidal, amphotericin B lipid complex, amphotericin B liposome, ampicillin, ampicillin-sulbactam, anidulafungin, atenolol, atracurium, aztreonam, bivalirudin, bleomycin, bumetanide, buprenorphine, butorphanol, calcium chloride/gluconate, caspofungin, ceFAZolin, cefepime, cefoperazone, cefotaxime, cefotetan, cefoxitin, ceftazidime, ceftizoxime, cefTRIAXone, cefuroxime, chloramphenicol, chlorproMAZINE, cimetidine, ciprofloxacin, cisatracurium, CISplatin, clindamycin, codeine, cyclophosphamide, cycloSPORINE, DAPTOmycin, DAUNOrubicin, dexamethasone, dexmedetomidine, dexrazoxane, digoxin, diltiazem, diphenhydrAMINE, DOBUTamine, docetaxel, DOPamine, DOXOrubicin, doxycycline, droperidol, enalaprilat, ePHEDrine, EPINEPHrine, ertapenem, erythromycin, esmolol, etoposide, famotidine, fenoldopam, fentaNYL, fluconazole, fludarabine, foscarnet, fosphenytoin, furosemide, ganciclovir, gatifloxacin, gemcitabine, gentamicin, glycopyrrolate, granisetron, haloperidol, heparin, hydrALAZINE, hydrocortisone, HYDROmorphone, hydrOXYzine, IDArubicin, ifosfamide, imipenem-cilastatin, inamrinone, insulin (regular), isoproterenol, ketorolac, labetalol, leucovorin, levofloxacin, levorphanol, lidocaine, linezolid, LORazepam, magnesium sulfate, mannitol, melphalan, meperidine, meropenem, mesna, metaraminol, methohexital, methotrexate, methyldopate, methylPREDNISolone, metoclopramide, metoprolol, metroNIDAZOLE, midazolam, milrinone, minocycline, mitomycin, mitoxantrone, morphine, nafcillin, nalbuphine, naloxone, nesiritide, nitroglycerin, nitroprusside, norepinephrine, octreotide, ofloxacin, ondansetron, oxaliplatin, paclitaxel, palonosetron, pancuronium, pemetrexed, pentamidine, pentazocine, PENTobarbital, PHENobarbital, phenylephrine, piperacillin, piperacillin-tazobactam, polymyxin B, potassium chloride/phosphates, procainamide, prochlorperazine, promethazine, propranolol, quiNIDine, quinupristin-dalfopristin, ranitidine, remifentanil, riTUXimab, sargramostim, sodium acetate/bicarbonate/phosphates, succinylcholine, SUFentanil, sulfamethoxazole-trimethoprim, tacrolimus, teniposide, theophylline, thiopental, thiotepa, ticarcillin, ticarcillin-clavulanate, tigecycline, tirofiban, tobramycin, tolazoline, topotecan, trastuzumab, trimethobenzamide, vancomycin, vasopressin, vecuronium, verapamil, vinBLAStine, vinCRIStine, vinorelbine, voriconazole, zidovudine, zoledronic acid

SIDE EFFECTS

CNS: Malaise, fatigue, lethargy, fever
EENT: Chelitis, dysphagia, esophagitis
GI: *Nausea, vomiting, anorexia, stomatitis,* hepatotoxicity, abdominal pain, diarrhea
HEMA: Thrombocytopenia, leukopenia, aplastic anemia
INTEG: *Rash,* alopecia, pain at inj site, folliculitis, acne, desquamation, extravasation
MS: Myalgia

PHARMACOKINETICS

Half-life 36 hr; IV onset 2-5 min; concentrates in kidneys, liver, spleen; does not cross blood-brain barrier; excreted in feces and urine

INTERACTIONS

Increase: toxicity—other antineoplastics, radiation

Drug/Lab Test

Increase: uric acid

NURSING CONSIDERATIONS

Assess:

- Bone marrow suppression: CBC, differential, platelet count weekly; withhold product if WBC is $<4000/mm^3$ or platelet count is $<75,000/mm^3$; notify prescriber
- Renal studies: BUN, serum uric acid, urine CCr, electrolytes before, during therapy
- I&O ratio; report fall in urine output to <30 ml/hr
- Monitor temp q4hr; fever may indicate beginning infection
- Hepatic studies before, during therapy: bilirubin, AST, ALT, alk phos as needed or monthly; check for jaundice of skin, sclera; dark urine; clay-colored stools; itchy skin; abdominal pain; fever; diarrhea
- Bleeding: hematuria, guaiac stools, bruising, petechiae, mucosa or orifices q8hr
- Food preferences; list likes, dislikes
- Effects of alopecia on body image; discuss feelings about body changes
- Inflammation of mucosa, breaks in skin
- Buccal cavity q8hr for dryness, sores, ulceration, white patches, oral pain, bleeding, dysphagia

⚠ **Symptoms indicating severe allergic reaction:** rash, pruritus, urticaria, purpuric skin lesions, itching, flushing

- GI symptoms: frequency of stools, cramping, nausea, vomiting, anorexia
- Acidosis, signs of dehydration: rapid respirations, poor skin turgor, decreased urine output, dry skin, restlessness, weakness, sunken eyeballs in children

Perform/provide:

- Liquid diet: carbonated beverages; gelatin may be added if patient is not nauseated or vomiting
- Rinsing of mouth tid-qid with water, club soda; brushing of teeth bid-qid with soft brush or cotton-tipped applicators for stomatitis; use unwaxed dental floss to prevent injury
- Storage in cool, dark environment; do not expose to bright light or freeze
- Fluid increase to 3 L/day

Evaluate:

- Therapeutic response: decreased tumor size, spread of malignancy

Teach patient/family:

Black Box Warning: That reliable contraception is needed during treatment and for 4-6 mo after discontinuing therapy (pregnancy D); not to breastfeed

- To avoid vaccinations without order from prescriber
- That hair may be lost during treatment after 1-2 wk and that wig or hairpiece may make patient feel better; that new hair may be different in color, texture
- To avoid foods with citric acid, hot or rough texture when stomatitis is present

• To report any bleeding, white spots, ulcerations in mouth to prescriber; to examine mouth daily
• To avoid crowds, persons with known infection when granulocyte count is low

dalfampridine (Rx)

(dal-fam′pri-deen)

Ampyra

Func. class.: Neurological agent—MS
Chem. class.: Broad spectrum potassium channel blocker

ACTION: Mechanism of action is not fully understood; a broad-spectrum potassium channel blocker that inhibits potassium channels and increased action potential conduction in demyelinated axions

USES: For improved walking in patients with multiple sclerosis

CONTRAINDICATIONS: Renal failure (CCr <50 ml/min), seizures
Precautions: Pregnancy (C), breastfeeding, geriatric patients, renal disease

DOSAGE AND ROUTES

• **Adult: PO** 10 mg q12hr
Renal dose
• **Adult: PO** CCr 51-80 ml/min, no dosage adjustment needed but seizure risk unknown; CCr ≤50 ml/min, do not use
Available forms: Ext rel tab 10 mg
Administer:
• Do not break, crush, or chew; give without regard to meals
• Do not give closer together than q12hr; seizures may occur
• Do not double doses; if a dose is missed, skip it

SIDE EFFECTS

CNS: Seizures, paresthesias, headache, dizziness, asthenia, insomnia
GI: Nausea, constipation, dyspepsia
GU: Urinary tract infection
MS: Back pain

PHARMACOKINETICS

Bioavailability 96%; peak 3-4 hr (fasting), longer if taken with food; largely unbound to plasma proteins; 96% recovered in urine

INTERACTIONS

• Do not use with fampridine, other 4-aminopyridine (4-AP)–containing products

NURSING CONSIDERATIONS

Assess:
• **Multiple sclerosis:** improved walking, including speed
• **Seizures:** more common in those with previous seizure disorder
Evaluate:
• Therapeutic response: ability to walk at improved speed in MS
Teach patient/family:
• To notify prescriber if pregnancy is planned or suspected; not to breastfeed
• Expected results; side effects, including seizures

⚠ HIGH ALERT

dalteparin (Rx)

(dahl′ta-pear-in)

Fragmin

Func. class.: Anticoagulant
Chem. class.: Low-molecular-weight heparin

ACTION: Inhibits factor Xa/IIa (thrombin), resulting in anticoagulation

USES: Unstable angina/non–Q-wave MI; prevention of deep venous thrombosis in abdominal surgery, hip replacement, or in those with restricted mobility during acute illness, PE
Unlabeled uses: Antiphospholipid antibody, arterial thromboembolism (after heart valve surgery), cerebral thromboembolism

CONTRAINDICATIONS: Hypersensitivity to this product, heparin, or pork products, benzyl alcohol; active major bleeding, hemophilia, leukemia with bleeding, thrombocytopenic purpura, cerebrovascular hemorrhage, cerebral aneurysm; those undergoing regional anesthesia for unstable angina, non–Q-wave MI, dalteparin-induced thrombocytopenia

Precautions: Pregnancy (B), breastfeeding, children, recent childbirth, geriatric patients; hepatic disease; severe renal disease; blood dyscrasias; bacterial endocarditis; acute nephritis; uncontrolled hypertension; recent brain, spine, eye surgery; congenital or acquired disorders; severe cardiac disease; peptic ulcer disease; hemorrhagic stroke; history of HIT; pericarditis; pericardial effusion; recent lumbar puncture; vasculitis; other diseases in which bleeding is possible

Black Box Warning: Epidural anesthesia

DOSAGE AND ROUTES

Hip replacement surgery/DVT prophylaxis

- **Adult: SUBCUT** 2500 international units 2 hr prior to surgery and 2nd dose in the evening on the day of surgery (4-8 hr postop), then 5000 international units **SUBCUT** 1st postop day and daily × 5-10 days

Unstable angina/non–Q-wave MI

- **Adult: SUBCUT** 120 international units/kg q12hr × 5-8 days, max 10,000 international units q12hr × 5-8 days with concurrent aspirin; continue until stable

DVT, prophylaxis for abdominal surgery

- **Adult: SUBCUT** 2500 international units 1-2 hr before surgery; repeat daily × 5-10 days; for high-risk patients, 5000 international units should be used

DVT/pulmonary embolism in cancer patients

- **Adult: SUBCUT** 200 international units/kg daily during 1st month (max single dose 18,000 international units), then 150 international units/kg daily for months 2-6 (max single dose 18,000 international units), use prefilled syringe that is closest to calculated dose; if platelets are 50,000-100,000/mm^3, reduce dose by 2500 international units until platelets ≥100,000 mm^3; if platelets <50,000/mm^3, discontinue until >50,000/mm^3

Renal dose

- **Adult: SUBCUT** cancer patient with CCr <30 ml/min, monitor anti-factor Xa during extended treatment

APLA (unlabeled)

- **Adult (female): SUBCUT** Antepartum 5000 international units/day with aspirin; maintain anti-factor Xa of 0.2-0.6 international units/ml

Cerebral thromboembolism (unlabeled)

- **Adult: SUBCUT** 120 international units/kg (max 10,000 international units) q12hr × 5-8 days, usually with aspirin therapy

Arterial thromboembolism prophylaxis (unlabeled)

- **Adult: SUBCUT** LMWH in combination with oral anticoagulants until INR is in therapeutic range × 2 consecutive days

Available forms: Prefilled syringes, 2500, 5000 international units/0.2 ml; 7500 international units/0.3 ml; 10,000, 25,000 international units/ml

Administer:

- Cannot be used interchangeably (unit for unit) with unfractionated heparin or LMWHs
- Do not give IM or IV product route; approved is SUBCUT only; do not mix with other inj or sol
- Have patient sit or lie down; SUBCUT inj may be 2 inches from umbilicus in a U-shape, upper outer side of thigh, around navel, or upper outer quadrangle of the buttocks; rotate inj sites
- Changing needles not recommended; change inj site daily; use at same time of day

SIDE EFFECTS

CNS: Intracranial bleeding
HEMA: Thrombocytopenia
INTEG: Pruritus, superficial wound infection
SYST: Hypersensitivity, hemorrhage, anaphylaxis possible

PHARMACOKINETICS

87% absorbed, excreted by kidneys, elimination half-life 3-5 hr, peak 4 hr, onset 1-2 hr, duration >12 hr

INTERACTIONS

Increase: bleeding risk—aspirin, oral anticoagulants, platelet inhibitors, NSAIDs, salicylates, thrombolytics
Drug/Lab Test
Increase: AST, ALT

NURSING CONSIDERATIONS

Assess:

- Blood studies (Hct/Hgb, CBC, platelets, anti-Xa, stool guaiac) during treatment because bleeding can occur

⚠ **Bleeding:** Bleeding gums, petechiae, ecchymosis, black tarry stools, hematuria, epistaxis, decrease in Hct, B/P; may indicate bleeding, possible hemorrhage; notify prescriber immediately, product should be discontinued

⚠ **Epidural anesthesia:** Neurologic impairment frequently in those when neuraxial anesthesia has been used, spinal/epidural hematomas can occur, with paralysis

- **Hypersensitivity:** fever, skin rash, urticaria; notify prescriber immediately
- Needed dosage change q1-2wk; dose may need to be decreased if bleeding occurs

Evaluate:

- Therapeutic response: absence of DVT

Teach patient/family:

- To avoid OTC preparations that contain aspirin; other anticoagulants, serious product interaction may occur unless approved by prescriber
- To use soft-bristle toothbrush to avoid bleeding gums; to avoid contact sports; use electric razor; to avoid IM inj
- To report any signs of bleeding (gums, under skin, urine, stools), unusual bruising

TREATMENT OF OVERDOSE:

Protamine sulfate 1% given IV; 1 mg protamine/100 anti-Xa international units of dalteparin given

dantrolene (Rx)

(dan′troe-leen)

Dantrium, Revonto

Func. class.: Skeletal muscle relaxant, direct acting
Chem. class.: Hydantoin

Do not confuse:
Dantrium/danazol

ACTION: Interferes with intracellular release of calcium from the sarcoplasmic reticulum necessary to initiate contraction; slows catabolism in malignant hyperthermia

USES: Spasticity in multiple sclerosis, stroke, spinal cord injury, cerebral palsy, malignant hyperthermia
Unlabeled uses: Neuroleptic malignant syndrome

CONTRAINDICATIONS: Hypersensitivity, compromised pulmonary function, impaired myocardial function

Black Box Warning: Active hepatic disease

Precautions: Pregnancy (C), breastfeeding, geriatric patients, peptic ulcer disease, cardiac/renal/hepatic disease, stroke, seizure disorder, diabetes mellitus, ALS, COPD, MS, mannitol/gelatin hypersensitivity, labor, lactase deficiency, extravasation

Black Box Warning: Females

DOSAGE AND ROUTES

Spasticity

• **Adult: PO** 25 mg/day; may increase to 25-100 mg bid-qid, max 400 mg/day

• **Child: PO** 0.5 mg/kg/day given in divided doses bid; dosage may increase gradually, max 400 mg/day

Prevention of malignant hyperthermia

• **Adult and child: PO** 4-8 mg/kg/day in 3-4 divided doses × 1-2 days prior to procedure, give last dose 4 hr preop; **IV** 2.5 mg/kg prior to anesthesia

Malignant hyperthermia

• **Adult and child: IV** 1 mg/kg, may repeat to total dose of 10 mg/kg; **PO** 4-8 mg/kg/day in 4 divided doses × 3 days to prevent further hyperthermia; post-crisis follow up 4-8 mg/kg/day for 1-3 days

Neuroleptic malignant syndrome (unlabeled)

• **Adult: PO** 100-300 mg/day in divided doses; **IV** 1.25-1.5 mg/kg

Available forms: Caps 25, 50, 100 mg; powder for inj 20 mg/vial

Administer:

• Avoid use with other CNS depressants

PO route

• Do not crush or chew caps

• Caps may be opened, mixed with juice and swallowed

• With meals for GI symptoms

IV route

• IV after diluting 20 mg/60 ml sterile water for inj without bacteriostatic agent (333 mcg/ml); shake until clear; give by rapid IV push through Y-tube or 3-way stopcock; follow with prescribed doses immediately; may also give by intermittent inf over 1 hr prior to anesthesia

SIDE EFFECTS

CNS: *Dizziness, weakness, fatigue, drowsiness,* headache, disorientation, insomnia, paresthesias, tremors, seizures

CV: Hypotension, chest pain, palpitations

EENT: Nasal congestion, blurred vision, mydriasis

GI: Hepatic injury, *nausea,* constipation, vomiting, increased AST, alk phos, abdominal pain, dry mouth, anorexia, hepatitis, dyspepsia

GU: Urinary frequency, nocturia, impotence, crystalluria

HEMA: Eosinophilia, aplastic anemia, leukopenia

INTEG: Rash, pruritus, photosensitivity, extravasation (tissue necrosis)

RESP: Pleural effusion

PHARMACOKINETICS

PO: Peak 5 hr, highly protein bound, half-life 8 hr, metabolized in liver, excreted in urine (metabolites), absorption poor (35%)

INTERACTIONS

• Considered incompatible in sol or syringe; compatibility unknown

Increase: dysrhythmias—verapamil

Increase: hepatotoxicity—estrogens, other hepatotoxics

Increase: CNS depression—alcohol, tricyclics, opiates, barbiturates, sedatives, hypnotics, antihistamines

NURSING CONSIDERATIONS

Assess:

• **Seizures:** increased seizure activity, ECG in epilepsy patient; poor seizure control has occurred

• I&O ratio; check for urinary retention, frequency, hesitancy, especially geriatric patients

Black Box Warning: **Active hepatic disease:** hepatic function by frequent determination of AST, ALT, bilirubin, alk phos, GGTP; renal function studies, BUN, creatinine, CBC

• **Allergic reactions:** rash, fever, respiratory distress

• Severe weakness, numbness in extremities; prescriber should be notified and product discontinued

• Tolerance: increased need/more frequent requests for medication, increased pain

• CNS depression: dizziness, drowsiness, insomnia, psychiatric symptoms

⚠ **Signs of hepatotoxicity:** jaundice, yellow sclera, pain in abdomen, nausea, fever; prescriber should be notified, product discontinued

Perform/provide:

• Storage in tight container at room temp; protect diluted sol from light, use reconstituted sol within 6 hr

• Gum, frequent sips of water for dry mouth

• Assistance with ambulation if dizziness, drowsiness occurs

Evaluate:

• Therapeutic response: decreased pain, spasticity

Teach patient/family:

• Not to discontinue medication quickly because hallucinations, spasticity, tachycardia will occur; product should be tapered off over 1-2 wk; to notify prescriber of abdominal pain, jaundiced sclera, clay-colored stools, change in color of urine

• That, if improvement does not occur within 6 wk, prescriber may discontinue product

• To avoid hazardous activities if drowsiness, dizziness occurs

• To avoid using OTC medications: cough preparations, antihistamines, other CNS depressants, alcohol unless directed by prescriber

• To use sunscreen or stay out of the sun to prevent burns

TREATMENT OF OVERDOSE:

Activated charcoal, supportive care

dapiprazole ophthalmic

See Appendix B

DAPTOmycin (Rx)

(dap′toe-mye-sin)

Cubicin

Func. class.: Antiinfective—miscellaneous

Chem. class.: Lipopeptides

D

ACTION: A new class of antiinfective; it binds to the bacterial membrane and results in a rapid depolarization of the membrane potential, thereby leading to inhibition of DNA, RNA, and protein synthesis

USES: Complicated skin, skin-structure infections caused by *Staphylococcus aureus* including methicillin-resistant strains, *Streptococcus pyogenes, Streptococcus agalactiae, Streptococcus dysgalactiae, Enterococcus faecalis* (vancomycin-susceptible strains)

Unlabeled uses: Bacteremia, endocarditis, UTI, vancomycin-resistant enterococci (VRE), *Corynebacterium jeikeium, Staphylococcus haemolyticus, Enterococcus facium*

CONTRAINDICATIONS: Hypersensitivity

Precautions: Pregnancy (B), breastfeeding, children, geriatric patients, GI/renal disease, myopathy, ulcerative/pseudomembranous colitis, rhabdomyolysis, eosinophilic pneumonia

DOSAGE AND ROUTES

• **Adult: IV INF** 4-6 mg/kg over ½ hr diluted in 0.9% NaCl, give q24hr × 7-14 days

• **Adolescent/child/infant ≥5 mo (unlabeled): IV** 4-6 mg/kg/day

Renal dose

• **Adult: IV INF** CCr <30 ml/min, hemodialysis, CAPD 4 mg/kg q48hr

Bacteremia, endocarditis, UTI (unlabeled)

• **Adult: IV** 6 mg/kg/day

VRE (unlabeled)
- **Adult:** IV 4 mg/kg/day

Available forms: Lyophilized powder for inj 500 mg

Administer:

IV route
- After reconstitution with 5 ml 0.9% NaCl (250 mg/5 ml) or 10 ml 0.9% NaCl (500 mg/10 ml); further dilution is needed with 0.9 NaCl; infuse over ½ hr or give reconstituted sol (50 mg/ml) by IV inj over 2 min, do not use dextrose-containing solutions

Y-site compatibilities: Alfentanil, amifostine, amikacin, aminocaproic acid, aminophylline, amiodarone, amphotericin B liposome, ampicillin, ampicillin-sulbactam, argatroban, arsenic trioxide, atenolol, atracurium, azithromycin, aztreonam, bivalirudin, bleomycin, bumetanide, buprenorphine, busulfan, butorphanol, calcium chloride/gluconate, CARBOplatin, carmustine, caspofungin, ceFAZolin, cefepime, cefotaxime, cefotetan, cefoxitin, ceftazidime, ceftizoxime, cefTRIAXone, cefuroxime, chloramphenicol, chlorproMAZINE, cimetidine, ciprofloxacin, cisatracurium, CISplatin, clindamycin, cyclophosphamide, cycloSPORINE, dacarbazine, DACTINomycin, DAUNOrubicin, dexamethasone, dexmedetomidine, dexrazoxane, diazepam, digoxin, diltiazem, diphenhydrAMINE, DOBUTamine, docetaxel, dolasetron, DOPamine, doripenem, doxacurium, DOXOrubicin, DOXOrubicin liposomal, doxycycline, droperidol, enalaprilat, ePHEDrine, EPINEPHrine, epirubicin, eptifibatide, ertapenem, erythromycin, esmolol, etoposide, famotidine, fenoldopam, fentaNYL, fluconazole, fludarabine, fluorouracil, foscarnet, fosphenytoin, furosemide, ganciclovir, gentamicin, glycopyrrolate, granisetron, haloperidol, heparin, hydrALAZINE, hydrocortisone, HYDROmorphone, hydrOXYzine, IDArubicin, ifosfamide, inamrinone, insulin (regular), irinotecan, isoproterenol, ketorolac, labetalol, leucovorin, levofloxacin, lidocaine, linezolid, LORazepam, magnesium sulfate, mannitol, mechlorethamine, melphalan, meperidine, meropenem, mesna, metaraminol, methyldopate, methylPREDNISolone, metoclopramide, metoprolol, midazolam, milrinone, mitoxantrone, mivacurium, morphine, moxifloxacin, mycophenolate mofetil, nafcillin, nalbuphine, naloxone, niCARdipine, nitroprusside, norepinephrine, octreotide, ondansetron, oxaliplatin, oxytocin, paclitaxel, palonosetron, pamidronate, pancuronium, pemetrexed, pentamidine, PHENobarbital, phenylephrine, piperacillin-tazobactam, polymyxin B, potassium acetate/chloride/phosphates, procainamide, prochlorperazine, promethazine, propranolol, quinupristin-dalfopristin, ranitidine, rocuronium, sodium acetate/bicarbonate/citrate/phosphates, succinylcholine, sulfamethoxazole-trimethoprim, tacrolimus, teniposide, theophylline, thiotepa, ticarcillin, ticarcillin-clavulanate, tigecycline, tirofiban, tobramycin, topotecan, trimethobenzamide, vasopressin, vecuronium, verapamil, vinBLAStine, vinCRIStine, vinorelbine, voriconazole, zidovudine, zoledronic acid

Solution compatibilities: 0.9% NaCl, LR

SIDE EFFECTS

CNS: Headache, insomnia, dizziness, confusion, anxiety, fatigue, fever

CV: Hypo/hypertension, **heart failure,** chest pain

GI: Nausea, constipation, diarrhea, vomiting, dyspepsia, **pseudomembranous colitis,** abdominal pain

GU: Nephrotoxicity

HEMA: Leukocytosis, anemia, **thrombocytopenia**

INTEG: Rash, pruritus

MISC: Fungal infections, UTI, anemia

MS: Muscle pain or weakness, arthralgia, pain, **rhabdomyolysis**

RESP: Cough, **eosinophilic pneumonia**

SYST: Anaphylaxis

PHARMACOKINETICS

Site of metabolism unknown, protein binding 92%, terminal half-life 8-9 hr, 78% excreted unchanged (urine)

INTERACTIONS

Increase: myopathy—HMG-CoA reductase inhibitors

Drug/Lab Test

Increase: CPK, AST, ALT, BUN, creatinine, albumin

NURSING CONSIDERATIONS

Assess:

- I&O ratio: report hematuria, oliguria, serum creatinine, BUN; nephrotoxicity may occur
- **Eosinophilic pneumonia:** dyspnea, fever, cough, shortness of breath; if left untreated, can lead to respiratory failure and death

⚠ **Nephrotoxicity:** any patient with compromised renal system, toxicity may occur; BUN, creatinine

- Blood studies: CBC, CPK
- C&S; product may be given as soon as culture taken
- B/P during administration; hypo/hypertension may occur
- Signs of infection
- Respiratory status: rate, character, wheezing
- Allergies before treatment, reaction of each medication

Evaluate:

- Therapeutic response: negative culture

Teach patient/family:

- About allergies before treatment, reaction to each medication
- To report sore throat, fever, fatigue; could indicate superinfection

darbepoetin (Rx)

(dar'bee-poh'eh-tin)

Aranesp

Func. class.: Hematopoietic agent

Chem. class.: Recombinant human erythropoietin

D

ACTION: Stimulates erythropoiesis by the same mechanism as endogenous erythropoietin; in response to hypoxia, erythropoietin is produced in the kidney and released into the bloodstream, where it interacts with progenitor stem cells to increase red-cell production

USES: Anemia associated with chronic renal failure, in patients on and not on dialysis, and anemia in nonmyeloid malignancies for patients receiving coadministered chemotherapy

CONTRAINDICATIONS: Hypersensitivity to mammalian-cell–derived products or human albumin; uncontrolled hypertension; red-cell aplasia

Precautions: Pregnancy (C), breastfeeding, children, seizure disorder, porphyria, hypertension, sickle cell disease; vit B_{12}, folate deficiency; chronic renal failure, dialysis; latex hypersensitivity, CABG, angina, anemia

Black Box Warning: Hgb >12 g/dl, surgery

DOSAGE AND ROUTES

Correction of anemia in chronic renal failure

- **Adult: SUBCUT/IV** 0.45 mcg/kg as a single inj; every week, titrate max target Hgb of 12 g/dl

Chemotherapy treatment

- **Adult: SUBCUT** 2.25 mcg/kg/wk or 500 mcg q3wk

Epoetin alfa to darbepoetin conversion

- **Adult: SUBCUT/IV** (epoetin alfa <2500 units/wk) 6.25 mcg/wk; (epoetin alfa 2500-4999 units/wk) 12.5 mcg/

wk; (epoetin alfa 5000-10,999 units/wk) 25 mcg/wk; (epoetin alfa 11,000-17,999 units/wk) 40 mcg/wk; (epoetin alfa 18,000-33,999 units/wk) 60 mcg/wk; (epoetin alfa 34,000-89,999 units/wk) 100 mcg/wk; (epoetin alfa >90,000 units/wk) 200 mcg/wk

Available forms: Sol for inj 25, 40, 60, 100, 150, 200, 300, 500 mcg/ml

Administer:

SUBCUT/IV route

- Without shaking; check for discoloration, particulate matter, do not use if present; do not dilute, do not mix with other products or sol, discard unused portion, do not pool unused portions
- Subcut typically used for those not requiring dialysis
- IV given direct undiluted or bolus into IV tubing or venous line after completion of dialysis; watch for clotting of line
- Adjust dosage every month or more

SIDE EFFECTS

CNS: Seizures, sweating, headache, dizziness, stroke

CV: *Hypo/hypertension,* cardiac arrest, *angina pectoris,* thrombosis, CHF, acute MI, dysrhythmias, chest pain, transient ischemic attacks, edema

GI: *Diarrhea, vomiting, nausea, abdominal pain, constipation*

HEMA: Red-cell aplasia

MISC: *Infection, fatigue, fever,* death, *fluid overload,* vascular access hemorrhage, dehydration, sepsis

MS: *Bone pain, myalgia, limb pain, back pain*

RESP: *URI, dyspnea, cough, bronchitis,* PE

SYST: Allergic reactions, anaphylaxis

PHARMACOKINETICS

IV: Onset of increased reticulocyte count 2-6 wk; distributed to vascular space; absorption slow and rate limiting; terminal half-life 49 hr (SUBCUT), 21 hr (IV); peak concentration at 34 hr; increased Hgb levels not generally observed until 2-6 wk after treatment initiated

INTERACTIONS

⚠ Do not use epoetin alfa with product

Increase: darbepoetin-alfa effect—androgens

Drug/Lab Test

Increase: WBC, platelets

Decrease: bleeding time

NURSING CONSIDERATIONS

Assess:

- Symptoms of anemia: fatigue, dyspnea, pallor

⚠ **Serious allergic reactions:** rash, urticaria; if anaphylaxis occurs, stop product, administer emergency treatment (rare)

- Renal studies: urinalysis, protein, blood, BUN, creatinine; monitor dialysis shunts; during dialysis, heparin may need to be increased

Black Box Warning: Blood studies: ferritin, transferrin monthly; transferrin saturation ≥20%, ferritin ≥100 ng/ml; Hgb 2×/wk until stabilized in target range (30%-33%) then at regular intervals; those with endogenous erythropoietin levels of <500 units/L respond to this agent; iron stores should be corrected before beginning therapy

- B/P: check for rising B/P as Hgb rises; antihypertensives may be needed

⚠ CV status: hypertension may occur rapidly, leading to **hypertensive encephalopathy;** Hgb >12 g/dl may lead to death, do not administer

- I&O; report drop in output to <50 ml/hr
- **Seizures:** if Hgb is increased by 4 pts within 2 wk, institute seizure precautions
- CNS symptoms: sweating, pain in long bones
- **Dialysis patients:** thrill, bruit of shunts, monitor for circulation impairment

Evaluate:

- Therapeutic response: increase in reticulocyte count, Hgb/Hct; increased appetite, enhanced sense of well-being

Teach patient/family:
- To avoid driving or hazardous activity during beginning of treatment
- To monitor B/P, Hgb
- To take iron supplements, vit B_{12}, folic acid as directed
- To report side effects to prescriber; to comply with treatment regimen
- That menses and fertility may return; to use contraception
- About home administration procedures, if appropriate

darunavir (Rx)

(dar-ue′na-vir)

Prezista

Func. class.: Antiretroviral

Chem. class.: Protease inhibitor

ACTION: Inhibits human immunodeficiency virus (HIV-1) protease; this prevents maturation of the virus

USES: HIV-1 in combination with ritonavir and other antiretrovirals

CONTRAINDICATIONS: Hypersensitivity

Precautions: Pregnancy (B), breastfeeding, children, geriatric patients, renal/hepatic disease, history of renal stones, diabetes, hypercholesterolemia, sulfonamide hypersensitivity, antimicrobial resistance, bleeding, immune reconstitution syndrome, pancreatitis

DOSAGE AND ROUTES

Treatment-Naive Patients
- **Adult: PO** 800 mg with ritonavir 100 mg daily

Treatment-Experienced Patients
- **Adult/adolescent >40 kg/child ≥6 yr: PO** 600 mg bid; with ritonavir 100 mg bid with food; 800 mg daily with ritonavir 100 mg with food (without darunavir resistance)
- **Adolescent ≥30 kg, <40 kg and child ≥6 yr: PO** 450 mg bid with ritonavir 60 mg bid
- **Adolescent ≥20 kg, <30 kg and child ≥6 yr: PO** 375 mg bid with ritonavir 50 mg bid
- **Child 3 to <6 yr (14 kg to <15 kg: PO** 280 mg (with ritonavir 48 mg) bid with food
- **Child 3 to <6 yr (13 kg to <14 kg: PO** 260 mg (with ritonavir 40 mg) bid with food
- **Child 3 to <6 yr (12 kg to <13 kg: PO** 240 mg (with ritonavir 40 mg) bid with food
- **Child 3 to <6 yr (11 kg to <12 kg: PO** 220 mg (with ritonavir 32 mg) bid with food
- **Child 3 to <6 yr (10 kg to <11 kg: PO** 200 mg (with ritonavir 32 mg) bid with food

Available forms: Tabs 75, 150, 400, 600 mg

Administer:
- With food and ritonavir
- Water to 1.5 L/day minimum to prevent nephrolithiasis
- Tab should be swallowed whole

SIDE EFFECTS

CNS: *Headache, insomnia,* dizziness, somnolence

GI: *Diarrhea, abdominal pain, nausea, vomiting,* anorexia, dry mouth, hepatitis, **hepatotoxicity**

GU: Nephrolithiasis

INTEG: Rash, **angioedema, Stevens-Johnson syndrome, toxic epidermal necrolysis**

MS: Pain

OTHER: Asthenia, **insulin-resistant hyperglycemia,** hyperlipidemia, **ketoacidosis,** lipodystrophy

PHARMACOKINETICS

95% protein binding; metabolized by CYP3A; peak 2.5-4 hr; terminal half-life 15 hr; excreted in feces 79.5%, urine 13.9%

INTERACTIONS

⚠ **Life-threatening dysrhythmias: ergots, midazolam, rifampin, pimozide, triazolam; do not use concurrently**

Increase: myopathy—HMG-CoA reductase inhibitors (atorvastatin, lovastatin, simvastatin)
Increase: darunavir levels—CYP3A4 inhibitors: (ketoconazole, itraconazole)
Increase: levels of both products—clarithromycin, zidovudine
Decrease: darunavir levels—CYP3A4 inducers (carBAMazepine, phenytoin, fosphenytoin, PHENobarbital), rifamycins, fluconazole, nevirapine, efavirenz
Decrease: levels of oral contraceptives

Drug/Herb

Decrease: darunavir levels—St. John's wort; avoid concurrent use
Increase: myopathy, rhabdomyolysis risk—red yeast rice

Drug/Food

Increase: darunavir absorption

NURSING CONSIDERATIONS

Assess:

- Complaints of lower back, flank pain; indicates kidney stones
- Signs of infection, anemia, the presence of other sexually transmitted diseases
- **Serious skin reactions:** angioedema, Stevens-Johnson syndrome, toxic epidermal necrolysis; discontinue immediately, notify prescriber
- **Hepatotoxicity:** hepatic studies (ALT, AST, bilirubin, amylase); all may be elevated in those with underlying liver disease
- Viral load, CD4, HIV RNA during treatment
- Bowel pattern before, during treatment; if severe abdominal pain with bleeding occurs, product should be discontinued; monitor hydration
- Skin eruptions: rash, urticaria, itching
- Allergies before treatment, reaction to each medication; place allergies on chart
- **Hyperlipidemia:** cholesterol, triglycerides, LDL may be elevated; monitor serum cholesterol, lipid panel throughout treatment

Evaluate:

- Therapeutic response: decreased viral load, increased CD4 count

Teach patient/family:

- To use nonhormonal birth control; not to breastfeed
- To take as prescribed; if dose is missed, to take as soon as remembered up to 1 hr before next dose; not to double dose
- That product must be taken at same time of day to maintain blood levels for duration of therapy

⚠ That **hyperglycemia** may occur; watch for increased thirst, weight loss, hunger, dry, itchy skin; to notify prescriber if these occur

- To increase fluids to prevent kidney stones; if stone formation occurs, that treatment may need to be interrupted
- That product does not cure AIDS, only controls symptoms; not to donate blood; not to share; to notify all health care providers of use; not to use with any other products without prescriber's approval

dasatinib (Rx)

(da-si′ti-nib)

Sprycel

Func. class.: Antineoplastic—miscellaneous
Chem. class.: Protein-tyrosine kinase inhibitor

ACTION: Inhibits BCR-ABL, SRC, LKC, YES, FYN, C-KIT, $EPHA_2$, and PDGFR-β tyrosine kinase created in chronic myeloid leukemia (CML)

USES: Treatment of accelerated, chronic blast phase CML or acute lymphoblastic leukemia (ALL); chronic phase CML with resistance or intolerance to prior therapy; Philadelphia chromosome-positive CML in chronic phase

CONTRAINDICATIONS: Pregnancy (D), hypersensitivity
Precautions: Breastfeeding, children, geriatric patients, QT prolongation, infection, thrombocytopenia, accidental exposure, edema, infertility, lactase deficiency, neutropenia

DOSAGE AND ROUTES

Accelerated or myeloid/lymphoid blast phase CML with resistance/ intolerance to prior therapy

- **Adult: PO** 140 mg daily titrated up to 180 mg daily in those resistant to therapy

Chronic phase CML with resistance/intolerance to prior therapy

- Adult: **PO** 100 mg daily either AM or PM

Dosage reduction for those taking a strong CYP3A4 inhibitor

- **Adult: PO** 20 mg daily

Available forms: Tabs 20, 50, 70, 100 mg

Administer:

- Do not break, crush, or chew tab
- After meal and with large glass of water

SIDE EFFECTS

CNS: CNS hemorrhage, headache, dizziness, insomnia, neuropathy, asthenia

CV: Dysrhythmias, chest pain, CHF, pericardial effusion, congestive cardiomyopathy, decreased injection fraction, QT prolongation

GI: *Nausea,* vomiting, *anorexia, abdominal pain,* constipation, diarrhea, **GI bleeding,** muscositis, stomatitis

HEMA: Neutropenia, thrombocytopenia, bleeding

INTEG: *Rash, pruritus*

META: Fluid retention, edema, hypocalcemia, hypophosphatemia

MISC: Increased/decreased weight

MS: Pain, arthralgia, myalgia

RESP: Cough, dyspnea, pulmonary edema/hypertension, pneumonia, upper respiratory tract infection, **pleural effusion**

PHARMACOKINETICS

Metabolized by CYP3A4; 96% protein bound; peak 0.5-6 hr; excreted in feces (85%), small amount in urine (4%); terminal half-life 1.3-5 hr

INTERACTIONS

- Altered action of CYP3A4 substrates: alfentanil, cycloSPORINE, ergots, fentanyl, pimozide, quiNIDine, sirolimus, tacrolimus

Increase: dasatinib concentrations—CYP3A4 inhibitors: ketoconazole, itraconazole, erythromycin, clarithromycin, nefazodone, protease inhibitors, telithromycin

Increase: plasma concentrations of simvastatin

Increase: QT prolongation—class IA/III antidysrhythmics and other products that increase QT prolongation

Decrease: dasatinib concentrations—CYP3A4 inducers (dexamethasone, phenytoin, carBAMazepine, rifampin, PHENobarbital), H_2 blockers (famotidine), proton pump inhibitors (omeprazole)

Drug/Herb

Decrease: dasatinib concentration—St. John's wort

NURSING CONSIDERATIONS

Assess:

- **Myelosuppression:** ANC, platelets; in chronic phase, if ANC $<1 \times 10^9$/L and/or platelets $<50 \times 10^9$/L, stop until ANC $>1.5 \times 10^9$/L and platelets $>75 \times 10^9$/L; in accelerated phase/blast crisis, if ANC $<0.5 \times 10^9$/L and/or platelets $<10 \times 10^9$/L, determine whether cytopenia is related to biopsy/aspirate, if not, reduce dose by 200 mg, if cytopenia continues, reduce dose by another 100 mg; if cytopenia continues for 4 wk, stop product until ANC $\geq 1 \times 10^9$/L
- **Hepatotoxicity:** monitor LFTs before treatment and monthly; if liver transaminases $>5 \times$ IULN, withhold until transaminase levels return to $<2.5 \times$ IULN
- **Signs of fluid retention, edema:** weigh, monitor lung sounds, assess for edema; some fluid retention is dose dependent, may result in CHF, congestive cardiomyopathy, decreased injection failure

Perform/provide:

- Nutritious diet with iron, vitamin supplement
- Storage at 25° C (77° F)

Evaluate:
• Therapeutic response: decrease in leukemic cells or size of tumor

Teach patient/family:
• To report adverse reactions immediately: SOB, swelling of extremities, bleeding
• About reason for treatment, expected results
• To use contraception (pregnancy category D), to avoid breastfeeding

⚠ HIGH ALERT

DAUNOrubicin (Rx)

(daw-noe-roo′bi-sin)

Cerubidine

DAUNOrubicin citrate liposomal (Rx)

DaunoXome

Func. class.: Antineoplastic, antibiotic
Chem. class.: Anthracycline glycoside

Do not confuse:
DAUNOrubicin/DOXOrubicin

ACTION: Inhibits DNA synthesis, primarily; derived from *Streptomyces coerulorubidus;* replication is decreased by binding to DNA, which causes strand splitting; cell-cycle specific (S phase); a vesicant

USES: Acute lymphocytic leukemia (ALL), acute myelogenous leukemia (AML); *liposomal:* Kaposi's sarcoma
Unlabeled uses: *Liposomal:* multiple myeloma, AML, breast cancer, non-Hodgkin's lymphoma

CONTRAINDICATIONS: Pregnancy (D), breastfeeding, hypersensitivity, systemic infections, cardiac disease, bone marrow depression
Precautions: Tumor lysis syndrome, MI, infection, thrombocytopenia, renal/hepatic disease; gout

Black Box Warning: Bone marrow suppression, cardiac disease, extravasation, renal failure

DOSAGE AND ROUTES

Use decreased dose for those >60 yr

DAUNOrubicin
• **Adult: IV** 45-60 mg/m^2/day × 3 days then 2 days of subsequent courses in combination, max 400-600 mg/m^2 total cumulative dose
• **Child: IV** 30-40 mg/m^2/day depending on cycle (AML); ≤2 yr or <0.5 m^2: 1 mg/kg on day 1 weekly in combination with vinCRIStine and predniSONE, base dose on body weight not surface area (ALL); >2 yr or 0.5 m^2: 25 mg/m^2 day 1 weekly in combination with vinCRIStine and predniSONE (ALL)

DAUNOrubicin citrate liposomal
• **Adult: IV** 40 mg/m^2 q2wk (Kaposi's sarcoma); 100 mg/m^2 q3wk (multiple myeloma, unlabeled); **IV** 100-140 mg/m^2 q3wk (non-Hodgkin's lymphoma, unlabeled; metastatic breast cancer, unlabeled); IV escalating doses of 75, 100, 125, 135, 150 mg/m^2/day × 3 days (AML, unlabeled)

Renal dose
• **Adult: IV** serum CCr >3 mg/dl, reduce dose by 50%

Hepatic dose
• **Adult: IV** serum bilirubin 1.2-3 mg/dl, reduce dose by 50%; bilirubin >3 mg/dl, reduce dose by 75%; bilirubin >5 mg/dl, omit dose

Available forms: Inj 20 mg powder/vial, *liposomal:* solution for inj 2 mg/ml

Administer:
• Antiemetic 30-60 min before giving product and 6-10 hr after treatment to prevent vomiting

Black Box Warning: Do not give by IM/subcut injection

IV route (Cerubidine)
Do not confuse with liposome
• Use cytotoxic handling precautions
• After diluting 20 mg/4 ml sterile water for inj (5 mg/ml), rotate, further dilute in 10-15 ml 0.9% NaCl; give over 3-5 min by

direct IV through Y-tube or 3-way stopcock of inf of D_5 or 0.9% NaCl; or dilute in 50 ml 0.9% NaCl and give over 10-15 min; or dilute in 100 ml and give over 30 min
• Hydrocortisone for extravasation; apply ice compress after stopping inf

Solution compatibilities: $D_{3.3}$%/0.3% NaCl, D_5W, Normosol R, LR, 0.9% NaCl
Y-site compatibilities: Amifostine, anidulafungin, atenolol, bivalirudin, bleomycin, CARBOplatin, caspofungin, CISplatin, codeine, cyclophosphamide, cytarabine, DACTINomycin, DAPTOmycin, dexmedetomidine, etoposide, fenoldopam, filgrastim, gemcitabine, gemtuzumab, granisetron, melphalan, meperidine, methotrexate, nesiritide, octreotide, ondansetron, oxaliplatin, paclitaxel, palonosetron, quinupristin-dalfopristin, riTUXimab, sodium acetate/bicarbonate, teniposide, thiotepa, tigecycline, trastuzumab, vinCRIStine, vinorelbine, voriconazole, zoledronic acid
IV route (DaunoXome)
• Dilute with D_5W to (1 mg/ml), give over 1-2 hr, do not use in-line filter, reconstituted sol may be stored ≤6 hr refrigerated; do not admix

IV compatibilities: Anidulafungin, bivalirudin, meperidine, octreotide, sodium acetate, tirofiban, trastuzumab

SIDE EFFECTS

DAUNOrubicin
CNS: Fever, chills
CV: **CHF, pericarditis, myocarditis, peripheral edema, fatal myocarditis, left ventricular failure, QT prolongation, ST-T wave changes, QRS voltage changes, tachycardia, SVT, PVCs**
GI: *Nausea, vomiting, anorexia, mucositis,* **hepatotoxicity**
GU: Impotence, sterility, amenorrhea, gynecomastia
HEMA: **Thrombocytopenia, leukopenia, anemia**
INTEG: *Rash,* extravasation, dermatitis, reversible alopecia, cellulitis, thrombophlebitis at inj site
SYST: **Anaphylaxis, tumor lysis syndrome**
DAUNOrubicin citrate liposomal
CNS: *Fatigue, headache,* depression, insomnia, dizziness, *malaise, neuropathy*
CV: Chest pain, edema
GI: Abdominal pain, stomatitis, *nausea, vomiting, diarrhea,* constipation
INTEG: *Alopecia, pruritus,* sweating
MISC: *Allergic reactions, chest pain, fever,* edema, flulike symptoms
MS: *Rigors,* arthralgia, back pain
RESP: *Cough, dyspnea, rhinitis, sinusitis*

PHARMACOKINETICS

Half-life 18½ hr, liposome 55½ hr; metabolized by liver; crosses placenta; excreted in breast milk, urine, bile

INTERACTIONS

Increase: QT prolongation, torsades de pointes—arsenic trioxide, chloroquine, clarithromycin, class IA, class III antidysrhythmics, dasatinib, dolasetron, droperidol, erythromycin, flecainide, halofantrine, haloperidol, levomethadyl, methadone, ondansetron, palonosetron, pentamidine, some phenothiazines, propafenone, risperidone, sparfloxacin; tricyclic antidepressants (high doses); vorinostat, ziprasidone
Increase: bleeding risk—NSAIDs, salicylates, anticoagulants, platelet inhibitors, thrombolytics
Increase: toxicity—other antineoplastics, radiation, cyclophosphamide
Decrease: DAUNOrubicin effects—hematopoietic progenitor cells given within 24 hr
Decrease: antibody reaction—live virus vaccines
Drug/Lab Test
Increase: uric acid

NURSING CONSIDERATIONS

Assess:

Black Box Warning: CBC, differential, platelet count weekly, leukocyte nadir within 2 wk after administration, recovery within 3 wk; do not administer if absolute granulocyte count is <750/mm^3 (liposome)

- **Acute renal failure, uric acid nephropathy:** renal studies: BUN, urine CCr, electrolytes, uric acid baseline before each dose; I&O ratio; report fall in urine output to <30 ml/hr; provide aggressive alkalinization of urine and use of allopurinol; can prevent urate nephropathy
- Monitor temp q4hr; fever may indicate beginning infection
- **Hepatotoxicity:** monitor hepatic studies baseline before each dose: bilirubin, AST, ALT, alk phos; check for jaundice of skin, sclera; dark urine, clay-colored stools; itchy skin, abdominal pain, fever; diarrhea

Black Box Warning: Chest x-ray, echocardiography, radionuclide angiography, MUGA, ECG; watch for ST-T wave changes, low QRS and QT prolongation, possible dysrhythmias (sinus tachycardia, heart block, PVCs); watch for CHF (jugular vein distention, weight gain, edema, crackles), may occur after 2-6 mo of treatment

- Bleeding: hematuria, guaiac stools, bruising, petechiae, mucosa or orifices q8hr
- Effects of alopecia on body image; discuss feelings about body changes
- Buccal cavity q8hr for dryness, sores, ulceration, white patches, oral pain, bleeding, dysphagia
- **Tumor lysis syndrome:** hyperkalemia, hyperphosphatemia, hyperuricemia, hypocalcemia

Black Box Warning: Extravasation: swelling, pain, decreased blood return; if extravasation occurs, stop infusion, remove tubing, attempt to aspirate the drug prior to removing the needle, elevate area, treat with ice pack

- GI symptoms: frequency of stools, cramping

Perform/provide:

- Increased fluid intake to 2-3 L/day to prevent urate and calculi formation
- Rinsing of mouth tid-qid with water, club soda; brushing of teeth bid-qid with soft brush or cotton-tipped applicators for stomatitis; use unwaxed dental floss

Evaluate:

- Therapeutic response: decreased tumor size, spread of malignancy

Teach patient/family:

- To report signs of infection, bleeding, bruising, SOB, swelling, change in heart rate
- That hair may be lost during treatment; that wig or hairpiece may make patient feel better; that new hair may be different in color, texture
- To avoid pregnancy (D) while taking product and for 4 mo thereafter; not to breastfeed
- To avoid foods with citric acid, hot or rough texture if stomatitis is present
- To report any bleeding, white spots, ulcerations in mouth; to examine mouth daily
- That urine and other body fluids may be red-orange for 48 hr
- To avoid vaccines, alcohol, aspirin, NSAIDs while taking this product
- To avoid crowds, those with known infections

decitabine (Rx)

(de-sit′a-been)

Dacogen

Func. class.: Antineoplastic, antimetabolite

Chem. class.: Pyrimidine analog

ACTION: Incorporated into DNA and inhibits DNA methylation, thus halting growth and rapid proliferation of blasts

USES: Treatment of naïve and experienced myelodysplasic syndrome

Unlabeled uses: Chronic myelogenous leukemia (CML)

CONTRAINDICATIONS:

Pregnancy (D), breastfeeding, children, hypersensitivity to this product, severe neurotoxicity, severe blood dyscrasias

Precautions: Men (men should not father a child while receiving treatments or for 2 mo after treatment ends), severe renal/hepatic disease, dental work, infections, thrombocytopenia

DOSAGE AND ROUTES

• **Adult: CONT IV** 1st treatment cycle: 15 mg/m^2 over 3 hr q8hr × 3 days; subsequent treatment cycles: repeat above cycle q6wk for at least 4 cycles; a partial or complete response may take more than 4 cycles

Available forms: Powder for inj, lyophilized 50 mg, in single-dose vial

Administer:

• Use procedures for handling and disposal of products

SIDE EFFECTS

CNS: *Headache, anxiety, dizziness, hypoesthesia, insomnia,* confusion

CV: *Edema, murmur, hypotension*

GI: *Nausea, anorexia, vomiting, diarrhea, constipation, stomatitis,* abdominal pain, dyspepsia

HEMA: **Neutropenia, thrombocytopenia, leukopenia, anemia**

INTEG: *Alopecia, ecchymosis, erythema, pallor, petechiae, pruritus, rash, swelling face, urticaria,* hematoma, cellulitis

META: *Decreased potassium, sodium, magnesium, albumin; increased bilirubin, increased/decreased glucose*

MS: *Myalgia, arthralgia, back pain, chest wall pain, pain in limbs*

RESP: *Cough, crackles,* ***hypoxia,*** *pharyngitis,* ***pneumonia, pulmonary edema***

PHARMACOKINETICS

Protein binding <1%; may be metabolized by the liver, granulocytes, intestinal epithelium, whole blood; terminal half-life 0.2-0.8 hr; data is limited

INTERACTIONS

• Do not use with live virus vaccines

NURSING CONSIDERATIONS

Assess:

• **Bone marrow suppression:** CBC (RBC, Hct, Hgb), differential, platelet count weekly; withhold product if WBC <4000/mm^3, platelets <75,000/mm^3, or RBC, Hct, Hgb is low; notify prescriber of results

• Renal studies: BUN, serum uric acid, urine CCr, electrolytes before and during therapy

• **Infection:** Treat all infections before treatment; monitor temp q4hr; fever may indicate beginning infection; no rectal temps

• Hepatic studies before and during treatment: bilirubin, AST, ALT, alk phos as needed or monthly

• **Bleeding:** hematuria, heme-positive stools, bruising, petechiae, mucosa or orifices daily; blood dyscrasias can occur

• Dyspnea, crackles, unproductive cough, chest pain, tachypnea, fatigue, increased pulse, pallor, lethargy, personality changes

• Buccal cavity daily for dryness, ulceration, white patches, oral pain, bleeding, dysphagia

• GI symptoms: frequency of stools, cramping; if severe diarrhea occurs, electrolytes may need to be given

Perform/provide:

• Rinsing of mouth tid-qid with water or club soda; brushing teeth tid with soft toothbrush or cotton-tipped applicator for stomatitis; use unwaxed dental floss

• Storage at room temp, away from light

Evaluate:

• Therapeutic response: decreased blast count

Teach patient/family:

• To report bleeding; not to use commercial mouthwashes, razors

• To report signs of **infection:** increased temp, sore throat, flulike symptoms

• To report signs of **anemia:** fatigue, headache, faintness, SOB, irritability

• To avoid citric acid, rough-textured foods if stomatitis is present
• To notify prescriber if **pregnancy** is suspected or planned; to use contraception while taking this product; that men should not father a child while taking this product (pregnancy category D); to avoid breastfeeding while taking this product
• Not to operate machinery or perform other hazardous activities while taking this product
• To inform prescriber of renal/hepatic disease
• Not to receive vaccinations while taking this product
• To drink 2-3 L of fluids per day unless contraindicated

RARELY USED

deferasirox (Rx)

(def-a′sir-ox)

Exjade

Func. class.: Heavy metal chelating agent

USES: Chronic iron overload, transfusion hemosiderosis

CONTRAINDICATIONS: Breastfeeding, children, hypersensitivity, severe renal/hepatic disease, GI hemorrhage

DOSAGE AND ROUTES

• **Adult and child >2 yr: PO** 20-30 mg/kg/day; oral dispersion tablet is dissolved in water <1 g in 3.5 oz; >1 g in 7 oz or more; give on empty stomach at least 30 min before meals

RARELY USED

deferoxamine (Rx)

(de-fer-ox′a-meen)

Desferal

Func. class.: Heavy metal chelator

Do not confuse:
deferoxamine/cefuroxime

USES: Acute, chronic iron intoxication; hemochromatosis, hemosiderosis

CONTRAINDICATIONS: Children <3 yr, hypersensitivity, anuria, severe renal disease

DOSAGE AND ROUTES

Acute iron toxicity
• **Adult and child: IM/IV** 1 g, then 500 mg q4hr × 2 doses, then 500 mg q4-12hr as needed, max 15 mg/kg/hr or 6 g/24 hr

Chronic iron toxicity
• **Adult and child: IM** 500 mg-1 g/day plus **IV INF** 2 g given by separate line with each unit of blood, max 15 mg/kg/hr or 6 g/24 hr; **SUBCUT** 1-2 g over 8-24 hr by SUBCUT inf pump

Iron overload due to transfusion-dependent anemias
• **Adult: IM** 0.5-1 g/day plus **IV** 2 g per unit of blood, max 1 g/day with no blood; 6 g/day with 3 or more units of blood or packed RBCs

Aluminum toxicity (unlabeled)
• **Adult: IV/IM/SUBCUT** 1 g q1-2×/wk

delavirdine (Rx)

(de-la-veer′deen)

Rescriptor

Func. class.: Antiretroviral

Chem. class.: Nonnucleoside reverse transcriptase inhibitor (NNRTI)

ACTION: Binds directly to reverse transcriptase; blocks RNA-, DNA-dependent polymerase activities, causing a disruption of the enzyme's site

USES: HIV-1 in combination with at least 2 other antiretrovirals

CONTRAINDICATIONS: Hypersensitivity

Precautions: Pregnancy (C), breastfeeding, children, hepatic disease, achlorhydria, antimicrobial resistance, exfoliative dermatitis, hepatitis, immune reconstitution syndrome

DOSAGE AND ROUTES

- **Adult and adolescent ≥16 yr: PO** 400 mg tid, max 1200 mg/day

Available forms: Tabs 100, 200 mg

Administer:

- 100-mg tab: dispersion by adding 4 tab/3-4 oz water, let stand, stir, swallow, rinse glass, swallow; use only 100-mg tabs for dispersion; 200-mg tab take as intact tab
- Do not give within 1 hr of antacids or didanosine

SIDE EFFECTS

CNS: Headache, fatigue, anxiety, insomnia, fever

GI: Diarrhea, abdominal pain, nausea, anorexia, vomiting, dyspepsia, **hepatotoxicity**

GU: **Nephrotoxicity**

HEMA: **Neutropenia, leukopenia, thrombocytopenia, anemia, granulocytopenia**

INTEG: Rash, pruritus

MISC: Cough

MS: Pain, myalgia

SYST: **Stevens-Johnson syndrome; immune reconstitution syndrome (combination therapy)**

PHARMOCOKINETICS

98% protein bound, half-life 5.8 hr, peak 1 hr, duration 8 hr, extensively metabolized by CYP3A4, excreted in urine, feces

INTERACTIONS

⚠ **Serious life-threatening adverse reaction: amphetamines, ergots, benzodiazepines, calcium channel blockers, sedative/hypnotics, antidysrhythmics, sildenafil, pimozide, cisapride, alprazolam, astemizole, midazolam, terfenadine, opiates, triazolam**

Increase: levels of alprazolam, clarithromycin, dapsone, ergots, felodipine, midazolam, NIFEdipine, indinavir, saquinavir, lovastatin, simvastatin, atorvastatin, other CYP3A4, 2D6 inhibitors

Increase: delavirdine levels—fluoxetine, ketoconazole

Increase: levels of both products—quiNIDine, warfarin, clarithromycin

Decrease: delavirdine levels—antacids, anticonvulsants, rifamycins, protease inhibitors, didanosine

Decrease: action of oral contraceptives, didanosine

Drug/Herb

Decrease: delavirdine level—St. John's wort

NURSING CONSIDERATIONS

Assess:

- **HIV:** obtain hepatitis B virus (HBV) screening to ensure proper treatment, if coinfected, a fully suppressive antiretroviral regimen with products against both; CBC, blood chemistry, plasma HIV RNA, absolute CD41/CD81/cell counts/%, serum β-2 microglobulin, serum ICD124 antigen levels
- **Immune reconstitution syndrome:** when treated with combination therapy; development of opportunistic infections (*Mycobacterium avium complex* [MAC], cytomegalovirus [CMV], *Pneumocystis carinii* pneumonia [PCP], TB)
- Signs of infection, anemia
- Hepatic studies: ALT, AST; renal studies
- Bowel pattern before, during treatment; if severe abdominal pain with bleeding occurs, product should be discontinued; monitor hydration
- Allergies before treatment, reaction to each medication; place allergies on chart
- Plasma delavirdine concentrations (trough 10 micromolar)
- **Toxicity:** severe nausea/vomiting, maculopapular rash
- **Serious skin reactions:** Stevens-Johnson syndrome; rash may occur within 1-3 wk of beginning treatment; if rash is not severe, manage with diphenhydrAMINE, hydrOXYzine, topical corticosteroids

Evaluate:

- Therapeutic response: increased CD4 cell count, decreased viral load, improvement in symptoms of HIV

Teach patient/family:
- To take as prescribed; if dose is missed, to take as soon as remembered up to 1 hr before next dose; not to double dose
- That tabs may be dissolved in 1/2 cup of water; to stir; when dissolved, drink right away; to rinse cup with water and drink to get all medication
- To make sure health care provider knows about all medications being taken
- That, if severe rash, mouth sores, swelling, aching muscles/joints, or eye redness occur, to notify health care provider
- Not to breastfeed if taking this product
- That this product is not a cure, only controls symptoms

demecarium ophthalmic

See Appendix B

denileukin diftitox (Rx)

(den-ih-loo′kin dif′tih-tox)

Ontak

Func. class.: Antineoplastic—miscellaneous

Chem. class.: Fusion protein

ACTION: A recombinant DNA-derived cytotoxic protein that interacts with high-affinity IL-2 receptors on the cell surface and inhibits cellular protein synthesis

USES: Cutaneous T-cell lymphoma that expresses CD25 component of the IL-2 receptor

Unlabeled uses: Non-Hodgkin's lymphoma, psoriasis

CONTRAINDICATIONS: Hypersensitivity to denileukin, diphtheria toxin, IL-2

Precautions: Pregnancy (C), breastfeeding, children, geriatric patients, CAD, *Escherichia coli,* protein hypersensitivity, immunosuppression, peripheral vascular disease

Black Box Warning: Capillary leak syndrome, infusion-related reactions, visual disturbances

DOSAGE AND ROUTES

- **Adult: IV** 9 or 18 mcg/kg/day given for 5 days q21days, infused over ≥15 min

Available forms: Sol for inj, frozen 150 mcg/ml

Administer:
- Antiemetic 30-60 min before product to prevent vomiting
- Premedicate with acetaminophen or NSAID and diphenhydrAMINE 15-30 min prior to inf; use dexamethasone (20 mg PO or 8 mg IV)

Intermittent IV INF route
- Use cytotoxic handling precautions
- Bring to room temp; after thawing, a haze may be visible, should be clear at room temp
- Do not shake vigorously, mix gently by swirling
- Prepare and hold sol in plastic syringes or soft plastic IV bags only, no glass containers
- Draw calculated dose from vial, inject into empty IV inf bag; for each 1 ml of product removed from vial, no more than 9 ml of sterile saline without preservative should be added to IV bag; infuse over ≥15 min; do not give by bolus; do not admix with other products; do not use a filter; use within 6 hr, discard unused portions

SIDE EFFECTS

CNS: *Dizziness, paresthesia, nervousness, confusion, insomnia*

CV: *Hypotension, vasodilation, tachycardia, thrombosis, hypertension, dysrhythmias,* capillary leak syndrome

EENT: Persistent visual impairment

GI: *Nausea, anorexia, vomiting, diarrhea, constipation, dyspepsia, dysphagia*

GU: Hematuria, albuminuria, pyuria, creatinine increase

HEMA: Thrombocytopenia, leukopenia, anemia

INTEG: *Rash, pruritus, sweating*
META: *Hypoalbuminemia, edema, hypocalcemia,* weight decrease, dehydration, hypokalemia
MISC: *Fever, chills, asthenia, infection, pain, headache, chest pain,* flulike symptoms, **serious infection, capillary leak syndrome**
MS: *Myalgia,* arthralgia
RESP: *Dyspnea, cough, pharyngitis, rhinitis*

PHARMACOKINETICS

Concentrates in liver/kidneys, metabolized by proteolytic degradation

INTERACTIONS

Increase: bone marrow depression—radiation, other antineoplastics
Decrease: antibody reaction—live vaccines

NURSING CONSIDERATIONS

Assess:

- CBC, differential, platelet count weekly; withhold product if WBC $<4000/mm^3$ or platelet count $<75,000/mm^3$; notify prescriber of results
- Monitor temp q4hr; fever may indicate beginning infection
- Hepatic studies before, during therapy (bilirubin, AST, ALT, LDH) as needed or monthly
- Bleeding: hematuria, guaiac, bruising petechiae of mucosa or orifices q8hr
- Jaundice of skin, sclera; dark urine, clay-colored stools; itchy skin; abdominal pain; fever; diarrhea

Black Box Warning: For capillary leak syndrome after 2 wk of treatment (hypotension, edema, hypoalbuminemia); monitor weight, B/P, serum albumin, edema

- Obtain CD25 expression on skin biopsy samples, obtain serum albumin levels; should be ≥ 3 g/dl prior to administration

Black Box Warning: Infusion-related reactions, may be fatal; visual disturbances may be permanent, monitor visual acuity, color vision

Perform/provide:

- Storage in light-resistant container, dry area
- Warm compresses at inf site for inflammation

Evaluate:

- Therapeutic response: decreased tumor size, spread of malignancy

Teach patient/family:

- To report signs of **infection:** fever, sore throat, flulike symptoms
- To report signs of **anemia:** fatigue, headache, faintness, SOB, irritability
- To report **bleeding;** to avoid use of razors, commercial mouthwash
- To avoid use of aspirin products, NSAIDs, or ibuprofen
- To use reliable contraception; not to breastfeed

denosumab (Rx)

(den-oh'sue-mab)

Prolia, Xgeva

Func. class.: Bone resorption inhibitor
Chem. class.: Monoclonal antibody, bone resorption

ACTION:

Neutralizes activity of receptor activator nuclear factor kappa-B ligand (RANKL) by binding to it and blocking its interaction with cell-surface receptors; use of a RANKL inhibitor may reduce bone turnover and decrease tumor burden

USES:

Osteoporosis in postmenopausal women at high risk for fractures; prevention of skeletal-related events in bone metastases from solid tumors

CONTRAINDICATIONS:

Hypersensitivity, hypocalcemia
Precautions: Pregnancy (C), breastfeeding, child/infant/neonate, anemia, coagulopathy, diabetes mellitus, dialysis,

eczema, hypoparathyroidism, immunosuppression, latex hypersensitivity, malabsorption syndrome, neoplastic disease, pancreatitis, parathyroid disease, dental/renal/thyroid disease, TB, vit D deficiency

DOSAGE AND ROUTES

Postmenopausal osteoporosis

• **Adult female: SUBCUT** 60 mg q6mo with 1000 mg calcium and 400 international units vitamin D, max 60 mg q6mo

Bone metastases from solid tumors

• **Adult: SUBCUT** 120 mg q4wk, max 120 mg q4wk; administer with calcium and vitamin D as necessary to prevent hypocalcemia

Prevention of skeletal-related events with bone metastases from solid tumors

• **Adult: SUBCUT** (Xgeva): 120 mg q4wk

Available forms: Sol for inj 60 mg/ml (Prolia); 120 mg/1.7 ml (Xgeva)

Administer:

SUBCUT route

• Give acetaminophen before and for 72 hr after to decrease pain

• Do not use if particulate matter or discoloration is present; sol is clear and colorless to slightly yellow with small white/opalescent particles; remove from refrigerator and allow to warm to room temp (15-30 min)

• **Use of prefilled syringe with needle safety guard:** leave green guard in original position until after administration, remove and discard needle cap immediately before inj, give by subcut inj in upper arm/thigh or abdomen; after inj, point needle away from people and slide green guard over needle

• **Use of single-use vials:** use 27G needle, give in upper arm/thigh or abdomen, do not re-insert needle in vial, discard supplies as appropriate

SIDE EFFECTS

CNS: Chills, fever, flushing, headache, vertigo, neuropathic pain

CV: Angina, atrial fibrillation

GI: Abdominal pain, constipation, *diarrhea,* flatulence, GERD, *vomiting, nausea*

GU: Cystitis, lactation suppression

HEMA: Anemia, neutropenia

INTEG: Atopic dermatitis, pruritus

META: Hypercholesterolemia, hypocalcemia, hypophosphatemia

MS: Back, bone pain; MS pain, myalgia, osteonecrosis of the jaw

RESP: Cough, *dyspnea*

SYST: Infection, secondary malignancy

PHARMACOKINETICS

Terminal half-life 25.4 days, bioavailability 62%, max serum concentration 3-21 days, steady state 6 mo

INTERACTIONS

Increase: infection, possible—immunosupressives, corticosteroids

Increase: osteonecrosis of the jaw, possible—antineoplastics, corticosteroids

NURSING CONSIDERATIONS

Assess:

• **Acute acute-phase reaction:** fever, myalgia, headache, flulike symptoms for 72 hr after inj, usually resolves after 72 hr

• **Blood tests:** serum calcium, creatitine, BUN, magnesium, phosphate

• **Hypocalcemia:** paresthesia, twitching, laryngospasm, Chvostek's and Trouseau's signs; preexisting hypocalcemia should be corrected prior to treatment; patient with vit D deficiency may require higher doses of vit D

• **Hypercalcemia:** nausea, vomiting, anorexia, weakness, thirst, constipation, dysrhythmias

• **Dental status:** correct dental complications prior to product use; good oral hygiene should be maintained; if dental work is to be performed, antiinfectives should be given to prevent osteonecrosis of the jaw

• **Infection:** do not start treatment in patients with active infections; infections should be resolved first

Perform/provide:
• Storage and use out of direct sunlight/heat; do not freeze, use within 14 days after removal from refrigerator, store unopened containers in refrigerator
Evaluate:
• Therapeutic response: increased/maintained bone density, decreased calcium levels
Teach patient/family:
• To report hypercalcemic relapse: nausea, vomiting, bone pain, thirst
• To continue with dietary recommendations, including additional calcium and vit D
• To avoid use during pregnancy and breastfeeding; to notify prescriber if pregnancy is planned, suspected
• To use acetaminophen before and for 72 hr after inj to lessen bone pain
• About the purpose of this product and its expected results
• To avoid OTC, Rx medications and herbs and supplements unless approved by prescriber
• To exercise regularly, stop smoking, and avoid alcohol to maintain bone health
• To inform all health care providers of product use; to avoid dental procedures/surgery if possible; to practice good oral hygiene
• That lab tests and follow-up exams will be required

desipramine (Rx)

(dess-ip′ra-meen)

Apo-Desipramine ✦, Norpramin, PMS-Desipramine ✦

Func. class.: Antidepressant, tricyclic
Chem. class.: Dibenzazepine, secondary amine

ACTION: Blocks reuptake of norepinephrine, serotonin into nerve endings, thereby increasing action of norepinephrine, serotonin in nerve cells

USES: Depression
Unlabeled uses: Chronic pain, postherpetic neuralgia, ADHD, bulimia, diabetic neuropathy, panic disorder, social phobia

CONTRAINDICATIONS: Hypersensitivity to tricyclics, closed-angle glaucoma, acute MI
Precautions: Pregnancy (C), breastfeeding, geriatric patients, severe depression, increased intraocular pressure, seizure disorder, CV disease, urinary retention, cardiac dysrhythmias, cardiac conduction disturbances, family history of sudden death, prostatic hypertrophy, thyroid disease

Black Box Warning: Children <18 yr, suicidal patients

DOSAGE AND ROUTES

Major depression
• **Adult: PO** 50-75 mg/day in 1-4 divided doses, titrate by 25-50 mg weekly up to 300 mg/day in single or divided doses
• **Geriatric: PO** 25 mg/day at bedtime, titrate weekly, may increase to 150 mg/day
• **Adolescent: PO** 25-50 mg/day in divided doses, max 150 mg/day
• **Child 6-12 yr: PO** 1-3 mg/kg/day in divided doses; give >3 mg/kg/day with close medical monitoring; max 5 mg/kg/day
ADHD/bulimia nervosa (unlabeled)
• **Adult: PO** 25 mg tid, may titrate to 200 mg/day by 25-50 mg/day at weekly intervals
Neuropathic pain/postherpetic neuralgia (unlabeled)
• **Adult: PO** 10-25 mg at bedtime, titrate to relief
Diabetic neuropathy (unlabeled)
• **Adult: PO** 75-150 mg
Available forms: Tabs 10, 25, 50, 75, 100, 150 mg
Administer:
• Increased fluids, bulk in diet for constipation, especially in geriatric patients; with food or milk for GI symptoms; crushed if patient is unable to swallow medication whole

• Dosage at bedtime if oversedation occurs during day; may take entire dose at bedtime; geriatric patients may not tolerate once-daily dosing
• Gum, hard candy, frequent sips of water for dry mouth

SIDE EFFECTS

CNS: *Dizziness, drowsiness,* confusion, headache, anxiety, tremors, stimulation, weakness, insomnia, nightmares, EPS (geriatric patients), increased psychiatric symptoms, paresthenia, suicidal ideation
CV: *Orthostatic hypotension, ECG changes, tachycardia, hypertension,* palpitations
EENT: *Blurred vision,* tinnitus, mydriasis, ophthalmoplegia
GI: *Diarrhea, dry mouth,* nausea, vomiting, paralytic ileus, increased appetite, cramps, epigastric distress, jaundice, hepatitis, stomatitis, constipation, weight gain
GU: *Retention,* acute renal failure
HEMA: Agranulocytosis, thrombocytopenia, eosinophilia, leukopenia
INTEG: Rash, urticaria, sweating, pruritus, photosensitivity

PHARMACOKINETICS

Well absorbed, widely distributed, protein binding 92%, extensively metabolized in the liver to active metabolite of imipramine, half-life 7-60 hr

INTERACTIONS

Increase: serotonin syndrome, neuroleptic malignant syndrome—SSRIs, SNRIs, serotonin-receptor agonists, other tricyclic antidepressants
Increase: CNS depression—alcohol, barbiturates, opioids, CNS depressants
Increase: desipramine level—cimetidine, diltiazem, fluvoxamine, FLUoxetine, paroxetine, sertraline, verapamil
Increase: life-threatening B/P elevations, do not use concurrently—cloNIDine
Increase: hypertension—EPINEPHrine, norepinephrine
Increase: hyperpyrexia, seizures, excitation; do not use within 14 days of MAOIs
Increase: QT interval—tricyclics, sunitinib, vorinostat, ziprasidone, gatifloxacin, levofloxacin, moxifloxacin, sparfloxacin, class IA/III antidysrhythmics
Drug/Herb
Increase: serotonin syndrome, avoid concurrent use—St. John's wort
Increase: CNS depression—kava, valerian
Drug/Lab Test
Increase: serum bilirubin, blood glucose, alk phos

NURSING CONSIDERATIONS

Assess:
• B/P (lying, standing), pulse q4hr; if systolic B/P drops 20 mm Hg, hold product, notify prescriber; take VS q4hr in patients with cardiovascular disease
• Hepatic studies: AST, ALT, bilirubin; thyroid function studies
• Weight weekly; appetite may increase with product
• **ECG** for flattening T wave, bundle branch block, AV block, dysrhythmias in cardiac patients
• **EPS** primarily in geriatric patients: rigidity, dystonia, akathisia
• **Seizure activity** in those with a history of seizures
• Mental status: mood, sensorium, affect, **suicidal tendencies**, increase in psychiatric symptoms (depression, panic)
• Urinary retention, constipation; constipation most likely in children
• **Withdrawal symptoms:** headache, nausea, vomiting, muscle pain, weakness; not usual unless product discontinued abruptly
• Alcohol consumption; if consumed, hold dose until morning
Perform/provide:
• Storage at room temp
• Assistance with ambulation during beginning of therapy for drowsiness/dizziness
• Safety measures, primarily in geriatric patients

• Check to confirm that PO medication is swallowed

Evaluate:

• Therapeutic response: decreased depression

Teach patient/family:

• That therapeutic effects may take 2-3 wk

• That suicidal thoughts/behaviors may occur; to notify prescriber immediately

• To use caution when driving, performing other activities requiring alertness because of drowsiness, dizziness, blurred vision

• To avoid alcohol, other CNS depressants

• Not to discontinue medication abruptly after long-term use because this may cause nausea, headache, malaise

• To wear sunscreen or large hat because photosensitivity occurs

TREATMENT OF OVERDOSE:

ECG monitoring; lavage, activated charcoal; administer anticonvulsant

desloratadine (Rx)

(des′lor-at′ah-deen)

Clarinex, Clarinex RediTabs

Func. class.: Antihistamine, 2nd generation

Chem. class.: Selective histamine (H_1)-receptor antagonist

ACTION: Binds to peripheral histamine receptors, thus providing antihistamine action without sedation

USES: Seasonal/perennial allergic rhinitis, chronic idiopathic urticaria, pruritus

CONTRAINDICATIONS: Hypersensitivity, infants/neonates

Precautions: Pregnancy (C), breastfeeding, child, asthma, renal/hepatic impairment

DOSAGE AND ROUTES

• **Adult and child ≥12 yr: PO** 5 mg/day

• **Child 6-11 yr: PO** 2.5 mg/day

• **Child 2-5 yr: PO** 1.25 mg/day

• **Child 6-11 mo: PO** 1 mg/day (urticaria, only)

Hepatic/renal dose

• **Adult: PO** 5 mg every other day

Available form: Tabs 5 mg; orally disintegrating tabs 2.5, 5 mg (Reditabs); syr 0.5 mg/ml

Administer:

• Without regard to meals

• Do not remove RediTabs from blister until ready to use

• RediTabs directly on tongue; may take with or without water

SIDE EFFECTS

CNS: Sedation (more common with increased doses), headache, psychomotor hyperactivity, **seizures**, fatigue

GI: **Hepatitis**, nausea, dry mouth

MISC: Flulike symptoms

PHARMACOKINETICS

Onset antihistamine effect 1 hr, relief as early as 1 day, duration up to 24 hr, peak 1½ hr, elimination half-life 8½-28 hr, metabolized in liver to active metabolites, excreted in urine

INTERACTIONS

Increase: CNS depression (rare)—alcohol, opiates, sedative/hypnotics, H_1 blockers, antipsychotics, tricyclic antidepressants, anxiolytics

Increase: desloratadine, nilotinib, etravirine

NURSING CONSIDERATIONS

Assess:

• **Allergy:** hives, rash, rhinitis; monitor respiratory status; test interaction, antigen skin test

Perform/provide:

• Storage in tight container at room temp

Evaluate:
- Therapeutic response: absence of running or congested nose, other allergy symptoms

Teach patient/family:
- To avoid driving, other hazardous activities if drowsiness occurs; to use caution until product's effects are known
- That product may cause photosensitivity; to use sunscreen or stay out of the sun to prevent burns

desmopressin (Rx)

(des-moe-press'in)

Apo-Desmopressin ♣, DDAVP, Minirin, Octostim ♣, Stimate

Func. class.: Pituitary hormone

Chem. class.: Synthetic antidiuretic hormone

ACTION:
Promotes reabsorption of water by action on renal tubular epithelium; causes smooth muscle constriction, increase in plasma factor VIII levels, which increases platelet aggregation, thereby resulting in vasopressor effect; similar to vasopressin

USES:
Hemophilia A, von Willebrand's disease type 1, nonnephrogenic diabetes insipidus, symptoms of polyuria/polydipsia caused by pituitary dysfunction, nocturnal enuresis

Unlabeled uses: Cardiopulmonary bypass, sickle cell disease, uremic bleeding

CONTRAINDICATIONS:
Hypersensitivity, nephrogenic diabetes insipidus, severe renal disease

Precautions: Pregnancy (B), breastfeeding, coronary artery disease, hypertension, cystic fibrosis, thrombus

DOSAGE AND ROUTES

Primary nocturnal enuresis
- **Adult and child ≥6 yr: PO** 0.2 mg at bedtime, max 0.6 mg at bedtime; intranasal 0.2 ml at bedtime, half in each nostril

Diabetes insipidus
- **Adult: INTRANASAL** 0.1-0.4 ml/day in divided doses (1-4 sprays with pump); **IV/SUBCUT** 0.5-1 ml/day in divided doses
- **Child 3 mo to 12 yr: INTRANASAL** 0.05-0.3 ml/day in divided doses

Hemophilia/von Willebrand's disease
- **Adult and child >3 mo: IV** 0.3 mcg/kg in 0.9% NaCl over 15-30 min; may repeat if needed

Antihemorrhagic
- **Adult and child >3 mo: IV** 0.3 mcg/kg
- **Adult and child <50 kg: INTRANASAL** 1 spray in 1 nostril
- **Adult and child >50 kg:** 1 spray in each nostril

Cardiopulmonary bypass (unlabeled)
- **Adult: IV** 0.3 mcg/kg with aminocaproic acid given as a single postop dose

Sickle cell disease (unlabeled)
- **Adult: SUBCUT/IV** 0.3 mcg/kg with a high fluid intake

Uremic bleeding (unlabeled)
- **Adult: SUBCUT/IV** 0.2-0.4 mcg/kg/dose

Available forms: Inj 4, 15 mcg/ml; Rhihal Tube delivery 2.5 mg/vial (0.1 mg/ml); tabs 0.1, 0.2 mg; nasal spray pump 10 mcg/spray (0.1 mg/ml); nasal sol 1.5 mg/ml (150 mcg/dose)

Administer:

Direct IV route
- Undiluted over 1 min for diabetes insipidus

Intermittent IV INF route
- Diluted single dose/50 ml of 0.9% NaCl (adult and child >10 kg), single dose/10 ml as IV inf over 15-30 min for von Willebrand's disease or hemophilia A

SIDE EFFECTS

CNS: Drowsiness, headache, lethargy, flushing, seizures

CV: Increased B/P, palpitations, tachycardia

EENT: Nasal irritation, congestion, rhinitis

GI: Nausea, heartburn, cramps
GU: Vulval pain
META: Hyponatremia, hyponatremia-induced seizures
SYST: **Anaphylaxis (IV)**

PHARMACOKINETICS

PO: Onset 1 hr, peak 4-7 hr
INTRANASAL: Onset 1 hr; peak 1-4 hr; duration 8-20 hr; half-life 8 min, 76 min (terminal)
IV: Onset 1 min, peak ½ hr, duration >3 hr

INTERACTIONS

Increase: antidiuretic action—carBAMazepine, chlorproPAMIDE, clofibrate
Decrease: antidiuretic action—lithium, alcohol, demeclocycline, heparin, large doses of EPINEPHrine

NURSING CONSIDERATIONS

Assess:

- Pulse, B/P when giving IV or SUBCUT
- I&O ratio, weight daily; check for edema in extremities; if water retention severe, diuretic may be prescribed
- **Water intoxication:** lethargy, behavioral changes, disorientation, neuromuscular excitability
- Intranasal use: nausea, congestion, cramps, headache; usually decreased with decreased dose; for nasal mucosa changes: congestion, edema, discharge, scarring (nasal route)

⚠ **For severe allergic reaction, including anaphylaxis (IV route)**

- Urine volume/osmolality and plasma osmolality (diabetes insipidus)
- Factor VIII coagulant activity, bleeding time before using for hemostasis
- **Nocturnal enuresis:** frequency of enuresis before and during treatment

Perform/provide:

- Storage in refrigerator or cool environment

Evaluate:

- Therapeutic response: absence of severe thirst, decreased urine output, decreased osmolality

Teach patient/family:

- About the proper technique for nasal instillation: to insert tube into nostril to instill product
- To avoid OTC products (cough, hay fever) because these preparations may contain EPINEPHrine, decrease product response; not to use with alcohol because adverse reactions may occur
- To wear emergency ID specifying therapy
- That, if dose is missed, to take when remembered up to 1 hr before next dose; not to double dose; to avoid fluids from 1 hr to up to 8 hr after PO dose
- To report upper respiratory infection, nasal congestion to prescriber

desonide topical

See Appendix B

desoximetasone topical

See Appendix B

desoxyephedrine nasal agent

See Appendix B

desvenlafaxine

Pristiq

Func. class.: Antidepressant, serotonin-receptor norepinephrine reuptake inhibitor (SNRI)

ACTION:

May work by blocking the central presynaptic reuptake of 5-HT and NE, resulting in an increased sustained level of these neurotransmitters.

USES:

Major depressive disorder
Unlabeled uses: Vasomotor symptoms (hot flashes) associated with menopause

CONTRAINDICATIONS:

Hypersensitivity to this product or *venlafaxine, MAOI therapy*

Precautions:

CNS depression, abrupt discontinuation, hypertension, hepatic/renal disease, hyponatremia, geriatric patients, pregnancy (C), labor and delivery, breastfeeding, angina, bleeding, cardiac dysrhythmias, MI, stroke, mania, hypovolemia, dehydration

Black Box Warning: Children, suicidal ideation

DOSAGE AND ROUTES

- **Adult: PO** Initially, 50 mg/day; max 400 mg/day with adjustments as needed

Vasopastic effects of menopause (unlabeled)

- **Adult: PO** 100-150 mg/day

Available forms:

Extended release tabs 50, 100 mg

Administer:

- Without regard to food, food may minimize GI symptoms
- Extended release tab: do not crush, break, or chew

SIDE EFFECTS

CNS: *Dizziness,* drowsiness, *headache,* tremor, paresthesias, asthenia, worsening of depression, suicidal thoughts/behaviors, seizures, fatigue, chills, yawning, hot flashes, flushing, *irritability, insomnia, anxiety, abnormal dreams, fatigue*

CV: Palpitations, sinus tachycardia, increased blood pressure, orthostatic hypotension

EENT: Blurred vision, mydriasis, tinnitus

GI: *Nausea,* xerostomia, *diarrhea,* constipation, vomiting, anorexia, weight loss, dysgeusia, hypercholesterolemia, hypertriglyceridemia

GU: Urinary retention/hesitancy, orgasm dysfunction, decreased libido, impotence, proteinuria

HEMA: Impaired platelet aggregation

INTEG: Photosensitivity, hyperhidrosis, diaphoresis

SYST: Serotonin syndrome, neuroleptic malignant syndrome-like symptoms, toxic epidermal necrolysis, rash, Stevens-Johnson syndrome, erythema multiforme, angioedema; neonatal abstinence syndrome (fetal exposure)

PHARMACOKINETICS

Protein binding 30%, elimination half-life 11 hrs; elimination half-life is increased (hepatic/renal disease)

INTERACTIONS

Increase: serotonin syndrome, neuroleptic malignant syndrome-like reactions—SSRIs, other SNRIs, serotonin receptor agonists (almotriptan, eletriptan, frovatriptan, naratriptan, rizatriptan, sumatriptan, zolmitriptan), TCAs, trazadone, sibutramine, sumatriptan, ergots, dexfenfluramine, fenfluramine, lithium, nefazodone, meperidine, phentermine, MAOIs, dextromethorphan, linezolid, promethazine, methylphenidate, dexmethylphenidate, mirtazapine, pentazocine, tryptophan; do not administer concurrently

Increase: bleeding risk—salicylates, thrombolytics, NSAIDs, platelet inhibitors, anticoagulants

Increase: CNS depression—alcohol, opioids, antihistamines, sedatives/hypnotics

Increase: hallucinations, delusions, disorientation—zolpidem

Drug/Herb

Increase: desvenlafaxine action—kava, valerian

NURSING CONSIDERATIONS

Assess:

- Suicidal thoughts/behaviors: mental status and mood, identify suicidal ideation
- **Serotonin syndrome, neuroleptic malignant syndrome-like symptoms:** assess for nausea/vomiting, sedation, dizziness, diaphoresis (sweating), facial flush, hallucinations, mental status changes, myoclonia, restlessness, shiver-

ing, elevated blood pressure, hyperthermia, muscle rigidity, autonomic instability, mental status changes; if serotonin syndrome occurs discontinue desvenlafaxine, and any other serotonergic agents
• Monitor B/P baseline and periodically during treatment
• Appetite and nutritional intake, weight loss is common, change diet as need to support weight

Perform/provide:
• Store at room temperature

Evaluate:
• Decreased depression; increased sense of well-being, renewed interest in activities

Teach patient/family:
• To take as directed, not to double or skip doses; if a dose is missed, take as soon as remembered unless close to next dose; do not discontinue abruptly, decreased gradually
• To report immediately suicidal thoughts/behaviors, have family members look for symptoms of suicidal ideation
• Not to operate machinery or engage in hazardous activities until reaction is known, may cause dizziness, drowsiness
• To avoid all other products unless approval by prescriber
• To report if pregnancy is planned or suspected (pregnancy category C) or if breastfeeding
• To report immediately allergic reactions, including rash, hives, difficulty breathing, or swelling of face, lips
• That continuing follow-up exams will be needed

dexamethasone (Rx)
(dex-ah-meth'a-sone)

Apo-Dexamethasone ✱, Baycadron, Decadron, Dexasone ✱, DexPak, Maxidex ✱, PMS-Dexamethasone ✱, ratio-Dexamethasone ✱, Zena-Pak

dexamethasone sodium phosphate (Rx)

Func. class.: Corticosteroid, synthetic
Chem. class.: Glucocorticoid, long acting

Do not confuse:
Decadron/Percodan

ACTION: Decreases inflammation by suppression of migration of polymorphonuclear leukocytes, fibroblasts, reversal of increased capillary permeability and lysosomal stabilization

USES: Inflammation, allergies, neoplasms, cerebral edema, septic shock, collagen disorders

Unlabeled uses: ARDS, bone pain, bronchopulmonary dysplasia (BPD), Churg-Strauss syndrome, endophthalmitis, hyaline membrane disease prophylaxis, infertility with clomiPHENE, laryngeal edema prophylaxis, mixed connective-tissue disease, polychondritis, polyarteritis nodosa, pulmonary edema, temporal arteritis, Wegener's granulomatosis, pediatric bacterial meningitis, cancer chemotherapy (nausea/vomiting), croup

CONTRAINDICATIONS: Children <2 yr, psychosis, hypersensitivity to corticosteroids or benyl alcohol; idiopathic thrombocytopenia, acute glomerulonephritis, amebiasis, fungal infections, nonasthmatic bronchial disease, AIDS, TB, ocular infection, glaucoma

Precautions: Pregnancy (C), breastfeeding, diabetes mellitus, osteoporosis, seizure disorders, ulcerative colitis, CHF, myasthenia gravis, renal disease, peptic ulcer, esophagitis

DOSAGE AND ROUTES

Inflammation

- **Adult: PO** 0.75-9 mg/day in divided doses q6-12hr or phosphate **IM** 0.5-9 mg/day divided q6-12hr
- **Child: PO** 0.024-0.34 mg/kg/day in divided doses q6-12hr

Anaphylactic shock

- **Adult: IV** (Phosphate) single dose 1-6 mg/kg or **IV** 40 mg q2-6hr as needed up to 72 hr

Cerebral edema

- **Adult: IV** (Phosphate) 10 mg, then 4-6 mg **IM** q6hr × 2-4 days, then taper over 1 wk
- **Child:** Loading dose 1-2 mg/kg **(PO/IM/IV)** then 1-1.5 mg/kg/day, max 16 mg/day divided q4-6hr for 2-4 days, then taper down weekly

Adrenocortical insufficiency

- **Adult: PO** 0.75-9 mg/day in divided doses
- **Child: PO** 0.03-0.3 mg/kg/day in 2-4 divided doses

Suppression test

- **Adult: PO** 1 mg at 11 PM or 0.5 mg q6hr × 48 hr

ARDS (unlabeled)

- **Adult: IM/IV** (phosphate) 0.5-9 mg/day in 2-4 divided doses
- **Child: IM/IV** 0.06-0.3 mg/kg/day or 1.2-10 mg/m^2 in divided doses q6-12hr

Bone pain (unlabeled)

- **Adult: PO/IV** 12-20 mg/day in divided doses

Pediatric bacterial meningitis (unlabeled)

- **Child and infant >2 mo: IV** 0.15 mg/kg qid × first 2 days of antibiotics

Croup (unlabeled)

- **Child: PO** 0.024-0.34 mg/kg/day or 0.66-10 mg/m^2/day in 2-4 divided doses; single dose of 0.6 mg/kg has been used for mild to moderate croup; **IM/IV** 0.06-0.3 mg/kg/day or 1.2-10 mg/m^2/day in divided doses q6-12hr, single dose of 0.6 mg/kg IM has been used for severe croup

Available forms: *Dexamethasone:* tabs 0.25, 0.5, 0.75, 1, 1.5, 2, 4, 6 mg; elix 0.5 mg/5 ml; oral sol 0.5 mg/5 ml, 1 mg/1 ml; *inj phosphate:* 4, 10, 20, 24 mg/ml

Administer:

PO route

- Titrated dose; use lowest effective dose
- With food or milk to decrease GI symptoms

IM route

- IM inj deeply in large muscle mass; rotate sites; avoid deltoid; use 21G needle
- In 1 dose in AM to prevent adrenal suppression; avoid SUBCUT administration, may damage tissue

Direct IV route

- Undiluted direct over ≤1 min

Intermittent IV INF route

- Diluted with 0.9% NaCl or D_5W, give as IV inf at prescribed rate
- After shaking suspension (parenteral); do not give suspension IV

Dexamethasone sodium phosphate

Syringe compatibilities: Caffeine, dimenhydrAMINE, furosemide, granisetron, ketamine, metoclopramide, octreotide, oxycodone, palonosetron, ranitidine, sufentanil, tramadol

Y-site compatibilities: Acyclovir, alfentanil, allopurinol, amifostine, amikacin, aminocaproic acid, aminophylline, amphotericin B cholesteryl, amphotericin B lipid complex, amphotericin B liposome, amsacrine, anidulafungin, ascorbic acid injection, atenolol, atracurium, atropine, aztreonam, benztropine, bivalirudin, bleomycin, bumetanide, buprenorphine, butorphanol, caffeine, CARBOplatin, cefamandole, ceFAZolin, cefepime, cefmetazole, cefonicid, cefoperazone, cefotaxime, cefotetan, cefoxitin, cefpirome, ceftazidime, ceftizoxime, ceftobiprole, cefTRIAXone, cephalothin, cephapirin, chloramphenicol, cimetidine, cisatracurium, CISplatin, cladribine, clindamycin, codeine, cyanocobalamin, cyclophosphamide, cycloSPORINE, cytarabine, DACTINomycin, DAPTOmycin, dexmedetomidine, digoxin, diltiazem, docetaxel, DOPamine, doripenem, doxacurium, DOXOrubicin, DOXOrubicin liposomal, enalaprilat, ePHEDrine, EPINEPHrine, epoetin alfa, eptifibatide, ertapenem, etoposide, famotidine, fentaNYL, filgrastim, fluconazole, fludarabine, fluorouracil, folic acid, foscarnet, furosemide, ganciclovir, gatifloxacin, gemcitabine, glycopyrrolate, granisetron, heparin, hydrocortisone, HYDROmorphone, ifosfamide, imipenem-cilastatin, indomethacin, insulin (regular), irinotecan, isoproterenol, ketorolac, lansoprazole, levofloxacin, lidocaine, linezolid, LORazepam, LR, mannitol, mechlorethamine, melphalan, meropenem, metaraminol, methadone, methicillin, methoxamine, methyldopate, methylPREDNISolone, metoclopramide, metoprolol, metroNIDAZOLE, mezlocillin, miconazole, milrinone, morphine, moxalactam, multiple vitamins injection, nafcillin, nalbuphine, naloxone, nitroglycerin, nitroprusside, norepinephrine, octreotide, ondansetron, oxacillin, oxaliplatin, oxycodone, oxytocin, paclitaxel, palonosetron, pamidronate, pancuronium, pemetrexed, penicillin G potassium/sodium, PENTobarbital, PHENObarbital, phenylephrine, phytonadione, piperacillin, piperacillin-tazobactam, potassium chloride, procainamide, propofol, propranolol, pyridoxine, ranitidine, remifentanil, Ringer's, ritodrine, riTUXimab, sargramostim, sodium acetate/bicarbonate, succinylcholine, SUFentanil, tacrolimus, teniposide, theophylline, thiamine, thiotepa, ticarcillin, ticarcillin-clavulanate, tigecycline, tirofiban, TNA, tolazoline, topotecan, trastuzumab, trimetaphan, urokinase, vancomycin, vasopressin, vecuronium, verapamil, vinCRIStine, vinorelbine, vitamin B complex/C, voriconazole, zidovudine, zoledronic acid

SIDE EFFECTS

CNS: *Depression, flushing, sweating,* headache, mood changes, euphoria, psychosis, **seizures,** insomnia
CV: *Hypertension,* **circulatory collapse, thrombophlebitis, embolism, tachycardia,** edema, cardiomyopathy
EENT: Fungal infections, increased intraocular pressure, blurred vision, cataracts, glaucoma
ENDO: HPA suppression, hyperglycemia, sodium, fluid retention
GI: *Diarrhea, nausea, abdominal distention,* **GI hemorrhage,** *increased appetite,* **pancreatitis**
HEMA: **Thrombocytopenia,** transient leukocytosis, **thromboembolism**
INTEG: Acne, poor wound healing, ecchymosis, petechiae, hirsutism
META: Hypokalemia
MS: Fractures, osteoporosis, weakness, arthralgia, myopathy

PHARMACOKINETICS

Half-life 36-54 hr
PO: Onset 1 hr, peak 1-2 hr, duration $2^1/_2$ days
IM: Duration 2 days-3 wk

INTERACTIONS

Increase: side effects—alcohol, salicylates, amphotericin B, digoxin, cycloSPORINE, diuretics, NSAIDs
Increase: dexamethasone action—salicylates, estrogens, indomethacin, hormonal contraceptives, ketoconazole, macrolide antiinfectives
Increase: tendinitis tendon rupture risk—quinolones
Increase: effect of—antidiabetics
Decrease: dexamethasone action—cholestyramine, colestipol, barbiturates, rifampin, ePHEDrine, phenytoin, theophylline, antacids
Decrease: anticoagulant effect, anticonvulsants, antidiabetics, ambenonium, neostigmine, isoniazid, toxoids, vaccines, anticholinesterases, salicylates, somatrem

Drug/Lab Test
Increase: cholesterol, sodium, blood glucose, uric acid, calcium, urine glucose
Decrease: calcium, K, T_4, T_3, thyroid ^{131}I uptake test, urine 17-OHCS, 17-KS, PBI
False negative: skin allergy tests

NURSING CONSIDERATIONS

Assess:
- Potassium, blood, urine glucose while receiving long-term therapy; hypo/hyperglycemia
- Weight daily; notify prescriber of weekly gain >5 lb
- B/P q4hr, pulse; notify prescriber of chest pain
- I&O ratio; be alert for decreasing urinary output, increasing edema
- Plasma cortisol levels during long-term therapy (normal: 138-635 nmol/L SI units when drawn at 8 AM); prolonged use can cause cushingoid symptoms
- **Infection:** fever, WBC even after withdrawal of medication; product masks infection
- **Potassium depletion:** paresthesias, fatigue, nausea, vomiting, depression, polyuria, dysrhythmias, weakness
- Edema, hypertension, cardiac symptoms
- Mental status: affect, mood, behavioral changes, aggression

Perform/provide:
- Assistance with ambulation for patients with bone-tissue disease to prevent fractures

Evaluate:
- Therapeutic response: decreased inflammation

Teach patient/family:
- That ID as corticosteroid user should be carried
- To contact prescriber if surgery, trauma, stress occurs because dose may need to be adjusted
- To notify prescriber if therapeutic response decreases because dosage adjustment may be needed

⚠ Not to discontinue abruptly because **adrenal crisis** can result
- About symptoms of adrenal insufficiency: nausea, anorexia, fatigue, dizziness, dyspnea, weakness, joint pain
- To avoid OTC products: salicylates, alcohol in cough products, cold preparations unless directed by prescriber
- About all aspects of product usage, including cushingoid symptoms; to notify health care provider of infection
- To avoid exposure to chickenpox or measles, persons with infection

dexamethasone ophthalmic

See Appendix B

dexamethasone topical

See Appendix B

dexlansoprazole (Rx)

(dex-lan-so-prey′zole)

Dexilant

Func. class.: Antiulcer, proton pump inhibitor
Chem. class.: Benzimidazole

ACTION: Suppresses gastric secretion by inhibiting hydrogen/potassium ATPase enzyme system in gastric parietal cell; characterized as gastric acid pump inhibitor because it blocks final step of acid production

USES: Gastroesophageal reflux disease (GERD), severe erosive esophagitis, heartburn

CONTRAINDICATIONS: Hypersensitivity
Precautions: Pregnancy (B), breastfeeding, children, proton pump hypersensitivity, gastric cancer, hepatic disease, vit B_{12} deficiency

DOSAGE AND ROUTES

Erosive esophagitis

- **Adult: PO** 60 mg daily for up to 8 wk; maintenance: **PO** 30 mg daily for up to 6 mo

GERD

- **Adult: PO** 30 mg daily × 4 wk

Available forms: Del rel caps 30, 60 mg

Administer:

- Swallow caps whole; do not crush, chew caps; caps may be opened, contents sprinkled on food, use immediately; do not chew contents of capsule, give without regard to food

SIDE EFFECTS

CNS: Headache, dizziness, confusion, agitation, amnesia, depression, anxiety, seizures, insomnia, migraine

CV: Chest pain, angina, bradycardia, palpitations, CVA, hypertension, MI

EENT: Tinnitus

GI: Diarrhea, abdominal pain, vomiting, nausea, constipation, flatulence, colitis, dysgeusia

HEMA: Anemia, neutropenia, thrombocytopenia, pernicious anemia, thrombosis

INTEG: Rash, urticaria, pruritus

META: Gout

MS: Arthralgia, mylagia

RESP: Upper respiratory infections, cough, epistaxis, dyspnea, pneumonia

SYST: Anaphylaxis, Stevens-Johnson syndrome, toxic epidermal necrolysis, exfoliative dermatitis

PHARMACOKINETICS

Absorption 57%-64%; plasma half-life 1-2 hr; protein binding 96.1%-98.8%; extensively metabolized in liver; excreted in urine, feces; clearance decreased in geriatric patients, renal/hepatic impairment; peak dual 1-2 hr, 4-5 hr

INTERACTIONS

Increase: dexlansoprazole effect—CYP2C19, 3A4 inhibitors (fluvoxamine, voriconazole)

- Dexlansoprazole absorption: sucralfate

Decrease: absorption of ketoconazole, itraconazole, iron, delavirdine, ampicillin, calcium carbonate

NURSING CONSIDERATIONS

Assess:

- GI system: bowel sounds q8hr, abdomen for pain, swelling, anorexia, monitor serum magnesium
- **Hepatotoxicity:** hepatitis, jaundice, monitor hepatic studies (AST, ALT, alk phos) if hepatic adverse reactions occur
- **Anaphylaxis, serious skin disorders:** require emergency intervention

Evaluate:

- Therapeutic response: absence of epigastric pain, swelling, fullness

Teach patient/family:

- To report severe diarrhea; product may have to be discontinued
- That diabetic patient should know that hypoglycemia may occur
- To avoid hazardous activities; dizziness may occur
- To avoid alcohol, salicylates, ibuprofen; may cause GI irritation

dexmedetomidine (Rx)

(dex-med-eh-tom′o-deen)

Precedex

Func. class.: Sedative, α_2-adrenoceptor agonist

ACTION: Produces α_2-agonist activity seen at low and moderate doses, also α_1 at high doses

USES: Sedation in mechanically ventilated, intubated patients in ICU

CONTRAINDICATIONS: Hypersensitivity, chronic hypertension

Precautions: Pregnancy (C), breastfeeding, children, geriatric patients, respiratory depression, severe respiratory disorders, cardiac dysrhythmias, hypovolemia, diabetes, CV/renal/hepatic disease

DOSAGE AND ROUTES

• **Adult: IV** Loading dose of 1 mcg/kg over 10 min then 0.2-0.7 mcg/kg/hr; do not use for more than 24 hr

• **Child and infant (unlabeled): IV** 0.28 mcg/kg/hr for 24 hr to mechanically ventilated patients

Available forms: Inj 100 mcg/ml

Administer:

Continuous IV INF route

• After diluting with 0.9% NaCl, withdraw 2 ml of product and add to 48 ml of 0.9% NaCl to a total of 50 ml (4 mcg/ml), shake gently to mix well, use controlled inf device

• Give loading dose over 10 min by continuous IV inf; do not give by bolus or rapid IV inj; use for ≤24hr

• Only with resuscitative equipment available

• Only by qualified persons trained in ICU sedation

Solution compatibilities: LR, D_5W, 0.9% NaCl

Additive compatibilities: Mannitol

Y-site compatibilities: Acyclovir, alfentanil, allopurinol, amifostine, amikacin, aminocaproic acid, aminophylline, amiodarone, amphotericin B liposome, ampicillin, ampicillin-sulbactam, anidulafungin, atenolol, atracurium, atropine, azithromycin, aztreonam, bivalirudin, bleomycin, bumetanide, buprenorphine, busulfan, butorphanol, calcium chloride/gluconate, CARBOplatin, carmustine, caspofungin, ceFAZolin, cefepime, cefoperazone, cefotaxime, cefotetan, cefoxitin, ceftazidime, ceftizoxime, cefTRIAXone, cefuroxime, chlorproMAZINE, cimetidine, ciprofloxacin, cisatracurium, CISplatin, clindamycin, cyclophosphamide, cycloSPORINE, cytarabine, dacarbazine, DACTINomycin, DAPTOmycin, DAUNOrubicin, dexamethasone, dexrazoxane, digoxin, diltiazem, diphenhydrAMINE, DOBUTamine, docetaxel, dolasetron, DOPamine, doxacurium, DOXOrubicin, doxycycline, droperidol, enalaprilat, ePHEDrine, EPINEPHrine, ertapenem, erythromycin, esmolol, etomidate, etoposide, famotidine, fenoldopam, fentaNYL, fluconazole, fludarabine, fluorouracil, foscarnet, fosphenytoin, furosemide, ganciclovir, gatifloxacin, gemcitabine, gentamicin, glycopyrrolate, granisetron, haloperidol, heparin, hydrocortisone, HYDROmorphone, hydrOXYzine, IDArubicin, ifosfamide, imipenem-cilastatin, inamrinone, insulin (regular), isoproterenol, ketorolac, labetalol, leucovorin, levofloxacin, levorphanol, lidocaine, linezolid, LORazepam, magnesium sulfate, mannitol, mechlorethamine, meperidine, meropenem, mesna, methohexital, methotrexate, methylPREDNISolone, metoclopramide, metoprolol, metroNIDAZOLE, midazolam, milrinone, minocycline, mitomycin, mitoxantrone, mivacurium, morphine, mycophenolate mofetil, nalbuphine, naloxone, nesiritide, niCARdipine, nitroglycerin, nitroprusside, norepinephrine, octreotide, ofloxacin, ondansetron, oxaliplatin, oxytocin, paclitaxel, palonosetron, pamidronate, pancuronium, pemetrexed, pentamidine, PENTobarbital, PHENobarbital, phenylephrine, piperacillin, piperacillin-tazobactam, potassium chloride/phosphates, procainamide, prochlorperazine, promethazine, propofol, propranolol, quinupristin-dalfopristin, ranitidine, rapacuronium, remifentanil, rocuronium, sodium acetate/bicarbonate/ phosphates, succinylcholine, SUFentanil, sulfamethoxazole-trimethoprim, tacrolimus, teniposide, theophylline, thiopental, thiotepa, ticarcillin, ticarcillin-clavulanate, tigecycline, tirofiban, tobramycin, topotecan, vancomycin, vasopressin, vecuronium, verapamil, vinBLAStine, vinCRIStine, vinorelbine, voriconazole, zidovudine, zoledronic acid

SIDE EFFECTS

CV: *Bradycardia, hypotension,* hypertension, **atrial fibrillation, infarction, cardiac arrest**

GI: *Nausea,* thirst

GU: Oliguria
HEMA: Leukocytosis, anemia
MISC: Hyperkalemia
RESP: **Pulmonary edema, pleural effusion, hypoxia, respiratory acidosis**

PHARMACOKINETICS

Rapid distribution, excreted in urine, metabolized in liver, protein binding 94%, elimination half-life 2 hr

INTERACTIONS

Increase: CNS depression—alcohol, opioids, sedative/hypnotics, antipsychotics, skeletal muscle relaxants, inhalational anesthetics
Increase: hypotension—antihypertensives

NURSING CONSIDERATIONS

Assess:
- Inj site: phlebitis, burning, stinging
- Cardiac status: B/P, heart rate, ECG for changes: atrial fibrillation, monitor geriatric patients more closely
- CNS changes: movement, jerking, tremors, dizziness, LOC, pupil reaction
- Respiratory dysfunction: respiratory depression, character, rate, rhythm; notify prescriber if respirations are <10/min

Perform/provide:
- Safety measures: side rails, night-light, call bell within easy reach

Evaluate:
- Therapeutic response: induction of anesthesia

Teach patient/family:
- About reason for treatment, expected results

dexmethylphenidate (Rx)

(dex′meth-ul-fen′ih-dayt)

Focalin, Focalin XR

Func. class.: Central nervous system (CNS) stimulant, psychostimulant

Controlled Substance Schedule II

D

ACTION: Increases release of norepinephrine and DOPamine into the extraneuronal space, also blocks the reuptake of norepinephrine and DOPamine into the presynaptic neuron; mode of action for treating attention-deficit/hyperactivity disorder (ADHD) is unknown

USES: ADHD

CONTRAINDICATIONS: Breastfeeding, children <6 yr, hypersensitivity to methylphenidate, anxiety, history of Gilles de la Tourette's syndrome, tics, psychosis, glaucoma, concurrent treatment with MAOIs or within 14 days of discontinuing treatment with MAOIs
Precautions: Pregnancy (C), hypertension, depression, seizures, CV disorders, alcoholism

Black Box Warning: Substance abuse

DOSAGE AND ROUTES

- **Adult/adolescent/child >6 yr: PO** 2.5 mg bid with doses at least 4 hr apart, gradually increase to a maximum of 20 mg/day (10 mg bid); for those taking methylphenidate, use ½ of methylphenidate dose initially then increase as needed to a max of 20 mg/day
- **Adolescent and child ≥6 yr: EXT REL** 5 mg/day, may adjust to 20 mg/day in 5-mg increments, max 30 mg/day
- **Adult: PO EXT REL** 10 mg/day, may adjust to 20 mg/day in 10-mg increments, max 40 mg/day

Available forms: Tabs 2.5, 5, 10 mg; ext rel caps 5, 10, 20 mg (Focalin XR)

Administer:

- Twice daily at least 4 hr apart; ext rel once a day; in the morning, ext rel cap may be opened and contents sprinkled onto applesauce and consumed without chewing
- Without regard to meals
- Do not break, crush, or chew ext rel product

SIDE EFFECTS

CNS: Dizziness, headache, drowsiness, nervousness, insomnia, toxic psychosis, neuroleptic malignant syndrome (rare), Tourette's syndrome

CV: Palpitations, B/P changes, angina, dysrhythmias, tachycardia, MI, stroke

GI: *Nausea, anorexia*, abnormal hepatic function, hepatic coma, *abdominal pain*

HEMA: Leukopenia, anemia, thrombocytopenic purpura

INTEG: Exfoliative dermatitis, urticaria, rash, erythema multiforme

MISC: *Fever*, arthralgia, scalp hair loss

PHARMACOKINETICS

Readily absorbed, elimination half-life 2.2 hr, metabolized by liver, excreted by kidneys

PO: Peak 1½ hr, onset ½-1 hr, duration 4 hr

PO-ER: Onset unknown, peak 4 hr, duration 8 hr

INTERACTIONS

⚠ **Increase:** hypertensive crisis—MAOIs or within 14 days of MAOIs, vasopressors

Increase: sympathomimetic effect—decongestants, vasoconstrictors

Increase: effects of anticonvulsants, tricyclics, SSRIs, coumarin

Decrease: effects of antihypertensives

Drug/Herb

- Synergistic effect: melatonin

NURSING CONSIDERATIONS

Assess:

Black Box Warning: Substance abuse, past or current

- VS, B/P; may reverse antihypertensives; check patients with cardiac disease more often for increased B/P
- CBC, differential platelet counts during long-term therapy, urinalysis; with diabetes: blood glucose, urine glucose; insulin changes may have to be made because eating will decrease
- Height, growth rate q3mo in children; growth rate may be decreased
- Mental status: mood, sensorium, affect, stimulation, insomnia, aggressiveness, hostility

⚠ Withdrawal symptoms: headache, nausea, vomiting, muscle pain, weakness

- Appetite, sleep, speech patterns
- For attention span, decreased hyperactivity in persons with ADHD

Evaluate:

- Therapeutic response: decreased hyperactivity or ability to stay awake

Teach patient/family:

- To decrease caffeine consumption (coffee, tea, cola, chocolate); may increase irritability, stimulation
- To take early in day to prevent insomnia
- To avoid OTC preparations unless approved by prescriber; to avoid alcohol ingestion
- To taper off product over several wk to avoid depression, increased sleeping, lethargy
- To avoid hazardous activities until stabilized on medication
- To get needed rest; patients will feel more tired at end of day
- To notify all health care workers, including school nurse, of medication and schedule
- About information, instructions provided in patient information section

TREATMENT OF OVERDOSE:

Administer fluids; hemodialysis or peritoneal dialysis; antihypertensive for increased B/P; administer short-acting barbiturate before lavage

dextran 40 (Rx)

(deks'tran)

Gentran 40

dextran 70/75 (Rx)

Gentran 70

Func. class.: Plasma volume expander

Chem. class.: Low-molecular-weight polysaccharide

ACTION: Similar to human albumin, which expands plasma volume by drawing fluid from interstitial space to intravascular space

USES: Expand plasma volume, prophylaxis of embolism, thrombosis

CONTRAINDICATIONS: Hypersensitivity

Precautions: Pregnancy (C), active hemorrhage, sodium restriction, bowel surgery, thrombocytopenia, renal failure, CHF (severe), extreme dehydration, pulmonary edema, bleeding disorders

DOSAGE AND ROUTES

Dextran 40

Shock

- **Adult: IV INF** 500 ml over 15-30 min, total dose in 24 hr, max 20 ml/kg; subsequent doses given slowly; if given >24 hr, max 10 ml/kg/day; max therapy ≤5 days
- **Child: IV** Total dose ≤20 ml/kg during first 24 hr then ≤10 ml/kg/day if needed

Thrombosis/embolism

- **Adult: IV INF** 500-1000 ml, then 500 ml/day × 3 days, then 500 ml q2-3 days × 2 wk if needed

Dextran 70/75

- **Adult: IV INF** 500-1000 ml not to exceed 20-40 ml/min, max 10 ml/kg/24 hr if therapy >24 hr

Available forms: 10% dextran 40/D_5W, 10% dextran 40/0.9% NaCl, 70/75 dextran in 0.9% NaCl, D_5%

Administer:

IV route

- After prescribed dilution; may give initial 500 mg at 15-30 min; distribute remainder of daily dose over 8-24 hr
- After crossmatch is drawn if blood also to be given
- D_5W sol in patients with heart failure as ordered

SIDE EFFECTS

CV: Hypotension, **cardiac arrest, CHF**

GI: Nausea, vomiting, increased AST, ALT

GU: **Osmotic nephrosis, renal failure,** stasis, hyponatremia

HEMA: Decreased hematocrit, platelet function; **increased bleeding/coagulation times, thrombocytopenia**

INTEG: Rash, urticaria, pruritus, angioedema, chills, fever, flushing

RESP: Wheezing, dyspnea, **bronchospasm, pulmonary edema**

SYST: **Anaphylaxis**

PHARMACOKINETICS

Dextran 40

IV: Expands blood vol 1-2× amount infused, excreted in urine, feces

Dextran 70/75

IV: Onset within mins, duration 12 hr, expands blood vol 1-2× amount infused; excreted in urine, feces

INTERACTIONS

- Incompatible with chlortetracycline, phytonadione, promethazine

Drug/Lab Test

False increase: blood glucose, urinary protein, bilirubin, total protein

Interference: Rh test, blood typing/crossmatching

NURSING CONSIDERATIONS

Assess:

- VS q5min × 30 min; Hgb/Hct if falling by 30%, notify prescriber

• CVP during inf (5-10 cm water—normal range)
• Urine output q1hr; watch for increase in urinary output (common); if output does not increase, decrease or discontinue inf
• I&O ratio and specific gravity, urine osmolarity; if specific gravity very low, renal clearance low, product should be discontinued
• Allergy: rash, urticaria, pruritus, wheezing, dyspnea, bronchospasm, product should be discontinued immediately
⚠ **Circulatory overload:** increased pulse, respirations, SOB, wheezing, chest tightness, chest pain
• Dehydration after infusion: decreased output, decreased specific gravity of urine, increased temp, poor skin turgor, increased specific gravity, dry skin

Perform/provide:
• Storage at constant temp (15° C-30° C [59° F-86° F]); discard unused portions, protect from freezing

Evaluate:
• Therapeutic response: increased plasma volume

Teach patient/family:
• About signs of bleeding: bruising, blood in urine or black, tarry stools

dextroamphetamine (Rx)

(dex-troe-am-fet′a-meen)

Dexedrine, ProCentra

Func. class.: Cerebral stimulant
Chem. class.: Amphetamine

Controlled Substance Schedule II

ACTION:
Increases release of norepinephrine, DOPamine in cerebral cortex to reticular activating system

USES:
Narcolepsy, attention-deficit/hyperactivity disorder (ADHD)
Unlabeled uses: Obesity

CONTRAINDICATIONS:
Hypersensitivity to sympathomimetic amines, hyperthyroidism, hypertension, glaucoma, severe arteriosclerosis, substance abuse, anxiety, anorexia nervosa, tartrazine dye hypersensitivity

Black Box Warning: Symptomatic CV disease, substance abuse

Precautions: Pregnancy (C), breastfeeding, children <3 yr, depression, Gilles de la Tourette's disorder, cardiomyopathy, bipolar disorder

DOSAGE AND ROUTES

Narcolepsy
• **Adult: PO** 5 mg bid, titrate daily dose by no more than 10 mg/wk, max 60 mg/day
• **Child 6-12 yr: PO** 5 mg/day, titrate daily dose by no more than 5 mg/day at weekly intervals

ADHD
• **Adult: PO** 5-60 mg/day in divided doses
• **Child 3-5 yr: PO** 2.5 mg/day increasing by 2.5 mg/day at weekly intervals, max 40 mg/day
• **Child >6-12 yr: PO** 5 mg daily-bid increasing by 5 mg/day at weekly intervals

Obesity, exogenous (unlabeled)
• **Adult and adolescent: PO** 5-30 mg/dose given 30-60 min before meals, use for 3-6 wk only

Available forms: Tabs 5, 10 mg; oral sol 5 mg/5 ml

Administer:
• At least 6 hr before bedtime to avoid sleeplessness
• Use calibrated measuring device for oral sol

SIDE EFFECTS

CNS: *Hyperactivity, insomnia, restlessness, talkativeness,* dizziness, headache, chills, stimulation, dysphoria, irritability, aggressiveness, tremor, dependence, addiction

CV: *Palpitations, tachycardia,* hypertension, decrease in heart rate, dysrhythmias

GI: *Anorexia,* dry mouth, diarrhea, constipation, weight loss, metallic taste

GU: Impotence, change in libido

INTEG: Urticaria

PHARMACOKINETICS

Onset 1 hr; peak 2 hr; duration 4-20 hr; metabolized by liver; urine excretion pH dependent; crosses placenta, breast milk; half-life 6-8 hr (child), 10-12 hr (adult)

INTERACTIONS

⚠ Hypertensive crisis: MAOIs or within 14 days of MAOIs

Increase: serotonin syndrome, neuroleptic malignant syndrome, SSRIs, SNRIs, do not use concurrently

Increase: dextroamphetamine effect—acetaZOLAMIDE, antacids, sodium bicarbonate

Increase: CNS effect—haloperidol, tricyclics, phenothiazines

Decrease: absorption of barbiturates, phenytoin

Decrease: dextroamphetamine effect—ascorbic acid, ammonium chloride, guanethidine

Decrease: effect of adrenergic blockers, antidiabetics, antihypertensives, antihistamines

Drug/Herb

- Serotonin syndrome: St. John's wort

Decrease: stimulant effect—eucalyptus

Drug/Food

Increase: amine effect—caffeine (cola, coffee, tea [green/black])

Drug/Lab Test

Increase: plasma corticosteroids, urinary steroids

NURSING CONSIDERATIONS

Assess:

Black Box Warning: VS, B/P; product may reverse antihypertensives; check patients with cardiac disease often

- CBC, urinalysis; with diabetes: blood glucose, urine glucose; insulin changes may be required because eating will decrease
- Height, growth rate in children; growth rate may be decreased, weight
- Mental status: mood, sensorium, affect, stimulation, insomnia, irritability
- Tolerance or dependency: increased amount may be used to get same effect; will develop after long-term use
- **Overdose:** pain, fever, dehydration, insomnia, hyperactivity

Perform/provide:

- Gum, hard candy, frequent sips of water for dry mouth
- Storage of tabs and caps at room temp; store oral sol at room temp, protect from light

Evaluate:

- Therapeutic response: increased CNS stimulation, decreased drowsiness

Teach patient/family:

- To take before meals (obesity)
- To decrease caffeine consumption (coffee, tea, cola, chocolate); may increase irritability, stimulation
- To avoid OTC preparations unless approved by prescriber
- To taper product over several wk; depression, increased sleeping, lethargy may occur
- To avoid alcohol ingestion
- To avoid hazardous activities until stabilized on medication
- To get needed rest; patient will feel more tired at end of day

TREATMENT OF OVERDOSE:

Administer fluids, hemodialysis, or peritoneal dialysis; antihypertensive for increased B/P, ammonium Cl for increased excretion

dextromethorphan (OTC)

(dex-troe-meth-or′fan)

Balminil ♣, Benylin ♣, Buckley's DM, Bukley's Mixture, Cough Suppressant Long-Acting, Delsym 12-Hour, ElixSure Cough, Koffex ♣, PediaCare Children's Long-Acting Cough, PediaCare Long-Acting Cough, Robafan, Robitussin, Robitussin Cough with honey, Robitussin Maximum Strength, Scot-Tussin Diabetes CF, Silphen-DM, Top Care Day Time Cough, Top Care Tussin Cough Suppressant Long-Acting, Triaminic Long Acting Cough, Tylenol Childrens Simply Cough, Vicks Formula 44, Wal-Tussin

Func. class.: Antitussive, nonopioid
Chem. class.: Levorphanol derivative

ACTION: Depresses cough center in medulla by direct effect

USES: Nonproductive cough caused by colds or inhaled irritants

CONTRAINDICATIONS: Hypersensitivity

Precautions: Pregnancy (C), fever, hepatic disease, asthma/emphysema, chronic cough

DOSAGE AND ROUTES

- **Adult and child ≥12 yr: PO** 10-20 mg q4hr or 30 mg q6-8hr, max 120 mg/day; **SUS-REL LIQ** 60 mg q12hr, max 120 mg/day
- **Child 6-12 yr: PO** 5-10 mg q4hr; **SUS REL LIQ** 30 mg bid, **LOZ** 5-10 mg q1-4hr; max 60 mg/day
- **Child 4-6 yr: PO** 2.5-7.5 mg q4-8hr, max 30 mg/day; **SUS REL LIQ** 15 mg bid
- **Child <4 yr:** Not recommended

Available forms: Liq 7.5, 15 mg/5 ml; syr 10 mg/5 ml, 15 mg/5 ml, 30 mg/15 ml; gel caps 15 mg; caps 15 mg; ext rel susp: 30 mg/5 ml

Administer:

- **Chew tabs:** chew well; **syrup:** use calibrated measuring device; **ext rel susp:** shake well, use calibrated measuring device
- Decreased dose for geriatric patients; metabolism may be slowed

SIDE EFFECTS

CNS: *Dizziness,* sedation, confusion, ataxia, fatigue
GI: *Nausea*

PHARMACOKINETICS

PO: Onset 15-30 min, duration 3-6 hr
SUS: Duration 12 hr, terminal half-life 11 hr, metabolized by the liver, excreted via kidneys

INTERACTIONS

- Do not give with MAOIs or within 2 wk of MAOIs; avoid furazolidone, linezolid, procarbazine (MAOI activity)

Increase: CNS depression—alcohol, antidepressants, antihistamines, opioids, sedative/hypnotics
Increase: adverse reactions—amiodarone, quiNIDine, serotonin receptor agonist, sibutramine, SSRI

NURSING CONSIDERATIONS

Assess:

- **Cough:** type, frequency, character, including sputum

Perform/provide:

- Increased fluids to liquify secretions
- Humidification of patient's room

Evaluate:

- Therapeutic response: absence of cough

Teach patient/family:

- To avoid driving, other hazardous activities until stabilized on medication
- To avoid smoking, smoke-filled rooms, perfumes, dust, environmental pollutants, cleaners that increase cough

• To avoid alcohol, CNS depressants
• To notify prescriber if cough persists over a few days

dextrose (D-glucose) (Rx)

Func. class.: Caloric, parenteral solution

ACTION: Needed for adequate utilization of amino acids; decreases protein, nitrogen loss; prevents ketosis

USES: Increases intake of calories; increases fluids in patients unable to take adequate fluids, calories orally; acute hypoglycemia

CONTRAINDICATIONS: Hyperglycemia, delirium tremens, hemorrhage (cranial/spinal), CHF, anuria, allergy to corn products
Precautions: Cardiac/renal/hepatic disease, diabetes mellitus, carbohydrate intolerance

DOSAGE AND ROUTES

• **Adult and child: IV** Depends on individual requirements

Hypoglycemia

• **Adult: PO/IV** 10-25 mg

Available forms: Inj 2.5%, 5%, 10%, 20%, 25%, 30%, 38.5%, 40%, 50%, 60%, 70%; oral gel 40%; chew tab 5 g

Administer:

• Only (4%) protein and dextrose (up to 12.5%) via peripheral vein; stronger sol: central IV administration
• May be given undiluted via prepared sol; give 10% sol, 5 ml/15 sec; 10% sol, 1000 ml/3 hr or more; 20% sol, 500 ml/½-1 hr; 50% sol, 10 ml/min; control rate, rapid inf may cause fluid shifts, do not use same inf set as used for blood
• Oral glucose preparations (gel, chew tabs) to be used in conscious patients only; check serum blood glucose 10 min after 1st dose
• After changing IV catheter, dressing q24hr with aseptic technique

SIDE EFFECTS

CNS: Confusion, **loss of consciousness,** dizziness
CV: Hypertension, **CHF, pulmonary edema, intracranial hemorrhage**
ENDO: Hyperglycemia, rebound hypoglycemia, hyperosmolar syndrome, hyperglycemic nonketotic syndrome, aluminum toxicity, hypokalemia, hypomagnesium
GI: Nausea
GU: Glycosuria, osmotic diuresis
INTEG: Chills, flushing, warm feeling, rash, urticaria, extravasation necrosis
RESP: Pulmonary edema

INTERACTIONS

Increase: fluid retention/electrolyte excretion—corticosteroids

NURSING CONSIDERATIONS

Assess:

• Electrolytes (K, Na, Ca, Cl, Mg), blood glucose, ammonia, phosphate
• Inj site for extravasation: redness along vein, edema at site, necrosis, pain; hard, tender area; site should be changed immediately
• Monitor temp q4hr for increased fever, indicating infection; if infection suspected, discontinue inf, culture tubing, bottle, catheter tip cultured
• Serum glucose in patients receiving hypotonic glucose 50% and over
• Nutritional status: calorie count by dietitian

Evaluate:

• Therapeutic response: increased weight

Teach patient/family:

• About the reason for dextrose inf
• To review hypoglycemia/hyperglycemia symptoms
• To review blood glucose monitoring procedures

diazepam (Rx)

(dye-az′-e-pam)

Apo-Diazepam ✱, Diastat, Valium

Func. class.: Antianxiety, anticonvulsant, skeletal muscle relaxant, central acting

Chem. class.: Benzodiazepine, long-acting

Controlled Substance Schedule IV

Do not confuse:
diazepam/Ditropan/LORazepam

ACTION: Potentiates the actions of GABA, especially in the limbic system, reticular formation; enhances presympathetic inhibition, inhibits spinal polysynaptic afferent paths

USES: Anxiety, acute alcohol withdrawal, adjunct for seizure disorders; preoperatively as a relaxant for skeletal muscle relaxation; rectally for acute repetitive seizures

Unlabeled uses: Agitation, benzodiazepine withdrawal, chloroquine overdose, insomnia, seizure prophylaxis

CONTRAINDICATIONS: Pregnancy (D), hypersensitivity to benzodiazepines, closed-angle glaucoma, coma, myasthenia gravis, ethanol intoxication, hepatic disease, sleep apnea

Precautions: Breastfeeding, children <6 mo, geriatric patients, debilitation, renal disease, asthma, bipolar disorder, COPD, CNS depression, labor, Parkinson's disease, neutropenia, psychosis, seizures, substance abuse, smoking

DOSAGE AND ROUTES

Anxiety/seizure disorders

- **Adult: PO** 2-10 mg bid-tid; **IM/IV** 2-10 mg q3-4hr
- **Geriatric: PO** 1-2 mg daily-bid, increase slowly as needed
- **Child >6 mo: IM/IV** 0.04-0.3 mg/kg/dose q2-4hr, max 0.6 mg/kg in an 8-hr period

Precardioversion

- **Adult: IV** 5-15 mg 5-10 min precardioversion

Preendoscopy

- **Adult: IV** 2.5-20 mg; **IM** 5-10 mg ½ hr preendoscopy

Muscle relaxation

- **Adult: PO** 2-10 mg tid-qid or **EXT REL** 15-30 mg/day; **IV/IM** 5-10 mg, repeat in 2-4 hr
- **Geriatric: PO** 2-5 mg bid-qid; **IV/IM** 2-5 mg, may repeat in 2-4 hr

Tetanic muscle spasms

- **Child >5 yr: IM/IV** 5-10 mg q3-4hr prn
- **Infant >30 days: IM/IV** 1-2 mg q3-4hr prn

Status epilepticus

- **Adult: IV/IM** 5-10 mg, 2 mg/min, may repeat q10-15min, max 30 mg; may repeat in 2-4 hr if seizures reappear
- **Child >5 yr: IM** 1 mg q2-5min; **IV** 1 mg slowly
- **Child 1 mo-5 yr: IV** 0.2-0.5 mg slowly; **IM** 0.2-0.5 mg slowly q2-5min up to 5 mg, may repeat in 2-4 hr prn

Seizures other than status epilepticus

- **Adult: RECT** 0.2 mg/kg, may repeat in 4-12 hr
- **Child 6-11 yr: RECT** 0.3 mg/kg, may repeat in 4-12 hr
- **Child 2-5 yr: RECT** 0.5 mg/kg, may repeat in 4-12 hr

Alcohol withdrawal

- **Adult: IV** 10 mg initially then 5-10 mg q3-4hr prn

Benzodiazepine withdrawal (unlabeled)

- **Adult: PO** Taper 0.5-2 mg over 4-16 wk

Febrile seizure prophylaxis (unlabeled)

- **Child 6 mo-5 yr: PO** 0.33 mg/kg q8hr until afebrile for ≥24 hr

Available forms: Tabs 2, 5, 10 mg; inj 5 mg/ml; oral sol 5 mg/5 ml, 5 mg/ml; gel, rectal delivery system 10 mg, twin packs; ext rel cap 15 mg

Administer:

- With food or milk for GI symptoms; crushed if patient is unable to swallow medication whole
- Sugarless gum, hard candy, frequent sips of water for dry mouth
- Reduced opioid dose by 1/3 if given concomitantly with diazepam
- Concentrate: use calibrated dropper only; mix with water, juice, pudding, applesauce; to be consumed immediately

Rectal route

- Do not use more than 5×/mo or for an episode q5days

Direct IV route

- Into large vein; give IV 5 mg or less/1 min or total dose over 3 min or more (children, infants); continuous inf is not recommended; inject as close to vein insertion as possible; do not dilute or mix with other products

Y-site compatibilities: DAUNOrubicin, DAPTOmycin, docetaxel, fentanyl, methadone, piperacillin/tazobactam, teniposide

Y-site incompatibilities: Acetaminophen, acyclovir, alemtuzumab, alfentanil, amikacin, aminophylline, amphotericin B cholesteryl, amphotericin B colloidal, amphotericin B liposome, ampicillin, ampicillin/sulbactam, anidulafungin, ascorbic acid, atracurium, atropine, azaTHIOprine, aztreonam, bivalirudin, bumetanide, buprenorphine, butorphanol, calcium chloride/gluconate, CARBOplatin, caspofungin, ceFAZolin, cefepime, cefonicid, cefoperazone, cefotaxime, cefotetan, cefoxitin, ceftazidime, ceftizoxime, cefTRIAXone, cefuroxime, chloramphenicol, chlorproMAZINE, cimetidine, CISplatin, clindamycin, cyanocobalamin, cyclophosphamide, cycloSPORINE, cytarabine, DACTINomycin, dantrolene, dexamethasone, dexmedetomidine, diazoxide, digoxin, diltiazem, diphenhydrAMINE, DOPamine, doripenem, doxacurium, DOXOrubicin, doxycycline, enalaprilat, ePHEDrine, EPINEPHrine, epirubicin, epoetin alfa, eptifibatide, erythromycin, esmolol, etoposide, etoposide phosphate, famotidine, fenoldopam, fluconazole, fludarabine, fluorouracil, folic acid, foscarnet, furosemide, ganciclovir, gemcitabine, gentamicin, glycopyrrolate, granisetron, haloperidol, heparin, hydrALAZINE, hydrocortisone, hydrOXYzine, IDArubicin, ifosfamide, imipenem/cilastatin, inamrinone, indomethacin, insulin, isoproterenol, ketorolac, labetalol, levofloxacin, lidocaine, linezolid, magnesium chloride, mannitol, mechlorethamine, meperidine, meropenem, metaraminol, methotrexate, methoxamine, methyldopate, methylPREDNISolone, metoclopramide, metoprolol, metroNIDAZOLE, midazolam, milrinone, mitoxantrone, multivitamin, nalbuphine, naloxone, nesiritide, nitroglycerin, nitroprusside, norepinephrine, octreotide, oxacillin, oxaliplatin, oxytocin, paclitaxel, palonosetron, pancuronium, pantoprazole, papaverine, pemetrexed, penicillin G, pentamidine, pentazocine, PENTobarbital, PHENobarbital, phentolamine, phenylephrine, phenytoin, phytonadione, potassium chloride, procainamide, prochlorperazine, promethazine, propofol, propranolol, protamine, pyridoxime, quinupristin/dalfopristin, ranitidine, rocuronium, sodium acetate, sodium bicarbonate, succinylcholine, tacrolimus, theophylline, thiamine, thiotepa, ticarcillin/clavulanate, tigecycline, tirofiban, tobramycin, tolazoline, trimetaphan, trimethoprim/sulfamethoxazole, urokinase, vancomycin, vasopressin, vecuronium, verapamil, vinCRIStine, vinorelbine, vitamin B complex with C, voriconazole, zoledronic acid

SIDE EFFECTS

CNS: *Dizziness, drowsiness,* confusion, headache, anxiety, tremors, stimulation, fatigue, depression, insomnia, hallucinations, ataxia, fatigue

CV: *Orthostatic hypotension,* **ECG changes, tachycardia,** hypotension

EENT: *Blurred vision,* tinnitus, mydriasis, nystagmus
GI: Constipation, dry mouth, nausea, vomiting, anorexia, diarrhea
HEMA: Neutropenia
INTEG: Rash, dermatitis, itching
RESP: Respiratory depression

PHARMACOKINETICS

Metabolized by liver via CYP2C19, CYP3A4; excreted by kidneys; crosses placenta; excreted in breast milk; crosses the blood-brain barrier; half-life 20-50 hr; more reliable by mouth; 99% protein binding
PO: Rapidly absorbed, onset ½ hr, duration 2-3 hr
IM: Onset 15-30 min, duration 1-1½ hr, absorption slow and erratic
RECT: Peak 1.5 hr
IV: Onset immediate, duration 15 min-1 hr

INTERACTIONS

Increase: toxicity—barbiturates, SSRIs, cimetidine, CNS depressants, valproic acid, CYP3A4 inhibitors
Increase: CNS depression—CNS depressants, alcohol
Decrease: diazepam metabolism—oral contraceptives, valproic acid, disulfiram, isoniazid, propranolol
Decrease: diazepam effect—CYP3A4 inducers (rifampin, barbiturates, carBAMazepine, ethotoin, phenytoin, fosphenytoin)
Drug/Lab Test
Increase: AST/ALT, serum bilirubin
Decrease: RAIU
False increase: 17-OHCS

NURSING CONSIDERATIONS

Assess:
- B/P (lying, standing), pulse; respiratory rate; if systolic B/P drops 20 mm Hg, hold product, notify prescriber; respirations q5-15min if given IV
- Blood studies: CBC during long-term therapy; blood dyscrasias (rare); hepatic studies: AST, ALT, bilirubin, creatinine, LDH, alk phos
- **Degree of anxiety;** what precipitates anxiety and whether product controls symptoms
- **Alcohol withdrawal symptoms,** including hallucinations (visual, auditory), delirium, irritability, agitation, fine to coarse tremors
- Seizure control and type, duration, intensity of seizures
- For muscle spasms; pain relief
- IV site for thrombosis or phlebitis, which may occur rapidly
- Mental status: mood, sensorium, affect, sleeping pattern, drowsiness, dizziness, suicidal tendencies
- **Physical dependency, withdrawal symptoms:** headache, nausea, vomiting, muscle pain, weakness after long-term use

Perform/provide:
- Assistance with ambulation during beginning therapy, for drowsiness, dizziness, safety measures
- Check to confirm PO medication swallowed

Evaluate:
- Therapeutic response: decreased anxiety, restlessness, insomnia

Teach patient/family:
- That product may be taken with food
- That product not to be used for everyday stress or for > 4 mo unless directed by prescriber; to take no more than prescribed amount; that product may be habit forming
- To avoid OTC preparations unless approved by prescriber
- To avoid driving, activities that require alertness; drowsiness may occur
- To avoid alcohol, other psychotropic medications unless directed by prescriber; that smoking may decrease diazepam effect by increasing diazepam metabolism
- Not to discontinue medication abruptly after long-term use; to gradually taper
- To rise slowly or fainting may occur, especially in geriatric patients

- That drowsiness may worsen at beginning of treatment
- To avoid use during pregnancy

TREATMENT OF OVERDOSE:
Lavage, VS, supportive care, flumazenil

dibucaine topical
See Appendix B

diclofenac epolamine (Rx)
(dye-kloe′fen-ak)

Flector

diclofenac potassium (Rx)
Cambia, Cataflam, Rapide ♣, Zipsor

diclofenac sodium (Rx)
Apo-Dilo ♣, Novo-Difenac ♣, Nu-Diclo ♣, PENNSAID, Sandoz Diclofenac ♣, Solaraze Topical Gel, Voltaren, Voltaren Topical Gel, Voltaren XR

Func. class.: Nonsteroidal antiinflammatory products (NSAIDs), nonopioid analgesic

Chem. class.: Phenylacetic acid

Do not confuse:
Cataflam/Catapres

ACTION: Inhibits COX-1, COX-2 by blocking arachidonate resulting in analgesic, antiinflammatory, antipyretic

USES: Acute, chronic RA; osteoarthritis; ankylosing spondylitis; analgesia; primary dysmenorrhea; patch: mild to moderate pain

Unlabeled uses: Arthralgia, headache, migraine, bone pain, myalgia

CONTRAINDICATIONS: Hypersensitivity to aspirin, iodides, other NSAIDs, asthma, serious CV disease, pregnancy (D) 3rd trimester

Black Box Warning: Treatment of perioperative pain (CABG), surgery

Precautions: Pregnancy (C) 1st trimester, breastfeeding, children, not recommended in 2nd half of pregnancy, bleeding disorders, GI disorders, cardiac disorders, hypersensitivity to other antiinflammatory agents, CCr <30 ml/min

Black Box Warning: GI bleeding, MI, stroke

DOSAGE AND ROUTES

Osteoarthritis
- **Adult: PO** (Cataflam) 50 mg bid-tid, max 150 mg/day; **DEL REL** (Voltaren) 50 mg bid-tid or 75 mg bid, max 150 mg/day; **EXT REL** (Voltaren-XR) 100 mg daily, max 150 mg/day; **TOP GEL** 1% (Voltaren gel) 4 g for each of lower extremities qid, max 16 g/day; 2 g for each of upper extremities qid, max 8 g/day; **TOP SOL** (Pennsaid) apply 40 drops to each affected knee qid; apply 10 drops at a time, spread over entire knee

Rheumatoid arthritis
- **Adult: PO** (Cataflam) 50 mg tid-qid, max 200 mg/day; **DEL REL** (Voltaren) 50 mg tid-qid or 75 mg bid, max 200 mg/day; **EXT REL** (Voltaren-XR) 100 mg daily, may increase to 200 mg/day, max 200 mg/day

Ankylosing spondylitis
- **Adult: PO DEL REL** (Voltaren) 25 mg qid and 25 mg at bedtime, max 125 mg/day

Acute migraine with/without aura
- **Adult: PO** (powder for oral sol) (Cambia) 50 mg as a single dose, mix contents of packet in 1-2 oz water

Mild to moderate pain
- **Adult: PO** (Zipsor) 25 mg qid

Dysmenorrhea or nonrheumatic inflammatory conditions
- **Adult: PO** (Cataflam) 50 mg tid or 100 mg initially then 50 mg tid, max 200 mg 1st day then 150 mg/day

Pain of strains/sprains

• **Adult: TOP PATCH** (Flector) apply patch to area bid

Actinic keratosis

• **Adult: TOP GEL** (Solaraze) apply to area bid

Prevention of heterotropic ossification (unlabeled)

• **Adult: PO** 50 mg tid × 3 wk

Renal dose

• **Avoid:** Use of topical gel, patch, sol, potassium oral tab for advanced renal disease

Available forms: *Epolamine:* topical patch 1.3%; *potassium:* tabs 50 mg; tabs liquid filled 25 mg; oral powder for sol 50 mg; *sodium:* delayed rel tabs (enteric-coated) 25, 50, 75, 100 mg; Pennsaid: top sol 1.5%, ext rel 100 mg; topical gel 1%, 3%

Administer:

PO route

• Do not break, crush, or chew enteric products

• Take with a full glass of water to enhance absorption, remain upright for ½ hr; if dose missed, take as soon as remembered within 2 hr if taking 1-2×/day; do not double doses

Topical patch route (Flector)

• Wash hands before handling patch

• Remove and release liner before administration

• Use only on normal, intact skin

• Remove before bath, shower, swimming

• Discard removed patch in trash away from children, pets

Topical gel route

• Apply to intact skin

• Use only for osteoarthritis, mild to moderate pain

Topical solution route

• Apply to clean, dry skin

• Wait until dry before applying clothing, other creams/lotions

• Wait ≥30 min after use before bathing, swimming

SIDE EFFECTS

CNS: *Dizziness, headache,* drowsiness, fatigue, tremors, confusion, insomnia, anxiety, depression, nervousness, paresthesia, muscle weakness

CV: CHF, tachycardia, peripheral edema, palpitations, dysrhythmias, hypo/hypertension, fluid retention, MI, stroke

EENT: Tinnitus, hearing loss, blurred vision, laryngeal edema

GI: Nausea, anorexia, vomiting, diarrhea, jaundice, cholestatic hepatitis, constipation, flatulence, cramps, dry mouth, peptic ulcer, GI bleeding, hepatotoxicity

GU: Nephrotoxicity: dysuria, hematuria, oliguria, azotemia, cystitis, UTI

HEMA: Blood dyscrasias, epistaxis, bruising

INTEG: Purpura, rash, pruritus, sweating, erythema, petechiae, photosensitivity, alopecia

RESP: Dyspnea, hemoptysis, pharyngitis, bronchospasm, rhinitis, SOB

SYST: Anaphylaxis

PHARMACOKINETICS

PO: Peak 2-3 hr; **TOP Patch:** peak 12 hr; elimination half-life 2.5 hr, 99% bound to plasma proteins, metabolized in liver to metabolite, excreted in urine

INTERACTIONS

• Hyperkalemia: potassium-sparing diuretics

• Need for dosage adjustment: antidiabetics

Increase: anticoagulant effect—anticoagulants, NSAIDs, platelet inhibitors, salicylates, thrombolytics, SSRIs

Increase: toxicity—phenytoin, lithium, cycloSPORINE, methotrexate

Increase: GI side effects—aspirin, other NSAIDs, bisphosphonates, corticosteroids

Decrease: antihypertensive effect—β-blockers, diuretics, ACE inhibitors

NURSING CONSIDERATIONS

Assess:

• **Pain:** location, character, aggravating/alleviating factors, ROM before and 1 hr after dose

• Patients with asthma, aspirin hypersensitivity, nasal polyps; may develop hypersensitivity

• LFTs (may be elevated), uric acid (may be decreased—serum; increased—urine) periodically; also BUN, creatinine, electrolytes (may be elevated)

⚠ **Blood dyscrasias (thrombocytopenia):** bruising, fatigue, bleeding, poor healing; blood counts during therapy; watch for decreasing platelets; if low, therapy may need to be discontinued, restarted after hematologic recovery; stool guaiac

Perform/provide

• Storage of patches at room temp in resealable envelope provided

Evaluate:

• Therapeutic response: decreased inflammation in joints, after cataract surgery

Teach patient/family:

• That product must be continued for prescribed time to be effective; to contact prescriber prior to surgery regarding when to discontinue this product

• To report bleeding, bruising, fatigue, malaise; **blood dyscrasias** do occur

• To avoid aspirin, alcoholic beverages, NSAIDs, or other OTC medications unless approved by prescriber

• To take with food, milk, or antacids to avoid GI upset; to swallow whole

• To use caution when driving; drowsiness, dizziness may occur

• To report **hepatotoxicity:** flulike symptoms, nausea, vomiting, jaundice, pruritus, lethargy

• To use sunscreen to prevent photosensitivity

• To report respiratory difficulty, trouble swallowing

• To notify all providers of product use

diclofenac ophthalmic

See Appendix B

didanosine (Rx)

(dye-dan′oh-seen)

ddI, Videx Pediatric Powder, Videx EC

Func. class.: Antiretroviral

Chem. class.: Nucleoside reverse transcriptase inhibitor (NRTI)

ACTION: Nucleoside analog incorporating into cellular DNA by viral reverse transcriptase, thereby terminating the cellular DNA chain

USES: HIV-1 infection in combination with at least 2 other antiretrovirals

Unlabeled uses: HIV prophylaxis

CONTRAINDICATIONS: Hypersensitivity, lactic acidosis, pancreatitis, phenylketonuria

Precautions: Pregnancy (B), breastfeeding, children, renal disease, sodium-restricted diets, elevated amylase, preexisting peripheral neuropathy, hyperuricemia, gout, CHF, noncirrhotic portal hypertension

Black Box Warning: Hepatic disease, lactic acidosis, pancreatitis

DOSAGE AND ROUTES

• **Adult >60 kg: PO DEL REL** caps 400 mg/day; 200 mg bid preferred

• **Adult <60 kg: PO DEL REL** caps 250 mg/day; 125 mg bid preferred

• **Child: PO** (child BSA 1.1-1.4 m^2); reconstitute pediatric powder 125 mg q8-12hr; **PO** (child BSA 0.8-1 m^2); reconstitute pediatric powder 94 mg q8-12hr; **PO** (child BSA 0.5-0.7 m^2); reconstitute pediatric powder 62 mg q8-12hr; **PO** (child BSA <0.4 m^2); reconstitute pediatric powder 31 mg q8-12hr

Renal dose

- **Adult >60 kg: PO** (Videx EC cap) CCr 30-59 ml/min, 200 mg/day; CCr 10-29 ml/min, 125 mg/day; CCr <10 ml/min, 125 mg/day
- **Adult <60 kg: PO** (Videx EC cap) CCr 30-59 ml/min, 125 mg/day; CCr 10-29 ml/min, 125 mg/day; CCr <10 ml/min, avoid use

Available forms: Powder for oral sol 10 mg/ml; del rel caps 125, 200, 250, 400 mg

Administer:

- Pediatric powder for oral sol after preparation by pharmacist; dilution required using purified USP water then antacid (10 mg/ml), refrigerate, shake before use
- On an empty stomach ≥30 min before or 2 hr after meals
- Adjust dose with renal impairment

SIDE EFFECTS

CNS: Peripheral neuropathy, seizures, confusion, *anxiety,* hypertonia, abnormal thinking, asthenia, *insomnia,* CNS depression, pain, dizziness, chills, fever

CV: Hypertension, vasodilation, dysrhythmia, syncope, CHF, palpitation

EENT: Ear pain, otitis, photophobia, visual impairment, retinal depigmentation

GI: Pancreatitis, *diarrhea, nausea,* vomiting, *abdominal pain,* constipation, stomatitis, dyspepsia, liver abnormalities, flatulence, taste perversion, dry mouth, oral thrush, melena, increased ALT/AST, alk phos, amylase, hepatic failure, noncirrhotic portal hypertension

GU: Increased bilirubin, uric acid

HEMA: Leukopenia, granulocytopenia, thrombocytopenia, anemia

INTEG: *Rash, pruritus,* alopecia, ecchymosis, hemorrhage, petechiae, sweating

MS: Myalgia, arthritis, myopathy, muscular atrophy

RESP: Cough, pneumonia, dyspnea, asthma, epistaxis, hypoventilation, sinusitis

SYST: Lactic acidosis, anaphylaxis

PHARMACOKINETICS

PO: Peak 0.67 hr, del rel 2 hr; elimination half-life 1.62 hr; extensive metabolism thought to occur; administration within 5 min of food will decrease absorption (50%); excreted urine, feces

INTERACTIONS

Increase: didanosine level—allopurinol, tenofovir; do not use together

Increase: side effects from magnesium, aluminum antacids

Decrease: absorption—ketoconazole, dapsone

Decrease: concentrations of fluoroquinolones, other antiretrovirals, itraconazole, tetracyclines

Decrease: didanosine level—methadone

- Do not use with these products PO: gatifloxacin, gemifloxacin, grepafloxacin, levofloxacin, lomefloxacin, moxifloxacin, norfloxacin, sparfloxacin, trovafloxacin

Drug/Food

- Any food decreases rate of absorption 50%
- Do not use with acidic juices

NURSING CONSIDERATIONS

Assess:

- **Peripheral neuropathy:** tingling or pain in hands and feet, distal numbness; onset usually occurs 2-6 mo after beginning treatment, may persist if product not discontinued

⚠ **Lactic acidosis, severe hepatomegaly, pancreatitis:** abdominal pain, nausea, vomiting, elevated hepatic enzymes; product should be discontinued because condition can be fatal

- For anaphylaxis, lactic acidosis
- Children by dilated retinal exam q6mo to rule out retinal depigmentation
- CBC, differential, platelet count monthly; withhold product if WBC is <4000 or platelet count is <75,000; notify prescriber of results; alk phos, monitor amylase; viral load, CD4 count
- Renal studies: BUN, serum uric acid, urine CCr before, during therapy

⚠ Nurse Alert

• Temp q4hr, may indicate beginning infection
• Hepatic studies before, during therapy (bilirubin, AST, ALT) as needed, monthly

Perform/provide:
• Clean up of powdered products; use wet mop or damp sponge
• Storage of tabs, caps in tightly closed bottle at room temp; store oral sol after dissolving at room temp ≤4 hr

Evaluate:
• Therapeutic response: absence of infection; symptoms of HIV

Teach patient/family:
• To avoid use with alcohol
• To report numbness/tingling in extremities
• To take on an empty stomach; not to take dapsone at same time as ddI; not to mix powder with fruit juice; chew tab or crush and dissolve in water; to drink powder immediately after mixing
• To report signs of **infection:** increased temp, sore throat, flulike symptoms
• To report signs of **anemia:** fatigue, headache, faintness, SOB, irritability
• To report **bleeding;** to avoid use of razors, commercial mouthwash
• That hair may be lost during therapy (rare); that a wig or hairpiece may make patient feel better
• That product does not cure, only controls symptoms

RARELY USED

diflunisal (Rx)

(dye-floo′ni-sal)

Dolobid

Func. class.: Nonsteroidal anti-inflammatory/analgesic (nonopioid)

USES: Mild to moderate pain or fever including arthritis; 3-4× more potent than aspirin

CONTRAINDICATIONS: Pregnancy (3rd trimester), children <12 yr, hypersensitivity to salicylates, bleeding disorders, vit K deficiency, Reye's syndrome, anemia, dehydration

Black Box Warning: GI bleeding, perioperative pain of CABG, MI, stroke

DOSAGE AND ROUTES

• **Adult: PO** Loading dose 1 g then 250-1000 mg/day in 2 divided doses q12hr not to exceed 1500 mg/day
• **Geriatric: PO** 1/2 adult dose

difluprednate ophthalmic

See Appendix B

HIGH ALERT

digoxin (Rx)

(di-jox′in)

APO-Digoxin ♣, Lanoxin, PMS-Digoxin ♣

Func. class.: Cardiac glycoside, inotropic, antidysrhythmic

Chem. class.: Digoxin preparation

Do not confuse:
Lanoxin/Lasix/Lonox/Lomotil/Xanax/Levoxine

ACTION: Inhibits the sodium-potassium ATPase pump, which makes more calcium available for contractile proteins, thereby resulting in increased cardiac output (positive inotropic effect); increases force of contractions; decreases heart rate (negative chronotropic effect); decreases AV conduction speed

USES: Heart failure, atrial fibrillation, atrial flutter, atrial tachycardia, cardiogenic shock, paroxysmal atrial tachycardia, rapid digitalization in these disorders

Unlabeled uses: Atrial flutter, paroxysmal supraventricular tachycardia (PSVT) treatment/prophylaxis

CONTRAINDICATIONS:
Hypersensitivity to digoxin, ventricular fibrillation, ventricular tachycardia, carotid sinus syndrome, 2nd- or 3rd-degree heart block

Precautions: Pregnancy (C), breastfeeding, geriatric patients, renal disease, acute MI, AV block, severe respiratory disease, hypothyroidism, sinus nodal disease, hypokalemia

DOSAGE AND ROUTES

Loading dose (IV or oral dosage—capsules)

- **Adult: PO/IV** 10-15 mcg/kg in 3 divided doses q6-8hr, with first dose equaling about 1/2 of total
- **Child >10 yr: PO/IV** 8-12 mcg/kg in 3 or more divided doses, with the first dose equaling about 1/2 of total; give other doses q6-8hr
- **Child 6-10 yr: PO/IV** 15-30 mcg/kg in 3 or more divided doses, with the first dose equaling about 1/2 of total; give other doses q6-8hr
- **Child 2-5 yr: PO/IV** 25-35 mcg/kg in 3 or more divided doses with of the first dose equaling about 1/2 of total; give other doses q6-8hr
- **Child <2 yr and infant: PO/IV** 30-50 mcg/kg in 3 or more divided doses with the first dose equaling about 1/2 of the total; give other doses q6-8hr
- **Full-term neonate: PO/IV** 20-30 mcg/kg in 3 or more divided doses with the first dose equaling about 1/2 of the total; give other doses q6-8hr
- **Premature neonate: PO/IV** 15-25 mcg/kg in 3 or more divided doses with the first dose equaling about 1/2 of the total; give other doses q6-8hr

Maintenance dose (IV or oral dosage—capsules)

- **Adult: PO/IV** 125-350 mcg, depending on CCr and lean body weight, in 1 or 2 divided doses
- **Child >10 yr: PO/IV** 2-3 mcg/kg/day in single daily dose
- **Child 5-10 yr: PO/IV** 4-8 mcg/kg/day in 2 daily doses
- **Child 2-5 yr: PO/IV** 6-9 mcg/kg/day in 2 daily doses
- **Child <2 yr and infant: PO/IV** 7.5-12 mcg/kg/day in 2 daily doses
- **Full-term neonate: PO/IV** 5-8 mcg/kg/day in 2 daily doses
- **Preterm neonate: PO/IV** 4-6 mcg/kg/day in 2 daily doses

Loading dose (oral dosage—elixir or tablets)

- **Adult, adolescent, child >10 yr: PO** 10-15 mcg/kg in 3 or more divided doses with the first dose equaling about 1/2 of the total; give other doses q6-8hr
- **Child 5-10 yr: PO** 20-35 mcg/kg in 3 divided doses q6-8hr
- **Child 2-5 yr: PO** 30-40 mcg/kg in 3 divided doses q6-8hr
- **Child <2 yr and infant: PO** 35-60 mcg/kg in 3 divided doses q6-8hr
- **Full-term neonate: PO** 25-35 mcg/kg in 3 divided doses q6-8hr
- **Premature neonate: PO** 20-30 mcg/kg in 3 divided doses q6-8hr

Maintenance dose (oral dosage—elixir or tablets)

- **Adult: PO** 125-500 mcg q day, depending on CCr and lean body weight
- **Child >10 yr: PO** 2.5-5 mcg/kg q day
- **Child 5-10 yr: PO** 5-10 mcg/kg/day in 2 divided doses
- **Child 2-5 yr: PO** 7.5-10 mcg/kg/day in 2 divided doses
- **Child <2 yr and infant: PO** 10-15 mcg/kg/day in 2 divided doses
- **Full-term neonate: PO** 6-10 mcg/kg/day in 2 divided doses
- **Preterm neonate: PO** 5-7.5 mcg/kg/day in 2 divided doses

Renal dose

Oral dosage (capsules) or IV

- **PO/IV** CCr 50-59 ml/min, LBW 50-69 kg: 150 mcg q day
- **PO/IV** CCr 50-59 ml/min, LBW 70-89 kg: 200 mcg q day
- **PO/IV** CCr 20-49 ml/min, LBW 50-59 kg: 100 mcg q day

Oral dosage (elixir or tablets)
- **PO** CCr 50-59 ml/min, LBW 50-69 kg: 188 mcg/day
- **PO** CCr 50-59 ml/min, LBW 70-89 kg: 250 mcg/day
- **PO** CCr 20-49 ml/min, LBW 50-59 kg: 125 mcg/day

Available forms: Caps 0.05, 0.1, 0.2 mg; elix 0.05 mg/ml; tabs 0.125, 0.25, 0.5 mg; inj 0.5 ✤, 0.25 mg/ml; pediatric inj 0.1 mg/ml

Administer:

PO route
- Do not break, crush, or chew caps
- PO with/without food; may crush tabs, only mix with food, fluids
- Potassium supplements (if ordered for potassium levels <3) or foods high in potassium: bananas, orange juice

IV route
- Undiluted or 1 ml of product/4 ml sterile water, D_5, or NS; give >5 min through Y-tube or 3-way stopcock; during digitalization, close monitoring is necessary

Additive compatibilities: Cimetidine, floxacillin, furosemide, lidocaine, potassium chloride, ranitidine, verapamil

Syringe compatibilities: Heparin, milrinone

Y-site compatibilities: Acyclovir, alfentanil, amikacin, aminocaproic acid, aminophylline, amphotericin B lipid complex, anidulafungin, ascorbic acid injection, atenolol, atracurium, atropine, aztreonam, benztropine, bivalirudin, bleomycin, bumetanide, buprenorphine, butorphanol, calcium chloride/gluconate, CARBOplatin, cefamandole, ceFAZolin, cefmetazole, cefonicid, cefoperazone, cefotaxime, cefotetan, cefoxitin, ceftazidime, ceftizoxime, ceftobiprole, cefTRIAXone, cefuroxime, cephalothin, cephapirin, chloramphenicol, chlorproMAZINE, cimetidine, ciprofloxacin, cisatracurium, CISplatin, clindamycin, codeine, cyanocobalamin, cyclophosphamide, cycloSPORINE, cytarabine, DACTINomycin, DAPTOmycin, dexamethasone, dexmedetomidine, diltiazem, diphenhydrAMINE, DOBUTamine, docetaxel, DOPamine, doripenem, doxacurium, doxycycline, enalaprilat, ePHEDrine, EPINEPHrine, epirubicin, epoetin alfa, eptifibatide, ertapenem, erythromycin, esmolol, etoposide, famotidine, fenoldopam, fentaNYL, fludarabine, fluorouracil, folic acid, furosemide, ganciclovir, gatifloxacin, gemcitabine, gentamicin, glycopyrrolate, granisetron, heparin, hydrocortisone, HYDROmorphone, hydrOXYzine, ifosfamide, imipenem-cilastatin, indomethacin, irinotecan, isoproterenol, ketorolac, labetalol, levofloxacin, lidocaine, linezolid, LORazepam, LR, magnesium sulfate, mannitol, mechlorethamine, meperidine, meropenem, metaraminol, methicillin, methotrexate, methoxamine, methyldopate, methylPREDNISolone, metoclopramide, metoprolol, metroNIDAZOLE, mezlocillin, miconazole, midazolam, milrinone, morphine, moxalactam, multiple vitamins injection, mycophenolate mofetil, nafcillin, nalbuphine, naloxone, nesiritide, metilmicin, nitroglycerin, nitroprusside, norepinephrine, octreotide, ondansetron, oxacillin, oxaliplatin, oxytocin, palonosetron, pamidronate, pancuronium, pantoprazole, papaverine, pemetrexed, penicillin G potassium/sodium, pentazocine, PENTobarbital, PHENobarbital, phenylephrine, phytonadione, piperacillin, piperacillin-tazobactam, polymyxin B, potassium chloride, procainamide, prochlorperazine, promethazine, propranolol, protamine, pyridoxine, quiNIDine, ranitidine, remifentanil, Ringer's, ritodrine, riTUXimab, rocuronium, sodium acetate/bicarbonate, succinylcholine, SUFentanil, tacrolimus, teniposide, theophylline, thiamine, thiotepa, ticarcillin, ticarcillin-clavulanate, tigecycline, tirofiban, TNA, tobramycin, tolazoline, TPN, trastuzumab, trimetaphan, urokinase, vancomycin, vasopressin, vecuronium, verapamil, vinCRIStine, vinorelbine, vitamin B complex, voriconazole, zoledronic acid

SIDE EFFECTS

CNS: *Headache,* drowsiness, apathy, confusion, disorientation, fatigue, depression, hallucinations
CV: Dysrhythmias, *hypotension,* bradycardia, AV block
EENT: Blurred vision, yellow-green halos, photophobia, diplopia
GI: Nausea, vomiting, anorexia, abdominal pain, diarrhea

PHARMACOKINETICS

Half-life 1.5 days, excreted in urine, protein binding 20%-30%
PO: Onset ½-2 hr, peak 6-8 hr, duration 3-4 days
IV: Onset 5-30 min, peak 1-5 hr, duration variable

INTERACTIONS

Increase: hypercalcemia, hypomagnesemia, digoxin toxicity—thiazides, parenteral calcium
Increase: hypokalemia, digoxin toxicity—diuretics, amphotericin B, carbenicillin, ticarcillin, corticosteroids
Increase: digoxin levels—propantheline, quiNIDine, verapamil, amiodarone, anticholinergics, diltiazem, NIFEdipine
Increase: bradycardia—β-adrenergic blockers, antidysrythmics
Increase: cardiac dysrhythmia risk—sympathomimetics
Decrease: digoxin absorption—antacids, kaolin/pectin
Decrease: digoxin level—thyroid agents, cholestyramine, colestipol, metoclopramide
Drug/Lab Test
Increase: CPK

NURSING CONSIDERATIONS

Assess:
- Apical pulse for 1 min before giving product; if pulse <60 in adult or <90 in infant, take again in 1 hr; if <60 in adult, call prescriber; note rate, rhythm, character; monitor ECG continuously during parenteral loading dose
- Electrolytes: K, Na, Cl, Mg, Ca; renal function studies: BUN, creatinine; blood studies: ALT, AST, bilirubin, Hct, Hgb before initiating treatment and periodically thereafter
- I&O ratio, daily weights; monitor turgor, lung sounds, edema
- Monitor product levels; therapeutic level 0.5-2 ng/ml
- Cardiac status: apical pulse, character, rate, rhythm

Perform/provide:
- Storage protected from light

Evaluate:
- Therapeutic response: decreased weight, edema, pulse, respiration, crackles; increased urine output; serum digoxin level (0.5-2 ng/ml)

Teach patient/family:
- Not to stop product abruptly; about all aspects of product; to take exactly as ordered; how to monitor heart rate
- To avoid OTC medications, herbal remedies because many adverse product interactions may occur; not to take antacid at same time
- To notify prescriber of loss of appetite, lower stomach pain, diarrhea, weakness, drowsiness, headache, blurred or yellow vision, rash, depression, toxicity
- About the toxic symptoms of this product; when to notify prescriber
- To maintain a sodium-restricted diet as ordered
- To report shortness of breath, difficulty breathing, weight gain, edema, persistent cough

TREATMENT OF OVERDOSE:

Discontinue product; give potassium; monitor ECG; give adrenergic-blocking agent, digoxin immune FAB

digoxin immune FAB (ovine) (Rx)

(di-jox'in im-myoon' FAB)

DigiFab

Func. class.: Antidote—digoxin specific

ACTION: Antibody fragments bind to free digoxin or digitoxin to reverse toxicity by not allowing digoxin or digitoxin to bind to sites of action

USES: Life-threatening digoxin toxicity

CONTRAINDICATIONS: Mild digoxin toxicity, hypersensitivity to this product, papain or ovine protein

Precautions: Pregnancy (C), breastfeeding, children, geriatric patients, renal/cardiac disease, allergy to ovine proteins, hypocalcemia, heart failure

DOSAGE AND ROUTES

1 (38-mg) vial binds 0.5 mg digoxin; 1 (40 mg) DigiFab binds 0.5 mg digoxin

Digoxin toxicity (known amount) (tabs, oral sol, IM)

- **Adult and child: IV** dose (mg) = dose ingested (mg) × 0.8/1000 × 38- or 40-mg vial

Toxicity (known amount) (cap, IV)

- **Adult and child: IV** dose = dose ingested (mg)/0.5 × 38- or 40-mg vial

Toxicity (known amount) by serum digoxin concentrations (SDCs)

- **Adult and child: IV** SDC (ng/ml) × kg of weight/100 × 38- or 40-mg vial

Digoxin toxicity (unknown amount)

- **Adult and child >20 kg: IV** 228 mg (6 vials)
- **Infant and child <20 kg: IV** 38 mg (1 vial)

Acute ingestion

- **Adult: IV** 380 mg (10 vials)

Life-threatening ingestion

- **Adult: IV** 760 mg (20 vials)

Skin test

- **Adult: ID** 9.5 mcg

Available forms: Inj 38 mg/vial (binds 0.5 mg digoxin), 40 mg/vial (binds 0.5 mg digoxin)

Administer:

- Test doses proven to be ineffective in the general population; only use test dose in those with known allergies or those previously treated with digoxin immune FAB
- **For test dose** dilute 0.1 ml of reconstituted product (9.5 mg/ml) in 9.9 ml sterile isotonic saline, inj 0.1 ml (1:100 dilution) ID and observe for wheal with erythema; read in 20 min
- **For scratch test,** place 1 gtt of sol on skin, make a scratch through the drop with a sterile needle; read in 20 min
- After diluting 38 mg/4 ml of sterile water for inj 10 mg/ml mix; may be further diluted with normal saline; sol should be clear, colorless
- By bolus if cardiac arrest is imminent or IV over 30 min using a 0.22-μm filter

SIDE EFFECTS

CV: CHF, ventricular rate increase, atrial fibrillation, low cardiac output, hypotension

INTEG: *Hypersensitivity,* allergic reactions, facial swelling, redness, phlebitis

META: Hypokalemia

MISC: Anaphylaxis (rare)

RESP: Impaired respiratory function, rapid respiratory rate

PHARMACOKINETICS

IV: Peaks after completion of inf; onset 30 min (variable); not known if crosses placenta, breast milk; half-life biphasic: 14-20 hr, prolonged with renal disease; excreted by kidneys

INTERACTIONS

- Considered incompatible with all products in syringe or sol

Drug/Lab Test Interference: immunoassay digoxin

NURSING CONSIDERATIONS

Assess:

- **Hypokalemia:** ST depression, flat T waves, presence of U wave, ventricular dysrhythmia; potassium levels may decrease rapidly
- **CHF:** dyspnea, crackles, peripheral edema, B/P, volume overload

Perform/provide:

- Storage of reconstituted sol for up to 4 hr in refrigerator
- Do not freeze DigiFab

Evaluate:

- Therapeutic response: correction of digoxin toxicity; check digoxin levels 0.5-2 ng/ml; digitoxin level 9-25 ng/ml

Teach patient/family:

- About the purpose of medication; to report delayed hypersensitivity: fever, chills, itching, swelling, dyspnea

⚠ HIGH ALERT

diltiazem (Rx)

(dil-tye′a-zem)

Cardizem, Cardizem CD, Cardizem LA, Cartia XT, Dilacor-XR, Dilt-CD, Diltia XR, Diltia XT, Diltzac, Gen-Diltiazem ✦, ratio-Diltiazem ✦, Sandoz Diltiazem ✦, Taztia XT, Tiazac

Func. class.: Calcium channel blocker, antiarrhythmic class IV, antihypertensive

Chem. class.: Benzothiazepine

Do not confuse:
Cardizem/Cardene

ACTION: Inhibits calcium ion influx across cell membrane during cardiac depolarization; produces relaxation of coronary vascular smooth muscle, dilates coronary arteries, slows SA/AV node conduction times, dilates peripheral arteries

USES: **PO** Angina pectoris due to coronary artery spasm, hypertension, **IV** atrial fibrillation, flutter, paroxysmal supraventricular tachycardia

Unlabeled uses: Unstable angina, proteinuria, cardiomyopathy, diabetic neuropathy

CONTRAINDICATIONS: Sick sinus syndrome, AV heart block, hypotension <90 mm Hg systolic, acute MI, pulmonary congestion, cardiogenic shock

Precautions: Pregnancy (C), breastfeeding, children, geriatric patients, CHF, aortic stenosis, bradycardia, GERD, hepatic disease, hiatal hernia, ventricular dysfunction

DOSAGE AND ROUTES

Prinzmetal's or variant angina, chronic stable angina

- **Adult: PO** 30 mg qid, increasing dose gradually to 180-360 mg/day in divided doses or (SR) 60-120 mg bid; may increase to 240-360 mg/day or 120 or 180 mg **EXT REL** (LA, CD, XT, XR products) **PO** daily

Atrial fibrillation/flutter, paroxysmal supraventricular tachycardia

- **Adult: IV BOL** 0.25 mg/kg over 2 min initially then 0.35 mg/kg may be given after 15 min; if no response, may give **CONT INF** 5-15 mg/hr for up to 24 hr

Hypertension

- **Adult: PO** or 120-240 mg **(EXT REL once-daily dosing)** daily or 60-120 mg bid **(SUS REL twice-daily dosing)**

Rapid ventricular rate secondary to dysrhythmias (unlabeled)

- **Adolescent/child/infant >7 mo: IV BOL** 0.25 mg/kg over 5 min then **CONT IV INF** 0.11 mg/kg/hr

Available forms: Tabs 30, 60, 90, 120 mg; ext rel tabs 120, 180, 240, 300, 360, 420 mg; ext rel caps 60, 90, 120, 180, 240, 300, 360, 420 mg; inj 5 mg/ml (5, 10 ml)

Administer:

PO route

- **Cardiazem LA** ext rel tab 24 hr: give daily, either AM or PM, without regard to meals
- **Dilacor XR/Diltia XT** ext rel cap 24 hr: give daily; take on empty stomach; swallow whole; do not cut, crush, chew, open
- **Tiazac, Tiztia XT:** give daily without regard to meals
- **Conventional regular-rel tab:** give before meals, at bedtime
- **Cardizem CD or equivalent (Cartia XT):** generic ext rel cap 24 hr: give daily, without regard to meals
- May crush, sprinkle regular tab on applesauce for administration

Oral suspension (unlabeled)

- Grind 16 90-mg diltiazem regular rel tab into fine powder
- In separate container, mix 60 ml Ora-Sweet and 60 ml Ora-Plus
- Add small amount of sol to powder to form paste, add geometric amounts of base to achieve desired vol, place in amber container

Direct IV route

- IV undiluted over 2 min

Continuous IV INF route

- Diluted 125 mg/100 ml, 250 mg/250 ml of D_5W, 0.9% NaCl, D_5/0.45% NaCl, give 10 mg/hr, may increase by 5 mg/hr to 15 mg/hr, continue inf up to 24 hr

Y-site compatibilities: Albumin, amikacin, amphotericin B, aztreonam, bumetanide, ceFAZolin, cefotaxime, cefotetan, cefoxitin, ceftazidime, cefTRIAXone, cefuroxime, cimetidine, ciprofloxacin, clindamycin, digoxin, DOBUTamine, DOPamine, doxycycline, EPINEPHrine, erythromycin, esmolol, fentaNYL, fluconazole, gentamicin, hetastarch, HYDROmorphone, imipenem-cilastatin, labetalol, lidocaine, LORazepam, meperidine, metoclopramide, metroNIDAZOLE, midazolam, milrinone, morphine, multivitamins, niCARdipine, nitroglycerin, norepinephrine, oxacillin, penicillin G potassium, pentamidine, piperacillin, potassium chloride, potassium phosphates, ranitidine, sodium nitroprusside, theophylline, ticarcillin, ticarcillin/clavulanate, tobramycin, trimethoprim-sulfamethoxazole, vancomycin, vecuronium

SIDE EFFECTS

CNS: *Headache, fatigue, drowsiness,* dizziness, depression, weakness, insomnia, tremor, paresthesia

CV: Dysrhythmia, *edema,* CHF, bradycardia, hypotension, palpitations, heart block

GI: *Nausea,* vomiting, diarrhea, gastric upset, *constipation*, increased LFTs

GU: Nocturia, polyuria, acute renal failure

INTEG: *Rash,* flushing, photosensitivity, burning, pruritus at inj site

RESP: Rhinitis, dyspnea, pharyngitis

PHARMACOKINETICS

Onset 30-60 min; peak 2-3 hr immediate rel, 10-14 hr ext rel, 6-11 hr sus rel; half-life 3½-9 hr; metabolized by liver; excreted in urine (96% as metabolites)

INTERACTIONS

Increase: effect, toxicity—theophylline

Increase: effects of β-blockers, digoxin, lithium, carBAMazepine, cycloSPORINE, anesthetics, HMG-CoA reductase inhibitors, benzodiazepines, lovastatin, methylPREDNISolone

Increase: effects of diltiazem—cimetidine

Drug/Food

Increase: hypotensive effects—grapefruit juice

NURSING CONSIDERATIONS

Assess:

- **CHF:** dyspnea, weight gain, edema, jugular venous distention, rales; monitor I&O ratios daily, weight
- **Angina:** location, duration, alleviating factors, activity when pain starts
- **Dysrhythmias:** cardiac status: B/P, pulse, respiration, ECG and intervals PR,

QRS, QT; if systolic B/P <90 mm Hg or HR <50 bpm, hold dose, notify prescriber

Perform/provide:
- Storage in tight container at room temp

Evaluate:
- Therapeutic response: decreased anginal pain, decreased B/P

Teach patient/family:
- How to take pulse, B/P before taking product; that a record or graph should be kept
- To avoid hazardous activities until stabilized on product, dizziness is no longer a problem
- To limit caffeine consumption; to avoid grapefruit juice
- To avoid OTC products unless directed by prescriber
- About the importance of complying with all areas of medical regimen: diet, exercise, stress reduction, product therapy
- To change position slowly
- ⚠ To report dizziness, SOB, palpitations
- Not to discontinue abruptly

TREATMENT OF OVERDOSE:
Atropine for AV block, vasopressor for hypotension

dinoprostone (Rx)
(dye-noe-prost′one)

Cervidil, Prepidil, Prostin E-2

Func. class.: Oxytocic, abortifacient

Chem. class.: Prostaglandin E_2

Do not confuse:
Prepidil/bepridil

ACTION: Stimulates uterine contractions, causing abortion; acts within 30 hr for complete abortion

USES: Abortion during 2nd trimester, benign hydatidiform mole, expulsion of uterine contents in fetal deaths to 28 wk, missed abortion, to efface and dilate the cervix in pregnancy at term

CONTRAINDICATIONS: Hypersensitivity, C-section, surgery

Precautions: Pregnancy (C), cardiac/renal/hepatic disease, asthma, anemia, jaundice, diabetes mellitus, seizure disorders, hypertension, glaucoma, uterine fibrosis, cervical stenosis, pelvic surgery, pelvic inflammatory disease, respiratory disease

Black Box Warning: Hypotension, diarrhea, fever, vomiting

DOSAGE AND ROUTES

Abortifacient/2nd trimester/missed abortion/benign hydatidiform mole/intrauterine fetal death
- **Adult:** **VAG SUPP** 20 mg, repeat q3-5hr until abortion occurs, max dose is 240 mg

Cervical ripening
- **Adult:** **GEL** warm to room temp, choose correct-length shielded catheter (10 or 20 mm), fill catheter by pushing plunger; patient should remain recumbent for 15-30 min; **INSERT** one 10-mg insert

Available forms: Vag supp 20 mg; gel 0.5 mg/3 g (prefilled syringe); vag insert 10 mg

Administer:
- **By gel:** after warming to room temp, remove seal from end of syringe, remove protective end cap and insert into plunger stopper assembly; make sure patient is in dorsal position; **insert:** must be kept frozen until use
- Antiemetic/antidiarrheal before administration of this product

SIDE EFFECTS

CNS: *Headache,* dizziness, chills, fever, flushing
CV: Hypotension, dysrhythmias, DIC
EENT: Blurred vision
SYST: Anaphylactoid syndrome of pregnancy
FETAL: Bradycardia (i.e., deceleration)
GI: *Nausea, vomiting, diarrhea*
GU: Vaginitis, vaginal pain, vulvitis, vaginismus

INTEG: Rash, skin color changes
MS: *Leg cramps, joint swelling,* weakness
GEL: Uterine contractile abnormality, GI side effects, back pain, fever
INSERT: Uterine hyperstimulation, fever, nausea, vomiting, diarrhea, abdominal pain
SUPPOSITORY: Uterine rupture, anaphylaxis

INTERACTIONS

Increase: effect—other oxytocics
Decrease: oxytocic effect—alcohol

PHARMACOKINETICS

Metabolized in spleen, kidney, lungs; excreted in urine
GEL: Onset 10 min, peak 30-45 min
SUPP: Onset 10 min, duration 2-3 hr

NURSING CONSIDERATIONS

Assess:

- **Cervical ripening:** dilation, effacement of cervix and uterine contraction, fetal heart tones, check for contractions over 1 min
- For fever that occurs ½ hr after suppository insertion (abortion)
- Respiratory rate, rhythm, depth; notify prescriber of abnormalities, pulse, B/P, temp
- **Vaginal discharge:** check for itching, irritation; indicates vaginal infection

Evaluate:

- Therapeutic response: expulsion of fetus

Teach patient/family:

- To remain supine for 10-15 min after insertion of supp, 2 hr after insert, 15-30 min after gel
- To report excessive cramping, bleeding, chills, fever
- About some methods of pain, comfort control
- To avoid intercourse, tub baths, douches, tampon use for at least 2 wk

diphenhydrAMINE (OTC, Rx)

(dye-fen-hye′dra-meen)

Allerdryl ♣, AllerMax ♣, Altaryl, Banophen, Benadryl, Benadryl Allergy, Benadryl Allergy Dye Free, Benadryl Children's Allergy, Buckley's Bedtime, Diphedryl, Diphenhist, Dytan, ElixSure Allergy, Equaline Allergy, Equaline Children's Allergy, Equate Allergy, Equate Children's Allergy, Genahist, Good Sense Children's Allergy Relief, Good Sense Diphedryl, Leader Complete Allergy, Nytol, PediaCare Children's Allergy, PediaCare Nighttime Cough, Q-Dryl Allergy, Select Brand Allergy, Siladryl, Silphen, Simply Sleep, Sleepinal, Sleep Tabs, Sominex, Top Care Allergy, Top Care Children's Allergy, Unisom ♣, Valu-Dryl, Wal-dryl Allergy, Wal-dryl Allergy Dye Free, Wal-dryl Children's Allergy, Walgreen's Sleep Aid, Walgreen's Sleep II, Wal-Som

Func. class.: Antihistamine (1st generation, nonselective)
Chem. class.: Ethanolamine derivative, H_1-receptor antagonist

Do not confuse:
diphenhydrAMINE/dicyclomine
diphenhydrAMINE/dimenhyDRINATE

ACTION: Acts on blood vessels, GI, respiratory system by competing with histamine for H_1-receptor site; decreases allergic response by blocking histamine

USES: Allergy symptoms, rhinitis, motion sickness, antiparkinsonism, nighttime sedation, infant colic, nonproductive cough, insomnia in children

Unlabeled uses: Nystagmus

CONTRAINDICATIONS:

Hypersensitivity to H_1-receptor antagonist, acute asthma attack, lower respiratory tract disease, neonates

Precautions: Pregnancy (B), breastfeeding, children <2 yr, increased intraocular pressure, cardiac/renal disease, hypertension, bronchial asthma, seizure disorder, stenosed peptic ulcers, hyperthyroidism, prostatic hypertrophy, bladder neck obstruction

DOSAGE AND ROUTES

- **Adult and child >12 yr: PO** 25-50 mg q4-6hr, max 300 mg/day; **IM/IV** 10-50 mg, max 300 mg/day
- **Child 6-12 yr: PO/IM/IV** 5 mg/kg/day in 4 divided doses, max 300 mg/day

Nighttime sleep aid

- **Adult and child ≥12 yr: PO** 25-50 mg at bedtime

Antitussive (syrup only)

- **Adult and child ≥12 yr: PO** 25 mg q4hr, max 150 mg/24 hr
- **Child 6-12 yr: PO** 12.5 mg q4hr, max 75 mg/24 hr

Renal disease

- CCr >50 ml/min, dose q6hr; CCr 10-50 ml/min, dose q6-12hr; CCr <10 ml/min, dose q12-18hr

Peripheral vestibular nystagmus (unlabeled)

- **Adult: PO** 25-50 mg q4-6hr up to 48 hr

Available forms: Caps 25, 50 mg; tabs 25, 50 mg; chew tabs 12.5 mg; elix 12.5 mg/5 ml; syr 12.5 mg/5 ml; inj 10, 50 mg/ml; orally disintegrating tabs 12.5, 25 mg

Administer:

⚠ Avoid use in children <2 yr; death has occurred; overdose has occurred with topical gel taken orally (adult/child)

- With meals for GI symptoms; absorption rate may slightly decrease
- Deep IM in large muscle; rotate site
- At bedtime only if using for sleep aid

Direct IV route

- Undiluted; give 25 mg/1 min

Intermittent IV INF route

- Dilute with 0.9% NaCl, 0.45% NaCl, D_5W, 0.9% NaCl, $D_{10}W$, LR, Ringer's

Syringe compatibilities: Atropine, butorphanol, chlorproMAZINE, cimetidine, dimenhyDRINATE, droperidol, fentaNYL, fluphenazine, glycopyrrolate, HYDROmorphone, hydrOXYzine, meperidine, metoclopramide, midazolam, morphine, nalbuphine, pentazocine, perphenazine, prochlorperazine, promazine, promethazine, ranitidine, scopolamine, SUFentanil

Y-site compatibilities: Abciximab, aldesleukin, alfentanil hydrochloride, amifostine, amikacin sulfate, aminocaproic acid, amphotericin B lipid complex (Abelcet), amphotericin B liposome (AmBisome), amsacrine, anidulafungin, argatroban, ascorbic acid injection, atenolol, atracurium besylate, atropine sulfate, azithromycin, benztropine mesylate, bivalirudin, bleomycin, bumetanide, buprenorphine, butorphanol, calcium chloride/gluconate, CARBOplatin, caspofungin, ceftazidime, ceftizoxime, chlorproMAZINE, cimetidine, ciprofloxacin, cisatracurium, CISplatin, cladribine, clindamycin, codeine, cyanocobalamin, cyclophosphamide, cycloSPORINE, cytarabine, DACTINomycin, DAPTOmycin, digoxin, diltiazem, DOBUTamine, docetaxel, DOPamine, doripenem, doxacurium, DOXOrubicin, DOXOrubicin liposomal, doxycycline, enalaprilat, ePHEDrine, EPINEPHrine, epirubicin, epoetin alfa, eptifibatide, ertapenem, erythromycin, esmolol, etoposide, famotidine, fenoldopam, fentaNYL, filgrastim, fluconazole, fludarabine, folic acid, gallium, gatifloxacin, gemcitabine, gemtuzumab, gentamicin, glycopyrrolate, granisetron, HYDROmorphone, hydrOXYzine, IDArubicin, ifosfamide, imipenem-cilastatin, irinotecan, isoproterenol, labetalol, levofloxacin, lidocaine, linezolid, LORazepam, LR, magnesium sulfate, mannitol, mechlorethamine, melphalan, meperidine, meropenem, metaraminol, methadone, methicillin, methotrexate, methoxamine, methyldopate, metoclopramide, metoprolol, metroNIDAZOLE, miconazole, midazolam, minocycline, mitoxantrone, morphine, multiple vitamins injection, mycophenolate, nalbuphine, naloxone, nesiritide, netilmicin, nitroglycerin, norepinephrine, octreotide, ondansetron, oxaliplatin, oxytocin, paclitaxel, palonosetron, pamidronate, pancuronium, papaverine, pemetrexed, penicillin G potassium/sodium, pentamidine, pentazocine, phenylephrine, phytonadione, piperacillin, piperacillin-tazobactam, polymyxin B, potassium chloride, procainamide, prochlorperazine, promethazine, propofol, propranolol, protamine, pyridoxine, quiNIDine, quinupristin-dalfopristin, ranitidine, remifentanil, Ringer's, ritodrine, riTUXimab, rocuronium, sargramostim, sodium acetate, succinylcholine, SUFentanil, tacrolimus, teniposide, theophylline, thiamine, thiotepa, ticarcillin, ticarcillin-clavulanate, tigecycline, tirofiban, TNA, tobramycin, tolazoline, TPN, trastuzumab, trimetaphan, urokinase, vancomycin, vasopressin, vecuronium, verapamil, vinCRIStine, vinorelbine, vitamin B complex/C, voriconazole, zoledronic acid

SIDE EFFECTS

CNS: *Dizziness, drowsiness,* poor coordination, fatigue, anxiety, euphoria, confusion, paresthesia, neuritis, seizures
CV: Hypotension, palpitations
EENT: Blurred vision, dilated pupils, tinnitus, nasal stuffiness, dry nose, throat, mouth
GI: Nausea, anorexia, diarrhea
GU: *Retention,* dysuria, frequency
HEMA: **Thrombocytopenia, agranulocytosis, hemolytic anemia**
INTEG: Photosensitivity
MISC: **Anaphylaxis**
RESP: Increased thick secretions, wheezing, chest tightness

PHARMACOKINETICS

Metabolized in liver, excreted by kidneys, crosses placenta, excreted in breast milk, half-life 2-7 hr
PO: Peak 1-3 hr, duration 4-7 hr
IM: Onset ½ hr, peak 1-4 hr, duration 4-7 hr
IV: Onset immediate, duration 4-7 hr

INTERACTIONS

Increase: CNS depression—barbiturates, opiates, hypnotics, tricyclics, alcohol
Increase: diphenhydrAMINE effect—MAOIs
Drug/Lab Test
False negative: skin allergy tests

NURSING CONSIDERATIONS

Assess:
- Urinary retention, frequency, dysuria; product should be discontinued
- CBC during long-term therapy; blood dyscrasias may occur
- Respiratory status: rate, rhythm, increase in bronchial secretions, wheezing, chest tightness

Perform/provide:
- Hard candy, gum, frequent rinsing of mouth for dryness
- Storage in tight container at room temp

Evaluate:
- Therapeutic response: absence of running or congested nose or rashes, improved sleep

Teach patient/family:
- About all aspects of product use; to notify prescriber of confusion, sedation, hypotension
- To avoid driving, other hazardous activity if drowsiness occurs
- That photosensitivity may occur
- To avoid concurrent use of alcohol, other CNS depressants
- To avoid breastfeeding

TREATMENT OF OVERDOSE:

Administer diazepam, vasopressors, phenytoin IV

diphenoxylate/atropine (Rx)

(dye-fen-ox′ee-late/a′troe-peen)

Lomotil, Lonox

difenoxin/atropine (Rx)

(dye-fen-ox′in/a′troe-peen)

Motofen

Func. class.: Antidiarrheal

Chem. class.: Phenylpiperidine derivative opiate agonist

Controlled Substance Schedule V

diphenoxylate/atropine

Controlled Substance Schedule IV

difenoxin/atropine (US)

Do not confuse:

Lomotil/LaMICtal/LamISIL/Lanoxin/Lasix/Ludomil

ACTION: Inhibits gastric motility by acting on mucosal receptors responsible for peristalsis

USES: Acute nonspecific and acute exacerbations of chronic functional diarrhea

CONTRAINDICATIONS: Children <2 yr, hypersensitivity, pseudomembranous colitis, severe electrolyte imbalances, diarrhea associated with organisms that penetrate intestinal mucosa

Precautions: Pregnancy (C), breastfeeding, hepatic disease, ulcerative colitis, severe hepatic disease, substance abuse, dehydration

DOSAGE AND ROUTES

Diphenoxylate/atropine

- **Adult: PO** 5 mg qid titrated to patient response needed, max 8 tabs/day
- **Child 2-12 yr: PO** (liquid only) 0.3-0.4 mg/kg/day in 4 divided doses

Difenoxin/atropine

- **Adult: PO** 2 tabs then 1 tab after each loose stool or q3-4hr prn, max 8 tabs/day

Available forms: *Diphenoxylate/atropine:* tabs 2.5 mg with atropine 0.025 mg; liquid 2.5 mg with atropine 0.025 mg/5 ml; *difenoxin/atropine:* tabs 1 mg difenoxin/0.025 atropine

Administer:

- For 48 hr only; if no response, product should be discontinued

SIDE EFFECTS

CNS: *Dizziness, drowsiness, lightheadedness, headache,* fatigue, nervousness, insomnia, confusion

EENT: Burning eyes, blurred vision

GI: *Nausea, vomiting, dry mouth, epigastric distress,* constipation, paralytic ileus, toxic megacolon

MISC: Anaphylaxis, angioedema

RESP: Respiratory depression

PHARMACOKINETICS

PO: Onset 40-60 min, peak 2 hr, duration 3-4 hr, terminal half-life 12-14 hr, metabolized in liver to active metabolite; excreted in urine and feces

INTERACTIONS

- Do not use with MAOIs; hypertensive crisis may occur

Increase: action of alcohol, opioids, barbiturates, other CNS depressants, anticholinergics

Decrease: GI motility, possible toxic megacolon—amantadine, antimuscarinics, amoxapine, diphenhydrAMINE, clozapine, clemastine, cyclobenzaprine, loperamide, maprotiline, phenothiazines, tricyclics, disopyramide, olanzapine

NURSING CONSIDERATIONS

Assess:

- Electrolytes (K, Na, Cl) if receiving long-term therapy
- Bowel pattern before; for rebound

constipation after termination of medication; bowel sounds
- Response after 48 hr; if none, product should be discontinued
- **Abdominal distention, toxic megacolon;** may occur in ulcerative colitis
- Hepatic studies if receiving long-term therapy

Evaluate:
- Therapeutic response: decreased diarrhea

Teach patient/family:
- To avoid OTC products unless directed by prescriber (may contain alcohol); not to use alcohol or CNS depressants
- Not to exceed recommended dose
- That product may be habit forming
- Not to engage in hazardous activities; that drowsiness may occur; not to use for longer than 48 hr for acute diarrhea

dipivefrin ophthalmic
See Appendix B

dipyridamole (Rx)
(dye-peer-id′a-mole)

Apo-Dipyridamole ♣, Persantine

Func. class.: Coronary vasodilator, antiplatelet agent

Chem. class.: Nonnitrate

ACTION:
Inhibits adenosine uptake, which produces coronary vasodilation; increases oxygen saturation in coronary tissues, coronary blood flow; acts on small resistance vessels with little effect on vascular resistance; may increase development of collateral circulation; decreases platelet aggregation by the inhibition of phosphodiesterase (an enzyme)

USES:
Prevention of transient ischemic attacks, inhibition of platelet adhesion to prevent myocardial reinfarction, thromboembolism, with warfarin in prosthetic heart valves, prevention of coronary bypass graft occlusion with aspirin; IV form used to evaluate CAD; used as alternative to exercise with thallium myocardial perfusion imaging to evaluate CAD

Unlabeled uses: Cardiomyopathy, MI prophylaxis, proteinuria, TIA, valvular heart disease

CONTRAINDICATIONS:
Hypersensitivity

Precautions: Pregnancy (B), breastfeeding, hypotension

DOSAGE AND ROUTES

Inhibition of platelet adhesion
- **Adult: PO** 75-100 mg qid in combination with aspirin or warfarin

Thallium myocardial perfusion imaging
- **Adult: IV** 570 mcg/kg

TIA with aspirin (unlabeled)
- **Adult: PO** 225-400 mg/day max 400 mg/day

Available forms: Tabs 25, 50, 75 mg; inj 10 mg/2 ml

Administer:

PO route
- On empty stomach: 1 hr before meals or 2 hr after; give with 8 oz water for better absorption

IV route
- IV after diluting to at least 1:2 ratio using D_5W, 0.45% NaCl, or 0.9% NaCl to a total vol of 20-50 ml; give over 4 min; do not give undiluted

SIDE EFFECTS

CNS: *Headache, dizziness, weakness, fainting, syncope;* IV: transient cerebral ischemia, weakness

CV: *Postural hypotension;* IV: MI

GI: *Nausea, vomiting,* anorexia, diarrhea

INTEG: *Rash,* flushing

RESP: IV: Bronchospasm

PHARMACOKINETICS

PO: Peak 1.25 hr, duration 6 hr, therapeutic response may take several months, metabolized in liver, excreted in bile, undergoes enterohepatic recirculation, protein binding 91%-99%, terminal half-life 12 hr

INTERACTIONS

- Prevention of coronary vasodilation: theophylline

Increase: digoxin effect—digoxin
Increase: bleeding risk—NSAIDs, cefamandole, cefotetan, cefoperazone, plicamycin, valproic acid, salicylates, sulfinpyrazole, anticoagulants, thrombolytics

NURSING CONSIDERATIONS

Assess:
- B/P, pulse during treatment until stable; take B/P lying, standing; orthostatic hypotension is common
- Cardiac status: chest pain; what aggravates, ameliorates condition

Perform/provide:
- Storage at room temp

Evaluate:
- Therapeutic response: decreased platelet adhesion

Teach patient/family:
- That medication is not a cure; may have to be taken continuously in evenly spaced doses only as directed
- To avoid hazardous activities until stabilized on medication; dizziness may occur
- To rise slowly from sitting or lying to prevent orthostatic hypotension
- Not to use alcohol or OTC medications unless approved by prescriber

disopyramide (Rx)

(dye-soe-peer'a-mide)

Norpace, Norpace CR, Rythmodan ✱

Func. class.: Antidysrhythmic (Class IA)

Chem. class.: Nonnitrate

Do not confuse:
disopyramide/desipramine

ACTION: Decreases myocardial conduction, velocity, excitability, and contracting by inhibiting the influx of sodium by fast channels in myocardial cell membranes with increased recovery after repolarization

USES: PVCs, ventricular tachycardia, supraventricular tachycardia

Unlabeled uses: Atrial flutter, fibrillation

CONTRAINDICATIONS: Hypersensitivity, 2nd- or 3rd-degree block, cardiogenic shock, CHF (uncompensated), sick sinus syndrome

Black Box Warning: QT prolongation

Precautions: Pregnancy (C), breastfeeding, children, geriatric patients, diabetes mellitus, renal/hepatic disease, myasthenia gravis, closed-angle glaucoma, cardiomyopathy, conduction abnormalities, potassium imbalance

Black Box Warning: Arrhythmias, MI, torsades de pointes

DOSAGE AND ROUTES

- **Adult >18 yr and >50 kg: PO** 150-200 mg q6hr; **EXT REL CAP** 300 mg q12hr
- **Adult >18 yr and <50 kg: PO** 100 mg q6hr; **EXT REL CAP** 200 mg q12hr
- **Adolescent 12-18 yr: PO** 6-15 mg/kg/day in divided doses q6hr
- **Child 5-12 yr: PO** 10-15 mg/kg/day in divided doses q6hr
- **Child 1-4 yr: PO** 10-20 mg/kg/day in divided doses q6hr
- **Child <1 yr: PO** 10-30 mg/kg/day in divided doses q6hr

Renal dose
- **Adult: PO** CCr >40 ml/min, 100 mg q6hr or 200 mg q12hr (ext rel); CCr 30-40 ml/min, dose q8hr; CCr 15-30 ml/min, dose q12hr; CCr <15 ml/min, dose q24hr

Hepatic dose

• **Adult: PO** 400 mg/day in divided doses (q6hr for regular release, q12hr for ext rel)

Conversion to/maintenance of sinus rhythm in atrial fibrillation/flutter (unlabeled)

• **Adult: PO EXT REL** 400-800 mg/day in divided doses q12hr; **REG REL** 200 mg q4-6hr, max 800 mg/day

Available forms: Caps 100, 150 mg; ext rel caps (CR) 100, 150 mg; ext rel tabs 150 mg ✤

Administer:

• Do not break, crush, or chew sus rel cap; give 1 hr before or 2 hr after meals

• Sugar-free gum, frequent sips of water for dry mouth

SIDE EFFECTS

CNS: *Headache, dizziness,* psychosis, fatigue, depression, paresthesias, insomnia

CV: *Hypotension, bradycardia,* angina, PVCs, tachycardia, increased QRS, QT segments, cardiac arrest, edema, weight gain, AV block, CHF, syncope, chest pain, torsades de pointes

EENT: *Blurred vision; dry nose, throat, eyes;* angle-closure glaucoma

GI: *Dry mouth, constipation,* nausea, anorexia, flatulence, diarrhea, vomiting

GU: *Urinary retention, hesitancy,* impotence

HEMA: Thrombocytopenia, agranulocytosis, anemia (rare), decreased Hgb, Hct

INTEG: Rash, pruritus, urticaria

META: Hypoglycemia, hypokalemia

MS: Weakness, pain in extremities

PHARMACOKINETICS

PO: Onset 30 min-3 hr; duration 6-12 hr; half-life 4-10 hr; metabolized in liver; excreted in feces, urine, breast milk; crosses placenta

INTERACTIONS

Increase: QT prolongation: class IA/IC/III antidysrhythmics, arsenic trioxide, chloroquine, droperidol, grepafloxacin, halofantrine, levomethadyl, methadone, pentamidine, some phenothiazines, pimozide, probucol, sparfloxacin, ziprasidone

Increase: disopyramide effect—quinidine, procainamide, propranolol, lidocaine, atenolol, other antidysrhythmics, erythromycin

Increase: side effects, urinary retention—anticholinergics

Decrease: disopyramide effect—phenytoin, rifampin, PHENobarbital

Drug/Lab Test

Increase: hepatic enzymes, lipids, BUN, creatinine

Decrease: Hgb/Hct, blood glucose

NURSING CONSIDERATIONS

Assess:

• B/P, apical pulse for 1 min; if <60, check again in 1 hr; if still <60, notify prescriber; for rebound hypertension after 1-2 hr

Black Box Warning: QT prolongation, ECG; check for increased QT, widening QRS; product should be discontinued

⚠ **CHF:** crackles, jugular venous distention, weight gain, peripheral edema, dyspnea

• Dehydration or hypovolemia, I&O ratio, electrolytes (Na, K, Cl)

• Renal, hepatic studies (AST, ALT, bilirubin, BUN, creatinine) during treatment

• Diabetics for signs of hypoglycemia (rare)

• **Constipation:** increased bulk in diet; water, stool softeners, or laxatives needed

• Cardiac rate, respiration: rhythm, character

• Urinary hesitancy, frequency, change in I&O ratio; check for edema daily; check for toxicity

Evaluate:

• Therapeutic response: decreased dysrhythmias

Teach patient/family:

• To take product exactly as prescribed; if dose is missed, take within 3-4 hr of next dose; not to double dose; may take with food or milk to prevent gastric upset

• To avoid alcohol because severe hypotension may occur; to avoid OTC products because serious drug interactions may occur
• To make position changes slowly during early therapy to prevent orthostatic hypotension
• To avoid hazardous activities if dizziness or blurred vision occurs; to use a medical alert bracelet
• About the importance of complying with product regimen; that product does not cure condition

TREATMENT OF OVERDOSE:
O_2, artificial ventilation, ECG, DOPamine for circulatory depression; diazepam or thiopental for seizures

DOBUTamine (Rx)
(doe-byoo′ta-meen)
Func. class.: Adrenergic direct-acting β_1-agonist, cardiac stimulant
Chem. class.: Catecholamine

Do not confuse:
DOBUTamine/DOPamine

ACTION: Causes increased contractility, increased cardiac output without marked increase in heart rate by acting on β_1-receptors in heart; minor α and β_2 effects

USES: Cardiac decompensation due to organic heart disease or cardiac surgery
Unlabeled uses: Cardiogenic shock in children; congenital heart disease in children undergoing cardiac catheterization

CONTRAINDICATIONS: Hypersensitivity, idiopathic hypertrophic subaortic stenosis
Precautions: Pregnancy (B), breastfeeding, children, hypertension, CAD, MI, hypovolemia, dysrhythmias

DOSAGE AND ROUTES
• **Adult and child: IV INF** 2-20 mcg/kg/min; may increase to 40 mcg/kg/min if needed
Available forms: Inj 12.5 mg/ml, 250 mg/20 ml
Administer:
IV route
• Dilute each 250 mg/10 ml of sterile water or D_5W for inj; may be further diluted in ≤50 ml given at prescribed rate; should be gradually increased to desired rate; use a CVP catheter or large peripheral vein, use inf pump, titrate to patient response
• Standard concentrations: 250 mcg/ml to 1000 mcg/ml, max 5 mg of DOBUTamine/ml

Y-site compatibilities: Alfentanil, alprostadil, amifostine, amikacin, aminocaproic acid, amiodarone, anidulafungin, argatroban, ascorbic acid injection, atenolol, atracurium, atropine, aztreonam, benztropine, bleomycin, bumetanide, buprenorphine, butorphanol, calcium chloride/gluconate, CARBOplatin, caspofungin, chlorproMAZINE, cimetidine, ciprofloxacin, cisatracurium, CISplatin, cladribine, clarithromycin, cloNIDine, codeine, cyanocobalamin, cyclophosphamide, cycloSPORINE, cytarabine, DACTINomycin, DAPTOmycin, dexmedetomidine, digoxin, diltiazem, diphenhydrAMINE, docetaxel, DOPamine, doripenem, doxacurium, DOXOrubicin, DOXOrubicin liposomal, doxycycline, enalaprilat, ePHEDrine, EPINEPHrine, epirubicin, epoetin alfa, eptifibatide, erythromycin, esmolol, etoposide, famotidine, fenoldopam, fentaNYL, fluconazole, fludarabine, gatifloxacin, gemcitabine, gentamicin, glycopyrrolate, granisetron, HYDROmorphone, hydrOXYzine, IDArubicin, ifosfamide, irinotecan, isoproterenol, labetalol, levofloxacin, lidocaine, linezolid, LORazepam, LR, magnesium sulfate, mannitol, mechlorethamine, meperidine, meropenem, metaraminol, methoxamine, methyldopate, methylPREDNISolone, metoclopramide, metoprolol, metroNIDAZOLE, miconazole, milrinone, minocycline, mitoxantrone, morphine, multiple vitamins injection, mycophenolate mofetil, nafcillin, nalbuphine, naloxone, netilmicin, niCARdipine, nitroglycerin, norepinephrine, octreotide, ondansetron, oxaliplatin, oxytocin, paclitaxel, palonosetron, pamidronate, pancuronium, papaverine, pentamidine, pentazocine, phenylephrine, polymyxin B, potassium chloride, procainamide, prochlorperazine, promethazine, propofol, propranolol, protamine, pyridoxine, quiNIDine, ranitidine, remifentanil, Ringer's, ritodrine, riTUXimab, rocuronium, sodium acetate, succinylcholine, SUFentanil, tacrolimus, temocillin, teniposide, theophylline, thiamine, thiotepa, tigecycline, tirofiban, TNA, tobramycin, tolazoline, TPN, trastuzumab, trimetaphan, urokinase, vancomycin, vasopressin, vecuronium, verapamil, vinCRIStine, vinorelbine, voriconazole, zidovudine, zoledronic acid

SIDE EFFECTS

CNS: *Anxiety,* headache, dizziness, fatigue
CV: Palpitations, tachycardia, hyper/hypotension, PVCs, angina
ENDO: Hypokalemia
GI: Heartburn, nausea, vomiting
MS: Muscle cramps (leg)
RESP: Dyspnea

PHARMACOKINETICS

IV: Onset 1-2 min, peak 10 min, half-life 2 min, metabolized in liver (inactive metabolites), excreted in urine

INTERACTIONS

Increase: severe hypertension—guanethidine
Increase: dysrhythmias—general anesthetics
Increase: pressor effect, dysrhythmias—atomoxetine, COMT inhibitors, tricyclics, MAOIs, oxytocics
Decrease: DOBUTamine action—other β-blockers

NURSING CONSIDERATIONS

Assess:

- **Hypovolemia;** if present, correct first; administer cardiac glycoside before DOBUTamine
- **Oxygenation/perfusion deficit:** check B/P, chest pain, dizziness, loss of consciousness
- **Heart failure:** S_3 gallop, dyspnea, neck venous distention, bibasilar crackles in patients with CHF, cardiomyopathy, palpate peripheral pulses; report if extremities become cold or mottled or if peripheral pulses decrease
- **ECG** during administration continuously; if B/P increases, product is decreased; CVP or PCWP, cardiac output during inf; report changes
- Serum electrolytes, urine output

⚠ **Sulfite sensitivity,** which may be life threatening

Perform/provide:

- Storage of reconstituted sol for 24 hr if refrigerated

Evaluate:

- Therapeutic response: increased B/P with stabilization, increased urine output

Teach patient/family:

- About the reason for product administration; to report dyspnea, chest pain, numbness of extremities, headache, IV site discomfort

TREATMENT OF OVERDOSE:

Administer a β_1-adrenergic blocker; reduce IV or discontinue, ensure oxygenation/ventilation; for severe tachydysrhythmias (ventricular), give lidocaine or propranolol

docetaxel (Rx)

(doe-se-tax′el)

Taxotere

Func. class.: Antineoplastic—miscellaneous
Chem. class.: Taxane

Do not confuse:
Taxotere/Taxol

ACTION: Inhibits reorganization of microtubule network needed for interphase and mitotic cellular functions; also causes abnormal bundles of microtubules during cell cycle and multiple esters of microtubules during mitosis

USES: Locally advanced or metastatic breast cancer, non–small-cell lung cancer, androgen-independent metastatic prostate cancer, postsurgery operable node-positive breast cancer, induction treatment of locally advanced squamous cell of the head and neck, adjuvant treatment of breast cancer with CARBOplatin and trastuzumab, gastric adenocarcinoma

Unlabeled uses: Malignant melanoma, ovarian cancer, front-line use with bevacizumab for metastatic breast cancer

CONTRAINDICATIONS: Pregnancy (D), breastfeeding, hypersensitivity to this product or severe hepatic disease, bilirubin exceeding upper normal limit or severely elevated ALT, AST, alk phos

Black Box Warning: Other products with polysorbate 80, neutropenia of <1500/mm^3

Precautions: Children, cardiovascular disease, pulmonary disorders, bone marrow depression, herpes zoster, pleural effusion

Black Box Warning: Edema, hepatic disease, lung cancer, taxane hypersensitivity

DOSAGE AND ROUTES:

- Other regimens are used

Locally advanced or metastatic breast cancer after failure of other chemotherapy

- **Adult: IV** 60-100 mg/m^2 given over 1 hr q3wk; if neutrophil count is <500 cells/mm^3 for >1 wk, reduce dose by 25%

Operable node-positive breast cancer

- **Adult: IV** (TAC regimen) 75 mg/m^2 1 hr after DOXOrubicin 50 mg/m^2 and cyclophosphamide 500 mg/m^2 q3wk × 6 cycles

Adjuvant treatment of operable stage I-III invasive breast cancer in combination with cyclophosphamide

- **Adult: IV** (TAC regimen) docetaxel 75 mg/m^2 with cyclophosphamide 600 mg/m^2 q21days × 4 cycles

Locally advanced or metastatic non–small-cell lung cancer after failure of CISplatin chemotherapy

- **Adult: IV** 75 mg/m^2 over 1 hr q3wk; if neutrophil count is <500 cells/mm^3 for >1 wk, reduce dose to 55 mg/m^2; if patient develops grade 3 peripheral neuropathy, stop product

Unreactable, locally advanced, or metastatic non–small-cell lung cancer previously treated with chemotherapy

- **Adult: IV** 75 mg/m^2 over 1 hr then CISplatin 75 mg/m^2 **IV** given over 30-60 min q3wk; reduce dose to 65 mg/m^2 in those with hematologic or non-hematologic toxicities

Androgen-independent metastatic prostate cancer

- **Adult: IV** 75 mg/m^2 given over 1 hr q3wk with 5 mg predniSONE **PO** bid continuously; give dexamethasone 8 mg **PO** at 12 hr, 3 hr, and 1 hr prior to docetaxel; if neutrophil count is <500 cells/mm^3 for more than 1 wk or other toxicities occur, reduce dose to 60 mg/m^2

Adjuvant postsurgery treatment of operable node-positive breast cancer

- **Adult: IV** 75 mg/m^2 over 1 hr given 1 hr after DOXOrubicin 50 mg/m^2, cyclophosphamide 500 mg/m^2 q3wk × 6 cycles

Squamous cell of head and neck

- **Adult: IV** 75 mg/m^2 over 1 hr, then CISplatin 75 mg/m^2 over 1 hr on day 1, then 5FU 750 mg/m²/day **CONT INF** × 5 days, repeat cycle q3wk

Gastric adenocarcinoma

• **Adult: IV** 75 mg/m² q3wk, given with CISplatin, fluorouracil

Advanced ovarian cancer/ metastatic melanoma (unlabeled)

• **Adult: IV** 100 mg/m² over 1 hr q3wk

Available forms: Inj 20 mg/0.5 ml, 20 mg/ml, 80 mg/2 ml, 80 mg/4 ml

Administer:

• Premedicate with dexamethasone 8 mg **PO** bid × 3 days starting 1 day prior to treatment

• Antiemetic 30-60 min before product and prn

Intermittent IV INF route

• Use cytotoxic handling procedures

• Allow vials to warm to room temp; withdraw all diluent, inject in vial of docetaxel; rotate gently to mix; allow to stand to decrease foaming, then withdraw the required amount (10 mg/ml), inject in 250 ml of 0.9% NaCl, D_5W; mix gently; give over 1 hr

Y-site compatibilities: Acyclovir, alfentanil, allopurinol, amifostine, amikacin, aminocaproic acid, aminophylline, amiodarone, amphotericin B lipid complex, ampicillin, ampicillin-sulbactam, anidulafungin, atenolol, atracurium, azithromycin, aztreonam, bivalirudin, bleomycin, bumetanide, buprenorphine, busulfan, butorphanol, calcium chloride/gluconate, CARBOplatin, carmustine, caspofungin, ceFAZolin, cefepime, cefonicid, cefoperazone, cefotaxime, cefotetan, cefoxitin, ceftazidime, ceftizoxime, cefTRIAXone, cefuroxime, cephapirin, chloramphenicol, chlorproMAZINE, cimetidine, ciprofloxacin, cisatracurium, CISplatin, clindamycin, codeine, cyclophosphamide, cycloSPORINE, cytarabine, dacarbazine, DACTINomycin, DAPTOmycin, dexamethasone, dexmedetomidine, dexrazoxane, diazepam, digoxin, diltiazem, diphenhydrAMINE, DOBUTamine, DOPamine, doripenem, doxacurium, DOXOrubicin, doxycycline, droperidol, enalaprilat, ePHEDrine, EPINEPHrine, epirubicin, ertapenem, erythromycin, esmolol, etoposide, famotidine, fenoldopam, fentaNYL, fluconazole, fludarabine, fluorouracil, foscarnet, fosphenytoin, furosemide, ganciclovir, gatifloxacin, gemcitabine, gentamicin, glycopyrrolate, granisetron, haloperidol, heparin, hydrALAZINE, hydrocortisone, HYDROmorphone, hydrOXYzine, ifosfamide, imipenem-cilastatin, inamrinone, insulin (regular), irinotecan, isoproterenol, ketorolac, labetalol, leucovorin, levofloxacin, levorphanol, lidocaine, linezolid, LORazepam, LR, magnesium sulfate, mannitol, meperidine, meropenem, mesna, methotrexate, methyldopate, metoclopramide, metoprolol, metroNIDAZOLE, midazolam, milrinone, minocycline, mitoxantrone, mivacurium, morphine, nafcillin, naloxone, nesiritide, netilmicin, niCARdipine, nitroglycerin, nitroprusside, norepinephrine, octreotide, ofloxacin, ondansetron, oxaliplatin, palonosetron, pamidronate, pancuronium, pantoprazole, pemetrexed, pentamidine, pentazocine, PENTobarbital, PHENobarbital, phenylephrine, piperacillin, piperacillin-tazobactam, polymyxin B, potassium chloride/phosphates, procainamide, prochlorperazine, promethazine, propranolol, quiNIDine, quinupristin-dalfopristin, ranitidine, remifentanil, riTUXimab, rocuronium, sodium acetate/bicarbonate/phosphates, succinylcholine, SUFentanil, sulfamethoxazole-trimethoprim, tacrolimus, teniposide, theophylline, thiopental, thiotepa, ticarcillin, ticarcillin-clavulanate, tigecycline, tirofiban, tobramycin, tolazoline, trastuzumab, trimethobenzamide, vancomycin, vasopressin, vecuronium, verapamil, vinCRIStine, vinorelbine, voriconazole, zidovudine, zoledronic acid

SIDE EFFECTS

CNS: Seizures

CV: *Hypotension,* fluid retention, peripheral edema, flushing, MI, sinus tachycardia

GI: *Nausea, vomiting, diarrhea,* hepatotoxicity, stomatitis, colitis
HEMA: Neutropenia, leukopenia, thrombocytopenia, anemia, bleeding, infections, myelosuppression
INTEG: *Alopecia,* nail pain, rash, skin eruptions
MISC: Amenorrhea, fever of unknown origin, secondary malignancy, Stevens-Johnson syndrome
MS: *Arthralgia, myalgia,* back pain
NEURO: *Peripheral neuropathy*
RESP: Dyspnea, pulmonary edema, fibrosis, embolism
SYST: *Hypersensitivity reactions,* AML, death

PHARMACOKINETICS

Metabolized in liver, excreted in feces, terminal half-life 11.1 hr

INTERACTIONS

- Altered docetaxel levels: cycloSPORINE, erythromycin, ketoconazole, troleadomycin

Increase: myelosuppression—other antineoplastics, radiation
Decrease: immune response—live virus vaccines

NURSING CONSIDERATIONS

Assess:

Black Box Warning: CBC, differential, platelet count before treatment and weekly; withhold product if WBC is <1500/mm³ or platelet count is <100,000/mm³; notify prescriber

- Monitor temp q4hr; fever may indicate beginning of infection
- CV status: B/P, edema, flushing
- **Hepatic disease:** hepatic studies before, during therapy (bilirubin, AST, ALT, LDH) prn or monthly; check for jaundiced skin and sclera, dark urine, clay-colored stools, itchy skin, abdominal pain, fever, diarrhea
- **CNS changes:** confusion, paresthesias, dysethenia, pain, weakness; if severe, product should be discontinued
- VS during 1st hr of inf, check IV site for signs of infiltration

⚠ **Hypersensitive reactions, anaphylaxis,** including hypotension, dyspnea, angioedema, generalized urticaria; discontinue infusion immediately

- **Bone marrow depression/bleeding:** hematuria, guaiac, bruising or petechiae, mucosa or orifices q8hr; obtain prescription for viscous lidocaine (Xylocaine); avoid invasive procedures
- Effects of alopecia on body image; discuss feelings about body changes

Perform/provide:

- Confirmation that dexamethasone was given 12 hr and 6 hr before inf begins
- Storage of prepared sol up to 27 hr in refrigerator

Evaluate:

- Therapeutic response: decreased tumor size, spread of malignancy

Teach patient/family:

- To report signs of **infection:** fever, sore throat, flulike symptoms
- To report signs of **anemia:** fatigue, headache, faintness, SOB, irritability
- To report **bleeding;** to avoid use of razors, commercial mouthwash
- To avoid use of aspirin, ibuprofen
- To report any complaints or side effects to nurse or prescriber
- That hair may be lost during treatment; that a wig or hairpiece may make patient feel better; that new hair may be different in color and texture
- That pain in muscles and joints 2-5 days after inf is common
- To use barrier contraception during and for several months after treatment, pregnancy (D); to avoid breastfeeding
- To avoid receiving vaccinations while taking product

docosanol topical

See Appendix B

docusate calcium (OTC)

(dok'yoo-sate cal'see-um)

Kao-Tin, ratio-Docusate Calcium ♣, Stool Softener DC, Sur-Q-Lax, Walgreen's Stool Softener

docusate sodium (OTC)

Apo-Docusate ♣, Colace, Correctol, Diocto, Doc-Q-Lace, Docu DOK, Doculace, Enemeez, Equaline Stool Softener, Good Sense Stool Softener, Leader Stool Softener, Phillip's Stool Softener, ratio-Docusate Sodium ♣, Regulex ♣, Select Brand Docusate Sodium, Selex ♣, Silace, Soflax ♣, Top Care Stool Softener, Walgreen's Stool Softener

Func. class.: Laxative, emollient; stool softener

Chem. class.: Anionic surfactant

ACTION: Increases water, fat penetration in intestine; allows for easier passage of stool

USES: Prevention of dry, hard stools

CONTRAINDICATIONS: Hypersensitivity, obstruction, fecal impaction, nausea/vomiting

Precautions: Pregnancy (C), breastfeeding

DOSAGE AND ROUTES

- **Adult: PO** 50-300 mg/day (sodium) or 240 mg (calcium) prn; **ENEMA** 4 ml
- **Child >12 yr: ENEMA** 2 ml
- **Child 6-12 yr: PO** 40-150 mg/day (sodium) in divided doses
- **Child 3-6 yr: PO** 20-60 mg/day (sodium) in divided doses
- **Child <3 yr: PO** 10-40 mg/day (sodium) in divided doses

Available forms: *Calcium:* 240 mg; *sodium:* caps 50, 100, 250 mg; tabs 100 mg; syr 20 mg/5 ml, 50 mg/15 ml, 100 mg/30 ml, 150 mg/15 ml; oral sol 10, 50 mg/ml; enema 283 mg/3.9 cap

Administer:

- Swallow tabs whole; do not break, crush, or chew
- Oral sol: diluted in milk, fruit juice to decrease bitter taste
- In morning or evening (oral dose)

SIDE EFFECTS

EENT: Bitter taste, throat irritation

GI: Nausea, anorexia, cramps, diarrhea

INTEG: Rash

PHARMACOKINETICS

Onset 12-72 hr

INTERACTIONS

- **Toxicity:** mineral oil

Drug/Herb

Increase: laxative action—flax, senna

NURSING CONSIDERATIONS

Assess:

- **Cause of constipation;** identify whether fluids, bulk, or exercise missing from lifestyle; constipating products
- Cramping, rectal bleeding, nausea, vomiting; if these occur, product should be discontinued

Perform/provide:

- Storage in cool environment; do not freeze

Evaluate:

- Therapeutic response: decrease in constipation

Teach patient/family:

- That normal bowel movements do not always occur daily
- Not to use in presence of abdominal pain, nausea, vomiting
- To notify prescriber if constipation unrelieved or if symptoms of electrolyte imbalance occur: muscle cramps, pain, weakness, dizziness, excessive thirst
- That product may take up to 3 days to soften stools

• To take oral preparations with a full glass of water (unless on fluid restrictions) and to increase fluid intake

dofetilide (Rx)

Tikosyn

Func. class.: Antidysrhythmic (Class III)

ACTION: Blocks cardiac ion channel carrying the rapid component of delayed potassium current; no effect on sodium channels

USES: Atrial fibrillation, flutter, maintenance of normal sinus rhythm

CONTRAINDICATIONS: Children, hypersensitivity, digoxin toxicity, aortic stenosis, pulmonary hypertension, severe renal disease

Black Box Warning: QT prolongation, torsades de pointes, renal failure

Precautions: Pregnancy (C), breastfeeding, AV block, bradycardia, electrolyte imbalance

Black Box Warning: Renal disease, arrhythmias

DOSAGE AND ROUTES

• **Adult: PO** 125-500 mcg bid depending on CCr, initial dose is based on renal function and QTc, may be adjusted q2-3hr to get appropriate increase in QTc

Renal dose

• **Adult: PO** CCr >60 ml/min, 500 mcg bid; CCr 40-60 ml/min, 250 mcg bid; CCr 20-39 ml/min, 125 mcg bid; CCr <20 ml/min, do not use

Available forms: Caps 125, 250, 500 mcg

Administer:

• For 3 days hospitalized

• Give dofetilide after withholding class I, III antidysrhythmic for 3 half-lives of dofetilide

• Do not open caps

SIDE EFFECTS

CNS: *Syncope, dizziness,* headache

CV: *Hypotension, postural hypotension, bradycardia,* angina, PVCs, substernal pressure, transient hypertension, precipitation of angina, QT prolongation, torsades de pointes, ventricular dysrhythmias

GI: *Nausea, vomiting,* severe diarrhea, anorexia

RESP: Dyspnea, respiratory infections

PHARMACOKINETICS

Well absorbed, max plasma conc 2-3 hr, steady state 2-3 days, half-life 10 hr, metabolized by liver, excreted by kidneys

INTERACTIONS

• Do not use with cimetidine, ketoconazole, verapamil, prochlorperazine, trimethoprim-sulfamethoxazole, megestrol, hydrochlorothiazide

Increase: QT prolongation, torsades de pointes—class IA/III antidysrhythmics, arsenic trioxide, chloroquine, clarithromycin, droperidol, erythromycin, halofantrine, haloperidol, levomethadyl, methadone, pentamidine, some phenothiazines, ziprasidone

Increase: hypokalemia—potassium-depleting diuretics

Increase: toxicity—amiloride metFORMIN, entecavir, lamivudine, memantine, triamterene, procainamide, trospium

Increase: dofetilide levels—antiretroviral protease inhibitors

Drug/Food

• Do not use with grapefruit juice

NURSING CONSIDERATIONS

Assess:

Black Box Warning: ECG continuously for a minimum of 3 days or 12 hr after conversion to determine product effectiveness, PVCs, other dysrhythmias; renal function, QTc at baseline; reassess QTc interval 2-3 hr after each dose; if QTc >440 msec or 500 msec if ventricular conduction disturbance, discontinue until QTc at starting level; product only available to facilities educated in its administration; patient must be hospitalized

- AF patients should receive anticoagulation prior to cardioversion
- Cardiac status: rate, rhythm, character, continuously; B/P

Black Box Warning: **Severe renal impairment CCr <20 ml/min:** do not use for mild to moderate renal disease; monitor BUN/creatinine; adjust dose based on creatinine clearance

Perform/provide:
- Place patient in supine position unless otherwise ordered; assist with ambulation

Evaluate:
- Therapeutic response: control of atrial fibrillation

Teach patient/family:
- To make position changes slowly; orthostatic hypotension may occur
- To notify prescriber if fast heartbeats with fainting or dizziness occur
- To notify all prescribers of all medications, supplements taken
- That, if dose is missed, not to double; to take next dose at usual time
- To avoid breastfeeding

dolasetron (Rx)

(do-la′se-tron)

Anzemet

Func. class.: Antiemetic

Chem. class.: 5-HT3 receptor antagonist

ACTION: Prevents nausea, vomiting by blocking serotonin peripherally, centrally, and in the small intestine

USES: Prevention of nausea, vomiting associated with cancer chemotherapy, radiotherapy; prevention of postoperative nausea, vomiting

Unlabeled uses: Radiotherapy-induced nausea/vomiting

CONTRAINDICATIONS: Hypersensitivity

Precautions: Pregnancy (B), breastfeeding, children, geriatric patients, hypokalemia, electrolyte imbalances; granisetron/ondansetron/palonosetron hypersensitivity, QT prolongation

DOSAGE AND ROUTES

Prevention of nausea and vomiting during cancer chemotherapy
- **Adult: PO** 100 mg 1 hr prior to chemotherapy
- **Child 2-16 yr: PO** 1.8 mg/kg prior to chemotherapy; max 100 mg

Prevention of postoperative nausea and vomiting
- **Adult: IV** 12.5 mg as single dose 15 min before cessation of anesthesia; **PO** 100 mg 2 hr before surgery (prevention only)
- **Child 2-16 yr: IV** 0.35 mg/kg as single dose 15 min before cessation of anesthesia; **PO** 1.2 mg/kg 2 hr before surgery (prevention only)

Available forms: Tabs 50, 100 mg; inj 20 mg/ml (12.5 mg/0.625 ml)

Administer:

PO route
- Do not mix product for oral administration in apple or apple-grape juice until immediately before administration; diluted product can be kept for 2 hr at room temp

Intermittent IV INF route
- By inj 100 mg/30 sec or more or diluted in 50 ml compatible sol; give over 15 min

Y-site compatibilities: Anidulafungin, atenolol, azithromycin, bivalirudin, caspofungin, cyclophosphamide, cytarabine, DAPTOmycin, dexmedetomidine, doxacurium, DOXOrubicin, epirubicin, eptifibatide, ertapenem, fenoldopam, ifosfamide, irinotecan, levofloxacin, linezolid, mechlorethamine, meperidine, mycophenolate, nesiritide, octreotide, oxaliplatin, oxytocin, pamidronate, pancuronium, pemetrexed, quinupristin-dalfopristin, rocuronium, sodium acetate, tacrolimus, tigecycline, tirofiban, vecuronium, vinCRIStine, voriconazole, zoledronic acid

SIDE EFFECTS

CNS: *Headache,* dizziness, fatigue, drowsiness
CV: Dysrhythmias, ECG changes, hypo/hypertension, tachycardia, bradycardia; ventricular tachycardia/fibrillation, QT prolongation, torsades de pointes, cardiac arrest (IV)
GI: *Diarrhea,* constipation, increased AST/ALT, abdominal pain, anorexia
GU: Urinary retention, oliguria
MISC: Rash, bronchospasm

PHARMACOKINETICS

Well absorbed, metabolized to active metabolite, half-life of active metabolite 8 hr, max concentrations after 1 hr

INTERACTIONS

Increase: dysrhythmias—antidysrhythmics
Increase: dolasetron levels—cimetidine
Increase: QT prolongation—thiazide/loop diuretics, antidysrhythmics—class IA, III, arsenic trioxide, chloroquine, clarithromycin, droperidol, erythromycin, halofantrine, haloperidol, levomethadyl, methadone, pentamidine, some phenothiazines, ziprasidone
Decrease: dolasetron levels—rifampin

NURSING CONSIDERATIONS

Assess:

- For absence of nausea, vomiting during chemotherapy
- **Hypersensitivity reaction:** rash, bronchospasm
- Cardiac conduction conditions, electrolyte imbalances, dysrhythmias, heart rate

Perform/provide:

- Storage at room temp 48 hr after dilution

Evaluate:

- Therapeutic response: absence of nausea, vomiting during cancer chemotherapy

Teach patient/family:

- To report diarrhea, constipation, nausea, vomiting, rash, or changes in respirations
- May cause headache; use analgesic

donepezil (Rx)

(don-ep-ee′zill)

Aricept, Aricept ODT

Func. class.: Anti-Alzheimer's agent
Chem. class.: Reversible cholinesterase inhibitor

ACTION:

Elevates acetylcholine concentrations (cerebral cortex) by slowing degradation of acetylcholine released in cholinergic neurons; does not alter underlying dementia

USES:

Mild to severe dementia with Alzheimer's disease
Unlabeled uses: Subcortical, vascular dementia; dementia with Lewy bodies

CONTRAINDICATIONS:

Hypersensitivity to this product or piperidine derivatives
Precautions: Pregnancy (C), breastfeeding, children, sick sinus syndrome, history of ulcers, GI bleeding, hepatic disease, bladder obstruction, asthma, seizures, COPD, abrupt discontinuation, AV block, GI obstruction, Parkinson's disease, surgery

DOSAGE AND ROUTES

- **Adult: PO** 5 mg/day at bedtime; may increase to 10 mg/day after 4-6 wk, may increase to 23 mg/day after 3 mo of 10 mg/day

Available forms: Tabs 5, 10, 23 mg; orally disintegrating tabs (Aricept ODT) 5, 10 mg

Administer:

- Daily in the evening prior to bedtime; swallow whole; do not cut, break, chew, or crush tab
- Dosage adjusted to response no more than q4-6wk; oral dosage forms are interchangeable
- Orally disintegrating tabs: allow to dissolve on tongue before swallowing; may be given with/without water

SIDE EFFECTS

CNS: Dizziness, *insomnia,* somnolence, *headache,* fatigue, abnormal dreams, syncope, seizures, drowsiness, agitation, depression, confusion, fever, hallucinations

CV: Atrial fibrillation, hypo/hypertension, sinus bradycardia, AV block

GI: *Nausea, vomiting,* anorexia, *diarrhea,* abdominal pain, GI bleeding, weight loss

GU: Urinary frequency, UTI, incontinence

INTEG: Rash, flushing, diaphoresis, bruising

META: Hyperlipidemia

MS: Cramps, arthritis, arthralgia

RESP: Rhinitis, URI, cough, pharyngitis, dyspnea

PHARMACOKINETICS

Well absorbed PO; metabolized by CYP2D6, CYP3A4; elimination half-life 10 hr single dose, 70 hr multiple doses; protein binding 96%

INTERACTIONS

Increase: donepezil effects—CYP2D6, CYP3A4 inhibitors

Increase: synergistic effect—succinylcholine, cholinesterase inhibitors, cholinergic agonists

Increase: gastric acid secretions—NSAIDs

Decrease: donepezil effects—CYP2D6, CYP3A4 inducers

Decrease: action of anticholinergics

Decrease: donepezil effect—carBAMazepine, dexamethasone, phenytoin, PHENObarbital, rifampin

Drug/Herb

Decrease: donepezil—St. John's wort

NURSING CONSIDERATIONS

Assess:

- B/P: hypo/hypertension, heart rate
- Mental status: affect, mood, behavioral changes, depression, complete suicide assessment; neurologic status
- GI status: nausea, vomiting, anorexia, diarrhea; monitor weight
- GU status: urinary frequency, incontinence, I&O

Perform/provide:

- Assistance with ambulation during beginning therapy; dizziness, ataxia may occur

Evaluate:

- Therapeutic response: decrease in confusion, improved mood

Teach patient/family:

- To report side effects: twitching, nausea, vomiting, sweating, dizziness; indicates cholinergic crisis or overdose
- To use product exactly as prescribed
- To notify prescriber of nausea, vomiting, diarrhea (dose increase or beginning treatment), or rash
- Not to increase or abruptly decrease dose; serious consequences may result
- That product is not a cure, relieves symptoms

⚠ HIGH ALERT

DOPamine (Rx)

(doe′pa-meen)

Func. class.: Adrenergic

Chem. class.: Catecholamine

Do not confuse:

DOPamine/DOBUTamine

ACTION:
Causes increased cardiac output; acts on β_1- and α-receptors, causing vasoconstriction in blood vessels; low dose causes renal and mesenteric vasodilation; β_1 stimulation produces inotropic effects with increased cardiac output

USES:
Shock, increased perfusion, hypotension, cardiogenic/septic shock

Unlabeled uses: Bradycardia, cardiac arrest, CPR, acute renal failure, cirrhosis, barbiturate intoxication

CONTRAINDICATIONS:
Hypersensitivity, ventricular fibrillation, tachydysrhythmias, pheochromocytoma, hypovolemia

Precautions: Pregnancy (C), breastfeeding, geriatric patients, arterial embolism, peripheral vascular disease, sulfite hypersensitivity, acute MI

Black Box Warning: Extravasation

DOSAGE AND ROUTES

Shock

- **Adult: IV INF** 2-5 mcg/kg/min, titrate upward in 5-10 mcg/kg/min increments, max 50 mcg/kg/min; titrate to patient's response
- **Child: IV** 1-5 mcg/kg/min initially; usual dosage range, 2-20 mcg/kg/min

COPD

- **Adult: IV** 4 mcg/kg/min

CHF

- **Adult: IV** 3-10 mcg/kg/min

Bradycardia (unlabeled)

- **Adult: IV** 2-10 mcg/kg/min, titrate as needed

Available forms: Inj 40 mg, 80 mg, 160 mg/ml; conc for IV inf 0.8, 1.6, 3.2 mg/ml in 250, 500 ml D_5W

Administer:

IV route

- IV after diluting 200-400 mg/250-500 ml of D_5W, D_5 0.45% NaCl, D_5 0.9% NaCl, D_5LR, LR; use large vein
- After reconstituting, use inf pump; give at rate of 0.5-5 mcg/kg/min, increase by 1-4 mcg/kg/min at 10-30 min intervals until desired response

Y-site compatibilities: Alfentanil, alprostadil, amifostine, amikacin, aminocaproic acid, aminophylline, amiodarone, anidulafungin, argatroban, ascorbic acid injection, atenolol, atracurium, atropine, aztreonam, benztropine, bivalirudin, bleomycin, bumetanide, buprenorphine, butorphanol, calcium chloride/gluconate, CARBOplatin, caspofungin, cefamandole, cefmetazole, cefonicid, cefotaxime, cefotetan, cefoxitin, cefpirome, ceftazidime, ceftizoxime, cefTRIAXone, cefuroxime, chlorproMAZINE, cimetidine, ciprofloxacin, cisatracurium, CISplatin, cladribine, clarithromycin, clindamycin, cloNIDine, codeine, cyanocobalamin, cyclophosphamide, cycloSPORINE, cytarabine, DACTINomycin, DAPTOmycin, dexamethasone, dexmedetomidine, digoxin, diltiazem, diphenhydrAMINE, DOBUTamine, docetaxel, doripenem, doxacurium, DOXOrubicin, DOXOrubicin liposomal, doxycycline, droperidol, enalaprilat, ePHEDrine, EPINEPHrine, epirubicin, epoetin alfa, eptifibatide, ertapenem, erythromycin, esmolol, etoposide, famotidine, fenoldopam, fentaNYL, fluconazole, fludarabine, fluorouracil, folic acid, foscarnet, gatifloxacin, gemcitabine, gemtuzumab, gentamicin, glycopyrrolate, granisetron, heparin, hydrocortisone, HYDROmorphone, hydrOXYzine, IDArubicin, ifosfamide, imipenem-cilastatin, irinotecan, isoproterenol, ketorolac, labetalol, levofloxacin, lidocaine, linezolid, LORazepam, LR, magnesium sulfate, mannitol, mechlorethamine, meperidine, metaraminol, methicillin, methoxamine, methyldopate, methylPREDNISolone, metoclopramide, metoprolol, metroNIDAZOLE, mezlocillin, micanfungin, miconazole, midazolam, milrinone, minocycline, mitoxantrone, morphine, moxalactam, multiple vitamins injection, mycophenolate, nafcillin, nalbuphine, naloxone, netilmicin, niCARdipine, nitroglycerin, nitroprusside, norepinephrine, octreotide, ondansetron, oxacillin, oxaliplatin, oxytocin, paclitaxel, palonosetron, pamidronate, pancuronium, pantoprazole, papaverine, pemetrexed, penicillin G potassium/sodium, pentamidine, pentazocine, PENTobarbital, PHENobarbital, phenylephrine, phytonadione, piperacillin, piperacillin-tazobactam, polymyxin B, potassium chloride, procainamide, prochlorperazine, promethazine, propofol, propranolol, protamine, pyridoxine, quiNIDine, ranitidine, remifentanil, Ringer's, ritodrine, riTUXimab, rocuronium, sargramostim, sodium acetate, succinylcholine, SUFentanil, tacrolimus, temocillin, teniposide, theophylline, thiamine, thiotepa, ticarcillin, ticarcillin-clavulanate, tigecycline, tirofiban, TNA, tobramycin, tolazoline, TPN, trastuzumab, trimetaphan, urokinase, vancomycin, vasopressin, vecuronium, verapamil, vinCRIStine, vinorelbine, vitamin B complex/C, voriconazole, warfarin, zidovudine, zoledronic acid

SIDE EFFECTS

CNS: *Headache,* anxiety
CV: *Palpitations, tachycardia, hypertension, ectopic beats, angina, wide QRS complex,* peripheral vasoconstriction, hypotension
GI: *Nausea, vomiting, diarrhea*
INTEG: Necrosis, tissue sloughing with extravasation, gangrene
RESP: Dyspnea

PHARMACOKINETICS

IV: Onset 5 min; duration <10 min; metabolized in liver, kidney, plasma; excreted in urine (metabolites); half-life 2 min

INTERACTIONS

- Do not use within 2 wk of MAOIs; hypertensive crisis may result

Increase: bradycardia, hypotension—phenytoin
Increase: dysrhythmias—general anesthetics
Increase: severe hypertension—ergots
Increase: B/P—oxytocics
Increase: pressor effect—tricyclics, MAOIs
Decrease: DOPamine action—β-/α-blockers
Drug/Lab Test
Increase: urinary catecholamine, serum glucose

NURSING CONSIDERATIONS

Assess:

- Hypovolemia; if present, correct first
- **Oxygenation/perfusion deficit:** check B/P, chest pain, dizziness, loss of consciousness
- **Heart failure:** S_3 gallop, dyspnea, neck venous distention, bibasilar crackles in patients with CHF, cardiomyopathy, palpate peripheral pulses
- I&O ratio: if urine output decreases without decrease in B/P, product may need to be reduced
- **ECG** during administration continuously; if B/P increases, product should be decreased; PCWP, CVP during inf
- B/P, pulse q5min
- Paresthesias and coldness of extremities; peripheral blood flow may decrease
- Inj site: tissue sloughing; if this occurs, administer phentolamine mixed with NS

Perform/provide:

- Storage of reconstituted sol for up to 24 hr if refrigerated
- Do not use discolored sol; protect from light

Evaluate:

- Therapeutic response: increased B/P with stabilization; increased urine output

Teach patient/family:

- About the reason for product administration

TREATMENT OF OVERDOSE:

Discontinue IV, may give a short-acting α-adrenergic blocker

doripenem (Rx)

(dore-i-pen′em)
Doribax
Func. class.: Antiinfective—miscellaneous
Chem. class.: Carbapenem

ACTION: Bactericidal; interferes with cell-wall replication of susceptible organisms; osmotically unstable cell wall swells, bursts from osmotic pressure

USES: Serious infections caused by *Acinetobacter baumannii, Bacteroides caccae, Bacteroides fragilis, Bacteroides thetaiotaomicron, Bacteroides uniformis, Bacteroides vulgatus, Escherichia coli, Klebsiella pneumoniae, Peptostreptococcus micros, Proteus mirabilis, Pseudomonas aeruginosa, Streptococcus constellatus, Streptococcus intermedius*; complicated urinary tract infections, pyelonephritis, complicated intraabdominal infections

CONTRAINDICATIONS: Hypersensitivity to carbapenems (meropenem, doripenem, imipenem), penicillin, β-lactam; viral infection

Precautions: Pregnancy (B), breastfeeding, geriatric patients, renal disease, seizure disorder, pseudomembranous colitis, nebulizer or inhalation use

DOSAGE AND ROUTES

• **Adult: IV** 500 mg q8hr × 5-14 days; if improvement occurs after 3 days, switch to appropriate oral product

Renal dose

• **Adult: IV** CCr 30-50 ml/min, 250 mg over 1 hr, q8hr; CCr >10 to <30 ml/min, 250 mg over 1 hr q12hr; CCr ≤10 ml/min, no data

Available forms: Powder for inj 250, 500 mg

Administer:

Intermittent IV INF route

• After C&S is taken

• 500-mg dose using 500-mg vial: constitute vial with 10 ml sterile water for inj or NaCl 0.9%; gently shake (50 mg/ml); sol must be further diluted using a 21G needle; withdraw susp, add to 100-ml inf bag of D_5W; gently shake until clear

• 250-mg dose using 500-mg vial: constitute vial with 10 ml sterile water for inj or NaCl 0.9%; gently shake (50 mg/ml); sol must be further diluted using a 21G needle; withdraw susp and add to 100-ml inf bag of D_5W; gently shake; remove 55 ml of sol; discard; remaining sol contains 250 mg doripenem (4.5 mg/ml)

• 250-mg dose using 250-mg vial: constitute vial with 10 ml sterile water for inj or NaCl 0.9%; gently shake (25 mg/ml); sol must be further diluted using a 21G needle; withdraw susp and add to 50 or 100 ml D_5W or NS, gently shake (4.2 mg/ml 50-ml inf bag, 2.3 mg/ml 100-ml inf bag)

• Infuse over 1 hr

• Storage: constituted sol may be held in vial for ≤1 hr before transfer/dilution in inf bag; diluted inf sol stable for ≤12 hr in NS, 4 hrs in D_5W at room temp; 73 hr in NS or 24 hr in D_5W refrigerated; do not freeze constituted sol; if Baxter Mini bag inf bags used, consult instructions from Baxter

• Do not mix with or physically add to sol containing other drugs

Y-site compatibilities: Acyclovir, amikacin, aminophylline, amiodarone, anidulafungin, atropine, azithromycin, bumetanide, calcium gluconate, CARBOplatin, caspofungin, ceftobiprole, cimetidine, ciprofloxacin, CISplatin, cyclophosphamide, cycloSPORINE, DAPTOmycin, dexamethasone, digoxin, diltiazem, diphenhydrAMINE, DOBUTamine, docetaxel, DOPamine, DOXOrubicin, enalaprilat, esmolol, esomeprazole, etoposide, famotidine, fentaNYL, fluconazole, fluorouracil, foscarnet, furosemide, gemcitabine, gentamicin, granisetron, heparin, hydrocortisone, HYDROmorphone, ifosfamide, insulin (regular), labetalol, levofloxacin, linezolid, LORazepam, magnesium sulfate, mannitol, meperidine, methotrexate, methylPREDNISolone, metoclopramide, metroNIDAZOLE, micafungin, midazolam, milrinone, morphine, moxifloxacin, norepinephrine, ondansetron, paclitaxel, pantoprazole, PHENobarbital, phenylephrine, potassium chloride, ranitidine, sodium bicarbonate/phosphates, tacrolimus, tigecycline, tobramycin, vancomycin, voriconazole, zidovudine

Solution compatibilities: D_5W, 0.9% NaCl, sterile water for inj

SIDE EFFECTS

CNS: Seizures, headache
GI: Diarrhea, nausea, vomiting, pseudomembranous colitis, hepatitis
HEMA: Neutropenia, leukopenia, anemia
INTEG: *Rash,* urticaria, phlebitis, erythema at inj site, Stevens-Johnson syndrome, toxic epidermal necrolysis, pruritus
SYST: Anaphylaxis

PHARMACOKINETICS

IV: Distributed to most body fluids/tissue, excreted mainly unchanged in urine, 70% recovered in 48 hr, half-life 1 hr, half-life extended in renal disease

INTERACTIONS

Increase: doripenem plasma levels—probenecid
Decrease: effect of valproic acid, divalproex sodium
Drug/Lab Test
Increase: AST, ALT, LDH, BUN, alk phos, bilirubin, creatinine
False positive: direct Coombs' test

NURSING CONSIDERATIONS

Assess:
- Sensitivity to carbapenem antibiotics, penicillins
- Renal disease: lower dose may be required
- Bowel pattern daily; if severe diarrhea occurs, product should be discontinued; may indicate pseudomembranous colitis
- For infection: temp; sputum; characteristics of wound before, during, and after treatment

⚠ **Allergic reactions, anaphylaxis:** rash, urticaria, pruritus; may occur few days after therapy begins
- **Overgrowth of infection:** perineal itching, fever, malaise, redness, pain, swelling, drainage, rash, diarrhea, change in cough, sputum

Evaluate:
- Therapeutic response: negative C&S; absence of symptoms and signs of infection

Teach patient/family:
- To report severe diarrhea; may indicate pseudomembranous colitis
- To report sore throat, bruising, bleeding, joint pain; may indicate blood dyscrasias (rare)
- To report overgrowth of infection: black, furry tongue; vaginal itching; foul-smelling stools
- To avoid breastfeeding; product is excreted in breast milk

TREATMENT OF HYPERSENSITIVITY: EPINEPHrine, antihistamines; resuscitate if needed (anaphylaxis)

dorzolamide ophthalmic

See Appendix B

doxazosin (Rx)

(dox-ay′zoe-sin)

Cardura, Cardura XL

Func. class.: Peripheral α_1-adrenergic receptor blocker
Chem. class.: Quinazoline

Do not confuse:
Cardura/Coumadin/Cardene/Ridaura

ACTION: Dilates peripheral blood vessels, lowers peripheral resistance; reduction in B/P results from peripheral α_1-adrenergic receptors being blocked

USES: Hypertension, urinary outflow obstruction, symptoms of benign prostatic hyperplasia

CONTRAINDICATIONS: Hypersensitivity to quinazolines
Precautions: Pregnancy (C), breastfeeding, children, hepatic disease

DOSAGE AND ROUTES

BPH

• **Adult: PO** 1 mg/day, increase in stepwise manner to 2, 4, 8 mg/day as needed at 1-2 wk intervals, max 8 mg

Hypertension

• **Adult: PO** 1 mg/day increasing up to 16 mg/day if required; usual range 4-16 mg/day

• **Geriatric: PO** 0.5 mg nightly, gradually increase

Available forms: Tabs 1, 2, 4, 8 mg; ext rel tabs 4, 8 mg

Administer:

• **Tabs** broken, crushed, or chewed; if chewed, will be bitter; do not break, crush, chew XL tabs

• **Immediate release tab:** without regard to meals; **ext rel tabs:** give with breakfast; when switching from immediate release to ext rel, the final evening dose of immediate release should not be taken

SIDE EFFECTS

CNS: *Dizziness*, headache, drowsiness, anxiety, depression, vertigo, weakness, fatigue, asthenia

CV: Palpitations, *orthostatic hypotension*, tachycardia, edema, dysrhythmias, chest pain

EENT: Epistaxis, tinnitus, dry mouth, red sclera, pharyngitis, rhinitis

GI: Nausea, vomiting, diarrhea, constipation, abdominal pain

GU: Incontinence, polyuria, priapism

PHARMACOKINETICS

PO: Onset 2 hr, peak 2-6 hr, duration 6-12 hr, half-life 22 hr, metabolized in liver, excreted via bile/feces (<63%) and in urine (9%), extensively protein bound (98%)

INTERACTIONS

Increase: hypotensive effects—alcohol, other antihypertensives, sildenafil, vardenafil, nitrates

Decrease: antihypertensive effects of cloNIDine

NURSING CONSIDERATIONS

Assess:

• **Hypertension:** B/P (lying, standing), pulse 2-6 hr after each dose, with each increase; postural effects may occur, crackles, dyspnea, orthopnea with B/P; pulse; jugular venous distention during beginning treatment

• **BPH:** urinary pattern changes (hesitancy, dribbling, incomplete bladder emptying, dysuria, urgency, nocturia, urgency incontinence, intermittency) before and during treatment

• I&O, weight daily; edema in feet, legs daily

Perform/provide:

• Storage in tight container in cool environment

Evaluate:

• Therapeutic response: decreased B/P; decreased symptoms of BPH

Teach patient/family:

• That fainting occasionally occurs after 1st dose; not to drive, operate machinery for 4 hr after 1st dose, after dosage increase; to take 1st dose at bedtime; may take 1-2 wk to respond with BPH

TREATMENT OF OVERDOSE:

Administer volume expanders or vasopressors; discontinue product; place patient in supine position

doxepin (Rx)

(dox′e-pin)

Apo-Doxepin ♣, Prudoxin Cream, Silenor, Zonalon Topical Cream

Func. class.: Antidepressant, tricyclic, antihistamine (topical)

Chem. class.: Dibenzoxepin, tertiary amine

ACTION: Blocks reuptake of norepinephrine, serotonin into nerve endings, increasing action of norepinephrine, serotonin in nerve cells

USES:
Major depression, anxiety; *topical:* lichen simplex, atopic dermatitis, eczema

Unlabeled uses: Topical pruritus, insomnia, migraine prophylaxis

CONTRAINDICATIONS:
Hypersensitivity to tricyclics, urinary retention, closed-angle glaucoma, prostatic hypertrophy, acute recovery from MI

Precautions: Pregnancy (C) (PO) (B) (topical), breastfeeding, geriatric patients, seizures

Black Box Warning: Children, suicidal patients

DOSAGE AND ROUTES

Depression/anxiety

- **Adult: PO** 50-75 mg/day, may increase to 300 mg/day for severely ill; give in divided doses if >150 mg/day
- **Geriatric: PO** 25-50 mg at bedtime, increase weekly by 25-50 mg to desired dose, max 150 mg/day

Pruritus

- **Adult: PO** 10 mg at bedtime, may increase to 25 mg at bedtime; **TOP** apply thin film qid at least 3 hr apart

Insomnia (Silenor)

- **Adult: PO** 6 mg 30 min before bedtime, 3 mg may be sufficient, max 6 mg/night

Available forms: Caps 10, 25, 50, 75, 100, 150 mg; oral conc 10 mg/ml; cream 5%; tabs (Silenor) 3, 6 mg

Administer:

- **Oral conc:** should be diluted with 120 ml water, milk or orange, grapefruit, tomato, prune, or pineapple juice; do not mix with grape juice
- Increased fluids, bulk in diet for constipation
- With food, milk for GI symptoms; do not give with carbonated beverages
- Dosage at bedtime to avoid oversedation during day; may take entire dose at bedtime; geriatric patients may not tolerate daily dosing
- Gum, hard candy, or frequent sips of water for dry mouth
- **Topical:** by applying to affected area, rub slightly; do not use occlusive dressings

SIDE EFFECTS

CNS: *Dizziness, drowsiness,* confusion, headache, anxiety, tremors, stimulation, weakness, insomnia, nightmares, EPS (geriatric patients), increased psychiatric symptoms, paresthesia, **suicidal ideation**

CV: *Orthostatic hypotension, ECG changes, tachycardia,* **hypertension, palpitations, dysrhythmias**

EENT: *Blurred vision,* tinnitus, mydriasis, ophthalmoplegia, glossitis

GI: *Diarrhea, dry mouth,* nausea, vomiting, **paralytic ileus,** increased appetite, cramps, epigastric distress, jaundice, **hepatitis,** stomatitis, constipation

GU: *Urinary retention,* **acute renal failure**

HEMA: **Agranulocytosis, thrombocytopenia, eosinophilia, leukopenia, pancytopenia,** purpuric disorder

INTEG: Rash, urticaria, sweating, pruritus, photosensitivity

PHARMACOKINETICS

PO: Steady state 2-8 days, metabolized by liver, excreted by kidneys, crosses placenta, excreted in breast milk, half-life 8-24 hr

INTERACTIONS

Increase: hyperpyretic crisis, seizures, hypertensive episode—MAOIs

Increase: hypertensive action—EPINEPHrine, norepinephrine

Increase: hypertensive crisis—cloNIDine; do not use together

Increase: doxepin effect—cimetidine, FLUoxetine, fluvoxamine, paroxetine, sertraline

Increase: CNS depression—barbiturates, benzodiazepines, sedative/hypnotics, alcohol, other CNS depressants

Increase: QT interval: class IC/III antiarrhythmics (propafenone, flecainide), quinolones

Serotonin syndrome
Increase: toxicity—SSRIs, SNRIs, serotonin-receptor agonists
Increase: anticholinergic effects—anticholinergics
Drug/Herb
• Serotonin syndrome: St. John's wort
Drug/Lab Test
Increase: serum bilirubin, blood glucose, alk phos, LFTs

NURSING CONSIDERATIONS

Assess:
• B/P (lying, standing), pulse q4hr; if systolic B/P drops 20 mm Hg, hold product, notify prescriber; VS q4hr in patients with CV disease
• Blood studies: CBC, leukocytes, differential, cardiac enzymes if patient is receiving long-term therapy
• Hepatic studies: AST, ALT, bilirubin
• Weight weekly; appetite may increase with product
• **ECG** for flattening of T wave, bundle branch block, AV block, dysrhythmias in cardiac patients; product should be discontinued gradually several days before surgery
• **EPS** primarily in geriatric patients: rigidity, dystonia, akathisia
• **Depression:** mood, sensorium, affect, suicidal tendencies, increase in psychiatric symptoms
• **Chronic pain:** location, severity, type before and during treatment, alleviating/aggravating factors
• Urinary retention, constipation; constipation most likely in children, geriatric patients
• **Withdrawal symptoms:** headache, nausea, vomiting, muscle pain, weakness; not usual unless product is discontinued abruptly
• Alcohol consumption; if alcohol is consumed, hold dose until morning
Perform/provide:
• Storage in tight container protected from direct sunlight
• Assistance with ambulation during beginning therapy, since drowsiness/dizziness occurs; safety measures primarily for geriatric patients
• Check to confirm that PO medication is swallowed
Evaluate:
• Therapeutic response: decreased anxiety, depression
Teach patient/family:
• That therapeutic effect (depression) may take 2-3 wk, antianxiety effects sooner
• To use caution when driving, during other activities requiring alertness because of drowsiness, dizziness, blurred vision
• To avoid alcohol, other CNS depressants; may potentiate effects
• Not to discontinue medication abruptly after long-term use; may cause nausea, headache, malaise
• To wear sunscreen or large hat, since photosensitivity occurs
• That clinical worsening and suicide may occur
• To immediately report urinary retention

TREATMENT OF OVERDOSE:

ECG monitoring; lavage, activated charcoal; administer anticonvulsant, sodium bicarbonate

doxercalciferol (Rx)

Hectorol
Func. class.: Parathyroid agent (calcium regulator)
Chem. class.: Vit D hormone

ACTION: Synthetic vit D analog; reduces parathyroid hormone

USES: To lower high parathyroid hormone levels in patients undergoing chronic kidney dialysis; for those in stages 3 or 4 of chronic renal disease prior to dialysis
Unlabeled uses: Renal osteodystrophy

CONTRAINDICATIONS:
Hypersensitivity, hyperphosphatemia, hypercalcemia, vit D toxicity

Precautions: Pregnancy (C), breastfeeding, renal calculi, CV disease, hepatic disease

DOSAGE AND ROUTES

Secondary hyperparathyroidism; renal osteodystrophy (unlabeled)

- **Adult: PO** 1 mcg/day, max 3.5 mcg/day; if iPTH level >70 pg/ml or >110 pg/ml, increase dose by 0.5 mcg q2wk as needed; if iPTH 35-70 pg/ml or 70-110 pg/ml, maintain dose; if iPTH <35 pg/ml or <70 pg/ml, hold dose for 1 wk, resume dose at 0.5 mcg lower than previous

Stage 5 chronic kidney disease in patient on dialysis

- **Adult: PO** 10 mcg 3×/wk at dialysis (iPTH >400 pg/ml), max 20 mcg 3×/wk; **IV BOL** 4 mcg 3×/wk end of dialysis (iPTH >400 pg/ml), max 6 mcg 3×/wk (initially); if iPTH decreases by <50% and >300 pg/ml, increase dose by 2.5 mcg **PO** or 1-2 mcg **IV** q8wk as needed; if iPTH decreases by >50% and <300 pg/ml, maintain **IV** dose; if iPTH are 150-300 pg/ml, maintain dose; if iPTH is 100-149 pg/ml, 2.5 mcg **PO** or 1 mcg **IV**, lower than previous dose

Available forms: Caps 0.5, 1, 2.5 mcg; inj 2 mcg/ml

Administer:

- Do not break, crush, or chew caps

SIDE EFFECTS

CNS: Drowsiness, headache, lethargy

GI: Nausea, diarrhea, vomiting, anorexia, dry mouth, constipation, cramps, metallic taste

GU: Polyuria, hypercalciuria, hyperphosphatemia, hematuria

MS: Myalgia, arthralgia, decreased bone development

RESP: SOB

PHARMACOKINETICS

Peak 11-12 hr, metabolized in liver, terminal half-life 32-37 hr

INTERACTIONS

Decrease: absorption of doxercalciferol—cholestyramine, magnesium antacids, mineral oil; do not use together

NURSING CONSIDERATIONS

Assess:

- BUN, urinary calcium, AST, ALT, cholesterol, creatinine, albumin, uric acid, electrolytes, urine pH, phosphate; may increase calcium, should be kept at 9-10 mg/dl, vit D 50-135 international units/dl, phosphate 70 mg/dl, intact parathyroid hormone conc (iPTH) target 150-300 pg/ml, serum calcium
- For increased drug level, since toxic reactions may occur rapidly
- For dry mouth, metallic taste, polyuria, bone pain, muscle weakness, headache, fatigue, change in LOC, dysrhythmias, increased respirations, anorexia, nausea, vomiting, cramps, diarrhea, constipation; may indicate hypercalcemia
- Renal status: decreased urinary output (oliguria, anuria), edema in extremities, weight gain 5-7 lb, periorbital edema
- Nutritional status, diet for sources of vit D (milk, some seafood), calcium (dairy products, dark green vegetables), phosphates (dairy products) must be avoided

Perform/provide:

- Storage protected from light, heat, moisture
- Restriction of sodium, potassium if required
- Restriction of fluids if required for chronic renal failure

Evaluate:

- Therapeutic response: calcium 9-10 mg/dl, decreasing symptoms of hypocalcemia, hypoparathyroidism

Teach patient/family:

- About the symptoms of hypercalcemia
- About foods rich in calcium; to avoid all preparations containing vit D

• To avoid products with sodium in chronic renal failure: cured meats, dairy products, cold cuts, olives, beets, pickles, soups, meat tenderizers
• To avoid products with potassium in chronic renal failure: oranges, bananas, dried fruit, peas, dark green leafy vegetables, milk, melons, beans
• To avoid OTC products containing calcium, potassium, sodium, and antacids in chronic renal failure
• To monitor weight weekly

⚠ HIGH ALERT

DOXOrubicin (Rx)

(dox-oh-roo′bi-sin)

Adriamycin, Adriamycin PFS ✱, Caelyx ✱

DOXOrubicin liposomal (Rx)

Doxil

Func. class.: Antineoplastic, antibiotic
Chem. class.: Anthracycline glycoside

Do not confuse:
DOXOrubicin/Idamycin/DAUNOrubicin
Adriamycin/Aredia/Idamycin

ACTION: Inhibits DNA synthesis primarily; derived from Streptomyces peucetius; replication is decreased by binding to DNA, which causes strand splitting; active throughout entire cell cycle; a vesicant

USES: Wilms' tumor; bladder, breast, liver, lung, ovarian, stomach, testicular, thyroid cancer; Hodgkin's disease; acute lymphoblastic leukemia; myeloblastic leukemia; neuroblastomas; lymphomas; sarcomas; *Doxil:* AIDS-related Kaposi's sarcoma, metastatic ovarian carcinoma
Unlabeled uses: Colorectal hepatocellular, pancreatic cancer, desmoid tumor, malignant melanoma, multiple myeloma

CONTRAINDICATIONS: Pregnancy (D) 1st trimester, breastfeeding, hypersensitivity, systemic infections, cardiac disorders
Precautions: Cardiac/renal disease, gout

Black Box Warning: Hepatic disease, bone marrow depression (severe), extravasation, heart failure, secondary malignancy

DOSAGE AND ROUTES

DOXOrubicin

ALL
• **Adult and child:** **IV** 30 mg/m²/wk × 4 wk or 30 mg/m² on day 1, 2, 14 of induction or 20 mg/m² on 15, 16, 17 as part multiregimen

AML
• **Adult and child:** **IV** 30 mg/m²/day × 3 days, may repeat q4wk

Ovarian cancer
• **Adult:** **IV** 40-50 mg/m²/mo

Hepatic dose
• **Adult:** **IV** Bilirubin 1.2-3 mg/dl, give 50% of dose; bilirubin 3.1-5 mg/dl, give 25% of dose

Gastric/pancreatic cancer (unlabeled)
• **Adult:** **IV** 30 mg/m²/dose on days 1 and 29 q8wk; given with fluorouracil/mitomycin

Multiple myeloma (unlabeled)
• **Adult:** **IV** 9 mg/m²/day as **CONT IV** × 4 days with vinCRIStine/dexamethasone (VAD regimen)

DOXOrubicin liposomal

Kaposi's sarcoma
• **Adult:** **IV** 20 mg/m² q3wk

Available forms: Inj 10, 20, 50, 100, 150 mg; liposomal dispersion for inj: (Doxil) 2 mg/ml

Administer:
• Antiemetic 30-60 min before product to prevent vomiting
• Allopurinol or sodium bicarbonate to maintain uric acid levels, alkalinization of urine
• Topical or systemic analgesics for pain
• Antispasmodic for GI symptoms

IV route

- Use cytotoxic handling procedures

⚠ **Do not interchange DOXOrubicin with DOXOrubicin liposomal**

Direct IV route (DOXOrubicin)

- IV after diluting 10 mg/5 ml of NaCl for inj; another 5 ml of diluent/10 mg is recommended; shake; give over 3-5 min; give through Y-tube of free-flowing 5% dextrose INF or NS

Y-site compatibilities: Alemtuzumab, alfentanil, amifostine, amikacin, anidulafungin, argatroban, aztreonam, bivalirudin, bleomycin, bumetanide, buprenorphine, butorphanol, calcium chloride/gluconate, CARBOplatin, carmustine, caspofungin, ceftizoxime, chlorproMAZINE, cimetidine, ciprofloxacin, CISplatin, cladribine, clindamycin, cyclophosphamide, cycloSPORINE, cytarabine, DACTINomycin, DAPTOmycin, dexamethasone, dexmedetomidine, dexrazoxane, diltiazem, diphenhydrAMINE, DOBUTamine, docetaxel, dolasetron, DOPamine, doripenem, doxycycline, droperidol, enalaprilat, ePHEDrine, EPINEPHrine, erythromycin, esmolol, etoposide, etoposide phosphate, famotidine, fenoldopam, fentaNYL, filgrastim, fluconazole, fludarabine, gemcitabine, gentamicin, granisetron, haloperidol, hydrocortisone, HYDROmorphone, ifosfamide, imipenem cilastatin, inamrinone, isoproterenol, ketorolac, labetalol, leucovorin, levorphanol, lidocaine, linezolid, LORazepam, mannitol, mechlorethamine, melphalan, meperidine, mesna, methotrexate, metoclopramide, metoprolol, metroNIDAZOLE, midazolam, milrinone, mitomycin, morphine, nalbuphine, naloxone, nesiritide, niCARdipine, nitroglycerin, nitroprusside, octreotide, ofloxacin, ondansetron, oxaliplatin, paclitaxel, palonosetron, pancuronium, phenylephrine, potassium chloride, procainamide, prochlorperazine, promethazine, propranolol, quinupristin-dalfopristin, ranitidine, sargramostim, sodium acetate, tacrolimus, teniposide, theophylline, thiotepa, ticarcillin/clavulanate, tigecycline, tirofiban, tobramycin, topotecan, trastuzumab, trimethobenzamide, vancomycin, vasopressin, vecuronium, verapamil, vinBLAStine, vinCRIStine, vinorelbine, zidovudine, zoledronic acid

Intermittent IV INF route (DOXOrubicin liposomal)

- Dilute dose up to 90 mg/250 ml D_5W, give over 1/2 hr; do not admix with other sol or meds
- Dose modifications for toxicity: Grade 1, redose unless patient has experienced previous grade 3 or 4; Grade 2, delay dosing up to 2 wk or until resolved to grade 0 or 1; Grade 3, delay dosing up to 2 wk or until resolved to grade 0 or 1, resume dose at 25% decrease, return to original dosing after interval; Grade 4, delay dosing up to 2 wk or until grade 0 or 1, resume dose at 25% decrease then return to original dose, discontinue if no resolution after 2 wk

Y-site compatibilities: Acyclovir, allopurinol, aminophylline, ampicillin, aztreonam, bleomycin, butorphanol, calcium gluconate, CARBOplatin, ceFAZolin, cefepime, cefoxitin, ceftizoxime, cefTRIAXone, chlorproMAZINE, cimetidine, ciprofloxacin, CISplatin, clindamycin, cyclophosphamide, cytarabine, dacarbazine, dexamethasone, diphenhydrAMINE, DOBUTamine, DOPamine, droperidol, enalaprilat, etoposide, famotidine, fluconazole, fluorouracil, furosemide, ganciclovir, gentamicin, granisetron, haloperidol, heparin, hydrocortisone, HYDROmorphone, ifosfamide, leucovorin, LORazepam, magnesium sulfate, mesna, methotrexate, methylPREDNISolone, metroNIDAZOLE, ondansetron, piperacillin, potassium chloride, prochlorperazine, ranitidine, ticarcillin/clavulanate, tobramycin, trimethoprim-sulfamethoxazole, vancomycin, vinBLAStine, vinCRIStine, vinorelbine, zidovudine

SIDE EFFECTS

CV: Increased B/P, sinus tachycardia, PVCs, chest pain, bradycardia, extrasystoles

GI: *Nausea, vomiting,* anorexia, *mucositis,* hepatotoxicity

GU: Impotence, sterility, amenorrhea, gynecomastia, hyperuricemia

HEMA: Thrombocytopenia, leukopenia, anemia

INTEG: *Rash, necrosis at inj site,* dermatitis, reversible *alopecia,* cellulitis, thrombophlebitis at inj site

PHARMACOKINETICS

Triphasic pattern of elimination; half-life 12 min, 3¹/₃ hr, 29²/₃ hr; metabolized by liver; crosses placenta; excreted in urine, bile, breast milk

INTERACTIONS

Increase: hepatotoxicity—mercaptopurine

Increase: toxicity—other antineoplastics or radiation, mercaptopurine

Increase: hemorrhagic cystitis risk, cardiac toxicity—cyclophosphamide

Decrease: antibody response—live virus vaccine

Decrease: antineoplastic effect—hematopoietic progenitor cell; do not use 24 hr before or after treatment

Drug/Lab Test

Increase: uric acid

NURSING CONSIDERATIONS

Assess:

Black Box Warning: Bone marrow depression: CBC, differential, platelet count weekly; withhold product if WBC is <4000/mm³ or platelet count is <75,000/mm³; notify prescriber of these results

- Renal studies: BUN, serum uric acid, urine CCr, electrolytes before, during therapy
- I&O ratio; report fall in urine output to <30 ml/hr
- Monitor temp q4hr; fever may indicate beginning infection

Black Box Warning: Hepatotoxicity: hepatic studies before, during therapy: bilirubin, AST, ALT, alk phos as needed or monthly; check for jaundice of skin and sclera, dark urine, clay-colored stools, itchy skin, abdominal pain, fever, diarrhea

Black Box Warning: Dysrhythmias: ECG; watch for ST-T wave changes, low QRS and T, possible dysrhythmias (sinus tachycardia, heart block, PVCs), ejection fraction before treatment, signs of irreversible cardiomyopathy, can occur up to 6 mo after treatment begins

- Bleeding: hematuria, guaiac, bruising, petechiae of mucosa or orifices q8hr
- Effects of alopecia on body image; discuss feelings about body changes; almost total alopecia is expected
- Inflammation of mucosa, breaks in skin
- Buccal cavity q8hr for dryness, sores, ulceration, white patches, oral pain, bleeding, dysphagia
- Alkalosis if severe vomiting is present
- **Extravasation:** local irritation, pain, burning at inj site; a vesicant; if extravasation occurs, stop drug, restart at another site, apply ice, elevate extremity to reduce swelling; if resolution does not occur, surgical debridement may be required
- GI symptoms: frequency of stools, cramping

Perform/provide:

- Liquid diet: carbonated beverages, gelatin may be added if patient is not nauseated or vomiting
- Increased fluid intake to 2-3 L/day to prevent urate, calculi formation
- Rinsing of mouth tid-qid with water, club soda; brushing of teeth bid-tid with soft brush or cotton-tipped applicators for stomatitis; use unwaxed dental floss
- Storage at room temp for 24 hr after reconstituting or 48 hr refrigerated

Evaluate:

- Therapeutic response: decreased tumor size, spread of malignancy

Teach patient/family:

- To add 2-3 L of fluids unless contraindicated prior to and for 24-48 hr after to decrease possible **hemorrhagic cystitis**
- To report any complaints, side effects to nurse or prescriber
- That hair may be lost during treatment; that wig or hairpiece may make patient feel better; that new hair may be different in color, texture
- To avoid foods with citric acid, hot or rough texture
- To report any bleeding, white spots, ulcerations in mouth to prescriber; to examine mouth daily
- That urine, other body fluids may be red-orange for 48 hr
- To avoid crowds and persons with infections when granulocyte count is low
- That barrier contraceptive measures are recommended during therapy and for 4 mo after (pregnancy [D]); to avoid breastfeeding
- To avoid vaccinations because reactions may occur; to avoid alcohol

doxycycline (Rx)

(dox-i-sye′kleen)

Oracea

doxycycline calcium

Vibramycin

doxycycline hyclate

Adoxa, Apo-Doxy ✱, Doryx, Doxy, Doxycaps, Doxycin ✱, Periostat, Vibramycin, Vibra-Tabs

doxycycline monohydrate

Adoxa, Monodox, Vibramycin

Func. class.: Antiinfective

Chem. class.: Tetracycline

Do not confuse:
doxycycline/doxepin/dicyclomine

ACTION: Inhibits protein synthesis, phosphorylation in microorganisms by binding to 30S ribosomal subunits, reversibly binding to 50S ribosomal subunits; bacteriostatic

USES: Syphilis, *Chlamydia trachomatis,* gonorrhea, *Rickettsia*, lymphogranuloma venereum, uncommon gram-negative/gram-positive organisms, malaria prophylaxis, chronic periodontitis, acne, anthrax, Lyme disease

Unlabeled uses: Traveler's diarrhea, prevention of chronic bronchitis, leptospirosis, pleural effusion, malaria (chloroquine-resistant *Plasmodium falciparum*)

CONTRAINDICATIONS: Pregnancy (D), children <8 yr, hypersensitivity to tetracyclines, esophageal ulceration

Precautions: Breastfeeding, hepatic disease, pseudomembranous colitis, ulcerative colitis

DOSAGE AND ROUTES

Most infections

- **Adult: PO/IV** 100 mg q12hr on day 1 then 100 mg/day; **IV** 200 mg in 1-2 inf on day 1 then 100-200 mg/day
- **Child >8 yr, ≥45 kg: PO** 100 mg q12hr on day 1 then 100 mg daily; severe infections 100 mg q12hr; **IV** 200 mg on day 1 then 100-200 mg daily, give 200 mg dose as 1 or 2 inf
- **Child ≥8 yr, <45 kg: PO** 2.2 mg/kg q12hr on day 1 then 2.2 mg/kg daily, severe infections 2.2 mg/kg q12hr; **IV** 4.4 mg/kg on day 1 then 2.2-4.4 mg/kg daily in 1 to 2 divided doses

Gonorrhea (uncomplicated) in patients allergic to penicillin

- **Adult: PO** 100 mg q12hr × 7 days or 300 mg followed 1 hr later by another 300 mg

Malaria prophylaxis

- **Adult: PO** 100 mg/day 1-2 days prior to travel, daily during travel, and for 4 wk after return
- **Adolescent/child ≥8 yr, <45 kg: PO** 2 mg/kg (up to 100 mg/day) begin 1-2

days prior to travel, continue for 4 wk after return

C. trachomatis

• **Adult: PO** 100 mg bid × 7 days

Syphilis

• **Adult: PO** 100 mg bid × 14 days

Anthrax

• **Adult and child >8 yr and ≥45 kg: IV** 100 mg q12hr; change to **PO** when able × 60 days

• **Adolescent/child ≥8 yr and <45 kg: PO** 2.2 mg/kg q12hr × 60 days; **IV** 100 mg q12hr, change to **PO** when able × 60 days

Lyme disease

• **Adult/adolescent/child ≥8 yr: PO** 100 mg bid × 10-21 days

Periodontitis

• **Adult:** 20 mg bid after scaling and root planing for ≤9 mo; give close to meal time AM or PM

Pleural effusion (unlabeled)

• **Adult: INTRACAVITARY** 500 mg diluted with 250 ml 0.9% NaCl given by chest tube lavage and drainage

Available forms: Doxycycline: cap 40 mg; doxycycline calcium: syrup 50 mg/5 ml; doxycycline hyclate: cap 50, 100 mg; pellet caps 75, 100 mg; inj 42.5, 100, 200 mg; tabs 20, 100 mg; doxycycline monohydrate: caps 50, 100 mg; tabs 50, 75, 100 mg; oral susp 25 mg/5 ml

Administer:

PO route

• Do not break, crush, or chew caps; may crush tabs and mix with food

• On empty stomach or with full glass of water 2 hr before or after meals; avoid dairy products, antacids, laxatives, iron-containing products; if these must be taken, give 2 hr before or after product; avoid giving oral products within 1 hr of bedtime, esophageal uleration may occur

Intermittent IV INF route

• After diluting 100 mg or less/10 ml of sterile water or NS for inj, further dilute with 100-1000 ml of NaCl, D_5, Ringer's, LR D_5LR, Normosol-M, Normosol-R in D_5W; run 100 mg or less over 1-4 hr; do not give; inf must be completed in 6 hr when diluted in LR sol or 12 hr with other sol; protect from light, heat

Y-site compatibilities: Acyclovir, alemtuzumab, alfentanil, amifostine, amikacin, aminophylline, amiodarone, anidulafungin, ascorbic acid, atracurium, atropine, aztreonam, bivalirudin, bumetanide, buprenorphine, butorphanol, calcium chloride/gluconate, CARBOplatin, caspofungin, cefonicid, cefotaxime, cefTRIAXone, chlorproMAZINE, cimetidine, cisatracurium, CISplatin, clindamycin, codeine, cyanocobalamin, cyclophosphamide, cycloSPORINE, cytarabine, DACTINomycin, DAPTOmycin, dexmedetomidine, digoxin, diltiazem, diphenhydrAMINE, DOBUTamine, docetaxel, DOPamine, doxacurium, DOXOrubicin, enalaprilat, ePHEDrine, EPINEPHrine, epirubicin, epoetin alfa, eptifibatide, ertapenem, esmolol, etoposide, etoposide phosphate, famotidine, fenoldopam, fentaNYL, filgrastim, fluconazole, fludarabine, gemcitabine, gemtuzumab, gentamicin, glycopyrrolate, granisetron, HYDROmorphone, IDArubicin, ifosfamide, imipenem/cilastatin, insulin, isoproterenol, labetalol, levofloxacin, lidocaine, linezolid, LORazepam, magnesium sulfate, mannitol, mechlorethamine, melphalan, meperidine, metaraminol, methoxamine, methyldopate, metoclopramide, metoprolol, metroNIDAZOLE, miconazole, midazolam, milrinone, mitoxantrone, morphine, multivitamins, nalbuphine, naloxone, nesiritide, netilmicin, nitroglycerin, nitroprusside, norepinephrine, octreotide, ondansetron, oxaliplatin, oxytocin, paclitaxel, pancuronium, pantoprazole, papaverine, pentamidine, pentazocine, perphenazine, phentolamine, phenylephrine, phytonadione, potassium chloride, procainamide, prochlorperazine, promethazine, propofol, propranolol, protamine, pyridoxime, quinupristin/dalfopristin, ranitidine, remifentanil, ritodrine, riTUXimab, rocuronium, sargramostim, sodium acetate, succinylcholine, SUFentanil, tacrolimus, telavancin, teniposide, theophylline, thiamine, thiotepa, tirofiban, tobramycin, tolazoline, TPN (2 in 1), trastuzumab, trimetaphan, urokinase, vancomycin, vasopressin, vecuronium, verapamil, vinCRIStine, vinorelbine, voriconazole, zoledronic acid

SIDE EFFECTS

CNS: Fever
CV: Pericarditis
EENT: Dysphagia, glossitis, decreased calcification of deciduous teeth, oral candidiasis, tooth discoloration
GI: *Nausea, abdominal pain, vomiting, diarrhea,* anorexia, enterocolitis, **hepatotoxicity**, flatulence, abdominal cramps, gastric burning, stomatitis
GU: *Increased BUN*
HEMA: **Eosinophilia, neutropenia, thrombocytopenia, hemolytic anemia**
INTEG: *Rash, urticaria, photosensitivity, increased pigmentation,* **exfoliative dermatitis**, pruritus
MS: Bone growth retardation (<8 yr old)
SYST: **Stevens-Johnson syndrome, angioedema, anaphylaxis**

PHARMACOKINETICS

PO: Well absorbed; widely distributed; peak 1½-4 hr; half-life 14-17 hr; excreted in urine, feces, bile; 23%-93% protein bound; crosses placenta; enters breast milk

INTERACTIONS

Increase: effect of—anticoagulants, digoxin
Decrease: doxycycline effect—antacids, $NaHCO_3$, dairy products, alkali products, iron, kaolin/pectin, barbiturates, carBAMazepine, phenytoin, cimetidine sucralfate, cholestyramine, colestipol, rifampin, bismuth; iron, magnesium, zinc, calcium, aluminum salts
Decrease: effects—penicillins, oral contraceptives, digoxin

Drug/Lab Test
Increase: BUN, alk phos, bilirubin, amylase, ALT, AST, eosinophils, WBC
Decrease: Hgb
False increase: urinary catecholamines

NURSING CONSIDERATIONS

Assess:
- I&O ratio
- Blood studies: PT, CBC, AST, ALT, BUN, creatinine
- Signs of infection
- **Allergic reactions:** rash, itching, pruritus, angioedema
- Nausea, vomiting, diarrhea; administer antiemetic, antacids as ordered
- **Overgrowth of infection:** fever, malaise, redness, pain, swelling, drainage, perineal itching, diarrhea, changes in cough or sputum
- IV site for phlebitis/thrombosis; product is highly irritating
- After C&S is obtained, do not wait for results

Perform/provide:
- Storage in tight, light-resistant container at room temp; IV stable for 12 hr at room temp, 72 hr refrigerated; discard if precipitate forms

Evaluate:
- Therapeutic response: decreased temp, absence of lesions, negative C&S

Teach patient/family:
- To avoid sun because burns may occur; that sunscreen does not seem to decrease photosensitivity
- That all prescribed medication must be taken to prevent superinfection; not to use outdated products because Fanconi syndrome may occur (reversible nephrotoxicity)
- That if children ≤8 yr old are undergoing tooth development, teeth will be permanently discolored

⚠ HIGH ALERT

dronedarone (Rx)

(drone′da′rone)

Multaq

Func. class.: Antidysrhythmic (class III)

Chem. class.: Iodinated benzofuran derivative

ACTION: Prolongs duration of action potential and effective refractory period, noncompetitive α- and β-adrenergic inhibition; increases RR and QT intervals, decreases sinus rate, decreases peripheral vascular resistance

USES: Atrial fibrillation, atrial flutter

CONTRAINDICATIONS: Pregnancy (X), breastfeeding; 2nd-, 3rd-degree AV block; bradycardia, severe sinus node dysfunction, hypersensitivity, heart failure, hepatic disease, QT prolongation

Black Box Warning: NYHA Class IV heart failure or Class II-III with recent decompensation requiring hospitalization, permanent atrial fibrillation (cannot restore sinus rhythm)

Precautions: Children, geriatric patients, Asian patients, females, electrolyte imbalances, atrial fibrillation/flutter

DOSAGE AND ROUTES

• **Adult: PO** 400 mg bid; discontinue class I, III antidysrhythmics or strong CYP3A4 inhibitors prior to beginning treatment; max 800 mg/day

Available forms: Tabs 400 mg

Administer:

PO route

• Give bid with morning, evening meals

• Give MedGuide; should be dispensed with each prescription, refill

SIDE EFFECTS

CV: *Bradycardia,* heart failure, QT prolongation, torsades de pointes

ENDO: Hypo/hyperthyroidism

GI: Nausea, vomiting, diarrhea, abdominal pain, severe hepatic injury, hepatic failure

INTEG: Rash, photosensitivity

PHARMACOKINETICS

Peak 3-6 hr, half-life 13-19 hr, metabolized by liver, excreted in feces (84%), via kidneys (6%), protein binding >98%

INTERACTIONS

Increase: dronedarone levels: CYP3A inhibitors/2D6 inhibitors

Decrease: dronedarone levels: 3A/2D6 inducers

Increase: 3A/2D6 substrate levels

Increase: bradycardia—β-blockers, calcium channel blockers

Increase: levels of cycloSPORINE, dextromethorphan, digoxin, disopyramide, flecainide, methotrexate, phenytoin, procainamide, quinidine, theophylline

Increase: anticoagulant effects—dabigatran, warfarin

Drug/Herb

Increase: anticoagulant effect—yohimbine

Decrease: dronedarone effect—St. John's wort

Drug/Food:

Increase: dronedarone effect, grapefruit; avoid use

Drug/Lab Test

Increase: T_4

NURSING CONSIDERATIONS

Assess:

• **ECG** to determine product effectiveness; measure PR, QRS, QT intervals; check for PVCs, other dysrhythmias, B/P continuously for hypo/hypertension; report dysrhythmias, slowing heart rate

• Serum creatinine, potassium, magnesium

• I&O ratio; electrolytes (potassium, creatinine, magnesium)

• Dehydration or hypovolemia

• Rebound hypertension after 1-2 hr

• **Hypothyroidism:** lethargy, dizziness,

constipation, enlarged thyroid gland, edema of extremities; cool, pale skin

- **Hyperthyroidism:** restlessness, tachycardia, eyelid puffiness, weight loss, frequent urination, menstrual irregularities, dyspnea; warm, moist skin
- Cardiac rate, respiration: rate, rhythm, character, chest pain; start with patient hospitalized and monitored up to 1 wk

Evaluate:

- Therapeutic response: atrial fibrillation, flutter

Teach patient/family:

- To take this product as directed; to avoid missed doses; not to use with grapefruit juice, to avoid all other products without approval of provider
- To immediately report weight gain, edema, difficulty breathing
- To use effective contraception during treatment (pregnancy X) not to breastfeed

TREATMENT OF OVERDOSE:

O_2, artificial ventilation, ECG, administer DOPamine for circulatory depression; administer diazepam or thiopental for seizures, isoproterenol

⚠ HIGH ALERT

droperidol (Rx)

(droe-per'i-dole)

Func. class.: Sedative/hypnotic
Chem. class.: Butyrophenone

ACTION: Acts on CNS at subcortical levels, produces tranquilization, sleep; antiemetic; mild α-blockade

USES: Premedication for surgery; induction, maintenance in general anesthesia; postoperatively for nausea, vomiting

Unlabeled uses: Anxiety, general anesthesia induction/maintenance, preanesthesia, sedation induction

CONTRAINDICATIONS: Breastfeeding, children <2 yr, hypersensitivity

Black Box Warning: QT prolongation, torsades de pointes

Precautions: Pregnancy (C), geriatric patients, CV disease (hypotension, bradydysrhythmias), renal/hepatic disease, Parkinson's disease, pheochromocytoma, CHF, hypokalemia, hypomagnesemia, cardiac hypertrophy

DOSAGE AND ROUTES

Induction, adjunct

- **Adult: IV/IM** 1.25-2.5 mg, may give additional 1.25 mg with caution
- **Child 2-12 yr: IV** 0.05-0.1 mg/kg, titrate to response

Premedication

- **Adult: IM** 2.5 mg ½-1 hr before surgery, may give 1.25-2.5 mg additionally
- **Child 2-12 yr: IM** 0.05-0.1 mg/kg

Available forms: Inj 2.5 mg/ml

Administer:

- Protect sol from light
- Anticholinergics (benztropine, diphenhydrAMINE) for EPS
- Only with crash cart, resuscitative equipment nearby
- IM deep in large muscle mass

Direct IV route

- Undiluted; give through Y-tube at 10 mg or less/min; titrate to patient response

Intermittent IV INF route

- May be given as inf by adding dose to 250 ml LR, D_5W, 0.9% NaCl; give slowly, titrate to patient response

Syringe compatibilities: Atropine, bleomycin, butorphanol, chlorproMAZINE, cimetidine, CISplatin, cyclophosphamide, dimenhyDRINATE, diphenhydrAMINE, DOXOrubicin, fentaNYL, glycopyrrolate, hydrOXYzine, meperidine, metoclopramide, midazolam, mitomycin, morphine, nalbuphine, pentazocine, perphenazine, prochlorperazine, promazine, promethazine, scopolamine, vinBLAStine, vinCRIStine

Y-site compatibilities: Amifostine, aztreonam, bleomycin, cisatracurium, CISplatin, cladribine, cyclophosphamide, cytarabine, DOXOrubicin, DOXOrubicin liposome, famotidine, filgrastim, fluconazole, fludarabine, granisetron, hydrocortisone, IDArubicin, melphalan, meperidine, metoclopramide, mitomycin, ondansetron, paclitaxel, potassium chloride, propofol, remifentanil, sargramostim, teniposide, thiotepa, vinBLAStine, vinCRIStine, vinorelbine, vit B/C

SIDE EFFECTS

CNS: EPS (dystonia, akathisia, flexion of arms, fine tremors); dizziness, anxiety, drowsiness, restlessness, hallucination, depression, seizures, neuroleptic malignant syndrome
CV: *Tachycardia, hypotension,* prolonged QT, torsades de pointes
EENT: Upward rotation of eyes, oculogyric crisis
INTEG: *Chills, facial sweating, shivering*
RESP: Laryngospasm, bronchospasm

PHARMACOKINETICS

IM/IV: Onset 3-10 min, peak $^1/_2$ hr, duration 3-6 hr, metabolized in liver, excreted in urine as metabolites, crosses placenta, half-life 2-3 hr

INTERACTIONS

Increase: CNS depression—alcohol, opiates, barbiturates, antihistamines, antipsychotics, or other CNS depressants
Increase: hypotension—nitrates, antihypertensives
Increase: side effects of lithium
Increase: QT prolongation—class IA/III antiarrhythmics, some phenothiazines, tricyclics, some quinolones, others
Drug/Herb
Increase: action—kava, valerian, hops, chamomile

NURSING CONSIDERATIONS

Assess:
- VS q10min during IV administration, q30min after IM dose
- EPS: dystonia, akathisia

⚠ For increasing heart rate or decreasing B/P, notify prescriber at once; do not place patient in Trendelenburg position because sympathetic blockade may occur, thereby causing respiratory arrest

Black Box Warning: ECG prior to and 2-3 hr after administration for serious arrhythmias

Evaluate:
- Therapeutic response: decreased anxiety, absence of vomiting during and after surgery

Teach patient/family:
- To rise slowly from sitting or standing to minimize orthostatic hypotension
- To avoid ambulation without assistance; drowsiness, dizziness may occur

drotrecogin (Rx)

(droh′treh-koh-jin al′fah)

Xigris

Func. class.: Biologic response modifier

Chem. class.: Recombinant human activated protein C

ACTION: Activated protein C exerts an antithrombotic effect by inhibiting factor Va/VIIIa

USES: Severe sepsis associated with organ dysfunction

CONTRAINDICATIONS: Hypersensitivity, internal active bleeding, intraspinal surgery, CNS neoplasms, ulcerative colitis, hypocoagulation, within 3 mo of hemorrhagic stroke, epidural catheter in place, cerebral embolism/thrombosis/hemorrhage, within 2 mo of major surgery, trauma
Precautions: Pregnancy (C), breastfeeding, children, within 6 wk of GI bleeding, PT−INR >3, use >96 hr, hepatic disease, within 3 mo of ischemic stroke

DOSAGE AND ROUTES

- **Adult: IV INF** 24 mcg/kg/hr × 96 hr based on actual body weight

Available forms: Powder for inj, lyophilized, 5, 20 mg

Administer:

Intermittent IV INF route

- Reconstitute 5-mg vial/2.5 ml; 20-mg vial/10 ml sterile water for inj to a concentration of 2 mg/ml; slowly add sterile water for inj, do not shake or invert, gently swirl until dissolved
- Further dilute with 0.9% NaCl, slowly withdraw prescribed amount, add to bag of 0.9% NaCl, direct stream to side of bag, gently invert bag; do not transport inf bag between locations using mechanical delivery systems
- Use immediately after reconstituting; may be held for only 3 hr at controlled room temp 59° F-86° F; must complete inf within 12 hr after preparation
- Do not use if discolored or if particulate is present
- If using inf pump, usual concentration is 100-200 mcg/ml; if using syringe pump, usual concentration is 100-1000 mcg/ml
- Use dedicated IV line or dedicated lumen of central venous catheter; may use only 0.9% NaCl, LR, dextrose, or dextrose/saline mixtures through same line
- Do not expose to heat or direct sunlight
- Discontinue 2 hr prior to invasive surgery or procedures introducing risk for bleeding; may be reinstated 12 hr after invasive procedures if hemostasis achieved; may restart immediately after less invasive procedures

SIDE EFFECTS

HEMA: Decreased Hct, **bleeding**

SYST: **GI, GU, intracranial, intraabdominal, intrathoracic, retroperitoneal bleeding; surface bleeding**

PHARMACOKINETICS

Inactivated by endogenous plasma protease inhibitors, half-life 1.6 hr

INTERACTIONS

- Bleeding potential: aspirin, indomethacin, phenylbutazone, anticoagulants, thrombolytics, glycoprotein IIb/IIIa inhibitors, cilostazol, clopidogrel, dipyridamole, ticlopidine, other NSAIDs

NURSING CONSIDERATIONS

Assess:

- ⚠ **For bleeding during treatment; hematuria, hematemesis, bleeding from mucous membranes, epistaxis, ecchymosis; may require transfusion (rare), continue to assess for bleeding**
- Blood studies (Hct, platelets, PTT, PT, TT, aPTT) before starting therapy; PT or aPTT must be $<2\times$ control before starting therapy; PTT or PT q3-4hr during treatment
- VS, B/P, pulse, respirations, neurologic signs, temp at least q4hr; temp $>104°$ F (40° C) indicates internal bleeding; systolic pressure increase >25 mm Hg should be reported to prescriber
- ⚠ **For neurologic changes that may indicate intracranial bleeding**
- ⚠ **Retroperitoneal bleeding: back pain, leg weakness, diminished pulses**

Perform/provide:

- Refrigerated storage at 2° C to 8° C (36° F to 46° F); do not freeze
- Protect unreconstituted vials from light; keep in carton until time of use

Evaluate:

- Therapeutic response: decreasing symptoms of sepsis, lack of mortality

Teach patient/family:

- About reason for therapy, expected results
- That bleeding may occur for up to 1 mo after therapy; about signs, symptoms of bleeding

DULoxetine (Rx)

(du-lox'uh-teen)

Cymbalta

Func. class.: Antidepressant

Chem. class.: Serotonin-norepinephrine reuptake inhibitor (SNRI)

ACTION: May potentiate serotonergic, noradrenergic activity in the CNS; in studies, DULoxetine is a potent inhibitor of neuronal serotonin and norepinephrine reuptake

USES: Major depressive disorder (MDD), neuropathic pain associated with diabetic neuropathy, generalized anxiety disorder, fibromyalgia, chronic low back pain, osteoarthritis pain

Unlabeled uses: Stress, urinary incontinence

CONTRAINDICATIONS: Alcohol intoxication, alcoholism, closed-angle glaucoma, hepatic disease, hepatitis, jaundice, hypersensitivity

Precautions: Pregnancy (C), breastfeeding, geriatric patients, mania, hypertension, renal/cardiac disease, seizures, increased intraocular pressure, anorexia nervosa, bleeding, dehydration, diabetes, hyponatremia, hypotension, hypovolemia, orthostatic hypotension, abrupt product withdrawal

Black Box Warning: Children, suicidal ideation

DOSAGE AND ROUTES

Depression

- **Adult: PO** 40-60 mg/day as single dose or 2 divided doses

Diabetic neuropathy

- **Adult: PO** 60 mg/day

Generalized anxiety disorder

- **Adult: PO** 60 mg/day, may start with 30 mg/day × 1 wk then increase to 60 mg/day; maintenance 60-120 mg/day

Fibromyalgia

- **Adult: PO** 30 mg/day × 1 wk then 60 mg/day

Musculoskeletal pain

- **Adult: PO** 60 mg/day

Renal dose

- **Adult: PO** Start with 20 mg, gradually increase; avoid use in severe renal disease

Available forms: Caps 20, 30, 60 mg

Administer:

- Swallow cap whole; do not break, crush, or chew; do not sprinkle on food or mix with liquid
- Without regard to food

SIDE EFFECTS

CNS: Insomnia, anxiety, dizziness, tremor, somnolence, fatigue, decreased appetite, decreased weight, agitation, diaphoresis, hallucinations, neuroleptic malignant-like syndrome reaction, aggression, seizures, *headache*

CV: Thrombophlebitis, peripheral edema, hypertension, palpitations, supraventricular dysrhythmia

EENT: *Abnormal vision*

ENDO: Hypo/hyperglycemia

GI: Constipation, diarrhea, dysphagia, *nausea,* vomiting, anorexia, dry mouth, colitis, gastritis, abdominal pain, hepatic failure

GU: Abnormal ejaculation, urinary hesitation/retention/frequency, ejaculation delayed, erectile dysfunction, gynecologic bleeding

INTEG: Photosensitivity, bruising, sweating, Stevens-Johnson syndrome

MS: Gait disturbance, muscle spasm, restless leg syndrome

SYST: Anaphylaxis, angioedema, serotonin syndrome

PHARMACOKINETICS

Well absorbed; extensively metabolized (CYP2D6, CYP1A2) in the liver to an active metabolite; 70% of product recovered in urine, 20% in feces; 90% protein binding; elimination half-life 9.2-19.1 hr

INTERACTIONS

- Narrow therapeutic index: CYP2D6 extensively metabolized products (flecainide, phenothiazines, propafenone, tricyclics, thioridazine)

⚠ Hyperthermia, rigidity, rapid fluctuations of vital signs, mental status changes, neuroleptic malignant syndrome—MAOIs, coadministration contraindicated within 14 days of MAOI use

Increase: CNS depression—opioids, antihistamines, sedative/hypnotics

Increase: serotonin syndrome, neuroleptic malignant syndrome—SSRIs, serotonin-receptor agonists

Increase: bleeding risk—anticoagulants, antiplatelets, salicylates, NSAIDs

Increase: action of DULoxetine—CYP1A2 inhibitors (fluvoxamine, quinolone anti-infectives); CYP2D6 inhibitors (FLUoxetine, quiNIDine, PARoxetine)

Increase: ALT, bilirubin—alcohol

Drug/Herb

- Serotonin syndrome: St. John's wort

Increase: CNS depression—kava, valerian

Drug/Lab Test

Increase: blood glucose

NURSING CONSIDERATIONS

Assess:

Black Box Warning: Depression: mood, sensorium, affect, **suicidal tendencies,** increase in psychiatric symptoms; depression, panic

- B/P lying, standing; pulse q4hr; if systolic B/P drops 20 mm Hg, hold product, notify prescriber; take VS q4hr in patients with CV disease
- Hepatic studies: AST, ALT, bilirubin
- Weight weekly; weight loss or gain; appetite may increase; peripheral edema may occur
- Sugarless gum, hard candy, frequent sips of water for dry mouth
- **Withdrawal symptoms:** headache, nausea, vomiting, muscle pain, weakness; not common unless product is discontinued abruptly

⚠ **Malignant neuroleptic-like syndrome reaction**

⚠ **Serotonin syndrome:** nausea/vomiting, dizziness, facial flush, shivering, sweating

- **Sexual dysfunction:** ejaculation dysfunction, erectile dysfunction, decreased libido, orgasm dysfunction

Perform/provide:

- Storage in tight container at room temp; do not freeze
- Assistance with ambulation during beginning therapy, since drowsiness, dizziness occur
- Confirmation that PO medication swallowed

Evaluate:

- Therapeutic response: decreased depression

Teach patient/family:

- To report urinary retention; about signs and symptoms of bleeding (GI bleeding, nosebleed, ecchymoses, bruising)
- To use with caution when driving, performing other activities requiring alertness because of drowsiness, dizziness, blurred vision
- To avoid alcohol ingestion, MAOIs, other CNS depressants
- Not to discontinue medication quickly after long-term use; may cause nausea, headache, malaise; taper

Black Box Warning: That clinical worsening and suicide risk may occur

- To wear sunscreen or large hat, since photosensitivity may occur
- To notify prescriber if pregnancy planned or suspected, or if breastfeeding
- Improvement may occur in 4-8 wk or in up to 12 wk (geriatric patients)

dutasteride (Rx)

(doo-tass′ter-ide)

Avodart

Func. class.: Androgen inhibitor

Chem. class.: Synthetic 5α-reductase inhibitor, 4-azasteroid compound

ACTION: Inhibits both type 1 and type 2 forms of a steroid enzyme that converts testosterone to 5α-dihydrotestosterone (DHT), which is responsible for the initial growth of prostatic tissue

USES: Treatment of benign prostatic hyperplasia (BPH) in men with an enlarged prostate gland; may be used in combination with tamsulosin

Unlabeled uses: Alopecia

CONTRAINDICATIONS: Pregnancy (X), breastfeeding, women, children, hypersensitivity

Precautions: Hepatic disease

DOSAGE AND ROUTES

Benign prostatic hyperplasia (BPH)

- **Adult: PO** 0.5 mg/day

Alopecia (unlabeled)

- **Adult: PO** 0.5-2.5 mg/day

Available form: Caps 0.5 mg

Administer:

- Swallow caps whole; do not break, crush, chew
- Without regard to meals

SIDE EFFECTS

GU: Decreased libido, impotence, gynecomastia, ejaculation disorders (rare), mastalgia, teratogenesis

INTEG: Serious skin infections

PHARMACOKINETICS

Peak 2-3 hr, protein binding 99%, metabolized in liver by CYP3A4, excreted in feces, half-life 5 wk at steady state

INTERACTIONS

Increase: dutasteride concentrations—ritonavir, ketoconazole, verapamil, diltiazem, cimetidine, ciprofloxacin, antiretroviral protease inhibitors, or other products metabolized by CYP3A4

Drug/Lab Test

Decrease: PSA

NURSING CONSIDERATIONS

Assess:

- **For decreasing symptoms of BPH:** decreasing urinary retention, frequency, urgency, nocturia
- PSA levels; digital rectal, urinary obstruction; determine the absence of urinary cancer before starting treatment
- Blood studies: ALT, AST, bilirubin, CBC with differential, serum creatinine, serum electrolytes

Evaluate:

- Therapeutic response: decreasing symptoms of BPH; decreased urinary retention, frequency, urgency, nocturia

Teach patient/family:

- To read patient information leaflet before starting therapy; to reread it upon prescription renewal
- To notify prescriber if therapeutic response decreases, if edema occurs
- Not to discontinue product abruptly
- About changes in sex characteristics
- That men taking dutasteride should not donate blood for at least 6 mo after last dose to prevent blood administration to pregnant female
- That caps should not be handled by a woman who is pregnant or who may become pregnant because product can be absorbed through skin
- That ejaculate volume may decrease during treatment; that product rarely interferes with sexual function

econazole topical
See Appendix B

ecothiophate ophthalmic
See Appendix B

RARELY USED

edetate calcium disodium (Rx)
(ee′de-tate)

Calcium Disodium Versenate

Func. class.: Heavy metal antagonist (antidote)

Do not confuse:
edetate calcium disodium/edetate disodium

USES: Lead poisoning, acute lead encephalopathy

CONTRAINDICATIONS: Hypersensitivity, anuria, poisoning of other metals, severe renal disease, hepatitis

Black Box Warning: Child <3 yr

DOSAGE AND ROUTES

Lead mobilization test (lead toxicity 25-45 mcg/dl)

- **Adult/adolescent: IV INF** 500 mg/m^2 over 1 hr or **IM**
- **Child: IV INF** 500 mg/m^2 over 1 hr or **IM** as single dose or 2 divided doses

Acute lead encephalopathy (blood levels >70 mcg/dl)

- **Adult/adolescent/child/infant: IM/IV** 1500 mg/m^2 as **IV INF** over 12-24 hr in combination with dimercaprol **IM,** give 1st dose ≥4 hr after initial dimercaprol, when urine flow established

RARELY USED

edetate disodium (Rx)
(ee′de-tate)

Endrate

Func. class.: Heavy metal antagonist (chelator)

Do not confuse:
edetate disodium/edetate calcium disodium

USES: Hypercalcemic crisis, control of ventricular dysrhythmias associated with digoxin toxicity

CONTRAINDICATIONS: Children <3 yr, hypersensitivity, anuria, hepatic insufficiency, poisoning of other metals, severe renal disease, seizure disorders, active/inactive TB

DOSAGE AND ROUTES

Digitalis glycoside toxicity/ ventricular dysrhythmias/ hypercalcemia crisis

- **Adult: IV** 50 mg/kg/day given over 3 hr or more/day × 5 days, skip 2 days, repeat as needed up to 15 doses, max 3 g/ day

efavirenz (Rx)
(ef-ah-veer′enz)

Sustiva

Func. class.: Antiretroviral

Chem. class.: Nonnucleoside reverse transcriptase inhibitor (NNRTI)

ACTION: Binds directly to reverse transcriptase and blocks RNA, DNA polymerase, thus causing a disruption of the enzyme's site

USES: HIV-1 in combination with at least 2 other antivirals

Unlabeled uses: HIV prophylaxis

CONTRAINDICATIONS:
Pregnancy (D), hypersensitivity

Precautions: Breastfeeding, children <3 yr, renal/hepatic disease, myelosuppression, depression, seizures

DOSAGE AND ROUTES

Given in combination with protease inhibitor or nucleoside analog reverse transcriptase inhibitors (NARTIs)

- **Adult and child >40 kg: PO** 600 mg/day at bedtime
- **Child 32.5-39.9 kg: PO** 400 mg/day at bedtime
- **Child 25-32.4 kg: PO** 350 mg/day at bedtime
- **Child 20-24.9 kg: PO** 300 mg/day at bedtime
- **Child 15-19.9 kg: PO** 250 mg/day at bedtime
- **Child 10-14.9 kg: PO** 200 mg/day at bedtime

Available forms: Caps 50, 100, 200 mg; 600-mg tabs

Administer:

- Give on empty stomach; give at bedtime to decrease CNS side effects
- Caps may be opened, added to grape jelly to disguise peppery taste

SIDE EFFECTS

CNS: Fatigue, impaired cognition, insomnia, abnormal dreams, depression, headache, dizziness, anxiety, drowsiness

GI: *Diarrhea,* abdominal pain, *nausea,* hyperlipidemia, constipation, increased LFTs

GU: Hematuria, kidney stones

INTEG: Rash, erythema multiforme, Stevens-Johnson syndrome, toxic epidermal necrolysis

PHARMACOKINETICS

Peak 3-5 hr, well absorbed, metabolized by liver; terminal half-life 52-76 hr; >99% protein binding, excreted in urine, feces; concentrations higher in females and those of African, Asian, and Hispanic descent

INTERACTIONS

- Do not give together with benzodiazepines, ergots, midazolam, triazolam, CISapride

Increase: CNS depression—alcohol, antidepressants, antihistamines, opioids

Increase: levels of both products—ritonavir, estrogens, anticonvulsants

Increase: levels of warfarin, ergots, midazolam, triazolam, statins (except pravastatin, fluvastatin)

Decrease: levels of indinavir, saquinavir, clarithromycin, methadone

Decrease: efavirenz metabolism—CYP3A4 inhibitors (conivaptan, ambrisentan, sorafenib)

Decrease: efavirenz effect—CYP3A4 inducers (carBAMazepine, rifamycins)

Drug/Herb

Decrease: efavirenz level—St. John's wort; do not use together

Drug/Food

Increase: absorption—high-fat foods

Drug/Lab Test

Increase: ALT

False positive: cannibinoids

NURSING CONSIDERATIONS

Assess:

- Signs of infection, anemia
- Hepatic studies: ALT, AST; renal studies
- Bowel pattern before, during treatment; if severe abdominal pain with bleeding occurs, product should be discontinued; monitor hydration
- **Serious skin reactions:** Stevens-Johnson syndrome, toxic epidermal necrolysis
- **HIV:** Monitor CBC, blood chemistry, plasma HIV RNA, absolute CD4+/CD8+ cell counts/%, serum β_2 microglobulin, serum ICD+24 antigen levels, cholesterol, hepatic enzymes
- **Signs of toxicity:** severe nausea/vomiting, maculopapular rash

Evaluate:

- Therapeutic response: increased CD4 cell counts; decreased viral load; slowing progression of HIV

Teach patient/family:
- To take as prescribed; if dose is missed, to take as soon as remembered; not to double dose; to take with water, juice; to take on empty stomach at bedtime
- To make sure health care provider knows all medications, supplements, OTC products taken
- That, if severe rash occurs, to notify health care provider; that adverse reactions (rash, dizziness, abnormal dreams, insomnia) lessen after 1 mo
- Not to breastfeed or become pregnant if taking this product; to use nonhormonal contraception because serious birth defects have occurred (pregnancy D)
- To avoid hazardous activities if dizziness, drowsiness occur
- That product does not cure disease but controls symptoms; that HIV can be transmitted to others even while taking this product; to continue with safe-sex practices

eletriptan (Rx)

(el-ee-trip′tan)

Relpax

Func. class.: Antimigraine agent, abortive

Chem. class.: 5-HT_1-1B/1D receptor agonist, triptan

ACTION: Binds selectively to the vascular 5-HT_1-receptor subtype; causes vasoconstriction in cranial arteries

USES: Acute treatment of migraine with/without aura

CONTRAINDICATIONS: Hypersensitivity, coronary artery vasospasm, peripheral vascular disease, hemiplegic/basilar migraine, uncontrolled hypertension; ischemic bowel, heart disease; severe renal/hepatic disease, acute MI, stroke, angina, CV disease

Precautions: Pregnancy (C), breastfeeding, children, geriatric patients, postmenopausal women, men >40 yr; risk factors of CAD, MI, or other cardiac disease; hypercholcsterolemia, obesity, diabetes, impaired renal/hepatic function

DOSAGE AND ROUTES

- **Adult: PO** 20 or 40 mg, may increase if needed, max 40 mg (single dose); may repeat in 2 hr if headache improves but returns, max 80 mg/24 hr

Available forms: Tabs 20, 40 mg

Administer:
- Swallow tabs whole; do not break, crush, or chew
- At beginning of headache; if headache returns, repeat dose after 2 hr of 1st dose if 1st dose is ineffective

SIDE EFFECTS

CNS: *Dizziness,* headache, anxiety, paresthesia, asthenia, somnolence, flushing, fatigue, hot/cold sensation, chills, vertigo, hypertonia, **seizures, serotonin syndrome**

CV: Chest pain, palpitations, hypertension, **MI, sinus tachycardia, stroke, ventricular fibrillation/tachycardia, atrial fibrillation, AV block, bradycardia, chest** pressure syndrome, **coronary vasospasm**

GI: Nausea, dry mouth

MS: *Weakness,* back pain

RESP: Chest tightness, pressure

PHARMACOKINETICS

Onset of pain relief 2 hr, metabolized in the liver, 70% excreted in urine and feces

INTERACTIONS

Increase: plasma concentration of eletriptan—CYP3A4 inhibitors (clarithromycin, erythromycin, itraconazole, ketoconazole, nelfinavir, ritonavir), propranolol, ergots

Increase: serotonin syndrome—SSRIs, SNRIs, serotonin-receptor agonists

NURSING CONSIDERATIONS

Assess:

- **Migraine:** pain location, character, intensity, nausea, vomiting, aura
- B/P; signs, symptoms of coronary vasospasms
- Tingling, hot sensation, burning, feeling of pressure, numbness, flushing
- Stress level, activity, recreation, coping mechanisms
- Neurologic status: LOC, blurring vision, nausea, vomiting, tingling in extremities preceding headache
- Ingestion of tyramine foods (pickled products, beer, wine, aged cheese), food additives, preservatives, colorings, artificial sweeteners, chocolate, caffeine, which may precipitate these types of headaches
- Patients with CAD risk factors; 1st dose should be administered in prescriber's office or medical facility

Perform/provide:

- Quiet, calm environment with decreased stimulation from noise, bright light, excessive talking

Evaluate:

- Therapeutic response: decrease in frequency, severity of migraine

Teach patient/family:

- To report any side effects to prescriber
- To use contraception while taking product; to inform prescriber if pregnant or intending to become pregnant
- To provide dark, quiet environment
- That product does not prevent or reduce number of migraine attacks

emedastine ophthalmic

See Appendix B

emtricitabine (Rx)

(em-tri-sit′uh-bean)

Emtriva

Func. class.: Antiretroviral

Chem. class.: Nucleoside reverse transcriptase inhibitor (NRTI)

ACTION: A synthetic nucleoside analog of cytosine; inhibits replication of HIV virus by competing with the natural substrate and then becoming incorporated into cellular DNA by viral reverse transcriptase, thereby terminating cellular DNA chain

USES: HIV-1 infection with other antiretroviral

Unlabeled uses: HBV (hepatitis B virus) infection with HIV, HIV prophylaxis

CONTRAINDICATIONS: Hypersensitivity

Black Box Warning: Lactic acidosis

Precautions: Pregnancy (B), breastfeeding, children, geriatric patients, renal disease

Black Box Warning: Hepatic insufficiency, chronic hepatitis B virus (HPV)

DOSAGE AND ROUTES

Oral cap and solution are not interchangeable

- **Adult: PO** Caps 200 mg/day; oral sol 240 mg (24 ml)/day
- **Adolescent/child >33 kg: PO** Caps 200 mg/day; **child 3 mo-17 yr:** oral sol 6 mg/kg/day, max 240 mg (24 ml)
- **Infants <3 mo: PO oral sol** 3 mg/kg daily, do not use caps

Renal dose

- **Adult: PO** Caps CCr 30-49 ml/min, 200 mg q48hr; oral sol 120 mg q24hr; caps CCr 15-29 ml/min, 200 mg q72hr; oral sol 80 mg q24hr; caps CCr <15 ml/min, 200 mg q96hr; oral sol 60 mg q24hr

Available forms: Cap 200 mg; oral sol 10 mg/ml

Administer:

- Give without regard to meals
- Oral cap and solution not interchangeable

SIDE EFFECTS

CNS: *Headache,* abnormal dreams, *depression,* dizziness, *insomnia,* neuropathy, paresthesia, *asthenia*
GI: *Nausea, vomiting, diarrhea, anorexia, abdominal pain, dyspepsia,* **hepatomegaly with steatosis (may be fatal)**
INTEG: *Rash,* skin discolorization
MS: Arthralgia, myalgia
RESP: *Cough*
SYST: Change in body fat distribution, **lactic acidosis**

PHARMACOKINETICS

Rapidly, extensively absorbed; peak 1-2 hr; protein binding <4%; excreted unchanged in urine (86%), feces (14%); half-life 10 hr

INTERACTIONS

- Do not use with efavirenz, tenofovir, lamiVUDine, treatment duplication

Decrease: emtricitabine level—interferons

- Complex interactions—ribavirin, cautious use

NURSING CONSIDERATIONS

Assess:

- Renal/hepatic function tests: AST, ALT, bilirubin, amylase, lipase, triglycerides periodically during treatment

⚠ **Lactic acidosis, severe hepatomegaly with steatosis;** if lab reports confirm these conditions, discontinue treatment; may be fatal

Perform/provide:

- Storage (caps) at 25° C (77° F); (oral sol) refrigerated, use within 3 mo

Evaluate:

- Therapeutic response: decreased signs, symptoms of HIV; decreased viral load, increased CP4 counts

Teach patient/family:

- That GI complaints resolve after 3-4 wk of treatment
- To report planned or suspected pregnancy; not to breastfeed while taking product
- That product must be taken at same time of day to maintain blood level
- That product will control symptoms but is not a cure for HIV; patient still infectious, may pass HIV virus on to others; that other products may be necessary to prevent other infections
- That changes in body fat distribution may occur

Black Box Warning: Lactic acidosis: to notify prescriber immediately if fatigue, muscle aches/pains, abdominal pain, difficulty breathing, nausea, vomiting, change in heart rhythm occur

Black Box Warning: Hepatotoxicity: to notify prescriber of dark urine, yellowing of skin/eyes, clay-colored stools, anorexia, nausea, vomiting

enalapril/enalaprilat (Rx)

(e-nal′a-pril)/(e-nal′a-pril-at)

Vasotec

Func. class.: Antihypertensive
Chem. class.: Angiotensin-converting enzyme (ACE) inhibitor

Do not confuse:
enalapril/ramipril/Anafranil/Eldepryl

ACTION:
Selectively suppresses renin-angiotensin-aldosterone system; inhibits ACE; prevents conversion of angiotensin I to angiotensin II, dilation of arterial, venous vessels

USES:
Hypertension, CHF, left ventricular dysfunction
Unlabeled uses: Diabetic nephropathy, hypertensive emergency/urgency, post-MI, proteinuria, renal crisis in scleroderma

CONTRAINDICATIONS:

Hypersensitivity, history of angioedema

Black Box Warning: Pregnancy (D)

Precautions: Breastfeeding, renal disease, hyperkalemia, hepatic failure, dehydration, bilateral renal artery stenosis

DOSAGE AND ROUTES

Hypertension

- **Adult: PO** 2.5-5 mg/day, may increase or decrease to desired response, range 10-40 mg/day; **IV** 0.625-1.25 mg q6hr over 5 min
- **Child: PO** 0.08 mg/kg/day in 1-2 divided doses, max 0.58 mg/kg/day
- **Child: IV** 5-10 mcg/kg/dose q8-24hr

CHF

- **Adult: PO** 2.5-20 mg/day in 2 divided doses, max 40 mg/day in divided doses

Renal disease

- **Adult: PO** 2.5 mg/day (CCr <30 ml/min), increase gradually; **IV** CCr >30 ml/min, 1.25 mg q6hr; CCr <30 ml/min, 0.625 mg as one-time dose, increase as per B/P

Hypertensive emergency/urgency (unlabeled)

- **Adult: PO** 2.5 mg bid, gradually titrate up to 20 mg bid

Available forms: *Enalapril:* tabs 2.5, 5, 10, 20 mg; *enalaprilat:* inj 1.25 mg/ml

Administer:

PO route

- Tab may be crushed, given without regard to meals

IV route

- Prepare in sterile environment using aseptic technique
- Dilute each dose with ≤50 ml compatible sol
- For 25 mcg/ml dilution often used for neonatal or pediatric patients, combine 1 ml enalaprilat 1.25 mg/ml and 49 ml compatible sol for IV

IV, Direct/Intermittent IV INF route

- Undiluted over ≥5 min, use diluent provided or 50 ml D_5W, 0.9% NaCl, 0.9% NaCl in D_5W or LR, Isolyte E; give through Y-tube of free-flowing inf of 0.9% NaCl, D_5W, LR, Isolyte E

Y-site compatibilities: Acyclovir, alemtuzumab, alfentanil, allopurinol, amifostine, amikacin, aminophylline, amphotericin B liposome, anidulafungin, ascorbic acid, atracurium, atropine, azaTHIOprine, aztreonam, benztropine, bivalirudin, bretylium, bumetanide, buprenorphine, butorphanol, calcium chloride/gluconate, CARBOplatin, ceFAZolin, cefonicid, cefoperazone, cefotaxime, cefotetan, cefoxitin, ceftazidime, ceftizoxime, cefTRIAXone, cefuroxime, cephalothin, cephapirin, chloramphenicol, cimetidine, cisatracurium, cladribine, clindamycin, cyanocobalamin, cyclophosphamide, cycloSPORINE, cytarabine, DACTINomycin, DAPTOmycin, dexamethasone, dexmedetomidine, dextran 40, digoxin, diltiazem, diphenhydrAMINE, DOBUTamine, docetaxel, DOPamine, doripenem, doxacurium, DOXOrubicin, DOXOrubicin liposome, doxycycline, ePHEDrine, EPINEPHrine, epirubicin, epoetin, ertapenem, erythromycin, esmolol, etoposide, etoposide phosphate, famotidine, fenoldopam, fentaNYL, filgrastim, fluconazole, fludarabine, fluorouracil, folic acid, furosemide, ganciclovir, gemcitabine, gentamicin, granisetron, heparin, hydrocortisone, HYDROmorphone, ifosfamide, imipenem-cilastatin, indomethacin, insulin, isoproterenol, ketorolac, labetalol, levofloxacin, lidocaine, linezolid, LORazepam, magnesium sulfate, mannitol, mechlorethamine, melphalan, meperidine, meropenem, metaraminol, methicillin, methotrexate, methoxamine, methyldopate, methylPREDNISolone, metoclopramide, metoprolol, metroNIDAZOLE, mezlocillin, miconazole, midazolam, milrinone, minocycline, mitoxantrone, morphine, moxalactam, multiple vitamin injection, nafcillin, nalbuphine, naloxone, netilmicin, niCARdipine, nitroglycerin, nitroprusside, norepinephrine, octreotide, ondansetron, oxacillin, oxaliplatin, oxytocin, paclitaxel, palonosetron, papaverine, pemetrexed, penicillin G potassium, pentamidine, pentazocine, PENTobarbital, PHENobarbital, phentolamine, phenylephrine, phytonadione, piperacillin-tazobactam, potassium chloride/phosphate, procainamide, prochlorperazine, promethazine, propofol, propranolol, protamine, pyridoxime, quinupristin-dalfopristin, ranitidine, remifentanil, ritodrine, riTUXimab, rocuronium, sodium acetate, sodium bicarbonate, succinylcholine, SUFentanil, tacrolimus, teniposide, tetracycline, theophylline, thiamine, thiotepa, ticarcillin/clavulanate, tigecycline, tirofiban, tobramycin, tolazoline, trastuzumab, trimetaphan, urokinase, vancomycin, vasopressin, vecuronium, verapamil, vinCRIStine, vinorelbine, voriconazole, zoledronic acid

Additive compatibilities: DOBUTamine, DOPamine, heparin, meropenem, nitroglycerin, nitroprusside, potassium chloride

SIDE EFFECTS

CNS: *Insomnia, dizziness,* paresthesias, headache, fatigue, anxiety

CV: *Hypotension,* chest pain, tachycardia, **dysrhythmias**, syncope, angina, **MI**, orthostatic hypotension

EENT: *Tinnitus;* visual changes; sore throat; double vision; dry, burning eyes

GI: Nausea, vomiting, colitis, cramps, diarrhea, constipation, flatulence, dry mouth, loss of taste

GU: Proteinuria, renal failure, increased frequency of polyuria or oliguria

HEMA: Agranulocytosis, neutropenia

INTEG: Rash, purpura, alopecia, hyperhidrosis, photosensitivity

META: Hyperkalemia

RESP: Dyspnea, dry cough, crackles

SYST: Toxic epidermal necrolysis, Stevens-Johnson syndrome, angioedema

PHARMACOKINETICS

Enalapril: PO: Onset 1 hr, peak 4-6 hr, duration ≥24 hr

Enalaprilat: IV: Onset 5-15 min, peak up to 4 hr, duration 4-6 hr, half-life 11 hr

Metabolized by liver to active metabolite, excreted in urine

INTERACTIONS

Increase: hypersensitivity—allopurinol

Increase: hypotension—diuretics, other antihypertensives, phenothiazines, nitrates, acute alcohol ingestion, general anesthesia

Increase: potassium levels—salt substitutes, potassium-sparing diuretics, potassium supplements, cycloSPORINE, indomethacin

Increase: levels of lithium, digoxin

Decrease: effects of enalapril—antacids, rifampin

Drug/Lab Test

Increase: ALT, AST, bilirubin, alk phos, glucose, uric acid

False positive: ANA titer

NURSING CONSIDERATIONS

Assess:

• **Bone marrow depression (rare):** neutrophils, decreased platelets; WBC with differential baseline, q3mo; if neutrophils <1000/mm^3, discontinue treatment (recommended with collagen-vascular disease)

• **Hypertension:** B/P, peak/trough level, orthostatic hypotension, syncope when used with diuretic, pulse q4hr; note rate, rhythm, quality

• Baselines of renal, hepatic studies before therapy begins and 1 wk into therapy; electrolytes: K, Na, Cl during 1st 2 wk of therapy

• Skin turgor, dryness of mucous membranes for hydration status; edema in feet, legs daily

• **Symptoms of CHF:** edema, dyspnea, wet crackles, weight gain, jugular venous distension, difficulty breathing

Evaluate:

• Therapeutic response: decreased B/P

Teach patient/family:

• Not to use OTC (cough, cold, or allergy) products unless directed by prescriber; to avoid potassium, salt substitutes

- To avoid sunlight or wear sunscreen for photosensitivity
- To comply with dosage schedule even if feeling better
- To notify prescriber of mouth sores, sore throat, fever, swelling of hands or feet, irregular heartbeat, chest pain, signs of angioedema
- That excessive perspiration, dehydration, vomiting, diarrhea may lead to fall in blood pressure; to consult prescriber if these occur
- That product may cause dizziness, fainting; that lightheadedness may occur during 1st few days of therapy
- That product may cause skin rash, impaired perspiration or angioedema; to discontinue if angioedema occurs
- Not to discontinue product abruptly
- That CV adverse reactions may reoccur
- To rise slowly to sitting or standing position to minimize orthostatic hypotension

Black Box Warning: To use contraception during treatment; pregnancy (D)

TREATMENT OF OVERDOSE:

Lavage, IV atropine for bradycardia, IV theophylline for bronchospasm, digoxin, O_2, diuretic for cardiac failure

enfuvirtide (Rx)

(en-fyoo′vir-tide)

Fuzeon

Func. class.: Antiretroviral

Chem. class.: Fusion Inhibitor

ACTION: Inhibitor of the fusion of HIV-1 with CD4+ cells

USES: Treatment of HIV-1 infection in combination with other antiretrovirals

Unlabeled uses: HIV prophylaxis after occupational exposure

CONTRAINDICATIONS: Breastfeeding, hypersensitivity

Precautions: Pregnancy (B), children <6 yr, liver disease, myelosuppression, infections

DOSAGE AND ROUTES

- **Adult: SUBCUT** 90 mg (1 ml) bid
- **Child 6-16 yr and <42.6 kg: SUBCUT** 2 mg/kg bid, max 90 mg bid; 11-15.5 kg 27 mg/0.3 ml bid; 15.6-20 kg 36 mg/0.4 ml bid; 20.1-24.5 kg 45 mg/0.5 ml bid; 24.6-29 kg 54 mg/0.6 ml bid; 29.1-33.5 kg 63 mg/0.7 ml bid; 33.6-38 kg 72 mg/0.8 ml bid; 38.1-42.5 kg 81 mg/0.9 ml bid

HIV prophylaxis (unlabeled)

- **Adult: SUBCUT** 90 mg bid added to PEP regimen

Available forms: Powder for inj, lyophilized 108 mg (90 mg/ml when reconstituted)

Administer:

SUBCUT route

- **Reconstitute** vial with 1.1 ml sterile water for inj; tap and roll to mix; allow to stand until completely dissolved, may take up to 45 min; after dissolved, immediately **inject** or refrigerate up to 24 hr
- Do not mix with other medications
- SUBCUT: give bid, rotate sites; preferred sites: upper arm, anterior thigh, abdomen

SIDE EFFECTS

CNS: Anxiety, peripheral neuropathy, taste disturbance, **Guillain-Barré syndrome**, insomnia, depression

GI: Abdominal pain, anorexia, constipation, pancreatitis

GU: Glomerulonephritis, renal failure

HEMA: Thrombocytopenia, neutropenia

INTEG: Inj site reactions

MISC: Influenza, cough, conjunctivitis, lymphadenopathy, myalgia, hyperglycemia, pneumonia, rhinitis, fatigue

PHARMACOKINETICS

Peak 8 hr, terminal half-life 3.8 hr, well absorbed, undergoes catabolism, 92% protein binding

NURSING CONSIDERATIONS

Assess:

- **Signs of infection, inj site reactions**
- **Glomerulonephritis/renal failure:** BUN, creatinine, renal failure may occur
- Bowel pattern before, during treatment; if severe abdominal pain or constipation occurs, notify prescriber; monitor hydration
- Skin eruptions, rash, urticaria, itching
- Allergies before treatment, reaction to each medication
- **HIV:** CBC, blood chemistry, plasma HIV RNA, absolute CD4+/CD8+ cell counts/%, serum β_2 microglobulin, serum ICD+24 antigen levels, cholesterol

Evaluate:

- Therapeutic response: increased CD4 cell counts; decreased viral load; slowing progression of HIV-1 infection

Teach patient/family:

- To notify prescriber if pregnancy is suspected or if breastfeeding
- That pneumonia may occur; to contact prescriber if cough, fever occur
- That hypersensitive reactions may occur; rash, pruritus; to stop product, contact prescriber
- That product is not a cure for HIV-1 infection but controls symptoms; HIV-1 can still be transmitted to others; that product is to be used in combination only with other antiretrovirals

⚠ HIGH ALERT

enoxaparin (Rx)

(ee-nox′a-par-in)

Lovenox

Func. class.: Anticoagulant, antithrombotic

Chem. class.: Low-molecular-weight heparin (LMWH)

Do not confuse:

enoxaparin/enoxacin

Lovenox/Lotronex

ACTION: Binds to antithrombin III inactivating factors Xa/IIa, thereby resulting in a higher ratio of anti-factor Xa to IIa

USES: Prevention of DVT (inpatient or outpatient), PE (inpatient) in hip and knee replacement, abdominal surgery at risk for thrombosis; unstable angina/non–Q-wave MI

Unlabeled uses: Antiphospholipid antibody syndrome, arterial thromboembolism prophylaxis, cerebral thromboembolism, percutaneous coronary intervention

CONTRAINDICATIONS: Hypersensitivity to this product, benzyl alcohol, heparin, pork; active major bleeding, hemophilia, leukemia with bleeding, peptic ulcer disease, thrombocytopenic purpura, heparin-induced thrombocytopenia

Precautions: Pregnancy (B), breastfeeding, children, geriatric patients, low weight men (<57 kg), women (<45 kg), severe renal/hepatic disease, blood dyscrasias, severe hypertension, subacute bacterial endocarditis, acute nephritis, recent burn, spinal surgery, indwelling catheters

Black Box Warning: Lumbar puncture, epidural anesthesia, spinal anesthesia

DOSAGE AND ROUTES

DVT prevention before hip or knee surgery

- **Adult: SUBCUT** 30 mg bid given 12-24 hr postop for 7-10 days until DVT risk is diminished

DVT prevention before hip replacement

- **Adult: SUBCUT** 40 mg/day started 9-15 hr preop or 30 mg q12hr started 12-24 hr postop, continued until DVT risk diminished or patient adequately on anticoagulant

DVT prophylaxis before abdominal surgery

• **Adult: SUBCUT** 40 mg/day starting 24 hr prior to surgery × 7-10 days to prevent thromboembolic complications

Treatment of DVT or PE

• **Adult: SUBCUT** 1 mg/kg q12hr (without PE, outpatient); 1 mg/kg q12hr or 1.5 mg/kg/day (with or without PE, inpatient); warfarin should be started within 72 hr, continued ≥5 days until INR is 2-3 (usually 7 days)

Prevention of ischemic complications in unstable angina or non–Q-wave MI

• **Adult: SUBCUT/IV** 1 mg/kg q12hr until stable with aspirin 100-325 mg/day × ≥2 days

Renal dose

• **Adult: SUBCUT** <30 ml/min 30 mg/day (thrombosis prophylaxis)

Available forms: Prefilled syringes/inj 30 mg/0.3 ml, 40 mg/0.4 ml, 60 mg/0.6 ml, 80 mg/0.8 ml, 100 mg/1 ml, 120 mg/0.8 ml, 150 mg/ml; multidose vials 100 mg/ml (3 ml)

Administer:

• Only after screening patient for bleeding disorders

• Do not mix with other products or inf fluids

⚠ **Only this product when ordered; not interchangeable with heparin or other LMWHs**

• At same time each day to maintain steady blood levels

• Avoid all IM inj that may cause bleeding

• Prepare in a sterile environment using aseptic technique

• Dilution may be stored for up to 4 wk in glass vial at room temp, up to 2 wk in TB syringes with rubber stoppers at room temp or refrigerated

SUBCUT route

• Do not give IM; begin 1 hr prior to surgery; do not aspirate; rotate sites; do not expel bubble from syringe before administration

• To recumbent patient, give SUBCUT; rotate inj sites (left/right anterolateral, left/right posterolateral abdominal wall)

• Insert whole length of needle into skin fold held with thumb and forefinger

• If withdrawing from multidose vial, use TB syringe for proper measurement

• Prefilled syringes (30, 40 mg) not graduated; do not use for partial doses

• Do not administer if particulate is present

Direct IV route

• Use multidose vial for IV administration; use TB syringe, other graduated syringe to measure dose; give IV BOL through IV line, flush after

SIDE EFFECTS

CNS: Fever, confusion
GI: Nausea
HEMA: **Hemorrhage, hypochromic anemia, thrombocytopenia, bleeding**
INTEG: Ecchymosis, inj site hematoma
META: Hyperkalemia in renal failure
SYST: Edema, peripheral edema

PHARMACOKINETICS

SUBCUT: 90% absorbed, maximum antithrombin activity (3-5 hr), elimination half-life 4½ hr, excreted in urine

INTERACTIONS

Increase: enoxaparin action—anticoagulants, salicylates, NSAIDs, antiplatelets, thrombolytics

Drug/Lab Test

Increase: AST, ALT
Decrease: platelet count

NURSING CONSIDERATIONS

Assess:

• Blood studies (Hct/Hgb, CBC, coagulation studies, platelets, occult blood in stools), anti-factor Xa (should be checked 4 hr after inj); thrombocytopenia may occur

• Renal studies: BUN/creatinine baseline and periodically

• **Bleeding:** gums, petechiae, ecchymosis, black tarry stools, hematuria; notify prescriber

Black Box Warning: Neurologic symptoms in patients who have received spinal anesthesia

Perform/provide:
• Storage at 77° F (25° C); do not freeze

Evaluate:
• Therapeutic response: prevention of DVT

Teach patient/family:
• To use soft-bristle toothbrush to avoid bleeding gums; to use electric razor
• To report any signs of bleeding: gums, under skin, urine, stools
• To avoid OTC products containing aspirin unless approved by prescriber

TREATMENT OF OVERDOSE:
Protamine SO_4 1% sol; dose should equal dose of enoxaparin

entacapone (Rx)
(en'ta-kah-pone)

Comtan

Func. class.: Antiparkinson agent
Chem. class.: COMT inhibitor

ACTION: Inhibits COMT (catechol *O*-methyltransferase) and alters the plasma pharmacokinetics of levodopa; given with levodopa/carbidopa

USES: Parkinson's disease for those experiencing end of dose; decreased effect as adjunct to levodopa/carbidopa

CONTRAINDICATIONS: Hypersensitivity

Precautions: Pregnancy (C), breastfeeding, children, renal/hepatic disease, affective disorders, psychosis

DOSAGE AND ROUTES
• **Adult: PO** 200 mg given with carbidopa/levodopa, max 1600 mg/day; may allow for 25% dosage reduction in levodopa therapy

Available forms: Tabs, film coated 200 mg

Administer:
• Only after MAOIs have been discontinued for 2 wk
• Give with dose of levodopa/carbidopa; product has no effect on its own

SIDE EFFECTS
CNS: *Involuntary choreiform movements, hand tremors, fatigue, headache, anxiety, twitching, numbness, dyskinesia, hypokinesia, hyperkinesia, weakness, confusion, agitation, nightmares,* psychosis, hallucination, hypomania, severe depression, dizziness, **neuroleptic malignant syndrome**

CV: *Orthostatic hypotension*

GI: *Nausea, vomiting, anorexia, abdominal distress, dry mouth, flatulence, bitter taste, diarrhea, constipation, dyspepsia,* gastritis, GI disorder

INTEG: Rash, sweating, alopecia

MISC: Dark urine and other body fluids, back pain, dyspnea, purpura, fatigue, asthenia, bacterial infection, **rhabdomyolysis**

PHARMACOKINETICS
Duration up to 8 hr; excreted in urine, feces; well absorbed; protein binding 98%; metabolized in liver extensively; enters breast milk; half-life of levodopa extended, half-life 0.5 hr initial, 2.5 hr second

INTERACTIONS
• Prevents catecholamine metabolism—nonselective MAOIs; do not use together

Increase: B/P, tachycardia, dysrhythmias, avoid use—bitolterol, DOPamine, DOBUTamine, EPINEPHrine, methyldopa, isoetharine, norepinephrine

Decrease: excretion of entacapone—ampicillin, chloramphenicol, probenecid, erythromycin, rifampin

Drug/Herb
Increase: B/P—ma huang
Decrease: effect—kava

NURSING CONSIDERATIONS

Assess:

⚠ **Neuroleptic malignant syndrome:** high temp, increased CPK, rigidity, change in LOC usually during rapid withdrawal

- **Involuntary movements of Parkinson's disease:** akinesia, tremors, staggering gait, muscle rigidity, drooling when given with levodopa/carbidopa
- B/P, respirations during initial treatment
- Mental status: affect, mood, behavioral changes, depression; complete suicide assessment
- **Rhabdomyolysis:** muscle pain, tenderness, weakness; swelling of affected muscles; may lead to decreased B/P, shock

Perform/provide:

- Assistance with ambulation during beginning therapy

Evaluate:

- Therapeutic response: decrease in akathisia, increased mood when given with levodopa/carbidopa

Teach patient/family:

- That hallucinations, mental changes, nausea, dyskinesia can occur; may mean patient is overmedicated
- To change positions slowly to prevent orthostatic hypotension; not to drive, operate machinery until stabilized on medication and mental performance not affected
- To use product exactly as prescribed; if dose is missed, to take as soon as remembered up to 2 hr before next dose; not to discontinue abruptly; to withdraw gradually
- That urine, sweat may darken
- To notify prescriber if pregnancy is suspected; if lactating, that product excreted in breast milk

entecavir (Rx)

(en-te′ka-veer)

Baraclude

Func. class.: Antiretroviral nucleoside reverse transcriptase inhibitor (NRTIs)
Chem. class.: Guanosine nucleoside analog

ACTION: Inhibits hepatitis B virus DNA polymerase by competing with natural substrates and by causing DNA termination after its incorporation into viral DNA; causes viral DNA death

USES: Chronic hepatitis B (HBV)

CONTRAINDICATIONS: Hypersensitivity

Precautions: Pregnancy (C), breastfeeding, children, geriatric patients, severe renal disease

Black Box Warning: Hepatic disease, hepatitis, HIV, lactic acidosis

DOSAGE AND ROUTES

Chronic hepatitis B (nucleoside treatment naive)

- **Adult and adolescent ≥16 yr: PO** 0.5 mg/day

Chronic hepatitis B with compensated liver disease and history of hepatitis B viremia while receiving lamivudine or known lamivudine/telbivudine-resistant mutations

- **Adult and adolescent ≥16 yr: PO** 1 mg/day

Renal dose

- **Adult: PO** CCr ≥50 ml/min, 0.5 mg/day; CCr 30-49 ml/min, 0.25 mg/day, 0.5 mg/day or 1 mg q48hr for lamivudine-refractory patient; CCr 10-29 ml/min, 0.15/day, 0.3 mg or 1 mg q72hr for lamivudine-refractory patient; CCr <10 ml/min, 0.05 mg/day, 0.1 mg/day or 1 mg q7days for lamivudine-refractory patient

Available forms: Tabs, film coated 0.5, 1 mg; oral sol 0.05 mg/ml

Administer:
- After hemodialysis
- By mouth on empty stomach 2 hr before or after food
- **Oral liquid:** use calibrated oral dosing spoon provided; may be used interchangeably with tabs

SIDE EFFECTS

CNS: *Headache,* fatigue, dizziness, insomnia
ENDO: Hyperglycemia
GI: *Dyspepsia,* nausea, vomiting, diarrhea, elevated liver function enzymes
INTEG: Alopecia, rash
SYST: **Lactic acidosis, severe hepatomegaly with stenosis**

PHARMACOKINETICS

Peak 0.5-1.5 hr, steady state 6-10 days, 100% bioavailability, extensively distributed to tissues, protein binding 13%, terminal half-life 128-149 hr, excreted unchanged (62%-73%) via kidneys

INTERACTIONS

Drug/Food
Decrease: absorption—high-fat meal
Drug/Lab Test
Increase: ALT, AST, total bilirubin, amylase, lipase, creatinine, blood glucose, urine glucose
Decrease: platelets, albumin

NURSING CONSIDERATIONS

Assess:
- For nephrotoxicity: increasing CCr, BUN

Black Box Warning: For HIV before beginning treatment because HIV resistance may occur in chronic hepatitis B patients; monitor HIV RNA

Black Box Warning: For lactic acidosis, severe hepatomegaly with stenosis; increased serum lactate, increased hepatic enzymes, palpate line; discontinue if present

- Geriatric patients more carefully; may develop renal, cardiac symptoms more rapidly

Black Box Warning: For exacerbations of hepatitis (jaundice, pruritus, fatigue) after discontinuing treatment, monitor LFTs

Perform/provide:
- Storage in cool environment; protect from light

Evaluate:
- Therapeutic response: decreased symptoms of chronic hepatitis B, improving LFTs

Teach patient/family:
- Not to take with food
- To take exactly as prescribed
- Not to stop medication without approval of prescriber
- That optimal duration of treatment is unknown
- To avoid use with other medications unless approved by prescriber
- To notify prescriber of decreased urinary output, blood in urine

Black Box Warning: Symptoms of lactic acidosis: muscle pain, severe tiredness, weakness, trouble breathing, stomach pain with nausea/vomiting, coldness in arms/legs, fast/irregular heartbeat, dizziness

Black Box Warning: Symptoms of hepatotoxicity: eyes/skin turning yellow, dark urine, light bowel movements, no appetite for days, nausea, stomach pain

- That product does not cure but lowers amount of HBV in body
- That product does not stop spread of HBV to others by sex, sharing needles, or being exposed to blood
- Not to breastfeed

ePHEDrine nasal agent

See Appendix B

epinastine ophthalmic

See Appendix B

⚠ HIGH ALERT

EPINEPHrine (Rx)

(ep-i-nef′rin)

Adrenaclick, Adrenalin, EpiPen, EpiPen Jr., Primatene Mist, Twinject, Walgreens Bronchial Mist

Func. class.: Bronchodilator nonselective adrenergic agonist, vasopressor

Chem. class.: Catecholamine

Do not confuse:
EPINEPHrine/ePHEDrine

ACTION: β_1- and β_2-agonist causing increased levels of cAMP, thereby producing bronchodilation, cardiac, and CNS stimulation; high doses cause vasoconstriction via α-receptors; low doses can cause vasodilation via β_2-vascular receptors

USES: Acute asthmatic attacks, hemostasis, bronchospasm, anaphylaxis, allergic reactions, cardiac arrest, adjunct in anesthesia, shock

Unlabeled uses: Bradycardia, chloroquine overdose

CONTRAINDICATIONS: Hypersensitivity to sympathomimetics, closed-angle glaucoma, nonanaphylactic shock during general anesthesia

Precautions: Pregnancy (C), breastfeeding, cardiac disorders, hyperthyroidism, diabetes mellitus, prostatic hypertrophy, hypertension, organic brain syndrome, local anesthesia of certain areas, labor, cardiac dilation, coronary insufficiency, cerebral arteriosclerosis, organic heart disease

DOSAGE AND ROUTES

Anaphylaxis/severe asthma exacerbation

- **Adult: IM/SUBCUT** 0.3-0.5 mg, may repeat q10-15min (anaphylaxis) or q20min-4 hr (asthma)

Severe allergic reactions type I

- **Adult/child ≥30 kg: IM** 0.3 mg (EpiPen/EpiPen 2-Pak, 1:1000)
- **Child <30 kg: IM** 0.15 mg (EpiPen Jr/EpiPen Jr 2-Pak 1:2000)
- **Adult/child ≥66 lb: IM/SUBCUT** 0.3 mg (0.3 ml) initially (Twinject 1.1 ml 1:1000, 1 mg/ml, containing 2 doses of 0.3 mg)
- **Adult/child 33-66 lb: IM/SUBCUT** 0.15 mg (0.15 ml) initially, may give another 0.15 mg after 10 min (Twinject 1.1 ml 1:1000 [1 mg/ml] containing 2 doses of 0.15 mg)

Status asthmaticus

- **Adult: IV** 0.3-0.5 mg SUBCUT (0.3-0.5 ml 1:1000 inj) q20min × 3 doses
- **Infant/child: IV** 0.01 mg/kg up to 0.5 mg SUBCUT q20min × 3 doses

Available forms: Nasal spray (sol) 1 mg/ml; sol for inj 1 mg/ml, 1:10,000, 1:1000; inh vapor (sol) 0.22 mg/actuation; pressurized inh (sol) 0.22 mg/actuation; sol for inj 0.15 mg/0.15 ml autoinjector, 0.3 mg/0.3 ml autoinjector, 0.15 mg/0.3 ml

Administer:

- Increased dose of insulin for diabetic patients if glucose is elevated
- Check for correct concentration, route, dosage before administering

IM/SUBCUT route

- Rotate inj sites, massage after inj, shake before using

Endotracheal route

- Give directly via endrotracheal tube, use 1:10,000 sol; for small dose, further dilute dose prior to administration, follow with quick insufflations

Inhalation route

- Place in nebulizer (10 gtt of a 1% base sol)
- Dilute racepinephrine 2.25% sol

IV route

- 1:10,000 sol can be given undiluted
- Parenteral dose slowly after reconstituting 1 mg (1:1000 sol)/10 ml or more 0.9% NaCl; to prepare a 1:10,000 sol for maintenance, may be further diluted in 500 ml D_5W; give 1 mg or less over ≥1 min through Y-tube or 3-way stopcock; 1 mg = 1 ml of 1:1000 or 10 ml of 1:10,000; protect from light, use large vein

Y-site compatibilities: Alfentanil, amikacin, amiodarone, amphotericin B liposome, anidulafungin, ascorbic acid, atracurium, atropine, aztreonam, benztropine, bivalirudin, bleomycin, bumetanide, buprenorphine, butorphanol, calcium chloride/gluconate, CARBOplatin, caspofungin, ceFAZolin, cefoperazone, cefotaxime, cefotetan, cefoxitin, ceftazidime, ceftizoxime, cefTRIAXone, cefuroxime, chloramphenicol, chlorproMAZINE, cimetidine, cisatracurium, CISplatin, clindamycin, cyanocobalamin, cyclophosphamide, cycloSPORINE, cytarabine, DACTINomycin, DAPTOmycin, dexamethasone, dexmedetomidine, digoxin, diltiazem, diphenhydrAMINE, DOBUTamine, docetaxel, DOPamine, DOXOrubicin, doxycycline, enalaprilat, epirubicin, epoetin alfa, ertapenem, erythromycin, esmolol, etoposide, etoposide phosphate, famotidine, fenoldopam, fentaNYL, fluconazole, fludarabine, folic acid, furosemide, gemcitabine, gentamicin, glycopyrrolate, granisetron, heparin, hydrocortisone, HYDROmorphone, ifosfamide, imipenem-cilastatin, isoproterenol, ketorolac, labetalol, levofloxacin, lidocaine, linezolid, LORazepam, magnesium sulfate, mannitol, mechlorethamine, meperidine, metaraminol, methicillin, methotrexate, methoxamine, methyldopa, methylPREDNISolone, metoclopramide, metoprolol, metroNIDAZOLE, midazolam, milrinone, minocycline, mitoxantrone, morphine, multiple vitamins, nafcillin, nalbuphine, naloxone, niCARdipine, nitroglycerin, nitroprusside, norepinephrine, octreotide, ondansetron, oxacillin, oxaliplatin, oxytocin, paclitaxel, palonosetron, pancuronium, pantoprazole, pemetrexed, penicillin G potassium, pentamidine, pentazocine, phentolamine, phenylephrine, phytonadione, piperacillin/tazobactam, potassium chloride, procainamide, prochlorperazine, promethazine, propofol, propranolol, protamine, pyridoxime, quinupristin/dalfopristin, ranitidine, remifentanil, ritodrine, rocuronium, sodium acetate, streptomycin, succinylcholine, SUFentanil, tacrolimus, teniposide, theophylline, thiamine, thiotepa, ticarcillin/clavulanate, tigecycline, tirofiban, tobramycin, tolazoline, trimethaphan, urokinase, vancomycin, vasopressin, vecuronium, verapamil, vinCRIStine, vinorelbine, vitamin B complex with C, voriconazole, warfarin, zoledronic acid

SIDE EFFECTS

CNS: *Tremors, anxiety,* insomnia, headache, *dizziness,* confusion, hallucinations, **cerebral hemorrhage**, weakness, drowsiness
CV: *Palpitations, tachycardia,* hypertension, *dysrhythmias,* increased T wave
GI: *Anorexia, nausea, vomiting*
MISC: Sweating, dry eyes
RESP: *Dyspnea*

PHARMACOKINETICS

Crosses placenta, metabolized in liver
SUBCUT: Onset 5-15 min, duration 20 min-4 hr
INH: Onset 1-5 min, duration 1-3 hr

INTERACTIONS

- Do not use with MAOIs or tricyclics; hypertensive crisis may occur
- Toxicity: other sympathomimetics

Decrease: hypertensive effects—β-adrenergic blockers
Drug/Herb

- Increased stimulation: coffee, tea, guarana, yerba maté

NURSING CONSIDERATIONS

Assess:

- **Asthma:** auscultate lungs, pulse, B/P, respirations, sputum (color, character); monitor pulmonary function studies before and during treatment
- **ECG** during administration continuously; if B/P increases, decrease dose; B/P, pulse q5min after parenteral route; CVP, ISVR, PCWP during inf if possible; inadvertent high arterial B/P can result in angina, aortic rupture, cerebral hemorrhage
- Inj site: tissue sloughing; administer phentolamine with NS
- **Sulfite sensitivity;** may be life-threatening
- Cardiac status, I&O; blood glucose in diabetes
- **Allergic reactions, bronchospasms:** withhold dose, notify prescriber

Perform/provide:

- Storage of reconstituted sol refrigerated ≤24 hr
- Do not use discolored sol

Evaluate:

- Therapeutic response: increased B/P with stabilization or ease of breathing

Teach patient/family:

- About the reason for product administration; how to administer
- To rinse mouth after use to prevent dryness after inhalation
- Not to take OTC preparations

TREATMENT OF OVERDOSE:
Administer α-blocker and β-blocker

EPINEPHrine/ epinephryl borate ophthalmic
See Appendix B

EPINEPHrine nasal agent
See Appendix B

⚠ HIGH ALERT

epirubicin (Rx)
(ep-ih-roo′bi-sin)

Ellence, Pharmorubicin ♣

Func. class.: Antineoplastic, antibiotic

Chem. class.: Anthracycline

ACTION:
Inhibits DNA synthesis primarily; replication is decreased by binding to DNA, which causes strand splitting; maximum cytotoxic effects at S and for G_2 phases; a vesicant

USES:
Adjuvant therapy for breast cancer with axillary node involvement after resection

Unlabeled uses: Used in combination for treatment of advanced forms of cancer: bladder, gastric, head and neck, hepatocellular, lung, ovarian, multiple myeloma, soft-tissue sarcoma

CONTRAINDICATIONS:
Pregnancy (D), breastfeeding, hypersensitivity to product, anthracyclines, anthracenediones, baseline neutrophil count <1500 cell/mm³, severe myocardial insufficiency, recent MI, systemic infections

Black Box Warning: Severe hepatic disease

Precautions: Children, geriatric patients, cardiac/renal/hepatic disease, gout, previous anthracycline use

Black Box Warning: Bone marrow depression (severe), heart failure, extravasation, secondary malignancy

DOSAGE AND ROUTES

- **Adult: IV INF** 100-120 mg/m² initially, given with other antineoplastics (cyclophosphamide, 5-fluorouracil); given in repeated 3-4 cycles

Epirubicin dosage adjustments

- **Adult: IV** 100 mg/m² on day 1 of each cycle; toxicity nadir platelet counts <50,000 mm³, ANC 250 mm³, neutropenic fever or grade 3 or 4 nonhematologic toxicity; next cycle give 75% of day 1 dose; delay next cycle until platelets are ≥100,000 mm^3, ANC ≥1500 mm^3, nonhematologic toxicities have recovered to < grade 1

Hepatic dose

• **Adult: IV** Bilirubin 1.2-3 mg/dl or AST 2-4× normal upper limit, 50% of starting dose; bilirubin >3-5 mg/dl or AST >4 × normal upper limit, 25% of starting dose

Available forms: Inj (2 mg/ml) 10 mg/5 ml, 50 mg/25 ml, 150 mg/75 ml, 200 mg/100 ml

Administer:

• Antiemetic 30-60 min before product to prevent vomiting

• Allopurinol or sodium bicarbonate to maintain uric acid levels, alkalinization of urine

IV route

• Use cytotoxic handling procedures; pregnant women must not handle product

• Reconstitute 50 mg and 200 mg powder for inj with 25 ml and 100 ml, respectively, of sterile water for inj (2 mg/ml); shake well

IV Injection route

• Given into tubing of free-flowing IV infusion (0.9% NaCl or D_5); give over 3-5 min

Intermittent IV INF route

Dilute in appropriate dose of 0.9% NaCl or D_5W; infuse over 30-60 min

• Do not mix with other products in syringe

Y-site compatibilities: Alfentanil, amifostine, amikacin, aminocaproic acid, anidulafungin, atracurium, aztreonam, bivalirudin, bleomycin, bumetanide, buprenorphine, butorphanol, calcium chloride/gluconate, CARBOplatin, caspofungin, ceFAZolin, cefotaxime, ceftizoxime, chlorproMAZINE, cimetidine, ciprofloxacin, cisatracurium, CISplatin, clindamycin, cyclophosphamide, cycloSPORINE, DAPTOmycin, dexrazoxane, digoxin, diltiazem, diphenhydrAMINE, DOBUTamine, docetaxel, dolasetron, DOPamine, doxacurium, doxycycline, droperidol, enalaprilat, ePHEDrine, EPINEPHrine, erythromycin, etoposide, famotidine, fenoldopam, fentaNYL, fluconazole, gatifloxacin, gemcitabine, gentamicin, granisetron, haloperidol, hydrocortisone, HYDROmorphone, hydrOXYzine, ifosfamide, imipenem-cilastatin, inamrinone, insulin (regular), isoproterenol, labetalol, levofloxacin, levorphanol, lidocaine, linezolid, LORazepam, mannitol, meperidine, mesna, methotrexate, metoclopramide, metoprolol, metroNIDAZOLE, midazolam, milrinone, minocycline, mitomycin, mivacurium, morphine, nalbuphine, naloxone, nesiritide, niCARdipine, nitroglycerin, nitroprusside, norepinephrine, octreotide, ofloxacin, ondansetron, oxaliplatin, paclitaxel, palonosetron, pamidronate, pancuronium, pentamidine, pentazocine, phenylephrine, potassium chloride, procainamide, prochlorperazine, promethazine, propranolol, quinupristin-dalfopristin, ranitidine, remifentanil, rocuronium, sodium acetate, succinylcholine, SUFentanil, tacrolimus, teniposide, theophylline, thiotepa, tirofiban, tobramycin, trimethobenzamide, vancomycin, vasopressin, vecuronium, verapamil, vinBLAStine, vinCRIStine, vinorelbine, voriconazole, zidovudine, zoledronic acid

SIDE EFFECTS

CV: Increased B/P, sinus tachycardia, PVCs, chest pain, bradycardia, extrasystoles

GI: *Nausea, vomiting, anorexia, mucositis, diarrhea*

GU: *Amenorrhea, hot flashes, hyperuricemia*

HEMA: Thrombocytopenia, leukopenia, anemia, neutropenia, secondary AML

INTEG: *Rash,* necrosis, *pain at inj site, reversible alopecia*

MISC: *Infection, febrile neutropenia, lethargy, fever, conjunctivitis,* tumor lysis syndrome

PHARMACOKINETICS

Triphasic pattern of elimination; half-life 3 min, 2.5 hr, 33 hr; metabolized by liver; crosses placenta; excreted in urine, bile, breast milk

INTERACTIONS

Increase: toxicity—other antineoplastics or radiation, cimetidine

Decrease: antibody response—live virus vaccine

NURSING CONSIDERATIONS

Assess:

Black Box Warning: Bone marrow depression (severe): CBC, differential, platelet count weekly; withhold product if baseline neutrophil $\leq$1500/mm^3; leukocyte nadir occurs 10-14 days after administration, recovery by day 21; notify prescriber of results

- Blood, urine uric acid levels; swelling, joint pain primarily in extremities; patient should be well hydrated to prevent urate deposits
- Renal disease: BUN, serum uric acid, urine CCr, electrolytes before, during therapy; I&O ratio; report fall in urine output to <30 ml/hr; dosage adjustment needed if serum creatinine >5 mg/dl

Black Box Warning: Hepatic studies before, during therapy: bilirubin, AST, ALT, alk phos as needed or monthly

Black Box Warning: Heart failure: B/P, pulse, character, rhythm, rate, ABGs, ECG, LVEF, MUGA scan, or ECHO; watch for ST-T wave changes, low QRS and T, possible dysrhythmias (sinus tachycardia, heart block, PVCs)

- Bleeding: hematuria, guaiac, bruising, or petechiae, mucosa or orifices q8hr
- Effects of alopecia on body image; discuss feelings about body changes

Black Box Warning: Extravasation (vesicant): local irritation, pain, burning, necrosis at inj site, discontinue and start at another site

- GI symptoms: frequency of stools, cramping

Perform/provide:

- Strict hand-washing technique, gloves, protective clothing
- Liquid diet: carbonated beverages, gelatin may be added if patient not nauseated or vomiting
- Increased fluid intake to 2-3 L/day to prevent urate, calculi formation

Evaluate:

- Therapeutic response: decreased tumor size, spread of malignancy

Teach patient/family:

- To report any complaints, side effects to nurse or prescriber
- That hair may be lost during treatment; that wig or hairpiece may make patient feel better; that new hair may be different in color, texture
- To avoid crowds, persons with infections when granulocyte count is low
- That contraceptive measures recommended during therapy and for 4 mo thereafter for men and women; pregnancy (D)
- To avoid vaccinations because reactions may occur; to avoid cimetidine during therapy
- That urine may appear red for 2 days
- To avoid OTC medications, supplements unless approved by prescriber
- That irreversible myocardial damage, leukopenia, menopause may occur

eplerenone (Rx)

(ep-ler-ee'known)

Inspra

Func. class.: Antihypertensive

Chem. class.: Selective aldosterone receptor antagonist

ACTION: Binds to mineralocorticoid receptor and blocks the binding of aldosterone, a component of the renin-angiotensin-aldosterone system (RAAS)

USES: Hypertension, alone or in combination with thiazide diuretics, CHF, post-MI

CONTRAINDICATIONS:

Hypersensitivity; increased serum creatinine >2 mg/dl (male), >1.8 mg/dl (female); potassium >5.5 mEq/L, type 2 diabetes with microalbuminuria, hepatic disease, CCr <30 ml/min; CCr <50 ml/min in hypertension

Precautions: Pregnancy (B), breastfeeding, child, geriatric patients, impaired renal/hepatic function, hyperkalemia

DOSAGE AND ROUTES

- **Adult: PO** 50 mg/day initially, may increase to 50 mg bid after 4 wk; start dose at 25 mg/day if patient is taking CYP3A4 inhibitors

CHF or post-MI

- **Adult: PO** 25 mg/day initially, may increase to 50 mg/day max after 4 wk

Available forms: Tabs 25, 50 mg

Administer:

- Without regard to food
- Do not use salt substitutes containing potassium

SIDE EFFECTS

CNS: Headache, dizziness, fatigue
CV: Angina, **MI**
GI: Increased GGT diarrhea, abdominal pain, increased ALT
GU: Increased BUN, creatinine, gynecomastia, mastodynia (males), abnormal vaginal bleeding
META: Hyperkalemia, hyponatremia, hypercholesteremia, hypertriglyceridemia, increased uric acid
RESP: Cough

PHARMACOKINETICS

Peak $1^1/_2$ hr; serum protein binding 50%; half-life 4-6 hr; metabolized in liver by CYP3A4 inhibitor; excreted in urine, feces

INTERACTIONS

Increase: hyperkalemia—ACE inhibitors, angiotensin II antagonists, NSAIDs, potassium supplements, potassium-sparing diuretics
Increase: serum levels of lithium
Increase: levels of eplerenone—CYP3A4 inhibitors (ketoconazole, itraconazole, saquinavir, erythromycin, verapamil, fluconazole); reduce dose of eplerenone
Decrease: antihypertensive effect—NSAIDs

Drug/Herb

Decrease: antihypertensive effect—ephedra

Drug/Food

- Grapefruit, grapefruit juice increase product level by 25%
- Do not use salt substitutes containing potassium

NURSING CONSIDERATIONS

Assess:

- **Hypertension:** B/P at peak/trough level of product, orthostatic hypotension, syncope when used with diuretic; monitor lithium level in those also taking lithium
- Renal studies: protein, BUN, creatinine; increased LFTs, uric acid may be increased
- Potassium levels, hyperkalemia may occur

Perform/provide:

- Storage in tight container at ≤86° F (30° C)

Evaluate:

- Therapeutic response: decreased B/P

Teach patient/family:

- Not to discontinue product abruptly
- Not to use OTC products (cough, cold, allergy) unless directed by prescriber; not to use salt substitutes containing potassium without consulting prescriber
- To comply with dosage schedule, even if feeling better
- That product may cause dizziness, fainting, lightheadedness; may occur during first few days of therapy
- How to take B/P; and about normal readings for age group

epoetin alfa (Rx)

(ee-poe′e-tin)

EPO, Epogen, Eprex ✱, Procrit

Func. class.: Antianemic, biologic modifier, hormone

Chem. class.: Amino acid polypeptide

ACTION: Erythropoietin is 1 factor controlling the rate of red cell production; product is developed by recombinant DNA technology

USES: Anemia caused by reduced endogenous erythropoietin production, primarily end-stage renal disease; to correct hemostatic defect in uremia; anemia due to AZT treatment in patients with HIV or those receiving chemotherapy; reduction of allogenic blood transfusion in surgery patients

Unlabeled uses: Anemia in premature preterm infants, anemia due to ribavirin and interferon-alfa therapy in hepatitic C

CONTRAINDICATIONS: Hypersensitivity to mammalian-cell–derived products, human albumin; uncontrolled hypertension

Precautions: Pregnancy (C), breastfeeding, children <1 mo, seizure disorder; multidose preserved formulation contains benzyl alcohol and should not be used in premature infants; porphyria, CV disease, hemodialysis, latex allergy, hypertension, history of CABG

Black Box Warning: Hgb >12 g/dl, surgery, neoplastic disease

DOSAGE AND ROUTES

Anemia related to chemotherapy (nonmyeloid malignancies)

• **Adult: SUBCUT** 150 units/kg 3×/wk, may increase after 2 mo up to 300 units/kg 3×/wk

Anemia with chronic renal failure

• **Adult: SUBCUT/IV** 50-100 units/kg 3×/wk then adjust to maintain target Hct of 30%-36%

• **Child: IV/SUBCUT** 50 units/kg 3×/wk

Anemia secondary to zidovudine treatment

• **Adult: SUBCUT/IV** 100 units/kg 3×/wk × 2 mo, may increase by 50-100 units/kg q1-2mo up to 300 units/kg 3×/wk

Surgery

• **Adult: SUBCUT** 300 units/kg/day × 10 days prior to surgery, the day of surgery, and for 4 days postsurgery or 600 units/kg at 3 wk, 2 wk, 1 wk prior to and on day of surgery

Anemia due to ribavirin/interferon-alfa therapy in hepatitic C (unlabeled)

• **Adult: SUBCUT** 40,000 units/wk; if Hgb has not increased by ≥1 g/dl after 4 wk, increase to 60,000 units/wk

Available forms: Inj 2000, 3000, 4000, 10,000, 20,000, 40,000 units/ml

Administer:

• Do not shake vial

• Use 1 single-use vial/dose, once syringe has entered single dose vial, sterility cannot be guaranteed, do not administer with other product, multidose vials can be stored in refrigerator up to 21 days once opened

SUBCUT route

• Before injecting preservative free-, single-dose formulation may be admixed using 0.9% NaCl with benzyl alcohol 0.9% at a 1:1 ratio to reduce inj site discomfort

Direct IV route

• Additional heparin to lower chance of clots

• By direct inj or bolus into IV tubing or venous line at end of dialysis

• Decrease dose by 25 units/kg if Hct increases by 4% in 2 wk; increase dose if Hct does not increase by 5-6 pts after 8 wk of therapy; suggested target Hct range 30%–36%

Solution compatibilities: Do not dilute or administer with other sol

SIDE EFFECTS

CNS: Seizures, coldness, sweating, headache

CV: *Hypertension,* hypertensive encephalopathy, CHF, edema, DVT

INTEG: Pruritus, rash, inj site reaction

MISC: Iron deficiency

MS: Bone pain

RESP: Cough

PHARMACOKINETICS

IV: Metabolized in body, extent of metabolism unknown, onset of increased reticulocyte count 2-6 wk, peak immediate

INTERACTIONS

- Need for increased heparin during hemodialysis

NURSING CONSIDERATIONS

Assess:

- Renal studies: urinalysis, protein, blood, BUN, creatinine; I&O, report drop in output $<$50 ml/hr

Black Box Warning: Blood studies: ferritin, transferrin, serum iron monthly; transferrin sat $\geq$20%, ferritin $\geq$100 ng/ml; Hct 2×/wk until stabilized in target range (30%-36%) then at regular intervals; those with endogenous erythropoietin levels of $<$500 units/L respond to product; monitor Hct 2×/wk with chronic renal failure; patients treated with zidovudine or patients with cancer should be monitored weekly then periodically after stabilization; death may occur with Hgb $>$12 g/dl

- B/P; check for rising B/P as Hct rises, antihypertensives may be needed; hypertension may occur rapidly, leading to hypertensive encephalopathy
- CNS symptoms: coldness, sweating, pain in long bones; for seizures if Hct is increased within 2 wk by 4 pts
- Hypersensitivity reactions: skin rashes, urticaria (rare), antibody development does not occur

⚠ **Pure cell aplasia (PRCA)** in absence of other causes; evaluate by testing sera for recombinant erythropoetin antibodies; any loss of response to epoetin should be evaluated

- Dialysis patients: thrill, bruit of shunts; monitor for circulation impairment
- **Seizures:** place patient on seizure precautions if increase of $\geq$4 points HCT in 2 wk, increased B/P; more common in chronic renal failure during the first 90 days of treatment

Evaluate:

- Therapeutic response: increase in reticulocyte count in 2-6 wk, Hgb/Hct; increased appetite, enhanced sense of well-being

Teach patient/family:

- To avoid driving or hazardous activities during beginning of treatment
- To monitor B/P
- To take iron supplements, vit B_{12}, folic acid as directed

eprosartan (Rx)

(ep-roh-sar'tan)

Teveten

Func. class.: Antihypertensive

Chem. class.: Angiotensin II–receptor antagonist (Subtype AT_1)

ACTION: Blocks the vasoconstrictive and aldosterone-secreting effects of angiotensin II; selectively blocks the binding of angiotensin II to the AT_1 receptor found in tissues

USES: Hypertension, alone or with other antihypertensives

CONTRAINDICATIONS: Hypersensitivity

Black Box Warning: Pregnancy (D) 2nd/3rd trimesters

Precautions: Pregnancy (C) 1st trimester, breastfeeding, children, geriatric patients, hypersensitivity to ACE inhibitors; renal/hepatic disease, angioedema

DOSAGE AND ROUTES

• **Adult: PO** 600 mg/day; dose may be divided, given bid, with total daily doses from 400-800 mg, max 900 mg/day

Available forms: Tabs 400, 600 mg

Administer:

• Without regard to meals

SIDE EFFECTS

CNS: *Dizziness,* depression, fatigue, headache

CV: Chest pain, hypotension

EENT: Sinusitis

GI: *Diarrhea, dyspepsia,* abdominal pain

GU: UTI

INTEG: Pruritus, angioedema

META: Hypertriglyceridemia

MS: Myalgia, arthralgia, rhabdomyolysis

RESP: *Cough, upper respiratory infection,* rhinitis, pharyngitis, viral infection

SYST: Anaphylaxis

PHARMACOKINETICS

Peak 1-2 hr, food delays absorption; protein binding 98%; moderate renal impairment increases product levels by 30%, hepatic impairment increases levels by 40%; excreted in urine and feces; half-life 5-9 hr

INTERACTIONS

Decrease: antihypertensive effect—NSAIDs, salicylates

Drug/Lab Test

Increase: ALT, AST, alk phos

Decrease: Hgb

NURSING CONSIDERATIONS

Assess:

• B/P with position changes, pulse q4hr; note rate, rhythm, quality

⚠ Hypersensitivity reactions, including anaphylaxis

⚠ Myalgia, arthralgia; may cause rhabdomyolysis

• Baselines of renal, hepatic studies before therapy begins

• Edema in feet, legs daily

• Skin turgor, dryness of mucous membranes for hydration status

Evaluate:

• Therapeutic response: decreased B/P

Teach patient/family:

• To comply with dosage schedule, even if feeling better

• To notify prescriber of fever; chest pain; swelling of hands, feet, face, lip, or tongue

• That excessive perspiration, dehydration, diarrhea may lead to fall in B/P; consult prescriber if these occur

• That product may cause dizziness; to avoid hazardous activities until effect is known

Black Box Warning: Not to take this product if pregnant or breastfeeding, or if have had an allergic reaction to product

• To take missed dose as soon as possible unless within 1 hr before next dose

• That therapeutic effect may take 2-3 wk

⚠ HIGH ALERT

eptifibatide (Rx)

(ep-tih-fib′ah-tide)

Integrilin

Func. class.: Antiplatelet agent

Chem. class.: Glycoprotein IIb/IIIa inhibitor

ACTION: Platelet glycoprotein antagonist; this agent reversibly prevents fibrinogen, von Willebrand's factor from binding to the glycoprotein IIb/IIIa receptor, thus inhibiting platelet aggregation

USES: Acute coronary syndrome including those undergoing percutaneous coronary intervention (PCI)

CONTRAINDICATIONS: Hypersensitivity, active internal bleeding; history of bleeding, stroke within 2 yr; major surgery with severe trauma, severe hypertension, history of intracranial bleeding, current or planned use of another parenteral GP IIb/IIIa inhibitor, dependence on renal dialysis, coagulopathy, AV malformation, aneurysm

Precautions: Pregnancy (B), breastfeeding, children, geriatric patients, bleeding, impaired renal function

DOSAGE AND ROUTES

Acute coronary syndrome

• **Adult: IV BOL** 180 mcg/kg as soon as diagnosed, max 22.6 mg, then **IV CONT** 2 mcg/kg/min until discharge or CABG up to 72 hr, max 15 mg/hr

PCI in patients without acute coronary syndrome

• **Adult: IV BOL** 180 mcg/kg given immediately before PCI then 2 mcg/kg/min × 18 hr and a second 180-mcg/kg bolus 10 min after 1st bolus; continue inf for up to 18-24 hr at rate of 1 mcg/kg/min

Renal dose

• **Adult: IV BOL** CCr <50 ml/min, 2-4 mg/dl same loading dose then ½ usual inf dose; CCr <10 ml/min, contraindicated

Available forms: Sol for inj 2 mg/ml (10 ml), 0.75 mg/ml (100 ml)

Administer:

• Aspirin and heparin may be given with this product; check for bleeding

• D/C heparin before removing femoral artery sheath, after PCI

Direct IV route

• After withdrawing bolus dose from 10-ml vial, give IV push over 1-2 min

Continuous IV INF route

• Follow bolus dose with continuous inf using pump; give product undiluted directly from 100-ml vial, spike 100-ml vial with vented inf set, use caution when centering spike on circle of stopper top

Y-site compatibilities: Alfentanil, alteplase, amikacin, aminophylline, amphotericin B lipid complex, amphotericin B liposome, ampicillin, ampicillin-sulbactam, anidulafungin, argatroban, atenolol, atracurium, atropine, azithromycin, aztreonam, bivalirudin, bumetanide, buprenorphine, butorphanol, calcium chloride/gluconate, ceFAZolin, cefepime, cefoperazone, cefotaxime, cefotetan, cefoxitin, ceftazidime, ceftizoxime, cefTRIAXone, cefuroxime, cimetidine, ciprofloxacin, cisatracurium, clindamycin, cycloSPORINE, DAPTOmycin, dexamethasone, D_5/NaCl 0.9%, diazepam, diltiazem, diphenhydrAMINE, DOBUTamine, dolasetron, DOPamine, doxycycline, droperidol, enalaprilat, ePHEDrine, EPINEPHrine, ertapenem, erythromycin, esmolol, famotidine, fentaNYL, fluconazole, fosphenytoin, ganciclovir, gatifloxacin, gentamicin, granisetron, haloperidol, heparin, hydrocortisone, HYDROmorphone, hydrOXYzine, imipenem-cilastatin, inamrinone, isoproterenol, ketorolac, labetalol, leucovorin, levofloxacin, levorphanol, lidocaine, linezolid, LORazepam, magnesium sulfate, mannitol, meperidine, meropenem, methylPREDNISolone, metoclopramide, metoprolol, metroNIDAZOLE, micafungin, midazolam, milrinone, minocycline, mivacurium, morphine, nalbuphine, naloxone, niCARdipine, nitroglycerin, nitroprusside, NS, octreotide, ofloxacin, ondansetron, oxytocin, palonosetron, pancuronium, pemetrexed, PENTobarbital, PHENobarbital, phenylephrine, piperacillin, piperacillin-tazobactam, potassium chloride/phosphates, procainamide, prochlorperazine, promethazine, propranolol, ranitidine, remifentanil, rocuronium, sodium bicarbonate/phosphates, succinylcholine, SUFentanil, sulfamethoxazole-trimethoprim, teniposide, theophylline, ticarcillin, ticarcillin-clavulanate, tigecycline, tirofiban, tobramycin, trimethobenzamide, vancomycin, vecuronium, verapamil, zidovudine, zoledronic acid

Solution compatibilities: 0.9% NaCl, D_5/0.9% NaCl

SIDE EFFECTS

CV: Stroke, hypotension

GU: Hematuria

HEMA: Thrombocytopenia

SYST: Bleeding, anaphylaxis

PHARMACOKINETICS

Onset within 1 hr, protein binding 25%, half-life 1.5-2 hr, steady state 4-6 hr, metabolism limited, excretion via kidneys

INTERACTIONS

• Do not give with glycoprotein inhibitors IIb, IIIa

Increase: bleeding—aspirin, heparin, NSAIDs, anticoagulants, ticlopidine, clopidogrel, dipyridamole, thrombolytics, valproate, abciximab

Drug/Herb

Increase: Bleeding risk—arnica, chamomile, clove, dong quai, feverfew, garlic, ginger, ginkgo, Panax ginseng

NURSING CONSIDERATIONS

Assess:

▲ **Thrombocytopenia:** platelets, Hgb, Hct, creatinine, PT/APTT baseline INR within 6 hr of loading dose, daily therafter, patients undergoing PCI should have ACT monitored; maintain APTT 50-70 sec unless PCI to be performed; during PCI, ACT should be 200-300 sec; if platelets drop $<100,000/mm^3$, obtain additional platelet counts; if thrombocytopenia is confirmed, discontinue product; draw Hct, Hgb, serum creatinine

▲ **Bleeding:** gums, bruising, ecchymosis, petechiae; from GI, GU tract, cardiac cath sites, IM inj sites

Perform/provide:

• Do not give discolored solutions, those with particulates; discard unused amount

• Discontinue product prior to CABG

• All medications PO if possible; avoid IM inj, all catheters

Teach patient/family:

• About reason for medication and expected results

• To report bruising, bleeding, chest pain immediately

ergotamine (Rx)

(er-got′a-meen)

Ergomar

dihydroergotamine

(dye-hye-droe-er-got′a-meen)

DHE45, Migranal

Func. class.: α-Adrenergic blocker, vascular headache suppressant

Chem. class.: Ergot alkaloid—amino acid

ACTION: Constricts smooth muscle in peripheral, cranial blood vessels; relaxes uterine muscle; blocks serotonin release

USES: Vascular headache (migraine, cluster histamine)

CONTRAINDICATIONS: Pregnancy (X), hypersensitivity to ergot preparations, occlusion (peripheral, vascular), renal/hepatic disease, peptic ulcer, intermittent claudication, glaucoma, CVA

Black Box Warning: Coronary artery disease, hypertension, Raynaud's disease, peripheral vascular disease, angina

Precautions: Breastfeeding, children, anemia, geriatric patients, basilar/hemiplegic migraine

Black Box Warning: MI, stroke, Buerger's disease, cardiac disease

DOSAGE AND ROUTES

Ergotamine

• **Adult: SL** 1 tab (2 mg), may use q30min, max 3 tabs (6 mg)/24 hr or 10 mg/wk

• **Adolescent/child ≥10 yr (unlabeled): SL** 1 mg, may repeat after 30 min, max 3 mg/24 hr or per attack

Dihydroergotamine

• **Adult: SUBCUT/IM/IV** 1 mg, may repeat after 1 hr to 3 mg, max 3 mg/day **(IM, SUBCUT)**, 2 mg **(IV)** or 6 mg/wk; **INTRANASAL** 1 spray in each nostril,

repeat after 15 min, max 3 mg/24 hr, 4 mg/wk
• **Child ≥6 yr: SUBCUT/IM** 0.5 mg, may repeat after 1 hr; **IV** 0.25 mg, may repeat after 1 hr

Available forms: *Ergotamine:* SL tabs 2 mg; tabs 1 mg; *dihydroergotamine:* inj 1 mg/ml; nasal spray 4 mg/ml

Administer:
• At beginning of headache; dose must be titrated to patient response
• Do not give to pregnant women; harm to fetus may occur

Intranasal route
• Prime nasal sprayer 4× before dose, use 1 spray in each nostril, wait 15 min, use another spray in each nostril; use nasal applicator for 4 treatments only, discard

Direct IV route
• Give dihydroergotamine undiluted over 1 min

SIDE EFFECTS

CNS: *Numbness in fingers, toes;* headache, weakness

CV: Transient tachycardia, chest pain, bradycardia, edema, claudication, increase or decrease in B/P, **MI**, peripheral vascular ischemia

GI: Nausea, vomiting, diarrhea, abdominal cramps

MS: Muscle pain

PHARMACOKINETICS

Metabolized in liver, excreted as metabolites in feces, crosses blood-brain barrier, excreted in breast milk, protein binding 90%-93%, half-life 2 hr

PO: Peak 30 min-3 hr, duration up to 48 hr

IM/SUBCUT: Peak (IM) 15-30 min, (SUBCUT) 30-60 min; duration (IM) 3-4 hr, (SUBCUT) 8 hr

IV: Peak 3 min, duration 8 hr

INTERACTIONS

Increase: toxicity—CYP4503A4 inhibitors (protease inhibitors, some macrolides, azole antifungals); do not use together

Increase: vasoconstriction—β-blockers, oral contraceptives, nicotine, vasoconstrictors, other migraine agents

NURSING CONSIDERATIONS

Assess:
• **Migraine characteristics:** duration, nausea, vomiting, change in vision, frequency before and at least 1 hr after administration
• **Ergotism:** nausea, vomiting, weakness, muscular pain, insensitivity to cold, paresthesia of extremities; product should be discontinued
• **Toxicity:** dyspnea; hypo/hypertension; rapid, weak pulse; delirium; nausea; vomiting
• For peripheral ischemia, GI side effects

Black Box Warning: CAD, hypertension, Raynaud's disease, angina, MI, stroke; do not administer to these patients

Perform/provide:
• Quiet, calm environment with decreased stimulation from noise, bright light, or excessive talking

Evaluate:
• Therapeutic response: decrease in frequency, severity of headache

Teach patient/family:
• Not to use OTC medications; serious product interactions may occur
• To maintain dose at approved level; not to increase even if product does not relieve headache
• To report side effects, including increased vasoconstriction starting with cold extremities, then paresthesia, weakness
• That an increase in headaches may occur when this product is discontinued after long-term use
⚠ To keep product out of reach of children; death may occur

TREATMENT OF OVERDOSE:

Induce emesis or gastric lavage if orally ingested; administer saline cathartic; keep warm

eribulin
(er'i-bu'lin)

Halaven

Func. class.: Antineoplastics—non-taxane

ACTION: Potent antimitotic agent, different from taxanes, vinca alkaloids, epothilones; blocks cell progression during G2-M phase; inhibits the growth phase of microtubules and sequesters tubules, leading to the disruption of mitotic spindles and apoptotic cell death

USES: Metastatic breast cancer in patients who have received at least 2 chemotherapy regimens

CONTRAINDICATIONS: Hypersensitivity, pregnancy (D)

Precautions: Breastfeeding, neonates, infants, children, bradycardia, electrolyte imbalances, heart failure, hypokalemia, hypomagnesemia, infertility, neutropenia, peripheral neuropathy, QT prolongation, hepatic/renal disease

DOSAGE AND ROUTES

• **Adult: IV** 1.4 mg/m^2 over 2-5 min on days 1 and 8, repeat q21days

• **Recommendations for dose delay:** for ANC <1000/mm^3, platelets <75,000/mm^3, or grade 3 or 4 nonhematologic toxicities: do not administer; the day 8 dose may be delayed a maximum of 1 wk; for the day 8 dose, if toxicities do not resolve to ≤ Grade 2 by day 15: omit the dose; for the day 8 dose, if toxicities resolve or improve to ≤ Grade 2 by day 15: administer eribulin at reduced dose (see below), initiate the next cycle no sooner than 2 wk later

• **Dose adjustments for hematologic toxicity:** ANC <500/mm^3 for >7 days or ANC <1000/mm^3 with fever or infection: permanently reduce dose to 1.1 mg/m^2; platelets <25,000/mm^3 or <50,000/mm^3 requiring transfusion: permanently reduce dose to 1.1 mg/m^2; if day 8 of previous cycle omitted or delayed: permanently reduce dose to 1.1 mg/m^2; while receiving 1.1 mg/m^2, if recurrence of hematologic event occurs, or if day 8 of previous cycle omitted or delayed: permanently reduce dose to 0.7 mg/m^2; while receiving 0.7 mg/m^2, if recurrence of hematologic event occurs, or if day 8 of previous cycle omitted or delayed: discontinue

• **Dose adjustments of eribulin for nonhematologic toxicity during treatment:** any Grade 3 or 4 nonhematologic toxicity: permanently reduce dose to 1.1 mg/m^2; if day 8 of previous cycle omitted or delayed: permanently reduce dose to 1.1 mg/m^2; while receiving 1.1 mg/m^2, if recurrence of Grade 3 or 4 nonhematologic toxicity occurs, or if day 8 of previous cycle omitted or delayed: permanently reduce dose to 0.7 mg/m^2; while receiving 0.7 mg/m^2, if recurrence of Grade 3 or 4 nonhematologic toxicity occurs, or if day 8 of previous cycle omitted or delayed: discontinue

Available forms: Sol for inj 1 mg/2 ml

Administer:

IV direct, intermittent route

• Visually inspect for particulate matter, discoloration as solution and container permit; withdraw required amount (0.5 mg/ml) from single-use vial, give undiluted over 2-5 min or diluted in 100 ml 0.9% NaCl and give as intermittent inf; do not give through line with dextrose or any other product

SIDE EFFECTS

CNS: Depression, dizziness, fatigue, fever, headache, insomnia, peripheral neuropathy

CV: QT prolongation, peripheral edema

GI: Abdominal pain, anorexia, constipation, diarrhea, dyspepsia, nausea, vomiting, weight loss

HEMA: Anemia, neutropenia, thrombocytopenia

INTEG: Alopecia, rash, stomatitis

META: Hypokalemia

MS: Arthralgia, myalgia, bone/back pain
RESP: Cough, dyspnea
SYST: Infection

PHARMACOKINETICS

Protein binding 49%-65%; inhibits CYP3A4; excreted in feces 82%; urine 9%; elimination half-life 40 hr; increased levels in hepatic/renal disease

INTERACTIONS

Increase: QT prolongation—arsenic trioxide, astemizole, bepridil, chloroquine, certain phenothiazines (chlorpromazine, mesoridazine, thioridazine), cisapride, clarithromycin, class IA antiarrhythmics (disopyramide, procainamide, quiNIDine), class III antiarrhythmics (amiodarone, bretylium, dofetilide, ibutilide, sotalol), dextromethorphan; quinidine, dronedarone, droperidol, erythromycin, halofantrine, haloperidol, levomethadyl, methadone, pentamidine, pimozide, posaconazole, probucol, propafenone, saquinavir, sparfloxacin terfenadine, troleandomycin, and ziprasidone; also to a lesser degree abarelix, alfuzosin, amoxapine, apomorphine, artemether; lumefantrine, asenapine, β-agonists, ofloxacin, clozapine, cyclobenzaprine, dasatinib, dolasetron, flecainide, gatifloxacin, gemifloxacin, halogenated anesthetics, iloperidone, lapatinib, levofloxacin, local anesthetics, lopinavir; ritonavir, magnesium sulfate; potassium sulfate; sodium sulfate, maprotiline, mefloquine, moxifloxacin, nilotinib, norfloxacin, octreotide, ciprofloxacin, olanzapine, ondansetron, paliperidone, palonosetron, some phenothiazines (fluphenazine, perphenazine, prochlorperazine, trifluoperazine), quetiapine, ranolazine, risperidone, sertindole, sunitinib, tacrolimus, telavancin, telithromycin, tetrabenazine, tricyclic antidepressants, venlafaxine, vardenafil, vorinostat

NURSING CONSIDERATIONS

Assess:

- **QT prolongatation:** assess for drug interactions that may occur; monitor ECG, heart rate
- **Bone marrow depression:** CBC, differential, serum creatinine, BUN, electrolytes, LFTs at baseline, periodically; increased AST/ALT >3 × ULN or total bilirubin >1.5 × ULN involve greater chance of Grade 4 or febrile neutropenia

Perform/provide:

- Storage at room temp for 4 hr or 24 hr refrigerated

Teach patient/family:

- About reason for product and expected results
- To report side effects to health care provider
- To avoid other medications, supplements unless approved by provider; serious drug interactions may occur
- About hair loss, use of wig or hairpiece
- To notify prescriber if pregnancy is planned or suspected (pregnancy [D]), to avoid breastfeeding

erlotinib (Rx)

(er-loe′tye-nib)

Tarceva

Func. class.: Antineoplastic—miscellaneous

Chem. class.: Epidermal growth factor receptor inhibitor

ACTION: Not fully understood; inhibits intracellular phosphorylation of cell-surface receptors associated with epidermal growth factor receptors

USES: Non–small-cell lung cancer (NSCLC), pancreatic cancer

Unlabeled uses: Squamous cell head and neck cancer

CONTRAINDICATIONS: Pregnancy (D), breastfeeding, hypersensitivity

Precautions: Children, geriatric patients, ocular/pulmonary/renal/hepatic disorders, tobacco smoking, radiation therapy, fever, dehydration, chemotherapy

DOSAGE AND ROUTES

Non–small-cell lung cancer (NSCLC)

- **Adult: PO** 150 mg/day

Pancreatic cancer

- **Adult: PO** 100 mg/day in combination with gemcitabine 1000 mg/m^2 cycle 1, days 1, 8, 15, 22, 29, 36, 43 of 8-wk cycle; cycle 2 and subsequent cycle, days 1, 8, 15 of 4-wk cycle

CYP3A4 inducers concurrently (e.g., rifampin, phenytoin)

- Dosage increase is advised

CYP3A4 inhibitors (atazanavir, clarithromycin, indinavir, itraconazole, ketoconazole, telithromycin, ritonavir, saquinavir, troleandomycin, nelfinavir)

- Dosage reduction may be needed

Head or neck cancer (unlabeled)

- **Adult: PO** 150 mg daily

Available forms: Tabs 25, 100, 150 mg

Administer:

- 1 hr before or 2 hr after food; at same time of day

SIDE EFFECTS

CNS: CVA, anxiety, depression, headache, rigors
CV: MI/ischemia
EENT: Ocular changes, *conjunctivitis, eye pain*
GI: *Nausea, diarrhea, vomiting, anorexia, mouth ulceration,* hepatic failure, GI perforation
GU: Renal impairment/failure
HEMA: Deep vein thrombosis
INTEG: *Rash,* Stevens-Johnson–like skin reaction, toxic epidermal necrolysis
MISC: *Fatigue, infection*
RESP: Interstitial lung disease, *cough, dyspnea,* ARDS, pulmonary fibrosis
SYST: Hepatorenal syndrome

PHARMACOKINETICS

Slowly absorbed (60%); peak 3-7 hr; excreted in feces (86%), urine (<4%); metabolized by CYP3A4; terminal half-life 36 hr; protein binding 93%

INTERACTIONS

Increase: erlotinib concentrations—CYP3A4 inhibitors (ketoconazole, itraconazole, erythromycin, clarithromycin, telithromycin)
Increase: plasma concentration of warfarin, metoprolol
Decrease: erlotinib levels—CYP3A4 inducers (phenytoin, rifampin, carBAMazepine, PHENobarbital)

Drug/Herb

Decrease: erlotinib levels—St. John's wort

Drug/Smoking

Decrease: erlotinib level; dose may need to be increased

Drug/Food

Increase: effect of erlotinib—grapefruit juice

NURSING CONSIDERATIONS

Assess:

⚠ **MI/ischemia, CVA** in patients with pancreatic cancer

⚠ **Pulmonary changes:** lung sounds, cough, dyspnea; interstitial lung disease may occur, may be fatal; discontinue therapy if confirmed

- **Ocular changes:** eye irritation, corneal erosion/ulcer, aberrant eyelash growth
- GI symptoms: frequency of stools; if diarrhea is poorly tolerated, therapy may be discontinued for ≤14 days
- Blood studies: INR, LFTs, PT
- **Hepatic failure:** interrupt dosing if severe changes to liver function occur (total bilirubin >3× ULN and/or transaminases >5× ULN when normal pretreatment LFTs)

Evaluate:

- Therapeutic response: decrease in NSCLC cells, pancreatic cancer cells

Teach patient/family:

⚠ To report adverse reactions immediately: SOB, severe abdominal pain, persistent diarrhea or vomiting, ocular changes, skin eruptions

- About reason for treatment, expected results
- To use reliable contraception during treatment (pregnancy D); to avoid breastfeeding

ertapenem (Rx)

(er-tah-pen′em)

Invanz

Func. class.: Antiinfective—miscellaneous

Chem. class.: Carbapenem

Do not confuse:

Invanz/Avinza

ACTION: Interferes with cell wall replication of susceptible organisms; osmotically unstable cell wall swells, bursts from osmotic pressure; bactericidal

USES: Adult patients with moderate to severe infections caused by the following organisms: intraabdominal infections—*Escherichia coli, Clostridium clostridioforme, Eubacterium lentum, Peptostreptococcus* sp., *Bacteroides fragilis, Bacteroides distasonis, Bacteroides ovatus, Bacteroides thetaiotaomicron, Bacteroides uniformis;* complicated skin/skin-structure infections—*Staphylococcus aureus* (methicillin-susceptible), *Streptococcus pyogenes, E. coli, Peptostreptococcus* sp.; community-acquired pneumonia—*Streptococcus pneumoniae* (penicillin-susceptible), *Haemophilus influenzae* (β-lactamase–negative), *Moraxella catarrhalis;* complicated UTI—*E. coli, Klebsiella pneumoniae;* acute pelvic infections—*Streptococcus agalactiae, E. coli, B. fragilis, Porphyromonas asaccharolytica, Peptostreptococcus* sp., *Prevotella bivia,* infection prophylaxis prior to elective colorectal surgery

CONTRAINDICATIONS: Hypersensitivity to this product, its components, amide-type local anesthetics (IM only); anaphylactic reactions to β-lactams

Precautions: Pregnancy (B), breastfeeding, children, geriatric patients, GI/renal/hepatic disease

DOSAGE AND ROUTES

Complicated intraabdominal infections

- **Adult/adolescent: IM/IV** 1 g/day × 5-14 days
- **Infant ≥3 mo/child: IM/IV** 15 mg/kg bid (max 1 g/day) × 5-14 days

Complicated skin/skin-structure infections

- **Adult: IM/IV** 1 g/day × 7-14 days
- **Child 3 mo-12 yr: IM/IV** 15 mg/kg bid × 7-14 days

Community-acquired pneumonia

- **Adult: IM/IV** 1 g/day × 10-14 days
- **Child 3 mo-12 yr: IM/IV** 15 mg/kg bid × 10-14 days

Complicated UTI

- **Adult: IM/IV** 1 g/day × 10-14 days
- **Child 3 mo-12 yr: IM/IV** 15 mg/kg bid × 10-14 days

Acute pelvic infections

- **Adult: IM/IV** 1 g/day × 3-10 days
- **Child 3 mo-12 yr: IM/IV** 15 mg/kg bid 3-10 days

Surgical infection prophylaxis (unlabeled)

- **Adult: IV** 1 g as a single dose 1 hr prior to surgical incision

Available form: Powder, lyophilized, 1 g

Administer:

- By IV or IM
- After C&S is taken

IM route

- Reconstitute 1-g vial of ertapenem with 3.2 ml of 1% lidocaine HCl without EPINEPHrine; shake well
- Withdraw contents, administer deep IM in large muscle mass, use within 1 hr

Intermittent IV IVF route

- Do not confuse or mix with other medications; do not use diluents containing dextrose
- **Reconstitute** 1-g vial of ertapenem with 10 ml of water for inj, 0.9% NaCl, or bacteriostatic water for inj (100 mg/ml)
- Shake well to dissolve, transfer contents of reconstituted vial to 50 ml 0.9% NaCl inj
- Complete inf within 6 hr

Y-site compatibilities: Acyclovir, alfentanil, amifostine, amikacin, aminocaproic acid, aminophylline, amphotericin B lipid complex, amphotericin B liposome, argatroban, arsenic trioxide, atenolol, atracurium, azithromycin, aztreonam, bivalirudin, bleomycin, bumetanide, buprenorphine, busulfan, butorphanol, calcium chloride/gluconate, CARBOplatin, carmustine, chloramphenicol, cimetidine, ciprofloxacin, cisatracurium, CISplatin, cyclophosphamide, cycloSPORINE, cytarabine, dacarbazine, DACTINomycin, DAPTOmycin, dexamethasone, dexmedetomidine, dexrazoxane, digoxin, diltiazem, diphenhydrAMINE, docetaxel, dolasetron, DOPamine, doxacurium, doxycycline, enalaprilat, ePHEDrine, EPINEPHrine, eptifibatide, erythromycin, esmolol, etoposide, famotidine, fenoldopam, fluconazole, fludarabine, fluorouracil, foscarnet, fosphenytoin, furosemide, ganciclovir, gatifloxacin, gemcitabine, gemtuzumab, gentamicin, glycopyrrolate, granisetron, haloperidol, heparin, hydrocortisone, HYDROmorphone, ifosfamide, inamrinone, insulin (regular), irinotecan, isoproterenol, ketorolac, labetalol, leucovorin, levofloxacin, lidocaine, linezolid, LORazepam, magnesium sulfate, mannitol, mechlorethamine, melphalan, meperidine, mesna, metaraminol, methotrexate, methyldopate, methylPREDNISolone, metoclopramide, metroNIDAZOLE, milrinone, mitomycin, mivacurium, morphine, moxifloxacin, nalbuphine, naloxone, nesiritide, nitroglycerin, nitroprusside, norepinephrine, octreotide, oxaliplatin, oxytocin, paclitaxel, pamidronate, pancuronium, pantoprazole, pemetrexed, PENTobarbital, PHENobarbital, phentolamine, phenylephrine, polymyxin B, potassium acetate/chloride/phosphates, procainamide, propranolol, ranitidine, remifentanil, rocuronium, sodium acetate/bicarbonate/phosphates, streptozocin, succinylcholine, SUFentanil, sulfamethoxazole-trimethoprim, tacrolimus, teniposide, theophylline, thiotepa, tigecycline, tirofiban, tobramycin, trimethobenzamide, vancomycin, vasopressin, vecuronium, vinBLAStine, vinCRIStine, vinorelbine, voriconazole, zidovudine

SIDE EFFECTS

CNS: Insomnia, seizures, dizziness, *headache*
CV: Tachycardia
GI: *Diarrhea, nausea, vomiting,* pseudomembranous colitis
GU: *Vaginitis*
INTEG: *Rash,* urticaria, *pruritus,* pain at inj site, *infused vein complication, phlebitis/thrombophlebitis,* erythema at inj site
RESP: Dyspnea, cough, pharyngitis, crackles, respiratory distress
SYST: Anaphylaxis

PHARMACOKINETICS

IV: Onset immediate; peak dose dependent; half-life 4 hr; metabolized by liver; excreted in urine, feces, breast milk

INTERACTIONS

Increase: ertapenem levels—probenecid; do not coadminister
Drug/Lab Test
Increase: hepatic enzymes

NURSING CONSIDERATIONS

Assess:

- Renal disease: lower dose may be required

• **Pseudomembranous colitis:** bowel pattern daily: if severe diarrhea occurs, product should be discontinued
• For infection: temp, sputum, characteristics of wound before, during, after treatment
⚠ **Allergic reactions, anaphylaxis;** rash, urticaria, pruritus; may occur a few days after therapy begins; sensitivity to carbapenem antibiotics, other β-lactam antibiotics, penicillins
• **Overgrowth of infection:** perineal itching, fever, malaise, redness, pain, swelling, drainage, rash, diarrhea, change in cough or sputum

Evaluate:
• Therapeutic response: negative C&S; absence of signs, symptoms of infection

Teach patient/family:
• To report severe diarrhea (may indicate **pseudomembranous colitis**), CNS side effects
• To report overgrowth of infection: black, furry tongue; vaginal itching; foul-smelling stools
• To avoid breastfeeding; product is excreted in breast milk

TREATMENT OF OVERDOSE:
EPINEPHrine, antihistamines; resuscitate if needed (anaphylaxis)

erythromycin base (Rx)
(eh-rith-roh-my′sin)

Apo-Erythro ♣, Ery-Tab, Novo-Rythro Encap ♣, PCE

erythromycin ethylsuccinate (Rx)
Apo-Erythro-Es ♣, E.E.S., Ery Ped, Novo-Rythro ♣

erythromycin lactobionate (Rx)
Erythrocin

erythromycin stearate (Rx)
Apo-Erythro-S ♣, My-E, Novo-Rythro ♣

Func. class.: Antiinfective
Chem. class.: Macrolide

Do not confuse:
erythromycin/azithromycin

ACTION: Binds to 50S ribosomal subunits of susceptible bacteria and suppresses protein synthesis

USES: Infections caused by *Neisseria gonorrhoeae;* mild to moderate respiratory tract, skin, soft-tissue infections caused by *Bordetella pertussis, Borrelia burgdorferi, Chlamydia trachomatis; Corynebacterium diphtheriae, Haemophilus influenzae* (when used with sulfonamides); *Legionella pneumophila,* Legionnaire's disease, *Listeria monocytogenes; Mycoplasma pneumoniae, Streptococcus pneumoniae,* syphilis: *Treponema pallidum*
Unlabeled uses: Bartonellosis, burn wound infection, chancroid, cholera, diabetic gastroparesis, endocarditis, prophylaxis, gastroenteritis, granuloma inguinale, Lyme disease, tetanus

CONTRAINDICATIONS: Hypersensitivity, preexisting hepatic disease (estolate)

Precautions: Pregnancy (B), breastfeeding, geriatric patients, hepatic disease, GI disease, QT prolongation, seizure disorder, myasthenia gravis

DOSAGE AND ROUTES

Lower/upper respiratory infections

- **Adult: PO** (base, stearate) 250-500 mg q6hr; **PO** (ethylsuccinate) 400-800 mg q6hr; **IV INF** (lactobionate) 15-20 mg/kg/day divided q6hr
- **Adolescent/child/infant: PO** 20-50 mg/kg/day divided q6hr, max adult dose
- **Neonates >7 days, weighing ≥1200 g:** 30 mg/day in divided doses q8hr
- **Neonates >7 days, weighing <1200 g: PO** 20 mg/kg/day divided q12hr
- **Neonates ≤7 days: PO** 20 mg/kg/day divided q12hr

Neisseria gonorrhoeae and PID

- **Adult: IV** (gluceptate, lactobionate) 500 mg q6hr × 3 days then **PO** (base, stearate) 250 mg or 400 mg (ethylsuccinate) q6hr × 1 wk

Pertussis (whooping cough) treatment/prophylaxis

- **Adult: PO** 500 mg qid (2 g total) × 14 days
- **Infant/child/adolescent: PO** 40-50 mg/kg/day, max 2 g/day, in 4 divided doses × 14 days

Syphilis

- **Adult: PO** 500 mg qid × 14 days

Chlamydia

- **Adult/adolescent: PO** 500 mg q6hr × 1 wk or 250 mg qid × 2 wk
- **Infant: PO** 50 mg/kg/day in 4 divided doses × 3 wk or more

Intestinal amebiasis

- **Adult: PO** (base, stearate) 250 mg q6hr × 10-14 days
- **Child: PO** (base, stearate) 30-50 mg/kg/day in divided doses q6hr × 10-14 days

Available forms: *Base:* enteric-coated tabs 250, 333, 500 mg; film-coated tabs 250, 500 mg; enteric-coated caps 250, 333 mg; *stearate:* film-coated tabs 250 mg; *ethylsuccinate:* granules for oral susp 200, 400 mg/5 ml; powder for inj 500 mg, 1 g (lactobionate), 1 g (as gluceptate)

Administer:

- Do not break, crush, or chew time rel cap or tab; chew only chewable tabs; enteric-coated tablets may be given with food
- Do not give by IM or IV push
- Oral product with full glass of water; do not give with fruit juice
- Give 1 hr before or 2 hr after meals
- Chew tab: crush or chew

IV route

- After **reconstituting** 500 mg or less/10 ml sterile water without preservatives; dilute further in 100-250 ml of 0.9% NaCl, LR, Normosol-R; may be **further diluted** to 1 mg/ml and **given** as cont inf; run 1 g or less/100 ml over ½-1 hr; cont inf over 6 hr, may require buffers to neutralize pH if dilution is <250 ml, use inf pump

Lactobionate

Y-site compatibilities: Acyclovir, alfentanil, amikacin, aminocaproic acid, aminophylline, amiodarone, anidulafungin, atenolol, atosiban, atracurium, atropine, azathioprine, benztropine, bivalirudin, bleomycin, bumetanide, buprenorphine, butorphanol, calcium chloride/gluconate, CARBOplatin, caspofungin, cefotaxime, ceftazidime, cefTRIAXone, cefuroxime, chlorproMAZINE, cimetidine, CISplatin, cyanocobalamin, cyclophosphamide, cycloSPORINE, cytarabine, DACTINomycin, DAPTOmycin, dexmedetomidine, digoxin, diltiazem, diphenhydrAMINE, DOBUTamine, docetaxel, DOPamine, doxacurium, doxapram, DOXOrubicin, enalaprilat, ePHEDrine, EPINEPHrine, epirubicin, epoetin alfa, eptifibatide, ertapenem, esmolol, etoposide, famotidine, fenoldopam, fentaNYL, fluconazole, fludarabine, fluorouracil, folic acid, foscarnet, gatifloxacin, gemcitabine, gentamicin, glycopyrrolate, granisetron, hydrocortisone, HYDROmorphone, hydrOXYzine, IDArubicin, ifosfamide, imipenem-cilastatin, insulin (regular), irinotecan, isoproterenol, labetalol, levofloxacin, lidocaine, LORazepam, LR, mannitol, mechlorethamine, meperidine, methicillin, methotrexate, methoxamine, methyldopate, methylPREDNISolone, metoclopramide, metroNIDAZOLE, miconazole, midazolam, milrinone, mitoxantrone, morphine, multiple vitamins injection, mycophenolate, nafcillin, nalbuphine, naloxone, nesiritide, netilmicin, niCARdipine, nitroglycerin, norepinephrine, octreotide, ondansetron, oxacillin, oxaliplatin, oxytocin, paclitaxel, palonosetron, pamidronate, pancuronium, papaverine, pentamidine, pentazocine, perphenazine, phenylephrine, phytonadione, piperacillin, piperacillin-tazobactam, polymyxin B, procainamide, prochlorperazine, promethazine, propranolol, protamine, pyridoxine, quiNIDine, ranitidine, Ringer's, ritodrine, sodium acetate/bicarbonate, succinylcholine, SUFentanil, tacrolimus, temocillin, teniposide, theophylline, thiamine, thiotepa, tigecycline, tirofiban, TNA, tobramycin, tolazoline, TPN, trimetaphan, urokinase, vancomycin, vasopressin, vecuronium, verapamil, vinCRIStine, vinorelbine, vitamin B complex/C, voriconazole, zidovudine, zoledronic acid

SIDE EFFECTS

CNS: Seizures
CV: Dysrhythmias, QT prolongation
EENT: Hearing loss, tinnitus
GI: *Nausea, vomiting, diarrhea,* hepatotoxicity, abdominal pain, stomatitis, heartburn, anorexia, pseudomembranous colitis
GU: *Vaginitis, moniliasis*
INTEG: Rash, urticaria, pruritus, thrombophlebitis (IV site)
SYST: Anaphylaxis

PHARMACOKINETICS

Peak 4 hr (base); ½-2½ hr (ethylsuccinate); half-life 1-2 hr; metabolized in liver; excreted in bile, feces; protein binding 75%-90%; inhibitor of CYP3A4 and P-glycoprotein

INTERACTIONS

⚠ Serious dysrhythmias—diltiazem, itraconazole, ketoconazole, nefazodone, pimozide, protease inhibitors, verapamil
Increase: action, toxicity of alfentanil, alprazolam, bromocriptine, busPIRone, carBAMazepine, cilostazol, clindamycin, clozapine, cycloSPORINE, diazepam, digoxin, disopyramide, ergots, felodipine, HMG-CoA reductase inhibitors, methylPREDNISolone, midazolam, quiNIDine, rifabutin, sildenafil, tacrolimus, tadalafil, theophylline, triazolam, vardenafil, vinBLAStine, warfarin

Drug/Lab Test
Increase: AST/ALT
Decrease: folate assay
False increase: 17-OHCS/17-KS

NURSING CONSIDERATIONS

Assess:

- **Infection:** temp, characteristics of wounds, urine, stools, sputum, WBCs at baseline and periodically
- I&O ratio; report hematuria, oliguria in renal disease
- Hepatic studies: AST, ALT if patient is receiving long-term therapy
- Hearing at baseline and after treatment
- Renal studies: urinalysis, protein, blood
- C&S before product therapy; product may be given as soon as culture is taken; C&S may be repeated after treatment
- **Pseudomembranous colitis:** diarrhea with blood, mucus; abdominal pain, fever; product should be discontinued immediately, notify prescriber
- **Anaphylaxis:** generalized hives, itching, flushing, swelling of lips, tongue, throat, wheezing; have emergency equipment nearby
- **QT prolongation:** may occur (IV >15 mg/min); those with electrolyte imbalances, congenital QT prolongation, elderly at greater risk; correct electrolyte imbalances before treatment, ECG

Perform/provide:

- Storage at room temp; store susp in refrigerator

• Adequate intake of fluids (2 L) during diarrhea episodes

Evaluate:

• Therapeutic response: decreased symptoms of infection

Teach patient/family:

• To report sore throat, fever, fatigue (could indicate superinfection), rhythm changes in the heart, hearing loss

• To notify nurse of diarrhea stools, dark urine, pale stools, jaundice of eyes or skin, severe abdominal pain

• To take at evenly spaced intervals; to complete dosage regimen; to take without food

TREATMENT OF HYPERSENSITIVITY:

Withdraw product; maintain airway; administer EPINEPHrine, aminophylline, O_2, IV corticosteroids

erythromycin ophthalmic

See Appendix B

erythromycin topical

See Appendix B

escitalopram (Rx)

(es-sit-tal′oh-pram)

Lexapro

Func. class.: Antidepressant, SSRI (selective serotonin reuptake inhibitor)

ACTION:

Inhibits CNS neuron uptake of serotonin but not of norepinephrine

USES:

General anxiety disorder; major depressive disorder in adults/adolescents

Unlabeled uses: Panic disorder, social phobia

CONTRAINDICATIONS:

Hypersensitivity to this product, citalopram

Precautions: Pregnancy (C), breastfeeding, geriatric patients, renal/hepatic disease, history of seizures

Black Box Warning: Children/adolescents ≤12 yr, suicidal ideation

DOSAGE AND ROUTES

• **Adult: PO** 10 mg/day in AM or PM; after 1 wk, if no clinical improvement is noted, dose may be increased to 20 mg/day PM; maintenance 10-20 mg/day; reassess to determine need for treatment

Hepatic dose/geriatric

• **Adult: PO** 10 mg/day

Available forms: Tabs 5, 10, 20 mg; oral sol 5 mg (as base)/5 ml (contains sorbitol)

Administer:

• With food or milk for GI symptoms, give with full glass of water

• Crushed if patient is unable to swallow medication whole

• Dosage at bedtime if oversedation occurs during the day

• Gum, hard candy, frequent sips of water for dry mouth

• Oral sol: measure with calibrated device

SIDE EFFECTS

CNS: *Headache, nervousness, insomnia,* suicidal ideation, *drowsiness, anxiety, tremor, dizziness, fatigue, sedation, poor concentration, abnormal dreams, agitation,* seizures, apathy, euphoria, hallucinations, delusions, psychosis, neuroleptic malignant-like syndrome

CV: *Hot flashes, palpitations,* angina pectoris, hemorrhage, hypertension, tachycardia, 1st-degree AV block, bradycardia, MI, thrombophlebitis, postural hypotension

EENT: Visual changes, ear/eye pain, photophobia, tinnitus

GI: *Nausea, diarrhea, dry mouth, anorexia, dyspepsia, constipation, cramps, vomiting, taste changes, flatulence, decreased appetite*

GU: *Dysmenorrhea, decreased libido, urinary frequency, UTI,* amenorrhea, cystitis, impotence, urine retention, ejaculation disorder
INTEG: *Sweating, rash, pruritus,* acne, alopecia, urticaria, photosensitivity
MS: *Pain,* arthritis, twitching
RESP: *Infection, pharyngitis, nasal congestion, sinus headache, sinusitis, cough, dyspnea, bronchitis,* asthma, hyperventilation, pneumonia
SYST: *Asthenia, viral infection, fever, allergy, chills,* serotonin syndrome

PHARMACOKINETICS

PO: Metabolized in liver; excreted in urine; 56% protein binding; metabolized by CYP2C19, 3A4, half-life 27-32 hr; half-life increased by 50% in geriatric patients

INTERACTIONS

• Paradoxical worsening of OCD: busPIRone
Increase: serotonin syndrome—tryptophan, amphetamines, busPIRone, lithium, amantadine, bromocriptine, SSRI, SNRIs, serotonin-receptor agonists, tramadol
⚠ Do not use pimozide, MAOIs, with or 14 days before escitalopram
Increase: CNS depression—alcohol, antidepressants, opioids, sedatives
Increase: side effects of escitalopram—highly protein-bound products
Increase: levels or toxicity of carBAMazepine, lithium, warfarin, phenytoin, antipsychotics, antidysrhythmics
Increase: levels of tricyclics, phenothiazines, haloperidol, diazepam
Increase: bleeding risk—NSAIDs, salicylates, anticoagulants, SSRIs, platelet inhibitors
Decrease: escitalopram effect—cyproheptadine

Drug/Herb
• St. John's wort: do not use together
Increase: CNS effect—kava, valerian

Drug/Food
• Grapefruit juice—increased escitalopram effect

Drug/Lab Test
Increase: serum bilirubin, blood glucose, alk phos
Decrease: VMA, 5-HIAA
False increase: urinary catecholamines

NURSING CONSIDERATIONS

Assess:

Black Box Warning: Mental status: mood, sensorium, affect, **suicidal tendencies,** increase in psychiatric symptoms, depression, panic

• Appetite with bulimia nervosa, weight daily; increase nutritious foods in diet, watch for bingeing and vomiting
• **Allergic reactions:** itching, rash, urticaria; product should be discontinued, may need to give antihistamine
• B/P (lying/standing), pulse q4hr; if systolic B/P drops 20 mm Hg, hold product, notify prescriber
• Blood studies: CBC, leukocytes, differential, cardiac enzymes if patient receiving long-term therapy; check platelets; bleeding can occur
• **Serotonin syndrome:** nausea, vomiting, sedation, dizziness, sweating, facial flushing, mental changes, shivering, increased B/P; discontinue product, notify prescriber
• Hepatic studies: AST, ALT, bilirubin, creatinine; thyroid function studies
• Weight weekly; appetite may decrease with product
• **ECG** for flattening of T wave, bundle branch, AV block, dysrhythmias in cardiac patients
• Alcohol consumption; if alcohol is consumed, hold dose until AM
• **Sexual dysfunction:** ejaculation dysfunction, erectile dysfunction, decreased libido, orgasm dysfunction, priapism

Perform/provide:
• Storage at room temp; do not freeze
• Assistance with ambulation during therapy, since drowsiness, dizziness occur; safety measures primarily for geriatric patients

Evaluate:
- Therapeutic response: decreased depression

Teach patient/family:
- That therapeutic effect may take 1-4 wk
- To use caution when driving, performing other activities requiring alertness because drowsiness, dizziness, blurred vision may occur
- To avoid alcohol, other CNS depressants; to avoid all OTC products unless approved by prescriber
- To notify prescriber if pregnant or planning to become pregnant or breastfeeding
- To change positions slowly, orthostatic hypotension may occur
- To report signs of urinary retention immediately

Black Box Warning: That clinical worsening and suicide risk may occur
- To use MedGuide provided

TREATMENT OF OVERDOSE:
Activated charcoal, supportive care, serotonin antagonist

esmolol (Rx)
(ez′moe-lole)

Brevibloc

Func. class.: β-Adrenergic blocker (antidysrhythmic II)

Do not confuse:
esmolol/Osmitrol
Brevibloc/Brevital

ACTION:
Competitively blocks stimulation of β_1-adrenergic receptors in the myocardium; produces negative chronotropic, inotropic activity (decreases rate of SA node discharge, increases recovery time), slows conduction of AV node, decreases heart rate, decreases O_2 consumption in myocardium; also decreases renin-aldosterone-angiotensin system at high doses; inhibits β_2-receptors in bronchial system at higher doses

USES:
Supraventricular tachycardia, noncompensatory sinus tachycardia, hypertensive crisis, intraoperative and postoperative tachycardia and hypertension

Unlabeled uses: Acute MI, ECT, thyroid storm, pheochromocytoma

CONTRAINDICATIONS:
2nd- or 3rd-degree heart block; cardiogenic shock, CHF, cardiac failure, hypersensitivity, severe bradycardia

Precautions: Pregnancy (C), breastfeeding, geriatric patients, hypotension, peripheral vascular disease, diabetes, hypoglycemia, thyrotoxicosis, renal disease, atrial fibrillation, bronchospasms, hyperthyroidism, myasthenia gravis

Black Box Warning: Abrupt discontinuation

DOSAGE AND ROUTES
- **Adult:** **IV** loading dose 500 mcg/kg/min over 1 min; maintenance 50 mcg/kg/min for 4 min; if no response after 5 min, give 2nd loading dose then increase inf to 100 mcg/kg/min for 4 min; if no response, repeat loading dose then increase maintenance inf by 50 mcg/kg/min (max of 200 mcg/kg/min); titrate to patient response
- **Child:** **IV** total loading dose of 600 mcg/kg over 2 min, maintenance **IV INF** 200 mcg/kg/min, titrate upward by 50-100 mcg/kg/min q5-10min until B/P, heart rate reduced by >10%

Available forms: Inj 10 mg, 20 mg/ml

Administer:
- Do not discontinue product suddenly

IV route
- Check that correct concentration being given
- 10 mg/ml inj sol needs no dilution, may be used as an IV loading dose using a handheld syringe

Continuous IV INF route
- Ready-to-use bags of premixed isotonic sol of 10 mg/ml and 20 mg/ml available in 100-, 250-ml bags; use controlled inf device, central line preferred; rate is based on patient's weight

Additive compatibilities: Aminophylline, atracurium, heparin, potassium chloride, sodium bicarbonate

Y-site compatibilities: Amikacin, aminophylline, amiodarone, atracurium, butorphanol, calcium chloride, ceFAZolin, ceftazidime, ceftizoxime, chloramphenicol, cimetidine, cisatracurium, clindamycin, diltiazem, DOPamine, enalaprilat, erythromycin, famotidine, fentaNYL, gentamicin, insulin (regular), labetalol, magnesium sulfate, methyldopate, metroNIDAZOLE, midazolam, morphine, nitroglycerin, nitroprusside, norepinephrine, pancuronium, penicillin G potassium, piperacillin, polymyxin B, potassium chloride, potassium phosphate, propofol, ranitidine, remifentanil, streptomycin, tacrolimus, tobramycin, trimethoprim-sulfamethoxazole, vancomycin, vecuronium, voriconazole, zoledronic acid

SIDE EFFECTS

CNS: Confusion, lightheadedness, paresthesia, somnolence, fever, dizziness, fatigue, headache, depression, anxiety, **seizures**

CV: Hypotension, bradycardia, chest pain, peripheral ischemia, SOB, **CHF**, conduction disturbances; 1st-, 2nd-, 3rd-degree heart block

GI: *Nausea,* vomiting, anorexia, gastric pain, flatulence, constipation, heartburn, bloating

GU: Urinary retention, impotence, dysuria

INTEG: *Induration, inflammation at site,* discoloration, edema, erythema, burning pallor, flushing, rash, pruritus, dry skin, alopecia

RESP: **Bronchospasm**, dyspnea, cough, wheeziness, nasal stuffiness, **pulmonary edema**

PHARMACOKINETICS

Onset very rapid, duration short, half-life 9 min, metabolized by hydrolysis of ester linkage, excreted via kidneys

INTERACTIONS

- Avoid use with MAOIs

Increase: antihypertensive effect—general anesthetics

Increase: digoxin levels—digoxin

Increase: α-adrenergic stimulation—ePHEDrine, EPINEPHrine, amphetamine, norepinephrine, phenylephrine, pseudoephedrine

Decrease: action of thyroid hormones

Decrease: action of esmolol—thyroid hormone

Drug/Herb

Increase: β-blocking effect—hawthorn

Decrease: antihypertensive effect—ephedra

Drug/Lab Test

Interference: glucose/insulin tolerance test

NURSING CONSIDERATIONS

Assess:

- **CHF:** I&O ratio, weight daily, jugular venous distention, weight gain, crackles, edema
- **Dysrhythmias:** B/P, pulse q4hr; note rate, rhythm, quality; rapid changes can cause shock; if systolic <100 or diastolic <60, notify prescriber before giving product; ECG continuously during inf, hypotension common
- Baselines in renal/hepatic studies, blood glucose before therapy begins
- **Bronchospasm:** breath sounds, respiratory pattern

Perform/provide:

- Storage protected from light, moisture; in cool environment

Evaluate:

- Therapeutic response: lower B/P immediately, lower heart rate

Teach patient/family:

- About reason for use, expected results
- To notify prescriber if chest pain, SOB, wheezing, hypotension, bradycardia, pain, swelling at IV site occurs

TREATMENT OF OVERDOSE:

Discontinue product

esomeprazole (Rx)

(es'oh-mep'rah-zohl)

Nexium

Func. class.: Antiulcer

Chem. class.: Proton pump inhibitor, benzimidazole

ACTION: Suppresses gastric secretions by inhibiting hydrogen/potassium ATPase enzyme system in gastric parietal cell; characterized as gastric acid pump inhibitor because it blocks the final step of acid production

USES: Gastroesophageal reflux disease (GERD), adult/child/infant; severe erosive esophagitis, adult/child; treatment of active duodenal ulcers in combination with antiinfectives for *Helicobacter pylori* infection; long-term use for hypersecretory conditions

CONTRAINDICATIONS: Hypersensitivity to proton pump inhibitors (PPIs)

Precautions: Pregnancy (B), breastfeeding, children, geriatric patients

DOSAGE AND ROUTES

Active duodenal ulcers associated with *H. pylori*

- **Adult: PO** 40 mg/day × 10 days in combination with clarithromycin 500 mg bid × 10 days and amoxicillin 1000 mg bid × 10 days

Hepatic dose

- **Adult: PO/IV** max 20 mg/day (severe hepatic disease)

GERD/erosive esophagitis

- **Adult: PO** 20 or 40 mg/day × 4-8 wk; no adjustment needed in renal/liver failure, geriatric patients; **IV** 20 or 40 mg/day up to 10 days
- **Adolescent and child 12-17 yr: PO** 20 or 40 mg/day 1 hr before meals for ≤8 wk
- **Child 1-11 yr and ≥20 kg: PO** 10 mg/day 1 hr before meals for ≤8 wk
- **Infant ≥1 mo: IV** 0.5 mg/day over 10-30 min
- **Infant 1-11 mo (>7.5-12 kg): PO** 10 mg daily × up to 6 wk
- **Infant 1-11 mo (>5-7.5 kg): PO** 5 mg daily × up to 6 wk
- **Infant 1-11 mo (3-5 kg): PO** 2.5 mg daily × up to 6 wk

Available forms: Del rel caps 20, 40 mg; powder for IV inj 20, 40 mg/vial; del rel powder for oral susp 10, 20, 40 mg

Administer:

- Swallow caps whole; do not crush or chew; cap may be opened and sprinkled over Tbsp of applesauce
- Same time daily, 1 hr before meal
- **Oral susp (del rel):** empty contents of packet into container with 1 Tbsp of water, let stand 2-3 min to thicken, restir, give within 30 min of mixing; any residual product should be flushed with more water, taken immediately
- **NG tube (del rel oral susp):** add 15 ml water to contents of packet in syringe, shake, leave 2-3 min to thicken, shake, inject through NG tube within 30 min

IV, direct route

- Reconstitute each vial with 5 ml 0.9% NaCl, D_5W, LR; give over 3 min

Intermittent IV INF route

- Dilute reconstituted sol to 50 ml, give over 30 min, do not admix, flush line with D_5W, 0.9% NaCl, LR after inf

Solution compatibilities: D_5W, LR, 0.9% NaCl

Y-site compatibilities: D_5W, doripenem, LR

SIDE EFFECTS

CNS: *Headache, dizziness*

GI: *Diarrhea, flatulence,* abdominal pain, constipation, dry mouth, **hepatic failure, hepatitis**

INTEG: *Rash,* dry skin

MISC: **Heart failure**

RESP: *Cough,* pneumonia

SYST: **Stevens-Johnson syndrome, toxic epidermal necrolysis, exfoliative dermatitis**

PHARMACOKINETICS

Well absorbed 90%; protein binding 97%; extensively metabolized in liver (CYP2C19); terminal half-life 1-1.5 hr; eliminated in urine as metabolites and in feces; in geriatric patients, elimination rate decreased, bioavailability increased

INTERACTIONS

Increase: effect, toxicity of diazepam, digoxin, penicillins, saquinavir
Decrease: effect—atazanavir, nelfinavir, dapsone, iron, itraconazole, ketoconazole, indinavir, calcium carbonate, vit B_{12}, clopidogrel
Drug/Lab Test
Increase: creatinine, bilirubin, uric acid, alk phos, AST, ALT
Interference: sodium, potassium, Hgb, WBC, platelets, thyroxine

NURSING CONSIDERATIONS

Assess:

- GI system: bowel sounds q8hr, abdomen for pain, swelling, anorexia
- **Hepatic failure, hepatitis:** AST, ALT, alk phos at baseline and periodically during treatment
- **Serious skin disorders:** Stevens-Johnson syndrome, toxic epidermal necrolysis, exfoliative dermatitis

Evaluate:

- Therapeutic response: absence of epigastric pain, swelling, fullness

Teach patient/family:

- To report severe diarrhea; abdominal pain; black, tarry stools; product may have to be discontinued
- That hypoglycemia may occur if diabetic
- To avoid hazardous activities; dizziness may occur
- To avoid alcohol, salicylates, NSAIDs; may cause GI irritation

estradiol (Rx)
(es-tra-dye′ole)
Estrace, Femtrace, Gynodiol

estradiol cypionate (Rx)
Depo-Estradiol

estradiol gel (Rx)
Divigel, Elestrin, Estrogel

estradiol spray (Rx)
Evamist

estradiol topical emulsion (Rx)
Estrasorb

estradiol valerate (Rx)
Delestrogen

estradiol transdermal system (Rx)
Alora, Climara, Menostar, Vivelle

estradiol vaginal tablet (Rx)
Vagifem

estradiol vaginal ring (Rx)
Estring, Femring

Func. class.: Estrogen, progestins

ACTION: Needed for adequate functioning of female reproductive system; affects release of pituitary gonadotropins; inhibits ovulation, adequate calcium use in bone

USES: Vasomotor symptoms (menopause), inoperable breast cancer (selected cases), prostatic cancer, atrophic vaginitis, kraurosis vulvae, hypogonadism, primary ovarian failure, prevention of osteoporosis, castration

CONTRAINDICATIONS: Pregnancy (X), breastfeeding, reproductive cancer, genital bleeding (abnormal, undiagnosed)

Black Box Warning: Breast/endometrial cancer, thromboembolic disorders, MI, stroke

Precautions: Hypertension, asthma, blood dyscrasias, gallbladder/bone/renal/hepatic disease, CHF, diabetes mellitus, depression, migraine headache, seizure disorders, family history of cancer of breast or reproductive tract, smoking, uterine fibroids, vaginal irritation/infection, accidental exposure of children, pets to topical product

Black Box Warning: Cardiac disease, dementia

DOSAGE AND ROUTES

Hormone replacement/menopause symptoms

• **Adult: TRANSDERMAL** 1 patch delivering 0.025, 0.0375, 0.05, 0.075, or 0.1 mg/day 2×/wk (Alora, Estraderm, Vivelle-Dot); 1 patch delivering 0.025, 0.0375, 0.05, 0.06, 0.075, or 0.1 mg/day replace q7days (Climara); 1 patch delivering 0.025 mg/day, replace q7days, may increase to 2 patches after 4-6 wk; **GEL** apply entire unit-dose packet to 5 × 7-inch area of upper thigh/day, alternate thighs; **SPRAY** (Evamist) 1 spray to inner surface of forearm/day in AM

Menopause/hypogonadism/castration/ovarian failure

• **Adult: PO** 1-2 mg/day, 3 wk on, 1 wk off or 5 days on, 2 days off; **IM** (cypionate) 1-5 mg q3-4wk; (valerate) 10-20 mg q4wk

• **Adult: TOP** (Estraderm) 0.05 mg/24 hr applied 2×/wk; (Climara) 0.05 mg/hr applied 1×/wk in cyclic regimen; women with hysterectomy may use continuously

Prostatic cancer (inoperable)

• **Adult: IM** (valerate) 30 mg q1-2wk; **PO** (oral estradiol) 1-2 mg bid-tid

Breast cancer (palliative treatment)

• **Adult: PO** 10 mg tid × 3 mo or longer

Atropic vaginitis/kraurosis vulvae

• **Adult: VAG CREAM** 2-4 g/day × 1-2 wk, then 1 g 1-3×/wk cycled; vag tab 1/day × 2 wk, maintenance 1 tab 2×/wk; **VAG RING** inserted, left in place continuously for 3 mo

Vasomotor symptoms

• **Adult: TOP** after cleaning and drying skin on left thigh, calf, rub in contents of pouch using both hands until completely absorbed; wash hands

Available forms: ***Estradiol:*** tabs 0.5, 1, 2 mg; ***valerate:*** inj 10, 20, 40 mg/ml; ***transdermal:*** 0.025, 0.0375, 0.05, 0.075, 0.1 mg/24 hr release rate; ***vag cream:*** 100 mcg/g; ***vag tab:*** 25 mcg; ***vag ring:*** 2 mg/90 days; ***topical emulsion:*** 2.5 mg; ***gel*** (Divigel) 0.1%; ***spray*** (Evamist) 1.53 mg/acuation

Administer:

• Titrated dose; use lowest effective dose

• IM inj deeply in large muscle mass

PO route

• With food or milk to decrease GI symptoms

Transdermal route

• Apply to trunk of body 2×/wk; press firmly, hold in place for 10 sec to ensure good contact

• On intermittent cycle schedule: 3 wk on then 1 wk off; if patch falls off, reapply

Topical route

• Use Evamist daily; spray to inner upper arm; may increase to 2-3×/day based on response; allow to dry for 2 min

Vaginal route

• Use applicator provided

SIDE EFFECTS

CNS: Dizziness, headache, migraines, depression, seizures

CV: Hypertension, thrombophlebitis, edema, thromboembolism, stroke, pulmonary embolism, MI, chest pain

EENT: Contact lens intolerance, increased myopia, astigmatism, throat swelling, eyelid edema

GI: *Nausea,* vomiting, diarrhea, anorexia, pancreatitis, cramps, constipation, increased appetite, increased weight, cholestatic jaundice, hepatic adenoma

GU: Amenorrhea, cervical erosion, breakthrough bleeding, dysmenorrhea, vaginal candidiasis, breast changes, *gynecomastia, testicular atrophy, impotence,* **increased risk of breast cancer, endometrial cancer,** changes in libido; **toxic shock, vaginal wall ulceration/erosion (vag ring)**

INTEG: Rash, urticaria, acne, hirsutism, alopecia, oily skin, seborrhea, purpura, melasma

META: Folic acid deficiency, hypercalcemia, hyperglycemia

PHARMACOKINETICS

PO/INJ/TRANSDERMAL: Degraded in liver, excreted in urine, crosses placenta, excreted in breast milk

INTERACTIONS

Increase: action of corticosteroids

Increase: toxicity—cycloSPORINE, dantrolene

Decrease: action of anticoagulants, oral hypoglycemics, tamoxifen

Decrease: estradiol action—anticonvulsants, barbiturates, phenylbutazone, rifampin, calcium

Drug/Herb

- Altered estrogen effect: black cohosh, DHEA

Decrease: estrogen effect—saw palmetto, St. John's wort

Drug/Food

Increase: estrogen level—grapefruit juice

Drug/Lab Test

Increase: BSP retention test, PBI, T_4, serum sodium, platelet aggregation, thyroxine-binding globulin (TBG), prothrombin; factors VII, VIII, IX, X; triglycerides

Decrease: serum folate, serum triglyceride, T_3 resin uptake test, glucose tolerance test, antithrombin III, pregnanediol, metyrapone test

False positive: LE prep, ANA

NURSING CONSIDERATIONS

Assess:

Black Box Warning: For previous breast/endometrial cancer, thrombo-embolic disorders, MI, stroke, dementia

- Blood glucose of diabetic patient; hyperglycemia may occur
- Weight daily; notify prescriber of weekly weight gain >5 lb; if increase, diuretic may be ordered
- B/P q4hr; watch for increase caused by water and sodium retention
- I&O ratio; decreasing urinary output, increasing edema, report changes
- Hepatic studies, including AST, ALT, bilirubin, alk phos at baseline, periodically; periodic folic acid level
- Hypertension, cardiac symptoms, jaundice, hypercalcemia
- Mental status: affect, mood, behavioral changes, aggression
- Female patient for intact uterus; if so, progesterone should be added to estrogen therapy to decrease risk of endometrial cancer

Evaluate:

- Therapeutic response: reversal of menopause symptoms; decrease in tumor size in prostatic, breast cancer

Teach patient/family:

- To weigh weekly; to report gain >5 lb

⚠ **To report breast lumps, vaginal bleeding, edema, jaundice, dark urine, clay-colored stools, dyspnea, headache, blurred vision, abdominal pain, numbness or stiffness in legs, chest pain; tenderness, redness, and swelling in extremities; males to report impotence, gynecomastia; to report dermal rash with transdermal patch**

RARELY USED

estramustine (Rx)

(ess-tra-muss'teen)

Emcyt

Func. class.: Antineoplastic alkylating agent

USES: Metastatic prostate cancer

CONTRAINDICATIONS: Pregnancy (D), hypersensitivity to estradiol, thromboembolic disorders, stroke, thrombophlebitis

DOSAGE AND ROUTES

- **Adult: PO** 14-16 mg/kg/day or 600 mg/m^2/day in 3-4 divided doses; treatment may continue for ≥3 mo

estrogens, conjugated (Rx)

Cenestin, Premarin

estrogens, conjugated synthetic B (Rx)

Enjuvia

Func. class.: Estrogen, hormone

Do not confuse:
Premarin/Provera

ACTION: Needed for adequate functioning of female reproductive system; affects release of pituitary gonadotropins, inhibits ovulation, adequate calcium use in bone

USES: Vasomotor symptoms (menopause), inoperable breast cancer, prostatic cancer, abnormal uterine bleeding, hypogonadism, primary ovarian failure, prevention of osteoporosis, castration
Unlabeled uses: Gender identity disorder

CONTRAINDICATIONS: Pregnancy (X), breastfeeding, thromboembolic disorders, reproductive cancer, genital bleeding (abnormal, undiagnosed), hypersensitivity, MI, stroke, thrombophlebitis

Black Box Warning: Endometrial cancer

Precautions: Hypertension, asthma, blood dyscrasias, CHF, diabetes mellitus, depression, migraine headache, seizure disorders, gallbladder/bone/hepatic/renal disease, family history of cancer of breast or reproductive tract, smoking, dementia, hypothyroidism, obesity, SLE

Black Box Warning: Cardiac disease, dementia

DOSAGE AND ROUTES

Estrogens conjugated

Vasomotor symptoms (menopause)
- **Adult: PO** 0.3-1.25 mg/day 3 wk on, 1 wk off

Prevention of osteoporosis
- **Adult: PO** 0.625 mg/day or in cycle

Atrophic vaginitis
- **Adult: VAG CREAM** 2-4 g/day × 21 days, off 7 days, repeat

Prostatic cancer
- **Adult: PO** 1.25-2.5 mg tid

Advanced inoperable breast cancer
- **Adult: PO** 10 mg tid × ≥3 mo

Abnormal uterine bleeding
- **Adult: IV/IM** 25 mg q6-12hr

Castration/primary ovarian failure
- **Adult: PO** 1.25 mg/day 3 wk on, 1 wk off

Hypogonadism
- **Adult: PO** 2.5-7.5 mg/day × 20 days/mo

Estrogens conjugated synthetic B

Vasomotor symptoms (menopause)
- **Adult: PO** 0.625 mg/day initially; may increase based on response

Available forms: Tabs 0.3, 0.45, 0.625, 0.9, 1.25, 2.5 mg; inj 25 mg/vial; vag cream 0.625 mg/g; *synthetic B:* tabs 0.625, 1.25 mg

Administer:
- Titrated dose; use lowest effective dose

PO route
- Give with or immediately after food to reduce nausea

IM route
- IM reconstitute after withdrawing 5 ml of air from container, inject sterile diluent on vial side, rotate to dissolve; give inj deep in large muscle mass, aspirate before inj

Vaginal route
- Use applicator provided, wash after use

Direct IV route
- IV, after reconstituting as for IM, inject into distal port of running IV line of D_5W, 0.9% NaCl at ≤5 mg/min

Y-site compatibilities: Heparin, hydrocortisone, potassium chloride, vit B/C

SIDE EFFECTS

CNS: Dizziness, headache, migraine, depression, seizures, mood disturbances
CV: Hypertension, thrombophlebitis, **edema, thromboembolism, stroke, pulmonary embolism, MI, chest pain**
EENT: Contact lens intolerance, increased myopia, astigmatism
GI: *Nausea,* vomiting, diarrhea, anorexia, pancreatitis, cramps, constipation, increased appetite, **cholestatic jaundice, hepatic adenoma**, weight gain/loss
GU: Amenorrhea, cervical erosion, breakthrough bleeding, dysmenorrhea, vaginal candidiasis, breast changes, *gynecomastia, testicular atrophy, impotence,* **increased risk of breast cancer, endometrial cancer**, libido changes
INTEG: Rash, urticaria, acne, hirsutism, alopecia, oily skin, seborrhea, purpura, melasma
META: Folic acid deficiency, hypercalcemia, hyperglycemia

PHARMACOKINETICS

PO/IM/IV: Degraded in liver, excreted in urine, crosses placenta, excreted in breast milk

INTERACTIONS

Increase: toxicity—cycloSPORINE, dantrolene
Increase: action of corticosteroids
Decrease: action of estrogens—anticonvulsants, barbiturates, phenylbutazone, rifampin
Decrease: action of anticoagulants, oral hypoglycemics, tamoxifen, thyroid

Drug/Food
Increase: estrogen level—grapefruit juice

Drug/Lab Test
Increase: BSP retention test, PBI, T_4, serum sodium, platelet aggregation, thyroxine-binding globulin (TBG), prothrombin; factors VII, VIII, IX, X; triglycerides
Decrease: serum folate, serum triglyceride, T_3 resin uptake test, glucose tolerance test, antithrombin III, pregnanediol, metyrapone test
False positive: LE prep, antinuclear antibodies

NURSING CONSIDERATIONS

Assess:
- Blood glucose if diabetic patient; hyperglycemia may occur
- Weight daily; notify prescriber of weekly weight gain >5 lb; if increase, diuretic may be ordered; check for edema; B/P baseline and periodically
- Hepatic studies: AST, ALT, bilirubin, alk phos
- Hypertension, cardiac symptoms, jaundice, hypercalcemia
- Mental status: affect, mood, behavioral changes, aggression
- Female patient for intact uterus; if so, progesterone should be added to estrogen therapy to decrease risk of endometrial cancer; abnormal uterine bleeding, breast exam; Pap smear

Evaluate:
- Therapeutic response: absence of breast engorgement, reversal of menopause symptoms, decrease in tumor size with prostatic cancer

Teach patient/family:

- To avoid breastfeeding, since product excreted in breast milk
- To weigh weekly; to report gain >5 lb

⚠ **To report breast lumps, vaginal bleeding, edema, jaundice, dark urine, clay-colored stools, dyspnea, headache, blurred vision, abdominal pain; leg pain and redness, numbness or stiffness; chest pain; males to report impotence or gynecomastia**

- To avoid sunlight or wear sunscreen; burns may occur
- To notify prescriber if pregnancy is suspected
- That vasomotor symptoms improve in 2 wk, max relief in 8 wk

eszopiclone (Rx)

(es-zop′i-klone)

Lunesta

Func. class.: Sedative/hypnotic, non-benzodiazepine

Chem. class.: Cyclopyrrolone

Controlled Substance Schedule IV

ACTION: Interacts with GABA receptors

USES: Insomnia

CONTRAINDICATIONS: Hypersensitivity, ethanol intoxication

Precautions: Pregnancy (C), breastfeeding, children, geriatric patients, severe hepatic disease, abrupt discontinuation, COPD, depression, labor, sleep apnea, substance abuse, suicidal ideation

DOSAGE AND ROUTES

- **Adult: PO** 2 mg immediately before bed, may increase to 3 mg if needed

Hepatic dose/CYP3A4 inhibitors

- **Adult: PO** 1 mg immediately before bed with severe hepatic disease

Available forms: Tabs 1, 2, 3 mg

Administer:

- Do not break, crush, or chew tab
- Immediately before bedtime; avoid use with food; for short-term use only
- Assistance with ambulation, night light, call bell within reach
- Check to see that product swallowed

SIDE EFFECTS

CNS: Worsening depression, hallucinations, headache, daytime drowsiness, **suicidal thoughts/actions**, migraine, restlessness, anxiety, sleep driving, sleepwalking

CV: Peripheral edema, chest pain

GI: Dry mouth, bitter taste (dysgeusia)

GU: Gynecomastia, dysmenorrhea

INTEG: Rash, **angioedema**

PHARMACOKINETICS

Onset rapid; peak 1 hr; duration 6 hr; extensively metabolized in the liver by CYP3A4, CYP2E1; excreted via kidneys; half-life 6 hr, geriatric patients 9 hr, protein binding 52%-59%

INTERACTIONS

Increase: CNS depression—CNS depressants

Increase: toxicity due to decreased eszopiclone elimination—CYP3A4 inhibitors (clarithromycin, itraconazole, ketoconazole, nefazodone, nelfinavir, ritonavir, troleandomycin, SSRIs)

Drug/Food

Decrease: product action—food

NURSING CONSIDERATIONS

Assess:

- **Sleep pattern:** ability to go to sleep, stay asleep, early morning awakenings, conservative methods used
- For abuse of this product, other products

Perform/provide:

- Alternative methods to improve sleep: reading, quiet environment, warm bath, milk

Evaluate:
- Therapeutic response: ability to fall asleep and stay asleep throughout the night

Teach patient/family:
- That daytime drowsiness may occur; not to engage in hazardous activities until effect is known; that memory problems may occur
- That all other medications and supplements should be avoided unless approved by prescriber; to avoid alcohol
- To notify prescriber if pregnancy is suspected or planned

etanercept (Rx)
(eh-tan′er-sept)
Enbrel
Func. class.: Antirheumatic agent (disease modifying)(DMARDs)
Chem. class.: Anti-TNF agent

ACTION: Binds tumor necrosis factor (TNF), which is involved in immune and inflammatory reactions

USES: Acute, chronic rheumatoid arthritis that has not responded to other disease-modifying agents, polyarticular course of juvenile rheumatoid arthritis (JRA), ankylosing spondylitis, plaque psoriasis, psoriatic arthritis
Unlabeled uses: Crohn's disease; plaque psoriasis (child ≥4 yr)

CONTRAINDICATIONS: Sepsis, active infections

Black Box Warning: Hypersensitivity to product, latex needle cap, benzyl alcohol

Precautions: Pregnancy (B), breastfeeding, children <4 yr, geriatric patients, malignancies, CHF, seizures, multiple sclerosis

Black Box Warning: Infection, lymphoma, neoplastic disease

DOSAGE AND ROUTES

Rheumatoid/psoriatic arthritis, ankylosing spondylitis
- **Adult: SUBCUT** 50 mg/wk or 25 mg 2×/wk, 3-4 days apart
- **Child 2-17 yr: SUBCUT** 0.8 mg/kg/wk, max 50 mg/wk

Plaque psoriasis
- **Adult: SUBCUT** 50 mg 2×/wk × 3 mo
- **Adolescent/child 4-17 yr (unlabeled): SUBCUT** 0.8 mg/kg/wk, max 50 mg/wk

Juvenile rheumatoid arthritis (JRA)
- **Adolescent/child 2-17 yr: SUBCUT** 0.8 mg/kg/wk, max 50 mg/wk

Available forms: Powder for inj 25 mg; inj 50 mg/ml; autoinjector, single use

Administer:
- After reconstituting 1 ml of supplied diluent, slowly inject diluent into vial, swirl contents; do not shake, sol should be clear/colorless, do not use if cloudy, discolored
- Do not admix with other sol or medications, do not use filter
- May be injected SUBCUT into upper arm, abdomen, thigh; rotate inj sites

SIDE EFFECTS

CNS: *Headache,* asthenia, dizziness
GI: Abdominal pain, dyspepsia, vomiting
HEMA: **Pancytopenia, anemia, thrombocytopenia, leukopenia, neutropenia**
INTEG: Rash, *inj site reaction,* keratoderma blenorrhagicum
RESP: *Pharyngitis, cough, URI, non-URI,* sinusitis, *rhinitis*
SYST: **Serious infections, sepsis, death, malignancies**

PHARMACOKINETICS

Elimination half-life 102 hr, 60% absorbed (SUBCUT)

INTERACTIONS

- **Increase:** neutropenia—sulfasalazine
- Do not give concurrently with vaccines; immunizations should be brought up to date before treatment

• Avoid use with anakinra, cyclophosphamide, rilonacept

NURSING CONSIDERATIONS

Assess:

• **RA:** pain, stiffness, ROM, swelling of joints before, during, after treatment
• For inj site pain, swelling; usually occurs after 2 inj (4-5 days)

Black Box Warning: Infection: patients using immunosuppressives, corticosteroids, methotrexate at greater risk; assess for fever

• **Hypersensitivity:** to this product, latex needle cap, benzyl alcohol; usual reactions to product last 3-5 days

Evaluate:

• Therapeutic response: decreased inflammation, pain in joints

Teach patient/family:

• That product must be continued for prescribed time to be effective
• To use caution when driving; dizziness may occur
• Not to receive live vaccinations during treatment
• About self-administration if appropriate: inj should be made in thigh, abdomen, upper arm; rotate sites at least 1 in from previous site
• To notify prescriber of possible infection (upper respiratory, other)

ethambutol (Rx)

(e-tham′byoo-tole)

Etibi ✦, Myambutol

Func. class.: Antitubercular

Chem. class.: Diisopropylethylene diamide derivative

Do not confuse:
ethambutol/Ethmozine

ACTION: Inhibits RNA synthesis, decreases tubercle bacilli replication

USES: Pulmonary TB as an adjunct, other mycobacterial infections

CONTRAINDICATIONS: Children <13 yr, hypersensitivity, optic neuritis

Precautions: Pregnancy (B), breastfeeding, renal disease, diabetic retinopathy, cataracts, ocular defects, hepatic and hematopoietic disorders

DOSAGE AND ROUTES

• **Adult/child >13 yr: PO** 15-25 mg/kg/day as single dose, 50 mg/kg 2×/wk, or 25-30 mg/kg 3×/wk

Renal disease

• CCr 10-50 ml/min, dose q24-36hr; CCr <10 ml/min, dose q48hr

Retreatment

• **Adult: PO** 25 mg/kg/day as single dose × 2 mo with at least 1 other product then decrease to 15 mg/kg/day as single dose, max 2.5 g/day
• **Child: PO** 15 mg/kg/day

Available forms: Tabs 100, 400 mg

Administer:

• With meals to decrease GI symptoms
• Antiemetic if vomiting occurs
• After C&S completed; monthly to detect resistance
• 2 hr before antacids

SIDE EFFECTS

CNS: *Headache, confusion,* fever, malaise, dizziness, *disorientation,* hallucinations, peripheral neuropathy

EENT: Blurred vision, optic neuritis, photophobia, decreased visual acuity

GI: *Abdominal distress, anorexia, nausea, vomiting*

INTEG: Dermatitis, pruritus, toxic epidermal necrolysis, erythema multiforme

META: *Elevated uric acid, acute gout,* impaired hepatic function

MISC: Thrombocytopenia, joint pain, anaphylaxis

PHARMACOKINETICS

Peak 2-4 hr, half-life 3 hr, metabolized in liver, excreted in urine (unchanged product/inactive metabolites, unchanged product in feces)

INTERACTIONS

- Delayed absorption of ethambutol: aluminum salts, separate by 4 hr
- Neurotoxicity: other neurotoxics

NURSING CONSIDERATIONS

Assess:

- Hepatic studies weekly × 2 wk then q2mo: ALT, AST, bilirubin; decreased appetite, jaundice, dark urine, fatigue
- Signs of anemia: Hct, Hgb, fatigue
- Mental status often: affect, mood, behavioral changes; psychosis may occur
- C&S, including sputum, before treatment
- Visual status: decreased activity, altered color perception
- **Serious skin reactions:** toxic epidermal necrolysis

Evaluate:

- Therapeutic response: decreased symptoms of TB, decrease in acid-fast bacteria

Teach patient/family:

- To avoid alcohol products
- That compliance with dosage schedule, duration is necessary
- That scheduled appointments must be kept or relapse may occur
- To report to prescriber any visual changes; rash; hot, swollen, painful joints; numbness, tingling of extremities

etidronate (Rx)

(eh-tih-droe′nate)

Didronel

Func. class.: Bone resorption inhibitor
Chem. class.: Bisphosphonate

Do not confuse:
etidronate/etretinate/etomidate

ACTION: Decreases bone resorption and new bone development (accretion)

USES: Paget's disease, heterotopic ossification, hypercalcemia of malignancy

Unlabeled uses: Osteoporosis, osteoporosis prophylaxis

CONTRAINDICATIONS: Achalasia, esophageal stricture, osteomalacia

Precautions: Pregnancy (C), breastfeeding, children, renal disease, restricted vit D, calcium, colitis, vit D deficiency, anemia, esophagitis, pathologic fractures, severe renal disease with creatinine >5 mg/dl, poor dentition, asthma, coagulopathy, dental disease or work, GERD, hiatal hernia, hyperthyroidism, infection, phosphate hypersensitivity

DOSAGE AND ROUTES

Paget's disease

- **Adult: PO** 5-10 mg/kg/day 2 hr before meals with water, max 20 mg/kg/day, max 6 mo or 11-20 mg/kg/day for max of 3 mo

Heterotopic ossification

- **Adult: PO** 20 mg/kg/day × 2 wk then 10 mg/kg/day for 10 wk for a total of 12 wk

Hypercalcemia

- **Adult: PO** 20 mg/kg/day × 30 days

Heterotopic ossification/hip replacement

- **Adult: PO** 20 mg/kg/day × 4 wk before and then for 3 mo after surgery (4 mo total)

Available forms: Tabs 200, 400 mg

Administer:

- On empty stomach with water 2 hr before meals; avoid simultaneous vitamins/mineral/antacids with calcium, iron, magnesium, or aluminum

SIDE EFFECTS

CNS: Headache
CV: Atrial fibrillation
GI: Nausea, constipation, diarrhea, gastritis, esophagitis
GU: Nephrotoxicity
MISC: Dyspnea, low magnesium, phosphorus, alopecia, Stevens-Johnson syndrome, angioedema

MS: Bone pain, hypocalcemia, decreased mineralization of nonaffected bones, **osteonecrosis of the jaw**, arthralgia, leg cramps

PHARMACOKINETICS

Absorbed poorly, not metabolized, excreted in urine/feces, therapeutic response 1-3 mo

INTERACTIONS

Increase: protime—warfarin
Decrease: absorption—calcium, aluminum, magnesium antacids/supplements, iron products
Drug/Food
Decrease: absorption—dairy products

NURSING CONSIDERATIONS

Assess:

- **Nephrotoxicity:** I&O ratio; check for decreased output in renal patients; patients with renal failure should not use this product
- BUN, creatinine, phosphate calcium, alk phos; calcium should be kept at 9-10 mg/dl, vit D 50-135 international units/dl
- For bone pain, weakness during treatment
- **Hypocalcemia:** muscle spasm, laryngospasm, paresthesias, facial twitching, colic
- Nutritional status, diet for sources of vit D (milk, some seafood), calcium (dairy products, dark green vegetables), phosphates—adequate intake is necessary
- Persistent nausea or diarrhea
- **Osteonecrosis of the jaw:** patients undergoing dental procedures (extraction), if required/appropriate, antiinfectives should be used

Evaluate:

- Therapeutic response: management of bone deficiencies, Paget's disease

Teach patient/family:

- To avoid OTC products
- That therapeutic response may take 1-3 mo; that effects persist for months after product is discontinued
- That adequate intake of calcium, vit D is necessary
- To report sudden onset of unexplained pain, restricted mobility, heat over bone; hypercalcemic relapse
- To perform good oral hygiene

RARELY USED

etomidate (Rx)

(e-tom′i-date)

Amidate

Func. class.: General anesthetic

USES:
Induction of general anesthesia

CONTRAINDICATIONS:
Hypersensitivity, labor/delivery

DOSAGE AND ROUTES

- **Adult/child >10 yr: IV** 0.2-0.6 mg/kg over $^1/_2$-1 min

HIGH ALERT

etoposide (Rx)

(e-toe-poe′side)

Toposar

etoposide phosphate (Rx)

Etopophos

Func. class.: Antineoplastic—miscellaneous

Chem. class.: Semisynthetic podophyllotoxin

ACTION:
Inhibits mitotic activity through metaphase to mitosis; also inhibits cells from entering mitosis, depresses DNA/RNA synthesis, cell-cycle–specific S and G_2; binds to a complex of DNA and topoisomerase II

USES:
Testicular cancer, small-cell carcinoma of the lung

Unlabeled uses: Leukemias (ALL, AML), desmoid tumor, gastric/ovarian cancer, bone marrow ablation, Hodgkin's/non-Hodgkin's lymphoma, malignant glioma, neuroblastoma, stem cell transplant preparation, trophoblastic disease

CONTRAINDICATIONS:

Pregnancy (D), breastfeeding, hypersensitivity, severe renal/hepatic disease

Precautions: Children, renal/hepatic disease, gout

Black Box Warning: Bone marrow depression, infection, bleeding

DOSAGE AND ROUTES

Testicular cancer

- **Adult: IV** 100 mg/m²/day on days 1, 2 in combination with methotrexate, leucovorin, actinomycin D, cyclophosphamide and vinCRIStine (EMA-CO regimen) q2-3wk

Small-cell carcinoma of the lung

- **Adult: IV** 35 mg/m²/day × 4 days to 50 mg/m²/day × 5 days in combination; resected stage IB-III (unlabeled) with CISplatin **IV** 100 mg/m² on days 1-3 with CISplatin 100 mg/m² on day 1 q21days ×4 cycles; **PO** 2× IV dose rounded to nearest 50 mg; given once a day if total dose ≤400 mg/day or in divided doses if >400 mg/day

Renal dose

- **Adult: IV** CCr 45-60 ml/min, reduce dose by 15%; CCr 30-44 ml/min, reduce dose by 20%; CCr <30 ml/min, reduce dose by 25%

Available forms: Inj 20 mg/ml; caps 50 mg

Administer:

- Antiemetic 30-60 min before product and prn to prevent vomiting
- **Urate nephropathy:** Allopurinol, aggressive alkalinization to maintain uric acid levels
- Antispasmodic, EPINEPHrine, corticosteroids, antihistamines for reactions

PO route

- Give without regard to food

Intermittent IV INF route (etoposide)

- Use cytotoxic handling procedures, use Luer-Lok fittings to prevent leakage
- After **diluting** 5-ml vial with 100 mg/250 ml or more D_5W or NaCl to 0.2-0.4 mg/ml, **infuse** over 30-60 min

Additive compatibilities: CARBOplatin, CISplatin, cytarabine, floxuridine, fluorouracil, hydrOXYzine, ifosfamide, ondansetron

Y-site compatibilities: Acyclovir, alfentanil, allopurinol, amifostine, amikacin, aminocaproic acid, aminophylline, amiodarone, amphotericin B colloidal, amphotericin B lipid complex, amphotericin B liposome, ampicillin, ampicillin-sulbactam, anidulafungin, atenolol, atracurium, aztreonam, bivalirudin, bleomycin, bumetanide, buprenorphine, butorphanol, calcium chloride/gluconate, CARBOplatin, caspofungin, ceFAZolin, cefoperazone, cefotaxime, cefotetan, cefoxitin, ceftazidime, ceftizoxime, cefTRIAXone, cefuroxime, chloramphenicol, chlorproMAZINE, cimetidine, ciprofloxacin, cisatracurium, CISplatin, cladribine, clindamycin, codeine, cyclophosphamide, cycloSPORINE, cytarabine, DACTINomycin, DAPTOmycin, DAUNOrubicin, dexamethasone, dexmedetomidine, dexrazoxane, digoxin, diltiazem, diphenhydrAMINE, DOBUTamine, docetaxel, DOPamine, doxacurium, DOXOrubicin, DOXOrubicin liposomal, doxycycline, droperidol, enalaprilat, ePHEDrine, EPINEPHrine, epirubicin, ertapenem, erythromycin, esmolol, famotidine, fenoldopam, fentaNYL, floxuridine, fluconazole, fludarabine, fluorouracil, foscarnet, fosphenytoin, furosemide, ganciclovir, gatifloxacin, gemcitabine, gentamicin, glycopyrrolate, granisetron, haloperidol, heparin, hydrALAZINE, hydrocortisone, HYDROmorphone, hydrOXYzine, ifosfamide, imipenem-cilastatin, inamrinone, insulin (regular), irinotecan, isoproterenol, ketorolac, labetalol, lansoprazole, leucovorin, levofloxacin, levorphanol, lidocaine, linezolid, LORazepam, magnesium sulfate, mannitol, mechlorethamine, melphalan, meperidine, meropenem, mesna, methohexital, methotrexate, methyldopate, methylPREDNISolone, metoclopramide, metoprolol, metroNIDAZOLE, micafungin, midazolam, milrinone, minocycline, mitoxantrone, mivacurium, morphine, nafcillin, nalbuphine, naloxone, nesiritide, nitroglycerin, nitroprusside, norepinephrine, NS, octreotide, ofloxacin, ondansetron, oxaliplatin, paclitaxel, palonosetron, pamidronate, pancuronium, pemetrexed, pentamidine, pentazocine, PENTobarbital, PHENobarbital, phenylephrine, piperacillin, piperacillin-tazobactam, polymyxin B, potassium chloride/phosphates, procainamide, prochlorperazine, promethazine, propranolol, quinupristin-dalfopristin, ranitidine, remifentanil, rocuronium, sargramostim, sodium acetate/bicarbonate/phosphates, succinylcholine, SUFentanil, sulfamethoxazole-trimethoprim, tacrolimus, teniposide, theophylline, thiotepa, ticarcillin, ticarcillin-clavulanate, tigecycline, tirofiban, tobramycin, topotecan, trimethobenzamide, vancomycin, vasopressin, vecuronium, verapamil, vinBLAStine, vinCRIStine, vinorelbine, voriconazole, zidovudine, zoledronic acid

Intermittent IV INF route (etoposide phosphate)

• **Reconstitute** each vial with 5 or 10 ml of D_5W, 0.9% NaCl for a concentration of 20 mg/ml or 10 mg/ml, respectively; may give diluted or undiluted to concentration of as little as 0.1 mg/ml, **give** over 5-210 min

Y-site compatibilities: Acyclovir, alfentanil, amifostine, amikacin, aminocaproic acid, aminophylline, amiodarone, ampicillin, ampicillin-sulbactam, anidulafungin, atenolol, atracurium, aztreonam, bivalirudin, bleomycin, bumetanide, buprenorphine, butorphanol, calcium acetate/chloride/gluconate, CARBOplatin, carmustine, caspofungin, ceFAZolin, cefonicid, cefoperazone, cefotaxime, cefotetan, cefoxitin, ceftazidime, ceftizoxime, cefTRIAXone, cefuroxime, chloramphenicol, cimetidine, ciprofloxacin, cisatracurium, CISplatin, clindamycin, codeine, cyclophosphamide, cycloSPORINE, cytarabine, dacarbazine, DACTINomycin, DAPTOmycin, DAUNOrubicin, dexamethasone, digoxin, diltiazem, diphenhydrAMINE, DOBUTamine, docetaxel, DOPamine, doripenem, doxacurium, DOXOrubicin, doxycycline, enalaprilat, ePHEDrine, EPINEPHrine, epirubicin, ertapenem, erythromycin, esmolol, famotidine, fenoldopam, fentaNYL, floxuridine, fluconazole, fludarabine, fluorouracil, foscarnet, fosphenytoin, furosemide, ganciclovir, gatifloxacin, gemcitabine, gentamicin, glycopyrrolate, granisetron, haloperidol, heparin, hydrALAZINE, hydrocortisone, HYDROmorphone, hydrOXYzine, IDArubicin, ifosfamide, inamrinone, insulin (regular), irinotecan, isoproterenol, ketorolac, labetalol, leucovorin, levofloxacin, levorphanol, lidocaine, linezolid, LORazepam, magnesium sulfate, mannitol, mechlorethamine, meperidine, meropenem, mesna, metaraminol, methotrexate, methyldopate, metoclopramide, metoprolol, metroNIDAZOLE, midazolam, milrinone, minocycline, mitoxantrone, mivacurium, morphine, nafcillin, nalbuphine, naloxone, nesiritide, netilmicin, nitroglycerin, nitroprusside, norepinephrine, octreotide, ofloxacin, ondansetron, oxaliplatin, paclitaxel, palonosetron, pamidronate, pancuronium, pemetrexed, pentamidine, pentazocine, PENTobarbital, PHENobarbital, phenylephrine, piperacillin, piperacillin-tazobactam, plicamycin, polymyxin B, potassium chloride/phosphates, procainamide, promethazine, propranolol, quiNIDine, quinupristin-dalfopristin, ranitidine, remifentanil, riTUXimab, rocuronium, sodium acetate/bicarbonate/phosphates, streptozocin, succinylcholine, SUFentanil, sulfamethoxazole-trimethoprim, tacrolimus, teniposide, theophylline, thiopental, thiotepa, ticarcillin,

ticarcillin-clavulanate, tigecycline, tirofiban, tobramycin, tolazoline, trastuzumab, trimethobenzamide, vancomycin, vasopressin, vecuronium, verapamil, vinBLAStine, vinCRIStine, vinorelbine, voriconazole, zidovudine, zoledronic acid

SIDE EFFECTS

CNS: Headache, *fever,* peripheral neuropathy, paresthesias, confusion, chills, fever
CV: *Hypotension,* MI, dysrhythmias
GI: *Nausea, vomiting, anorexia,* hepatotoxicity, dyspepsia, diarrhea, constipation
GU: Nephrotoxicity
HEMA: Thrombocytopenia, leukopenia, myelosuppression, anemia
INTEG: *Rash, alopecia,* phlebitis at IV site, radiation recall, Stevens-Johnson syndrome
RESP: Bronchospasm, pleural effusion
SYST: Anaphylaxis

PHARMACOKINETICS

Half-life 7 hr, metabolized in liver, excreted in urine, crosses placental barrier

INTERACTIONS

Increase: bone marrow depression—other antineoplastics, radiation, immunosuppressives
Increase: adverse reactions—live virus vaccines, toxoids
Increase: effect of etoposide, toxicity—voriconazole, conivaptan, cyclosporine, imatinib, nilotinib, etravirine, telithromycin
Increase: risk of bleeding—anticoagulants, NSAIDs, platelet inhibitors, thrombolytics, salicylate
Decrease: etoposide effect—sargramostim, filgrastim, separate by ≥24 hr

Drug/Food

- Decreased oral etoposide—grapefruit juice

NURSING CONSIDERATIONS

Assess:

Black Box Warning: **Bone marrow depression:** CBC, differential, platelet count weekly; withhold product if WBC is <1000 or platelet count is <50,000; notify prescriber

- **Nephrotoxicity:** BUN; serum uric acid; urine CCr; electrolytes before, during therapy; I&O ratio; report fall in urine output to <30 ml/hr; check B/P bid, report any significant decrease
- Monitor temp q4hr; fever may indicate beginning infection
- Hepatic studies before, during therapy (bilirubin, AST, ALT, LDH) as needed or monthly

Black Box Warning: **Bleeding:** hematuria, guaiac stools, bruising or petechiae, mucosa or orifices q8hr

- Effects of alopecia on body image; discuss feelings about body changes
- Jaundice of skin and sclera, dark urine, clay-colored stools, itchy skin, abdominal pain, fever, diarrhea
- B/P q15min during inf; if systolic reading <90 mm Hg, discontinue inf, notify prescriber
- Buccal cavity q8hr for dryness, sores or ulceration, white patches, oral pain, bleeding, dysphagia
- Local irritation, pain, burning, discoloration at inj site

⚠ **Symptoms indicating severe allergic reaction:** rash, pruritus, urticaria, purpuric skin lesions, itching, flushing, restlessness, coughing, difficulty breathing

- **Frequency of stools, characteristics:** cramping, acidosis; **signs of dehydration:** rapid respirations, poor skin turgor, decreased urine output, dry skin, restlessness, weakness
- **Geriatric patients:** increased alopecia, GI effects, infection, nephrotoxicity, myelosuppression

Perform/provide:

- Increased fluid intake to 2-3 L/day to prevent urate deposits, calculi formation

- Refrigerate oral product, do not freeze

Evaluate:

- Therapeutic response: decreased tumor size, spread of malignancy

Teach patient/family:

- To report any complaints or side effects to nurse or prescriber
- To report any changes in breathing or coughing
- That hair may be lost during treatment; that a wig or hairpiece may make patient feel better; that new hair may be different in color, texture
- That metallic taste may occur
- To report symptoms of infection; to avoid crowds, persons with known infections
- To avoid immunizations
- To use reliable contraception during and for several months after therapy; to avoid breastfeeding

etravirine (Rx)

(e-tra′veer-een)

INTELENCE

Func. class.: Antiretroviral

Chem. class.: Nonnucleoside reverse transcriptase inhibitor (NNRTI)

ACTION: Binds directly to reverse transcriptase, thus blocking the RNA- and DNA-dependent DNA polymerase action and causing a disruption of the enzyme's catalytic site

USES: In combination with other antiretroviral agents for HIV infection in treatment-experienced patients with evidence of HIV replication despite ongoing antiretroviral therapy

CONTRAINDICATIONS: Breastfeeding, hypersensitivity

Precautions: Pregnancy (B), children, geriatric patients, impaired hepatic function, antimicrobial resistance, hepatitis, hypercholesterolemia, hypertriglycerides, immune reconstitution syndrome

DOSAGE AND ROUTES

- **Adult: PO** 200 mg bid after a meal, max 400 mg/day; not established for treatment-naïve patients

Available forms: Tabs 100, 200 mg

Administer:

- In combination with other antiretrovirals with food or after a meal
- Tabs may be dispersed in water; once dispersed, stir well, give immediately, rinse glass, have patient drink to ensure all medication taken

SIDE EFFECTS

CNS: *Headache, insomnia,* amnesia, anxiety, confusion, fatigue, nightmares, peripheral neuropathy, **seizures, stroke,** tremor

CV: **Atrial fibrillation,** hypertension, MI

EENT: Blurred vision

GI: *Nausea, vomiting, diarrhea, anorexia,* abdominal pain, increased AST/ALT, constipation, flatulence, gastritis, GERD, **hematemesis, hepatitis,** hepatomegaly, **pancreatitis**

GU: **Renal failure**

HEMA: **Hemolytic anemia, neutropenia, thrombocytopenia, anemia**

INTEG: *Rash,* erythema multiforme, angioedema, **Stevens-Johnson syndrome**

MS: **Rhabdomyolysis**

OTHER: Diabetes mellitus, gynecomastia, hyperamylasemia, hypercholesterolemia, hyperglycemia, hyperlipidemia

RESP: Dyspnea, **bronchospasm**

PHARMACOKINETICS

99.9% plasma protein binding; metabolized by CYP3A4, 2C9, 2C19; half-life 21-61 hr; excreted in feces

INTERACTIONS

- Do not use concurrently with atazanavir, carBAMazepine, delavirdine, fosamprenavir, fosphenytoin, phenytoin, PHENobarbital, rifapentine, rifampin, tipranavir
- Altered effect of cycloSPORINE, tacrolimus, sirolimus

Increase: myopathy, rhabdomyolysis—HMG-CoA reductase inhibitors
Increase: etravirine levels—fluconazole, itraconazole, ketoconazole, lopinavir, posaconazole, ritonavir, voriconazole
Increase: withdrawal symptoms—methadone
Increase: levels of diazepam, rifampin, voriconazole, warfarin
Decrease: levels of amiodarone, atazanavir, clarithromycin, flecainide, fosamprenavir, lidocaine, mexiletine, propafenone, quiNIDine, sildenafil, tadalafil, vardenafil
Decrease: etravirine levels—darunavir, dexamethasone, disopyramide, efavirenz, nevirapine, ritonavir, saquinavir, tipranavir

Drug/Herb
Decrease: etravirine—St. John's wort

NURSING CONSIDERATIONS

Assess:

- **Symptoms of HIV, possible infections;** increased temp

⚠ **Fatal hypersensitivity reactions:** fever, rash, nausea, vomiting, fatigue, cough, dyspnea, diarrhea, abdominal discomfort; treatment should be discontinued and not restarted

- **Blood dyscrasias** (anemia, granulocytopenia): bruising, fatigue, bleeding, poor healing
- **Renal failure:** BUN, serum uric acid, CCr before, during therapy; may be elevated throughout treatment
- **Hepatitis/pancreatitis:** hepatic studies before and during therapy: bilirubin, AST, ALT, amylase, alk phos, creatine phosphokinase, creatinine, monthly
- HIV: monitor viral load, CD4 counts, plasma HIV RNA during treatment; watch for decreasing granulocytes, Hgb; if low, therapy may have to be discontinued and restarted after hematologic recovery; blood transfusions may be required; cholesterol/lipid profile

Perform/provide:

- Storage in cool environment; protect from light

Evaluate:

- Therapeutic response: increased CD4 count, decreased viral load

Teach patient/family:

- That product is not a cure but will control symptoms; that patient is still infective, may pass AIDS virus to others
- To notify prescriber of sore throat, swollen lymph nodes, malaise, fever; other infections may occur; to stop product and notify prescriber immediately if skin rash, fever, cough, SOB, GI symptoms occur; to advise all health care providers that allergic reaction has occurred with etravirine
- That follow-up visits must be continued, since serious toxicity may occur; blood counts must be performed
- To use contraception during treatment; that patient still able to transmit disease
- About information on medication guide and warning card; discuss points on guide
- That other products may be necessary to prevent other infections
- To take medication after a meal

everolimus (Rx)

(e-ve-ro'li-mus)

Afinitor, Zortress

Func. class.: Antineoplastic—miscellaneous
Chem. class.: Immunosuppressant, macrolide

ACTION: Proliferation signal inhibitor that inhibits mammalian target of rapamycin (mTOR); this pathway is dysregulated in cancer

USES: Renal cell cancer in those with failed treatment with sorafenib, kidney transplant rejection prophylaxis with cycloSPORINE, subependymal giant cell astrocytoma, progressive pancreatic neuroendocrine tumor (PNET) with unresectable locally advanced/metastatic disease

CONTRAINDICATIONS:

Breastfeeding; hypersensitivity to this product, rapamine, torisel, pregnancy (D)

Precautions: Children <13 yr, renal/hepatic disease; diabetes mellitus, hyperlipidemia, plural effusion

Black Box Warning: Immunosuppression, infection, renal artery thrombosis, renal impairment, renal vein thrombosis

DOSAGE AND ROUTES

Kidney transplant rejection prophylaxis (Zortress)

• **Adult: PO** 0.75 mg q12hr with cycloSPORINE in combination with basiliximab, corticosteroids, reduced doses of cycloSPORINE

Advanced renal cancer (Afinitor)

• **Adult: PO** 10 mg daily as long as clinically beneficial; with strong 3A4 inducers 10 mg daily then may increase by 5 mg increments to 20 mg daily

Progressive neuroendocrine tumor (PNET) (Afinitor only)

• **Adult: PO** 10 mg daily, reduce dose to 5 mg daily if intolerable adverse reactions occur

Subependymal giant-cell astrocytoma (SEGA) (Afinitor only)

• **Adult/adolescent/child ≥3 yr: PO** BSA ≥2.2 m^2, give 7.5 mg daily; BSA 1.3-2.1 m^2, give 5 mg daily; BSA 0.5-01.2 m^2, give 2.5 mg daily; adjust q2wk based on trough, clinical response

Hepatic dose

• **Adult: PO** (Child-Pugh B) Afinitor: 5 mg/day; Zortress: 0.75 mg/day divided q12hr

Available forms: Tabs 0.25, 0.5, 0.75 (Zortess); 2.5, 5, 10 mg (Afinitor)

Administer:

• Follow procedure for proper handling of antineoplastics

• Swallow tabs whole with a full glass of water; do not chew, crush, or break

• **Afinitor:** take at same time of day without regard to food; if unable to swallow, disperse in 30 ml of water

• **Zortress:** must take consistently with/without food, give at same time of day q12hr with cycloSPORINE

• Store protected from light at room temp

SIDE EFFECTS

CNS: *Headache, insomnia, paresthesia,* chills, fever

CV: Hypertension, *CHF,* peripheral edema

EENT: Blurred vision, photophobia

GI: Nausea, vomiting, diarrhea

GU: Renal failure

HEMA: Anemia, leukopenia, thrombocytopenia

INTEG: *Rash, acne*

META: Hyperglycemia, increased creatinine, *hyperlipemia,* hyperphosphatemia, weight loss

RESP: Pleural effusion, *dyspnea*

PHARMACOKINETICS

Rapidly absorbed; peak 1-2 hr; protein binding 74%; extensively metabolized by CYP3A4 enzyme system; half-life 30 hr; reduced by high-fat meal; excreted in feces (80%), urine (5%)

INTERACTIONS

Increase: blood levels—antifungals, calcium channel blockers, cimetidine, danazol, erythromycin, cycloSPORINE, HIV-protease inhibitors

Decrease: blood levels of everolimus—carBAMazepine, PHENobarbital, phenytoin, rifamycin, rifapentine

Decrease: effect of live vaccines

Drug/Herb

• St. John's wort: may decrease effect of everolimus

Drug/Food

• Alters bioavailability; use consistently with/without food; do not use with grapefruit juice

NURSING CONSIDERATIONS

Assess:

• Lipid profile: cholesterol, triglycerides, lipid-lowering agent may be needed; blood glucose

Black Box Warning: Blood studies: CBC with differential during treatment monthly; if leukocytes <3000/mm³ or platelets <100,000/mm³, product should be discontinued or reduced; decreased hemoglobulin level may indicate bone marrow suppression

- Hepatic/renal studies: AST, ALT, amylase, bilirubin, creatinine, phosphate, and for hepatotoxicity: dark urine, jaundice, itching, light-colored stools; product should be discontinued
- Obtain everolimus blood levels in kidney transplant, hepatic disease, CYP3A4 inducers, inhibitors

Evaluate:
- Therapeutic response

Teach patient/family:
- To report fever, rash, severe diarrhea, chills, sore throat, fatigue; serious infections may occur; to report clay-colored stools, cramping (hepatotoxicity)

Black Box Warning: To avoid crowds, persons with known infections to reduce risk for infection

- To use contraception before, during, and 12 wk after product discontinued; to avoid breastfeeding
- Not to use with grapefruit juice
- To avoid live vaccines
- That product may decrease male, female fertility
- That drinking alcohol is not recommended

exemestane (Rx)

(ex-em′eh-stane)

Aromasin

Func. class.: Antineoplastic

Chem. class.: Aromatase inhibitor

ACTION: Lowers serum estradiol concentrations; many breast cancers have strong estrogen receptors

USES: Advanced breast carcinoma not responsive to other therapy (postmenopausal)

CONTRAINDICATIONS: Pregnancy (X), breastfeeding, premenopausal women, hypersensitivity

Precautions: Children, geriatric patients, renal/hepatic disease

DOSAGE AND ROUTES

- **Adult: PO** 25 mg/day after meals; may need 50 mg/day if taken with a potent CYP3A4 inducer

Available forms: Tabs 25 mg

Administer:
- After meals at same time of day

SIDE EFFECTS

CNS: *Headache, depression, insomnia, anxiety, fatigue, hot flashes, diaphoresis*

CV: Hypertension

GI: *Nausea,* vomiting, diarrhea, constipation, abdominal pain, increased appetite

HEMA: *Lymphopenia*

MS: Fracture, bone loss

RESP: Cough, *dyspnea*

PHARMACOKINETICS

Half-life 24 hr; excreted in feces, urine

INTERACTIONS

Decrease: exemestane action—CYP3A4 inducers, estrogens

NURSING CONSIDERATIONS

Assess:
- B/P; hypertension may occur
- Bone mineral density, x-ray of thoracic or lumbar spine if bone changes suspected

Perform/provide:
- At room temp

Evaluate:
- Therapeutic response: decreased tumor size, spread of malignancy

Teach patient/family:
- To report any complaints, side effects to prescriber
- That hot flashes are reversible after discontinuing treatment

• To use reliable contraception (pregnancy X); not to breastfeed
• That vit D, calcium may be used for bone loss

exenatide (Rx)

(ex-en'a-tide)

Byetta

Func. class.: Antidiabetic
Chem. class.: Incretin mimetic

ACTION: Binds and activates known human GLP-1 receptor, mimics natural physiology for self-regulating glycemic control

USES: Type 2 diabetes mellitus given in combination with metFORMIN, a sulfonylurea, or a thiazolidinedione
Unlabeled uses: Once-weekly dosing

CONTRAINDICATIONS: Hypersensitivity
Precautions: Pregnancy (C), geriatric patients, severe renal/hepatic/GI disease, pancreatitis

DOSAGE AND ROUTES

• **Adult: SUBCUT** 5 mcg bid 1 hr before morning and evening meal; may increase to 10 mcg bid after 1 mo of therapy
Available forms: Inj 5, 10 mcg
Administer:
• May be used as monotherapy or combined with other products
• SUBCUT only, do not give IV/IM
• Pen needles must be purchased separately, compatible; prime prior to use; inject into thigh, abdomen, upper arm; rotate sites
• Product 1 hr before meals, approximately 6 hr apart; if patient is NPO, may need to hold dose to prevent hypoglycemia

SIDE EFFECTS

CNS: *Headache, dizziness,* feeling jittery, restlessness, weakness
ENDO: Hypoglycemia
GI: Nausea, vomiting, diarrhea, dyspepsia, anorexia, gastroesophageal reflux, weight loss

PHARMACOKINETICS

Peak 2.1 hr, elimination by glomerular filtration

INTERACTIONS

• May decrease effect of acetaminophen
• Do not use with erythromycin, metoclopramide
Increase: hypoglycemia—ACE inhibitors, disopyramide, sulfonylureas, androgens, fibric acid derivatives, alcohol
Increase: hyperglycemia—phenothiazines, corticosteroids, anabolic steroids
Decrease: action of digoxin, lovastatin, acetaminophen (elixir)
Decrease: hypoglycemia—niacin, dextrothyroxine, thiazide diuretics, triamterene, estrogens, progestins, oral contraceptives, MAOIs

NURSING CONSIDERATIONS

Assess:
• Fasting blood, glucose, A1c levels, postprandial glucose during treatment to determine diabetes control
• Renal studies: urinalysis, creatinine
• Hypo/hyperglycemic reaction that can occur soon after meals; for severe hypoglycemia, give IV $D_{50}W$ then IV dextrose solution
• Nausea, vomiting, ability to tolerate product
Perform/provide:
• Storage in refrigerator for unopened pen; may store at room temp after opening for up to 30 days
Evaluate:
• Therapeutic response: decrease in polyuria, polydipsia, polyphagia, clear sensorium, improving A1c, weight; absence of dizziness, stable gait
Teach patient/family:
• About the symptoms of hypo/hyperglycemia, what to do about each; to have glucagon emergency kit available; to

carry a glucose source (candy, sugar cube) to treat hypoglycemia
• That product must be continued on a daily basis; about consequences of discontinuing product abruptly
• That diabetes is a lifelong illness; product will not cure disease; to carry emergency ID with prescriber and medication information
• That all food in diet plan must be eaten to prevent hypoglycemia
• To continue weight control, dietary restrictions, exercise, hygiene
• That regular blood glucose monitoring and A1c testing is needed
• To notify prescriber if pregnant or intending to become pregnant
• About the importance of reading "Information for the Patient" and "Pen User Manual"; about self-injection

ezetimibe (Rx)

(ehz-eh-tim′bee)

Ezetrol ✹, Zetia

Func. class.: Antilipemic; cholesterol absorption inhibitor

ACTION: Inhibits absorption of cholesterol by the small intestine, causes reduced hepatic cholesterol stores

USES: Hypercholesterolemia, homozygous familial hypercholesterolemia (HoFH), homozygous sitosterolemia

CONTRAINDICATIONS: Hypersensitivity, severe hepatic disease

Precautions: Pregnancy (C), breastfeeding, children, hepatic disease

DOSAGE AND ROUTES

• **Adult/adolescent/child >10 yr: PO** 10 mg/day; may be given with HMG-CoA reductase inhibitor at same time; may be given with bile acid sequestrant; give ezetimibe 2 hr before or 4 hr after bile acid sequestrant

Available forms: Tabs 10 mg

Administer:
• Without regard to meals

SIDE EFFECTS

CNS: Fatigue, dizziness, headache
GI: Diarrhea, abdominal pain
MISC: Chest pain
MS: *Myalgias, arthralgias,* back pain, myopathy, rhabdomyolysis
RESP: Pharyngitis, sinusitis, cough, *URI*
SYST: Angioedema

PHARMACOKINETICS

Metabolized in small intestine, liver; excreted in feces 78%, urine 11%; peak 4-12 hr; half-life 22 hr

INTERACTIONS

Increase: action of ezetimibe—fibric acid derivatives, cycloSPORINE
Decrease: action of ezetimibe—antacids, cholestyramine
Drug/Lab Test
Increase: LFTs

NURSING CONSIDERATIONS

Assess:
• **Hypercholestrolemia:** diet history: fat content, lipid levels (triglycerides, LDL, HDL, cholesterol); LFTs at baseline, periodically during treatment
• **Myopathy/rhabdomyolysis:** increased CPK, myalgia, muscle cramps, musculoskeletal pain, lethargy, fatigue, fever; more common when combined with statins

Evaluate:
• Therapeutic response: decreased cholesterol, LDL; increased HDL

Teach patient/family:
• That compliance is needed
• That risk factors should be decreased: high-fat diet, smoking, alcohol consumption, absence of exercise
• To notify prescriber if pregnancy suspected, planned or if breastfeeding
• To notify prescriber if unexplained weakness, muscle pain present
• To notify prescriber of dietary/herbal supplements

ezogabine

(e-zog′a-been)

Potiga

Func. class.: Anticonvulsant

ACTION:

The exact mechanism of anticonvulsant effects is not fully known. However, studies indicate that the drug enhances transmembrane potassium currents, which may stabilize the resting membrane potential and reduce brain excitability. May also augment GABA-mediated currents.

USES:

Partial seizures

CONTRAINDICATIONS:

Hypersensitivity

Precautions: Suicidal ideation/behavior, prostatic hypertrophy, dementia, psychotic disorders, QT prolongation, congestive heart failure, ventricular hypertrophy, hypokalemia, hypomagnesemia, abrupt discontinuation, renal impairment, hepatic disease, geriatrics pregnancy category C, breastfeeding, neonates, infants, children, adolescents

DOSAGE AND ROUTES

- **Adult/geriatric patient ≤65 years of age: PO** Initially, 100 mg tid, increase by ≤50 mg tid per day at weekly intervals depending on response, up to a maintenance dose of 200-400 mg tid depending on response; max is 400 mg tid (1200 mg/day).
- **Geriatric patient > 65 years of age: PO** initially, 50 mg tid, increase by ≤ 50 mg tid per day at weekly intervals depending on response; max 250 mg tid (750 mg/day).

Available forms: Film-coated tabs 50, 200, 300, 400 mg

Administer:

- Tab should be swallowed whole without regard to meals
- Give in 3 equally divided doses

SIDE EFFECTS

CNS: Dizziness, drowsiness, memory impairment, tremor, vertigo, abnormal coordination, disturbance in attention, gait disturbance, aphasia, dysarthria, balance disorder, paresthesias, amnesia, dysphagia, myoclonia, hypokinesia, confusion, anxiety, hallucinations, suicidal thoughts/behaviors, fatigue, asthenia, malaise

EENT: Diplopia, blurred vision

GU: Urinary retention, hydronephrosis, dysuria, urinary hesitation, hematuria, chromaturia

GI: Nausea, constipation, dyspepsia, xerostomia, constipation, weight gain, appetite stimulation

MISC: Influenza, dyspnea, QT prolongation

MS: Muscle spasms, weakness

PHARMACOKINETICS

80% protein bound; extensively distributed in the body; extensively metabolized by glucuronidation and acetylation; inactive N-glucuronides are the primary metabolites; elimination half-lives of ezogabine and its N-acetyl metabolite are 7 hr and 11 hr, respectively; 36% excreted renally as exogabine, 18% as NAMR, 24% as the N-glururonides of ezogabine and NAMR, 14% fecal excretion; rapidly absorbed, peak 0.5-2 hr, bioavailability 60%; high-fat food increases peak concentration; increased in hepatic/renal disease, geriatric patients, young adult females

INTERACTIONS:

Increase: QT prolongation—arsenic trioxide, chloroquine, chlorproMAZINE, mesoridazine thioridazine, clarithromycin, Class IA antiarrhythmics (disopyramide, procainamide, quiNIDine), Class III antiarrhythmics (amiodarone, dofetilide, ibutilide, sotalol), dextromethorphan, dronedarone, droperidol, erythromycin, grepafloxacin, halofantrine, levomethadyl, methadone, pentamidine, pimozide, posaconazole, probucol, propafenone, quiNIDine, saquinavir, sparfloxacin, terfenadine, troleandomycin, ziprasidone

Decrease: effect of phenytoin

Decrease: effect of ezogabine—carBAMazepine

Increase: effect of digoxin

Increase: urinary retention—antimuscarinics, amantadine, H1-blockers

Increase: CNS depression—anxiolytics, sedatives, hypnotics, buprenorphine, butorphanol, dronabinol, mirtazapine, nabilone, nalbuphine, opiate agonists, pentazocine, pregabalin, skeletal muscle relaxants, tramadol, trazodone, ethanol

NURSING CONSIDERATIONS

Assess:

⚠ **Seizures:** Assess for type, duration, location, activity, presence of aura

⚠ **QT prolongation:** Monitor in those with known QT prolongation, congestive heart failure, ventricular hypertrophy, hypokalemia, hypomagnesemia, and in patients receiving medications known to cause QT prolongation. QT prolongation can occur within 3 hr of dose

⚠ **Abrupt withdrawal:** Withdraw gradually to minimize increased seizure frequency

⚠ **Suicidal thoughts/behaviors:** Assess for any unusual changes in moods or behaviors, including emotional lability or emerging or worsening depression and suicidal ideation

Teach patient/family:

- To avoid driving or operating machinery or performing other tasks that require mental alertness until reaction is known
- To avoid concurrent use of alcohol
- To avoid abruptly discontinuing this product

⚠ **Suicidal thought/behaviors:** Advise patient to notify prescriber immediately of suicidal thought/behaviors

⚠ ***HIGH ALERT***

factor VIIa, recombinant (Rx)

NovoSeven, NovoSeven RT

Func. class.: Antihemophilic

ACTION: Promotes hemostasis by activating the intrinsic pathway of coagulation

USES: Bleeding with hemophilia A or B, with inhibitors to factor VIII or IX, factor VII deficiency, acquired hemophilia

Unlabeled uses: Coumarin toxicity, von Willebrand's disease

CONTRAINDICATIONS: Hypersensitivity to this product or to mouse, hamster, or bovine products

Precautions: Pregnancy (C), breastfeeding, children, DIC, septicemia, intracranial hemorrhage

Black Box Warning: Thromboembolic disease (off-label use)

DOSAGE AND ROUTES

Bleeding prophylaxis or hemophilia with inhibitors to factor VIII/IX

- **Adult: IV BOL** 90 mcg/kg q2hr until hemostasis occurs or until therapy is deemed inadequate; posthemostatic doses q3-6hr may be required

Bleeding prophylaxis factor VII deficiency

- **Adult: IV BOL** 15-30 mcg/kg over 2-5 min q4-6hr

Acquired hemophilia

- **Adult/adolescent/child: IV BOL** 70-90 mcg/kg q2-3hr

Available forms: Lyophilized powder 1.2 mg/vial (1200 mcg/vial), 2.4 mg/vial (2400 mcg/vial), 4.8 mg/vial (4800 mcg/vial) recombinant human coagulation factor VIIa (rFVIIa); *NovoSevenRT:* 1 mg, 2, 5, 8 mg powder for inj

Administer:

IV route (NovoSeven)

• Bring to room temp; for 1.2 mg vial/2.2 ml sterile water for inj; for 4.8 mg vial/8.5 ml sterile water for inj

• Remove caps from stopper, cleanse stopper with alcohol, allow to dry; draw back plunger of sterile syringe and allow air into syringe, insert needle of syringe into sterile water for inj, inject air and withdraw amount required, insert syringe needle with diluent into product vial, aim to side so liquid runs down vial wall, gently swirl until dissolved, use within 3 hr, give by bol over 3-5 min

• Do not admix, keep refrigerated until ready to use, avoid sunlight

IV route (NovoSeven RT)

• May be stored in refrigerator or at room temp prior to reconstitution

• Reconstitute with hisitidine diluent 1.1 ml for 1-mg vial, 2.1 ml for 2-mg vial, 5.2 ml for 5-mg vial, 8.1 ml for 8-mg vial; allow diluent to run down side of vial; gently swirl until powder dissolved (1 mg/ml)

SIDE EFFECTS

CNS: Fever, headache, cerebral artery occlusion

CV: Ischemic heart disease, myocardial infarction, hypertension

INTEG: Pain, redness at inj site, pruritus, purpura, rash

SYST: Hemorrhage NOS, hemarthrosis, fibrinogen plasma decreased, hypertension, bradycardia, DIC, coagulation disorder, thrombosis, acute renal failure

PHARMACOKINETICS

Half-life 2.3 hr

INTERACTIONS

• Do not use with activated prothrombin complex concentrates or prothrombin complex concentrate

NURSING CONSIDERATIONS

Assess:

• VS, B/P, pulse, respirations, neurologic signs, temp at least q4hr; temp 104° F (40° C) or indicators of internal bleeding, cardiac rhythm

• PT, aPTT, plasma FVII clotting, clotting inhibitor titers

• For thrombosis, dose should be reduced or stopped

Evaluate:

• Therapeutic response: hemostasis

Teach patient/family:

• About the reason for use, expected results

⚠ HIGH ALERT

factor IX complex (human) (Rx)

Alpha-Nine SD, Bebulin VH, BeneFIX, Mononine, Profilnine SD

Func. class.: Hemostatic

Chem. class.: Factors II, VII, IX, X

ACTION: Causes an increase in blood levels of clotting factors II, VII, IX, X; factor IX (human) has IX activity

USES: Hemophilia B (Christmas disease), factor IX deficiency, anticoagulant reversal, control of bleeding in patients with factor VIII inhibitors, reversal of overdose of anticoagulants in emergencies

CONTRAINDICATIONS: Hypersensitivity to mouse or hamster protein, DIC, mild factor IX deficiency

Precautions: Pregnancy (C), neonates/infants, hepatic disease, elective surgery

DOSAGE AND ROUTES

Factor IX complex (human) bleeding in hemophilia B

• **Adult and child: IV** establish 25% of normal factor IX or 60-75 units/kg then 10-20 units/kg/day 1-2×/wk

Prophylaxis for bleeding in hemophilia B

• **Adult and child:** IV 10-20 units/kg 1-2×/wk

Bleeding in hemophilia A/inhibitors of factor VIII (Proplex T, Konyne 80)

• **Adult and child:** IV 75 units/kg, repeat after 12 hr

Oral anticoagulant reversal

• **Adult and child:** IV 15 units/kg

Factor VII deficiency (use Proplex T only)

• **Adult and child:** IV 0.5 units/kg × weight (kg) × desired factor IX increase (% of normal); repeat q4-6hr if needed

Factor IX (human) minor to moderate hemorrhage

Use only Alpha-Nine, Alpha-Nine SD

• **Adult and child:** IV dose to increase factor IX level to 20%-30% in one dose

Serious hemorrhage

• **Adult and child:** IV dose to increase factor IX to 30%-50% as daily inf

Minor hemorrhage (mononine only)

• **Adult and child:** IV dose to increase factor IX to 15%-25% (20-30 units/kg), repeat after 24 hr if needed

Major hemorrhage

• **Adult and child:** IV dose to increase factor IX to 25%-50% (75 units/kg) q18-30hr × ≤10 days

Available forms: Inj (number of units noted on label)

Administer:

• Hepatitis B vaccine before administration

• IV after warming to room temp ≤3 ml/min, with plastic syringe only; do not admix

• After dilution with provided diluent, 50 units/ml or 25 units/ml; do not exceed 10 ml/min; decrease rate if fever, headache, flushing, tingling occur

• After cross-matching if patient has blood type A, B, AB to determine incompatibility with factor

BeneFIX

• Allow vials of concentrate/diluent to warm to room temp

• After removing flip-top cap from vial, wipe top of vial with alcohol swab; allow to dry

• Peel back cover from vial adapter package; do not remove

• Place vial adapter over vial; press firmly until it snaps; attach plunger rod to diluent syringe and break plastic tip cap from diluent syringe

• Lift package away from adapter and connect diluent syringe; depress plunger; swirl contents

F

SIDE EFFECTS

CNS: Headache, dizziness, malaise, paresthesia, *lethargy, chills, fever, flushing*

CV: *Hypotension,* tachycardia, *MI,* **venous thrombosis, pulmonary embolism**

GI: Nausea, vomiting, abdominal cramps, **jaundice, viral hepatitis**

HEMA: Thrombosis, hemolysis, AIDS, DIC

INTEG: Rash, flushing, *urticaria,* inj site reactions

RESP: Bronchospasm

PHARMACOKINETICS

IV: Half-life factor IX: 22 hr; rapidly cleared from plasma

INTERACTIONS

• Incompatible with protein products

⚠ **Increase: thrombosis risk—aminocaproic acid; do not administer**

Decrease: effect of warfarin

NURSING CONSIDERATIONS

Assess:

• Blood studies: coagulation factor assays by % normal: 5% prevents spontaneous hemorrhage, 30%-50% for surgery, 80%-100% for severe hemorrhage; APTT, clotting inhibitor titers, D-dimer, factor IX, VII concentration, fibrin degradation products, fibrinogen, platelets, PT, thrombin time

• Increased B/P, pulse

• For bleeding q15-30min; immobilize and apply ice to affected joints

• I&O; if urine becomes orange or red, notify prescriber

• **Allergic or pyrogenic reaction:** fever, chills, rash, itching, slow inf rate if not severe

DIC: bleeding, ecchymosis, hypersensitivity, changes in coagulation tests

• For tingling sensation; if present, reduce rate

Perform/provide:

• Storage of reconstituted sol for 3 hr at room temp or for ≤2 yr with refrigeration (powder); check expiration date

Evaluate:

• Therapeutic response: prevention of hemorrhage

Teach patient/family:

• To report any signs of bleeding: gums, under skin, urine, stools, emesis; calf pain, joint pain, yellowing of eyes/skin

• About the risk for viral hepatitis, AIDS; to be tested q2-3mo for HIV, although low risk

• That immunization for hepatitis B may be given first

• To carry emergency ID identifying disease; to avoid salicylates, NSAIDs; to inform other health professionals of condition

famciclovir (Rx)

(fam-cy′clo-veer)

Famvir, Sandoz Famciclovir ✦

Func. class.: Antiviral

Chem. class.: Guanosine nucleoside

ACTION: Inhibits DNA polymerase and viral DNA synthesis by conversion of this guanosine nucleoside to penciclovir

USES: Treatment of acute herpes zoster (shingles), genital herpes; recurrent mucocutaneous herpes simplex virus (HSV) in patients with HIV; initial episodes of herpes genitalis; herpes labialis in the immunocompromised

Unlabeled uses: Bell's palsy, herpes labialis prophylaxis, postherpetic neuralgia prophylaxis

CONTRAINDICATIONS: Hypersensitivity to this product, penciclovir, acyclovir, ganciclovir, valacyclovir, valganciclovir

Precautions: Pregnancy (B), breastfeeding, renal disease

DOSAGE AND ROUTES

Herpes zoster

• **Adult: PO** 500 mg q8hr for 7 days

Renal dose

• **Adult: PO** CCr ≥60 ml/min, 500 mg q8hr; CCr 40-59 ml/min, 500 mg q12hr; CCr 20-39 ml/min, 500 mg q24hr; CCr <20 ml/min, 250 mg q24hr

Recurrent herpes simplex virus

• **Adult: PO** 125 mg q12hr × 5 days

Renal dose

• **Adult: PO** CCr <39 ml/min, 125 mg q24hr × 5 days

Suppression of recurrent herpes simplex virus

• **Adult: PO** 250 mg q12hr up to 1 yr

Renal dose

• **Adult: PO** CCr 20-39 ml/min, 125 mg q12hr × 5 days; CCr <20 ml/min, 125 mg q24hr × 5 days

Genital herpes/herpes labialis (recurrent)

• **Adult: PO** 125 mg bid × 5 days or 1000 mg bid for 1 day; begin treatment at 1st sign of recurrence

Suppression of recurrent genital herpes

• **Adult: PO** 250 mg bid for up to 1 yr

Herpes genitalis initial episodes

• **Adult: PO** 250 mg tid × 7-10 days

Bell's palsy (unlabeled)

• **Adult: PO** 750 mg tid × 7 days with predniSONE

Varicella-zoster virus (shingles); chickenpox (unlabeled)

• **Adult: PO** 500 mg q8hr × 7 days, preferably within 48 hr of onset

Herpes zoster in HIV (unlabeled)

• **Adult/adolescent: PO** 500 mg tid × 7-10 days

Available forms: Tabs 125, 250, 500 mg

Administer:

- Without regard to meals
- As soon as diagnosed; for herpes zoster within 72 hr

SIDE EFFECTS

CNS: *Headache, fatigue, dizziness,* paresthesia, somnolence, fever
GI: Nausea, vomiting, diarrhea, constipation, abdominal pain, anorexia
GU: Decreased sperm count
INTEG: *Pruritus*
MS: Back pain, arthralgia
RESP: Pharyngitis, sinusitis

PHARMACOKINETICS

Bioavailability 77%, 20% protein binding, 73% excreted via kidneys, terminal plasma half-life 2-3 hr

INTERACTIONS

Decrease: renal excretion—theophylline, probenecid, digoxin
Decrease: metabolism—cimetidine

NURSING CONSIDERATIONS

Assess:

- **Herpes zoster:** number, distribution of lesions; burning, itching, pain, which are early symptoms of herpes infection; assess daily during therapy
- Renal studies: urine CCr; BUN before and during treatment if decreased renal function; dose may have to be lowered
- Bowel pattern before, during treatment; diarrhea may occur
- Posttherapeutic neuralgia during and after treatment

Evaluate:

- Therapeutic response: decreased size, spread of lesions

Teach patient/family:

- How to recognize beginning infection
- How to prevent spread of infection; that this medication does not prevent spread to others; that condoms should be used
- About the reason for medication, expected results
- That women with genital herpes should have yearly Pap smears; that cervical cancer is more likely

famotidine (OTC, Rx)

(fa-moe′ti-deen)

Apo-Famotidine ✤, Equaline Heartburn Prevention, Gen-Famotidine ✤, Good Sense Acid Reducer, Heartburn Relief, Leader Acid Reducer, Nu-Famotidine ✤, Pepcid, Pepcid AC, Top Care Acid Reducer, Top Care Acid Reducer Maximum Strength, Walgreens Acid Controller

Func. class.: H_2-histamine receptor antagonist

ACTION: Competitively inhibits histamine at histamine H_2-receptor site, thus decreasing gastric secretion while pepsin remains at a stable level

USES: Short-term treatment of active duodenal ulcer, maintenance therapy for duodenal ulcer, Zollinger-Ellison syndrome, multiple endocrine adenomas, gastric ulcers; gastroesophageal reflux disease, heartburn
Unlabeled uses: GI disorders in those taking NSAIDs; urticaria; prevention of stress ulcers, aspiration pneumonitis, inactivation of oral pancreatic enzymes in pancreatic disorders

CONTRAINDICATIONS: Hypersensitivity
Precautions: Pregnancy (B), breastfeeding, children <12 yr, geriatric patients, severe renal/hepatic disease

DOSAGE AND ROUTES

Active ulcer

- **Adult: PO** 40 mg/day at bedtime × 4-8 wk then 20 mg/day at bedtime if needed (maintenance); **IV** 20 mg q12hr if unable to take **PO**

• **Child 1-16 yr: PO** 0.5 mg/kg/day at bedtime or divided bid, max 40 mg/day

Hypersecretory conditions

• **Adult: PO** 20 mg q6hr; may give 160 mg q6hr if needed; **IV** 20 mg q12hr if unable to take **PO**

Heartburn relief/prevention

• **Adult: PO** 10 mg with water or 15 min-1 hr before eating

Renal disease

• **Adult: PO** CCr <50 ml/min, decrease dose by 50% or extend interval to 36-48 hr

Available forms: Tabs 10, 20, 40 mg; gel cap 10 mg; powder for oral susp 40 mg/5 ml; inj 10 mg/ml, 20 mg/50 ml; chew tabs 10 mg

Administer:

• Antacids 1 hr before or 2 hr after famotidine; may be given with foods or liquids

• After shaking oral suspension

Direct IV route

• After diluting 2 ml of product (10 mg/ml) in 0.9% NaCl to total volume of 5-10 ml; inject over 2 min to prevent hypotension

Intermittent IV INF route

• After diluting 20 mg (2 ml) of product in 100 ml of LR, 0.9% NaCl, D_5W, $D_{10}W$; run over 15-30 min

Continuous IV INF route

• *Adults:* Dilute 40 mg of product in 250 ml D_5W, NS; infuse over 24 hr, run at 11 ml/hr, use inf device

Y-site compatibilities: Acyclovir, alfentanil, allopurinol, amifostine, amikacin, aminocaproic acid, aminophylline, amiodarone, amphotericin B lipid complex, amphotericin B liposome, amsacrine, anakinra, anidulafungin, ascorbic acid injection, atenolol, atracurium, atropine, aztreonam, benztropine, bivalirudin, bleomycin, bumetanide, buprenorphine, butorphanol, calcium chloride/gluconate, CARBOplatin, caspofungin, cefonicid, cefotaxime, ceftazidime, cefuroxime, chlorproMAZINE, cimetidine, cisatracurium, CISplatin, cladribine, clindamycin, codeine, cyanocobalamin, cyclophosphamide, cycloSPORINE, cytarabine, DACTINomycin, DAPTOmycin, dexamethasone, dexmedetomidine, digoxin, diltiazem, diphenhydrAMINE, DOBUTamine, docetaxel, DOPamine, doripenem, doxacurium, DOXOrubicin, DOXOrubicin liposomal, doxycycline, droperidol, enalaprilat, ePHEDrine, EPINEPHrine, epirubicin, epoetin alfa, eptifibatide, ertapenem, erythromycin, esmolol, etoposide, fenoldopam, fentaNYL, filgrastim, fluconazole, fludarabine, fluorouracil, folic acid, gatifloxacin, gemcitabine, gentamicin, glycopyrrolate, granisetron, heparin, hydrocortisone, HYDROmorphone, hydrOXYzine, IDArubicin, ifosfamide, imipenem-cilastatin, irinotecan, isoproterenol, ketorolac, labetalol, levofloxacin, lidocaine, linezolid, LORazepam, LR, magnesium sulfate, mannitol, mechlorethamine, melphalan, meperidine, metaraminol, methicillin, methotrexate, methoxamine, methyldopate, methylPREDNISolone, metoclopramide, metoprolol, metroNIDAZOLE, miconazole, midazolam, milrinone, mitoxantrone, morphine, moxalactam, multiple vitamins injection, mycophenolate, nafcillin, nalbuphine, naloxone, nesiritide, netil-micin, niCARdipine, nitroglycerin, nitroprusside, norepinephrine, 0.9% NaCl, octreotide, ondansetron, oxacillin, oxaliplatin, oxytocin, paclitaxel, palonosetron, pamidronate, pancuronium, papaverine, pemetrexed, penicillin G potassium/sodium, pentamidine, pentazocine, PENTobarbital, perphenazine, PHENObarbital, phenylephrine, phytonadione, polymyxin B, potassium chloride/phosphates, procainamide, prochlorperazine, promethazine, propofol, propranolol, protamine, pyridoxine, quiNIDine, ranitidine, remifentanil, Ringer's, ritodrine, riTUXimab, sargramostim, sodium acetate/bicarbonate, succinylcholine, SUFentanil, tacrolimus, teniposide, theophylline, thiamine, thiotepa, ticarcillin, ticarcillin-clavulanate, tigecycline, tirofiban, TNA, tobramycin, tolazoline, TPN, trastuzumab, trimetaphan, urokinase, vancomycin, vasopressin, vecuronium, verapamil, vinCRIStine, vinorelbine, voriconazole, zoledronic acid

SIDE EFFECTS

CNS: *Headache, dizziness,* paresthesia, depression, anxiety, somnolence, insomnia, fever, **seizures in renal disease**

CV: **Dysrhythmias, QT prolongation (impaired renal functioning)**

EENT: Taste change, tinnitus, orbital edema

GI: *Constipation,* nausea, vomiting, anorexia, cramps, abnormal hepatic enzymes, diarrhea

HEMA: **Thrombocytopenia, aplastic anemia**

INTEG: Rash, **toxic epidermal necrolysis, Stevens-Johnson syndrome**

MS: Myalgia, arthralgia

RESP: **Pneumonia**

PHARMACOKINETICS

Plasma protein binding 15%-20%, metabolized in liver 30% (active metabolites), 70% excreted by kidneys, half-life $2^1/_2$-$3^1/_2$ hr

PO: Onset 30-60 min, duration 6-12 hr, peak 1-3 hr, absorption 50%

IV: Onset immediate, peak 30-60 min, duration 8-15 hr

INTERACTIONS

Decrease: absorption—ketoconazole, itraconazole, cefpodoxime, cefditoren

Decrease: famotidine absorption—antacids

Decrease: effect of—atazanavir, delavirdine

NURSING CONSIDERATIONS

Assess:

- **Ulcers:** epigastric pain, adominal pain, frank or occult blood in emesis, stools
- Intragastric pH, serum creatinine/BUN baseline and periodically
- Blood counts during therapy; watch for decreasing platelets; if low, therapy may have to be discontinued, restarted after hematologic recovery
- For bleeding, hematuria, hematuresis, occult blood in stools; abdominal pain
- **Blood dyscrasias (thrombocytopenia):** bruising, fatigue, bleeding, poor healing

Perform/provide:

- Storage in cool environment (oral); IV sol stable for 48 hr at room temp; do not use discolored sol; discard unused oral sol after 1 mo
- Increase in bulk and fluids in diet to prevent constipation

Evaluate:

- Therapeutic response: decreased abdominal pain

Teach patient/family:

- That product must be continued for prescribed time in prescribed method to be effective; not to double dose
- To report bleeding, bruising, fatigue, malaise, since blood dyscrasias occur
- About possibility of decreased libido; that this is reversible after discontinuing therapy
- To avoid irritating foods, alcohol, aspirin, extreme-temp foods that may irritate GI system
- That smoking should be avoided because it diminishes effectiveness of product
- To avoid tasks requiring alertness because dizziness, drowsiness may occur

fat emulsions (Rx)

Intralipid 10%, Intralipid 20%, Liposyn II 10%, Liposyn II 20%, Liposyn III 10%, Liposyn III 20%, Soyacal 20%

Func. class.: Caloric

Chem. class.: Fatty acid, long chain; nutritional supplement

ACTION: Needed for energy, heat production; consist of neutral triglycerides, primarily unsaturated fatty acids

USES: Increase calorie intake, fatty acid deficiency, prevention

CONTRAINDICATIONS: Hypersensitivity to this product or eggs, soybeans, legumes; hyperlipemia, lipid necrosis, acute pancreatitis accompanied by hyperlipemia, hyperbilirubinemia of the newborn; renal insufficiency, hepatic damage

Precautions: Pregnancy (C), premature/term newborns, severe hepatic disease, diabetes mellitus, thrombocytopenia, gastric ulcers, sepsis

Black Box Warning: Preterm infants

DOSAGE AND ROUTES

Deficiency

- **Adult and child:** IV 8%-10% of required calorie intake (intralipid)

Adjunct to TPN

- **Adult:** IV 1 ml/min over 15-30 min (10%) or 0.5 ml/min over 15-30 min (20%); may increase to 500 ml over 4-8 hr if no adverse reactions occur; max 2.5 g/kg
- **Child:** IV 0.1 ml/min over 10-15 min (10%) or 0.05 ml/min over 10-15 min (20%); may increase to 1 g/kg over 4 hr if no adverse reactions occur; max 4 g/kg

Prevention of deficiency

- **Adult:** IV 500 ml 2×/wk (10%), given 1 ml/min for 30 min, max 500 ml over 6 hr
- **Child:** IV 5-10 ml/kg/day (10%), given 0.1 ml/min for 30 min, max 100 ml/hr

Available forms: Inj 10% (50, 100, 200, 250, 500 ml), 20% (50, 100, 200, 250, 500 ml)

Administer:

Intermittent IV INF route

- At 10% (1 ml/min) or 20% (0.5 ml/min) initially × 15-30 min, may increase 10% (120 ml/hr) or 20% (62.5 ml/hr) if no adverse reaction; do not give more than 500 ml on 1st day
- After changing IV tubing at each inf; infection may occur with old tubing
- With inf pump at prescribed rate; do not use in-line filter sized for lipid emulsion; clogging will occur

SIDE EFFECTS

CNS: Dizziness, headache, drowsiness, focal seizures

CV: Shock

GI: Nausea, vomiting, hepatomegaly

HEMA: Hyperlipemia, hypercoagulation, thrombocytopenia, leukopenia, leukocytosis

RESP: Dyspnea, fat in lung tissue

PHARMACOKINETICS

Completely absorbed, distributed to intravascular space, converted to triglycerides then to free fatty acids

NURSING CONSIDERATIONS

Assess:

- Triglycerides, free fatty acid levels, platelet counts daily to prevent fat overload, thrombocytopenia
- Hepatic studies: AST, ALT, Hct, Hgb; notify prescriber if abnormal
- Nutritional status: calorie count by dietitian; monitor weight daily

Perform/provide:

- Do not use mixed sol if separated or oily looking

Evaluate:

- Therapeutic response: increased weight

Teach patient/family:

- About the reason for use of lipids

febuxostat (Rx)

(feb-ux′oh-stat)

Uloric

Func. class.: Antigout drug, antihyperuricemic

Chem. class.: Xanthene oxidase inhibitor

ACTION: Inhibits the enzyme xanthine oxidase, thereby reducing uric acid synthesis; more selective for xanthine oxidase than allopurinol

USES: Chronic gout, hyperuricemia

CONTRAINDICATIONS:
Hypersensitivity

Precautions: Pregnancy (C), breastfeeding, children, renal/hepatic/cardiac/neoplastic disease, stroke, MI, organ transplant, Lesch-Nyhan syndrome

DOSAGE AND ROUTES

- **Adult: PO** 40 mg daily, may increase to 80 mg daily if uric acid levels are >6 mg/dl after 2 wk of therapy

Available forms: Tabs 40, 80 mg

Administer:

PO route

- Without regard to meals or antacids; may crush and add to foods or fluids
- A few days before antineoplastic therapy

SIDE EFFECTS

CNS: Weakness, flushing

CV: **MI, atrial fibrillation, atrial flutter, AV block,** bradycardia, hypo/hypertension, palpitations, **sinus tachycardia, stroke,** angina

EENT: Retinopathy, cataracts, epistaxis

GI: *Nausea, vomiting, anorexia,* constipation, diarrhea, dyspepsia, hematemesis, hepatitis, hepatomegaly, weight gain/loss, cholecystitis, cholelithiasis, melena

GU: Renal failure, urinary urgency/frequency/incontinence, nephrolithiasis, hematuria

HEMA: **Thrombocytopenia, anemia, pancytopenia, leukopenia, bone marrow suppression**

INTEG: Rash

MISC: Arthralgia, gout flare

PHARMACOKINETICS

Peak 1-1.5 hr; excreted in feces, urine; half-life 5-8 hr; protein binding 99.2%

INTERACTIONS

Increase: toxicity—azathioprine

Increase: xanthine nephropathy, calculi—rasburicase, antineoplastics

Increase: myelosuppression—mercaptopurine, theophylline

NURSING CONSIDERATIONS

Assess:

- **Hyperuricemia:** uric acid levels q2wk; uric acid levels should be ≤6 mg/dl
- CBC, AST, BUN, creatinine before starting treatment, periodically
- **Renal disease:** I&O ratio; increase fluids to 2 L/day to prevent stone formation and toxicity
- For rash, hypersensitivity reactions; discontinue
- **Gout:** joint pain, swelling; may use with NSAIDs for acute gouty attacks and gout flare

Evaluate:

- Therapeutic response: decreased pain in joints, decreased stone formation in kidneys, decreased uric acid levels

Teach patient/family:

- That tabs may be crushed
- To take as prescribed; if dose is missed, to take as soon as remembered; not to double dose
- To increase fluid intake to 2 L/day unless contraindicated
- To avoid alcohol, caffeine because they will increase uric acid levels
- To report cardiovascular events to prescriber immediately

RARELY USED

felbamate (Rx)

(fell′ba-mate)

Felbatol

Func. class.: Anticonvulsant

USES:
Partial seizures with or without generalization in adults; partial and generalized seizures in children with Lennox-Gastaut syndrome

CONTRAINDICATIONS:
Hypersensitivity to this product, other carbamates

Black Box Warning: Aplastic anemia, hepatic disease, anemia, agranulocytosis, bone marrow suppression, hematologic disease, hepatitis, leukopenia, neutropenia, thrombocytopenia

DOSAGE AND ROUTES

Adjunctive therapy

- **Adult and child >14 yr: PO** add 1.2 g/day in 3-4 divided doses; reduce other anticonvulsants (valproic acid, phenytoin, carBAMazepine and derivatives) by 20%-33% to control plasma concentrations; may increase felbamate by 1.2-g/day increments weekly up to 3.6 g/day

Monotherapy

- **Adult: PO** 1.2 g/day in 3-4 divided doses; titrate with close supervision; increase dose by 600-mg increments q2wk to 3.6 g/day if needed

Lennox-Gastaut syndrome adjunctive therapy

- **Child 2-14 yr: PO** add 15 mg/kg/day in 3-4 divided doses; reduce other anticonvulsants (valproic acid, phenytoin, carBAMazepine, and derivatives) by 20%-33% to control plasma concentrations; may increase felbamate 15 mg/kg/day per wk up to 45 mg/kg/day, max 3600 mg/day

felodipine (Rx)

(fe-loe′-di-peen)

Plendil ✱, Renedil ✱, Sandoz Felodipine ✱

Func. class.: Antihypertensive, calcium channel blocker, antianginal

Chem. class.: Dihydropyridine

Do not confuse:
Plendil/pindolol/Pletal/Prilosec/Prinivil

ACTION:
Inhibits calcium ion influx across cell membrane, resulting in the inhibition of the excitation and contraction of vascular smooth muscle

USES:
Essential hypertension alone or with other antihypertensives

Unlabeled uses: Hypertension in adolescents and children, angina pectoris; Prinzmetal's angina (vasospastic)

CONTRAINDICATIONS:
Hypersensitivity to this product or dihydropyridines, sick sinus syndrome, 2nd- or 3rd-degree heart block, hypotension <90 mm Hg systolic

Precautions: Pregnancy (C), breastfeeding, children, geriatric patients, CHF, hepatic injury, renal disease

DOSAGE AND ROUTES

- **Adult: PO** 5 mg/day initially; usual range 2.5-10 mg/day; max 10 mg/day; do not adjust dosage at intervals of <2 wk
- **Geriatric: PO** 2.5 mg/day

Hepatic disease

- **Adult: PO** 2.5-5 mg, max 10 mg/day

Hypertension in adolescent/child (unlabeled)

- **Adolescent and child: PO** 2.5 mg initially, titrate upward, max 10 mg/day

Available forms: Ext rel tabs 2.5, 5, 10 mg

Administer:

- Swallow whole; do not break, crush, or chew ext rel products
- Once daily with light meal; avoid grapefruit juice

SIDE EFFECTS

CNS: *Headache,* fatigue, drowsiness, dizziness, anxiety, depression, nervousness, insomnia, light-headedness, paresthesia, tinnitus, psychosis, somnolence, flushing

CV: Dysrhythmia, *edema,* CHF, hypotension, palpitations, MI, pulmonary edema, tachycardia, syncope, AV block, angina

GI: Nausea, vomiting, diarrhea, gastric upset, constipation, increased LFTs, dry mouth

GU: Nocturia, polyuria

HEMA: Anemia

INTEG: Rash, pruritus

MISC: Flushing, sexual difficulties, cough, nasal congestion, SOB, wheezing, epistaxis, respiratory infection, chest pain, **angioedema**, gingival hyperplasia

PHARMACOKINETICS

Peak plasma levels 2.5-5 hr, highly protein bound >99%, metabolized in liver, 0.5% excreted unchanged in urine, elimination half-life 11-16 hr

INTERACTIONS

Increase: bradycardia, CHF—β-blockers, digoxin, phenytoin, disopyramide

Increase: toxicity, hypotension—nitrates, alcohol, quiNIDine, zileuton, miconazole, diltiazem, delavirdine, quinupristin, dalfopristin, conivaptan, cycloSPORINE, cimetidine, clarithromycin, antiretroviral protease inhibitors, other antihypertensives, MAOIs, ketoconazole, erythromycin, itraconazole, propranolol

Decrease: antihypertensive effects—NSAIDs, carBAMazepine, barbiturates, phenytoin

Drug/Herb

Increase: antihypertensive effect—ginseng, ginkgo, hawthorn

Decrease: antihypertensive effect—ephedra, St. John's wort

Drug/Food

Increase: felodipine level—grapefruit juice

NURSING CONSIDERATIONS

Assess:

- **CHF:** I&O, weight daily; weight gain, crackles, dyspnea, edema, jugular venous distention
- Renal, hepatic studies
- Cardiac status: B/P, pulse, respiration; ECG periodically
- **Angina pain:** location, duration, intensity; ameliorating, aggravating factors

Evaluate:

- Therapeutic response: decreased B/P, decreased anginal attacks, increased activity tolerance

Teach patient/family:

- To avoid hazardous activities until stabilized on product, dizziness no longer a problem
- To avoid OTC products, alcohol unless directed by prescriber; to limit caffeine consumption
- About the importance of complying with all areas of medical regimen: diet, exercise, stress reduction, product therapy
- That tablets may appear in stools but are insignificant
- To report dyspnea, palpitations, irregular heart beat, swelling of extremities, nausea, vomiting, severe dizziness, severe headache
- To change positions slowly to prevent orthostatic hypotension
- To obtain correct pulse; to contact prescriber if pulse <50 bpm
- To use protective clothing, sunscreen to prevent photosensitivity

TREATMENT OF OVERDOSE:

Atropine for AV block, vasopressor for hypotension

fenofibrate (Rx)

(fen-oh-fee′brate)

Antara, Apo-Fenofibrate ♣, Apo-Feno-Micro ♣, Fenoglide, Gen-Fenofibrate ♣, Lipidil Micro ♣, Lipidil Supra Cap, Lipofen, Lofibra, PMS-Fenofibrate ♣, ratio-Fenofibrate ♣, Tricor, Triglide

Func. class.: Antilipemic

Chem. class.: Fibric acid derivative

ACTION: Increases lipolysis and elimination of triglyceride-rich particles from plasma by activating lipoprotein lipase, thereby resulting in changes in triglyceride size and composition of LDL, leading to rapid breakdown of LDL; mobilizes triglycerides from tissue; increases excretion of neutral sterols

USES: Hypercholesterolemia; types IV, V hyperlipidemia that do not respond to other treatment and that increase risk for pancreatitis; Fredrickson type IIa, IIb hypertriglyceridemia

CONTRAINDICATIONS:

Hypersensivity, severe renal/hepatic disease, primary biliary cirrhosis, preexisting gallbladder disease

Precautions: Pregnancy (C), breastfeeding, geriatric patients, peptic ulcer, pancreatitis, renal/hepatic disease

DOSAGE AND ROUTES

Hypertriglyceridemia

- **Adult: PO** (Antara) 43-130 mg/day; (Lofibra) 67-200 mg/day; (Tricor) 48-145 mg/day; (Triglide) 50-160 mg/day

Primary hypercholesterolemia/ mixed hyperlipidemia

- **Adult: PO** (Antara) 130 mg/day; (Lofibra) 200 mg/day; (Tricor) 145 mg/day; (Triglide) 160 mg/day

Renal dose (geriatric)

- **Adult: PO** (Tricor) CCr 30-80 ml/min, 48 mg/day; CCr <30 ml/min, contraindicated
- **Adult: PO** CCr 11-49 ml/min, 50 mg/day (Triglide, Liprofen), 43 mg/day (Antara), 67 mg/day (Lofibra); CCr <10 ml/min, contraindicated (Antara, Lipofen, Lofibra, Triglide)

Available forms: Tabs (Triglide) 50, 160 mg; (Tricor) 48, 145 mg; micronized cap (Antara) 43, 130 mg; (Lofibra) 67, 134, 200 mg; cap (Lipofen) 50, 100, 150 mg; tabs (Fenoglide) 40, 120 mg

Administer:

- Product with meals (Lipofen, Lofibra); Triglide without regard to food; may increase q4-8wk; brands are not interchangeable; therapy should be discontinued if there is not adequate response after 2 mo

SIDE EFFECTS

CNS: *Fatigue, weakness,* drowsiness, dizziness, insomnia, depression, vertigo
CV: Angina, dysrhythmias, hypertension
GI: *Nausea,* vomiting, dyspepsia, increased liver enzymes, flatulence, hepatomegaly, gastritis
GU: Dysuria, urinary frequency
HEMA: Anemia, leukopenia, thrombosis/pulmonary embolism
INTEG: *Rash,* urticaria, pruritus, photosensitivity
MISC: Polyphagia, weight gain, infection, flulike syndrome
MS: *Myalgias, arthralgias,* myopathy, rhabdomyolysis
RESP: Pharyngitis, bronchitis, cough

PHARMACOKINETICS

Peak 6-8 hr, protein binding 99%, converted to fenofibric acid, metabolized in liver, excreted in urine (60%), half-life 20 hr

INTERACTIONS

Increase: nephrotoxicity—cycloSPORINE

- Avoid use with HMG-CoA reductase inhibitors; rhabdomyolysis may occur

Increase: anticoagulant effects—oral anticoagulants
Increase: effects of—antidiabetics
Decrease: absorption of fenofibrate—bile acid sequestrants

Drug/Herb

Increase: effect—red yeast rice

Drug/Food

Increase: absorption

Drug/Lab Test

Increase: ALT, AST, BUN, CK, creatinine
Decrease: WBC, uric acid, Hgb

NURSING CONSIDERATIONS

Assess:

- **Diet history:** fat content; lipid levels (triglycerides, LDL, HDL, cholesterol), LFTs at baseline, periodically during treatment, CPK if muscle pain occurs, CBC, Hct, Hgb; PT with anticoagulant therapy
- **Pancreatitis, cholelithiasis renal failure, rhabdomyolysis** (when combined with HMG Co-A reductase inhibitors), myositis; product should be discontinued

Evaluate:
- Therapeutic response: decreased triglycerides, cholesterol levels

Teach patient/family:
- That compliance is needed
- That risk factors should be decreased: high-fat diet, smoking, alcohol consumption, absence of exercise
- To notify prescriber if pregnancy is suspected or planned
- To report GU symptoms: decreased libido, impotence, dysuria, proteinuria, oliguria, hematuria
- To notify prescriber of muscle pain, weakness, fever, fatigue, epigastric pain

fenofibric acid (Rx)

(fen′oh-fye′brick)

TriLipix, Fibricor

Func. class.: Antilipemic

Chem. class.: Fibric acid derivative

ACTION: An active metabolite of fenofibrate; increases lipolysis and elimination of triglyceride-rich particles from plasma by activating lipoprotein lipase, thereby resulting in changes in triglyceride size and composition of LDL, leading to rapid breakdown of LDL; mobilizes triglycerides from tissue; increases excretion of neutral sterols

USES: Hyperlipoproteinemia, hypertriglyceridemia

CONTRAINDICATIONS: Breastfeeding, hypertensivity, severe renal/hepatic disease, primary biliary cirrhosis, preexisting gallbladder disease

Precautions: Pregnancy (C), geriatric patients, pancreatitis, thromboembolic disease

DOSAGE AND ROUTES

Combination with HMG-CoA reductase inhibitors to reduce triglycerides and increase HDL-C in those with mixed dyslipidemia or coronary heart disease
- **Adult:** del rel cap **PO** 135 mg daily

Severe hypertriglyceridemia
- **Adult:** del rel cap **PO** 45-135 daily; tabs 35-105 mg daily

Renal dose
- **Adult: PO** CCr 30-80 ml/min, 35 mg (Fibricor), 45 mg (TriLipix) daily initially; CCr <30 ml/min, do not use

Available forms: Tabs, 35, 105 mg (Fibricor); caps, gastro-resistant pellet 45, 135 mg (TriLipix)

Administer:
- Without regard to meals
- Do not crush, break, chew caps

SIDE EFFECTS

CNS: Fatigue, weakness, drowsiness, dizziness, insomnia, depression, vertigo, asthenia, headache

CV: Hypertension

EENT: Blurred vision

GI: *Nausea,* vomiting, dyspepsia, increased liver enzymes, abdominal pain, cholecystitis, cholelithiasis, constipation, diarrhea, hepatitis, jaundice, pancreatitis

GU: Impotence, decreased libido

HEMA: Anemia, leukopenia, thrombosis/pulmonary embolism, agranulocytosis, eosinophilia

INTEG: *Rash,* urticaria, pruritus, Stevens-Johnson syndrome

MISC: Infection

MS: *Myalgias, arthralgias,* myopathy, back pain, musculoskeletal pain, rhabdomyolysis

RESP: Pharyngitis, cough

PHARMACOKINETICS

Peak (del rel cap) 4-5 hr, tabs 2.5 hr, protein binding 99%, converted to fenofibric acid, metabolized in liver, excreted in urine (60%), half-life 20 hr

INTERACTIONS

• Nephrotoxicity: cycloSPORINE
• Monitor use with HMG-CoA reductase inhibitors; rhabdomyolysis may occur
Increase: anticoagulant effects—oral anticoagulants
Decrease: absorption of fenofibrate—bile acid sequestrants
Drug/Food
Increase: absorption

NURSING CONSIDERATIONS

Assess:
• **Diet history:** fat content, lipid levels (triglycerides, LDL, HDL, cholesterol), LFTs at baseline, periodically during treatment, CBC with differential, CPK, serum bilirubin (direct/indirect)
• **Pancreatitis, cholelithiasis renal failure, rhabdomyolysis** (when combined with HMG-COA reductase inhibitors), myositis; product should be discontinued
Evaluate:
• Therapeutic response: decreased triglycerides
Teach patient/family:
• That compliance is needed
• That risk factors should be decreased: high-fat diet, smoking, alcohol consumption, absence of exercise
• To notify prescriber if pregnancy is suspected or planned
• To report GU symptoms: decreased libido, impotence
• To notify prescriber of muscle pain, weakness, fever, fatigue, epigastric pain

fenoldopam (Rx)

(feh-nahl′doh-pam)

Corlopam

Func. class.: Antihypertensive, vasodilator

ACTION:
Agonist at D_1-like DOPAmine receptors; binds to α_2-adrenoceptors; increases renal blood flow

USES:
Hypertensive crisis, malignant hypertension
Unlabeled uses: Prevention of contrast-agent–associated nephrotoxicity, postoperative hypertension

CONTRAINDICATIONS:
Hypersensitivity, sulfite sensitivity
Precautions: Pregnancy (B), breastfeeding, children, tachycardia, intraocular pressure, hypokalemia, CVA, CAD, CHF, increased intraocular pressure

DOSAGE AND ROUTES

• **Adult: IV** 0.1 mcg/kg/min, titrate upward or downward ≤15 min by 0.05-0.1 mcg/kg/min
• **Child: CONT IV** 0.2 mcg/kg/min with effects within 5 min; may increase dose to 0.3-0.5 mcg/kg/min q20-30min depending on response, max 0.8 mcg/kg/min
Available forms: Inj 10 mg/ml
Administer:
• To patient in recumbent position; keep patient in that position for 1 hr after administration
Adult
• After diluting contents of ampules in 0.9% NaCl or 5% dextrose inj (40 mcg/ml); then add 4 ml of conc (40 mg of product/1000 ml); 2 ml of conc (20 mg of product/500 ml); 1 ml of conc (10 mg of product/250 ml); do not admix
Child
• Use inf pump
• After dilution 3 ml (30 mg)/500 ml (60 mcg/ml); 1.5 ml (15 mg)/250 ml (60 mcg/ml); 0.6 ml (6 mg)/100 ml (60 mcg/ml)
Y-site compatibilities: Alfentanil, allopurinol, amifostine, aminocaproic acid, amiodarone, amphotericin B liposome, ampicillin-sulbactam, anidulafungin, argatroban, atenolol, atracurium, atropine, azithromycin, aztreonam, bivalirudin, bleomycin, buprenorphine, busulfan, butorphanol, calcium chloride/gluconate, CARBOplatin, carmustine, caspofungin, ceFAZolin, cefepime, cefoperazone, cefo-

taxime, cefotetan, ceftazidime, ceftizoxime, cefTRIAXone, cefuroxime, chloramphenicol, chlorproMAZINE, cimetidine, ciprofloxacin, cisatracurium, CISplatin, clindamycin, cyclophosphamide, cycloSPORINE, cytarabine, dacarbazine, DACTINomycin, DAPTOmycin, DAUNOrubicin, digoxin, diltiazem, diphenhydrAMINE, DOBUTamine, docetaxel, dolasetron, DOPamine, doxacurium, DOXOrubicin, doxycycline, droperidol, enalaprilat, ePHEDrine, EPINEPHrine, epirubicin, ertapenem, erythromycin, esmolol, etoposide, famotidine, fentaNYL, fluconazole, fludarabine, fluorouracil, foscarnet, gatifloxacin, gemcitabine, gentamicin, glycopyrrolate, granisetron hydrochloride, haloperidol, heparin, hydrALAZINE, hydrocortisone, HYDROmorphone, hydrOXYzine, IDArubicin, ifosfamide, imipenem-cilastatin, inamrinone, insulin (regular), irinotecan, isoproterenol, labetalol, leucovorin, levofloxacin, levorphanol, lidocaine, linezolid, LORazepam, magnesium sulfate, mannitol, mechlorethamine, meperidine, metaraminol, methotrexate, methyldopate, metoclopramide, metoprolol, metroNIDAZOLE, micafungin, midazolam, milrinone, minocycline, mitoxantrone, mivacurium, morphine, mycophenolate, nafcillin, nalbuphine, naloxone, niCARdipine, nitroglycerin, nitroprusside, norepinephrine, octreotide, ondansetron, oxaliplatin, oxytocin, paclitaxel, palonosetron, pamidronate, pancuronium, pemetrexed, pentamidine, pentazocine, PHENobarbital, phenylephrine, piperacillin, piperacillin-tazobactam, polymyxin B, potassium chloride/phosphates, procainamide, promethazine, propofol, propranolol, quiNIDine, quinupristin-dalfopristin, ranitidine, remifentanil, rocuronium, sodium acetate/phosphates, streptozocin, succinylcholine, SUFentanil, sulfamethoxazole-trimethoprim, tacrolimus, teniposide, theophylline, thiotepa, ticarcillin, ticarcillin-clavulanate, tigecycline, tirofiban, tobramycin, tolazoline, topotecan, trimethobenzamide, vancomycin, vasopressin, vecuronium, verapamil, vinBLAStine, vinCRIStine, vinorelbine, voriconazole, zidovudine, zoledronic acid

SIDE EFFECTS

CNS: Headache, anxiety, dizziness, insomnia
CV: **Hypotension, ST/T-wave changes**, angina pectoris, tachycardia, palpitations, **MI, ischemic heart disease, flushing**
GI: Nausea, vomiting, constipation, diarrhea
HEMA: **Leukocytosis, bleeding**
INTEG: Sweating
META: Hypokalemia

PHARMACOKINETICS

Adult: Onset 5 min, duration 15-30 min, elimination half-life 5-10 min, steady state 20 min, crosses placenta, conjugated in liver, protein binding 88%
Child 1 mo-12 yr: Elimination half-life 3-5 min

INTERACTIONS

Increase: hypotension—avoid use with β-blockers
Decrease: antihypertensive effects—metoclopramide, peripherally acting dopamine antagonists
Drug/Herb
Decrease: antihypertensive effect—ephedra

NURSING CONSIDERATIONS

Assess:
- **Hypertensive crisis/malignant hypertension:** B/P, pulse q5min until stabilized, then q1hr × 2 hr, then q4hr; pulse, jugular venous distention q4hr, ECG; expect tachycardia (dose dependent)
- Electrolytes, blood studies: K, Na, C1, CO_2, CBC, serum glucose
- IV site for extravasation

Perform/provide:
- Diluted sol stable in normal light/room temp for 24 hr

Evaluate:
- Therapeutic response: decreased B/P

Teach patient/family:
- To report dyspnea, chest pain, bleeding, pain at inj site
- About the reason for medication, expected results

⚠ HIGH ALERT

fentaNYL (Rx)

(fen′ta-nill)

ABSTRAL, Actiq, Fentora, Onsolis, RAN-Fentanyl ✤

fentaNYL transdermal (Rx)

Duragesic

fentaNYL nasal spray (Rx)

Lazanda

fentaNYL SL spray (Rx)

Subsys

Func. class.: Opioid analgesic

Chem. class.: Synthetic phenylpiperidine

Controlled Substance Schedule II

Do not confuse:
fentanyl/Sufenta

ACTION: Inhibits ascending pain pathways in CNS, increases pain threshold, alters pain perception by binding to opiate receptors

USES: Controls moderate to severe pain; preoperatively, postoperatively; adjunct to general anesthetic, adjunct to regional anesthesia; **FentaNYL:** anesthesia as premedication, conscious sedation; **Actiq:** breakthrough cancer pain

CONTRAINDICATIONS: Hypersensitivity to opiates, myasthenia gravis

Black Box Warning: Headache, migraine (Actiq, ABSTRAL, Fentora, Lazanda, Onsolis); emergency room use (ABSTRAL, Lazanda); outpatient surgeries (Duragesic TD); opioid-naive patients

Precautions: Pregnancy (C), breastfeeding, geriatric patients, increased intracranial pressure, seizure disorders, severe respiratory disorders, cardiac dysrhythmias

Black Box Warning: Accidental exposure, ambient temperature increase, fever, skin abrasion (TD patch), substance abuse, respiratory depression, surgery

DOSAGE AND ROUTES

Fentanyl

Anesthetic
- **Adult: IV** 25-100 mcg (0.7-2 mcg/kg) q2-3min prn

Anesthesia supplement
- **Adult and child >12 yr: IM/IV** 2-20 mcg/kg **IV INF** 0.025-0.25 mcg/kg/min

Induction and maintenance
- **Adult: IV BOL** 5-40 mcg/kg
- **Child 2-12 yr: IV** 2-3 mcg/kg

Preoperatively
- **Adult and child >12 yr: IM/IV** 0.05-0.1 mg q30-60min before surgery

Postoperatively
- **Adult and child >12 yr: IM/IV** 0.05-0.1 mg q1-2hr prn

Sedation/analgesia
- **Adult and child >12 yr: IV** 0.5-1 mcg/kg/dose; may repeat after 30-60 min
- **Child 1-12 yr: IV BOL** 1-2 mcg/kg/dose; may repeat q30-60min; **CONT IV** 1-5 mcg/kg/hr after IV bol dose
- **Neonate: IV BOL** 0.5-3 mcg/kg/dose; **CONT IV** 0.5-2 mcg/kg/hr after IV bol

Actiq
- **Adult: TRANSMUCOSAL** 200 mcg; redose if needed 15 min after completion of 1st dose; do not give more than 2 doses during titration period

Fentora
- **Adult: BUCCAL** 100 mcg placed above rear molar between upper cheek and gum

Onsolis

• **Adult: TRANSMUCOSAL** 200 mcg, titrate, max 1200 mcg/dose or 4 doses/day

ABSTRAL

• **Adult: SL** 100 mcg; another dose may be taken 30 min after 1st, max 2 doses per episode of breakthrough pain; ≥2 hr must elapse before treating again; titrate stepwise over consecutive episodes

FentaNYL transdermal

• **Adult:** 25 mcg/hr; may increase until pain relief occurs; apply patch to flat surface on upper torso and wear for 72 hr; apply new patch on different site for continued relief

FentaNYL nasal spray

• **Adult:** 100 mcg (1 spray in 1 nostril), may retreat after ≥2 hr, titrate upward until adequate analgesia; treat a max of 4 episodes daily

FentaNYL SL spray

• **Adult:** 100 mcg sprayed under tongue, titrate stepwise carefully

Available forms: Inj 0.05 mg/ml; lozenges 100, 200, 300, 400 mcg; lozenges on a stick 200, 400, 600, 800, 1200, 1600 mcg; buccal tab 100, 200, 400, 600, 800 mcg; oral dissolving film (Onsolis) 120, 200, 400, 600, 800 mcg; SL tab (ABSTRAL) 100, 200, 300, 400, 600, 800 mcg; *transdermal:* patch 12, 25, 50, 75, 100 mcg/hr; *SL spray:* 100, 200, 400, 600, 800, 1200, 1600 mcg/spray

Administer:

• By inj (IM, IV); give slowly to prevent rigidity

• Must have emergency equipment available, opioid antagonists, O_2; to be used only by those appropriately trained; IV products to be used in OR, ER, ICU

Transmucosal route

• Remove foil just before administration; instruct patient to place product between cheek and lower gum, moving it back and forth and sucking, not chewing (Actiq); place above rear molar (Fentora); place film on the inside of the cheek (Onsolis); all products not used or only partially used should be flushed down the toilet

Transdermal route

• q72hr for continuous pain relief; dosage adjusted after at least 2 applications; apply to clean, dry skin and press firmly

• Give short-acting analgesics until patch takes effect (8-24 hr); when reducing dosage or switching to alternative IV treatment, withdraw gradually; serum levels drop gradually, give ½ the equianalgesic dose of new analgesic 12-18 hr after removal as ordered

SL spray

• Open blister package with scissors immediately before use; spray contents of unit under tongue; dispose of each used unit after use by placing it into one of the disposable bags provided; seal bag, discard into a trash container out of reach of children

IV route

• IV undiluted by anesthesiologist or diluted with 5 ml or more sterile water or 0.9% NaCl given through Y-tube or 3-way stopcock at 0.1 mg or less/1-2 min

Additive compatibilities: Bupivacaine, caffeine citrate, cloNIDine, droperidol, EPINEPHrine, ketamine, lidocaine, ziconotide

Solution compatibilities: D_5W, 0.9% NaCl

Syringe compatibilities: Alprostadil, atracurium, atropine, bupivacaine/ketamine, butorphanol, chlorproMAZINE, cimetidine, clonidine/lidocaine, diphenhyDRINATE, diphenhydrAMINE, droperidol, heparin, hydromorphone, hydrOXYzine, lidocaine, meperidine, metoclopramide, midazolam, morphine, pentazocine, perphenazine, prochlorperazine, promazine, promethazine, ranitidine, scopolamine

Y-site compatibilities: Abciximab, acyclovir, alfentanil, alprostadil, amikacin, aminocaproic acid, aminophylline, amiodarone, amphotericin B cholesteryl, amphotericin B lipid complex, amphotericin B liposome, anidulafungin, argatroban, ascorbic acid injection, atenolol, atracurium, atropine, azathioprine, aztreonam, benztropine, bivalirudin, bleomycin, bumetanide, buprenorphine, butorphanol, calcium chloride/gluconate, CARBOplatin, caspofungin, cefamandole, ceFAZolin, cefmetazole, cefonicid, cefoperazone, cefotaxime, cefotetan, cefoxitin, ceftazidime, ceftizoxime, ceftobiprole, cefTRIAXone, cefuroxime, cephalothin, chloramphenicol, chlorproMAZINE, cimetidine, cisatracurium, CISplatin, clindamycin, cloNIDine, cyanocobalamin, cyclophosphamide, cycloSPORINE, cytarabine, DACTINomycin, DAPTOmycin, dexamethasone, dexmedetomidine, digoxin, diltiazem, diphenhydrAMINE, DOBUTamine, docetaxel, DOPamine, doripenem, doxacurium, doxapram, DOXOrubicin, doxycycline, enalaprilat, ePHEDrine, EPINEPHrine, epirubicin, epoetin alfa, eptifibatide, erythromycin, esmolol, etomidate, etoposide, famotidine, fenoldopam, fluconazole, fludarabine, fluorouracil, folic acid, furosemide, ganciclovir, gatifloxacin, gemcitabine, gentamicin, glycopyrrolate, granisetron, heparin, hydrocortisone, HYDROmorphone, hydrOXYzine, IDArubicin, ifosfamide, imipenem-cilastatin, inamrinone, insulin (regular), irinotecan, isoproterenol, ketorolac, labetalol, lansoprazole, levofloxacin, lidocaine, linezolid, LORazepam, LR, magnesium sulfate, mannitol, mechlorethamine, meperidine, metaraminol, methicillin, methotrexate, methotrimeprazine, methoxamine, methyldopate, methylPREDNISolone, metoclopramide, metoprolol, metroNIDAZOLE, mezlocillin, miconazole, midazolam, milrinone, minocycline, mitoxantrone, mivacurium, morphine, moxalactam, multiple vitamins injection, mycophenolate, nafcillin, nalbuphine, naloxone, nesiritide, netilmicin, niCARdipine, nitroglycerin, nitroprusside, norepinephrine, octreotide, ondansetron, oxacillin, oxaliplatin, oxytocin, paclitaxel, palonosetron, pamidronate, pancuronium, papaverine, pemetrexed, penicillin G potassium/sodium, pentamidine, pentazocine, PENTobarbital, PHENObarbital, phenylephrine, phytonadione, piperacillin, piperacillin-tazobactam, polymyxin B, potassium chloride, procainamide, prochlorperazine, promethazine, propofol, propranolol, protamine, pyridoxine, quiNIDine, quinupristin-dalfopristin, ranitidine, remifentanil, Ringer's, ritodrine, riTUXimab, rocuronium, sargramostim, scopolamine, sodium acetate/bicarbonate, succinylcholine, SUFentanil, tacrolimus, teniposide, theophylline, thiamine, thiopental, thiotepa, ticarcillin, ticarcillin-clavulanate, tigecycline, tirofiban, TNA, tobramycin, tolazoline, TPN, trastuzumab, trimetaphan, urokinase, vancomycin, vasopressin, vecuronium, verapamil, vinCRIStine, vinorelbine, vitamin B complex/C, voriconazole, zoledronic acid

SIDE EFFECTS

CNS: Dizziness, delirium, euphoria, sedation

CV: Bradycardia, arrest, hypo/hypertension

EENT: Blurred vision, miosis

GI: Nausea, vomiting, constipation

GU: Urinary retention

INTEG: Rash, diaphoresis

MS: Muscle rigidity

RESP: Respiratory depression, arrest, laryngospasm

PHARMACOKINETICS

Metabolized by liver, excreted by kidneys, crosses placenta, excreted in breast milk, half-life $1^1/_2$-6 hr, 80% bound to plasma proteins

IM: Onset 7-8 min, peak 30 min, duration 1-2 hr

IV: Onset 1 min, peak 3-5 min, duration $^1/_2$-1 hr

INTERACTIONS

Increase: fentaNYL effect with other CNS depressants—alcohol, opioids, sedative/hypnotics, antipsychotics, skeletal muscle relaxants

Decrease: fentaNYL effect—CYP3A4 inducers (carBAMazepine, phenytoin, PHENObarbital, rifampin)

Drug/Herb

Increase: action of fentaNYL—St. John's wort

Decrease: effect of fentaNYL—echinacea

Drug/Lab Test
Increase: amylase, lipase

NURSING CONSIDERATIONS

Assess:
- VS after parenteral route; note muscle rigidity, drug history, hepatic/renal function tests
- CNS changes: dizziness, drowsiness, hallucinations, euphoria, LOC, pupil reaction
- Allergic reactions: rash, urticaria

Black Box Warning: Respiratory dysfunction: respiratory depression, character, rate, rhythm; notify prescriber if respirations are <10/min

- **Headache/migraine:** ABSTRAL, Actiq, Fentora, Lazanda, Onsolis not to be used for this condition; ABSTRAL, Lazanda not to be used in ER; Duragesic TD not to be used for outpatient surgery patients
- **Apnea, respiratory arrest in opioid-naive patients:** do not use ABSTRAL, Actiq, Duragesic, Fentora, Lazanda, Onsolis; opioid-tolerant patients are those using ≥60 mg/day oral morphine, ≥30 mg/day oxycodone PO, 8 mg/day HYDROmorphone, 25 mcg TD fentaNYL/hr

Perform/provide:
- Storage in light-resistant area at room temp

Evaluate:
- Therapeutic response: induction of anesthesia, relief of breakthrough cancer pain, general pain relief
- Cancer pain, general pain relief

Teach patient/family:
- About coughing, turning, deep breathing for postoperative patients
- About safety measures: side rails, night-light, call bell within reach
- About CNS changes: physical dependence; not to use with alcohol, other CNS depressants
- **Accidental exposure:** Discuss the dangers of children or pets getting product

Transdermal route
- **Ambient temperature increase:** that excessive heat may increase absorption; do not use with heating pads, electric blankets, heat/tanning lamps, saunas, hot tubs, heated waterbeds, when sunbathing
- That excessive perspiration may alter adhesiveness
- To dispose of patch by placing sticky sides together and flushing down toilet
- That patient may need to clip hair before applying to ensure adhesion

ferrous fumarate (Rx)

Ferretts, Ferrimin, Ferro-Sequels, Hemocyte, Palafer ✱, Walgreens Finest Iron

ferrous gluconate (Rx)

Apo-Ferrous Gluconate ✱, Ferate, Walgreens Gold Seal Ferrous Gluconate

ferrous sulfate (Rx)

Apo-Ferrous Sulfate ✱, Equaline Ferrous Sulfate, Leader Ferrous Sulfate, Slow Release Iron, Walgreens Gold Seal Ferrous Sulfate

ferrous sulfate, dried (Rx)

Slow Fe

carbonyl iron (OTC)

(kar′bo-nil)

ICAR Pediatric, Iron Chews

iron polysaccharide (OTC)

iFerex, Niferex, Nu-Iron

Func. class.: Hematinic
Chem. class.: Iron preparation

ACTION: Replaces iron stores needed for red blood cell development as well as energy and O_2 transport and use; fumarate contains 33% elemental iron; gluconate, 12%; sulfate, 20%; iron, 30%; ferrous sulfate exsiccated

USES:
Iron deficiency anemia, prophylaxis for iron deficiency in pregnancy, nutritional supplementation

CONTRAINDICATIONS:
Sideroblastic anemia, thalassemia, hemosiderosis/hemochromatosis

Precautions: Pregnancy (B) (ferric gluconate complex), (C) (iron dextran, oral products), anemia (long term), ulcerative colitis/regional enteritis, peptic ulcer disease, hemolytic anemia, cirrhosis, sulfite sensitivity

Black Box Warning: Accidental exposure

DOSAGE AND ROUTES

Fumarate

- **Adult: PO** 50-100 mg tid
- **Child: PO** 3 mg/kg/day (elemental iron) tid-qid
- **Infant: PO** 10-25 mg/day (elemental iron) in 3-4 divided doses, max 15 mg/day

Gluconate

- **Adult: PO** 60 mg bid-qid
- **Child: PO** 3 mg/kg/day in divided doses

Sulfate

- **Adult: PO** 0.75-1.5 g/day in divided doses tid
- **Child 6-12 yr: PO** 3 mg/kg/day in divided doses

Pregnancy

- **Adult: PO** 300-600 mg/day in divided doses

Complex

- **Adult: IV INF** (125 mg) 10 ml/100 ml of NaCl for inj given over 1 hr

Iron polysaccharide

- **Adult: PO** 100-200 mg tid
- **Child: PO** 4-6 mg/kg/day in 3 divided doses (severe iron deficiency)

Available forms: *Fumarate:* tabs 63, 195, 200, 324, 325 mg; chewable tabs 100 mg; cont rel tabs 300 mg; oral susp 100 mg/5 ml, 45 mg/0.6 ml; *gluconate:* tabs 300, 320, 325 mg; caps 86, 325, 435 mg; film-coated tabs 300 mg; elix 300 mg/5 ml; *sulfate:* tabs 195, 300, 325 mg; enteric-coated tabs 325 mg; ext rel tabs, time-rel caps, 525 mg; ***dried:*** tabs 200 mg; ext rel tabs 160 mg; ext rel caps 160 mg; *iron polysaccharide:* tabs 50 mg; caps 150 mg; sol 100 mg/5 ml

Administer:

- Swallow tabs whole; not to break, crush, or chew unless labeled as chewable
- Between meals for best absorption; may give with juice; do not give with antacids or milk, delay at least 1 hr; if GI symptoms occur, give after meals even if absorption is decreased; eggs, milk products, chocolate, caffeine interfere with absorption
- Liquid through plastic straw to avoid discoloration of tooth enamel; dilute thoroughly
- At least 1 hr before bedtime, since corrosion may occur in stomach; ferrous gluconate is less irritating of GI tract than ferrous sulfate
- For <6 mo for anemia

SIDE EFFECTS

GI: *Nausea, constipation, epigastric pain, black and red tarry stools,* vomiting, diarrhea

INTEG: Temporarily discolored tooth enamel and eyes

SYST: Hypersensitivity reactions (Ferrlecit)

PHARMACOKINETICS

PO: Excreted in feces, urine, skin, breast milk; enters bloodstream; bound to transferrin; crosses placenta

INTERACTIONS

Increase: action of iron preparation—ascorbic acid, chloramphenicol

Decrease: absorption of penicillamine, levodopa, methyldopa, fluoroquinolones, L-thyroxine, tetracycline

Decrease: absorption of iron preparations—antacids, H_2-antagonists, proton pump inhibitors, cholestyramine, vit E

Drug/Food
Decrease: absorption—dairy products, caffeine, eggs
Drug/Lab Test
False positive: occult blood

NURSING CONSIDERATIONS

Assess:

• Blood studies: Hct, Hgb, reticulocytes, bilirubin before treatment, at least monthly; iron studies (Fe, TIBC, ferritin)
⚠ **Toxicity:** nausea, vomiting, diarrhea (green then tarry stools), hematemesis, pallor, cyanosis, shock, coma
• Elimination; if constipation occurs, increase water, bulk, activity
• **Nutrition:** amount of iron in diet (meat, dark green leafy vegetables, dried beans, dried fruits, eggs)
• Cause of iron loss or anemia, including salicylates, sulfonamides, antimalarials, quiNIDine
• **Hypersensitivity:** more common with Ferrlecit

Perform/provide:

• Storage in tight, light-resistant container

Evaluate:

• Therapeutic response: improvement in Hct, Hgb, reticulocytes; decreased fatigue, weakness

Teach patient/family:

• That iron will turn stools black or dark green
• That iron poisoning may occur if increased beyond recommended level
• **Accidental exposure:** to keep out of reach of children, pets
• Not to substitute 1 iron salt for another; that elemental iron content differs (e.g., 300 mg ferrous fumarate contains about 100 mg elemental iron; 300 mg ferrous gluconate contains only about 30 mg elemental iron)
• To avoid reclining position for 15-30 min after taking product to avoid esophageal corrosion
• To follow a diet high in iron; to avoid taking iron, dairy products, calcium supplements, and vit C together because they compete for absorption

TREATMENT OF OVERDOSE:

Induce vomiting; give eggs, milk until lavage can be done

ferumoxytol (Rx)

(fer′ue-mox′i-tol)
Feraheme
Func. class.: Hematinic

F

ACTION:
Iron is carried by transferrin to the bone marrow, where it is incorporated into hemoglobin

USES:
Iron deficiency anemia with chronic kidney disease
Unlabeled uses: MRI

CONTRAINDICATIONS:
Hypersensitivity, hemochromatosis
Precautions: Pregnancy (B), breastfeeding, children, geriatric patients, all anemias excluding iron deficiency anemia, iron overload, dialysis, hepatic disease, hypotension, MRI, siderblastic anemia, thalassemia

DOSAGE AND ROUTES

• **Adult: IV** 510 mg of elemental iron followed by a 2nd dose 3-8 days later; if giving during dialysis, give after B/P is stable and after 1 hr of hemodialysis

Available forms: 510 mg/17 ml solution for inj

Administer:

• Only with epinephrine, with Solu-medrol available in case of anaphylactic reaction during dose

IV route

• Give directly in dialysis line by slow inj or inf; give by slow inj at 1 ml/min (5 min/vial); inf dilute each vial exclusively in a maximum of 100 ml of 0.9% NaCl, give at rate of 100 mg of iron/15 min, discard unused portions

SIDE EFFECTS

CNS: Headache, dizziness
CV: Chest pain, hypo/hypertension, hypervolemia, edema

GI: *Nausea, vomiting, abdominal pain,* constipation, diarrhea
INTEG: Rash, pruritus, urticaria, fever
MS: Back pain
OTHER: Anaphylaxis
RESP: Dyspnea, cough

PHARMACOKINETICS

Half-life 15 hr

INTERACTIONS

Increase: toxicity—oral iron; do not use

NURSING CONSIDERATIONS

Assess:

- Blood studies: Hct, Hgb, reticulocytes, transferrin, plasma iron concentrations, ferritin, total iron binding, bilirubin before treatment, at least monthly
- **Allergy/anaphylaxis,** rash, pruritus, fever, wheezing; notify prescriber immediately, keep emergency equipment available
- Cardiac status: hypo/hypertension, hypervolemia
- **Toxicity:** nausea, vomiting, diarrhea, fever, abdominal pain (early symptoms), cyanotic-looking lips, nailbeds, seizures, CV collapse (late symptoms)

Perform/provide:

- Storage at room temp in cool environment; do not freeze

Evaluate:

- Therapeutic response: increased serum iron levels, Hct, Hgb

Teach patient/family:

- To report itching, rash, chest pain, headache, vertigo, nausea, vomiting, abdominal pain, joint/muscle pain, numbness, tingling
- That iron poisoning may occur if increased beyond recommended level; not to take oral iron preparation
- That product may alter MRI studies

TREATMENT OF OVERDOSE:

Discontinue product, treat allergic reaction, give diphenhydrAMINE or EPINEPHrine as needed; give iron-chelating product for acute poisoning

fesoterodine (Rx)

(fess′oh-ter-oh-deen)

Toviaz

Func. class.: Overactive bladder product

Chem. class.: Muscarinic receptor antagonist

ACTION:

Relaxes smooth muscles in urinary tract by inhibiting acetylcholine at postganglionic sites

USES:

Overactive bladder (urinary frequency, urgency), urinary incontinence

CONTRAINDICATIONS:

GI obstruction, ileus, pyloric stenosis, urinary retention, gastric retention, hypersensitivity, closed-angle glaucoma

Precautions: Pregnancy (C), breastfeeding, children, renal/hepatic disease, urinary tract obstruction, ambient temperature increase, autonomic neuropathy, constipation, contact lenses, hazardous activity, GERD, gastroparesis, myasthenia gravis, prostatic hypertrophy, toxic megacolon, ulcerative colitis, possible cross-sensitivity with tolterodine

DOSAGE AND ROUTES

- **Adult and geriatric: PO EXT REL** 4 mg/day, may increase to 8 mg/day based on response, max 4 mg/day in those taking potent CYP3A4 inhibitors

Renal dose

- **Adult: PO EXT REL** CCr <30 ml/min, max 4 mg/day in severe renal impairment

Available forms: Ext rel tabs 4, 8 mg

Administer:

- Do not break, crush, or chew ext rel product
- Give without regard to meals

SIDE EFFECTS

CV: Chest pain, angina, QT prolongation
EENT: Xerophthalmia

GI: *Nausea, vomiting,* abdominal pain, constipation, dry mouth
GU: Dysuria, urinary retention
INTEG: Rash, **angioedema**
MISC: Peripheral edema, insomnia
MS: Back pain
RESP: Cough
SYST: Infection

PHARMACOKINETICS

Peak 5 hr, rapidly absorbed, protein binding 50%, excreted in urine/feces, half-life 7 hr

INTERACTIONS

Increase: action of fesoterodine—antiretroviral protease inhibitors, macrolide antiinfectives, azole antifungals
Increase: anticholinergic effect—antimuscarinics, anticholinergics
Increase: urinary frequency—diuretics
Drug/Herb
Decrease: fesoterodine—caffeine, green tea, guarana
Drug/Food
Increase: fesoterodine level—grapefruit juice
Decrease: fesoterodine level—cola, coffee, tea
Drug/Lab Test
Increase: LFTs

NURSING CONSIDERATIONS

Assess:
- **Urinary patterns:** distention, nocturia, frequency, urgency, incontinence
- **Allergic reactions:** rash; if this occurs, product should be discontinued

Perform/provide:
- Storage at room temp; protect from moisture

Evaluate:
- Therapeutic response: absence of urinary frequency, urgency, incontinence

Teach patient/family:
- Not to drink liquids before bedtime
- About the importance of bladder maintenance

fexofenadine (Rx, OTC)

(fex-oh-fi′na-deen)

Allegra, Allegra ODT

Func. class.: Antihistamine—2nd generation

Chem. class.: Piperidine, peripherally selective

Do not confuse:
Allegra/Viagra

F

ACTION: Acts on blood vessels, GI, respiratory system by competing with histamine for H_1-receptor site; decreases allergic response by blocking pharmacologic effects of histamine, less sedating

USES: Rhinitis, allergy symptoms, chronic idiopathic urticaria

CONTRAINDICATIONS: Breastfeeding, newborn or premature infants, hypersensitivity, severe hepatic disease
Precautions: Pregnancy (C), children, geriatric patients, respiratory disease, closed-angle glaucoma, prostatic hypertrophy, bladder neck obstruction, asthma

DOSAGE AND ROUTES

- **Adult and child >12 yr: PO** Rx only, 60 mg bid or 180 mg/day; PO OTC only, 60 mg bid or 180 mg/day (self-treatment of allergic rhinitis)
- **Child 2-11 yr: PO** 30 mg bid; **ORALLY DISINTEGRATING TAB Child 6-11 yr:** 30 mg bid dissolved on tongue

Renal dose
- **Adult and child ≥12 yr: PO** CCr <80 ml/min, 60 mg/day
- **Child 2-11 yr: PO** CCr <80 ml/min, 30 mg q day
- **Child <2 yr: PO** CCr <80 ml/min, 15 mg q day

Available forms: Tabs 30, 60, 180 mg; oral susp 6 mg/ml, orally disintegrating tab 30 mg

Administer:

- Without regard to meals; caps/tabs should not be given with or right before grapefruit, orange, or apple juice
- **Orally disintegrating tab:** allow to dissolve, swallow; do not remove from blister pack until time of administration
- **Oral susp:** shake well, use calibrated measuring device

SIDE EFFECTS

CNS: Headache, stimulation, drowsiness, sedation, fatigue, confusion, blurred vision, tinnitus, restlessness, tremors, paradoxical excitation in children or geriatric patients

CV: Hypotension, palpitations, bradycardia, tachycardia, **dysrhythmias** (rare)

GI: Nausea, diarrhea, abdominal pain, vomiting, constipation

GU: Frequency, dysuria, urinary retention, impotence

HEMA: Hemolytic anemia, thrombocytopenia, leukopenia, agranulocytosis, pancytopenia

INTEG: Rash, eczema, photosensitivity, urticaria

RESP: Thickening of bronchial secretions, dry nose, throat

PHARMACOKINETICS

Well absorbed; onset 1 hr; peak 2-3 hr; duration 12-24 hr; 80% excreted in urine; half-life 14.5 hr, increased in renal disease

INTERACTIONS

Decrease: effect—magnesium-aluminum-containing antacids

Drug/Food

Decrease: absorption of product—apple, orange, grapefruit juice

Drug/Lab Test

False negative: skin allergy tests

NURSING CONSIDERATIONS

Assess:

- **Allergy:** itchy, runny, watery eyes; congested nose; before and during treatment
- I&O ratio: be alert for urinary retention, frequency, dysuria, especially among geriatric patients; product should be discontinued if these occur; serum creatinine/BUN at baseline and periodically during treatment
- Respiratory status: rate, rhythm, increase in bronchial secretions, wheezing, chest tightness

Perform/provide:

- Storage in tight, light-resistant container

Evaluate:

- Therapeutic response: absence of running or congested nose or rashes

Teach patient/family:

- About all aspects of product use; to notify prescriber if confusion, sedation, hypotension occur
- To avoid driving, other hazardous activity if drowsiness occurs
- To avoid alcohol, other CNS depressants
- Not to exceed recommended dose; that dysrhythmias may occur

TREATMENT OF OVERDOSE:

Lavage, diazepam, vasopressors, IV phenytoin

fidaxomicin

(fye-dax′oh-mye′sin)

Dificid

Func. class.: Antiinfective-macrolide

ACTION: Bactericidal against *Clostridium difficile;* is a fermentation product obtained from *Dactylosporangium aurantiacum;* inhibits RNA synthesis by inhibiting transcription of bacterial RNA polymerases; may act at the early stages of transcription

USES: Pseudomembraneous colitis *Clostridium difficile*-associated diarrhea

CONTRAINDICATIONS: Hypersensitivity

Precautions: Pregnancy (B), breastfeeding, children

DOSAGE AND ROUTES

- **Adult: PO** 200 mg bid × 10 days

Available forms: Tab 200 mg
Administer:

- Without regard to food

SIDE EFFECTS

GI: Nausea, vomiting, abdominal pain, GI bleeding
HEMA: Anemia, neutropenia

PHARMACOKINETICS

Minimal systemic absorption after oral administration; primarily transformed by hydrolysis to its main active metabolite, OP-1118, both fidaxomicin and OP-1118 are substrates of the P-glycoprotein (PGP) efflux transporter in the GI tract; half-life of fidaxomicin is 11.7 +/− 4.8 hr, and the half-life of OP-1118 is 11.2 hours +/− 3.01 hr; fidaxomicin Tmax is 2 hr (range 1-5 hr); OP-1118 Tmax 1.02 hr (range 1-5 hr); primarily excreted (feces >92%) as parent drug and OP-1118; (urine 0.59%) OP-1118

INTERACTIONS

Increase: fidaxomicin action—cycloSPORINE

NURSING CONSIDERATIONS

Assess:

- Pseudomembraneous colitis: for diarrhea, abdominal pain, fever, fatigue, anorexia, anemia, elevated WBC and low serum albumin; product may be used in place of vancomycin; monitor CBC with differential and stool culture (*Clostridium difficile*)

Perform/provide:

- Storage of tab at room temperature

Evaluate:

- Positive therapeutic response: resolution of *Clostridium difficile*

Teach patient/family:

- To report GI bleeding, or severe abdominal pain
- To report if pregnancy is planned or suspected or if breast feeding

filgrastim (Rx)

(fill-grass′stim)

G-CSF, granulocyte colony stimulator, Neupogen

Func. class.: Biologic modifier
Chem. class.: Granulocyte colony-stimulating factor

F

ACTION: Stimulates proliferation and differentiation of neutrophils

USES: To decrease infection in patients receiving antineoplastics that are myelosuppressive; to increase WBC in patients with product-induced neutropenia; bone marrow transplantation

Unlabeled uses: Neutropenia with HIV infection, aplastic anemia, ganciclovir-induced neutropenia, zidovudine-induced neutropenia

CONTRAINDICATIONS: Hypersensitivity to proteins of *Escherichia coli*

Precautions: Pregnancy (C), breast-feeding, cardiac conditions, children, myeloid malignancies, radiation therapy, sepsis, sickle cell disease, chemotherapy, respiratory disease

DOSAGE AND ROUTES

After myelosuppressive chemotherapy

- **Adult and child: IV/SUBCUT** 5 mcg/kg/day in a single dose × 14 days; may increase by 5 mcg/kg with each cycle

After bone marrow transplantation

- **Adult: IV/SUBCUT** 10 mcg/kg/day as **INF (IV)** over 4 hr or 24 hr, begin 24 hr after chemotherapy and 24 hr after bone marrow transplantation

Peripheral blood progenitor cell collection/therapy

- **Adult:** 10 mcg/kg/day as bolus or **CONT INF** × ≥4 days before leukapheresis, continue to last leukapheresis; may alter dose if WBC >100,000 cells/mm^3

Severe neutropenia (chronic), idiopathic/cyclical

• **Adult: SUBCUT** 5 mcg/kg daily

Available forms: Inj 300 mcg/ml, 480 mcg/1.6 ml, 480 mcg/0.8 ml, 3000 mcg/0.5 ml

Administer:

• Using single-use vials; after dose is withdrawn, do not reenter vial

• No sooner than 24 hr after antineoplastics, bone marrow inf

• Do not shake; may warm to room temp before using; discard any product left out for >24 hr

• For 2 wk or until ANC is 10,000/mm^3 after the expected chemotherapy neutrophil nadir

SUBCUT route

• May divide into 2 inj if amount to be given is >1 ml

IV route

• Dilute in D_5W to a conc of 5-15 mcg/ml; vial is for one-time use; give over 15-30 min (chemotherapy) or over 4-24 hr (bone marrow transplantation); do not use 0.9% NaCl to dilute product

Y-site compatibilities: Acyclovir, allopurinol, amikacin, aminophylline, ampicillin, ampicillin/sulbactam, aztreonam, bleomycin, bumetanide, buprenorphine, butorphanol, calcium gluconate, CARBOplatin, carmustine, ceFAZolin, cefotetan, ceftazidime, chlorproMAZINE, cimetidine, CISplatin, cyclophosphamide, cytarabine, dacarbazine, DAUNOrubicin, dexamethasone, diphenhydrAMINE, DOXOrubicin, doxycycline, droperidol, enalaprilat, famotidine, floxuridine, fluconazole, fludarabine, gallium, ganciclovir, granisetron, haloperidol, hydrocortisone, hydromorphone, hydrOXYzine, IDArubicin, ifosfamide, leucovorin, LORazepam, mechlorethamine, melphalan, meperidine, mesna, methotrexate, metoclopramide, miconazole, minocycline, mitoxantrone, morphine, nalbuphine, netilmicin, ondansetron, plicamycin, potassium chloride, promethazine, ranitidine, sodium bicarbonate, streptozocin, ticarcillin, ticarcillin/clavulanate, tobramycin, trimethoprim-sulfamethoxazole, vancomycin, vinBLAStine, vinCRIStine, vinorelbine, zidovudine

SIDE EFFECTS

CNS: Fever, headache

GI: *Nausea,* vomiting, diarrhea, mucositis, anorexia

HEMA: **Thrombocytopenia,** excessive leukocytosis

INTEG: Alopecia, exacerbation of skin conditions, urticaria, cutaneous vasculitis

MS: Osteoporosis, skeletal pain

OTHER: Chest pain, hypotension

RESP: **Acute respiratory distress syndrome,** wheezing, **alveolar hemorrhage**

PHARMACOKINETICS

SUBCUT: Onset 5-60 min, peak 2-8 hr, duration up to 1 wk

IV: Onset 5-60 min, peak 24 hr, duration up to 1 wk

INTERACTIONS

Increase: adverse reactions—do not use this product concomitantly with antineoplastics, lithium

Drug/Lab Test

Increase: uric acid, LDH, alk phos

NURSING CONSIDERATIONS

Assess:

• Blood studies: CBC, platelet count before treatment and twice weekly; neutrophil counts may be increased for 2 days after therapy

• B/P, respirations, pulse before and during therapy

• Bone pain; give mild analgesics

• CBC with differential, platelets

Perform/provide:

• Storage in refrigerator; do not freeze; may store at room temp up to 24 hr

Evaluate:

• Therapeutic response: absence of infection

Teach patient/family:

• About the technique for self-administration: dose, side effects, disposal of containers and needles; provide instruction sheet

finasteride (Rx)

(fin-ass′te-ride)

Propecia, Proscar

Func. class.: Hormone, androgen inhibitor, hair stimulant

Chem. class.: 5-α-Reductase inhibitor

Do not confuse:
finasteride/furosemide
Proscar/ProSom/Prozac

ACTION: Inhibits 5-α-reductase and reduction in DHT; DHT induces androgenic effects by binding to androgen receptors in the cell nuclei of the prostate gland, liver, skin; prevents development of BHP

USES: Symptomatic benign prostatic hyperplasia (Proscar); male-pattern baldness (Propecia)

Unlabeled uses: Hirsutism, prostate cancer prophylaxis

CONTRAINDICATIONS: Pregnancy (X), breastfeeding, children, women who are pregnant or who may become pregnant should not handle tabs, hypersensitivity

Precautions: Large residual urinary volume, severely diminished urinary flow, hepatic function abnormalities

DOSAGE AND ROUTES

BPH

- **Adult: PO** 5 mg/day × 6-12 mo (Proscar)

Male-pattern baldness

- **Adult: PO** 1 mg/day for 3 mo or more for results (Propecia)

Hirsutism (unlabeled)

- **Adult (nonpregnant): PO** 5 mg/day alone or in combination with oral contraceptives

Prostate cancer prophylaxis (unlabeled)

- **Adult (male): PO** 5 mg/day

Available forms: Tabs (Propecia) 1 mg, (Proscar) 5 mg

Administer:

- Without regard to meals
- For a minimum of 6 mo; not all patients will respond

SIDE EFFECTS

GU: Impotence, decreased libido, decreased volume of ejaculate

INTEG: Rash

MISC: Breast tenderness, **secondary malignancy**

PHARMACOKINETICS

Bioavailability 63%; readily absorbed from GI tract; plasma protein binding 90%; metabolized in the liver; excreted in urine (metabolites) 39%, feces (57%); crosses blood-brain barrier; peak 1-2 hr; duration 24 hr

INTERACTIONS

Decrease: finasteride effect—theophylline, adrenergic bronchodilators, anticholinergics

Drug/Lab Test

Decrease: PSA levels

NURSING CONSIDERATIONS

Assess:

- **BPH:** urinary patterns, residual urinary volume, severely diminished urinary flow
- PSA levels and digital rectal exam prior to initiating therapy and periodically thereafter
- Hepatic studies prior to treatment; extensively metabolized in liver

Perform/provide:

- Storage <86° F (30° C); protect from light; keep container tightly closed

Evaluate:

- Therapeutic response: increased urinary flow; decreased postvoiding dribbling, frequency, nocturia or hair growth within 3-6 mo; regression of prostate size

Teach patient/family:

⚠ **That pregnant women or women who may become pregnant should not touch crushed tabs or come into contact with the semen of a patient taking this product; that product may adversely affect developing male fetus**

- That volume of ejaculate may be decreased during treatment; that impotence and decreased libido may also occur
- That Propecia results may not occur for 3 mo
- That Proscar results may not occur for 6-12 mo

fingolimod (Rx)

(fin-gol'i-mod)

Gilenya

Func. class.: Biologic response modifier

Chem. class.: Sphingosine 1-phosphate receptor modulator

ACTION:

Binds with high affinity to sphingosine 1-phosphate receptors; blocks lymphocyte egress to lymph nodes, thereby reducing the number of peripheral blood lymphocytes; may reduce lymphocyte migration into the CNS

USES:

To reduce frequency of exacerbation, to delay physical disability of relapsing forms of MS

CONTRAINDICATIONS:

Hypersensitivity

Precautions: Pregnancy (C), breastfeeding, neonates/infants/children, AIDS, asthma, AV block, bradycardia, cardiac disease, COPD, diabetes mellitus, dysrhythmias, heart failure, hepatic disease, HIV, hypertension, immunosuppression, leukemia, lymphoma, QT prolongation, respiratory insufficiency, sick sinus syndrome, syncope, uveitis

DOSAGE AND ROUTES

- **Adult: PO** 0.5 mg/day

Hepatic dose

- **Adult: PO** Child-Pugh C, total score >10: closely monitor, fingolimod exposure is doubled

Available forms: Caps 0.5 mg

Administer:

PO route

- Watch patient for 6 hr after initial dose or if product not given for >2 wk for development of bradycardia
- Give without regard to food

SIDE EFFECTS

CNS: Asthenia, depression, fatigue, headache, dizziness, encephalopathy, migraine, paresthesias, **stroke**

CV: AV block, bradycardia, chest pain, hypertension, palpitations

EENT: Blurred vision, vision impairment, ocular pain, macular edema

GI: Abdominal pain, anorexia, diarrhea, jaundice, vomiting, weight loss

HEMA: **Leukopenia, lymphopenia, neutropenia**

INTEG: Alopecia, pruritus

MS: Back pain

RESP: Dyspnea, cough

SYST: Infection, influenza, **secondary malignancy**

PHARMACOKINETICS

Protein binding (99.7%), distributed to RBCs (86%), steady state 1-2 months, metabolized by CYP4F2 and CYP2D6 to a lesser extent, terminal half-life 6-9 days, excreted in urine (81% inactive metabolites), peak 12-16 hr

INTERACTIONS

Increase: immunosuppression—antineoplastics, immunosuppressants, immune modulating therapies

Increase: fingolimod effect—ketoconazole

Increase: infection risk—live vaccines

Decrease: effect of—inactive vaccines, toxoids

Increase: risk of torsades de pointes—Class Ia/III antidysrhythmics

NURSING CONSIDERATIONS

Assess:

- **Multiple sclerosis:** improving paresthesia, muscle weakness, clonus, muscle spasms, difficulty with moving, difficulty with coordination of balancc, speech, swallowing, vision problems, fatigue; prevention of increasing disability
- **Laboratory monitoring:** obtain before initial dose; CBC, LFTs, serum bilirubin, ophthalmologic exam, antibodies to VZV; if there is no history of chickenpox or no vaccination, may give VZV vaccination to antibody-negative patient before giving product, postpone for 1 mo after vaccination; obtain ECG for evidence of bradycardia, AV block

Perform/provide:

- Storage at room temp, protect from moisture

Evaluate:

- Therapeutic response: improved symptoms of multiple sclerosis and prevention of increasing disability

Teach patient/family:

- About use of product and expected results; provide med guide to patient
- That continuing follow-up exams and laboratory tests will be required on a regular basis
- To report any side effects of therapy
- To protect product from moisture
- To report chest pain, palpitations, jaundice

flavocoxid (Rx)

(flav-uh-kox′id)

Limbrel

Func. class.: Analgesic, nonopioid
Chem. class.: Flavanoid

ACTION: Exhibits antiinflammatory, analgesic properties; thought to result from the inhibition of prostaglandin synthesis via the inhibition of cyclooxygenase

USES: Dietary management of osteoarthritis

CONTRAINDICATIONS: Hypersensitivity

Precautions: Pregnancy (UK), breastfeeding, children <18 yr, history of stomach ulcers, angina, CAD, edema, geriatric patients, GI disease, rheumatoid arthritis, stroke, tachycardia/MI

DOSAGE AND ROUTES

- **Adult: PO** 250-500 mg with or without 50 mg of citrated zinc bisglycinate 250/50 mg or 500/50 mg q12hr

Available forms: Cap 250 mg

Administer:

- 1 hr before or after meals, food increases absorption

SIDE EFFECTS

MISC: Hypertension, increase in varicose veins, psoriasis

MS: Fluid accumulation in the knees

PHARMACOKINETICS

Metabolism primarily via glucuronidation and sulfation

NURSING CONSIDERATIONS

Assess:

- **Pain of rheumatoid arthritis, osteoarthritis;** check ROM, inflammation of joints, characteristics of pain
- For history of GI ulcers, bleeding; use fecal occult blood test to determine GI bleeding

Evaluate:

- Therapeutic response: decreased pain, inflammation in arthritic conditions

Teach patient/family:

- That product does not take the place of other products, including corticosteroids for osteoarthritis
- To notify prescriber if pregnancy is planned or suspected

flecainide (Rx)

(flek-ay′nide)

Tambocor

Func. class.: Antidysrhythmic (Class IC)

ACTION: Decreases conduction in all parts of the heart, with greatest effect on the His-Purkinje system, which stabilizes cardiac membrane

USES: Life-threatening ventricular dysrhythmias, sustained ventricular tachycardia, supraventricular tachydysrhythmias, paroxysmal atrial fibrillation/flutter associated with disabling symptoms

Unlabeled uses: Atrial fibrillation, single dose

CONTRAINDICATIONS: Hypersensitivity, severe heart block, cardiogenic shock, nonsustained ventricular dysrhythmias, frequent PVCs, non–life-threatening dysrhythmias

Precautions: Pregnancy (C), breastfeeding, children, geriatric patients, renal/hepatic disease, CHF, respiratory depression, myasthenia gravis, electrolyte abnormalities, atrial fibrillation, sick sinus syndrome, torsades de pointes

Black Box Warning: MI, cardiac arrhythmias

DOSAGE AND ROUTES

PSVT/PAT

- **Adult: PO** 50 mg q12hr; may increase q4days by 50 mg q12hr to desired response, max 300 mg/day

Life-threatening ventricular dysrhythmias

- **Adult: PO** 100 mg q12hr; may increase by 50 mg q12hr q4days, max 400 mg/day

Renal dose

- **Adult: PO** CCr <35 ml/min, 100 mg daily or 50 mg bid initially

Available forms: Tabs 50, 100, 150 mg

Administer:

- Reduced dosage as soon as dysrhythmia is controlled
- May give with meals for GI upset
- May adjust dose q4days

SIDE EFFECTS

CNS: *Headache, dizziness,* involuntary movement, confusion, psychosis, restlessness, irritability, paresthesias, ataxia, flushing, somnolence, depression, anxiety, malaise, fatigue, asthenia, tremors

CV: *Hypotension, bradycardia,* angina, PVCs, **heart block, cardiovascular collapse, arrest,** dysrhythmias, **CHF, fatal ventricular tachycardia,** palpitations, **QT prolongation, torsades de pointes**

EENT: Tinnitus, *blurred vision,* hearing loss, corneal deposits, dry eyes

GI: Nausea, vomiting, anorexia, constipation, abdominal pain, flatulence, change in taste, diarrhea

GU: Impotence, decreased libido, polyuria, urinary retention

HEMA: Leukopenia, thrombocytopenia

INTEG: Rash, urticaria, edema, swelling

RESP: Dyspnea, **respiratory depression**

PHARMACOKINETICS

Peak 3 hr, half-life 12-27 hr, metabolized by liver, excreted unchanged by kidneys (10%), excreted in breast milk

INTERACTIONS

Increase: of both products—propranolol

Increase: CV depressant action—β-blockers, disopyramide, verapamil

Increase: flecainide level—amiodarone, cimetidine, ritonavir

Increase: digoxin level—digoxin

Increase or decrease: effect—urinary, alkalinizing agents, acidifying agents

Drug/Lab Test

Increase: CPK

NURSING CONSIDERATIONS

Assess:

- I&O, daily weight

⚠ **CHF: edema, weight gain, dyspnea, jugular venous distention, crackles**

• **Electrolyte imbalances:** hypo/hyperkalemia before administration; correct electrolytes
• **Dysrhythmias:** B/P, ECG or Holter monitor continuously for fluctuations; watch for QRS widening, prolongation of QT and PR
• CNS effects: dizziness, confusion, psychosis, paresthesias, seizures; product should be discontinued
• Increased respiration, pulse; product should be discontinued

Evaluate:
• Therapeutic response: decreased dysrhythmias

Teach patient/family:
• To change position slowly from lying or sitting to standing to minimize orthostatic hypotension
• To take as prescribed; not to skip or double dose
• To avoid hazardous activities that require alertness until response is known
• To carry emergency ID with disorder, medications taken
• To notify all health care providers of treatment
• To report new or worsening cardiac symptoms

TREATMENT OF OVERDOSE:
O_2, artificial ventilation, ECG, DOPamine for circulatory depression, diazepam or thiopental for seizures, treat ventricular dysrhythmias

RARELY USED

floxuridine (Rx)
(flox-yoor′i-deen)
FUDR
Func. class.: Antineoplastic, antimetabolite

USES: Hepatocellular, colorectal cancer metastatic to liver

CONTRAINDICATIONS: Pregnancy (D), breastfeeding; hypersensitivity, poor nutritional status, serious infections

Black Box Warning: Myelosuppression, GI bleeding

DOSAGE AND ROUTES
• **Adult: INTRAARTERIAL** by cont inf 0.1-0.6 mg/kg/day × 1-6 wk

fluconazole (Rx)
(floo-kon′a-zole)
Apo-Fluconazole ✦, Diflucan, Gen-Fluconazole ✦
Func. class.: Antifungal, systemic; azole
Chem class: Triazole

Do not confuse:
Diflucan/Diprivan

ACTION: Inhibits ergosterol biosynthesis, causes direct damage to fungal membrane phospholipids

USES: Oropharyngeal candidiasis, chronic mucocutaneous candidiasis; systemic, vaginal, urinary candidiasis; cryptococcal meningitis; prevention of candidiasis in bone marrow transplant in those who receive chemotherapy and/or radiation therapy; cystitis, fungal prophylaxis, peritonitis, pneumonia, pyelonephritis
Unlabeled uses: Prophylaxis, systemic candidiasis in very-low-birthweight premature infants, blastomycosis, chemotherapy-induced neutropenia, coccidioidomycosis cryptococcosis prophylaxis, endocarditis, endophthalmitis, histoplasmosis infectious arthritis, myocarditis, osteomyelitis, pericarditis

CONTRAINDICATIONS: Hypersensitivity to this product or azoles, pregnancy (D)
Precautions: Breastfeeding, renal/hepatic disease, torsades de pointes

DOSAGE AND ROUTES

Vaginal candidiasis

- **Adult: PO** 150 mg as a single dose

Serious fungal infections

- **Adult: PO/IV** 50-400 mg initially then 200 mg/day for 4 wk
- **Child:** 6-12 mg/kg/day

Oropharyngeal candidiasis

- **Adult: PO/IV** 200 mg initially then 100 mg/day for ≥2 wk
- **Child: PO/IV** 6 mg/kg initially then 3 mg/kg/day for ≥2 wk

Prevention of candidiasis in bone marrow transplant

- **Adult: PO/IV** 400 mg/day

Renal disease

- **Adult: PO/IV** CCr ≤50 ml/min, after loading dose, give 50% of usual dose

Available forms: Tabs 50, 100, 150, 200 mg; inj 2 mg/ml; powder for oral susp 50, 200 mg/ml

Administer:

PO route

- Tap bottle to loosen powder, add 24 ml distilled or purified water to bottles with 0.35 or 1.4 g drug, shake well, conc 50 or 200 mg/5 ml, respectively
- Shake oral susp before each use

Intermittent IV INF route

- After diluting according to package directions; run at ≤200 mg/hr; do not use plastic containers in connections; check for bag leaks
- Use inf pump; check for extravasation and necrosis q2hr
- Do not use if cloudy or precipitated
- Do not admix; do not refrigerate

Y-site compatibilities: Acyclovir, aldesleukin, alfentanil, allopurinol, amifostine, amikacin, aminocaproic acid, aminophylline, amiodarone, anidulafungin, ascorbic acid injection, atenolol, atracurium, atropine, azathioprine, aztreonam, benztropine, bivalirudin, bleomycin, bumetanide, buprenorphine, butorphanol, calcium chloride, CARBOplatin, caspofungin, cefamandole, ceFAZolin, cefepime, cefmetazole, cefonicid, cefoperazone, cefotetan, cefoxitin, cefpirome, ceftazidime, ceftizoxime, ceftobiprole, cephalothin, cephapirin, chlorproMAZINE, cimetidine, cisatracurium, CISplatin, codeine, cyanocobalamin, cyclophosphamide, cycloSPORINE, cytarabine, DACTINomycin, DAPTOmycin, dexamethasone, diltiazem, dimenhyDRINATE, diphenhydrAMINE, DOBUTamine, docetaxel, DOPamine, doripenem, doxacurium, DOXOrubicin, DOXOrubicin liposomal, doxycycline, droperidol, drotrecogin alfa, enalaprilat, ePHEDrine, EPINEPHrine, epirubicin,epoetin alfa, eptifibatide, ertapenem, erythromycin, esmolol, etoposide, famotidine, fenoldopam, fentaNYL, filgrastim, fludarabine, fluorouracil, folic acid, foscarnet, gallium, ganciclovir, gatifloxacin, gemcitabine, gentamicin, glycopyrrolate, granisetron, heparin, hydrocortisone, HYDROmorphone, IDArubicin, ifosfamide, IV immune globulin, inamrinone, indomethacin, insulin (regular), irinotecan, isoproterenol, ketorolac, labetalol, lansoprazole, leucovorin, levofloxacin, lidocaine, linezolid, LORazepam, LR, magnesium sulfate, mannitol, mechlorethamine, melphalan, meperidine, meropenem, metaraminol, methicillin, methotrexate, methoxamine, methyldopate, methylPREDNISolone, metoclopramide, metoprolol, metroNIDAZOLE, mezlocillin, miconazole, midazolam, milrinone, minocycline, mitoxantrone, morphine, moxalactam, multiple vitamins injection, mycophenolate, nafcillin, nalbuphine, naloxone, nesiritide, nitroglycerin, nitroprusside, norepinephrine, octreotide, ondansetron, oxacillin, oxaliplatin, oxytocin, paclitaxel, palonosetron, pamidronate, pancuronium, papaverine, pemetrexed, penicillin G potassium/sodium, pentazocine, PENTobarbital, PHENobarbital, phenylephrine, phenytoin, phytonadione, piperacillin-tazobactam, polymyxin B, potassium chloride, procainamide, prochlorperazine, promethazine, propofol, propranolol, protamine, pyridoxine, quiNIDine, quinupristin-dalfopristin, ranitidine, remifentanil, Ringer's, ritodrine, riTUXimab, rocuronium, sargramostim, sodium acetate/bicarbonate, succinylcholine, SUFentanil, tacrolimus, temocillin, teniposide, theophylline, thiotepa, ticarcillin-clavulanate, tigecycline, tirofiban, TNA, tobramycin, tolazoline, TPN, trastuzumab, trimetaphan, urokinase, vancomycin, vasopressin, vecuronium, verapamil, vinCRIStine, vinorelbine, voriconazole, zidovudine, zoledronic acid

SIDE EFFECTS

CNS: Headache, **seizures**
CV: **QT prolongation, torsades de pointes**
GI: Nausea, vomiting, diarrhea, cramping, flatus, increased AST, ALT, **hepatotoxicity**
HEMA: **Agranulocytosis, eosinophilia, leukopenia, neutropenia, thrombocytopenia**
INTEG: **Stevens-Johnson syndrome, angioedema, anaphylaxis, exfoliative dermatitis, toxic epidermal necrolysis**

PHARMACOKINETICS

Peak 2-4 hr, bioavailability (PO) >90%, excreted unchanged in urine 80%, metabolized by CYP3A enzyme system at dose >200 mg/day, elimination half-life 30 hr

INTERACTIONS

Increase: hypoglycemia—oral antidiabetics
Increase: anticoagulation—warfarin
Increase: plasma concentrations—cycloSPORINE, phenytoin, theophylline, rifabutin, tacrolimus, sirolimus
Increase: myopathy, rhabdomyolysis risk—lovastatin, simvastatin
Increase: effect of zidovudine, methadone, SUFentanil, alfentanil, buprenorphine, saquinavir, fentaNYL, ergots
Decrease: effect of oral contraceptives, calcium channel blockers

NURSING CONSIDERATIONS

Assess:

• **Infection:** clearing of CSF and other culture during treatment, obtain C&S baseline and throughout treatment, product may be started as soon as culture is taken

⚠ **Hepatotoxicity: increasing AST, ALT, periodically alk phos, bilirubin; for renal status: BUN, creatinine**

Perform/provide:

• Storage protected from moisture and light; diluted sol stable 24 hr; do not freeze

Evaluate:

• Therapeutic response: decreasing oral candidiasis, fever, malaise, rash; negative C&S for infection organism

Teach patient/family:

• That long-term therapy may be needed to clear infection
• That medication may be taken with food to reduce GI effects
• To notify prescriber of nausea, vomiting, diarrhea, jaundice, anorexia, clay-colored stools, dark urine
• To use alternative method of contraception while taking this product, pregnancy (D)

RARELY USED

fludarabine (Rx)

(floo-dar′a-been)

Fludara, Oforta

Func. class.: Antineoplastic, antimetabolite

USES: Chronic lymphocytic leukemia, non-Hodgkin's lymphoma

CONTRAINDICATIONS: Pregnancy (D), breastfeeding, hypersensitivity

Black Box Warning: Hemolytic anemia, bone marrow suppression, coma, seizures, visual disturbances

DOSAGE AND ROUTES

• **Adult: IV** 25 mg/m^2 over 30 min × 5 days, may repeat q28days; reconstitute with 2 ml of sterile water for inj; dissolution should occur in <15 sec, adjust dose based on toxicity; **PO** 40 mg/m^2 × 5 days q28days

flumazenil (Rx)

(flu-maz′e-nill)

Anexate ✱, Romazicon

Func. class.: Antidote: benzodiazepine receptor antagonist

Chem. class.: Imidazobenzodiazepine derivative

ACTION: Antagonizes actions of benzodiazepines on CNS, competitively inhibits activity at benzodiazepine recognition site on GABA/benzodiazepine receptor complex

USES: Reversal of sedative effects of benzodiazepines

CONTRAINDICATIONS: Hypersensitivity to this product or benzodiazepines, serious cyclic antidepressant overdose, patients given benzodiazepine for control of life-threatening conditions

Precautions: Pregnancy (C), breastfeeding, children, geriatric patients, status epilepticus, head injury, labor/delivery, renal/hepatic disease, hypoventilation, panic disorder, drug and alcohol dependency, ambulatory patients

Black Box Warning: Benzodiazepine dependence, seizures

DOSAGE AND ROUTES

Reversal of conscious sedation or general anesthesia

- **Adult: IV** 0.2 mg given over 15 sec; wait 45 sec then give 0.2 mg if consciousness does not occur; may be repeated at 60-sec intervals prn (max 3 mg/hr) or 1 mg/5 min
- **Child: IV** 10 mcg (0.01 mg)/kg; cumulative dose of 1 mg or less

Management of suspected benzodiazepine overdose

- **Adult: IV** 0.2 mg given over 30 sec; wait 30 sec then give 0.3 mg over 30 sec if consciousness does not occur; further doses of 0.5 mg can be given over 30 sec at intervals of 1 min up to cumulative dose of 3 mg
- **Child: IV** 10 mcg (0.01 mg/kg), cumulative dose of <1 mg

Available forms: Inj 0.1 mg/ml

Administer:

- Check airway and IV access before administration
- Use large vein

Direct IV route

- Give undiluted or diluted with 0.9% NaCl, D_5W, LR; give over 15-30 sec into running IV
- Stable for 24 hr if drawn into a syringe or mixed with other solutions

SIDE EFFECTS

CNS: Dizziness, agitation, emotional lability, confusion, **seizures**, somnolence, panic attacks

CV: Hypertension, palpitations, cutaneous vasodilation, **dysrhythmias**, bradycardia, tachycardia, chest pain

EENT: Abnormal vision, blurred vision, tinnitus

GI: Nausea, vomiting, hiccups

SYST: Headache, inj site pain, increased sweating, fatigue, rigors

PHARMACOKINETICS

Terminal half-life 41-79 min, metabolized in liver, onset 1-2 min

INTERACTIONS

- Toxicity: mixed product overdosage
- Antagonize action of benzodiazepines, zaleplon, zolpidem

NURSING CONSIDERATIONS

Assess:

- Cardiac status using continuous monitoring
- For seizures; protect patient from in-

jury; most likely among those who are withdrawing from sedatives

- GI symptoms: nausea, vomiting; place patient in side-lying position to prevent aspiration
- **Allergic reactions:** flushing, rash, urticaria, pruritus

Black Box Warning: Seizures/benzodiazepine dependence: do not use in those who have used these products for IIP or status epilepticus; use in intensive care setting cautiously, there may be unrecognized benzodiazepine dependence

Evaluate:

- Therapeutic response: decreased sedation, respiratory depression, toxicity

Teach patient/family:

- That amnesia may continue
- Not to engage in hazardous activities for 18-24 hr after discharge
- Not to take any alcohol or non-prescription products for 18-24 hr

flunisolide nasal agent

See Appendix B

fluocinolone ophthalmic

See Appendix B

fluocinolone topical

See Appendix B

fluorometholone ophthalmic

See Appendix B

⚠ HIGH ALERT

fluorouracil (Rx)

(flure-oh-yoor′a-sil)

Adrucil, Carac, Efudex, 5-FU

Func. class.: Antineoplastic, antimetabolite

Chem. class.: Pyrimidine analog

Do not confuse:
fluorouracil/flucytosine

ACTION: Inhibits DNA, RNA synthesis; interferes with cell replication by competitively inhibiting thymidylate production, specific for S phase of cell cycle; vesicant

USES: *Systemic:* cancer of breast, colon, rectum, stomach, pancreas; *topical:* multiple actinic keratoses, superficial basal cell carcinomas

CONTRAINDICATIONS: Pregnancy (X), breastfeeding, hypersensitivity, poor nutritional status, serious infections, major surgery within 1 mo

Black Box Warning: Bone marrow suppression

Precautions: Children, renal/hepatic disease, angina

Black Box Warning: GI bleeding

DOSAGE AND ROUTES

Doses vary widely, based on actual body weight unless obese, then based on lean body weight

Advanced colorectal cancer

- **Adult:** IV 370 mg/m² given after leucovorin or 425 mg/m² given after leucovorin daily × 5 days; repeat q4-5wk

Other cancer

- **Adult:** IV 12 mg/kg/day × 4 days, max 800 mg/day; may repeat with 6 mg/kg on days 6, 8, 10, 12; maintenance is 10-15 mg/kg/wk as a single dose, max 1 g/wk

Actinic/solar keratoses

- **Adult:** TOP 1% cream/sol 1-2×/day or 2-5% sol for hands

Superficial basal cell carcinoma
- **Adult: TOP** 5% sol or cream 2×/day × 3-12 wk

Available forms: Inj 50 mg/ml; cream 1%, 5%; sol 1%, 2%, 5%

Administer:
- Antiemetic 30-60 min before product to prevent vomiting, for several days thereafter

Topical route
- Wear gloves when applying; may use with a loose dressing; use plastic or wooden applicator

IV route
- Prepared in biologic cabinet using gloves, gown, mask; use cytotoxic handling procedures
- Undiluted; may inject through Y-tube or 3-way stopcock; give over 1-3 min; may be diluted in NS, D_5W, given over 2-8 hr as IV INF

Y-site compatibilities: Acyclovir, alfentanil, allopurinol, amifostine, amikacin, amphotericin B lipid complex, amphotericin B liposome, ampicillin, ampicillin-sulbactam, anidulafungin, atenolol, atracurium, azithromycin, aztreonam, bivalirudin, bleomycin, bumetanide, butorphanol, calcium gluconate, CARBOplatin, ceFAZolin, cefepime, cefoperazone, cefotaxime, cefotetan, cefoxitin, ceftazidime, ceftizoxime, cefTRIAXone, cefuroxime, cimetidine, cisatracurium, CISplatin, clindamycin, codeine, cyclophosphamide, cycloSPORINE, DAPTOmycin, dexamethasone, digoxin, docetaxel, DOPamine, doripenem, DOXOrubicin liposomal, enalaprilat, ePHEDrine, ertapenem, erythromycin, esmolol, etoposide phosphate, famotidine, fenoldopam, fentaNYL, fluconazole, fludarabine, foscarnet, fosphenytoin, furosemide, ganciclovir, gatifloxacin, gemcitabine, gentamicin, granisetron, heparin, hydrocortisone, HYDROmorphone, ifosfamide, imipenem-cilastatin, inamrinone, isoproterenol, ketorolac, labetalol, leucovorin, levorphanol, lidocaine, linezolid, magnesium sulfate, mannitol, melphalan, meperidine, meropenem, mesna, methohexital, methotrexate, methylPREDNISolone, metoprolol, metroNIDAZOLE, milrinone, mitomycin, mitoxantrone, morphine sulfate, nalbuphine, naloxone, nesiritide, nitroglycerin, nitroprusside, octreotide, ofloxacin, paclitaxel, palonosetron, pamidronate, pancuronium, pantoprazole, pemetrexed, PENTobarbital, PHENobarbital, phenylephrine, piperacillin, piperacillin-tazobactam, potassium chloride/phosphates, procainamide, propofol, propranolol, ranitidine, remifentanil, riTUXimab, sargramostim, sodium acetate/bicarbonate/phosphates, succinylcholine, SUFentanil, sulfamethoxazole-trimethoprim, teniposide, theophylline, thiopental, thiotepa, ticarcillin, ticarcillin-clavulanate, tigecycline, tirofiban, tobramycin, trastuzumab, vasopressin, vecuronium, vinBLAStine, vinCRIStine, vitamin B complex/C, voriconazole, zidovudine, zoledronic acid

SIDE EFFECTS

Systemic use

CNS: Lethargy, malaise, weakness, acute cerebellar dysfunction

CV: Myocardial ischemia, angina

EENT: Epistaxis, light intolerance, lacrimation

GI: *Anorexia, stomatitis,* diarrhea, nausea, vomiting, **hemorrhage**, enteritis, glossitis

HEMA: **Thrombocytopenia, leukopenia, myelosuppression, anemia, agranulocytosis**

INTEG: *Rash,* fever, photosensitivity

PHARMACOKINETICS

Half-life 20 hr terminal; metabolized in liver; excreted in urine; crosses blood-brain barrier

INTERACTIONS

Increase: toxicity, bone marrow depression—radiation or other antineoplastics

Decrease: antibody response—live virus vaccines

Drug/Lab Test
Increase: AST, ALT, LDH, serum bilirubin, Hct, Hgb, WBC, platelets, 5-HIAA
Decrease: albumin

NURSING CONSIDERATIONS

Assess:

Black Box Warning: Bone marrow suppression: CBC, differential, platelet count daily (IV); withhold product if WBC is <3500/mm³ or platelet count is <100,000/mm³; notify prescriber of results; product should be discontinued; nadir of leukopenia within 2 wk, recovery 1 mo

- Renal studies: BUN, serum uric acid, urine CCr, electrolytes before, during therapy
- Hepatic studies before, during therapy: bilirubin, alk phos, AST, ALT, LDH before, during therapy
- **Bleeding:** hematuria, guaiac, bruising, petechiae, mucosa or orifices q8hr
- Inflammation of mucosa, breaks in skin; buccal cavity q8hr for dryness, sores or ulceration, white patches, oral pain, bleeding, dysphagia
- GI symptoms: frequency of stools, cramping, intractable vomiting, stomatitis

Perform/provide:

- Strict asepsis, protective isolation if WBC levels low
- Changing of IV site q48hr
- Rinsing of mouth tid-qid with water, club soda; brushing of teeth bid-tid with soft brush or cotton-tipped applicator for stomatitis; use unwaxed dental floss, give ice chips for mucositis
- Nutritious diet with iron, vitamin supplements, low fiber, few dairy products, especially when combined with radiotherapy as ordered

Evaluate:

- Therapeutic response: decreased tumor size, spread of malignancy

Teach patient/family:

- To avoid crowds, persons with known infection
- To avoid foods with citric acid, hot or rough texture if stomatitis is present; to drink adequate fluids
- To report stomatitis: any bleeding, white spots, ulcerations in mouth; that patient should examine mouth daily, report symptoms; viscous lidocaine may be used
- To report signs of **infection:** fever, sore throat, flulike symptoms
- To report signs of **anemia:** fatigue, headache, faintness, shortness of breath, irritability
- To report **bleeding:** to avoid razors, commercial mouthwash
- Not to use aspirin products or NSAIDs
- To use contraception during therapy (men and women), pregnancy (X); to avoid breastfeeding (topical use)
- Not to receive vaccinations during therapy
- To use sunscreen or stay out of the sun to prevent photosensitivity
- About hair loss; to explore use of wigs or other products until hair regrowth occurs
- To apply topically only to affected areas, being careful around mouth, nose, eyes

FLUoxetine (Rx)

(floo-ox′eh-teen)

Apo-Fluoxetine ✥, CO-Fluoxetine ✥, Gen-Fluoxetine ✥, Novo-Fluoxetine ✥, Nu-Fluoxetine ✥, PMS-Fluoxetine ✥, Prozac, Prozac Weekly, Sandoz Fluoxetine ✥, Sarafem, Selfemra

Func. class.: Antidepressant, SSRI (selective serotonin reuptake inhibitor)

Do not confuse:
Prozac/Proscar/ProSom/PriLOSEC
Sarafem/Serophene

ACTION: Inhibits CNS neuron uptake of serotonin but not of norepinephrine

USES:
Major depressive disorder, obsessive-compulsive disorder (OCD), bulimia nervosa; *Sarafem:* premenstrual dysphoric disorder (PMDD), panic disorder

Unlabeled uses: Alcoholism, anorexia nervosa, borderline personality disorder, obesity, posttraumatic stress disorder, autism, fibromyalgia, orthostatic hypotension, premature ejaculation

CONTRAINDICATIONS:
Hypersensitivity

Precautions: Pregnancy (C), breastfeeding, geriatric patients, diabetes mellitus, narrow-angle glaucoma, cardiac malformations in infants (exposed to FLUoxetine in utero)

Black Box Warning: Children, suicidal ideation

DOSAGE AND ROUTES

Depression/obsessive-compulsive disorder

• **Adult: PO** 20 mg/day in AM; after 4 wk, if no clinical improvement is noted, dose may be increased to 20 mg bid in AM, PM, max 80 mg/day; **PO** 90 mg/wk

• **Geriatric: PO** 5-10 mg/day, increase as needed

• **Child 8-18 yr: PO** 5-10 mg/day, max 20 mg/day

Premenstrual dysphoric disorder (Sarafem)

• **Adult: PO** 20 mg/day, may be taken daily 14 days before menses

Alcoholism (unlabeled)

• **Adult: PO** 20-80 mg/day

Anorexia nervosa (unlabeled)

• **Adult: PO** 10 mg every other day to 20 mg/day

Borderline personality disorder/fibromyalgia/autism/orthostatic hypotension/premature ejaculation/hot flashes (unlabeled)

• **Adult: PO** 20 mg/day, max 80 mg/day

Obesity (unlabeled)

• **Adult: PO** 60 mg/day after titration

Posttraumatic stress disorder (unlabeled)

• **Adult: PO** 10-80 mg/day

Available forms: Caps 10, 20, 40 mg; tabs 10, 20 mg; oral sol 20 mg/5 ml; del rel caps (PROzac Weekly) 90 mg; tab 10, 15, 20 mg (Sarafem)

Administer:

• Without regard to meals

• Crushed if patient is unable to swallow medication whole (tab only)

• Gum, hard candy, frequent sips of water for dry mouth

• **PROzac Weekly** on the same day each week, swallow whole; do not crush, cut, chew

• **Oral sol:** use oral syringe or calibrated measuring device

SIDE EFFECTS

CNS: *Headache, nervousness, insomnia, drowsiness, anxiety, tremor, dizziness, fatigue, sedation, poor concentration, abnormal dreams, agitation,* **seizures**, apathy, euphoria, hallucinations, delusions, psychosis, **suicidal ideation, neuroleptic malignant syndrome–like reactions**, serotonin syndrome

CV: *Hot flashes, palpitations,* angina pectoris, hypertension, **tachycardia, 1st-degree AV block, bradycardia, MI, thrombophlebitis**

EENT: Visual changes, ear/eye pain, photophobia, tinnitus

GI: *Nausea, diarrhea, dry mouth, anorexia, dyspepsia, constipation, cramps, vomiting, taste changes, flatulence, decreased appetite*

GU: *Dysmenorrhea, decreased libido, urinary frequency, UTI,* amenorrhea, cystitis, impotence, urine retention

HEMA: **Hemorrhage**

INTEG: *Sweating, rash, pruritus,* acne, alopecia, urticaria, **angioedema, exfoliative dermatitis, Stevens-Johnson syndrome, toxic epidermal necrolysis**

META: Hyponatremia

MS: *Pain,* arthritis, twitching

RESP: *Infection, pharyngitis, nasal congestion, sinus headache, sinusitis,*

cough, dyspnea, bronchitis, asthma, hyperventilation, pneumonia
SYST: *Asthenia, viral infection, fever, allergy, chills*

PHARMACOKINETICS

PO: Peak 6-8 hr, metabolized in liver, excreted in urine, terminal half-life 2-3 days, norfluoxetine active metabolite half-life 4-16 days, steady state 28-35 days, protein binding 94%

INTERACTIONS

Increase: serotonin syndrome—SSRIs, SNRIs, serotonin-receptor agonists, selegiline, busPIRone, tryptophan, phenothiazines, haloperidol, loxapine, thiothixene, tricyclics; do not use concurrently
Increase: bleeding risk—platelet inhibitors, thrombolytics, NSAIDs, salicylates, anticoagulants
⚠ Do not use MAOIs with or 14 days prior to FLUoxetine
Increase: levels or toxicity of carBAMazepine, lithium, digoxin, warfarin, phenytoin, diazepam, vinBLAStine, donepezil, antidiabetics, dorifenacin, paricalcitrol, budesonide, bosentan
Increase: CNS depression—alcohol, antidepressants, opioids, sedatives
Decrease: FLUoxetine effect—cyproheptadine

Drug/Herb

⚠ Do not use together; increased risk of serotonin syndrome: St. John's wort, SAM-e
Increase: CNS effect—hops, kava, lavender, valerian

Drug/Lab Test

Increase: serum bilirubin, blood glucose, alk phos, BUN, CK

NURSING CONSIDERATIONS

Assess:

Black Box Warning: Mental status: mood, sensorium, affect, suicidal tendencies (child/young adult), increase in psychiatric symptoms, depression, panic; monitor for seizures, seizure potential increased

- **Bulimia nervosa:** appetite, weight daily, increase nutritious foods in diet, watch for bingeing and vomiting

⚠ **Allergic reactions/serious skin reactions:** angioedema, exfoliative dermatitis, Stevens-Johnson syndrome, toxic epidermal necrolysis, itching, rash, urticaria; product should be discontinued, may need to give antihistamine

- B/P (lying/standing), pulse q4hr; if systolic B/P drops 20 mm Hg, hold product, notify prescriber; ECG for flattening of T wave, bundle branch, AV block, dysrhythmias in cardiac patients
- Blood studies: CBC, leukocytes, differential, cardiac enzymes if patient is receiving long-term therapy; check platelets; bleeding can occur, thyroid function, growth rate, weight
- Hepatic studies: AST, ALT, bilirubin, creatinine, weight weekly; appetite may decrease with product
- Alcohol consumption; if alcohol is consumed, hold dose until AM

Perform/provide:

- Storage at room temp; do not freeze
- Safety measures, primarily for geriatric patients

Evaluate:

- Therapeutic response: decreased depression, symptoms of OCD

Teach patient/family:

- That therapeutic effect may take 1-4 wk
- To use caution when driving, performing other activities requiring alertness because of drowsiness, dizziness, blurred vision
- To avoid alcohol, other CNS depressants
- To notify prescriber if pregnant, planning to become pregnant, or breastfeeding
- To change positions slowly because orthostatic hypotension may occur
- To avoid all OTC products unless approved by prescriber

Black Box Warning: That suicidal thoughts/behaviors may occur in young adults, children

fluphenazine decanoate (Rx)

(floo-fen′a-zeen)

Apo-Fluphenazine Decanoate ✤, Modecate ✤

fluphenazine hydrochloride (Rx)

Apo-Fluphenazine ✤

Func. class.: Antipsychotic

Chem. class.: Phenothiazine, piperazine

Do not confuse:
Prolixin/Proloid

ACTION: Depresses cerebral cortex, hypothalamus, limbic system, which control activity and aggression; blocks neurotransmission produced by DOPamine at synapse; exhibits strong α-adrenergic and anticholinergic blocking action; mechanism for antipsychotic effects is unclear

USES: Psychotic disorders, schizophrenia

CONTRAINDICATIONS: Hypersensitivity, circulatory collapse, hepatic damage, cerebral arteriosclerosis, coronary disease, severe hypo/hypertension, blood dyscrasias, coma, brain damage, closed-angle glaucoma, bone marrow depression, alcohol and barbiturate withdrawal

Precautions: Pregnancy (C), breastfeeding, children <12 yr, geriatric patients, seizure disorders, hypertension, cardiac/hepatic disease

Black Box Warning: Dementia

DOSAGE AND ROUTES

Decanoate

- **Adult and child >16 yr: IM/SUBCUT** 12.5-25 mg q1-3wk, may increase slowly
- **Child 12-16 yr: IM/SUBCUT** 6.25-18.75 mg, then repeat q1-3wk, then increase slowly; max 25 mg
- **Child 5-12 yr: IM/SUBCUT** 3.125-12.5 mg, then repeat q1-3wk, increase slowly

HCl

- **Adult: PO** 2.5-10 mg in divided doses q6-8hr, max 40 mg/day; **IM** initially 1.25 mg then 2.5-10 mg in divided doses q6-8hr
- **Child: PO** 0.25-3.5 mg/day in divided doses q4-6hr, max 10 mg/day

Available forms: *Decanoate:* inj 25 mg/ml; *HCl:* tabs 1, 2.5, 5, 10 mg; inj 2.5 mg/ml

Administer:

- **PO:** with food, milk, or full glass of water
- **Oral sol:** with juice, milk, or uncaffeinated drink
- Anticholinergic agent if EPS occur
- IM (HCL only) inj into large muscle mass; to minimize postural hypotension, give inj, have patient remain seated or recumbent for ½ hr
- Use dry needle or solution will become cloudy; use 21G or larger due to viscosity

SIDE EFFECTS

CNS: *EPS: pseudoparkinsonism, akathisia, dystonia, tardive dyskinesia, drowsiness, headache,* **seizures, neuroleptic malignant syndrome**

CV: *Orthostatic hypotension,* hypertension, **cardiac arrest,** ECG changes, **tachycardia**

EENT: Blurred vision, glaucoma, dry eyes

GI: *Dry mouth, nausea, vomiting, anorexia, constipation,* diarrhea, jaundice, weight gain, **paralytic ileus, hepatitis,** cholecystic jaundice

GU: Urinary retention, urinary frequency, enuresis, impotence, amenorrhea, gynecomastia

HEMA: Anemia, **leukopenia, leukocytosis, agranulocytosis, aplastic anemia, thrombocytopenia**

INTEG: *Rash,* photosensitivity, dermatitis

RESP: **Laryngospasm,** dyspnea, **respiratory depression**

PHARMACOKINETICS

Metabolized by liver, excreted in urine (metabolites), crosses placenta, enters breast milk, protein binding >90%, not dialyzable

PO/IM (HCl): Onset 1 hr, peak 2-4 hr, duration 6-8 hr, half-life 3.5-4 days

IM/SUBCUT (decanoate): Onset 1-3 days; peak 1-2 days, duration over 4 wk, single-dose half-life 6.8-9.6 days, multiple dose 14.3 days

INTERACTIONS

Increase: serotonin syndrome, neuroleptic malignant syndrome—SSRIs, SNRIs, serotonin-receptor agonists

Increase: QT prolongation, torsades de pointes (at higher doses)—amiodarone, arsenic trioxide, astemizole, dasatinib, disopyramide, dofetilide, droperidol, erythromycin, flecainide, gatifloxacin, ibutilide, levomethadyl, ondansetron, paliperidone, palonosetron, some antidepressants, vorinostat, ziprasidone

Increase: sedation—other CNS depressants, alcohol, barbiturate anesthetics, haloperidol, metyrosine, risperidone

Increase: toxicity—EPINEPHrine

Increase: anticholinergic effects—anticholinergics

Decrease: effects of levodopa, lithium

Decrease: fluphenazine effects—smoking, barbiturates

Drug/Lab Test

Increase: LFTs, cardiac enzymes, cholesterol, blood glucose, prolactin, bilirubin, cholinesterase

Decrease: hormones (blood and urine)

False positive: pregnancy tests, PKU urinary steroids, 17-OHCS

NURSING CONSIDERATIONS

Assess:

Black Box Warning: Dementia: deaths have occurred; not approved for this use

- **Serotonin syndrome, neuroleptic malignant syndrome:** severe EPS, increased CPK, altered mental state, sinus tachycardia, change in B/P, sweating, often occurs in young men, heat stress, physical exhaustion, dehydration, organic brain disease

⚠ **QT prolongation, torsades de pointes:** ECG for changes

- Swallowing of PO medication; check for hoarding, giving of medication to other patients
- I&O ratio; palpate bladder if low urinary output occurs, urinary retention may be the cause
- Bilirubin, CBC, LFTs monthly
- Urinalysis recommended before and during prolonged therapy
- Affect, orientation, LOC, reflexes, gait, coordination, sleep pattern disturbances
- B/P standing and lying; pulse and respirations q4hr during initial treatment; establish baseline before starting treatment; report drops of 30 mm Hg
- Dizziness, faintness, palpitations, tachycardia on rising
- **EPS** including akathisia (inability to sit still, no pattern to movements), tardive dyskinesia (bizarre movements of jaw, mouth, tongue, extremities), pseudoparkinsonism (rigidity, tremors, pill rolling, shuffling gait)
- Constipation, urinary retention daily; if these occur, increase bulk, water in diet

Perform/provide:

- Supervised ambulation until stabilized on medication; do not involve patient in strenuous exercise; fainting possible; patient should not stand still for long periods
- Increased fluids to prevent constipation
- Sips of water, candy, gum for dry mouth
- Storage in tight, light-resistant container in cool environment

Evaluate:

- Therapeutic response: decrease in emotional excitement, hallucinations, delusions, paranoia, reorganization of patterns of thought, speech

Teach patient/family:

- That orthostatic hypotension occurs often; to rise from sitting or lying position

F

gradually; to avoid hazardous activities until stabilized on medication

- To avoid hot tubs, hot showers, tub baths, since hypotension may occur; that, in hot weather, heat stroke may occur; to take extra precautions to stay cool

⚠ **To avoid abrupt withdrawal of this product or EPS may result; that product should be withdrawn slowly**

- To avoid OTC preparations (cough, hay fever, cold) unless approved by prescriber; that serious product interactions may occur; to avoid use with alcohol, CNS depressants; that increased drowsiness may occur
- To use a sunscreen to prevent burns
- About the importance of compliance with product regimen
- About EPS and the need for meticulous oral hygiene, since oral candidiasis may occur
- To report sore throat, malaise, fever, bleeding, mouth sores; if these occur, CBC should be drawn, product discontinued
- That urine may turn pink to reddish brown

TREATMENT OF OVERDOSE:

Lavage; if orally ingested, provide an airway; *do not induce vomiting*

flurandrenolide topical

See Appendix B

flurazepam (Rx)

(flure-az′e-pam)

Apo-Flurazepam ✱

Func. class.: Sedative/hypnotic

Chem. class.: Benzodiazepine, long-acting

Controlled Substance Schedule IV (USA), Targeted (CDSA IV) (Canada)

Do not confuse:
flurazepam/temazepam

ACTION: Produces CNS depression at the limbic, thalamic, hypothalamic levels of CNS; may be mediated by neurotransmitter γ-aminobutyric acid (GABA); results are sedation, hypnosis, skeletal muscle relaxation, anticonvulsant activity, anxiolytic action

USES: Insomnia, short term

Unlabeled uses: Anxiety

CONTRAINDICATIONS: Pregnancy (X), breastfeeding

Precautions: Children <15 yr, geriatric patients, anemia, renal/hepatic disease, suicidal individuals, drug abuse, psychosis, angioedema, pulmonary disease, suicidal ideation, hypersensitivity to benzodiazepines, intermittent porphyria, uncontrolled pain, sleep apnea

DOSAGE AND ROUTES

- **Adult: PO** 15-30 mg at bedtime; may repeat dose once if needed
- **Geriatric: PO** 15 mg at bedtime; may increase if needed

Hepatic dose

Dosage adjustment may be needed due to prolonged half-life

Available forms: Caps 15, 30 mg

Administer:

- ½-1 hr before bedtime for sleeplessness
- Caps may be opened and mixed with food
- Best to avoid in geriatric patients; long half-life

SIDE EFFECTS

CNS: *Lethargy, drowsiness, daytime sedation,* dizziness, confusion, lightheadedness, headache, anxiety, irritability, complex sleep-related reactions: sleep driving, sleep eating

CV: Chest pain, pulse changes, palpitations

GI: Nausea, vomiting, diarrhea, heartburn, abdominal pain, constipation

HEMA: Leukopenia, granulocytopenia (rare)

MISC: Physical, psychological dependence, blurred vision, **apnea**

PHARMACOKINETICS

PO: Onset 15-45 min, duration 7-8 hr, metabolized by liver, excreted by kidneys (inactive/active metabolites), crosses placenta, excreted in breast milk, half-life 47-100 hr, 97% protein binding

INTERACTIONS

Increase: flurazepam effects—cimetidine, disulfiram, probenicid, isoniazid, oral contraceptives, FLUoxetine, ketoconazole, propranolol, valproic acid, CYP3A4 inhibitors

Increase: CNS depression—alcohol, CNS depressants

Decrease: flurazepam effect—rifampin, barbiturates, theophylline

Drug/Herb

Decrease: flurazepam effect—St. John's wort

Drug/Lab Test

Increase: AST, ALT, serum bilirubin

Decrease: RAI uptake

False increase: urinary 17-OHCS

NURSING CONSIDERATIONS

Assess:

- Mental status: mood, sensorium, affect, memory (long, short); physical, psychological dependence or tolerance
- Type of sleep problem: falling asleep, staying asleep
- Withdrawal signs if discontinued abruptly
- For excessive sedation, impaired coordination, especially in geriatric patients

Perform/provide:

- Assistance with ambulation after receiving dose, safety measures: night-light, call bell within easy reach
- Storage in tight container in cool environment

Evaluate:

- Therapeutic response: ability to sleep at night, decreased amount of early morning awakening if taking product for insomnia

Teach patient/family:

- To avoid driving or other activities requiring alertness until product is stabilized
- To avoid alcohol, CNS depressants; serious CNS depression may result
- That effects may take 2 nights for benefits to be noticed; limit to 7-10 days of continuous use
- About alternative measures to improve sleep: reading, exercise several hours before bedtime, warm bath, warm milk, TV, self-hypnosis, deep breathing
- That hangover is common in geriatric patients
- To use contraceptives; pregnancy category (X)

TREATMENT OF OVERDOSE:

Lavage, activated charcoal; monitor electrolytes, VS

flurbiprofen ophthalmic

See Appendix B

flutamide (Rx)

(floo'ta-mide)

Apo-Flutamide ♣, Euflex ♣

Func. class.: Antineoplastic, hormone

Chem. class.: Antiandrogen

ACTION:

Interferes with androgen uptake in the nucleus or androgen activity in target tissues; arrests tumor growth in androgen-sensitive tissue (i.e., prostate gland)

USES:

Metastatic prostatic carcinoma, stage D_2 in combination with LHRH agonistic analogs (leuprolide), B_2-C in combination with goserelin and radiation

CONTRAINDICATIONS:

Pregnancy (D), hypersensitivity

Black Box Warning: Severe hepatic disease

Precautions: G6PD deficiency, hemoglobinopathy, lactase deficiency, polycystic ovary syndrome, tobacco smoking

DOSAGE AND ROUTES

- **Adult: PO** 250 mg q8hr for a daily dosage of 750 mg

Available forms: Caps 125, 250 ✱ mg

Administer:

- Do not break, crush, chew caps
- Flutamide must be taken with leuprolide; do not change dosing

SIDE EFFECTS

CNS: *Hot flashes,* drowsiness, confusion, depression, anxiety, paresthesia

GI: *Diarrhea, nausea, vomiting,* increased levels in hepatic studies, hepatitis, anorexia, hepatotoxicity, abdominal pain, cholestasis, **hepatic necrosis/failure**

GU: *Decreased libido, impotence, gynecomastia*

HEMA: Hemolytic anemia

INTEG: Irritation at site, rash, photosensitivity

MISC: Edema, neuromuscular and pulmonary symptoms, hypertension, secondary malignancy

PHARMACOKINETICS

Rapidly and completely absorbed; excreted in urine and feces as metabolites; half-life 6 hr, geriatric half-life 8 hr; 94% bound to plasma proteins

INTERACTIONS

Increase: PT—warfarin

Decrease: flutamide action—LHRH analog (leuprolide)

NURSING CONSIDERATIONS

Assess:

⚠ **Severe hepatic disease:** AST, ALT, alk phos, which may be elevated; if LFTs elevated, product may need to be discontinued; monitor CBC, bilirubin, creatinine

- CNS symptoms, including drowsiness, confusion, depression, anxiety

Evaluate:

- Therapeutic response: decrease in prostatic tumor size, decrease in spread of cancer

Teach patient/family:

- To report side effects: decreased libido, impotence, breast enlargement, hot flashes, diarrhea
- To report nausea, vomiting, yellow eyes or skin, dark urine, clay-colored stools; hepatotoxicity may be the cause
- Notify of yellow, green urine discoloration
- Avoid sun exposure, tanning beds
- To use contraception during treatment; pregnancy category (D)

fluticasone (Rx)

(floo-tic′a-sone)

Flovent HFA, Flovent Diskus

Func. class: Corticosteroids, inhalation; antiasthmatic

ACTION:
Decreases inflammation by inhibiting mast cells, macrophages, and leukotrienes; antiinflammatory and vasoconstrictor properties

USES:
Prevention of chronic asthma during maintenance treatment in those requiring oral corticosteroids; nasal symptoms of seasonal/perennial, allergic/nonallergic rhinitis

Unlabeled uses: COPD

CONTRAINDICATIONS:
Hypersensitivity to this product or milk protein, primary treatment in status asthmaticus

Precautions: Pregnancy (C), breastfeeding, active infections, glaucoma, diabetes, immunocompromised patients

DOSAGE AND ROUTES

Prevention of chronic asthma during maintenance treatment in those requiring oral corticosteroids

Flovent HFA

- **Adult and child ≥12 yr: INH** 88-660 mcg bid (in those previously taking bronchodilators alone); **INH** 88-220 mcg bid, max 440 mcg bid (in those previously taking inhaled corticosteroids); **INH** 440 mcg bid, max 880 mcg bid (in those previously taking oral corticosteroids)
- **Child 4-11 yr: INH** 88 mcg bid

Flovent Diskus

- **Adult and child ≥12 yr: INH** 100 mcg bid, max 500 mcg (in those previously taking bronchodilators alone); **INH** 100-250 mcg bid, max 500 mcg bid (in those previously taking inhaled corticosteroids); **INH** 500-1000 mcg bid, max 1000 mcg bid (in those previously taking oral corticosteroids)
- **Child 4-11 yr: INH** Initially 50 mcg bid, max 100 mcg bid (in those previously taking bronchodilators alone or inhaled corticosteroids)

Available forms: Oral inhalation aerosol 44, 110, 220 mcg; oral inhalation powder 50, 100, 250 mcg

Administer:

- Give at 1-min intervals; if a bronchodilator aerosol spray is used, use bronchodilator first, wait 5-15 min, then use fluticasone
- Decrease dose to lowest effective dose after desired effect; decrease dose at 2-4 wk intervals

Inhalation route (aerosol)

- Shake well, prime prior to 1st use, release 4 sprays into air away from face, prime using 1 spray if not used for ≥7 days; when the counter reads 000, discard; clean inhaler daily in warm water, dry; do not share inhaler with others
- In general, child <4 yr requires a face mask with spacer/VHC device for delivery; allow 3-5 INH per actuation; do not use spacer with Flovent Diskus

SIDE EFFECTS

CNS: Fever, headache, nervousness, dizziness, migraines, numbness in fingers

EENT: *Pharyngitis*, sinusitis, rhinitis, laryngitis, hoarseness, dry eyes, cataracts, nasal discharge, epistaxis

GI: Diarrhea, abdominal pain, nausea, vomiting, *oral candidiasis,* gastroenteritis

GU: UTI

INTEG: Urticaria, dermatitis

META: Hyperglycemia, growth retardation in children, cushingoid features

MISC: Influenza, **eosinophilic conditions, angioedema, Churg-Strauss syndrome, anaphylaxis, adrenal insufficiency (high** doses), bone mineral density reduction

MS: Osteoporosis, muscle soreness, joint pain

RESP: *Upper respiratory infection,* dyspnea, cough, bronchitis, **bronchospasm**

PHARMACOKINETICS

Absorption 30% aerosol, 13.5% powder; protein binding 91%; metabolized in liver after absorption in lung; half-life 7.8 hr; <5% excreted in urine and feces

Oral INH: Onset 24 hr, peak several days, duration 1-2 wk

INTERACTIONS

Increase: fluticasone levels—CYP3A4 inhibitors (ketoconazole, itraconazole), darunavir, nelfinavir, ritonavir, amprenavir, fosamprenavir, atazanavir, delavirdine, saquinavir

Increase: tendonitis, tendon rupture—quinolones

Decrease: effects of growth hormones—mecasermin

Drug/Lab Test

Increase: urine/serum glucose

NURSING CONSIDERATIONS

Assess:

- **Respiratory status:** lung sounds, pulmonary function tests during, for several months after change from systemic to inhalation corticosteroids

• Withdrawal symptoms from oral corticosteroids: depression, pain in joints, fatigue

⚠ **Adrenal insufficiency: nausea, weakness, fatigue, hypotension, hypoglycemia, anorexia; may occur when changing from systemic to inhalation corticosteroids; may be life-threatening; adrenal function tests periodically: hypothalamic–pituitary–adrenal axis suppression in long-term treatment**

• Growth rate in children; blood glucose, serum potassium for all patients

Evaluate:

• Therapeutic response: decreased severity of asthma

Teach patient/family:

• To use bronchodilator 1st, before using inhalation, if taking both

• Not to use for acute asthmatic attack; for acute asthma, may require oral corticosteroids

• To avoid smoking, smoke-filled rooms, those with URIs, those not immunized against chickenpox or measles

• To rinse mouth after inhaled product to decrease risk of oral candidiasis

fluticasone nasal agent

See Appendix B

fluticasone topical

See Appendix B

fluvastatin (Rx)

(flu′vah-stay-tin)

Lescol, Lescol XL

Func. class.: Antilipemic

Chem. class.: HMG-CoA reductase inhibitor

Do not confuse:

fluvastatin/FLUoxetine

ACTION: Inhibits HMG-CoA reductase enzyme, which reduces cholesterol synthesis

USES: As an adjunct for primary hypercholesterolemia (types Ia, Ib), coronary atherosclerosis in CAD; to reduce the risk for secondary prevention of coronary events in patients with CAD; as an adjunct to diet to reduce LDL, total cholesterol, apo B levels in heterozygous familial hyper-cholesterolemia (LDL-C ≥190 mg/dl) or LDL-C ≥160 mg/dl with history of premature CV disease

CONTRAINDICATIONS: Pregnancy (X), breastfeeding, hypersensitivity, active hepatic disease

Precautions: Previous hepatic disease, alcoholism, severe acute infections, trauma, hypotension, uncontrolled seizure disorders, severe metabolic disorders, electrolyte imbalance, myopathy, rhabdomyolysis

DOSAGE AND ROUTES

• **Adult: PO** 20-40 mg/day in PM initially, usual range 20-80 mg, max 80 mg; may be given in 2 doses (40 mg AM, 40 mg PM); dosage adjustments may be made at ≥4-wk intervals

Heterozygous familial hypercholesterolemia

• **Adolescent ≥1 yr postmenarche (10-16 yr): PO** 20 mg daily at bedtime, may increase q6wk, max 40 mg bid (cap) or 80 mg (ext rel)

Available forms: Caps 20, 40 mg; ext rel tab 80 mg

Administer:

• Do not break, crush, or chew ext rel tabs

• Bile acid sequestrant should be given at least 4 hr before fluvastatin

SIDE EFFECTS

CNS: Headache, dizziness, insomnia

EENT: Lens opacities

GI: *Abdominal pain, cramps, nausea, constipation, diarrhea, dyspepsia, flatus,* **hepatic dysfunction, pancreatitis**

HEMA: Thrombocytopenia, hemolytic anemia, leukopenia

INTEG: Rash, pruritus

MISC: Fatigue, influenza, photosensitivity
MS: Myalgia, **myositis, rhabdomyolysis,** *arthritis, arthralgia*
RESP: *Upper respiratory infection,* rhinitis, cough, pharyngitis, sinusitis, bronchitis

PHARMACOKINETICS

Peak response 3-4 wk, metabolized in liver, >98% protein bound, excreted primarily in feces, enters breast milk, half-life 1.2 hr, steady state 4-5 wk

INTERACTIONS

Increase: effects of warfarin, digoxin, phenytoin
Increase: myopathy—cycloSPORINE, niacin, colchicine, protease inhibitors, fibric acid derivatives
Increase: effects of fluvastatin—alcohol, cimetidine, ranitidine, omeprazole, phenytoin
Decrease: fluvastatin effect—cholestyramine
Drug/Herb
Increase: adverse reactions—red yeast rice
Drug/Food
• Grapefruit juice: possible increased toxicity

NURSING CONSIDERATIONS

Assess:
• **Hypercholesterolemia:** diet history: fats, fasting lipid profile (cholesterol, LDL, HDL, TG) before and q4-6wk, then q3-6mo when stable
• **Hepatotoxicity/pancreatitis:** monitor hepatic studies before, q12wk after dosage change, then q6mo; AST, ALT, LFTs may be increased
• Renal studies in patients with compromised renal system: BUN, I&O ratio, creatinine
⚠ **Myopathy, rhabdomyolysis: muscle pain, tenderness; obtain baseline CPK if elevated; if these occur, product should be discontinued**

Perform/provide:
• Storage in cool environment in tight container protected from light
Evaluate:
• Therapeutic response: decrease in sLDL, VLDL, total cholesterol; increased HDL, decreased triglycerides, slowing of CAD
Teach patient/family:
• That blood work will be necessary during treatment; to take product as prescribed
• To report severe GI symptoms, headache, muscle pain, weakness, tenderness
• That previously prescribed regimen will continue: low-cholesterol diet, exercise program, smoking cessation
• To report suspected pregnancy; not to use during pregnancy (X), breastfeeding

fluvoxamine (Rx)

(flu-vox′a-meen)

Apo-Fluvoxamine ✤, CO Fluvoxamine ✤, Luvox CR, PMS-Fluvoxamine ✤, ratio-Fluvoxamine ✤, Sandoz Fluvoxamine ✤

Func. class.: Antidepressant SSRI (selective serotonin reuptake inhibitor)

Do not confuse:
Luvox/Levoxyl/Lasix/Lovenox
Fluvoxamine/FLUoxetine/Fluphenazine

ACTION: Inhibits CNS neuron uptake of serotonin but not of norepinephrine

USES: Obsessive-compulsive disorder, social phobia
Unlabeled uses: Depression, bulimia nervosa, panic disorder, autism, anxiety, posttraumatic stress disorder (PTSD), premenstrual dysphoric disorder (PMDD)

CONTRAINDICATIONS: Hypersensitivity
Precautions: Pregnancy (C), breastfeeding, geriatric patients, hepatic/

cardiac disease, abrupt discontinuation, dehydration, ECT, hyponatremia, hypovolemia, bipolar disorder, seizure disorder

Black Box Warning: Children <8 yr, suicidal ideation

DOSAGE AND ROUTES

Obsessive-compulsive disorder (OCD)

- **Adult: PO** 50 mg at bedtime, increase by 50 mg at 4-7 day intervals, max 300 mg; doses over 100 mg should be divided; **EXT REL** 100 mg at bedtime, may titrate upward by 50 mg/wk, max 300 mg/day
- **Child 12-17 yr: PO** 25 mg at bedtime, increase by 25 mg/day q4-7days, max 300 mg/day; doses over 50 mg should be divided
- **Child 8-11 yr: PO** 25 mg/day at bedtime, may increase q4-7days, max 200 mg/day

Social anxiety disorder

- **Adult: PO EXT REL CAP** (Luvox CR) 100 mg at bedtime initially, titrate as needed by 50 mg/wk to 100-300 mg/day; **PO** 50 mg at bedtime, titrate as needed by 50 mg q4-7days to 50-300 mg/day
- **Child/adolescent 12-17 yr: PO** 25 mg at bedtime, titrate by 25-50 mg q4-7days, max 300 mg/day; if total daily dose >50 mg, divide equally

Hepatic dose/geriatric

- **Adult: PO** 25 mg at bedtime, may titrate upward slowly

Autism (unlabeled)

- **Adult: PO** up to 150 mg/day

Bulimia nervosa, depression (unlabeled)

- **Adult: PO** 50 mg at bedtime × 4-7 days, titrate by 25-50 mg/dose q4-7days as needed

Premenstrual dysphoric disorder (unlabeled)

- **Adult: PO** 50 mg/day, may titrate to 100 mg/day

Schizophrenia (unlabeled)

- **Adult: PO** 100 mg daily in combination with other agents

Posttraumatic stress disorder (PTSD) (unlabeled)

- **Adult: PO** 25-50 mg at bedtime × 4-7 days then titrate by 25-50 mg/dose q4-7days, range 25-300 mg/day single or divided dose × 3-12 wk

Available forms: Tabs 25, 50, 100 mg; ext rel cap 100, 150 mg

Administer:

- With food, milk for GI symptoms
- **Immediate release:** give at bedtime; doses >100 mg/day (or >50 mg/day in those aged 8-17 yr) in 2 divided doses; if doses are not equal, give larger dose at bedtime
- **Ext rel:** give at bedtime; do not break, crush, chew ext rel product

SIDE EFFECTS

CNS: *Headache, drowsiness, dizziness, seizures,* sleep disorders, insomnia, suicidal ideation (children/adolescents), neuroleptic-malignant-syndrome–like reactions, *weakness*

GI: *Nausea, anorexia, constipation,* hepatotoxicity, *vomiting, diarrhea,* dry mouth

GU: *Decreased libido,* anorgasmia

INTEG: *Rash, sweating*

PHARMACOKINETICS

Crosses blood-brain barrier, 77% protein binding, metabolism by the liver, terminal half-life 15.6 hr, peak 2-8 hr

INTERACTIONS

⚠ Fatal reaction—MAOIs

Increase: CNS depression—alcohol, barbiturates, benzodiazepines

Increase: effect of—ramelteon, thioridazine; do not use together

⚠ **Increase:** QT prolongation, death—pimozide, do not use together

Increase: fluvoxamine, toxicity levels—tricyclics, clozapine, alosetron, tizanidine; do not use together

Increase: metabolism, decrease effects—smoking

Increase: serotonin syndrome, neuroleptic malignant syndrome: SSRIs, SNRIs,

serotonin-receptor agonists, atypical antipsychotics
Increase: bleeding risk—anticoagulants, NSAIDs, salicylates, thrombolytics
• Avoid use with clopidogrel
Decrease: metabolism, increase action of propranolol, diazepam, lithium, theophylline, carBAMazepine, warfarin
Drug/Herb
Increase: CNS effect—kava, valerian
Increase: serotonin syndrome—tryptophan, St. John's wort; do not use together

NURSING CONSIDERATIONS

Assess:
• Hepatic studies: AST, ALT, bilirubin
• Mental status: mood, sensorium, affect, **suicidal tendencies;** increase in psychiatric symptoms: depression, panic, obsessive-compulsive symptoms
• Constipation; most likely in geriatric patients
⚠ **For toxicity: nausea, vomiting, diarrhea, syncope, increased pulse, seizures**
Perform/provide:
• Storage at room temp; do not freeze
Evaluate:
• Therapeutic response: decrease in depression
Teach patient/family:
• That therapeutic effects may take 2-3 wk
• To use caution when driving, performing other activities requiring alertness because drowsiness, dizziness may occur
• Not to use other CNS depressants, alcohol, barbiturates, benzodiazepines, St. John's wort, kava
• To notify prescriber if pregnancy is suspected, planned
• To notify prescriber of allergic reaction
• To increase bulk in diet if constipation occurs, especially in geriatric patients
Black Box Warning: That suicidal thoughts/behaviors may occur
• To stop taking MAOIs at least 14 days before starting product

TREATMENT OF OVERDOSE:

Activated charcoal, gastric lavage

folic acid (vit B_9) (OTC)

(foe′lik a′sid)

Apo-Folic ✦, Equaline Folic Acid, Folacin, Vitamin B_9, Walgreens Gold Seal Folic Acid

Func. class.: Vit B complex group, water-soluble vitamin

F

ACTION:
Needed for erythropoiesis; increases RBC, WBC, platelet formation with megaloblastic anemias

USES:
Megaloblastic or macrocytic anemia caused by folic acid deficiency; hepatic disease, alcoholism, hemolysis, intestinal obstruction, pregnancy to reduce risk for neural tube defects
Unlabeled uses: Reduce risk for heart disease, stroke, methotrexate toxicity prophylaxis

CONTRAINDICATIONS:
Hypersensitivity
Precautions: Pregnancy (A), anemias other than megaloblastic/macrocytic anemia, vit B_{12} deficiency anemia, uncorrected pernicious anemia

DOSAGE AND ROUTES

RDA
• **Adult and child ≥14 yr: PO** 400 mcg
• **Adult (pregnant/lactating): PO** 600 mcg/day
• **Child 9-13 yr: PO** 300 mcg
• **Child 4-8 yr: PO** 200 mcg
• **Child 1-3 yr: PO** 150 mcg
• **Infant 6 mo-1 yr: PO** 80 mcg
• **Neonate/infant <6 mo: PO** 65 mcg
Megaloblastic/macrocytic anemia due to folic acid or nutritional deficiency
• **Pregnant/lactating: PO** 800-1000 mcg
Therapeutic dose
• **Adult and child: PO/IM/SUBCUT/IV** up to 1 mg/day

Maintenance dose

- **Adult and child >4 yr: PO/IM/SUBCUT/IV** 0.4 mg/day
- **Pregnant and lactating: PO/IM/SUBCUT/IV** 0.8-1 mg/day
- **Child <4 yr: PO/IM/SUBCUT/IV** up to 0.3 mg/day
- **Infant: PO/IM/SUBCUT/IV** up to 0.1 mg/day

Prevention of neural tube defects during pregnancy

- **Adult: PO** 0.6 mg/day

Prevention of megaloblastic anemia during pregnancy

- **Adult: PO/IM/SUBCUT** up to 1 mg/day during pregnancy

Tropical sprue

- **Adult: PO** 3-15 mg/day

Available forms: Tabs 0.1, 0.4, 0.8, 1, 5 mg; inj 5, 10 mg/ml

Administer:

SUBCUT route

- Do not inject intradermally

IM route

- Inject deeply in large muscle mass, aspirate

Direct IV route

- Direct undiluted ≤5 mg/1 min or more

Continuous IV INF route

- May be added to most IV sol or TPN

Y-site compatibilities: Alfentanil, aminophylline, ascorbic acid injection, atracurium, atropine, azathioprine, aztreonam, benztropine, bumetanide, calcium gluconate, cefamandole, ceFAZolin, cefmetazole, cefonicid, cefoperazone, cefotaxime, cefotetan, cefoxitin, ceftazidime, ceftizoxime, cefTRIAXone, cefuroxime, cephalothin, cephapirin, chloramphenicol, cimetidine, clindamycin, cyanocobalamin, cycloSPORINE, dexamethasone, digoxin, diphenhydrAMINE, DOPamine, enalaprilat, ePHEDrine, EPINEPHrine, epoetin alfa, erythromycin, esmolol, famotidine, fentaNYL, fluconazole, furosemide, ganciclovir, glycopyrrolate, heparin, hydrocortisone, hydrOXYzine, imipenem-cilastatin, indomethacin, insulin (regular), ketorolac, labetalol, lidocaine, LR, magnesium sulfate, mannitol, meperidine, methicillin, methylPREDNISolone, metoclopramide, metoprolol, mezlocillin, midazolam, moxalactam, multiple vitamins injection, naloxone, nitroglycerin, nitroprusside, ondansetron, oxacillin, oxytocin, penicillin G potassium/sodium, PENTobarbital, PHENobarbital, phenylephrine, phytonadione, piperacillin, potassium chloride, procainamide, propranolol, ranitidine, Ringer's, ritodrine, sodium bicarbonate, succinylcholine, SUFentanil, theophylline, ticarcillin, ticarcillin-clavulanate, TPN, trimetaphan, urokinase, vancomycin, vasopressin

SIDE EFFECTS

CNS: Confusion, depression, excitability, irritability

GI: Anorexia, nausea

INTEG: Pruritus, rash, erythema

RESP: Bronchospasm

SYST: Anaphylaxis (rare)

PHARMACOKINETICS

PO: Peak ½-1 hr, bound to plasma proteins, excreted in breast milk, metabolized by liver, excreted in urine (small amounts)

INTERACTIONS

Increase: need for folic acid—estrogen, hydantoins, carBAMazepine, glucocorticoids

Decrease: folate levels—methotrexate, sulfonamides, sulfasalazine, trimethoprim

Decrease: phenytoin levels, fosphenytoin, may increase seizures

NURSING CONSIDERATIONS

Assess:

- Megaloblastic anemia: fatigue, dyspnea, weakness
- Hgb, Hct, reticulocyte count
- Nutritional status: bran, yeast, dried beans, nuts, fruits, fresh vegetables, asparagus
- Products currently taken: estrogen,

carBAMazepine, glucocorticoids, hydantoins; these products may cause increased folic acid use by body and contribute to a deficiency if taking other neurotoxic products

Perform/provide:

- Storage in light-resistant container

Evaluate:

- Therapeutic response: increased weight, oriented, well-being; absence of fatigue; increase in reticulocyte count within 5 days of beginning treatment, absence of neural tube defect

Teach patient/family:

- To take product exactly as prescribed; that periodic lab work is required
- To alter nutrition to include high–folic-acid foods: organ meats, vegetables, fruit
- That urine will turn bright yellow
- To notify prescriber of allergic reaction
- To avoid breastfeeding

⚠ HIGH ALERT

fondaparinux (Rx)

(fon-dah-pair′ih-nux)

Arixtra

Func. class.: Anticoagulant, antithrombotic

Chem. class.: Synthetic, selective factor Xa inhibitor

Do not confuse:

Arixtra/Anti-Xa

ACTION: Acts by antithrombin III (ATIII)-mediated selective inhibition of factor Xa; neutralization of factor Xa interrupts blood coagulation and inhibits thrombin formation; does not inactivate thrombin (activated factor II) or affect platelets

USES: Prevention/treatment of deep venous thrombosis, PE in hip and knee replacement, hip fracture or abdominal surgery

Unlabeled uses: Acute coronary syndrome

CONTRAINDICATIONS: Hypersensitivity to this product; hemophilia, leukemia with bleeding, peptic ulcer disease, hemorrhagic stroke, surgery, thrombocytopenic purpura, weight <50 kg, severe renal disease (CCr <30 ml/min), active major bleeding, bacterial endocarditis

Precautions: Pregnancy (B), breastfeeding, children, geriatric patients, alcoholism, hepatic disease (severe), blood dyscrasias, heparin-induced thrombocytopenia, uncontrolled severe hypertension, subacute bacterial endocarditis, acute nephritis, mild to moderate renal disease

Black Box Warning: Spinal/epidural anesthesia, lumbar puncture

DOSAGE AND ROUTES

Deep venous thrombosis/PE

- **Adult <50 kg: SUBCUT** 5 mg/day × ≥5 days until INR 2-3; may give warfarin within 72 hr of fondaparinux
- **Adult 50-100 kg: SUBCUT** 7.5 mg/day × ≥5 days until INR 2-3; may give warfarin within 72 hr of fondaparinux
- **Adult >100 kg: SUBCUT** 10 mg/day × ≥5 days until INR 2-3; may give warfarin within 72 hr of fondaparinux

Prevention of deep venous thrombosis

- **Adult: SUBCUT** 2.5 mg/day given 6 hr after surgery; continue for 5-9 days; for hip surgery, up to 32 days; for abdominal surgery, up to 24 days

Coronary artery thrombosis prophylaxis/acute coronary syndrome (unlabeled)

- **Adult: SUBCUT** 2.5 mg until hospital discharge or ≤8 days with standard treatment

Renal disease

- **Adult: SUBCUT** CCr <30 ml/min, do not use

Available forms: Inj 2.5 mg/0.5 ml, 5 mg/0.4 ml, 7.5 mg/0.6 ml, 10 mg/0.8 ml prefilled syringes

Administer:

- Alone; do not mix with other products or solutions; cannot be used interchangeably (unit to unit) with other anticoagulants
- For 5-9 days
- Only after screening patient for bleeding disorders

SUBCUT route

- SUBCUT only; do not give IM; do not give <6 hr after surgery
- Check for discolored sol or sol with particulate; if present, do not give
- Administer 6-8 hr after surgery; administer to recumbent patient, rotate inj sites (left/right anterolateral, left/right posterolateral abdominal wall)
- Wipe surface of inj site with alcohol swab, twist plunger cap and remove, remove rigid needle guard by pulling straight off needle; do not aspirate, do not expel air bubble from surface
- Insert whole length of needle into skinfold held with thumb and forefinger
- When product is injected, a soft click may be felt or heard
- Give at same time each day to maintain steady blood levels; observe inj site
- Avoid all IM inj that may cause bleeding

⚠ **Administer only this product when ordered; not interchangeable with heparin**

SIDE EFFECTS

CNS: *Fever*, confusion, headache, dizziness, *insomnia*

GI: *Nausea, vomiting*, diarrhea, dyspepsia, *constipation*, increased AST, ALT

GU: UTI, urinary retention

HEMA: *Anemia*, minor bleeding, purpura, hematoma, **thrombocytopenia, major bleeding (intracranial, cerebral, retroperitoneal hemorrhage), postoperative hemorrhage, heparin-induced thrombocytopenia**

INTEG: Increased wound drainage, bullous eruption, local reaction—*rash*, pruritus, inj site bleeding

META: Hypokalemia

OTHER: Hypotension, pain, *edema*

PHARMACOKINETICS

Rapidly, completely absorbed; peak steady state 3 hr; distributed primarily in blood; does not bind to plasma proteins except 94% to ATIII; metabolism unknown; eliminated unchanged in urine within 72 hr with normal renal function; terminal half-life 17-21 hr

INTERACTIONS

Increase: bleeding risk—salicylates, NSAIDs, abciximab, eptifibatide, tirofiban, clopidogrel, dipyridamole, quiNIDine, valproic acid

Drug/Herb

Increase: bleeding risk—feverfew, garlic, ginger, ginkgo, ginseng, green tea, horse chestnut, kava

NURSING CONSIDERATIONS

Assess:

Black Box Warning: Monitor patients who have received epidural/spinal anesthesia or lumbar puncture for neurological impairment

- Blood studies (CBC, anti-Xa, Hgb/Hct, prothrombin time, platelets, occult blood in stools), thrombocytopenia may occur; if platelets <100,000/mm^3, treatment should be discontinued; renal studies: BUN, creatinine
- For bleeding: gums, petechiae, ecchymosis, black tarry stools, hematuria; decreased Hct, notify prescriber
- For risk of hemorrhage if coadministering with other products that may cause bleeding
- For hypersensitivity: rash, fever, chills; notify prescriber

Perform/provide:

- Storage at 25° C (77° F); do not freeze

Evaluate:
• Therapeutic response: prevention of DVT

Teach patient/family:
• To use soft-bristle toothbrush to avoid bleeding gums; to use electric razor
• To report any signs of bleeding: gums, under skin, urine, stools
• To avoid OTC products containing aspirin

formoterol (Rx)

(for-moh'ter-ahl)

Foradil Aerolizer, Oxeze ♣, Perforomist

Func. class.: Bronchodilator

Chem. class.: β-Adrenergic agonist

Do not confuse:
Foradil/Toradol

ACTION: Has β_1 and β_2 action; relaxes bronchial smooth muscle and dilates the trachea and main bronchi by increasing levels of cAMP, which relaxes smooth muscles; causes increased contractility and heart rate by acting on β-receptors in heart

USES: Maintenance, treatment of asthma, COPD; prevention of exercise-induced bronchospasm

CONTRAINDICATIONS: Hypersensitivity to sympathomimetics, monotherapy for asthma

Precautions: Pregnancy (C), geriatric patients, cardiac disorders, hyperthyroidism, diabetes mellitus, prostatic hypertrophy, hypertension, African descendants

Black Box Warning: Asthma-related death

DOSAGE AND ROUTES

Maintenance, treatment of asthma
• **Adult and child ≥5 yr: INH** AM and PM long-term 1 cap (12 mcg) q12hr using aerolizer inhaler

Maintenance of COPD
• **Adult: INH** 12 mcg q12hr

Prevention of exercise-induced bronchospasm
• **Adult and child ≥12 yr: INH** prn occasionally 1 cap (12 mcg) ≥15 min before exercise, do not use additional doses for ≥12 hr

Available form: INH powder in cap 12 mcg; nebulizer sol for INH 20 mcg/2 ml

Administer:

Inhalation route
• Place cap in aerolizer inhaler; cap is punctured; do not wash aerolizer inhaler
• Pull off cover, twist mouthpiece to open, push buttons in; make sure the 4 pins are visible; remove cap from blister pack, place cap in chamber; twist to close, press (a click will be heard), release; patient should exhale, place inhaler in mouth, inhale rapidly

SIDE EFFECTS

CNS: *Tremors*, *anxiety*, insomnia, headache, dizziness, stimulation
CV: Palpitations, tachycardia, hypertension, chest pain
GI: Nausea, vomiting, xerostomia
RESP: Bronchial irritation, dryness of oropharynx, **bronchospasms** (overuse), infection, inflammatory reaction (child)

PHARMACOKINETICS

Onset 15 min; peak 1-3 hr; duration 12 hr; metabolized in liver, lungs, GI tract; half-life 10 hr

INTERACTIONS

⚠ **Increase: serious dysrhythmias—MAOIs, tricyclics**
Increase: hypokalemia—loop/thiazide diuretics
Increase: effects of both products—other sympathomimetics, thyroid hormones
Increase: QT prolongation—class IA/III antiarrhythmics, phenothiazines, pimozide, haloperidol, risperidone, sertindole, ziprasidone, amoxapine, arsenic trioxide, chloroquine, clarithromycin,

dasatinib, dolasetron, droperidol, erythromycin, halofantrine, halogenated anesthetics, levomethadyl, maprotiline, methadone, some quinolones, ondansetron, paliperidone, palonosetron, pentamidine, probucol, ranolazine, sunitinib, tricyclics, vorinostat

Decrease: action when used with β-blockers

NURSING CONSIDERATIONS

Assess:

- Respiratory function: B/P, pulse, lung sounds; note sputum color, character; respiratory function tests before, during treatment
- Cardiac status: hypertension, palpitations, tachycardia
- For paresthesias, coldness of extremities; peripheral blood flow may decrease

Perform/provide:

- Storage at room temp; protection from heat, moisture

Evaluate:

- Therapeutic response: ease of breathing

Teach patient/family:

Black Box Warning: Asthma-related death, severe asthma exacerbations; if wheezing worsens and cannot be relieved during an acute asthma attack, immediate medical attention should be sought

- To rinse mouth after use
- About correct use of inhaler/nebulizer (review package insert with patient); to avoid getting aerosol in eyes
- About all aspects of product; to avoid smoking, smoke-filled rooms, persons with respiratory infections; not to swallow caps

TREATMENT OF OVERDOSE:

Administration of β-blocker

fosamprenavir (Rx)

(fos-am-pren′a-veer)

Lexiva, Telzir ✱

Func. class.: Antiretroviral

Chem. class.: Protease inhibitor

ACTION: A prodrug of amprenavir; inhibits human immunodeficiency virus (HIV) protease, which prevents maturation of the infectious virus

USES: HIV-1 infection in combination with antiretrovirals

CONTRAINDICATIONS: Hypersensitivity to protease inhibitors

Precautions: Pregnancy (C), breastfeeding, geriatric patients, hepatic disease, hemolytic anemia, diabetes, sulfa sensitivity

DOSAGE AND ROUTES

Therapy-naive patients

- **Adult: PO** 1400 mg bid without ritonavir or fosamprenavir 1400 mg/day and with ritonavir 200 mg/day or fosamprenavir 700 mg bid and ritonavir 100 mg bid

Protease-experienced patients (PI)

- **Adult: PO** 700 mg bid and ritonavir 100 mg bid

Combination with efavirenz

- **Adult: PO** add another 100 mg/day of ritonavir for a total of 300 mg/day when all 3 products given

Hepatic dose

- **Adult: PO** (Child-Pugh 5-6) 700 mg bid without ritonavir (treatment-naive patients) or 700 mg bid with ritonavir 100 mg daily (treatment-naive or experienced patients); (Child-Pugh 7-9) 700 mg bid without ritonavir (treatment-naive patients) or 450 mg bid with ritonavir 100 mg daily (treatment-naive or experienced patients); (Child-Pugh 10-15) 350 mg bid without ritonavir (treatment-naive patients) or 300 mg bid with ritonavir

100 mg daily (treatment-naive or experienced patients)

Available forms: Tabs 700 mg (equivalent to 600 mg amprenavir); oral susp 50 mg/ml

Administer:

- **Tab:** without regard to food
- **Oral susp:** give without food (adult), with food (pediatric); if vomiting occurs within 30 min of dose, readminister; shake vigorously prior to dose, use calibrated device

SIDE EFFECTS

CNS: Headache, fatigue, depression, oral paresthesia

GI: *Nausea, diarrhea, vomiting, abdominal pain*

INTEG: Rash, pruritus

MISC: Redistribution or accumulation of body fat, hyperglycemia, **Stevens-Johnson syndrome**

PHARMACOKINETICS

Prodrug of amprenavir, peak 1½-4 hr; 90% protein binding; metabolized in liver by cytochrome P4503AY (CYP3A4); excretion of unchanged product minimal; half-life 7.7 hr

INTERACTIONS

Increase: effect of—warfarin

⚠ Serious life-threatening reactions: amiodarone, calcium channel blockers, lidocaine, pimozide, ergots, midazolam, triazolam, flecainide, lovastatin, simvastatin, propafenone

Increase: effect of—aripiprazole, rifbutin, ketoconazole, itraconazole, sildenafil, vardenafil

Increase: toxicity—HMG-CoA reductase inhibitors

Decrease: effect of oral contraceptives, methadone

Decrease: fosamprenavir levels—nevirapine, antacids, efavirenz, saquinavir, ranitidine, carbamazepine, phenytoin, lopinavir/ritonavir, barbiturates, proton-pump inhibitors, H_2-receptor antagonists, dexamethasone; avoid concurrent use

Drug/Herb

- Avoid use with St. John's wort

Drug/Lab Test

Increase: serum glucose, AST, ALT, triglycerides

NURSING CONSIDERATIONS

Assess:

- **HIV:** monitor CD4 + T cell count, plasma HIV RNA, serum cholesterol, serum lipid profile
- Bowel pattern before, during treatment; monitor hydration
- Skin eruptions, rash, urticaria, itching; allergy to sulfonamides; cross-sensitivity may occur

⚠ Stevens-Johnson syndrome; skin reactions, report immediately

Teach patient/family:

- To avoid taking with other medications unless directed by provider
- That product does not cure but does manage symptoms; that product does not prevent transmission of HIV to others
- To use a nonhormonal form of birth control while taking this product
- That if dose is missed, to take as soon as remembered up to 1 hr before next dose; not to double dose
- Not to alter dose or stop therapy without talking to physician
- To advise physician if patient has sulfa allergy
- To report all medications, including herbal supplements, to physician
- That patients receiving phosphodiesterase type 5 inhibitors may be at increased risk for PDE5 inhibitor adverse effects

foscarnet (Rx)

(foss-kar′net)

Func. class.: Antiviral

Chem. class.: Inorganic pyrophosphate organic analog

ACTION: Antiviral activity is produced by selective inhibition at the pyrophosphate binding site on virus-specific DNA polymerases and reverse transcriptases at concentrations that do not affect cellular DNA polymerases

USES: Treatment of CMV retinitis, HSV infections; used with ganciclovir for relapsing patients

CONTRAINDICATIONS: Hypersensitivity, CCr <0.4 ml/min/kg

Precautions: Pregnancy (C), breastfeeding, children, geriatric patients, seizure disorders, severe anemia

Black Box Warning: Renal disease, electrolyte/mineral imbalances

DOSAGE AND ROUTES

CMV retinitis

- **Adult: IV INF** 60 mg/kg given over ≥ 1 hr or 120 mg/kg given over 2 hr q8hr $\times$ 2-3 wk or 90 mg/kg q12hr; usually give with at least 750-1000 ml NS daily

HSV

- **Adult: IV** 40 mg/kg q8-12hr $\times$ 2-3 wk

Renal dose

- **Adult: IV**

Male:

$$\frac{\text{(kg) weight} \times 140 - \text{age}}{\text{(mg/dl) serum creatinine} \times 72} = \text{CCr}$$

Female: 0.85 × above value

Dose based on table provided in package insert

Available forms: Inj 6000 mg/250 ml, 12,000 mg/500 ml (24 mg/ml)

Administer:

- Increased fluids before and during product administration to induce diuresis, minimize renal toxicity

Intermittent IV INF route

- Using inf device at no more than 1 mg/kg/min; do not give by rapid or bolus IV; give by CVP or peripheral vein; standard 24 mg/ml sol may be used without dilution if using by CVP; dilute the 24 mg/ml sol to 12 mg/ml with D_5W or NS if using peripheral vein
- Manufacturer recommends product not be given with other medications in syringe or admixed

SIDE EFFECTS

CNS: *Fever*, dizziness, *headache*, seizures, *fatigue*, neuropathy, asthenia, encephalopathy, malaise, meningitis, *paresthesia*, depression, *confusion*, *anxiety*

CV: ECG abnormalities, 1st-degree AV block, nonspecific ST-T segment changes, cerebrovascular disorder, cardiomyopathy, cardiac arrest, atrial fibrillation, CHF, sinus tachycardia

GI: *Nausea*, *vomiting*, *diarrhea*, *anorexia*, abdominal pain, pancreatitis

GU: Acute renal failure, decreased CCr, increased serum creatinine, azotemia, diabetes insipidus, renal tubular disorders

HEMA: *Anemia*, granulocytopenia, leukopenia, thrombocytopenia, thrombosis, neutropenia, lymphadenopathy

INTEG: *Rash*, sweating, pruritus, skin discoloration

RESP: *Coughing*, *dyspnea*, pneumonia, pulmonary infiltration, pneumothorax, hemoptysis

SYST: *Hypokalemia*, *hypocalcemia*, *hypomagnesemia*; hypophosphatemia

PHARMACOKINETICS

14%-17% protein bound, half-life 18-88 hr in normal renal function, 79%-92% excreted via kidneys

INTERACTIONS

Increase: nephrotoxicity—acyclovir, cidofovir, CISplatin, gold compounds, penicillamine, tacrolimus, tenofovir, van-

comycin, aminoglycosides, amphotericin B, NSAIDs, lithium, cycloSPORINE
Increase: hypocalcemia—pentamidine

NURSING CONSIDERATIONS

Assess:

• **Renal tubular disorders:** I&O ratio, urine pH, serum creatinine at baseline, 3×/wk during initial therapy then 2×/wk thereafter; CCr at baseline, throughout treatment; if CCr <0.4 ml/min/kg, discontinue

• Blood counts q2wk; watch for decreasing granulocytes, Hgb; if low, therapy may have to be discontinued and restarted after hematologic recovery; blood transfusions may be required

• Lesions in HSV

• Electrolytes and minerals (calcium, phosphate, magnesium, potassium); watch closely for tetany during 1st administration

• GI symptoms: nausea, vomiting, diarrhea; severe symptoms may necessitate discontinuing product

⚠ **Blood dyscrasias** (anemia, granulocytopenia): bruising, fatigue, bleeding, poor healing

• **Allergic reactions:** flushing, rash, urticaria, pruritus

CMV retinitis

• Culture should be performed prior to treatment (blood, urine, throat); a negative culture does not rule out CMV

• Ophthalmic exam should confirm diagnosis

Perform/provide:

• Close monitoring during therapy for tingling, numbness, paresthesias; if these occur, stop inf, obtain lab sample for electrolytes

Evaluate:

• Therapeutic response: improvement in CMV retinitis

Teach patient/family:

• To call prescriber if sore throat, swollen lymph nodes, malaise, fever occur, since other infections may occur

• To report perioral tingling, numbness in extremities, and paresthesias

• That serious product interactions may occur if OTC products are ingested; check first with prescriber

• That product is not a cure but will control symptoms

fosinopril (Rx)

(foss′in-oh-pril)

Monopril

Func. class.: Antihypertensive

Chem. class.: Angiotensin-converting enzyme (ACE) inhibitor

Do not confuse:
Monopril/minoxidil/Accupril/Monoket

ACTION: Selectively suppresses renin-angiotensin-aldosterone system; inhibits ACE; prevents conversion of angiotensin I to angiotensin II; results in dilation of arterial, venous vessels

USES: Hypertension, alone or in combination with thiazide diuretics, systolic CHF

Unlabeled uses: Proteinuria in nondiabetic nephropathy

CONTRAINDICATIONS: Breastfeeding, children, hypersensitivity to ACE inhibitors, history of ACE-inhibitor–induced angioedema

Black Box Warning: Pregnancy (D)

Precautions: Geriatric patients, impaired hepatic function, hypovolemia, blood dyscrasias, CHF, COPD, asthma, angioedema, hyperkalemia, renal artery stenosis, renal disease

DOSAGE AND ROUTES

CHF

• **Adult: PO** 10 mg/day then up to 40 mg/day increased over several weeks; use lower dose for those diuresed before fosinopril

Hypertension

• **Adult: PO** 10 mg/day initially then 20-

40 mg/day divided bid or daily, max 80 mg/day

Available forms: Tabs 10, 20, 40 mg

Administer:

- May be taken without regard to meals

SIDE EFFECTS

CNS: *Headache, dizziness,* fatigue

CV: *Hypotension,* orthostatic hypotension, tachycardia

GI: *Nausea,* constipation, vomiting, diarrhea, **hepatotoxicity, cholestatic jaundice, fulminant hepatic necrosis, hepatic failure, death**

GU: Increased BUN, creatinine, azotemia, **renal artery stenosis**

HEMA: Decreased Hct, Hgb; **eosinophilia, leukopenia, neutropenia**

META: Hyperkalemia

RESP: Cough

SYST: Anaphylaxis, angioedema

PHARMACOKINETICS

Peak 3 hr, serum protein binding 97%, half-life 11.5-14 hr, metabolized by liver (metabolites excreted in urine, feces)

INTERACTIONS

Increase: hypotension—diuretics, other antihypertensives, ganglionic blockers, adrenergic blockers, nitrates, acute alcohol ingestion

Increase: toxicity—vasodilators, hydrALAZINE, prazosin, potassium-sparing diuretics, sympathomimetics, digoxin, lithium, NSAIDs

Decrease: absorption—antacids

Decrease: antihypertensive effect—salicylates

Drug/Herb

Increase: antihypertensive effect—hawthorn

Decrease: antihypertensive effect—ephedra

Drug/Lab Test

Increase: AST, ALT, alk phos, glucose, bilirubin, uric acid

False positive: urine acetone

Positive: ANA titer

NURSING CONSIDERATIONS

Assess:

- **Hypertension:** B/P, orthostatic hypotension, syncope
- Blood studies: neutrophils, decreased platelets; obtain WBC with differential baseline and monthly × 6 mo then q2-3mo × 1 yr; if neutrophils $<1000/mm^3$, discontinue (recommended with collagen–vascular disease)
- Renal studies: protein, BUN, creatinine; increased levels may indicate nephrotic syndrome
- Baselines of renal, hepatic studies before therapy begins
- Potassium levels, although hyperkalemia rarely occurs
- **CHF:** edema in feet, legs daily; weigh daily
- **Allergic reactions:** rash, fever, pruritus, urticaria; product should be discontinued if antihistamines fail to help

Perform/provide:

- Storage in tight container at ≤86° F (30° C)
- Supine position for severe hypotension

Evaluate:

- Therapeutic response: decrease in B/P

Teach patient/family:

- Not to discontinue product abruptly; to take at same time of day
- Not to use OTC products (cough, cold, allergy) unless directed by prescriber; not to use salt substitutes containing potassium without consulting prescriber
- About the importance of complying with dosage schedule, even if feeling better
- To rise slowly to sitting or standing position to minimize orthostatic hypotension
- To notify prescriber of mouth sores, sore throat, fever, swelling of hands or feet, irregular heartbeat, chest pain, nonproductive cough
- To report excessive perspiration, dehydration, vomiting, diarrhea; may lead to fall in B/P
- That product may cause dizziness, fainting, lightheadedness during first few days of therapy

- That product may cause skin rash or impaired perspiration
- How to take B/P; normal readings for age group

Black Box Warning: To notify prescriber if pregnancy is planned or suspected, pregnancy (D)

TREATMENT OF OVERDOSE:
0.9% NaCl IV inf, hemodialysis

fosphenytoin (Rx)
(foss-fen′i-toy-in)
Func. class.: Anticonvulsant
Chem. class.: Hydantoin, phosphate phenytoin ester

ACTION:
Inhibits spread of seizure activity in motor cortex by altering ion transport; increases AV conduction, prodrug of phenytoin

USES:
Generalized tonic-clonic seizures, status epilepticus, partial seizures

CONTRAINDICATIONS:
Pregnancy (D), hypersensitivity, psychiatric conditions, bradycardia, SA and AV block, Stokes-Adams syndrome, absence seizures

Precautions: Breastfeeding, allergies, renal/hepatic disease, myocardial insufficiency, hypoalbuminemia, hypothyroidism, Asian patients positive for HLA-B 1502

Black Box Warning: Rapid IV inf

DOSAGE AND ROUTES
All doses in PE (phenytoin sodium equivalent)

Status epilepticus

- **Adult and adolescent: IV** 15-20 mg PE/kg
- **Child <12 yr (unlabeled): IV** 15-20 mg PE/kg

Nonemergency/maintenance dosing

- **Adult and adolescent >16 yr: IM/IV** 10-20 mg PE/kg; 4-6 mg PE/kg/day (maintenance); start maintenance 12 hr after loading dose; give in 2-3 divided doses

Available forms: Inj 150 mg (100 mg phenytoin equiv), 750 mg (500 mg phenytoin equiv), 50-mg/ml vials

Administer:

IV, direct route

- Dilute product in D_5W or 0.9% NaCl (1.5-25 mg PE/ml)

Black Box Warning: Give at a rate of <150 mg PE/min (adult) or <3 mg PE/kg/min (child)

Y-site compatibilities: Aminocaproic acid, amphotericin B lipid complex, amphotericin B liposome, anidulafungin, atenolol, bivalirudin, bleomycin, CARBOplatin, CISplatin, cyclophosphamide, cytarabine, DACTINomycin, DAPTOmycin, dexmedetomidine, diltiazem, docetaxel, doxacurium, eptifibatide, ertapenem, etoposide, fludarabine, fluorouracil, gatifloxacin, gemcitabine, gemtuzumab, granisetron, ifosfamide, levofloxacin, linezolid, LORazepam, mechlorethamine, meperidine, methotrexate, metroNIDAZOLE, nesiritide, octreotide, oxaliplatin, oxytocin, paclitaxel, palonosetron, pamidronate, pantoprazole, pemetrexed, PHENobarbital, piperacillin-tazobactam, rocuronium, sodium acetate, tacrolimus, teniposide, thiotepa, tigecycline, tirofiban, vinCRIStine, vinorelbine, voriconazole, zoledronic acid

SIDE EFFECTS
CNS: Drowsiness, dizziness, insomnia, paresthesias, depression, **suicidal tendencies**, aggression, headache, confusion, paresthesia

CV: Hypo/hypertension, **ventricular fibrillation, CHF, shock**

EENT: Nystagmus, diplopia, blurred vision

GI: Nausea, vomiting, diarrhea, constipation, anorexia, weight loss, hepatitis, jaundice, gingival hyperplasia

HEMA: Agranulocytosis, leukopenia, aplastic anemia, thrombocytopenia, megaloblastic anemia

INTEG: Rash, lupus erythematosus, **Stevens-Johnson syndrome,** hirsutism, hypersensitivity, pruritus

SYST: Hyperglycemia, hypokalemia, SJS/TEN Asian patients positive for HLA-B 1502

PHARMACOKINETICS

Metabolized by liver, excreted by kidneys, protein binding 95%-99%, rapidly converted to phenytoin

INTERACTIONS

Increase: fosphenytoin level—cimetidine, amiodarone, chloramphenicol, estrogens, H_2 antagonists, phenothiazines, salicylates, sulfonamides, tricyclics, CYP1A2 inhibitors

Decrease: fosphenytoin effects—alcohol (chronic use), antihistamines, antacids, tramadol, antineoplastics, rifampin, folic acid, carBAMazepine, theophylline, CYP1A2 inducers

Drug/Herb

Increase: anticonvulsant effect—ginkgo

Decrease: anticonvulsant effect—ginseng, valerian

Drug/Lab Test

Increase: glucose, alk phos

Decrease: dexamethasone, metyrapone test serum, PBI, urinary steroids

NURSING CONSIDERATIONS

Assess:

- Drug level: target level 10-20 mcg/ml, toxic level 30-50 mcg/ml, wait >2 hr after dose before testing, 4 hr after IM dose
- Blood studies: CBC, platelets q2wk until stabilized, then monthly × 12 mo, then q3mo; discontinue product if neutrophils <1600/mm^3; serum calcium, albumin, phosphorus

⚠ Mental status: mood, sensorium, affect, memory (long, short), **suicidal thoughts/behaviors**

- Seizure activity including type, location, duration, character; provide seizure precaution
- Renal studies: urinalysis, BUN, urine creatinine
- Hepatic studies: ALT, AST, bilirubin, creatinine
- Allergic reaction: red, raised rash; product should be discontinued
- **Toxicity/bone marrow depression:** nausea, vomiting, ataxia, diplopia, cardiovascular collapse, slurred speech, confusion
- Respiratory depression: rate, depth, character of respirations

⚠ **Blood dyscrasias:** fever, sore throat, bruising, rash, jaundice

- Continuous monitoring of ECG, B/P, respiratory function
- Rash; discontinue as soon as rash develops, serious adverse reactions such as **Stevens-Johnson syndrome** can occur

Evaluate:

- Therapeutic response: decrease in severity of seizures

Teach patient/family:

- About the reason for, expected outcomes of treatment
- Not to use machinery or engage in hazardous activity, since drowsiness, dizziness may occur
- To carry emergency ID denoting product use, name of prescriber
- To notify prescriber of rash, bleeding, bruising, slurred speech, jaundice of skin or eyes, joint pain, nausea, vomiting, severe headaches
- To keep all medical appointments, including those for lab work, physical assessment
- To notify prescriber if pregnancy is planned, suspected
- To use contraception while using this product

⚠ HIGH ALERT

fospropofol (Rx)

(fos-proe′poe-fol)

Lusedra

Func. class.: General anesthetic

ACTION: Produces dose-dependent CNS depression by activation of GABA receptor

USES: Induction or maintenance of anesthesia as part of balanced anesthetic technique; sedation in mechanically ventilated patients

CONTRAINDICATIONS: Hypersensitivity to product

Precautions: Pregnancy (B), breastfeeding, children, geriatric patients, respiratory depression, severe respiratory disorders, cardiac dysrhythmias, labor/delivery, renal disease, hyperlipidemia

DOSAGE AND ROUTES

Induction/Maintenance

- **Adult <65 (healthy), >90 kg:** 577.5 **IV BOL,** may give supplemental doses up to max of 140 mg, give no more frequently than q4min; 61-89 kg 6.5 mg/kg (max 577.5 mg) **IV BOL** may give supplemental doses up to 1.6 mg/kg/dose (max 140 mg/dose; give no more frequently than q4min); <60 kg 385 mg **IV BOL,** may give supplemental doses up to max 105 mg/dose, give no more frequently than q4min
- **Adult: <65 yr (severe systemic disease), ≥90 kg** 437.5 mg **IV BOL,** give supplemental doses up to max 105 mg/dose, give no more frequently than q4min; 61-89 kg 4.875 mg/kg (max 437.5 mg) give supplemental doses of 75% of standard dose/up to 1.2 mg/kg/dose (max 105 mg/dose) give no more frequently than q4min; <60 kg 297.5 **IV BOL,** give supplemental doses up to max 70 mg/dose, give no more frequently than q4min
- **Geriatric ≥90 kg: IV BOL** 437.5 then supplemental doses up to max 105 mg; give no more frequently than q4min; 61-89 kg, **IV BOL** give 75% standard dosing regimen (4.875 mg/kg), give no more frequently than q4min (max 105 mg/dose)

Available forms: Inj 1050 mg/30 ml

Administer:

IV Bolus route

- Visually inspect for particulate matter and discoloration
- Each vial is single patient/single use
- Draw from vial, discard unused portion
- Do not mix with other drugs prior to use
- Give by IV BOL in free-flowing peripheral IV line of D_5W, 5% dextrose/0.2% NaCl, 5% dextrose/0.45% NaCl D_5LR, LR, 0.45% NaCl, NS, 5% dextrose/0.45% NaCl/20 mEq KCl; do not mix with other fluids, flush line with NS before and after administration
- No filtration needed
- Give only with resuscitative equipment available
- Only qualified persons trained in anesthesia should administer

SIDE EFFECTS

CNS: Involuntary movement, headache, jerking, fever, dizziness, shivering, tremor, confusion, somnolence, paresthesia, agitation, abnormal dreams, euphoria, fatigue, **increased intracranial pressure, impaired cerebral flow, seizures**

CV: *Bradycardia, hypotension,* hypertension, PVC, PAC, tachycardia, abnormal ECG, ST segment depression, **asystole, bradydysrhythmias**

EENT: Blurred vision, tinnitus, eye pain, strange taste, diplopia

GI: *Nausea, vomiting, abdominal cramping,* dry mouth, swallowing, hypersalivation, **pancreatitis**

GU: Urine retention, green urine, cloudy urine, oliguria

INTEG: *Flushing, phlebitis, hives, burning/stinging at inj site,* rash, pain of extremities

MS: Myalgia
RESP: Apnea, *cough, hiccups,* dyspnea, hypoventilation, sneezing, wheezing, tachypnea, hypoxia, respiratory acidosis

PHARMACOKINETICS

Onset 15-30 sec, rapid distribution, half-life 1-8 min, terminal half-life .81-.88 hr; 70% excreted in urine; metabolized in liver by conjugation to inactive metabolites, 95%-99% protein binding

INTERACTIONS

⚠ **Do not use within 10 days of MAOIs**
Increase: CNS depression—alcohol, opioids, sedative/hypnotics, antipsychotics, skeletal muscle relaxants, inhalational anesthetics
Drug/Herb
Increase: fospropofol effect—St. John's wort

NURSING CONSIDERATIONS

Assess:
- Inj site: phlebitis, burning, stinging
- **ECG** for changes: PVC, PAC, ST segment changes; monitor VS
- CNS changes: movement, jerking, tremors, dizziness, LOC, pupil reaction
- Allergic reactions: hives
- **Respiratory depression,** character, rate, rhythm; notify prescriber if respirations are <10/min; hypoxemia detectable by pulse oximetry

Perform/provide:
- Storage of unopened vials at room temp

Evaluate:
- Therapeutic response: induction of anesthesia

Teach patient/family:
- That this medication will cause dizziness, drowsiness, sedation

TREATMENT OF OVERDOSE:

Discontinue product; administer vasopressor agents or anticholinergics, artificial ventilation

frovatriptan (Rx)

(froh-vah-trip'tan)

Frova

Func. class.: Antimigraine agent
Chem. class.: 5-HT_1-Receptor agonist

ACTION:

Binds selectively to the vascular 5-HT_{1B}, 5-HT_{1D} receptor subtypes; exerts antimigraine effect; binds to benzodiazepine receptor sites, causes vasoconstriction in cranium

USES:

Acute treatment of migraine with/without aura

CONTRAINDICATIONS:

Hypersensitivity, angina pectoris, history of MI, documented silent ischemia, Prinzmetal's angina, ischemic heart disease; concurrent ergotamine-containing preparations; uncontrolled hypertension; basilar or hemiplegic migraine; ischemic bowel disease; peripheral vascular disease, severe hepatic disease, prophylactic migraine treatment
Precautions: Pregnancy (C), breastfeeding, children, geriatric patients, postmenopausal women, men >40 yr, risk factors for CAD, hypercholesterolemia, obesity, diabetes, impaired hepatic function, seizure disorder

DOSAGE AND ROUTES

- **Adult: PO** 2.5 mg; a 2nd dose may be taken after ≥2 hr; max 3 tabs (7.5 mg/day)

Available form: Tabs 2.5 mg
Administer:
- Swallow tabs whole; do not break, crush, or chew
- With fluids
- 2 days/wk or less; rebound headache may occur

SIDE EFFECTS

CNS: *Hot/cold sensation,* paresthesia, *dizziness,* headache, fatigue, insomnia, anxiety, somnolence, **seizures**

CV: *Flushing*, chest pain, palpitation
GI: Dry mouth, dyspepsia, abdominal pain, diarrhea, vomiting, nausea
MS: Skeletal pain

PHARMACOKINETICS

Onset of pain relief 2-3 hr, terminal half-life 25-29 hr, protein binding 15%, metabolized liver by CYP1A2

INTERACTIONS

Increase: frovatriptan levels—CYP1A2 inhibitors (cimetidine, ciprofloxacin, erythromycin), estrogen, propranolol, oral contraceptives
Increase: toxicity—SSRIs, other serotonin agonists (dextromethorphan, tramadol, antidepressants)

NURSING CONSIDERATIONS

Assess:
- **Migraine symptoms:** aura, unable to view light; ingestion of tyramine-containing foods (pickled products, beer, wine, aged cheese), food additives, preservatives, colorings, artificial sweeteners, chocolate, caffeine, which may precipitate these types of headaches
- B/P; signs, symptoms of coronary vasospasms
- For stress level, activity, recreation, coping mechanisms

Perform/provide:
- Quiet, calm environment with decreased stimulation from noise, bright light, excessive talking

Evaluate:
- Therapeutic response: decrease in frequency, severity of migraine

Teach patient/family:
- To report any side effects to prescriber
- To use contraception while taking product; to inform prescriber if pregnant or planning to become pregnant
- To consult prescriber if breastfeeding

fulvestrant (Rx)

(full-vess′trant)

Faslodex

Func. class.: Antineoplastic
Chem. class.: Estrogen-receptor antagonist

ACTION:
Inhibits cell division by binding to cytoplasmic estrogen receptors, downregulates estrogen receptors

USES:
Advanced breast carcinoma in estrogen-receptor–positive patients (usually postmenopausal)
Unlabeled uses: Loading dose for metastatic breast cancer

CONTRAINDICATIONS:
Pregnancy (D), breastfeeding, children, hypersensitivity
Precautions: Hepatic disease

DOSAGE AND ROUTES

- **Adult: IM** 500 mg as 5-ml injections on days 1, 15, 29 and monthly thereafter

Available forms: Inj 50 mg/ml
Administer:
IM route
- IM 5 ml as a single inj or give 2 inj of 2.5 ml; give slowly in buttock
- Antiemetic 30-60 min before product to prevent vomiting prn

SIDE EFFECTS

CNS: *Headache,* depression, dizziness, insomnia, paresthesia, anxiety
GI: *Nausea, vomiting,* anorexia, constipation, diarrhea, abdominal pain
HEMA: Anemia
INTEG: *Rash,* sweating, hot flashes, inj site pain
MS: Bone pain, arthritis, back pain
RESP: Pharyngitis, dyspnea, cough
SYST: Angioedema

PHARMACOKINETICS

Half-life 40 days, metabolized by CYP3A4, excretion in feces 90%

NURSING CONSIDERATIONS

Assess:

- For side effects; report to prescriber

Perform/provide:

- Liquid diet, if needed, including cola, gelatin; dry toast or crackers may be added if patient is not nauseated or vomiting
- Store in refrigerator, protect from light

Evaluate:

- Therapeutic response: decreased tumor size, spread of malignancy

Teach patient/family:

- To report any complaints, side effects to prescriber
- To report vaginal bleeding immediately
- That tumor flare (increase in size of tumor, increased bone pain) may occur, will subside rapidly; that analgesics may be taken for pain
- That premenopausal women must use mechanical birth control because ovulation may be induced; not to breastfeed
- To use contraception to prevent pregnancy; pregnancy category (D)

furosemide (Rx)

(fur-oh′se-mide)

Apo-Furosemide ✱, Lasix

Func. class.: Loop diuretic

Chem. class.: Sulfonamide derivative

Do not confuse:

furosemide/torsemide

Lasix/Luvox/Lomotil/Lanoxin

ACTION: Inhibits reabsorption of sodium and chloride at proximal and distal tubule and in the loop of Henle

USES: Pulmonary edema; edema with CHF, hepatic disease, nephrotic syndrome, ascites, hypertension

Unlabeled uses: Hypercalcemia with malignancy, hypertensive emergency/urgency, pulmonary edema or prevention of hemodynamic effects associated with blood product transfusion, ascites

CONTRAINDICATIONS: Breastfeeding, infants, anuria, hypovolemia, electrolyte depletion

Precautions: Pregnancy (C), diabetes mellitus, dehydration, severe renal disease, cirrhosis, ascites, hypersensitivity to sulfonamides/thiazides

DOSAGE AND ROUTES

Edema

- **Adult: PO** 20-80 mg/day in AM; may give another dose after 6 hr up to 600 mg/day; **IM/IV** 20-40 mg; increase by 20 mg q2hr until desired response
- **Child: PO/IM/IV** 2 mg/kg; may increase by 1-2 mg/kg q6-8hr up to 6 mg/kg

Acute pulmonary edema

- **Adult: IV** 40 mg given over several min, repeated after 1 hr; increase to 80 mg if needed
- **Child: IV/IM** 1-2 mg/kg q6-12hr, max 6 mg/kg/dose
- **Premature neonate >32 wk postconceptional age: IV/IM** 1-2 mg/kg q12-24hr
- **Premature neonate ≤32 wk postconceptional age: IV/IM** max 1 mg/kg initially

Antihypercalcemia

- **Adult: IM/IV** 80-100 mg q1-4hr or **PO** 120 mg/day or divided bid
- **Child: IM/IV** 25-50 mg, repeat q4hr if needed

Acute/chronic renal failure

- **Adult: PO** 80 mg/day, increase by 80-120 mg/day to desired response; **IV** 100-200 mg, max 600-800 mg

Hypertensive emergency/urgency (unlabeled)

- **Adult: IV** 40-80 mg

Pulmonary edema/prevention of adverse hemodynamic effects associated with blood product transfusion (unlabeled)

- **Adult: IV** 40 mg injected slowly then 80 mg injected slowly after 2 hr if needed
- **Child: IM/IV** 1-2 mg/kg q6-12hr

• **Premature neonate >32 wk postconceptional age: IM/IV** 1-2 mg/kg q12-24hr
• **Premature neonate ≤32 wk postconceptional age: IM/IV** Max 1 mg/kg, give no more frequently than q24hr

Available forms: Tabs 20, 40, 80 mg; oral sol 8 mg/ml, 10 mg/ml; inj 10 mg/ml

Administer:
• In AM to avoid interference with sleep if using product as diuretic
• Potassium replacement if potassium <3 mg/dl
• PO with food if nausea occurs; absorption may be decreased slightly; tabs may be crushed

IV route
• Undiluted; may be given through Y-tube or 3-way stopcock; give ≤20 mg/min; may be added to NS or D_5W; if large doses required and given as IV inf, max 4 mg/min; use inf pump

Y-site compatibilities: Acyclovir, alfentanil, allopurinol, alprostadil, amifostine, amikacin, aminocaproic acid, aminophylline, amphotericin B cholesteryl/lipid complex/liposome, anidulafungin, argatroban, ascorbic acid, atenolol, atropine, azathioprine, aztreonam, bivalirudin, bleomycin, bumetanide, calcium chloride/gluconate, CARBOplatin, cefamandole, ceFAZolin, cefepime, cefmetazole, cefonicid, cefoperazone, cefotaxime, cefotetan, cefoxitin, ceftazidime, ceftizoxime, ceftobiprole, cefTRIAXone, cefuroxime, cephalothin, cephapirin, chloramphenicol, CISplatin, cladribine, clindamycin, cyanocobalamin, cyclophosphamide, cycloSPORINE, cytarabine, DACTINomycin, DAPTOmycin, dexamethasone, dexmedetomidine, digoxin, docetaxel, doripenem, doxacurium, DOXOrubicin liposome, enalaprilat, ePHEDrine, EPINEPHrine, etoposide, fentaNYL, fludarabine, fluorouracil, folic acid, foscarnet, gallium nitrate, ganciclovir, granisetron, heparin, hydrocortisone, HYDROmorphone, ifosfamide, imipenem-cilastatin, indomethacin, insulin (regular), isosorbide, kanamycin, leucovorin, lidocaine, linezolid, LORazepam, LR, mannitol, mechlorethamine, melphalan, meropenem, methicillin, methotrexate, methylPREDNISolone, metoprolol, metroNIDAZOLE, mezlocillin, micafungin, miconazole, mitomycin, moxalactam, multiple vitamin injection, nafcillin, naloxone, nitroprusside, octreotide, oxacillin, oxaliplatin, oxytocin, paclitaxel, palonosetron, pamidronate, pantoprazole, pemetrexed, penicillin G, PENTobarbital, PHENobarbital, phytonadione, piperacillin, piperacillin-tazobactam, potassium chloride, procainamide, propofol, propranolol, ranitidine, remifentanil, Ringer's, ritodrine, sargramostim, sodium acetate/bicarbonate, succinylcholine, SUFentanil, temocillin, teniposide, theophylline, thiopental, thiotepa, ticarcillin, ticarcillin-clavulanate, tigecycline, tirofiban, TNA, tobramycin, urokinase, vit B/C, voriconazole, zoledronic acid

SIDE EFFECTS

CNS: Headache, fatigue, weakness, vertigo, paresthesias
CV: Orthostatic hypotension, chest pain, ECG changes, **circulatory collapse**
EENT: Loss of hearing, ear pain, tinnitus, blurred vision
ELECT: *Hypokalemia, hypochloremic alkalosis, hypomagnesemia, hyperuricemia, hypocalcemia, hyponatremia,* metabolic alkalosis
ENDO: *Hyperglycemia*
GI: *Nausea,* diarrhea, dry mouth, vomiting, anorexia, cramps, oral, gastric irritations, pancreatitis
GU: *Polyuria,* **renal failure**, glycosuria
HEMA: **Thrombocytopenia, agranulocytosis, leukopenia, neutropenia, anemia**
INTEG: *Rash, pruritus,* purpura, **Stevens-Johnson syndrome**, sweating, photosensitivity, urticaria
MS: Cramps, stiffness

PHARMACOKINETICS

PO: Onset 1 hr, peak 1-2 hr, duration 6-8 hr, absorbed 70%

IV: Onset 5 min; peak $\frac{1}{2}$ hr; duration 2 hr (metabolized by the liver 30%); excreted in urine, some as unchanged product, and feces; crosses placenta; excreted in breast milk; half-life $\frac{1}{2}$-1 hr

INTERACTIONS

Increase: toxicity—lithium, non-depolarizing skeletal muscle relaxants, digoxin
Increase: hypotensive action of antihypertensives, nitrates
Increase: ototoxicity—aminoglycosides, CISplatin, vancomycin
Increase: effects of anticoagulants, salicylates
Decrease: furosemide effect—probenecid

Drug/Lab Test
Interference: GTT
Increase: LDL

NURSING CONSIDERATIONS

Assess:

- **CHF:** weight, I&O daily to determine fluid loss; effect of product may be decreased if used daily
- **Hypertension:** B/P lying, standing; postural hypotension may occur
- Metabolic alkalosis: drowsiness, restlessness
- **Hypokalemia:** postural hypotension, malaise, fatigue, tachycardia, leg cramps, weakness
- Rashes, temp elevation daily
- Confusion, especially in geriatric patients; take safety precautions if needed
- **Hearing,** including tinnitus and hearing loss, when giving high doses for extended periods
- Rate, depth, rhythm of respiration, effect of exertion, lung sounds
- Electrolytes (potassium, sodium, chloride); include BUN, blood glucose, CBC, serum creatinine, blood pH, ABGs, uric acid
- Glucose in urine if patient diabetic
- Allergies to sulfonamides, thiazides

Perform/provide:

- Increased fluid intake 2-3 L/day unless contraindicated

Evaluate:

- Therapeutic response: improvement in edema of feet, legs, sacral area (CHF); increase urine output, decreased B/P; decreased calcium levels (hypercalcemia)

Teach patient/family:

- To discuss the need for a high-potassium diet or potassium replacement with prescriber
- To rise slowly from lying or sitting position because orthostatic hypotension may occur
- To recognize adverse reactions that may occur: muscle cramps, weakness, nausea, dizziness
- About the entire treatment regimen, including exercise, diet, stress relief for hypertension
- To take with food or milk for GI symptoms
- To use sunscreen or protective clothing to prevent photosensitivity
- To take early in the day to prevent sleeplessness
- To avoid OTC medications unless directed by prescriber

TREATMENT OF OVERDOSE:

Lavage if taken orally; monitor electrolytes; administer dextrose in saline; monitor hydration, CV, renal status

gabapentin (Rx)

(gab′a-pen-tin)

Apo-Gabapentin ♣, CO Gabapentin ♣, Gen-Gabapentin ♣, Gralise, Horizant, Neurontin, Novo-Gabapentin ♣, PMS-Gabapentin ♣, ratio-Gabapentin ♣

Func. class.: Anticonvulsant

Do not confuse:
Neurontin/Noroxin/Neoral

ACTION: Mechanism unknown; may increase seizure threshold; structurally similar to GABA; gabapentin binding sites in neocortex, hippocampus

USES: Adjunct treatment of partial seizures, with/without generalization in patients >12 yr; adjunct for partial seizures in children 3-12 yr, postherpetic neuralgia, primary restless leg syndrome in adults

Unlabeled uses: Tremors with multiple sclerosis (MS), neuropathic pain, bipolar disorder, migraine prophylaxis, diabetic neuropathy, nystagmus, pruritus, spasticity, menopause, hot flashes, ALS, MS

CONTRAINDICATIONS: Hypersensitivity to this product

Precautions: Pregnancy (C), breastfeeding, children <3 yr, geriatric patients, renal disease, hemodialysis, suicidal thoughts, depression

DOSAGE AND ROUTES

- **Adult and child >12 yr: PO** 900-1800 mg/day in 3 divided doses; may titrate by giving 300 mg on 1st day, 300 mg bid on 2nd day, 300 mg tid on 3rd day; may increase to 1800-2400 mg/day by adding 300 mg on subsequent days
- **Child 3-12 yr: PO** 10-15 mg/kg/day in 3 divided doses, initially titrate dose upward over approximately 3 days; 25-35 mg/kg/day; all given in 3 divided doses

Postherpetic neuralgia

- **Adult: PO** 300 mg on day 1, 600 mg/day divided bid on day 2, 900 mg/day divided tid, may titrate to 1800-3600 mg divided tid if needed; **EXT REL** (Gralise only) 300 mg on day 1, 600 mg on day 2, 900 mg on days 3-6, 1200 mg on days 7-10, 1500 mg on days 11-14, 1800 mg on day 15 and thereafter

Moderate to severe restless leg syndrome (RLS) (Horizant only)

- **Adult: PO EXT REL** 600 mg daily with food at about 5 PM; if dose missed, take next day at 5 PM

Renal dose

- **Adult and child >12 yr:** CCr 30-59 ml/min, 200-700 mg bid, CCr 15-29 ml/min, 200-700 mg/day, CCr <15 ml/min, 100-300 mg/day

Uremic pruritus in hemodialysis (unlabeled)

- **Adult: PO** 300 mg 3×/wk

Brachioradical pruritus (unlabeled)

- **Adult: PO** 300-1800 mg/day

ALS (unlabeled)

- **Adult: PO** 1000 mg/day in divided doses × 6 mo

Pendular/congenital nystagmus (unlabeled)

- **Adult: PO** 900 mg/day in divided doses initially, up to 2400 mg/day in divided doses

Spasticity in MS (unlabeled)

- **Adult: PO** 600-1200 mg/day in divided doses

Available forms: Caps 100, 300, 400 mg; tabs 600, 800 mg; Horizant: ext rel tab 600 mg; oral sol 250 mg/5 ml

Administer:

- Do not crush or chew caps, ext rel tabs; caps may be opened and contents put in applesauce or dissolved in juice; scored tabs may be cut in half
- 2 hr apart when giving antacids
- Give without regard to meals
- Gradually withdraw over 7 days; abrupt withdrawal may precipitate seizures

• **Oral sol:** Measure with calibrated device

• **Ext rel:** Give with food at about 5 PM, bioavailability increased with food; swallow whole; do not interchange Gralise with Horizant

SIDE EFFECTS

CNS: *Drowsiness, confusion,* dizziness, fatigue, anxiety, somnolence, ataxia, amnesia, abnormal thinking, unsteady gait, *depression;* children 3-12 yr old, emotional lability, aggression, thought disorder, hyperkinesia, hostility, seizures, suicidal ideation

CV: Vasodilation, peripheral edema, hypotension

EENT: Dry mouth, blurred vision, *diplopia,* nystagmus

GI: Constipation, increased appetite, dental abnormalities, nausea, vomiting

GU: Impotence, bleeding, *UTI*

HEMA: Leukopenia, decreased WBC

INTEG: Pruritus, abrasion, Stevens-Johnson syndrome

MS: Myalgia

RESP: *Rhinitis,* pharyngitis, cough

PHARMACOKINETICS

Protein binding <3% not metabolized; excreted in urine (unchanged); elimination half-life 5-7 hr, prolonged to 130 hr in ESRD

INTERACTIONS

Increase: CNS depression—alcohol, sedatives, antihistamines, all other CNS depressants

Increase: gabapentin levels—morphine

Decrease: gabapentin levels—antacids, sevelamar, cimetidine

Decrease: effect of—HYDROcodone

Drug/Lab Test

False positive: urinary protein using Ames N-multistix SG

NURSING CONSIDERATIONS

Assess:

• **Seizures:** aura, location, duration, activity at onset

• **Pain:** location, duration, characteristics if using for chronic pain, migraine

⚠ Mental status: mood, sensorium, affect, behavioral changes, **suicidal thoughts/behaviors;** if mental status changes, notify prescriber

• Eye problems, need for ophthalmic exam before, during, after treatment (slit lamp, funduscopy, tonometry)

• WBC, gabapentin level (therapeutic 5.9-21 mcg/ml, toxic >85 mcg/ml)

Perform/provide:

• Storage at room temp away from heat and light

• **Seizure precautions:** padded side rails; move objects that may harm patient

• Increased fluids, bulk in diet for constipation

Evaluate:

• Therapeutic response: decreased seizure activity; decrease in chronic pain

Teach patient/family:

• To carry emergency ID stating patient's name, products taken, condition, prescriber's name and phone number

• To avoid driving, other activities that require alertness because dizziness, drowsiness may occur

• Not to discontinue medication quickly after long-term use; to taper over ≥1 wk because withdrawal-precipitated seizures may occur; not to double doses if dose is missed; to take if 2 hr or more before next dose

• To notify prescriber if pregnancy planned or suspected; to avoid breastfeeding

• Not to use within 2 hr of antacid

galantamine (Rx)

(gah-lan'tah-meen)

Razadyne, Razadyne ER, Reminyl ✦

Func. class.: Anti-Alzheimer agent

Chem. class.: Centrally acting cholinesterase inhibitor

ACTION:
Enhances cholinergic functioning by increasing acetylcholine in cerebral cortex

USES:
Mild to moderate dementia of Alzheimer's disease

Unlabeled uses: Vascular dementia, dementia with Lewy bodies, Pick's disease

CONTRAINDICATIONS:
Hypersensitivity to this product, GI bleeding, jaundice, renal failure, breastfeeding, children

Precautions: Pregnancy (B), geriatric patients, respiratory/renal/hepatic/cardiac disease, seizure disorder, peptic ulcer, asthma, bradycardia, heart block, surgery, urinary tract obstruction

DOSAGE AND ROUTES

• **Adult: PO** 4 mg bid with morning and evening meals; after 4 wk or more, may increase to 8 mg bid; may increase to 12 mg bid after another 4 wk, usual dose 16-24 mg/day in 2 divided doses; **EXT REL** 8 mg/day in AM; may increase to 16 mg/day after 4 wk and 24 mg/day after another 4 wk

Hepatic dose

• **Adult: PO** Child-Pugh 7-9, max 16 mg/day; Child-Pugh 10-15, avoid use

Renal dose

• **Adult: PO** CCr 10-70 ml/min, max 16 mg/day; CCr $<$9 ml/min, avoid use

Available forms: Tabs 4, 8, 12 mg; ext rel tabs 8, 16, 24 mg; oral sol 4 mg/ml

Administer:

• With meals; take with morning and evening meal (immediate rel); morning (ext rel)

• Dose increase after minimum of 4 wk at prior dose; if dose is interrupted for $\geq$ 3 days, restart at lower dose, titrate to current dose

• Ext rel in AM with food; do not crush, open, or chew

• Oral sol: use pipette provided

SIDE EFFECTS

CNS: *Tremors, insomnia,* depression, dizziness, headache, somnolence, fatigue

CV: Bradycardia, chest pain

GI: *Nausea, vomiting, anorexia, abdominal distress, flatulence,* diarrhea

GU: Urinary incontinence, bladder outflow obstruction, hematuria

HEMA: Anemia

META: Weight decrease

MS: Asthenia

RESP: Upper respiratory tract infection, rhinitis

PHARMACOKINETICS

Rapidly and completely absorbed; metabolized by CYP2D6, 3A4; excreted via kidneys; clearance is lower in geriatric patients, hepatic disease; clearance is 20% lower in females; elimination half-life 7 hr; 18% protein binding

INTERACTIONS

• Synergistic effect: cholinomimetics, other cholinesterase inhibitors

Increase: galantamine effect—CYP3A4, CYP2D6 inhibitors (antiretroviral protease inhibitors, ketoconazole, erythromycin, conivaptan, delaviridine, diltiazem, efavirenz, fluconazole, fluroxamine, imatinib, itraconazole, clarithromycin, troleandomycin, nefazodone, niCARdipine, verapamil, voriconazole, zafirlukast)

Increase: GI effects—NSAIDs

Decrease: galantamine effect—CYP3A4, CYP2D6 inducers (bosentan, carBAMazepine, nevirapine, oxcarbazepine, phenytoin, fosphenytoin/rifabutin, rifampin, rifapentine, troglitazone)

Drug/Herb

Decrease: galantamine effect—St. John's wort

NURSING CONSIDERATIONS

Assess:

Alzheimer's disease: mental status: affect, mood, behavioral changes, depression, attention, confusion; neurologic status: long- and short-term memory, cognitive functioning

- Hepatic/renal studies: AST, ALT, alk phos, LDH, bilirubin, CBC; BUN, creatinine
- For severe GI effects: nausea, vomiting, anorexia, weight loss
- B/P, heart rate, respiration during initial treatment: bradycardia may occur
- Fluid status: ensure adequate hydration

Perform/provide:

- Assistance with ambulation during beginning therapy

Evaluate:

- Therapeutic response: decreased confusion

Teach patient/family:

- To notify all prescribers of use
- About correct procedure for giving oral sol using instruction sheet provided
- To notify prescriber of severe GI effects; hypo/hypertension, slow heart rate
- That product is not a cure but relieves symptoms
- That results may take several weeks or months to occur

ganciclovir (Rx)

(gan-sye'kloe-vir)

Cytovene, Vitrasert

Func. class.: Antiviral

Chem. class.: Synthetic nucleoside analog

Do not confuse:

Cytovene/Cytosar

ACTION: Inhibits replication of herpesviruses; competitively inhibits human CMV DNA polymerase and is incorporated, resulting in termination of DNA elongation

USES: Cytomegalovirus (CMV) retinitis in immunocompromised persons, including those with AIDS, after indirect ophthalmoscopy confirms diagnosis; prophylaxis for CMV in transplantation

Unlabeled uses: CMV pneumonia in organ transplant patients; CMV gastroenteritis, esophagitis, colitis; CMV pneumonitis, congenital CMV disease; Epstein-Barr virus; herpes simplex types 1, 2; varicella-zoster, hepatitis B

CONTRAINDICATIONS: Hypersensitivity to acyclovir, ganciclovir, famciclovir, penciclovir, valacyclovir, valganciclovir

Black Box Warning: Absolute neutrophil count <500, platelet count <25,000 (intravitreal)

Precautions: Pregnancy (C), breastfeeding, children <6 mo, geriatric patients, preexisting cytopenias, renal function impairment, radiation therapy

Black Box Warning: Secondary malignancy, bone marrow suppression, anemia, infertility, neutropenia

DOSAGE AND ROUTES

Prevention of CMV

- **Adult/adolescent (unlabeled): IV** 5 mg/kg/dose over 1 hr q12hr × 1-2 wk, then 5 mg/kg/day 7 day/wk, then 6 mg/kg/day × 5 days/wk; **PO** 1000 mg tid starting 10 days posttransplant × 14 wk

Induction treatment

- **Adult: IV** 5 mg/kg/dose given over 1 hr, q12hr × 2-3 wk

Maintenance treatment

- **Adult: IV INF** 5 mg/kg given over 1 hr, daily × 7 days/wk or 6 mg/kg/day × 5 days/wk; **PO** 1000 mg tid with food or 500 mg q3hr while awake for 6 doses; **INTRAVITREAL** 4.5 mg implant

Renal dose

- **Adult:** **IV** CCr 50-69 ml/min, reduce to 2.5 mg/kg q12hr (induction), 2.5 mg/kg q24hr (maintenance); **PO** 1500 mg/day or 500 mg tid; **IV** CCr 25-49 ml/min, reduce to 2.5 mg q24hr (induction); 1.25 mg/kg q24hr (maintenance); **PO** 1000 mg/day or 500 mg bid; **IV** CCr 10-24 ml/min, reduce to 1.25 mg/kg q24hr (induction); 0.625 mg/kg q24hr (maintenance); **PO** 500 mg/day; **IV** CCr <10 ml/min, reduce to 1.25 mg/kg 3×/wk after hemodialysis (induction); 0.625 mg/kg 3×/wk after hemodialysis (maintenance); **PO** 500 mg 3×/wk after hemodialysis

Available forms: Powder for inj 500 mg/vial; caps 250, 500 mg; implant, intraviteral 4.5 mg

Administer:

PO route

- With food
- Do not open, crush capsules

IV route

- Mixed in biologic cabinet using gown, gloves, mask; use cytotoxic handling procedures

Intermittent IV INF route

- IV after reconstituting 500 mg/10 ml sterile water for inj (50 mg/ml); shake; further dilute in 50-250 ml D_5W, 0.9% NaCl, LR, Ringer's and run over 1 hr; use inf pump, in-line filter
- Do not give by bolus IV, IM, SUBCUT inj
- Use reconstituted sol within 24 hr; do not refrigerate or freeze

Y-site compatibilities: Allopurinol, amphotericin B cholesteryl, CISplatin, cyclophosphamide, DOXOrubicin liposome, enalaprilat, etoposide, filgrastim, fluconazole, gatifloxacin, granisetron, linezolid, melphalan, methotrexate, paclitaxel, propofol, remifentanil, tacrolimus, teniposide, thiotepa

Intravitreal implant route

- Implanted by surgeon only
- Handle carefully to prevent damage to coating

Intravitreal inj route (unlabeled)

- Reconstitute and dilute IV powder to 2 mg/0.1 ml or 5 mg/0.1 ml, depending on dose; injected using TB syringe

SIDE EFFECTS

CNS: *Fever,* chills, coma, *confusion*, abnormal thoughts, dizziness, bizarre dreams, *headache*, psychosis, tremors, somnolence, *paresthesia*, *weakness,* **seizures**, peripheral neuropathy

CV: Dysrhythmia, hypo/hypertension

EENT: Retinal detachment in CMV retinitis, ocular hypertension, ocular pain, conjunctival scarring, cataracts

GI: *Abnormal LFTs, nausea, vomiting, anorexia, diarrhea, abdominal pain,* **hemorrhage, perforation, pancreatitis**

GU: **Hematuria**, *increased creatinine,* BUN

HEMA: **Granulocytopenia, thrombocytopenia, irreversible neutropenia, anemia, eosinophilia, pancytopenia**

INTEG: *Rash*, alopecia, *pruritus*, urticaria, pain at site, phlebitis

RESP: Dyspnea

PHARMACOKINETICS

Half-life 3-4½ hr; excreted by kidneys (unchanged); crosses blood-brain barrier, CSF, increased bioavailability with fatty foods

INTERACTIONS

⚠ **Severe granulocytopenia: zidovudine, antineoplastics, radiation; do not give together**

Increase: ganciclovir toxicity—adriamycin, amphotericin B, cycloSPORINE, dapsone, DOXOrubicin, flucytosine, pentamidine, probenecid, trimethoprim-sulfamethoxazole combinations, vinBLAStine, vinCRIStine, other nucleoside analogs, mycophenolate, tenofovir, tacrolimus, aminoglycosides, NSAIDs

Increase: seizures—imipenem/cilastatin

Increase: didanosine effect—didanosine

NURSING CONSIDERATIONS

Assess:

- **CMV retinitis:** culture should be completed before starting treatment (urine, blood, throat), ophthalmic exam
- **Infection:** increased temp, sore throat, chills, fever; report to prescriber
- **Leukopenia/neutropenia/thrombocytopenia:** CBC, WBCs, platelets q2days during 2×/day dosing and then q1wk for leukopenia with daily WBC count in patients with prior leukopenia with other nucleoside analogs or for whom leukopenia counts are <1000 cells/mm^3 at start of treatment
- Serum creatinine or CCr ≥q2wk, BUN; LFTs; ophthalmic exam
- For seizures, dysrhythmias

Evaluate:

- Therapeutic response: decreased symptoms or prevention of CMV

Teach patient/family:

- That product does not cure condition; that regular blood tests, ophthalmologic exams are necessary
- That major toxicities may necessitate discontinuing product
- To use contraception during treatment and that infertility may occur; to use barrier contraception for 90 days after treatment
- To take PO with food

⚠ **To report infection:** fever, chills, sore throat; blood dyscrasias: bruising, bleeding, petechiae; to avoid crowds, persons with respiratory infections

ganciclovir ophthalmic

See Appendix B

ganirelix (Rx)

Orgalutran ✤

Func. class.: Gonadotropin-releasing hormone antagonist

Chem. class.: Synthetic decapeptide

ACTION: Inhibitor of pituitary gonadotropin secretion; initially increases LH and FSH, induces a rapid suppression of gonadotropin secretion

USES: For inhibition of premature LH surges in women undergoing controlled ovarian hyperstimulation

CONTRAINDICATIONS: Pregnancy (X), breastfeeding, hypersensitivity, latex allergy

DOSAGE AND ROUTES

- **Adult:** Give FSH on day 2 or 3 of cycle then **SUBCUT** 250 mcg/day during mid-to-late portion follicular phase; continue until the day of hCG administration

Available forms: Inj 250 mcg/0.5 ml

Administer:

- SUBCUT using abdomen around navel or upper thigh; swab inj area with disinfectant; clean a 2-in circle and allow to dry; pinch up area between thumb and finger; insert needle at 45-90 degrees to surface; if positioned correctly, no blood will be drawn back into syringe; if blood is drawn into syringe, reposition needle without removing it, inject slowly; prefilled syringe for 1-time use

SIDE EFFECTS

CNS: Headache

ENDO: Ovarian hyperstimulation syndrome, abdominal pain (GYN)

GI: Nausea

GU: *Spotting, breakthrough bleeding,* decreased urine, fetal death

INTEG: Pain on inj

SYST: Fetal death

PHARMACOKINETICS

Excreted in feces/urine, half-life 13-16 hr, metabolized to metabolites, protein binding 82%

NURSING CONSIDERATIONS

Assess:

- For suspected pregnancy (X), latex allergy; product should not be used
- Reproductive tests: serum gonadotropin, serum progesterone, LH, estradiol, ovarian ultrasound, pelvic exam at baseline and during treatment

Perform/provide:

- Protection from light

Evaluate:

- Therapeutic response: pregnancy

Teach patient/family:

- To report abdominal pain, vaginal bleeding

gatifloxacin ophthalmic

See Appendix B

gemcitabine (Rx)

(jem-sit′a-been)

Gemzar

Func. class.: Antineoplastic—miscellaneous

Chem. class.: Nucleoside analog

Do not confuse:

Gemzar/Zinecard

ACTION: Exhibits antitumor activity by killing cells undergoing DNA synthesis (S phase) and blocking G1/S-phase boundary

USES: Adenocarcinoma of the pancreas (nonresectable stage II, III, or metastatic stage IV); in combination with CISplatin for inoperable, advanced, or metastatic non–small-cell lung cancer; advanced breast cancer in combination with paclitaxel; with CARBOplatin for ovarian cancer; biliary tract cancer

Unlabeled uses: Bladder cancer, mesothelioma, adjuvant treatment of pancreatic cancer, ovarian cancer single agent, biliary tract cancer

CONTRAINDICATIONS: Pregnancy (D), breastfeeding, hypersensitivity

Precautions: Children, geriatric patients, myelosuppression, radiation therapy, renal/hepatic disease

DOSAGE AND ROUTES

Pancreatic carcinoma (nonresectable stage II, III, IV)

- **Adult: IV** 1000 mg/m^2 given over 30 min/wk up to 7 wk then 1 wk rest period; subsequent cycles should be infused 1×/wk × 3 wk out of every 4 wk depending on hematologic toxicity

Non–small-cell lung cancer

- **Adult: IV** (4-wk schedule) 1000 mg/m^2 given over 30 min on days 1, 8, 15, of each 28-day cycle; give CISplatin **IV** 100 mg/m^2 on day 1 after gemcitabine; 3-wk schedule: 1250 mg/m^2 given over 30 min on days 1, 8 of each 21-day cycle; give CISplatin **IV** 100 mg/m^2 after the inf of gemcitabine on day 1

Advanced breast cancer

- **Adult: IV** 1250 mg/m^2 over 30 min on days 1 and 8 of 21-day cycle; give with paclitaxel 175 mg/m^2 over 3 hr prior to gemcitabine on day 1

Recurrent ovarian cancer (single agent) (unlabeled)

- **Adult: IV** 1 g/m^2, days 1, 8, 15 of 28-day cycle

Adjuvant treatment of pancreatic cancer (unlabeled)

- **Adult: IV** 1000 mg/m^2 over 30 min on days 1, 8, 15 q28days × 6 cycles

Available forms: Lyophilized powder for inj 20 mg/ml

Administer:

IV route

- Prepare in biologic cabinet using gown, mask, gloves; use cytotoxic handling procedures

G

• After reconstituting with 0.9% NaCl 5 ml/200-mg vial of product or 25 ml/1-g vial of product (38 mg/ml) shake; may be further diluted with 0.9% NaCl to conc as low as 0.1 mg/ml; discard unused portions, give over 30 min, do not admix

Y-site compatibilities: Amifostine, amikacin, aminophylline, ampicillin, aztreonam, bleomycin, bumetanide, butorphanol, calcium gluconate, cefoxitin, ceftazidime, ceftizoxime, cefTRIAXone, chlorproMAZINE, cimetidine, ciprofloxacin, CISplatin, clindamycin, cyclophosphamide, cytarabine, DACTINomycin, DAUNOrubicin, diphenhydrAMINE, DOBUTamine, docetaxel, DOPamine, DOXOrubicin, droperidol, enalaprilat, etoposide, famotidine, floxuridine, fluconazole, fludarabine, fluorouracil, gentamicin, granisetron, haloperidol, heparin, hydrocortisone, HYDROmorphone, IDArubicin, ifosfamide, leucovorin, linezolid, LORazepam, mannitol, meperidine, mesna, metoclopramide, metroNIDAZOLE, minocycline, mitoxantrone, morphine, nalbuphine, ondansetron, paclitaxel, promethazine, ranitidine, streptozocin, teniposide, thiotepa, ticarcillin, tobramycin, topotecan, trimethoprim/sulfamethoxazole, vancomycin, vinBLAStine, vinCRIStine, vinorelbine, zidovudine, zoledronic acid

SIDE EFFECTS

GI: Diarrhea, nausea, vomiting, anorexia, constipation, stomatitis

GU: Proteinuria, hematuria

HEMA: **Leukopenia, anemia, neutropenia, thrombocytopenia**

INTEG: Irritation at site, rash, alopecia

OTHER: Dyspnea, fever, **hemorrhage**, infection, flulike symptoms, paresthesia, peripheral edema, myalgia

PHARMACOKINETICS

Half-life 42-379 min, crosses placenta, excretion: renal, 92%-98%

INTERACTIONS

Increase: bleeding—NSAIDs, alcohol, salicylates, anticoagulants

Increase: myelosuppression, diarrhea—other antineoplastics, radiation

Decrease: antibody response—live virus vaccines

Drug/Lab Test

Increase: BUN, AST, ALT, alk phos, bilirubin, creatinine

NURSING CONSIDERATIONS

Assess:

• **Bone marrow depression:** CBC, differential, platelet count before each dose; single agent: absolute granulocyte count >1000 and platelets >100,000, give complete dose; absolute granulocyte count 500-999, platelets 50,000-99,999, give 75%; absolute granulocyte count <500 or platelets <50,000, do not give; combination with paclitaxel for breast cancer: absolute granulocyte count >1200 and platelets >75,000, give complete dose; absolute granulocyte count 1000-1199 or platelets 50,000-75,000, give 75%; absolute granulocyte 700-999 or platelets ≥50,000, give 50%; granulocyte count <700 or platelet <50,000, do not give; combination with CARBOplatin for ovarian cancer: absolute granulocyte count >1500 and platelet count >100,000, give complete dose; absolute granulocyte count 1000-1499 or platelets 75,000-99,000, give 75%; absolute granulocyte count <1000 or platelets <75,000, do not give

• **Blood dyscrasias:** bruising, bleeding, petechiae

• I&O, nutritional intake; food preferences: list likes, dislikes

• Renal, hepatic studies before and during treatment; may increase AST, ALT, alk phos, bilirubin, BUN, creatinine

• Buccal cavity for dryness, sores, ulceration, white patches, oral pain, bleeding, dysphagia

• GI symptoms: frequency of stools, cramping

• Signs of dehydration: rapid respirations, poor skin turgor, decreased urine output, dry skin, restlessness, weakness

Perform/provide:

• Increased fluid intake to 2-3 L/day to prevent dehydration unless contraindicated

• Rinsing of mouth tid-qid with water, club soda; brushing of teeth bid-tid with soft brush or cotton-tipped applicator for stomatitis; use unwaxed dental floss

• Nutritious diet with iron, low fiber, few dairy products

• Antiemetic agents

Evaluate:

• Therapeutic response: decrease in tumor size; decrease in spread of cancer; symptom relief

Teach patient/family:

• To avoid foods with citric acid or hot or rough texture if stomatitis is present; to drink adequate fluids; to avoid use with NSAIDs, alcohol, salicylates

• To report stomatitis and any bleeding, white spots, ulcerations in mouth; to examine mouth daily, report symptoms

• To report signs of anemia: fatigue, headache, faintness, SOB, irritability; hematuria, dysuria

• To use contraception during therapy and for 4 mo after; pregnancy (D)

• Not to receive vaccinations during treatment

• About possible hair loss and what can be done

• To report flulike symptoms, swelling of feet/legs

• To report bruising, bleeding: gums, blood in urine, stool, emesis

• To avoid crowds, persons with known upper-respiratory infections

• To avoid use of hard-bristle toothbrush, electric razor

gemfibrozil (Rx)

(jem-fi′broe-zil)

Apo-Gemfibrozil ♣, Gen-Gemfibrozil ♣, Lopid, PMS-Gemfibrozil ♣

Func. class.: Antilipemic

Chem. class.: Fibric acid derivative

Do not confuse:

Lopid/Levbid/Slo-bid

G

ACTION:
Inhibits biosynthesis of VLDL, decreases triglycerides, increases HDL

USES:
Type IIb, IV, V hyperlipidemia as adjunct with diet therapy, hypertriglyceridemia

CONTRAINDICATIONS:
Severe renal/hepatic disease, preexisting gallbladder disease, primary biliary cirrhosis, hypersensitivity

Precautions: Pregnancy (C), breastfeeding; monitor hematologic and hepatic function

DOSAGE AND ROUTES

• **Adult: PO** 600 mg bid 30 min before AM, PM meal

Hepatic/renal dose

• Avoid use

Available forms: Tabs 600 mg; caps 300 mg ♣

Administer:

• Should not be used with repaglinide or itraconazole

• 30 min before AM, PM meals

• Discontinue product if response does not occur within 3 mo

SIDE EFFECTS

CNS: Fatigue, vertigo, headache, paresthesia, dizziness, somnolence

GI: *Dyspepsia, diarrhea, abdominal pain,* nausea, vomiting

HEMA: **Leukopenia, anemia, eosinophilia, thrombocytopenia**

INTEG: Rash, urticaria, pruritus
MISC: Taste perversion
MS: Myopathy, rhabdomyolysis
SYST: Angioedema, exfoliative dermatitis

PHARMACOKINETICS

Peak 1-2 hr; plasma protein binding >90%; half-life $1^1/_2$ hr; 70% excreted in urine mostly unchanged; metabolized in liver (minimal)

INTERACTIONS

Increase: hypoglycemic effect—sulfonylureas, repaglinide
Increase: anticoagulant properties—warfarin
Increase: risk of myositis, myalgia—HMG-CoA reductase inhibitors
Decrease: effect of cycloSPORINE
Decrease: effect of gemfibrozil—bile acid sequestrants, separate by >2 hr
Drug/Lab Test
Increase: LFTs, CK
Decrease: Hgb, Hct, WBC, potassium

NURSING CONSIDERATIONS

Assess:

- Hyperlipidemia: diet history: fats, triglycerides, cholesterol; if lipids increase, product should be discontinued; LDL, VLDL baseline and periodically
- **Myopathy, rhabdomyolysis:** For muscle pain, tenderness; obtain baseline CPK; if elevated or if these occur, product should be discontinued
- Renal, hepatic studies, CBC, blood glucose if patient is receiving long-term therapy; if LFTs increase, therapy should be discontinued
- Bowel pattern daily; watch for increasing diarrhea (common)

Evaluate:

- Therapeutic response: decreased cholesterol, triglyceride levels; HDL, cholesterol ratios improved

Teach patient/family:

- That compliance is needed for positive results; not to double or skip dose
- That risk factors should be decreased: high-fat diet, smoking, alcohol consumption, absence of exercise
- To notify prescriber of diarrhea, nausea, vomiting, chills, fever, sore throat, muscle cramps, abdominal cramps, severe flatulence
- To avoid driving, hazardous activities if dizziness, blurred vision occur

gemifloxacin (Rx)

(gem-ah-flox′a-sin)

Factive

Func. class.: Antiinfective
Chem. class.: Fluoroquinolone

ACTION: Inhibits DNA gyrase, which is an enzyme involved in replication, transcription, and repair of bacterial DNA

USES: Acute bacterial exacerbation of chronic bronchitis caused by *Streptococcus pneumoniae, Haemophilus influenzae, Haemophilus parainfluenzae, Moraxella catarrhalis;* community-acquired pneumonia caused by *Streptococcus pneumoniae* including multiproduct-resistant strains, *H. influenzae, M. catarrhalis, Mycoplasma pneumoniae, Chlamydia pneumoniae, Klebsiella pneumoniae*
Unlabeled uses: *Actinetobacter iwoffii,* cystitis, *Klebsiella oxytoca, Legionella pneumophilia, Proteus vulgaris,* pyelonephritis, sinusitis, *Streptococcus pyogenes* (group A β-hemolytic streptococci), urinary tract infection

CONTRAINDICATIONS: Hypersensitivity to quinolones
Precautions: Pregnancy (C), breastfeeding, children, geriatric patients, hypokalemia, hypomagnesium, renal disease, seizure disorders, excessive exposure to sunlight, psychosis, increased intracranial pressure, history of QT interval prolongation, dysrhythmias, myasthenia gravis, torsades de pointes

Black Box Warning: Tendon pain/rupture, tendinitis

DOSAGE AND ROUTES

• **Adult: PO** 320 mg/day × 5-10 days depending on type of infection

Renal dose

• **Adult: PO** CCr ≤40 ml/min, 160 mg q24hr

Available forms: Tabs 320 mg

Administer:

• 2 hr before or 3 hr after aluminum/magnesium antacids, iron, zinc products, or buffered 2 hr before sucralfate

SIDE EFFECTS

CNS: *Dizziness, headache,* somnolence, depression, insomnia, nervousness, confusion, agitation, **seizures**

CV: QT prolongation, vasodilation

EENT: Visual disturbances

GI: Diarrhea, *nausea,* vomiting, anorexia, flatulence, heartburn, dry mouth; increased AST, ALT; constipation, abdominal pain, oral thrush, glossitis, stomatitis, **pseudomembranous colitis**

GU: Crystalluria (rare)

HEMA: Thrombocytopenia, neutropenia

INTEG: Rash, pruritus, urticaria, *photosensitivity*

MS: Tendinitis, tendon rupture

SYST: Anaphylaxis, Stevens-Johnson syndrome

PHARMACOKINETICS

Rapidly absorbed; bioavailability 71%; peak 1-2 hr; half-life 4-12 hr; excreted in urine as active product, metabolites

INTERACTIONS

Increase: CNS stimulation—NSAIDs

Increase: toxicity of gemifloxacin—probenecid

⚠ **Increase: QT prolongation—class IA, III antidysrhythmics, tricyclics, amoxapine, maprotiline, phenothiazines, haloperidol, pimozide, risperidone, sertindole, ziprasidone, β-blockers, chloroquine, clozapine, dasatinib, dolasetron, droperidol, dronedarone, flecainide, halogenated/local anesthetics, local anesthetics, lapatinib, methadone, erythromycin, telithromycin, troleandomycin, octreotide, ondansetron, palonosetron, pentamidine, propafenone, ranolazine, sunitinib, tacrolimus, vardenafil, vorinostat**

Decrease: absorption antacids containing aluminum, magnesium, sucralfate, zinc, iron, give 2 hr before or 3 hr after meals

Drug/Herb

• Do not use acidophilus with antiinfectives; separate by several hours

NURSING CONSIDERATIONS

Assess:

• Renal, hepatic studies: BUN, creatinine, AST, ALT; I&O ratio

• CNS symptoms: insomnia, vertigo, headache, agitation, confusion

⚠ **Allergic reactions and anaphylaxis: rash, flushing, urticaria, pruritus, chills, fever, joint pain; may occur a few days after therapy begins; epinephrine and resuscitation equipment should be available for anaphylactic reaction**

• **Pseudomembranous colitis:** bowel pattern daily; if severe diarrhea, fever, abdominal pain occur, product should be discontinued

• **Overgrowth of infection:** perineal itching, fever, malaise, redness, pain, swelling, drainage, rash, diarrhea, change in cough, sputum

⚠ **Tendon rupture: tendon pain, inflammation; if present, discontinue use**

Evaluate

• Therapeutic response: negative C&S, absence of signs, symptoms of infection

Teach patient/family:

• To take with/without food

• That fluids must be increased to 2 L/day to avoid crystallization in kidneys

• That, if dizziness or lightheadedness occurs, to perform activities with assistance

• To complete full course of product therapy

- To contact prescriber if adverse reactions occur
- To avoid iron- or mineral-containing supplements or aluminum/magnesium antacids, buffered products within 2 hr before and 3 hr after dosing, 2 hr before sucralfate
- That photosensitivity may occur and sunscreen should be used
- To use frequent rinsing of mouth, sugarless candy or gum for dry mouth
- To avoid other medication unless approved by prescriber

gentamicin (Rx)

(jen-ta-mye′sin)

Func. class.: Antiinfective

Chem. class.: Aminoglycoside

Do not confuse:
gentamicin/kanamycin

ACTION: Interferes with protein synthesis in bacterial cell by binding to ribosomal subunit, thus causing misreading of genetic code; inaccurate peptide sequence forms in protein chain, thereby causing bacterial death

USES: Severe systemic infections of CNS, respiratory, GI, urinary tract, bone, skin, soft tissues caused by susceptible strains of *Pseudomonas aeruginosa, Proteus, Klebsiella, Serratia, Escherichia coli, Enterobacter, Citrobacter, Staphylococcus, Shigella, Salmonella, Acinetobacter, Bacillus anthracis,* acute PID

CONTRAINDICATIONS: Hypersensitivity to this product, other aminoglycosides; fungal/viral/mycobacterial infection

Black Box Warning: Pregnancy (D), severe renal disease

Precautions: Breastfeeding, neonates, geriatric patients

Black Box Warning: Mild renal disease, hearing deficits, myasthenia gravis, Parkinson's disease, infant botulism

DOSAGE AND ROUTES

Severe systemic infections

- **Adult: IV INF** 3-5 mg/kg/day in divided doses q8hr; dilute in 50-200 ml 0.9% NaCl or D_5W given over 30 min-1 hr; **IV** (pulse dosing, once-daily dosing) (unlabeled) 5-7 mg/kg; **IM** 3 mg/kg/day in divided doses q8hr
- **Child: IM/IV** 2-2.5 mg/kg q8hr; **IV** (pulse dosing, once daily dosing) (unlabeled) 5 mg/kg
- **Neonate and infant: IM/IV** 2.5 mg/kg q8-12hr
- **Neonate <1 wk: IV** 2.5 mg/kg q12-24hr

Renal dose

- **Adult: IM/IV** CCr 70-100 ml/min, reduce dose by multiplying maintenance dose by 0.85, give q8-12hr; CCr 50-69 ml/min, reduce as above, give q12hr; CCr 25-49 ml/min, reduce as above, give q24hr; CCr <25 ml/min, reduce as above, give based on serum concentrations

Available forms: Inj 10, 40 mg/ml; premixed inj 40, 60, 70, 80, 100 mg/50 ml

Administer:

IM route

- IM inj in large muscle mass; rotate inj sites
- Product in evenly spaced doses to maintain blood level

Intermittent IV INF route

- After diluting in 50-200 ml NS, D_5W; decrease vol of diluent in child; maintain 0.1% sol run over ½-1 hr (adults) or up to 2 hr (children); flush IV line with NS, D_5W after administration

Syringe compatibilities: Clindamycin, methicillin, penicillin G sodium

Y-site compatibilities: Amifostine, amiodarone, amsacrine, atracurium, aztreonam, cefpirome, ciprofloxacin, cyclophosphamide, cytarabine, diltiazem, enalaprilat, esmolol, famotidine, filgrastim, fluconazole, fludarabine, foscarnet, granisetron, HYDROmorphone, IL-2, insulin, labetalol, LORazepam, magnesium sulfate, melphalan, meperidine, meropenem, midazolam, morphine, multivitamins, ondansetron, paclitaxel, pancuronium, perphenazine, sargramostim, tacrolimus, teniposide, theophylline, thiotepa, tolazine, vecuronium, vinorelbine, vit B/C, zidovudine

SIDE EFFECTS

CNS: Confusion, depression, numbness, tremors, **seizures**, muscle twitching, **neurotoxicity**, dizziness, vertigo

CV: Hypo/hypertension, palpitations, edema

EENT: **Ototoxicity**, *deafness*, visual disturbances, tinnitus

GI: *Nausea, vomiting, anorexia;* increased ALT, AST, bilirubin; hepatomegaly, **hepatic necrosis**, splenomegaly

GU: **Oliguria, hematuria, renal damage, azotemia, renal failure, nephrotoxicity,** proteinuria

HEMA: **Agranulocytosis, thrombocytopenia, leukopenia,** eosinophilia, anemia

INTEG: *Rash,* burning, urticaria, dermatitis, alopecia, photosensitivity

PHARMACOKINETICS

Not metabolized, excreted unchanged in urine, crosses placental barrier

IM: Onset rapid, peak 1-2 hr

IV: Onset immediate; peak 1-2 hr; plasma half-life 1-2 hr, infants 6-7 hr; duration 6-8 hr

INTERACTIONS

- Do not use at the same time or physically mix with penicillins

Increase: ototoxicity, neurotoxicity, nephrotoxicity—other aminoglycosides, amphotericin B, polymyxin, vancomycin, ethacrynic acid, furosemide, mannitol, methoxyflurane, CISplatin, cephalosporins, penicillins, cidofovir, acyclovir

Increase: effects—nondepolarizing neuromuscular blockers

Drug/Lab Test

Increase: LDH, AST, ALT, bilirubin, BUN, creatinine, eosinophils

Decrease: Hgb, WBC, platelet, granulocytes

NURSING CONSIDERATIONS

Assess:

Black Box Warning: Neuromuscular disease (myasthenia gravis, Parkinson's disease, infant botulism): paresthesias, tetany, positive Chvostek's/Trousseau's signs, confusion (adults), tetany, muscle weakness (infants); correct electrolyte imbalance

- Weight before treatment; calculation of dosage is usually based on ideal body weight but may be calculated on actual body weight

Black Box Warning: Renal disease: I&O ratio, urinalysis daily for proteinuria, cells, casts; report sudden change in urine output; urine pH if product is used for UTI; urine should be kept alkaline; urine for CCr testing, BUN, serum creatinine; lower dosage should be given with renal impairment (CCr <80 ml/min); toxicity is increased in patients with decreased renal function if high doses are given

- VS during inf; watch for hypotension, change in pulse
- IV site for thrombophlebitis, including pain, redness, swelling q30min, change site if needed; discontinue, apply warm compresses to site
- Serum peak drawn at 30-60 min after IV inf or 60 min after IM inj and trough level drawn just before next dose; blood level should be 2-4 times bacteriostatic level; peak (5-10 mcg/ml), trough (0.5-2 mcg/ml), depending on type of infection

Black Box Warning: Hearing deficits: eighth cranial nerve dysfunction by audiometric testing; also ringing, roaring in ears, vertigo; assess hearing before, during, after treatment

- Dehydration: high specific gravity, decrease in skin turgor, dry mucous membranes, dark urine

- **Overgrowth of infection:** fever, malaise, redness, pain, swelling, perineal itching, diarrhea, stomatitis, change in cough or sputum
- C&S before starting treatment to identify infecting organism
- **Vestibular dysfunction:** nausea, vomiting, dizziness, headache; product should be discontinued if severe
- Inj sites for redness, swelling, abscesses; use warm compresses at site

Perform/provide:

- Adequate fluids of 2-3 L/day unless contraindicated to prevent irritation of tubules
- Supervised ambulation, other safety measures with vestibular dysfunction

Evaluate:

- Therapeutic response: absence of fever, draining wounds, negative C&S after treatment

Teach patient/family:

- To report headache, dizziness, symptoms of overgrowth of infection, renal impairment
- To report loss of hearing; ringing, roaring in ears; feeling of fullness in head

gentamicin ophthalmic

See Appendix B

gentamicin topical

See Appendix B

glatiramer (Rx)

(glah-tear′a-meer)

Copaxone

Func. class.: Multiple sclerosis agent

ACTION: Unknown; may modify the immune responses responsible for multiple sclerosis (MS)

USES: Reduction of the frequency of relapses in patients with relapsing or remitting MS after first clinical episode with MRI results consistent with MS

CONTRAINDICATIONS: Hypersensitivity to this product or mannitol

Precautions: Pregnancy (B), breastfeeding, children <18 yr, immune disorders, renal disease

DOSAGE AND ROUTES

- **Adult: SUBCUT** 20 mg/day

Available forms: Inj, premixed 20 mg/ml

Administer:

SUBCUT route

- If refrigerated, allow to warm for 20 min; visually inspect for particulate or cloudiness, if present discard; prefilled syringe contents is for single use; administer SUBCUT into hip, thigh, arm; discard unused portion
- Use SUBCUT route only; do not give IM or IV

SIDE EFFECTS

CNS: *Anxiety, hypertonia, tremor, vertigo,* speech disorder, *agitation,* confusion, flushing

CV: *Migraine, palpitations, syncope, tachycardia, vasodilation,* chest pain, hypertension

EENT: *Ear pain, blurred vision*

GI: *Nausea, vomiting, diarrhea, anorexia, gastroenteritis*

GU: *Urinary urgency, dysmenorrhea, vaginal moniliasis*

HEMA: *Ecchymosis, lymphadenopathy*

INTEG: *Pruritus, rash, sweating, urticaria, erythema,* inj site reaction

META: Edema, weight gain

MS: *Arthralgia, back pain, neck pain,* increased muscle tone

RESP: *Bronchitis, dyspnea, laryngismus, rhinitis*

PHARMACOKINETICS

May be hydrolyzed locally, may reach regional lymph nodes

NURSING CONSIDERATIONS

Assess:

- CNS symptoms: anxiety, confusion, vertigo
- GI status: diarrhea, vomiting, abdominal pain, gastroenteritis
- Cardiac status: tachycardia, palpitations, vasodilation, chest pain

Evaluate:

- Therapeutic response: decreased symptoms of MS

Teach patient/family:

- With written, detailed instructions about product; provide initial and return demonstrations on inj procedure; give information about use and disposal of product, inj site reaction (hives, rash, irritation, severe pain, flushing, chest pain)
- That blurred vision, sweating may occur
- That irregular menses, dysmenorrhea, metrorrhagia, breast pain may occur; to use contraception during treatment
- That, if pregnancy is suspected or if nursing, to notify prescriber
- Not to change dosing or stop taking product without advice of prescriber
- About immediate postinjection reaction: flushing, chest pain, palpitations, anxiety, dyspnea, laryngeal constriction, urticaria; does not usually require treatment

glimepiride (Rx)

(glye-me′pi-ride)

Amaryl, CO Glimepiride ✤, ratio-Glimepiride ✤, Sandoz Glimepiride ✤

glipiZIDE (Rx)

(glip-i′zide)

Glucotrol, Glucotrol XL

Func. class.: Antidiabetic

Chem. class.: Sulfonylurea (2nd generation)

Do not confuse:

glipiZIDE/Glucotrol/glyBURIDE

ACTION:

Causes functioning β cells in pancreas to release insulin, leading to drop in blood glucose levels; may improve insulin binding to insulin receptors or increase the number of insulin receptors with prolonged administration; may also reduce basal hepatic glucose secretion; not effective if patient lacks functioning β cells

USES:

Type 2 diabetes mellitus

CONTRAINDICATIONS:

Hypersensitivity to sulfonylureas, type 1 diabetes, diabetic ketoacidosis

Precautions: Pregnancy (C), geriatric patients, cardiac disease, severe renal/hepatic disease, G6PD deficiency

DOSAGE AND ROUTES

Glimepiride

- **Adult: PO** 1-2 mg/day with breakfast, then increase by ≤2 mg/day q1-2wk, max 8 mg/day
- **Geriatric: PO** 1 mg/day; may increase if needed

Renal dose

- **Adult: PO** 1 mg/day with breakfast; may titrate upward as needed

GlipiZIDE

- **Adult: PO** 5 mg initially before breakfast then increase by 2.5-5 mg after several days to desired response; max 40 mg/day in divided doses or 15 mg/dose; **PO** (XL) 5 mg/day with breakfast, may increase to 10 mg/day, max 20 mg/day
- **Geriatric: PO** 2.5 mg/day; may increase if needed

Hepatic disease

- **Adult: PO** 2.5 mg initially then increase to desired response; max 40 mg/day in divided doses or 15 mg/dose

Available forms: *Glimepiride:* tabs 1, 2, 4 mg; *glipiZIDE:* tabs, scored 5, 10 mg; ext rel tab (XL) 2.5, 5, 10 mg

Administer:

- Do not break, crush, or chew ext rel tabs; may crush tabs and mix with fluids if unable to swallow whole

• **GlipiZIDE:** product 30 min before meals (regular release); with breakfast (ext rel); **Glimepiride:** with breakfast; if patient is NPO, may need to hold dose to prevent hypoglycemia
• Gradual conversion from other oral hypoglycemics to these products is not needed; insulin ≥20 units/day, convert using 25% reduction in insulin dose every day or every other day

SIDE EFFECTS

CNS: *Headache, weakness, dizziness, drowsiness,* tinnitus, fatigue, vertigo
ENDO: Hypoglycemia
GI: Hepatotoxicity, cholestatic jaundice, nausea, vomiting, diarrhea, heartburn
HEMA: Leukopenia, thrombocytopenia, agranulocytosis, aplastic anemia; increased AST, ALT, alk phos; pancytopenia, hemolytic anemia
INTEG: Rash, allergic reactions, pruritus, urticaria, eczema, photosensitivity, erythema, allergic vasculitis

PHARMACOKINETICS

PO: Completely absorbed by GI route; **glipiZIDE:** onset 1-1½ hr, peak 1-3 hr, duration 10-24 hr, half-life 2-4 hr; **glimepiride:** peak 2-3 hr, half-life 5 hr; metabolized in liver, excreted in urine, 90%-95% plasma-protein bound

INTERACTIONS

• May mask symptoms of hypoglycemia: β-blockers
Increase: action of digoxin, glycosides
Increase: hypoglycemic effects—insulin, MAOIs, cimetidine, chloramphenicol, guanethidine, methyldopa, NSAIDs, salicylates, probenecid, androgens, anticoagulants, clofibrate, fenfluramine, fluconazole, gemfibrozil, histamine H_2 antagonists, magnesium salts, phenylbutazone, sulfinpyrazone, sulfonamides, tricyclics, urinary acidifiers, clarithromycin, fibric acid derivatives, voriconazole
Decrease: hypoglycemic effect—thiazide diuretics, rifampin, isoniazid, cholestyramine, diazoxide, hydantoins, urinary alkalinizers, charcoal, corticosteroids

Drug/Herb
Increase: antidiabetic effect—garlic, horse chestnut
Decrease: hypoglycemic effect—green tea

Drug/Lab Test
Increase: AST, ALT, LDH, BUN, creatinine

NURSING CONSIDERATIONS

Assess:
• **Hypo/hyperglycemic reaction** that can occur soon after meals; for severe hypoglycemia give IV $D_{50}W$, then IV dextrose solution
• Blood glucose, A1c levels during treatment to determine diabetes control
⚠ Blood dyscrasias: CBC at baseline and throughout treatment; report decreased blood count

Perform/provide:
• Storage in tight, light-resistant container at room temp

Evaluate:
• Therapeutic response: decrease in polyuria, polydipsia, polyphagia; clear sensorium; absence of dizziness; stable gait; improved serum glucose, A1c

Teach patient/family:
• Not to drink alcohol; about disulfiram reaction (nausea, headache, cramps, flushing, hypoglycemia)
• To report bleeding, bruising, weight gain, edema, SOB, weakness, sore throat
• To check for symptoms of cholestatic jaundice: dark urine, pruritus, yellow sclera; prescriber should be notified
• About symptoms of hypo/hyperglycemia, what to do about each; to have glucagon emergency kit available; to carry sugar packets
• That product must be continued on daily basis; about consequences of discontinuing product abruptly; to take product in morning to prevent hypoglycemic reactions at night
• To use sunscreen or stay out of the sun, wear protective clothing (photosensitivity)

- To avoid OTC medications unless ordered by prescriber
- That diabetes is a lifelong illness; product will not cure disease
- That all food in diet plan must be eaten to prevent hypoglycemia; to continue weight control, dietary restrictions, exercise, hygiene
- To carry emergency ID with prescriber and medication information
- To test using blood glucose meter while taking this product
- That ext rel tab may appear in stool

TREATMENT OF OVERDOSE:

Glucose 25 g IV via dextrose 50% sol, 50 ml, 1 mg glucagon, or carbohydrate depending on severity

glucarpidase

(glu-car-pie′dase)

Voraxaze

Func. class.: Recombinant bacterial enzyme

ACTION: A recombinant bacterial enzyme that hydrolyzes glutamate residue from methotrexate and provides an alternate nonrenal pathway for methotrexate elimination in patients with renal dysfunction during high-dose methotrexate treatment. As a result of its enzymatic action, converts methotrexate to its inactive metabolites

USES: The treatment of methotrexate toxicity (methotrexate plasma concentration >1 micromole/liter) in those with delayed methotrexate clearance due to impaired renal function

Precautions: Pregnancy (C), breastfeeding

DOSAGE AND ROUTES

- **Adult/adolescent/child:** **IV** 50 Units/kg over 5min; continue to give leucovorin, IV hydration, urinary alkalinization as needed

Available forms: Sol for IV

Administer:

IV direct route

- Visually inspect parenteral products for particulate matter and discoloration prior to administration
- Reconstitution: add 1 ml of sterile saline for injection to vial, roll and tilt the vial gently to mix; do not shake; flush the IV line then inject as a bolus inj over 5 min; flush the IV line again
- Do not administer to patients who exhibit the expected clearance of methotrexate (plasma methotrexate concentrations within 2 standard deviations of the mean methotrexate excretion curve specific for the dose of methotrexate administered)
- Do not administer to patients with normal or mildly impaired renal function because of the potential risk of subtherapeutic exposure to methotrexate
- Continue to administer leucovorin after glucarpidase, but do not administer leucovorin within 2 hr before or after a glucarpidase. For the first 48 hr after glucarpidase administration, administer the same leucovorin dose as given before glucarpidase. After 48 hr after glucarpidase, administer leucovorin based on the measured methotrexate concentration. Do not discontinue therapy with leucovorin based on the determination of a single methotrexate concentration below the leucovorin treatment threshold. Continue leucovorin until the methotrexate concentration has been maintained below the leucovorin treatment threshold for a minimum of 3 days; use of a chromatographic method to determine methotrexate concentrations is needed for the first 48 hr after glucarpidase receipt
- Continue hydration and alkalinization of the urine as needed

SIDE EFFECTS

CNS: Paresthesias, headache

CV: Hypo/hypertension

EENT: Throat irritation or tightness

GI: Nausea, vomiting

INTEG: Flushing, hot, burning sensation; rash, hypersensitivity, serious allergic reactions
SYST: Antibody formation

PHARMACOKINETICS

Elimination half-life of 5.6 hr, methotrexate concentration reduced 97% within 15 min

INTERACTIONS

Decrease: elucarpidase level—pemetrexed, pralatrexate; avoid concurrent use

NURSING CONSIDERATIONS

Assess:

- Continue monitoring of methotrexate blood levels, renal status (creatinine/BUN) after glucarpidase is given. Methotrexate concentrations within 48 hr of glucarpidase are only reliable measure by a chromatographic method. Leucovorin receipt is needed until methotrexate level has been maintained below leucovorin treatment threshold for a minimum of 3 days

Perform/provide:

- Storage of reconstituted solution refrigerated ≤4 hr; discard any unused product, no preservative is present

Evaluate:

- For resolution of methotrexate toxicity

Teach patient/family:

- To immediately report any infusion-related reactions: fever, chills, flushing, feeling hot, rash, hives, itching, throat tightness or breathing problems, tingling, numbness, or headache

glyBURIDE (Rx)

(glye′byoor-ide)

Apo-Glyburide ✦, DiaBeta, Glynase PresTab, Novo-Glyburide ✦, Nu-Glyburide ✦, PMS-Glyburide ✦, ratio-Glyburide ✦, Sandoz Glyburide ✦

Func. class.: Antidiabetic
Chem. class.: Sulfonylurea (2nd generation)

Do not confuse:
glyBURIDE/Glucotrol/glipiZIDE
DiaBeta/Zebeta

ACTION: Causes functioning β cells in pancreas to release insulin, thereby leading to a drop in blood glucose levels; may improve insulin binding to insulin receptors and increase number of insulin receptors with prolonged administration; may also reduce basal hepatic glucose secretion; not effective if patient lacks functioning β cells

USES: Type 2 diabetes mellitus
Unlabeled use: Gestational diabetes not controlled by diet

CONTRAINDICATIONS: Hypersensitivity to sulfonylureas, type 1 diabetes, diabetic ketoacidosis, renal failure
Precautions: Pregnancy (C), geriatric patients, cardiac/thyroid disease, severe renal/hepatic disease, severe hypoglycemic reactions, sulfonamide/sulfonylurea hypersensitivity, G6PD deficiency

DOSAGE AND ROUTES

DiaBeta

- **Adult: PO** 1.25-5 mg initially then increase to desired response at weekly intervals up to 20 mg/day; may be given as a single or divided dose
- **Geriatric: PO** 1.25 mg initially then increase to desired response; max 20 mg/day, maintenance 1.25-20 mg/day

Glynase PresTab (micronized)

• **Adult: PO** 1.5-3 mg/day initially, may increase by 1.5 mg/wk, max 12 mg/day
• **Geriatric: PO** 0.75-3 mg/day, may increase by 1.5 mg/wk

Gestational diabetes (unlabeled)

• **Adult (pregnant female): PO** 2.5 mg/day titrated up to 20 mg/day (conventional glyBURIDE)

Available forms: Tabs (DiaBeta) 1.25, 2.5, 5 mg; (Glynase PresTab) 1.5, 3, 6 mg

Administer:

• With breakfast as single or divided dose, hold dose if patient NPO to avoid hypoglycemia, take at same time each day
• Gradual conversion from other oral hypoglycemics to product is not needed; insulin ≥20 units/day; convert using 25% reduction in insulin dose every day
• Micronized glyBURIDE/nonmicronized glyBURIDE not equivalent

SIDE EFFECTS

CNS: *Headache, weakness,* paresthesia, tinnitus, fatigue, vertigo
EENT: Blurred vision
ENDO: **Hypoglycemia**
GI: Nausea, fullness, heartburn, **hepatotoxicity, cholestatic jaundice,** vomiting, diarrhea, **hepatic failure**
HEMA: **Leukopenia, thrombocytopenia, agranulocytosis, aplastic anemia (rare),** increased AST, ALT, alk phos
INTEG: Rash, allergic reactions, pruritus, urticaria, eczema, photosensitivity, erythema
MS: Joint pain

PHARMACOKINETICS

PO: Completely absorbed by GI route; onset 2 hr; peak 2-4 hr; duration 24 hr; half-life 10 hr; metabolized in liver; excreted in urine, feces (metabolites); crosses placenta; 99% plasma-protein bound

INTERACTIONS

Increase: masking symptoms of hypoglycemia—β-blockers
Increase: level—digoxin
Increase: hypoglycemic effects—insulin, MAOIs, oral anticoagulants, chloramphenicol, guanethidine, methyldopa, NSAIDs, salicylates, probenecid, androgens, fenfluramine, fluconazole, gemfibrozil, histamine H_2 antagonists, magnesium salts, phenylbutazone, sulfinpyrazone, sulfonamides, tricyclics, urinary acidifiers, β-blockers, clarithromycin
Increase: LFTs—bosentan; avoid concurrent use
Increase: triglyceride levels—colesevelam
Increase: action of—cycloSPORINE
Decrease: both products' effects—diazoxide
Decrease: glyBURIDE action—thiazide diuretics, rifampin, isoniazid, cholestyramine, hydantoins, urinary alkalinizers, charcoal, corticosteroids, phenothiazines; oral contraceptives, estrogens, thyroid, voriconazole

Drug/Herb

Increase: antidiabetic effect—garlic, horse chestnut
Decrease: hypoglycemic effect—green tea

Drug/Lab Test

Increase: AST, ALT, LDH, BUN, creatinine

NURSING CONSIDERATIONS

Assess:

• Hypo/hyperglycemic reaction that can occur soon after meals; for severe hypoglycemia, give IV $D_{50}W$ then IV dextrose sol
• Blood glucose; A1c levels during treatment

⚠ **Blood dyscrasias: CBC at baseline, throughout treatment; report decreased blood counts**

Perform/provide:

• Storage in tight container in cool environment

Evaluate:
- Therapeutic response: decrease in polyuria, polydipsia, polyphagia; clear sensorium; absence of dizziness; stable gait; improved serum glucose, A1c

Teach patient/family:
- To check for symptoms of cholestatic jaundice: dark urine, pruritus, jaundiced sclera; if these occur, notify prescriber
- To use a blood glucose meter for testing while taking this product
- About the symptoms of hypo/hyperglycemia, what to do about each
- That product must be continued on a daily basis; about consequences of discontinuing product abruptly
- To take product in morning to prevent hypoglycemic reactions at night if taking once a day
- To avoid OTC medications unless ordered by prescriber
- To report bleeding, bruising, weight gain, edema, SOB, weakness, sore throat
- That diabetes is a lifelong illness; that product will not cure disease
- That all food included in diet plan must be eaten to prevent hypoglycemia; to have glucagon emergency kit, sugar packets always available
- To use sunscreen or stay out of the sun, wear protective clothing (photosensitivity)
- To carry an emergency ID with prescriber and medication information

TREATMENT OF OVERDOSE:
Glucose 25 g IV via dextrose 50% sol, 50 ml, 1 mg glucagon, or carbohydrate depending on severity

RARELY USED

glycerin (OTC)
(gli′ser-in)

Sani-Supp

Func. class.: Laxative, hyperosmotic

USES: Constipation

CONTRAINDICATIONS: Hypersensitivity

DOSAGE AND ROUTES
Laxative
- **Adult and child >6 yr: RECT SUPP** 3 g; **ENEMA** 5-15 ml
- **Child <6 yr: RECT SUPP** 1-1.8 g; **ENEMA** 2-5 ml

glycopyrrolate (Rx)
(glye-koe-pye′roe-late)

Cuvposa, Robinul, Robinul-Forte

Func. class.: Cholinergic blocker, antispasmodic

Chem. class.: Quaternary ammonium compound

ACTION: Inhibits the action of acetylcholine at receptor sites in parasympathetic nervous system, which controls secretions, free acids in stomach

USES: Decreased secretions before surgery, reversal of neuromuscular blockade, peptic ulcer disease, irritable bowel syndrome, bradycardia, drooling

CONTRAINDICATIONS: Children <3 yr, hypersensitivity, closed-angle glaucoma, myasthenia gravis, GI/GU obstruction, tachycardia, myocardial ischemia, hepatic disease, ulcerative colitis, toxic megacolon, prostatic hypertrophy

Precautions: Pregnancy (B), breastfeeding, geriatric patients, pulmonary/

renal disease, CHF, hyperthyroidism, CAD, Down syndrome, hiatal hernia, hypertension

DOSAGE AND ROUTES

Preoperatively

- **Adult: IM** 4 mcg/kg 30 min-1 hr before surgery, max 0.1 mg
- **Child >2 yr (unlabeled): IM** 4 mcg/kg 30-60 min before procedure
- **Child <2 yr (unlabeled): IM** 4-9 mcg/kg

Intraoperative

- **Adult: IV** 0.1 mg; may repeat q2-3min prn
- **Child: IM/IV** 4 mcg/kg q2-3min prn; max 0.1 mg/dose

Reversal of neuromuscular blockade

- **Adult/child: IV** 200 mcg for each 1 mg of neostigmine or 5 mg **IV** of pyridostigmine simultaneously

GI disorders

- **Adult: PO** 1-2 mg bid-tid, max 6 mg/day; **IM/IV** 100-200 mcg tid-qid, titrated to patient response

Antidysrhythmic

- **Adult: IV** 100 mcg, may repeat q2min
- **Child: IV** 4.4 mcg/kg, may repeat q2min, max 100 mcg

Secretion control

- **Child: PO** 40-100 mcg/kg/dose tid-qid; **IM/IV** 4-10 mcg/kg/dose q3-4hr; max 0.2 mg/dose or 0.8 mg/24 hr

Chronic drooling

- **Child/adolescent 3-16 yr: PO (oral sol)** 0.02 mg/kg tid, titrate by 0.02 mg/kg/dose q5-7days, max 0.1 mg/kg/dose tid or 13-17 kg, 1.5 mg/dose; 18-22 kg, 2 mg/dose; 23-27 kg, 2.5 mg/dose, ≥28 kg, 3 mg/dose
- **Child: IM/IV** (unlabeled) 4-9 mcg/kg q3-4hr

Available forms: Tabs 1, 2 mg; inj 200 mcg (0.2 mg)/ml; oral sol 1 mg/5 ml

Administer:

PO route

- With or after meals to prevent GI upset; may give with fluids other than water

IM/IV route

- Parenteral dose with patient recumbent to prevent postural hypotension
- Parenteral dose slowly; keep patient in bed for ≥1 hr after dose
- After checking dose carefully; even slight overdose may lead to toxicity

Direct IV route

- Undiluted; give through a Y-tube or 3-way stopcock; give ≤0.2 mg over 1-2 min

Syringe compatibilities: Atropine, benzquinamide, chlorproMAZINE, cimetidine, codeine, diphenhydrAMINE, droperidol, HYDROmorphone, hydrOXYzine, levorphanol, lidocaine, meperidine, midazolam, morphine, nalbuphine, neostigmine, oxymorphone, procaine, prochlorperazine, promazine, promethazine, pyridostigmine, ranitidine, scopolamine, triflupromazine, trimethobenzamide

Y-site compatibilities: Morphine, propofol

Solution compatibilities: D_5W, 0.9% NaCl, Ringer's, D_5/0.45% NaCl

SIDE EFFECTS

CNS: Confusion, anxiety, restlessness, irritability, delusions, hallucinations, headache, sedation, depression, incoherence, dizziness, lethargy, flushing, weakness, **seizures**

CV: Palpitations, tachycardia, postural hypotension, paradoxical bradycardia

EENT: Blurred vision, photophobia, dilated pupils, difficulty swallowing, increased intraocular pressure, mydriasis, cycloplegia

GI: *Dryness of mouth, constipation,* nausea, vomiting, abdominal distress, paralytic ileus, altered taste perception

GU: Urinary hesitancy, retention, impotence

INTEG: Urticaria, allergic reactions

MISC: Suppression of lactation, nasal congestion, decreased sweating, **malignant hyperthermia**

SYST: Anaphylaxis

PHARMACOKINETICS

Excreted in urine (>80% unchanged), half-life 1-2 hr
PO: Peak 1 hr, duration 8-12 hr
IM: Peak 30-45 min, duration 2-7 hr
IV: Peak 10-15 min, duration 2-7 hr

INTERACTIONS

Increase: anticholinergic effect—alcohol, antihistamines, phenothiazines, amantadine, tricyclics
Decrease: glycopyrrolate absorption—antacids, antidiarrheals

NURSING CONSIDERATIONS

Assess:
- B/P, respirations, heart rate before and during IM/IV administration
- I&O ratio; retention commonly causes decreased urinary output
- Urinary hesitancy, retention: palpate bladder if retention occurs
- Constipation, abdominal distention, bowel sounds; increase fluids, bulk if this occurs

Perform/provide:
- Storage at room temp

Evaluate:
- Therapeutic response: decreased secretions; decreased pain in GI disorders; reversal of neuromuscular blockers

Teach patient/family:
- To use hard candy, frequent drinks, sugarless gum to relieve dry mouth; to perform good oral hygiene
- Not to discontinue this product abruptly; to taper off over 1 wk; to take PO 30 min-1 hr before meals
- To avoid driving, other hazardous activities because drowsiness, blurred vision may occur
- To avoid OTC medication: cough, cold preparations with alcohol, antihistamines unless directed by prescriber
- To avoid hot temp, since sweating is decreased, heat stroke is possible
- To change positions slowly to prevent orthostatic hypotension
- To notify prescriber of eye pain, blurred vision, light sensitivity; cardiac dysrhythmias

golimumab (Rx)

(goal-lim′yu-mab)

Simponi

Func. class.: Antirheumatic agent (disease modifying), immunomodulator

Chem. class.: Monoclonal antibody, DMARD, tumor necrosis factor (TNF-α) modifier

ACTION: Monoclonal antibody specific for human tumor necrosis factor (TNF); elevated levels of TNF are found in patients with rheumatoid arthritis

USES: Rheumatoid arthritis (RA), ankylosing spondylitis, psoriatic arthritis

CONTRAINDICATIONS: Hypersensitivity, active infections

Precautions: Pregnancy (B), breastfeeding, children, geriatric patients, CNS demyelinating disease, Guillain-Barré syndrome, CHF, hepatitis B carriers, blood dyscrasias, surgery, MS, neurologic disease, diabetes, immunosuppression

Black Box Warning: Infection, neoplastic disease

DOSAGE AND ROUTES

- **Adult: SUBCUT** 50 mg q month; for RA, give with methotrexate

Available form: Inj 50 mg/0.5 ml prefilled syringe, SmartJect Auto Injector

Administer:

SUBCUT route
- Visually inspect sol for particulate or discoloration, sol should be clear to slightly opalescent and colorless to slightly yellow, there may be tiny white particles; do not shake
- **SmartJect autoinjector:** Allow to reach room temp for 30 min prior to use;

remove cap, and inject within 5 min of removing cap, do not put cap back on, place open end against the inj site at a 90-degree angle without pushing button, push the injector firmly against the skin, press the button once and release, listen for the first click, wait for the second click or 15 sec, then remove injector; do not rub site

• **Prefilled syringe:** Allow to warm to room temp for 30 min, remove needle cover by pulling straight off, do not twist or recap, inject within 5 min of needle cover removal, hold syringe in one hand like a pencil and use other hand to pinch the skin, inject needle at a 45-degree angle, push plunger down as far as it will go, keep pressure on plunger head and remove needle from skin, remove pressure from plunger head, needle guard will cover needle; do not rub site

SIDE EFFECTS

CNS: Dizziness, paresthesia, **CNS demyelinating disorder,** weakness
CV: Hypertension, **CHF**
GI: **Hepatitis**
HEMA: **Agranulocytosis, aplastic anemia, leukopenia, polycythemia, thrombocytopenia, pancytopenia**
INTEG: Psoriasis
MISC: **Increased cancer risk,** antibody development to this drug; **risk for infection (TB, invasive fungal infections, other opportunistic infections), may be fatal,** inj site reactions

PHARMACOKINETICS

Terminal half-life 2 wk, lower

INTERACTIONS

• Do not give concurrently with vaccines; immunizations should be brought up to date before treatment

• Dosage change may be needed: warfarin, cycloSPORINE, theophylline

Increase: infection—abatacept, etanercept, rilonacept, rituximab, adalimumab, anakinra, immunosuppressants, infliximab

NURSING CONSIDERATIONS

Assess:

• **Pain,** stiffness, ROM, swelling of joints during treatment

• Inj site pain, swelling; usually occur after 2 inj (4-5 days)

⚠ **Blood dyscrasias:** CBC, differential prior to and periodically during treatment

Black Box Warning: Infection: fever, flulike symptoms, dyspnea, change in urination, redness/ swelling around any wounds; stop treatment if present; some serious infections including sepsis may occur, may be fatal; patients with active infections should not be started on this product

• LFTs; hepatitis B serology, may reactivate HBV

• **CHF:** B/P, pulse, edema, SOB

• **Psoriasis:** may occur or worsen

Perform/provide:

• Refrigerate, do not freeze; allow to warm to room temp before using

Evaluate:

• Therapeutic response: decreased inflammation, pain in joints, decreased joint destruction

Teach patient/family:

• About self-administration if appropriate: inj should be made in thigh, abdomen, upper arm; rotate sites at least 1 inch from old site, do not inject in areas that are bruised, red, hard

• That, if medication not taken when due, to inject next dose as soon as remembered and then the following dose as scheduled

• Not to receive any live virus vaccines during treatment

• To report signs, symptoms of infection, allergic reaction, or lupuslike syndrome

goserelin (Rx)

(goe′se-rel-lin)

Zoladex

Func. class.: Gonadotropin-releasing hormone, antineoplastic (hormone)

Chem. class.: Synthetic decapeptide analog of LHRH

ACTION:

Inhibitor of pituitary gonadotropin secretion; initially increases LH and FSH, with increases in testosterone, reduction in sex steroid levels (substitute serum testosterone levels)

USES:

Advanced prostate cancer stage B2-C (10.8 mg), endometriosis, advanced breast cancer, endometrial thinning (3.6 mg)

CONTRAINDICATIONS:

Pregnancy (D) (breast cancer), (X) (endometriosis), breastfeeding, children, nondiagnosed vaginal bleeding; hypersensitivity to LHRH, LHRH-agonist analogs; 10.8 mg dose contraindicated in women

Precautions: Spinal cord decompression, renal disease, bone mineral density loss

DOSAGE AND ROUTES

- **Adult: SUBCUT** 3.6 mg q28days or 10.8 mg q12wk

Endometrial thinning

- **Adult: SUBCUT** 1-2 depot inj, usually 1 depot, surgery performed at 4 wk; if 2 depots, surgery performed 2-4 wk after 2nd depot

Available forms: Depot inj 3.6, 10.8 mg

Administer:

Depot

- SUBCUT using implant, inserted by qualified person into upper subcutaneous tissue in abdominal wall q28days or q12wk (10.8 mg); do not attempt to remove air bubbles from syringe

SIDE EFFECTS

CNS: *Headaches,* spinal cord compression, *anxiety, depression, dizziness, insomnia, lethargy,* hot flashes, emotional lability

CV: Dysrhythmia, cerebrovascular accident, hypertension, chest pain, CHF; MI, sudden cardiac death, stroke (men)

ENDO: Gynecomastia, breast tenderness, hot flashes; hyperglycemia, diabetes (men)

GI: *Nausea,* vomiting, constipation, diarrhea, ulcer

GU: *Spotting, breakthrough bleeding, decreased libido,* renal insufficiency, urinary obstruction, urinary tract infection, *impotence*

INTEG: Rash, pain on inj, diaphoresis

MS: Osteoneuralgia

RESP: COPD, URI

PHARMACOKINETICS

Peak serum concentrations in 14-28 days, half-life 4½ hr

INTERACTIONS

Drug/Lab Test

Increase: alk phos, estradiol, FSH, LH, testosterone levels

Decrease: testosterone levels, progesterone

NURSING CONSIDERATIONS

Assess:

- **Reproductive studies:** pelvic ultrasound, pelvic exam, PSA, serum estradiol/testosterone, pregnancy test prior to therapy
- I&O ratios; palpate bladder for distention in urinary obstruction
- **Cancer metastases:** for relief of bone pain (back pain), change in motor function
- Blood studies: acid phosphatase; calcium breast/prostate cancer, hypercalcemia may occur

Evaluate:

- Therapeutic response: more normal levels of PSA, acid phosphatase, alk phos;

testosterone level of <25 ng/dl; thinning of endometrial lining

Teach patient/family:

- To continue with appointments monthly
- That hyperglycemia may occur in diabetic patients
- That gynecomastia and postmenopausal symptoms may occur but will decrease when treatment is discontinued
- That bone pain may increase then decrease
- To notify prescriber of difficulty urinating, hot flashes
- Not to breastfeed; to use effective nonhormonal contraception; to notify prescriber if menstrual period continues

granisetron (Rx)

(grane-iss′e-tron)

Granisol, Kytril, Sancuso

Func. class.: Antiemetic

Chem. class.: 5-HT_3 receptor antagonist

ACTION: Prevents nausea, vomiting by blocking serotonin peripherally, centrally, and in the small intestine

USES: Prevention of nausea, vomiting associated with cancer chemotherapy, including high-dose CISplatin, radiation

Unlabeled uses: Acute nausea, vomiting after surgery

CONTRAINDICATIONS: Hypersensitivity to this product, benzyl alcohol

Precautions: Pregnancy (B), breastfeeding, children, geriatric patients, ondansetron/palonosetron/dolasetron hypersensitivity, cardiac dysrhythmias, cardiac/hepatic disease, electrolyte imbalances

DOSAGE AND ROUTES

Nausea, vomiting in chemotherapy

- **Adult and child ≥2 yr: IV** 10 mcg/kg over 5 min, 30 min before the start of cancer chemotherapy; **TD** apply 1 patch (3.1 mg/24 hr) to upper outer arm 24-48 hr before chemotherapy, patch may be worn up to 7 days
- **Adult: PO** 1 mg bid, give 1st dose 1 hr before chemotherapy and next dose 12 hr after 1st or 2 mg as a single dose anytime within 1 hr prior to chemotherapy

Nausea, vomiting in radiation therapy

- **Adult: PO** 2 mg/day 1 hr prior to radiation

Available forms: Inj 1 mg/ml; tab 1 mg; oral sol 2 mg/10 ml; patch TD 3.1 mg/24 hr

Administer:

- Chemotherapy/radiation: given on day of chemotherapy or radiation

PO route

- Give dose 1 hr prior to chemotherapy/radiation and another 12 hr after 1st dose

Direct IV route

- May give undiluted over 30 sec via Y-site

Intermittent IV INF route

- Dilute in 0.9% NaCl for inj or D_5W (20-50 ml); give over 5-15 min 30 min before chemotherapy

Additive compatibilities: Dexamethasone, methylPREDNISolone

Solution compatibilities: D_5W, 0.9% NaCl

Y-site compatibilities: Acyclovir, allopurinol, amifostine, amikacin, aminophylline, amphotericin B cholesteryl, ampicillin, ampicillin/sulbactam, amsacrine, aztreonam, bleomycin, bumetanide, buprenorphine, butorphanol, calcium gluconate, CARBOplatin, carmustine, ceFAZolin, cefepime, cefonicid, cefoperazone, cefotaxime, cefotetan, cefoxitin, ceftazidime, ceftizoxime, cefTRIAXone, cefuroxime, chlorproMAZINE, cimetidine, ciprofloxacin, CISplatin, cladribine, clindamycin, cyclophosphamide, cytarabine, dacarbazine, DACTINomycin, DAUNOrubicin, dexamethasone, diphenhydrAMINE, DO-

BUTamine, DOPamine, DOXOrubicin, DOXOrubicin liposome, doxycycline, droperidol, enalaprilat, etoposide, famotidine, filgrastim, fluconazole, fluorouracil, floxuridine, fludarabine, furosemide, gallium, ganciclovir, gentamicin, haloperidol, heparin hydrocortisone, HYDROmorphone, hydrOXYzine, IDArubicin, ifosfamide, imipenem-cilastatin, leucovorin, lorazepam, magnesium sulfate, melphalan, meperidine, mesna, methotrexate, methylPREDNISolone, metoclopramide, metroNIDAZOLE, mezlocillin, miconazole, minocycline, mitomycin, mitoxantrone, morphine, nalbuphine, netilmicin, ofloxacin, paclitaxel, piperacillin, piperacillin/tazobactam, plicamycin, potassium chloride, prochlorperazine, promethazine, propofol, ranitidine, sargramostim, sodium bicarbonate, streptozocin, teniposide, thiotepa, ticarcillin, ticarcillin/clavulanate, tobramycin, trimethoprim-sulfamethoxazole, vancomycin, vinBLAStine, vinCRIStine, vinorelbine, zidovudine

Transdermal route

• Apply to dry, clean, intact skin of upper outer arm 24-48 hr prior to chemotherapy, firmly press on skin, keep on during chemotherapy; can bathe, avoid swimming, whirlpool; remove ≥24 hr after chemotherapy completion

SIDE EFFECTS

CNS: *Headache, asthenia,* anxiety, dizziness

CV: Hypertension, QT prolongation

GI: Diarrhea, *constipation,* increased AST, ALT, *nausea*

HEMA: Leukopenia, anemia, thrombocytopenia

MISC: Rash, bronchospasm

PHARMACOKINETICS

Metabolized in liver to an active metabolite, half-life 10-12 hr, protein binding 65%

INTERACTIONS

Increase: EPS—antipsychotics

Increase: QT prolongation—amoxapine, β-blockers, chloroquine, class IA, III antidysrhythmics, clozapine, dasatinib, dolasetron, dronedarone, droperidol, erythromycin, flecainide, halogenated/local anesthetics, haloperidol, lapatinib, maprotiline, methadone, octreotide, ondansetron, palonosetron, pentamidine, phenothiazines, pimozide, propafenone, ranolazine, risperidone, sertindole, sunitinib, tacrolimus, telithromycin, tricyclics, troleandomycin, vardenafil, vorinostat, ziprasidone

NURSING CONSIDERATIONS

Assess:

• For absence of nausea, vomiting during chemotherapy

• **Hypersensitivity reaction:** rash, bronchospasm

Perform/provide:

• Storage at room temp for 24 hr after dilution

Evaluate:

• Therapeutic response: absence of nausea, vomiting during cancer chemotherapy

Teach patient/family:

• To report diarrhea, constipation, rash, changes in respirations

• That headache requiring an analgesic is common

guaiFENesin (OTC, Rx)

(gwye-fen′e-sin)

Alfen, Altarussin, Balminil ✱, Bidex, Diabetic Tussin, Elix Sure EX, Equaline Non-Drowsy Tussin, Equate Tussin Cough, Ganidin NR, Good Sense Mucus Relief, Good Sense Tussin Chest Congestion, Guaifenesin NR, Guiatuss, Humibid, Iophen NR, Liquibid, Miltuss EX, Mucinex, Mucinex Children's Mucus Relief, Mucinex Junior Strength, Naldecon Senior EX, Organ-1NR, Organidin NR, Q-Tussin, Robafen, Robitussin Guaifenesin ✱, Scot-Tussin Expectorant, Siltussin DAS, Siltussin SA, Top Care Children's Mucus Relief, Top Care Tussin Chest Congestion Solution, Wal-Tussin Expectorant, XPect

Func. class.: Expectorant

ACTION: Increases the volume and reduces the viscosity of secretions in the trachea and bronchi to facilitate secretion removal

USES: Productive and nonproductive cough

CONTRAINDICATIONS: Hypersensitivity; chronic, persistent cough

Precautions: Pregnancy (C), breastfeeding, CHF, asthma, emphysema, fever

DOSAGE AND ROUTES

- **Adult and adolescent: PO** 200-400 mg q4hr; **EXT REL** 600-1200 mg q12hr, max 2.4 g/day
- **Child 6-11 yr: PO** 100-200 mg q4hr; **EXT REL** 600 mg q12hr, max 1.2 g/day
- **Child 2-5 yr: PO** 50-100 mg q4hr; max 600 mg/day; ext rel 300 mg q12hr, max 600 mg/day

Available forms: Tabs 200, 400 mg; oral sol 100 mg/5 ml; ext rel tabs 600, 1200 mg; syrup 100 mg/5 ml; oral granules 50, 100 mg/packet

Administer:

- Do not break, crush, chew ext rel tabs

SIDE EFFECTS

CNS: Drowsiness, headache, dizziness

GI: Nausea, anorexia, vomiting, diarrhea

PHARMACOKINETICS

Half-life 1 hr, excreted in urine (metabolites)

NURSING CONSIDERATIONS

Assess:

- **Cough:** type, frequency, character, including sputum; fluids should be increased to 2 L/day

Perform/provide:

- Storage at room temp
- Increased fluids, room humidification to liquefy secretions

Evaluate:

- Therapeutic response: productive cough, thinner secretions

Teach patient/family:

- To avoid driving, other hazardous activities if drowsiness occurs (rare)
- To avoid smoking, smoke-filled room, perfumes, dust, environmental pollutants, cleansers
- To consult health provider if cough lasts >7 days

halcinonide topical

See Appendix B

haloperidol (Rx)

(hal-oh-pehr'ih-dol)

Apo-Haloperidol ✦

haloperidol decanoate (Rx)

Haldol Decanoate

haloperidol lactate (Rx)

Haldol

Func. class.: Antipsychotic, neuroleptic

Chem. class.: Butyrophenone

Do not confuse:
haloperidol/Halotestin
Haldol/Stadol

ACTION: Depresses cerebral cortex, hypothalamus, limbic system, which control activity and aggression; blocks neurotransmission produced by DOPamine at synapse; exhibits strong α-adrenergic, anticholinergic blocking action; mechanism for antipsychotic effects unclear

USES: Psychotic disorders, control of tics, vocal utterances in Gilles de la Tourette's syndrome, short-term treatment of hyperactive children showing excessive motor activity, prolonged parenteral therapy in chronic schizophrenia, organic mental syndrome with psychotic features, hiccups (short-term), emergency sedation of severely agitated or delirious patients, ADHD

Unlabeled uses: Nausea, vomiting during surgery; autism; migraine

CONTRAINDICATIONS: Children <3 yr, hypersensitivity, blood dyscrasias, coma, brain damage, bone marrow depression, alcohol and barbiturate withdrawal states, Parkinson's disease, angina, epilepsy, urinary retention, closed-angle glaucoma

Precautions: Pregnancy (C), breastfeeding, geriatric patients, seizure disorders, hypertension, pulmonary/cardiac/hepatic disease

Black Box Warning: Dementia

DOSAGE AND ROUTES

Acute psychosis

- **Adult: IM/IV** (lactate) 2-10 mg, may repeat q1hr, convert to **PO** as soon as possible, **PO** should be 150% of total parenteral dose required
- **Child 6-12 yr: IM/IV** (lactate) (unlabeled) 1-3 mg q4-8hr, max 0.15 mg/kg/day, switch to **PO** as soon as possible

Chronic schizophrenia

- **Adult: IM** (decanoate) 50-100 mg q4wk, max 100 mg for 1st inj
- **Child 3-12 yr: PO/IM** 0.05-0.15 mg/kg/day

Tourette's syndrome

- **Adult and adolescent: PO** 0.5-2 mg bid-tid, increase until desired response occurs
- **Child 3-12 yr or weighing 15-40 kg: PO** 0.25-0.5 mg/day in 2-3 divided doses, increase by 0.25-0.5 mg q5-7days, max 0.15 mg/kg/day

ADHD

- **Child 3-12 yr: PO** 0.25-0.5 mg/day in 2-3 divided doses, may increase by 0.025-0.5 mg q5-7days; maintenance 0.01-0.03 mg/kg/day as a single dose

Autism (unlabeled)

- **Child: PO** 0.04 mg/kg/day or 1-3 mg/day, max 4 mg/day

Migraine (unlabeled)

- **Adult: PO/IM** (lactate) 5 mg at onset, may repeat once

Available forms: Tabs 0.5, 1, 2, 5, 10, 20 mg; *lactate:* oral sol 2 mg/ml; inj 5 mg/ml, *decanoate:* 50 mg/ml, 100 mg/ml

Administer:

- Reduced dose to geriatric patients
- Antiparkinsonian agent if EPS occurs
- Avoid use with CNS depressants

PO route

- Oral liquid: use calibrated device; do not mix in coffee or tea
- PO with food or milk

IM route

- IM inj into large muscle mass, use 21G, 2-in needle; give no more than 3 ml/inj site; patient should remain recumbent for 30 min

IV route (lactate)

- Give undiluted for psychotic episode at 5 mg/min

Intermittent IV INF route

- Dilute in 30-50 ml of D_5W, give over 30 min

Y-site compatibilities: Amifostine, amsacrine, cisatracurium, cladribine, DOXOrubicin liposome, filgrastim, fludarabine, granisetron, LORazepam, melphalan, milrinone, paclitaxel, palonosetron, pamidronate, pancuronium, propofol, remifentanil, riTUXimab, rocuronium, tacrolimus, teniposide, thiotepa, tigecycline, tirofiban, TPN, trastuzumab, vecuronium, vinCRIStine, vinorelbine, voriconazole, zoledronic acid

SIDE EFFECTS

CNS: *EPS: pseudoparkinsonism, akathisia, dystonia, tardive dyskinesia, drowsiness, headache,* **seizures, neuroleptic malignant syndrome,** confusion

CV: *Orthostatic hypotension,* hypertension, **cardiac arrest,** ECG changes, tachycardia, **QT prolongation, sudden death, torsades de pointes**

EENT: Blurred vision, glaucoma, dry eyes

GI: *Dry mouth, nausea, vomiting, anorexia, constipation,* diarrhea, jaundice, weight gain, **ileus, hepatitis**

GU: Urinary retention, dysuria, urinary frequency, enuresis, impotence, amenorrhea, gynecomastia

INTEG: *Rash,* photosensitivity, dermatitis

RESP: **Laryngospasm, dyspnea, respiratory depression**

SYST: **Risk for death (dementia)**

PHARMACOKINETICS

Metabolized by liver; excreted in urine, bile; crosses placenta; enters breast milk; protein binding 92%; terminal half-life 12-36 hr (metabolites)

PO: Onset erratic, peak 2-6 hr, half-life 24 hr

IM: Onset 15-30 min, peak 15-20 min, half-life 21 hr

IM (Decanoate): Peak 4-11 days, half-life 3 wk

INTERACTIONS

Increase: serotonin syndrome, neuroleptic malignant syndrome—SSRIs, SNRIs

Increase: QT prolongation—class IA, III antidysrhythmics, tricyclics, amoxapine, maprotiline, phenothiazines, pimozide, risperidone, sertindole, ziprasidone, β-blockers, chloroquine, clozapine, dasatinib, dolasetron, droperidol, dronedarone, flecainide, halogenated/local anesthetics, lapatinib, methadone, erythromycin, telithromycin, troleandomycin, octreotide, ondansetron, palonosetron, pentamidine, propafenone, ranolazine, sunitinib, tacrolimus, vardenafil, vorinostat

Increase: oversedation—other CNS depressants, alcohol, barbiturate anesthetics

Increase: toxicity—EPINEPHrine, lithium

Increase: both drugs effects—β-adrenergic blockers, alcohol

Increase: anticholinergic effects—anticholinergics

Decrease: effects—lithium, levodopa

Decrease: haloperidol effects—PHENObarbital, carBAMazepine

Drug/Lab Test

Increase: LFTs, cardiac enzymes, cholesterol, blood glucose, prolactin, bilirubin, PBI, cholinesterase, alk phos

Decrease: hormones (blood, urine), PT

False positive: pregnancy tests, PKU

False negative: urinary steroids

NURSING CONSIDERATIONS

Assess:

• Swallowing of PO medication; check for hoarding or giving of medication to other patients

• Prolactin, CBC, urinalysis, ophthalmic exam before and during prolonged therapy

Black Box Warning: Dementia, affect, orientation, LOC, reflexes, gait, coordination, sleep pattern disturbances

• B/P standing, lying; take pulse, respirations q4hr during initial treatment; establish baseline before starting treatment; report drops of 30 mm Hg

• Dizziness, faintness, palpitations, tachycardia on rising

• **EPS** including akathisia (inability to sit still, no pattern to movements), tardive dyskinesia (bizarre movements of jaw, mouth, tongue, extremities), pseudoparkinsonism (rigidity, tremors, pill rolling, shuffling gait)

⚠ **Neuroleptic malignant syndrome/serotonin syndrome:** hyperthermia, muscle rigidity, altered mental status, increased CPK, seizures, hypo/hypertension, tachycardia; notify prescriber immediately

• Constipation, urinary retention daily; if these occur, increase bulk, water in diet

Perform/provide:

• Supervised ambulation until patient stabilized on medication; do not involve patient in strenuous exercise program, fainting is possible; patient should not stand still for long periods

• Sips of water, sugarless candy, gum for dry mouth

• Storage in tight, light-resistant container

Evaluate:

• Therapeutic response: decrease in emotional excitement, hallucinations, delusions, paranoia, reorganization of patterns of thought, speech; improvement in specific behaviors

Teach patient/family:

• That orthostatic hypotension occurs often; to rise from sitting or lying position gradually; to remain lying down after IM inj for at least 30 min

• To avoid hazardous activities until stabilized on medication

• To avoid hot tubs, hot showers, tub baths, since hypotension may occur

• To avoid abrupt withdrawal of this product because EPS may result; to withdraw slowly

• To avoid OTC preparations (cough, hay fever, cold) unless approved by prescriber, since serious product interactions may occur; to avoid use with alcohol, increased drowsiness may occur

• To use a sunscreen to prevent burns

• About compliance with product regimen

• About EPS and necessity of meticulous oral hygiene, since oral candidiasis may occur

• To report impaired vision, jaundice, tremors, muscle twitching

• That, in hot weather, heat stroke may occur; to take extra precautions to stay cool

TREATMENT OF OVERDOSE:

Activated charcoal, lavage if orally ingested; provide an airway; do not induce vomiting

⚠ HIGH ALERT

heparin (Rx)

(hep′a-rin)

Hepalean ✤, Heparin Leo ✤, Hep-Lock, Hep-Lock U/P, Monoject Prefill

Func. class.: Anticoagulant, antithrombotic

Do not confuse:

heparin/Hespan

ACTION: Prevents conversion of fibrinogen to fibrin and prothrombin to thrombin by enhancing inhibitory effects of antithrombin III

USES: Prevention of deep venous thrombosis, PE, MI, open heart surgery, disseminated intravascular clotting syndrome, atrial fibrillation with embolization, as an anticoagulant in transfusion and dialysis procedures, prevention of DVT/PE, to maintain patency of indwelling venipuncture devices; diagnosis, treatment of DIC

CONTRAINDICATIONS: Hypersensitivity, hemophilia, leukemia with bleeding, peptic ulcer disease, severe thrombocytopenic purpura, severe renal/hepatic disease, blood dyscrasias, severe hypertension, subacute bacterial endocarditis, acute nephritis; benzyl alcohol products in neonates/infants/pregnancy/lactation

Precautions: Pregnancy (C), children, geriatric patients, alcoholism, hyperlipidemia, diabetes, renal disease

DOSAGE AND ROUTES

Deep venous thrombosis/pulmonary embolism

- **Adult: IV BOL** 80 international units/kg then maintenance **IV INF** 18 international units/kg/hr; if aPTT <35 (1.2× normal), increase **IV INF** rate by 4 international units/kg/hr and rebolus with 80 international units/kg; if aPTT 35-45 (1.2-1.5× normal), increase **IV INF** by 2 international units/kg/hr and rebolus with 40 international units/kg; if aPTT 46-70 (1.5-2.3× normal), maintain **IV INF;** if aPTT 71-90 (2.3-3× normal), decrease **IV INF** by 2 international units/kg/hr; if aPTT >90 (>3× normal), hold **IV INF** for 1 hr then decrease rate 3 international units/kg/hr
- **Child/infant/neonate: IV** loading dose 75 international units/kg
- **Child >1 yr:** 20 international units/kg/hr
- **Infant/neonate <1 yr:** 28 international units/kg/hr as initial maintenance dose

Thrombosis prophylaxis (open heart/CV surgery)

- **Adult: IV** ≥150 international units/kg; procedures <60 min, up to 300 international units/kg; procedures >60 min, up to 400 international units/kg based on ACT

Thrombosis prophylaxis (PCI, not receiving abciximab)

- **Adult: IV BOL** weight adjusted with 60-100 international units/kg, maintain ACT within 250-300 sec (HemoTec) or 300-350 sec (Hemochron)
- **Child/infant/neonate: IV BOL** 100-150 international units/kg

Prophylaxis for DVT/PE

- **Adult: SUBCUT** 5000 units q8-12hr

IV catheter occlusion prophylaxis

- **Adult/child: IV** 10-100 units/ml
- **Infant <10 kg: IV** 10 units/ml

Available forms: Sol for inj 10, 100, 1000, 5000, 7500, 10,000, 20,000, 40,000 units/ml; premixed 1000 units/500 ml, 2000 units/1000 ml, 12,500 units/250 ml, 25,000 units/250 ml, 25,000 units/500 ml; lock flush preparations 10 units/ml

Administer:

- Cannot be used interchangeably (unit for unit) with LMWHs or heparinoids
- At same time each day to maintain steady blood levels

Heparin Lock route

⚠ Do not mistake heparin sodium inj 10,000 units/ml and Hep-Lock U/P 10 units/ml; they have similar blue labeling; deaths in pediatric patients have occurred when heparin sodium inj vials were confused with heparin flush vials

SUBCUT route

- **Give** deeply with 25G 3/8-in needle; do not massage area or aspirate when giving SUBCUT inj; give in abdomen between pelvic bones, rotate sites; do not pull back on plunger; leave in for 10 sec; apply gentle pressure for 1 min
- Changing needles is not recommended
- Avoid all IM inj that may cause bleeding, hematoma

H

Direct IV route

- Give loading dose undiluted, over ≥1 min, use before continuous inf

Continuous IV INF route

- Dilute 25,000 units/250-500 ml 0.9 NaCl or D_5W, (50-100 units) solutions are premixed and ready for use
- When product is added to inf sol for cont IV, invert container at least 6 times to ensure adequate mixing

Additive compatibilities: Avoid adding to sol, even if compatible; rate of heparin inf times may need to be changed

Y-site compatibilities: Acyclovir, allopurinol, amifostine, aminophylline, atropine, aztreonam, betamethasone, bleomycin, calcium gluconate, ceFAZolin, cefotetan, ceftazidime, cefTRIAXone, chlordiazepoxide, cimetidine, CISplatin, cladribine, clindamycin, conjugated estrogens, cyanocobalamin, cyclophosphamide, cytarabine, dexamethasone, digoxin, DOPamine, DOXOrubicin liposome, edrophonium, enalaprilat, EPINEPHrine, esmolol, ethacrynate, etoposide, famotidine, fentaNYL, fluconazole, fludarabine, fluorouracil, foscarnet, furosemide, gallium, gemcitabine, granisetron, hydrocortisone, HYDROmorphone, insulin (regular), isoproterenol, kanamycin, leucovorin, linezolid, lidocaine, LORazepam, magnesium sulfate, melphalan, menadiol, meropenem, methotrexate, methoxamine, methyldopate, methylergonovine, metoclopramide, metroNIDAZOLE, midazolam, milrinone, minocycline, mitomycin, morphine, nafcillin, neostigmine, nitroglycerin, nitroprusside, norepinephrine, ondansetron, oxacillin, oxytocin, paclitaxel, pancuronium, penicillin G potassium, phytonadione, piperacillin, piperacillin/tazobactam, potassium chloride, prednisoLONE, procainamide, propofol, propranolol, pyridostigmine, ranitidine, remifentanil, sargramostim, scopolamine, sodium bicarbonate, succinylcholine, tacrolimus, theophylline, thiopental, thiotepa, ticarcillin, ticarcillin/clavulanate, tirofiban, trimethobenzamide, trimethaphan, vecuronium, vinBLAStine, warfarin, zidovudine, zoledronic acid

SIDE EFFECTS

CNS: *Fever,* chills, headache

GU: Hematuria

HEMA: **Hemorrhage, thrombocytopenia, anemia**

INTEG: *Rash,* dermatitis, urticaria, pruritus, delayed transient alopecia, hematoma, cutaneous necrosis (SUBCUT)

META: Hyperkalemia, hypoaldosteronism

SYST: **Anaphylaxis**

PHARMACOKINETICS

Half-life 1½ hr; excreted in urine; 95% bound to plasma proteins; does not cross placenta or alter breast milk; removed from the system via the lymph and spleen; partially metabolized in kidney, liver; excreted in urine (<50% unchanged)

SUBCUT: Onset 20-60 min, duration 8-12 hr, well absorbed >35,000 international units/24 hr

IV: Peak 5 min, duration 2-6 hr

INTERACTIONS

Increase: heparin action—oral anticoagulants, salicylates, dextran, NSAIDs, platelet inhibitors, cephalosporins, penicillins, ticlopidine, dipyridamole, antineoplastics, clopidogrel, presgrel, SSRIs, SNRIs

Decrease: heparin action—digoxin, tetracyclines, antihistamines, cardiac glycosides, nicotine

Drug/Lab Test

Increase: ALT, AST, INR, PT, PTT, potassium

Decrease: platelets, triglycerides, cholesterol, plasma free fatty acids

NURSING CONSIDERATIONS

Assess:

- ⚠ **Bleeding, hemorrhage: gums, petechiae, ecchymosis, black tarry stools, hematuria, epistaxis, decrease in Hct, B/P; HIT may occur after product discontinuation**

• Blood studies (Hct, occult blood in stools) q3mo
• Partial prothrombin time, which should be 1.5-2.5× control; for continuous IV inf, check aPTT baseline 6 hr after initiation and 6 hr after any dose change; use aPTT for dosing adjustments; after therapeutic aPTT has been measured 2×, check aPTT daily
• Platelet count q2-3days; thrombocytopenia may occur on 4th day of treatment
• **Hypersensitivity:** rash, chills, fever, itching; report to prescriber

Perform/provide:
• Storage at room temp

Evaluate:
• Therapeutic response: decrease of DVT, adequate anticoagulation based on aPTT

Teach patient/family:
• To avoid OTC preparations that may cause serious product interactions unless directed by prescriber
• That product may be held during active bleeding (menstruation), depending on condition
• To use soft-bristle toothbrush to avoid bleeding gums; to avoid contact sports; to use an electric razor, to avoid IM inj
• To carry emergency ID identifying product taken
• To report to prescriber any signs of bleeding: gums, under skin, urine, stools
• To report to prescriber any signs of hypersensitivity: rash, chills, fever, itching

TREATMENT OF OVERDOSE:
Withdraw product, protamine 1 mg protamine/100 units heparin

hepatitis B immune globulin (Rx)

HepaGam B, Hyper HEP B S/D, Nabi-HB

Func. class.: Immune globulin

ACTION:
Provides passive immunity to hepatitis B

USES:
Prevention of hepatitis B virus in exposed patients, including passive immunity in neonates born to HBsAg-positive mother, prevention of hepatitis B recurrence after liver transplant in HBsAg-positive patients

CONTRAINDICATIONS:
Hypersensitivity to immune globulins, coagulation disorders

Precautions: Pregnancy (C), breastfeeding, children, geriatric patients, hemophilia, active infection, IgA deficiency

DOSAGE AND ROUTES
• **Adult and child: IM** 0.06 ml/kg (usual 3-5 ml) within 7 days of exposure; repeat 28 days after exposure if patient wishes to not receive hepatitis B vaccine

Neonates born to hepatitis B surface-antigen–positive persons
• **Neonate: IM** 0.5 ml within 12 hr of birth

Prevention of hepatitis B infection recurrence after liver transplant
• **Adult: IV** (HepaGam B only) 20,000 international units concurrent with grafting transplanted liver, then 20,000 international units/day on days 1-7, then 20,000 international units q2wk starting on day 14, then 20,000 international units/mo starting with mo 4

Available forms: Inj 1-, 4-, 5-ml vials; neonatal syringe 0.5 ml; HepaGam B sol for inj 312 units/ml; Hyper HEP B S/D 217 units/ml

Administer:

IM route
• After rotating vial; do not shake
• Only with EPINEPHrine 1:1000 on unit to treat laryngospasm
• In deltoid for better absorption (adult)

IV route (HepaGam B only)
• Calculate volume needed for each 20,000 international-unit dose using measured potency of each lot; potency stamped on label
• Promptly use after vial entered; discard unused product

• Give at 2 ml/min through separate IV line, use inf pump, decrease to 1 ml/min if inf-related event occurs, patient becomes uncomfortable

SIDE EFFECTS

CNS: Headache, dizziness, fever
GI: Nausea, vomiting
INTEG: Soreness at inj site, urticaria, erythema, swelling
SYST: Induration, anaphylaxis, angioedema

INTERACTIONS

• Do not use within 3 mo of hepatitis B immune globulin, MMR, varicella, or rotavirus vaccines even after discontinuing product

NURSING CONSIDERATIONS

Assess:

• History of allergies, skin conditions (eczema, psoriasis, dermatitis), reactions to vaccinations
• Skin reactions: rash, induration, urticaria
⚠ **Anaphylaxis:** inability to breathe, bronchospasm, hypotension, wheezing, diaphoresis, fever, flushing

Perform/provide:

• Written record of immunization

Evaluate:

• Prevention of hepatitis B

Teach patient/family:

• That discomfort may occur at site
• To report any rash, wheezing, inability to breathe immediately

homatropine ophthalmic

See Appendix B

hydrALAZINE (Rx)

(hye-dral′a-zeen)

Apresoline ♣, Apo-HydrALAZINE ♣

Func. class.: Antihypertensive, direct-acting peripheral vasodilator

Chem. class.: Phthalazine

Do not confuse:
hydrALAZINE/hydrOXYzine
Apresoline/allopurinol

ACTION: Vasodilates arteriolar smooth muscle by direct relaxation; reduction in blood pressure with reflex increases in heart rate, stroke volume, cardiac output

USES: Essential hypertension; severe essential hypertension
Unlabeled uses: CHF

CONTRAINDICATIONS: Hypersensitivity to hydrALAZINEs, mitral valvular rheumatic heart disease, CAD
Precautions: Pregnancy (C), breastfeeding, geriatric patients, CVA, advanced renal disease, hepatic disease, SLE, dissecting aortic aneurysm

DOSAGE AND ROUTES

Hypertension

• **Adult: PO** 10 mg qid 2-4 days, then 25 mg for rest of 1st wk, then 50 mg qid individualized to desired response, max 300 mg/day
• **Child: PO** 0.75-1 mg/kg/day in 2-4 divided doses, max 25 mg/dose, increase over 3-4 wk to max 7.5 mg/kg/day or 200 mg, whichever is less

Hypertensive crisis

• **Adult: IV BOL** 10-20 mg q4-6hr, administer **PO** as soon as possible; **IM** 10-50 mg q4-6hr
• **Child: IV BOL** 0.1-0.6 mg/kg q4hr; **IM** 0.1-0.6 mg/kg q4-6hr, max 1.7-3.5 mg/kg/day

CHF

• **Adult: PO** 10-25 mg tid, max 75 mg tid

Available forms: Inj 20 mg/ml; tabs 10, 25, 50, 100 mg

Administer:

PO route

• Give with meals (PO) to enhance absorption

IM route

• Do not admix

• No dilution needed, inject deeply in large muscle, aspirate

Direct IV route

• IV undiluted; give through Y-tube or 3-way stopcock, give each 10 mg over ≥1 min

• To recumbent patient, keep recumbent for 1 hr after administration

Y-site compatibilities: Alemtuzumab, anidulafungin, argatroban, atenolol, bivalirudin, bleomycin, DACTINomycin, DAPTOmycin, dexrazoxone, diltiazem, docetaxel, etoposide, fludarabine, gatifloxacin, gemcitabine, granisetron, HYDROmorphone, IDArubicin, irinotecan, leucovorin, linezolid, mechlorethamine, metroNIDAZOLE, milrinone, mitoxantrone, octreotide, oxaliplatin, paclitaxel, palonosetron, pancuronium, potassium chloride, tacrolimus, teniposide, thiotepa, tirofiban, vecuronium, vinorelbine, vitamin B/C, voriconazole

Solution compatibilities: D_5LR, D_5W, $D_{10}W$, $D_{10}LR$, 0.45% NaCl, 0.9% NaCl, Ringer's, LR

SIDE EFFECTS

CNS: *Headache, tremors, dizziness, anxiety,* peripheral neuritis, depression, fever, chills

CV: *Palpitations, reflex tachycardia, angina,* **shock**, rebound hypertension, orthostatic hypotension

GI: *Nausea, vomiting, anorexia, diarrhea,* constipation, paralytic ileus

GU: Urinary retention, glomerulonephritis, hematuria

HEMA: Leukopenia, agranulocytosis, anemia, thrombocytopenia

INTEG: Rash, pruritus, urticaria

MISC: Nasal congestion, muscle cramps, *lupuslike symptoms,* flushing, edema, dyspnea

PHARMACOKINETICS

Half-life 3-7 hr, metabolized by liver, 12%-14% excreted in urine, protein binding 89%

PO: Onset 20-30 min, peak 1-2 hr, duration 2-4 hr

IM: Onset 10-30 min, peak 1 hr, duration 2-6 hr

IV: Onset 5-30 min, peak 10-80 min, duration 2-6 hr

INTERACTIONS

Increase: severe hypotension—MAOIs

Increase: tachycardia, angina—sympathomimetics (EPINEPHrine, norepinephrine)

Increase: hypotension—other antihypertensives, alcohol, levodopa, thiazide diuretics

Increase: effects of β-blockers

Decrease: hydrALAZINE effects—NSAIDs, estrogens

Drug/Lab Test

Decrease: Hgb, WBC, RBC, platelets, neutrophils

Positive: ANA titer

NURSING CONSIDERATIONS

Assess:

• Cardiac status: B/P q5min × 2 hr, then q1hr × 2 hr, then q4hr; pulse, jugular venous distention q4hr

• Electrolytes, blood studies: K, Na, Cl, CO_2, CBC, serum glucose, LE prep, ANA titer before, during treatment; assess for fever, joint pain, rash, sore throat (lupuslike symptoms); notify prescriber

• Weight daily, I&O

• Edema in feet, legs daily, skin turgor, dryness of mucous membranes for hydration status

• Crackles, dyspnea, orthopnea

• IV site for extravasation, rate

• Mental status: affect, mood, behavior, anxiety; check for personality changes

Evaluate:
- Therapeutic response: decreased B/P

Teach patient/family:
- To take with food to increase bioavailability (PO)
- To avoid OTC preparations unless directed by prescriber
- To notify prescriber if chest pain, severe fatigue, fever, muscle or joint pain occurs
- To rise slowly to prevent orthostatic hypotension
- To notify prescriber if pregnancy is suspected

TREATMENT OF OVERDOSE:
Administer vasopressors, volume expanders for shock; if PO, lavage or give activated charcoal, digitalization

hydrochlorothiazide (Rx)

(hye-droe-klor-oh-thye′a-zide)

Apo-Hydro ✤, Diovan HCT ✤, Ezide, Neo-Codema ✤, PMS-Hydrochlorothiazide ✤

Func. class.: Thiazide diuretic, antihypertensive

Chem. class.: Sulfonamide derivative

ACTION: Acts on distal tubule and ascending limb of loop of Henle by increasing excretion of water, sodium, chloride, potassium

USES: Edema, hypertension, diuresis, CHF; edema in corticosteroid, estrogen, NSAIDs; idiopathic lower extremity edema therapy

Unlabeled uses: Diabetes insipidus, hypercalciuria, nephrolithiasis, premenstrual syndrome, renal calculus

CONTRAINDICATIONS: Hypersensitivity to thiazides or sulfonamides, anuria, renal decompensation, hypomagnesemia

Precautions: Pregnancy (B), breastfeeding, hypokalemia, renal/hepatic disease, gout, COPD, LE, diabetes mellitus, hyperlipidemia, CCr $<$30 ml/min

DOSAGE AND ROUTES
- **Adult: PO** 12.5-25 mg/day, may increase to 50 mg/day in 1-2 divided doses
- **Child >6 mo: PO** 1-2 mg/kg/day in divided doses
- **Child <6 mo: PO** up to 2-3.3 mg/kg/day in divided doses

Available forms: Tabs 12.5, 25, 50 mg; caps 12.5 mg

Administer:
- In AM to avoid interference with sleep if using product as a diuretic; tab may be crushed, mixed with food
- Potassium replacement if potassium $<$3 mg/dl
- With food; if nausea occurs, absorption may be decreased slightly

SIDE EFFECTS
CNS: Drowsiness, paresthesia, depression, headache, *dizziness, fatigue, weakness,* fever

CV: Irregular pulse, orthostatic hypotension, palpitations, volume depletion, allergic myocarditis

EENT: Blurred vision

ELECT: *Hypokalemia,* hypercalcemia, hyponatremia, hypochloremia, hypomagnesemia

GI: *Nausea, vomiting, anorexia,* constipation, diarrhea, cramps, pancreatitis, GI irritation, hepatitis

GU: *Urinary frequency,* polyuria, uremia, glucosuria, hyperuricemia

HEMA: Aplastic anemia, hemolytic anemia, leukopenia, agranulocytosis, thrombocytopenia, neutropenia

INTEG: *Rash,* urticaria, purpura, photosensitivity, alopecia, erythema multiforme

META: *Hyperglycemia, hyperuricemia,* increased creatinine, BUN

PHARMACOKINETICS
PO: Onset 2 hr, peak 4 hr, duration 6-12 hr, half-life 6-15 hr, excreted unchanged by kidneys, crosses placenta, enters breast milk

INTERACTIONS

Increase: hyperglycemia, hyperuricemia, hypotension—diazoxide
Increase: hypokalemia—glucocorticoids, amphotericin B
Increase: toxicity—lithium, non-depolarizing skeletal muscle relaxants, cardiac glycosides
Increase: renal failure risk—NSAIDs
Increase: effects—loop diuretics
Decrease: antidiabetics effects
Decrease: thiazides absorption—cholestyramine, colestipol

Drug/Lab Test
Increase: amylase, parathyroid test

NURSING CONSIDERATIONS

Assess:
- Weight, I&O daily to determine fluid loss; effect of product may be decreased if used daily
- Rate, depth, rhythm of respiration, effect of exertion
- B/P lying, standing; postural hypotension may occur
- Blood studies: BUN, blood glucose, CBC, serum creatinine, blood pH, ABGs, uric acid, electrolytes
- **Signs of metabolic alkalosis:** drowsiness, restlessness
- **Signs of hypokalemia:** postural hypotension, malaise, fatigue, tachycardia, leg cramps, weakness, dehydration
- Confusion, especially in geriatric patients; take safety precautions if needed

Evaluate:
- Therapeutic response: improvement in edema of feet, legs, sacral area daily, decreased B/P

Teach patient/family:
- To increase fluid intake to 2-3 L/day unless contraindicated; to rise slowly from lying or sitting position
- To notify prescriber of muscle weakness, cramps, nausea, dizziness; hypokalemia is common
- That product may be taken with food or milk
- To use sunscreen for photosensitivity
- That blood glucose may be increased in diabetics
- To take early in day to avoid nocturia
- To avoid alcohol, OTC meds unless approved by prescriber

TREATMENT OF OVERDOSE:

Lavage if taken orally; monitor electrolytes; administer dextrose in saline; monitor hydration, CV, renal status

HYDROcodone (Rx)

(hye-droe-koe′done)

Hycodan ✦, Tussigon

HYDROcodone/acetaminophen (Rx)

Co-Gesic, Dolorex Forte, Duocet, Hycet, Lorcet, Lortab, Margesic H, Liquicet, Maxidone, Norco, Polygesic, Stagesic, Vanacet, Vicodin, Vicodin ES, Vicodin HP, Xodol, Zamicet, Zydone

HYDROcodone/ibuprofen (Rx)

Ibudone, Reprexain, Vicoprofen

Func. class.: Antitussive opioid analgesic/nonopioid analgesic

Controlled Substance Schedule III

Do not confuse:
HYDROcodone/hydrocortisone
Hycodan/Vicodin

ACTION: Acts directly on cough center in medulla to suppress cough; binds to opiate receptors in CNS to reduce pain

USES: Hyperactive and nonproductive cough, mild to moderate pain

CONTRAINDICATIONS: Acne rosacea/vulgaris, Cushing's syndrome, measles, perioral dermatitis, varicella, abrupt discontinuation; hypersensitivity to this product, benzyl

Precautions: Pregnancy (C), breastfeeding, neonates, addictive personality, increased intracranial pressure, MI (acute), severe heart disease, respiratory depression, renal/hepatic disease, bowel impaction, urinary retention, viral infection, ulcerative colitis, seizures, sulfite hypersensitivity, psychosis, hypertension, hyperthyroidism

DOSAGE AND ROUTES

Analgesic

• **Adult: PO** 2.5-10 mg q3-6hr prn, max 60 mg/day

Antitussive

• **Adult: PO** 5 mg q4-6hr prn, max 30 mg/24 hr

Available forms: ***HYDROcodone:*** bulk powder; ***HYDROcodone/acetaminophen:*** 5 mg HYDROcodone/500 mg acetaminophen (Co-Gesic, Lorcet, Lortab 5/500, Stagesic, Vicodin); 7.5 mg HYDROcodone/400 mg acetaminophen (Zydone), 7.5 mg HYDROcodone/500 mg acetaminophen (Lortab 7.5/500), 7.5 mg HYDROcodone/750 mg acetaminophen (Vicodin ES), 5 mg HYDROcodone/325 acetaminophen, 10 mg HYDROcodone/325 acetaminophen (Norco), 10 mg HYDROcodone/500 mg acetaminophen (Lortab 10/500), 10 mg HYDROcodone/650 mg acetaminophen (Lorcet 10/650, Vicodin HP), 10 mg HYDROcodone/660 acetaminophen (Vicodin HP); caps 5 mg HYDROcodone/500 mg acetaminophen (Stagesic, Zydone); ***HYDROcodone/ibuprofen:*** tabs 7.5 mg HYDROcodone/200 mg ibuprofen (Vicoprofen)

Administer:

• Do not break, crush, or chew tabs; only scored tabs can be broken

• With antiemetic after meals if nausea or vomiting occurs

• Do not exceed 4 g acetaminophen with combination product

• Give with food or milk to prevent gastric upset

SIDE EFFECTS

CNS: *Drowsiness*, dizziness, light-headedness, confusion, headache, sedation, euphoria, dysphoria, weakness, hallucinations, disorientation, mood changes, dependence, seizures

CV: Palpitations, tachycardia, bradycardia, change in B/P, circulatory depression, syncope; cardiac arrest (children)

EENT: Tinnitus, blurred vision, miosis, diplopia

GI: *Nausea, vomiting, anorexia, constipation*, cramps, dry mouth, ulcers

GU: Increased urinary output, dysuria, urinary retention

INTEG: Rash, urticaria, flushing, pruritus

RESP: Respiratory depression; pulmonary edema, bronchopneumonia, respiratory arrest (children)

PHARMACOKINETICS

Onset 10-20 min, duration 4-6 hr, half-life $3\frac{1}{2}$-$4\frac{1}{2}$ hr, metabolized in liver, excreted in urine, crosses placenta

INTERACTIONS

Increase: CNS depression—alcohol, opioids, sedative/hypnotics, phenothiazines, skeletal muscle relaxants, general anesthetics, tricyclics

Increase: severe reactions—MAOIs

Drug/Herb

Increase: CNS depression—lavender, valerian

Drug/Lab Test

Increase: amylase, lipase

NURSING CONSIDERATIONS

Assess:

• **Pain:** intensity, type, location, other characteristics before, 1 hr after giving product; titrate upward by 25% until pain reduced by half; need for pain medication, physical dependence, opioid is more effective before pain is severe

• **CNS changes:** dizziness, drowsiness, hallucinations, euphoria, LOC, pupil reaction

• B/P, pulse, respirations before, periodically; if respirations <10/min, dose

may need to be reduced, oversedation may occur
• Bowel status: constipation; provide fluids, fiber in diet, may need stimulate laxatives
• **Allergic reactions:** rash, urticaria
• Cough and respiratory dysfunction: respiratory depression, character, rate, rhythm
• History of ulcers if using ibuprofen combination product

Perform/provide:
• Storage in light-resistant area at room temp
• Safety measures: night-light, call bell within easy reach; assistance with ambulation

Evaluate:
• Therapeutic response: decrease in pain or cough

Teach patient/family:
• To report any symptoms of CNS changes, allergic reactions
• That physical dependency may result when used for extended periods
• That withdrawal symptoms may occur: nausea, vomiting, cramps, fever, faintness, anorexia
• To avoid driving, other hazardous activities because drowsiness occurs
• To avoid other CNS depressants; they will enhance sedating properties of this product
• To change positions slowly to reduce orthostatic hypotension

TREATMENT OF OVERDOSE:
Naloxone HCl (Narcan) 0.2-0.8 mg IV, O_2, IV fluids, vasopressors

hydrocortisone (Rx)
(hy-dro-kor′tih-sone)

Cortef, Colocort, Cortenema

hydrocortisone acetate (Rx)
Anucort, Anusol, Cortifoam, Hemril, Proctocort, Rectasol

hydrocortisone sodium succinate (Rx)
A-hydroCort, Solu-Cortef

Func. class.: Corticosteroid
Chem. class.: Short-acting glucocorticoid

Do not confuse:
hydrocortisone/HYDROcodone

ACTION: Decreases inflammation by suppression of migration of polymorphonuclear leukocytes, fibroblasts, reversal of increased capillary permeability, and lysosomal stabilization

USES: Severe inflammation, adrenal insufficiency, ulcerative colitis, collagen disorders

Unlabeled uses: Carpal tunnel syndrome, Churg-Strauss syndrome, endophthalmitis, mixed connective-tissue disease, multiple myeloma, polyarteritis nodosa, polychondritis, pulmonary edema, temporal arteritis, Wegener's granulomatosis

CONTRAINDICATIONS: Children <2 yr, psychosis, hypersensitivity, idiopathic thrombocytopenia (IM), acute glomerulonephritis, amebiasis, fungal infections, nonasthmatic bronchial disease, AIDS, TB, recent MI (associated with left ventricular rupture)

Precautions: Pregnancy (C), breastfeeding, diabetes mellitus, glaucoma, osteoporosis, seizure disorders, ulcerative colitis, CHF, myasthenia gravis, renal disease, esophagitis, peptic ulcer, metastatic carcinoma

DOSAGE AND ROUTES

Adrenal insufficiency/inflammation

• **Adult: PO** 20-240 mg daily; **IM/IV** 100-500 mg (succinate)

Shock prevention

• **Adult: IM/IV** (succinate) 50 mg/kg repeated after 4 hr, repeat q24hr as needed

Colitis

• **Adult: PO** 20-240 mg (base)/day in 2-4 divided doses; **ENEMA** 100 mg nightly for 21 days

• **Child: PO** 2-8 mg (base)/kg/day or 60-240 mg (base)/m^2/day in 3-4 divided doses

Available forms: Tabs 5, 10, 20 mg; inj 25, 50 mg/ml; enema 100 mg/60 ml; **acetate:** inj 25 ✱, 50 mg/ml ✱, rectal 10% aerosol foam; supp 25, 30 mg; **succinate:** inj 100 mg, 250 mg, 500 mg, 1000 mg/vial

Administer:

• Daily dose in AM for better results

• In one dose in AM to prevent adrenal suppression; avoid SUBCUT administration, may damage tissue

• Do not use acetate or susp for IV

PO route

• With food or milk for GI symptoms

Rectal route

• Tell patient to retain for 1 hr if possible

IM route

• IM inj deep in large muscle mass; rotate sites; avoid deltoid; use 21G needle

IV route

• **Succinate:** IV in mix-o-vial or reconstitute ≤250 mg/2 ml bacteriostatic water for inj; mix gently; give direct IV over ≥1 min; may be further diluted in 100, 250, 500, or 1000 ml of D_5W, D_5 0.9%, NaCl 0.9% given over ordered rate

Sodium succinate preparations

Y-site compatibilities: Acyclovir, allopurinol, amifostine, aminophylline, amphotericin B cholesteryl, ampicillin, amrinone, amsacrine, atracurium, atropine, aztreonam, betamethasone, calcium gluconate, cefepime, cefmetazole, cephalothin, cephapirin, chlordiazepoxide, chlorproMAZINE, cisatracurium, cladribine, cyanocobalamin, cytarabine, dexamethasone, digoxin, diphenhydrAMINE, DOPamine, DOXOrubicin liposome, droperidol, edrophonium, enalaprilat, EPINEPHrine, esmolol, estrogens conjugated, ethacrynate, famotidine, fentaNYL, fentaNYL/droperidol, filgrastim, fludarabine, fluorouracil, foscarnet, furosemide, gallium, granisetron, heparin, hydrALAZINE, insulin (regular), isoproterenol, kanamycin, lidocaine, LORazepam, magnesium sulfate, melphalan, menadiol, meperidine, methicillin, methoxamine, methylergonovine, minocycline, morphine, neostigmine, norepinephrine, ondansetron, oxacillin, oxytocin, paclitaxel, pancuronium, penicillin G potassium, pentazocine, phytonadione, piperacillin/tazobactam, prednisoLONE, procainamide, prochlorperazine, propofol, propranolol, pyridostigmine, remifentanil, scopolamine, sodium bicarbonate, succinylcholine, tacrolimus, teniposide, theophylline, thiotepa, trimethaphan, trimethobenzamide, vecuronium, vinorelbine

SIDE EFFECTS

CNS: *Depression, flushing, sweating,* headache, mood changes, **pseudotumor cerebri**

CV: *Hypertension,* **circulatory collapse, thrombophlebitis, embolism,** tachycardia, edema

EENT: Fungal infections, increased intraocular pressure, blurred vision

GI: *Diarrhea, nausea,* abdominal distention, **GI hemorrhage,** increased appetite, **pancreatitis**

HEMA: Thrombocytopenia

INTEG: Acne, poor wound healing, ecchymosis, petechiae

MS: Fractures, osteoporosis, weakness

PHARMACOKINETICS

Metabolized by liver, excreted in urine (17-OHCS, 17-KS), crosses placenta

PO: Peak 1-2 hr, duration 1-1½ days

IM/IV: Onset 20 min, peak 4-8 hr, duration 1-1½ days

RECT: Onset 3-5 days

INTERACTIONS

Increase: GI bleeding risk—salicylates, NSAIDs

Increase: side effects—alcohol, amphotericin B, digoxin, cycloSPORINE, diuretics

Decrease: hydrocortisone action—bosentan, cholestyramine, colestipol, barbiturates, rifampin, ePHEDrine, phenytoin, theophylline

Decrease: anticoagulant effects, anticonvulsants, antidiabetics, calcium supplements, toxoids, vaccines

Drug/Lab Test

Increase: cholesterol, sodium, blood glucose, uric acid, calcium, glucose

Decrease: calcium, potassium, T_4, T_3, thyroid ^{131}I uptake test, urine 17-OHCS, 17-KS

False negative: skin allergy tests

NURSING CONSIDERATIONS

Assess:

- Potassium, blood glucose, urine glucose while patient receiving long-term therapy; hypokalemia and hyperglycemia; potassium depletion: paresthesias, fatigue, nausea, vomiting, depression, polyuria, dysrhythmias, weakness
- B/P, pulse; notify prescriber of chest pain
- I&O ratio; be alert for decreasing urinary output, increasing edema; weight daily, notify prescriber of weekly gain >5 lb
- **Adrenal insufficiency (cushingoid symptoms):** nausea, anorexia, SOB, moon face, fatigue, dizziness, weakness, joint pain before and during treatment; plasma cortisol levels during long-term therapy (normal level: 138-635 nmol/L SI units when drawn at 8 AM)
- **Infection:** increased temp, WBC even after withdrawal of medication; product masks infection
- Mental status: affect, mood, behavioral changes, aggression
- **GI effects:** nausea, vomitting, anorexia or appetite stimulation, diarrhea, constipation, abdominal pain, hiccups, gastritis, pancreatitis, GI bleeding/perforation with long-term treatment

Perform/provide:

- Assistance with ambulation for patient with bone-tissue disease to prevent fractures

Evaluate:

- Therapeutic response: decreased inflammation, GI symptoms

Teach patient/family:

- That emergency ID as corticosteroid user should be carried
- To immediately report abdominal pain, black tarry stools because GI bleeding/perforation can occur
- To notify prescriber if therapeutic response decreases; that dosage adjustment may be needed; about signs of infection
- Not to discontinue abruptly because adrenal crisis can result; that product should be tapered
- That supplemental calcium/vit D may be needed if patient receiving long-term therapy
- That product can mask infection and cause hypoglycemia (diabetic)
- To avoid OTC products: salicylates, alcohol in cough products, cold preparations unless directed by prescriber
- About cushingoid symptoms of adrenal insufficiency: nausea, anorexia, fatigue, dizziness, dyspnea, weakness, joint pain, moon face
- To avoid live-virus vaccines if using steroids long term

hydrocortisone nasal

See Appendix B

hydrocortisone topical

See Appendix B

H

⚠ HIGH ALERT

HYDROmorphone (Rx)

(hye-droe-mor′fone)

Dilaudid, Dilaudid HP, Exalgo, Hydromorph Contin ✦, PMS-Hydromorphone ✦

Func. class.: Opiate analgesic

Chem. class.: Semisynthetic phenanthrene

Controlled Substance Schedule II

Do not confuse:
HYDROmorphone/meperidine/morphine
Dilaudid/Demerol

ACTION: Inhibits ascending pain pathways in CNS, increases pain threshold, alters pain perception

USES: Moderate to severe pain, nonproductive cough

CONTRAINDICATIONS: Hypersensitivity

Black Box Warning: Respiratory depression, opioid-naive patients

Precautions: Pregnancy (C), breastfeeding, children <18 yr, addictive personality, increased intracranial pressure, MI (acute), severe heart disease, renal/hepatic disease, bowel impaction, abrupt discontinuation, COPD

Black Box Warning: Substance abuse

DOSAGE AND ROUTES

Analgesic

- **Adult: PO** (oral solution) 2.5-10 mg q3-6hr or (tabs) 2-4 mg q4-6hr; **EXT REL** (Exalgo): convert to **EXT REL** by giving total daily dose of immediate release/day, if needed titrate **EXT REL** q3-4days until adequate pain relief; use 25-50% increase for each titration step, if more than 2 doses of rescue medication needed in 24 hr consider titration; **IM/SUBCUT/IV** 1-2 mg q4-6hr prn, may be increased; **RECT** 3 mg q6-8hr prn
- **Geriatric: PO** 1-2 mg q4-6hr
- **Child >50 kg (unlabeled): PO** 2-4 mg q3-4hr in opioid-naive patients, titrate
- **Infant >6 mo/child <50 kg (unlabeled): PO** 0.04-0.08 mg/kg q3-4hr in opioid-naive patients, titrate

Available forms: Inj 1, 2, 4, 10 mg/ml; tabs 2, 4, 8 mg; supp 3 mg; oral sol 5 mg/5 ml; ext rel tab 8, 12, 16 mg

Administer:

PO route

- Give with food or milk for GI irritation
- **Ext rel (Exalgo):** discontinue all other ext rel opioids, give q24hr; do not crush, break, chew
- When pain is beginning to return; determine interval by response

Black Box Warning: Do not use ext rel products in opioid-naïve patients

Extended release

- **Converting from oral opioids;** conversion ratios are approximate; initiate ext rel tabs at 50% of calculated total daily equivalent dose of ext rel, give q24hr; max increase q3-4days, consider titration increases of 25-50% with each step
- **Converting from transdermal patch (fentanyl):** initiate ext rel tabs 18 hr after removal of patch; for each 25 mcg/hr dose of transdermal fentanyl dose is 12 mg q24hr, start dose at 50% of calculated HYDROmorphone ext rel dose q24hr; titrate no more often than q3-4days, consider dose increases of 25-50% with each step; if more than 2 rescue doses are required in 24 hr, consider titration

Subcut route

- Use short 30G needle, make sure not to inject ID
- Rotate inj sites

IV route

- **Direct,** diluted with 5 ml sterile water or NS; give through Y-connector or 3-way stopcock; give ≤2 mg over 3-5 min

• **IV INF:** Dilute each 0.1-1 mg/ml NS (0.1-1 mg/ml), deliver by opioid syringe infusor; may be diluted in D_5W, D_5/NaCl, 0.45% NaCl, NS for larger amounts, delivery through inf pump

Additive compatibilities: Bupivacaine, cloNIDine, fluorouracil, heparin, midazolam, ondansetron, potassium chloride, promethazine, verapamil, ziconotide

Solution compatibilities: D_5W, D_5/0.45% NaCl, D_5/0.9% NaCl, D_5/LR, D_5/Ringer's sol, 0.45% NaCl, 0.9% NaCl, Ringer's and lactated Ringer's sol

Syringe compatibilities: Atropine, bupivacaine, ceftazidime, chlorproMAZINE, cimetidine, dimenhyDRINATE, diphenhydrAMINE, fentaNYL, glycopyrrolate, hydrOXYzine, LORazepam, midazolam, pentazocine, promethazine, ranitidine, scopolamine, tetracaine, thiethylperazine, trimethobenzamide

Y-site compatibilities: Acyclovir, allopurinol, amifostine, amikacin, amsacrine, aztreonam, cefamandole, ceFAZolin, cefepime, cefmetazole, cefoperazone, cefotaxime, cefoxitin, ceftazidime, ceftizoxime, cefuroxime, cephalothin, cephapirin, chloramphenicol, cisatracurium, CISplatin, cladribine, clindamycin, cyclophosphamide, cytarabine, diltiazem, DOBUTamine, DOPamine, DOXOrubicin, DOXOrubicin liposome, doxycycline, EPINEPHrine, erythromycin lactobionate, famotidine, fentaNYL, filgrastim, fludarabine, foscarnet, furosemide, gentamicin, granisetron, heparin, kanamycin, labetalol, LORazepam, magnesium sulfate, melphalan, methotrexate, metroNIDAZOLE, mezlocillin, midazolam, milrinone, morphine, moxalactam, nafcillin, niCARdipine, nitroglycerin, norepinephrine, ondansetron, oxacillin, paclitaxel, penicillin G potassium, piperacillin, piperacillin/tazobactam, propofol, ranitidine, remifentanil, teniposide, thiotepa, ticarcillin, tobramycin, trimethoprim-sulfamethoxazole, vancomycin, vecuronium, vinorelbine

SIDE EFFECTS

CNS: *Drowsiness, dizziness, confusion, headache, sedation, euphoria,* mood changes, **seizures**

CV: Palpitations, bradycardia, change in B/P, hypotension, tachycardia, peripheral vasodilation

EENT: Tinnitus, blurred vision, miosis, diplopia

GI: *Nausea, vomiting, anorexia, constipation, cramps,* dry mouth, **paralytic ileus**

GU: Increased urinary output, dysuria, urinary retention

INTEG: *Rash,* urticaria, bruising, flushing, diaphoresis, pruritus

RESP: **Respiratory depression**, dyspnea

PHARMACOKINETICS

Onset 15-30 min, peak ½-1 hr, duration 4-5 hr, metabolized by liver, excreted by kidneys, crosses placenta, excreted in breast milk, half-life 2-3 hr

INTERACTIONS

Increase: effects—other CNS depressants (alcohol, opiates, sedative/hypnotics, antipsychotics, skeletal muscle relaxants)

⚠ **Increase: severe CNS, respiratory depression—MAOIs**

Decrease: HYDROmorphone effects—opiate antagonists

Drug/Herb

Increase: action—chamomile, hops, kava, lavender, St. John's wort, valerian

Drug/Lab Test

Increase: amylase

NURSING CONSIDERATIONS

Assess:

Black Box Warning: Respiratory dysfunction: respiratory depression, character, rate, rhythm; notify prescriber if respirations <10/min

• I&O ratio; check for decreasing output; may indicate urinary retention

• CNS changes: dizziness, drowsiness, hallucinations, euphoria, LOC, pupil reaction

- Bowel function, constipation
- Allergic reactions: rash, urticaria
- Need for pain medication, physical dependence
- **Pain:** control, sedation by scoring on 0-10 scale, ATC dosing is best for pain control

Perform/provide:

- Storage in light-resistant area at room temp
- Assistance with ambulation
- Safety measures: side rails, night-light, call bell within easy reach

Evaluate:

- Therapeutic response: decrease in pain

Teach patient/family:

- To report any symptoms of CNS changes, allergic reactions
- That physical dependency may result when used for extended periods; that withdrawal symptoms may occur: nausea, vomiting, cramps, fever, faintness, anorexia
- To avoid driving, other hazardous activities because drowsiness occurs

TREATMENT OF OVERDOSE:

Naloxone (Narcan) 0.2-0.8 mg IV, O_2, IV fluids, vasopressors

hydroxychloroquine (Rx)

(hye-drox-ee-klor′oh-kwin)

Apo-Hydroxyquine ✱, Gen-Hydroxychloroquine ✱, Plaquenil

Func. class.: Antimalarial, antirheumatic (DMARDs)

Chem. class.: 4-Aminoquinoline derivative

ACTION: Impairs complement-dependent antigen–antibody reactions

USES: Malaria caused by susceptible strains of *Plasmodium vivax, P. malariae, P. ovale, P. falciparum* (some strains); SLE, rheumatoid arthritis

Unlabeled uses: SLE in children

CONTRAINDICATIONS: Hypersensitivity to this product or chloroquine; retinal field changes

Black Box Warning: Children (long term), ocular disease

Precautions: Pregnancy (C), breastfeeding, blood dyscrasias, severe GI disease, neurologic disease, alcoholism, hepatic disease, G6PD deficiency, psoriasis, eczema

DOSAGE AND ROUTES

Malaria

- **Adult: PO** *Suppression or prevention:* 400 mg/wk, begin 1-2 wk before travel, continue 4 wk after returning; *treatment:* 800 mg, then 400 mg after 6-8 hr, then 400 mg/day on 2nd and 3rd day, total dose 2 g
- **Child: PO** *Suppression or prevention:* 6.4 mg/kg (5 mg/kg base) weekly, begin 1-2 wk before travel, continue 4 wk after returning; *treatment:* 10 mg/kg, 6.4 mg/kg (5 mg/kg base) at 6, 18, 24 hr after 1st dose

Lupus erythematosus

- **Adult: PO** 400 mg (310 mg base) daily-bid; length depends on patient response; maintenance 200-400 mg/day
- **Child (unlabeled): PO** 5 mg/kg/day, max 400 mg/day; long-term therapy is contraindicated

Rheumatoid arthritis

- **Adult: PO** 400-600 mg/day for 4-12 wk then 200-300 mg/day after good response

Available forms: Tabs 200 mg

Administer:

- Tabs may be crushed and mixed with food, fluids
- With food or milk; at same time each day to maintain product level
- For malaria, prophylaxis should be started 2 wk prior to exposure, continued for 4-6 wk after leaving exposure area

SIDE EFFECTS

CNS: Headache, stimulation, fatigue, irritability, **seizures**, bad dreams, dizziness, confusion, psychosis, decreased reflexes
CV: Hypotension, heart block, **asystole with syncope**
EENT: *Blurred vision, corneal changes, retinal changes, difficulty focusing,* tinnitus, vertigo, deafness, photophobia, corneal edema
GI: *Nausea, vomiting, anorexia,* diarrhea, cramps
HEMA: **Thrombocytopenia, agranulocytosis, leukopenia, aplastic anemia**
INTEG: Pruritus, pigmentation changes, skin eruptions, lichen-planus–like eruptions, eczema, **exfoliative dermatitis**, alopecia, **Stevens-Johnson syndrome**, photosensitivity

PHARMACOKINETICS

Peak 3 hr; terminal half-life 32-50 days; metabolized in liver; excreted in urine, feces, breast milk; crosses placenta, protein binding 45%

INTERACTIONS

Increase: digoxin, methotrexate levels
Increase: antibody titer—rabies vaccine
Decrease: hydroxychloroquine action—Mg or Al compounds
Decrease: effect of—live virus vaccines, botulinum toxoids

NURSING CONSIDERATIONS

Assess:

- **SLE, malaria symptoms:** before treatment and daily
- **Rheumatoid arthritis:** pain, swelling, ROM, temp of joints
- Ophthalmic exam at baseline and q6mo if long-term treatment or product dosage >150 mg/day
- Hepatic studies q wk: AST, ALT, bilirubin if patient receiving long-term treatment
- **Blood dyscrasias:** blood studies: CBC, platelets; WBC, RBC, platelets may be decreased; if severe, product should be discontinued; assess for malaise, fever, bruising, bleeding (rare)
- For decreased reflexes: knee, ankle
- **ECG** during therapy: watch for depression of T waves, widening of QRS complex
- **Allergic reactions:** pruritus, rash, urticaria
- **For ototoxicity** (tinnitus, vertigo, change in hearing); audiometric testing should be done before, after treatment

⚠ **For toxicity: blurring vision, difficulty focusing, headache, dizziness, knee, ankle reflexes; product should be discontinued immediately**

Perform/provide:

- Storage in tight, light-resistant container at room temp; keep inj in cool environment

Evaluate:

- Therapeutic response: decreased symptoms of malaria, SLE, rheumatoid arthritis

Teach patient/family:

- To use sunglasses in bright sunlight to decrease photophobia; to wear protective clothing (photosensitivity)
- That urine may turn rust or brown; that skin may become blue-black
- To report hearing, visual problems, fever, fatigue, bruising, bleeding, which may indicate blood dyscrasias

TREATMENT OF OVERDOSE:

Induce vomiting; gastric lavage; administer barbiturate (ultrashort acting), vasopressor, ammonium chloride; tracheostomy may be necessary

hydroxyurea (Rx)

(hye-drox′ee-yoo-ree-ah)

Apo-Hydroxyurea ✱, Droxia, Hydrea

Func. class.: Antineoplastic, antimetabolite

Chem. class.: Synthetic urea analog

ACTION: Acts by inhibiting DNA synthesis without interfering with RNA or protein synthesis; incorporates thymidine into DNA, thereby causing direct damage to DNA strands; specific for S phase of cell cycle

USES:
Melanoma, chronic myelogenous leukemia, recurrent or metastatic ovarian cancer, squamous cell carcinoma of the head and neck, sickle cell anemia

Unlabeled uses: Psoriasis, acute myelogenous leukemia (AML), astrocytoma, HIV, lung cancer, malignant glioma, polycythemia vera, thrombocytosis

CONTRAINDICATIONS:
Pregnancy (D), breastfeeding, hypersensitivity

Black Box Warning: Leukopenia (<2500/mm^3), thrombocytopenia (<100,000/mm^3), anemia (severe)

Precautions: Renal disease (severe)

DOSAGE AND ROUTES

Ovarian cancer, malignant melanoma

- **Adult: PO** 80 mg/kg as a single dose q3days or 20-30 mg/kg as a single dose daily

Ovarian cancer in combination with radiation

- **Adult: PO** 80 mg/kg as a single dose q3days

Chronic myelogenous leukemia (CML)/acute myelogenous leukemia (unlabeled)

- **Adult: PO** WBC >100,000/mm^3, 50-75 mg/kg/day; WBC <100,000/mm^3, 10-30 mg/kg/day; adjust for WBCs
- **Child: PO** 10-20 mg/kg/day, adjust to hematologic response

Sickle cell anemia

- **Adult: PO** 15 mg/kg/day, may increase by 5 mg/kg/day q12wk, max 35 mg/kg/day

Renal/hepatic disease

- Reduce dose

Available forms: Caps 200, 300, 400, 500 mg

Administer:

- Gloves should be worn when handling bottles or caps, including by caregivers
- Do not crush or chew caps; caps can be opened and contents mixed with water
- Antiemetic 30-60 min before product and prn

SIDE EFFECTS

CNS: Headache, confusion, hallucinations, dizziness, **seizures**

CV: Angina, ischemia

GI: Nausea, vomiting, anorexia, diarrhea, stomatitis, constipation, **hepatotoxicity**

GU: Increased BUN, uric acid, creatinine, temporary renal function impairment

HEMA: **Leukopenia, anemia, thrombocytopenia, megaloblastic erythropoiesis**

INTEG: *Rash,* urticaria, pruritus, dry skin, facial erythema

META: Hyperphosphatemia, hyperuricemia, hypocalcemia

MISC: Fever, chills, malaise, **secondary** cancers, tumor lysis syndrome

PHARMACOKINETICS

Readily absorbed when taken orally; peak level in 1-4 hr; degraded in liver; excreted in urine, almost totally eliminated within 24 hr; readily crosses blood-brain barrier; eliminated as CO_2; terminal half-life 3.5-4.5 hr

INTERACTIONS

Increase: pancreatitis—didanosine, stavudine

Increase: toxicity—radiation or other antineoplastics

Increase: bleeding risk—NSAIDs, anticoagulants, thrombolytics, salicylates, platelet inhibitors

- Do not use with live virus vaccines
- Do not use hematopoietic progenitor cells (sargramostim, filgrastim) 24 hr before or after antineoplastic

Drug/Lab Test

Increase: renal studies

NURSING CONSIDERATIONS

Assess:

- **Bone marrow suppression:** CBC, differential, platelet count weekly; withhold product if WBC is <2500/mm³ or platelet count is <100,000/mm³; notify prescriber; product should be discontinued
- Renal studies: BUN, serum uric acid, urine CCr, electrolytes before, during therapy
- **Tumor lysis syndrome;** hyperkalemia, hyperphosphatemia, hyperuricemia, hypocalcemia; uric acid nephropathy, acute renal failure, metabolic acidosis can also occur; aggressive alkalinization of urine, allopurinol can prevent this
- I&O ratio; report fall in urine output to <30 ml/hr
- Monitor temp q4hr; fever may indicate beginning infection
- Hepatic studies before, during therapy: bilirubin, alk phos, AST, ALT, LDH; prn or q mo
- B/P q3-4hr; check for chest pain; angina, ischemia may occur
- **Bleeding:** hematuria, guaiac, bruising or petechiae, mucosa or orifices q8hr
- Inflammation of mucosa, breaks in skin
- Buccal cavity for dryness, sores or ulceration, white patches, oral pain, bleeding, dysphagia
- **Symptoms indicating severe allergic reaction:** rash, urticaria, itching, flushing
- **Neurotoxicity:** headaches, hallucinations, seizures, dizziness

Perform/provide:

- Rinsing of mouth tid-qid with water, club soda; brushing of teeth bid-tid with soft brush or cotton-tipped applicators for stomatitis; use unwaxed dental floss

Evaluate:

- Therapeutic response: decreased tumor size, spread of malignancy

Teach patient/family:

- To report signs of infection: elevated temp, sore throat, flulike symptoms
- To report signs of anemia: fatigue, headache, faintness, SOB, irritability
- To report bleeding: to avoid use of razors, commercial mouthwash
- To avoid use of aspirin products, ibuprofen (thrombocytopenia)
- To avoid foods with citric acid, hot or rough texture if stomatitis is present
- To report stomatitis: any bleeding, white spots, ulcerations in the mouth; to examine mouth daily, report symptoms
- That contraceptive measures are recommended during therapy; pregnancy (D)
- To notify prescriber of fever, chills, sore throat, nausea, vomiting, anorexia, diarrhea, bleeding, bruising; may indicate blood dyscrasias

H

hydrOXYzine (Rx)

(hye-drox′i-zeen)

ANX, Apo-Hydroxyzine ✦, Vistaril

Func. class.: Antianxiety/antihistamine/sedative/hypnotic, antiemetic

Chem. class.: Piperazine derivative

Do not confuse:

hydrOXYzine/hydrALAZINE

Vistaril/Versed

ACTION: Depresses subcortical levels of CNS, including limbic system, reticular formation; competes with H_1-receptor sites

USES: Anxiety preoperatively, postoperatively to prevent nausea, vomiting; to potentiate opioid analgesics; sedation; pruritus, ethanol withdrawal

Unlabeled uses: Insomnia, allergic rhinitis, generalized anxiety disorder

CONTRAINDICATIONS: Pregnancy 1st trimester, breastfeeding; hypersensitivity to this product or cetirizine; acute asthma

Precautions: Pregnancy (C) (2nd/3rd trimester), geriatric patients, debilitated, renal/hepatic disease, closed-angle glaucoma, COPD, prostatic hypertrophy, asthma

DOSAGE AND ROUTES

Anxiety

- **Adult: PO** 50-100 mg qid, max 600 mg/day; **IM** 50-100 mg q4-6hr
- **Geriatric: PO** max 50 mg/day
- **Child >6 yr: PO** 50-100 mg/day in divided doses
- **Child <6 yr: PO** 50 mg/day in divided doses

Alcohol withdrawal

- **Adult: IM** 50-100 mg q4-6hr

Preoperatively/postoperatively (nausea/vomiting)

- **Adult: IM** 25-100 mg q4-6hr
- **Child: IM** 1.1 mg/kg as a single dose

Pruritus

- **Adult: PO** 25 mg tid-qid; **IM** 50-100 mg then q4-6hr prn, switch to **PO** as soon as feasible
- **Child ≥6 yr: PO** 50-100 mg/day in divided doses; **IM** 0.5-1 mg/kg/dose q4-6hr prn, use **PO** when possible
- **Child <6 yr: PO** 50 mg/day in divided doses

Insomnia (unlabeled)

- **Adult: PO** 50-100 mg 30-60 min before bedtime; **IM** 50 mg 30-60 min before bedtime

Renal dose

- **Adult: PO** CCr <50 ml/min, give 50% of dose

Available forms: Tabs 10, 25, 50 mg; caps 25, 50, 100 mg; oral sol 10 mg/ 5 ml; inj 25, 50 mg/ml; oral susp 25 mg/ 5 ml

Administer:

PO route

- With food or milk for GI symptoms
- Crushed if patient is unable to swallow medication whole
- Gum, hard candy, frequent sips of water for dry mouth

IM route

- Does not need to be diluted; give by Z-track inj in large muscle to decrease pain, chance of necrosis, never give IV/ SUBCUT

Additive compatibilities: CISplatin, cyclophosphamide, cytarabine, dimenhyDRINATE, etoposide, lidocaine, mesna, methotrexate, nafcillin

Syringe compatibilities: Atropine, butorphanol, chlorproMAZINE, cimetidine, codeine, diphenhydrAMINE, doxapram, droperidol, fentaNYL, fluphenazine, glycopyrrolate, HYDROmorphone, lidocaine, meperidine, metoclopramide, midazolam, morphine, nalbuphine, oxymorphone, pentazocine, perphenazine, procaine, prochlorperazine, scopolamine, SUFentanil

SIDE EFFECTS

CNS: *Dizziness, drowsiness,* confusion, headache, tremors, fatigue, depression, seizures

CV: Hypotension

GI: Dry mouth, increased appetite, nausea, diarrhea, weight gain

PHARMACOKINETICS

PO: Onset 15-60 min, duration 4-6 hr, half-life 3 hr, metabolized by liver, excreted by kidneys

INTERACTIONS

Increase: CNS depressant effect—barbiturates, opioids, analgesics, alcohol, sedative/hypnotics, other CNS depressants

Increase: anticholinergic effects—phenothiazines, quiNIDine, disopyramide, antihistamines, antidepressants, atropine, haloperidol, MAOIs

NURSING CONSIDERATIONS

Assess:

- B/P (lying, standing), pulse; if systolic B/P drops 20 mm Hg, hold product, notify prescriber
- Mental status: mood, sensorium, affect, anxiety, behavior, increased sedation

Perform/provide:

- Assistance with ambulation during beginning therapy, since drowsiness, dizziness occurs
- Safety measures, including side rails

• Checking to confirm that PO medication has been swallowed

Evaluate:

• Therapeutic response: decreased anxiety

Teach patient/family:

• That medication is not to be used for everyday stress or for >4 mo
• To avoid OTC preparations (cold, cough, hay fever) unless approved by prescriber
• To avoid driving, activities that require alertness
• To avoid alcohol, psychotropic medications
• Not to discontinue medication quickly after long-term use
• To rise slowly because fainting may occur

TREATMENT OF OVERDOSE:

Lavage if orally ingested; VS, supportive care; IV norepinephrine for hypotension

hyoscyamine (Rx)

(hye-oh-sye′a-meen)

Anaspaz, Colidrops, Colytrol Pediatric, Cystospaz-M, ED-SPAZ, HydroMax-DT, HydroMax-FT, HydroMax-SR, HyoMax, HyoMax SL, Hyosyne, Levbid, Levsin, Medispax, NuLev, Spacol, Spasdel, Symax

Func. class.: Anticholinergic/antispasmodics

Chem. class.: Belladonna alkaloid

ACTION: Inhibits muscarinic actions of acetylcholine at postganglionic parasympathetic neuroeffector sites; reduces rigidity, tremors, hyperhidrosis of parkinsonism

USES: Treatment of peptic ulcer disease in combination with other products; other GI disorders, other spastic disorders, IBS, urinary incontinence

CONTRAINDICATIONS: Hypersensitivity to anticholinergics, closed-angle glaucoma, GI obstruction, myasthenia gravis, paralytic ileus, GI atony, toxic megacolon, prostatic hypertrophy, urinary tract obstruction

Precautions: Pregnancy (C), geriatric patients, hyperthyroidism, dysrhythmias, CHF, ulcerative colitis, hypertension, hiatal hernia, renal/hepatic disease, urinary retention, CAD

DOSAGE AND ROUTES

• **Adult/adolescent/child ≥12 yr: PO/SL** 0.125-0.25 mg q4hr; **EXT REL** 0.375-0.75 mg q12hr; **adult: IM/SUBCUT/IV** 0.25-0.5 mg in a single dose or 2-4×/day q6hr
• **Geriatric:** Max 1.5 mg/day in divided doses or max 4 biphasic tabs
• **Child 2-12 yr: PO** SL 0.0625-0.125 q4hr

Available forms: Tabs 0.125, 0.15 mg; ext rel caps 0.375 mg; sol 0.125 mg/ml; elix 0.125 mg/5 ml; sol for inj 0.5 mg/ml; SL tab 0.125 mg; tab, biphasic 0.125, 0.375 mg; orally disintegrating tab 0.125 mg

Administer:

• Do not break, crush, or chew ext rel caps
• ½ hr before meals for better absorption
• Decreased dose to geriatric patients; metabolism may be slowed
• Gum, hard candy, frequent rinsing of mouth for dryness of oral cavity

SIDE EFFECTS

CNS: *Confusion, stimulation in geriatric patients,* headache, insomnia, dizziness, drowsiness, anxiety, weakness, hallucination

CV: *Palpitations,* tachycardia

EENT: *Blurred vision,* photophobia, mydriasis, cycloplegia, increased ocular tension

GI: *Dry mouth, constipation, paralytic ileus,* heartburn, nausea, vomiting, dysphagia, absence of taste

H

GU: *Urinary hesitancy, retention,* impotence
INTEG: Urticaria, rash, pruritus, anhidrosis, fever, allergic reactions

PHARMACOKINETICS

PO: Duration 4-6 hr, metabolized by liver, excreted in urine, half-life 3.5 hr

INTERACTIONS

Increase: anticholinergic effect—amantadine, tricyclics, MAOIs, H_1-antihistamines
Decrease: hyoscyamine effect—antacids
Decrease: effect of phenothiazines, levodopa, ketoconazole

NURSING CONSIDERATIONS

Assess:
- VS, cardiac status: checking for dysrhythmias, increased rate, palpitations
- I&O ratio; check for urinary retention or hesitancy
- GI complaints: pain, nausea, vomiting, anorexia

Perform/provide:
- Storage in tight container protected from light
- Increased fluids, bulk, exercise to decrease constipation

Evaluate:
- Therapeutic response: absence of epigastric pain, bleeding, nausea, vomiting

Teach patient/family:
- To avoid driving, other hazardous activities until stabilized on medication
- To avoid alcohol or other CNS depressants; they will enhance sedating properties of this product
- To avoid hot environments because heat stroke may occur; that product suppresses perspiration
- To use sunglasses when outside to prevent photophobia; that product may cause blurred vision

ibandronate (Rx)

(eye-ban′dro-nate)
Boniva
Func. class.: Bone-resorption inhibitor, electrolyte modifier
Chem. class.: Bisphosphonate

ACTION: Inhibits bone resorption, apparently without inhibiting bone formation and mineralization; absorbs calcium phosphate crystals in bone and may directly block dissolution of hydroxyapatite crystals of bone; more potent than other products

USES: Osteoporosis and prophylaxis
Unlabeled uses: Hypercalcemia of malignancy, osteolytic metastases, Paget's disease, osteoporosis (treatment/prevention) in those taking anastrozole

CONTRAINDICATIONS: Achalasia, esophageal stricture, hypocalcemia, intraarterial administration, renal failure, hypersensitivity to bisphosphonates
Precautions: Pregnancy (C), breastfeeding, children, geriatric patients, anemia, chemotherapy, coagulopathy, dental disease, diabetes mellitus, dysphagia, GI/renal disease, GERD, hypertension, infection, multiple myeloma, phosphate hypersensitivity, vit D deficiency

DOSAGE AND ROUTES

Postmenopausal osteoporosis
- **Adult: PO** 2.5 mg/day or 150 mg/mo; **IV BOL** 3 mg q3mo

Prophylaxis
- **Adult: PO** 2.5 mg/day or 150 mg/mo

Paget's disease (unlabeled)
- **Adult: IV** 2 mg as a single dose

Osteoporosis in those taking anastrozole (unlabeled)
- **Postmenopausal women: PO** 150 mg/mo

Osteolytic metastases (unlabeled)
- **Adult: IV** 6 mg over 1 hr × 3 days, repeat q4wk

Hypercalcemia (unlabeled)
• **Adult: IV INF** 2-4 mg over 2 hr
Renal dose
• **Adult: PO** CCr <30 ml/min, avoid use
Available forms: Tabs 2.5, 150 mg; sol for inj 1 mg/ml
Administer:
PO route
• Give early AM with a glass of water; if monthly, give on same day of each month
Direct IV route
• Use single-dose prefilled syringe; discard unused portion; give over 15-30 sec; give q3mo

SIDE EFFECTS

CNS: Fever, insomnia, dizziness, headache
CV: Hypertension, atrial fibrillation
EENT: Ocular pain/inflammation, uveitis
GI: Constipation, nausea, vomiting, diarrhea, dyspepsia
INTEG: Rash, inj site reaction
META: *Hypomagnesemia, hypophosphatemia, hypocalcemia,* hypercholesterolemia
MS: Bone pain, myalgia, osteonecrosis of the jaw

PHARMACOKINETICS

Half-life 5-60 hr, 86%-99% protein binding; taken up mainly by bones, primarily in areas of high bone turnover; eliminated primarily by kidneys

INTERACTIONS

Increase: neurotoxicity—aminoglycosides, cycloSPORINE, tacrolimus, NSAIDs, radiopaque contrast agents, vancomycin
Increase: hypocalcemia—loop diuretics
Decrease: ibandronate effect—calcium/vit D/iron/aluminum/magnesium salts; separate by 1 hr
Drug/Food
• Do not take with food, calcium
Drug/Lab Test
Decrease: Alk phos

NURSING CONSIDERATIONS

Assess:
• **Osteoporosis:** before and during treatment; DEXA scan for bone mineral density
• Atrial fibrillation
• **Dental health;** before dental extraction, give antiinfectives
• Blood studies: electrolytes, calcium, magnesium, phosphate; creatinine/BUN, vit D: correct deficiencies prior to treatment
• For bone pain; use analgesics
Perform/provide:
• Storage at room temp
Evaluate:
• Therapeutic response: increased bone mineral density
Teach patient/family:
• **To report hypercalcemic relapse:** nausea, vomiting, bone pain, thirst, unusual muscle twitching, muscle spasms, severe diarrhea, constipation
• To continue with dietary recommendations, including calcium, vit D
• To obtain an analgesic from provider for bone pain
• That, if nausea, vomiting occur, small, frequent meals may help
• To report vision symptoms: blurred vision, edema, inflammation
• To report if pregnancy is planned or suspected or if planning to breastfeed
• To exercise regularly, stop smoking, decrease alcohol intake
• To take PO first thing in AM at least 60 min before other medications, food, beverages
• To sit upright for ≥60 min after PO

ibritumomab (Rx)

(ee-brit-u-moe′mab)
Zevalin
Func. class.: Radiopharmaceutical
Chem. class.: Monoclonal antibody

ACTION: High affinity for indium-111, yttrium-90; induces CD20+ B-cell lines

USES:
Non-Hodgkin's lymphoma, B-cell NHL

CONTRAINDICATIONS:
Pregnancy (D), hypersensitivity to murine proteins, prior murine antibody exposure

Black Box Warning: Hypersensitivity to this product, neutropenia, thrombocytopenia

Precautions: Breastfeeding, children, geriatric patients, cardiac conditions, immunizations after therapy

Black Box Warning: Altered biodistribution, infusion-related reaction

DOSAGE AND ROUTES

Step 1

- **Adult: IV** rituximab 250 mg/m^2 given first; premedicate with acetaminophen 650 mg and diphenhydrAMINE 50 mg

Step 2

- **Adult (baseline platelets ≥150,000/mm^3):** 7-9 days after step 1, give a second dose of rituximab 250 mg/m^2; within 4 hr of completing rituximab inf, give Y-90 ibritumomab tiuxetan 0.4 mCi/kg (14.8 MBq/kg) IV over 10 min, the dose given should be within 10% of actual prescribed dose of Y-90 ibritumomab tiuxetan, total dose given max 32 mCi (1184 MBq) regardless of patient's weight
- **Adult (baseline platelets 100,000-149,000/mm^3):** 7-9 days after step 1, give a second dose of rituximab 250 mg/m^2 IV; within 4 hr of completing rituximab inf, give Y-90 ibritumomab tiuxetan 0.3 mCi/kg (11.1 MBq/kg) IV over 10 min; the dose given should be within 10% of actual prescribed dose of Y-90 ibritumomab tiuxetan, total dose given max 32 mCi (1184 MBq) regardless of patient's weight
- **Adult (baseline platelets <100,000/mm^3):** do not use

Available forms: Inj 3.2 mg/2 ml

Administer:

- Do not use as bolus or direct IV
- See manufacturer's product labeling for preparation

SIDE EFFECTS

CV: Cardiac dysrhythmias

GI: *Nausea, vomiting, anorexia,* abdominal pain, diarrhea

GU: Renal failure

HEMA: Leukopenia, neutropenia, thrombocytopenia, anemia

INTEG: *Irritation at site, rash,* fatal mucocutaneous infections (rare)

OTHER: Fever, chills, asthenia, headache, angioedema, hypotension, myalgia, bronchospasm, hemorrhage, infections, cough, dyspnea, dizziness, anxiety

SYST: Stevens-Johnson syndrome, secondary malignancies (AML, MDS), fatal infections

PHARMACOKINETICS

Half-life 30 hr

NURSING CONSIDERATIONS

Assess:

Black Box Warning: Fatal inf reaction: hypoxia, pulmonary infiltrates, ARDS, MI, ventricular fibrillation, cardiogenic shock; most fatal inf reactions occur with 1st inf; potentially fatal

- Biodistribution: 1st image 2-24 hr, 2nd image 48-72 hr, 3rd image 90-120 hr (optimal)
- For infection; murine antibody titers

Black Box Warning: Severe mucocutaneous reactions: Stevens-Johnson syndrome, lichenoid dermatitis, toxic epidermal lysis; occur 1-13 wk after product given

Black Box Warning: Tumor lysis syndrome: acute renal failure requiring hemodialysis, hyperkalemia, hypocalcemia, hyperuricemia, hyperphosphatemia

Black Box Warning: Bone marrow depression: CBC, differential, platelet count weekly; withhold product if WBC <3500/mm^3, or platelet count <150,000/mm^3; notify prescriber

• GI symptoms: frequency of stools
• Signs of dehydration: rapid respirations, poor skin turgor, decreased urine output, dry skin, restlessness, weakness

Perform/provide:

• Increased fluid intake to 2-3 L/day to prevent dehydration unless contraindicated
• Emergency equipment nearby with EPINEPHrine, antihistamines, corticosteroids

Evaluate:

• Therapeutic response: improvement in blood counts, decreased evidence of disease

Teach patient/family:

• To report adverse reactions
• To use contraception during and for 12 months after therapy; pregnancy (D)
• About radiation safety precautions, disposal of bodily fluids
• About symptoms of infection
• About neutropenia and bleeding precautions

ibuprofen (OTC, Rx)

(eye-byoo-proe′fen)

Advil, Advil Children's, Advil Infants' Concentrated, Advil Junior Strength, Apo-Ibuprofen ✤, Caldolor, ElixSure IB, Equaline Ibuprofen, Genpril, GoodSense Ibuprofen Junior Strength, Ibren, IBU, Infants Leader Ibu-drops, Leader Ibuprofen Jr, Midol Cramps and Body Aches Formula, Motrin ✤, Motrin IB, Motrin Infant's, Motrin Junior Strength, Pamprin IB ✤, Samson-8 Select Brand, Top Care Infant, Walgreens Ibuprofen, Wal-Profen

ibuprofen lysine (Rx)

NeoProfen

Func.class.: Nonsteroidal antiinflammatory, antipyretic, nonopioid analgesics

Chem. class.: Propionic acid derivative

Do not confuse:
Nuprin/Lupron

ACTION: Inhibits COX-1, COX-2 by blocking arachidonate; analgesic, antiinflammatory, antipyretic

USES: Rheumatoid arthritis, osteoarthritis, primary dysmenorrhea, gout, dental pain, musculoskeletal disorders, fever, migraine
Unlabeled uses: Ankylosing spondylitis, bone pain, cystic fibrosis, gouty arthritis, psoriatic arthritis

CONTRAINDICATIONS: Pregnancy (D) 3rd trimester; hypersensitivity to this product, NSAIDs, salicylates; asthma; severe renal/hepatic disease

Black Box Warning: Perioperative pain in CABG

Precautions: Pregnancy (B) 1st and 2nd trimesters, breastfeeding, children, geriatric patients, bleeding disorders, GI disorders, cardiac disorders, hypersensitivity to other antiinflammatory agents, CHF, CCr $<$25 ml/min

Black Box Warning: GI bleeding, MI, stroke

DOSAGE AND ROUTES

Self-treatment of minor aches/pains

- **Adult/adolescent: PO** (OTC product) 200 mg q4-6hr, may increase to 400 mg q4-6hr if needed, max 1200 mg/day

Analgesic

- **Adult: PO** 200-400 mg q4-6hr, max 3.2 g/day; OTC use max 1200 mg/day
- **Child: PO** 4-10 mg/kg/dose q6-8hr

Moderate to severe pain (hospitalized patients) (Caldolor)

- **Adult: IV** 400-800 mg q6hr as an adjunct to opiate-agonist therapy

Dysmenorrhea

- **Adult: PO** 400 mg q4hr, max 1200 mg/day

Antipyretic

- **Child 6 mo-12 yr: PO** 5 mg/kg (temp $<$102.5° F or 39.2° C), 10 mg/kg (temp $>$102.5° F), may repeat q6-8hr, max 40 mg/kg/day

Antiinflammatory

- **Adult: PO** 400-800 mg tid-qid, max 3.2 g/day
- **Child: PO** 30-40 mg/kg/day in 3-4 divided doses, max 50 mg/kg/day

Patent ductus arteriosus (PDA) (NeoProfen)

- **Premature neonate $\leq$32 wk gestation who weighs 500-1500 g: IV** 10 mg/kg initially, then, if needed, 2 doses of 5 mg/kg at 24-hr intervals; if oliguria occurs, hold dose

Available forms: Tabs 100, 200, 400, 600, 800 mg; cap, liq gels 200 mg; oral susp 100 mg/5 ml; liq 100 mg/5 ml; chew tabs 50, 100 mg; drops 50 mg/1.25 ml; inj 10 mg/ml (NeoProfen); inj (Caldolor) 100 mg/ml

Administer:

PO route

- With food, milk, or antacid to decrease GI symptoms; if nausea and vomiting occur or persist, notify prescriber
- Shake susp well before use

IV route

- Patient must be well hydrated prior to administration
- Dilute to $\leq$4 mg/ml with 0.9% NaCl, LR, D_5; infuse over $\geq$30 min; do not give IM
- Discard unused portion
- Visually inspect for particulate
- **Ibuprofen lysine:** dilute with dextrose or saline to appropriate volume (10 mg/kg of ibuprofen is recommended); give within 30 min of preparation; give via IV port nearest insertion site; give over 15 min
- Check for extravasation; do not give in same line with TPN; interrupt TPN for 15 min before and after product administration

SIDE EFFECTS

CNS: *Headache,* dizziness, drowsiness, fatigue, tremors, confusion, insomnia, anxiety, depression

CV: Tachycardia, peripheral edema, palpitations, dysrhythmias, CV thrombotic events, MI, stroke

EENT: Tinnitus, hearing loss, blurred vision

GI: Nausea, *anorexia,* vomiting, diarrhea, jaundice, hepatitis, constipation, flatulence, cramps, dry mouth, peptic ulcer, GI bleeding, ulceration, necrotizing enterocolitis, GI perforation

GU: Nephrotoxicity: dysuria, hematuria, oliguria, azotemia

HEMA: Blood dyscrasias, increased bleeding time

INTEG: Purpura, rash, pruritus, sweating, urticaria, nectrotizing fasciitis

SYST: Anaphylaxis, Stevens-Johnson syndrome

PHARMACOKINETICS

PO: Onset ½ hr, peak 1-2 hr, half-life 1.8-2 hr, metabolized in liver (inactive metabolites), excreted in urine (inactive metabolites), 90%-99% plasma protein binding, does not enter breast milk, well absorbed

INTERACTIONS

Increase: bleeding risk—valproic acid, thrombolytics, antiplatelets, anticoagulants, salicylates
Increase: blood dyscrasia risk—antineoplastics, radiation
Increase: toxicity—lithium, oral anticoagulants, cycloSPORINE, methotrexate
Increase: GI reactions—aspirin, corticosteroids, NSAIDs, alcohol, tobacco
Increase: hypoglycemia—oral antidiabetics
Decrease: effect of antihypertensives, thiazides, furosemide
Decrease: ibuprofen action—aspirin
Drug/Herb
Increase: bleeding risk—feverfew, garlic, ginger, ginkgo, ginseng *(Panax)*

NURSING CONSIDERATIONS

Assess:
- Renal, hepatic, blood studies: BUN, creatinine, AST, ALT, Hgb, stool guaiac, before treatment, periodically thereafter
- **Pain:** note type, duration, location, intensity with ROM 1 hr after administration
- Audiometric, ophthalmic exam before, during, after long-term treatment; for eye, ear problems: blurred vision, tinnitus; may indicate toxicity
- **Infection,** may mask symptoms; fever: temp before and 1 hr after administration
- Cardiac status: edema (peripheral), tachycardia, palpitations; monitor B/P, pulse for character, quality, rhythm, especially in patients with cardiac disease, geriatric patients
- For history of peptic ulcer disorder; asthma, aspirin, hypersensitivity; check closely for hypersensitivity reactions

Perform/provide:
- Storage at room temp

Evaluate:
- Therapeutic response: decreased pain, stiffness in joints; decreased swelling in joints; ability to move more easily; reduction in fever or menstrual cramping

Teach patient/family:
- To report blurred vision, ringing, roaring in ears (may indicate toxicity); that eye and hearing tests should be done during long-term therapy
- To avoid driving, other hazardous activities if dizziness or drowsiness occurs

⚠ **Nephrotoxicity: to report change in urinary pattern, increased weight, edema, increased pain in joints, fever, blood in urine**
- That therapeutic inflammatory effects may take up to 1 mo

⚠ **To avoid alcohol, NSAIDs, salicylates; bleeding may occur**
- To report use of this product to all health care providers

TREATMENT OF OVERDOSE:

Lavage, activated charcoal, induce diuresis

⚠ *HIGH ALERT*

ibutilide (Rx)

(eye-byoo′tih-lide)

Corvert

Func. class.: Antidysrhythmic (class III)

ACTION: Prolongs duration of action potential and effective refractory period

USES: For rapid conversion of atrial fibrillation/flutter, including within 1 wk of coronary artery bypass or valve surgery

CONTRAINDICATIONS: Hypersensitivity

Precautions: Pregnancy (C), breastfeeding, children <18 yr, geriatric patients, sinus node dysfunction, 2nd- or 3rd-degree AV block, electrolyte imbalances, bradycardia, renal/hepatic disease, CHF

Black Box Warning: QT prolongation, torsades de pointes, ventricular arrhythmias, ventricular tachycardia, cardiac dysrhythmias

DOSAGE AND ROUTES

Atrial fibrillation/flutter

- **Adult ≥60 kg: IV INF** 1 vial (1 mg) given over 10 min, may repeat same dose after 10 min
- **Adult <60 kg: IV INF** 0.01 mg/kg given over 10 min, may repeat same dose after 10 min

Available forms: Inj 0.1 mg/ml

Administer:

IV route

- Undiluted or diluted in 50 ml 0.9% NaCl, or D_5W (0.017 mg/ml); give over 10 min
- Solution is stable for 48 hr refrigerated or 24 hr at room temp
- Do not admix with other sol, products
- Reduce dosage slowly with ECG monitoring

SIDE EFFECTS

CNS: *Headache*

CV: *Hypotension, bradycardia,* **sinus arrest, CHF, dysrhythmias, torsades de pointes,** hypertension, extrasystoles, ventricular tachycardia, bundle branch block, AV block, palpitations, supraventricular extrasystoles, syncope, **prolonged QT interval**

GI: Nausea

PHARMACOKINETICS

Elimination half-life 6 hr, metabolized by liver, excreted by kidneys

INTERACTIONS

Increase: prodysrhythmia—phenothiazines, tricyclics, tetracyclics, antidepressants, H_1-receptor antagonists, antihistamines

Increase: masking of cardiotoxicity—digoxin

- Do not use within 5 hr of ibutilide: class Ia antidysrhythmics (disopyramide, quiNIDine, procainamide), class III agents (amiodarone, sotalol)

NURSING CONSIDERATIONS

Assess:

Black Box Warning: ECG continuously for ≥4 hr to determine product effectiveness; measure PR, QRS, QT intervals, check for PVCs, other dysrhythmias; discontinue if atrial fibrillation/flutter ceases; continue until QT interval corrected for heart rate (QTc) returned to baseline

- I&O ratio; electrolytes: K, Na, Cl
- Hepatic studies: AST, ALT, bilirubin, alk phos
- Dehydration or hypovolemia
- Rebound hypertension after 1-2 hr
- Cardiac rate, respiration: rate, rhythm, character, chest pain

Evaluate:

- Therapeutic response: decrease in atrial fibrillation/flutter

Teach patient/family:

- To report side effects immediately
- About reason for medication

⚠ HIGH ALERT

IDArubicin (Rx)

(eye-dah-roob′ih-sin)

Idamycin PFS

Func. class.: Antineoplastic, antibiotic

Chem. class.: Anthracycline glycoside

Do not confuse:

IDArubicin/DOXOrubicin/DAUNOrubicin/epirubicin

Idamycin/Adriamycin

ACTION: Non–cell-cycle specific; topoisomerase II inhibitor; vesicant

USES: Used in combination with other antineoplastics for acute myelocytic leukemia in adults

Unlabeled uses: Breast cancer, liquid tumors, non-Hodgkin's lymphoma, ALL, CLL, AML

CONTRAINDICATIONS:
Pregnancy (D), breastfeeding, hypersensitivity

Black Box Warning: Myelosuppression, bilirubin >5 mg/dl

Precautions: Children, gout, bone marrow depression, preexisting CV disease

Black Box Warning: Renal/hepatic disease, heart failure

DOSAGE AND ROUTES

- **Adult: IV** 8-12 mg/m²/day × 3 days in combination with cytarabine (induction)
- **Adolescent/child (unlabeled): IV** 10-12 mg/m²/day × 3 days

Renal/hepatic dose

- **Adult: IV** CCr >2.5 mg/dl, reduce dose; bilirubin 2.5-5 mg/dl, reduce dose by 50%; bilirubin >5 mg/dl, do not use

Available forms: Inj 1 mg/ml

Administer:

- Ice compress after stopping inf for extravasation

Intermittent IV INF route

- Do not give IM/SUBCUT
- Use cytotoxic handling procedures after preparing in biologic cabinet wearing gown, gloves, mask
- Antiemetic 30-60 min before product and 6-10 hr after treatment to prevent vomiting
- After reconstituting 5-mg vial with 5 ml 0.9% NaCl (1 mg/1 ml); give over 10-15 min through Y-tube or 3-way stopcock of inf of D_5 or NS; discard unused portion; use caution when needle inserted into vial (negative pressure)

Y-site compatibilities: Amifostine, amikacin, aztreonam, cimetidine, cladribine, cyclophosphamide, cytarabine, diphenhydrAMINE, droperidol, erythromycin, filgrastim, granisetron, imipenem/CISplatin, magnesium sulfate, mannitol, melphalan, metoclopramide, potassium chloride, ranitidine, sargramostim, thiotepa, vinorelbine

SIDE EFFECTS

CNS: Fever, chills, *headache,* **seizures**
CV: **Dysrhythmias, CHF, pericarditis, myocarditis,** peripheral edema, angina, **MI, myocardial toxicity**
GI: *Nausea, vomiting, abdominal pain, mucositis, diarrhea,* **hepatotoxicity**
GU: **Nephrotoxicity,** red urine
HEMA: **Thrombocytopenia, leukopenia,** anemia
INTEG: Rash, extravasation, dermatitis, *reversible alopecia,* urticaria; thrombophlebitis and tissue necrosis at inj site; radiation recall
SYST: **Infection,** tumor lysis syndrome

PHARMACOKINETICS

Half-life 22 hr; metabolized by liver; crosses placenta; excreted in bile, urine (primarily as metabolites); 97% protein binding

INTERACTIONS

Increase: toxicity—other antineoplastics or radiation
Decrease: antibody response—live virus vaccines

Drug/Lab Test
Increase: uric acid

NURSING CONSIDERATIONS

Assess:

- CBC, differential, platelet count weekly; withhold product if WBC is <4000/mm³ or platelet count is <75,000/mm³; notify prescriber of results
- Renal studies: BUN, serum uric acid, urine CCr, electrolytes before, during therapy
- ⚠ **Tumor lysis syndrome: hyperkalemia, hyperphosphatemia, hyperuricemia, hypocalcemia**
- I&O ratio; report fall in urine output to <30 ml/hr
- Monitor temp; fever may indicate beginning infection

• Hepatic studies before, during therapy: bilirubin, AST, ALT, alk phos prn or monthly; check for jaundice of skin and sclera, dark urine, clay-colored stools, itchy skin, abdominal pain, fever, diarrhea

Black Box Warning: Cardiac toxicity: CHF, dysrythmias, cardiomyopathy; cardiac studies before and periodically during treatment: ECG, chest x-ray, MUGA; ECG: watch for ST-T wave changes, low QRS and T, possible dysrhythmias (sinus tachycardia, heart block, PVCs)

• Bleeding: hematuria, guaiac stools, bruising or petechiae, mucosa or orifices
• Effects of alopecia on body image; discuss feelings about body changes
• Inflammation of mucosa, breaks in skin
• Buccal cavity for dryness, sores, ulceration, white patches, oral pain, bleeding, dysphagia
⚠ Local irritation, pain, burning at inj site; extravasation (vesicant)
• GI symptoms: frequency of stools, cramping

Perform/provide:
• Strict hand-washing technique, gloves, protective clothing
• Increase fluid intake to 2-3 L/day to prevent urate and calculi formation
• Rinsing of mouth tid-qid with water, club soda; brushing of teeth tid-qid with soft brush or cotton-tipped applicators for stomatitis; use unwaxed dental floss
• Storage at room temp for 3 days after reconstituting or 7 days refrigerated

Evaluate:
• Therapeutic response: decreased liquid tumor, spread of malignancy

Teach patient/family:
• To report signs of CHF, cardiac toxicity, beginning infection
• That hair may be lost during treatment; that wig or hairpiece may make patient feel better; that new hair may be different in color, texture
• To avoid foods with citric acid, hot or rough texture
• To avoid crowds, persons with upper respiratory illness
• To report any bleeding, white spots, ulcerations in mouth; to examine mouth daily
• That urine may be red-orange for 48 hr
• To use contraception during treatment, for ≥4 mo after treatment
• That all body fluids will change color

⚠ **HIGH ALERT**

ifosfamide (Rx)

(i-foss′fa-mide)

Ifex

Func. class.: Antineoplastic alkylating agent

Chem. class.: Nitrogen mustard

Do not confuse:
ifosfamide/cyclophosphamide

ACTION: Alkylates DNA, RNA, inhibits enzymes that allow synthesis of amino acids in proteins; also responsible for cross-linking DNA strands; activity is not cell-cycle–stage specific

USES: Testicular cancer

Unlabeled uses: Soft-tissue sarcoma, Ewing's sarcoma, non-Hodgkin's lymphoma, lung/pancreatic sarcoma

CONTRAINDICATIONS: Pregnancy (D), hypersensitivity

Black Box Warning: Bone marrow suppression

Precautions: Breastfeeding, children, renal/hepatic disease

Black Box Warning: Coma, hemorrhagic cystitis

DOSAGE AND ROUTES

• **Adult: IV** 1.2-2 g/m^2/day × 5 days, repeat course q3wk, given with mesna

Renal dose
• **Adult: IV** CCr 31-60 ml/min, give 75% of dose; CCr 10-30 ml/min, give 50% of dose; CCr <10 ml/min, do not give

Available forms: Inj 1-, 3-g vials

Administer:

• Antiemetic 30-60 min before product to prevent vomiting

• Always give with mesna to prevent ifosfamide-induced hemorrhagic cystitis; hydrate before and after inf

IV route

• After reconstituting 1 g/20 ml or 3 g/60 ml sterile or bacteriostatic water for inj with parabens or benzyl only; shake; may be diluted further with D_5W, LR, NS, sterile water for inj (concentrations 0.6-20 mg/ml); give over ≥30 min

Additive compatibilities: CARBOplatin, CISplatin, etoposide, fluorouracil, mesna

Y-site compatibilities: Allopurinol, amifostine, amphotericin B cholesteryl, aztreonam, DOXOrubicin liposome, filgrastim, fludarabine, gallium, granisetron, melphalan, ondansetron, paclitaxel, piperacillin/tazobactam, propofol, sargramostim, sodium bicarbonate, teniposide, thiotepa, vinorelbine

SIDE EFFECTS

CNS: Facial paresthesia, fever, malaise, somnolence, confusion, depression, hallucinations, dizziness, disorientation, **seizures, coma, cranial nerve dysfunction**

GI: Nausea, vomiting, anorexia, **hepatotoxicity**, stomatitis, constipation, diarrhea

GU: **Hematuria, nephrotoxicity, hemorrhagic cystitis**, dysuria, urinary frequency

HEMA: **Thrombocytopenia, leukopenia, anemia**

INTEG: Dermatitis, alopecia, pain at inj site, hyperpigmentation

META: Metabolic acidosis

PHARMACOKINETICS

Metabolized by liver, saturation occurs at high doses, excreted in urine, half-life 7-15 hr, depends on dose

INTERACTIONS

Increase: myelosuppression—other antineoplastics, radiation

Increase: toxicity—CYP3A4 inducers, barbiturates, allopurinol

Increase: bleeding risk—NSAIDs, anticoagulants, salicylates, thrombolytics

Decrease: antibody response—live virus vaccines

Decrease: effect of ifosfamide—CYP3A4 inhibitors

NURSING CONSIDERATIONS

Assess:

• Hepatic studies before, during therapy (bilirubin, AST, ALT, LDH) monthly or as needed; jaundice of skin and sclera, dark urine, clay-colored stools, itchy skin, abdominal pain, fever, diarrhea

Black Box Warning: CBC, differential, platelet count weekly; withhold product if WBC <2000 or platelet count <50,000; notify prescriber; severe myelosuppression may occur

• Monitor temp (may indicate beginning infection)

• Blood dyscrasias (anemia, granulocytopenia); bruising, fatigue, bleeding, poor healing

• Allergic reactions: dermatitis, exfoliative dermatitis, pruritus, urticaria

Black Box Warning: I&O ratio; monitor for hematuria; hemorrhagic cystitis can occur; increase fluids to 3 L/day; urinalysis prior to each dose

Black Box Warning: Neurologic symptoms: hallucinations, confusion, disorientation, coma; product should be discontinued

• Bleeding: hematuria, guaiac, bruising or petechiae, mucosa or orifices

Perform/provide:

• Storage of powder at room temp

• Increased fluid intake to ≥2 L/day to prevent hemorrhagic cystitis

• Warm compresses at inj site for inflammation

Evaluate:

• Therapeutic response: decrease in size and spread of tumor

Teach patient/family:

• To notify prescriber of sore throat, swollen lymph nodes, malaise, fever; other infections may occur

• Not to have vaccinations during or after treatment
• That hair may be lost during treatment; that wig or hairpiece may make the patient feel better; that new hair may be different in color, texture
• To report signs of anemia: fatigue, headache, faintness, SOB, irritability
• To report bleeding; to avoid use of razors, commercial mouthwash
• To avoid use of aspirin products, NSAIDs, ibuprofen because hemorrhage can occur
• To use contraceptive measures during therapy; not to breastfeed
• To avoid crowds, persons with infections
• To report confusion, hallucinations, extreme drowsiness, numbness, tingling; to avoid alcohol use for ≥4 mo after treatment

iloperidone (Rx)

(ill-o-pehr′ih-dohn)

Fanapt

Func. class.: Antipsychotic

Chem. class.: Benzisoxazole derivative

ACTION: Unknown; may be mediated through both dopamine type 2 (D2) and serotonin type 2 (5-HT2) antagonism

USES: Schizophrenia

CONTRAINDICATIONS: Breastfeeding, hypersensitivity

Precautions: Pregnancy (C), children, geriatric patients, renal/hepatic disease, breast cancer, Parkinson's disease, dementia with Lewy bodies, seizure disorder, QT prolongation, bundle branch block, acute MI, ambient temperature increase, AV block, stroke, substance abuse, suicidal ideation, tardive dyskinesia, torsade de pointes, blood dyscrasias

Black Box Warning: Dementia

DOSAGE AND ROUTES

• **Adult: PO** 1 mg bid day 1, 2 mg bid day 2, 4 mg bid day 3, 6 mg bid day 4, 8 mg bid day 5, 10 mg bid day 6, 12 mg bid day 7; max 24 mg/day in 2 divided doses; reduce dose by 50% in patient who is a poor metabolizer of CYP2D6 or when used with strong CYP2D6/CYP3A4 inhibitors

Available forms: Tabs 1, 2, 4, 6, 8, 10, 12 mg; titration pack

Administer:

• Use without regard to meals
• Reduced dose in geriatric patients
• Anticholinergic agent for EPS
• Avoid use with CNS depressants

SIDE EFFECTS

CNS: *EPS, pseudoparkinsonism, akathisia, dystonia, tardive dyskinesia; drowsiness,* **seizures, neuroleptic malignant syndrome,** dizziness, delirium, depression, paranoia, fatigue, hostility, lethargy, restlessness, vertigo, tremor

CV: Orthostatic hypotension, **heart failure, AV block, QT prolongation,** tachycardia

EENT: Blurred vision, cataracts, nystagmus, tinnitus

GI: *Nausea,* vomiting, *anorexia, constipation,* jaundice, weight gain/loss, abdominal pain, stomatitis

GU: Hyperprolactinemia, urinary retention/incontinence, testicular pain, **renal failure**

HEMA: Agranulocytosis, leukopenia, neutropenia

MISC: Renal artery occlusion

PHARMACOKINETICS

PO: Extensively metabolized by liver to major active metabolite by CYP2D6, CYP3A4; protein binding 95%; peak 2-4 hr; excreted in urine and feces; terminal half-life 18 hr in extensive metabolizers; 33 hr in poor metabolizers

INTERACTIONS

Increase: serotonin syndrome, neuroleptic malignant syndrome—SSRIs, SNRI

Increase: sedation—other CNS depressants, alcohol
Increase: iloperidone effect, decreased clearance—CYP2D6, CYP3A4 inhibitors (delavirdine, indinavir, isoniazid, itraconazole, dalfopristin, ritonavir, tipranavir)
Increase: QT prolongation—class IA/ III antidysrhythmics, some phenothiazines, β-agonists, local anesthetics, tricyclics, haloperidol, methadone, chloroquine, clarithromycin, droperidol, erythromycin, pentamidine
Decrease: iloperidone action—CYP2D6, CYP3A4 inducers (carBAMazepine, barbiturates, phenytoins, rifampin)
Drug/Lab Test
Increase: prolactin levels

NURSING CONSIDERATIONS

Assess:

- Mental status before initial administration
- Swallowing of PO medication; check for hoarding or giving of medication to other patients
- I&O ratio; palpate bladder if urinary output is low
- Bilirubin, CBC, hepatic studies monthly
- Urinalysis before, during prolonged therapy
- Affect, orientation, LOC, reflexes, gait, coordination, sleep-pattern disturbances
- B/P standing and lying; pulse, respirations; q4hr during initial treatment; establish baseline before starting treatment; report drops of 30 mm Hg; watch for ECG changes; QT prolongation may occur; dizziness, faintness, palpitations, tachycardia on rising
- EPS, including akathisia, tardive dyskinesia (bizarre movements of the jaw, mouth, tongue, extremities), pseudoparkinsonism (rigidity, tremors, pill rolling, shuffling gait)

Black Box Warning: Serious reactions in the geriatric patient: fatal pneumonia, heart failure, sudden death

Black Box Warning: Neuroleptic malignant syndrome: hyperthermia, increased CPK, altered mental status, muscle rigidity

- Constipation, urinary retention daily; if these occur, increase bulk and water in diet
- Weight gain, hyperglycemia, metabolic changes in diabetes

Perform/provide:

- Supervised ambulation until patient is stabilized on medication; do not involve patient in strenuous exercise program because fainting is possible; patient should not stand still for a long time
- Sips of water, candy, gum for dry mouth
- Storage in tight, light-resistant container (PO); unopened vials in refrigerator, protect from light; do not freeze

Evaluate:

- Therapeutic response: decrease in emotional excitement, hallucinations, delusions, paranoia; reorganization of patterns of thought, speech

Teach patient/family:

- That orthostatic hypotension may occur; to rise from sitting or lying position gradually
- To avoid hot tubs, hot showers, tub baths because hypotension may occur; that heat stroke may occur in hot weather; to take extra precautions to stay cool
- To avoid abrupt withdrawal of product because EPS may result; that product should be withdrawn slowly
- To avoid OTC preparations (cough, hay fever, cold) unless approved by prescriber because serious product interactions may occur; to avoid use of alcohol because increased drowsiness may occur
- To avoid hazardous activities if drowsy or dizzy
- To comply with product regimen
- To report impaired vision, tremors, muscle twitching
- To use contraception; to inform prescriber if pregnancy is planned or suspected

TREATMENT OF OVERDOSE:
Lavage if orally ingested; provide airway; *do not induce vomiting*

imatinib (Rx)
(im-ah-tin′ib)

Gleevec

Func. class.: Antineoplastic—miscellaneous

Chem. class.: Protein-tyrosine kinase inhibitor

ACTION:
Inhibits Bcr-Abl tyrosine kinase created in patients with chronic myeloid leukemia (CML)

USES:
Treatment of chronic myeloid leukemia (CML); Philadelphia-chromosome–positive patients in blast-cell crisis or patients in chronic failure after treatment failure with interferon alfa; gastrointestinal stromal tumors (GIST) positive for Kit; chronic eosinophilic leukemia, acute lymphocytic leukemia, dermatofibrosarcoma protuberans, myelodysplastic syndrome, systemic mastocytosis

Unlabeled uses: Desmoid tumor

CONTRAINDICATIONS:
Pregnancy (D), hypersensitivity

Precautions: Breastfeeding, children, geriatric patients, cardiac/renal/hepatic/dental disease, GI bleeding, bone marrow suppression, infection, thrombocytopenia, neutropenia, immunosuppression

DOSAGE AND ROUTES

Acute lymphocytic leukemia (ALL)
- **Adult: PO** 600 mg/day

CML, chronic phase
- **Adult: PO** 400-600 mg/day
- **Adolescent/child >2 yr: PO** 340 mg/m²/day, max 600 mg/day

CML, accelerated phase/blast crisis
- **Adult: PO** 600-800 mg/day

GI stromal tumor (GIST)
- **Adult: PO** 400-600 mg/day

Renal dose
- **Adult: PO** CCr 40-59 ml/min, max 600 mg/day; CCr 20-39 ml/min, decrease initial dose by 50%, max 400 mg/day; CCr <20 ml/min, use with caution, 100 mg/day

Hepatic dose
- **Adult: PO** Total bilirubin 1.5-3 × ULN and any AST, decrease initial dose to 400 mg/day; total bilirubin >3 × ULN and any AST, decrease initial dose to 300 mg/day

Available forms: Tabs 100, 400 mg

Administer:
- With meal and large glass of water to decrease GI symptoms; doses of 800 mg should be given as 400 mg bid
- Tab may be dispersed in a glass of water or apple juice, use 50 ml of liquid for 100-mg tab, 200 ml liquid for 400-mg tab

SIDE EFFECTS
CNS: CNS hemorrhage, headache, dizziness, insomnia

CV: Hemorrhage, heart failure, cardiac tamponade, hypereosinophilia, cardiac toxicity

EENT: Blurred vision, conjunctivitis

GI: *Nausea,* hepatotoxicity, vomiting, dyspepsia, GI hemorrhage, *anorexia, abdominal pain,* GI perforation, diarrhea

HEMA: Neutropenia, thrombocytopenia, bleeding

INTEG: *Rash, pruritus,* alopecia, photosensitivity

META: Fluid retention, hypokalemia, edema

MISC: Fatigue, epistaxis, pyrexia, night sweats, increased weight, flulike symptoms, hypothyroidism

MS: Cramps, pain, arthralgia, myalgia

RESP: Cough, dyspnea, nasopharyngitis, pneumonia, upper respiratory tract infection, pleural effusion, edema

PHARMACOKINETICS
Well absorbed (98%); protein binding 95%; metabolized by CYP3A4; excreted in feces, small amount in urine; peak 2-4

hr; duration 24 hr (imatinib), 40 hr (metabolite); half-life 18-40 hr

INTERACTIONS

Increase: hepatotoxicity—acetaminophen

Increase: imatinib concentrations—CYP3A4 inhibitors (ketoconazole, itraconazole, erythromycin, clarithromycin)

Increase: plasma concentrations of simvastatin, calcium channel blockers, ergots

Increase: plasma concentration of warfarin; avoid use with warfarin; use low-molecular-weight anticoagulants instead

Decrease: imatinib concentrations—CYP3A4 inducers (dexamethasone, phenytoin, carbamazepine, rifampin, PHENobarbital)

Drug/Food

Increase: imatinib effect—grapefruit juice; avoid use while taking product

Drug/Herb

Decrease: imatinib concentration—St. John's wort

NURSING CONSIDERATIONS

Assess:

- **Bone marrow suppression:** ANC, platelets; during chronic phase, if ANC $<1 \times 10^9$/L and/or platelets $<50 \times 10^9$/L, stop until ANC $>1.5 \times 10^9$/L and platelets $>75 \times 10^9$/L; during accelerated phase/blast crisis, if ANC $<0.5 \times 10^9$/L and/or platelets $<10 \times 10^9$/L, determine whether cytopenia related to biopsy/aspirate; if not, reduce dose by 200 mg; if cytopenia continues, reduce dose by another 100 mg; if cytopenia continues for 4 wk, stop product until ANC $\geq 1 \times 10^9$/L
- **Renal toxicity:** if bilirubin $>3 \times$ IULN, withhold imatinib until bilirubin levels return to $<1.5 \times$ IULN
- **Hepatotoxicity:** monitor LFTs, before treatment, q mo; if liver transaminases $>5 \times$ IULN, withhold imatinib until transaminase levels return to $<2.5 \times$ IULN
- Signs of fluid retention, edema: weigh, monitor lung sounds, assess for edema; some fluid retention is dose dependent

Perform/provide:

- Nutritious diet with iron, vit supplement, low fiber, few dairy products
- Storage at 25° C (77° F)

Evaluate:

- Therapeutic response: decrease in leukemic cells or size of tumor

Teach patient/family:

- To report adverse reactions immediately: shortness of breath, swelling of extremities, bleeding
- About reason for treatment, expected results
- That effect on male infertility is unknown

imipenem/cilastatin (Rx)

(i-me-pen′em sye-la-stat′in)

Primaxin IM, Primaxin IV

Func. class.: Antiinfective—miscellaneous

Chem. class.: Carbapenem

Do not confuse:

imipenem/Omnipen

Primaxin/Premarin

ACTION: Interferes with cell-wall replication of susceptible organisms; osmotically unstable cell wall swells, bursts from osmotic pressure; addition of cilastatin prevents renal inactivation that occurs with high urinary concentrations of imipenem

USES: Serious infections caused by gram-positive *Streptococcus pneumoniae,* group A β-hemolytic streptococci, *Staphylococcus aureus,* enterococcus; gram-negative *Klebsiella, Proteus, Escherichia coli, Acinetobacter, Serratia, Pseudomonas aeruginosa, Salmonella, Shigella, Haemophilus influenzae, Listeria* sp.

CONTRAINDICATIONS: Hypersensitivity to this product or amide local anesthetics, or carbapenems; AV block, shock (IM)

Precautions: Pregnancy (C), breastfeeding, children, geriatric patients, seizure disorders, renal disease, head trauma; hypersensitivity to cephalosporins, penicillins; pseudomembranous colitis, ulcerative colitis

DOSAGE AND ROUTES

• **Adult: IV** 250-500 mg q6-8hr; severe infections may require 1 g q6-8hr; may give **IM** q12hr (total daily **IM** dosage >1500 mg not recommended); mild to moderate infections

• **Child: IV** 60-100 mg/kg/day in divided doses, max 4 g/day; **IM** 10-15 mg/kg q6hr

Renal dose

• **Adult ≥70 kg (reduce normal dose of 1 g/day to): IV** CCr 41-70 ml/min, 250 mg q8hr; CCr 6-40 ml/min, 250 mg q12hr; *(reduce normal dose of 1.5 g/day to):* CCr 41-70 ml/min, 250 mg q6hr; CCr 21-40 ml/min, q8hr; CCr 6-20 ml/min, 250 mg q12hr; *(reduce normal dose of 2 g/day to):* CCr 41-70 ml/min, 500 mg q8hr; CCr 21-40 ml/min, 250 mg q6hr; CCr 6-20 ml/min, 250 mg q12hr

Available forms: Powder for sol inj 250, 500 mg; powder for susp 500 mg

Administer:

• After C&S is taken

IM route

• Reconstitute 500 mg/2 ml lidocaine without EPINEPHrine; shake

• Inject deeply in large muscle, aspirate, **product for IM is not for IV use**

IV route

• After reconstitution of 250 or 500 mg with 10 ml of diluent and shake; add to ≥100 ml of same inf sol

• 250-500 mg over 20-30 min; ≥750 mg over 40-60 min; give through Y-tube or 3-way stopcock; do not give by IV bolus or if cloudy

Y-site compatibilities: Acyclovir, amifostine, aztreonam, cefepime, cisatracurium, diltiazem, famotidine, fludarabine, foscarnet, granisetron, IDArubicin, insulin (regular), melphalan, methotrexate, ondansetron, propofol, remifentanil, tacrolimus, teniposide, thiotepa, vinorelbine, zidovudine

SIDE EFFECTS

CNS: Fever, somnolence, **seizures,** confusion, dizziness, weakness, myoclonus

CV: Hypotension, palpitations, tachycardia

GI: *Diarrhea, nausea, vomiting,* **pseudomembranous colitis, hepatitis,** glossitis

GU: Renal toxicity/failure

HEMA: Eosinophilia, neutropenia, decreased Hgb, Hct

INTEG: Rash, urticaria, pruritus, pain at inj site, phlebitis, erythema at inj site

RESP: Chest discomfort, dyspnea, hyperventilation

SYST: Anaphylaxis, Stevens-Johnson syndrome

PHARMACOKINETICS

IV: Onset immediate, peak ½-1 hr, half-life 1 hr, 70%-80% excreted unchanged in urine

INTERACTIONS

Increase: imipenem plasma levels—probenecid

Increase: antagonistic effect—β-lactam antibiotics

Increase: seizure risk—ganciclovir, theophylline, aminophylline, cycloSPORINE

Decrease: effect of valproic acid

Drug/Lab Test

Increase: AST, ALT, LDH, BUN, alk phos, bilirubin, creatinine

False positive: direct Coombs' test

NURSING CONSIDERATIONS

Assess:

• Renal studies: creatinine/BUN

• **Infection:** increased temp, WBC, characteristics of wounds, sputum, urine or stool culture

• Sensitivity to penicillin—may have sensitivity to this product

• Renal disease: lower dose may be required
• Bowel pattern daily; if severe diarrhea occurs, product should be discontinued; may indicate pseudomembranous colitis
⚠ **Allergic reactions, anaphylaxis: rash, urticaria, pruritus, wheezing, laryngeal edema; may occur a few days after therapy begins; have epinephrine, antihistamine, emergency equipment available**
• **Overgrowth of infection:** perineal itching, fever, malaise, redness, pain, swelling, drainage, rash, diarrhea, change in cough, sputum

Evaluate:
• Therapeutic response: negative C&S; absence of signs and symptoms of infection

Teach patient/family:
⚠ **To report severe diarrhea; may indicate pseudomembranous colitis**
⚠ **To report sore throat, bruising, bleeding, joint pain; may indicate blood dyscrasias (rare)**

TREATMENT OF ANAPHYLAXIS: EPINEPHrine, antihistamines; resuscitate if needed

imipramine (Rx)

(im-ip′ra-meen)

Apo-Imipramine ✦, Tofranil, Tofranil PM

Func. class.: Antidepressant, tricyclic
Chem. class.: Dibenzazepine, tertiary amine

Do not confuse:
imipramine/desipramine

ACTION: Blocks reuptake of norepinephrine, serotonin into nerve endings, thereby increasing action of norepinephrine, serotonin in nerve cells

USES: Depression, enuresis in children
Unlabeled uses: Chronic pain, migraine headaches, cluster headaches as adjunct, incontinence, ADHD, neuralgia, bulimia, neuropathic pain, social phobia

CONTRAINDICATIONS: Pregnancy (D), hypersensitivity to tricyclics, AV block, bundle branch block, ileus, QT prolongation, acute MI
Precautions: Breastfeeding, geriatric patients, suicidal patients, severe depression, increased intraocular pressure, closed-angle glaucoma, urinary retention, cardiac/hepatic disease, hyperthyroidism, electroshock therapy, elective surgery, seizure disorders, prostatic hypertrophy, MI

Black Box Warning: Children other than for enuresis; suicidal ideation

DOSAGE AND ROUTES

• **Adult: PO** 75-100 mg/day in divided doses, may increase by 25-50 mg to 200 mg/day (outpatients), 300 mg/day (inpatients); may give daily dose at bedtime
• **Geriatric: PO** 25-50 mg at bedtime, may increase to 100 mg/day in divided doses
• **Child ≥6 yr (unlabeled): PO** 1.5 mg/kg/day in divided doses, max 2.5 mg/kg/day

Enuresis
• **Child 6-12 yr: PO** 10-25 mg at bedtime, max 50 mg

Neuropathic pain (unlabeled)
• **Adult: PO** 10-150 mg/day

Social phobia/panic disorder (unlabeled)
• **Adult: PO** 10 mg at bedtime, titrate q2-4days to 100-200 mg/day

Overactive bladder (OAB) (unlabeled)
• **Adult: PO** 10-50 mg daily, may titrate to 150 mg/day

Available forms: Tabs 10, 25, 50 mg; caps 75, 100, 125, 150 mg

Administer:
PO route
• Not to break, crush, or chew caps
• With food or milk for GI symptoms

• Dosage at bedtime if oversedation occurs during day; may take entire dose at bedtime; geriatric patients may not tolerate once daily dosing
• Sugarless gum, hard candy, or frequent sips of water for dry mouth

SIDE EFFECTS

CNS: *Dizziness, drowsiness,* confusion, seizures, headache, anxiety, tremors, stimulation, weakness, insomnia, nightmares, EPS (geriatric patients), increased psychiatric symptoms, paresthesia
CV: *Orthostatic hypotension, ECG changes, tachycardia,* hypertension, palpitations, dysrhythmias
EENT: Blurred vision, tinnitus, mydriasis
GI: *Diarrhea, dry mouth,* nausea, vomiting, paralytic ileus; increased appetite; cramps, epigastric distress, jaundice, hepatitis, stomatitis, constipation, taste change
GU: *Retention,* acute renal failure
HEMA: Agranulocytosis, thrombocytopenia, eosinophilia, leukopenia
INTEG: Rash, urticaria, sweating, pruritus, photosensitivity; hyperpigmentation (rare)

PHARMACOKINETICS

Steady state 2-5 days; metabolized to desipramine by liver; excreted in urine, breast milk, feces; crosses placenta; half-life 6-20 hr

INTERACTIONS

⚠ Hyperpyretic crisis, seizures, hypertensive episode: MAOIs, cloNIDine
⚠ **Increase:** serotonin syndrome, neuroleptic malignant syndrome—SSRIs, SNRIs, serotonin-receptor agonists; avoid concurrent use
Increase: QT interval—class IA/III antidysrhythmics, tricyclics, gatifloxacin, levofloxacin, moxifloxacin, ziprasidone
Increase: effects of direct-acting sympathomimetics (EPINEPHrine), alcohol, barbiturates, benzodiazepines, CNS depressants
Decrease: effects of guanethidine, cloNIDine, indirect-acting sympathomimetics (ePHEDrine)
Drug/Herb
Increase: serotonin syndrome—SAM-e, St. John's wort
Drug/Lab Test
Increase: serum bilirubin, alk phos, blood glucose
Decrease: 5-HIAA, VMA, urinary catecholamines

NURSING CONSIDERATIONS

Assess:
• B/P (lying, standing), pulse q4hr; if systolic B/P drops 20 mm Hg, hold product, notify prescriber; take vital signs q4hr in patients with CV disease
• Blood studies: CBC, leukocytes, differential, cardiac enzymes, serum imipramine levels (125-250 ng/ml) if patient is receiving long-term therapy
• Hepatic studies: AST, ALT, bilirubin
• Weight weekly; appetite may increase with product
⚠ **QT prolongation:** ECG for flattening of T wave, bundle branch block, AV block, dysrhythmias in cardiac patients
• EPS primarily in geriatric patients: rigidity, dystonia, akathisia
• Mental status: mood, sensorium, affect, suicidal tendencies; increase in psychiatric symptoms: depression, panic
• Urinary retention, constipation; constipation is more likely to occur in children, geriatric patients; increase fluids, bulk in diet
⚠ **Withdrawal symptoms:** headache, nausea, vomiting, muscle pain, weakness, diarrhea, insomnia, restlessness; not usual unless product is discontinued abruptly
• Alcohol consumption; if alcohol is consumed, hold dose until morning

Perform/provide:
- Storage in tight container at room temp; do not freeze
- Assistance with ambulation during beginning therapy, since drowsiness, dizziness, orthostatic hypotension occurs
- Safety measures, primarily for geriatric patients

Evaluate:
- Therapeutic response: decreased depression, enuresis, pain

Teach patient/family:
- That therapeutic effects may take 2-3 wk
- That product is dispensed in small amounts because of suicide potential, especially at beginning of therapy
- To use caution when driving, performing other activities requiring alertness because of drowsiness, dizziness, blurred vision
- To report urinary retention immediately
- To avoid alcohol, other CNS depressants during treatment
- Not to discontinue medication abruptly after long-term use; may cause nausea, headache, malaise
- To wear sunscreen or large hat because photosensitivity occurs
- To rise slowly, orthostatic hypotension may occur

TREATMENT OF OVERDOSE:

ECG monitoring; lavage, activated charcoal; administer anticonvulsant

immune globulin IM (IMIG/IGIM) (Rx)

Bay Gam 15%, Flebogamma 5%, Flebogamma DIF 5%, Gammagard, Gamunex 10%, Privigen 10%, Vivaglobin 10%

immune globulin IV (IGIV, IVIG) (Rx)

Bay Gam 15%, Carimune NF, Flebogamma 5%, Flebogamma 10% DIF, Gammagard S/D, Gammaked, Gammaplex, Gammar-P IV, Gamunex, Iveegam EN, Polygam S/D, Privigen, Vivaglobin

immune globulin SC (SCIG/IGSC)

Bay Gam 15%, Flebogamma 5%, Flebogamma DIF 5%, Gammagard 10%, Gammaked, Gammaplex, Gamunex 10%, Privigen 10%, Vivaglobin

Func. class.: Immune serum
Chem. class.: IgG

ACTION: Provides passive immunity to hepatitis A, measles, varicella, rubella, immune globulin deficiency; contains gamma globulin antibodies (IgG)

USES: Immunodeficiency syndrome; B-cell chronic lymphocytic leukemia; Kawasaki syndrome; bone marrow transplantation; pediatric HIV infection; agammaglobulinemia; hepatitis A, B exposure; measles exposure; measles vaccine complications; purpura; rubella exposure; chickenpox exposure; chronic inflammatory demyelinating polyneuropathy
Unlabeled uses: IV posttransfusion purpura, Guillain-Barré syndrome, refractory pemphigus vulgaris, West Nile virus, meningitis, myasthenia gravis, thrombocytopenia encephalitis, HIV, cy-

tomegalovirus, neonatal jaundice, RSV infection, primary humoral immunodeficiency, refractory pemphigus vulgaris

CONTRAINDICATIONS:
Coagulopathy, hemophilia, IgA deficiency, thrombocytopenia

Precautions: Pregnancy (C), breastfeeding, children, agammaglobulinemia, bleeding, hypogammaglobulinemia, infection, IV, viral infection

DOSAGE AND ROUTES

Immune globulin IM (IMIG, IGIM)

Hepatitis A prophylaxis

• **Adult/geriatric/adolescent/child/infant (unlabeled):** **IM** 0.02 ml/kg for those who have not received hepatitis A vaccine and been exposed during the prior 2 wk

Measles prophylaxis (exposed during prior 6 days)

• **Adult:** **IM** 0.25 ml/kg (immunocompetent)

• **Child (unlabeled):** **IM** 0.5 ml/kg as a single dose, max 15 ml (immunocompromised)

Varicella prophylaxis

• **Adult:** **IM** 0.6-1.2 ml/kg as soon as possible and if varicella-zoster immune globulin is not available

Rubella prophylaxis in exposed/susceptible individual who will not consider a therapeutic abortion

• **Adult pregnant women:** **IM** 0.55 ml/kg

Immunoglobulin deficiency

• **Adult:** **IM** 1.32 ml/kg then 0.66 ml/kg (≥100 mg/kg) q3-4wk

Immune globulin IV (IVIG, IGIV)

Primary immunodeficiency

Gammagard S/D

• **Adult/adolescent/child:** **IV** 300-600 mg/kg q3-4wk

Polygam S/D

• **Adult/adolescent/child:** **IV** 100 mg/kg/mo; initially 200-400 mg/kg may be used

Gammar-P IV

• **Adult:** **IV** 200-400 mg/kg q3-4wk

• **Adolescent/child:** **IV** 200 mg/kg q3-4wk

Gamunex

• **Adult/adolescent/child:** **IV INF** 300-600 mg/kg (3-6 ml/kg) q3-4wk, initial inf rate 1 mg/kg/min (max 8 mg/kg/min)

Iveegam EN

• **Adult/adolescent/child:** **IV** 200 mg/kg q mo, max 800 mg/kg/mo

Panglobulin NF/Carimune NF

• **Adult/adolescent/child:** **IV** 200 mg/kg/mo

Gamagard liquid/Flebogamma 5%

• **Adult/adolescent/child:** **IV** 300-600 mg/kg q3-4wk

Privigen

• **Adult/adolescent/child ≥3 yr:** **IV** 200-800 mg q3wk

Idiopathic thrombocytopenic purpura (ITP)

Panglobulin NF/Carimune NF

• **Adult/child:** **IV** 400 mg/kg daily × 2-5 days; with acute ITP of childhood, only 2 of 5 days are needed if initial platelets are 30,000-50,000 mcl after 2 doses

Gammagard S/D/Polygam S/D

• **Adult/adolescent/child:** **IV** 1000 mg/kg as a single dose; may give on alternate days for up to 3 doses

Gamunex

• **Adult/adolescent/child:** **IV INF** total dose of 2000 mg/kg divided as 1000 mg/kg (10 ml/kg), give on 2 consecutive days; initial rate is 1 mg/kg/min (max 8 mg/kg/min); if after 1st dose adequate platelets are observed after 24 hr, may withhold 2nd dose

Privigen

• **Adult/adolescent ≥15 yr:** **IV** 1 g/kg/day × 2 days

Kawasaki disease

Iveegam EN

• **Child:** **IV** 400 mg/kg daily × 4 consecutive days or a single dose of 2000 mg/kg over 10 hr, given with aspirin 100 mg/kg/day through 14th day of illness, then 3-5 mg/kg each day thereafter for 5 wk

Gammagard S/D/Polygam S/D

- **Infant/child: IV** 1000 mg/kg as a single dose or 400 mg/kg/day × 4 days beginning within 7 days of fever onset, with aspirin 80-100 mg/kg/day × 4 divided doses

Immune globulin SC (SCIG/IGSC)

- **Adult/child >2 yr: SUBCUT INF** 100-200 mg/kg q wk, **Vivaglobin** brand of SCIG 160 mg IgG/ml, **SUBCUT** inj 15 ml/inj site, given at max of 20 ml/hr

Available forms: IM: Inj 2-, 10-ml vial (Bay Gam); **IV:** 5%, 10% sol (Gamimune N); powder for inj 1-, 3-, 6-, 12-g vials (Carimune NF); 50 mg protein/ml in 2.5-, 5-, 10-g vials (Gammagard S/D); 1-, 2.5-, 5-, 10-g vials (Gammar-P IV); 500 mg, 1-, 2.5-, 5-g vials (Iveegam); 6-, 12-g vials (Panglobulin); 2.5-, 5-, 10-g vials (Polygam S/D); sol for inj 1-, 2.5-, 5-, 10-, 20-g vials (Gamunex); Human sol for inj: Flebogamma 5%, 10% DIF

Administer:

- IM ≤3 ml at 1 site; use large muscle mass
- Only with EPINEPHrine 1:1000, resuscitative equipment available
- Only within 2 wk of exposure to hepatitis A

IV route

- **Gamimune N:** IV undiluted or dilute with D_5; give 0.01 ml/kg/min; may increase to 0.02-0.04 ml/kg/min
- **Venoglobulin-I:** (50 mg/ml sol) give 0.01-0.02 ml/kg/min; if no adverse reaction within ½ hr, increase to 0.04 ml/kg/min; store at room temp
- **Gammagard:** reconstitute with sterile water for inj (50 mg protein/ml); give 0.5 ml/kg/hr, may increase to 4 ml/kg/hr; use inf set provided
- **Gammar-IV:** give 0.01 ml/kg/min (50 mg/ml sol) × 15-30 min, may increase to 0.02 ml/kg/min, may increase to 0.03-0.06 ml/kg/min

Y-site compatibilities: Fluconazole, sargramostim

SIDE EFFECTS

CNS: Headache, fatigue, malaise
GI: Abdominal pain
HEMA: **Thromboembolism (Vivaglobin)**
INTEG: Pain at inj site, rash, pruritus, chills
MS: Arthralgia, chest pain
SYST: Lymphadenopathy, **anaphylaxis**

INTERACTIONS

- Do not administer live virus vaccines within 3 mo of this product

Drug/Lab Test
Interference: glucose testing system

NURSING CONSIDERATIONS

Assess:

- Exposure date: this product should be given within 6 days of measles, 7 days of hepatitis B, 14 days of hepatitis A
- Anaphylaxis: diaphoresis, wheezing, chest tightness, hypotension

Perform/provide:

- Storage at 36° F-46° F (2° C-8° C)

Evaluate:

- Prevention of infection, increased platelets

Teach patient/family:

- That passive immunity is temporary
- About the treatment of anaphylaxis: EPINEPHrine, diphenhydrAMINE, oxygen, vasopressors, corticosteroids

HIGH ALERT

inamrinone (Rx)

(in-am′rih-nohn)

Func. class.: Inotropic
Chem. class.: Bipyrimidine derivative

Discontinued

Do not confuse:
inamrinone/amiodarone

ACTION: Positive inotropic agent with vasodilator properties; reduces preload and afterload by direct relaxation of vascular smooth muscle, increases cardiac output

USES: Short-term management of CHF that has not responded to other medication (diuretics, other vasodilators); can be used with digoxin

CONTRAINDICATIONS: Hypersensitivity to this product or bisulfites; severe aortic disease, severe pulmonic valvular disease, acute MI

Precautions: Pregnancy (C), breastfeeding, children, geriatric patients, renal/hepatic disease, atrial flutter/fibrillation, asthma

DOSAGE AND ROUTES

- **Adult and child: IV BOL** 0.75 mg/kg given over 2-3 min; start inf of 5-10 mcg/kg/min; may give another bol 30 min after start of therapy, max 10 mg/kg total daily dose
- **Adolescent/child/infant (unlabeled): IV** 0.75-1 mg/kg over 5 min, may repeat × 2, then **IV INF** 2-20 mcg/kg/min

Renal dose

- **Adult: IV** CCr >10 ml/min, 100% of dose; CCr <10 ml/min, 50%-75% of dose

Discontinued

Available forms: Inj 5 mg/ml

Administer:

IV route

- Sol should be clear yellow; do not mix directly with dextrose solutions; chemical reaction occurs over 24 hr; precipitate forms if inamrinone and furosemide come in contact
- May give undiluted over 2-3 min or dilute with 0.9%, 0.45% NaCl to 1-3 mg/ml; run at prescribed rate by continuous inf; by inf pump for doses other than bolus
- Potassium supplements if ordered for potassium levels <3.0; correct before using amrinone

Syringe compatibilities: Propranolol, verapamil

Y-site compatibilities: Alfentanil, aminocaproic acid, anidulafungin, argatroban, atracurium, atropine, benztropine, bivalirudin, bleomycin, buprenorphine, calcium chloride, CARBOplatin, caspofungin, cisatracurium, CISplatin, cyclophosphamide, cytarabine, DACTINomycin, DAPTOmycin, dexmedetomidine, diltiazem, docetaxel, doxacurium, DOXOrubicin, ePHEDrine, epirubicin, eptifibatide, ertapenem, etoposide, fenoldopam, fentaNYL, fluconazole, fludarabine, fluorouracil, gatifloxacin, glycopyrrolate, granisetron, hydrOXYzine, IDArubicin, ifosfamide, irinotecan, labetalol, lidocaine, linezolid, mechlorethamine, metaraminol, metroNIDAZOLE, midazolam, minocycline, mitoxantrone, mycophenolate, naloxone, nitroprusside, oxaliplatin, paclitaxel, palonosetron, pamidronate, pantoprazole, propofol, propranolol, protamine, remifentanil, tacrolimus, teniposide, thiotepa, tolazoline, trimetaphan, vasopressin, verapamil, vinCRIStine, vinorelbine, voriconazole

SIDE EFFECTS

CV: Dysrhythmias, *hypotension*, chest pain

Discontinued

GI: *Nausea, vomiting, anorexia,* abdominal pain, hepatotoxicity (rare), ascites, jaundice, hiccups

HEMA: Thrombocytopenia

INTEG: Allergic reactions, burning at inj site

RESP: Pleuritis, pulmonary densities, hypoxemia

PHARMACOKINETICS

IV: Onset 2-5 min, peak 10 min, duration ½ = 2 hr, terminal half-life 4-6 hr, metabolized in liver, excreted in urine as product and metabolites 10-40%, half-life 4.6 hr, protein binding 40%

INTERACTIONS

- Excessive hypotension: antihypertensives, disopyramide
- Additive effect: cardiac glycosides

Drug/Lab Test

Increase: hepatic enzymes

Decrease: serum K

NURSING CONSIDERATIONS

Assess:

• B/P and pulse q5min during inf; if B/P drops 30 mm Hg, stop inf, call prescriber
• Electrolytes: K, S, Cl, Ca; renal studies: BUN, creatinine; blood studies: platelet count; ALT, AST, bilirubin daily; monitor fluid status (CVP) of geriatric patients
• I&O ratio and weight daily; diuresis should increase with continuing therapy
⚠ If platelets are <150,000/mm³, product is usually discontinued and another product started
• Extravasat **Discontinued** q48hr

Evaluate:

• Therapeutic response: increased cardiac output, decreased PCWP, adequate CVP; decreased dyspnea, fatigue, edema, ECG

Teach patient/family:

• That burning may occur at IV site
• To report adverse reactions promptly
• Not to breastfeed unless approved by prescriber

TREATMENT OF OVERDOSE:

Discontinue product, support circulation

indacaterol

(in-da-kat'er-ol)

Arcapta Neohaler

Func. class.: Beta-2 agonist, long acting respiratory

ACTION:

An agonist at β-2 receptors. These receptors are present in large numbers in the lungs and are located on bronchiolar smooth muscle. Stimulation of β-2 receptors in the lung causes relaxation of bronchial smooth muscle, which produces bronchodilation and an increase in bronchial airflow. These effects may be mediated, in part, by increased activity of adenyl cyclase, an intracellular enzyme responsible for the formation of cyclic-3′,5′-adenosine monophosphate (cAMP); has >24-fold agonist activity at β-2 receptors (primarily in the lung) compared to β-1 receptors (primarily in the heart)

USES:

Bronchitis, chronic obstructive pulmonary disease (COPD), emphysema

CONTRAINDICATIONS:

Acute bronchospasm, acute asthma attack, status asthmaticus, acute respiratory insufficiency, monotherapy of asthma

Precautions:

Ischemic cardiac disease (coronary artery disease), hypertension, cardiac arrhythmias, tachycardia, QT prolongation, congenital long QT syndrome, torsades de pointes history, hyperthyroidism (thyrotoxicosis, thyroid disease), pheochromocytoma, unusual responsiveness to other sympathomimetic amines, seizure disorder, diabetes mellitus, hypokalemia, milk protein hypersensitivity, severe hepatic disease; not indicated for neonates, infants, children, or adolescents under the age of 18 years, pregnancy (category C), breastfeeding

DOSAGE AND ROUTES

• **Adult: NH** 75 mcg (contents of 1 capsule) inhaled once daily; administer at the same time every day, max 1 dose in 24 hours

Available forms: Powder for inhalation 75 mcg

Administer:

Inhalation route

• For oral inhalation use only. Instruct patients NOT to swallow the capsules; always use the Neohaler Inhaler to administer capsules; this inhaler should not be used with any other medication. Do NOT use with a spacer.
• To administer, use dry hands to remove a capsule from the blister pack immediately before use and place into the capsule chamber of the Neohaler Inhaler; click the inhaler closed; do not place capsule into the mouthpiece; then, holding the inhaler upright, depress buttons fully once to pierce capsule, a click will be heard; have patient breathe out

fully away from inhaler, place inhaler in the mouth with buttons positioned to the left and right (not up and down), close lips around mouthpiece, then breathe deeply, rapidly, and steadily in through the inhaler. A whirring sound should be heard; if no sound is heard, check the chamber because the capsule may be stuck. Gently tap the base of the device to loosen capsule, if necessary. After inhalation, patient should hold the breath as long as comfortable while removing inhaler from the mouth; check the chamber to see if any powder remains in the capsule; repeat inhalation steps until no powder remains. Most patients empty the capsule in 1 or 2 inhalations. After administration, open chamber and discard empty capsule.

- Advise all patients that coughing after administration is not problematic; as long as the capsule is empty the full dose has been administered
- Occasionally the gelatin capsule might break into very small pieces that pass through the inhaler screen and reach the mouth. Accidental inhalation or ingestion of these pieces is harmless; piercing capsule more than once increases risk of shattering capsule. Do not wash in inhaler; keep it dry; although cleaning is not necessary, if desired, a clean, dry, lint-free cloth may be used to wipe out the inhaler.
- Use the new inhaler provided with each new prescription
- To avoid the spread of infection, do not share inhaler

SIDE EFFECTS

CNS: Headache tremor

CV: Sinus tachycardia, hypertension, QT prolongation and ST-T wave changes, prolonged QTc (an increase of >60 ms from baseline), non-sustained ventricular tachycardia, supraventricular tachycardia (SVT) episodes, intermittent ectopic atrial rhythm

ENDO: Hyperglycemia

GI: Nausea, dry mouth (xerostomia)

META: Hypokalemia

MS: Muscle cramps/spasm, musculoskeletal pain

RESP: Paradoxical bronchospasm, cough, dyspnea, sputum purulence or volume, wheezing nasopharyngitis, pneumonia, sinusitis and upper respiratory tract infection

PHARMACOKINETICS:

Protein binding 94%-96%, approximately 1/3 of total drug-related AUC over 24 hours, a hydroxylated derivative, glucuronate and dealkylate metabolites are present; metabolized by CYP3A4, CYP1A1, CYP2D6, UGT1A1; elimination multiphasic with terminal half-life of 45.5-126 hours; excreted renally (2%-6%), fecally (>90%); onset 5 min, peak 15 min, steady state 12-15 days

INTERACTIONS:

Increase QT prolongation: Class IA/III antiarrhythmics, flecainide, propafenone some antipsychotics (phenothiazines, pimozide, haloperidol risperidone, sertindole ziprasidone), amoxapine, arsenic trioxide, astemizole, bepridil, cisapride, citalopram, chloroquine, clarithromycin, dasatinib, dolasetron, dronedarone, droperidol, erythromycin, halofantrine, halogenated anesthetics, levomethadyl, maprotiline, methadone, some quinolones (ofloxacin, gatifloxacin, gemifloxacin, grepafloxacin, levofloxacin, moxifloxacin, sparfloxacin), ondansetron, paliperidone, palonosetron, pentamidine, probucol, propafenone, ranolazine, sunitinib, terfenadine, thioridazine, tricyclic antidepressants, troleandomycin, vorinostat, tetrabenazine

Increase hypokalemia: theophylline, aminophylline, corticosteroids

Increase cardiovascular reactions: MAOIs, furazolidone, procarbazine, rasagiline

NURSING CONSIDERATIONS

Assess

- COPD, emphysema, bronchospasm: monitor pulmonary function tests
- QT prolongation: monitor ECG, ejection fraction for QT prolongation
- Paradoxical bronchospasm: if paradoxical bronchospasm occurs, discontinue product immediately, use a short-acting β-agonist for rescue therapy, as appropriate

Teach patient/family

- To report dyspnea, wheezing, bronchospasm
- Not to use with other products unless approved by prescriber; there are many interactions

indapamide (Rx)

(in-dap′a-mide)

Apo-Indapamide ♣, Gen-Indapamide ♣, Lozide ♣, PMS-Indapamide ♣

Func. class.: Diuretic—thiazide-like, antihypertensive

Chem. class.: Indoline

ACTION: Acts on proximal section of distal renal tubule by inhibiting reabsorption of sodium; may act by direct vasodilation caused by blocking of calcium channels

USES: Edema of CHF, hypertension

CONTRAINDICATIONS: Hypersensitivity to this product or sulfonamides; anuria, hepatic coma, pregnancy (D)

Precautions: Breastfeeding, hypokalemia, dehydration, ascites, hepatic disease, severe renal disease, CCr <30 ml/min (not effective), diabetes mellitus, gout

DOSAGE AND ROUTES

Edema

- **Adult: PO** 2.5 mg/day in AM; may be increased to 5 mg/day if needed after 1 wk

Antihypertensive

- **Adult: PO** 1.25-5 mg/day; may increase to 5 mg/day over 8 wk

Available forms: Tabs 1.25, 2.5 mg

Administer:

- In AM to avoid interference with sleep
- With food if nausea occurs; absorption may be decreased slightly

SIDE EFFECTS

CNS: *Headache,* dizziness, fatigue, weakness, nervousness, agitation, extremity numbness, depression

CV: Orthostatic hypotension, volume depletion, palpitations, dysrhythmias, PVCs, vasculitis

EENT: Blurred vision, nasal congestion, increased intraocular pressure

ELECT: *Hypochloremic alkalosis, hypomagnesemia, hyperuricemia, hypercalcemia, hyponatremia,* hypokalemia, hyperglycemia

GI: *Nausea,* diarrhea, dry mouth, vomiting, anorexia, cramps, constipation, abdominal pain

GU: *Polyuria,* nocturia, urinary frequency, impotence

INTEG: *Rash, pruritus*

MS: Cramps

PHARMACOKINETICS

Well absorbed (PO); widely distributed; metabolized by liver; excreted by kidney (small amounts); onset 1-2 hr; peak 2 hr; duration up to 36 hr; excreted in urine, feces; half-life 14-18 hr

INTERACTIONS

Increase: hyperglycemia—diazoxide

Increase: toxicity of muscle relaxants, steroids, lithium, digoxin

Increase: hypokalemia—corticosteroids, amphotericin B, loop diuretics, thiazide diuretics

Decrease: effects—antidiabetics, antigout agents, anticoagulants

Decrease: absorption—cholestyramine, colestipol

Decrease: hypotensive effect—indomethacin, NSAIDs

Drug/Herb
• Severe photosensitivity: St. John's wort
Drug/Lab Test
Increase: calcium, parathyroid test, glucose, uric acid

NURSING CONSIDERATIONS

Assess:
• Weight, I&O daily to determine fluid loss; effect of product may be decreased if used daily
• Rate, depth, rhythm of respirations, effect of exertion
• B/P lying, standing; postural hypotension may occur
• Electrolytes: potassium, magnesium, sodium, chloride: include BUN, CBC, serum creatinine, blood pH, ABGs, uric acid, Ca, glucose
• Signs of metabolic alkalosis, hypokalemia
• Rashes, fever daily; allergy to sulfa products
• Confusion, especially in geriatric patients; take safety precautions if needed
• Hydration: skin turgor, thirst, dry mucous membranes
Evaluate:
• Therapeutic response: improvement in edema of feet, legs, sacral area daily; decreased B/P
Teach patient/family:
• To consume diet high in potassium; to rise slowly from lying or sitting position
• To recognize adverse reactions: muscle cramps, weakness, nausea, dizziness
• To take with food, milk for GI symptoms; to take early in day to prevent nocturia
• To notify prescriber if urinary output decreases; to monitor daily weight

TREATMENT OF OVERDOSE:

Lavage if taken orally; monitor electrolytes, administer IV fluids; monitor hydration, CV, renal status

indinavir (Rx)

(en-den′a-veer)

Crixivan

Func. class.: Antiretroviral
Chem. class.: Protease inhibitor

Do not confuse: indinavir/Denavir

ACTION:
Inhibits human immunodeficiency virus (HIV-1) protease; this prevents the maturation of the virus

USES:
HIV-1 in combination with at least 2 other antiretrovirals
Unlabeled uses: Prevention of HIV-1 after exposure

CONTRAINDICATIONS:
Hypersensitivity, breastfeeding
Precautions: Pregnancy (C), children, renal/hepatic disease, history of renal stones, diabetes, hypercholesterolemia, hemophilia

DOSAGE AND ROUTES

• **Adult: PO** 800 mg q8hr; 400 mg bid with ritonavir 400 mg bid or 800 mg bid with ritonavir 100-200 mg bid; decrease dose to 600 mg bid when given with lopinavir, ritonavir
Mild to moderate hepatic impairment
• **Adult: PO** 600 mg q8h
Available forms: Caps 100, 200, 333, 400 mg
Administer:
• Do not break, crush, or chew caps
• With water, 1 hr before or 2 hr after meals; may be given with other liquids or small meal; do not give with high-fat, high-protein meals
• Dosage adjustment will need to be considered when given with efavirenz
• Increase water to 1.5 L/day minimum to prevent nephrolithiasis

SIDE EFFECTS

CNS: *Headache, insomnia,* dizziness, somnolence

GI: *Diarrhea, abdominal pain, nausea, vomiting,* anorexia, dry mouth
GU: Nephrolithiasis
INTEG: Rash
MS: Pain
OTHER: Asthenia, **insulin-resistant hyperglycemia**, hyperlipidemia, **ketoacidosis**, lipodystrophy

PHARMACOKINETICS

Terminal half-life 2 hr; 60% protein binding; metabolized liver; excreted <20% unchanged in urine, 83% in feces

INTERACTIONS

⚠ **Life-threatening dysrhythmias: ergots, midazolam, rifampin, triazolam, amiodarone, pimozide, alfazosin**
Increase: myopathy—statins (atorvastatin, lovastatin, simvastatin)
Increase: indinavir levels—CYP3A4 inhibitors (arepitant, protease inhibitors, azole antifungals, nefazodone, verapamil); phosphodiesterase-5 inhibitors (sildenafil, tadalafil, vardenafil)
Increase: levels of both products—clarithromycin, zidovudine
Increase: levels of isoniazid, oral contraceptives
Decrease: indinavir levels—CYP3A4 inducers (barbiturates, carBAMazepine, nonnucleoside reverse transcriptase inhibitors, phenytoins, rifamycins, modafinil)
Decrease: effect of both products—anticonvulsants
Decrease: effect—CYP3A4 substrates (calcium channel blockers, immunosuppressants, benzodiazepines, azole antifungals, macrolides, SSRIs, statins)

Drug/Herb
Decrease: indinavir levels—St. John's wort; avoid concurrent use

Drug/Food
Decrease: indinavir absorption—grapefruit juice; high-fat, high-protein foods

Drug/Lab Test
Increase: AST, ALT, amylase, total bilirubin

NURSING CONSIDERATIONS

Assess:
- Complaints of lower back, flank pain; indicates kidney stones
- Signs of infection, anemia, presence of other sexually transmitted diseases
- Blood/hepatic studies: ALT, AST; total bilirubin, amylase, blood glucose, serum cholesterol/lipid profile, may be elevated
- Plasma HIV RNA, viral load, CD4 during treatment
- Bowel pattern before, during treatment; if severe abdominal pain with bleeding occurs, product should be discontinued; monitor hydration
- Skin eruptions; rash, urticaria, itching
- Allergies before treatment, reaction of each medication; place allergies on chart

Teach patient/family:
- To take as prescribed; if dose is missed, to take as soon as remembered up to 1 hr before next dose; not to double dose
- That product must be taken in equal intervals around the clock to maintain blood levels for duration of therapy

⚠ **That hyperglycemia may occur; to watch for increased thirst, weight loss, hunger, and dry, itchy skin; to notify prescriber**
- To increase fluids to prevent kidney stones; if stone formation occurs, that treatment may need to be interrupted
- That product does not cure AIDS, only controls symptoms; not to donate blood

indomethacin (Rx)

(in-doe-meth'a-sin)

Apo-Indomethacin ✤, Indocin, Nu-Indo ✤

Func. class.: Nonsteroidal antiinflammatory product (NSAID), antirheumatic
Chem. class.: Propionic acid derivative

Do not confuse:
Indocin/Endocet/minocin/Vicodin

ACTION: Inhibits prostaglandin synthesis by decreasing enzyme needed for biosynthesis; analgesic, antiinflammatory, antipyretic

USES: RA, ankylosing spondylitis, osteoarthritis, bursitis, tendinitis, acute gouty arthritis; closure of patent ductus arteriosus in premature infants (IV)

Unlabeled uses: Bone pain, headache, heterotopic ossification, juvenile rheumatoid arthritis, pericarditis

CONTRAINDICATIONS: Pregnancy (D) 3rd trimester, neonates, aortic coarctation, bleeding salicylate/NSAID hypersensitivity, ulcer disease

Black Box Warning: Perioperative pain in CABG

Precautions: Pregnancy (B) 1st trimester, breastfeeding, children, bleeding disorders, GI disorders, cardiac disorders, depression, renal/hepatic disease, asthma, diabetes, acute bronchospasm, ulcerative colitis, seizures, Parkinson's disease

Black Box Warning: Stroke, GI bleeding, MI

DOSAGE AND ROUTES

Arthritis/antiinflammatory

- **Adult: PO** 25-50 mg bid-tid; max 200 mg/day; **EXT REL** 75 mg/day, may increase to 75 mg bid

Acute gouty arthritis

- **Adult: PO** 50 mg tid; use only for acute attack then reduce dose

Patent ductus arteriosus

Longer or repeated treatment courses may be necessary for very premature infants

- **Infant <2 days: IV** 0.2 mg/kg then 0.1 mg/kg × 2 doses after 12, 24 hr
- **Infant 2-7 days: IV** 0.2 mg/kg then 0.2 mg/kg × 2 doses after 12, 24 hr
- **Infant >7 days: IV** 0.2 mg/kg then 0.25 mg/kg × 2 doses after 12, 24 hr

Available forms: Caps 25, 50 mg; ext rel caps 75 mg; inj 1-mg vial; supp 50 mg; oral susp 5 mg/ml

Administer:

PO route

- Do not break, crush, or chew sus rel cap or reg caps
- With food to decrease GI symptoms and prevent ulcerations
- Shake susp; do not mix with other liquids

IV route

- After reconstituting 1-2 mg/ml or more NS or sterile water for inj without preservative; infuse over 20-30 min, avoid extravasation; do not inj/inf via umbilical catheter to avoid dramatic shift in cerebral blood flow

Y-site compatibilities: Furosemide, insulin (regular), potassium chloride, sodium bicarbonate, sodium nitroprusside

SIDE EFFECTS

CNS: Dizziness, drowsiness, fatigue, tremors, confusion, insomnia, anxiety, depression, *headache*

CV: Tachycardia, peripheral edema, palpitations, dysrhythmias, hypertension, **CV thrombotic events, MI, stroke**

EENT: Tinnitus, hearing loss, blurred vision

GI: *Nausea,* anorexia, *vomiting,* diarrhea, jaundice, **cholestatic hepatitis,** *constipation,* flatulence, cramps, dry mouth, peptic ulcer, **ulceration, perforation, GI bleeding**

GU: Nephrotoxicity: dysuria, hematuria, oliguria, azotemia

HEMA: Blood dyscrasias, prolonged bleeding

INTEG: Purpura, rash, pruritus, sweating

PHARMACOKINETICS

PO: Onset 1-2 hr; peak 3 hr; duration 4-6 hr; metabolized in liver, kidneys; excreted in urine 60%, feces 33%; crosses placenta; excreted in breast milk; 99% protein binding; half-life 1 hr 1st pass, 2.6-11.2 hr 2nd pass

INTERACTIONS

Increase: hyperkalemia—potassium-sparing diuretics
Increase: toxicity—lithium, methotrexate, cycloSPORINE, zidovudine, probenecid
Increase: effect of—digoxin, penicillamine, phenytoin, aminoglycosides
Increase: bleeding risk—anticoagulants, abciximab, cefamandole, cefoperazone, cefotetan, clopidogrel, eptifibatide, plicamycin, ticlopidine, tirofiban, valproic acid, thrombolytics, aspirin, SSRIs, SNRIs
Decrease: effect of—antihypertensives

NURSING CONSIDERATIONS

Assess:

- Arthritis symptoms: ROM, pain, swelling before and 2 hr after treatment

Black Box Warning: Cardiac disease, CV, thrombotic events (MI, stroke) before administration

- Patent ductus arteriosus: respiratory rate, character, heart sounds
- Renal, hepatic, blood studies: BUN, creatinine, AST, ALT, Hgb before treatment, periodically thereafter; if renal function has decreased, do not give subsequent doses
- Eye/ear problems: blurred vision, tinnitus; may indicate toxicity; audiometric, ophthalmic exam before, during, after treatment if patient receiving long-term therapy
- Confusion, mood changes, hallucinations, especially among geriatric patients
- Asthma, nasal polyps, aspirin sensitivity, may develop hypersensitivity to indomethacin

Perform/provide:

- Storage at room temp

Evaluate:

- Therapeutic response: decreased pain, stiffness, swelling in joints; ability to move more easily

Teach patient/family:

- To report blurred vision, ringing, roaring in ears; may indicate toxicity
- To avoid driving, other hazardous activities if dizziness, drowsiness occurs
- To report change in urine pattern, increased weight, edema, increased pain in joints, fever, blood in urine; may indicate nephrotoxicity
- To report mood changes: anxiety, depression
- That therapeutic antiinflammatory effects may take up to 1 mo
- To avoid alcohol, NSAIDs, salicylates because bleeding may occur
- To report use to all health care providers

inFLIXimab (Rx)

(in-fliks′ih-mab)

Remicade

Func. class.: Biologic response modifiers

Chem. class.: Tumor necrosis factor modifiers

ACTION: Monoclonal antibody that neutralizes the activity of tumor necrosis factor alpha (TNFα) found in Crohn's disease; decreased infiltration of inflammatory cells

USES: Crohn's disease, fistulizing (moderate to severe); RA, given with methotrexate; plaque psoriasis, ankylosing spondylitis, ulcerative colitis, psoriasis

Unlabeled uses: Psoriatic arthritis, Behçet's syndrome, uveitis, juvenile arthritis

CONTRAINDICATIONS: Hypersensitivity to murines, moderate to severe CHF (NYHA class III/IV)

Precautions: Pregnancy (B), breastfeeding, children, geriatric patients, COPD, hepatotoxicity, hemalologic abnormalities, hepatitis B, Guillain-Barré syndrome, seizures, multiple sclerosis

Black Box Warning: Infection, neoplastic disease, TB

DOSAGE AND ROUTES

Crohn's disease (moderate to severe)/(fistulizing)

• **Adult/adolescent/child ≥6 yr: IV INF** 5 mg/kg initially then at 2 wk, 6 wk, q8wk thereafter; may increase to 10 mg/kg/dose if needed (adults)

Rheumatoid arthritis

• **Adult: IV** 3 mg/kg initially then at 2 wk, 6 wk, q8wk thereafter; max 10 mg/kg/dose

Available forms: Powder for inj 100 mg

Administer:

Intermittent IV INF route

• Pretreat with diphenhydrAMINE, acetaminophen, predniSONE if a reaction is inf related

• Give immediately after reconstitution; reconstitute each vial with 10 ml sterile water for inj; further dilute total dose/250 ml of 0.9% NaCl inj to a total conc of 0.4-4 mg/ml; use 21G or smaller needle for reconstitution; direct sterile water at glass wall of vial; gently swirl; do not shake; may foam; allow to stand for 5 min, give within 3 hr

• Give over ≥2 hr, use polyethylene-lined inf with in-line, sterile, low-protein-bind filter

• Do not admix

SIDE EFFECTS

CNS: *Headache, dizziness, depression, vertigo, fatigue, anxiety, fever,* seizures, *chills, flulike symptoms,* demyelinating disease

CV: Chest pain, hypo/hypertension, tachycardia, CHF, acute coronary syndrome

GI: *Nausea, vomiting, abdominal pain, stomatitis, constipation, dyspepsia, flatulence*

GU: Dysuria, urinary frequency

HEMA: Anemia, leukopenia, thrombocytopenia, pancytopenia

INTEG: *Rash, dermatitis, urticaria,* dry skin, sweating, flushing, hematoma, pruritus, keratoderma blenorrhagicum

MS: Myalgia, back pain, arthralgia

RESP: URI, pharyngitis, bronchitis, cough, dyspnea, sinusitis

SYST: Anaphylaxis, fatal infections, sepsis, malignancies, immunogenicity, Stevens-Johnson syndrome, toxic epidermal necrolysis

PHARMACOKINETICS

Distributed to vascular compartment, half-life 9.5 days

INTERACTIONS

• Do not administer live vaccines concurrently

NURSING CONSIDERATIONS

Assess:

• For RA, ROM, pain

• GI symptoms: nausea, vomiting, abdominal pain

• Periodic blood counts (CBC), ANA titer, LFTs

• CV status: B/P, pulse, chest pain

⚠ **Allergic reaction, anaphylaxis:** rash, dermatitis, urticaria, dyspnea, hypotension, fever, chills; discontinue if severe, administer EPINEPHrine, corticosteroids, antihistamines; assess for allergies to murine proteins before starting therapy

Black Box Warning: Fatal infections: discontinue if infection occurs, do not administer to patients with active infection; identify TB before beginning treatment; a TB test should be obtained; if present, TB should be treated before patient receives product; exercise caution when switching from 1 DMARD to another

• Report suspected adverse reactions to the FDA (1-800-FDA-1088)

Black Box Warning: For neoplastic disease in those <18 yr, including hepatosplenic T-cell lymphoma

Perform/provide:

• Refrigerated storage, do not freeze

Evaluate:

• Therapeutic response: absence of fever, mucus in stools

Teach patient/family:

- Not to breastfeed while taking this product
- To notify prescriber of GI symptoms, hypersensitivity reactions, heart symptoms
- Not to operate machinery, drive if dizziness, vertigo occur
- To avoid live virus vaccinations

HIGH ALERT

INSULINS

Rapid Acting

insulin glulisine (Rx)

Apidra, Apidra SoloStar

insulin aspart (Rx)

Novolog, Novolog Flexpen, Novolog Pen Fill, NovoMix 30 ♣, Novo Rapid ♣

insulin lispro (Rx)

Humalog

Short Acting

insulin, regular (OTC)

Humulin R, Novolin R, ReliOn R

insulin, regular concentrated (Rx)

Humulin R U-500

Intermediate Acting

insulin, isophane suspension (NPH) (OTC)

Humulin N, Novolin ge NPH ♣, Novolin N, Novolin N Prefilled, ReliOn N

Long Acting

insulin detemir (Rx)

Levemir

insulin glargine (Rx)

Lantus

Mixtures

insulin, isophane suspension and regular insulin (Rx)

Humulin 70/30, Humulin 30/70 ♣, Novolin 70/30 Prefilled, ReliOn 70/30

isophane insulin suspension (NPH) and insulin mixtures (Rx)

Humulin 50/50

insulin lispro mixture (Rx)

Humalog KwikPen Mix 50/50, Humalog Mix 25 ♣, Humalog Mix 50 ♣, Humalog Mix 75/25, Humalog Mix 50/50

insulin aspart mixture (Rx)

Novolog 70/30, Novolog Mix Flexpen Prefilled Syringe 70/30

Func.class.: Antidiabetic, pancreatic hormone

Chem. class.: Modified structures of endogenous human insulin

Do not confuse:
Lantus/lente
Novolin 70/30 PenFill/Novolin 70/30 Prefilled

ACTION: Decreases blood glucose; by transport of glucose into cells and the conversion of glucose to glycogen, indirectly increases blood pyruvate and lactate, decreases phosphate and potassium; insulin may be human (processed by recombinant DNA technologies)

USES: Type 1 diabetes mellitus, type 2 diabetes mellitus, gestational diabetes; insulin lispro may be used in combination with sulfonylureas in children >3 yr

CONTRAINDICATIONS: Hypersensitivity to protamine; creosol (aspart)

Precautions: Pregnancy (B) lispro, (regular) aspart; (C) all others

DOSAGE AND ROUTES

Insulin glulisine

• **Adult/adolescent/child ≥4 yr: SUBCUT** dosage individualized, give within 15 min before or 20 min after starting a meal; **Adult: IV** dilute to 1 unit/ml in inf systems with 0.9% NaCl, use PVC Viaflex inf bags and PVC tubing, use dedicated line

Insulin aspart

• **Adult/adolescent/child ≥6 yr: INTERMITTENT SUBCUT** Total daily dose is given as 2-4 inj/day just prior to beginning of meal; in general, 50%-70% of total daily insulin may be given as insulin aspart, remainder should be intermediate-or long-acting insulin; **CONTINUOUS SUBCUT** used with external insulin pump via cont SUBCUT insulin inf (CSII), insulin dose should be based on insulin dose from previous regimen

Insulin lispro

• **Adult/adolescent/child ≥3 yr: SUBCUT** 15 min before meals; **CONT SUBCUT INF (external insulin pump):** total daily dose should be based on insulin dose from previous regimen, 50% of total dose can be given as meal-related boluses, remainder as basal inf

Human regular

• **Adult: SUBCUT** ½-1 hr before meals

Insulin, isophane suspension

• **Adult: SUBCUT** dosage individualized by blood, urine glucose; usual dose 7-26 units; may increase by 2-10 units/day if needed

Insulin detemir

• **Adult: SUBCUT** 1-2×/day; if 1×, give with evening meal

Insulin glargine

• **Adult and child ≥6 yr: SUBCUT** 10 international units/day, range 2-100 international units/day

Regular insulin (ketoacidosis)

• **Adult: IV** 5-10 units, then 5-10 units/hr until desired response, then switch to **SUBCUT** dose; **IV/INF** 2-12 units (50 units/500 ml of normal saline)

• **Child: IV** 0.1 units/kg

Replacement

• **Adult and child: SUBCUT** 0.5-1 units/kg/day qid given 30 min before meals

• **Adolescent: SUBCUT** 0.8-1.2 mg/kg/day; this dosage is used during rapid growth

Available forms: ***NPH*** Inj 100 units/ml; ***regular*** inj 100 units/ml, cartridges 100 units/ml; ***insulin analog*** inj 100 units/ml; ***isophane insulin*** inj 100 units/ml, cartridges 100 units/ml; ***insulin lispro*** 100 units/ml, 1.5-ml cartridges, ***insulin lispro*** Humalog Pen sol for inj 100 units/ml; ***insulin glulisine*** inj 100 units/ml; ***insulin glargine*** inj 100 units/ml; ***insulin detemir*** inj 100 units/ml in 10 vials, 3-ml cartridges; ***insulin aspart*** inj 100 mg/ml (Flexpen, Pen Fill)

Administer:

SUBCUT route

• After warming to room temp by rotating in palms to prevent injecting cold insulin; use only insulin syringes with markings or syringe matching units/ml; rotate inj sites within one area: abdomen, upper back, thighs, upper arm, buttocks; keep record of sites

• Increased dosages if tolerance occurs

• Premixed insulins, NPH are cloudy suspensions

• Regular human insulin, rapid-acting analogs, long-acting analogs are clear; do not use if cloudy, thick, or discolored

CONT SUBCUT route (insulin infusion CSII)

• Do not mix with other insulins when using a pump

• Insulin lispro 3-ml cartridges to be used in Disetronic H-TRON plus V100 pump using Disetronic rapid inf sets; inf set and cartridge adapter should be changed q3days; replace 3-ml cartridge q6days

IV route (insulin glulisine only)

• Dilute to 1 international unit/ml in inf systems with 0.9% NaCl using PVC viaflex inf bags and PVC tubing; use dedicated line; do not admix

IV route (regular only)

⚠ **When regular insulin is administered IV, monitor glucose, potassium often to prevent fatal hypoglycemia, hypokalemia**

• IV direct, undiluted via vein, Y-site, 3-way stopcock; give at ≤50 units/min

• By cont inf after diluting with IV sol and run at prescribed rate; use IV inf pump for correct dosing; give reduced dose at serum glucose level of 250 mg/100 ml

Additive compatibilities: Cimetidine, lidocaine, meropenem, ranitidine, verapamil

Y-site compatibilities: Amiodarone, ampicillin, ampicillin/sulbactam, aztreonam, ceFAZolin, cefotetan, DOBUTamine, esmolol, famotidine, gentamicin, heparin, heparin/hydrocortisone, imipenem/cilastatin, indomethacin, magnesium sulfate, meperidine, meropenem, midazolam, morphine, nitroglycerin, oxytocin, PENTobarbital, potassium chloride, propofol, ritodrine, sodium bicarbonate, sodium nitroprusside, tacrolimus, terbutaline, ticarcillin, ticarcillin/clavulanate, tobramycin, vancomycin, vit B/C

SIDE EFFECTS

EENT: Blurred vision, dry mouth

INTEG: Flushing, rash, urticaria, warmth, lipodystrophy, lipohypertrophy, swelling, redness

META: *Hypoglycemia,* rebound hyperglycemia (Somogyi effect 12-72 hr or longer)

MISC: Peripheral edema

SYST: **Anaphylaxis**

PHARMACOKINETICS

Rapid acting

Insulin glulisine: Onset 15-30 min, peak ½-1½ hr, duration 3-4 hr

Insulin aspart: Onset 10-20 min, peak 1-3 hr, duration 3-5 hr

Insulin lispro: Onset 15-30 min, peak ½-1½ hr, duration 3-5 hr

Short acting

Insulin regular: Onset 30 min, peak 2.5-5 hr, duration up to 7 hr

Intermediate acting

Insulin, isophane suspension (NPH): Onset 1.5-4 hr, peak 4-12 hr, duration ≤24 hr

Long acting

Insulin detemir: Onset 0.8-2 hr, peak unknown, duration ≤24 hr (conc dependent)

Insulin glargine: Onset 1.5 hr, no peak identified, duration ≥24 hr

Mixtures

Insulin, isophane suspension and regular insulin (70/30): Onset 10-20 min, peak 2.4 hr, duration ≤24 hr

Insophane insulin suspension (NPH) and insulin mixtures (50/50): Onset ½-1 hr, peak dual, duration 10-16 hr

INTERACTIONS

Increase: hypoglycemia—salicylate, alcohol, β-blockers, anabolic steroids, fenfluramine, phenylbutazone, sulfinpyrazone, guanethidine, oral hypoglycemics, MAOIs, tetracycline

Decrease: hypoglycemia—thiazides, thyroid hormones, oral contraceptives, corticosteroids, estrogens, DOBUTamine, EPINEPHrine

Drug/Lab Test

Increase: VMA

Decrease: potassium, calcium

Interference: LFTs, thyroid function studies

NURSING CONSIDERATIONS

Assess:

• Fasting blood glucose; A1c may be drawn to identify treatment effectiveness q3mo

• Urine ketones during illness; insulin requirements may increase during stress, illness, surgery

• Hypoglycemic reaction that can occur during peak time (sweating, weakness, dizziness, chills, confusion, headache, nausea, rapid weak pulse, fatigue, tachy-

cardia, memory lapses, slurred speech, staggering gait, anxiety, tremors, hunger)
• Hyperglycemia: acetone breath; polyuria; fatigue; polydipsia; flushed, dry skin; lethargy

Perform/provide:
• Store at room temp for <1 mo (some insulins); keep away from heat and sunlight; refrigerate all other supply; NPH, premixed insulins are cloudy; regular, rapid-acting analogs, long-acting analogs are clear; do not freeze—IV route, regular only

Evaluate:
• Therapeutic response: decrease in polyuria, polydipsia, polyphagia; clear sensorium; absence of dizziness; stable gait

Teach patient/family:
• That blurred vision occurs; not to change corrective lens until vision is stabilized after 1-2 mo
• To keep insulin, equipment available at all times; to carry a glucagon kit, candy, or lump of sugar to treat hypoglycemia
• That product does not cure diabetes but controls symptoms
• To carry emergency ID as diabetic
• To recognize hypoglycemia reaction: headache, tremors, fatigue, weakness
• To recognize hyperglycemia reaction: frequent urination, thirst, fatigue, hunger
• About the dosage, route, mixing instructions, diet restrictions (if any), disease process
• About the symptoms of ketoacidosis: nausea; thirst; polyuria; dry mouth; decreased B/P; dry, flushed skin; acetone breath; drowsiness; Kussmaul respirations
• That a plan is necessary for diet, exercise; that all food on diet should be eaten; that exercise routine should not vary
• About blood glucose testing; how to determine glucose level
• To avoid OTC products unless directed by prescriber

TREATMENT OF OVERDOSE:
Glucose 25 g IV, via dextrose 50% sol, 50 ml or glucagon 1 mg

interferon alfa-2b (recombinant) (Rx)

Intron A

Func. class.: Antineoplastic—miscellaneous

Chem. class.: Protein product

Do not confuse:
Roferon-A/Imferon

ACTION:
Antiviral action inhibits viral replication by reprogramming virus; antitumor action suppresses cell proliferation; immunomodulating action phagocytizes target cells; may also inhibit virus replication in virus-infested cells

USES:
Hairy-cell leukemia in persons >18 yr; condylomata acuminata; chronic hepatitis C, hepatitis B; malignant melanoma; non-Hodgkin's lymphoma

Unlabeled uses: Bladder cancer, carcinoid tumors, Kaposi's sarcoma, chronic myelogenous leukemia, hemangioma, hypereosinophilic syndrome, multiple myeloma, ovarian/renal cell cancer, St. Louis encephalitis, West Nile virus infection

CONTRAINDICATIONS:
Hypersensitivity

Precautions: Pregnancy (C), breastfeeding, children, severe hypotension, dysrhythmia, tachycardia, severe renal/hepatic disease, seizure disorder, optic neuritis, ocular/pulmonary/thyroid disease

Black Box Warning: Autoimmune disorders, cardiac disease, infection, depression

DOSAGE AND ROUTES

Hairy-cell leukemia
• **Adult: SUBCUT/IM** 2 million international units/m^2 3×/wk up to 6 mo

Condylomata acuminata

• **Adult: INTRALESIONAL** 1 million international units (0.1 ml) inj into each lesion 3×/wk on alternating days for 3 wk, treat ≤5 warts per course

Chronic hepatitis B

• **Adult: SUBCUT/IM** 30-35 million international units/wk × 16 wk given 5 million international units/day or 10 million international units 3×/wk

Kaposi's sarcoma

• **Adult: SUBCUT/IM** 30 million international units/m^2 3×/wk

Renal cell cancer (unlabeled)

• **Adult: SUBCUT** 5-18 million international units/m^2/day 3×/wk alone or in combination with interleukin-2, 5-fluorouracil, or vinBLASTine

Available forms: Inj 3, 5, 10, 18, 25 million units/vial, powder for inj 10, 18, 50 million units/vial

Administer:

• IM/SUBCUT after reconstituting 3-5 million international units/1 ml, 10 million international units/2 ml, 25 million international units/5 ml of diluent provided; mix gently, do not shake

• Each brand has different dilution directions; check package insert

• Intralesional: after reconstituting 10 million international units/1 ml bacteriostatic water for inj; ≤5 lesions can safely be treated at a time

• At bedtime to minimize side effects

• Acetaminophen as ordered to alleviate fever and headache

SIDE EFFECTS

CNS: *Dizziness, confusion, numbness, paresthesias,* hallucinations, **seizures,** **coma,** amnesia, anxiety, mood changes, depression, somnolence, paranoia, irritability, hostility, encephalopathy

CV: *Edema, hypotension,* hypertension, chest pain, palpitations, dysrhythmias, **CHF, MI, CVA,** tachycardia, syncope

GI: *Weight loss, taste changes,* nausea, anorexia, diarrhea, xerostomia

GU: *Impotence*

HEMA: **Neutropenia, thrombocytopenia**

INTEG: *Rash, dry skin, itching, alopecia,* flushing, photosensitivity, **serious skin infection**

MISC: *Flulike syndrome; fever, fatigue, myalgias, headache, chills,* optic neuritis, **anaphylaxis, angioedema**

PHARMACOKINETICS

Half-life 2-7 hr, peak 6-8 hr

INTERACTIONS

Increase: aminophylline levels—aminophylline

Increase: neutropenia—clozapine, warfarin, zidovudine

Drug/Lab Test

Interference: AST, ALT, LDH, alk phos, WBC, platelets, granulocytes, creatinine

NURSING CONSIDERATIONS

Assess:

• Symptoms of infection; chills, fever, headache; may be masked by product fever

• CNS reaction: LOC, mental status, dizziness, confusion, paresthesia, slurred speech, anxiety, depression, paranoia, hallucinations, suicidal thoughts

• Cardiac status: lung sounds; ECG before and during treatment, especially in those with cardiac disease; MI, CHF, CVA, hypo/hypertension may occur; LFTs, thyroid function tests

• Bone marrow depression: bruising, bleeding, blood in stools, urine, sputum, emesis

• CBC with differential before and during treatment, nadirs of leukopenia/thrombocytopenia occur after 18-19 days (alfa-2a); recovery after 3-4 wk; if granulocytes <750/mm^3 or platelets <50,000/mm^2, reduce by 50%; if granulocytes <500/mm^3 or platelets <30,000/mm^2, discontinue product

Perform/provide:

• Reconstituted sol must be used within 24 hr

• Increased fluid intake to 2-3 L/day

Evaluate:
- Therapeutic response: improved blood counts; improvement or slowed disease progression

Teach patient/family:
- To take acetaminophen for fever
- To avoid hazardous tasks, since confusion, dizziness may occur; to avoid prolonged sunlight; to use sunscreen
- That brands of this product should not be changed; that each form is different, with different doses
- That fatigue is common; that activity may have to be altered; to take at bedtime to minimize flulike symptoms
- Not to become pregnant while taking product; possible mutagenic effects
- To report signs of infection: sore throat, fever, diarrhea, vomiting, sore or white patches in mouth
- That impotence may occur during treatment but is temporary
- That suicidal ideation is common; notify prescriber if severe or incapacitating

interferon alfacon-1 (Rx)

(in-ter-feer′on al′fa-kon)

Infergen

Func. class.: Recombinant type 1 interferon

ACTION: Induces biologic responses and has antiviral, antiproliferative, and immunomodulatory effects

USES: Chronic hepatitis C infections in those ≥18 yr with compensated liver disease who have anti-HCV antibodies or HCV RNA, may use in combination with ribavirin

Unlabeled uses: Hairy-cell leukemia when used with G-CSF

CONTRAINDICATIONS: Hypersensitivity to α-interferons or products from *Escherichia coli;* decompensated hepatic disease, autoimmune hepatitis

Precautions: Pregnancy (C), breastfeeding, children <18 yr, geriatric patients, thyroid disorders, myelosuppression, hepatic disease, seizure disorder, alcoholism, hepatitis

Black Box Warning: Cardiac disease, autoimmune disease, infection, depression

DOSAGE AND ROUTES

- **Adult: SUBCUT monotherapy** 9 mcg as single inj 3×/wk × 24 wk; leave ≥48 hr between injections; for patients who did not respond or relapsed after discontinuation, give 15 mcg 3×/wk × 48 wk; **combination: SUBCUT** 15 mcg daily with ribavirin 1000 mg/day PO (<75 kg), 1200 mg/day PO (≥75 kg); give in 2 divided doses for up to 48 wks, use stepwise dose reduction of the interferon dose from 15 mcg to 9 mcg to 6 mcg for serious adverse reactions

Available forms: Inj 9 mcg/0.3 ml, 15 mcg/0.5 ml

Administer:
- Premedicate with acetaminophen or ibuprofen
- Do not shake vial; use 1 dose per vial; discard unused portion; use proper inj sites; rotate sites
- Do not miss doses

SIDE EFFECTS

CNS: Depression, headache, fatigue, fever, rigors, insomnia, dizziness, agitation, nervousness, anxiety, lability, abnormal thinking

CV: Hypertension, palpitation, tachycardia

EENT: Tinnitus, earache, conjunctivitis, eye pain

GI: Abdominal pain, nausea, diarrhea, anorexia, dyspepsia, vomiting, constipation, flatulence, hemorrhoids, decreased salivation

GU: Dysmenorrhea, vaginitis, menstrual disorders

HEMA: **Granulocytopenia, thrombocytopenia, leukopenia,** ecchymosis, **aplastic anemia**

INTEG: Alopecia, pruritus, rash, erythema, dry skin

MISC: Anaphylaxis, angioedema, flulike illness
MS: Back, limb, neck skeletal pain; rigors
RESP: Pharyngitis, upper respiratory infection, cough, sinusitis, rhinitis, respiratory tract congestion, epistaxis, dyspnea, bronchitis

PHARMACOKINETICS

Peak 1-4 hr, peak biologic response 24-36 hr

INTERACTIONS

Increase: myelosuppression—myelosuppressives
Increase: toxicity—aldesleukin, IL-2 eflornithine, theophylline
Decrease: effect of—antiretrovirals (NNRTIs, NRTIs, protease inhibitors)

NURSING CONSIDERATIONS

Assess:

- Past or present history of depression, seizures; use with caution with these disorders
- Ophthalmologic status; report periodically
- CBC, LFTs, ECG, platelet counts, heme concentration, ANC, serum creatinine, albumin, bilirubin, TSH, T_4, triglycerides at baseline and periodically
- Myelosuppression: hold dose if neutrophil count is $<500 \times 10^6$/L or if platelets are $<50 \times 10^9$/L
- For hypersensitivity: discontinue immediately if hypersensitivity occurs

Evaluate:

- Therapeutic response: decreased chronic hepatitis C signs/symptoms

Teach patient/family:

- With detailed written information about product
- To report signs, symptoms of infection, thyroid/liver dysfunction, changes in behavior

interferon alfa-n3 (Rx)

(in-ter-feer'on)

Alferon N

Func. class.: Antineoplastic, antiviral
Chem. class.: Human interferon α-protein

ACTION: Binds interferon to membrane receptors on cell surface with high specificity; inhibition of virus replication, suppression of cell proliferation, increased phagocytosis

USES: Condylomata acuminata (venereal/genital warts), papillomavirus
Unlabeled uses: Adenovirus, coronavirus, encephalomyocarditis virus, hepatitis B virus, hepatitis C infection/virus, hepatitis D, herpes simplex type 1 and 2, HIV, HTLV-I, poliovirus, rhinovirus, varicella-zoster virus, variola virus, vesicular stomatitis virus

CONTRAINDICATIONS: Hypersensitivity to this product, egg protein, IgG, neomycin, murine protein
Precautions: Pregnancy (C), breastfeeding, children, CHF, angina (unstable), COPD, diabetes mellitus with ketoacidosis, hemophilia, PE, thrombophlebitis, bone marrow depression, seizure disorder, hepatic/thyroid disease, suicidal ideation, albumin hypersensitivity, infection

DOSAGE AND ROUTES

External condylomata acuminata

- **Adult: INTRALESIONAL** 0.05 ml (250,000 international units) per wart, given 2×/wk × 8 wk; not to exceed 0.5 ml (2.5 million international units); inject into base of wart

Chronic hepatitis C (unlabeled)

- **Adult: SUBCUT/IM** 10 million international units 3×/wk × 6 mo (monotherapy); 3 million international units 3×/wk plus ribavirin 1000 mg **PO** daily × 6 mo (combination)

Available forms: Inj 5 million international units/ml vial

Administer:

• Acetaminophen to alleviate fever and headache

SIDE EFFECTS

CNS: *Fever, headache,* sweating, vasovagal reaction, chills, fatigue, dizziness, insomnia, sleepiness, depression, suicidal ideation
CV: *Chest pain, hypotension*
GI: *Nausea, vomiting, heartburn, diarrhea, constipation, anorexia, stomatitis, dry mouth,* taste disturbance
INTEG: *Pain at inj site, pruritus,* pyrosis
MISC: Flulike symptoms
MS: *Myalgias, arthralgia, back pain*

PHARMACOKINETICS

Unable to detect

INTERACTIONS

Increase: toxicity—aldesleukin, IL-2, eflornithine, theophylline
Decrease: effect of—antiretrovirals (NNRTs, NRTIs, protease inhibitors)
Drug/Lab Test
Interference: AST, ALT, LDH, alk phos, WBC, platelets, granulocytes, creatinine

NURSING CONSIDERATIONS

Assess:

• For flulike symptoms; may be masked by drug fever
• CNS reaction: LOC, mental status, dizziness, confusion, insomnia, depression, suicidal ideation
• For body image disturbance

Perform/provide:

• Storage of reconstituted sol for 1 mo in refrigerator
• Increased fluid intake to 2-3 L/day

Evaluate:

• Therapeutic response: decrease in wart size

Teach patient/family:

• To avoid hazardous tasks, since confusion, dizziness may occur
• That brands of this product should not be changed; that each form is different, with different doses
• That fatigue is common; activity may have to be altered
• Not to become pregnant while taking product; possible mutagenic effects
• To report signs of infection: sore throat, fever, diarrhea, vomiting
• To recognize signs of hypersensitivity: liver, urticaria, wheezing, dyspnea; to notify prescriber immediately
• That suicidal thoughts/behaviors may occur

interferon beta-1a (Rx)

(in-ter-feer′on)

Avonex, Rebif

interferon beta-1b (Rx)

Betaseron, Extavia

Func. class.: Multiple sclerosis agent, immune modifier

Chem. class.: Interferon, *Escherichia coli* derivative

ACTION: Antiviral, immunoregulatory; action not clearly understood; biologic response-modifying properties mediated through specific receptors on cells, inducing expression of interferon-induced gene products

USES: Ambulatory patients with relapsing or remitting MS

Unlabeled uses: May be useful for treatment of AIDS, AIDS-related Kaposi's sarcoma, malignant melanoma, metastatic renal cell carcinoma, cutaneous T-cell lymphoma, acute non-A/non-B hepatitis, chronic hepatitis C

CONTRAINDICATIONS: Hypersensitivity to natural or recombinant interferon-β or human albumin, hamster protein, rotovirus vaccine

Precautions: Pregnancy (C), breastfeeding, children <18 yr, chronic progressive MS, depression, mental disorders, seizure disorder, latex allergy, autoimmune disorders, bone marrow suppression, hepatotoxicity, cardiac disease, alcoholism, chickenpox, herpes zoster

DOSAGE AND ROUTES

Interferon beta-1a

Remitting or relapsing multiple sclerosis

- **Adult: IM** (Avonex) 30 mcg/wk
- **Adult: SUBCUT** (Rebif) 22 or 44 mcg 3×/wk with each dose 48 hr apart, titrate to full dose over 4-wk period

Chronic hepatitis C (unlabeled)

- **Adult: SUBCUT** (Rebif) 44 mcg 3×/wk × 24 wk

Interferon beta-1b

Relapsing or remitting multiple sclerosis

- **Adult: SUBCUT** 0.0625 mg every other day for wk 1 and 2, then 0.125 mg every other day for wk 3 and 4, then 0.1875 mg every other day for wk 5 and 6, then 0.25 mg every other day thereafter; higher doses should not be used

Available forms: *beta-1a:* (Avonex) 30 mcg (6.6 million international units/vial); (Rebif) 22 mcg, 44 mcg/0.5 ml; *beta-1b:* powder for inj 0.3 mg (9.6 m international units) Kit

Administer:

- Acetaminophen for fever, headache
- Products are not interchangeable
- In evening to minimize adverse effects

SIDE EFFECTS

CNS: *Headache, fever, pain, chills, mental changes, depression,* hypertonia, suicide attempts, seizures

CV: *Migraine, palpitations, hypertension,* tachycardia, peripheral vascular disorders

EENT: *Conjunctivitis,* blurred vision

GI: *Diarrhea, constipation, vomiting, abdominal pain*

GU: *Dysmenorrhea, irregular menses, metrorrhagia,* cystitis, breast pain

HEMA: Decreased lymphocytes, ANC, WBC; *lymphadenopathy,* anemia

INTEG: *Sweating, inj site reaction*

MS: *Myalgia,* myasthenia

RESP: *Sinusitis,* dyspnea

PHARMACOKINETICS

β-1a: Onset ≤12 hr, peak 48 hr, duration 4 days, half-life 8.6 hr

β-1b: Onset rapid, peak 2-8 hr, duration unknown, half-life 8 min-4.3 hr

INTERACTIONS

Increase: hepatic damage—antiretrovirals (NNRTIs, NRTIs, protease inhibitors)

Increase: myelosuppression—antineoplastics

Decrease: clearance of zidovudine

Drug/Herb

- Change in immunomodulation: astragalus, echinacea, melatonin

Drug/Lab Test

Interference: vaccines, toxoids; avoid concurrent use

Increase: LFTs

NURSING CONSIDERATIONS

Assess:

- Blood, hepatic studies: CBC, differential, platelet counts, BUN, creatinine ALT, urinalysis; if absolute neutrophil count <750/mm^3 or if AST/ALT is 10× normal, discontinue product
- CNS symptoms: headache, fatigue, depression
- GI status: diarrhea or constipation, vomiting, abdominal pain
- Cardiac status: increased B/P, tachycardia
- Mental status: depression, depersonalization, suicidal thoughts, insomnia
- Multiple sclerosis symptoms

Interferon β-1a

- Reconstitute with 1.1-ml diluent, swirl, give within 6 hr, warm to room temp before administration

Interferon β-1b

- Reconstitute by injecting diluent provided (1.2 ml) into vial; swirl (8 m international units/ml); use 27G needle for inj

Perform/provide:

- Storage in refrigerator; do not freeze

Evaluate:

- Therapeutic response: decreased symptoms of multiple sclerosis

Teach patient/family:

- With written, detailed information about product
- That blurred vision, sweating may occur
- That female patients may experience irregular menses, dysmenorrhea or metrorrhagia, breast pain
- To use sunscreen to prevent photosensitivity
- To notify prescriber if pregnancy is suspected
- About inj technique, care of equipment
- To notify prescriber of increased temp, chills, muscle soreness, fatigue, depression, symptoms of hepatotoxicity

interferon gamma-1b (Rx)

(in-ter-feer'on)

Actimmune

Func. class.: Biologic response modifier

Chem. class.: Lymphokine, interleukin type

ACTION: Species-specific protein synthesized in response to viruses, effects; can mediate killing of *Staphylococcus aureus, Toxoplasma gondii, Leishmania donovani, Listeria monocytogenes, Mycobacterium avium intracellulare;* enhances oxidative metabolism of macrophages, enhances antibody-dependent cellular cytotoxicity

USES: Serious infections associated with chronic granulomatous disease, osteopetrosis

Unlabeled uses: *Mycobacterium avium* complex (MAC), pulmonary fibrosis

CONTRAINDICATIONS: Hypersensitivity to interferon-γ, *Escherichia coli*–derived products

Precautions: Pregnancy (C), breastfeeding, children <1 yr, cardiac disease, seizure disorders, CNS disorders, myelosuppression

DOSAGE AND ROUTES

- **Adult: SUBCUT** 50 mcg/m^2 (1.5 million units/m^2) for patients with surface area >0.5 m^2; 1.5 mcg/kg/dose for patients with surface area <0.5 m^2; give Monday, Wednesday, Friday for 3×/wk dosing

Available forms: Inj 100 mcg (2 million units)/single-dose vial

Administer:

- At bedtime to minimize adverse reactions; give acetaminophen for fever, headache
- 50% of dose if severe reactions occur or discontinue treatment until reactions subside
- In right and left deltoid and anterior thigh
- Warm to room temp before use; do not leave at room temp >12 hr (unopened vial)

SIDE EFFECTS

CNS: *Headache, fatigue,* depression, fever, chills

GI: *Nausea, anorexia,* abdominal pain, weight loss, diarrhea, vomiting, colitis

HEMA: Leukopenia, thrombocytopenia, neutropenia

INTEG: Rash, pain at inj site, Stevens-Johnson syndrome

MS: Myalgia, arthralgia

PHARMACOKINETICS

SUBCUT: Dose absorbed 89%, elimination half-life 5.9 hr, peak 7 hr

INTERACTIONS

Increase: myelosuppression—other myelosuppressive agents

Increase: level of theophylline, aminophylline

Increase: liver toxicity—protease inhibitors, nucleoside reverse transcriptase inhibitors (NRTIs), nonnucleoside reverse transcriptase inhibitors (NNRTIs)

NURSING CONSIDERATIONS

Assess:

- Blood, renal, hepatic studies: CBC, differential, platelet counts, BUN, creatinine, ALT, urinalysis
- CNS symptoms: headache, fatigue, depression

Perform/provide:

- Storage in refrigerator upon receipt; do not freeze; do not shake

Evaluate:

- Therapeutic response: decreased serious infections; improvement in existing infections and inflammatory conditions

Teach patient/family:

- About the method of administration if family members will be giving medication
- With written, detailed information about product

ipilimumab

(ip-i-lim′ue-mab)

Yervoy

Func. class.: Antineoplastic; biologic response modifier

ACTION: A recombinant, human monoclonal antibody that binds to the cytotoxic T-lymphocyte-associated antigen 4 (CTLA-4); action is indirect, possibly through T-cell–mediated anti-tumor immune responses

USES: Treatment of unresectable or metastatic malignant melanoma

CONTRAINDICATIONS Hypersensitivity

Precautions: Pregnancy, breastfeeding, Crohn's disease, hepatitis, immunosuppression, inflammatory bowel disease, iritis, ocular disease, organ transplant, pancreatitis, renal disease, rheumatoid arthritis, sarcoidosis, systemic lupus erythematosus, thyroid disease, ulcerative colitis, uveitis

Black Box Warning: Adrenal insufficiency, diarrhea, Guillain-Barré syndrome, hepatic disease, myasthenia gravis, hypo/hyperthyroidism, hypopituitarism, peripheral neuropathy, serious rash

DOSAGE AND ROUTES

- **Adult/geriatric: IV** 3 mg/kg over 90 min q3wk × 4 doses; permanently discontinue if the full treatment course is not completed within 16 wk from 1st dose or for severe or life-threatening adverse reactions; withhold a dose for any moderate endocrine or immune-mediated adverse reactions; if the moderate adverse reaction completely or partially resolves (Grade 0-1) and if the patient is receiving <7.5 mg predniSONE or equivalent/day, resume at a dose of 3 mg/kg IV q3wk until all 4 planned doses or 16 wk from 1st dose, whichever occurs earlier; if moderate adverse reactions are persistent or if the corticosteroid dose cannot be reduced to 7.5 mg predniSONE or equivalent/day, permanently discontinue

Available forms: Sol for inj 50 mg/10 ml, 200 mg/40 ml

Administer:

Intermittent IV INF route

- Visually inspect parenteral products for particulate matter and discoloration before using whenever sol and container permit; sol may have a pale yellow color and have translucent to white, amorphous particles; discard the vial if sol is cloudy, if there is pronounced discoloration, or if particulate matter is present
- Allow vials to stand at room temperature for 5 min before inf preparation; withdraw the required volume and transfer into an IV bag; discard partially used vials or empty vials; dilute with 0.9% sodium chloride injection or 5% dextrose injection to a final conc (1-2 mg/ml); mix diluted sol by gentle inversion; do not admix

• Give inf over 90 min through an IV line with a low-protein binding in-line filter, do not give with other products; after each inf, flush the line with 0.9% sodium chloride injection or 0.5% dextrose injection

SIDE EFFECTS

CNS: Severe and fatal immune-mediated neuropathies, fatigue, headache, fever
EENT: Uveitis, iritis, episcleritis
ENDO: Severe and fatal immune-mediated endocrinopathies
GI: Severe and fatal immune-mediated enterocolitis, hepatitis, pancreatitis, abdominal pain, nausea, diarrhea, appetite decreased, vomiting, constipation, colitis
INTEG: Severe and fatal immune-mediated dermatitis pruritus, rash, urticaria
MISC: Cough, dyspnea, anemia, eosinophilia, nephritis
SYST: Antibody formation, Stevens-Johnson syndrome, toxic epidermal necrolysis

PHARMACOKINETICS:

Steady state by 3rd dose; terminal half-life 14.7 days

NURSING CONSIDERATIONS

• Serious skin disorders: Stevens-Johnson syndrome, toxic epidermal necrolysis: permanently discontinue in these or rash complicated by full thickness dermal ulceration or necrotic, bullous, or hemorrhagic manifestations like bullous rash; give systemic corticosteroids at a dose of 1-2 mg/kg/day of predniSONE or equivalent; when dermatitis is controlled, taper corticosteroids over a period of at least 1 mo, withhold in patients with moderate to severe reactions; for mild to moderate dermatitis (localized rash and pruritus), give topical or systemic corticosteroids
• Hepatotoxicity: monitor liver functions tests baseline and before each dose to rule out infectious or malignant causes, increase the frequency of liver function test monitoring until resolution, permanently discontinue in patients with Grade 3-5, give systemic corticosteroids at a dose of 1-2 mg/kg/day of predniSONE or equivalent
• Neuropathy: monitor for motor or sensory neuropathy (unilateral or bilateral weakness, sensory alterations, or paresthesias) before each dose; permanently discontinue if severe neuropathy (interfering with daily activities), such as Guillain-Barré–like syndromes, occur
• Endocrinopathy: monitor thyroid function tests at baseline and before each dose; monitor hypophysitis, adrenal insufficiency, adrenal crisis, hypo/hyperthyroidism (fatigue, headache, mental status changes, abdominal pain, unusual bowel habits, hypotension, or nonspecific symptoms that may resemble other causes)

Perform/provide:
• Storage once diluted for no more than 24 hr refrigerated or at room temperature

Evaluate:
Decreasing spread of malignant melanoma

Teach patient/family:
• To immediately report allergic reactions, skin rash, severe abdominal pain, yellowing of skin or eyes, tingling of extremities, change in bowel habits
• About the reason for treatment and expected results

ipratropium (Rx)

(i-pra-troe′pee-um)

Atrovent HFA

Func. class.: Anticholinergic, bronchodilator
Chem. class.: Synthetic quaternary ammonium compound

Do not confuse:
Atrovent/Alupent

ACTION: Inhibits interaction of acetylcholine at receptor sites on the bronchial smooth muscle, thereby resulting in decreased cGMP and bronchodilation

USES:
COPD; rhinorrhea (nasal spray)

CONTRAINDICATIONS:
Hypersensitivity to this product, atropine, bromide, soybean or peanut products

Precautions: Breastfeeding, children <12 yr, angioedema, heart failure, surgery, acute bronchospasm, bladder obstruction, closed-angle glaucoma, prostatic hypertrophy, urinary retention, pregnancy (B)

DOSAGE AND ROUTES

- **Adult: INH** 2 sprays (17 mcg/spray) 3-4×/day, max 12 **INH**/24 hr; **SOL** 500 mcg (1 unit dose) given 3-4×/day by nebulizer; nasal spray: 2 sprays (42 mcg/spray) 3-4×/day
- **Child 5-11 yr: INH** 4-8 inhalations q20min as needed for ≤3 hr (asthma, unlabeled); **NEB** 250-500 mcg q20min as needed for ≤3 hr (asthma, unlabeled)
- **Child 5-12 yr: INTRANASAL** 2 sprays in each nostril 3×/day

Available forms: Aerosol 17 mcg/actuation; nasal spray 0.03%, 0.06%; sol for inh 0.0125% ♣, 0.02%

Administer:

Nebulizer route

- Use sol in nebulizer with a mouthpiece rather than a face mask

Intranasal route

- Priming pump initially requires 7 actuations of pump; priming again is not necessary if used regularly

SIDE EFFECTS

CNS: *Anxiety, dizziness, headache,* nervousness

CV: Palpitation

EENT: Dry mouth, blurred vision, nasal congestion

GI: *Nausea, vomiting, cramps*

INTEG: Rash

RESP: *Cough, worsening of symptoms,* bronchospasms

PHARMACOKINETICS

Half-life 2 hr, does not cross blood-brain barrier

INTERACTIONS

Increase: toxicity—other bronchodilators (INH)

Increase: anticholinergic action—phenothiazines, antihistamines, disopyramide

Drug/Herb

Increase: anticholinergic effect—belladonna

Increase: bronchodilator effect—green tea (large amts), guarana

NURSING CONSIDERATIONS

Assess:

- Palpitations; if severe, product may have to be changed
- Tolerance over long-term therapy; dose may have to be increased or changed
- Atropine sensitivity; patient may also be sensitive to this product
- Respiratory status: rate, rhythm, auscultate breath sounds prior to and after administration

Perform/provide:

- Storage at room temp
- Hard candy, frequent drinks, sugarless gum to relieve dry mouth

Evaluate:

- Therapeutic response: ability to breathe adequately

Teach patient/family:

- That compliance is necessary with number of inhalations/24 hr or overdose may occur; about spacer device for geriatric patients; that max therapeutic effects may take 2-3 mo
- To shake before using
- About the correct method of inhalation; how to clean equipment daily

irbesartan (Rx)

(er-be-sar′tan)

Avapro

Func. class.: Antihypertensive

Chem. class.: Angiotensin II receptor blocker (Type AT_1)

Do not confuse:
Avapro/Anaprox

ACTION: Blocks the vasoconstrictor and aldosterone-secreting effects of angiotensin II; selectively blocks the binding of angiotensin II to the AT_1 receptor found in tissues

USES: Hypertension, alone or in combination; nephropathy in type 2 diabetic patients; proteinuria

Unlabeled uses: Heart failure

CONTRAINDICATIONS: Hypersensitivity

Black Box Warning: Pregnancy (D) 2nd/3rd trimester

Precautions: Pregnancy (C) 1st trimester, breastfeeding, children <6 yr, geriatric patients, hypersensitivity to ACE inhibitors; hepatic/renal disease; renal artery stenosis

DOSAGES AND ROUTES

Hypertension

• **Adult: PO** 150 mg/day; may be increased to 300 mg/day, volume-depleted patients: start with 75 mg/day

Nephropathy in type 2 diabetic patients

• **Adult: PO** maintenance dose 300 mg/day, start 75 mg/day

Available forms: Tabs 75, 150, 300 mg

Administer:

• Without regard to meals

SIDE EFFECTS

CNS: *Dizziness,* anxiety, headache, fatigue

CV: Hypotension

GI: Diarrhea, dyspepsia

MISC: Edema, chest pain, rash, tachycardia, UTI, angioedema, hyperkalemia

RESP: *Cough, upper respiratory tract infection,* sinus disorder, pharyngitis, rhinitis

PHARMACOKINETICS

Peak 1.5-2 hr, extensively metabolized, half-life 11-15 hr, highly bound to plasma proteins, excreted in urine and feces, protein binding 90%

INTERACTIONS

Increase: hyperkalemia: potassium-sparing diuretics, potassium salt substitutes, ACE inhibitors

Increase: irbesartan level—CYP2C9 inhibitors (amiodarone, delavirdine, fluconazole, fluoxetine, fluvastatin, fluvoxamine, imatinib, sulfonamides, sulfinpyrazone, voriconazole, zafirlukast)

Decrease: antihypertensive effect—NSAIDs

Drug/Herb

Increase: antihypertensive effect—black cohosh, goldenseal, hawthorn, kelp

Increase or decrease: antihypertensive effect—astragalus, cola tree

Decrease: antihypertensive effect—guarana, khat, licorice, yohimbe

NURSING CONSIDERATIONS

Assess:

• B/P, pulse q4hr; note rate, rhythm, quality

• Baselines of renal/hepatic studies before therapy begins; periodically monitor LFTs, total/direct bilirubin

• Skin turgor, dryness of mucous membranes for hydration status; edema in feet, legs daily

Evaluate:

• Therapeutic response: decreased B/P

Teach patient/family:

• To comply with dosage schedule, even if feeling better; that max therapeutic effects may take 2-3 mo

• That product may cause dizziness, fainting, lightheadedness

• To rise slowly to sitting or standing position to minimize orthostatic hypotension

Black Box Warning: To notify prescriber if pregnancy is suspected; discontinue if pregnant

⚠ HIGH ALERT

irinotecan (Rx)

(ear-een-oh-tee′kan)

Camptosar

Func. class.: Antineoplastic

Chem. class.: Camptothecin analog

ACTION: Cytotoxic by producing damage to single-strand DNA during DNA synthesis; binds to topoisomerase I

USES: Metastatic carcinoma of the colon or rectum or 1st-line treatment in combination with 5-FU and leucovorin for metastatic colon or rectal carcinomas

Unlabeled uses: Cervical, gastric, lung, ovarian, pancreatic cancer, malignant glioma, rhabdomyosarcoma

CONTRAINDICATIONS: Pregnancy (D), hypersensitivity

Precautions: Breastfeeding, children, geriatric patients, irradiation, hepatic disease

Black Box Warning: Myelosuppression, diarrhea

DOSAGE AND ROUTES

Single agent

• **Adult: IV** 125 mg/m^2 given over 1$^1/_2$ hr weekly × 4 wk, q6wk

Combination dosage schedules

• **Regimen 1:** Irinotecan 75-125 mg/m^2, leucovorin 20 mg/m^2, 5-FU 300-500 mg/m^2, depending on dosing levels

• **Regimen 2:** Irinotecan 120-180 mg/m^2, leucovorin 200 mg/m^2, 5-FU BOL 240-400 mg/m^2, 5-FU inf 360-600 mg/m^2

Available forms: Inj 20 mg/ml

Administer:

• Antiemetics and dexamethasone 10 mg at least $^1/_2$ hr before antineoplastics

• Use cytotoxic handling procedures after preparing in biologic cabinet using gloves, mask, gown

• Early diarrhea and other cholinergic symptoms can be treated with atropine

• Late diarrhea must be treated promptly with loperimide; late diarrhea can be life-threatening

Intermittent IV INF route

• By intermittent inf after diluting with 0.9% NaCl, D_5W (0.12-2.8 mg/ml); give over 1$^1/_2$ hr

• Do not admix with other sol or products

• Stable for 24 hr at room temp; 48 hr if refrigerated

SIDE EFFECTS

CNS: Fever, headache, chills, dizziness

CV: Vasodilation, edema, thromboembolism

GI: Severe diarrhea, *nausea, vomiting,* anorexia, constipation, cramps, flatus, stomatitis, dyspepsia, hepatotoxicity

HEMA: Leukopenia, anemia, neutropenia

INTEG: Irritation at site, rash, sweating, alopecia

MISC: Edema, asthenia, weight loss, back pain

RESP: Dyspnea, increased cough, rhinitis

PHARMACOKINETICS

Rapidly and completely absorbed, excreted in urine and bile as metabolites, half-life 6-12 hr, bound to plasma proteins 30%-68%, increased risk for toxicity in patients homozygous for UGT1A1 28

INTERACTIONS

Increase: toxicity—fluorouracil

Increase: bleeding risk—NSAIDs, anticoagulants

Increase: irinotecan levels—some CYP3A4 inhibitors (ketoconazole)

Increase: myelosuppression, diarrhea—other antineoplastics, radiation

Increase: lymphocytopenia, hyperglycemia—dexamethasone
Increase: akathisia—prochlorperazine
Increase: dehydration—diuretics
Decrease: irinotecan levels—CYP3A4 inducers (phenytoin, carBAMazepine, PHENobarbital)

Drug/Herb

Decrease: product level—St. John's wort; avoid concurrent use

Drug/Lab Test

Increase: alk phos, AST

NURSING CONSIDERATIONS

Assess:

• CNS symptoms: fever, headache, chills, dizziness

Black Box Warning: CBC, differential, platelet count weekly; use colony-stimulating factor if WBC <2000/mm³ or platelet count <100,000/mm³, Hgb ≤9 g/dl, neutrophil ≤1000/mm³; notify prescriber of results; product should be discontinued and colony-stimulating factor given

• Buccal cavity for dryness, sores or ulceration, white patches, oral pain, bleeding, dysphagia

Black Box Warning: GI symptoms: frequency of stools; cramping; severe, life-threatening diarrhea may occur with fluid and electrolyte imbalances

• Signs of dehydration: rapid respirations, poor skin turgor, decreased urine output, dry skin, restlessness, weakness
• Bone marrow depression: bruising, bleeding, blood in stools, urine, sputum, emesis

Perform/provide:

• Increased fluid intake to 2-3 L/day to prevent dehydration unless contraindicated
• Rinsing of mouth tid-qid with water, club soda; brushing of teeth bid-tid with soft brush or cotton-tipped applicator for stomatitis; use unwaxed dental floss
• Nutritious diet with iron, low fiber, few dairy products; avoid raw fruits, vegetables, herbal products

Evaluate:

• Therapeutic response: decrease in tumor size, spread of cancer

Teach patient/family:

• To avoid foods with citric acid or hot or rough texture if stomatitis is present; to drink adequate fluids
• To report stomatitis; any bleeding, white spots, ulcerations in mouth; to examine mouth daily, report symptoms
• To report signs of anemia: fatigue, headache, faintness, SOB, irritability
• To use contraception during therapy
• To avoid salicylates, NSAIDs, alcohol because bleeding may occur
• About alopecia; that, when hair grows back, it will be different texture, thickness
• To avoid vaccinations while taking this product

⚠ To report diarrhea that occurs 24 hr after administration; severe dehydration can occur rapidly

TREATMENT OF OVERDOSE:

Induce vomiting, provide supportive care, prevent dehydration

iron dextran (Rx)

DexFerrum, INFeD

Func. class.: Hematinic

Chem. class.: Ferric hydroxide complex with dextran

ACTION:

Iron is carried by transferrin to the bone marrow, where it is incorporated into hemoglobin

USES:

Iron-deficiency anemia

CONTRAINDICATIONS:

Black Box Warning: Hypersensitivity

Precautions: Pregnancy (C), breastfeeding, neonates, infants <4 mo, children, acute renal disease, asthma, rheumatoid arthritis (IV), ankylosing spondylitis, lupus, hypotension, all anemias excluding iron-deficiency anemia, hepatic/cardiac/renal disease

DOSAGE AND ROUTES

- **Adult and child: IM** 0.5 ml as a test dose by Z-track then no more than the following/day:
- **Adult <50 kg: IM** 100 mg
- **Adult >50 kg: IM** 250 mg
- **Child <5-9 kg: IM** 50 mg
- **Infant <5 kg: IM** 25 mg
- **Adult: IV** 0.5 ml (25 mg) test dose then 100 mg/day after 2-3 days; give 25 mg test dose, wait 5 min, then infuse over 6-12 hr or use equation that follows:

$$\frac{0.3 \times \text{wt (lb)} \times 100\text{-Hgb (g/dl)} \times 100}{14.8} = \text{mg iron}$$

Patient weighing <30 lb (66 kg) should be given 80% of above formula dose

Available forms: Inj 50 mg/ml (2-ml, 10-ml vials)

Administer:

- D/C oral iron before parenteral; give only after test dose of 25 mg by preferred route; wait at least 1 hr before giving remaining portion
- IM deeply in large muscle mass; use Z-track method, 19-20G 2-3–in needle; ensure needle long enough to place product deep in muscle; change needles after withdrawing product and before injecting to prevent skin, tissue staining

⚠ Only with EPINEPHrine available in case of anaphylactic reaction during dose

IV route

- IV after flushing with 10 ml 0.9% NaCl; give undiluted; may be diluted in 50-250 ml NS for inf; give ≤1 ml (50 mg) over ≥1 min; flush line after use with 10 ml 0.9% NaCl; patient should remain recumbent for 1/2-1 hr
- IV inj requires single-dose vial without preservative; verify on label that IV use approved

Solution compatibility: TPN No. 211

SIDE EFFECTS

CNS: Headache, paresthesia, dizziness, shivering, weakness, seizures

CV: Chest pain, shock, hypotension, tachycardia

GI: *Nausea,* vomiting, metallic taste, abdominal pain

HEMA: Leukocytosis

INTEG: Rash, pruritus, urticaria, fever, sweating, chills, brown skin discoloration, pain at inj site, necrosis, sterile abscesses, phlebitis

OTHER: Anaphylaxis

RESP: Dyspnea

PHARMACOKINETICS

IM: Excreted in feces, urine, bile, breast milk; crosses placenta; most absorbed through lymphatics; can be gradually absorbed over weeks/months from fixed locations

INTERACTIONS

Increase: toxicity—oral iron; do not use

Decrease: reticulocyte response—chloramphenicol

Drug/Lab Test

False increase: serum bilirubin

False decrease: serum calcium

False positive: ^{99m}Tc diphosphate bone scan, iron test (large doses >2 ml)

NURSING CONSIDERATIONS

Assess:

- Observe for 1 hr after test dose
- Blood studies: Hct, Hgb, reticulocytes, transferrin, plasma iron concentrations, ferritin, total iron binding, bilirubin before treatment, at least monthly

Black Box Warning: Allergy: anaphylaxis, rash, pruritus, fever, chills, wheezing; notify prescriber immediately, keep emergency equipment available

- Cardiac status: anginal pain, hypotension, tachycardia
- Nutrition: amount of iron in diet (meat, dark green leafy vegetables, dried beans, dried fruits, eggs)
- Cause of iron loss or anemia, including use of salicylates, sulfonamides
- Toxicity: nausea, vomiting, diarrhea, fever, abdominal pain (early symptoms),

cyanotic-looking lips, nailbeds, seizures, CV collapse (late symptoms)

Perform/provide:

• Storage at room temp in cool environment

• Recumbent position 30 min after IV inj to prevent orthostatic hypotension

• Therapeutic response: increased serum iron levels, Hct, Hgb

Teach patient/family:

• That iron poisoning may occur if increased beyond recommended level; not to take oral iron preparation or vitamins containing iron

• That delayed reaction may occur 1-2 days after administration and last 3-4 days (IV), 3-7 days (IM); to report fever, chills, malaise, muscle, joint aches, nausea, vomiting, backache

• To avoid breastfeeding

• That stools may become dark

TREATMENT OF OVERDOSE:

Discontinue product, treat allergic reaction, give diphenhydrAMINE or EPINEPHrine as needed, give iron-chelating product for acute poisoning

iron sucrose (Rx)

Venofer

Func. class.: Hematinic

Chem. class.: Ferric hydroxide complex with dextran

ACTION: Iron is carried by transferrin to the bone marrow, where it is incorporated into hemoglobin

USES: Iron-deficiency anemia

Unlabeled uses: Dystrophic epidermolysis bullosa (DEB)

CONTRAINDICATIONS: Hypersensitivity, all anemias excluding iron-deficiency anemia, iron overload

Precautions: Pregnancy (B), breastfeeding, children, geriatric patients, abdominal pain, anaphylactic shock, arthralgia, chest pain, cough, diarrhea, dizziness, dyspnea, edema, increased LFTs, fever, headache, heart failure, hypo/hypertension, infection, MS pain nausea/vomiting, seizures, weakness

DOSAGE AND ROUTES

• **Adult:** **IV** 5 ml (100 mg of elemental iron) given during dialysis; most will need 1000 mg of elemental iron over 10 sequential dialysis sessions

Available forms: Inj 20 mg/ml

Administer:

⚠ Only with EPINEPHrine, Solu-medrol available in case of anaphylactic reaction during dose

IV route

• Give directly in dialysis line by slow inj or inf; give by slow inj at 1 ml/min (5 min/vial); inf dilute each vial exclusively in ≤100 ml 0.9% NaCl, give at 100 mg of iron/15 min; discard unused portions

SIDE EFFECTS

CNS: Headache, dizziness

CV: Chest pain, hypo/hypertension, hypervolemia

GI: *Nausea, vomiting, abdominal pain*

INTEG: Rash, pruritus, urticaria, fever, sweating, chills

OTHER: Anaphylaxis

RESP: Dyspnea, pneumonia, cough

PHARMACOKINETICS

Excreted in urine, half-life 6 hr

INTERACTIONS

Increase: toxicity—oral iron, dimercaprol, do not use

Decrease: iron sucrose effect—chloramphenicol

NURSING CONSIDERATIONS

Assess:

• Blood studies: Hct, Hgb, reticulocytes, transferrin, plasma iron concentrations, ferritin, total iron binding; bilirubin before treatment, at least monthly

• Allergy: anaphylaxis, rash, pruritus, fever, chills, wheezing; notify prescriber

immediately, keep emergency equipment available
- Cardiac status: hypo/hypertension, hypervolemia
- Toxicity: nausea, vomiting, diarrhea, fever, abdominal pain (early symptoms), cyanotic-looking lips, nailbeds, seizures, CV collapse (late symptoms)

Perform/provide:
- Storage at room temp in cool environment, do not freeze

Evaluate:
- Therapeutic response: increased serum iron levels, Hct, Hgb

Teach patient/family:
- To report itching, rash, chest pain, headache, vertigo, nausea, vomiting, abdominal pain, joint/muscle pain, numbness, tingling
- That iron poisoning may occur if dosage increased beyond recommended level; not to take oral iron preparation

TREATMENT OF OVERDOSE:

Discontinue product, treat allergic reaction, give diphenhydrAMINE or EPINEPHrine as needed, give iron-chelating product for acute poisoning

isoflurophate ophthalmic

See Appendix B

isoniazid (Rx)

(eye-soe-nye′a-zid)

Isotamine ✦

Func. class.: Antitubercular

Chem. class.: Isonicotinic acid hydrazide

ACTION: Bactericidal interference with lipid, nucleic acid biosynthesis

USES: Treatment, prevention of TB

CONTRAINDICATIONS: Hypersensitivity

Black Box Warning: Acute hepatic disease

Precautions: Pregnancy (C), renal disease, diabetic retinopathy, cataracts, ocular defects, IV drug users, >35 yr, postpartum, HIV, neuropathy

Black Box Warning: Alcoholism, females (African descent/Hispanics)

DOSAGE AND ROUTES

- **Adult/adolescent with/without HIV: PO/IM** 5 mg/kg/day ≤300 mg/day or 15 mg/kg 2-3×/wk, max 900 mg 2-3×/wk
- **Child/infant with HIV: PO/IM** 10-15 mg/kg/day, max 300 mg/day

Available forms: Tabs 100, 300 mg; inj 100 mg/ml

Administer:
- PO with meals to decrease GI symptoms; better to take on empty stomach 1 hr before or 2 hr after meals
- Antiemetic if vomiting occurs
- After C&S is completed; monthly to detect resistance
- IM deep in large muscle mass; massage; rotate inj site; warm inj to room temp to dissolve crystals

SIDE EFFECTS

CNS: *Peripheral neuropathy, dizziness,* memory impairment, **toxic encephalopathy, seizures, psychosis,** slurred speech

EENT: Blurred vision, optic neuritis

GI: *Nausea, vomiting,* epigastric distress, **jaundice, fatal hepatitis**

HEMA: Agranulocytosis, hemolytic, aplastic anemia, thrombocytopenia, eosinophilia, methemoglobinemia

Hypersensitivity: Fever, skin eruptions, lymphadenopathy, vasculitis

MISC: Dyspnea, B_6 deficiency, pellagra, hyperglycemia, metabolic acidosis, gynecomastia, rheumatic syndrome, SLE-like syndrome

PHARMACOKINETICS

Metabolized in liver, excreted in urine (metabolites), crosses placenta, excreted in breast milk
PO: Peak 1-2 hr
IM: Peak 45-60 min

INTERACTIONS

Increase: toxicity—tyramine foods, alcohol, cycloSERINE, ethionamide, rifampin, carBAMazepine, warfarin, phenytoin, benzodiazepines, meperidine
Increase: serotonin syndrome—SSRIs, SNRIs
Decrease: absorption—aluminum antacids
Decrease: effectiveness of BCG vaccine, ketoconazole
Drug/Food
• Do not give with high-tyramine foods, alcohol

NURSING CONSIDERATIONS

Assess:

Black Box Warning: Hepatic studies weekly: ALT, AST, bilirubin; increased test results may indicate hepatitis; hepatic status: decreased appetite, jaundice, dark urine, fatigue

• Mental status often: affect, mood, behavioral changes; psychosis may occur
• Paresthesia in hands, feet

Evaluate:
• Therapeutic response: decreased symptoms of TB

Teach patient/family:
• That compliance with dosage schedule, duration is necessary; not to skip or double dose
• That scheduled appointments must be kept or relapse may occur
⚠ To avoid alcohol while taking product; may increase risk for hepatic injury
• That, if diabetic, to use blood glucose monitor to obtain correct result
⚠ To report weakness, fatigue, loss of appetite, nausea, vomiting, jaundice of skin or eyes, tingling/numbness of hands/feet

TREATMENT OF OVERDOSE:
Pyridoxine

isosorbide dinitrate (Rx)
(eye-soe-sor′bide)

Apo-ISDN ✱, Dilatrate-SR, Isochron, IsoDitrate, Isordil

isosorbide mononitrate (Rx)

Apo-ISMN ✱, Imdur, Monoket
Func. class.: Antianginal, vasodilator
Chem. class.: Nitrate

Do not confuse:
Monoket/Monopril
Imdur/Imuran/Inderal/K-Dur

ACTION: Relaxation of vascular smooth muscle, which leads to decreased preload, afterload, which is responsible for decreasing left ventricular end-diastolic pressure, systemic vascular resistance, and reducing cardiac oxygen demand

USES: Treatment, prevention of chronic stable angina pectoris
Unlabeled uses: Diffuse esophageal spasm, heart failure (dinitrate)

CONTRAINDICATIONS: Hypersensitivity to this product or nitrates; severe anemia, increased intracranial pressure, cerebral hemorrhage, acute MI
Precautions: Pregnancy (C), breastfeeding, children, postural hypotension, MI, CHF, severe renal/hepatic disease

DOSAGE AND ROUTES

Dinitrate
• **Adult: PO** 5-20 mg bid-tid initially, maintenance 10-40 mg bid-tid; **SL,** buccal 2.5-5 mg, may repeat q5-10min × 3 doses; **EXT REL** 40-80 mg q8-12hr, max 160 mg/day

Mononitrate
• **Adult: PO** (Monoket) 10-20 mg bid, 7 hr apart; (Imdur) initiate at 30-60 mg/

day as a single dose, increase q3days as needed, may increase to 120 mg/day, max 240 mg/day

Available forms: *Dinitrate:* sus rel caps (SR) 40 mg, SR tabs 40 mg; tabs 5, 10, 20, 30, 40 mg; SL tabs 2.5, 5 mg; *mononitrate:* tabs (Monoket) 10, 20 mg; ext rel (Imdur) 30, 60, 120 mg

Administer:
- Do not break, crush, or chew sus rel caps, SL tabs
- After checking expiration date
- PO with 8 oz water on empty stomach
- SL tabs should be placed under the tongue until dissolved; avoid smoking, eating, drinking until dissolved

SIDE EFFECTS

CNS: *Vascular headache, flushing, dizziness,* weakness, faintness
CV: *Postural hypotension,* tachycardia, collapse, syncope, palpitations
GI: Nausea, vomiting, diarrhea
INTEG: Pallor, sweating, rash
MISC: Twitching, hemolytic anemia, methemoglobinemia, tolerance

PHARMACOKINETICS

Dinitrate
Metabolized by liver, excreted in urine as metabolites (80%-100%)
PO: Onset 15-30 min, duration 4-6 hr
SUS REL: Onset ≤4 hr, duration 6-8 hr
SL: Onset 2-5 min, duration 1-4 hr
Mononitrate
SUS REL: Onset 30-60 min, peak 1-4 hr, duration 6-8 hr

INTERACTIONS

⚠ Fatal hypotension: sildenafil, tadalafil, vardenafil
Increase: hypotension—β-blockers, diuretics, antihypertensives, alcohol, calcium channel blockers, phenothiazines

NURSING CONSIDERATIONS

Assess:
- **Anginal pain:** duration, time started, activity being performed, character
- B/P, pulse, respirations during beginning therapy
- Tolerance if taken over long period
- Headache, lightheadedness, decreased B/P; may indicate a need for decreased dosage

Evaluate:
- Therapeutic response: decrease or prevention of anginal pain

Teach patient/family:
- To leave tabs in original container
- To avoid alcohol, OTC products unless approved by prescriber
- That product may cause headache; that taking with meals may reduce or eliminate headache; to take no later than 7 PM (last dose)
- To avoid hazardous activities if dizziness occurs
- About the importance of complying with complete medical regimen
- To make position changes slowly to prevent orthostatic hypotension

I

RARELY USED

isotretinoin (Rx)
(eye-soe-tret′i-noyn)
Amnesteem, Claravis, Sotret
Func. class.: Antiacne agent, retinoid

USES: Severe recalcitrant nodulocystic acne

CONTRAINDICATIONS: Hypersensitivity, inflamed skin
Black Box Warning: Pregnancy (X)

DOSAGE AND ROUTES

- **Adult: PO** 0.5-2 mg/kg/day in 2 divided doses × 15-20 wk; if relapse occurs, repeat after 2 mo off product

isradipine (Rx)

(is-ra′di-peen)

DynaCirc CR

Func. class.: Antihypertensive, antianginal (calcium channel blocker)

Chem. class.: Dihydropyridine

Do not confuse:
DynaCirc/Dynabac/Dynacin

ACTION:
Inhibits calcium ion influx across cell membrane during cardiac depolarization; produces relaxation of coronary vascular smooth muscle, peripheral vascular smooth muscle; dilates coronary vascular arteries

USES:
Essential hypertension

Unlabeled uses: Angina pectoris; hypertension in children/adolescents

CONTRAINDICATIONS:
Hypersensitivity to this product or dihydropyridines

Precautions: Pregnancy (C), breastfeeding, children, geriatric patients, CHF, hypotension, renal/hepatic disease, acute MI, bradycardia, cardiogenic shock, GERD, hiatal hernia, ventricular dysfunction

DOSAGE AND ROUTES

- **Adult: PO** 2.5 mg bid, increase at 2-4–wk intervals up to 5 mg bid or 10 mg/day; **CONT REL** 5 mg/day, increase q2-4wk, max 20 mg/day
- **Child/adolescent (unlabeled): PO** (hypertension) 0.15-0.2 mg/kg/day in divided doses q6-8hr, max 0.8 mg/kg/day or 20 mg/day

Available forms: Caps 2.5, 5 mg; cont rel tabs (CR) 5, 10 mg

Administer:

- Do not break, crush, or chew cont rel tabs
- Without regard to meals

SIDE EFFECTS

CNS: *Headache,* fatigue, dizziness, fainting, sleep disturbances, weakness, depression, drowsiness

CV: Peripheral edema, tachycardia, hypotension, chest pain, **dysrhythmias**, syncope

GI: Nausea, vomiting, diarrhea, gastric upset, constipation, **hepatitis**, abdominal pain, distention, dry mouth

GU: Nocturia, urinary frequency

HEMA: **Leukopenia**

INTEG: Rash, pruritus, urticaria, **angioedema**

MISC: Flushing

PHARMACOKINETICS

Metabolized in liver; metabolites excreted in urine, feces; secreted in breast milk; peak 1.5 hr immediate rel, 7-18 hr cont rel; half-life biphasic 1-1½ hr, 8hr; protein binding 95%

INTERACTIONS

Increase: additive/synergistic effect—β-blockers

Increase: bradycardia, conduction defects—disopyramide

Increase: hypotension—nitrates, fentanyl, other antihypertensives

Increase: serum concentration of isradipine—rifampin, CYP3A4 inhibitors

Decrease: serum concentration of isradipine—cimetidine, ranitidine, CYP3A4 inducers

Decrease: concentration—lovastatin

Decrease: antihypertensive action—NSAIDs, salicylates

Drug/Food

- Avoid grapefruit juice

Drug/Herb

Increase: antihypertensive effect—ginkgo, ginseng, hawthorn

Decrease: antihypertensive effect—St. John's wort

NURSING CONSIDERATIONS

Assess:

- I&O ratio, daily weight, watch for CHF:

edema, dyspnea, weight gain, crackles, jugular venous distention

• Renal/hepatic studies, electrolytes prior to and during treatment

• Cardiac status: B/P, pulse, respiration, ECG; assess anginal pain, precipitating, ameliorating factors

Evaluate:

• Therapeutic response: decreased anginal pain, decreased B/P

Teach patient/family:

• To avoid hazardous activities until stabilized on product, dizziness is no longer a problem

• To limit caffeine consumption

• To avoid OTC products unless directed by prescriber

• About the importance of compliance with all areas of regimen: diet, exercise, stress reduction

• To notify prescriber of irregular heartbeat, SOB, swelling of feet/hands, pronounced dizziness, constipation, nausea, hypotension

TREATMENT OF OVERDOSE:

Defibrillation, β-agonists, IV calcium inotropic agents, diuretics, atropine for AV block, vasopressor for hypotension

itraconazole (Rx)

(it-ra-con′a-zol)

Sporanox

Func. class.: Antifungal, systemic

Chem. class.: Triazole derivative

ACTION: Alters cell membranes; inhibits several fungal enzymes

USES: Histoplasmosis, blastomycosis (pulmonary and extrapulmonary), aspergillosis, onychomycosis of toenail/fingernail

Unlabeled uses: Dermatomycosis, histoplasmosis, chromoblastomycosis, coccidioidomycosis, pityriasis versicolor, sebopsoriasis, vaginal candidiasis, cryptococcus, subcutaneous mycoses, dimorphic infections, fungal keratitis, zygomycosis, superficial mycoses (dermatophytoses), chronic mucocutaneous candidiasis

CONTRAINDICATIONS: Hypersensitivity, fungal meningitis; onychomycosis or dermatomycosis with cardiac dysfunction, in females

Black Box Warning: Heart failure, ventricular dysfunction, coadministration with other products

Precautions: Pregnancy (C), breastfeeding, children, cardiac/renal/hepatic disease, achlorhydria or hypochlorhydria (product-induced), dialysis

DOSAGE AND ROUTES

Dose varies with type of infection

• **Adult: PO** 200 mg/day with food; may increase to 400 mg/day if needed; life-threatening infections may require a loading dose of 200 mg tid × 3 days; **IV** 200 mg bid × 4 doses; then 200 mg/day, give each dose over 1 hr; maintenance **PO** 200-400 mg/day

• **Child: PO** 3-5 mg/kg/day

Available forms: Caps 100 mg; oral sol 10 mg/ml; inj 10 mg/ml

Administer:

• In the presence of acid products only; do not use alkaline products, antacids within 2 hr of product; may give coffee, tea, acidic fruit juices

PO route

• Swallow caps whole; do not break, crush, or chew caps

• Give caps after full meal to ensure absorption

• Oral sol: patient should swish in mouth vigorously, use on empty stomach

• Oral sol and caps are not interchangeable on mg/mg basis

IV route

• After adding full contents of 25-50–ml bag of 0.9% NaCl, mix, use inf pump, give at a rate of 1 ml/min, flush line with 0.9% NaCl after inf; do not give by bolus

SIDE EFFECTS

CNS: *Headache, dizziness,* insomnia, somnolence, depression
CV: Hypertension
GI: *Nausea, vomiting, anorexia, diarrhea,* cramps, abdominal pain, flatulence, **GI bleeding, hepatotoxicity**
GU: Gynecomastia, impotence, decreased libido
INTEG: *Pruritus,* fever, *rash,* **toxic epidermal necrolysis**
MISC: *Edema, fatigue,* malaise, hypokalemia, tinnitus, **rhabdomyolysis**

PHARMACOKINETICS

PO: Peak 3-5 hr; half-life 21 hr; metabolized in liver; excreted in bile, feces, urine 40%; requires acid pH for absorption; distributed poorly to CSF; 99.8% protein bound; inhibits CYP4503A4

INTERACTIONS

⚠ **Life-threatening CV reactions: pimozide, quiNIDine, dofetilide, levomethadyl**
Increase: tinnitus, hearing loss—quiNIDine
Increase: hepatotoxicity—other hepatotoxic products
Increase: edema—calcium channel blockers
Increase: severe hypoglycemia—oral hypoglycemics
Increase: sedation—alprazolam, clorazepine, diazepam, estazolam, flurazepam, triazolam, oral midazolam
Increase: levels, toxicity—busPIRone, busulfan, clarithromycin, cycloSPORINE, diazepam, digoxin, felodipine, fentaNYL, atorvastatin, carBAMazepine, disopyramide, indinavir, isradipine, niCARdipine, niFEDipine, nimodipine, phenytoin, quiNIDine, quetiapine, ritonavir, saquinavir, tacrolimus, warfarin
Decrease: effect of oral contraceptives
Decrease: itraconazole action—antacids, H_2-receptor antagonists, rifamycins, didanosine, carBAMazepine, isoniazid, proton pump inhibitors

Drug/Food

- Food increases absorption
- Grapefruit juice decreases itraconazole level

NURSING CONSIDERATIONS

Assess:

- **CHF:** if present, discontinue product
- Type of infection; may begin treatment prior to obtaining results
- **Infection:** temp, WBC, sputum at baseline and periodically
- I&O ratio, potassium levels
- Hepatic studies (ALT, AST, bilirubin) if patient receiving long-term therapy
- Allergic reaction: rash, photosensitivity, urticaria, dermatitis

⚠ **Hepatotoxicity: nausea, vomiting, jaundice, clay-colored stools, fatigue**

Perform/provide:

- Storage in tight container at room temp, do not freeze

Evaluate:

- Therapeutic response: decreased fever, malaise, rash, negative C&S for infecting organism

Teach patient/family:

- That long-term therapy may be needed to clear infection (1 wk-6 mo, depending on infection)
- To avoid hazardous activities if dizziness occurs
- To take 2 hr before administration of other products that increase gastric pH (antacids, H_2-blockers, omeprazole, sucralfate, anticholinergics); to avoid grapefruit juice; to notify health care provider of all medications taken; to take after a full meal (caps) or on empty stomach (oral sol)
- About the importance of compliance with product regimen; to use alternative methods of contraception
- To notify prescriber of GI symptoms; signs of hepatic dysfunction (fatigue, nausea, anorexia, vomiting, dark urine, pale stools); heart failure (trouble breathing, unusual weight gain, fatigue, swelling); hearing changes

ixabepilone (Rx)

(ix-ab-ep′i-lone)

Ixempra

Func. class.: Antineoplastic—miscellaneous

Chem. class.: Epothilone

ACTION: Microtubule stabilizing agent; microtubules are needed for cell division

USES: Breast cancer

CONTRAINDICATIONS: Pregnancy (D), breastfeeding, hypersensitivity to products with polyoxyethylated castor oil, neutropenia of $<1500/mm^3$, thrombocytopenia

Black Box Warning: Hepatic disease

Precautions: Children, geriatric patients, alcoholism, bone marrow suppression, cardiac dysrhythmias, cardiac/renal disease, diabetes mellitus, peripheral neuropathy, ventricular dysfunction

DOSAGE AND ROUTES

Breast cancer, metastatic or locally advanced given with capecitabine and resistant to anthracycline, taxane

- **Adult: IV INF** 40 mg/m^2 over 3 hr q3wk plus capecitabine **PO** 2000 mg/m^2/day in 2 divided doses on days 1-14 q21days; in those with BSA >2.2 m^2, dose should be calculated for a BSA of 2.2 m^2

Breast cancer, metastatic or locally advanced resistant/refractory to anthracycline, taxane, capecitabine

- **Adult: IV INF** 40 mg/m^2 over 3 hr q3wk; in those with BSA >2.2 m^2, dose should be calculated for a BSA of 2.2 m^2

Dosage reduction in those taking a strong CYP3A4 inhibitor

- **Adult: IV INF** 20 mg/m^2 over 3 hr q3wk

Available forms: Powder for inj 15, 45 mg

Administer:

- Antiemetic 30-60 min before product and prn

IV route

- Let kit stand at room temp for 30 min; to reconstitute, withdraw supplied diluent (8 ml for 15-mg vials, 23.5 ml for 45-mg vials); slowly inject sol into vial; gently swirl and invert to mix, final conc 2 mg/ml; further dilute in LR in DEHP-free bags, final conc should be between 0.2 and 0.6 mg/ml; after added, mix by manual rotation
- Diluted sol stable for 6 hr at room temp; inf must be completed within 6 hr
- Use in-line filter, 0.2-1.2 micron
- Give over 3 hr

SIDE EFFECTS

CNS: *Peripheral neuropathy,* impaired cognition, chills, fatigue, fever, flushing, headache, insomnia, *asthenia*

CV: Bradycardia, *hypotension,* abnormal ECG, angina, atrial flutter, cardiomyopathy, chest pain, edema, MI, vasculitis

GI: *Nausea, vomiting, diarrhea,* abdominal pain, anorexia, colitis, constipation, gastritis, jaundice, GERD, hepatic failure, trismus

GU: Renal failure

HEMA: Neutropenia, thrombocytopenia, anemia, infections, coagulopathy

INTEG: *Alopecia,* rash, hot flashes

META: Hypokalemia, metabolic acidosis

MS: *Arthralgia, myalgia*

RESP: Bronchospasm, cough, dyspnea

SYST: *Hypersensitivity reactions,* anaphylaxis, dehydration, radiation recall reaction

PHARMACOKINETICS

Metabolized in liver by P45CYP3A4; excreted in feces (65%) and urine (21%); terminal half-life 52 hr

INTERACTIONS

Increase: ixabepilone level—CYP3A4 inhibitors (amiodarone, amprenavir, apre-

pitant, atazanavir, chloramphenicol, clarithromycin, conivaptan, cycloSPORINE, danazol, darunavir, dalforpistin, delavirdine, diltiazem, erythromycin, estradiol, fluconazole, fluvoxamine, fosamprenavir, imatinib, indinavir, isoniazid, itraconazole, ketoconazole, lopinavir, miconazole, nefazodone, nelfinavir, propoxyphene, ritonavir, RU-486, saquinavir, tamoxifen, telithromycin, troleandomycin, verapamil, voriconazole, zafirlukast)
Decrease: ixabepilone levels—CYP3A4 inducers (aminoglutethimide, barbiturates, bexarotene, bosentan, carBAMazepine, dexamethasone, efavirenz, griseofulvin, modafinil, nafcillin, nevirapine, OXcarbazepine, phenytoin, rifamycin, topiramate)
Drug/Herb
- Avoid use with St. John's wort

Drug/Food
- Avoid use with grapefruit products

NURSING CONSIDERATIONS

Assess:
- CBC, differential, platelet count prior to treatment and weekly; withhold product if WBC is $<1500/mm^3$ or platelet count is $<100,000/mm^3$, notify prescriber
- Monitor temp q4hr (may indicate beginning infection)

Black Box Warning: Liver function tests before, during therapy (bilirubin, AST, ALT, LDH) prn or monthly; check for jaundiced skin and sclera, dark urine, clay-colored stools, itchy skin, abdominal pain, fever, diarrhea

- VS during 1st hr of infusion; check IV site for signs of infiltration

⚠ **Hypersensitivity reactions, anaphylaxis** including hypotension, dyspnea, angioedema, generalized urticaria; discontinue inf immediately; keep emergency equipment available
- Effects of alopecia on body image; discuss feelings about body changes

Evaluate:
- Therapeutic response: decreased tumor size, spread of malignancy

Teach patient/family:
- To report signs of infection: fever, sore throat, flulike symptoms
- To report signs of anemia: fatigue, headache, faintness, SOB
- To report any complaints or side effects to nurse or prescriber
- That hair may be lost during treatment; that a wig or hairpiece may make patient feel better; that new hair may be different in color, texture
- That pain in muscles and joints 2-5 days after inf is common
- To use nonhormonal type of contraception
- To avoid receiving vaccinations while receiving product

ketoconazole (Rx)

(kee-toe-koe′na-zole)
Func. class.: Antifungal
Chem. class.: Imidazole derivative

ACTION: Alters cell membrane permeability and inhibits several fungal enzymes, thereby leading to cell death

USES: Systemic candidiasis, chronic mucocandidiasis, oral thrush, candiduria, coccidioidomycosis, histoplasmosis, chromomycosis, paracoccidioidomycosis, blastomycosis; tinea cruris, tinea corporis, tinea versicolor, *Pityrosporum ovale*
Unlabeled uses: Cushing's syndrome, advanced prostatic cancer, candidiasis/fungal prophylaxis, fungal keratitis, leishmaniasis

CONTRAINDICATIONS: Breastfeeding, hypersensitivity, fungal meningitis

Black Box Warning: Coadministration with other products

Precautions: Pregnancy (C), children <2 yr, renal disease, achlorhydria (product-induced)

Black Box Warning: Hepatic disease

DOSAGE AND ROUTES

- **Adult: PO** 200-400 mg/day for 1-2 wk (candidiasis), 6 wk (other infections)
- **Child ≥2 yr: PO:** 3.3-6.6 mg/kg/day as a single daily dose

Prostate cancer (unlabeled)

- **Adult: PO** 400 mg tid

Available forms: Tabs 200 mg; oral susp 100 mg/5 ml ✦

Administer:

- In the presence of acid products only; do not use alkaline products, proton pump inhibitors, H_2-antagonists, antacids within 2 hr of product; may give coffee, tea, acidic fruit juices, cola
- With food to decrease GI symptoms
- With HCl if achlorhydria is present; dissolve tab/4 ml of aqueous sol 0.2 N hydrochloric acid; use straw to avoid contact; rinse with water afterward and swallow

SIDE EFFECTS

CNS: Headache, dizziness, somnolence
GI: Nausea, vomiting, anorexia, diarrhea, abdominal pain, **hepatotoxicity**
GU: Gynecomastia, impotence
HEMA: **Thrombocytopenia, leukopenia, hemolytic anemia**
INTEG: Pruritus, fever, chills, photophobia, rash, dermatitis, purpura, urticaria
SYST: **Anaphylaxis**

PHARMACOKINETICS

PO: Peak 1-2 hr; half-life 2 hr, terminal 8 hr; metabolized in liver; excreted in bile, feces; requires acid pH for absorption; distributed poorly to CSF; highly protein bound

INTERACTIONS

Decrease: effect of—theophylline

- Inhibited metabolism: paclitaxel

Increase: hepatotoxicity—other hepatotoxic products, alcohol

Increase: anticoagulant effect—warfarin, anticoagulants

Decrease: CYP3A4 pathway, toxicity: alfentanil, alprazolam, amprenavir, aripiprazole, atorvastatin, calcium channel blockers, carBAMazepine, cerivastatin, clarithromycin, corticosteroids, cyclophosphamide, cycloSPORINE, donepezil, eletriptan, erythromycin, fentanyl, ifosfamide, indinavir, lovastatin, midazolam, nelfinavir, nisoldipine, quiNIDine, ritonavir, saquinavir, sildenafil, simvastatin, sufentanil, tamoxifen, triazolam, vinBLAStine, vinca alkaloids, vinCRIStine, zolpidem

Decrease: action of ketoconazole—antacids, H_2-receptor antagonists, anticholinergics, phenytoin, isoniazid, rifampin, ddI, gastric acid pump inhibitors

Decrease: effect of oral contraceptives

NURSING CONSIDERATIONS

Assess:

- Infection symptoms before and after treatment
- C&S before starting treatment
- Allergic reaction: rash, photosensitivity, urticaria, dermatitis

Black Box Warning: Hepatotoxicity: nausea, vomiting, jaundice, clay-colored stools, fatigue; hepatic studies (ALT, AST, bilirubin) if patient receiving long-term therapy

Perform/provide:

- Storage in tight container at room temp

Evaluate:

- Therapeutic response: decreased fever, malaise, rash, negative C&S for infectious organism, absence of scaling

Teach patient/family:

- That long-term therapy may be needed to clear infection (1 wk-6 mo, depending on infection)
- To avoid hazardous activities if dizziness occurs
- To take 2 hr before administration of other products that increase gastric pH (antacids, H_2-blockers, omeprazole, sucralfate, anticholinergics)
- About the importance of compliance with product regimen

K

Black Box Warning: To notify prescriber of GI symptoms, signs of hepatic dysfunction (fatigue, nausea, anorexia, vomiting, dark urine, pale stools)

• To use sunglasses to prevent photophobia

• To use alternative method of contraception while taking this product

ketoconazole topical

See Appendix B

ketoprofen (OTC, Rx)

(ke-toe-proe′fen)

Apo-Keto ♣

Func. class.: Nonsteroidal antiinflammatory product (NSAID), antirheumatic

Chem. class.: Propionic acid derivative

ACTION: Inhibits COX-1, COX-2; analgesic, antiinflammatory, antipyretic

USES: Mild to moderate pain, osteoarthritis, rheumatoid arthritis, dysmenorrhea; OTC relief of minor aches, pains

Unlabeled uses: Ankylosing spondylitis, bone pain, gouty arthritis

CONTRAINDICATIONS: Pregnancy (D) 2nd/3rd trimester, hypersensitivity to this product, NSAIDs, salicylates; asthma, severe renal/hepatic disease, ulcer disease

Black Box Warning: Perioperative pain with CABG

Precautions: Pregnancy (B) 1st trimester, breastfeeding, children, geriatric patients, bleeding, GI/cardiac disorders, hypersensitivity to other antiinflammatory agents

Black Box Warning: GI bleeding, MI, stroke

DOSAGE AND ROUTES

Antiinflammatory

• **Adult: PO** 50 mg qid or 75 mg tid, max 300 mg/day or **EXT REL** 200 mg/day

Analgesic

• **Adult: PO** 25-50 mg q6-8hr, max 300 mg/day

Available forms: Caps 50, 75 mg; ext rel cap 200 mg

Administer:

• Do not break, crush, or chew ext rel caps

• With food to decrease GI symptoms

SIDE EFFECTS

CNS: Dizziness, drowsiness, fatigue, tremors, confusion, insomnia, anxiety, depression, headache

CV: Tachycardia, peripheral edema, palpitations, dysrhythmias, hypertension, CV thrombotic events, MI, stroke

EENT: Tinnitus, hearing loss, blurred vision

GI: *Nausea, anorexia, vomiting, diarrhea,* jaundice, hepatitis, constipation, flatulence, cramps, dry mouth, peptic ulcer, GI bleeding

GU: Nephrotoxicity: dysuria, hematuria, oliguria, azotemia

HEMA: Blood dyscrasias

INTEG: Purpura, rash, pruritus, sweating

SYST: Anaphylaxis

PHARMACOKINETICS

PO: Peak 1.2 hr; ext rel 6.8 hr, half-life 2-4 hr; 5.4 hr ext rel, metabolized in liver, urine (metabolites), breast milk; 99% plasma protein binding

INTERACTIONS

Increase: serotonin syndrome—SSRIs, SNRIs

Increase: hypoglycemia—insulin, sulfonylureas

Increase: toxicity—cycloSPORINE, lithium, methotrexate, phenytoin, alcohol

Increase: bleeding risk—anticoagulants, clopidogrel, eptifibatide, plicamycin, thrombolytics, ticlopidine, tirofiban, valproic acid

Increase: ketoprofen levels—aspirin, probenecid
Increase: adverse GI reactions—aspirin, corticosteroids, NSAIDs, alcohol
Increase: hematologic toxicity—radiation, antineoplastics
Decrease: effect of diuretics, antihypertensives
Drug/Herb
Increase: bleeding risk—feverfew, garlic, ginger, ginkgo
Drug/Lab Test
Increase: potassium, BUN, alk phos, AST, ALT, LDH, creatinine, bleeding time
Decrease: blood glucose, HCT, Hgb, platelets, CCr, leukocyte
Interference: urine albumin, 17 KS, 17-hydroxycorticosteroid, bilirubin

NURSING CONSIDERATIONS

Assess:

- **Pain:** type, location, intensity, ROM before and 1-2 hr after treatment
- Renal, hepatic, blood studies: BUN, creatinine, AST, ALT, Hgb before treatment, periodically thereafter

⚠ Aspirin sensitivity, asthma; these patients may be more likely to develop hypersensitivity to NSAIDs

- Audiometric, ophthalmic exam before, during, after treatment
- For eye/ear problems: blurred vision, tinnitus; may indicate toxicity

Black Box Warning: GI bleeding: blood in sputum, emesis, stools

Black Box Warning: CV thrombotic events: MI, stroke

Perform/provide:

- Storage at room temp

Evaluate:

- Therapeutic response: decreased pain, stiffness, swelling in joints; ability to move more easily; decreased fever

Teach patient/family:

- To report blurred vision, ringing, roaring in ears; may indicate toxicity
- To avoid driving, other hazardous activities if dizziness, drowsiness occurs, especially in geriatric patients
- To report change in urine pattern, increased weight, edema, increased pain in joints, fever, blood in urine (indicate nephrotoxicity); rash, itching, blurred vision, ringing in ears, flulike symptoms
- That therapeutic effects may take up to 1 mo; to take with 8 oz water; to sit upright for ½ hr after administration to prevent GI irritation
- To avoid aspirin, alcohol, corticosteroids, acetaminophen, other medications, supplements unless approved by prescriber
- To wear sunscreen to prevent photosensitivity
- To report product use to all health care providers

ketorolac (Rx)

(kee-toe′role-ak)

Apo-Ketorolac ♣, ratio-Ketorolac ♣, Toradol ♣

Func. class.: Nonsteroidal antiinflammatory/nonopioid analgesic

Chem. class.: Acetic acid

ACTION: Inhibits prostaglandin synthesis by decreasing an enzyme needed for biosynthesis; analgesic, antiinflammatory, antipyretic effects

USES: Mild to moderate pain (short term); seasonal allergic conjunctivitis (ophthalmic)

CONTRAINDICATIONS: Pregnancy (D) 3rd trimester, hypersensitivity, asthma, hepatic disease, peptic ulcer disease, CV bleeding

Black Box Warning: Breastfeeding, severe renal disease, L&D, perioperative pain in CABG, prior to major surgery, epidural/intrathecal administration, GI bleeding, hypovolemia

Precautions: Pregnancy (C), GI/cardiac disorders, hypersensitivity to other antiinflammatory agents, CCr <25 ml/min

Black Box Warning: Children, geriatric patients, bleeding, MI, stroke

DOSAGE AND ROUTES

• **Adult/adolescent >17 yr and ≥50 kg:** **PO** continuation from **IM/IV** only 20 mg then 10 mg q4-6hr prn, max 40 mg/day
• **Adult/adolescent >17 yr and <50 kg:** **IM** (single dose) 30-60 mg, **IV** 15-30 mg; **IM/IV** (multiple dosing) 15-30 mg q6hr, max 60 mg/day × 5 days combined either **PO/IM/IV**

Available forms: Inj 15, 30 mg/ml (prefilled syringes); tab 10 mg

Administer:
• Not to exceed 5 days

IM route
• IM inj deeply in large muscle mass

IV route
• Give undiluted over ≥15 sec

Solution compatibility: D_5W, 0.9% NaCl, LR, D_5, Plasma-Lyte A

Syringe compatibilities: SUFentanil

Y-site compatibilities: Cisatracurium, remifentanil, SUFentanil

SIDE EFFECTS

CNS: Dizziness, *drowsiness,* tremors, seizures

CV: Hypertension, flushing, syncope, pallor, edema, vasodilation, CV thrombotic events, MI, stroke

EENT: Tinnitus, hearing loss, blurred vision

GI: Nausea, anorexia, vomiting, diarrhea, constipation, flatulence, cramps, dry mouth, peptic ulcer, GI bleeding, perforation, taste change, hepatitis, hepatic failure

GU: Nephrotoxicity: dysuria, hematuria, oliguria, azotemia

HEMA: Blood dyscrasias, prolonged bleeding

INTEG: Purpura, rash, pruritus, sweating, angioedema, Stevens-Johnson syndrome, toxic epidermal necrolysis

PHARMACOKINETICS

Half-life 6 hr, enters breast milk, <50% metabolized by liver, excreted by kidneys

PO: Peak 2-3 hr, duration 4-6 hr
IM: Peak 50 min

INTERACTIONS

Increase: toxicity—methotrexate, lithium, cycloSPORINE, pentoxifylline, probenecid

Increase: bleeding risk—anticoagulants, cefamandole, cefoperazone, cefotetan, clopidogrel, eptifibatide, plicamycin, salicylates, ticlopidine, tirofiban, thrombolytics, valproic acid, SSRIs, SNRIs

Increase: renal impairment—ACE inhibitors

⚠ **Increase:** ketorolac levels—aspirin, other NSAIDs; contraindicated

Increase: GI effects—corticosteroids, alcohol, aspirin, NSAIDs

Decrease: effects—antihypertensives, diuretics

Drug/Lab Test

Increase: AST, ALT, LDH, alk phos, bleeding time, BUN, creatinine, potassium

Decrease: blood glucose, Hct/Hgb, platelets

NURSING CONSIDERATIONS

Assess:

• Aspirin sensitivity, asthma: patients may be more likely to develop hypersensitivity to NSAIDs; monitor for hypersensitivity
• Pain: type, location, intensity, ROM before and 1 hr after treatment

Black Box Warning: Renal, hepatic, blood studies: BUN, creatinine, AST, ALT, Hgb before treatment, periodically thereafter; check for dehydration

Black Box Warning: Bleeding times; check for bruising, bleeding, occult blood in urine

• Eye/ear problems: blurred vision, tinnitus (may indicate toxicity)

⚠ Hepatic dysfunction: jaundice, yellow sclera and skin, clay-colored stools

Black Box Warning: CV thrombotic events: MI, stroke

• Audiometric, ophthalmic exam before, during, after treatment

⚠ Nurse Alert

Perform/provide:
• Storage at room temp, protect from light

Evaluate:
• Therapeutic response: decreased pain, stiffness, swelling in joints, ability to move more easily

Teach patient/family:
• To report blurred vision, ringing/roaring in ears (may indicate toxicity)
• To avoid driving, other hazardous activities if dizziness or drowsiness occurs

Black Box Warning: To report change in urine pattern, weight increase, edema; pain increase in joints, fever, blood in urine (indicates nephrotoxicity); bruising, black tarry stools (indicates bleeding)

• To avoid alcohol, salicylates, other NSAIDs, acetaminophen
• To report product use to all health care providers

Black Box Warning: Not to breastfeed

ketorolac ophthalmic
See Appendix B

ketotifen ophthalmic
See Appendix B

labetalol (Rx)
(la-bet′a-lole)

Apo-Labetalol ✱, Trandate

Func. class.: Antihypertensive, antianginal

Chem. class.: α-1/β-Blocker

Do not confuse:
Trandate/Tridrate

ACTION: Produces decreases in B/P without reflex tachycardia or significant reduction in heart rate through mixture of α-blocking, β-blocking effects; elevated plasma renins are reduced

USES: Mild to moderate hypertension; treatment of severe hypertension (IV)

Unlabeled uses: Hypertension in patients with pheochromocytoma, hypertension during cloNIDine withdrawal, pediatric hypertension

CONTRAINDICATIONS: Hypersensitivity to β-blockers, cardiogenic shock, heart block (2nd or 3rd degree), sinus bradycardia, CHF, bronchial asthma

Precautions: Pregnancy (C), breastfeeding, geriatric patients, major surgery, diabetes mellitus, thyroid/renal/hepatic disease, COPD, well-compensated heart failure, CAD, nonallergic bronchospasm, peripheral vascular disease

Black Box Warning: Abrupt discontinuation

DOSAGE AND ROUTES

Hypertension
• **Adult: PO** 100 mg bid; may be given with diuretic; may increase to 200 mg bid after 2 days; may continue to increase q1-3days; max 2400 mg/day in divided doses
• **Child/adolescent (unlabeled): PO** 1-3 mg/kg/day, titrate to max 10-20 mg/kg/day based on B/P; **IV** 0.2-1 mg/kg over 2 min, max 40 mg/dose; **IV INF** 0.25-3 mg/kg/hr

Hypertensive crisis
• **Adult: IV INF** 200 mg/160 ml D_5W, run at 2 mg/min or 1.6 ml/min; stop inf at desired response, repeat q6-8hr as needed; **IV BOL** 20-80 mg over 2 min, may repeat q10min, not to exceed 300 mg

Available forms: Tabs 100, 200, 300 mg; inj 5 mg/ml

Administer:
• PO before meals, at bedtime; tab may be crushed or swallowed whole; give with meals to increase absorption
• Reduced dosage for renal dysfunction
• Do not discontinue prior to surgery

Direct IV route
• Give undiluted (5 mg/ml) over 2 min

Continuous IV INF route

• Diluted in LR, D_5W, D_5 in 0.2%, 0.9%, 0.33% NaCl, Ringer's inj; inf is titrated to patient response; 200 mg of product/160 ml sol = 1 mg/ml; 300 mg of product/240 ml sol = 1 mg/ml; 200 mg of product/250 ml sol = 2 mg/3 ml; use inf pump

• Keep patient recumbent during and for 3 hr after administration; monitor VS q5-15min

Y-site compatibilities: Amikacin, aminophylline, amiodarone, ampicillin, butorphanol, calcium gluconate, ceftazidime, ceftizoxime, cimetidine, diltiazem, DOBUTamine, DOPamine, enalaprilat, EPINEPHrine, erythromycin, esmolol, famotidine, fentaNYL, gentamicin, HYDROmorphone, lidocaine, LORazepam, magnesium sulfate, meperidine, metroNIDAZOLE, midazolam, milrinone, morphine, niCARdipine, nitroglycerin, norepinephrine, nitroprusside, oxacillin, potassium chloride, potassium phosphate, propofol, ranitidine, sodium acetate, tobramycin, vancomycin, vecuronium

SIDE EFFECTS

CNS: Dizziness, mental changes, drowsiness, fatigue, headache, catatonia, depression, anxiety, nightmares, paresthesias, lethargy

CV: *Orthostatic hypotension, bradycardia,* CHF, chest pain, ventricular dysrhythmias, AV block, scalp tingling

EENT: *Tinnitus,* visual changes; sore throat; double vision; dry, burning eyes, floppy iris syndrome

GI: *Nausea, vomiting, diarrhea,* dyspepsia, taste distortion

GU: Impotence, dysuria, ejaculatory failure

HEMA: Agranulocytosis, thrombocytopenia, purpura (rare)

INTEG: Rash, alopecia, urticaria, pruritus, fever, exfoliative dermatitis

RESP: Bronchospasm, dyspnea, wheezing

PHARMACOKINETICS

Half-life 2.5-8 hr, metabolized by liver (metabolites inactive), excreted in urine, crosses placenta, excreted in breast milk, protein binding 50%

PO: Onset 30 min, peak 2-4 hr, duration 8-12 hr

IV: Onset 5 min, peak 15 min, duration 2-4 hr

INTERACTIONS

• Do not use within 2 wk of MAOIs

Increase: myocardial depression—hydantoins, general anesthetics, verapamil, class I antidysrhythmics

Increase: tremor—tricyclic antidepressants

Increase: hypotension—diuretics, other antihypertensives, cimetidine, nitroglycerin, alcohol, nitrates

Decrease: effects of—sympathomimetics, lidocaine, theophylline, β-blockers, bronchodilators, xanthines

Decrease: antihypertensive effect—NSAIDs, salicylates

Increase or decrease: effects of—antidiabetics

Drug/Herb

Increase: antihypertensive effect—hawthorn

Decrease: antihypertensive effect—ephedra

Drug/Lab Test

Increase: ANA titer, blood glucose, alk phos, LDH, AST, ALT, BUN, potassium, triglyceride, uric acid, serum lipoprotein

False increase: urinary catecholamines

NURSING CONSIDERATIONS

Assess:

• **Hypertension:** B/P during beginning treatment, periodically thereafter; note pulse, rate, rhythm, quality; apical/radial pulse before administration; notify prescriber of any significant changes

⚠ CHF: I&O, weight daily; fluid overload: weight gain, jugular venous distention, edema, crackles in lungs

Black Box Warning: Abrupt discontinuation: product should be tapered to prevent adverse reactions

• Baselines of renal/hepatic studies before therapy begins

Perform/provide:

• Storage in dry area at room temp; do not freeze

Evaluate:

• Therapeutic response: decreased B/P after 1-2 wk

Teach patient/family:

Black Box Warning: Not to discontinue product abruptly; to taper over 2 wk; may cause precipitate angina

• Not to use OTC products containing α-adrenergic stimulants (nasal decongestants, OTC cold preparations) unless directed by prescriber
• To report bradycardia, dizziness, confusion, depression, fever
• To take pulse at home; advise when to notify prescriber
• To avoid alcohol, smoking, increased sodium intake
• To comply with weight control, dietary adjustments, modified exercise program
• To carry emergency ID to identify product, allergies
• To avoid hazardous activities if dizziness is present
• **To report symptoms of CHF:** difficulty breathing, especially on exertion or when lying down; night cough; swelling of extremities
• To take medication at bedtime to prevent effect of orthostatic hypotension; to rise slowly
• To avoid driving or other hazardous activities until response is known; dizziness, drowsiness, may occur
• To wear support hose to minimize effects of orthostatic hypotension

TREATMENT OF OVERDOSE:
Lavage, IV glucagonor atropine for bradycardia, IV theophylline for bronchospasm; digoxin, O_2, diuretic for cardiac failure; hemodialysis useful for removal/hypotension; administer vasopressor

lacosamide (Rx)
(la-koe′sa-mide)

Vimpat

Func. class.: Anticonvulsant
Chem. class.: Functionalized amino acid

ACTION: May act through action at sodium channels; exact action is unknown

USES: Adjunctive therapy for partial seizures

CONTRAINDICATIONS: Hypersensitivity

Precautions: Pregnancy (C), breastfeeding, children <17 yr, geriatric patients, allergies, cardiac/renal/hepatic disease, acute MI, atrial fibrillation/flutter, AV block, bradycardia, CHD, dehydration, depression, dialysis, hazardous activity, electrolyte imbalance, heart failure, labor, PR prolongation, sick sinus syndrome, substance abuse, suicidal ideation, syncope, torsades de pointes

DOSAGE AND ROUTES
• **Adult and adolescent ≥17 yr: PO** 50 mg bid, may increase weekly by 100 mg bid to 200-400 mg/day; **IV** 50 mg bid, infuse over 30-60 min, may be increased by 100 mg/day weekly up to 200-400 mg/day maintenance

Renal/hepatic dose

• **Adult: PO/IV** max 300 mg/day for mild to moderate hepatic disease or CCr ≤30 ml/min

Available forms: Film-coated tabs 50, 100, 150, 200 mg; IV 20 ml single-use vials (200 mg/20 ml); oral sol 10 mg/ml

Administer:

PO route

• **Tablet:** give without regard to meals
• **Oral sol:** measure with calibrated measuring device

L

IV route

- May give undiluted or mixed in 0.9%NaCl, D_5, or LR
- Infuse over 30-60 min
- Do not use if discolored or if particulates are present; discard unused portions

SIDE EFFECTS

CNS: Dizziness, syncope, tremor, vertigo, ataxia, drowsiness, fever, hypoesthesia, paresthesias, depression, fatigue, headache, confusion, irritability, psychologic dependence, **suicidal ideation**

CV: **Atrial fibrillation/flutter, AV block, bradycardia, myocarditis, orthostatic hypotension, palpitations, PR prolongation**

EENT: Diplopia, blurred vision, nystagmus, tinnitus

GI: Nausea, constipation, vomiting, **hepatitis**, diarrhea, dyspepsia

HEMA: **Anemia, neutropenia**

INTEG: Rash, erythema, inj site reaction, pruritus, xerostomia

MS: Asthenia, dysarthria

SYST: **Drug reaction with eosinophilia, systemic symptoms (DRESS)**

PHARMACOKINETICS

Metabolized by liver; excreted by kidneys, 95%; protein binding <15%

PO: Peak 1-4 hr

IV: Peak 30-60 min; half-life 13 hr; elimination half-life 15-23 hr

INTERACTIONS

⚠ **Increase:** PR prolongation—beta-blockers, calcium channel blockers, atazanavir, dronedarone, digoxin, lopinavir, ritonavir

⚠ **Increase:** lincosamide effect—CYP2C19 inhibitors (fluconazole, isoniazid, miconazole)

Drug/Lab Test

Increase: LFTs

NURSING CONSIDERATIONS

Assess:

- **Seizures:** duration, type, intensity precipitating factors
- Renal function: albumin concentration
- CV status: orthostatic hypotension, PR prolongation; monitor cardiac status throughout treatment
- Mental status: mood, sensorium, affect, memory (long, short term), depression, suicidal ideation, psychologic dependence
- Rash, hypersensitivity reactions

Perform/provide:

- Storage of PO products/IV vials at room temp; sol is stable for 24 hr when mixed with compatible diluents in glass or PVC bags at room temp

Evaluate:

- Therapeutic response: decrease in severity of seizures

Teach patient/family:

- Not to discontinue product abruptly; to taper over 1 week because seizures may occur
- To avoid hazardous activities until stabilized on product
- To carry emergency ID stating product use
- To notify prescriber of suicidal thoughts/behaviors, syncope, cardiac changes
- To notify prescriber if pregnancy is planned or suspected
- That interactions with other medications may occur
- To consult MedGuide for proper use, risks

lactulose (Rx)

(lak′tyoo-lose)

Apo-Lactulose ♣, Constulose, Enulose, Generlac, Kristalose, PMS-Lactulose ♣, ratio-Lactulose ♣

Func. class.: Laxative; ammonia detoxicant (hyperosmotic)

Chem. class.: Lactose synthetic derivative

ACTION:

Prevents absorption of ammonia in colon by acidifying stool; increases water, softens stool

USES:
Chronic constipation, portal-systemic encephalopathy in patients with hepatic disease

CONTRAINDICATIONS:
Hypersensitivity, low-galactose diet

Precautions: Pregnancy (B), breastfeeding, geriatric patients, debilitated patients, diabetes mellitus

DOSAGE AND ROUTES

Constipation

- **Adult: PO** 15-30 ml/day (10-20 g), may increase to 60 ml/day prn
- **Child: PO** 7.5 ml/day

Hepatic encephalopathy

- **Adult: PO** 30-45 ml (20-30 g) tid or qid until stools soft; **RETENTION ENEMA** 300 ml (200 g) diluted
- **Child: PO** 40-90 ml/day in 3-4 divided doses
- **Infant: PO** 2.5-10 ml/day in divided doses

Available forms: Oral sol (encephalopathy) 10 g/15 ml; oral sol (constipation) 10 g/15 ml

Administer:

PO route

- With 8 oz fruit juice, water, milk to increase palatability of oral form; for rapid effect, give on empty stomach
- Kristalose: dissolve contents of packet/4 oz water

Rectal route

- **Retention enema** by diluting 300 ml lactose/700 ml of water; administer by rectal balloon catheter
- Increased fluids to 2 L/day; do not give with other laxatives; if diarrhea occurs, reduce dosage

SIDE EFFECTS

GI: *Nausea, vomiting, anorexia, abdominal cramps,* diarrhea, flatulence, distention, belching

META: Hypernatremia

PHARMACOKINETICS

Metabolized in colon, excreted by kidneys, onset 1-2 days, peak unknown, duration unknown

INTERACTIONS

- Do not use with other laxatives (hepatic encephalopathy)

Increase: GI obstruction—NIFEdipine ext-rel tabs

Decrease: lactulose effects—neomycin, other oral antiinfectives, antacids

Drug/Herb

Increase: laxative action—flax, senna

Drug/Lab Test

Increase: blood glucose (diabetic patients)

Decrease: blood ammonia

NURSING CONSIDERATIONS

Assess:

- **Stool:** amount, color, consistency
- **Cause of constipation;** determine whether fluids, bulk, or exercise is missing from lifestyle; use of constipating products
- **Hepatic encephalopathy:** blood ammonia level (30-70 mg/100 ml); may decrease ammonia level by 25%-50%; clearing of confusion, lethargy, restlessness, irritability if portal-systemic encephalopathy
- Blood, urine electrolytes if product used often; may cause diarrhea, hypokalemia, hyponatremia
- I&O ratio to identify fluid loss
- Cramping, rectal bleeding, nausea, vomiting; if these symptoms occur, product should be discontinued

Evaluate:

- Therapeutic response: decreased constipation, decreased blood ammonia level, clearing of mental state

Teach patient/family:

- Not to use laxatives long term
- To dilute with water or fruit juice to counteract sweet taste
- To store in cool environment; not to freeze

L

• To take on an empty stomach for rapid action
• To report diarrhea; may indicate overdose

lamiVUDine 3TC (Rx)

(lam-i-voo′deen)

Epivir, Epivir HBV, Heptovir

Func. class.: Antiretroviral

Chem. class.: Nucleoside reverse transcriptase inhibitor (NRTI)

Do not confuse:
lamiVUDine/lamoTRIgine

ACTION:
Inhibits replication of HIV virus by incorporating into cellular DNA by viral reverse transcriptase, thereby terminating cellular DNA chain

USES:
HIV-1 infection in combination with at least 2 other antiretrovirals; chronic hepatitis B (Epivir-HBV)

Unlabeled uses: Prophylaxis of HIV: postexposure with indinavir and zidovudine

CONTRAINDICATIONS:
Hypersensitivity

Black Box Warning: Lactic acidosis

Precautions: Pregnancy (C), breastfeeding, children, geriatric patients, granulocyte count <1000/mm³ or Hgb <9.5 g/dl, renal disease, pancreatitis, peripheral neuropathy

Black Box Warning: Severe hepatic dysfunction

DOSAGE AND ROUTES

HIV

• **Adult and adolescent >16 yr: PO** 150 mg bid or 300 mg/day
• **Child 3 mo-16 yr: PO** 4 mg/kg bid, max 150 mg bid

Chronic hepatitis B

• **Adult: PO** 100 mg/day
• **Child and adolescent 2-17 yr: PO** 3 mg/kg/day, max 100 mg

Renal dose

• **Adult: PO** CCr 30-49 ml/min: Epivir 150 mg/day; Epivir HBV 100 mg 1st dose then 50 mg/day; CCr 15-29 ml/min: Epivir 150 mg 1st dose then 100 mg/day; Epivir HBV 100 mg 1st dose then 25 mg/day; CCr 5-14 ml/min: Epivir 150 mg 1st dose then 50 mg/day; Epivir HBV 35 mg 1st dose then 15 mg/day; CCr <5 ml/min: Epivir 50 mg 1st dose then 25 mg/day; Epivir HBV 35 mg 1st dose then 10 mg/day

Available forms: (Epivir) oral sol 10 mg/ml; tabs 150, 300 mg; **(Epivir HBV)** oral sol 5 mg/ml; tabs 100 mg

Administer:

• PO daily or bid, without regard to meals
• Epivir and Epivir HBV are not interchangeable

SIDE EFFECTS

CNS: *Fever, headache, malaise, dizziness, insomnia, depression, fatigue, chills,* seizures, peripheral neuropathy, paresthesias

EENT: Taste change, hearing loss, photophobia

GI: *Nausea, vomiting, diarrhea,* anorexia, cramps, dyspepsia, hepatomegaly with steatosis, pancreatitis

HEMA: Neutropenia, anemia, thrombocytopenia

INTEG: *Rash*

MS: *Myalgia, arthralgia, pain*

RESP: *Cough*

SYST: Lactic acidosis, anaphylaxis, Stevens-Johnson syndrome

PHARMACOKINETICS

Rapidly absorbed, distributed to extravascular space, excreted unchanged in urine, protein binding <36%, terminal half-life 5-7 hr

INTERACTIONS

Decrease: both products—zalcitabine; avoid concurrent use

Increase: lamiVUDine level—trimethoprim-sulfamethoxazole, amiloride,

dofetilide, entecavir, metformin, memantine, procainamide, trospium
• Do not use with emtricitabine, duplication
Decrease: lamiVUDine effect—interferons
Drug/Lab Test
Increase: ALT, bilirubin
Decrease: Hgb, neutrophil, platelet count

NURSING CONSIDERATIONS

Assess:
• **HIV:** blood counts q2wk; watch for neutropenia, thrombocytopenia, Hgb, CD4, viral load; if low, therapy may have to be discontinued and restarted after hematologic recovery; blood transfusions may be required; assess for lessening of symptoms
• **Hepatitis B:** fatigue, anorexia, pruritus, jaundice during and for several months after discontinuation; AST, ALT, bilirubin; amylase, lipase, triglycerides, periodically during treatment
• **Children for pancreatitis:** abdominal pain, nausea, vomiting, neuropathy

Black Box Warning: Lactic acidosis, severe hepatomegaly with steatosis: obtain baseline LFTs, if elevated, discontinue treatment; discontinue even if LFTs are normal if lactic acidosis, severe hepatomegaly develops, may be fatal

Perform/provide:
• With other antiretrovirals only
• Storage in cool environment; protect from light
Evaluate:
• Blood dyscrasias: bruising, fatigue, bleeding, poor healing
Teach patient/family:
• That GI complaints, insomnia resolve after 3-4 wk of treatment
• That product is not a cure for HIV but will control symptoms; that compliance is necessary; to take as directed; to complete full course of treatment even if feeling better
• To notify prescriber of sore throat, swollen lymph nodes, malaise, fever, peripheral neuropathy; other infections may occur
• That patient is still infective, may pass HIV virus on to others
• That follow-up visits must be continued since serious toxicity may occur; that blood counts must be done
• That other products may be necessary to prevent other infections
• That product may cause fainting or dizziness

lamoTRIgine (Rx)

(la-moe′tri-geen)

Apo-Lamotrigine ✦, Gen-Lamotrigine ✦, Lamictal, Lamictal CD, Lamictal ODT, Lamictal XR, PMS-Lamotrigine ✦, ratio-Lamotrigine ✦

Func. class.: Anticonvulsant—miscellaneous
Chem. class.: Phenyltriazine

Do not confuse:
lamoTRIgine/lamiVUDine
LaMICtal/Lomotil/LamiSIL

ACTION: Inhibits voltage-sensitive sodium channels, thus decreasing seizures

USES: Adjunct for the treatment of partial, tonic-clonic seizures; children with Lennox-Gastaut syndrome, bipolar disorder
Unlabeled uses: Absence, seizures

CONTRAINDICATIONS: Hypersensitivity
Precautions: Pregnancy (C) (cleft lip/palate during 1st trimester), breastfeeding, geriatric patients, cardiac/renal/hepatic disease, severe depression, suicidal, blood dyscrasias

Black Box Warning: Children <16 yr

DOSAGE AND ROUTES

Seizures: monotherapy
• **Adult and adolescent ≥16 yr: PO** 50 mg/day while receiving 1 enzyme-induc-

ing AED (carBAMazepine, PHENobarbital, phenytoin, primidone but not valproic acid) wk 1-2, then increase to 100 mg divided bid wk 3-4; maintenance 300-500 mg/day; EXT REL 50 mg/day × 1-2 wk, then 100 mg/day wk 3-4, then 200 mg/day wk 5, then 300 mg/day wk 6, then 400 mg/day wk 7; after wk 7, range is 400-600 mg/day

• **Adolescent <16 yr and child: PO** 0.3 mg/kg/day wk 1-2, then 0.6 mg/kg/day wk 3-4; depends on use of AED; usual dose 4.5-7.5 mg/kg/day, max 300 mg/day

Monotherapy for patients taking valproate

• **Adult and adolescent ≥1 yr receiving lamoTRIgine and valproate without enzyme-inducing drug: PO** (immediate release) stabilize on valproate, target dose of 200 mg/day lamoTRIgine; if patient is not taking lamoTRIgine 200 mg/day, increase dose by 25-50 mg/day q1-2wk to reach 200 mg/day; while maintaining lamoTRIgine 200 mg/day, decrease valproate to 500 mg/day by ≤500 mg/day/wk, maintain valproate at 500 mg/day × 1 wk, then increase lamoTRIgine to 300 mg/day while decreasing valproate 250 mg/day × 1 wk, then discontinue valproate and increase lamoTRIgine by 100 mg/day/wk to maintenance of 500 mg/day

Seizures: multiple therapy with valproate

• **Adult and adolescent ≥16 yr: PO** 25 mg every other day then 25 mg/day wk 3-4, increase by 25-50 mg q1-2wk, maintenance 100-400 mg/day

• **Adolescent <16 yr and child: PO** 0.1-0.2 mg/kg/day initially then increase q2wk as needed to 1-5 mg/kg/day or 200 mg/day

Bipolar disorder (escalation regimen for those not taking carBAMazepine, other enzyme-inducing drugs, or valproate)

• **Adult and adolescent ≥16 yr: PO** wk 1-2, 25 mg/day; wk 3-4, 50 mg/day; wk 5, 100 mg/day; wk 6-7, 200 mg/day; for patients taking valproic acid: wk 1-2, 25 mg every other day; wk 3-4, 25 mg/day; wk 5, 50 mg/day; wk 6, 100 mg/day; wk 7, 100 mg/day

Hepatic dose

• **Adult: PO** moderate hepatic impairment or severe without ascites: reduce by 25%; severe hepatic impairment with ascites: reduce by 50%

Absence seizures (unlabeled)

• **Adolescent and child 3-13 yr: PO** 0.5 mg/kg/day in 2 divided doses × 2 wk then 1 mg/kg/day in 2 divided doses × 2 wk, adjusted q5days

Available forms: Tabs 25, 100, 150, 200 mg; PO ext rel 25-50-100, 50-100-200 mg titration kit; PO 25-100 mg starter kit; ext rel 25, 50, 100, 250 mg; chew dispersible tabs 5, 25 mg; oral disintegrating tab 25, 50, 100, 200 mg; oral disintegrating tab 25-50, 50-100 mg, 25-50-100 mg titration kit

Administer:

• Correct starter kit; errors have occurred

• Discontinue all products gradually over ≥2 wk; abrupt discontinuation can increase seizures

• **Chewable dispersible tab:** may be swallowed whole, chewed, mixed in water or fruit juice; to mix, add to small amount of liquid in glass or spoon; tabs will dissolve in 1 min, then mix in more liquid and swirl and swallow immediately

• **Orally disintegrating tabs:** place on tongue, move around in mouth, when disintegrated, swallow; examine blister pack before use, do not use if blisters are torn or missing

• **Extended-release tabs:** swallow whole, do not cut, break, chew

SIDE EFFECTS

CNS: *Dizziness,* ataxia, *headache,* fever, insomnia, tremor, depression, anxiety, suicidal ideation

EENT: Nystagmus, *diplopia, blurred vision*

GI: *Nausea, vomiting, anorexia, abdominal pain,* hepatotoxicity
GU: *Dysmenorrhea*
HEMA: Anemia, DIC, leukopenia, thrombocytopenia
INTEG: Rash (potentially life-threatening), alopecia, photosensitivity
SYST: **Stevens-Johnson syndrome, angioedema, toxic epidermal necrolysis**

PHARMACOKINETICS

Half-life varies depending on dose; terminal half-life 24 hr, 15 hr with enzyme inducers; rapidly, completely absorbed; metabolized by glucuronic acid conjunction; protein binding 55%; peak 1.4-2.3 hr; crosses placenta; excreted in breast milk

INTERACTIONS

Decrease: metabolic clearance of lamoTRIgine—valproic acid, CYP3A4 inhibitors
Decrease: lamoTRIgine serum concentration—carBAMazepine, rifamycins, oral contraceptives, acetaminophen, phenytoin, primodone, PHENobarbital, oxcarbazepine, succinimides, estrogen
Drug/Herb
Increase: anticonvulsant effect—ginkgo
Decrease: anticonvulsant effect—ginseng

NURSING CONSIDERATIONS

Assess:
- **Seizure:** duration, type, intensity, halo before seizure

⚠ **Rash (Stevens-Johnson syndrome, toxic epidermal necrolysis) in pediatric patients; product should be discontinued at first sign of rash**

⚠ **Bipolar disorder:** **suicidal thoughts/behaviors**

Evaluate:
- Therapeutic response: decrease in severity of seizures or of bipolar symptoms

Teach patient/family:
- To take PO doses divided, with or after meals to decrease adverse effects; not to discontinue product abruptly because seizures may occur
- To avoid hazardous activities until stabilized on product
- To carry emergency ID; to notify prescriber of skin rash, increased seizure activity; to use sunscreen, protective clothing if photosensitivity occurs
- To notify prescriber if pregnant, intending to become pregnant
- To notify prescriber immediately of suicidal thoughts/behaviors

lansoprazole (Rx, OTC)

(lan-so-prey′zole)

Prevacid, Prevacid SoluTab

Func. class.: Antiulcer, proton pump inhibitor

Chem. class.: Benzimidazole

Do not confuse:
Prevacid/Pravachol/Prinivil

ACTION: Suppresses gastric secretion by inhibiting hydrogen/potassium ATPase enzyme system in gastric parietal cell; characterized as gastric acid pump inhibitor because it blocks the final step of acid production

USES: Gastroesophageal reflux disease (GERD), severe erosive esophagitis, poorly responsive systemic GERD, pathologic hypersecretory conditions (Zollinger-Ellison syndrome, systemic mastocytosis, multiple endocrine adenomas); possibly effective for treatment of duodenal, gastric ulcers, maintenance of healed duodenal ulcers
Unlabeled uses: GERD (infants/neonates)

CONTRAINDICATIONS: Hypersensitivity
Precautions: Pregnancy (B), breastfeeding, children

DOSAGE AND ROUTES

Frequent heartburn

• **Adult: PO (OTC)** 15 mg daily up to 14 days

Duodenal ulcer

• **Adult: PO** 15 mg/day before eating for 4 wk then 15 mg/day to maintain healing of ulcers; associated with *Helicobacter pylori*: 30 mg lansoprazole, 500 mg clarithromycin, 1 g amoxicillin bid × 14 days or 30 mg lansoprazole, 1 g amoxicillin tid × 14 days

Pathologic hypersecretory conditions

• **Adult: PO** 60 mg/day, may give up to 90 mg bid, administer doses of >120 mg/day in divided doses

GERD/esophagitis

• **Adult and adolescent: PO** 15-30 mg/day × 8 wk

• **Child 1-11 yr (>30 kg): PO** 30 mg/day ≤12 wk

• **Child 1-11 yr (≤30 kg): PO** 15 mg/day ≤12 wk

• **Infant (unlabeled): PO** 1-1.74 mg/kg/day; limited data available

• **Neonate (unlabeled): PO** 0.5-1 mg/kg/day

Stress gastric prophylaxis

• **Adult: NG** Use 30 mg oral cap or 30 mg disintegrating tab

Available forms: Del rel caps 15, 30 mg; orally disintegrating tabs 15, 30 mg

Administer:

PO route

• Swallow caps whole 30 min before eating; do not crush or chew caps; caps may be opened and contents sprinkled on food

NG route

• **Oral cap:** open cap and pour 1/4 of granules into NG feeding syringe with plunger removed, slowly add water and depress plunger, repeat until all granules used; flush tube with 15 ml water

• **Oral disintegrating tab:** mix 30 mg tab in 10 ml water, give via NG tube, flush tube with 10 ml sterile water, clamp for 60 min

SIDE EFFECTS

CNS: Headache, dizziness, confusion, agitation, amnesia, depression

CV: Chest pain, angina, tachycardia, bradycardia, palpitations, CVA, hypo/hypertension, MI, shock, vasodilation

EENT: Tinnitus, taste perversion, deafness, eye pain, otitis media

GI: Diarrhea, abdominal pain, vomiting, nausea, constipation, flatulence, acid regurgitation, anorexia, irritable colon, microscopic colitis

GU: Hematuria, glycosuria, impotence, kidney calculus, breast enlargement

HEMA: Hemolysis, anemia

INTEG: Rash, urticaria, pruritus, alopecia

META: Weight gain/loss, gout

RESP: Upper respiratory infections, cough, epistaxis, asthma, bronchitis, dyspnea, pneumonia

PHARMACOKINETICS

Absorption after granules leave stomach 80%; plasma half-life 1½-2 hr; protein binding 97%; extensively metabolized in liver; excreted in urine, feces; clearance decreased in geriatric patients, renal/hepatic impairment

INTERACTIONS

Decrease: antiplatelets, effect of—clopidogrel

Increase: lansoprazole, toxicity—fluroxamine, voriconazole

Decrease: lansoprazole absorption—sucralfate

Decrease: absorption of ketoconazole, itraconazole, iron salts, calcium carbonate, atazanavir, ampicillin

Increase: hypomagnesemia—loop/thiazide diuretics

Decrease: lansoprazole effect—antimuscarinics, octreotide, H_2-blockers, misoprostol

Decrease: release of ext rel amphetamine/dextroamphetamine

• Avoid use with dasatinib, delavirdine

Drug/Herb

• Avoid use with red yeast rice

Drug/Lab Test
Increase: AST, ALT, alk phos, creatinine, LDH, gastrin, bilirubin

NURSING CONSIDERATIONS

Assess:
- GI system: bowel sounds q8hr, abdomen for pain, swelling, anorexia, blood in stool, emesis
- Hepatic studies: AST, ALT, alk phos during treatment
- INR and prothrombin time when taking warfarin

Evaluate:
- Therapeutic response: absence of epigastric pain, swelling, fullness

Teach patient/family:
- To report severe diarrhea; product may have to be discontinued
- That hypoglycemia may occur if diabetic
- To avoid hazardous activities; that dizziness may occur
- To avoid alcohol, salicylates, ibuprofen; may cause GI irritation

RARELY USED

lanthanum (Rx)
(lan′-tha-num)
Fosrenol
Func. class.: Phosphate binder

USES: End-stage renal disease

CONTRAINDICATIONS: Hypophosphatemia, hypersensitivity

DOSAGE AND ROUTES

- **Adult: PO** 750-1500 mg/day in divided doses with meals; titrate dose q2-3wk until an acceptable phosphate level is reached; tabs should be chewed completely before swallowing; intact tabs should not be swallowed; maintenance dose 1500-3000 mg/day divided with meals

⚠ HIGH ALERT

lapatinib (Rx)
(la-pa′tin-ib)
Tykerb
Func. class.: Antineoplastic—miscellaneous
Chem. class.: Biologic response modifier, signal transduction inhibitor (STIs)

ACTION: Reverses tyrosine kinase of both the epidermal growth factor receptor (ERbB1) and the human epidermal receptor type 2 (HER2) (ERbB2)

USES: Advanced metastatic breast cancer patients with tumor that overexpresses HER2 protein and who have received previous chemotherapy; those for whom hormonal therapy is indicated

CONTRAINDICATIONS: Pregnancy (D), breastfeeding, hypersensitivity, torsades de pointes
Precautions: Geriatric patients, cardiac disease, bradycardia, hypertension, hypokalemia, hypomagnesemia, QT prolongation
Black Box Warning: Hepatic disease

DOSAGE AND ROUTES

Advanced/metastatic breast cancer with HER2 overexpression who have received previous therapy
- **Adult: PO** 1250 mg (5 tabs)/day 1 hr before or after food on days 1-21 plus capecitabine 2000 mg/m^2/day in 2 divided doses on days 1-14 in a repeating 21-day cycle; continue until therapeutic response or toxicity occurs

Metastatic breast cancer with HER2 overexpression for whom hormonal therapy is indicated
- **Adult: PO** 1500 mg (6 tabs) 1 hr before food with letrozole 2.5 mg/day

L

Hepatic dose
- **Adult: PO** (Child-Pugh C) 750 mg/day (with capecitabine); 1000 mg/day (with letrozole)

Available forms: Tabs 250 mg
Administer:
- Once a day with water on an empty stomach, 1 hr before or after food
- Do not use with grapefruit products

SIDE EFFECTS

CNS: Fatigue, insomnia, palmar-plantar erythrodysesthesia (hand/foot syndrome)
CV: Heart failure, palpitations, QT prolongation
GI: Anorexia, diarrhea, dyspepsia, mouth ulcerations, nausea, vomiting, xerosis
HEMA: Anemia, neutropenia, thrombocytopenia
INTEG: Rash
RESP: Dyspnea, pneumonitis

PHARMACOKINETICS

Bioavailability incomplete; peak 4 hr; >99% protein bound; extensively metabolized in the liver by P450 enzymes CYP3A4, CYP3A5; elimination half-life 24 hr; steady state 6-7 days; increased half-life in hepatic disease

INTERACTIONS

⚠ **Increase:** effect of lapatinib—CYP3A4 inhibitors (amiodarone, amprenavir, aprepitant, atazanavir, chloramphenicol, clarithromycin, conivaptan, dalfopristin, danazol, darunavir, delavirdine, diltiazem, efavirenz, erythromycin, estradiol, fluconazole, fluvoxamine, imatinib, indinavir, isoniazid, itraconazole, ketoconazole, miconazole, mifepristone, nefazodone, nelfinavir, propoxyphene, quinupristin, ritonavir, RU-486, saquinavir, telithromycin, troleandomycin, verapamil, voriconazole, zafirlukast); avoid concurrent use
⚠ **Increase:** QT prolongation—CYP3A4 inhibitors (amiodarone, clarithromycin, erythromycin, telithromycin, troleandomycin); class IA/III antidysrhythmics, arsenic trioxide, chlorproMAZINE, chloroquine, haloperidol, levomethadyl, mesoridazine, pentamine, thioridazine, CYP3A4 substrates (methadone, pimozide, quetiapine, quiNIDine, risperidone, terfenadine, ziprasidone)

NURSING CONSIDERATIONS

Assess:
- Cardiac status: ECG for QT prolongation, ejection fraction; chest pain, palpitations, dyspnea
- Hepatic status: liver function tests; jaundice of sclera, skin; dose should be reduced in hepatic disease

⚠ **Skin toxicities** NCI CTC grade ≥2 discontinue use in those with decreased left ventricular ejection fraction (LVEF) or for a LVEF that drops below institution's lower limit of normal; product may be restarted after 2 wk if LVEF recovers to normal at 1000 mg/day; restart at 1250 mg/day when toxicity improves to grade 1 or better

Perform/provide:
- Storage at room temp, away from heat

Evaluate:
- Therapeutic response: decrease in breast cancer progression

Teach patient/family:
- To take with a full glass of water, once a day, 1 hr before or after food; not to take with food or grapefruit products
- To take as directed only; if a dose is missed, to take as soon as remembered; if it is close to the next dose, to take only that dose; not to double

⚠ To report chest pain, difficulty breathing, fever, chills, sore throat, bleeding, bruising, yellow skin or eyes, severe fatigue, dizziness, palpitations to prescriber
- That other side effects that may occur, but do not need to be reported: nausea, diarrhea, heartburn, mouth sores, rash, numbness/pain in hands/feet

⚠ To use adequate contraception because the fetus could be damaged by this product (D)

latanoprost ophthalmic

See Appendix B

leflunomide (Rx)

(leh-floo′noh-mide)

Arava

Func. class.: Antirheumatic (DMARDs)

Chem. class.: Immune modulator, pyrimidine synthesis inhibitor

ACTION: Inhibits an enzyme involved in pyrimidine synthesis; has antiproliferative, antiinflammatory effect

USES: RA: to reduce disease process and symptoms

Unlabeled uses: Juvenile RA

CONTRAINDICATIONS: Breastfeeding, hypersensitivity, jaundice, lactase deficiency, hepatic disease

Black Box Warning: Pregnancy (X)

Precautions: Children, renal disorders, vaccinations, infection, alcoholism, immunosuppression

Black Box Warning: Hepatic disease

DOSAGE AND ROUTES

Rheumatoid arthritis

- **Adult: PO** Loading dose 100 mg/day × 3 days, maintenance 20 mg/day; may be decreased to 10 mg/day if not well tolerated

Juvenile rheumatoid arthritis (unlabeled)

- **Adolescent and child >40 kg: PO** 20 mg
- **Adolescent and child 20-40 kg: PO** 15 mg
- **Adolescent and child 10-19.9 kg: PO** 10 mg

Available forms: Tabs 10, 20 mg

Administer:

- Give loading dose of 100 mg/day × 3, then 20 mg/day; decrease to 10 mg/day if poorly tolerated
- With food for GI upset
- **Drug elimination:** give cholestyramine 8 g tid × 11 days, check levels

SIDE EFFECTS

CNS: *Headache,* dizziness, insomnia, depression, paresthesia, anxiety, migraine, neuralgia

CV: Palpitations, hypertension, chest pain, angina pectoris, peripheral edema

EENT: Pharyngitis, oral candidiasis, stomatitis, dry mouth, blurred vision

GI: *Nausea, anorexia, vomiting, constipation, flatulence, diarrhea, elevated LFTs,* **hepatotoxicity**

HEMA: Anemia, ecchymosis, hyperlipidemia

INTEG: Rash, pruritus, alopecia, acne, hematoma, herpes infections

RESP: Pharyngitis, rhinitis, bronchitis, cough, respiratory infection, pneumonia, sinusitis, **interstitial lung disease**

SYST: **Opportunistic/fatal infections**

PHARMACOKINETICS

Metabolized in liver to active metabolite, half-life of metabolite 2 wk, excreted in urine

INTERACTIONS

Increase: NSAID effect—NSAIDs

Increase: leflunomide side effects—hepatotoxic agents, methotrexate

Increase: rifampin levels—rifampin

Decrease: antibody response—live virus vaccines

Decrease: leflunomide effect—activated charcoal, cholestyramine

NURSING CONSIDERATIONS

Assess:

- Screen for latent TB before starting treatment; if TB is present, pretreat before using product
- **Interstitial lung disease:** increased or worsening cough, SOB, fever; product may need to be discontinued
- **Arthritic symptoms:** ROM, mobility, swelling of joints at baseline and during treatment

Black Box Warning: Hepatic studies: if ALT elevations are > 2× ULN, reduce dose to 10 mg/day

- CBC with differential q6mo then q6-8mo thereafter; pregnancy test; serum electrolytes

⚠ **Infections:** fatal infections can occur

- B/P, weight; edema can occur

Evaluate:

- Therapeutic response: decreased inflammation, pain in joints

Teach patient/family:

- That product must be continued for prescribed time to be effective
- To take with food, milk, or antacids to avoid GI upset; to take at same time of day
- To use caution when driving because drowsiness, dizziness may occur
- To take with a full glass of water to enhance absorption

Black Box Warning: Not to become pregnant while taking this product; not to breastfeed while taking this product; men should also discontinue product and begin leflunomide removal protocol if pregnancy is planned

- That hair may be lost; review alternatives
- To avoid live virus vaccinations during treatment
- To notify prescriber of weight loss
- Overdose treatment: give cholestyramine tid × 24 hr or activated charcoal

lenalidomide (Rx)

(len-a-lid′o-mide)

Revlimid

Func. class.: Antianemic, biologic response modifier, hormone

Chem. class.: Thalidomide derivative/TNF modifier

ACTION: Decreases secretion of inflammatory cytokines; increases secretion of antiinflammatory cytokines, COX-2 inhibition

USES: Transfusion-dependent anemia due to low- or intermediate-1-risk myelodysplastic syndrome (MDS); multiple myeloma in combination with dexamethasone

CONTRAINDICATIONS: Breastfeeding, hypersensitivity

Black Box Warning: Pregnancy (X), females

Precautions: Children, geriatric patients, accidental exposure, bone marrow suppression, dental disease, uterine bleeding, fungal/viral infections, smoking

Black Box Warning: Neutropenia/thrombocytopenia, thromboembolic disease

DOSAGE AND ROUTES

Transfusion-dependent anemia due to low- or intermediate-1-risk myelodysplastic syndrome (MDS) associated with a deletion 5q cytogenetic abnormality with/without additional cytogenetic abnormalities

- **Adult: PO** 10 mg/day; continue/adjust based on clinical toxicity, laboratory findings

Multiple myeloma in combination with dexamethasone in patients who have failed to respond to at least 1 prior therapy

- **Adult: PO** 25 mg/day on days 1-21 along with dexamethasone 40 mg/day **PO** on days 1-4, 9-12, and 17-20 of each 28-day cycle for the first 4 therapy cycles; starting with cycle 5, lenalidomide dose stays the same but give only dexamethasone 40 mg/day **PO** on days 1-4 q28days; continue/adjust dosing based on clinical and laboratory findings

Dosage adjustments for hematologic toxicities (myelodysplastic syndrome [MDS])

- **Thrombocytopenia or neutropenia that develops within 4 wk of starting at 10 mg/day PO:** reduce dose from 10 mg/day **PO** to 5 mg/day **PO**; withhold lenalidomide if platelet count <50,000/mm^3 from a baseline of at least 100,000/mm^3, if platelet count falls to 50% of baseline value if baseline is <100,000/mm^3, if absolute neutrophil count (ANC) <750/mm^3 from baseline of at least 1000/mm^3, or if <500/mm^3 from baseline of <1000/mm^3; new dose of 5 mg/day **PO** may begin when platelet count is at least 50,000/mm^3 (30,000/mm^3 if the baseline <60,000/mm^3) and when the ANC returns to at least 1000/mm^3 or 500/mm^3 for patients with a baseline of <1000/mm^3

• **Thrombocytopenia or neutropenia that develops after 4 wk of starting at 10 mg/day PO:** Reduce dose from 10 mg/day **PO** to 5 mg/day **PO**; withhold lenalidomide if platelet count <30,000/mm^3, if platelet count <50,000/mm^3 and platelet transfusion occurs, if neutrophils <500/mm^3 for at least 7 days, or if neutrophils <500/mm^3 and temp of ≥38.5° C present; new dose of 5 mg/day **PO** may begin when platelet count at least 30,000/mm^3 without hemostatic failure and ANC at least 500/mm^3

• **Thrombocytopenia or neutropenia that develops while taking 5 mg/day PO:** Reduce dose from 5 mg/day **PO** to 5 mg/day **PO** every other day; withhold lenalidomide if platelet count <30,000/mm^3, platelet count <50,000/mm^3 and platelet transfusion occurs, neutrophils <500/mm^3 for at least 7 days, or if neutrophils <500/mm^3 and a temp of ≥38.5° C present; new dose of 5 mg **PO** every other day may begin when platelet count is at least 30,000/mm^3 without hemostatic failure and ANC is at least 500/mm^3

Dosage adjustments for toxicities (multiple myeloma)

• **Thrombocytopenia:** Reduce dose from 25 mg/day **PO** to 15 mg/day **PO**; withhold lenalidomide if platelet count <30,000/mm^3; check CBC weekly; new dose of 15 mg/day **PO** may begin when platelet count is at least 30,000/mm^3; withhold lenalidomide each time platelet count is <30,000/mm^3; new dose of 5 mg < previous dose should be started when platelet count is at least 30,000/mm^3; do not dose below 5 mg/day **PO**

• **Neutropenia without other toxicity:** Hold dose; withhold lenalidomide and add G-CSF if neutrophils <1000/mm^3; check CBC weekly; resume lenalidomide at 25 mg/day **PO** when neutrophils are at least 1000/mm^3 and neutropenia is only toxicity

• **Neutropenia with other toxicity:** Reduce dose from 25 mg/day **PO** to 15 mg/day **PO**; withhold lenalidomide, add G-CSF if neutrophils <1000/mm^3; check CBC weekly; resume lenalidomide at 15 mg/day **PO** when neutrophils are at least 1000/mm^3; withhold lenalidomide, add G-CSF each time the neutrophils are <1000/mm^3; if other toxicity is present, new dose of 5 mg < previous dose should be started when neutrophils are at least 1000/mm^3; do not dose below 5 mg/day **PO**

• **Other grade 3 or 4 toxicity judged to be related to lenalidomide:** Reduce dose from 25 mg/day **PO** to 15 mg/day **PO**; withhold lenalidomide and resume lenalidomide at 15 mg/day **PO** when toxicity has resolved to grade ≤2; withhold lenalidomide each time grade 3 or 4 toxicity occurs; new dose of 5 mg < previous dose should be started when toxicity has resolved to grade ≤2; do not dose below 5 mg/day **PO**

Renal dose

• **Adult: PO** CCr 30-59 ml/min, 5 mg q24hr (MDS); 10 mg q24hr (multiple myeloma); CCr <30 ml/min (not requiring dialysis), 5 mg q48hr (MDS), 15 mg q48hr (multiple myeloma)

Available forms: Caps 5, 10, 15, 25 mg

Administer:

• PO, with dexamethasone for multiple myeloma
• Do not crush or open caps
• All persons involved must comply with conditions of rev assist program

SIDE EFFECTS

CNS: Depression, dizziness, fatigue, fever, headache, sweating, peripheral enuropathy

CV: Chest pain, hypotension, palpitations
GI: Abdominal pain, anorexia, constipation, diarrhea, nausea/vomiting, dysgeusia, xerosis
HEMA: Anemia, leukopenia, neutropenia, pancytopenia, thrombocytopenia
META: Hypokalemia, hypomagnesemia
MS: Arthralgia, back pain, myalgia
RESP: Cough, dyspnea, pulmonary embolism, epistaxis, rhinitis
SYST: Angioedema, secondary malignancy

PHARMACOKINETICS

Rapid absorption, elimination half-life 3 hr

INTERACTIONS

Increase: bleeding risk—anticoagulants, salicylates, NSAIDs, thrombolytics, platelet inhibitors
Decrease: immune response—vaccines/toxoids

NURSING CONSIDERATIONS

Assess:

Black Box Warning: Blood studies: Hct, Hgb, electrolytes

- B/P for hypotension

Black Box Warning: For hypersensitivity reactions: skin rashes, urticaria (rare)

Black Box Warning: For pregnancy before treatment, pregnancy category (X)

Evaluate:

- Therapeutic response: increase in reticulocyte count

Teach patient/family:

- To avoid driving or hazardous activity during beginning of treatment

⚠ HIGH ALERT

lepirudin (Rx)

(lep-ih-roo′din)

Refludan

Func. class.: Anticoagulant

Chem. class.: Thrombin inhibitor, hirudin

ACTION: Direct inhibitor of thrombin that is highly specific

USES: Anticoagulation in those with heparin-induced thrombocytopenia (HIT) and other thromboembolic conditions
Unlabeled uses: Adjunct therapy for unstable angina, acute MI without ST elevation; prevention of DVT, PCI

CONTRAINDICATIONS: Hypersensitivity to hirudins
Precautions: Pregnancy (B), breastfeeding, children, geriatric patients, women, intracranial bleeding, hepatic disease, recent major surgery, hemorrhagic diathesis bacterial endocarditis, severe uncontrolled hypertension, advanced renal disease, recent active peptic ulcer, recent CVA, stroke, intracerebral surgery

DOSAGE AND ROUTES

Heparin-induced thrombocytopenia (not receiving thrombolytic therapy concurrently)

- **Adult: IV BOL** 0.4 mg/kg over 15-20 sec then 0.15 mg/kg/hr as a **CONT INF** for ≥2-10 days

Concomitant use with thrombolytic therapy

- **Adult: IV BOL** 0.2 mg/kg initially then **CONT IV INF** 0.1 mg/kg/hr

Renal dose

- **Adult: IV BOL** 0.2 mg/kg over 15-20 sec, then, if CCr 45-60 ml/min, 0.075 mg/kg/hr; CCr 30-44 ml/min, 0.045 mg/kg/hr; CCr 15-29 ml/min, 0.0225 mg/kg/hr

Available forms: Powder for inj 50 mg

Administer:

- Avoid all IM inj, venipunctures if possible

IV Direct route

- Reconstitute each vial with 1 ml sterile water or 0.9% NaCl; shake gently; transfer content of vial into 10-ml syringe, dilute to a volume of 10 ml with sterile water for inj, D_5W, or 0.9% NaCl; final conc 5 mg/ml

Continuous IV INF route

- Reconstitute 2 vials with 1 ml each of sterile water for inj or 0.9% NaCl; transfer contents into inf bag containing 250 or 500 ml 0.9% NaCl or D_5W for a conc of 0.2 mg/ml or 0.4 mg/ml, respectively; infuse at 0.15 mg/kg/hr; use inf pump

Y-site compatibilities: amiodarone

SIDE EFFECTS

CNS: *Fever,* **intracranial bleeding**

CV: **Heart failure, pericardial effusion, ventricular fibrillation**

GI: GI bleeding, abnormal LFTs

GU: **Hematuria,** abnormal kidney function, vaginal bleeding

HEMA: **Hemorrhage, thrombocytopenia, anemia**

INTEG: Allergic skin reactions

RESP: Pneumonia, stridor, dyspnea, **bronchospasm**

SYST: **Multiorgan failure, sepsis, anaphylaxis**

PHARMACOKINETICS

Distributed to extracellular fluid, metabolized by release of amino acids during catabolism, 50% unchanged in urine; terminal half-life 1.3 hr, longer with renal disease

INTERACTIONS

Increase: bleeding risk—warfarin derivatives, thrombolytics, NSAIDs, plicamycin, cefamandole, cefotetan, cefoperazone, aspirin, clopidogrel, dipyridamole, eptifibatide, ticlopidine, tirofiban, valproic acid

NURSING CONSIDERATIONS

Assess:

- **Anticoagulation:** obtain baseline aPTT before treatment; do not start treatment if aPTT ratio ≥2.5, then obtain aPTT 4 hr after initiation of treatment and at least daily thereafter; if aPTT above target, stop inf for 2 hr then restart at 50%, take aPTT in 4 hr; if below target, increase inf rate by 20%, take aPTT in 4 hr, max rate of 0.21 mg/kg/hr without checking for coagulation abnormalities
- aPTT, which should be 1.5-2.5× control

⚠ **Bleeding/hemorrhage: bleeding gums, petechiae, ecchymosis, black tarry stools, hematuria, epistaxis, B/P, vaginal bleeding and possible hemorrhage**

- Hct, Hgb, platelets, serum creatinine, urinalysis, stool guaiac
- **Hypersensitivity:** fever, skin rash, urticaria

Evaluate:

- Therapeutic response: anticoagulation, aPTT 1.5-2.5, absence of bleeding

Teach patient/family:

- To use soft-bristle toothbrush to avoid bleeding gums; to avoid contact sports; to use an electric razor; to avoid IM inj
- To report any signs of bleeding: gums, under skin, in urine or stools
- Overdose treatment: stop product, draw aPTT, Hct; provide blood transfusion

letrozole (Rx)

(let′tro-zohl)

Femara

Func. class.: Antineoplastic, nonsteroidal aromatase inhibitor

ACTION: Binds to the heme group of aromatase; inhibits conversion of androgens to estrogens to reduce plasma estrogen levels

USES: Early, advanced, or metastatic breast cancer in postmenopausal women

Unlabeled uses: Infertility, idiopathic short stature, constitutional delayed puberty

CONTRAINDICATIONS:

Pregnancy (D), premenopausal females, hypersensitivity

Precautions: Respiratory/hepatic disease, osteoporosis

DOSAGE AND ROUTES

• **Adult: PO** 2.5 mg/day

Infertility (unlabeled)

• **Adult: PO** 2.5, 5, 7.5 mg/day × 5 days, usually days 3-7 of menstrual cycle

Idiopathic short stature, constitutional delayed puberty (unlabeled)

• **Adolescent and child ≥9 (male): PO** 2.5 mg/day; use with testosterone for delayed puberty

Available forms: Tabs 2.5 mg

Administer:

• Without regard to meals; with small glass of water

• May administer biphosphates to increase bone density

SIDE EFFECTS

CNS: *Headache, lethargy,* somnolence, dizziness, depression, anxiety

CV: Angina, MI, CVA, thromboembolic events, hypertension, peripheral edema

GI: *Nausea, vomiting, anorexia,* constipation, heartburn, diarrhea

GU: Endometrial cancer, vaginal bleeding, endometrial proliferation disorders

INTEG: *Rash, pruritus,* alopecia, sweating

MISC: Hot flashes, night sweats, second malignancies, anaphylaxis, angioedema

MS: Arthralgia, arthritis, bone fracture, myalgia, osteoporosis

RESP: Dyspnea, cough

PHARMACOKINETICS

Metabolized in liver, excreted in urine, peak 2 days, terminal half-life 48 hr, steady state 2-6 wk

INTERACTIONS

Decrease: letrozole effect—estrogens, oral contraceptives

NURSING CONSIDERATIONS

Assess:

• Hepatic studies before, during therapy (bilirubin, AST, ALT, LDH) as needed or monthly

Evaluate:

• Therapeutic response: decrease in size of tumor

Teach patient/family:

• To report allergic reactions (rash; hives; difficulty breathing; tightness in chest; swelling of mouth, face, lips, tongue)

• To report vaginal bleeding, diarrhea, chest/bone pain

• To use adequate contraception in perimenopausal, recently postmenopausal women; pregnancy (D)

leucovorin (Rx)

(loo-koe-vor′in)

Func. class.: Vitamin, folic acid/methotrexate antagonist antidote

Chem. class.: Tetrahydrofolic acid derivative

Do not confuse:

leucovorin/Leukeran/leukine

folinic acid/folic acid

ACTION:

Needed for normal growth patterns; prevents toxicity during antineoplastic therapy by protecting normal cells

USES:

Megaloblastic or macrocytic anemia caused by folic acid deficiency, overdose of folic acid antagonist, methotrexate/pyrimethamine/ trimetrexate/trimethoprim toxicity, pneumocystosis, toxoplasmosis

CONTRAINDICATIONS:

Hypersensitivity to this product or folic acid, benzyl alcohol; anemias other than megaloblastic not associated with vit B_{12} deficiency

Precautions: Pregnancy (C), neonates, breastfeeding, geriatric patients, seizures, stomatitis, vomiting

DOSAGE AND ROUTES

Megaloblastic anemia caused by enzyme deficiency

- **Adult and child: PO/IV/IM** up to 6 mg/day

Megaloblastic anemia caused by deficiency of folate

- **Adult and child: IM** ≤1 mg/day until adequate response

Methotrexate toxicity/leucovorin rescue

- **Adult and child: PO/IM/IV Normal elimination** given 6 hr after dose of methotrexate (10 mg/m^2) until methotrexate $<5 \times 10^{-8}$ m, CCr >50% above prior level, or methotrexate level 5×10^{-8} m at 24 hr or $>9 \times 10^{-8}$ m at 48 hr; give leucovorin 100 mg/m^2 q3hr until level drops to $<10^{-8}$ m

Pyrimethamine/trimethoprim toxicity

- **Adult and child: PO/IM** 5-15 mg/day

Advanced colorectal cancer

- **Adult: IV** 200 mg/m^2, then 5-FU 370 mg/m^2 or leucovorin 20 mg/m^2, then 5-FU 425 mg/m^2; give daily × 5 days q4-5wk

Available forms: Tabs 5, 10, 15, 25 mg; inj 3, 5 mg/ml; powder for inj 10 mg/ml

Administer:

- Within 1 hr of folic acid antagonist
- Do not give concurrently with systemic methotrexate

IM route

- No reconstitution needed
- For treatment of megaloblastic anemia

IV route

- Reconstitute 50 mg/5 ml bacteriostatic or sterile water for inj (10 mg/ml) or (100 mg/10 ml); use immediately if sterile water used

Direct IV route

- Give over 160 mg/min or less (16 ml of 10 mg/ml sol/min)

Intermittent IV INF route

- Give after diluting in 100-500 ml of 0.9% NaCl, D_5W, $D_{10}W$, LR, Ringer's sol

Y-site compatibilities: Amifostine, aztreonam, bleomycin, cefepime, CISplatin, cladribine, cyclophosphamide, DOXOrubicin, DOXOrubicin liposome, filgrastim, fluconazole, fluorouracil, furosemide, granisetron, heparin, methotrexate, metoclopramide, mitomycin, piperacillin/tazobactam, tacrolimus, teniposide, thiotepa, vinBLAStine, vinCRIStine

SIDE EFFECTS

HEMA: Thrombocytosis (intraarterial)

INTEG: Rash, pruritus, erythema, urticaria

RESP: Wheezing

INTERACTIONS

Increase: metabolism of barbiturates, hydantoins, primidone

Decrease: effect of—sulfamethoxazole, trimethoprim

NURSING CONSIDERATIONS

Assess:

- CCr, creatinine before leucovorin rescue, daily to detect nephrotoxicity; methotrexate level
- I&O; urine pH q6hr, maintain >7 to prevent neurotoxicity; watch for nausea and vomiting
- **Other products taken:** alcohol, hydantoins, trimethoprim may cause increased folic acid use by body
- Neurologic status (rescue): weakness, fatigue
- Monitor calcium levels
- Megaloblastic anemia, plasma lactic acid, leticulocyte count, Hct, Hgb
- **Hypersensitivity:** rash, urticaria, wheezing; notify prescriber

Perform/provide:

- Increased fluid intake if used to treat folic acid inhibitor overdose
- Protection from light and heat

Evaluate:

- Therapeutic response: increased weight; improved orientation, well-being;

absence of fatigue; reversal of toxicity (methotrexate, folic acid antagonist overdose)

Teach patient/family:

- **For leucovorin rescue** to drink 3 L fluid/day of rescue
- **For folic acid deficiency,** to eat folic-acid–rich foods: bran; yeast; dried beans; nuts; fresh, green leafy vegetables
- To take product exactly as prescribed
- To notify prescriber of side effects
- To report signs of hyposensitivity reaction immediately
- To avoid breastfeeding

⚠ HIGH ALERT

leuprolide (Rx)

(loo-proe′lide)

Eligard, Lupron Depot, Viadur

Func. class.: Antineoplastic hormone

Chem. class.: Gonadotropin-releasing hormone

Do not confuse:

Lupron/Nuprin/Lopurin

ACTION: Causes initial increase in circulating levels of LH, FSH; continuous administration results in decreased LH, FSH; in men, testosterone is reduced to castrate levels; in premenopausal women, estrogen is reduced to menopausal levels

USES: Metastatic prostate cancer (inj implant), management of endometriosis, central precocious puberty, uterine leiomyomata (fibroids)

Unlabeled uses: Breast cancer, recurrent priapism, benign prostatic hyperplasia

CONTRAINDICATIONS: Pregnancy (X), breastfeeding, hypersensitivity to GnRH or analogs, thromboembolic disorders, undiagnosed vaginal bleeding; Viadur implant or Eligard should not be used in women, children

Precautions: Edema, hepatic disease, CVA, MI, seizures, hypertension, diabetes mellitus, CHF, depression, osteoporosis, spinal cord compression, urinary tract obstruction

DOSAGE AND ROUTES

Prostate cancer

- **Adult: SUBCUT** 1 mg/day; **IM** 7.5 mg/dose monthly; Viadur implant (72 mg) yearly; or **IM** 22.5 mg q3mo; or **IM** 30 mg q4mo; or IM 45 mg q6mo

Endometriosis/fibroids

- **Adult: IM** 3.75 mg q mo for 6 mo or 11.25 q3mo for 6 mo or 30 mg q4mo

Central precocious puberty

- **Child: SUBCUT** 50 mcg/kg/day; may increase by 10 mcg/kg/day as needed
- **Child >37.5 kg: IM** 15 mg q4wk
- **Child 25-37.5 kg: IM** 11.25 mg q4wk
- **Child ≤25 kg:** 7.5 mg q4wk

Benign prostatic hyperplasia (BPH) (unlabeled)

- **Adult: SUBCUT** (sol for inj) 1 mg/day, must be cont; IM (inj susp) 3.75 mg q28day × 24 wk

Available forms: Powder for inj depot 1 mo 3.75 mg, depot 3 mo/1.25 mg, 22.5 mg; depot 4 mo 30 mg; depot 6 mo 45 mg; depot-ped 7.5, 11.25, 15 mg; sol for inj 1 mg/0.2 ml; susp for inj 7.5, 22.5, 30, 45 mg; implant (Viadur) 65 mg

Administer:

- **SUBCUT:** No dilution needed if patient self-administering; make sure patient using syringes provided by manufacturer
- **Viadur DUROS Implant:** Insert in inner aspect of arm, remove after 12 mo
- **SUBCUT: Eligard:** bring to room temperature, once mixed, give within 30 mins, prepare the 2 syringes for mixing, join the 2 syringes together by pushing in and twisting until secure; mix the product by pushing the contents of both syringes back and forth between syringes until uniform; should be light tan to tan, hold syringes vertically with syringe B on the bottom, draw entire mixed product into syringe B (short, wide syringe) by depressing the syringe A plunger and

slightly withdrawing syringe B plunger, uncouple syringe A, while pushing down on syringe A plunger, small air bubbles will remain, hold syringe B upright, remove pink cap, attach needle cartridge to the end of syringe B, remove needle cover, give by subcut

IM route

• **Monthly:** reconstitute single-use vial with 1 ml of diluent; if multiple vials used, withdraw 0.5 ml, inject into each vial (1 ml); withdraw all, inject

• **3-month:** reconstitute microspheres using 1.5 ml of diluent, inject into vial; shake, withdraw, inject

• **12-month:** insert into upper arm; at the end of 12 months, implant must be removed

SIDE EFFECTS

CNS: Memory impairment, depression, **seizures**

CV: **MI, PE, dysrhythmias**, peripheral edema

GI: Nausea, vomiting, anorexia, diarrhea, **GI bleeding**

GU: Edema, hot flashes, impotence, decreased libido, amenorrhea, vaginal dryness, gynecomastia, **profuse vaginal bleeding**

INTEG: Alopecia

MS: Bone pain

PHARMACOKINETICS

SUBCUT: Onset 1-2 wk; peak 2-4 wk; absorbed rapidly (SUBCUT), slowly (IM depot); half-life 3 hr

INTERACTIONS

Increase: antineoplastic action—flutamide, megestrol

NURSING CONSIDERATIONS

Assess:

• **Prostate cancer:** increased bone pain for first 4 wk of treatment; those with metastases in spinal column may exhibit severe back pain

• **Symptoms of endometriosis** (lower abdominal pain)/**fibroids** (pelvic pain, excessive vaginal bleeding, bloating) before, during, after treatment

• **Central precocious puberty (CPP)** diagnosis should have been confirmed by secondary S_4 characteristics in children <9 yr, estradiol/testosterone levels, GnRH test, tomography of head, adrenal steroids, chorionic gonadotropin, wrist x-ray, height, weight

• Hepatic studies before, during therapy (bilirubin, AST, ALT, LDH) monthly, as needed; PSA, calcium, testosterone with prostate cancer; bone mineral density; blood glucose, HbA1c

• Pituitary gonadotropic and gonadal function during therapy and 4-8 wk after therapy decreased

• Tumor flare: worsening of signs and symptoms; normal during beginning therapy

• Fatigue, increased pulse, pallor, lethargy; edema in feet, joints; stomach pain

⚠ **Severe allergic reaction: rash, pruritus, urticaria, purpuric skin lesions, itching, flushing**

Perform/provide:

• Storage in tight container at room temp

Evaluate:

• Therapeutic response: decreased tumor size and spread of malignancy; decrease in lesions, pain with endometriosis, fibroids, correction of CPP; increased follicle maturation

Teach patient/family:

• To notify prescriber if menstruation continues; menstruation should stop

• To use a nonhormonal method of contraception during therapy

• That bone pain will disappear after 1 wk

• To report any complaints, side effects to nurse, prescriber; hot flashes may occur; record weight, report gain of >2 lb/day

• How to prepare, give; to rotate sites for SUBCUT inj

• To keep accurate records of dose

• **That tumor flare may occur:** increase in size of tumor, increased bone pain, will subside rapidly; may take analgesics for pain

- That premenopausal women must use mechanical birth control; that ovulation may be induced
- Not to breastfeed while taking product
- That voiding problems may increase during beginning of therapy but will decrease in several weeks

levalbuterol (Rx)

(lev-al-byoo′ter-ole)

Xopenex, Xopenex HFA

Func. class.: Bronchodilator, adrenergic β_2-agonist

ACTION: Causes bronchodilation by action on β_2 (pulmonary) receptors by increasing levels of cAMP, which relaxes smooth muscle; produces bronchodilation, CNS, cardiac stimulation as well as increased diuresis and gastric acid secretion

USES: Treatment or prevention of bronchospasm (reversible obstructive airway disease)

CONTRAINDICATIONS: Hypersensitivity to sympathomimetics, this product, albuterol

Precautions: Pregnancy (C), breastfeeding, hyperthyroidism, diabetes mellitus, hypertension, prostatic hypertrophy, angle-closure glaucoma, seizures, renal disease, QT prolongation, tachydysrhythmias, severe cardiac disease, hypokalemia

DOSAGE AND ROUTES

- **Adult/child ≥12 yr: INH** 0.63 mg tid q6-8hr by nebulization, may increase 1.25 mg q8hr
- **Adult/adolescent/child >4 yr:** (HFA, metered dose) 90 mcg (2 **INH**) q4-6hr
- **Child 6-11 yr: INH** 0.31 mg tid by nebulization, max 0.63 mg tid

Available forms: Sol, inh pediatric 0.31/3 ml; 0.63 mg, 1.25 mg/3 ml; 45 mcg per actuation (HFA)

Administer:

- By nebulization q6-8hr; wait ≥1 min between inhalation of aerosols

SIDE EFFECTS

CNS: *Tremors, anxiety,* insomnia, *headache,* dizziness, stimulation, *restlessness,* irritability, weakness

CV: Palpitations, tachycardia, hypertension, angina, hypotension, dysrhythmias, QT prolongation

EENT: Dry nose, irritation of nose and throat, rhinitis

GI: Heartburn, nausea, vomiting, diarrhea

INTEG: Rash

META: *Hypokalemia, hyperglycemia*

MS: Muscle cramps

RESP: Cough

SYST: Anaphylaxis, angioedema

PHARMACOKINETICS

Metabolized in the liver and tissues; crosses placenta, breast milk, blood-brain barrier; half-life 3.3-4 hr

INH sol: Onset 10-17 min, peak 1½ hr, duration 5-6 hr; **INH aerosol:** onset 4.5-10.2 min, peak 76-78 min, duration ≤6 hr

INTERACTIONS

Increase: action of aerosol bronchodilators

Increase: levalbuterol action—tricyclics, MAOIs, other adrenergics

Decrease: levalbuterol action—other β-blockers

Drug/Herb

Increase: stimulation—black/green tea, coffee, cola nut, guarana, yerba maté

NURSING CONSIDERATIONS

Assess:

- **Respiratory function:** vital capacity, forced expiratory volume, ABGs, lung sounds, heart rate and rhythm (baseline); character of sputum: color, consistency, amount

- Cardiac status: palpitations, increase/decrease in B/P, dysrhythmias

⚠ For evidence of allergic reactions, paradoxic bronchospasm, anaphylaxis, angioedema

Evaluate:

- Therapeutic response: absence of dyspnea, wheezing after 1 hr; improved airway exchange, ABGs

Teach patient/family:

- Not to use OTC medications because excess stimulation may occur
- To avoid getting aerosol in eyes because blurring may result
- To avoid smoking, smoke-filled rooms, persons with respiratory infections

⚠ That paradoxic bronchospasm may occur; to stop product immediately, contact prescriber

- To limit caffeine products such as chocolate, coffee, tea, colas, and herbs such as cola nut, guarana, yerba maté
- To use this product first if using other inhalers; to wait 5 min or more between products; to rinse mouth with water after each dose to prevent dry mouth

TREATMENT OF OVERDOSE:
Administer a β_1-adrenergic blocker

levetiracetam (Rx)
(lev-eh-teer-ass′eh-tam)

Keppra, Keppra XR

Func. class.: Anticonvulsant

Do not confuse:
Keppra/Kaletra

ACTION: Unknown; may inhibit nerve impulses by limiting influx of sodium ions across cell membrane in motor cortex

USES: Adjunctive therapy for partial-onset seizures, primary generalized tonic-clonic seizures

Unlabeled use: Pediatrics

CONTRAINDICATIONS: Hypersensitivity, breastfeeding

Precautions: Pregnancy (C), children, geriatric patients, renal/cardiac disease, psychosis

DOSAGE AND ROUTES

Adjunctive treatment of partial seizures

- **Adult/adolescent ≥16 yr: IV** 500 mg bid, may be titrated by 1000 mg/day q2wk, max 3000 mg/day in divided doses; **EXT REL** 1000 mg/day, may increase q2wk, max 3000 mg/day
- **Adolescent <16 yr/child/infant: PO** 10 mg/kg bid, increase daily dose q2wk by 20 mg/kg to dose of 30 mg/kg bid; if patient unable to tolerate, may reduce dose

Myoclonic seizures/tonic-clonic seizures/partial seizures

- **Adult/adolescent ≥16 yr: PO/IV** 500 mg bid, may increase by 1000 mg/day q2wk, max 3000 mg/day

Renal dose

- **Adult: PO** CCr 50-80 ml/min, 500-1000 mg q12hr or **EXT REL** 1000-2000 q24hr, max 2000 mg/day; CCr 30-49 ml/min, 250-750 mg q12hr or **EXT REL** 500-1500 mg q24hr, max 1500 mg/day; CCr <30 ml/min, 250-500 mg q12hr or **EXT REL** 500-1000 q24hr, max 1000 mg/day

Available forms: Tabs 250, 500, 750, 1000 mg; oral sol 100 mg/ml; sol for inj 100 mg/ml; ext rel tab 500, 750 mg

Administer:

PO route

- Swallow tab whole; do not break, crush, or chew
- With food, milk to decrease GI symptoms (rare)
- **Child:** <20 kg should be given oral solution; use calibrated device

Intermittent IV INF route

- Single-use vials: dilute in 100 ml of 0.9% NaCl, D_5, LR; give over 15 min, discard unused vial contents, do not use product with particulates or discoloration

Additive compatibilities: diazepam, LORazepam, valproate

SIDE EFFECTS

CNS: Dizziness, somnolence, asthenia, psychosis, suicidal ideation
HEMA: Lowered Hct, Hgb, RBC, infection
MISC: Infection, abdominal pain, pharyngitis

PHARMACOKINETICS

Rapidly absorbed; not protein bound; excreted via kidneys 66% unchanged; half-life 6-8 hr, longer in geriatric patients or with renal disease

INTERACTIONS

- Avoid use with alcohol
- Possible increased carBAMazepine toxicity: carBAMazepine

Decrease: levetiracetam absorption—sevelamer; separate by 1 hr before, 3 hr after sevelamer

NURSING CONSIDERATIONS

Assess:

- **Seizures:** type, location, duration, character; provide seizure precautions
- Renal studies: urinalysis, BUN, urine creatinine q3mo
- Blood studies: RBC, Hct, Hgb
- Description of seizures

⚠ Mental status: mood, sensorium, affect, behavioral changes, **suicidal thoughts/behaviors;** if mental status changes, notify prescriber

Perform/provide:

- Storage at room temp (PO)
- Diluted preparation stable for 24 hr at room temp in polyvinyl bags
- Assistance with ambulation during early part of treatment; dizziness occurs

Evaluate:

- Therapeutic response: decreased seizure activity; document on patient's chart

Teach patient/family:

- To carry emergency ID stating patient's name, products taken, condition, prescriber's name, phone number
- How to use oral sol; if trouble swallowing, measure oral sol in medicine cup or dropper, do not use teaspoon
- To notify prescriber if pregnant, intending to become pregnant
- To avoid driving, other activities that require alertness
- Not to discontinue medication quickly after long-term use because withdrawal seizure may occur
- Not to breastfeed, excreted in breast milk

levobetaxolol ophthalmic

See Appendix B

levobunolol ophthalmic

See Appendix B

levocabastine ophthalmic

See Appendix B

levocetirizine (Rx)

(lee-voh-she-teer′ah-zeen)

Xyzal

Func. class.: Antihistamine, low sedating

Chem. class.: H_1 histamine blocker, low sedating

ACTION: Acts on blood vessels, GI, respiratory system by competing with histamine for H_1-receptor site; decreases allergic response by blocking pharmacologic effects of histamine; minimal anticholinergic action

USES: Perennial or seasonal rhinitis, allergy symptoms, chronic idiopathic urticaria

CONTRAINDICATIONS:
Breast-feeding; children 6-11 yr with renal disease; end-stage renal disease; dialysis; hypersensitivity to this product, cetirizine, hydrOXYzine

Precautions: Pregnancy (B), driving, renal disease

DOSAGE AND ROUTES

- **Adult and child ≥12 yr: PO** 2.5-5 mg/day in the evening
- **Child 6-11 yr: PO** (oral solution) 2.5 mg/day in the evening
- **Child 2-5 yr: PO** (oral solution) 1.25 mg/day in the evening
- **Geriatric: PO** 2.5-5 mg/day in the evening

Renal dose

- **Adult: PO** CCr 50-80 ml/min, 2.5 mg/day; CCr 30-50 ml/min, 2.5 mg every other day; CCr 10-30 ml/min, 2.5 mg 2×/wk; CCr <10 ml/min, do not use

Available forms: Tabs 5 mg; oral sol 2.5 mg/15 ml

Administer:

- Without regard to meals in the evening; tabs scored, may be broken in half

SIDE EFFECTS

CNS: *Drowsiness, fatigue,* asthenia, dizziness, depression, **seizures, suicidal ideation,** insomnia, hallucinations, orofacial dyskinesia (rare)

CV: Hypotension, palpitations, sinus tachycardia

GI: Dry mouth, increase LFTs, **hepatitis**

HEMA: Hemolytic anemia, thrombocytopenia (rare)

INTEG: Rash, transient; **anaphylaxis, angioedema,** fixed drug eruption, pruritus

OTHER: Stillbirth (rare)

RESP: Dyspnea, cough

PHARMACOKINETICS

Rapid absorption; peak 0.9 hr; protein binding 91%-92%; half-life 8 hr; excreted in urine 85.4%, feces 12.9%

INTERACTIONS

Increase: CNS depression—alcohol, other CNS depressants

Increase: anticholinergic/sedative effect—MAOIs, phenothiazines, tricyclics

Decrease: clearance of levocetirizine—ritonavir

Drug/Lab Test

False negative: Skin allergy tests

NURSING CONSIDERATIONS

Assess:

- Allergy symptoms: pruritus, urticaria, watering eyes at baseline, during treatment
- Respiratory status: rate, rhythm, increase in bronchial secretions, wheezing, chest tightness
- Liver function tests, serum creatinine, BUN

Perform/provide:

- Storage in tight, light-resistant container

Evaluate:

- Therapeutic response: absence of running or congested nose or rashes

Teach patient/family:

- About all aspects of product use; to notify prescriber if confusion, sedation, hypotension occur
- To avoid driving, other hazardous activities if drowsiness occurs
- To avoid alcohol, other CNS depressants
- That product not recommended while breastfeeding

TREATMENT OF OVERDOSE:
Administer diazepam, vasopressors, IV phenytoin

levofloxacin (Rx)

(lee-voh-floks'a-sin)

Levaquin, Novo-Levofloxacin ❋

Func. class.: Antiinfective

Chem. class.: Fluoroquinolone

ACTION:
Interferes with conversion of intermediate DNA fragments into high-

L

molecular-weight DNA in bacteria; DNA gyrase inhibitor; inhibits topoisomerase IV

USES:
Acute sinusitis, acute chronic bronchitis, community-acquired pneumonia, uncomplicated skin infections, complicated UTI, cellulitis, PID, prostatitis, inhalational anthrax (postexposure); acute pyelonephritis caused by *Streptococcus pneumoniae, Haemophilus influenzae, Haemophilis parainfluenzae, Moraxella catarrhalis, Escherichia coli, Serratia marcescens, Klebsiella pneumoniae, Chlamydia pneumoniae, Legionella pneumophilia, Mycoplasma pneumoniae, Enterococcus faecalis, Staphylococcus epidermidis, Staphylococcus pyogenes;* inhalation anthrax in children

Unlabeled uses: Adnexitis, Bartholin abscess, bartholinitis, cervicitis, epididymis, gastroenteritis, *H. pylori* eradication, mastitis, MAC, nongonococcal urethritis, obstetric infections, PID, plague, SARS, shigellosis, TB, typhoid fever, gonococcal infections, disseminated; otitis media, otitis externa, tonsillitis, pharyngitis, sialadenitis

CONTRAINDICATIONS:
Hypersensitivity to quinolones

Precautions: Pregnancy (C), breastfeeding, children, photosensitivity, acute MI, atrial fibrillation, colitis, dehydration, diabetes, QT prolongation, myasthenia gravis, renal disease, seizure disorder, syphilis

Black Box Warning: Tendon pain/rupture, tendinitis

DOSAGE AND ROUTES

Acute bacterial exacerbation of chronic bronchitis
- **Adult: PO/IV** 500 mg q24hr × 7 days

Acute bacterial sinusitis
- **Adult: PO** 500 mg q24hr × 10-14 days or 750 mg q24hr × 5 days

Acute pyelonephritis
- **Adult: PO** 250 mg q24hr × 10 days or 750 mg q24hr × 5 days

Chronic bacterial prostitis
- **Adult: PO** 500 mg q24hr × 28 days

Postexposure inhalational anthrax
- **Adult/adolescent/child >50 kg: PO/IV** 500 mg q24hr × 60 days
- **Infant >6 mo/child <50 kg: IV** 8 mg/kg q12hr × 60 days, max 250 mg/dose

Pneumonia, community acquired
- **Adult: PO/IV** 500 mg q24hr × 7-14 days or 750 mg q24hr × 5 days

Pneumonia, nosocomial
- **Adult: PO/IV** 750 mg q24hr × 7-14 days

Skin/skin-structure infections, complicated
- **Adult: PO/IV** 750 mg q24hr × 7-14 days

Skin/skin-structure infections, uncomplicated
- **Adult: PO** 500 mg q24hr × 7-10 days

UTI, complicated
- **Adult: PO/IV** 250 mg q24hr × 10 days

UTI, uncomplicated
- **Adult: PO** 250 mg q24hr × 3 days

Gonococcal infection, disseminated (unlabeled)
- **Adult: IV** 250 mg q24hr × 24-48 hr then **PO** 500 mg/day × 7 days

PID
- **Adult: IV** 500 mg q24hr × 14 days

Otitis media (unlabeled)
- **Adult: PO** 100-200 mg bid-tid × 3-14 days
- **Child 6 mo-14 yr: PO** 10 mg/kg bid × ≥10 days

Renal disease
- **Adult: PO/IV** CCr 20-49 ml/min, initial 500 mg then 250 mg q24hr; CCr 10-19 ml/min, 250 or 500 mg, depending on condition, then 250 mg q48hr

Available forms: Single-use vials 500, 750 mg; premixed flexible containers 250 mg/50 ml D_5W, 500 mg/100 ml D_5W, 750 mg/150 ml D_5W; tabs 250, 500, 750 mg; oral sol 25 mg/ml

Administer:

• PO 4 hr before or 2 hr after antacids, iron, calcium, zinc

• Do not use theophylline with this product; toxicity may result

Intermittent IV INF route

• Discard any unused sol in single-dose vial

• Dilute with 0.9% NaCl, D5W to 5 mg/ml; give over 60 min/250 mg or 90 min/750 mg or using premix; tear outer wrap at notch and remove sol container; check for leaks; close control clamps; remove cover from port at bottom of container; insert pin into port with a twist; suspend container from hanger; squeeze, release drip chamber to proper fluid level; open flow control to expel air, close clamp; regulate rate with flow control clamps

Y-site compatibilities: Alfentanil, amifostine, amikacin, aminocaproic acid, aminophylline, ampicillin, anidulafungin, atenolol, atracurium, aztreonam, bivalirudin, bleomycin, bumetanide, buprenorphine, busulfan, butorphanol, caffeine citrate, calcium gluconate, CARBOplatin, carmustine, caspofungin, cefepime, cefotetan, ceftazidime, ceftizoxime, cefTRIAXone, cefuroxime, chlorproMAZINE, cimetidine, cisatracurium, CISplatin, clindamycin, cyclophosphamide, cycloSPORINE, cytarabine, DACTINomycin, DAPTOmycin, dexamethasone, dexrazoxane, digoxin, diltiazem, diphenhydrAMINE, DOBUTamine, docetaxel, dolasetron, DOPamine, doripenem, doxacurium, doxycycline, droperidol, enalaprilat, ePHEDrine, EPINEPHrine, epirubicin, ertapenem, erythromycin, esmolol, etoposide, famotidine, fenoldopam, fentaNYL, filgrastim, floxuridine, fluconazole, fludarabine, fosphenytoin, gemcitabine, gentamicin, granisetron, haloperidol, hydrocortisone, HYDROmorphone, IDArubicin, ifosfamide, imipenem-cilastatin, isoproterenol, labetalol, leucovorin, levorphanol, lidocaine, linezolid, magnesium sulfate, mannitol, mechlorethamine, meperidine, mesna, methylPREDNISolone, metoclopramide, metroNIDAZOLE, midazolam, milrinone, mitomycin, mitoxantrone, morphine, nalbuphine, naloxone, nesiritide, octreotide, ondansetron, oxacillin, oxaliplatin, oxytocin, paclitaxel, palonosetron, pancuronium, pemetrexed, penicillin G sodium, pentamidine, phenylephrine, plicamycin, potassium chloride, promethazine, propranolol, ranitidine, remifentanil, rocuronium, sargramostim, succinylcholine, SUFentanil, tacrolimus, teniposide, theophylline, thiotepa, tirofiban, tobramycin, trimethoprim-sulfamethoxazole, vancomycin, vasopressin, vecuronium, verapamil, vinBLAStine, vinCRIStine, vinorelbine, voriconazole, zidovudine

Solution compatibilities: 0.9% NaCl, D_5W, $D_5/0.9\%$ NaCl, D_5LR, $D_5/0.45\%$ NaCl, sodium lactate, plasma-lyte $56/D_5W$

L

SIDE EFFECTS

CNS: *Headache,* dizziness, *insomnia,* anxiety, **seizures, encephalopathy,** paresthesia

CV: Chest pain, palpitations, vasodilation, **QT prolongation**

EENT: Dry mouth, visual impairment

GI: *Nausea,* flatulence, *vomiting,* diarrhea, abdominal pain, **pseudomembranous colitis, hepatotoxicity**

GU: Vaginitis, crystalluria

HEMA: Eosinophilia, **hemolytic anemia,** lymphopenia

INTEG: Rash, pruritus, *photosensitivity,* **epidermal necrolysis**

MISC: Hypoglycemia, hypersensitivity, **tendinitis, tendon rupture**

RESP: Pneumonitis

SYST: **Anaphylaxis, multisystem organ failure, Stevens-Johnson syndrome**

PHARMACOKINETICS

Metabolized in liver, excreted in urine unchanged, half-life 6-8 hr, peak 1-2 hr

INTERACTIONS

• Do not use with magnesium in same IV line

Increase: levofloxacin levels—probenecid
Increase: CNS stimulation, seizures—NSAIDs, foscarnet
Increase: bleeding risk—warfarin
Decrease: levofloxacin absorption—antacids containing aluminum, magnesium; sucralfate, zinc, iron, calcium
Decrease: clearance of theophylline; toxicity may result

Drug/Lab Test
Decrease: glucose, lymphocytes

NURSING CONSIDERATIONS

Assess:
- Previous sensitivity reaction
- **Signs, symptoms of infection:** characteristics of sputum, WBC >10,000/mm^3, fever; obtain baseline information before, during treatment
- C&S before beginning product therapy to identify if correct treatment initiated

⚠ **Allergic reactions, anaphylaxis:** rash, urticaria, pruritus, chills, fever, joint pain; may occur a few days after therapy begins; EPINEPHrine and resuscitation equipment should be available for anaphylactic reaction

- **Pseudomembranous colitis:** bowel pattern daily; if severe diarrhea, fever occurs, product should be discontinued

⚠ **Overgrowth of infection:** perineal itching, fever, malaise, redness, pain, swelling, drainage, rash, diarrhea, change in cough, sputum

- Renal function (BUN/creatinine)

Perform/provide:
- Increased fluid intake to 2 L/day to prevent crystalluria

Evaluate:
- Therapeutic response: absence of signs, symptoms of infection (WBC <10,000/mm^3, temp WNL)

Teach patient/family:
- To contact prescriber if vaginal itching; loose, foul-smelling stools; furry tongue occur (may indicate superinfection); to report itching, rash, pruritus, urticaria
- To notify prescriber of diarrhea with blood or pus
- To take product 4 hr before or 2 hr after antacids, iron, calcium, zinc products
- To complete full course of therapy
- To avoid hazardous activities until response is known
- To use frequent rinsing of mouth, sugarless candy or gum for dry mouth
- To avoid other medication unless approved by prescriber
- To prevent sun exposure or to use sunscreen to prevent phototoxicity

levofloxacin ophthalmic

See Appendix B

levoleucovorin (Rx)

(lee-voe-loo-koe-voe′rin)

Fusilev

Func. class.: Chemotherapy protectant

Chem. class.: Tetrahydrofolic acid derivative

ACTION: Acts as a replacement to rescue cells from the effects of folate antagonists

USES: For methotrexate toxicity prophylaxis, colorectal cancer (to potentiate fluorouracil therapy)

CONTRAINDICATIONS: Hypersensitivity to this product, folic acid, mannitol; intrathecal administration

Precautions: Pregnancy (C), breastfeeding, children <6 yr, megaloblastic/pernicious anemia, seizure disorder, vitamin B_{12} deficiency

DOSAGE AND ROUTES

For levoleucovorin rescue after high-dose methotrexate treatment for osteosarcoma
- **Adult and child >6 yr: IV** 7.5 mg (approximately 5 mg/m^2) q6hr × 10 doses starting 24 hr after beginning methotrex-

ate inf; do not give >16 ml (160 mg) of reconstituted sol/min

For inadvertent overdose of methotrexate

- **Adult and child >6 yr: IV** 7.5 mg q6hr until serum methotrexate conc <0.01 micromolar; do not give >16 ml (160 mg) of reconstituted sol/min

Colorectal cancer

- **Adult: IV** 100 mg/m^2 over ≥3 min, then fluorouracil 370 mg/m^2 IV each day × 5 days or levoleucovorin 10 mg/m^2 IV then fluorouracil 425 mg/m^2 IV each day × 5 days; course may be repeated q28 days × 2 then repeated q28-35–day intervals if complete recovery from toxic effects has occurred

Available forms: Powder for inj 50 mg

Administer:

- Within 1 hr of folic acid antagonist
- Do not give concurrently with systemic methotrexate

IV route

- For IV, reconstitute 50 mg vial/5.3 ml normal saline (10 mg/ml)

Intermittent IV INF route

- Further dilute to final conc of 0.5 mg/ml-5 mg/ml
- Give max 160 mg/min

SIDE EFFECTS

CNS: Seizures, syncope
GI: Nausea, vomiting, stomatitis
GU: Abnormal renal function
INTEG: *Rash, pruritus,* anaphylaxis, *urticaria*
RESP: Dyspnea
SYST: Anaphylaxis

INTERACTIONS

Increase: metabolism of barbiturates, hydantoins
Increase: toxicity—fluorouracil, capecitabine, floxuridine
Decrease: effects of methotrexate, pyrimethamine, trimethoprim, trimetrexate

NURSING CONSIDERATIONS

Assess:

- CCr, creatinine before levoleucovorin rescue and daily to detect methotrexate level
- CBC with differential
- Other products taken: hydantoins, trimethoprim may cause increased folic acid use by body
- **Neurologic status (rescue):** weakness, fatigue
- Anaphylaxis: dyspnea, rash, temperature changes, pruritus when given with methotrexate regimen

Perform/provide:

- Increased fluid intake if used to treat folic-acid–inhibitor overdose
- Protection from light and heat

Evaluate:

- Therapeutic response: prevention of methotrexate toxicity

Teach patient/family:

- For folic acid deficiency, to eat folic-acid–rich foods: bran; yeast; dried beans; nuts; fresh, green leafy vegetables
- To notify prescriber of side effects
- To report signs of hyposensitivity reaction immediately
- To avoid breastfeeding

L

levothyroxine (T_4) (Rx)

(lee-voe-thye-rox′een)

Eltroxin ✦, Levothroid, Levoxyl, Synthroid, Tirosint, Unithroid

Func. class.: Thyroid hormone
Chem. class.: Levoisomer of thyroxine

Do not confuse:
Synthroid/Symmetrel

ACTION: Increases metabolic rate; controls protein synthesis; increases cardiac output, renal blood flow, O_2 consumption, body temp, blood volume, growth, development at cellular level via action on thyroid hormone receptors

USES:
Hypothyroidism, myxedema coma, thyroid hormone replacement, thyrotoxicosis, congenital hypothyroidism, some types of thyroid cancer, pituitary TSH suppression

CONTRAINDICATIONS:
Adrenal insufficiency, recent MI, thyrotoxicosis, hypersensitivity to beef, alcohol intolerance (inj only)

Black Box Warning: Obesity treatment

Precautions: Pregnancy (A), breastfeeding, geriatric patients, angina pectoris, hypertension, ischemia, cardiac disease, diabetes

DOSAGE AND ROUTES

Hypothyroidism

- **Adult ≤50 yr: PO** 1.7 mcg/kg/day, 6-8 wk, average dose 100-200 mcg/day; max 200 mcg/day **IM/IV** 50-100 mcg/day as single dose or 50% of usual oral dosage
- **Adult >50 yr without heart disease or <50 yr with heart disease: PO** 25-50 mcg/day, titrate q6-8wk
- **Adult >50 yr with heart disease: PO** 12.5-25 mcg/day, titrate by 12.5-25 mcg q6-8wk
- **Child >12 yr: PO** 2-3 mcg/kg/day as single dose in AM
- **Child 6-12 yr: PO** 4-5 mcg/kg/day as single dose in AM
- **Child 1-5 yr: PO** 5-6 mcg/kg/day as single dose in AM
- **Child 6-12 mo: PO** 6-8 mcg/kg/day as single dose in AM
- **Child to 6 mo: PO** 8-10 mcg/kg/day as single dose in AM

Myxedema coma

- **Adult: IV** 200-500 mcg, may increase by 100-300 mcg after 24 hr; give oral medication as soon as possible

Subclinical hypothyroidism

- **Adult: PO** 1 mcg/kg/day may be sufficient

Available forms: Powder for inj 200, 500 mcg/vial; tabs 25, 50, 88, 100, 112, 125, 137, 150, 175, 200, 300 mcg; cap (liquid filled) 13, 25, 50, 75, 88, 100, 112, 125, 137, 150 mcg

Administer:

PO route

- In AM if possible as single dose to decrease sleeplessness; at same time each day to maintain product level; take on empty stomach
- Only for hormone imbalances; not to be used for obesity, male infertility, menstrual conditions, lethargy
- Lowest dose that relieves symptoms; lower dose to geriatric patients and for those with cardiac diseases
- Crush and mix with water; nonsoy formula or breast milk for infants, children
- Separate antacids, iron, calcium products by 4 hr

Direct IV route

- IV after diluting with provided diluent 500 mcg/5 ml, 200 mcg/2 ml; shake; give through Y-tube or 3-way stopcock; give ≤100 mcg/1 min; do not add to IV inf
- Considered to be incompatible in syringe with all other products

SIDE EFFECTS

CNS: *Anxiety, insomnia, tremors,* headache, thyroid storm, excitability

CV: *Tachycardia, palpitations, angina, dysrhythmias,* hypertension, cardiac arrest

GI: Nausea, diarrhea, increased or decreased appetite, cramps

MISC: Menstrual irregularities, weight loss, sweating, heat intolerance, fever, alopecia, decreased bone mineral density

PHARMACOKINETICS

Half-life euthyroid 6-7 days, hypothyroid 9-10 days, hyperthyroid 3-4 days, distributed throughout body tissues

PO: Onset 3-5 days, peak 6-8 wk, duration 1-3 wk

IV: Onset 6-8 hr, peak 24 hr, duration unknown

INTERACTIONS

Increase: cardiac insufficiency risk—EPINEPHrine products

Increase: effects of anticoagulants, sympathomimetics, tricyclics
Decrease: levothyroxine absorption—bile acid sequestrants, orlistat, ferrous sulfate
Decrease: levothyroxine effect—estrogens, antacids, sucralfate, aluminum, magnesium, calcium, iron, rifampin, rifabutin
Drug/Herb
Decrease: thyroid hormone effect—soy
Drug/Lab Test
Increase: CPK, LDH, AST, blood glucose
Decrease: thyroid function tests

NURSING CONSIDERATIONS

Assess:
- B/P, pulse periodically during treatment
- Weight daily in same clothing, using same scale, at same time of day
- Height, growth rate of child
- T_3, T_4, FTIs, which are decreased; radioimmunoassay of TSH, which is increased; radio uptake, which is increased if patient receiving too low a dose of medication
- PT may require decreased anticoagulant; check for bleeding, bruising
- Increased nervousness, excitability, irritability, which may indicate too high a dose of medication, usually after 1-3 wk of treatment
- Cardiac status: angina, palpitation, chest pain, change in VS

Perform/provide:
- Storage in tight, light-resistant container; sol should be discarded if not used immediately
- Withdrawal of medication 4 wk before RAIU test

Evaluate:
- Therapeutic response: absence of depression; increased weight loss, diuresis, pulse, appetite; absence of constipation, peripheral edema, cold intolerance; pale, cool, dry skin; brittle nails, alopecia, coarse hair, menorrhagia, night blindness, paresthesias, syncope, stupor, coma, rosy cheeks

Teach patient/family:
- That hair loss will occur in child, is temporary; that hypothyroid child will show almost immediate behavior/personality change
- To report excitability, irritability, anxiety, which indicate overdose
- Not to switch brands unless approved by prescriber
- That product may be discontinued after giving birth; that thyroid panel should be evaluated after 1-2 mo
- That product is not to be taken to reduce weight
- To avoid OTC preparations with iodine; to read labels; to separate antacids, iron, calcium products by 4 hr
- To avoid iodine-rich food, iodized salt, soybeans, tofu, turnips, high-iodine seafood, some bread
- That product is not a cure but controls symptoms; that treatment is lifelong, full effect may take up to 6 wk

⚠ *HIGH ALERT*

lidocaine (parenteral) (Rx)

(lye′doe-kane)

LidoPen Auto-Injector, Xylocaine, Xylocard ♣

Func. class.: Antidysrhythmic (Class Ib)
Chem. class.: Aminoacyl amide

ACTION: Increases electrical stimulation threshold of ventricle, His-Purkinje system, which stabilizes cardiac membrane, decreases automaticity

USES: Ventricular tachycardia, ventricular dysrhythmias during cardiac surgery, digoxin toxicity, cardiac catheterization
Unlabeled uses: Attenuation of intracranial pressure increases during intubation/endotracheal tube suctioning

CONTRAINDICATIONS:

Hypersensitivity to amides, severe heart block, supraventricular dysrhythmias, Adams-Stokes syndrome, Wolff-Parkinson-White syndrome

Precautions: Pregnancy (B), breastfeeding, children, geriatric patients, renal/hepatic disease, CHF, respiratory depression, malignant hyperthermia, myasthenia gravis, weight <50 kg

DOSAGE AND ROUTES

• **Adult: IV BOL** 50-100 mg (1-1.5 mg/kg) 25-50 mg/min, repeat q3-5min, max 300 mg in 1 hr; begin **IV INF; IV INF** 1-4 mg/min (20-50 mcg/kg/min); **IM** 200-300 mg (4.3 mg/kg) in deltoid muscle, may repeat after 1-1½ hr if needed

Available forms: ***IV INF*** 0.2% (2 mg/ml), 0.4% (4 mg/ml), 0.8% (8 mg/ml); IV ad 4% (40 mg/ml), 10% (100 mg/ml), 20% (200 mg/ml); ***IV dir*** 1% (10 mg/ml), 2% (20 mg/ml); ***IM*** 10% 300 mg/ml

Administer:

• IM inj in deltoid; aspirate to avoid intravascular administration; check IV site daily for infiltration or extravasation

IV route

• Bolus undiluted (1%, 2% only), give ≤50 mg/1 min or dilute 1 g/250-500 ml D_5W; titrate to patient response; use inf pump; pediatric inf 120 mg lidocaine/100 ml D_5W; 1-2.5 ml/kg/hr = 20-50 mcg/kg/min; use only 1%, 2% sol for IV bol

Y-site compatibilities: Alemtuzumab, alteplase, amikacin, aminophylline, amiodarone, argatroban, atropine, aztreonam, bivalirudin, bumetanide, calcium chloride/gluconate, ceFAZolin, cefotaxime, cefoxitin, ceftazidime, ceftizoxime, cefTRIAXone, cefuroxime, chloramphenicol, cimetidine, ciprofloxacin, cisatracurium, clindamycin, cycloSPORINE, DAPTOmycin, dexamethasone, dexmedetomidine, digoxin, diltiazem, diphenhydrAMINE, DOBUTamine, DOPamine, doxycycline, enalaprilat, EPINEPHrine, eptifibatide, ertapenem, erythromycin, esmolol, etomidate, famotidine, fenoldopam, fentaNYL, fluconazole, furosemide, gentamicin, granisetron, haloperidol, heparin, hydrocortisone, imipenem/cilastatin, inamrinone, insulin, isoproterenol, ketorolac, labetalol, levofloxacin, linezolid, LORazepam, magnesium sulfate, meperidine, methylPREDNISolone sodium succinate, metoclopramide, metoprolol, metroNIDAZOLE, micafungin, midazolam, morphine, nafcillin, niCARdipine, nitroglycerin, nitroprusside, norepinephrine, ondansetron, palonosetron, penicillin G potassium, phenylephrine, phytonadione, piperacillin/tazobactam, potassium chloride, procainamide, prochlorperazine, promethazine, propofol, propranolol, protamine, quinupristin/dalfopristin, ranitidine, remifentanil, sodium bicarbonate, streptokinase, tacrolimus, theophylline, ticarcillin/clavulanate, tigecycline, tirofiban, tobramycin, vancomycin, vasopressin, verapamil, vitamin B complex with C, voriconazole, warfarin

SIDE EFFECTS

CNS: *Headache, dizziness,* involuntary movement, confusion, tremor, drowsiness, euphoria, **seizures, shivering**

CV: *Hypotension, bradycardia,* **heart block, CV collapse, arrest**

EENT: Tinnitus, blurred vision

GI: Nausea, vomiting, anorexia

HEMA: Methemoglobinemia

INTEG: Rash, urticaria, edema, swelling, petechiae, pruritus

MISC: Febrile response, phlebitis at inj site

RESP: Dyspnea, **respiratory depression**

PHARMACOKINETICS

Half-life 8 min, 1-2 hr (terminal); metabolized in liver; excreted in urine; crosses placenta

IM: Onset 5-15 min, duration 1½ hr

IV: Onset 2 min, duration 20 min

INTERACTIONS

Increase: cardiac depression, toxicity—amiodarone, phenytoin, procainamide, propranolol
Increase: hypotensive effects—MAOIs, antihypertensives
Increase: neuromuscular blockade—neuromuscular blockers, tubocurarine
Increase: lidocaine effects—cimetidine, beta blockers, protease inhibitors, ritonavir
Decrease: lidocaine effects—barbiturates, ciprofloxacin, voriconazole
Decrease: effect of—cycloSPORINE
Decrease: effect—coltsfoot
Drug/Lab Test
Increase: CPK

NURSING CONSIDERATIONS

Assess:

⚠ ECG continuously to determine increased PR or QRS segments; if these develop, discontinue or reduce rate; watch for increased ventricular ectopic beats, may have to rebolus; B/P

- Blood levels: therapeutic level, 1.5-5 mcg/ml
- I&O ratio, electrolytes (K, Na, Cl)

⚠ Malignant hyperthermia: tachypnea, tachycardia, changes in B/P, increased temp

- Respiratory status: rate, rhythm, lung fields for crackles, watch for respiratory depression; lung fields, bilateral crackles may occur with CHF; increased respiration, pulse; product should be discontinued
- CNS effects: dizziness, confusion, psychosis, paresthesias, convulsions; product should be discontinued

Evaluate:

- Therapeutic response: decreased dysrhythmias

Teach patient/family:

- About the use of automatic lidocaine injection device if ordered for personal use
- To report signs of toxicity

TREATMENT OF OVERDOSE:

O_2, artificial ventilation, ECG; administer DOPamine for circulatory depression, diazepam or thiopental for seizures; decrease product if needed

lidocaine topical

See Appendix B

linagliptin

(lin′a-glip′tin)

Tradjenta

Func. class.: Antidiabetic

Chem. class.: Didipeptidyl peptidase-4 inhibitor

ACTION: Slows the inactivation of incretin hormones. Concentrations of the active, intact hormones are increased thereby increasing and prolonging the action of these hormones. Incretin hormones are released by the intestine throughout the day, and levels are increased in response to a meal

USES: Type 2 diabetes mellitus

CONTRAINDICATIONS: *Hypersensitivity to linagliptin,* type 1 diabetes mellitus, diabetic ketoacidosis (DKA)

Precautions: Pregnancy (category B), breastfeeding, adolescents or children <18 yr, debilitated physical condition, malnutrition, uncontrolled adrenal insufficiency, pituitary insufficiency, hypo/hyperthyroidism, diarrhea, gastroparesis, GI obstruction, ileus, female hormonal changes, high fever, severe psychological stress, uncontrolled hypercortisolism

DOSAGE AND ROUTES

- **Adult: PO** 5 mg daily; when used in with a sulfonylurea, a lower dose of the sulfonylurea may be necessary to minimize the risk of hypoglycemia

Available forms: Tab 5 mg
Administer:
- Once daily; may give without regard to food

SIDE EFFECTS

CNS: Headache
EENT: Nasopharyngitis
ENDO: Hypoglycemia, hyperuricemia
GI: Body weight loss, pancreatitis
INTEG: Hypersensitivity reactions, urticaria, angioedema, exfoliative dermatitis
MISC: Arthralgia, back pain
RESP: Bronchial hyperreactivity (with bronchospasm), nasopharyngitis, cough

PHARMACOKINETICS

Extensively distributed in the tissues, protein binding is concentration-dependent, a weak to moderate inhibitor of CYP3A4, plasma terminal half life of >100 hr; effective half-life 12 hr, 90% excreted unchanged, 85% excreted via the enterohepatic system (80%) or in urine (5%) within 4 days of dosing, rapidly absorbed, peak in 1.5 hr; bioavailability 30%

INTERACTIONS

- Increased or prolonged hypoglycemia: sulfonylureas, beta blockers, ACE inhibitors, Angiotensin II receptor antagonists, disopyramide, guanethidine, cloNIDine, octreotide, fenfluramine, dexfenfluramine, fibric acid derivatives, monoamine oxidase inhibitors (MAOIs), fluoxetine, salicylates
- Increased masking of the signs and symptoms of hypoglycemia: reserpine
- Increased need for dosing change: cisapride, metoclopramide, tegaserod, androgens, alcohol, lithium, quinolones

Decrease: hypoglycemic effect—dextrothyroxine, bumetanide, furosemide, ethacrynic acid, torsemide, estrogens, progestins, oral contraceptives, thyroid hormones, glucocorticoids, glucagon, carbonic anhydrase inhibitors, phenytoin, fosphenytoin, or ethotoin; atypical antipsychotics (aripiprazole, clozapine, OLANZapine, quetiapine, risperidone, and ziprasidone), phenothiazine, niacin (nicotinic acid), triamterene, thiazide diuretics
Decrease: effect of linagliptin—CYP3A4 inducers (topiramate, rifabutin, pioglitazone, OXcarbazepine, carBAMazepine, nevirapine, modafinil, metyrapone, etravirine, efavirenz, bosentan, barbiturates, aprepitant, fosaprepitant
Drug/Herb:
Decrease: linagliptin effect—St. John's wort

NURSING CONSIDERATIONS

Assess
- Hypo/hyperglycemia: reaction may occur after meals, for severe hypoglycemia use IV Dextrose
- Monitor blood glucose, A1c, during treatment to determine diabetes control
- CBC baseline and periodically during treatment, report decreased blood counts

Perform/provide:
- Storage at room temperature

Evaluate:
- Improving blood glucose level, A1c; decreasing polydipsia, polyphagia, polyuria, clear sensorium, absence of dizziness

Teach patient/family:
- About the symptoms of hypo/hyperglycemia and what to do about each; to have glucagon emergency kit available, to carry sugar packets
- That product must be continued on a daily basis, about the consequences of discontinuing product abruptly; to take only as directed
- To avoid OTC products unless approved by prescriber
- That diabetes is a life-long illness, that product will not cure diabetes
- That all food in diet plan must be eaten to prevent hypoglycemia
- To carry emergency ID with prescriber, condition and medications taken
- To immediately report skin disorders, swelling, difficulty breathing, or severe abdominal pain

lindane (Rx)

(lin′dane)

Hexit ✦, PMS-Lindane ✦

Func. class.: Scabicide, pediculicide

Chem. class.: Chlorinated hydrocarbon (synthetic)

ACTION: Stimulates nervous system of arthropods, resulting in seizures, death

USES: Scabies, lice (head/pubic/body), nits in those intolerant to or who do not respond to other agents

CONTRAINDICATIONS: Hypersensitivity, patients with known seizure disorders, Norwegian (crusted) scabies

Black Box Warning: Premature neonate; inflammation of skin, abrasions, skin breaks; seizure disorder

Precautions: Pregnancy (C), breastfeeding, infants, children <10 yr, avoid contact with eyes

DOSAGE AND ROUTES

Lice

• **Adult and child: CREAM/LOTION** shampoo using 30 ml: work into lather, rub for 5 min, rinse, dry with towel; comb with fine-toothed comb to remove nits; most require 1 oz, max 2 oz

Scabies

• **Adult and child: TOP** apply 1% cream/lotion to skin, from neck to bottom of feet, toes; wash area with soap, water; remove visible crusts; apply to skin surfaces; remove with soap, water in 8-12 hr; repeat after 1 wk prn; most require 1 oz, max 2 oz

Available forms: Lotion, shampoo, cream (1%)

Administer:

• Caregivers applying these products to another person should wear gloves less permeable to lindane, thoroughly clean hands after application; avoid natural latex gloves

• **Cream/ointment/lotion:** use for scabies only; skin should be clean without other products on it, wait 1 hr after bathing or showering before application, shake well, apply under fingernails after trimming; toothbrush can be used to apply; after application wrap toothbrush in paper and throw away; use only a single application, apply as thin layer over all skin from neck down, close bottle containing leftover lotion, throw away

• Do not cover, wash off after 8-12 hr

• Use warm, not hot, water; do not leave on >12hr

• **Shampoo:** for lice only; do not use other hair products before use; shake well; hair should be completely dry; use only enough shampoo to lightly coat hair and scalp, work into hair, do not use water; allow to remain only 4 min, rinse, lather away, towel briskly

• To scalp only; do not apply to face, lips, mouth, eyes, any mucous membrane, anus, or meatus

• Topical corticosteroids as ordered to decrease contact dermatitis; antihistamines

• Lotions of menthol or phenol to control itching

• Topical antibiotics for infection

SIDE EFFECTS

CNS: Tremors, **seizures**, **CNS toxicity**, stimulation, dizziness (chronic inhalation of vapors), anxiety, insomnia

CV: **Ventricular fibrillation** (chronic inhalation of vapors)

GI: *Nausea, vomiting, diarrhea,* liver damage (inhalation of vapors)

GU: **Kidney damage** (chronic inhalation of vapors)

HEMA: **Aplastic anemia** (chronic inhalation of vapors), **myelosuppression**

INTEG: *Pruritus, rash, irritation, contact dermatitis*

PHARMACOKINETICS

Peak 6 hr, half-life 18-22 hr

INTERACTIONS

• Oils may increase absorption; if oil-based hair dressing used, shampoo, rinse, dry hair before applying lindane shampoo

NURSING CONSIDERATIONS

Assess:

Black Box Warning: Skin for abrasions, breaks, inflammation; do not use on these areas

• **Infestation:** head, hair for lice, nits before and after treatment; if scabies present, check all skin surfaces; identify source of infection: school, family, sexual contacts

Perform/provide:

• Isolation until areas on skin, scalp have cleared, treatment completed
• Removal of nits with fine-toothed comb rinsed in vinegar after treatment; use gloves

Evaluate:

• Therapeutic response: decreased crusts, nits, brownish trails on skin, itching papules in skin folds, decreased itching after several weeks

Teach patient/family:

• To wash all inhabitants' clothing using insecticide; that preventive treatment may be required of all persons living in same house using lotion or shampoo to decrease spread of infection; to use rubber gloves when applying product
• That itching may continue for 4-6 wk
• That product must be reapplied if accidently washed off or treatment will be ineffective
• Not to apply to face; if accidental contact with eyes occurs, flush with water
• To remove product after specified time to prevent toxicity
• To treat sexual contacts simultaneously
• To check for CNS toxicity: dizziness, cramps, anxiety, nausea, vomiting, seizures

linezolid (Rx)

(line-zoe′lide)

Zyvox

Func. class.: Broad-spectrum antiinfective

Chem. class.: Oxazolidinone

Do not confuse:

Zyvox/Ziox/Zosyn

ACTION: Inhibits protein synthesis by interfering with translation; binds to bacterial 23S ribosomal RNA of the 50S subunit, thus preventing formation of the bacterial translation process in primarily gram-positive organisms

USES: Vancomycin-resistant *Enterococcus faecium* infections, nosocomial pneumonia, uncomplicated or complicated skin and skin-structure infections, community-acquired pneumonia

CONTRAINDICATIONS: Hypersensitivity

Precautions: Pregnancy (C), breastfeeding, children, thrombocytopenia, bone marrow suppression, hypertension, hyperthyroidism, pheochromocytoma, seizure disorder, ulcerative colitis, MI, PKU, renal/GI disease

DOSAGE AND ROUTES

Vancomycin-resistant *Enterococcus faecium* infections

• **Adult/adolescent/child ≥12 yr: IV/PO** 600 mg q12hr × 14-28 days; max 1200 mg/day
• **Child <12 yr/infant/term neonate: IV/PO** 10 mg/kg q8hr × 14-28 days

Nosocomial pneumonia/complicated skin infections/community-acquired pneumonia/concurrent bacterial infection

• **Adult: IV/PO** 600 mg q12hr × 10-14 days; max 1200 mg/day
• **Child: birth-11 yr: PO** 10 mg/kg q8hr × 10-14 days

Uncomplicated skin infections
- **Adult: PO** 400 mg q12hr × 10-14 days; max 1200 mg/day
- **Adolescent: PO** 600 mg q12hr × 10-14 days; max 1200 mg/day
- **Infant preterm <7 days old: PO** 10 mg/kg q12hr × 10-14 days

Available forms: Tabs 600 mg; oral sus 100 mg/5 ml; inj 2 mg/ml

Administer:

PO route
- With/without food
- Store reconstituted oral susp at room temp, use within 3 wk

Intermittent IV INF route
- Premixed sol ready to use (2 mg/ml), give over 30-120 min; do not use IV inf bag in series connections; do not use with additives in sol; do not use with another product, administer separately, flush line before and after use

Y-site compatibilities: acyclovir, alfentanil, amikacin, aminophylline, ampicillin, aztreonam, buprenorphine, butorphanol, calcium gluconate, CARBOplatin, ceFAZolin, cefoperazone, cefotetan, cefoxitin, ceftazidime, ceftizoxime, cefuroxime, cimetidine, ciprofloxacin, cisatracurium, CISplatin, clindamycin, cyclophosphamide, cycloSPORINE, cytarabine, digoxin, furosemide, ganciclovir, gemcitabine, gentamicin, heparin, HYDROmorphone, ifosfamide, labetalol, leucovorin, levofloxacin, lidocaine, LORazepam, magnesium sulfate, mannitol, meperidine, meropenem, mesna, methotrexate, methylPREDNISolone, metoclopramide, metroNIDAZOLE, midazolam, minocycline, mitoxantrone, morphine, nalbuphine, naloxone, nitroglycerin, ofloxacin, ondansetron, paclitaxel, PENTobarbital, PHENobarbital, piperacillin, potassium chloride, prochlorperazine, promethazine, propranolol, ranitidine, remifentanil, SUFentanil, theophylline, ticarcillin, tobramycin, vancomycin, vecuronium, verapamil, vinCRIStine, zidovudine

Solution compatibilities: D_5, 0.9% NaCl, LR

SIDE EFFECTS

CNS: *Headache,* dizziness, insomnia

GI: *Nausea, diarrhea,* **pseudomembranous colitis,** increased ALT/AST, *vomiting,* taste change, tongue-color change

HEMA: **Myelosuppression**

MISC: Vaginal moniliasis, fungal infection, oral moniliasis, **lactic acidosis, anaphylaxis, angioedema, Stevens-Johnson syndrome**

PHARMACOKINETICS

Peak 1-2 hr, terminal half-life 4-5 hr, rapidly and extensively absorbed, protein binding 31%, metabolized by oxidation of the morpholine ring

INTERACTIONS

⚠ **Do not use with MAOIs (or within 2 wk) or with products that possess MAOI-like action (furazolidone, isoniazid, INH, procarbazine); hypertensive crisis may occur**

⚠ **Increase: hypertensive crisis, seizures, coma—amoxapine, maprotiline, mirtazapine, trazodone, cyclobenzaprine, tricyclics, methyldopa**

Increase: serotonin syndrome—SSRIs, SNRIs, serotonin receptor agonists

Increase: effects of adrenergic agents (DOPamine, EPINEPHrine, pseudoephedrine)

Drug/Herb
- Avoid use with green tea, valerian, ginseng, yohimbine, kava, guarana, St. John's wort

Drug/Food
- Tyramine foods: avoid; increased pressor response

NURSING CONSIDERATIONS

Assess:
- CBC with differential weekly, assess for myelosuppression (anemias, leukopenia, pancytopenia, thrombocytopenia)
- **Serotonin syndrome:** at least 2 wk should elapse between discontinuing linezolid and starting serotonergic agents; assess for increased heart rate, shivering, sweating, dilated pupils, tremor, high B/P, hyperthermia, headache, confusion;

if these occur, stop linezolid, administer a serotonin antagonist if needed

- **Lactic acidosis:** repeated nausea/vomiting, unexplained acidosis, low bicarbonate level; notify prescriber immediately
- **Anaphylaxis/angioedema/Stevens-Johnson syndrome:** rash, pruritus, difficulty breathing, fever; have emergency equipment nearby
- CNS symptoms: headache, dizziness
- Hepatic studies: AST, ALT
- Allergic reactions: fever, flushing, rash, urticaria, pruritus

⚠ **Pseudomembranous colitis:** diarrhea, abdominal pain, fever, fatigue, anorexia, possible anemia, elevated WBC, low serum albumin; stop product, usually either vancomycin or IV metroNIDAZOLE given

- Lactic acidosis: nausea, vomiting, low bicarbonate levels

Evaluate:

- Therapeutic response: decreased symptoms of infection, blood cultures negative

Teach patient/family:

- If dizziness occurs, to ambulate, perform activities with assistance
- To complete full course of product therapy
- To contact prescriber if adverse reaction occurs
- To inform prescriber if SSRIs or cold products, decongestants being used
- To inform prescriber of history of hypertension
- To avoid large amounts of high-tyramine foods, drinks; provide list

liothyronine (T_3) (Rx)

(lye-oh-thye′roe-neen)

Cytomel, *l*-triiodothyronine, Triostat

Func. class.: Thyroid hormone
Chem. class.: Synthetic T_3

Do not confuse:
Cytomel/Cytotec

ACTION: Increases metabolic rates, cardiac output, O_2 consumption, body temp, blood volume, growth, development at cellular level; exact mechanism unknown

USES: Hypothyroidism, myxedema coma, thyroid hormone replacement, congenital hypothyroidism, nontoxic goiter, T_3 suppression test

CONTRAINDICATIONS: Adrenal insufficiency, MI, thyrotoxicosis, untreated hypertension

Black Box Warning: Obesity treatment

Precautions: Pregnancy (A), breastfeeding, geriatric patients, angina pectoris, hypertension, ischemia, cardiac disease, diabetes

DOSAGE AND ROUTES

- **Adult: PO** 25 mcg/day, increase by 12.5-25 mcg q1-2wk until desired response, maintenance dose 25-75 mcg/day, max 100 mcg/day
- **Geriatric: PO** 5 mcg/day, increase by 5 mcg/day q1-2wk, maintenance 25-75 mcg/day

Congenital hypothyroidism

- **Child >3 yr: PO** 50-100 mcg/day
- **Child <3 yr: PO** 5 mcg/day, increase by 5 mcg q3-4days titrated to response, infant maintenance 20 mcg/day; 1-3 yr 50 mcg/day

Myxedema, severe hypothyroidism

- **Adult: PO** 25-50 mcg then may increase by 5-10 mcg q1-2wk; maintenance dose 50-100 mcg/day

Myxedema coma/precoma

- **Adult: IV** 25-50 mcg initially, 5 mcg in geriatric patients, 10-20 mcg with cardiac disease; give doses q4-12hr

Nontoxic goiter

- **Adult: PO** 5 mcg/day, increase by 12.5-25 mcg q1-2wk; maintenance dose 75 mcg/day

Suppression test

- **Adult: PO** 75-100 mcg/day × 1 wk; radioactive ^{131}I given before and after 1-wk dose

Available forms: Tabs 5, 25, 50 mcg; inj 10 mcg/ml

Administer:

- In AM if possible as a single dose to decrease sleeplessness
- At same time each day to maintain product level
- Only for hormone imbalances; do not use for obesity, male infertility, menstrual conditions, lethargy
- Lowest dose that relieves symptoms
- Liothyronine after discontinuing other thyroid preparations
- Do not give with calcium, iron, aluminum, magnesium, soy products

SIDE EFFECTS

CNS: *Insomnia, tremors,* headache, thyroid storm

CV: *Tachycardia, palpitations, angina, dysrhythmias,* hypertension, cardiac arrest

GI: Nausea, diarrhea, increased or decreased appetite, cramps

MISC: Menstrual irregularities, weight loss, sweating, heat intolerance, fever, alopecia

PHARMACOKINETICS

PO/IV: Peak 2-3 days, duration 72 hr, half-life 2.5 days

INTERACTIONS

Increase: effects of—anticoagulants, sympathomimetics, tricyclics, amphetamines, decongestants, vasopressors

Decrease: absorption of liothyronine—cholestyramine; colestipol; calcium, iron, aluminum, magnesium products

Decrease: effects of liothyronine—estrogens

Drug/Herb

Decrease: thyroid hormone effect—soy

Drug/Lab Test

Increase: CPK, LDH, AST, PBI, blood glucose

Decrease: thyroid function tests

NURSING CONSIDERATIONS

Assess:

- B/P, pulse periodically during treatment
- Weight daily in same clothing, using same scale, at same time of day
- Height, growth rate of child
- T_3, T_4, which are decreased; radioimmunoassay of TSH, which is increased; radio uptake, which is increased if patient receiving too low a dose of medication
- PT may require decreased anticoagulant; check for bleeding, bruising
- Increased nervousness, excitability, irritability, which may indicate too high a dose of medication, usually after 1-3 wk of treatment
- Cardiac status: angina, palpitation, chest pain, change in VS

Perform/provide:

- Removal of medication 4 wk before RAIU test

Evaluate:

- Therapeutic response: absence of depression; increased weight loss, diuresis, pulse, appetite; absence of constipation, peripheral edema, cold intolerance; pale, cool, dry skin; brittle nails; alopecia, coarse hair; menorrhagia; night blindness; paresthesia; syncope, stupor, coma; rosy cheeks

Teach patient/family:

- That hair loss will occur in child but is temporary
- To report excitability, irritability, anxiety, which indicate overdose
- Not to switch brands unless approved by prescriber
- That hypothyroid child will show almost immediate behavior/personality change
- That product is not to be taken to reduce weight
- To avoid OTC preparations with iodine; to read labels; not to take with calcium, iron, aluminum, magnesium products
- To avoid iodine-rich food, iodized salt, soybeans, tofu, turnips, high iodine seafood, some bread

L

• That product controls symptoms but does not cure; that treatment is lifelong

liotrix (Rx)

(lye'oh-trix)

Thyrolar, T_3/T_4

Func. class.: Thyroid hormone

Chem. class.: Levothyroxine/liothyronine (synthetic T_4, T_3)

Do not confuse:
Thyrolar/Thyrar

ACTION: Increases metabolic rates, cardiac output, O_2 consumption, body temp, blood volume, growth, development at cellular level; exact mechanism unknown

USES: Hypothyroidism, thyroid hormone replacement

CONTRAINDICATIONS: Adrenal insufficiency, MI, thyrotoxicosis

Black Box Warning: Obesity treatment

Precautions: Pregnancy (A), breastfeeding, geriatric patients, angina pectoris, hypertension, ischemia, cardiac disease, diabetes

DOSAGE AND ROUTES

• **Adult: PO** single dose of Thyrolar, 1/4 or 1/2 of adult dose, adjust as needed at 2-wk intervals

• **Geriatric: PO** 1/4 tab initially, adjust q6-8wk

Available forms: Tabs: Levothyroxine 12.5 mcg/liothyronine 3.1 mcg; levothyroxine 25 mcg/liothyronine 6.25 mcg (Thyrolar-1/2); levothyroxine 50 mcg/liothyronine 12.5 mcg (Thyrolar-1); levothyroxine 100 mcg/liothyronine 25 mcg (Thyrolar-2); levothyroxine 150 mcg/liothyronine 37.5 mcg (Thyrolar-3)

Administer:

• Separate products containing calcium, iron by ≥4 hr

• In AM if possible as a single dose to decrease sleeplessness

• At same time each day to maintain product level

• Only for hormone imbalances; do not use for obesity, male infertility, menstrual conditions, lethargy

• Lowest dose that relieves symptoms

SIDE EFFECTS

CNS: *Insomnia, tremors,* headache, thyroid storm, nervousness

CV: *Tachycardia, palpitations, angina, dysrhythmias,* hypertension, cardiac arrest

GI: Nausea, vomiting, diarrhea, increased or decreased appetite, cramps

MISC: Menstrual irregularities, weight loss, sweating, heat intolerance, fever

PHARMACOKINETICS

PO (T_4): Onset unknown, peak 1-3 wk, duration 1-3 wk, terminal half-life 6-7 days

PO (T_3): Onset unknown, peak 24-72 hr, duration 72 hr, terminal half-life 1-2 days

INTERACTIONS

Increase: effects of amphetamines, decongestants, vasopressors, anticoagulants, sympathomimetics, tricyclics, catecholamines

Decrease: absorption of liotrix—cholestyramine, colestipol

Decrease: effects of liotrix—estrogens, phenytoin, carBAMazepine, rifampin

Drug/Herb

Decrease: thyroid hormone effect—soy

Drug/Lab Test

Increase: CPK, LDH, AST, PBI, blood glucose

Decrease: thyroid function tests

NURSING CONSIDERATIONS

Assess:

• B/P, pulse periodically during treatment

• Weight daily in same clothing, using same scale, at same time of day

• Height, growth rate of child

• T_3, T_4, FTIs, which are decreased; radioimmunoassay of TSH, which is in-

creased; radio uptake, which is increased if patient is receiving too low a dose of medication
- May require decreased anticoagulant; check for bleeding, bruising
- Increased nervousness, excitability, irritability, which may indicate too high a dose of medication, usually after 1-3 wk of treatment
- Cardiac status: angina, palpitation, chest pain, change in VS

Perform/provide:
- Withdrawal of medication 4 wk before RAIU test
- Storage in airtight, light-resistant container

Evaluate:
- Therapeutic response: absence of depression; increased weight loss, diuresis, pulse, appetite; absence of constipation, peripheral edema, cold intolerance; pale, cool, dry skin; brittle nails; coarse hair; menorrhagia; night blindness; paresthesias; syncope, stupor, coma; rosy cheeks

Teach patient/family:
- That hair loss will occur in child, is temporary
- To report excitability, irritability, chest pain, increased pulse rate, palpitations, excessive sweating, heat intolerance, nervousness, anxiety, which indicate overdose
- Not to switch brands unless approved by prescriber
- That hypothyroid child will show almost immediate behavior/personality change
- That product is not to be taken to reduce weight
- To avoid OTC preparations with iodine; read labels; separate products containing calcium, iron by ≥4 hr
- To avoid iodine food, iodized salt, soybeans, tofu, turnips, high iodine seafood, some bread
- That product does not cure, but controls symptoms; treatment is lifelong

liraglutide (Rx)
(lir′a-gloo′tide)

Victoza

Func. class.: Antidiabetic agent
Chem. class.: Incretin mimetics

ACTION: Improved glycemic control and potential weight loss via activation of the glucagon-like peptide-1 (GLP-1) receptor

USES: Type 2 diabetes mellitus in combination with diet/exercise

CONTRAINDICATIONS: Hypersensitivity

Black Box Warning: Medullary thyroid carcinoma (MTC), multiple endocrine neoplasia syndrome type 2 (MEN 2), thyroid cancer

Precautions: Breastfeeding, children, geriatric patients, alcoholism, burns, cholelithiasis, type 1 diabetes mellitus, ketoacidosis, diarrhea, fever, gastroparesis, hepatic/renal disease, hypoglycemia, infection, pancreatitis, surgery, thyroid disease, trauma, vomiting

DOSAGES AND ROUTES
- **Adult: SUBCUT** 0.6 mg/day × 1 wk, then increase to 1.2 mg/day, max 1.8 mg/day

Available forms: Solution for injection 18 mg/3 ml pre-filled pen

Administer:

Subcut route
- Give subcut only, inspect for particulate matter, discoloration; do not use if unusually viscous, cloudy, discolored, or if particles present; give daily anytime, without regard to meals; pen needles must be purchased separately, use Novo Nordisk needle; prior to first use, prime, see manual for directions; give in thigh, abdomen, or upper arm; lightly pinch fold of skin, insert needle at 90-degree angle (45-degree angle if thin), release

skin; aspiration is not needed, give over 6 sec, rotate injection sites

SIDE EFFECTS

CNS: Dizziness, headache
CV: Hypertension
ENDO: Hypoglycemia
EENT: Sinusitis
GI: Abdominal pain, anorexia, constipation, diarrhea, dyspepsia, nausea, vomiting, **pancreatitis**
INTEG: **Angioedema**, erythema, injection site reaction, urticaria
MS: Back pain
SYST: Antibody formation, infection, influenza, **secondary thyroid malignancy**

INTERACTIONS

Increase: hypoglycemic reactions—angiotensin II receptor antagonists, ACE inhibitors, other antidiabetics, beta blockers, dexfenfluramine, fenfluramine, disopyramide, fluoxetine, fibric acid derivatives, mecasermin, MAOIs, octreotide, pegvisomant, salicylates
Increase: hyperglycemic reactions—protease inhibitors, phenothiazines, baclofen, atypical antipsychotics, corticosteroids, cycloSPORINE, tacrolimus, carbonic anhydrase inhibitors, dextrothyroxine, diazoxide, phenytoin, fosphenytoin, ethotoin, isoniazid, INH, niacin, nicotine, estrogens, progestins, oral contraceptives, growth hormones, sympathomimetics
Increase or decrease: hypoglycemic reactions—androgens, bortezomib, quinolones, cloNIDine, alcohol, lithium, pentamidine
Increase or decrease: effects of—torvastatin, acetaminophen, griseofulvin

PHARMACOKINETICS

Protein binding (98%); half-life 12-13 hr; binds to albumin, then released into circulation; peak 8-12 hr; body weight significantly affects pharmacokinetics

NURSING CONSIDERATIONS

Assess:

Black Box Warning: Thyroid C-cell tumors; monitor during treatment

• Hypoglycemic reactions that may occur soon after meals: hunger, sweating, weakness, dizziness, tremors, restlessness, tachycardia
• Hypersensitivity to this product
• Serum glucose, A1c, CBC during treatment
• **Stress:** those diabetic patients exposed to stress, surgery, fever, infections may require insulin administration temporarily
⚠ **Serious skin reactions:** angioedema, pancreatitis, secondary thyroid malignancy

Perform/Provide:

• Storage: do not store pen with needle attached; avoid direct heat and sunlight; discard 30 days after first use; after first use may be stored at room temp or refrigerated, do not freeze

Evaluate:

• Therapeutic response: stable and improved serum glucose, A1C, weight loss

Teach patient/family:

• About symptoms of hypo/hyperglycemia, what to do for each; to have glucagon emergency kit available; to carry a carbohydrate source at all times
• About side effects associated with therapy, such as nausea and vomiting; that upward dose titration can be delayed or ignored, depending on tolerance
• That diabetes is a life-long illness; that product does not cure disease and must be continued on a daily basis
• To carry emergency ID with prescriber's phone number and medications taken
• To continue with other recommendations: diet, exercise, hygiene
• To test blood glucose using a blood glucose meter
• To avoid other medications, herbs, supplements unless approved by prescriber

⚠ To report serious skin effects, abdominal pain with nausea/vomiting
• Provide patient with written instructions if self-administration is ordered

lisdexamfetamine (Rx)

(lis-dex'am-fet'a-meen)

Vyvanse

Func. class.: CNS stimulant
Chem. class.: Amphetamine

Controlled Substance Schedule II

ACTION: Increases release of norepinephrine, dopamine in cerebral cortex to reticular activating system

USES: Attention-deficit/hyperactivity disorder (ADHD)

CONTRAINDICATIONS: Breastfeeding, hyperthyroidism, hypertension, glaucoma, severe arteriosclerosis, CV disease, hypersensitivity to sympathomimetic amines

Black Box Warning: Substance abuse

Precautions: Pregnancy (C), children <6 yr, Gilles de la Tourette's disorder, depression, anorexia nervosa, psychosis, seizure disorder, suicidal ideation, MI, heart failure, alcoholism, aortic stenosis, bipolar disorder

DOSAGE AND ROUTES

• **Child 6-12 yr: PO** 30 mg/day, may increase by 10-20 mg/day at weekly intervals, max 70 mg/day

Available forms: Caps 30, 50, 70 mg

Administer:
• Give daily in AM
• Without regard to meals
• Caps: may take whole or opened and contents dissolved in water

SIDE EFFECTS

CNS: *Hyperactivity, insomnia, restlessness, talkativeness,* dizziness, headache, dysphoria, irritability, aggressiveness, CNS tumor, dependence, addiction, mild euphoria, somnolence, lability, psychosis, mania, hallucinations, aggression

CV: *Palpitations, tachycardia,* hypertension, decrease in heart rate, dysrhythmias, MI, cardiomyopathy

EENT: Blurred vision, mydriasis, dyplopia

ENDO: Growth inhibition

GI: *Anorexia,* dry mouth, diarrhea, weight loss

GU: Impotence, change in libido

INTEG: Urticaria, angioedema, Stevens-Johnson syndrome, toxic epidermal necrolysis

PHARMACOKINETICS

Metabolized by liver; urine excretion pH dependent; crosses placenta, breast milk; half-life <1hr

INTERACTIONS

⚠ Hypertensive crisis: MAOIs or within 14 days of MAOIs

Increase: serotonin syndrome, neuroleptic malignant syndrome—SSRIs, SNRIs, serotonin-receptor agonists

Increase: lisdexamfetamine effect—acetaZOLAMIDE, antacids, sodium bicarbonate, urinary alkalinizers

Increase: CNS effect—haloperidol, tricyclics, phenothiazines, modafinil, meperidine, PHENobarbital, phenytoin

Increase: CNS stimulation—melatonin

Decrease: absorption of phenytoin

Decrease: lisdexamfetamine effect—ascorbic acid, ammonium chloride, urinary acidifiers

Decrease: effect of—adrenergic blockers, antidiabetics

Drug/Herb
• Serotonin syndrome: St. John's wort

Increase: stimulant effect—khat, melatonin, green tea, guarana

Decrease: stimulant effect—eucalyptus

Drug/Food

Increase: amine effect—caffeine

NURSING CONSIDERATIONS

Assess:

• VS, B/P; product may reverse antihypertensives; check patients with cardiac disease often

• CBC, urinalysis; in diabetes: blood glucose; insulin changes may be required because eating may decrease

• Height, growth rate in children; growth rate may be decreased

• Mental status: mood, sensorium, affect, stimulation, insomnia, irritability

⚠ **Serotonin syndrome, neuroleptic malignant syndrome:** increased heart rate, shivering, sweating, dilated pupils, tremors, high B/P, hyperthermia, headache, confusion; if these occur, stop product, administer serotonin antagonist if needed; at least 2 wk should elapse between discontinuation of serotonergic agents and start of product

• **Tolerance or dependency:** increased amount of product may be used to get same effect; will develop after long-term use

• Overdose: pain, fever, dehydration, insomnia, hyperactivity

Black Box Warning: Before giving this product, identify presence of substance abuse; high potential for abuse

Perform/provide:

• Gum, hard candy, frequent sips of water for dry mouth

Evaluate:

• Therapeutic response: increased CNS stimulation, decreased drowsiness

Teach patient/family:

• To decrease caffeine consumption (coffee, tea, cola, chocolate); may increase irritability, stimulation

• To avoid OTC preparations unless approved by prescriber

• To taper product over several weeks; depression, increased sleeping, lethargy may occur

• To avoid alcohol ingestion

• To avoid breastfeeding

• To avoid hazardous activities until stabilized on medication

• To get needed rest; patient will feel more tired at end of day

• To use as part of a comprehensive treatment program

TREATMENT OF OVERDOSE:

Administer fluids, antihypertensive for increased B/P, ammonium chloride for increased excretion, chlorproMAZINE for antagonizing CNS effects

lisinopril (Rx)

(lyse-in′oh-pril)

Prinivil, Zestril

Func. class.: Antihypertensive, angiotensin-converting enzyme 1 (ACE) inhibitor

Chem. class.: Enalaprilat lysine analog

Do not confuse:

lisinopril/Risperdal

Prinivil/Plendil/Proventil/Prilosec

ACTION: Selectively suppresses renin-angiotensin-aldosterone system; inhibits ACE, thereby preventing conversion of angiotensin I to angiotensin II

USES: Mild to moderate hypertension, adjunctive therapy of systolic CHF, acute MI

CONTRAINDICATIONS: Hypersensitivity, angioedema

Black Box Warning: Pregnancy (D), 2nd/3rd trimesters

Precautions: Breastfeeding, renal disease, hyperkalemia, renal artery stenosis, CHF, pregnancy (C) 1st trimester

DOSAGE AND ROUTES

Hypertension

• **Adult: PO** 10-40 mg/day; max 80 mg/day

• **Child ≥6 yr: PO** 0.07 mg/kg/day up to 5 mg/day; titrate q1-2wk up to 0.6 mg/kg/day or 40 mg/day

• **Geriatric: PO** 2.5-5 mg/day, increase q7days

CHF

• **Adult: PO** 5 mg initially with diuretics, range 5-40 mg

• **Acute myocardial infarction in adults who are hemodynamically stable: PO** give 5 mg within 24 hr of onset of symptoms, then 5 mg after 24 hr, 10 mg after 48 hr, then 10 mg daily

Renal dose

• **Adult: PO** CCr <30 ml/min, reduce dose by 50%, initially 5 mg/day, max 40 mg/day; CCr <10 ml/min, 2.5 mg/day, max 40 mg/day

Available forms: Tabs 2.5, 5, 10, 20, 30, 40 mg

Administer:

• Severe hypotension may occur after 1st dose of product; may be prevented by reducing or discontinuing diuretic therapy 3 days before beginning lisinopril therapy

SIDE EFFECTS

CNS: *Vertigo,* depression, stroke, insomnia, paresthesias, headache, *fatigue,* asthenia, dizziness

CV: Chest pain, hypotension, sinus tachycardia

EENT: Blurred vision, nasal congestion

GI: Nausea, vomiting, anorexia, constipation, flatulence, GI irritation, diarrhea, **hepatic failure, hepatic necrosis**

GU: **Proteinuria, renal insufficiency,** sexual dysfunction, impotence

INTEG: Rash, pruritus

MISC: Muscle cramps, hyperkalemia

RESP: Dry cough, dyspnea

SYST: **Angioedema, anaphylaxis, toxic epidermal necrolysis**

PHARMACOKINETICS

Onset 1 hr, peak 6-8 hr, duration 24 hr, excreted unchanged in urine, half-life 12 hr

INTERACTIONS

Increase: hyperkalemia—potassium salt substitutes, potassium-sparing diuretics, potassium supplements, cycloSPORINE

Increase: possible toxicity—lithium

Increase: hypotensive effect—diuretics, other antihypertensives, probenecid, phenothiazines, nitrates, acute alcohol ingestion

Increase: hypersensitivity—allopurinol

Decrease: lisinopril effects—aspirin, indomethacin, NSAIDs

Drug/Food

• High-potassium diet (bananas, orange juice, avocados, nuts, spinach) should be avoided; hyperkalemia may occur

Drug/Lab Test

Interference: glucose/insulin tolerance tests, ANA titer

NURSING CONSIDERATIONS

Assess:

⚠ **Blood studies, platelets; WBC with differential at baseline, periodically q3mo; if neutrophils <1000/mm³, discontinue treatment (recommended with collagen-vascular disease)**

• Baselines of renal, hepatic studies before therapy begins, periodically; LFTs, uric acid, glucose may be increased

• **Angioedema: anaphylaxis, toxic epidermal necrolysis,** facial swelling, dyspnea, tongue swelling (rare)

• Pregnancy before starting treatment; pregnancy (D)

• **Hypertension:** B/P, pulse q4hr during beginning treatment and periodically thereafter; note rate, rhythm, quality; apical/pedal pulse before administration; notify prescriber of any significant changes

• Electrolytes: K, Na, Cl

• **CHF:** edema in feet, legs daily; weight daily; dyspnea, wet crackles

• Skin turgor, dryness of mucous membranes for hydration status

Evaluate:

• Therapeutic response: decreased B/P, CHF symptoms

L

Teach patient/family:
- Not to discontinue product abruptly; to taper
- To rise slowly to sitting or standing position to minimize orthostatic hypotension
- To avoid increasing potassium in the diet
- To report dry cough

Black Box Warning: To report if pregnancy is planned or suspected; pregnancy (D) 2nd/3rd trimesters

TREATMENT OF OVERDOSE:
Lavage, IV atropine for bradycardia, IV theophylline for bronchospasm, digoxin, O_2, diuretic for cardiac failure

lithium (Rx)
(li'thee-um)

Apo-Lithium Carbonate ✱, Carbolith ✱, Duralith ✱, Lithobid, PMS-Lithium Carbonate ✱

Func. class.: Antimanic, antipsychotic
Chem. class.: Alkali metal ion salt

ACTION: May alter sodium, potassium ion transport across cell membrane in nerve, muscle cells; may balance biogenic amines of norepinephrine, serotonin in CNS areas involved in emotional responses

USES: Bipolar disorders (manic phase), prevention of bipolar manic-depressive psychosis

CONTRAINDICATIONS: Pregnancy (D), breastfeeding, children <12 yr, hepatic disease, brain trauma, organic brain syndrome, schizophrenia, severe cardiac/renal disease, severe dehydration

Precautions: Geriatric patients, thyroid disease, seizure disorders, diabetes mellitus, systemic infection, urinary retention

Black Box Warning: Lithium level >1.5 mmol/L

DOSAGE AND ROUTES
- **Adult: PO** 300-600 mg tid, maintenance 300 mg tid or qid; **SLOW REL TABS** 300 mg bid; dose should be individualized to maintain blood levels at 0.5-1.5 mEq/L
- **Geriatric: PO** 300 mg bid, increase q7days by 300 mg to desired dose
- **Child: PO** 15-20 mg/kg/day in 3-4 divided doses; increase as needed; do not exceed adult doses; maintain blood levels at 0.4-0.5 mEq/L

Renal dose
- **Adult: PO** CCr 10-50 ml/min, 50%-75% of dose; CCr <10 ml/min, 25%-50% of dose

Available forms: Caps 150, 300, 600 mg; tabs 300 mg; ext rel tabs 300, 450 mg; syr 300 mg/5 ml (8 mEq/5 ml); slow rel caps 150, 300 mg ✱

Administer:
- Do not break, crush, chew caps, ext rel tabs
- Reduced dose to geriatric patients
- With meals to avoid GI upset
- Adequate fluids (2-3 L/day) to prevent dehydration during initial treatment, 1-2 L/day during maintenance

SIDE EFFECTS
CNS: *Headache, drowsiness, dizziness,* tremors, twitching, ataxia, seizure, slurred speech, restlessness, confusion, stupor, memory loss, clonic movements, fatigue
CV: *Hypotension,* ECG changes, dysrhythmias, circulatory collapse, edema
EENT: Tinnitus, blurred vision
ENDO: Hyponatremia, goiter, hyperglycemia, hypo/hyperthyroidism
GI: *Dry mouth, anorexia, nausea, vomiting, diarrhea,* incontinence, abdominal pain, metallic taste
GU: Polyuria, glycosuria, proteinuria, albuminuria, urinary incontinence, polydipsia
HEMA: Leukocytosis

INTEG: Drying of hair, alopecia, rash, pruritus, hyperkeratosis, acneiform lesions, folliculitis
MS: Muscle weakness

PHARMACOKINETICS

PO: Onset rapid, peak ½-12 hr, half-life 18-36 hr depending on age, crosses blood-brain barrier, 80% of filtered lithium reabsorbed by renal tubules, excreted in urine, crosses placenta, enters breast milk, well absorbed by oral method

INTERACTIONS

• Neurotoxicity: haloperidol, thioridazine
Increase: hypothyroid effects—antithyroid agents, calcium iodide, potassium iodide, iodinated glycerol
Increase: effects of neuromuscular blocking agents, phenothiazines
Increase: renal clearance—sodium bicarbonate, acetaZOLAMIDE, mannitol, aminophylline
Increase: masking of lithium toxicity—beta-blockers used for lithium tremor
Increase: toxicity—indomethacin, diuretics, NSAIDs, losartan
Increase: lithium effect/toxicity—carBAMazepine, FLUoxetine, methyldopa, thiazide diuretics, probenecid
Decrease: lithium effects—theophyllines, urea, urinary alkalinizers

Drug/Herb

• Avoid use with kava, St. John's wort, valerian
Decrease: lithium levels—black/green tea, guarana

Drug/Food

• Significant changes in sodium intake alter lithium excretion

Drug/Lab Test

Increase: potassium excretion, urine glucose, blood glucose, protein, BUN
Decrease: VMA, T_3, T_4, PBI, ^{131}I

NURSING CONSIDERATIONS

Assess:

• **Mental status:** manic symptoms, mood, behavior before, during treatment
• **Lithium toxicity:** diarrhea, vomiting, tremor, twitching
• Weight daily; check for, report edema in legs, ankles, wrists
• Sodium intake; decreased sodium intake with decreased fluid intake may lead to lithium retention; increased sodium, fluids may decrease lithium retention
• Skin turgor at least daily
• Urine for albuminuria, glycosuria, uric acid during beginning treatment, q2mo thereafter
• Neurologic status: LOC, gait, motor reflexes, hand tremors

Black Box Warning: serum lithium levels 2×/wk initially then q2mo (therapeutic level: 0.5-1.5 mEq/L); toxic level >1.5 mcg/L

• ECG in those >50 yr with CV disease

Evaluate:

• Therapeutic response: decrease in excitement, manic phase

Teach patient/family:

• About **the symptoms of minor toxicity:** vomiting, diarrhea, poor coordination, fine motor tremors, weakness, lassitude; **major toxicity:** coarse tremors, severe thirst, tinnitus, diluted urine
• To monitor urine specific gravity, emphasize need for follow-up care to determine lithium levels; to monitor lithium levels to ensure effective levels and treatment
• That contraception is necessary because lithium may harm fetus (pregnancy [D]); not to breastfeed
• Not to operate machinery until lithium levels stable
• That beneficial effects may take 1-3 wk
• About products that interact with lithium (provide list); about need for adequate, stable intake of salt and fluids; not to use OTC products unless approved by prescriber

TREATMENT OF OVERDOSE:

Induce emesis or lavage, maintain airway, respiratory function; dialysis for severe intoxication

Iodoxamide ophthalmic

See Appendix B

loperamide (OTC, Rx)

(loe-per'a-mide)

Anti-Diarrheal, Apo-Loperamide ✤, Equaline Anti-Diarrheal, Good Sense Anti-Diarrheal, Imodium ✤, Imodium A-D, Riva-Loperamide ✤, RxChoice Loperamide, Sandoz Loperamide ✤, Select Brand Anti-Diarrheal, Top Care Anti-Diarrheal, Walgreens Anti-Diarrheal

Func. class.: Antidiarrheal
Chem. class.: Piperidine derivative

Do not confuse:
Imodium/Indocin
Loperamide/furosemide

ACTION: Direct action on intestinal muscles to decrease GI peristalsis; reduces volume, increases bulk; electrolytes not lost

USES: Diarrhea (cause undetermined), travelers' diarrhea, chronic diarrhea, to decrease amount of ileostomy discharge

Unlabeled uses: Irinotecan-induced diarrhea, irritable bowel syndrome

CONTRAINDICATIONS: Hypersensitivity, pseudomembranous colitis, constipation, dysentery, GI bleeding/obstruction/perforation, ileus, vomiting

Precautions: Pregnancy (C), breastfeeding, children <2 yr, hepatic disease, dehydration, gastroenteritis, toxic megacolon, geriatric patients, severe ulcerative colitis

DOSAGE AND ROUTES

- **Adult: PO** 4 mg then 2 mg after each loose stool, max 16 mg/day
- **Child 9-11 yr: PO** 2 mg then 1 mg after each loose stool, max 6 mg/24 hr
- **Child 6-8 yr: PO** 2 mg then 0.1 mg/kg after each loose stool, max 4 mg/day
- **Child 2-5 yr: PO** 1 mg then 0.1 mg/kg after each loose stool, max 4 mg/24 hr

Irinotecan-induced diarrhea (unlabeled)

- **Adult: PO** 4 mg at first sign of late diarrhea (≥24 hr after irinotecan) then 2 mg q2hr × ≥12 hr; at night, 4 mg q4hr

Available forms: Caps 2 mg; liq 1 mg/5 ml; tabs 2 mg

Administer:

- Do not break, crush, or chew caps
- For 48 hr only
- Do not mix oral sol with other sol

SIDE EFFECTS

CNS: Dizziness, drowsiness, fatigue
GI: *Nausea, dry mouth, vomiting, constipation,* abdominal pain, anorexia, toxic megacolon, bacterial enterocolitis, flatulence
INTEG: Rash
MISC: Hyperglycemia
SYST: Anaphylaxis, angioedema, toxic epidermal necrolysis

PHARMACOKINETICS

PO: Onset 1-3 hr, duration 4-5 hr, half-life 9-14 hr, metabolized in liver, excreted in feces as unchanged product, small amount in urine

INTERACTIONS

Increase: CNS depression—alcohol, antihistamines, analgesics, opioids, sedative/hypnotics

Drug/Herb

Increase: CNS depression—chamomile, hops, kava, valerian

NURSING CONSIDERATIONS

Assess:

- **Stools:** volume, color, characteristics, frequency; bowel pattern before product; rebound constipation
- Electrolytes (K, Na, Cl) if receiving long-term therapy

• Skin turgor q8hr if dehydration is suspected; fluid replacement
• Response after 48 hr; if no response, product should be discontinued
• Dehydration, CNS problems in children, those with hepatic disease
• Abdominal distention, toxic megacolon; may occur with ulcerative colitis

Perform/provide:
• Storage in tight container

Evaluate:
• Therapeutic response: decreased diarrhea (48 hr); decreased chronic diarrhea (10 days)

Teach patient/family:
• To avoid OTC products unless directed by prescriber
• That ileostomy patient may take product for extended time
• If drowsiness occurs, not to operate machinery
• To use hard candy, sips of water for dry mouth

loratadine (OTC, Rx)

(lor-a′ti-deen)

Alavert, Apo-Loratadine ✱, Claritin, Claritin Children's, Claritin RediTabs, Clear-Atadine, Dimetapp, Equaline Non-Drowsy, Equate Allergy Relief, Good Sense Non-Drowsy, Leader Allergy Relief, Leader Loratadine, Tavist ND, Walgreens Loratadine, Wal-itin Aller-Melts, Wal-vert

Func. class.: Antihistamine, 2nd generation

Chem. class.: Selective histamine (H_1)-receptor antagonist

Do not confuse:
loratadine/lovastatin/LORazepam/losartan

ACTION: Binds to peripheral histamine receptors, thereby providing antihistamine action without sedation

USES: Seasonal rhinitis, chronic idiopathic urticaria for those ≥2 yr

CONTRAINDICATIONS: Hypersensitivity, acute asthma attacks, lower respiratory tract disease

Precautions: Pregnancy (B), breastfeeding, increased intraocular pressure, bronchial asthma, hepatic/renal disease

DOSAGE AND ROUTES

• **Adult and child ≥6 yr: PO** 10 mg/day
• **Child 2-5 yr: PO** 5 mg/day

Renal/hepatic dose
• **Adult: PO** CCr <30 ml/min or hepatic disease, 10 mg every other day

Available forms: Tabs 10 mg; rapid-disintegrating tabs 10 mg; orally disintegrating tabs 10 mg; syr 1 mg/ml; susp 5 mg/ml

Administer:
• **Rapid-disintegrating tabs** by placing on tongue, to be swallowed after disintegrated with/without water
• Use within 6 mo of opening pouch and immediately after opening blister pack
• On empty stomach daily

SIDE EFFECTS

CNS: Sedation (more common with increased doses), headache, fatigue, restlessness
CV: Sinus tachycardia
RESP: Wheezing

PHARMACOKINETICS

Onset 1-3 hr, peak 8-10 hr, duration 24 hr, metabolized in liver to active metabolites, excreted in urine, active metabolite desloratadine half-life 20 hr

INTERACTIONS

Increase: antihistamine effects—MAOIs
Increase: CNS depressant effects—alcohol, antidepressants, other antihistamines, sedative/hypnotics
Increase: loratadine level—cimetidine, ketoconazole, macrolides (clarithromycin, erythromycin)

Drug/Lab Test
False negative: skin allergy tests (discontinue antihistamine 3 days before testing)

NURSING CONSIDERATIONS

Assess:

- **Allergy:** hives, rash, rhinitis; monitor respiratory status
- LFTs, serum creatinine/BUN

Perform/provide:

- Storage in tight container at room temp
- Increased fluids to 2 L/day to decrease secretions

Evaluate:

- Therapeutic response: absence of running or congested nose, other allergy symptoms

Teach patient/family:

- To avoid driving, other hazardous activities if drowsiness occurs
- To use sunscreen or to stay out of sun to prevent photosensitivity
- To avoid use of other CNS depressants
- To increase fluids to 2 L/day to decrease secretions

LORazepam (Rx)

(lor-a′ze-pam)

Apo-Lorazepam ♣, Ativan, PMS-Lorazepam ♣

Func. class.: Sedative, hypnotic; antianxiety

Chem. class.: Benzodiazepine, short acting

Controlled Substance Schedule IV

Do not confuse:
LORazepam/ALPRAZolam/clonazePAM

ACTION: Potentiates the actions of GABA, especially in the limbic system and the reticular formation

USES: Anxiety, irritability with psychiatric or organic disorders, preoperatively; insomnia; adjunct for endoscopic procedures, status epilepticus
Unlabeled uses: Antiemetic prior to chemotherapy, rectal use, alcohol withdrawal, seizure prophylaxis, agitation, insomnia, sedation maintenance

CONTRAINDICATIONS: Pregnancy (D), breastfeeding, hypersensitivity to benzodiazepines, benzyl alcohol; closed-angle glaucoma, psychosis, history of drug abuse, COPD, sleep apnea
Precautions: Children <12 yr, geriatric patients, debilitated, renal/hepatic disease, addiction, suicidal ideation, abrupt discontinuation

DOSAGE AND ROUTES

Anxiety

- **Adult/adolescent: PO** 2-3 mg/day in divided doses, max 10 mg/day
- **Geriatric: PO** 1-2 mg/day in divided doses or 0.5-1 mg at bedtime

Preoperatively

- **Adult: IM** 50 mcg/kg 2 hr prior to surgery; **IV** 44 mcg/kg 15-20 min prior to surgery, max 2 mg 15-20 min prior to surgery
- **Child ≥12 yr: IV** 0.05 mg/kg

Status epilepticus

- **Neonate: IV** 0.05 mg/kg
- **Child: IV** 0.1 mg/kg up to 4 mg/dose; **RECT** (unlabeled) 0.05-0.1 mg × 2; wait 7 min before giving 2nd dose

Alcohol withdrawal (unlabeled)

- **Adult: PO** 2 mg q6hr × 4 doses then 1 mg q6hr for 8 doses

Insomnia (unlabeled)

- **Adult: PO** 2-4 mg at bedtime; only minimally effective after 2 wk continuous therapy
- **Geriatric: PO** 0.5-1 mg initially

Available forms: Tabs 0.5, 1, 2 mg; inj 2, 4 mg/ml; conc oral sol 2 mg/ml
Administer:
PO route

- With food or milk for GI symptoms; crushed if patient is unable to swallow medication whole

- Sugarless gum, hard candy, frequent sips of water for dry mouth
- Give largest dose before bedtime if giving in divided doses
- Concentrate: use calibrated dropper; add to food/drink; consume immediately

IM route

- Deep into large muscle mass

Direct IV route

- Prepare immediately before use; short stability time
- IV after diluting in equal vol sterile water, 5% dextrose, or 0.9% NaCl for inj; give through Y-tube or 3-way stopcock; give at ≤2 mg/1 min, do not give rapidly

Y-site compatibilities: Acyclovir, albumin, allopurinol, amifostine, amikacin, amoxicillin, amoxicillin/clavulanate, amphotericin B cholesteryl, amsacrine, atenolol, atracurium, bivalirudin, bleomycin, bumetanide, butorphanol, calcium chloride/gluconate, CARBOplatin, ceFAZolin, cefepime, cefotaxime, cefotetan, cefoxitin, ceftazidime, ceftizoxime, ceftobiprole, cefTRIAXone, cefuroxime, chloramphenicol, chlorproMAZINE, cimetidine, ciprofloxacin, cisatracurium, CISplatin, cladribine, clindamycin, cloNIDine, cyclophosphamide, cycloSPORINE, cytarabine, DACTINomycin, DAPTOmycin, dexamethasone, dexmedetomidine, diltiazem, DOBUTamine, docetaxel, DOPamine, doripenem, DOXOrubicin, DOXOrubicin liposomal, droperidol, enalaprilat, ePHEDrine, EPINEPHrine, epirubicin, eptifibatide, erythromycin, esmolol, etomidate, famotidine, fenoldopam, fentaNYL, filgrastim, fluconazole, fludarabine, fosphenytoin, furosemide, ganciclovir, gatifloxacin, gemcitabine, gentamicin, glycopyrrolate, granisetron, haloperidol, heparin, hydrocortisone, HYDROmorphone, hydrOXYzine, ifosfamide, inamrinone, insulin (regular), irinotecan, isoproterenol, ketorolac, labetalol, lidocaine, linezolid, magnesium sulfate, mannitol, mechlorethamine, melphalan, meropenem, metaraminol, methadone, methotrexate, methyldopate, methylPREDNISolone, metoclopramide, metoprolol, metroNIDAZOLE, micafungin, midazolam, milrinone, minocycline, mitoxantrone, morphine, mycophenolate, nafcillin, nalbuphine, naloxone, nesiritide, niCARdipine, nitroglycerin, nitroprusside, norepinephrine, octreotide, oxaliplatin, oxytocin, paclitaxel, palonosetron, pamidronate, pancuronium, pemetrexed, pentamidine, PENTobarbital, PHENobarbital, piperacillin, piperacillin-tazobactam, polymyxin B, potassium chloride, propofol, ranitidine, remifentanil, tacrolimus, teniposide, theophylline, thiotepa, ticarcillin, ticarcillin-clavulanate, tigecycline, tirofiban, tobramycin, TPN, trastuzumab, trimethobenzamide, trimethoprim-sulfamethoxazole, vancomycin, vasopressin, vecuronium, verapamil, vinCRIStine, vinorelbine, voriconazole, zidovudine

SIDE EFFECTS

CNS: *Dizziness, drowsiness,* confusion, headache, anxiety, tremors, stimulation, fatigue, depression, insomnia, hallucinations, weakness, unsteadiness

CV: *Orthostatic hypotension,* **ECG changes, tachycardia, hypotension;** apnea, cardiac arrest (IV, rapid)

EENT: *Blurred vision,* tinnitus, mydriasis

GI: Constipation, dry mouth, nausea, vomiting, anorexia, diarrhea

INTEG: Rash, dermatitis, itching

MISC: Acidosis

PHARMACOKINETICS

Metabolized by liver; excreted by kidneys; crosses placenta, excreted in breast milk; half-life 14 hr

PO: Onset ½ hr, peak 1-6 hr, duration 12-24 hr

IM: Onset 15-30 min, peak 1-1½ hr, duration 6-8 hr

IV: Onset 5-15 min, peak unknown, duration 6-8 hr

INTERACTIONS

Increase: LORazepam effects—CNS depressants, alcohol, disulfiram, oral contraceptives

Decrease: LORazepam effects—valproic acid

Drug/Herb

Increase: CNS depression—chamomile, kava, valerian

Drug/Lab Test

Increase: AST, ALT, serum bilirubin

Decrease: RAIU

False increase: 17-OHCS

NURSING CONSIDERATIONS

Assess:

⚠ **Anxiety:** decrease in anxiety; mental status: mood, sensorium, affect, sleeping pattern, drowsiness, dizziness, suicidal tendencies

• Renal/hepatic/blood status if receiving high-dose therapy

• **Physical dependency, withdrawal symptoms:** headache, nausea, vomiting, muscle pain, weakness, tremors, seizures, after long-term, excessive use

Perform/provide:

• Assistance with ambulation during beginning therapy, since drowsiness, dizziness occurs

• Check to confirm that PO medication has been swallowed

• Refrigerate parenteral form

Evaluate:

• Therapeutic response: decreased anxiety, restlessness, insomnia

Teach patient/family:

• That product may be taken with food

• Not to use product for everyday stress or for >4 mo unless directed by prescriber

• Not to take more than prescribed amount; may be habit forming

• To avoid OTC preparations (cough, cold, hay fever) unless approved by prescriber

• To avoid driving, activities that require alertness, since drowsiness may occur

• To avoid alcohol, other psychotropic medications unless directed by prescriber

• Not to discontinue medication abruptly after long-term use

• To rise slowly because fainting may occur, especially among geriatric patients

• That drowsiness may worsen at beginning of treatment

• To use birth control if of child-bearing age (pregnancy [D])

TREATMENT OF OVERDOSE:

Lavage, VS, supportive care, flumazenil

losartan

(lo-zar′tan)

Cozaar

Func. class.: Antihypertensive

Chem. class.: Angiotensin II receptor (type AT_1) antagonist

Do not confuse:

losartan/valsartan

Cozaar/Zocor

ACTION: Blocks the vasoconstrictor and aldosterone-secreting effects of angiotensin II; selectively blocks the binding of angiotensin II to the AT_1 receptor found in tissues

USES: Hypertension, alone or in combination; nephropathy in type 2 diabetes; proteinuria; stroke prophylaxis for hypertensive patients with left ventricular hypertrophy

CONTRAINDICATIONS: Hypersensitivity

Black Box Warning: Pregnancy (D) 2nd/3rd trimesters

Precautions: Pregnancy (C) 1st trimester, breastfeeding, children, geriatric patients; hypersensitivity to ACE inhibitors; hepatic disease, angioedema, renal artery stenosis, those of African-American descent

DOSAGE AND ROUTES

Hypertension

• **Adult: PO** 50 mg/day alone or 25 mg/day in combination with diuretic; maintenance 25-100 mg/day

• **Child ≥6 yr: PO** 0.7 mg/kg/day, max 50 mg/day

Hypertension with left ventricular hypertrophy (benefit does not apply to those of African-American descent)

• **Adult: PO** 50 mg/day; add hydrochlorothiazide 12.5 mg/day and/or increase losartan to 100 mg/day then increase hydrochlorothiazide to 25 mg/day

Nephropathy in type 2 diabetic patients/proteinuria

• **Adult: PO** 50 mg/day, may increase to 100 mg/day

Hepatic dose

• **Adult: PO** 25 mg/day as starting dose

Available forms: Tabs 25, 50, 100 mg

Administer:

• Without regard to meals

SIDE EFFECTS

CNS: *Dizziness, insomnia,* anxiety, confusion, abnormal dreams, migraine, tremor, vertigo, headache, malaise, depression

CV: Angina pectoris, 2nd-degree AV block, **cerebrovascular accident,** hypotension, **MI,** *dysrhythmias*

EENT: Blurred vision, burning eyes, conjunctivitis

GI: *Diarrhea, dyspepsia,* anorexia, constipation, dry mouth, flatulence, gastritis, vomiting

GU: Impotence, nocturia, urinary frequency, UTI, **renal failure**

HEMA: Anemia, **thrombocytopenia**

INTEG: Alopecia, dermatitis, dry skin, flushing, photosensitivity, rash, pruritus, sweating, **angioedema**

META: Gout

MS: Cramps, myalgia, pain, stiffness

RESP: *Cough, upper respiratory infection,* congestion, dyspnea, bronchitis

PHARMACOKINETICS

Peak 1-4 hr, extensively metabolized, half-life 2 hr, metabolite 6-9 hr, excreted in urine/feces, protein binding 98.7%

INTERACTIONS

Increase: lithium toxicity—lithium

Increase: antihypertensive effect—fluconazole

Increase: hyperkalemia—potassium-sparing diuretics, potassium supplements, ACE inhibitors

Decrease: antihypertensive effect—NSAIDs, PHENobarbital, rifamycin, salicylates

NURSING CONSIDERATIONS

Assess:

• B/P with position changes, pulse before and periodically during treatment; note rate, rhythm, quality

• Baselines of renal, hepatic studies before therapy begins and periodically thereafter

• Skin turgor, dryness of mucous membranes for hydration status

⚠ **Angioedema: facial swelling, dyspnea, wheezing; may occur rapidly; tongue swelling (rare)**

• **CHF:** jugular venous distention; edema in feet/legs, weight daily

• **Blood dyscrasias:** thrombocytopenia, anemia (rare)

Black Box Warning: Pregnancy before starting treatment; pregnancy (D) 2nd/3rd trimester

Evaluate:

• Therapeutic response: decreased B/P, slowing diabetic neuropathy

Teach patient/family:

• To avoid sunlight or to wear sunscreen if in sunlight; that photosensitivity may occur

• To comply with dosage schedule, even if feeling better; not to discontinue abruptly

• To notify prescriber of mouth sores, fever, swelling of hands or feet, irregular heartbeat, chest pain

• That excessive perspiration, dehydration, vomiting, diarrhea may lead to fall in B/P; to consult prescriber if these occur

• That product may cause dizziness, fainting, lightheadedness

• To rise slowly to sitting or standing position to minimize orthostatic hypotension

Black Box Warning: To use contraception while taking this product; pregnancy (D) 2nd/3rd trimesters

• To avoid salt substitutes, alcohol, grapefruit juice, OTC products unless approved by prescriber

loteprednol ophthalmic

See Appendix B

lovastatin (Rx)

(loh-vah-stat′in)

Altoprev, Mevacor

Func. class.: Antilipemic

Chem. class.: HMG-CoA reductase inhibitor

Do not confuse:
lovastatin/Lotensin/Leustatin
Mevacor/mivacron

ACTION: Inhibits HMG-CoA reductase enzyme, which reduces cholesterol synthesis

USES: As an adjunct for primary hypercholesterolemia (types IIa, IIb), atherosclerosis; heterozygous familial hypercholesterolemia (adolescents)

CONTRAINDICATIONS: Pregnancy (X), breastfeeding, hypersensitivity, active hepatic disease

Precautions: Children, past hepatic disease, alcoholism, severe acute infections, trauma, hypotension, uncontrolled seizure disorders, severe metabolic disorders, electrolyte imbalances, visual disorder

DOSAGE AND ROUTES

• **Adult: PO** 20 mg/day with evening meal; may increase to 20-80 mg/day in single or divided doses, max 40 mg/day; **EXT REL** 20-60 mg/day at bedtime, max 40 mg/day

Heterozygous familial hypercholesterolemia

• **Adolescent 10-17 yr: PO** 10-40 mg with evening meal

Renal dose

• **Adult: PO** CCr <30 mg/min, max 20 mg/day unless titrated

Available forms: Tabs 10, 20, 40 mg; ext rel tab (Altocor) 10, 20, 40, 60 mg

Administer:

• In evening with meal; if dose is increased, take with breakfast and evening meal

• Altroprev not equivalent to Mevacor

SIDE EFFECTS

CNS: *Dizziness, headache, tremor,* insomnia, paresthesia

EENT: *Blurred vision,* lens opacities

GI: *Flatus, nausea, constipation, diarrhea, dyspepsia, abdominal pain, heartburn,* hepatic dysfunction, vomiting, acid regurgitation, dry mouth, dysgeusia

HEMA: Thrombocytopenia, hemolytic anemia, leukopenia

INTEG: *Rash, pruritus,* photosensitivity

MS: *Muscle cramps, myalgia,* myositis, rhabdomyolysis; leg, shoulder, or localized pain

PHARMACOKINETICS

PO: Peak 2 hr; peak response 4-6 wk, ext rel peak 14 hr; metabolized in liver (metabolites); highly protein bound; excreted in urine 10%, feces 83%; crosses blood-brain barrier, placenta; excreted in breast milk; half-life 1 hr

INTERACTIONS

Increase: myalgia, myositis, rhabdomyolysis—azole antifungals, clarithromycin, clofibrate, cycloSPORINE, dalfopristin, danazol, diltiazem, erythromycin, gemfibrozil, niacin, protease inhibitors, quinupristin, telithromycin, verapamil

Increase: bleeding—warfarin

Increase: lovastatin effects—diltiazem
Decrease: effects of lovastatin—bile acid sequestrants, exonatide, bosentan

Drug/Herb

Decrease: effect—pectin, St. John's wort
Increase: adverse reactions—red yeast rice

Drug/Food

• Possible toxicity: grapefruit juice
Increase: levels of lovastatin with food; must be taken with food
Decrease: absorption—oat bran

Drug/Lab Test

Increase: CK, LFTs

NURSING CONSIDERATIONS

Assess:

• Diet; obtain diet history including fat, cholesterol in diet
• Fasting cholesterol, LDL, HDL, triglycerides periodically during treatment
• Hepatic studies at initiation, 6 wk, 12 wk after initiation or change in dose, periodically thereafter; AST, ALT, LFTs may increase
• Renal function in patients with compromised renal system: BUN, creatinine, I&O ratio

Perform/provide:

• Storage in cool environment in airtight, light-resistant container

Evaluate:

• Therapeutic response: decreased triglycerides, sLDL, total cholesterol; increased HDL; slowing CAD

Teach patient/family:

• To report suspected pregnancy (pregnancy [X]); not to breastfeed
• That blood work, ophthalmic exam will be necessary during treatment
• To report blurred vision, severe GI symptoms, dizziness, headache, muscle pain, weakness
• To use sunscreen or to stay out of the sun to prevent photosensitivity
• That previously prescribed regimen will continue: low-cholesterol diet, exercise program, smoking cessation
• That product should be taken with food

loxapine (Rx)

(lox′a-peen)

Loxapac ✦, Loxitane

Func. class.: Antipsychotic, neuroleptic

Chem. class.: Dibenzoxazepine

Do not confuse:
Loxitane/Soriatane

ACTION:
Depresses cerebral cortex, hypothalamus, limbic system, which control activity and aggression; blocks neurotransmission produced by DOPamine at synapse; exhibits strong α-adrenergic, anticholinergic blocking action; mechanism for antipsychotic effects is unclear

USES:
Psychotic disorders, nonpsychotic symptoms associated with dementia

Unlabeled uses: Depression, anxiety

CONTRAINDICATIONS:
Hypersensitivity, blood dyscrasias, coma, brain damage, bone marrow depression, alcohol and barbiturate withdrawal states, severe CNS depression, closed-angle glaucoma

Precautions: Pregnancy (C), breastfeeding, children <16 yr, geriatric patients, seizure disorders, cardiac/renal/hepatic disease, prostatic hypertrophy, cardiac conditions

Black Box Warning: Dementia

DOSAGE AND ROUTES

• **Adult: PO** 10 mg bid-qid initially, may be rapidly increased depending on severity of condition, maintenance 60-100 mg/day
• **Geriatric: PO** 5-10 mg daily-bid, increase q4-7days by 5-10 mg, max 250 mg/day

Available forms: Caps 5, 10, 25, 50 mg; tabs 5, 10, 25, 50 mg; conc 25 mg/ml

Administer:
- Reduced dose to geriatric patients
- Anticholinergic agent if EPS symptoms occur

PO route
- Concentrate mixed in orange or grapefruit juice

SIDE EFFECTS

CNS: *EPS: pseudoparkinsonism, akathisia, dystonia, tardive dyskinesia, drowsiness, headache,* **seizures**, confusion, **neuroleptic malignant syndrome**
CV: *Orthostatic hypotension,* **cardiac arrest**, ECG changes, tachycardia
EENT: Blurred vision, glaucoma
GI: *Dry mouth, nausea, vomiting, anorexia, constipation,* diarrhea, jaundice, weight gain
GU: Urinary retention, urinary frequency, enuresis, impotence, amenorrhea, gynecomastia
HEMA: **Anemia, leukopenia, leukocytosis, agranulocytosis**
INTEG: *Rash,* photosensitivity, dermatitis
RESP: **Laryngospasm, dyspnea, respiratory depression**

PHARMACOKINETICS

Metabolized by liver, excreted in urine, crosses placenta, enters breast milk, initial half-life 5 hr, terminal half-life 19 hr
PO: Onset 20-30 min, peak 2-4 hr, duration 12 hr

INTERACTIONS

Increase: toxicity—EPINEPHrine
Increase: EPS—other antipsychotics
Increase: CNS depression—MAOIs, antidepressants, alcohol
Decrease: effects—guanadrel, guanethidine, levodopa

Drug/Herb
Increase: CNS depression—chamomile, cola tree, hops, kava, nettle, nutmeg, skullcap, valerian
Increase: EPS—betel palm, kava

NURSING CONSIDERATIONS

Assess:
- Mental status before initial administration
- Swallowing of PO product; check for hoarding, giving of product to other patients
- I&O ratio; palpate bladder if low urinary output occurs, urinary retention may be present
- Bilirubin, CBC, LFTs q mo
- Urinalysis recommended before and during prolonged therapy
- Affect, orientation, LOC, reflexes, gait, coordination, sleep-pattern disturbances
- B/P standing and lying; pulse, respirations q4hr during initial treatment; establish baseline before starting treatment; report drops of 30 mm Hg
- Dizziness, faintness, palpitations, tachycardia on rising
- **EPS** including akathisia (inability to sit still, no pattern to movements), tardive dyskinesia (bizarre movements of jaw, mouth, tongue, extremities), pseudoparkinsonism (rigidity, tremors, pill rolling, shuffling gait)

⚠ **Neuroleptic malignant syndrome:** **muscle rigidity, increased CPK, altered mental status, hyperthermia**
- Constipation, urinary retention daily; if these occur, increase bulk, water in diet

Perform/provide:
- Decreased sensory input by dimming lights, avoiding loud noises
- Supervised ambulation until stabilized on medication; do not involve patient in strenuous exercise program because fainting is possible; patient should not stand still for long periods
- Increased fluids to prevent constipation
- Sips of water, candy, gum for dry mouth
- Storage in airtight, light-resistant container

Evaluate:
- Therapeutic response: decrease in emotional excitement, hallucinations, delusions, paranoia; reorganization of patterns of thought, speech

Teach patient/family:
- That orthostatic hypotension may occur; to rise from sitting or lying position gradually
- To avoid hot tubs, hot showers, tub baths because hypotension may occur; that, in hot weather, heat stroke may occur; to take extra precautions to stay cool
- To avoid abrupt withdrawal of product because EPS may result; that product should be withdrawn slowly
- To avoid OTC preparations (cough, hay fever, cold) unless approved by prescriber; that serious product interactions may occur; to avoid use with alcohol, CNS depressants; that increased drowsiness may occur
- To avoid hazardous activities until stabilized on medication
- To use sunscreen during sun exposure to prevent burns
- About necessity for meticulous oral hygiene because oral candidiasis may occur
- To report impaired vision, jaundice, tremors, muscle twitching

TREATMENT OF OVERDOSE:
Lavage; provide an airway

lubiprostone (Rx)
(loo-bee-pros′tone)

Amitiza

Func. class.: Gastrointestinal agent —miscellaneous

ACTION: Locally acting chloride channel activator; enhances a chloride-rich intestinal fluid secretion without altering other electrolytes; increases motility in the intestine, thereby increasing softening and passage of stool

USES: Chronic idiopathic constipation, constipation-predominant irritable bowel syndrome in women >18 yr

CONTRAINDICATIONS: Hypersensitivity, GI obstruction

Precautions: Pregnancy (C), breastfeeding, children, diarrhea, inflammatory bowel disease, abdominal pain, cholelithiasis, fecal impaction, GI/hepatic disease

DOSAGE AND ROUTES
Chronic idiopathic constipation
- **Adult: PO** 24 mcg bid with food, water

IBS with constipation (females)
- **Adult and adolescent ≥18 yr: PO** 8 mcg bid with food, water

Hepatic dose
- **Adult: PO For chronic constipation:** 16 mcg bid (Child-Pugh B); 8 mcg bid (Child-Pugh C); **for irritable bowel:** 8 mcg daily (Child-Pugh C), may be increased if tolerated

Available forms: Caps 8, 24 mcg

Administer:
- With food bid

SIDE EFFECTS
CNS: *Headache,* dizziness, depression, fatigue, insomnia

CV: Hypertension, chest pain

GI: *Nausea, abdominal pain, eructation,* abdominal distention, constipation, diarrhea, dry mouth, dyspepsia, flatulence, gastroenteritis viral, gastroesophageal reflux disease, vomiting, fecal incontinence, fecal urgency

GU: UTI

MISC: Chest pain, peripheral edema, influenza, pyrexia, viral infection

MS: Back pain, arthralgia, muscle cramps, pain in extremities

RESP: Bronchitis, cough, dyspnea, nasopharyngitis, sinusitis, upper respiratory tract infection

PHARMACOKINETICS
Peak 1.14 hr; 94% protein binding; half-life 0.9-1.4 hr; metabolism rapid, extensively in stomach, jejunum

INTERACTIONS
Decrease: effect by antidiarrheals and anticholinergics

• Do not use with sodium phosphate monobasic monohydrate, sodium phosphate dibasic anhydrous or with other laxative, purgatives when evacuating bowel prior to radiologic exam or surgery
• Possible GI obstruction: NIFEdipine ext rel tab

NURSING CONSIDERATIONS

Assess:
• **GI symptoms:** nausea, abdominal pain, diarrhea
• Need for continued treatment periodically

Perform/provide:
• Storage at room temp

Evaluate:
• Therapeutic response: decreased constipation

Teach patient/family:
• To notify prescriber of GI symptoms, diarrhea, hypersensitivity reactions

lurasidone (Rx)

(loo-ras'i-done)

Latuda

Func. class.: Atypical antipsychotic
Chem. class.: Benzoisothiazol derivative

ACTION: May modulate central dopaminergic and serotonergic activity; high affinity for dopamine-D2 receptors, serotonin 5-HT2A receptors; partial agonist at serotonin 5-HT1A receptor

USES: Schizophrenia

CONTRAINDICATIONS: Hypersensitivity

Precautions: Pregnancy (B), breastfeeding, children, geriatric patients, abrupt discontinuation, ambient temperature increase, breast cancer, cardiac disease, dehydration, diabetes, ketoacidosis, driving, operating machinery, dysphagia, heart failure, hematologic/hepatic/renal disease, hypotension, hypovolemia, MI, infertility, obesity, Parkinson's disease, seizures, strenuous exercise, stroke, substance abuse, suicidal ideation, syncope, tardive dyskinesia

Black Box Warning: Dementia: antipsychotics (e.g., as lurasidone) not approved for treatment of dementia-related psychosis in geriatric patients; may increase risk of death in this population

DOSAGE AND ROUTES

• **Adult: PO** 40 mg/day, range 40-80 mg/day; for those receiving CYP3A4 inhibitors (max 40 mg/day), do not use with strong CYP3A4 inducers/inhibitors

Hepatic/renal dose
• **Adult: PO** Child-Pugh class B/C; CCr ≥10 ml/min, ≤50 ml/min, max 40 mg/day

Available forms: Tabs 40, 80 mg

Administer:
• Give with meal of ≥350 calories

SIDE EFFECTS

CNS: Agitation, akathisia, anxiety, dizziness, drowsiness, fatigue, hyperthermia, insomnia, dystonic reactions; neuroleptic malignant syndrome (rare), pseudoparkinsonism, restlessness, seizures, suicidal ideation, syncope, tardive dyskinesia, vertigo
CV: Angina, AV block, bradycardia, hypertension, orthostatic hypotension, sinus tachycardia, stroke
EENT: Blurred vision
ENDO: Diabetes mellitus, ketoacidosis, hyperglycemia, hyperprolactinemia
GI: Abdominal pain, diarrhea, dyspepsia, nausea, vomiting, gastritis, weight gain/loss
GU: Amenorrhea, breast enlargement, dysmenorrhea, impotence, dysuria, renal failure
HEMA: Agranulocytosis, anemia, leucopenia, neutropenia
INTEG: Pruritus, rash
MS: Back pain, dysarthria; rhabdomyolysis (rare)
SYST: Angioedema

PHARMACOKINETICS

99% protein binding; excreted 80% in feces, 9% in urine; elimination half-life 18 hr; 9-19% absorbed; peak 1-3 hr, steady state 7 days

INTERACTIONS

Increase: lurasidone effect—strong CYP3A4 inhibitors; do not use concurrently

Increase: serotonin syndrome, neuroleptic malignant syndrome—SSRIs, SNRIs

NURSING CONSIDERATIONS

Assess:

- **Schizophrenia:** hallucinations, delusions, agitation, social withdrawal; monitor orientation, behavior, mood prior to and periodically during therapy
- **Neuroleptic malignant syndrome (rare):** fever, dyspnea, tachycardia, seizures, sweating, hypo/hypertension, muscle stiffness, pallor; report immediately
- **Blood dyscrasias:** CBC periodically; blood dyscrasias may occur
- **Serious cardiac symptoms:** AV block, stroke, bradycardia may occur
- **EPS:** restlessness, difficulty speaking, loss of balance, pill rolling, mask-like face, shuffling gait, rigidity, tremors, muscle spasms; monitor prior to and periodically during therapy; report tardive dyskinesia immediately

Perform/provide:

- Storage at room temp, protection from moisture

Evaluate:

- Therapeutic response: decreasing hallucinations, delusions, agitation, social withdrawal

Teach patient/family:

- About reason for treatment, expected results
- To report EPS symptoms, blood dyscrasias: sore throat, fever, unusual bleeding/bruising

lymphocyte immune globulin (antithymocyte, equine) (Rx)

Atgam

Func. class.: Immune globulins—immunosuppressant

ACTION: Produces immunosuppression by inhibiting the function of lymphocytes (T)

USES: Organ transplants to prevent rejection, aplastic anemia

Unlabeled uses: MS; myasthenia gravis; immunosuppressant in liver, bone marrow, heart, and other organ transplants; pure red-cell aplasia; scleroderma

CONTRAINDICATIONS: Hypersensitivity to this product or equine/leporine protein; acute viral illness

Precautions: Pregnancy (C), breastfeeding, children, severe renal/hepatic disease, leukopenia, thrombocytopenia

Black Box Warning: Infection, neoplastic disease

DOSAGE AND ROUTES

Renal allograft rejection

- **Adult/child:** IV 10-30 mg/kg/day × 14 days

Prevent renal allograft rejection

- **Adult:** IV 15 mg/kg/day × 7-14 days then every other day × 14 days for total of 21 doses in 28 days

Aplastic anemia

- **Adult:** IV 10-20 mg/kg/day × 8-14 days then every other day for ≤21 total doses

Available forms: Inj 50 mg equine gamma globulin/ml

Administer:

- Do not infuse <4 hr; usually given over 4-8 hr

L

Aplastic anemia

• Skin testing must be completed prior to treatment; use intradermal inj of 0.1 ml of a 1:1000 dilution (5 mcg horse IgG) in 0.9% NaCl; if wheal or rash >10 mm or both, use caution during inf

• Dilute in saline sol before inf; invert IV bag so undiluted product does not contact air inside; conc should not be >1 mg/ml; do not shake

• Keep emergency equipment nearby for severe allergic reaction

SIDE EFFECTS

Renal transplant

CNS: Fever, chills, headache, dizziness, weakness, faintness, seizures
CV: Chest pain, hypo/hypertension, tachycardia
GI: Diarrhea, nausea, vomiting, epigastric pain, GI bleeding
INTEG: Rash, pruritus, urticaria, wheal
SYST: Anaphylaxis

Aplastic anemia

CNS: Fever, chills, headache, seizures, lightheadedness, encephalitis, postviral encephalopathy
CV: Bradycardia, myocarditis, irregularity
GI: Nausea, LFTs abnormality
HEMA: Thrombocytopenia

PHARMACOKINETICS

Onset rapid, half-life 5-7 days

NURSING CONSIDERATIONS

Assess:

• **Infection:** if infection occurs, evaluation will be needed to continue therapy

• Renal studies: BUN, creatinine at least monthly during treatment, for 3 mo after treatment

• Hepatic studies: alk phos, AST, ALT, bilirubin

• CBC with differential

Evaluate:

• Therapeutic response: absence of rejection; hematologic recovery (aplastic anemia)

Teach patient/family:

• To report fever, chills, sore throat, fatigue, since serious infections may occur

• To use contraceptive measures during treatment, for 12 wk after therapy

mafenide topical

See Appendix B

MAGNESIUM SALTS

magnesium chloride (Rx)

Mag-64

magnesium citrate (OTC)

Walgreens Magnesium Citrate

magnesium gluconate (OTC)

Mag-G, Magtrate

magnesium oxide (OTC)

Mag-Ox 400, Uro-Mag

magnesium hydroxide (OTC)

Ex-Lax Milk of Magnesia, Freelax, Good Sense Milk of Magnesia, Leader Milk of Magnesia, MOM, Phillips' Milk of Magnesia, TopCare Milk of Magnesia, Walgreens Milk of Magnesia

magnesium sulfate (OTC, Rx)

epsom salts; magnesium sulfate (IV)—HIGH ALERT

Func. class.: Electrolyte; anticonvulsant; saline laxative, antacid

ACTION: Increases osmotic pressure, draws fluid into colon, neutralizes HCl

USES: Constipation; bowel preparation before surgery or exam; anticonvulsant for preeclampsia, eclampsia (magnesium sulfate); electrolyte

Unlabeled uses: *Magnesium sulfate:* persistent pulmonary hypertension of the newborn (PPHN), cardiac arrest, CPR, digitoxin/digoxin toxicity, premature labor, seizure prophylaxis, status asthmaticus, torsades de pointes, ventricular fibrillation/tachycardia

CONTRAINDICATIONS: Hypersensitivity, abdominal pain, nausea/vomiting, obstruction, acute surgical abdomen, rectal bleeding, heart block, myocardial damage

Precautions: Pregnancy (A); (B) (magnesium sulfate), renal/cardiac disease

DOSAGE AND ROUTES

Laxative

- **Adult: PO** (Milk of Magnesia) 15-60 ml at bedtime
- **Adult and child >12 yr: PO** (magnesium sulfate) 15 g in 8 oz water; **PO** (Concentrated Milk of Magnesia) 5-30 ml; **PO** (magnesium citrate) 5-10 oz at bedtime
- **Child 2-6 yr: PO** (Milk of Magnesia) 5-15 ml/day

Prevention of magnesium deficiency

- **Adult and child ≥10 yr: PO** (male) 350-400 mg/day; (female) 280-300 mg/day; (breastfeeding) 335-350 mg/day; (pregnancy) 320 mg/day
- **Child 8-10 yr: PO** 170 mg/day
- **Child 4-7 yr: PO** 120 mg/day

Magnesium sulfate deficiency

- **Adult: PO** 200-400 mg in divided doses tid-qid; **IM** 1 g q6hr × 4 doses; **IV** 5 g (severe)
- **Child 6-12 yr: PO** 3-6 mg/kg/day in divided doses tid-qid

Pre-eclampsia/eclampsia (magnesium sulfate)

- **Adult: IM/IV** 4-5 g IV inf; with 5 g **IM** in each gluteus, then 5 g q4hr or 4 g **IV INF**, then 1-2 g/hr **CONT INF**, max 40 g/day or 20 g/48 hr in severe renal disease

Persistent pulmonary hypertension of the newborn (PPHN) in mechanically ventilated neonates (unlabeled)

- **Premature infants >33 wk and term neonates: IV** (magnesium sulfate) 200 mg/kg over 20-30 min then **CONT IV INF** 20-150 mg/kg/hr to maintain blood magnesium levels at 3.5-5.5 mmol/L

Status asthmaticus (unlabeled)

- **Adult: IV** (magnesium sulfate) 2 g
- **Child: IV INF** (PALS) (magnesium sulfate) 25-50 mg/kg diluted in D_5W, given over 10-20 min, max 2 g/dose

Premature labor (unlabeled)

- **Adult: IV INF** (magnesium sulfate) 4-6 g given as a loading dose over 20-30 min then 2-4 g/hr **CONT INF;** use infusion pump until contractions cease; continue inf at lowest dose over 12-24 hr; **PO** (magnesium chloride/gluconate/oxide) 648-1200 mg/day elemental magnesium in divided doses

Torsades de pointes/cardiac dysrhythmias with hypomagnesemia (unlabeled)

- **Adult: IV** (magnesium sulfate) use ACLS guidelines or 1-2 g in 50-100 ml D_5W given over 5-20 min in emergent cases or over 5-60 min

Available forms: *Chloride:* sus rel tabs 535 mg (64 mg Mg); enteric tabs 833 mg (100 mg Mg); *citrate:* oral sol 240-, 296-, 300-ml bottles (77 mEq/100 ml); *oxide:* tabs 400 mg; caps 140 mg; *hydroxide:* liq 400 mg/5 ml; conc liq 800 mg/5 ml; chew tabs 300, 600 mg; *sulfate:* powder for oral, bulk packages; epsom salts, bulk packages; inj 10%, 12.5%, 25%, 50%

Administer:

PO route

- With 8 oz water
- Refrigerate magnesium citrate before giving
- Shake susp before using as antacid at least 2 hr after meals
- Tablets should be chewed thoroughly before patient swallows; give 4 oz of water afterwards
- **Laxative:** give on empty stomach

M

IM route (magnesium sulfate)
- Give deeply in gluteal site

IV route (magnesium sulfate)
- Only when calcium gluconate available for magnesium toxicity

Direct IV route
- Dilute 50% sol to ≤20%, give at ≤150 mg/min

Continuous IV INF route
- May dilute to 20% sol, infuse over 3 hr
- IV at less than 125 mg/kg/hr; circulatory collapse may occur; use inf pump

Y-site compatibilities: Acyclovir, aldesleukin, amifostine, amikacin, ampicillin, aztreonam, ceFAZolin, cefoperazone, cefotaxime, cefoxitin, cephalothin, cephapirin, chloramphenicol, cisatracurium, DOBUTamine, doxycycline, DOXOrubicin liposome, enalaprilat, erythromycin, esmolol, famotidine, fludarabine, gallium, gentamicin, granisetron, heparin, HYDROmorphone, IDArubicin, insulin, kanamycin, labetalol, meperidine, metroNIDAZOLE, minocycline, morphine, moxalactam, nafcillin, ondansetron, oxacillin, paclitaxel, penicillin G potassium, piperacillin, piperacillin/tazobactam, potassium chloride, propofol, remifentanil, sargramostim, thiotepa, ticarcillin, tobramycin, trimethoprim-sulfamethoxazole, vancomycin, vit B complex/C

SIDE EFFECTS

CNS: Muscle weakness, flushing, sweating, confusion, sedation, depressed reflexes, flaccid paralysis, hypothermia
CV: Hypotension, heart block, circulatory collapse, vasodilation
GI: *Nausea, vomiting, anorexia, cramps,* diarrhea
HEMA: Prolonged bleeding time
META: Electrolyte, fluid imbalances
RESP: Respiratory depression/paralysis

PHARMACOKINETICS

PO: Onset 1-2 hr
IM: Onset 1 hr, duration 4 hr
IV: Duration $^1/_2$ hr
Excreted by kidney, effective anticonvulsant serum levels 2.5-7.5 mEq/L

INTERACTIONS

Increase: effect of neuromuscular blockers
Increase: hypotension—antihypertensives
Decrease: absorption of tetracyclines, fluoroquinolones, nitrofurantoin
Decrease: effect of digoxin

NURSING CONSIDERATIONS

Assess:
- **Laxative:** cause of constipation; lack of fluids, bulk, exercise; cramping, rectal bleeding, nausea, vomiting; product should be discontinued

⚠ **Eclampsia:** seizure precautions, B/P, ECG (magnesium sulfate); **magnesium toxicity:** thirst, confusion, decrease in reflexes; I&O ratio; check for decrease in urinary output

Evaluate:
- Therapeutic response: decreased constipation; absence of seizures (eclampsia), normal serum calcium levels

Teach patient/family:
- Not to use laxatives for long-term therapy because bowel tone will be lost
- That chilling improves taste of magnesium citrate
- To shake suspension well
- Not to give at bedtime as a laxative; may interfere with sleep
- To give citrus fruit after administering to counteract unpleasant taste
- About reason for product, expected results

mannitol (Rx)

(man′i-tole)

Osmitrol, Resectisol

Func. class.: Diuretic, osmotic
Chem. class.: Hexahydric alcohol

ACTION: Acts by increasing osmolarity of glomerular filtrate, which inhibits reabsorption of water and electrolytes and increases urinary output

USES: Edema; promotion of systemic diuresis in cerebral edema; decrease in intraocular/intracranial pressure; improved renal function in acute renal failure, chemical poisoning

CONTRAINDICATIONS: Active intracranial bleeding, hypersensitivity, anuria, severe pulmonary congestion, edema, severe dehydration, progressive heart, renal failure

Precautions: Pregnancy (C), breastfeeding, geriatric patients, dehydration, severe renal disease, CHF, electrolyte imbalances

DOSAGE AND ROUTES

Oliguria, prevention

• **Adult: IV** after initial test dose; if urine output is 30-50 ml/hr × 2 hr, give 20-100 g over a 24-hr period of 15% or 20% sol

Oliguria, treatment

• **Adult: IV** after initial test dose; give balance of 50 g of a 20% sol over 1 hr then 5% via **CONT IV INF** to maintain output at 50 ml/hr

• **Child (unlabeled): IV** 0.5-2 g/kg as 15%-20% sol, run over 30-60 min; maintenance 0.25-0.5 g/kg q4-6hr

Intraocular pressure

• **Adult: IV** 1.5-2 g/kg of 15%-25% sol over 30-60 min

ICP

• **Adult: IV** 1-2 g/kg then 0.25-1 g/kg q4hr

Diuresis with drug intoxication

• **Adult and child >12 yr:** 5%-10% sol continuously up to 200 g **IV** while maintaining 100-500 ml urine output/hr

Available forms: Inj 5%, 10%, 15%, 20%, 25%; GU irrigation: 5%

Administer:

IV route

• In 15%-25% sol with filter; rapid inf may worsen CHF; warm in hot water, shake to dissolve if crystals are present

• **Test dose** with severe oliguria, 0.2 g/kg over 3-5 min; if continued oliguria, give 2nd test dose; if no response, reassess patient

Y-site compatibilities: Acyclovir, aldesleukin, alemtuzumab, amifostine, amikacin, ampicillin, atropine, aztreonam, bivalirudin, bumetanide, calcium gluconate, caspofungin, ceFAZolin, cefotaxime, cefoxitin, ceftazidime, ceftizoxime, chloramphenicol, cimetidine, cisatracurium, clindamycin, DAPTOmycin, dexmedetomidine, digoxin, diltiazem, diphenhydrAMINE, DOBUTamine, docetaxel, DOPamine, DOXOrubicin liposome, doxycycline, enalaprilat, EPINEPHrine, ertapenem, esmolol, famotidine, fenoldopam, fentaNYL, fluconazole, fludarabine, gentamicin, granisetron, heparin, HYDROmorphone, hydrOXYzine, IDArubicin, imipenem/cilastatin, insulin, isoproterenol, ketorolac, labetalol, levofloxacin, lidocaine, linezolid, LORazepam, meperidine, metoclopramide, metoprolol, metroNIDAZOLE, micafungin, midazolam, milrinone, morphine, nafcillin, niCARdipine, nitroglycerin, nitroprusside, norepinephrine, ondansetron, oxaliplatin, paclitaxel, palonosetron, pantoprazole, penicillin G potassium, phenylephrine, piperacillin/tazobactam, potassium chloride, procainamide, prochlorperazine, promethazine, propofol, propranolol, protamine, quinupristin/dalfopristin, ranitidine, remifentanil, sargramostim, sodium bicarbonate, tacrolimus, thiotepa, ticarcillin/clavulanate, tirofiban, tobramycin, trimethoprim/sulfamethoxazole, vancomycin, vasopressin, verapamil, vit B complex with C, voriconazole

SIDE EFFECTS

CNS: Dizziness, headache, seizures, rebound increased ICP, confusion

CV: Edema, thrombophlebitis, hypo/hypertension, tachycardia, angina-like chest pains, fever, chills, CHF, circulatory overload

EENT: Loss of hearing, blurred vision, nasal congestion, decreased intraocular pressure

ELECT: Fluid, electrolyte imbalances, *acidosis,* electrolyte loss, dehydration, hypo/hyperkalemia

M

GI: *Nausea, vomiting,* dry mouth, diarrhea
GU: Marked diuresis, urinary retention, thirst
RESP: Pulmonary congestion

PHARMACOKINETICS

IV: Onset 1-3 hr for diuresis, ½-1 hr for intraocular pressure, 15 min for cerebrospinal fluid; duration 4-6 hr for intraocular pressure, 3-8 hr for cerebrospinal fluid; excreted in urine; half-life 100 min

INTERACTIONS

Increase: elimination of mannitol—lithium
Increase: excretion of salicylates, barbiturates, imipramine, bromides
Increase: hypokalemia—arsenic trioxide, cardiac glycosides, levomethadyl
Drug/Lab Test
Interference: inorganic phosphorus, ethylene glycol

NURSING CONSIDERATIONS

Assess:

- Weight, I&O daily to determine fluid loss; effect of product may be decreased if used daily; output every hr prn
- Rate, depth, rhythm of respiration, effect of exertion
- B/P lying, standing; postural hypotension may occur
- Electrolytes: potassium, sodium, chloride; include BUN, CBC, serum creatinine, blood pH, ABGs, CVP, PAP
- **Metabolic acidosis:** drowsiness, restlessness
- **Hypokalemia:** postural hypotension, malaise, fatigue, tachycardia, leg cramps, weakness, or hyperkalemia
- Rashes, temp daily
- Confusion, especially in geriatric patients; take safety precautions if needed
- Hydration including skin turgor, thirst, dry mucous membranes
- Blurred vision, pain in eyes before, during treatment **(increased intraocular pressure);** neurologic checks, intracranial pressure during treatment **(increased intracranial pressure)**

Evaluate:

- Therapeutic response: improvement in edema of feet, legs, sacral area daily if medication being used with CHF; decreased intraocular pressure, prevention of hypokalemia, increased excretion of toxic substances; decreased ICP

Teach patient/family:

- To rise slowly from lying or sitting position
- About the reason for, method of treatment
- To report signs of electrolyte imbalance, confusion

TREATMENT OF OVERDOSE:

Discontinue inf; correct fluid, electrolyte imbalances; hemodialysis; monitor hydration, CV status, renal function

maraviroc (Rx)

(mah-rav′er-rock)

Selzentry

Func. class.: Antiretroviral
Chem. class.: Fusion inhibitor, CCR5-receptor antagonist

ACTION:
Interferes with entry into HIV-1 by inhibiting the fusion of the virus and the cell membrane

USES:
CCR5-tropic HIV in combination with other antiretroviral agents for treating experienced patients

CONTRAINDICATIONS:
Hypersensitivity

Precautions: Pregnancy (B), Asian patients, breastfeeding, renal/hepatic/cardiac disease, electrolyte imbalance, dehydration, immune reconstitution syndrome, infection, MI, orthostatic hypotension, children, geriatric patients

Black Box Warning: Hepatitis

DOSAGE AND ROUTES

Those not taking any CYP3A inducers/inhibitors

- **Adult: PO** 300 mg bid

Those taking CYP3A4 inhibitors with/without a CYP3A inducer

- **Adult: PO** 150 mg bid

Those taking CYP3A4 inducers without a strong CYP3A inhibitor

- **Adult: PO** 600 mg bid

Available forms: Tabs 150, 300 mg

Administer:

- May give without regard to meals, with 8 oz water; swallow whole, do not crush, chew, break

SIDE EFFECTS

CV: **MI, cardiac ischemia, orthostatic hypotension**

CNS: Dizziness, depression, **viral meningitis**, disturbances in consciousness, peripheral neuropathy, paresthesia, dysesthesia, fever

EENT: Gingival hyperplasia

GI: Diarrhea, constipation, dyspepsia, **pseudomembranous colitis, hepatotoxicity**

INTEG: Rash, urticaria, pruritus, folliculitis

MS: Joint pain, leg pain, muscle cramps

RESP: Cough, upper respiratory tract infection, sinusitis, bronchitis, pneumonia, **bronchospasm, obstruction**

SYST: Herpes virus

PHARMACOKINETICS

Metabolized by P450 system; CYP3A metabolism; excreted 20% urine, 76% feces; protein binding 76%; terminal half-life 14-18 hr

INTERACTIONS

Increase: maraviroc levels—CYP3A inhibitors (amiodarone, aprepitant, chloramphenicol, clarithromycin, conivaptan, cycloSPORINE, dalfopristin, danazol, diltiazem, erythromycin, estradiol, fluconazole, fluvoxamine, imatinib, isoniazid, itraconazole, ketoconazole, miconazole, nefazodone, niCARdipine, propoxyphene, RU-486, tamoxifen, telithromycin, troleandomycin, verapamil, voriconazole, zafirlukast)

Decrease: maraviroc levels—CYP3A4 inducers (efavirenz, aminoglutethimide, barbiturates, bexaroten, bosentan, carBAMazepine, dexamethasone, griseofulvin, modafinil, nafcillin, OXcarbazepine, phenytoin, fosphenytoin, rifabutin, rifampin, rifapentine, topiramate, tipranavir)

Drug/Herb

- Decreased maraviroc effect: St. John's wort

Drug/Food

- High-fat meal decreases absorption 33%

NURSING CONSIDERATIONS

Assess:

- HIV: CD_4, T-cell count, plasma HIV RNA, CCR5-tropic HIV-1; assess for changes in symptoms, other infections during treatment
- Renal studies: serum creatinine
- Bowel pattern before, during treatment
- **Allergies:** skin eruptions: rash, urticaria, itching; discontinue product

Black Box Warning: Hepatitis: dark urine; abdominal pain, vomiting; yellowing of skin, eyes; hepatomegaly; discontinue product; monitor liver function tests

Perform/provide:

- Storage at room temp

Evaluate:

- Therapeutic response: improvement in CD4, viral load, T-cell count

Teach patient/family:

- To take as prescribed; if dose is missed, to take as soon as remembered up to 1 hr before next dose; not to double dose; that product does not cure condition, should not be shared with others
- That product does not cure infection, just controls symptoms and does not prevent infecting others

⚠ To report sore throat, fever, fatigue **(may indicate superinfection)**; yellow

M

skin/eyes, abdominal pain, vomiting **(hepatitis)**; itching, SOB **(allergic reaction)**
• That product must be taken in equal intervals around the clock to maintain blood levels for duration of therapy
• To avoid all OTC products unless approved by prescriber
• To avoid driving, other hazardous activities until reaction is known; that dizziness may occur
• To make position changes slowly to prevent postural hypotension
• To notify prescriber if pregnancy is planned or suspected

mecasermin (Rx)

(mec-a′sir-men)

Increlex

Func. class.: Biologic response modifier; insulin-like growth factor

ACTION: Stimulates growth; IGF-1 is the principal hormonal mediator of statural growth; GH binds to its receptor in the liver and other tissues

USES: Growth failure in children with severe primary insulin-like growth factor-1 (IGF-1) deficiency (primary IGFD) or with growth hormone (GH) gene deletion who have developed neutralizing antibodies to GH

Unlabeled uses: ALS

CONTRAINDICATIONS: Hypersensitivity, benzyl alcohol, closed epiphyses, active/suspected neoplasia, IV use

Precautions: Pregnancy (C), breastfeeding, children <2 yr, diabetes mellitus, hypothyroidism, lymphoid tissue hypertrophy, increased intracranial pressure, malnutrition, scoliosis, sleep apnea

DOSAGE AND ROUTES

• **Child: SUBCUT** 0.04-0.08 mg/kg (40-80 mcg/kg) bid; if well tolerated for 1 wk, may increase by 0.04 mg/kg/dose, max 0.12 mg/kg bid

Available forms: Inj 10 mg/ml

Administer:

SUBCUT route

• Give within 20 min of meal or snack
• Rotate inj site; use sterile, disposable syringe/needles; use small-volume syringe for accurate measurement

SIDE EFFECTS

CNS: Headache, seizures, dizziness, cardiac valvulopathy, increased intracranial pressure
CV: Cardiac murmur
EENT: Ear pain, otitis media, abnormal tympanometry, papilledema, visual impairment, tonsillar hypertrophy
ENDO: **Hypoglycemia**, ketosis, hypothyroidism, hypercholesterolemia, hypertriglyceridemia
INTEG: Pruritus, urticaria, **anaphylaxis, angioedema**
GI: Vomiting, nausea
HEMA: Thymus hypertrophy
MISC: Bruising, lipohypertrophy, inj site reaction
MS: Arthralgia, joint pain, slipped upper femoral epiphysis
RESP: Snoring, apnea
SYST: Antibodies to growth hormone, secondary malignancy

PHARMACOKINETICS

Bioavailability almost 100%, metabolized in liver/kidney, half-life 5.8 hr

INTERACTIONS

Increase: hypoglycemia—antidiabetics, corticosteroids
Decrease: growth suppression possible—psychostimulants

NURSING CONSIDERATIONS

Assess:

• Monitor preprandial glucose at beginning of treatment and until well tolerated
• By funduscopic exam at beginning and periodically during treatment
• Allergic reactions; if present, interrupt treatment and notify prescriber

- Growth rate of child at intervals during treatment
- Serious skin disorders: angioedema, anaphylaxis

Perform/provide:

- Storage in refrigerator before opening, avoid freezing; after opening, stable for 30 days after initial vial entry, store in refrigerator; do not use if particulate matter is present, avoid direct light, do not use after expiration date

Evaluate:

- Therapeutic response: growth in children

Teach patient/family:

- That treatment may continue for years; that regular assessments are required
- To avoid hazardous activities, driving within 2-3 hr of dosing
- About correct administration, needle disposal

meclizine (OTC, Rx)

(mek'li-zeen)

Antivert, Bonamine ♣, Bonine, Dramamine Less Drowsy Formula, Medivert, Travel Sickness, Wal-Dram II

Func. class.: Antiemetic, antihistamine, anticholinergic

Chem. class.: H_1-receptor antagonist, piperazine derivative

ACTION: Acts centrally by blocking chemoreceptor trigger zone, which in turn acts on vomiting center

USES: Vertigo, motion sickness

CONTRAINDICATIONS: Hypersensitivity to cyclizines, shock

Precautions: Pregnancy (B), breastfeeding, children, geriatric patients, closed-angle glaucoma, urinary retention, prostatic hypertrophy, CV disease, hypertension, seizure disorder

DOSAGE AND ROUTES

Vertigo

- **Adult/adolescent: PO** 25-100 mg/day in divided doses

Motion sickness

- **Adult/adolescent: PO** 25-50 mg 1 hr before traveling, repeat dose q24hr prn

Available forms: Tabs 12.5, 25, 50 mg; chew tabs 25 mg; caps 25, 30 mg

Administer:

PO route

- Tablets may be swallowed whole, chewed, allowed to dissolve; give with food to decrease GI upset
- Lowest possible dose for geriatric patients; anticholinergic effects

SIDE EFFECTS

CNS: *Drowsiness,* fatigue, restlessness, headache, insomnia

CV: Hypotension

EENT: Dry mouth, blurred vision

GI: Nausea, anorexia, constipation, increased appetite

GU: Urinary retention

M

PHARMACOKINETICS

PO: Onset 1 hr, duration 8-24 hr, half-life 6 hr

INTERACTIONS

Increase: anticholinergic effects—other antihistamines, atropine, antidepressants, phenothiazines

Increase: effect of alcohol, opioids, other CNS depressants

Drug/Lab Test

False negative: allergy skin testing (allergen extracts)

NURSING CONSIDERATIONS

Assess:

- **Vertigo/motion sickness:** nausea, vomiting after 1 hr; assess vertigo periodically

⚠ Signs of toxicity of other products, masking of symptoms of disease: brain tumor, intestinal obstruction

• Observe for drowsiness, dizziness, level of consciousness

Evaluate:

• Therapeutic response: absence of dizziness, vomiting

Teach patient/family:

• That a false-negative result may occur with skin testing for allergies; that these procedures should not be scheduled for ≤4 days after discontinuing use

• To avoid hazardous activities, activities requiring alertness because dizziness may occur; to request assistance with ambulation

• To avoid alcohol, other depressants; not to breastfeed

medroxyPROGESTERone (Rx)

(me-drox′ee-proe-jess′te-rone)

Depo-Provera, Gen-Medroxy ✱, Provera

Func. class.: Antineoplastic, hormone, contraceptive

Chem. class.: Progesterone derivative

Do not confuse:
medroxyPROGESTERone/methylPREDNISolone
Provera/Premarin/Covera

ACTION: Inhibits secretion of pituitary gonadotropins, which prevents follicular maturation and ovulation; stimulates growth of mammary tissue; antineoplastic action against endometrial cancer

USES: Uterine bleeding (abnormal); secondary amenorrhea; prevention of endometrial changes associated with estrogen replacement therapy (ERT); contraceptive; inoperable, recurrent, metastatic endometrial/ renal cancer

Unlabeled uses: Hot flashes; symptoms of menopause; paraphilia (men); hot flashes (men) with prostate cancer

CONTRAINDICATIONS: Pregnancy (X), hypersensitivity, reproductive cancer, genital bleeding (abnormal, undiagnosed), missed abortion

Black Box Warning: Breast cancer, MI, stroke, thromboembolic disease, thrombophlebitis

Precautions: Breastfeeding, hypertension, asthma, blood dyscrasias, gallbladder disease, CHF, diabetes mellitus, bone disease, depression, migraine headache, seizure disorders, renal/hepatic disease, family history of cancer of breast or reproductive tract, bone mineral density loss, ocular disorders

Black Box Warning: Cardiac disease, dementia, osteoporosis

DOSAGE AND ROUTES

Secondary amenorrhea

• **Adult: PO** 5-10 mg/day × 5-10 days

Uterine bleeding

• **Adult: PO** 5-10 mg/day × 5-10 days starting on 16th or 21st day of menstrual cycle

With ERT

• **Adult: PO** 5-10 mg daily × 10-14 or more days/mo (sequential estrogen); 2.5-5 mg daily (continuous estrogen)

Contraceptive

• **Adult: IM** (contraceptive inj) 150 mg q12wk; **SUBCUT** (depot SUBCUT Provera 104 inj) 104 mg q3mo

Endometrial/renal cancer

• **Adult: IM** 400 mg-1 g (using 400 mg/ml depot inj susp) q wk

Hot flashes/symptoms of menopause (unlabeled)

• **Adult (female): PO** 20 mg/day; **IM** 150 mg q mo

Hot flashes (men) in prostate cancer (unlabeled)

• **Adult (male): IM** Depot 150 or 400 mg

Available forms: Tabs 2.5, 5, 10 mg; inj susp 50, 150, 400 mg/ml; depot-SUBCUT inj: 104 mg/0.65 ml

Administer:

- Titrated dose; use lowest effective dose
- Oil solution deep in large muscle mass (IM); rotate sites
- With food or milk to decrease GI symptoms (PO)

SIDE EFFECTS

CNS: Dizziness, headache, migraines, depression, fatigue, nervousness
CV: Hypotension, thrombophlebitis, edema, **thromboembolism, stroke, PE, MI**
EENT: Diplopia
GI: *Nausea,* vomiting, anorexia, cramps, increased weight, **cholestatic jaundice,** abdominal pain
GU: Amenorrhea, cervical erosion, breakthrough bleeding, dysmenorrhea, vaginal candidiasis, breast changes, *gynecomastia, testicular atrophy, impotence,* endometriosis, **spontaneous abortion**
INTEG: Rash, urticaria, acne, hirsutism, alopecia, oily skin, seborrhea, purpura, melasma, photosensitivity
META: Hyperglycemia
MS: Decreased bone density
SYST: **Angioedema, anaphylaxis**

PHARMACOKINETICS

PO: Duration 24 hr; excreted in urine and feces; metabolized in liver

INTERACTIONS

Decrease: medroxyPROGESTERone action—aminoglutethimide
Drug/Lab Test
Increase: alk phos, sodium (urine), pregnanediol, amino acids
Decrease: GTT, HDL

NURSING CONSIDERATIONS

Assess:

- Pelvic exam, Pap smear before treatment, periodically
- ⚠ **Severe allergic reaction, angioedema;** have EPINEPHrine and rescusitative equipment available
- Weight daily; notify prescriber of weekly weight gain >5 lb; bone mineral density
- B/P at beginning of treatment and periodically
- I&O ratio; be alert for decreasing urinary output, increasing edema
- Hepatic studies: ALT, AST, bilirubin periodically during long-term therapy
- Edema, hypertension, cardiac symptoms, jaundice
- Mental status: affect, mood, behavioral changes, depression

Black Box Warning: This product should not be given to those with breast cancer, MI, stroke, thromboembolic disorders

Black Box Warning: Use of product shown to increase dementia in women ≥65 yr old; use may increase osteoporosis in long-term treatment; those at greater risk also smoke; adequate calcium and vit D should be taken

Perform/provide:

- Storage in dark area

Evaluate:

- Therapeutic response: decreased abnormal uterine bleeding, absence of amenorrhea

Teach patient/family:

- To avoid sunlight or to use sunscreen; photosensitivity can occur
- ⚠ **To report breast lumps, vaginal bleeding, edema, jaundice, dark urine, clay-colored stools, dyspnea, headache, blurred vision, abdominal pain, sudden change in speech/coordination, numbness or stiffness in legs, chest pain; males to report impotence, gynecomastia**
- To report suspected pregnancy (X); fertility returns 6-12 mo after discontinuing

Black Box Warning: Long-term use decreases bone density; exercise, calcium supplements can help lessen osteoporosis

medrysone ophthalmic

See Appendix B

M

megestrol (Rx)

(me-jess'trole)

Apo-Megestrol ✱, Megace, Megace ES

Func. class.: Antineoplastic hormone

Chem. class.: Progestin

Do not confuse:
Megace/Reglan

ACTION: Affects endometrium with antiluteinizing effect; thought to bring about cell death

USES: Breast, endometrial cancer; renal cell cancer; cachexia, anorexia, weight loss with AIDS

Unlabeled uses: Hot flashes in women (menopause) or men (prostate cancer), unexplained weight loss in geriatric patients, endometriosis, renal cell cancer (palliative), endometrial cancer, breast cancer (metastatic)

CONTRAINDICATIONS: Pregnancy (D) tabs, (X) susp; hypersensitivity

Precautions: Diabetes, thrombosis, adrenal insufficiency

DOSAGE AND ROUTES

Endometrial/ovarian carcinoma

• **Adult: PO** 40-320 mg/day in divided doses

Breast carcinoma

• **Adult: PO** 40 mg qid or 160 mg/day

Anorexia (AIDS)

• **Adult: PO** 800 mg/day (oral susp) or 625 mg/day (ES)

Hot flashes (unlabeled)

• **Adult: PO** 20 mg bid

Metastatic breast/prostate/renal cell cancer (unlabeled)

• **Adult: PO** 40 mg qid × ≥2 mo

Metastatic endometrial cancer (unlabeled)

• **Adult: PO** 40-320 mg/day in divided doses × ≥2 mo

Prostate cancer (unlabeled)

• **Adult: PO** 120 mg as single daily dose in combination with diethylstilbesterol 0.1 mg

Available forms: Tabs 20, 40 mg; oral susp 40, 125 mg/ml

Administer:

• Oral susp for AIDS patients; shake well
• Tablets for carcinoma

SIDE EFFECTS

CNS: Mood swings, insomnia
CV: Thrombophlebitis, thromboembolism, hypertension
ENDO: Adrenal insufficiency
GI: Nausea, vomiting, diarrhea, abdominal cramps, weight gain, flatus, indigestion
GU: Gynecomastia, fluid retention, hypercalcemia, vaginal bleeding, discharge, impotence, decreased libido
INTEG: Alopecia, rash, pruritus, purpura, itching, sweating
META: Hyperglycemia

PHARMACOKINETICS

PO: Duration 1-3 days; half-life 60 min; metabolized in liver; excreted in feces, breast milk; food increases bioavailability of oral sol

INTERACTIONS

• Do not use with dofetilide

Decrease: megestrol effect—antidiabetics

Drug/Lab Test

Increase: alk phos, urinary sodium, urinary pregnanediol, plasma amino acids
Decrease: HDL, glucose tolerance test
False positive: urine glucose

NURSING CONSIDERATIONS

Assess:

• PSA levels in men (prostate cancer); blood glucose, LFTs, serum calcium, weight
• Effects of alopecia on body image; feelings about body changes
• Frequency of stools, characteristics: cramping, acidosis, signs of dehydration

(rapid respirations, poor skin turgor, decreased urine output, dry skin, restlessness, weakness)

• Anorexia, nausea, vomiting, constipation, weakness, loss of muscle tone

⚠ **Thrombophlebitis:** Homans' sign, edema; pain in calf, thigh; notify prescriber immediately

Perform/provide:

• Storage in tight container at room temp

Evaluate:

• Therapeutic response: decreased tumor size, spread of malignancy; weight gain in AIDS patients; resolved dysfunctional uterine bleeding

Teach patient/family:

• To report vaginal bleeding

• That nonhormonal contraception should be used during and for 4 mo after treatment; pregnancy (D) tabs, (X) susp

• That gynecomastia, alopecia can occur; reversible after discontinuing treatment

⚠ To recognize signs of fluid retention, thromboemboli; to report these immediately

• To monitor blood glucose if diabetic

meloxicam (Rx)

(mel-ox′i-kam)

Apo-Meloxicam ♣, CO Meloxicam ♣, Gen-Meloxicam ♣, Mobic, Mobicox ♣, Novo-Meloxicam ♣, PMS-Meloxicam ♣, ratio-Meloxicam ♣

Func. class.: Nonsteroidal antiinflammatory drugs (NSAIDs)/nonopioid analgesics

Chem. class.: Oxicam

ACTION: Inhibits COX-1 and COX-2 by blocking arachidonate; inhibits prostaglandin synthesis by decreasing an enzyme needed for biosynthesis; analgesic, anti-inflammatory, antipyretic effects

USES: Osteoarthritis, RA, juvenile arthritis

CONTRAINDICATIONS: Pregnancy (D) after 30 wk; breastfeeding; hypersensitivity, asthma, severe renal/hepatic disease, peptic ulcer disease, L&D, CV bleeding

Black Box Warning: Perioperative pain with CABG surgery

Precautions: Pregnancy (C) prior to 30 wk; children, geriatric patients, bleeding disorders, GI disorders, cardiac disorders, hypersensitivity to other anti-inflammatory agents, CCr <25 ml/min

Black Box Warning: GI bleeding, MI, stroke

DOSAGE AND ROUTES

• **Adult: PO** 7.5 mg/day, may increase to 15 mg/day; max 15 mg/day

Juvenile rheumatoid arthritis

• **Child ≥2 yr: PO** 0.125 mg/kg, max 7.5 mg/day

Available forms: Tabs 7.5, 15 mg; susp 7.5 mg/5 ml

Administer:

• Susp; tabs interchangeable

• May take without regard to meals; take with food for GI upset

• Take with full glass of water and sit upright for ½ hr (tab); shake susp before using

SIDE EFFECTS

CNS: Dizziness, drowsiness, tremors, headache, nervousness, malaise, fatigue, insomnia, depression, **seizures**

CV: Hypertension, angina, **cardiac failure, MI**, hypotension, palpitations, **dysrhythmias**, tachycardia, stroke

EENT: Tinnitus, hearing loss, blurred vision

GI: Pancreatitis, nausea, colitis, GERD, vomiting, diarrhea, constipation, flatulence, cramps, dry mouth, peptic ulcer, **GI bleeding, perforation, jaundice**

GU: Nephrotoxicity: dysuria, hematuria, oliguria, azotemia

M

HEMA: Blood dyscrasias, anemia, prolonged bleeding
INTEG: Rash, urticaria, photosensitivity
SYST: **Angioedema, anaphylaxis, Stevens-Johnson syndrome, toxic epidermal necrolysis**

PHARMACOKINETICS

PO: Peak 4-5 hr
IM: Peak 50 min
Half-life 15-20 hr; enters breast milk; <50% metabolized by liver; excreted by kidneys, feces; protein binding 99.4%

INTERACTIONS

Increase: nephrotoxicity—cycloSPORINE, tacrolimus
Increase: meloxicam action—sulfonamides, salicylates
Increase: action of aminoglycosides, diuretics, anticoagulants, lithium, methotrexate
Decrease: meloxicam action—cholestyramine
Decrease: action of β-blockers, ACE inhibitors, thiazides, other antihypertensives
Drug/Herb
Decrease: meloxicam effect—feverfew, ginkgo
Increase: bleeding risk—garlic

NURSING CONSIDERATIONS

Assess:
- **Pain:** ROM, intensity, duration, location
- Renal, hepatic, blood studies: BUN, creatinine, AST, ALT, Hgb before treatment, periodically thereafter

Black Box Warning: Check for GI bleeding, perforation, stool guaiac

⚠ **Anaphylaxis and angioedema;** emergency equipment should be nearby, those with asthma, aspirin-induced allergic and nasal polyps at greater risk for developing hypersensitivity
⚠ Fatal fulminant hepatitis, hepatic necrosis, hepatic failure: jaundice, yellow sclera and skin, clay-colored stools; monitor liver function studies; hepatic reactions more common among those with liver dysfunction
- Audiometric, ophthalmic exam before, during, after treatment

Black Box Warning: Hypertension, MI, stroke, cardiac conditions

Perform/provide:
- Storage at room temp

Evaluate:
- Therapeutic response: decreased pain, stiffness, swelling in joints; ability to move more easily

Teach patient/family:
- To report blurred vision or ringing, roaring in ears (may indicate toxicity)
- To avoid driving, other hazardous activities if dizziness or drowsiness occurs
- To report change in urine pattern, weight increase, edema, pain increase in joints, fever, blood in urine (indicates nephrotoxicity); to report rash, black stools, or continuing headache
- To avoid alcohol, aspirin, acetaminophen, NSAIDs without consulting prescriber; to report use to all health care providers

⚠ **HIGH ALERT**

melphalan (Rx)

(mel'fa-lan)
Alkeran
Func. class.: Antineoplastic, alkylating agent
Chem. class.: Nitrogen mustard

Do not confuse:
melphalan/Myleran

ACTION: Responsible for cross-linking DNA strands, thereby leading to cell death; activity is not cell-cycle–phase specific

USES: Multiple myeloma, malignant melanoma, advanced ovarian cancer
Unlabeled uses: Breast, testicular, prostate carcinoma; osteogenic sarcoma,

chronic myelogenous leukemia, non-Hodgkin's lymphoma, pediatric rhabdomyosarcoma, stem cell transplant, bone marrow ablation, AML, myelodysplastic syndrome

CONTRAINDICATIONS:

Pregnancy (D), breastfeeding, other nitrogen mustards

Black Box Warning: Hypersensitivity to this product

Precautions: Children, radiation therapy, infections, renal disease

Black Box Warning: Bone marrow depression, secondary malignancy

DOSAGE AND ROUTES

Multiple myeloma

- **Adult: PO** 6 mg daily × 2-3 wk, adjust dose based on blood counts or 10 mg daily × 7-10 day and 2 mg daily when WBC >4000 cells/mm^3, platelets >100,000 cells/mm^3, then 2-4 mg/day or 7 mg/m^2 × 5 day q5-6wk
- **Adult: IV INF** 16 mg/m^2, reduce with renal insufficiency, give over 15-20 min, give at 2-wk intervals × 4 doses then at 4-wk intervals

Ovarian carcinoma

- **Adult: PO** 200 mcg/kg/day × 5 days q4-5wk

Testicular cancer/breast cancer/non-Hodgkin's lymphoma/osteogenic sarcoma (unlabeled)

- **Adult: PO** 150 mcg/kg/day × 7 days q4wk; when leukocytes normal, give 50 mcg/kg/day maintenance

Pediatric rhabdomyosarcoma (unlabeled)

- **Child: IV** 10-35 mg/m^2 q21-28days

Stem cell transplant/bone marrow ablation/acute myelogenous leukemia/myelodysplastic syndrome (unlabeled)

- **Adult and child: IV** 140 mg/m^2 on day 1 or divided over 2 days prior to SCT

Available forms: Tabs 2 mg, powder for inj 50 mg

Administer:

- Antiemetic 30-60 min before product to prevent vomiting

PO route

- Give on empty stomach

Intermittent IV INF route

- Use gloves during administration; if skin exposure occurs, wash immediately with soap and water
- Give after reconstituting with 10 ml diluent provided (5 mg/ml); shake, dilute dose with 0.9% NaCl (≤0.45 mg/ml), give within 1 hr, run over ≥15 min

Y-site compatibilities: Acyclovir, amikacin, aminophylline, ampicillin, aztreonam, bleomycin, bumetanide, buprenorphine, butorphanol, calcium gluconate, CARBOplatin, carmustine, ceFAZolin, cefepime, cefoperazone, cefotaxime, cefotetan, ceftazidime, ceftizoxime, cefTRIAXone, cefuroxime, cimetidine, CISplatin, clindamycin, cyclophosphamide, cytarabine, dacarbazine, DACTINomycin, DAUNOrubicin, dexamethasone, diphenhydrAMINE, DOXOrubicin, doxycycline, droperidol, enalaprilat, etoposide, famotidine, floxuridine, fluconazole, fludarabine, fluorouracil, furosemide, gallium, ganciclovir, gentamicin, granisetron, haloperidol, heparin, hydrocortisone, hydrocortisone sodium phosphate, HYDROmorphone, hydrOXYzine, IDArubicin, ifosfamide, imipenem-cilastatin, LORazepam, mannitol, mechlorethamine, meperidine, mesna, methotrexate, methylPREDNISolone, metoclopramide, metroNIDAZOLE, miconazole, minocycline, mitomycin, mitoxantrone, morphine, nalbuphine, netilmicin, ondansetron, pentostatin, piperacillin, plicamycin, potassium chloride, prochlorperazine, promethazine, ranitidine, sodium bicarbonate, streptozocin, teniposide, thiotepa, ticarcillin, ticarcillin/clavulanate, tobramycin, trimethoprim-sulfamethoxazole, vancomycin, vinBLAStine, vinCRIStine, vinorelbine, zidovudine

M

SIDE EFFECTS

GI: *Nausea, vomiting,* stomatitis, diarrhea, hepatitis
GU: Amenorrhea, hyperuricemia, gonadal suppression, hyperuricemia
HEMA: Thrombocytopenia, neutropenia, leukopenia, anemia
INTEG: Rash, urticaria, alopecia, pruritus
RESP: Fibrosis, dysplasia, dyspnea, pneumonitis
SYST: Anaphylaxis, allergic reactions, secondary malignancies, edema

PHARMACOKINETICS

Metabolized in liver, excreted in urine, half-life $1^1/_2$ hr, protein binding 80%-90%

INTERACTIONS

- Avoid administration of sargramostim, GM-CSF, filgrastim, G-CSF 14 hr before or 24 hr after product

Increase: toxicity—antineoplastics, radiation
Increase: pulmonary toxicity—carmustine
Increase: renal failure risk—cycloSPORINE
Increase: enterocolitis risk—nalidixic acid
Increase: bleeding risk—NSAIDs, anticoagulants, salicylates, thrombolytics, platelet inhibitors
Decrease: antibody response—live virus vaccines

NURSING CONSIDERATIONS

Assess:

Black Box Warning: Bone marrow depression: CBC, differential, platelet count weekly; withhold product if WBC is <3000/mm³ or platelet count is <100,000/mm³; notify prescriber; recovery usually occurs in 6 wk

- Renal studies: BUN, serum uric acid before, during therapy
- I&O ratio; report fall in urine output to 30 ml/hr
- **Infection:** fever, cough, temp, chills, sore throat; notify prescriber
- Hepatic studies before, during therapy (bilirubin, AST, ALT, LDH) as needed
- **Bleeding:** hematuria, guaiac, bruising or petechiae, mucosa or orifices q8hr
- Jaundiced skin and sclera, dark urine, clay-colored stools, itchy skin, abdominal pain, fever, diarrhea
- Buccal cavity q8hr for dryness, sores, ulceration, white patches, oral pain, bleeding, dysphagia
- Local irritation, pain, burning, discoloration at inj site
- **Hyperuricemia:** joint pain, edema, increased uric acid, increase fluids to >2 L unless contraindicated

⚠ **Severe allergic reaction:** rash, pruritus, urticaria, purpuric skin lesions, itching, flushing; assess allergy to chlorambucil; cross-sensitivity may occur

Perform/provide:

- Storage in airtight, light-resistant container
- Increase fluid intake to 2-3 L/day to prevent urate deposits, calculi formation
- Diet low in purines: organ meats (kidney, liver), dried beans, peas to maintain alkaline urine
- Rinsing of mouth tid-qid with water, club soda; brushing of teeth bid-tid with soft brush or cotton-tipped applicators for stomatitis; use unwaxed dental floss
- Warm compresses at inj site for inflammation

Evaluate:

- Therapeutic response: decreased tumor size, spread of malignancy

Teach patient/family:

- That usually sterility, amenorrhea occur; reversible after discontinuing treatment
- To avoid foods with citric acid, hot or rough texture
- To report any bleeding, white spots, or ulcerations in mouth to prescriber; to examine mouth daily
- To report signs of infection: fever, sore throat, flulike symptoms

• To report suspected pregnancy; to use contraception during treatment; pregnancy (D)
• To report signs of anemia: fatigue, headache, faintness, SOB, irritability
• To avoid use of razors, commercial mouthwash
• To avoid use of aspirin products, NSAIDs, alcohol

memantine (Rx)

(me-man′teen)

Ebixa ✦, Namenda, Namenda XR

Func. class.: Anti-Alzheimer agent

Chem. class.: NMDA receptor antagonist

ACTION:

Antagonist action of CNS NMDA receptors that may contribute to the symptoms of Alzheimer's disease

USES:

Moderate to severe dementia in Alzheimer's disease

Unlabeled uses: Vascular dementia, acquired pendular nystagmus

CONTRAINDICATIONS:

Children, hypersensitivity

Precautions: Pregnancy (B), breastfeeding, renal disease, GU conditions that raise urine pH, seizures, severe hepatic disease, renal failure

DOSAGE AND ROUTES

• **Adult: PO** 5 mg/day, may increase dose in 5-mg increments ≥1 wk intervals; recommended target dose of 20 mg/day as 10 mg bid

Available forms: Tabs 5, 10 mg; tab titration pak 5, 10 mg; oral sol 2 mg/ml (10 mg/5 ml)

Administer:

• Can be taken without regard to meals
• Twice a day if dose >5 mg
• Dosage adjusted to response no more than q1wk
• **Ext rel caps:** do not crush, chew, divide; swallow whole or open and sprinkle on applesauce
• **Oral sol** using device provided; remove dosing syringe, green cap, plastic tube from plastic; attach tube to green cap; open cap by pushing down on cap, turning counterclockwise; remove unscrewed cap; carefully remove seal from bottle, discard; insert plastic tube fully into bottle, screw green cap tightly onto bottle by turning cap clockwise; keeping bottle upright on table, remove lid; with plunger fully depressed, insert tip of syringe into cap; while holding syringe, gently pull up on plunger; remove syringe; invert syringe, slowly press plunger to level that removes large air bubbles; keep plunger in inverted position; few small air bubbles may be present

SIDE EFFECTS

CNS: *Dizziness, confusion,* somnolence, headache, hallucinations
CV: Hypertension
GI: Vomiting, constipation
HEMA: Anemia
INTEG: Rash
MISC: Back pain, fatigue, pain
RESP: Coughing, dyspnea

PHARMACOKINETICS

Rapidly absorbed PO, 44% protein binding, very little metabolism, 57%-82% excreted unchanged in urine, terminal elimination half-life 60-80 hr

INTERACTIONS

• May alter levels of both products: hydrochlorothiazide, triamterene, cimetidine, quiNIDine, ranitidine, nicotine

Increase: effect—levodopa, some ergots

Decrease: clearance of memantine—products that make urine alkaline (sodium bicarbonate, carbonic anhydrase inhibitors)

NURSING CONSIDERATIONS

Assess:

• Alzheimer's dementia: affect, mood, behavioral changes; hallucinations, confusion, attention, orientation, memory

M

Perform/provide:

• Assistance with ambulation during beginning therapy; dizziness may occur

Evaluate:

• Therapeutic response: decrease in confusion, improved mood, maintenance of function, even with no improvement in symptoms

Teach patient/family:

• To report side effects: restlessness, psychosis, visual hallucinations, stupor, LOC; may indicate overdose

• To use product exactly as prescribed; that product not a cure

• To use oral sol dispenser

menotropins (Rx)

(men-oh-troe′pins)

Menopur, Repronex

Func. class.: Gonadotropin

Chem. class.: Exogenous gonadotropin

ACTION:

In women, increases follicular growth, maturation; in men, when given with hCG, stimulates spermatogenesis

USES:

Infertility, anovulation in women, stimulates spermatogenesis in men

CONTRAINDICATIONS:

Pregnancy (X), primary ovarian failure, abnormal bleeding, thyroid/adrenal dysfunction, organic intracranial lesion, ovarian cysts, primary testicular failure, high FSH, neoplastic disease

Precautions: Ascites, children, geriatric patients, endometriosis, polycystic ovary syndrome, thromboembolic disease, uterine leiomyomata, smoking

DOSAGE AND ROUTES

Infertility

• **Men: IM** 1 ampule 3×/wk with hCG 2000 units 2×/wk × 4 mo

• **Women: IM** 75 international units FSH, LH daily × 7-12 days then 10,000 units hCG 1 day after these products; repeat × 2 menstrual cycles, then increase to 150 international units FSH, LH daily × 9-12 days then 10,000 units hCG 1 day after these products × 2 menstrual cycles

Anovulation

• **Women: IM** (Humegon) 75 international units FSH, LH daily × 7-12 days then 10,000 units hCG 1 day after last dose of these products; repeat × 1-3 menstrual cycles; **IM/SUBCUT** (Repronex only) 75 international units FSH/LH activity daily × 5 days, adjust dose by no more than 75-150 international units/day q2days

Available forms: Powder for inj lyophilized 75 international units FSH, LH activity 150 international units FSH, LH activity

Administer:

IM route

• After reconstituting with 1-2 ml sterile saline for inj as per manufacturer; use immediately

SIDE EFFECTS

CNS: Fever, hot flashes, dizziness

CV: Hypovolemia, tachycardia

GI: *Nausea,* vomiting, diarrhea, anorexia

GU: Ovarian hyperstimulation syndrome (OHSS), *abdominal distention/pain,* multiple births, sudden ovarian enlargement, ascites with/without pain, ectopic pregnancy, gynecomastia in men

HEMA: Hemoperitoneum, arterial thromboembolism

INTEG: Rash, swelling of inj site

RESP: ARDS, PE, pulmonary infarction, pleural effusion, atelectasis, dyspnea, tachypnea

SYST: Anaphylaxis

NURSING CONSIDERATIONS

Assess:

• Weight daily; notify prescriber if weight increases rapidly

• Estrogen excretion level; if >100 mcg/24 hr, product is withheld; serum

progesterone, LH, estradiol level, pelvic exam, ovarian ultrasound; serum/urinary gonadotropin, testosterone, sperm count in males
- I&O ratio; be alert for decreasing urinary output
- Ovarian enlargement; abdominal distention, pain

Evaluate:
- Therapeutic response: ovulation, pregnancy

Teach patient/family:
- To report abdominal pain, distention
- That multiple births possible; if pregnancy occurs, usually will be 4-6 wk after start of treatment
- To keep daily appointments during treatment

⚠ HIGH ALERT

meperidine (Rx)

(me-per'i-deen)

Demerol, Meperitab

Func. class.: Opioid analgesic

Chem. class.: Phenylpiperidine derivative

Controlled Substance Schedule II

Do not confuse:
meperidine/HYDROmorphone/meprobamate/morphine
Demerol/Dilaudid/Desyrel/Demulen

ACTION: Depresses pain impulse transmission at the spinal cord level by interacting with opioid receptors

USES: Moderate to severe pain preoperatively, postoperatively

Unlabeled uses: Obstetric/regional analgesic, acute severe headache/migraine, shaking chills induced by IV amphotericin B or postoperative shivering

CONTRAINDICATIONS: Hypersensitivity

Precautions: Pregnancy (C), breastfeeding, children <18 yr, geriatric patients, addictive personality, increased intracranial pressure, MI (acute), severe heart disease, respiratory depression, renal/hepatic disease, seizure disorder, abrupt discontinuation, chronic pain

DOSAGE AND ROUTES

Moderate to severe pain
- **Adult: PO/SUBCUT/IM** 50-150 mg q3-4hr prn; **IV** 15-35 mg/hr as **CONT INF;** PCA 10 mg then 1- to 5-mg incremental dose; lockout interval 6-10 min
- **Child: PO/SUBCUT/IM** 1-1.8 mg/kg q3-4hr prn, max 100 mg q4hr

Labor analgesia
- **Adult: SUBCUT/IM** 50-100 mg given when contractions regularly spaced, repeat q1-3hr prn

Preoperatively
- **Adult: IM/SUBCUT** 50-100 mg 30-90 min before surgery
- **Child: IM/SUBCUT** 1-2.2 mg/kg 30-90 min before surgery, max 100 mg

Shaking, chills induced by amphotericin B or postoperative shivering (unlabeled)
- **Adult: IV** 25-50 mg as a single dose
- **Child and adolescent: IV** 0.35-1 mg/kg, max 50 mg; use lowest effective dose

Available forms: Inj 10, 25, 50, 75, 100 mg/ml; tabs 50, 100 mg; oral sol 50 mg/5 ml

Administer:

PO route
- May give with food or milk to decrease GI irritation
- Oral liquid: dilute in 4 oz water

IM/SUBCUT route
- Patient should remain recumbent for 1 hr after IM/SUBCUT route
- With antiemetic for nausea, vomiting
- When pain beginning to return; determine dosage interval by patient response
- In gradually decreasing dose after long-term use; withdrawal symptoms may occur
- Inject IM into large muscle mass; IM preferred route for multiple inj

Direct IV route

• Dilute to conc of 10 mg/ml with sterile water for inj or NS
• Inject slowly ≤25 mg/min
• Have emergency equipment and opiate antagonist on hand

Continuous IV INF route

• Dilute to conc of 1 mg/ml
• Infuse using inf pump

Syringe compatibilities: Butorphanol, chlorproMAZINE, cimetidine, dimenhyDRINATE, diphenhydrAMINE, droperidol, fentaNYL, glycopyrrolate, hydrOXYzine, ketamine, metoclopramide, midazolam, pentazocine, perphenazine, prochlorperazine, promazine, promethazine, ranitidine, scopolamine

Y-site compatibilities: Amifostine, amikacin, ampicillin, atenolol, aztreonam, bumetanide, ceFAZolin, cefotaxime, cefotetan, cefoxitin, ceftazidime, ceftizoxime, cefTRIAXone, cefuroxime, cephalothin, cephapirin, chloramphenicol, cisatracurium, cladribine, clindamycin, dexamethasone, diltiazem, diphenhydrAMINE, DOBUTamine, DOPamine, DOXOrubicin liposome, doxycycline, droperidol, erythromycin, famotidine, filgrastim, fluconazole, fludarabine, gallium, gentamicin, granisetron, heparin, hydrocortisone, insulin (regular), kanamycin, labetalol, lidocaine, methyldopate, magnesium sulfate, melphalan, methylPREDNISolone, metoclopramide, metoprolol, metroNIDAZOLE, moxalactam, ondansetron, oxacillin, oxytocin, paclitaxel, penicillin G potassium, piperacillin, potassium chloride, propofol, propranolol, ranitidine, remifentanil, sargramostim, teniposide, thiotepa, ticarcillin, ticarcillin/clavulanate, tobramycin, trimethoprim-sulfamethoxazole, vancomycin, verapamil, vinorelbine

Continuous intrathecal INF route

• Use controlled inf device; implantable controlled micro inf device used for highly concentrated inf, monitor for several days after implantation
• Filling of inf reservoir should only be done by those fully qualified
• To prevent pain, depletion of reservoir should be avoided

SIDE EFFECTS

CNS: *Drowsiness, dizziness, confusion, headache, sedation, euphoria,* **increased intracranial pressure, seizures,** serotonin syndrome
CV: Palpitations, bradycardia, hypotension, change in B/P, tachycardia (IV)
EENT: Tinnitus, blurred vision, miosis, diplopia, depressed corneal reflex
GI: Nausea, vomiting, anorexia, constipation, cramps, biliary spasm, paralytic ileus
GU: Urinary retention, dysuria
INTEG: Rash, urticaria, bruising, flushing, diaphoresis, pruritus
RESP: Respiratory depression
SYST: Anaphylaxis

PHARMACOKINETICS

Metabolized by liver (to active/inactive metabolites), excreted by kidneys; crosses placenta, excreted in breast milk; half-life 3-4 hr; toxic by-product accumulation can result from regular use or renal disease; protein binding 65%-75%
PO: Onset 15 min, peak ½-1 hr, duration 2-4 hr, absorption 50%
SUBCUT/IM: Onset 10 min, peak ½-1 hr, duration 2-4 hr, well absorbed
IV: Onset 5 min, duration 2 hr

INTERACTIONS

⚠ **May cause fatal reaction: MAOIs, procarbazine**
Increase: serotonin syndrome, neuroleptic malignant syndrome, SSRIs, SNRIs, serotonin-receptor agonists
Increase: effects with other CNS depressants, alcohol, opioids, sedative/hypnotics, antipsychotics, skeletal muscle relaxants
Increase: adverse reactions—protease inhibitor antiretrovirals
Decrease: meperidine effect—phenytoin
Drug/Herb
Increase: CNS depression—St. John's wort

Drug/Lab Test
Increase: amylase, lipase

NURSING CONSIDERATIONS

Assess:

- **Pain:** location, type, character; give product before pain becomes extreme; reassess after 60 min (IM, SUBCUT, PO) and 5-10 min (IV)
- Renal function prior to initiating therapy; poor renal function can lead to accumulation of toxic metabolite and seizures
- I&O ratio; check for decreasing output; may indicate urinary retention
- For constipation; increase fluids, bulk in diet; give stimulant laxatives if needed
- CNS changes: dizziness, drowsiness, hallucinations, euphoria, LOC, pupil reactions with chronic or high-dose use
- Allergic reactions: rash, urticaria

⚠ **Respiratory dysfunction:** depression, character, rate, rhythm; notify prescriber if respirations are <12/min

- CNS stimulation: with chronic or high doses

Perform/provide:

- Storage in light-resistant container at room temp
- Safety measures: night-light, call bell within easy reach

Evaluate:

- Therapeutic response: decrease in pain

Teach patient/family:

- To report any symptoms of CNS changes, allergic reactions
- That physical dependency may result from extended use
- That drowsiness, dizziness may occur; to call for assistance
- That withdrawal symptoms may occur: nausea, vomiting, cramps, fever, faintness, anorexia
- To make position changes slowly; orthostatic hypotension can occur
- To avoid OTC medications, alcohol unless directed by prescriber

TREATMENT OF OVERDOSE:

Naloxone (Narcan) 0.2-0.8 mg IV, O_2, IV fluids, vasopressors

mercaptopurine (6-MP) (Rx)

(mer-kap-toe-pyoor′een)

Purinethol

Func. class.: Antineoplastic-antimetabolite
Chem. class.: Purine analog

ACTION:

Inhibits purine metabolism at multiple sites, which inhibits DNA and RNA synthesis; specific for S phase of cell cycle

USES:

Chronic myelocytic or acute lymphoblastic leukemia in children
Unlabeled uses: Polycythemia vera, psoriatic arthritis, ulcerative colitis, Crohn's disease, AML, CML, lymphoma

M

CONTRAINDICATIONS:

Pregnancy (D), breastfeeding, patients with prior product resistance, leukopenia, thrombocytopenia, anemia
Precautions: Renal/hepatic disease, tumor lysis syndrome, dental disease, herpes, radiation therapy

DOSAGE AND ROUTES

Acute lymphocytic leukemia

- **Adult: PO** 2.5-5 mg/kg/day or 80-100 mg/m^2/day, maintenance 1.5-2.5 mg/kg/day
- **Child: PO** 2.5-5 mg/kg/day, maintenance 1.5-2.5 mg/kg/day or 70-100 mg/m^2/day

Acute myelogenous leukemia (unlabeled)

- **Adult and child: PO** 2.5 mg/kg/day

Chronic myelogenous leukemia (unlabeled)

- **Adult: PO** chronic phase 60-75 mg/m^2/day; blast crisis 100 mg/m^2 q12hr × 5-7 days

Crohn's disease/ulcerative colitis (unlabeled)
- **Adult: PO** 1.5-2 mg/kg/day

Available forms: Tabs 50 mg
Administer:
- Give product after evening meal, before bedtime, on an empty stomach
- Allopurinol or sodium bicarbonate to maintain uric acid levels, alkalinization of urine

SIDE EFFECTS

CNS: Weakness
GI: *Nausea, vomiting, anorexia, diarrhea, stomatitis,* hepatotoxicity (high doses), jaundice, gastritis, pancreatitis
GU: Renal failure, hyperuricemia, oliguria, crystalluria, hematuria
HEMA: Thrombocytopenia, leukopenia, myelosuppression, anemia
INTEG: *Rash,* dry skin, urticaria, alopecia

PHARMACOKINETICS

Incompletely absorbed when taken orally, metabolized in liver, excreted in urine, peak 1-2 hr, terminal half-life 1-1.5 hr

INTERACTIONS

Increase: effects—radiation or other antineoplastics, immunosuppressants
Increase: bone marrow depression—allopurinol, sulfamethoxazole-trimethoprim
Increase: anticoagulant action—anticoagulants, NSAIDs, thrombolytics, platelet inhibitors, salicylates
Decrease: antibodies—live virus vaccines

NURSING CONSIDERATIONS

Assess:
⚠ **Bone marrow suppression:** CBC, differential, platelet count weekly; withhold product if WBC is <3500 or platelet count is <100,000; notify prescriber; product should be discontinued
- Renal studies: BUN, serum uric acid, urine CCr, electrolytes before, during therapy
- I&O ratio; report fall in urine output to <30 ml/hr
- Monitor temp; fever may indicate beginning infection; no rectal temp
- Hepatic studies before, during therapy: bilirubin, alk phos, AST, ALT, weekly during beginning therapy
- **Bleeding:** hematuria, guaiac, bruising, petechiae, mucosa or orifices
- **Stomatitis:** buccal cavity for dryness, sores, ulceration, white patches, oral pain, bleeding, dysphagia

⚠ **Severe allergic reaction:** rash, urticaria, itching, flushing, laryngeal edema
Perform/provide:
- Strict medical asepsis, protective isolation if WBC levels low
- Increase fluid intake to 2-3 L/day to prevent urate deposits, calculi formation, unless contraindicated
- Diet low in purines: absence of organ meats (kidney, liver), dried beans, peas to maintain alkaline urine
- Rinsing of mouth tid-qid with water, club soda; brushing of teeth bid-tid with soft brush or cotton-tipped applicators for stomatitis; use unwaxed dental floss
- Storage in tightly closed container in cool environment

Evaluate:
- Therapeutic response: decreased size of tumor, spread of malignancy

Teach patient/family:
- To avoid foods with citric acid, hot or rough texture for stomatitis; to report stomatitis: any bleeding, white spots, ulcerations in mouth; to examine mouth daily, report symptoms
- That contraceptive measures recommended during therapy; to avoid breastfeeding
- To drink 10-12 8-oz glasses of fluid/day
- To notify prescriber of fever, chills, sore throat, nausea, vomiting, anorexia, diarrhea, bleeding, bruising, which may indicate blood dyscrasias

• To report signs of infection: fever, sore throat, flulike symptoms
• To report signs of anemia: fatigue, headache, faintness, SOB, irritability
• To report bleeding; to avoid use of razors, commercial mouthwash
• To avoid use of aspirin products, NSAIDs
• To take entire dose at one time

meropenem (Rx)

(mer-oh-pen'em)

Merrem

Func. class.: Antiinfective—miscellaneous

Chem. class.: Carbapenem

ACTION: Bactericidal; interferes with cell-wall replication of susceptible organisms; osmotically unstable cell wall swells, bursts from osmotic pressure

USES: Serious infections caused by gram-positive bacteria: *Streptococcus pneumoniae,* group A β-hemolytic streptococci, enterococcus; gram-negative: *Klebsiella, Proteus, Escherichia coli, Pseudomonas aeruginosa;* appendicitis, peritonitis caused by *viridans* group streptococci; *Bacteroides fragilis, Bacteroides thetaiotaomicron,* bacterial meningitis (≥3 mo)

Unlabeled uses: Febrile, neutropenic, community-acquired pneumonia

CONTRAINDICATIONS: Hypersensitivity to this product, carbapenems, cephalosporins, penicillins

Precautions: Pregnancy (B), breastfeeding, geriatric patients, renal disease, seizure disorder

DOSAGE AND ROUTES

Intraabdominal infections

• **Adult: IV** 1 g q8hr given over 15-30 min or as **IV BOL** 5-20 ml given over 3-5 min
• **Adolescent <50 kg/child ≥3 mo: IV** 20-40 mg/kg q8hr (max 2 g q8hr for meningitis)
• **Child >50 kg: IV** 1 g q8hr (intraabdominal infection) or 2 g q8hr (meningitis) given over 15-30 min or as **IV BOL** 5-20 ml over 3-5 min; max 2 g q8hr

Renal disease

• **Adult: IV** CCr 26-50 ml/min, give dose q12hr; CCr 10-25 ml/min, give ½ dose q12hr; CCr <10 ml/min, give ½ dose q24hr

Febrile neutropenia (unlabeled)

• **Adult: IV** 1 g q8hr

Community-acquired pneumonia (CAP) (unlabeled)

• **Adult: IV** 1 g q8hr with ciprofloxacin or with aminoglycoside plus fluoroquinolone

Available forms: Powder for inj 500 mg, 1 g

Administer:

• After C&S is taken

Direct IV route

• Reconstitute 500-mg or 1-g vials with 10, 20 ml of sterile water for inj, respectively; shake to dissolve, let stand until clear (average conc 50 mg/ml); reconstituted sol may be stored for 2 hr at room temp or for 12 hr refrigerated; inject up to 1 g in 5-20 ml over 3-5 min

Intermittent IV INF route

• Vials may be directly reconstituted with compatible inf fluid (NS, D_5W) to 2.5-50 mg/ml; vials with NS can be stored 2 hr at room temp or for ≤18 hr refrigerated, (D_5W solutions) may be stored for up to 1 hr at room temp or ≤8 hr refrigerated; infuse over 15-30 min

Y-site compatibilities: Aminophylline, atenolol, atropine, cimetidine, dexamethasone, digoxin, diphenhydrAMINE, enalaprilat, fluconazole, furosemide, gentamicin, heparin, insulin (regular), metoclopramide, morphine, norepinephrine, PHENobarbital, vancomycin

M

SIDE EFFECTS

CNS: Fever, somnolence, seizures, dizziness, weakness, myoclonia, *headache,* confusion

CV: Hypotension, palpitations, tachycardia

GI: Diarrhea, nausea, vomiting, pseudomembranous colitis, hepatitis, glossitis

HEMA: Eosinophilia, neutropenia, decreased Hgb, Hct, agranulocytosis

INTEG: *Rash,* urticaria, *pruritus,* pain at inj site, phlebitis, erythema at inj site

RESP: Chest discomfort, dyspnea, hyperventilation, PE

SYST: Anaphylaxis, Stevens-Johnson syndrome, angioedema

PHARMACOKINETICS

IV: Onset immediate, peak dose dependent, half-life 1 hr, excreted unchanged in urine (70%)

INTERACTIONS

Increase: meropenem plasma levels—probenecid

Decrease: effect of valproic acid

Drug/Lab Test

Increase: AST, ALT, LDH, BUN, alk phos, bilirubin, creatinine

False positive: direct Coombs' test

NURSING CONSIDERATIONS

Assess:

- Sensitivity to carbapenem antibiotics, penicillins
- Renal disease: lower dose may be required; monitor serum creatinine/BUN before, during therapy
- **Pseudomembranous colitis:** bowel pattern daily; if severe diarrhea, fever, abdominal pain, fatigue occurs, product should be discontinued
- **Infection:** temp, sputum, characteristics of wound before, during, and after treatment

⚠ **Allergic reactions, anaphylaxis:** rash, laryngeal edema, wheezing, urticaria, pruritus; may occur immediately or several days after therapy begins

- Overgrowth of infection: perineal itching, fever, malaise, redness, pain, swelling, drainage, rash, diarrhea, change in cough, sputum

Evaluate:

- Therapeutic response: negative C&S; absence of symptoms and signs of infection

Teach patient/family:

- **Pseudomembranous colitis:** to report severe diarrhea
- To report sore throat, bruising, bleeding, joint pain; may indicate blood dyscrasias (rare)
- To report overgrowth of infection: black, furry tongue; vaginal itching; foul-smelling stools
- To avoid breastfeeding; product is excreted in breast milk

TREATMENT OF ANAPHYLAXIS: EPINEPHrine, antihistamines; resuscitate if necessary

mesalamine, 5-ASA (Rx)

(mez-al′a-meen)

Apriso, Asacol, Asacol HD, Canasa, Lialda, Pentasa, Rowasa Salofalk 🍁, sf Rowasa

Func. class.: GI antiinflammatory

Chem. class.: 5-Aminosalicylic acid

Do not confuse:

Asacol/Ansaid/Os-Cal

ACTION: May diminish inflammation by blocking cyclooxygenase, inhibiting prostaglandin production in colon; local action only

USES: Mild to moderate active distal ulcerative colitis, proctosigmoiditis, proctitis

Unlabeled uses: Crohn's disease

CONTRAINDICATIONS: Hypersensitivity to this product or salicylates, 5-aminosalicylates

Precautions: Pregnancy (B), breastfeeding, children, geriatric patients, renal disease, sulfite sensitivity, pyloric stenosis

DOSAGE AND ROUTES

Treatment of ulcerative colitis

• **Adult: RECT** 60 ml (4 g) at bedtime, retained for 8 hr × 3-6 wk; **DEL REL TAB (Lialda)** 2.4-4.8 g/day × 8 wk; **DEL REL TAB (Asacol)** 800 mg tid × 6 wk; **CONTROLLED REL CAP (Pentasa)** 1 g qid up to 8 wk; **EXT REL** cap **(Apriso)** 1500 mg (4 caps) QAM daily up to 6 mo, **RECT SUPP** 500 mg bid retained for 1-3 hr × 3-6 wk until remission, may increase tid if needed

Maintenance of remission

• **Adult: PO** (del rel tab: Asacol) 800 mg bid or 400 mg qid; **PO** (del rel cap: Apriso) 1500 mg (4 caps) each AM; **PO** (del rel tab: Lialda) 2.4 g (2 tabs) daily with meal

Available forms: Enema 4 g/60 ml (Rowasa, sf Rowasa); ext rel tab 500 mg; ext rel cap 250, 500 mg (Pentasa); 0.375 g (Apriso); del rel tab 400 mg (Asacol), 800 mg (Asacol HD); del rel tab (Lialda) 1.2 g; rectal supp 1000 mg (Canasa)

Administer:

PO route

• Swallow tabs whole; do not break, crush, or chew tabs

• **Lialda:** take with meal

• **Apriso caps:** take without regard to meals in AM

Rectal suspension

• Product should be given at bedtime, retained until morning (8 hr); empty bowel before insertion, shake well

Rectal suppository

• Moisten prior to insertion; suppository should be retained for 1-3 hr

SIDE EFFECTS

CNS: *Headache, fever, dizziness,* insomnia, asthenia, weakness, fatigue

CV: Pericarditis, myocarditis, chest pain, palpitations

EENT: Sore throat, cough, pharyngitis, rhinitis

GI: *Cramps, gas, nausea, diarrhea,* rectal pain, constipation

INTEG: *Rash, itching,* acne

SYST: *Flulike symptoms, malaise,* back pain, peripheral edema, leg and joint pain, arthralgia, dysmenorrhea, anaphylaxis, acute intolerance syndrome

PHARMACOKINETICS

RECT: Primarily excreted in feces but some in urine as metabolite; half-life 1 hr, metabolite half-life 5-10 hr

INTERACTIONS

• Do not give H_2 blockers with Apriso

Increase: nephrotoxicity—NSAIDs

Increase: action of azathioprine

Decrease: digoxin level—digoxin

Decrease: mesalamine absorption—lactulose, antacids

Decrease: effect of—warfarin

Drug/Lab Test

Increase: AST, ALT, alk phos, LDH, GGTP, amylase, lipase

M

NURSING CONSIDERATIONS

Assess:

• **Allergy to salicylates, sulfonamides;** if allergic reactions occur, discontinue product

• Renal studies: BUN, creatinine before, during treatment; renal toxicity may occur

• **Bowel disorders:** cramps, gas, nausea, diarrhea, rectal pain; if severe, product should be discontinued

• I&O ratios, increase fluids to 1500 ml daily to prevent crystalluria

Perform/provide:

• Storage at room temp

Evaluate:

• Therapeutic response: absence of pain, bleeding from GI tract, decrease in number of diarrhea stools

Teach patient/family:

• That usual course of therapy is 3-6 wk

• To shake bottle well (rectal susp)

• About method of rectal administration

• To inform prescriber of GI symptoms
• To report abdominal cramping, pain, diarrhea with blood, headache, fever, rash, chest pain; product should be discontinued

metformin (Rx)

(met-for′min)

Apo-Metformin ✤, CO Metformin ✤, Fortamet, Gen-Metformin ✤, Glucophage, Glucophage XR, Glumetza, Novo-Metformin ✤, Nu-Metformin ✤, PMS-Metformin ✤, RAN-Metformin ✤, ratio-Metformin ✤, Riomet, Sandoz Metformin ✤

Func. class.: Antidiabetic, oral
Chem. class.: Biguanide

ACTION:
Inhibits hepatic glucose production and increases sensitivity of peripheral tissue to insulin

USES:
Type 2 diabetes mellitus

Unlabeled uses: Precocious puberty or early-normal onset of puberty to delay menarche; polycystic ovary syndrome, infertility

CONTRAINDICATIONS:
Hypersensitivity; hepatic disease; creatinine >1.5 mg/ml (males), ≥1.4 (females); alcoholism; cardiopulmonary disease; acidemia; acute MI; cardiogenic shock; diabetic ketoacidosis; metabolic acidosis

Black Box Warning: History of lactic acidosis

Precautions: Pregnancy (B), breastfeeding, geriatric patients, previous hypersensitivity, thyroid disease, CHF, type 1 diabetes mellitus

DOSAGE AND ROUTES

Type 2 diabetes mellitus

• **Adult: PO** 500 mg bid or 850 mg/day initially then 500 mg weekly or 850 mg q2wk up to 2000 mg/day in divided doses with morning meal, with dosage increased every other wk, max 2550 mg/day, **EXT REL** (Glucophage XR) 500 mg daily with evening meal, may increase by 500 mg per wk, max 2000 mg/day; (Glumetza) 1000 mg daily with food, preferably with PM meal, may increase by 500 mg per wk, max 2000 mg daily; (Fortamet) 500-1000 mg daily with PM meal, may increase by 500 mg per wk, max 2550 mg daily; regular rel or oral sol 2000-2500 mg/day for ext rel tab, depending on formulation
• **Geriatric: PO** Use lowest effective dose

To delay early menarche and to prolong pubertal growth with early onset of puberty (unlabeled)

• **Child 8-9 yr: PO** 825 mg/day with PM meal

To delay clinical puberty and early menarche in precocious puberty (unlabeled)

• **Child >6 yr: PO** 425 mg/day with PM meal

Polycystic ovary syndrome/ infertility related to hyperinsulinemia secondary to polycystic ovary syndrome (unlabeled)

• **Adult (female): PO** 500 mg tid

Available forms: Tabs 500, 850, 1000 mg; ext rel tab 500, 750, 1000 mg; oral sol 500 mg/5 ml

Administer:

PO route

• **Immediate rel product:** twice a day given with meals to decrease GI upset, and provide the best absorption; immediate rel tabs crushed, mixed with meal, fluids for patients with difficulty swallowing
• **Ext rel product** may also be taken as single dose; titrate slowly to therapeutic response, side effect tolerance
• Ext rel tabs: do not chew, break, crush

SIDE EFFECTS

CNS: *Headache, weakness, dizziness, drowsiness,* tinnitus, fatigue, vertigo, *agitation*

CV: Heart failure
ENDO: Lactic acidosis, hypoglycemia
GI: *Nausea, vomiting, diarrhea,* heartburn, anorexia, metallic taste
HEMA: Thrombocytopenia, decreased vit B_{12} levels
INTEG: Rash

PHARMACOKINETICS

Excreted by kidneys unchanged 35%-50%, half-life 1½-5 hr, terminal 6-20 hr, peak 1-3 hr

INTERACTIONS

- Do not give with radiologic contrast media; may cause renal failure
- Do not use with dofetilide; may cause lactic acidosis

Increase: metformin level—cimetidine, digoxin, morphine, procainamide, quiNIDine, ranitidine, triamterene, vancomycin
Increase: hypoglycemia—cimetidine, calcium channel blockers, corticosteroids, estrogens, oral contraceptives, phenothiazines, sympathomimetics, diuretics, phenytoin
Drug/Herb
Increase: hyperglycemia—glucosamine
Increase: hypoglycemia—garlic, green tea, horse chestnut

NURSING CONSIDERATIONS

Assess:

- **Hypoglycemic reactions** (sweating, weakness, dizziness, anxiety, tremors, hunger); hyperglycemic reactions soon after meals; these occur rarely with product, may occur when product combined with sulfonylureas
- CBC (baseline, q3mo) during treatment; check LFTs periodically, AST, LDH, renal studies: BUN, creatinine during treatment; glucose, A1c; folic acid, vit B_{12} q1-2yr

Black Box Warning: Lactic acidosis: malaise, myalgia, abdominal distress; risk increases with age, poor renal function; monitor electrolytes, lactate, pyruvate, blood pH, ketones, glucose

Perform/provide:

- Conversion from other oral hypoglycemic agents; change may be made without gradual dosage change; monitor serum glucose, urine ketones tid during conversion
- Storage in tight container in cool environment

Evaluate:

- Therapeutic response: decrease in polyuria, polydipsia, polyphagia; clear sensorium; absence of dizziness; stable gait; blood glucose, A1c at normal level

Teach patient/family:

Black Box Warning: Lactic acidosis: hyperventilation, fatigue, malaise, chills, myalgia, somnolence; to notify prescriber immediately

- To regularly self-monitor blood glucose with blood-glucose meter
- About symptoms of hypo/hyperglycemia, what to do about each (rare)
- That product must be continued on daily basis; about consequences of discontinuing product abruptly
- To avoid OTC medications, alcohol unless approved by prescriber
- That diabetes is a lifelong illness; that product is not a cure, only controls symptoms
- To carry emergency ID and glucagon emergency kit
- That Glucophage XR tab may appear in stool
- To take with meals
- About signs, symptoms of hypo/hyperglycemic reactions

M

⚠ HIGH ALERT

methadone (Rx)

(meth'a-done)

Dolophine, Metadol ♣, Methadose

Func. class.: Opioid analgesic

Chem. class.: Synthetic diphenylheptane derivative

Controlled Substance Schedule II

Do not confuse:
methadone/methylphenidate

ACTION:

Depresses pain impulse transmission at the spinal cord level by interacting with opioid receptors; produces CNS depression

USES:

Severe pain, opioid withdrawal

CONTRAINDICATIONS:

Hypersensitivity to this product or chlorobutanol (inj); asthma, ileus

Black Box Warning: Respiratory depression

Precautions: Pregnancy (C), breastfeeding, children <18 yr, geriatric patients, addictive personality, increased intracranial pressure, MI (acute), severe heart disease, respiratory depression, pulmonary/renal/hepatic disease, respiratory insufficiency, torsades de pointes, COPD

Black Box Warning: QT prolongation, pain

DOSAGE AND ROUTES

Severe pain

- **Adult: PO/SUBCUT/IM/IV** 2.5-10 mg q8-12hr prn

Opioid withdrawal

- **Adult including pregnant woman:** 20-30 mg initially unless low opioid tolerance expected; additional 5-10 mg q2-4hr as needed after initial dose; if symptoms continue, may give for ≤5 days

Renal disease

- **Adult:** may need to be modified

Available forms: Inj 10 mg/ml; tabs 5, 10 mg; oral sol 5, 10 mg/5 ml, 10 mg/ml

Administer:

- With antiemetic if nausea, vomiting occurs
- When pain is beginning to return; determine dosage interval by patient response
- Rotating inj sites, give deep in large muscle mass (IM)

SIDE EFFECTS

CNS: *Drowsiness, dizziness, confusion, headache, sedation,* euphoria, seizures

CV: Palpitations, bradycardia, change in B/P, cardiac arrest, shock, hypotension, torsades de pointes, QT prolongation

EENT: Tinnitus, blurred vision, miosis, diplopia

GI: *Nausea, vomiting, anorexia, constipation, cramps,* biliary tract spasm

GU: Increased urinary output, dysuria, urinary retention, impotence

INTEG: *Rash,* urticaria, bruising, flushing, diaphoresis, pruritus

RESP: Respiratory depression, respiratory arrest

PHARMACOKINETICS

Metabolized by liver; excreted by kidneys; crosses placenta; excreted in breast milk; half-life 8-59 hr, extended interval with continued dosing; 90% bound to plasma proteins

PO: Onset 30-60 min, peak 1-1.5 hr, duration 6-8 hr, cumulative 22-48 hr; PO half as active as INJ

SUBCUT/IM: Onset 10-20 min, peak $1^{1}/_{2}$-2 hr, duration 4-6 hr, cumulative 22-48 hr

INTERACTIONS

⚠ Unpredictable reactions: MAOIs; do not use together

• Do not use within 2 wk of selegiline

Increase: effects with other CNS depressants—alcohol, opiates, sedative/hypnotics, antipsychotics, skeletal muscle relaxants

Increase: toxicity—CYP3A4 inhibitors (aprepitant, antiretroviral protease inhibitors, clarithromycin, danazol, delavirdine, diltiazem, erythromycin, fluconazole, fluoxetine, fluroxamine, imatinib, ketoconazole, mibefradil, nefazodone, telithromycin, voriconazole)

Increase: QT prolongation—class IA antiarrhythmics (disopyramide, procainamide, quiNIDine), class III antiarrhythmics (amiodarone, dofetilide, ibutilide, sotalol), astemizole, arsenic trioxide, cisapride, chloroquine, clarithromycin, levomethadye, pentamidine, some phenothiazines, pimozide, terfenadine

Decrease: analgesia—rifampin, phenytoin, nalbuphine, pentazine

Decrease: methadone effect—CYP3A4 inducers (barbiturates, bosentan, carBAMazepine, efavirenz, phenytoins, nevirapine, rifabutin, rifampin)

Drug/Herb

• Avoid use with St. John's wort; withdrawal may result

Increase: CNS depression—chamomile, hops, kava, valerian

Drug/Lab Test

Increase: amylase, lipase

NURSING CONSIDERATIONS

Assess:

• **Pain:** type, location, intensity, grimacing before, 1½-2 hr after administration; use pain scoring

• I&O ratio; check for decreasing output; may indicate urinary retention

• CNS changes: dizziness, drowsiness, hallucinations, euphoria, LOC, pupil reaction

• Allergic reactions: rash, urticaria

Black Box Warning: Respiratory dysfunction: respiratory depression, character, rate, rhythm; notify prescriber if respirations are <10/min

• Opioid detoxification: no analgesia occurs, only prevention of withdrawal symptoms

Black Box Warning: B/P, pulse, ECG; QT prolongation, hypotension, palpitations may occur

• Bowel changes, bulk, fluids, laxatives should be used for constipation

Perform/provide:

• Storage in light-resistant container at room temp

• Assistance with ambulation

• Safety measures: night-light, call bell within easy reach

Evaluate:

• Therapeutic response: decrease in pain, successful opioid withdrawal

Teach patient/family:

• To report any symptoms of CNS changes, allergic reactions

• That physical dependency may result from extended use

⚠ That withdrawal symptoms may occur: nausea, vomiting, cramps, fever, faintness, anorexia

• To maintain proper hydration; to avoid alcohol use

TREATMENT OF OVERDOSE:

Naloxone (Narcan) 0.2-0.8 mg IV, O_2, IV fluids, vasopressors

methimazole (Rx)

(meth-im′a-zole)

Tapazole

Func. class.: Thyroid hormone antagonist (antithyroid)

Chem. class.: Thioamide

Do not confuse:

methimazole/metoprolol/minoxidil

ACTION: Inhibits synthesis of thyroid hormones by decreasing iodine use in manufacture of thyroglobin and iodothyronine; does not affect circulatory T_4, T_3

M

USES:
Hyperthyroidism, preparation for thyroidectomy, thyrotoxic crisis; thyroid storm when PTU is contraindicated

CONTRAINDICATIONS:
Pregnancy (D), breastfeeding, hypersensitivity

Precautions: Infection, bone marrow suppression, hepatic disease, bleeding disorders

DOSAGE AND ROUTES

Hyperthyroidism

- **Adult: PO** 15 mg/day (mild hyperthyroidism); 30-40 mg/day (moderate to severe); 60 mg/day (severe); maintenance 5-15 mg/day; may be divided
- **Child: PO** 0.4 mg/kg/day in divided doses q8hr; continue until euthyroid; maintenance dose 0.2 mg/kg/day in divided doses q8hr, max 30 mg/24 hr; may be divided

Preparation for thyroidectomy

- **Adult and child: PO** same as above; iodine may be added × 10 days before surgery

Thyrotoxic crisis

- **Adult and child: PO** same as hyperthyroidism with iodine and propranolol

Available forms: Tabs 5, 10, 15, 20 mg

Administer:

- With meals to decrease GI upset
- At same time each day to maintain product level
- Lowest dose that relieves symptoms; discontinue before RAIU

SIDE EFFECTS

CNS: *Drowsiness, headache, vertigo, fever,* paresthesias, neuritis

ENDO: *Enlarged thyroid*

GI: *Nausea, diarrhea, vomiting,* jaundice, hepatitis, loss of taste

GU: Nephritis

HEMA: Agranulocytosis, leukopenia, thrombocytopenia, hypothrombinemia, lymphadenopathy, bleeding, vasculitis

INTEG: *Rash, urticaria, pruritus, alopecia, hyperpigmentation,* lupuslike syndrome

MS: Myalgia, arthralgia, nocturnal muscle cramps

PHARMACOKINETICS

Onset 12-18 hr; duration 36-72 hr; half-life 4-12 hr; excreted in urine, breast milk; crosses placenta

INTERACTIONS

- Agranulocytosis: phenothiazines

Increase: bone marrow depression—radiation, antineoplastic agents

Increase: response to digoxin

Decrease: effectiveness—amiodarone, potassium iodide

Decrease: Anticoagulant effect—warfarin

Drug/Lab Test

Increase: PT, AST, ALT, alk phos

NURSING CONSIDERATIONS

Assess:

- **Hyperthyroidism:** palpitation, nervousness, loss of hair, insomnia, heat intolerance, weight loss, diarrhea
- **Hypothyroidism:** constipation, dry skin, weakness, fatigue, headache, intolerance to cold, weight gain; adjustment may be needed
- Pulse, B/P, temp
- I&O ratio; check for edema: puffy hands, feet, periorbits; these indicate hypothyroidism
- Weight daily; same clothing, scale, time of day
- T_3, T_4, which are increased; serum TSH, which is decreased; free thyroxine index, which is increased if dosage too low; discontinue product 3-4 wk before RAIU

⚠ **Blood dyscrasias:** CBC, leukopenia, thrombocytopenia, agranulocytosis; if these occur, product should be discontinued and other treatment initiated

- **Hypersensitivity:** rash, enlarged cervical lymph nodes; product may have to be discontinued
- **Hypoprothrombinemia:** bleeding, petechiae, ecchymosis

⚠ Nurse Alert

• **Clinical response:** after 3 wk should include increased weight; decreased T_4, pulse

⚠ **Bone marrow suppression:** sore throat, fever, fatigue

Perform/provide:

• Storage in light-resistant container

• Increased fluids to 3-4 L/day unless contraindicated

Evaluate:

• Therapeutic response: weight gain, decreased pulse, decreased T_4, B/P

Teach patient/family:

• Not to breastfeed

• To take pulse daily

• To report redness, swelling, sore throat, mouth lesions, fever, which indicate blood dyscrasias

• To keep graph of weight, pulse, mood

• To avoid OTC products, seafood that contains iodine, other iodine products

• Not to discontinue product abruptly because thyroid crisis may occur; stress patient response

• That response may take several months if thyroid is large

• **Symptoms and signs of overdose:** periorbital edema, cold intolerance, mental depression

• **Symptoms of inadequate dose:** tachycardia, diarrhea, fever, irritability

• To take medication as prescribed; not to skip or double dose

methocarbamol (Rx)

(meth-oh-kar′ba-mole)

Robaxin

Func. class.: Skeletal muscle relaxant, central acting

Chem. class.: Carbamate derivative

Do not confuse:

Robaxin/Reglan/Relafen/Rolephin

ACTION: Depresses multisynaptic pathways in the spinal cord, thereby causing skeletal muscle relaxation

USES: Adjunct for relief of spasm and pain in musculoskeletal conditions, tetanus

CONTRAINDICATIONS: Hypersensitivity to this product or PEG 300 (inj); children <12 yr, intermittent porphyria, renal disease (IM/IV)

Precautions: Pregnancy (C), breastfeeding, renal/hepatic disease, addictive personality, myasthenia gravis, epilepsy

DOSAGE AND ROUTES

Muscle spasm

• **Adult: PO** 1.5 g qid × 2-3 days then 1 g qid; **IM** 500 mg in each gluteal region, may repeat q8hr; **IV BOL** 1-3 g/day, max 3 ml/min; **IV INF** 1 g/250 ml D_5W or NS, max 3 g/day

• **Geriatric: PO** 500 mg qid, titrate to needed dose

Tetanus management

• **Adult: IV direct** 1-2 g or **IV INF** 1-3 g q6hr, max 3 g

• **Child: IV** 15 mg/kg q6hr prn, max 1.8 g/m^2/day for 3 consecutive days, max 3 ml/min IV

Available forms: Tabs 500, 750 mg; inj 100 mg/ml

Administer:

PO route

• With meals for GI symptoms

IM route

• IM deep in large muscle mass; rotate sites

• Do not give SUBCUT

• Considered incompatible with any product in sol or syringe

Direct IV route

• IV undiluted over ≥1 min; give ≤300 mg/≥1 min

• By slow IV to prevent phlebitis; keep patient recumbent for 15 min to prevent orthostatic hypotension; check for extravasation

Intermittent IV INF route

• May be diluted in ≤250 ml D_5W or NS sol for slow IV inf

• Considered incompatible with any product in sol or syringe

SIDE EFFECTS

CNS: *Dizziness, weakness, drowsiness,* headache, tremor, depression, confusion, syncope, flushing, insomnia; seizures (IV, IM use)
CV: Postural hypotension, bradycardia
EENT: Diplopia, temporary loss of vision, blurred vision, nystagmus, conjunctivitis, nasal congestion
GI: *Nausea,* vomiting, hiccups, anorexia, metallic taste, dyspepsia, jaundice
GU: Brown, black, green urine
HEMA: Hemolysis, increased hemoglobin, leukopenia (IV only)
INTEG: Rash, pruritus, fever, facial flushing, urticaria, phlebitis, extravasation
SYST: Anaphylaxis, angioneurotic edema (IM, IV)

PHARMACOKINETICS

Metabolized in liver, excreted in urine unchanged, crosses placenta
PO: Onset $^1/_2$ hr, peak 1-2 hr, half-life 1-2 hr
IM/IV: Onset rapid

INTERACTIONS

Increase: CNS depression—alcohol, tricyclics, opioids, barbiturates, sedatives, hypnotics

Drug/Herb

Increase: CNS depression—chamomile, hops, kava, skullcap, St. John's wort, valerian

Drug/Lab Test

False increase: VMA, urinary 5-HIAA

NURSING CONSIDERATIONS

Assess:

- **Pain, spasm:** ROM, ADLs, pain characteristics before and after treatment
- **Blood dyscrasias:** CBC, WBC, differential
- During and after inj: CNS effects, rash, conjunctivitis, nasal congestion may occur
- Hepatic studies: AST, ALT, alk phos; hepatitis may occur; renal studies: BUN, creatinine with IV use
- EEG in epileptic patients; poor seizure control has occurred
- **Allergic reactions:** rash, fever, respiratory distress
- Severe weakness, numbness in extremities
- **Tolerance:** increased need for medication, more frequent requests for medication, increased pain
- CNS depression: dizziness, drowsiness, psychiatric symptoms

Perform/provide:

- Storage in tight container at room temp
- Assistance with ambulation if dizziness, drowsiness occurs
- Recumbent position during and 10-15 min after IV administration

Evaluate:

- Therapeutic response: decreased pain, spasticity

Teach patient/family:

- Not to discontinue medication quickly; that insomnia, nausea, headache, spasticity, tachycardia will occur; that product should be tapered off over 1-2 wk
- That urine may turn green, black, or brown
- Not to take with alcohol, other CNS depressants
- To avoid altering activities while taking product
- To avoid hazardous activities if drowsiness, dizziness occurs
- To avoid using OTC medication, cough preparations, antihistamines unless directed by prescriber

TREATMENT OF OVERDOSE:

Activated charcoal, dialysis; have EPINEPHrine, antihistamines, and corticosteroids available; enhance elimination with osmotic diuresis, IV fluids for hypotension

⚠ HIGH ALERT

methotrexate (Rx)

(meth-oh-trex′ate)

Rheumatrex, Trexall

Func. class.: Antineoplastic-antimetabolite (vesicant)

Chem. class.: Folic acid antagonist

Do not confuse:
methotrexate/metolazone/mitoxantrone

ACTION: Inhibits an enzyme that reduces folic acid, which is needed for nucleic acid synthesis in all cells; specific to S phase of cell cycle; immunosuppressive

USES: Acute lymphocytic leukemia; in combination for breast, lung, head, neck carcinoma; lymphosarcoma, gestational choriocarcinoma, hydatidiform mole, psoriasis, RA, mycosis fungoides, osteosarcoma

Unlabeled uses: Burkitt's lymphoma, bladder or ovarian cancer, carcinomatous meningitis, desmoid tumor, fibromatosis, asthma, active Crohn's disease, ulcerative colitis, GVHD prophylaxis, ectopic pregnancy, pregnancy termination, psoriatic arthritis, pruritus due to cholestasis or primary biliary cirrhosis, SLE, sarcoidosis

CONTRAINDICATIONS: Hypersensitivity, leukopenia ($<3500/mm^3$), thrombocytopenia ($<100,000/mm^3$), anemia; psoriatic patients with severe renal disease, alcoholism, HIV

Black Box Warning: Pregnancy (X), hepatic disease

Precautions: Breastfeeding, children

Black Box Warning: Renal disease, ascites, diarrhea, exfoliative dermatitis, infection, intrathecal administration, lymphoma, pleural effusion, pulmonary disease, radiation therapy, stomatitis, tumor lysis syndrome

DOSAGE AND ROUTES

Acute lymphocytic leukemia

• **Adult and child: PO/IM/IV** 3.3 mg/m²/day × 4-6 wk until remission then 20-30 mg/m² **PO/IM** q wk in 2 divided doses or 2.5 mg/kg **IV** × 2 wk

Choriocarcinoma

• **Adult and child: PO/IM** 15-30 mg/day × 5 days then off 1 wk; may repeat

Meningeal leukemia

• **Adult and child:** 12 mg/m² **INTRATHECALLY** q2-5days until CSF is normal then 1 additional dose, max 15 mg

Lymphosarcoma (stage III)

• **Adult: PO/IM/IV** 0.625-2.5 mg/kg/day

Osteosarcoma

• **Adult and child: IV** 12 g/m² given over 4 hr then leucovorin rescue

Mycosis fungoides

• **Adult: PO** 2.5-10 mg/day until cleared (may be many months); **IM** 50 mg/wk or 15-37.5 mg 2×/wk

Psoriasis

• **Adult: PO/IM/IV** 10-25 mg/wk or 2.5 mg **PO** q12hr × 3 doses/wk, may increase to 25 mg/wk

Breast cancer

• **Adult: IV** 40-60 mg/m² on day 1 of every 21-28 days with other antineoplastics

Rheumatoid arthritis

• **Adult: PO** 7.5 mg/wk or in divided doses of 2.5 mg q12hr × 3 given per wk; max 20 mg/wk

Polyarticular-course juvenile RA

• **Child: PO/IM** 10 mg/m²/wk

Burkitt's lymphoma (stages I, II, III)

• **Adult/adolescent/child:** many different combination regimens exist

Bladder cancer (unlabeled)

• **Adult: IV** 30 mg/m² on days 1, 15, 22 q28days in combination with vinBLAStine, DOXOrubicin, CISplatin (MVAC) regimen

Desmoid tumor/fibromatosis (unlabeled)

• **Adult and child: IV** 20-30 mg/m²/wk in combination with vinBLAStine

Ovarian cancer (unlabeled)

• **Adult: IV** 40 mg/m² on days 1, 8 q28

M

days with hexamethylmelamine, cyclophosphamide, fluorouracil

Active Crohn's disease/ulcerative colitis (unlabeled)

- **Adult: IM** 25 mg/wk; **SUBCUT** 15 mg/kg/wk × 16 wk

GVHD prophylaxis (unlabeled)

- **Adult and child: IV** 15 mg/m^2 on day 1 after transplant then 10 mg/m^2 on days 3, 6, 11

Ectopic pregnancy (unlabeled)

- **Adult: IM** 50 mg/m^2 may be used in combination with mifepristone

Pregnancy termination prior to 63rd day of pregnancy (unlabeled)

- **Adult: IM** 50 mg/m^2 then intravaginal misoprostol 5-7 days later

Psoriatic arthritis (unlabeled)

- **Adult: PO** 5-7.5 mg q wk

Available forms: Tabs 2.5, 5, 7.5, 10, 15 mg; inj 25 mg/ml; powder for inj 20 mg, 1 g

Administer:

- Using chemotherapeutic handling
- Antiemetic 30-60 min before product
- Allopurinol or sodium bicarbonate to maintain uric acid levels, alkalinization of urine (pH >6.5), adequate fluids

Direct IV route

- After diluting 5 mg/2 ml of sterile water for inj; give through Y-tube or 3-way stopcock

Intermittent/Continuous IV INF route

- Further dilute in D5W, D5NS, NS, prior to infusion check patency of vein, flush with 5-10 ml of D5W, NS, infuse at 4-20 mg/hr or prescribed rate

⚠ **Leucovorin rescue:** leucovorin calcium within 24 hr of product to prevent tissue damage; check agency policy, continue until methotrexate level <10^{-8} m

IV INF intermediate or high dose (500 mg/m^2 over <4 hr or >1 g/m^2 over >4 hr): confirm WBC >1500/mm^3, neutrophils >200/mm^3, platelets >75,000/mm^3, serum bilirubin <1.2 mg/dl, serum creatinine WNL, SGPT <450 U, creatinine clearance >60 ml/min

⚠ Give sodium bicarbonate tabs or IV fluids to prevent precipitation of product at high doses; urine pH should be >7; may need to reduce dosage if BUN 20-30 mg/dl or creatinine is 1.2-2 mg/dl; stop product if BUN >30 mg/dl or creatinine >2 mg/dl

Additive compatibilities: Cephalothin, cyclophosphamide, cytarabine, fluorouracil, hydrOXYzine, mercaptopurine, ondansetron, sodium bicarbonate, vinCRIStine

Solution compatibilities: Amino acids, 4.25%/D_{25}, D_5W, sodium bicarbonate 0.05 mol/L, sodium chloride 0.9%

Syringe compatibilities: Bleomycin, CISplatin, cyclophosphamide, doxapram, DOXOrubicin, fluorouracil, furosemide, heparin, leucovorin, mitomycin, vinBLAStine, vinCRIStine

Y-site compatibilities: Allopurinol, amifostine, amphotericin B cholesteryl, asparaginase, aztreonam, bleomycin, cefepime, cefTRIAXone, cimetidine, CISplatin, cyclophosphamide, cytarabine, DAUNOrubicin, dexchlorpheniramine, diphenhydrAMINE, DOXOrubicin, DOXOrubicin liposome, etoposide, famotidine, filgrastim, fludarabine, fluorouracil, furosemide, gallium, ganciclovir, granisetron, heparin, HYDROmorphone, imipenem-cilastatin, leucovorin, LORazepam, melphalan, mesna, methylPREDNISolone, metoclopramide, mitomycin, morphine, ondansetron, oxacillin, paclitaxel, piperacillin/tazobactam, prochlorperazine, ranitidine, sargramostim, teniposide, thiotepa, vinBLAStine, vinCRIStine, vinorelbine

Intrathecal route

- Use preservative-free sol, reconstitute with NS; dose should be drawn into 5- to 10-ml syringe after LP, vol of CSF should be withdrawn equal to vol of methotrexate; allow CSF to flow into syringe and mix, inject over 15-30 sec with bevel of needle upward

SIDE EFFECTS

CNS: Dizziness, seizures, leukoencephalopathy, headache, confusion, hemiparesis, malaise, fatigue, chills, fever; arachnoiditis (intrathecal)

EENT: Blurred vision, optic neuropathy
GI: *Nausea, vomiting, anorexia, diarrhea, ulcerative stomatitis,* **hepatotoxicity,** cramps, ulcer, gastritis, **GI hemorrhage,** abdominal pain, hematemesis, **hepatic fibrosis, acute toxicity**
GU: Urinary retention, **renal failure,** menstrual irregularities, defective spermatogenesis, **hematuria, azotemia, uric acid nephropathy**
HEMA: **Leukopenia, thrombocytopenia, myelosuppression, anemia**
INTEG: *Rash, alopecia,* dry skin, urticaria, photosensitivity, folliculitis, vasculitis, petechiae, ecchymosis, acne, alopecia, **severe fatal skin reaction**
RESP: **Methotrexate-induced lung disease**
SYST: **Sudden death,** *Pneumocystis jiroveci,* **tumor lysis syndrome**

PHARMACOKINETICS

Not metabolized; excreted in urine (unchanged); crosses placenta, blood-brain barrier; 50% plasma protein bound; terminal half-life 10-12 hr
PO: Readily absorbed
PO/IM/IV: Onset, duration unknown
IT: Onset, peak, duration unknown

INTERACTIONS

Increase: toxicity—salicylates, sulfa products, other antineoplastics, radiation, alcohol, probenecid, NSAIDs, phenylbutazone, theophylline, penicillins
Increase: hypoprothrombinemia—oral anticoagulants
Decrease: effect of oral digoxin, vaccines, phenytoin, fosphenytoin
Decrease: effect of methotrexate—folic acid supplements

NURSING CONSIDERATIONS

Assess:

- Make sure product is taken weekly in RA, JRA

⚠ **CBC, differential, platelet count weekly; withhold product if WBC is <3500/mm³ or platelet count is <100,000/mm³; notify prescriber; WBC, platelet nadirs occur on day 7**

Black Box Warning: Renal disease: avoid use in renal failure, BUN, serum uric acid, urine CCr, electrolytes before, during therapy; I&O ratio; report fall in urine output to <30 ml/hr

- Monitor temp; fever may indicate beginning infection; no rectal temp
- Hepatic studies before and during therapy: bilirubin, alk phos, AST, ALT; liver biopsy should be done before start of therapy (psoriasis)
- Bleeding time, coagulation time during treatment; bleeding: hematuria, guaiac, bruising, or petechiae in mucosa or orifices
- Effects of alopecia on body image; discuss feelings about body changes

Black Box Warning: Pulmonary toxicity: those with ascites or pleural effusion at greater risk for toxicity; fluid should be removed before treatment; monitor plasma methotrexate levels

Black Box Warning: Tumor lysis syndrome: hyperkalemia, hyperphosphatemia, hyperuricemia, hypocalcemia, decreased urine output; use aggressive hydration, allopurinol to correct severe electrolyte imbalances, renal toxicity

⚠ **Hepatotoxicity: jaundiced skin and sclera, dark urine, clay-colored stools, pruritus, abdominal pain, fever, diarrhea**

- Monitor methotrexate levels, adjust leucovorin dose based on level
- Buccal cavity for dryness, sores, ulceration, white patches, oral pain, bleeding, dysphagia

⚠ **Severe allergic reaction:** rash, urticaria, itching, flushing

- **Rheumatoid arthritis:** ROM, pain, joint swelling before, during treatment
- **Psoriasis:** skin lesions before, during treatment

Perform/provide:

- Increased fluid intake to 2-3 L/day to prevent urate deposits, calculi formation unless contraindicated

M

• Rinsing of mouth tid-qid with water, club soda; brushing of teeth bid-tid with soft brush or cotton-tipped applicators for stomatitis; use unwaxed dental floss
• Storage in tightly closed container in cool environment; store injection, powder for inj in dark, dry area

Evaluate:
• Therapeutic response: decreased tumor size, spread of malignancy; decreased joint inflammation, pain in RA

Teach patient/family:
• To report any complaints, side effects to nurse or prescriber: black tarry stools, chills, fever, sore throat, bleeding, bruising, cough, SOB, dark or bloody urine, seizures
• That hair may be lost during treatment; that wig or hairpiece may make patient feel better; that new hair may be different in color, texture (alopecia rare)
• To avoid foods with citric acid, hot or rough texture if stomatitis is present
• To report stomatitis and any bleeding, white spots, ulcerations in mouth to prescriber; to examine mouth daily; to report symptoms to nurse; to use good oral hygiene

Black Box Warning: That contraceptive measures are recommended during therapy and for at least 8 wk after cessation of therapy; to discontinue breastfeeding; that toxicity to infant may occur; pregnancy (X)

• To drink 10-12 glasses of fluid/day
• To avoid alcohol, salicylates, live vaccines
• To avoid use of razors, commercial mouthwash
• To use sunblock to prevent burns

methoxy polyethylene glycol-epoetin beta (Rx)

(meth-ox′ee pol′ee-eth′i-leen glye′kol-e-poe′e-tin bay′ta)

Mircera

Func. class.: Antianemic, biologic modifier, hormone

Chem. class.: Amino acid polypeptide

ACTION: Erythropoietin is 1 factor that controls the rate of red cell production; product is developed with recombinant DNA technology

USES: Anemia caused by reduced endogenous erythropoietin production, primarily end-stage renal disease; to correct hemostatic defect of uremia for all dosages

CONTRAINDICATIONS: Red cell aplasia, neoplastic disease, hypersensitivity to mannitol, uncontrolled hypertension

Black Box Warning: Hgb >12 g/dl

Precautions: Pregnancy (C), breastfeeding, children <1 mo, multidose preserved formulation contains benzyl alcohol and should not be used in premature infants, seizure disorder, porphyria, CV disease, hemodialysis, latex allergy, surgery, hypertension, history of CABG

Black Box Warning: Neoplastic disease

DOSAGE AND ROUTES

For all dosages

• **Adult and geriatric:** reduce by 25% if Hgb >1 g/dl during any 2-wk period or if Hgb close to 12 g/dl; if Hgb continues to rise after decrease, hold until Hgb starts to decrease

Treatment of anemia in chronic renal failure (dialysis dependent/independent), not currently using ESA

• **Adult and geriatric: IV/SUBCUT** 0.6 mcg q2wk

Using >80 mcg/wk darbepoetin or >16,000 units/wk epoetin
- **Adult and geriatric: IV/SUBCUT** 180 mcg q2wk or 360 mcg q4wk

Using 40-80 mcg/wk darbepoetin or 8000-16,000 units/wk epoetin
- **Adult and geriatric: IV/SUBCUT** 100 mcg q2wk or 200 mcg q4wk

Using <40 mcg/wk darbepoetin or <8000 units/wk epoetin
- **Adult and geriatric: IV/SUBCUT** 60 mcg q2wk or 120 mcg q4wk

Administer:
- Do not shake vial
- Iron supplements as needed; adequate iron stores are needed for product to work properly

SUBCUT route
- Inject into outer aspect of upper arms, abdomen (except for 2 inches around navel) or front aspect of middle thigh; do not inject in areas that have stretch marks or that are scarred or bruised
- Rotate inj sites

Direct IV route
- Additional heparin to lower chance of clots
- By direct inj or bolus into venous line at end of dialysis

Solution compatibilities: Do not dilute or administer with other solutions

SIDE EFFECTS

CNS: Seizures, encephalopathy, headache
CV: *Hypertension,* edema, heart failure, hypotension, sinus tachycardia, stroke, MI
GI: Diarrhea
HEMA: Anemia, red cell aplasia, thrombocytopenia, thromboembolism, thrombosis
INTEG: Pruritus, rash, erythema, inj site reaction
MS: Muscle spasms, back pain
SYST: Antibody formation

PHARMACOKINETICS

SUBCUT: Half-life 139 6 67 hr; rise in reticulocytes on day 7, rise in Hgb after 7-14 days
IV: Half-life 134 6 65 hr

INTERACTIONS

- Adverse reactions: other erythropoiesis-stimulating agents (ESA) (epoetin, darbepoetin)

Increase: action of methoxy polyethylene glycol-epoetin—androgens

NURSING CONSIDERATIONS

Assess:
- Renal studies: urinalysis, protein, blood, BUN, creatinine; I&O, report drop in output <50 ml/hr

Black Box Warning: CBC, blood studies: ferritin, transferrin monthly; transferrin ≥20%, ferritin ≥100 ng/ml; Hct 2×/wk until stabilized in target range (30%-36%) then at regular intervals; those with endogenous erythropoietin levels of <500 units/L respond to this product; monitor Hct 2×/wk in patients with chronic renal failure; patients treated with zidovudine or patients with cancer should be monitored weekly then periodically after stabilization

⚠ Death may occur with Hgb >12 g/dl
- B/P; check for rising B/P as Hct rises, antihypertensives may be needed; hypertension may occur rapidly, leading to hypertensive encephalopathy
- CNS symptoms: for seizures if Hct is increased within 2 wk by 4 pts
- **Hypersensitivity reactions:** skin rashes, urticaria (rare), antibody development

⚠ **Pure cell aplasia** in absence of other causes, evaluate by testing sera for recombinant erythropoetin antibodies; any loss of response to epoetin should be evaluated
- Dialysis patients: thrill, bruit of shunts; monitor for circulation impairment

Evaluate:
• Therapeutic response: increase in reticulocyte count after 2-6 wk, Hgb/Hct; increased appetite, enhanced sense of wellbeing
Teach patient/family:
• To avoid driving or hazardous activity during beginning of treatment
• To monitor B/P
• To take iron supplements, vit B_{12}, folic acid as directed

methylcellulose (OTC)

(meth-ill-sell′yoo-lose)

Citrucel, Equaline Fiber Therapy, Fiber Therapy, Leader Fiber Therapy, Walgreens Fiber Therapy

Func. class.: Laxative, bulk forming
Chem. class.: Hydrophilic semisynthetic cellulose derivative

Do not confuse:
Citrucel/Citracal

ACTION: Attracts water, expands in intestine to increase peristalsis; absorbs excess water in stool; decreases diarrhea

USES: Chronic constipation

CONTRAINDICATIONS: Hypersensitivity, GI obstruction, hepatitis

DOSAGE AND ROUTES

• **Adult: PO** ≤6 g/day in divided doses
• **Child 6-12 yr: PO** 3 g/day in divided doses

Available forms: Powder 105 mg/g, 196 mg/g; tab 500 mg
Administer:
PO route
• Alone for better absorption; do not take within 1 hr of other products
• In AM or PM (oral dose)

SIDE EFFECTS

GI: Obstruction, abdominal distention

PHARMACOKINETICS

PO: Onset 12-24 hr, peak 1-3 days

INTERACTIONS

Decrease: absorption—digoxin, nitrofurantoin, salicylates, tetracyclines, oral anticoagulants
Drug/Herb
Increase: laxative action—flax senna

NURSING CONSIDERATIONS

Assess:
• Blood, urine electrolytes if used often
• I&O ratio to identify fluid loss
• Cause of constipation; lack of fluids, bulk, exercise, constipating products
• Cramping, rectal bleeding, nausea, vomiting; product should be discontinued
Evaluate:
• Therapeutic response: decrease in constipation
Teach patient/family:
• To mix powder in water, take with full glass of water
• To increase fluid intake
• That normal bowel movements do not always occur daily
• Not to use in presence of abdominal pain, nausea, vomiting
• To notify prescriber if constipation unrelieved or if symptoms of electrolyte imbalance occur: muscle cramps, pain, weakness, dizziness, excessive thirst

methyldopa/ methyldopate (Rx)

(meth-ill-doe′pa)

Apo-Methyldopa ✱

Func. class.: Antihypertensive
Chem. class.: Centrally acting α-adrenergic inhibitor

Do not confuse:
methyldopa/L-dopa/levodopa

ACTION: Stimulates central inhibitory α-adrenergic receptors or acts as false transmitter, resulting in reduction of arterial pressure

USES:
Hypertension, hypertensive crisis

CONTRAINDICATIONS:
Active hepatic disease, hypersensitivity

Precautions: Pregnancy (B), geriatric patients, cardiac disease, autoimmune disease, depression, dialysis, hemolytic anemia, Parkinson's disease, pheochromocytoma, sulfite hypersensitivity

DOSAGE AND ROUTES

- **Adult: PO** 250-500 mg bid or tid then adjusted q2days as needed, 0.5-2 g/day in 2-4 divided doses (maintenance), max 3 g/day; **IV** 250-500 mg in 100 ml D_5W q6hr, run over 30-60 min, max 1 g q6hr, switch to oral as soon as possible
- **Geriatric: PO** 125 mg bid-tid, increase q2days as needed, max 3 g/day
- **Child: PO** 10 mg/kg/day in 2-4 divided doses, max 65 mg/kg or 3 g/day, whichever is less; **IV** 20-40 mg/kg/day in 4 divided doses, max 65 mg/kg or 3 g, whichever is less

Available forms: *Methyldopa:* tabs 250, 500 mg; *methyldopate:* inj 50 mg/ml

Administer:

Intermittent IV INF route

- After diluting with 100 ml D_5W; run over 1/2-1 hr

Y-site compatibilities: Alfentanil, amikacin, aminophylline, anidulafungin, ascorbic acid, atenolol, atracurium, atropine, aztreonam, benztropine, bivalirudin, bleomycin, bumetanide, buprenorphine, butorphanol, calcium chloride/gluconate, caspofungin, cefamandole, ceFAZolin, cefmetazole, cefonicid, cefotaxime, cefotetan, cefoxitin, ceftazidime, ceftizoxime, cefTRIAXone, cefuroxime, cephalothin, chlorproMAZINE, cimetidine, clindamycin, cyanocobalamin, cycloSPORINE, DACTINomycin, DAPTOmycin, dexamethasone, digoxin, diltiazem, diphenhydrAMINE, docetaxel, DOPamine, doxycycline, enalaprilat, ePHEDrine, EPINEPHrine, epoetin alfa, ertapenem, erythromycin, esmolol, etoposide, etoposide phosphate, famotidine, fenoldopam, fentaNYL, fluconazole, fludarabine, gatifloxacin, gemcitabine, gentamicin, glycopyrrolate, granisetron, heparin, hydrocortisone, HYDROmorphone, hydrOXYzine, IDArubicin, insulin (regular), irinotecan, isoproterenol, labetalol, lidocaine, linezolid, LORazepam, magnesium sulfate, mannitol, mechlorethamine, meperidine, metaraminol, methicillin, methoxamine, methylPREDNISolone, metoclopramide, metoprolol, metroNIDAZOLE, mezlocillin, miconazole, midazolam, milrinone, minocycline, mitoxantrone, morphine, moxalactam, multiple vitamins, mycophenolate mofetil, nafcillin, nalbuphine, naloxone, netilmicin, nitroglycerin, nitroprusside, norepinephrine, octreotide, ondansetron, oxacillin, oxaliplatin, oxytocin, paclitaxel, palonosetron, pamidronate, pancuronium, pantoprazole, papaverine, pemetrexed, penicillin G potassium/sodium, pentazocine, phentolamine, phenylephrine, phytonadione, piperacillin, polymyxin B, potassium chloride, procainamide, prochlorperazine, promethazine, propranolol, protamine, pyridoxine, quiNIDine, ranitidine, ritodrine, sodium bicarbonate, succinylcholine, SUFentanil, tacrolimus, teniposide, theophylline, thiamine, thiotepa, ticarcillin, ticarcillin-clavulanate, tigecycline, tirofiban, tobramycin, tolazoline, trimetaphan, urokinase, vancomycin, vasopressin, vecuronium, verapamil, vinorelbine, voriconazole, zoledronic acid

M

SIDE EFFECTS

CNS: *Drowsiness, weakness, dizziness, sedation, headache,* depression, psychosis paresthesias, parkinsonism, Bell's palsy, nightmares

CV: Bradycardia, **myocarditis,** orthostatic hypotension, angina, edema, weight gain, **CHF,** paradoxic pressor response (IV)

EENT: Nasal congestion

ENDO: Breast enlargement, gynecomastia, amenorrhea
GI: Nausea, vomiting, diarrhea, constipation, **hepatic dysfunction**, sore or "black" tongue, **pancreatitis**, colitis, flatulence
GU: Impotence, failure to ejaculate
HEMA: **Leukopenia, thrombocytopenia, hemolytic anemia, granulocytopenia,** positive Coombs' test
INTEG: Rash, **toxic epidermal necrolysis,** lupuslike syndrome

PHARMACOKINETICS

PO: Peak 2-4 hr, duration 12-24 hr
IV: Peak 2 hr, duration 10-16 hr
Metabolized by liver, excreted in urine, half-life 2 hr

INTERACTIONS

- Lithium toxicity: lithium

⚠ **Increase: pressor effect—sympathomimetic amines, MAOIs; do not use concurrently with MAOIs**
Increase: hypotension, CNS toxicity—levodopa
Increase: hypotension—diuretics, other antihypertensives
Increase: psychosis—haloperidol
Increase: CNS depression—alcohol, antihistamines, antidepressants, analgesics, sedative/hypnotics
Increase: B/P—phenothiazines, β-blockers, amphetamines, NSAIDs, tricyclics, barbiturates
Increase: hypoglycemia—TOLBUTamide
Decrease: methyldopa absorption—iron
Drug/Lab Test
Interference: urinary uric acid, serum creatinine, AST
False increase: urinary catecholamines

NURSING CONSIDERATIONS

Assess:

- Blood studies: neutrophils, decreased platelets
- Direct Coombs' test before, after 6, 12 mo of therapy
- Baselines of renal, hepatic studies before therapy begins
- B/P when beginning treatment, periodically thereafter; report significant changes
- **Allergic reaction:** rash, fever, pruritus, urticaria; product should be discontinued if antihistamines fail to help
- CNS symptoms, especially in geriatric patients; depression, change in mental status
- **CHF:** edema, dyspnea, wet crackles, B/P
- Renal symptoms: polyuria, oliguria, urinary frequency; I&O ratio, weight; report weight gain >5 lb

Perform/provide:

- Storage of tabs in tight container

Evaluate:

- Therapeutic response: decrease in B/P with hypertension

Teach patient/family:

- To avoid hazardous activities
- Not to discontinue product abruptly because withdrawal symptoms may occur: anxiety, increased B/P, headache, insomnia, increased pulse, tremors, nausea, sweating
- Not to use OTC (cough, cold, allergy) products unless directed by prescriber
- To comply with dosage schedule even if feeling better
- To rise slowly to sitting or standing position to minimize orthostatic hypotension
- To notify prescriber of mouth sores, sore throat, fever, swelling of hands or feet, irregular heartbeat, chest pain, signs of angioedema
- That excessive perspiration, dehydration, vomiting, diarrhea may lead to fall in B/P; to consult prescriber
- That dizziness, fainting, lightheadedness may occur during first few days of therapy
- That compliance is necessary; not to skip or stop product unless directed by prescriber
- That product may cause skin rash or impaired perspiration

TREATMENT OF OVERDOSE:

Gastric evacuation, sympathomimetics may be indicated; if severe, hemodialysis

methylergonovine (Rx)

(meth-ill-er-goe-noe′veen)

Methergine

Func. class.: Oxytocic

Chem. class.: Ergot alkaloid

ACTION: Stimulates uterine, vascular, and smooth muscle, thereby causing contractions; decreases bleeding; arterial vasoconstriction

USES: Treatment of hemorrhage postpartum or postabortion, uterine contractions

CONTRAINDICATIONS: Pregnancy, hypertension, PID, respiratory/cardiac disease, peripheral vascular disease, angina, arteriosclerosis, CAD, dysfunctional uterine bleeding, eclampsia, MI, neonates, Raynaud's disease, sepsis, stroke, Buerger's disease, thrombophlebitis, hypersensitivity to ergot preparations

Precautions: Pregnancy (C), severe renal/hepatic disease, jaundice, diabetes mellitus, seizure disorders, sepsis, CAD

DOSAGE AND ROUTES

- **Adult: PO** 200 mcg tid-qid × ≤7 days; **IM/IV** 200 mcg q2-4hr × 1-5 doses

Available forms: Inj 200 mcg/ml; tabs 200 mcg

Administer:

- Only during 4th stage of labor; not to be used to augment labor
- IM in deep muscle mass; rotate inj sites for additional doses

Direct IV route

- Undiluted through Y-tube or 3-way stopcock; give ≤0.2 mg/min or diluted in 5 ml 0.9% NaCl given through Y-site
- With crash cart available on unit; IV route used only in emergencies

Y-site compatibilities: Heparin, hydrocortisone sodium succinate, potassium chloride, vit B/C

SIDE EFFECTS

CNS: *Headache, dizziness,* seizures

CV: Hypotension, chest pain, palpitation, **hypertension, dysrhythmias, CVA (IV)**

EENT: Tinnitus

GI: *Nausea, vomiting*

GU: Cramping

INTEG: Sweating, rash, allergic reactions

RESP: Dyspnea

PHARMACOKINETICS

Metabolized in liver, excreted in urine

PO: Onset 5-25 min, duration 3 hr

IM: Onset 2-5 min, duration 3 hr

IV: Onset immediate, duration 45 min

INTERACTIONS

Increase: vasoconstriction—vasopressors, nicotine

NURSING CONSIDERATIONS

Assess:

- B/P, pulse, character and amount of vaginal bleeding; watch for indications of hemorrhage
- Uterine relaxation; observe for severe cramping

⚠ **Ergot toxicity: tinnitus, hypertension, palpitations, chest pain, nausea, vomiting, weakness; cold, numb extremities**

Perform/provide:

- Refrigerated storage of ampules; protect from light; give only if solution is clear, colorless

Evaluate:

- Therapeutic response: absence of hemorrhage

Teach patient/family:

- To report increased blood loss, severe abdominal cramps, fever or foul-smelling lochia
- To avoid smoking
- Not to breastfeed while taking this product

M

methylnaltrexone (Rx)

(meth-il-nal-trex′one)

Relistor

Func. class.: Opioid antagonist

ACTION: Peripheral μ-opioid receptor antagonist that reduces constipation associated with opiate agonists

USES: Treatment of opioid-induced constipation in patients with advanced illness who are receiving palliative care when response to laxative therapy has been insufficient

Unlabeled uses: Pruritus; nausea, vomiting related to morphine; urinary retention from opioids

CONTRAINDICATIONS: Hypersensitivity, GI obstruction, IV route

Precautions: Pregnancy (B), breastfeeding, children, geriatric patients, renal disease, diarrhea, driving, operating machinery, neoplastic disease, Crohn's disease, peptic ulcer, ulcerative colitis

DOSAGE AND ROUTES

Opiate-agonist–induced constipation

- **Adult >114 kg: SUBCUT** 0.15 mg/kg every other day prn
- **Adult 62-114 kg: SUBCUT** 12 mg every other day prn
- **Adult 38-<62 kg: SUBCUT** 8 mg every other day prn
- **Adult <38 kg: SUBCUT** 0.15 mg/kg every other day prn

Renal dose

- **Adult: SUBCUT** CCr <30 ml/min, reduce normal adult dose by 50%

Pruritus, nausea, and vomiting related to morphine (unlabeled) (oral dose investigational)

- **Adult: PO** 19.2 mg/kg 20 min prior to morphine

Available forms: Sol for inj 12 mg/0.6 ml

Administer:

- SUBCUT only; oral dose investigational, not currently available
- Do not give IV; IV dosing for urinary retention investigational

SUBCUT route

- Inspect sol before use; should be clear, colorless to pale yellow aqueous sol; do not use if particulate matter or discoloration are present
- Withdraw needed amount of sol into sterile syringe; if immediate administration is impossible, syringe may be kept at room temp for ≤24 hr; syringe does not need to be kept away from light during the 24-hr period; immediately discard any unused portion in vial; no preservatives are present
- Administer into upper arm, abdomen, or thigh ≤1×/24 hr; rotate inj sites; do not inject same spot each time; do not inject into areas where skin is tender, bruised, red, or hard; avoid areas with scars or stretch marks
- If using with retractable needle, slowly push down on plunger past resistance point until the syringe is empty and click is heard

SIDE EFFECTS

CNS: Dizziness

GI: Nausea, vomiting, diarrhea, flatulence, abdominal pain

INTEG: Hyperhidrosis

PHARMACOKINETICS

Terminal half-life 8 hr, protein binding 11%-15.3%; renal impairment has marked effect on renal excretion of methylnaltrexone; dose adjustment is required for patients with CCr <30 ml/min; renal clearance decreased and total systemic exposure increased in patients with severe renal impairment who receive single SUBCUT dose of 0.3 mg/kg

SUBCUT: Peak 30 min

NURSING CONSIDERATIONS

Assess:
- Serum creatinine
- Stool characteristics, bowel sounds during treatment

Perform/provide:
- Storage at 15° C-30° C (59° F-86° F); do not freeze
- Storage away from light

Evaluate:
- Therapeutic response: decreasing constipation

Teach patient/family:
- Not to drive or operate machinery until effect is known
- That, after 30 min, to remain near toilet facilities because bowel relaxation occurs
- To notify prescriber of abdominal pain, continuous or severe diarrhea, nausea, vomiting

methylphenidate (Rx)

(meth-ill-fen′i-date)

Apo-Methylphenidate ✱, Biphentin ✱, Concerta, Daytrana, Metadate CD, Metadate ER, Methylin, PMS-Methylphenidate ✱, Ritalin, Ritalin LA, Ritalin SR

Func. class.: Cerebral stimulant
Chem. class.: Piperidine derivative

Controlled Substance Schedule II

Do not confuse:
methylphenidate/methadone

ACTION: Increases release of norepinephrine, dopamine in cerebral cortex to reticular activating system; exact action not known

USES: Attention deficit disorder (ADD), attention-deficit/hyperactivity disorder (ADHD); narcolepsy (except Concerta, Metadate CD, Ritalin LA)

CONTRAINDICATIONS: Children <6 yr, hypersensitivity, anxiety, history of Gilles de la Tourette's syndrome; glaucoma, anorexia nervosa, tartrazine dye hypersensitivity

Precautions: Pregnancy (C), breastfeeding, hypertension, depression, seizures

Black Box Warning: Substance abuse

DOSAGE AND ROUTES

Attention-deficit/hyperactivity disorder (ADHD) initial treatment, not currently on methylphenidate

Regular release: Ritalin, Methylin, Methylin oral sol, Methylin chew tabs
- **Adult: PO** 20-30 mg/day, range 10-60 mg/day in 2-3 divided doses, 30-45 min before meals
- **Child ≥6 yr: PO** 5 mg bid initially, increase 5-10 mg/day weekly, usual dose 0.3-2 mg/kg/day, max 60 mg/day

Extended release: Ritalin SR, Metadate ER, Methylin ER
- **Adult/adolescent/child ≥6 yr: PO** max 20-30 mg tid

Extended-release once-daily tabs: Concerta
- **Adult: PO** 18-36 mg/day initially then adjust by 18 mg/wk, max 72 mg/day
- **Adolescent: PO** 18 mg/day initially then adjust by 18 mg/wk, max 72 mg/day
- **Child ≥6 yr: PO** 18 mg/day initially then adjust by 18 mg/wk, max 54 mg/day

Extended-release once-daily capsules: Ritalin LA
- **Adult/adolescent/child ≥6 yr: PO** 20 mg q day in AM initially, adjust by 10 mg/wk, max 60 mg/day

Extended-release once-daily capsules: Metadate CD
- **Adult/adolescent/child ≥6 yr: PO** 20 mg/day in AM, adjust by 20 mg/wk, max 60 mg/day

Transdermal: Daytrana

• **Adolescent/child ≥6 yr: TD** wk 1: 10 mg/day (9-mg patch); wk 2: 15 mg/day (9-mg patch); wk 3: 20 mg/day (9-mg patch); wk 4: 30 mg/day (9-mg patch)

Conversion to once-daily treatment from other forms for ADHD

Extended-release once-daily capsules: Metadate CD

• **Adult/adolescent/child ≥6 yr: PO** give no more than total daily dose of other forms, may adjust by 20 mg/wk, max 60 mg/day

Extended-release once-daily capsules: Ritalin LA

• **Adult/adolescent/child ≥6 yr: PO** give no more than total daily dose of other forms, may adjust by 10 mg/wk, max 60 mg/day

Extended-release once-daily tablets: Concerta

• **Adult/adolescent/child ≥6 yr (currently on 10-15 mg/day): PO** 18 mg q AM initially, adjust by 18 mg/wk, max 72 mg/day (adult); max 72 mg/day, 2 mg/kg/day (adolescent); 54 mg/day (child) mg/day

• **Adult/adolescent/child ≥6 yr (currently receiving 20-30 mg/day): PO** 36 mg every AM, adjust by 18 mg/wk, max 72 mg/day (adult); 72 mg/day, 2 mg/kg/day (adolescent); 54 mg/day (child)

• **Adult/adolescent/child ≥6 yr (currently receiving 30-45 mg/day): PO** 54 mg every AM, adjust by 18 mg/wk, max 72 mg/day (adult); 72 mg/day, 2 mg/kg/day (adolescent); 54 mg/day (child)

• **Adult/adolescent/child ≥6 yr (currently receiving 40-60 mg/day): PO** 72 mg every AM, 72 mg/day

Transdermal: Daytrana

• **Adolescent and child ≥6 yr: TD** wk 1: 10 mg/day (9-mg patch); wk 2: 15 mg/day (9-mg patch); wk 3: 20 mg/day (9-mg patch); wk 4: 30 mg/day (9-mg patch)

Narcolepsy

Immediate release: Ritalin, Methylin oral sol, Methylin chew tabs

• **Adult: PO** 20-30 mg/day, range 10-60 mg/day in 2-3 divided doses

• **Child ≥6 yr: PO** 5 mg bid, may increase by 5-10 mg/wk, max 60 mg/day

Extended-release tabs: Ritalin SR, Metadate ER

• **Adult/adolescent/child ≥6 yr: PO** max 20 mg tid

Poststroke depression; major depression (unlabeled)

• **Adult and geriatric: PO** (immediate rel tabs) 2.5 mg bid, may increase by 2.5-5 mg q2-3days

Available forms: Tabs 5, 10, 20 mg; ext rel tabs 10, 20, mg; ext rel tabs (Concerta) 18, 27, 36, 54 mg; ext rel caps 10, 20, 30, 40 mg; oral sol 5 mg, 10 mg/ml; chew tabs (Methylin) 2.5, 5, 10 mg; transdermal patch 12.5 cm^2 (10 mg), 18.75 cm^2 (15 mg), 25 cm^2 (20 mg), 37.5 cm^2 (30 mg)

Administer:

PO route

• Do not crush, chew ext rel product; caps may be opened, beads sprinkled over spoonful of applesauce; give without regard to meals

• Gum, hard candy, frequent sips of water for dry mouth

• Give immediate rel dose 30-45 min before meals

• Chew tab with adequate water to prevent choking; contains phenylalanine

• Avoid metadate CD on day of surgery

Transdermal route

• Place on clean, dry area of hip; avoid waist; remove 9 hr after application; fold after removal, flush down toilet

• If patch falls off, apply new patch to different site; total wear time should be 9 hr

SIDE EFFECTS

CNS: *Hyperactivity, insomnia, restlessness, talkativeness,* dizziness, drowsiness, toxic psychosis, headache, akathisia, dyskinesia, masking or worsening of

Gilles de la Tourette's syndrome, seizures, hallucinations, **malignant neuroleptic syndrome, aggression; cerebral vasculitis, hemorrhage, stroke (rare)**
CV: *Palpitations, tachycardia,* B/P changes, **angina, dysrhythmias**
ENDO: Growth retardation
GI: Nausea, anorexia, dry mouth, weight loss, abdominal pain
HEMA: Leukopenia, anemia, thrombocytopenic purpura
INTEG: Exfoliative dermatitis, urticaria, rash, erythema multiforme, **hypersensitivity reactions**
MISC: Fever, arthralgia, scalp hair loss

PHARMACOKINETICS

PO: Onset ½-1 hr, duration 4-6 hr, metabolized by liver, excreted by kidneys, half-life 3-4 hr

INTERACTIONS

- Hypertensive crisis: MAOIs or within 14 days of MAOIs, vasopressors

Increase: effects of tricyclics, SSRIs, anticonvulsants, SNRIs, CNS stimulants
Decrease: effect of antihypertensives
Drug/Herb
Increase: CNS stimulation—cola nut, guarana, horsetail, yerba maté, yohimbe
Drug/Food
Increase: stimulation—caffeine

NURSING CONSIDERATIONS

Assess:

- **ADHD:** attention span, decreased hyperactivity
- VS, B/P; may reverse antihypertensives; check patients with cardiac disease more often for increased B/P
- CBC with differential, platelets, LFTs, urinalysis; in diabetes: blood glucose, urine glucose; insulin changes may have to be made because eating will decrease
- Height, growth rate q3mo in children; growth rate may be decreased
- Mental status: mood, sensorium, affect, stimulation, insomnia, aggressiveness

⚠ **Withdrawal symptoms: headache, nausea, vomiting, muscle pain, weakness**

- Appetite, sleep, speech patterns
- **Narcolepsy:** identify frequency, length of narcoleptic episodes

Evaluate:

- Therapeutic response: decreased hyperactivity (ADHD); increased ability to stay awake (narcolepsy)

Teach patient/family:

- To decrease caffeine consumption (coffee, tea, cola, chocolate), may increase irritability, stimulation; not to use guarana, yerba maté, cola nut
- To avoid OTC preparations unless approved by prescriber
- To taper off product over several weeks because depression, increased sleeping, lethargy will occur
- To avoid driving, hazardous activities if dizziness, blurred vision occur
- To avoid alcohol
- To avoid hazardous activities until stabilized on medication
- To get needed rest; patients will feel more tired at end of day
- That shell of Concerta tab may appear in stools
- To take regular tab at least 6 hr prior to sleep, 10 hr for ext rel, use dosing syringe to measure liquid; do not use household teaspoon
- That, for transdermal patch, after tray is opened, use within 2 mo; do not store patches without protective patch

TREATMENT OF OVERDOSE:

Administer fluids; hemodialysis or peritoneal dialysis; antihypertensive for increased B/P; administer short-acting barbiturate before lavage

methylPREDNISolone (Rx)

(meth-il-pred-niss′oh-lone)

A-Methapred, Depo-Medrol, Medrol, Solu-Medrol

Func. class.: Corticosteroid, synthetic

Chem. class.: Glucocorticoid, immediate acting

Do not confuse:
methylPREDNISolone/predniSONE/medroxyPROGESTERone/methylTESTOSTERone

ACTION: Decreases inflammation by suppression of migration of polymorphonuclear leukocytes, fibroblasts; reversal of increased capillary permeability and lysosomal stabilization

USES: Severe inflammation, shock, adrenal insufficiency, collagen disorders, management of acute spinal cord injury, multiple sclerosis

Unlabeled uses: Multiple myeloma, bronchospasm prophylaxis, airway-obstructing hemangioma, noncardiogenic pulmonary edema, idiopathic pulmonary fibrosis, carpal tunnel syndrome, temporal arteritis, Churg-Strauss syndrome, mixed connective-tissue disease, polyarteritis nodosa, relapsing polychondritis, polymyalgia rheumatica, vasculitis, Wegener's granulomatosis, *Pneumocystis jiroveci* pneumonia in AIDS patients, acute spinal cord injury, severe acute respiratory syndrome (SARS), acute interstitial nephritis

CONTRAINDICATIONS: Hypersensitivity, Cushing's syndrome, measles, varicella, fungal infections

Precautions: Pregnancy (C), breastfeeding, diabetes mellitus, glaucoma, osteoporosis, seizure disorders, ulcerative colitis, CHF, myasthenia gravis, renal disease, esophagitis, peptic ulcer, tartrazine, benzyl alcohol, corticosteroid hypersensitivity, viral infection, TB, traumatic brain injury

DOSAGE AND ROUTES

Adrenal insufficiency/inflammation

- **Adult: PO** 4-48 mg in 4 divided doses; **IM** 10-80 mg (acetate); **IM/IV** 10-250 mg (succinate); **INTRAARTICULAR** 4-80 mg (acetate)
- **Child: IV** 0.5-1.7 mg/kg in 3-4 divided doses (succinate)

Shock

- **Adult: IV** 100-250 mg q2-6hr or 30 mg/kg then q4-6hr prn for 2-3 days (succinate)

Multiple sclerosis

- **Adult: PO** 160 mg/day × 1 wk then 64 mg every other day × 30 days

Multiple myeloma/temporal arteritis/Churg-Strauss syndrome/mixed connective-tissue disease/polyarteritis nodosa/relapsing polychondritis/polymyalgia rheumatica/vasculitis/Wegener's granulomatosis (unlabeled)

- **Adult: PO** 4-48 mg/day in 4 divided doses; **IM** 10-120 mg (acetate); **IV** 10-40 mg over several min (sodium succinate)
- **Child: PO/IM** 0.5-1.7 mg/kg or 5-25 mg/m^2/day in divided doses q6-12hr

Bronchospasm prophylaxis (unlabeled)

- **Adult and adolescent: PO/IV** 40-80 mg/day in 1-2 divided doses
- **Child: PO/IV** 1 mg/kg in 2 divided doses (max 60 mg)

Airway-obstructing hemangioma (unlabeled)

- **Child: PO** 0.5-1.7 mg/kg or 5-25 mg/m^2/day in divided doses q6-12hr

Idiopathic pulmonary fibrosis (unlabeled)

- **Adult: IV** 1-2 g/wk or every other week

Carpal tunnel syndrome (unlabeled)

- **Adult: INJ** (local) 40-80 mg as a single inj

Available forms: Tabs 2, 4, 8, 16, 24, 32 mg; inj 20, 40, 80 mg/ml acetate; inj

40, 125, 500, 1000, 2000 mg/vial succinate

Administer:

• Titrated dose; use lowest effective dose

PO route

• With food or milk to decrease GI symptoms (PO)

IM route

• IM inj deep in large muscle mass; rotate sites; avoid deltoid; use 21G needle; after shaking suspension (parenteral)

• In one dose in AM to prevent adrenal suppression; avoid SUBCUT administration; may damage tissue

⚠ **Do not give Solu-Medrol intrathecally**

Direct IV route

• Use only methylPREDNISolone sodium succinate (Solu-Medrol) IV, never use methylPREDNISolone acetate suspension IV

• After diluting with diluent provided; agitate slowly; give ≤500 mg/≥1 min

Intermittent/continuous INF route

• Dilute further in D5W, NS, D5NS; haze may form, give over 15-60 min; large dose (≥500 mg) should be given over 30-60 min

Syringe compatibilities: Granisetron, metoclopramide

Y-site compatibilities: Acyclovir, amifostine, amphotericin B cholesteryl, amrinone, aztreonam, cefepime, CISplatin, cladribine, cyclophosphamide, cytarabine, DOPamine, DOXOrubicin, enalaprilat, famotidine, fludarabine, granisetron, heparin, melphalan, meperidine, methotrexate, metroNIDAZOLE, midazolam, morphine, piperacillin/tazobactam, remifentanil, sodium bicarbonate, tacrolimus, teniposide, theophylline, thiotepa

SIDE EFFECTS

CNS: Depression, flushing, sweating, headache, mood changes

CV: Hypertension, **circulatory collapse, thrombophlebitis, embolism,** tachycardia

EENT: Fungal infections, increased intraocular pressure, blurred vision, cataracts

GI: Diarrhea, nausea, abdominal distention, **GI hemorrhage,** increased appetite, pancreatitis

HEMA: **Thrombocytopenia**

INTEG: Acne, poor wound healing, ecchymosis, petechiae

MS: Fractures, osteoporosis, weakness

PHARMACOKINETICS

Half-life >3½ hr (plasma), 18-36 hr (tissue); crosses placenta, enters breast milk in small amounts; metabolized in liver; excreted by kidneys (unchanged)

PO: Peak 1-2 hr, duration 1½ days, well absorbed

IM: Peak 4-8 days, duration 1-4 wk, well absorbed

Intraarticular: Peak 1 wk

INTERACTIONS

Increase: side effects—amphotericin B, diuretics

Increase: methylPREDNISolone action—oral contraceptives

Increase: adrenal suppression—CYP3A4 inhibitors (aprepitant, antiretroviral protease inhibitors, clarithromycin, danazol, delavirdine, diltiazem, erythromycin, fluconazole, FLUoxetine, fluvoxamine, imatinib, ketoconazole, mibefradil, nefazodone, telithromycin, voriconazole)

Decrease: methylPREDNISolone effect—CYP3A4 inducers (barbiturates, bosentan, carBAMazepine, efavirenz, phenytoins, nevirapine, rifabutin, rifampin)

Decrease: effects of antidiabetics, vaccines, somatrem

Drug/Herb

• Avoid use with St. John's wort

Drug/Food

• Do not use with grapefruit juice; level of methylPREDNISolone will be increased

Drug/Lab Test

Increase: cholesterol, sodium, blood glucose, uric acid, calcium, urine glucose

Decrease: Ca, K, T_4, T_3, thyroid ^{131}I uptake test, urine 17-OHCS, 17-KS

False negative: skin allergy tests

M

NURSING CONSIDERATIONS

Assess:

- Potassium depletion: parethesias, fatigue, nausea, vomiting, depression, polyuria, dysrhythmias, weakness
- Edema, hypertension, cardiac symptoms
- Mental status: affect, mood, behavioral changes, aggression
- Potassium, blood glucose, urine glucose while receiving long-term therapy; hypokalemia and hyperglycemia
- Joint mobility, pain, edema if product given intraarticularly
- B/P q4hr, pulse; notify prescriber of chest pain, crackles
- I&O ratio; be alert for decreasing urinary output, increasing edema; weight daily; notify prescriber of weekly gain >5 lb

⚠ **Adrenal insufficiency:** weight loss, nausea, vomiting, confusion, anxiety, hypotension, weakness; plasma cortisol levels during long-term therapy (normal level: 138-635 nmol/L SI units when drawn at 8 AM)

- Growth in children receiving long-term treatment
- **Infection:** increased temp, WBC, even after withdrawal of product; product masks infection

Perform/provide:

- Assistance with ambulation in patient with bone-tissue disease to prevent fractures

Evaluate:

- Therapeutic response: ease of respirations, decreased inflammation; decreased symptoms of adrenal insufficiency

Teach patient/family:

- To increase intake of potassium, calcium, protein
- To carry emergency ID as corticosteroid user
- To notify prescriber if therapeutic response decreases; that dosage adjustment may be needed

⚠ Not to discontinue abruptly because adrenal crisis can result

- To avoid OTC products: salicylates, alcohol in cough products, cold preparations unless directed by prescriber; to avoid vaccinations because immunosuppression occurs
- To recognize symptoms of adrenal insufficiency: nausea, anorexia, fatigue, dizziness, dyspnea, weakness, joint pain

metipranolol ophthalmic

See Appendix B

metoclopramide (Rx)

(met-oh-kloe-pra′mide)

Apo-Metoclop ✦, Metozolv ODT, Nu-Metoclopramide ✦, Reglan

Func. class.: Cholinergic, antiemetic

Chem. class.: Central DOPamine receptor antagonist

Do not confuse:
metoclopramide/metolazone
Reglan/Megace/Renagel

ACTION: Enhances response to acetylcholine of tissue in upper GI tract, which causes the contraction of gastric muscle; relaxes pyloric, duodenal segments; increases peristalsis without stimulating secretions; blocks dopamine in chemoreceptor trigger zone of CNS

USES: Prevention of nausea, vomiting induced by chemotherapy, radiation, delayed gastric emptying, gastroesophageal reflux

Unlabeled uses: Hiccups, migraines, breastfeeding induction, lung cancer

CONTRAINDICATIONS: Hypersensitivity to this product, procaine, or procainamide; seizure disorder, pheochromocytoma, breast cancer (prolactin dependent), GI obstruction

Precautions: Pregnancy (B), breastfeeding, GI hemorrhage, CHF, Parkinson's disease

Black Box Warning: Tardive dyskinesia

DOSAGE AND ROUTES

Nausea/vomiting (chemotherapy)

- **Adult: IV** 1-2 mg/kg 30 min before administration of chemotherapy, then q2hr × 2 doses, then q3hr × 3 doses
- **Child (unlabeled): IV** 1-2 mg/kg/dose

Facilitate small-bowel intubation for radiologic exams

- **Adult and child >14 yr: IV** 10 mg over 1-2 min
- **Child <6 yr: IV** 0.1 mg/kg
- **Child 6-14 yr: IV** 2.5-5 mg

Diabetic gastroparesis

- **Adult: PO** 10 mg 30 min before meals, at bedtime × 2-8 wk
- **Geriatric: PO** 5 mg 30 min before meals, at bedtime, increase to 10 mg if needed

Gastroesophageal reflux

- **Adult: PO** 10-15 mg qid 30 min before meals and at bedtime
- **Child: PO** 0.4-0.8 mg/kg/day in 4 divided doses

Renal dose

- **Adult:** CCr <40 ml/min 50% of dose

Lactation induction (unlabeled)

- **Adult: PO** 10 mg bid-tid, may increase to 20-45 mg/day in divided doses

Non–small-cell lung cancer (NSCLC) radiation sensitizer (unlabeled)

- **Adult: IV** (Sensamide IV) 2 mg/kg given 1 hr prior to radiation therapy 3×/wk

Hiccups (unlabeled)

- **Adult: PO/IM/IV** 10 mg q6hr

Available forms: Tabs 5, 10 mg; syr 5 mg/5 ml; inj 5 mg/ml; conc sol 10 mg/ml; orally disintegrating tab 5, 10 mg

Administer:

PO route

- ½-1 hr before meals for better absorption
- Gum, hard candy, frequent rinsing of mouth for dry oral cavity
- **Oral disintegrating:** place on tongue, allow to dissolve, swallow, remove from bottle immediately before use

IM route

- Give for post-operative nausea, vomiting prior to end of surgery

Direct IV route

- DiphenhydrAMINE IV for EPS
- Undiluted if dose ≤10 mg; give over 2 min

Intermittent IV INF route

- >10 mg may be diluted in ≥50 ml D_5W, NaCl, Ringer's, LR, given over ≥15 min

Y-site compatibilities: Alfentanil, amifostine, amikacin, aminophylline, ascorbic acid, atracurium, atropine, azaTHIOprine, aztreonam, bivalirudin, bleomycin, bumetanide, buprenorphine, butorphanol, calcium chloride/gluconate, CARBOplatin, caspofungin, ceFAZolin, cefonicid, cefoperazone, cefotaxime, cefotetan, cefoxitin, ceftazidime, ceftizoxime, cefTRIAXone, cefuroxime, chloramphenicol, chlorproMAZINE, cimetidine, ciprofloxacin, cisatracurium, CISplatin, cladribine, clindamycin, cyanocobalamin, cyclophosphamide, cycloSPORINE, cytarabine, DACTINomycin, DAPTOmycin, dexamethasone, dexmedetomidine, digoxin, diltiazem, diphenhydrAMINE, DOBUTamine, docetaxel, DOPamine, doripenem, doxapram, DOXOrubicin hydrochloride, doxycycline, droperidol, enalaprilat, ePHEDrine, EPINEPHrine, epirubicin, epoetin alfa, ertapenem, erythromycin, esmolol, etoposide, etoposide phosphate, famotidine, fenoldopam, fentaNYL, filgrastim, fluconazole, fludarabine, folic acid, foscarnet, gallium nitrate, gemcitabine, gentamicin, glycopyrrolate, granisetron, heparin, hydrocortisone, HYDROmorphone, IDArubicin, ifosfamide, imipenem/cilastatin, indomethacin, insulin, isoproterenol, ketorolac, labetalol, leucovorin, levofloxacin, lidocaine, linezolid, LORazepam, magnesium sulfate, mannitol, mechlorethamine, melphalan, meperidine, meropenem, metaraminol, methadone, methotrexate, methoxamine, methyldopate, methylPREDNISolone, metoprolol, metroNIDAZOLE, miconazole, mid-

M

azolam, milrinone, minocycline, mitomycin, morphine, moxalactam, multiple vitamins, nafcillin, nalbuphine, naloxone, nesiritide, nitroglycerin, nitroprusside, norepinephrine, octreotide, ondansetron, oxaliplatin, oxytocin, paclitaxel, palonosetron, pantoprazole, papaverine, pemetrexed, penicillin G, pentamidine, pentazocine, PENTobarbital, PHENobarbital, phentolamine, phenylephrine, phytonadione, piperacillin/tazobactam, potassium chloride, procainamide, prochlorperazine, promethazine, propranolol, protamine, pyridoxine, quinupristin/dalfopristin, ranitidine, remifentanil, riTUXimab, rocuronium, sargramostim, sodium acetate/bicarbonate, succinylcholine, SUFentanil, tacrolimus, teniposide, theophylline, thiamine, thiotepa, ticarcillin/clavulanate, tigecycline, tirofiban, tobramycin, tolazoline, topotecan, trastuzumab, trimethaphan, urokinase, vancomycin, vasopressin, vecuronium, verapamil, vinBLAStine, vinCRIStine, vinorelbine, voriconazole, zidovudine

SIDE EFFECTS

CNS: *Sedation, fatigue, restlessness, headache, sleeplessness, dystonia,* dizziness, drowsiness, **suicidal ideation, seizures,** EPS, **neuroleptic malignant syndrome; tardive dyskinesia (>3 mo, high doses)**

CV: Hypotension, supraventricular tachycardia

GI: Dry mouth, constipation, nausea, anorexia, vomiting, diarrhea

GU: Decreased libido, prolactin secretion, amenorrhea, galactorrhea

HEMA: **Neutropenia, leukopenia, agranulocytosis**

INTEG: Urticaria, rash

PHARMACOKINETICS

Metabolized by liver, excreted in urine, half-life 4 hr

PO: Onset ½-1 hr, duration 1-2 hr

IM: Onset 10-15 min, duration 1-2 hr

IV: Onset 1-3 min, duration 1-2 hr

INTERACTIONS

- Avoid use with MAOIs

Increase: sedation—alcohol, other CNS depressants

Increase: risk for EPS—haloperidol, phenothiazines

Decrease: action of metoclopramide—anticholinergics, opiates

Drug/Lab Test

Increase: prolactin, aldosterone, thyrotropin

NURSING CONSIDERATIONS

Assess:

Black Box Warning: EPS, tardive dyskinesia; more likely to occur in geriatric patients

- **Neuroleptic malignant syndrome:** hyperthermia, change in B/P, pulse, tachycardia, sweating, rigidity, altered consciousness
- Mental status: depression, anxiety, irritability
- GI complaints: nausea, vomiting, anorexia, constipation

Perform/provide:

- Protect from light with aluminum foil during inf
- Discard open ampules

Evaluate:

- Therapeutic response: absence of nausea, vomiting, anorexia, fullness

Teach patient/family:

- To avoid driving, other hazardous activities until stabilized on product
- To avoid alcohol, other CNS depressants that will enhance sedating properties of this product

metolazone (Rx)

(me-tole′a-zone)

Zaroxolyn

Func. class.: Diuretic, antihypertensive

Chem. class.: Thiazide-like quinazoline derivative

Do not confuse:
metolazone/methotrexate/metoclopramide

ACTION:
Acts on distal tubule by increasing excretion of water, sodium, chloride, potassium, magnesium, bicarbonate

USES:
Edema, hypertension

Unlabeled uses: Heart failure, nephrotic syndrome

CONTRAINDICATIONS:
Hypersensitivity to thiazides, sulfonamides; anuria, coma

Black Box Warning: Hepatic encephalopathy

Precautions: Pregnancy (B), breastfeeding, geriatric patients, hypokalemia, renal/hepatic disease, gout, COPD, lupus erythematosus, diabetes mellitus, hypotension, history of pancreatitis; hypersensitivity to sulfonamides, thiazides; electrolyte imbalance

DOSAGE AND ROUTES

Edema

- **Adult: PO** 5-10 mg/day; max 20 mg/day

Hypertension

- **Adult: PO** 2.5-5 mg/day

Available forms: Tabs 2.5, 5, 10 mg

Administer:

- In AM to avoid interference with sleep if using product as diuretic
- Potassium replacement if potassium <3 mg/dl
- With food if nausea occurs; absorption may be decreased slightly
- Extended product is Zaroxolyn, prompt product is Mykrox; they are not interchangeable

SIDE EFFECTS

CNS: Anxiety, depression, *headache, dizziness, fatigue, weakness*

CV: Orthostatic hypotension, palpitations, volume depletion, hypotension, chest pain

EENT: Blurred vision

ELECT: *Hypokalemia,* hypercalcemia, hyponatremia

GI: *Nausea, vomiting, anorexia,* constipation, diarrhea, cramps, pancreatitis, GI irritation, dry mouth, jaundice

GU: *Urinary frequency,* polyuria, uremia, glucosuria, nocturia, impotence

HEMA: Aplastic anemia, hemolytic anemia, leukopenia, agranulocytosis, neutropenia

INTEG: *Rash,* urticaria, purpura, photosensitivity, fever, dry skin

META: *Hyperglycemia,* increased creatinine, BUN

MS: Muscle cramps, joint pain, swelling

PHARMACOKINETICS

Onset 1 hr, peak 2 hr, duration 12-24 hr, excreted unchanged by kidneys, crosses placenta, enters breast milk, half-life 14 hr

INTERACTIONS

Increase: hypokalemia—mezlocillin, piperacillin, amphotericin B, glucocorticoids, digoxin, stimulant laxatives

Increase: hypotension—alcohol (large amounts), nitrates, antihypertensives, barbiturates, opioids

Increase: toxicity—lithium

Increase: metolazone effects—loop diuretics

Decrease: action of metolazone—NSAIDs, salicylates

M

NURSING CONSIDERATIONS

Assess:

- Weight, I&O daily to determine fluid loss; effect of product may be decreased if used daily
- **CHF:** improvement in edema of feet, legs, sacral area daily if product being used
- Rate, depth, rhythm of respiration, effect of exertion
- **Hypertension:** B/P lying, standing; postural hypotension may occur
- Electrolytes: potassium, magnesium, sodium, chloride; include BUN, blood glucose, CBC, serum creatinine, blood pH, ABGs, uric acid, calcium
- Improvement in CVP q8hr
- Signs of metabolic alkalosis: drowsiness, restlessness
- **Hypokalemia:** postural hypotension, malaise, fatigue, tachycardia, leg cramps, weakness
- Rashes, fever daily
- Confusion, especially among geriatric patients; take safety precautions if needed

Black Box Warning: Hepatic encephalopathy: do not use in hepatic coma or pre-coma; fluctuations in electrolytes can occur rapidly and precipitate hepatic coma; use caution in patients with impaired hepatic function

Evaluate:

- Therapeutic response: decreased edema, B/P

Teach patient/family:

- To increase fluid intake to 2-3 L/day unless contraindicated; to rise slowly from lying or sitting position
- To notify prescriber of muscle weakness, cramps, nausea, dizziness
- That product may be taken with food or milk
- To use sunscreen for photosensitivity
- That blood glucose may be increased in diabetics
- To take early in day to avoid nocturia
- To avoid alcohol
- To avoid sodium foods, to increase potassium foods in diet

TREATMENT OF OVERDOSE:

Lavage if taken orally; monitor electrolytes; administer dextrose in saline; monitor hydration, CV, renal status

metoprolol (Rx)

(meh-toe′proe-lole)

Apo-Metoprolol ✤, Betaloc ✤, Gen-Metoprolol ✤, Lopressor, Novo-Metoprolol ✤, Nu-Metop ✤, PMS-Metoprolol ✤, Sandoz Metoprolol ✤, Toprol-XL

Func. class.: Antihypertensive, antianginal

Chem. class.: β_1-Blocker

Do not confuse:
metoprolol/misoprostol

ACTION:

Lowers B/P by β-blocking effects; reduces elevated renin plasma levels; blocks β_2-adrenergic receptors in bronchial, vascular smooth muscle only at high doses; negative chronotropic effect

USES:

Mild to moderate hypertension, acute MI to reduce cardiovascular mortality, angina pectoris, NYHA class II, III heart failure

Unlabeled uses: Migraine prevention, heart rate control for atrial fibrillation/flutter without accessory pathway, essential tremor, unstable angina

CONTRAINDICATIONS:

Hypersensitivity to β-blockers, cardiogenic shock, heart block (2nd, 3rd degree), sinus bradycardia, pheochromocytoma, sick sinus syndrome

Precautions: Pregnancy (C), breastfeeding, geriatric patients, major surgery, diabetes mellitus, thyroid/renal/hepatic disease, COPD, CAD, nonallergic bronchospasm, CHF, bronchial asthma, CVA, children, depression, vasospastic angina

Black Box Warning: Abrupt discontinuation

DOSAGE AND ROUTES

Hypertension

• **Adult: PO** 50 mg bid or 100 mg/day; may give up to 200-450 mg in divided doses; **EXT REL** 25-100 mg daily, titrate at weekly intervals; max 400 mg/day

• **Geriatric: PO** 25 mg/day initially, increase weekly as needed

• **Child and adolescent 6-16 yr: PO ER** 1 mg/kg up to 50 mg daily

Myocardial infarction

• **Adult: IV BOL** (early treatment) 5 mg q2min × 3 then 50 mg **PO** 15 min after last dose and q6hr × 48 hr; (late treatment) **PO** maintenance 50-100 mg bid for 1-3 yr

Heart failure (NYHA class II/III)

• **Adult: PO EXT REL** 25 mg daily × 2 wk (class II); 12.5 mg daily (class III); **PO** (unlabeled) 5 mg bid, titrate to 100-150 mg/day in 2-3 divided doses

Angina

• **Adult: PO** 100 mg/day as a single dose or in 2 divided doses, increase weekly prn or 100 mg **EXT REL** daily, max 400 mg/day ext rel

Migraine prevention (unlabeled)

• **Adult: PO** 25-100 mg bid-qid; 50-200 mg daily (XL)

Heart rate control for atrial fibrillation/flutter without accessory pathway (unlabeled)

• **Adult: IV BOL** (acute setting) 2.5-5 mg over 2 min, may repeat dose × 3; **PO** (nonacute setting) 25-100 mg bid

Essential tremor (unlabeled)

• **Adult: PO** 50 mg/day, may increase, max 300 mg/day in divided doses; **EXT REL** 100 mg/day, max 400 mg/day

Available forms: Tabs 50, 100 mg; inj 1 mg/ml; ext rel tab (succinate) (XL) 25, 50, 100, 200 mg; ext rel tabs, tartrate: 100 mg

Administer:

PO route

• Do not break, crush, or chew ext rel tabs

• Regular release tab after meals, at bedtime; tab may be crushed or swallowed whole; take at same time each day

Direct IV route

• IV, undiluted, give over 1 min × 3 doses at 2 to 5-min intervals; start **PO** 15 min after last IV dose

Y-site compatibilities: Abciximab, acyclovir, alemtuzumab, alfentanil, alteplase, amikacin, aminophylline, amiodarone, amphotericin B liposome, anidulafungin, argatroban, ascorbic acid, atracurium, atropine, azaTHIOprine, aztreonam, benztropine, bivalirudin, bleomycin, bumetanide, buprenorphine, butorphanol, calcium chloride/gluconate, CARBOplatin, caspofungin, ceFAZolin, cefonicid, cefoperazone, cefotaxime, cefotetan, cefoxitin, ceftazidime, ceftizoxime, cefTRIAXone, cefuroxime, chloramphenicol, chlorproMAZINE, cimetidine, CISplatin, clindamycin, cyanocobalamin, cyclophosphamide, cycloSPORINE, cytarabine, DACTINomycin, DAPTOmycin, dexamethasone, dexmedetomidine, digoxin, diltiazem, diphenhydrAMINE, DOBUTamine, docetaxel, DOPamine, doxacurium, DOXOrubicin, doxycycline, enalaprilat, ePHEDrine, EPINEPHrine, epirubicin, epoetin alfa, eptifibatide, esmolol, etoposide, etoposide phosphate, famotidine, fenoldopam, fentaNYL, fluconazole, fludarabine, fluorouracil, folic acid, furosemide, ganciclovir, gemcitabine, gentamicin, glycopyrrolate, granisetron, heparin, hydrocortisone, HYDROmorphone, IDArubicin, ifosfamide, imipenem/cilastatin, indomethacin, insulin, isoproterenol, ketorolac, labetalol, linezolid, LORazepam, magnesium sulfate, mannitol, mechlorethamine, meperidine, metaraminol, methotrexate, methoxamine, methyldopate, methylPREDNISolone, metoclopramide, metroNIDAZOLE, midazolam, milrinone, mitoxantrone, morphine, multivitamins, nafcillin, nalbuphine, naloxone, nitroprusside, norepinephrine, octreotide, ondansetron, oxacillin, oxaliplatin, oxytocin, paclitaxel, palonosetron, pancuronium, papaverine, pemetrexed, penicillin G, pentamidine, pentazocine, PENTobarbital, PHENobarbital, phentolamine, phenylephrine, phytonadione, piperacillin/tazobactam, potassium chloride, procainamide, prochlorperazine, promethazine, propranolol, protamine, pyridoxime, quinupristin/dalfopristin, ranitidine, rocuronium, sodium bicarbonate, succinylcholine, SUFentanil, tacrolimus, teniposide, theophylline, thiamine, thiotepa, ticarcillin/clavulanate, tigecycline, tirofiban, tobramycin, tolazoline, trimetaphan, urokinase, vancomycin, vasopressin, vecuronium, verapamil, vinCRIStine, vinorelbine, voriconazole

SIDE EFFECTS

CNS: *Insomnia, dizziness,* mental changes, hallucinations, depression, anxiety, headaches, nightmares, confusion, fatigue

CV: *Hypotension,* **bradycardia,** CHF, *palpitations,* dysrhythmias, **cardiac arrest, AV block, pulmonary/peripheral edema, chest pain**

EENT: Sore throat; dry, burning eyes

GI: *Nausea, vomiting,* colitis, cramps, *diarrhea,* constipation, flatulence, dry mouth, *hiccups*

GU: Impotence

HEMA: **Agranulocytosis, eosinophilia, thrombocytopenia, purpura**

INTEG: Rash, purpura, alopecia, dry skin, urticaria, pruritus

RESP: **Bronchospasm,** dyspnea, wheezing

PHARMACOKINETICS

Half-life 3-4 hr, metabolized in liver (metabolites), excreted in urine, crosses placenta, enters breast milk

PO: Peak 2-4 hr, duration 13-19 hr

PO-ER: Peak 6-12 hr, duration 24 hr

IV: Onset immediate, peak 20 min, duration 6-8 hr

INTERACTIONS

• Do not use with MAOIs

Increase: hypotension, bradycardia—reserpine, hydrALAZINE, methyldopa, prazosin, amphetamines, EPINEPHrine, H_2-antagonists, calcium channel blockers

Increase: hypoglycemic effects—insulin, oral antidiabetics

Increase: metoprolol level—cimetidine

Increase: effects of benzodiazepines

Decrease: antihypertensive effect—salicylates, NSAIDs

Decrease: metoprolol level—barbiturates

Decrease: effects of—xanthines

Drug/Food

Increase: absorption with food

Drug/Lab Test

Increase: BUN, potassium, ANA titer, serum lipoprotein, triglycerides, uric acid, alk phos, LDH, AST, ALT

NURSING CONSIDERATIONS

Assess:

• ECG directly when giving IV during initial treatment

• I&O, weight daily; check for CHF (weight gain, jugular venous distention, crackles, edema, dyspnea)

• B/P during initial treatment, periodically thereafter; pulse q4hr; note rate, rhythm, quality

• Apical/radial pulse before administration; notify prescriber of any significant changes or pulse <50 bpm

• Baselines of renal, hepatic studies before therapy begins

• Skin turgor, dryness of mucous membranes for hydration status

Perform/provide:

• Storage in dry area at room temp; do not freeze

Evaluate:

• Therapeutic response: decreased B/P after 1-2 wk, decreased anginal pain

Teach patient/family:

• To take immediately after meals; to take medication at bedtime to prevent effect of orthostatic hypotension

Black Box Warning: Not to discontinue product abruptly; to taper over 2 wk; may cause precipitate angina

• Not to use OTC products containing α-adrenergic stimulants (nasal decongestants, OTC cold preparations) unless directed by prescriber; to avoid alcohol, smoking, sodium intake

- To report bradycardia, dizziness, confusion, depression, fever, sore throat, SOB, decreased vision to prescriber
- To take pulse, B/P at home; when to notify prescriber
- To comply with weight control, dietary adjustments, modified exercise program
- To carry emergency ID to identify product, allergies
- To monitor blood glucose closely if diabetic
- To avoid hazardous activities if dizziness is present
- To report symptoms of CHF: difficult breathing, especially on exertion or when lying down; night cough; swelling of extremities
- To wear support hose to minimize effects of orthostatic hypotension
- To report Raynaud's symptoms

TREATMENT OF OVERDOSE:

Lavage, IV atropine for bradycardia, IV theophylline for bronchospasm, digoxin, O_2, diuretic for cardiac failure, hemodialysis, administer vasopressor

metroNIDAZOLE (Rx)

(me-troe-ni′da-zole)

Flagyl, Flagyl 375, Flagyl ER, Flagyl IV, Flagyl IV RTU, Florazone ER ♣, Novo-Nidazol ♣

Func. class.: Antiinfective—miscellaneous

Chem. class.: Nitroimidazole derivative

ACTION: Direct-acting amebicide/trichomonacide binds and disrupts DNA structure, thereby inhibiting bacterial nucleic acid synthesis

USES: Intestinal amebiasis, amebic abscess, trichomoniasis, refractory trichomoniasis, bacterial anaerobic infections, giardiasis, septicemia, endocarditis; bone, joint, lower respiratory tract infections; rosacea

Unlabeled uses: Crohn's disease, urethritis, amebiasis due to *Dientamoeba fragilis, Entamoeba polecki,* giardiasis, pruritus; gastric ulcer, dyspepsia *(H. pylori),* pseudomembranous colitis, guinea worm disease, periodontitis

CONTRAINDICATIONS: Pregnancy 1st trimester, breastfeeding, hypersensitivity to this product

Precautions: Pregnancy (B) 2nd/3rd trimesters, geriatric patients, *Candida* infections, heart failure, fungal infection, dental disease, bone marrow suppression, hematologic disease, GI/renal/hepatic disease, contracted visual or color fields, blood dyscrasias, CNS disorders

Black Box Warning: Secondary malignancy

DOSAGE AND ROUTES

Trichomoniasis

- **Adult: PO** 500 mg bid × 7 days or 2 g as single dose; do not repeat treatment for 4-6 wk
- **Child (unlabeled): PO** 15 mg/kg/day in 3 divided doses × 7-10 days
- **Infant (unlabeled): PO** 10-30 mg/kg/day × 5-8 days

Refractory trichomoniasis

- **Adult: PO** 250 mg bid × 10 days

Amebic hepatic abscess

- **Adult: PO** 500-750 mg tid × 5-10 days
- **Child: PO** 35-50 mg/kg/day in 3 divided doses × 10 days

Intestinal amebiasis

- **Adult: PO** 750 mg tid × 5-10 days
- **Child: PO** 35-50 mg/kg/day in 3 divided doses × 10 days then oral iodoquinol

Anaerobic bacterial infections

- **Adult: IV INF** 15 mg/kg over 1 hr then 7.5 mg/kg **IV** or **PO** q6hr, not to exceed 4 g/day; 1st maintenance dose should be administered 6 hr after loading dose

M

Bacterial vaginosis
• **Adult: PO** regular rel 500 mg bid or 250 mg tid × 7 days; ext rel 750 mg/day × 7 days
Persistent urethritis (unlabeled)
• **Adult and adolescent: PO** 2 g as single dose with azithromycin
Dientamoeba fragilis **(unlabeled)**
• **Child: PO** 250 mg tid × 7 days
Entamoeba polecki **(unlabeled)**
• **Adult: PO** 750 mg tid × 10 days
• **Child: PO** 30-50 mg/kg/day in 3 divided doses × 5-10 days
Guinea worm disease (unlabeled)
• **Adult: PO** 250 mg tid × 10 days
• **Child: PO** 25 mg/kg/day in 3 divided doses × 10 days
Crohn's disease (unlabeled)
• **Adult: PO** 250 mg tid-qid
Giardiasis (unlabeled)
• **Adult: PO** 250 mg tid × 5-7 days
• **Child: PO** 15 mg/kg/day in 3 divided doses × 5 days
Antibiotic-associated pseudomembranous colitis (unlabeled)
• **Adult: PO** 250-500 mg 3-4×/day × 7-14 days
• **Child: PO** 20 mg/kg/day (max 2 g) divided q6hr

Available forms: Tabs 250, 500 mg; ext rel tab (ER) 750 mg; caps 375 mg; inj 500 mg/100 ml; powder for inj 500-mg single dose

Administer:

PO route
• Do not break, crush, or chew ext rel product
• PO with or after meals to avoid GI symptoms, metallic taste; crush tabs if needed

IV route

Intermittent INF ([Flagyl] IV RTU)
• Prediluted, ready to use; inf over 30-60 min
• Lyophilized vials: dilute with 4.4 ml sterile water, 0.9% NaCl; must be diluted further with ≥8 mg/ml 0.9% NaCl, D_5W, or LR; must neutralize with 5 mEq $NaCO_3$/500 mg; CO_2 gas will be generated and may require venting; run over ≥1 hr; primary IV must be discontinued; may be given as cont inf; do not use aluminum products; IV may require venting
• Do not use aluminum needles or other products to prepare product

Y-site compatibilities: Acyclovir, alemtuzumab, alfentanil, allopurinol, amifostine, amikacin, aminophylline, amiodarone, ampicillin, ampicillin/sulbactam, anidulafungin, atracurium, bivalirudin, bumetanide, buprenorphine, busulfan, butorphanol, calcium acetate/chloride/gluconate, CARBOplatin, ceFAZolin, cefepime, cefoperazone, cefotaxime, cefotetan, cefTRIAXone, cefuroxime, chloramphenicol, chlorproMAZINE, cimetidine, ciprofloxacin, cisatracurium, CISplatin, clindamycin, codeine, cyclophosphamide, cycloSPORINE, cytarabine, DACTINomycin, dexamethasone, dexmedetomidine, dexrazoxane, digoxin, diltiazem, dimenhyDRINATE, diphenhydrAMINE, DOBUTamine, docetaxel, DOPamine, doripenem, doxacurium, doxapram, DOXOrubicin, DOXOrubicin liposome, doxycycline, droperidol, enalaprilat, ePHEDrine, EPINEPHrine, epirubicin, eptifibatide, ertapenem, erythromycin, esmolol, etoposide, etoposide phosphate, famotidine, fenoldopam, fentaNYL, fluconazole, fludarabine, fluorouracil, foscarnet, fosphenytoin, furosemide, gemcitabine, gentamicin, glycopyrrolate, granisetron, haloperidol, heparin, hydrALAZINE, hydrocortisone, HYDROmorphone, IDArubicin, ifosfamide, imipenem/cilastatin, inamrinone, insulin, isoproterenol, ketorolac, labetalol, leucovorin, levofloxacin, lidocaine, linezolid, LORazepam, magnesium sulfate, mannitol, mechlorethamine, melphalan, meperidine, meropenem, mesna, metaraminol, methotrexate, methyldopate, methylPREDNISolone, metoclopramide, metoprolol, midazolam, milrinone, mitoxantrone, morphine, nafcillin, nalbuphine, naloxone, nesiritide, niCARdipine, nitroglycerin, nitroprusside, norepinephrine, octreotide, ondansetron, oxaliplatin, oxytocin, paclitaxel, palonosetron, pancuronium, pentamidine, pentazocine, PENTobarbital, perphenazine, PHENObarbital, phentolamine, phenylephrine, piperacillin/tazobactam, potassium chloride/phosphates, prochlorperazine, promethazine, propranolol, ranitidine, remifentanil, riTUXimab, rocuronium, sargramostim, sodium acetate/bicarbonate/phosphates, streptozocin, succinylcholine, SUFentanil, tacrolimus, teniposide, theophylline, thiopental, thiotepa, ticarcillin/clavulanate, tigecycline, tiro-fiban, tobramycin, trastuzumab, trimethobenzamide, trimethoprim/sulfamethoxazole, vancomycin, vasopressin, vecuronium, verapamil, vinCRIStine, vinorelbine, voriconazole, zidovudine, zoledronic acid

SIDE EFFECTS

CNS: *Headache, dizziness,* confusion, irritability, restlessness, ataxia, depression, fatigue, drowsiness, insomnia, paresthesia, peripheral neuropathy, seizures, incoordination, depression, encephalopathy, **aseptic meningitis**

CV: Flattening of T waves

EENT: Blurred vision, sore throat, retinal edema, dry mouth, metallic taste, furry tongue, glossitis, stomatitis, photophobia, optic neuritis

GI: *Nausea, vomiting, diarrhea,* epigastric distress, *anorexia,* constipation, *abdominal cramps,* **pseudomembranous colitis**

GU: Darkened urine, vaginal dryness, polyuria, **albuminuria**, dysuria, cystitis, decreased libido, **nephrotoxicity**, incontinence, dyspareunia, candidiasis

HEMA: Leukopenia, bone marrow, depression, aplasia, thrombocytopenia

INTEG: Rash, pruritus, urticaria, flushing, **Stevens-Johnson syndrome**

PHARMACOKINETICS

Crosses placenta, enters breast milk, metabolized by liver 30%-60%, excreted in urine (60%-80%), half-life 6-8 hr

PO: Peak 1-2 hr, absorbed 80%-85%

IV: Onset immediate, peak end of inf

INTERACTIONS

- Avoid use with zalcitabine, bortezomib, norfloxacin
- Do not use with amprenavir

Decrease: metroNIDAZOLE half-life—barbiturates

Decrease: metroNIDAZOLE—cholestyramine

Increase: disulfiram reaction—alcohol

Increase: busulfan toxicity—busulfan; avoid concurrent use

Increase: metroNIDAZOLE level—cimetidine

Increase: lithium, CYP3A4 substrates

Increase: action of warfarin, phenytoin, lithium, fosphenytoin

Increase: leukopenia—azathioprine, fluorouracil

Drug/Lab Test

Altered: AST, ALT, LDH

Decrease: WBC, neutrophils

False decrease: triglycerides

NURSING CONSIDERATIONS

Assess:

- **Infection:** WBC, wound symptoms, fever, skin or vaginal secretions; start treatment after C&S; for opportunistic fungal infections; superinfection: fever, monilial growth, fatigue, malaise
- Stools during entire treatment; should be clear at end of therapy; stools should be free of parasites for 1 yr before patient considered cured (amebiasis)
- Vision by ophthalmic exam during, after therapy; vision problems often occur

⚠ Neurotoxicity: peripheral neuropathy, seizures, dizziness, uncoordination, pruritus, joint pain; product may be discontinued

- **Allergic reaction:** fever, rash, itching, chills; product should be discontinued if these occur
- Renal, reproductive dysfunction: dysuria, polyuria, impotence, dyspareunia, decreased libido, I&O; weight daily

Black Box Warning: Secondary malignancy: used only when indicated; avoid unnecessary use

M

Perform/provide:

- Storage in light-resistant container; do not refrigerate

Evaluate:

- Therapeutic response: decreased symptoms of infection

Teach patient/family:

- That urine may turn dark reddish brown; that product may cause metallic taste
- About proper hygiene after bowel movement; hand-washing technique
- To notify physician about numbness or tingling of extremities
- To avoid hazardous activities because dizziness can occur
- About need for compliance with dosage schedule, duration of treatment
- To use condoms if treatment for trichomoniasis or cross-contamination may occur; to notify prescriber if pregnant or planning to become pregnant; that treatment of both partners is necessary for trichomoniasis
- To use frequent sips of water, sugarless gum, candy for dry mouth
- Not to drink alcohol or use preparations containing alcohol during use or for 48 hr after use of product; disulfiram-like reaction can occur

metroNIDAZOLE topical/vaginal

See Appendix B

micafungin (Rx)

(my-ca-fun′gin)

Mycamine

Func. class.: Antifungal, systemic

Chem. class.: Echinocandin

ACTION:
Inhibits an essential component of fungal cell walls; causes direct damage to fungal cell wall

USES:
Treatment of esophageal candidiasis; prophylaxis for *Candida* infections in patients undergoing hematopoietic stem-cell transplantation (HSCT); susceptible *Candida* sp.: *C. albicans, C. glabrata, C. krusei, C. parapsilosis, C. tropicalis*

Unlabeled uses: *Aspergillus* sp., pediatrics to prevent candidiasis, endocarditis, endophthalmitis, infectious arthritis, myocarditis, osteomyelitis, pericarditis, pneumonia, sinusitis, tracheobronchitis

CONTRAINDICATIONS:
Hypersensitivity to this product or other echinocandins

Precautions: Pregnancy (C), breastfeeding, children, geriatric patients, severe hepatic disease

DOSAGE AND ROUTES

Esophageal candidiasis

- **Adult: IV INF** 150 mg/day given over 1 hr

Candidemia/acute disseminated candidiasis, abscess/peritonitis

- **Adult: IV** 100 mg/day over 1 hr

Prophylaxis for *Candida* infections

- **Adult: IV INF** 50 mg/day given over 1 hr
- **Adolescent/child/infant ≥6 mo (unlabeled): IV INF** 1 mg/kg/day, max 50 mg/day

***Aspergillus* sp. (unlabeled)**

- **Adult: IV INF** 25-150 mg/day × ≥30 days

Available forms: Powder for inj 50 mg, in single-dose vials 50-, 100-mg vial

Administer:

- Do not use if cloudy or precipitated; do not admix; by IV inf only
- Flush line before, and after administration with 0.9% NaCl

IV route

- Flush line before and after use with 0.9% NaCl
- **For *Candida* prevention,** reconstitute with provided dilutent 0.9% NaCl without bacteriostatic product; 50-mg vial/5 ml (10 mg/ml), swirl to dissolve, do not shake; further dilute with 100 ml 0.9% NaCl only; run over 1 hr

• **For *Candida* infection:** reconstitute with provided diluent 50 mg/5 ml (10 mg/ml); further dilute 3 reconstituted vials in 100 ml 0.9% NaCl, run over 1 hr

Y-site compatibilities: Aminophylline, bumetanide, calcium chloride/gluconate, cycloSPORINE, DOPamine, eptifibatide, esmolol, fenoldopam, furosemide, heparin, HYDROmorphone, lidocaine, LORazepam, magnesium sulfate, milrinone, nitroglycerin, nitroprusside, norepinephrine, phenylephrine, potassium chloride, potassium phosphate, tacrolimus, vasopressin

SIDE EFFECTS

CNS: Seizures, dizziness, *headache, somnolence,* fever, anxiety
CV: Flushing, hypertension, phlebitis, tachycardia
GI: Abdominal pain, *nausea, anorexia, vomiting, diarrhea, increased AST, ALT, alk phos, blood dehydrogenase, hyperbilirubinemia*
HEMA: **Neutropenia, thrombocytopenia, leukopenia, coagulopathy, anemia, hemolytic anemia**
INTEG: *Rash, pruritus, inj site pain*
META: Hypokalemia, hypocalcemia, hypomagnesemia
MS: *Rigors*

PHARMACOKINETICS

Metabolized in liver; excreted in feces, urine; terminal half-life 14-17.2 hr; protein binding 99%

INTERACTIONS

Increase: plasma concentrations—itraconazole, sirolimus, NIFEdipine; may need dosage reduction

NURSING CONSIDERATIONS

Assess:
• **Infection,** clearing of cultures during treatment; obtain culture at baseline and during treatment; product may be started as soon as culture is taken (esophageal candidiasis); monitor cultures during HSCT for prevention of *Candida* infections
• CBC (RBC, Hct, Hgb), differential, platelet count periodically; notify prescriber of results
• Renal studies: BUN, urine CCr, electrolytes before and during therapy
• Hepatic studies before and during treatment: bilirubin, AST, ALT, alk phos as needed
• **Bleeding:** hematuria, heme-positive stools, bruising, or petechiae, mucosa or orifices; blood dyscrasias can occur
• **For hypersensitivity:** rash, pruritus, facial swelling, phlebitis
• For hemolytic anemia
• GI symptoms: frequency of stools, cramping; if severe diarrhea occurs, electrolytes may need to be given

Perform/provide:
• Storage at room temp, away from light, do not freeze; discard unused sol

Evaluate:
• Therapeutic response: prevention of *Candida* infection with HSCT or decreased symptoms of *Candida* infection, negative culture

Teach patient/family:
• To notify prescriber if pregnancy is suspected or planned; to use nonhormonal form of contraception while taking this product
• To avoid breastfeeding while taking this product
• To inform prescriber of kidney or liver disease
• To report bleeding, facial swelling, wheezing, difficulty breathing, itching, rash, hives, increasing warmth, flushing
• To report signs of infection: increased temp, sore throat, flulike symptoms
• To notify prescriber of nausea, vomiting, diarrhea, jaundice, anorexia, clay-colored stools, dark urine; hepatotoxicity may occur

miconazole topical

See Appendix B

M

miconazole vaginal antifungal

See Appendix B

midazolam (Rx)

(mid'ay-zoe-lam)

Func. class.: Sedative, hypnotic, antianxiety

Chem. class.: Benzodiazepine, short-acting

Controlled Substance Schedule IV

ACTION: Depresses subcortical levels in CNS; may act on limbic system, reticular formation; may potentiate γ-aminobutyric acid (GABA) by binding to specific benzodiazepine receptors

USES: Preoperative sedation, general anesthesia induction, sedation for diagnostic endoscopic procedures, intubation, anxiety

Unlabeled uses: Refractory status epilepticus

CONTRAINDICATIONS: Pregnancy (D), hypersensitivity to benzodiazepines, acute closed-angle glaucoma, status asthmaticus

Precautions: Breastfeeding, children, geriatric patients, COPD, CHF, chronic renal failure, chills, debilitated, hepatic disease, shock, coma, alcohol intoxication

Black Box Warning: Neonates (contains benzyl alcohol), IV administration, respiratory depression/insufficiency

DOSAGE AND ROUTES

Preoperative sedation

- **Adult and child ≥12 yr: IM** 0.07-0.08 mg/kg 1/2-1 hr before general anesthesia
- **Child 6 yr-11 yr: IV** 0.025-0.05 mg/kg; total dose of 0.4 mg/kg may be necessary
- **Child 6 mo-5 yr: IV** 0.05-0.1 mg/kg; total dose of 0.6 mg/kg may be necessary
- **Child 1-6 mo: IM** 0.1-0.15 mg/kg; may give up to 0.5 mg/kg if needed, max 10 mg

Induction of general anesthesia

- **Adult >55 yr:** (ASA I/II) **IV** 150-300 mcg/kg over 30 sec; (ASA III/IV) limit dose to 250 mcg/kg (nonpremedicated) or 150 mcg/kg (premedicated)
- **Adult <55 yr: IV** 200-350 mcg/kg over 20-30 sec; if patient has not received premedication, may repeat by giving 20% of original dose; if patient has received premedication, reduce dose by 50 mcg/kg
- **Child:** No safe and effective dose established; however, doses of 50-200 mcg/kg **IV** have been used

Continuous infusion for intubation (critical care)

- **Adult: IV** 0.01-0.05 mg/kg over several min; repeat at 10- to 15-min intervals until adequate sedation then 0.02-0.10 mg/kg/hr maintenance; adjust as needed
- **Child: IV** 0.05-0.2 mg/kg over 2-3 min then 0.06-0.12 mg/kg/hr by cont inf; adjust as needed
- **Neonate: IV** 0.03-0.06 mg/kg/hr, titrate using lowest dose

Status epilepticus (unlabeled)

- **Child and infant >2 mo: IV** 0.15 mg/kg then **CONT IV** 1 mcg/kg/min, titrate upward q5min until seizures controlled

Available forms: Inj 1, 5 mg/ml, syr 2 mg/ml

Administer:

PO route

- Remove cap of press-in bottle adaptor, push adaptor into neck of bottle; close with cap; remove cap, insert tip of dispenser, insert into adaptor; turn upside-down, withdraw correct dose; place in mouth

IM route

- IM deep into large muscle mass

IV route

- May be given diluted or undiluted
- After diluting with D_5W or 0.9% NaCl to 0.25 mg/ml; give over 2 min (conscious sedation) or over 30 sec (anesthesia induction)

Y-site compatibilities: Abciximab, alfentamil, amikacin, amiodarone, argatroban, atracurium, atropine, aztreonam, benzotropine, calcium gluconate, ceFAZolin, cefotaxime, cefoxitine, cefTRIAXone, cimetidine, ciprofloxacin, CISplatin, clindamycin, cloNIDine, cyanocobalamin, cycloSPORINE, DACTINomycin, digoxin, diltiazem, diphenhydrAMINE, docetaxal, DOPamine, doxycyclin, enalaprilat, EPINEPHrine, erythromycin, esmolol, etomidate, etoposide, famotidine, fentaNYL, fluconazole, folic acid, gatifloxacin, gemcitabine, gentamicin, glycopyrrolate, granisetron, heparin, hetastarch, HYDROmorphone, hydrOXYzine, inamrinone, isoproterenol, labetalol, lactated Ringer's, levofloxacin, lidocaine, linezolid, LORazepam, magnesium, mannitol, meperdine, methadone, methyldopa, methylPREDNISolone, metoclopromide, metomolol, metroNIDAZOLE, milrinone, morphine, nalbuphine, naloxone, niCARdipine, nitroglycerin, nitroprusside, norepinephrine, ondansetron, oxacillin, oxytocin, paclitaxel, palonasetron, pancuronium, papaverin, phytonadione, piperacillin, potassium chloride, propanolol, protamine, pyridoxine, ranitidine, remifentanil, sodium nitroprusside, succinylcholine, SUFentanil, teniposide, theophylline, thiotepa, ticarcillin, tobramycin, vancomycin, vasopressin, vecuronium, verapamil, voriconazole

SIDE EFFECTS

CNS: Retrograde amnesia, euphoria, confusion, headache, anxiety, insomnia, slurred speech, paresthesia, tremors, weakness, chills, agitation, paradoxic reactions

CV: Hypotension, PVCs, tachycardia, bigeminy, nodal rhythm, **cardiac arrest**

EENT: Blurred vision, nystagmus, diplopia, loss of balance

GI: *Nausea, vomiting,* increased salivation, hiccups

INTEG: Urticaria; pain, swelling, pruritus at inj site; rash

RESP: Coughing, **apnea, bronchospasm, laryngospasm, dyspnea, respiratory depression**

PHARMACOKINETICS

Protein binding 97%; half-life 1.8-6.4 hr, metabolized in liver; metabolites excreted in urine; crosses placenta, blood-brain barrier

PO: Onset 20-30 min

IM: Onset 15 min, peak $^1/_2$-1 hr, duration 2-3 hr

IV: Onset 3-5 min, onset of anesthesia $1^1/_2$-$2^1/_2$ min, duration 2 hr

INTERACTIONS

Increase: hypotension—antihypertensives, opiates, alcohol, nitrates

Increase: extended half-life—CYP3A4 inhibitors (cimetidine, erythromycin, ranitidine)

Increase: respiratory depression—other CNS depressants, alcohol, barbiturates, opiate analgesics, verapamil, ritonavir, indinavir, fluvoxamine

Decrease: midazolam metabolism—CYP3A4 inducers (azole antifungals, theophylline)

Drug/Herb

Increase: sedation—kava, valerian

Decrease: midazolam effect—St. John's wort

Drug/Food

Increase: (PO) midazolam effect—grapefruit juice

NURSING CONSIDERATIONS

Assess:

- B/P, pulse, respirations during IV; emergency equipment should be nearby
- Inj site for redness, pain, swelling
- Degree of amnesia in geriatric patients; may be increased
- Anterograde amnesia

• Vital signs for recovery period in obese patients, since half-life may be extended

Black Box Warning: Respiratory depression insufficiency: apnea, respiratory depression that may be increased in geriatric patients

Perform/provide:

• Assistance with ambulation until drowsy period ends

• Storage at room temp; protect from light

• Immediate availability of resuscitation equipment, O_2 to support airway; do not give by rapid bolus

Evaluate:

• Therapeutic response: induction of sedation, general anesthesia

Teach patient/family:

• That amnesia occurs; that events may not be remembered

TREATMENT OF OVERDOSE:
Flumazenil, O_2

mifepristone

(mif-ee-press′tone)

Mifeprex

Func. class.: Abortifacient

Chem. class.: Antiprogestational

ACTION: Stimulates uterine contractions to cause complete abortion

USES: Abortion through 49 days' gestation

Unlabeled uses: Postcoital contraception/contragestation, intrauterine fetal death, endometriosis, Cushing's syndrome, unresectable meningioma

CONTRAINDICATIONS: Severe respiratory/cardiac/renal/hepatic disease, IUD, ectopic pregnancy, chronic adrenal failure, bleeding disorder, inherited porphyrias, PID; hypersensitivity to this product, misoprostol, or prostaglandins

Precautions: Pregnancy (C), asthma, anemia, jaundice, diabetes mellitus, convulsive disorders, women >35 yr who smoke ≥10 cigarettes/day, past uterine surgery

Black Box Warning: Infection, sepsis, vaginal bleeding

DOSAGE AND ROUTES

• **Adult: PO** 600 mg day 1 unless complete termination is confirmed, give 400 mcg misoprostol day 3 if needed

Advanced breast cancer/ unresectable or malignant meningioma (unlabeled)

• **Adult: PO** 200-400 mg/day

Uterine leiomyomata (unlabeled)

• **Adult: PO** 25-50 mg/day

Endometriosis (unlabeled)

• **Adult: PO** 50 mg/day

Available forms: Tabs 200 mg

SIDE EFFECTS

CNS: Dizziness, insomnia, anxiety, syncope, fainting, headache

GI: *Nausea, vomiting, diarrhea,* dyspepsia

GU: Uterine cramping, uterine hemorrhage, vaginitis, pelvic pain

MISC: Fatigue, back pain, fever, viral infections, chills, sinusitis

PHARMACOKINETICS

Rapidly absorbed, peak 90 min, 98% bound to plasma proteins, albumin, glycoprotein; excretion via feces, urine

INTERACTIONS

• Do not use with anticoagulants, long-term corticosteroids

Decrease: metabolism of erythromycin, ketoconazole, itraconazole

Drug/Herb

Decrease: by St. John's wort

Drug/Food

Decrease: metabolism of mifepristone—grapefruit juice

NURSING CONSIDERATIONS

Assess:

- B/P, pulse; watch for change that may indicate hemorrhage
- Respiratory rate, rhythm, depth; notify prescriber of abnormalities
- For length, duration of contraction; notify prescriber of contractions of ≥1 min or absence of contractions

⚠ **Incomplete abortion:** pregnancy must be terminated by another method; product is teratogenic

Perform/provide:

- Emotional support before and after abortion

Evaluate:

- Therapeutic response: expulsion of fetus

Teach patient/family:

⚠ **Sepsis:** to report increased blood loss, increased temp, foul-smelling lochia, weakness, nausea or vomiting, diarrhea

- About some methods of comfort control and pain control
- To continue with follow up
- That cramping and vaginal bleeding will occur

miglitol (Rx)

(mig′lih-tol)

Glyset

Func. class.: Oral hypoglycemic

Chem. class.: α-Glucosidase inhibitor

ACTION: Delays digestion and absorption of ingested carbohydrates, which results in a smaller rise in blood glucose after meals; does not increase insulin production

USES: Type 2 diabetes mellitus

CONTRAINDICATIONS: Hypersensitivity, diabetic ketoacidosis, cirrhosis, inflammatory bowel disease, colonic ulceration, partial intestinal obstruction, chronic intestinal disease, ileus

Precautions: Pregnancy (B), breastfeeding, children, renal/hepatic disease

DOSAGE AND ROUTES

- **Adult: PO** 25 mg tid initially, with 1st bite of meal; maintenance dose may be increased to 50 mg tid; may be increased to 100 mg tid if needed with dosage adjustment at 4- to 8-wk intervals

Available forms: Tabs 25, 50, 100 mg

Administer:

- Tid with first bite of each meal

SIDE EFFECTS

GI: *Abdominal pain, diarrhea, flatulence,* **hepatotoxicity**

HEMA: Low iron

INTEG: Rash

PHARMACOKINETICS

Peak 2-3 hr, not metabolized, excreted in urine as unchanged product, half-life 2 hr

INTERACTIONS

Decrease: levels of digoxin, propranolol, ranitidine

Decrease: miglitol levels—digestive enzymes, intestinal adsorbents; do not use together

Drug/Food

Increase: diarrhea—carbohydrates

NURSING CONSIDERATIONS

Assess:

- **Hypo/hyperglycemia;** even though product does not cause hypoglycemia, if patient receiving sulfonylureas or insulin, hypoglycemia may be additive (rare)
- Blood glucose levels, hemoglobin, A1c LFTs; if hypoglycemia occurs with monotherapy, treat with glucose

Perform/provide:

- Storage in tight container at room temp

Evaluate:

- Therapeutic response: decreased signs, symptoms of diabetes mellitus (polyuria, polydipsia, polyphagia; clear sensorium, absence of dizziness; stable gait); improved blood glucose, A1c

Teach patient/family:

- About the symptoms of hypo/hyperglycemia, what to do about each; that, during periods of stress, infection, or surgery, insulin may be required
- That medication must be taken as prescribed; about consequences of discontinuing medication abruptly
- To avoid OTC medications unless approved by health care provider
- That diabetes is lifelong; that product is not a cure
- To carry ID for emergency purposes
- That diet and exercise regimen must be followed
- About GI side effects

HIGH ALERT

milrinone (Rx)

(mill′rih-nohn)

Func. class.: Inotropic/vasodilator agent with phosphodiesterase activity

Chem. class.: Bipyridine derivative

ACTION:

Positive inotropic agent; increases contractility of cardiac muscle with vasodilator properties; reduces preload and afterload by direct relaxation on vascular smooth muscle

USES:

Short-term management of advanced heart failure that has not responded to other medication

Unlabeled uses: Adolescents, children, infants

CONTRAINDICATIONS:

Hypersensitivity to this product, severe aortic disease, severe pulmonic valvular disease, acute MI

Precautions: Pregnancy (C), breastfeeding, children, geriatric patients, renal/hepatic disease, atrial flutter/fibrillation

DOSAGE AND ROUTES

- **Adult: IV BOL** 50 mcg/kg given over 10 min; start inf of 0.375-0.75 mcg/kg/min
- **Adolescent/child/infant (unlabeled): IV** 50-75 mcg/kg over 10-60 min then 0.5-0.75 mcg/kg/min

Renal dose

- **Adult: IV** CCr 41-50 ml/min, 0.43 mcg/kg/min, titrate up; CCr 31-40 ml/min, 0.38 mcg/kg/min, titrate up; CCr 21-30 ml/min, 0.33 mcg/kg/min, titrate up; CCr 11-20 ml/min, 0.08 mcg/kg/min; CCr 6-10 ml/min, 0.23 mcg/kg/min; CCr ≤5 ml/min, 0.20 mcg/kg/min; max for all doses 0.75 mcg/kg/min

Available forms: Inj 1 mg/ml; premixed inj 200 mcg/ml in D_5W

Administer:

- Potassium supplements if ordered for potassium levels <3 mg/dl

Direct IV route

- Give IV loading dose undiluted over 10 min, use inf device

Continuous IV route

- Dilute 20-mg vial with 80, 113, 180 ml of 0.45% NaCl, 0.9% NaCl, or D_5W to a conc of 200, 150, 100 mcg/ml respectively
- Titrate rate based on hemodynamic and clinical response, use inf device
- Precipitation will form when furosemide is injected into line with milrinone

Y-site compatibilities: Acyclovir, alfentanil, allopurinol, amifostine, amikacin, aminocaproic acid, aminophylline, amiodarone, amphotericin B liposome, ampicillin, ampicillin-sulbactam, anidulafungin, argatroban, atenolol, atracurium, aztreonam, bivalirudin, bleomycin, bumetanide, buprenorphine, busulfan, butorphanol, calcium chloride/gluconate, CARBOplatin, caspofungin, ceFAZolin, cefepime, cefotaxime, cefotetan, cefoxitin, ceftazidime, ceftizoxime, cefTRIAXone, cefuroxime, chloramphenicol, chlorproMAZINE, cimetidine, ciprofloxacin, cisatracurium, CISplatin, clindamycin, cyclophosphamide, cycloSPORINE, cytarabine, DACTINomycin, DAPTOmycin, dexamethasone, digoxin, diltiazem, DOBUTamine, docetaxel, DOPamine, doripenem, doxacurium, DOXOrubicin, doxycycline, droperidol, enalaprilat, ePHEDrine, EPINEPHrine, epirubicin, eptifibatide, ertapenem, erythromycin, etoposide, famotidine, fenoldopam, fentaNYL, fluconazole, fludarabine, fluorouracil, gallium, ganciclovir, gatifloxacin, gemcitabine, gentamicin, glycopyrrolate, granisetron, haloperidol, heparin, hydrALAZINE, hydrocortisone, HYDROmorphone, IDArubicin, ifosfamide, insulin (regular), irinotecan, isoproterenol, ketorolac, labetalol, levofloxacin, linezolid, LORazepam, magnesium sulfate, mannitol, mechlorethamine, melphalan, meperidine, meropenem, methohexital, methotrexate, methyldopate, methylPREDNISolone, metoclopramide, metoprolol, metroNIDAZOLE, micafungin, midazolam, mitoxantrone, morphine, mycophenolate, nafcillin, nalbuphine, naloxone, nesiritide, niCARdipine, nitroglycerin, nitroprusside, norepinephrine, octreotide, oxacillin, oxaliplatin, oxytocin, paclitaxel, palonosetron, pamidronate, pancuronium, pemetrexed, pentamidine, pentazocine, PENTobarbital, PHENobarbital, phenylephrine, piperacillin, piperacillin-tazobactam, polymyxin B, potassium chloride/phosphates, prochlorperazine, promethazine, propofol, propranolol, quiNIDine, quinupristin-dalfopristin, ranitidine, remifentanil, rocuronium, sodium acetate/bicarbonate/phosphates, streptozocin, succinylcholine, SUFentanil, sulfamethoxazole-trimethoprim, tacrolimus, teniposide, theophylline, thiopental, thiotepa, ticarcillin, ticarcillin-clavulanate, tigecycline, tirofiban, tobramycin, torsemide, vancomycin, vasopressin, vecuronium, verapamil, vinCRIStine, vinorelbine, voriconazole, zidovudine, zoledronic acid

SIDE EFFECTS

CV: **Dysrhythmias**, hypotension, chest pain, *PVCs*

GI: Nausea, vomiting, anorexia, abdominal pain, **hepatotoxicity, jaundice**

HEMA: **Thrombocytopenia**

MISC: Headache, hypokalemia, tremor, inj site reactions

PHARMACOKINETICS

IV: Onset 2-5 min, peak 10 min, duration variable; terminal half-life 2.3 hr; metabolized in liver; excreted in urine as product (83%), metabolites (12%)

INTERACTIONS

Increase: effects of antihypertensives, diuretics

NURSING CONSIDERATIONS

Assess:

⚠ **ECG continuously during IV; ventricular dysrhythmia can occur**

- B/P, pulse q5min during inf; if B/P drops 30 mm Hg, stop inf, call prescriber
- Electrolytes: potassium, sodium, chloride, calcium; renal studies: BUN, creatinine; blood studies: platelet count
- ALT, AST, bilirubin daily
- I&O ratio, weight daily; diuresis should increase with continuing therapy
- If platelets are $<150,000/mm^3$, product is usually discontinued and another product started
- Extravasation; change site q48hr

Evaluate:

- Therapeutic response: increased cardiac output, decreased PCWP, adequate CVP; decreased dyspnea, fatigue, edema, ECG

Teach patient/family:

- To report angina immediately during inf
- To report headache, which can be treated with analgesics

TREATMENT OF OVERDOSE:

Discontinue product, support circulation

minocycline (Rx)

(min-oh-sye'kleen)

Apo-Minocycline ♣, Arestin, Dynacin, Gen-Minocycline ♣, Minocin, ratio-Minocycline ♣, Sandoz Minocycline ♣, Soledyn

Func. class.: Broad-spectrum antiinfective

Chem. class.: Tetracycline

ACTION: Inhibits protein synthesis, phosphorylation in microorganisms by binding to ribosomal subunits, reversibly binding to ribosomal subunits; bacteriostatic

USES: Syphilis, *Chlamydia trachomatis,* gonorrhea, lymphogranuloma venereum, rickettsial infections, inflammatory acne, *Neisseria meningitidis, Neisseria gonorrhoeae, Treponema pallidum, Chlamydia trachomatis, Ureaplasma urealyticum, Mycoplasma pneumoniae, Nocardia,* periodontitis, methicillin-resistant *S. aureus* (MRSA) infection, non-nodular moderate to severe acne vulgaris

Unlabeled uses: Rheumatoid arthritis, bullous pemphigoid, dental infection, prostatis, pleural effusion

CONTRAINDICATIONS: Pregnancy (D), children <8 yr, hypersensitivity to tetracyclines

Precautions: Hepatic disease, breastfeeding

DOSAGE AND ROUTES

- **Adult: PO/IV** 200 mg then 100 mg q12hr, max 400 mg/24 hr **IV; SUBGINGIVAL** inserted into periodontal pocket
- **Child >8 yr: PO/IV** 4 mg/kg then 4 mg/kg/day **PO** in divided doses q12hr

Gonorrhea

- **Adult: PO** 200 mg then 100 mg q12hr × ≥4 days

Chlamydia trachomatis

- **Adult: PO** 100 mg bid × 7 days

Syphilis

- **Adult: PO** 200 mg then 100 mg q12hr × 10-15 days

Uncomplicated gonococcal urethritis in men

- **Adult: PO** 100 mg q12hr × 5 days

Acne vulgaris (Solodyn only)

- **Adult/adolescent/child ≥12 yr:** ext rel 1 mg/kg/day × 12 wk or those weighing 126-136 kg—135 mg/day; 111-125 kg—115 mg/day; 97-110 kg—105 mg/day; 85-96 kg—90 mg/day; 72-84 kg—80 mg/day; 60-71 kg—65 mg/day; 50-59 kg—55 mg/day

Acne vulgaris (all except Solodyn)

- **Adult/adolescent/child ≥12 yr:** ext rel 1 mg/kg × 12 wk or 91-136 kg, 35 mg/day; 60-90 kg, 90 mg/day; 45-59 kg, 45 mg/day

Rheumatoid arthritis (unlabeled)

- **Adult: PO** 100 mg bid for ≤48 wk

Bullous pemphigus (unlabeled)

- **Adult: PO** 50 mg/day; may increase to 100 mg/day after 1-2 wk

Available forms: Caps 50, 75, 100 mg; oral susp 50 mg/5 ml; powder for inj 100 mg; caps, pellet filled 50, 100 mg; tabs 50, 75, 100 mg; ext rel tabs 45, 65, 90, 115, 135 mg

Administer:

- After C&S obtained

PO route

- With full glass of water; with food for GI symptoms
- 2 hr before or after laxative or ferrous products; 3 hr after antacid

IV route

- After diluting 100 mg/5 ml sterile water for inj; further dilute in 500-1000 ml of NaCl, dextrose sol, LR, Ringer's sol; run 100 mg/6 hr

Y-site compatibilities: Alfentanil, amikacin, atracurium, benztropine, buprenorphine, butorphanol, calcium chloride, CARBOplatin, caspofungin, cefonicid, chlorpromazine, cimetidine, cisatracurium, codeine, cyclophosphamide, cycloSPORINE, cytarabine, DACTINomycin, dexmedetomidine, diltiazem, diphenhydrAMINE, DOBUTamine, docetaxel, doxacurium, doxycycline, enalaprilat, ePHEDrine, EPINEPHrine, eptifibatide, etoposide, fenoldopam, fentaNYL, filgrastim, fludarabine, gatafloxacin, gemcitabine, gentamicin, glycopyrrolate, granisetron, heparin, hetastarch, IDArubicin, ifosfamide, inamrinone, isoproterenol, labetalol, levofloxacin, lidocaine, linezolid, LORazepam, magnesium sulfate, mannitol, melphalan, metaraminol, methotrexate, methyldopa, metoclopramide, metoprolol, midazolam, mitoxantrone, nalbuphine, naloxone, perphenazine, potassium chloride, remifentanil, sargramostim, teniposide, vinorelbine, vit B/C

SIDE EFFECTS

CNS: *Dizziness*, fever, lightheadedness, vertigo, **seizures, increased intracranial pressure**

CV: Pericarditis

EENT: Dysphagia, glossitis, decreased calcification of deciduous teeth, permanent discoloration of teeth, oral candidiasis

GI: *Nausea,* abdominal pain, *vomiting, diarrhea,* anorexia, enterocolitis, **hepatotoxicity,** flatulence, abdominal cramps, epigastric burning, stomatitis, **pseudomembranous colitis**

GU: *Increased BUN,* polyuria, polydipsia, **renal failure, nephrotoxicity**

HEMA: Eosinophilia, neutropenia, thrombocytopenia, hemolytic anemia, pancytopenia

INTEG: *Rash, urticaria, photosensitivity, increased pigmentation,* **exfoliative dermatitis,** pruritus, blue-gray color of skin, mucous membranes

MS: Myalgia, arthritis, bone discoloration, joint stiffness

SYST: Angioedema, Stevens-Johnson syndrome

PHARMACOKINETICS

PO: Peak 1-4 hr, half-life 11-22 hr; excreted in urine, feces, breast milk; crosses placenta; 70%-75% protein bound

INTERACTIONS

Increase: effect of warfarin, digoxin, insulin, oral anticoagulants, theophylline, neuromuscular blockers

Increase: chance of pseudomotor cerebri—retinoids; do not use concurrently

Decrease: effect of minocycline—antacids, sodium bicarbonate, alkali products, iron, kaolin/pectin, cimetidine, quinapril, sucralfate

Decrease: effect of barbiturates, carBAMazepine, phenytoin, penicillins, oral contraceptives, calcium

Drug/Lab Test

False negative: urine glucose with Clinistix or Tes-Tape

NURSING CONSIDERATIONS

Assess:

⚠ **Pseudomembranous colitis: diarrhea, abdominal cramps, fever; may start up to 2 mo after treatment ends**

- I&O ratio
- Age and tooth development
- Blood tests: PT, CBC, AST, ALT, BUN, creatinine
- Signs of anemia: Hct, Hgb, fatigue

⚠ **Allergic reactions: rash, itching, pruritus, angioedema**

- Nausea, vomiting, diarrhea; administer antiemetic, antacids as ordered

⚠ **Overgrowth of infection: fever, malaise, redness, pain, swelling, drainage, perineal itching, diarrhea; changes in cough or sputum; black, furry tongue**

Perform/provide:

- Storage in airtight, light-resistant container at room temp

Evaluate:

- Therapeutic response: decreased temp, absence of lesions, negative C&S

Teach patient/family:

- To avoid sunlight, wear protective clothing; sunscreen does not seem to decrease photosensitivity
- That all prescribed medication must be taken to prevent superinfection; not to use outdated product because Fanconi's syndrome may occur

M

• To avoid taking antacids, iron, cimetidine; use 2 hr before, 6 hr after this product; absorption may be decreased
• That teeth discoloration, joint or muscle pain may occur

minoxidil (Rx, OTC)

(mi-nox'i-dill)

Loniten, Rogaine (topical)

Func. class.: Antihypertensive

Chem. class.: Vasodilator, peripheral

Do not confuse:
minoxidil/Monopril
Loniten/Lipitor

ACTION: Directly relaxes arteriolar smooth muscle, causing vasodilation; reduces peripheral vascular resistance, decreases B/P

USES: Severe hypertension unresponsive to other therapy (use with diuretic and β-blocker); topically to treat alopecia

Unlabeled uses: Scleroderma renal crisis (SRC) to control hypertension

CONTRAINDICATIONS: Dissecting aortic aneurysm, hypersensitivity, pheochromocytoma

Black Box Warning: Acute MI

Precautions: Pregnancy (C), breastfeeding, children, geriatric patients, renal disease, CVD

Black Box Warning: CAD, CHF, cardiac disease, cardiac tamponade, edema, hypotension, orthostatic hypotension, pericardial effusion

DOSAGE AND ROUTES

Severe hypertension

• **Adult: PO** 2.5-5 mg/day in 1-2 divided doses; max 100 mg/day; usual range 10-40 mg/day in single dose
• **Geriatric: PO** 2.5 mg/day, may be increased gradually
• **Child <12 yr: PO** (initial) 0.1-0.2 mg/kg/day; (effective range) 0.25-1 mg/kg/day; (max) 50 mg/day

Alopecia

• **Adult: TOP** 1 ml bid, rub into scalp daily, max 2 ml/day

Scleroderma renal crisis (unlabeled)

• **Adult: PO** 5 mg/day in 1-2 divided doses, increase after 3 days by 10-20 mg/day to reach desired B/P, max 100 mg/day

Available forms: Tabs 2.5, 10 mg; topical 2%, 5% sol; topical foam 5%

Administer:

PO route

• With meals for better absorption, to decrease GI symptoms
• With β-blocker and/or diuretic for hypertension

Topical route

• 1 ml no matter how much balding has occurred; increasing dosage does not speed growth

SIDE EFFECTS

Systemic

CNS: Headache, fatigue

CV: *Severe rebound hypertension on withdrawal in children,* tachycardia, angina, increased T wave, CHF, pulmonary edema, pericardial effusion, edema, sodium, water retention, hypotension

GI: Nausea, vomiting

GU: Breast tenderness

HEMA: Hct, Hgb; erythrocyte count may decrease initially

INTEG: Pruritus, Stevens-Johnson syndrome, rash, hirsutism

PHARMACOKINETICS

PO: Onset 30 min, peak 2-3 hr, duration 48-120 hr; half-life 4.2 hr; metabolized in liver; metabolites excreted in urine, feces; protein binding minimal

INTERACTIONS

Increase: hypotension—antihypertensives, MAOIs

Decrease: antihypertensive effect—NSAIDs, salicylates, estrogens

Drug/Herb

Increase: antihypertensive effect—hawthorn

Drug/Lab Test

Increase: renal studies

Decrease: Hgb/Hct/RBC

NURSING CONSIDERATIONS

Assess:

⚠ Monitor closely; usually given with β-blocker to prevent tachycardia and increased myocardial workload; usually given with diuretic to prevent serious fluid accumulation; patient should be hospitalized during beginning treatment

- Nausea, edema in feet, legs daily
- Skin turgor, dryness of mucous membranes for hydration status
- Crackles, dyspnea, orthopnea
- Electrolytes: potassium, sodium, chloride, CO_2
- Renal studies: catecholamines, BUN, creatinine
- Hepatic studies: AST, ALT, alk phos
- B/P, pulse
- Weight daily, I&O

Perform/provide:

- Storage protected from light and heat

Evaluate:

- Therapeutic response: decreased B/P, increased hair growth

Teach patient/family:

- That body hair will increase but is reversible after discontinuing treatment
- Not to discontinue product abruptly
- To report pitting edema, dizziness, weight gain >5 lb, SOB, bruising or bleeding, heart rate >20 beats/min over normal, severe indigestion, dizziness, lightheadedness, panting, new or aggravated symptoms of angina
- To take product exactly as prescribed because serious side effects may occur

Topical

- That, for topical use, treatment must continue for the long term or new hair will be lost
- Not to use except on scalp

TREATMENT OF OVERDOSE:

Administer normal saline IV, vasopressors

mirtazapine (Rx)

(mer-ta′za-peen)

CO Mirtazapine ♣, Gen-Mirtazapine ♣, Novo-Mirtazapine ♣, PMS-Mirtazapine ♣, ratio-Mirtazapine ♣, Remeron, Remeron Soltab, Sandoz Mirtazapine ♣

Func. class.: Antidepressant

Chem. class.: Tetracyclic

ACTION: Blocks reuptake of norepinephrine and serotonin into nerve endings, thereby increasing action of norepinephrine and serotonin in nerve cells; antagonist of central α_2-receptors; blocks histamine receptors

USES: Depression; dysthymic disorder; bipolar disorder: depressed, agitated depression

Unlabeled uses: Resting tremor, benign familial tremor, levodopa-induced dyskinesias, pruritus

CONTRAINDICATIONS: Hypersensitivity to tricyclics, recovery phase of MI, agranulocytosis, jaundice

Precautions: Pregnancy (C), geriatric patients, suicidal patients, severe depression, increased intraocular pressure, closed-angle glaucoma, urinary retention, cardiac/renal/hepatic disease, hypo/hyperthyroidism, electroshock therapy, elective surgery, seizure disorder, bone marrow suppression, thrombocytopenia

Black Box Warning: Suicidal ideation, children

M

DOSAGE AND ROUTES

- **Adult: PO** 15 mg/day at bedtime, maintenance to continue for 6 mo, titrate up to 45 mg/day; **ORALLY DISINTEGRATING** tabs: open blister pack, place tab on tongue, allow to disintegrate, swallow
- **Geriatric: PO** 7.5 mg at bedtime, increase by 7.5 mg q1-2wk to desired dose, max 45 mg/day

Resting tremor/benign familial tremor/levodopa-induced dyskinesias (unlabeled)

- **Adult: PO** titrate up to 30 mg at bedtime

Pruritus (unlabeled)

- **Adult: PO** 15-30 mg/day

Available forms: Tabs 7.5, 15, 30, 45 mg; orally disintegrating tab (soltab) 15, 30, 45 mg

Administer:

- Increased fluids, bulk in diet for constipation, especially for geriatric patients
- With food, milk for GI symptoms
- Dosage at bedtime if oversedation occurs during day; may take entire dose at bedtime; geriatric patients may not tolerate once daily dosing
- Gum, hard candy, or frequent sips of water for dry mouth
- *Orally disintegrating tab:* no water needed; allow to dissolve on tongue, do not split

SIDE EFFECTS

CNS: *Dizziness, drowsiness,* confusion, headache, anxiety, tremors, stimulation, weakness, nightmares, EPS (geriatric patients), increased psychiatric symptoms, seizures

CV: *Orthostatic hypotension, ECG changes, tachycardia,* hypertension, palpitations

EENT: *Blurred vision,* tinnitus, mydriasis

GI: *Diarrhea, dry mouth,* nausea, vomiting, paralytic ileus, increased appetite, cramps, epigastric distress, constipation, jaundice, hepatitis, stomatitis, weight gain

GU: *Urinary retention,* acute renal failure

HEMA: Agranulocytosis, thrombocytopenia, eosinophilia, leukopenia

INTEG: Rash, urticaria, sweating, pruritus, photosensitivity

SYST: Flulike symptoms, increased cholesterol levels

PHARMACOKINETICS

PO: Peak 2 hr, metabolized by CYP1A2, 2D6, 3A4 in liver; excreted in urine, feces; crosses placenta; half-life 20-40 hr, protein binding 85%

INTERACTIONS

⚠ Increase: hyperpyretic crisis, seizures, hypertensive episode—MAOIs

Increase: CNS depression—alcohol, barbiturates, benzodiazepines, other CNS depressants

Increase: serotonin syndrome—SSRIs, SNRIs, serotonin-receptor agonists, fenfluramine, dexfenfluramine, sibutramine, nefazodone

Decrease: effects of cloNIDine, indirect-acting sympathomimetics (ePHEDrine)

Drug/Herb

- Serotonin syndrome: St. John's wort

Increase: CNS depression—kava

Drug/Lab Test

Increase: serum bilirubin, blood glucose, alk phos

Decrease: VMA, 5-HIAA

False increase: urinary catecholamines

NURSING CONSIDERATIONS

Assess:

- B/P (lying, standing), pulse q4hr; if systolic B/P drops 20 mm Hg, hold product, notify prescriber; vital signs q4hr in patients with CV disease
- Blood studies: CBC, leukocytes, differential, cardiac enzymes, lipid profile, blood glucose if patient is receiving long-term therapy
- Hepatic studies: AST, ALT, bilirubin, creatinine
- Weight weekly; appetite may increase with product

• ECG for flattening of T wave, bundle branch block, AV block, dysrhythmias in cardiac patients

Black Box Warning: Mental status: mood, sensorium, affect, suicidal tendencies (especially among adolescents, young adults), increase in psychiatric symptoms: depression, panic; EPS primarily in geriatric patients: rigidity, dystonia, akathisia

⚠ **Serotonin syndrome:** hyperthermia, hypertension, myoclonus, rigidity, delirium, coma; if using other serotonergic products

• Alcohol consumption; if alcohol consumed, hold dose until morning

Perform/provide:

• Storage in tight container at room temp; do not freeze

• Assistance with ambulation during beginning therapy, since drowsiness, dizziness occurs

• Safety measures, including side rails, primarily for geriatric patients

Evaluate:

• Therapeutic response: decreased depression

Teach patient/family:

• That therapeutic effects may take 2-3 wk; to take at bedtime; that there is decreased sedation with increased doses

• To use caution when driving, performing other activities requiring alertness because of drowsiness, dizziness, blurred vision

• To immediately report urinary retention, worsening of depression, suicidal thoughts/behaviors

• To avoid alcohol, other CNS depressants

• About how to take orally disintegrating tabs; dissolve on tongue, swallow

• Not to use within 14 days of MAOIs

TREATMENT OF OVERDOSE:

ECG monitoring, lavage, activated charcoal; administer anticonvulsant, IV fluids

misoprostol (Rx)

(mye-soe-prost′ole)

Apo-Misoprostol ✦, Cytotec

Func. class.: Gastric mucosa protectant, antiulcer

Chem. class.: Prostaglandin E_1 analog

Do not confuse:

misoprostol/metoprolol

Cytotec/Cytoxan

ACTION: Inhibits gastric acid secretion; may protect gastric mucosa; can increase bicarbonate, mucus production

USES: Prevention of NSAID-induced gastric ulcers

Unlabeled uses: Pregnancy termination, postpartum hemorrhage, cervical ripening/labor induction (vaginal), active duodenal/gastric ulcer, kidney transplant rejection prophylaxis

CONTRAINDICATIONS: Hypersensitivity to this product or prostaglandins

Black Box Warning: Pregnancy (X), females

Precautions: Breastfeeding, children, geriatric patients, renal/CV disease, abnormal fetal position, cardiac/renal/inflammatory bowel disease, C-section, dehydration, diarrhea, fever, ectopic pregnancy, fetal distress, sepsis, vaginal bleeding

DOSAGE AND ROUTES

• **Adult: PO** 200 mcg qid with food for duration of NSAID therapy, with last dose given at bedtime; if 200 mcg is not tolerated, 100 mcg may be given

Active duodenal/gastric ulcer (unlabeled)

• **Adult: PO** 100-200 mcg qid with meals at bedtime × 4-8 wk

Pregnancy termination prior to 63rd day (unlabeled)
• **Adult: INTRAVAGINALLY** 800 mcg 5-7 days after methotrexate IM
Cervical ripening induction for term pregnancy (unlabeled)
• **Adult: INTRAVAGINALLY** 25 mcg q3-6hr
Available forms: Tabs 100, 200 mcg
Administer:
• PO with meals for prolonged product effect; avoid use of magnesium antacids

SIDE EFFECTS

GI: *Diarrhea,* nausea, vomiting, flatulence, constipation, dyspepsia, abdominal pain
GU: Spotting, cramps, hypermenorrhea, menstrual disorders

PHARMACOKINETICS

PO: Peak 12 min, plasma steady state achieved within 2 days, excreted in urine

INTERACTIONS

Drug/Food
Decrease: maximum concentrations when taken with food

NURSING CONSIDERATIONS

Assess:
• GI symptoms: hematemesis, occult or frank blood in stools, gastric aspirate, cramping, severe diarrhea
• Obtain a negative pregnancy test; miscarriages are common
Perform/provide:
• Storage at room temp
Evaluate:
• Therapeutic response: absence of pain or GI complaints; prevention of ulcers
Teach patient/family:
• To take only as directed; to read patient information leaflet

Black Box Warning: Not to take if pregnant (can cause miscarriage) (X); not to become pregnant while taking product; if pregnancy occurs during therapy, discontinue product, notify prescriber; not to breastfeed

• Not to give product to anyone else or to take for more than 4 wk unless directed by prescriber
• To avoid OTC preparations: aspirin, cough, cold products; condition may worsen

⚠ HIGH ALERT

mitomycin (Rx)

(mye-toe-mye′sin)
Func. class.: Antineoplastic, antibiotic

Do not confuse:
mitomycin/mithramycin/mitotane/mitoxantrone

ACTION: Inhibits DNA synthesis, primarily; derived from *Streptomyces caespitosus;* appears to cause cross-linking of DNA; vesicant

USES: Pancreatic, stomach, colorectal, bladder cancer
Unlabeled uses: Palliative treatment of anal, bladder, head, neck, colon, breast, biliary, cervical, lung malignancies; bone marrow ablation, desmoid tumor, mesothelioma, stem cell transplant preparation

CONTRAINDICATIONS: Pregnancy (D) 1st trimester, breastfeeding, hypersensitivity, as single agent, coagulation disorders

Black Box Warning: Thrombocytopenia

Precautions: Accidental exposure, acute bronchospasm, anemia, children, dental disease/work, extravasation, females, infection, radiation therapy, surgery, vaccines, renal/respiratory disease

Black Box Warning: Bone marrow suppression, hemolytic-uremic syndrome

DOSAGE AND ROUTES

• **Adult: IV** 10-20 mg/m^2 q6-8wk
Available forms: Inj 5, 20, 40 mg/vial

Administer:

Direct IV route

- Use port, if possible
- Antiemetic 30-60 min before product to prevent vomiting
- IV after diluting 5 mg/10 ml, 20 mg/ 40 ml, 40 mg/80 ml (0.5 mg/ml) sterile water for inj; shake, allow to stand, give through Y-tube or 3-way stopcock; give slow IV push or infuse over 15-30 min; color of reconstituted sol is gray

Y-site compatibilities: Allopurinol, amifostine, bleomycin, CISplatin, cyclophosphamide, DOXOrubicin, droperidol, fluorouracil, furosemide, granisetron, heparin, leucovorin, melphalan, methotrexate, metoclopramide, ondansetron, teniposide, thiotepa, vinBLAStine, vinCRIStine

SIDE EFFECTS

CNS: Fever, headache, confusion, drowsiness, syncope, fatigue

EENT: Blurred vision

GI: *Nausea, vomiting, anorexia, stomatitis,* **hepatotoxicity**, diarrhea

GU: Urinary retention, **renal failure**, edema

HEMA: **Thrombocytopenia, leukopenia, anemia**

INTEG: *Rash,* alopecia, **extravasation**, nail discoloration

MISC: **Hemolytic uremic syndrome, CHF**

RESP: **Fibrosis, pulmonary infiltrate**, dyspnea

PHARMACOKINETICS

Half-life 1 hr, metabolized in liver, 10% excreted in urine (unchanged)

INTERACTIONS

Increase: toxicity—other antineoplastics, radiation

Increase: bleeding risk—NSAIDs, anticoagulants

Drug/Herb

- Avoid use with black cohosh

NURSING CONSIDERATIONS

Assess:

Black Box Warning: Bone marrow suppression: CBC, differential, platelet count weekly; withhold product if WBC is <2000/mm³, granulocyte count <1000/mm³, or platelet count is <100,000/mm³; notify prescriber; bleeding: hematuria, guaiac, bruising, petechiae, mucosa or orifices

- Pulmonary function tests; chest x-ray before, during therapy; chest x-ray should be obtained q2wk during treatment

Black Box Warning: Fatal hemolytic-uremic syndrome: hypertension, thrombocytopenia, microangiopathic hemolytic anemia; occurs in those receiving long-term therapy

- Renal studies: BUN, serum uric acid, urine CCr, electrolytes before, during therapy, adjust dose based on renal function
- I&O ratio; report fall in urine output to <30 ml/hr
- Monitor temp q4hr; fever may indicate beginning infection
- Hepatic studies before, during therapy: bilirubin, AST, ALT, alk phos as needed or monthly; check for jaundiced skin and sclera, dark urine, clay-colored stools, itchy skin, abdominal pain, fever, diarrhea

⚠ **Pulmonary fibrosis:** bronchospasm, dyspnea, crackles, unproductive cough; chest pain, tachypnea, fatigue, increased pulse, pallor, lethargy

- Effects of alopecia on body image; discuss feelings about body changes
- Inflammation of mucosa, breaks in skin
- Buccal cavity q8hr for dryness, sores, ulceration, white patches, oral pain, bleeding, dysphagia
- Local irritation, pain, burning at inj site
- GI symptoms: frequency of stools, cramping

M

• **Acidosis, signs of dehydration:** rapid respirations, poor skin turgor, decreased urine output, dry skin, restlessness, weakness

Perform/provide:

• Adequate fluids 2-3 L/day unless contraindicated

• Rinsing of mouth tid-qid with water; brushing of teeth with baking soda bid-tid with soft brush or cotton-tipped applicators for stomatitis; use unwaxed dental floss

• Storage at room temp for 1 wk after reconstituting or for 2 wk refrigerated

Evaluate:

• Therapeutic response: decreased tumor size, spread of malignancy

Teach patient/family:

• That hair may be lost during treatment; that wig or hairpiece may make patient feel better; that new hair may be different in color, texture

• To avoid foods with citric acid, hot or rough texture

• To report any bleeding, white spots, ulcerations in mouth; to examine mouth daily

• To avoid crowds, persons with infections if granulocyte count is low

• To immediately report urine retention, absence of urine, dyspnea, bleeding, jaundice

HIGH ALERT

mitoxantrone (Rx)

(mye-toe-zan'trone)

Novantrone

Func. class.: Antineoplastic, antiinfective, immunomodulator

Chem. class.: Synthetic anthraquinone

Do not confuse:
mitoxantrone/mitomycin/mithramycin/mitotane

ACTION: DNA reactive agent; cytocidal effect on both proliferating and nonproliferating cells; topoisomerase II inhibitor (vesicant)

USES: Acute myelogenous leukemia (adult), relapsed leukemia, breast cancer; used with steroids to treat bone pain (advanced prostate cancer), multiple sclerosis (MS)

Unlabeled uses: Liver malignancies, non-Hodgkin's lymphoma, breast cancer, ALL

CONTRAINDICATIONS: Pregnancy (D), hypersensitivity

Precautions: Breastfeeding, children; myelosuppression, renal/cardiac/hepatic disease; gout

Black Box Warning: Secondary malignancy, neutropenia, intrathecal administration, extravasation, heart failure

DOSAGE AND ROUTES

Acute myelogenous leukemia/induction

• **Adult: IV INF** 12 mg/m^2/day on days 1-3 and 100 mg/m^2 cytarabine × 7 days as continuous 24-hr inf

Consolidation

• **Adult: IV** 12 mg/m^2 given as short 5- to 15-min inf

Advanced prostate cancer

• **Adult: IV** 12-14 mg/m^2 as single dose or short inf q21days

Multiple sclerosis, relapsing

• **Adult: IV INF** 12 mg/m^2 as 5- to 15-min inf q3mo

Available forms: Inj 2, 10, 12.5, 15 mg/ml

Administer:

• Medications by oral route if possible; avoid IM, SUBCUT, IV routes

• Antiemetic 30-60 min before product to prevent vomiting

Direct IV route

• IV after diluting with ≥50 ml NS or D_5W; give over 3-5 min into running IV of D_5W or NS; check for extravasation; do not give IM, SUBCUT, or intraarterially

Intermittent IV INF route
- May be diluted further in D_5W, NS, run over 15-30 min

Continuous IV INF route
- Give over 24 hr

Y-site compatibilities: Allopurinol, amifostine, cladribine, filgrastim, fludarabine, granisetron, melphalan, ondansetron, sargramostim, teniposide, thiotepa, vinorelbine

SIDE EFFECTS

CNS: Headache, **seizures**, fatigue
CV: **CHF, cardiopathy, dysrhythmias**
EENT: Conjunctivitis, blue/green sclera, blurred vision
GI: *Nausea, vomiting, diarrhea, anorexia, mucositis,* **hepatotoxicity**
GU: Amenorrhea, menstrual disorders
HEMA: **Thrombocytopenia, leukopenia, myelosuppression, anemia, secondary leukemia**
INTEG: *Rash, necrosis at inj site,* dermatitis, thrombophlebitis at inj site, alopecia
MISC: Fever
RESP: Cough, dyspnea

PHARMACOKINETICS

Protein binding 78%; metabolized in liver; excreted via renal, hepatobiliary systems; half-life 23-215 hr

INTERACTIONS

- Do not mix with heparin; precipitate will form
- Do not mix with any other product

Increase: bone marrow depression toxicity—radiation, other antineoplastics
Increase: adverse reactions—live virus vaccines
Increase: bleeding risk—NSAIDs, anticoagulants

NURSING CONSIDERATIONS

Assess:
- CBC, differential, platelet count weekly; withhold product if WBC is <4000/mm^3 or platelet count is <75,000/mm^3; neutrophil count or ANC; notify prescriber of results
- Hepatic studies before, during therapy: bilirubin, AST, ALT, alk phos prn or monthly; dose reduction needed with hepatic disease
- Renal studies: BUN, serum uric acid, urine CCr, electrolytes before, during therapy
- Bleeding, hematuria, guaiac, bruising or petechiae, mucosa or orifices q8hr
- Jaundiced skin and sclera, dark urine, clay-colored stools, itchy skin, abdominal pain, fever, diarrhea

Black Box Warning: ECG, ECHO, chest x-ray, MUGA, RAI angiography; assess ejection fraction before and during treatment; cardiotoxic may develop during treatment or months to years after treatment; use vigilant cardiac monitoring in MS

- Acidosis, signs of dehydration: rapid respirations, poor skin turgor, decreased urine output, dry skin, restlessness, weakness

Black Box Warning: Secondary acute myelogenous leukemia (AML) that can develop after taking this product

⚠ **For MS: obtain MUGA, LVEF baselines; repeat LVEF if symptoms of CHF occur or if cumulative dose is >100 mg/m^2; do not administer to patients who have received lifetime dose of ≥140 mg/m^2 or if LVEF <50% or significant LVEF**

- Do not administer to patients with MS if neutrophils <1500 cells/mm^3, except in AML
- Obtain pregnancy test for all women of childbearing age, even if birth control is used

Perform/provide:
- Rinsing of mouth tid-qid with water, club soda; brushing of teeth bid-qid with soft brush or cotton-tipped applicators for stomatitis; use unwaxed dental floss
- Increased fluids to 2-3 L/day unless contraindicated

Evaluate:
- Therapeutic response: decreased tumor size, spread of malignancy

Teach patient/family:
• To immediately report bleeding, dyspnea, possible infections, seizure, jaundice
• To avoid hot foods or those with citric acid, rough texture
• To report any bleeding, white spots, ulcerations in mouth; to examine mouth daily
• To avoid crowds, persons with infections
• That sclera, urine may turn blue or green; that hair loss may occur
• To notify prescriber if pregnancy is suspected or planned; to use effective contraception

modafinil (Rx)

(mo-daf′i-nil)

Alertec ✱, Apo-Modafinil ✱, Provigil

Func. class.: CNS stimulant
Chem. class.: Racemic compound

Controlled Substance IV

ACTION: Similar action as that of sympathomimetics; does not alter release of dopamine, norepinephrine

USES: Narcolepsy, shift-work sleep disturbance, obstructive sleep apnea

CONTRAINDICATIONS: Hypersensitivity, ischemic heart disease, left ventricular hypertrophy, chest pain, dysrhythmias
Precautions: Pregnancy (C), breastfeeding, child <16 yr, geriatric patients, unstable angina, history of MI, severe hepatic disease

DOSAGE AND ROUTES

• **Adult and adolescent ≥16 yr: PO** 200 mg daily
Hepatic dose (severe hepatic disease)
• **Adult: PO** 100 mg daily

Available forms: Tabs 100, 200 mg
Administer:
• Give 1 hr before start of shift work or in AM for those with narcolepsy or sleep apnea

SIDE EFFECTS

CNS: *Headache,* anxiety, cataplexy, depression, dizziness, insomnia, amnesia, confusion, ataxia, tremors, paresthesia, dyskinesia, **suicidal ideation**
CV: Dysrhythmias, hypo/hypertension, chest pain, vasodilation
EENT: Change in vision, *rhinitis,* pharyngitis, epistaxis
GI: Nausea, vomiting, changes in LFTs, anorexia, diarrhea, thirst, mouth ulcers
GU: Ejaculation disorder, urinary retention, albuminuria
HEMA: Eosinophilia
INTEG: Rash, dry skin, herpes simplex, **Stevens-Johnson syndrome**
MISC: Infection, hyperglycemia, neck pain
RESP: *Dyspnea*, lung changes

PHARMACOKINETICS

Absorbed rapidly, 60% protein binding, metabolized by the liver (90%), half-life 15 hr, peak 2-4 hr

INTERACTIONS

Increase: effects of—diazepam, tricylic antidepressants, phenytoin, propranolol, warfarin
Decrease: effects of—cycloSPORINE, hormonal contraceptives, theophylline, estrogens
Drug/Herb
Increase: stimulation—cola nut, guarana, yerba maté, coffee, tea
Drug/Lab Test
Increase: LFTs, glucose, eosinophils

NURSING CONSIDERATIONS

Assess:
• Narcolepsy, shift work, history of sleep apnea
• Depression, suicidal ideation

• Monitor B/P in those with hypertension

Perform/provide:

• Storage at room temp

Evaluate:

• Ability to stay awake

Teach patient/family:

• To take only as directed; that product may be taken with/without food

• To use other form of contraception during and for ≥30 days after discontinuing medication if using hormonal birth control; to notify prescriber if pregnancy is planned or suspected or if breastfeeding

• To notify prescriber of allergic reaction, tremors, confusion

• To avoid all OTC medications unless approved by prescriber

• To avoid hazardous activities until drug effect is known

moexipril (Rx)

(moe-ex′ih-prill)

Univasc

Func. class.: Antihypertensive

Chem. class.: Angiotensin-converting enzyme inhibitor

ACTION: Selectively suppresses renin-angiotensin-aldosterone system; inhibits ACE; prevents conversion of angiotensin I to angiotensin II; results in dilation of arterial, venous vessels

USES: Hypertension, alone or in combination with thiazide diuretics

CONTRAINDICATIONS: Breastfeeding, children, hypersensitivity, heart block, bilateral renal stenosis, history of angioedema

Black Box Warning: Pregnancy (D)

Precautions: Dialysis patients, hypovolemia, leukemia, scleroderma, lupus erythematosus, blood dyscrasias, CHF, diabetes mellitus, thyroid/renal disease, COPD, asthma, potassium-sparing diuretics

DOSAGE AND ROUTES

• **Adult: PO** 7.5 mg 1 hr before meals initially; may be increased or divided depending on B/P response; maintenance dosage 7.5-30 mg/day in 1-2 divided doses 1 hr before meals

Renal dose

• **Adult: PO** CCr <40 ml/min, 3.75 mg/day; titrate to desired dose; max 15 mg/day

Available forms: Tabs 7.5, 15 mg

Administer:

• 1 hr before meals

• Do not use with potassium-sparing diuretics, sympathomimetics, potassium supplements

SIDE EFFECTS

CNS: Fever, chills, fatigue, headache

CV: Hypotension, postural hypotension

GI: Loss of taste, **hepatic failure/necrosis,** hepatitis

GU: Impotence, dysuria, nocturia, proteinuria, **nephrotic syndrome,** acute reversible renal failure, polyuria, oliguria, frequency

HEMA: **Neutropenia**

INTEG: Rash, photosensitivity

META: Hypokalemia, hyperkalemia, hyponatremia

MS: Myalgia

RESP: **Bronchospasm,** dyspnea, dry cough, pneumonitis

SYST: **Angioedema, anaphylaxis**

PHARMACOKINETICS

Peak 1.5 hr, metabolized by liver (metabolites); excreted in feces (52%), urine; crosses placenta, excreted in breast milk, protein binding 50%-70%, half-life 2-10 hr

INTERACTIONS

• Do not use with potassium-sparing diuretics, sympathomimetics, potassium supplements

M

Increase: hypotension—diuretics, other antihypertensives, ganglionic blockers, adrenergic blockers, phenothiazines
Increase: toxicity—digoxin, lithium
Increase: hyperkalemia—cycloSPORINE, potassium-sparing diuretics
Increase: myelosuppression—azaTHIOprine
Decrease: antihypertensive effect—NSAIDs

Drug/Herb
Increase: antihypertensive effect—hawthorn
Decrease: antihypertensive effect—yohimbe

Drug/Lab Test
False positive: urine acetone

NURSING CONSIDERATIONS

Assess:
- Blood tests: neutrophils, decreased platelets
- Renal studies: protein, BUN, creatinine; watch for increased levels that may indicate nephrotic syndrome
- Baselines of renal, hepatic studies before therapy begins
- Potassium levels, although hyperkalemia rarely occurs
- Edema in feet, legs daily
- Allergic reaction: rash, fever, pruritus, urticaria; product should be discontinued if antihistamines fail to help
- Symptoms of CHF; edema, dyspnea, wet crackles, B/P, difficulty breathing
- Renal symptoms: polyuria, oliguria, frequency

Perform/provide:
- Storage in tight container at ≤86° F (30° C)

Evaluate:
- Therapeutic response: decrease in B/P with hypertension

Teach patient/family:
- To take 1 hr before meals
- Not to discontinue product abruptly
- Not to use OTC (cough, cold, allergy) products unless directed by prescriber
- To comply with dosage schedule even if feeling better
- To rise slowly to sitting or standing position to minimize orthostatic hypotension
- To notify prescriber of mouth sores, sore throat, fever, swelling of hands or feet, irregular heartbeat, chest pain, signs of angioedema
- That excessive perspiration, dehydration, vomiting, diarrhea may lead to fall in B/P; to consult prescriber if these occur
- That dizziness, fainting, lightheadedness may occur during 1st few days of therapy
- That skin rash or impaired perspiration may occur
- How to take B/P

Black Box Warning: Notify prescriber if pregnancy is planned or suspected

TREATMENT OF OVERDOSE:
0.9% NaCl IV inf, hemodialysis

montelukast (Rx)
(mon-teh-loo′kast)

Singulair

Func. class.: Bronchodilator
Chem. class.: Leukotriene receptor antagonist, cysteinyl

ACTION: Inhibits leukotriene (LTD_4) formation; leukotrienes exert their effects by increasing neutrophil, eosinophil migration; aggregation of neutrophils, monocytes; smooth muscle contraction, capillary permeability; these actions further lead to bronchoconstriction, inflammation, edema

USES: Chronic asthma in adults and children, seasonal allergic rhinitis, bronchospasm prophylaxis

CONTRAINDICATIONS: Hypersensitivity
Precautions: Pregnancy (B), breastfeeding, children <6 yr, acute attacks of asthma, alcohol consumption, severe he-

patic disease, corticosteroid withdrawal, phenylketonuria

DOSAGE AND ROUTES

• **Adult and child ≥15 yr: PO** 10 mg/day in PM
• **Child 6-14 yr: PO** 5-mg chew tab/day in PM
• **Child 2-5 yr: PO** (chew tab/granules) 4 mg/day

Asthma

• **Child 12-23 mo: PO** 1 packet (4 mg) granules taken in PM

Exercise-induced bronchoconstriction

• **Adult and adolescent ≥15 yr: PO** 10 mg 2 hr prior to exercise; do not take another dose within 24 hr

Available forms: Tabs 10 mg; chew tabs 4, 5 mg; oral granules 4 mg/packet

Administer:

PO route

• In PM daily for all uses except exercise-induced bronchoconstriction; then take 2 hr prior to exercise
• Granules directly in mouth or mixed with spoonful of soft food (carrots, applesauce, ice cream, rice)
• Do not open granules packet until ready to use; mix whole dose; give within 15 min

SIDE EFFECTS

CNS: *Dizziness, fatigue, headache,* behavior changes, **suicidal ideation, suicide,** hallucinations, **seizures,** agitation, anxiety, depression, fever, drowsiness
GI: *Abdominal pain,* dyspepsia, nausea, vomiting, diarrhea, **pancreatitis**
HEMA: Thrombocytopenia
INTEG: Rash, pruritus, erythema
MS: Asthenia, myalgia, muscle cramps
RESP: *Influenza, cough,* nasal congestion
SYST: Anaphylaxis, angioedema, Churg-Strauss syndrome

PHARMACOKINETICS

Rapidly absorbed; peak 3-4 hr; half-life 2.7-5.5 hr; protein binding 99%; metabolized by liver; excreted via bile

INTERACTIONS

Decrease: montelukast levels—barbiturates, rifabutin, rifapentine, carBAMazepine, fosphenytoin, phenytoin, rifampin

Drug/Herb

Increase: stimulation—black, green tea, guarana

Drug/Lab Test

Increase: ALT, AST

NURSING CONSIDERATIONS

Assess:

⚠ **Churg-Strauss syndrome: adult patients carefully for symptoms: eosinophilia, vasculitic rash, worsening pulmonary symptoms, cardiac complications, neuropathy**
• CBC, blood chemistry during treatment
• Respiratory rate, rhythm, depth; auscultate lung fields bilaterally; notify prescriber of abnormalities
• Allergic reactions: rash, urticaria; product should be discontinued

⚠ **For behavior changes and suicidal ideation, other neuropsychiatric reactions**

Evaluate:

• Therapeutic response: ability to breathe more easily

Teach patient/family:

• To check OTC medications, current prescription medications for ePHEDrine, which will increase stimulation; to avoid alcohol
• To avoid hazardous activities; dizziness may occur
• That product is not to be used for acute asthma attacks
• If aspirin sensitivity is known, not to take NSAIDs while taking this product
• To continue to use inhaled β-agonists if exercise-induced asthma occurs

Black Box Warning: To notify prescriber of suicidal thoughts/behaviors

M

⚠ HIGH ALERT

morphine (Rx)

(mor′feen)

Astramorph PF, Avinza, Depo Dur, Infumorph PF, Kadian, M.O.S. ✤, MS Contin, MSIR ✤, Oramorph SR, PMS-Morphine Sulfate ✤, ratio-Morphine ✤, ratio-Morphine SR ✤

Func. class.: Opioid analgesic
Chem. class.: Alkaloid

Controlled Substance Schedule II

Do not confuse:
morphine/HYDROmorphone
MS Contin/oxycontin

ACTION: Depresses pain impulse transmission at the spinal cord level by interacting with opioid receptors

USES: Moderate to severe pain

CONTRAINDICATIONS: Hypersensitivity, addiction (opioid), hemorrhage, bronchial asthma, increased intracranial pressure, paralytic ileus, hypovolemia, shock

Black Box Warning: Respiratory depression

Precautions: Pregnancy (C), breastfeeding, children <18 yr, geriatric patients, addictive personality, acute MI, severe heart disease, renal/hepatic disease, bowel impaction

Black Box Warning: Abrupt discontinuation, accidental exposure, epidural/intrathecal administration, opioid-naive patients, substance abuse

DOSAGE AND ROUTES

- **Adult: SUBCUT/IM** 5-10 mg q4hr (opiate naive), 5-20 mg q4hr (prior opiate use); **PO** 10-30 mg q4hr prn; **EXT REL** 15-30 mg q8-12hr; **RECT** 10-20 mg q4hr prn; **IV** 2.5-15 mg diluted in 4-5 ml water for inj over 5 min; **SUS REL** caps (Kadian), **EXT REL** caps (Avinza) give total daily dose q24hr; for those with no tolerance to opioids, 30 mg/day; may adjust by no more than 30 mg q4days (MS Contin may be given in divided doses)
- **Child: SUBCUT/IV** 0.05-0.2 mg/kg, max 15 mg; **PO** 0.2-0.5 mg/kg q4-6hr (reg rel), q12hr (sus rel)

Available forms: Inj 0.5, 1, 2, 4, 5, 8, 10, 15, 25, 50 mg/ml; oral sol 10, 20 mg/5 ml, 10 mg/0.5 ml, 100 mg/5 ml; oral tabs 15, 30 mg; rect supp 5, 10, 20, 30 mg; ext rel tabs 15, 30, 60, 100, 200 mg; cont rel cap pellets (Kadian) 10, 20, 30, 50, 60, 80, 100, 200 mg; ext rel caps (Avinza) 30, 45, 60, 75, 90, 120 mg

Administer:

- May be given by patient: controlled analgesia
- Epidural cautiously in geriatric patients
- Kadian is not bioequivalent to other controlled-rel forms
- Kadian caps may be opened and sprinkled on applesauce immediately before use; pellets in cap should not be chewed, crushed, or dissolved, may lead to overdose; adjustments may need to be made when converting from another form of morphine

PO route

- Do not break, crush, or chew controlled or sus rel products
- With antiemetic for nausea, vomiting
- When pain is beginning to return; determine dosage interval by response; continuous dosing is more effective than prn
- 20 mg/ml concentrated oral sol for opioid-tolerant patients only

IV route

- Give after diluting with ≥5 ml sterile water or NS; give ≤15 mg/4-5 min; give through Y-tube or 3-way stopcock; may be added to IV sol; each 0.1-1 mg diluted in 1 ml D_5W, $D_{10}W$, 0.9% NaCl, 0.45% NaCl, Ringer's sol, LR, given with inf pump titrated to patient response

Syringe compatibilities: Atropine, benzquinamide, bupivacaine, butorphanol, cimetidine, dimenhyDRINATE, diphenhydrAMINE, droperidol, fentaNYL, glycopyrrolate, hydrOXYzine, ketamine, metoclopramide, midazolam, milrinone, pentazocine, perphenazine, promazine, ranitidine, scopolamine

Y-site compatibilities: Allopurinol, amifostine, amikacin, aminophylline, amiodarone, ampicillin, ampicillin/sulbactam, amsacrine, atenolol, atracurium, aztreonam, bumetanide, calcium chloride, cefamandole, ceFAZolin, cefmetazole, cefoperazone, cefotaxime, cefotetan, cefoxitin, ceftazidime, ceftizoxime, cefTRIAXone, cefuroxime, cephalothin, cephapirin, chloramphenicol, cisatracurium, CISplatin, cladribine, clindamycin, cyclophosphamide, cytarabine, dexamethasone, digoxin, diltiazem, DOBUTamine, DOPamine, doxycycline, enalaprilat, EPINEPHrine, erythromycin, esmolol, etomidate, famotidine, fentaNYL, filgrastim, fluconazole, fludarabine, foscarnet, gentamicin, granisetron, heparin, hydrocortisone, HYDROmorphone, IL-2, insulin (regular), kanamycin, labetalol, lidocaine, LORazepam, magnesium sulfate, melphalan, meropenem, methotrexate, methyldopate, methylPREDNISolone, metoclopramide, metoprolol, metroNIDAZOLE, mezlocillin, midazolam, milrinone, moxalactam, nafcillin, niCARdipine, nitroglycerin, norepinephrine, ondansetron, oxacillin, oxytocin, paclitaxel, pancuronium, penicillin G potassium, piperacillin, piperacillin/tazobactam, potassium chloride, propofol, propranolol, ranitidine, remifentanil, sodium bicarbonate, sodium nitroprusside, teniposide, thiotepa, ticarcillin, ticarcillin/clavulanate, tobramycin, trimethoprim-sulfamethoxazole, vancomycin, vecuronium, vinorelbine, vit B/C, warfarin, zidovudine

SIDE EFFECTS

CNS: Drowsiness, dizziness, confusion, headache, sedation, euphoria, insomnia, **seizures**

CV: Palpitations, **bradycardia**, change in B/P, **shock**, **cardiac arrest**, chest pain, hypo/hypertension, edema, **tachycardia**

EENT: Tinnitus, blurred vision, miosis, diplopia

GI: Nausea, vomiting, anorexia, constipation, cramps, biliary tract pressure

GU: Urinary retention

HEMA: **Thrombocytopenia**

INTEG: Rash, urticaria, bruising, flushing, diaphoresis, pruritus

RESP: **Respiratory depression, respiratory arrest, apnea**

PHARMACOKINETICS

PO: Onset variable, peak variable, duration variable

IM: Onset $^1/_2$ hr, peak 50-90 min, duration 3-7 hr

SUBCUT: Onset 15-20 min, peak 50-90 min, duration 3-5 hr

IV: Peak 20 min

RECT: Peak $^1/_2$-1 hr, duration 4-5 hr

Intrathecal: Onset rapid, duration ≤24 hr

Metabolized by liver, crosses placenta; excreted in urine, breast milk; half-life $1^1/_2$-2 hr

M

INTERACTIONS

- Unpredictable reaction, avoid use: MAOIs

Increase: effects with other CNS depressants—alcohol, opiates, sedative/hypnotics, antipsychotics, skeletal muscle relaxants

Decrease: morphine action—rifampin

Drug/Herb

Increase: anticholinergic effect—corkwood

Increase: CNS depression—chamomile, hops, kava, St. John's wort, valerian

Drug/Food

Decrease: morphine effect—cranberry juice (excessive amounts), oats

Drug/Lab Test

Increase: amylase

NURSING CONSIDERATIONS

Assess:

- **Pain:** location, type, character; give dose before pain becomes severe
- Bowel status; constipation common, use stimulant laxative if needed
- I&O ratio; check for decreasing output; may indicate urinary retention
- B/P, pulse, respirations (character, depth, rate)
- CNS changes: dizziness, drowsiness, hallucinations, euphoria, LOC, pupil reaction

Black Box Warning: Abrupt discontinuation: gradually taper to prevent withdrawal symptoms; decrease by 50% q1-2days; avoid use of narcotic antagonists

- Allergic reactions: rash, urticaria

Black Box Warning: Accidental exposure: if Duramorph or Infumorph gets on skin, remove contaminated clothing, rinse affected area with water

- **Respiratory dysfunction:** depression, character, rate, rhythm; notify prescriber if respirations are <12/min; accidental overdose has occurred with high-potency oral sols

Perform/provide:

- Storage in light-resistant container at room temp
- Assistance with ambulation
- Safety measures: side rails, night-light, call bell within easy reach
- Gradual withdrawal after long-term use

Evaluate:

- Therapeutic response; decrease in pain intensity

Teach patient/family:

- To change position slowly; orthostatic hypotension may occur
- To report any symptoms of CNS changes, allergic reactions
- That physical dependency may result from long-term use
- To avoid use of alcohol, CNS depressants
- That withdrawal symptoms may occur: nausea, vomiting, cramps, fever, faintness, anorexia

TREATMENT OF OVERDOSE:

Naloxone (Narcan) 0.2-0.8 mg IV, O_2, IV fluids, vasopressors

moxifloxacin (Rx)

Avelox, Avelox IV

Func. class.: Antiinfective

Chem. class.: Fluoroquinolone

ACTION: Interferes with conversion of intermediate DNA fragments into high-molecular-weight DNA in bacteria; DNA gyrase inhibitor

USES: Acute bacterial sinusitis: *Streptococcus pneumoniae, Haemophilus influenzae, Moraxella catarrhalis;* acute bacterial exacerbation of chronic bronchitis: *S. pneumoniae, H. influenzae, Haemophilus parainfluenzae, Klebsiella pneumoniae, Staphylococcus aureus, M. catarrhalis;* community-acquired pneumonia: *S. pneumoniae, H. influenzae, Mycoplasma pneumoniae, Chlamydia pneumoniae, M. catarrhalis;* uncomplicated skin/skin-structure infections: *S. aureus, Streptococcus pyogenes;* complicated intraabdominal infections including polymicrobial infections: *E. coli, Bacterioides fragilis, S. anginosus, S. constellatus, Enterococcus faecalis, Proteus mirabilis, Clostridium perfringens, Bacteroides thetaiotaomicron, Peptostreptococcus* sp; complicated skin, skin-structure infections caused by methicillin-susceptible: *S. aureus, E. coli, K. pneumoniae, Enterobacter cloacae*

CONTRAINDICATIONS: Hypersensitivity to quinolones

Precautions: Pregnancy (C), breastfeeding, children, hepatic/cardiac/renal/GI disease, epilepsy, uncorrected hypokalemia, prolonged QT interval; patients receiving class IA, III antidysrhythmics; seizure disorder

Black Box Warning: Tendon pain, rupture; tendinitis

DOSAGE AND ROUTES

Acute bacterial sinusitis

• **Adult: PO/IV** 400 mg q24hr × 10 days

Acute bacterial exacerbation of chronic bronchitis

• **Adult: PO/IV** 400 mg q24hr × 5 days

Community-acquired pneumonia

• **Adult: PO/IV** 400 mg q24hr × 7-14 days

Uncomplicated skin/skin-structure infections

• **Adult: PO/IV** 400 mg q24hr × 7 days

Complicated intraabdominal infections

• **Adult: IV** 400 mg/day × 5-14 days

Complicated skin, skin-structure infections

• **Adult: PO/IV** 400 mg/day × 7-21 days

Available forms: Tabs 400 mg; inj premix 400 mg/250 ml

Administer:

PO route

• 4 hr before or 8 hr after antacids, zinc, iron, calcium

IV route

• Discontinue primary IV while administering moxifloxacin, give over 60 min
• Do not give SUBCUT, IM
• Available as premixed sol; may be diluted at ratios from 1:10 to 10:1; do not refrigerate; give by direct inf or through Y-type inf set; do not add other medications to sol or inf through same IV line at same time

Solution compatibilities: 0.9% NaCl, D_5, D_{10}, LR, sterile water for inj

SIDE EFFECTS

CNS: *Headache,* dizziness, fatigue, insomnia, depression, *restlessness,* seizures, confusion, increased intracranial pressure, peripheral neuropathy

CV: Prolonged QT interval, dysrhythmias, torsades de pointes, tachycardia

EENT: Blurred vision, tinnitus, taste changes

GI: *Nausea, diarrhea,* increased ALT, AST, flatulence, heartburn, *vomiting,* oral candidiasis, dysphagia, pseudomembranous colitis

INTEG: *Rash,* pruritus, urticaria, photosensitivity, flushing, fever, chills

MS: Tremor, arthralgia, tendinitis, tendon rupture, myalgia

SYST: Anaphylaxis, Stevens-Johnson syndrome

PHARMACOKINETICS

Excreted in urine as active product, metabolites; parent product excreted in urine (20%), feces (25%); terminal half-life PO 12-16 hr, IV 8-15 hr

INTERACTIONS

Increase: moxifloxacin serum levels—probenecid

Increase: warfarin, cycloSPORINE effect

Increase: seizure risk—NSAIDs

⚠ **Increase:** tendon rupture—corticosteroids

Decrease: moxifloxacin absorption—magnesium antacids, aluminum hydroxide, zinc, iron, sucralfate, calcium, enteral feeding, didanosine

M

NURSING CONSIDERATIONS

Assess:

• CNS symptoms: headache, dizziness, fatigue, insomnia, depression, seizures
• Renal, hepatic studies: BUN, creatinine, AST, ALT
• I&O ratio, urine pH <5.5 is ideal

⚠ **Allergic reactions, Stevens-Johnson syndrome, toxic epidermal necrolysis, anaphylaxis:** fever, flushing, rash, urticaria, pruritus, sore throat, fatigue, ulcers, other lesions; keep EPINEPHrine, emergency equipment nearby for anaphylaxis

Black Box Warning: Tendon pain, rupture, tendinitis; if tendon becomes inflamed, product should be discontinued

⚠ **Cardiac status:** prolonged QT or use of products that increase QT prolongation

⚠ **Pseudomembranous colitis:** assess for diarrhea, abdominal pain, fever, fatigue, anorexia; possible anemia, elevated WBC, low serum albumin; stop product; usually either vancomycin or IV metroNIDAZOLE given

Perform/provide:

- Limited intake of alkaline foods, products: milk, dairy products, alkaline antacids, sodium bicarbonate
- Increased fluids to 3 L/day to avoid crystallization in kidneys

Evaluate:

- Therapeutic response: decreased pain, C&S; absence of infection

Teach patient/family:

- Not to take any products containing magnesium or calcium (such as antacids), iron, or aluminum with this product or 4 hr before or 8 hr after
- That photosensitivity may occur; to avoid sunlight or use sunscreen to prevent burns
- To use frequent rinsing of mouth, sugarless candy or gum for dry mouth
- To take as prescribed; not to double or miss doses
- If dizziness occurs, to ambulate, perform activities with assistance
- To complete full course of product therapy
- To contact prescriber if abnormal heart rhythm or seizures occur or if inflammation or pain in tendon occurs

moxifloxacin ophthalmic

See Appendix B

multivitamins (OTC, Rx)

Many brands available

Func. class.: Vitamins, multiple

Do not confuse:

Theragran/Phenergan

ACTION: Needed for adequate metabolism

USES: Prevention and treatment of vitamin deficiencies

Precautions: Pregnancy (A)

DOSAGE AND ROUTES

- **Adult and child: PO/IV** depends on brand

Available forms: Many

Administer:

- Liquid multivitamins diluted or dropped into patient's mouth using dropper provided with some brands
- Chew tabs should be chewed, not swallowed whole
- Give by cont IV inf only after diluting 5- to 10-ml multivitamins/500-1000 ml of D_5W, $D_{10}W$, $D_{20}W$, LR, D_5/LR, D_5/0.9% NaCl, 0.9% NaCl, 3% NaCl
- Do not use sol with crystals, precipitate, or color other than bright yellow

Additive compatibilities: Cefoxitin, isoproterenol, methyldopate, metoclopramide, metroNIDAZOLE, netilmicin, norepinephrine, sodium bicarbonate, verapamil

Y-site compatibilities: Acyclovir, ampicillin, ceFAZolin, cephalothin, cephapirin, diltiazem, erythromycin, fludarabine, gentamicin, tacrolimus

SIDE EFFECTS

None known at recommended dosage

NURSING CONSIDERATIONS

Assess:

- Vitamin deficiency: usually more than one vitamin is deficient

Evaluate:

- Therapeutic response: check each individual vitamin for guidelines

Teach patient/family:

- That adequate nutrition must be maintained to prevent further deficiencies
- To comply with regimen
- To avoid presenting flavored multivitamins as candy because child may overdose
- To store out of children's reach

mupirocin topical

See Appendix B

muromonab-CD3 (Rx)

(mur-oo-mone′ab)

Orthoclone OKT3

Func. class.: Immunosuppressant

Chem. class.: Murine monoclonal antibody

ACTION: Recognizes and reacts with T_3 antigens on T lymphocytes; leads to cytokine release, blocks T-cell function

USES: Acute allograft rejection in renal/cardiac/hepatic transplant patients

CONTRAINDICATIONS: CHF, uncontrolled hypertension, hypersensitivity to murine origin, breastfeeding, pregnancy (C)

Black Box Warning: Fluid overload, seizures

Precautions: Children <2 yr, fever, cerebral edema, thrombus, CV/vascular disease, MI, seizure disorder, lymphoma, human antimurine antibody (HAMA), pulmonary edema, infection

Black Box Warning: Angioedema, immunosuppression

DOSAGE AND ROUTES

- **Adult: IV BOL** 5 mg/day × 10-14 days
- **Child ≤30 kg: IV** 2.5 mg daily × 10-14 days

Cardiac/hepatic allograft rejection, steroid resistant

- **Adult: IV BOL** 5 mg/day × 10-14 days; begin when confirmed that rejection not reversed by steroids

Available forms: Inj 5 mg/5 ml

Administer:

- Pretreat with corticosteroids, acetaminophen, antihistamines

IV route

- IV undiluted; withdraw with 0.2-0.22 low-protein-binding μm filter, discard, use new needle for administration; give over 1 min
- Incompatible with any product in syringe or sol; do not admix

SIDE EFFECTS

CNS: *Pyrexia, chills, tremors,* aseptic meningitis, *fever,* headache, encephalopathy, seizures

CV: *Chest pain,* sinus tachycardia, hypertension, angina

EENT: Vision impairment, irreversible, blindness

GI: *Vomiting, nausea, diarrhea*

MISC: Infection, cytokine release syndrome, anaphylaxis, malaise, secondary malignancy

MS: Myalgia, arthralgia

RESP: *Dyspnea, wheezing,* pulmonary edema

PHARMACOKINETICS

Trough-level steady state 3-14 days

INTERACTIONS

Increase: immunosuppression—immunosuppressants

Increase: infection risk—cycloSPORINE, corticosteroids, azathioprine

Increase: CNS symptoms—indomethacin

Decrease: immune response—vaccines

Drug/Herb

- Interference with immunosuppression: astragalus, echinacea, melatonin

Decrease: effect—ginseng, St. John's wort

NURSING CONSIDERATIONS

Assess:

⚠ **Cytokine release syndrome (CRS):** nausea, vomiting, chills, fever, joint pain, weakness, dizziness, diarrhea, tremors, abdominal pain; usually occur within 30-48 hr, may last 6 hr; treat with antihistamines, acetaminophen

⚠ **Hypersensitivity, anaphylaxis:** dyspnea, bronchospasm, urticaria, tachycar-

M

dia, angioedema; emergency equipment must be available

- Blood studies: Hgb, WBC, platelets during treatment monthly; if leukocytes are <3000/mm^3, product should be discontinued; CD3, CD4, CD8, CD3 ≤25 cells/mm^3
- Hepatic studies: alk phos, AST, ALT, bilirubin

⚠ Hepatotoxicity: dark urine, jaundice, itching, light-colored stools; product should be discontinued

- Infection: sore throat, fever, chills, temp; notify prescriber immediately

⚠ Aseptic meningitis: fever, headache, photophobia

⚠ Fluid overload: increased weight, I&O, edema, crackles, B/P

Evaluate:

- Therapeutic response: absence of graft rejection

Teach patient/family:

- To report fever, chills, sore throat, fatigue, since serious infection may occur; rash, dyspnea, fast heartbeat; change in mental status
- To use contraceptive measures during treatment and for several months after; not to breastfeed
- To report cytokine-release syndrome; provide list of symptoms
- To avoid vaccinations during treatment
- To avoid persons with infections, crowds; infections may occur

mycophenolate mofetil (Rx)

(mye-koe-phen′oh-late)

CellCept, Myfortic

Func. class.: Immunosuppressant

ACTION: Inhibits inflammatory responses that are mediated by the immune system

USES: Prophylaxis for organ rejection in allogenic cardiac, hepatic, renal transplants

Unlabeled uses: Refractory uveitis, second-line therapy for Churg-Strauss syndrome, diffuse proliferative lupus nephritis (in combination), rheumatoid arthritis, psoriasis, GVHD, kidney disease, myasthenia gravis, atopic dermatitis

CONTRAINDICATIONS: Hypersensitivity to this product or mycophenolic acid

Black Box Warning: Pregnancy (D)

Precautions: Breastfeeding, lymphomas, neutropenia, renal disease, accidental exposure, anemia

Black Box Warning: Infection, neoplastic disease

DOSAGE AND ROUTES

Renal transplant

- **Adult: PO** mycophenolate mofetil or 720 mg mycophenolate sodium; 1 g or 720 mg bid given to renal transplant patients in combination with corticosteroids, cycloSPORINE
- **Child: PO-ER** 400 mg/m^2 bid, max 720 mg bid

Renal dose

- **Adult: PO/IV** GFR <25 ml/min, max 2 g/day

Cardiac transplant

- **Adult: PO/IV** 1.5 g bid, **IV** can be started ≤24 hr after transplant, switch to **PO** when able

Hepatic transplant

- **Adult: PO** 1.5 g bid; **IV** 1 g over ≥2 hr

Refractory acute kidney transplant rejection (unlabeled)

- **Adult: PO** 1.5 g (Mofetil) bid

Rheumatoid arthritis (unlabeled)

- **Adult: PO** 250 mg-2 g/day (Mofetil)

GVHD (unlabeled)

- **Adult: PO** 2 g/day (Mofetil) with cycloSPORINE and prednisoLONE

Diffuse proliferative lupus nephritis (unlabeled)

- **Adult: PO** 1 g/day (Mofetil)

Uveitis (unlabeled)

- **Adult: PO** 1 g (Mofetil) bid × 6-41 mo

Atopic dermatitis (unlabeled)
- **Adult: PO** 1 g (Mofetil) bid × 4 wk, then 500 mg bid × 4 wk
- **Adolescent/child ≥2 yr: PO** 30-50 mg/kg/day (Mofetil) in 2 divided doses

Available forms: Caps 250 mg; tabs 500 mg; inj (powder) 500 mg/20-ml vial; powder for oral susp 200 mg/ml; ext rel tab (Myfortic) 180, 360 mg

Administer:
- May be given in combination with corticosteroids, cycloSPORINE
- Del rel tab, cap, oral susp, tab are not interchangeable

PO route
- Do not break, crush, or chew tabs; do not open caps
- Give at same time each day
- Avoid inhalation or direct contact with skin, mucous membranes; teratogenic in animals
- Oral susp: tap closed bottle several times to loosen powder, use 94 ml of water in graduated cylinder, add 1/2 total amount of water for constitution and shake the closed bottle, add remaining water and shake; again, remove child-resistant cap, push adapter into neck of bottle, close tightly
- Give alone for better absorption

Intermittent IV INF route
- Reconstitute each vial with 14 ml D_5W, shake gently, further dilute to 6 mg/ml, dilute 1 g/140 ml D_5W, 1.5 g/210 ml D_5W; give by slow IV inf ≥2 hr, never give by bolus or rapid IV inj
- Do not give with other medications or sol

Y-site compatibilities: Alemtuzumab, alfentanil, amikacin, anidulafungin, argatroban, bivalirudin, caspofungin, cefepime, DAPTOmycin, DOPamine, norepinephrine, octreotide, oxytocin, tacrolimus, tigecycline, tirofiban, vancomycin

SIDE EFFECTS

CNS: *Tremor, dizziness, insomnia, headache, fever,* anxiety, pain, **progressive multifocal leukoencephalopathy**

CV: *Hypertension, chest pain,* hypotension

GI: *Diarrhea, constipation, nausea, vomiting,* stomatitis, **GI bleeding,** abdominal pain, anorexia, dyspepsia

GU: *UTI, hematuria,* **renal tubular necrosis, polyomavirus-associated nephropathy**

HEMA: **Leukopenia, thrombocytopenia, anemia, pancytopenia, pure red cell aplasia**

INTEG: *Rash*

META: *Peripheral edema, hypercholesterolemia, hypophosphatemia, edema, hyperkalemia, hypokalemia, hyperglycemia,* hypocalcemia, hypomagnesemia

MS: Arthralgia, muscle wasting, back pain, weakness

RESP: *Dyspnea, respiratory infection, increased cough, pharyngitis, bronchitis, pneumonia*

SYST: **Lymphoma,** *nonmelanoma skin carcinoma,* **sepsis**

PHARMACOKINETICS

Rapidly and completely absorbed; metabolized to active metabolite (MPA); excreted in urine, feces; protein binding (MPA) 97%; half-life (MPA) 17.9 hr

INTERACTIONS

- Avoid administration with azathioprine
- Increased bleeding risk: anticoagulants, NSAIDs, thrombolytics, salicylates

Increase: effects of phenytoin, theophylline

Increase: concentration of both products—acyclovir, ganciclovir

Increase: mycophenolate levels—probenecid

Decrease: mycophenolate levels—antacids, cholestyramine, colestipol

Decrease: protein binding of phenytoin, theophylline

Decrease: effect of live attenuated vaccines, oral contraceptives

Drug/Herb

Interference with immunosuppression: astragalus, echinacea, melatonin

M

Drug/Food
Decrease: absorption if taken with food
Drug/Lab Test
Increase: serum creatitine, BUN
• Abnormal LFTs

NURSING CONSIDERATIONS

Assess:

⚠ **Progressive multifocal leukoencephalopathy,** may be fatal; ataxia, confusion, apathy, hemiparesis, visual problems, weakness; side effects should be reported to FDA
• Blood studies: CBC during treatment monthly
• Hepatic studies: alk phos, AST, ALT, bilirubin
• Renal studies: BUN, CCr, electrolytes
• Pregnancy test within 1 wk prior to initiation of treatment; confirm negative pregnancy test

Evaluate:
• Therapeutic response: absence of graft rejection

Teach patient/family:
• To report fever, rash, severe diarrhea, chills, sore throat, fatigue because serious infections may occur
• To reduce risk of infection by avoiding crowds
• About the need for repeated lab tests
• To limit exposure to sunlight, UV light
• To use 2 forms of contraception before, during, and for 6 wk after therapy
• To take at same time each day

nabilone (Rx)

(nab′ih-lohn)

Cesamet

Func. class.: Antiemetic
Chem. class.: Cannabinoid—miscellaneous

ACTION: Orally, active cannabinoid, chemically related to marijuana; may decrease nausea by action on cannabinoid receptors in the CNS

USES: Prevention of nausea, vomiting associated with cancer chemotherapy in those who have not responded to other treatment; not to be used on an as-needed basis

CONTRAINDICATIONS: Hypersensitivity to this product or cannabinoids

Precautions: Pregnancy (C), breastfeeding, depression, mental disorders, severe renal/hepatic disease, hypertension, tachycardia, CV disorders, history of alcoholism/drug abuse

DOSAGE AND ROUTES

• **Adult: PO** 1-2 mg bid; give initial dose 1-3 hr prior to chemotherapy; start with lower dose and increase as needed; may give dose of 1-2 mg the night before chemotherapy; may give 2-3×/day during chemotherapy cycle

Available forms: Caps 1 mg

Administer:
• PO; not to be used on an as-needed basis

SIDE EFFECTS

CNS: *Headache, ataxia, drowsiness, dysphoria, euphoria, sleep disturbance, vertigo, asthenia, concentration difficulties, depression,* syncope, hallucinations, weakness
CV: Chest discomfort, tachycardia, orthostatic hypotension
GI: *Dry mouth,* nausea, *anorexia,* increased appetite
INTEG: Allergic reactions, rash, photosensitivity, pruritus
MS: Back, joint, muscle, neck pain

PHARMACOKINETICS

Absorption rapid, 10%-20% absorbed, duration is unpredictable, psychiatric symptoms may occur for ≤72 hr after treatment is concluded, terminal peak 2 hr, metabolized by liver, excreted via biliary system in feces

INTERACTIONS

Increase: hypomanic reaction—disulfiram and possibly FLUoxetine
Increase: hypertension, tachycardia, and possibly cardiotoxicity—sympathomimetics (amphetamines, cocaine)
Increase: tachycardia, drowsiness—anticholinergics (antihistamines, atropine, scopolamine)
Increase: drowsiness, CNS depression—CNS depressants (alcohol, barbiturates, benzodiazepines, busPIRone, lithium, muscle relaxants, opioids)
Increase: nabilone action—naltrexone
Increase: action of both—opioids
Increase: tachycardia, hypertension, drowsiness—tricyclics
Decrease: metabolism of theophylline

NURSING CONSIDERATIONS

Assess:

- Absence of nausea and vomiting during chemotherapy
- **CNS symptoms:** headache, depression, ataxia, drowsiness, dysphoria, euphoria, sleep disturbances, concentration difficulties
- CV symptoms, cardiac status: tachycardia, orthostatic hypo/hypertension
- Psychiatric symptoms: euphoria, depression, sleep disturbance

Perform/provide:

- Storage of capsules at room temp, away from light and moisture

Evaluate:

- Therapeutic response: decreased nausea, vomiting associated with chemotherapy

Teach patient/family:

- That mood, behavioral changes may occur while taking this product
- To notify prescriber if pregnancy is suspected; to avoid breastfeeding while taking product
- Not to use alcohol or other CNS depressants unless approved by prescriber
- Not to operate machinery or perform other hazardous activities while taking product; to remain under supervision of responsible adult during initial use, after dosage changes

nabumetone (Rx)

(na-byoo′me-tone)

Apo-Nabumetone ♣, Gen-Nabumetone ♣

Func. class.: Nonsteroidal antiinflammatory

Chem. class.: Acetic acid derivative

ACTION: Metabolite inhibits COX-1, COX-2 by blocking arachidonate; analgesic, antiinflammatory, antipyretic

USES: Osteoarthritis, rheumatoid arthritis, acute or chronic treatment

CONTRAINDICATIONS: Pregnancy (D) 3rd trimester; hypersensitivity to this product or aspirin, iodides, NSAIDs

Black Box Warning: Perioperative pain with CABG surgery

Precautions: Pregnancy (C), breastfeeding, children, geriatric patients, bleeding/GI/cardiac/renal disorders, hepatic dysfunction, asthma, bone marrow suppression, lupus (SLE), ulcerative colitis, blood dyscrasias

Black Box Warning: MI, stroke, GI bleeding

DOSAGE AND ROUTES

- **Adult: PO** 1 g as single dose or divided bid; max 2 g/day if needed

Available forms: Tabs 500, 750 mg

Administer:

- With food or antacids

SIDE EFFECTS

CNS: Dizziness, headache, drowsiness, fatigue, tremors, confusion, insomnia, anxiety, depression, nervousness
EENT: Tinnitus
CV: Tachycardia, peripheral edema, palpitations, dysrhythmias, **CHF, MI, stroke**

GI: Nausea, anorexia, vomiting, diarrhea, jaundice, cholestatic hepatitis, constipation, flatulence, cramps, dry mouth, peptic ulcer, gastritis, ulceration, perforation, bleeding
GU: Nephrotoxicity, dysuria, hematuria, oliguria, azotemia, cystitis
HEMA: Blood dyscrasias
INTEG: Purpura, rash, pruritus, sweating, photosensitivity
RESP: Dyspnea, pharyngitis, bronchospasm
SYST: Anaphylaxis, angioneurotic edema

PHARMACOKINETICS

PO: Peak $2^1/_2$-4 hr; protein binding >99%; half-life 24 hr; metabolized in liver to active metabolite; excreted in urine (metabolites), breast milk

INTERACTIONS

Increase: bleeding risk—anticoagulants, thrombolytics, valproic acid, cefamandole, cefotetan, cefoperazone, plicamycin, clopidogrel, eptifibatide, ticlopidine, SSRIs, SNRIs
Increase: hematologic toxicity—antineoplastics, radiation
Increase: GI reactions—salicylates, NSAIDs, alcohol, potassium, corticosteroids
Increase: effect of—lithium, methotrexate
Decrease: effect of diuretics, antihypertensives

Drug/Lab Test
Increase: bleeding time, K, BUN, AST, ALT, LDH, alk phos, creatinine
Decrease: CCr, blood glucose, Hct, Hgb

NURSING CONSIDERATIONS

Assess:

Black Box Warning: Cardiac status: CV thrombotic events, MI, stroke; may be fatal, not to be used in perioperative pain after CABG

Black Box Warning: GI status: ulceration, bleeding, perforation; may be fatal

- **Pain:** frequency, intensity, characteristics; relief of pain after taking product
- Asthma, aspirin sensitivity, or nasal polyps; increased hypersensitivity reactions
- Renal, hepatic studies: BUN, creatinine, AST, ALT, Hgb, LDH, blood glucose, WBC, platelets; CCr before treatment, periodically thereafter
- Audiometric, ophthalmic exam before, during, after treatment
- For eye, ear problems: blurred vision, tinnitus; may indicate toxicity

Perform/provide:
- Storage at room temp

Evaluate:
- Therapeutic response: decreased pain and stiffness in joints

Teach patient/family:
- To avoid alcoholic beverages and aspirin
- ⚠ To report blurred vision, ringing, roaring in ears; may indicate toxicity
- To avoid driving, other hazardous activities if dizziness, drowsiness occur
- ⚠ To report change in urine pattern, increased weight, edema, increased pain in joints, fever, blood in urine; indicates nephrotoxicity
- That therapeutic effects may take up to 1 mo
- To take with a full glass of water and food or antacids to enhance absorption; to sit upright for 30 min
- To report dark stools; may indicate GI bleeding
- To use sunscreen, wear protective clothing if in the sun
- To report use to all health care providers, to avoid all other products unless approved by prescriber

nadolol (Rx)

(nay-doe'lole)

Apo-Nadol ✱, Corgard

Func. class.: Antihypertensive, antianginal

Chem. class.: β-Adrenergic receptor blocker

Do not confuse:
Corgard/Cognex/Coreg
Nadolol/Mandol

ACTION: Long-acting, nonselective β-adrenergic receptor blocking agent, blocks β_1 in the heart and β_2 in the lungs, uterus, and circulatory system; mechanism is similar to that of propranolol

USES: Chronic stable angina pectoris, mild to moderate hypertension

Unlabeled uses: Tachydysrhythmias, anxiety, tremors, esophageal varices (rebleeding only), prophylaxis of migraine headaches, portal hypertension

CONTRAINDICATIONS: Hypersensitivity to this product, cardiac failure, cardiogenic shock, 2nd/3rd degree heart block, bronchospastic disease, sinus bradycardia, CHF, COPD

Precautions: Pregnancy (C), breastfeeding, diabetes mellitus, renal disease, hyperthyroidism, peripheral vascular disease, myasthenia gravis, major surgery, nonallergic bronchospasm

Black Box Warning: Abrupt discontinuation

DOSAGE AND ROUTES

- **Adult: PO** 40 mg/day, increase by 40-80 mg q3-7days; maintenance 40-240 mg/day for angina, 40-320 mg/day for hypertension
- **Geriatric: PO** 20 mg/day, may increase by 20 mg until desired dose

Renal dose

- **Adult: PO** CCr 31-50 ml/min, give q24-36hr; CCr 10-30 ml/min, give q24-48hr; CCr <10 ml/min, give q40-60hr

Migraine prevention (unlabeled)

- **Adult: PO** 80-240 mg/day × 2-18 mo

Available forms: Tabs 20, 40, 80 mg

Administer:

- With 8 oz water, check apical pulse prior to use, if <60 bpm, withhold; call prescriber

SIDE EFFECTS

CNS: Depression, dizziness, *fatigue,* lethargy, paresthesias, headache, *weakness,* insomnia, memory loss, nightmares

CV: **Bradycardia,** *hypotension,* **CHF,** palpitations, **AV block,** chest pain, peripheral ischemia, flushing, edema, vasodilation, conduction disturbances

EENT: Blurred vision, dry eyes, nasal congestion

ENDO: Hyperglycemia, hypoglycemia

GI: Nausea, vomiting, diarrhea, colitis, constipation, cramps, dry mouth, flatulence, hepatomegaly, **pancreatitis,** taste distortion

GU: *Impotence,* decreased libido

HEMA: **Agranulocytosis, thrombocytopenia**

INTEG: Rash, pruritus, fever, alopecia

RESP: Dyspnea, respiratory dysfunction, **bronchospasm,** cough, wheezing, **pulmonary edema,** pharyngitis, **laryngospasm**

PHARMACOKINETICS

PO: Onset variable, peak 3-4 hr, duration 17-24 hr; half-life 20-24 hr; not metabolized; excreted in urine (unchanged), bile, breast milk; protein binding 30%

INTERACTIONS

- Do not use with MAOIs; bradycardia may occur
- Peripheral ischemia: ergots

Increase: bradycardia—digoxin

Increase: hypotension, bradycardia—cloNIDine, EPINEPHrine

N

Increase: hypotensive effects—other hypotensive agents, phenothiazines
Decrease: β-blocking effect—thyroid hormones
Decrease: antihypertensive effect—NSAIDs

Drug/Lab Test
Increase: serum potassium, serum uric acid, ALT, AST, alk phos, LDH, blood glucose, cholesterol, ANA, triglycerides

NURSING CONSIDERATIONS

Assess:
- B/P, pulse, respirations during beginning therapy; orthostatic hypotension may occur
- Weight daily; report gain of 5 lb
- I&O ratio, CCr if kidney damage diagnosed; crackles, jugular venous distention, fatigue, dyspnea
- **Pain:** duration, time started, activity being performed, character
- Headache, lightheadedness, decreased B/P; may indicate a need for decreased dosage

Black Box Warning: Abrupt discontinuation: can result in MI, myocardial ischemia, ventricular dysrhythmias, severe hypertension; withdraw slowly by tapering

Evaluate:
- Therapeutic response: decreased B/P, heart rate, symptoms of angina

Teach patient/family:
- That product may mask signs of hypoglycemia or alter blood glucose in diabetics
- To avoid OTC products unless prescriber approves
- To avoid hazardous activities if dizziness occurs
- **Hypertension:** to comply with complete medical regimen; to report weight gain of >5 lb, swelling, unusual bruising, bleeding
- To rise slowly to prevent orthostatic hypotension
- About how and when to check B/P, pulse; to hold dose, contact prescriber if pulse ≤60 bpm, systolic B/P <90 mm Hg

Black Box Warning: Not to discontinue abruptly, may cause life-threatening cardiac changes

nafarelin (Rx)

(naf-ah-rell′in)

Synarel

Func. class.: Gonadotropin
Chem. class.: Analog of gonadotropin-releasing hormone

ACTION: Stimulates the release of LH and FSH, which increases ovarian steroid production; repeated dosing prevents stimulation of the pituitary gland

USES: Endometriosis, gonadotropin-central precocious puberty

CONTRAINDICATIONS: Pregnancy (X), breastfeeding, hypersensitivity to this product, GnRH, sorbitol; undiagnosed abnormal vaginal bleeding
Precautions: Children, females, menstruation, osteoporosis, pituitary insufficiency

DOSAGE AND ROUTES

- **Adult: NASAL** 400 mcg/day as 1 spray (200 mcg) into 1 nostril in morning and 1 spray into other nostril in evening; start treatment between days 2 and 4 of menstrual cycle; may increase to 800 mcg/day (1 spray into each nostril 2×/day); recommended duration of treatment, 6 mo
- **Child: NASAL** 2 sprays in each nostril AM and PM, may increase to 3 sprays alternating nostrils tid

Available forms: Nasal spray 2 mg/ml (200 mcg/spray)

Administer:
- Repeated doses may be necessary to elevate pituitary gonadotropin reserve; endometriosis treatment continues for ≤6 mo

• Tilt patient's head back slightly; wait 30 sec between sprays; do not use decongestant until 12 hr later
• Discontinue with onset of normal puberty; assess normal puberty signs

SIDE EFFECTS

CNS: *Headache,* flushing, depression, insomnia, *emotional lability,* hot flashes
CV: MI, stroke, thromboembolism, DVT, TIA
GU: *Decreased libido, vaginal dryness,* breast tenderness, increased pubic hair, *impaired fertility, reduction in breast size, absence of menses,* impotence, irregular periods
INTEG: *Acne*
META: Decreased bone density, increased cholesterol, triglycerides, diabetes mellitus
MISC: Body odor, seborrhea, rhinitis, *nasal irritation*
SENSITIVITY: Shortness of breath, chest pain, urticaria, pruritus

PHARMACOKINETICS

Rapidly absorbed, peak 10-40 min, half-life 3 hr; 80% bound to plasma proteins

INTERACTIONS

• Do not use with some antipsychotics, cimetidine, methyldopa, metoclopramide, reserpine
Decrease: nafarelin absorption—nasal decongestants (nasal sprays)
Drug/Herb
• Avoid black cohosh, chasteberry, DHEA

NURSING CONSIDERATIONS

Assess:
• Abdominal pain **(endometriosis)** during treatment
• **Central precocious puberty:** endocrine studies, bone age, sex steroids, RHCg, GnRH, baseline q8wk
• **Precocious puberty,** including secondary sex characteristics
• Test results: pituitary/hypothalamus dysfunction (decreased LH); postmenopausal (increased LH)
Perform/provide:
• Storage at room temp; protect from light
Evaluate:
• Therapeutic response: decreased symptoms of endometriosis; adequate resolution of central precocious puberty
Teach patient/family:
• To use nonhormonal contraception
• **About correct nasal use;** 1 spray in right nostril AM, 1 in left nostril PM for endometriosis; 2 sprays in each nostril in AM and PM for central precocious puberty
• That medication may cause hot flashes, decreased libido, vaginal dryness
• To avoid use of nasal decongestants or to separate from product by 12 hr
• That growth of facial hair, increased body odor and vaginal discharge may occur in females

nafcillin (Rx)

(naf-sill′in)
Func. class.: Antiinfective, broad-spectrum
Chem. class.: Penicillinase-resistant penicillin

N

ACTION:

Bacteriocidal, interferes with cell wall replication of susceptible organisms; cell lysis mediated by cell wall autolytic enzymes

USES:

Effective for gram-positive cocci *(Staphylococcus aureus, Streptococcus viridans, Streptococcus pneumoniae),* infections caused by penicillinase-producing *Staphylococcus*

CONTRAINDICATIONS:

Hypersensitivity to penicillins or corn
Precautions: Pregnancy (B), breastfeeding, neonates; hypersensitivity to cephalosporins or carbapenems; GI disease, asthma

DOSAGE AND ROUTES

- **Adult:** IV 500-2000 mg q4hr
- **Child and infant >1 mo:** IV 50-200 mg/kg/day in divided doses q4-6hr
- **Neonates >7 days (weight >2000 g):** IV 25 mg/kg q6hr
- **Neonates ≤7 days (weight <2000 g):** IV 25 mg/kg q8hr

Meningitis

- **Adult:** IV 100-200 mg/kg/day in divided doses q4-6hr, max 12 g/day
- **Neonates >7 days (weight >2000 g):** IV 50 mg/kg q6hr
- **Neonates ≤7 days (weight <2000 g):** IV 50 mg/kg q12hr

Available forms: Powder for inj 1, 2 g, premixed or Add-Vantage vials

Administer:

- Product after C&S has been drawn, begin therapy while waiting for results

IM route

- Reconstitute vials: add 1.7 (1.8 nafcil), 3, 4, or 6.4 ml (6.6 ml NaCl) (sterile water for inj, 0.9% NaCl, bacteriostatic water for inj with benzyl alcohol or parabens) to vials with 500 mg, 1 g, 2 g of nafcillin, respectively (250 mg/ml)
- No further dilution needed; after reconstitution, inject in deep muscle mass

IV route

- Reconstitute vials: add 1.7 (1.8 nafcil), 3, 4, or 6.4 ml (6.6 ml NaCl) sterile water for inj, 0.9% NaCl, bacteriostatic water for inj with benzyl alcohol or parabens) to vials with 500 mg, 1 g, 2 g of nafcillin, respectively (250 mg/ml)
- **Nallpen piggyback units:** reconstitute 1 or 2 g with 50-100 ml or 99 ml, respectively, of sterile water for inj, 0.45% NaCl, 0.9% NaCl
- **Unipen piggyback units:** reconstitute according to manufacturer

Direct Intermittent IV INJ route

- Further dilute reconstituted sol in 15-30 ml sterile water inj, 0.45% NaCl, 0.9% NaCl; inj slowly over 5-10 min into tubing of free-flowing compatible IV solution

Intermittent IV INF route

- Vials, further dilute reconstituted sol to 2-40 mg/ml for peripheral vein inf ≤20 mg/ml (preferred); piggyback unit, no further dilution needed; infuse ≥30-60 min, make sure entire dose is given before ≥10% of sol is inactivated

Y-site compatibilities: Acyclovir, atropine, cyclophosphamide, diazepam, enalaprilat, esmolol, famotidine, fentaNYL, fluconazole, foscarnet, heparin, HYDROmorphone, magnesium sulfate, morphine, perphenazine, propofol, theophylline, zidovudine

SIDE EFFECTS

CNS: Lethargy, hallucinations, anxiety, depression, twitching, coma, seizures

GI: *Nausea, vomiting, diarrhea,* increased AST, ALT, abdominal pain, glossitis, pseudomembranous colitis

GU: Oliguria, proteinuria, hematuria, vaginitis, moniliasis, glomerulonephritis, interstitial nephritis

HEMA: Anemia, increased bleeding time, bone marrow depression, neutropenia

SYST: Anaphylaxis, serum sickness, Stevens-Johnson syndrome

PHARMACOKINETICS

Half-life 1 hr; metabolized by liver; excreted in bile, urine

INTERACTIONS

- Avoid use with tetracyclines

Increase: nafcillin concentrations—probenecid

Decrease: effect of cycloSPORINE—warfarin

Decrease: nafcillin effect—chloramphenicol, macrolides, sulfonamides, tetracyclines

Drug/Food

Decrease: absorption—food, carbonated drinks, citrus fruit juices

Drug/Lab Test

False positive: urine glucose, urine protein

NURSING CONSIDERATIONS

Assess:

- I&O ratio; report hematuria, oliguria, high doses are nephrotoxic
- **Pseudomembranous colitis:** assess for diarrhea, abdominal pain, fever, fatigue, anorexia; possible anemia, elevated WBC, low serum albumin; stop product; usually either vancomycin or IV metroNIDAZOLE given
- Hepatic studies: AST, ALT
- Blood studies: CBC with differential bleeding time

⚠ Renal studies: urinalysis, BUN, creatinine; abnormal urinalysis may indicate nephrotoxicity

- C&S before product therapy; product may be given as soon as culture is taken
- Respiratory status: rate, character, wheezing, tightness in chest

⚠ Allergies before initiation of treatment; monitor for anaphylaxis, dyspnea, rash, laryngeal edema; stop product; keep emergency equipment nearby; skin eruptions after administration of penicillin to 1 wk after discontinuing product

- Differential WBC 2 × per wk in patients receiving long-term therapy

Perform/provide:

- Extravasation management with cold packs, hyaluronidase

Evaluate:

- Therapeutic response: absence of fever, draining wounds

Teach patient/family:

⚠ To report sore throat, fever, fatigue (may indicate superinfection); CNS reactions, pseudomembraneous colitis (diarrhea, fever, abdominal pain, fatigue)

- To wear or carry emergency ID if allergic to penicillins

TREATMENT OF ANAPHYLAXIS: Withdraw product; maintain airway; administer EPINEPHrine, aminophylline, O_2, IV corticosteroids

⚠ HIGH ALERT

nalbuphine (Rx)

(nal′byoo-feen)

Func. class.: Opioid analgesic

Chem. class.: Synthetic opioid agonist, antagonist

ACTION: Depresses pain impulse transmission at the spinal cord level by interacting with opioid receptors

USES: Moderate to severe pain

CONTRAINDICATIONS: Hypersensitivity, addiction (opiate)

Precautions: Pregnancy (C), breastfeeding, addictive personality, increased intracranial pressure, MI (acute), severe heart disease, respiratory depression, renal/hepatic disease, bowel impaction

DOSAGE AND ROUTES

Analgesic

- **Adult: SUBCUT/IM/IV** 10 mg q3-6hr prn (based on 70-kg body weight), max 160 mg/day (IV/IM/SUBCUT); 20 mg/dose if opiate naïve (IV/IM/SUBCUT)

Balanced anesthesia adjunct

- **Adult: IV** 0.3-3 mg/kg given over 10-15 min, may give 0.25-0.5 mg/kg as needed for maintenance

Available forms: Inj 10, 20 mg/ml

Administer:

- With antiemetic if nausea, vomiting occur
- When pain beginning to return; determine dosage interval by response

IM route

- IM deep in large muscle mass, rotate inj sites, protect from light

Direct IV route

- Undiluted ≤10 mg over 3-5 min into free-flowing IV line of D_5W, NS, or LR

Syringe compatibilities: Atropine, cimetidine, diphenhydrAMINE, droperidol, glycopyrrolate, hydrOXYzine, lidocaine, midazolam, prochlorperazine, ranitidine, scopolamine, trimethobenzamide

Y-site compatibilities: Amifostine, aztreonam, cefmetazole, cisatracurium, cladribine, filgrastim, fludarabine, granisetron, melphalan, paclitaxel, propofol, remifentanil, teniposide, thiotepa, vinorelbine

SIDE EFFECTS

CNS: *Drowsiness, dizziness, confusion, headache, sedation, euphoria,* dysphoria (high doses), hallucinations, dreaming, tolerance, physical, psychologic dependency

CV: Palpitations, bradycardia, change in B/P, orthostatic hypotension, cardiac arrest

EENT: Tinnitus, blurred vision, miosis, diplopia

GI: *Nausea, vomiting, anorexia, constipation, cramps,* abdominal pain, dyspepsia, xerostomia, bitter taste

GU: Increased urinary output, dysuria, urinary retention, urgency

INTEG: *Rash,* urticaria, bruising, flushing, diaphoresis, pruritus

RESP: Respiratory depression, pulmonary edema

PHARMACOKINETICS

SUBCUT/IM/IV: Peak 30 min, onset 2-15 min, duration 3-6 hr, metabolized by liver, excreted by kidneys, half-life 3-6 hr

INTERACTIONS

⚠ Avoid use with MAOIs; unpredictable reactions may occur

Increase: effects with other CNS depressants—alcohol, opiates, sedative/hypnotics, antipsychotics, skeletal muscle relaxants

Drug/Lab Test

Increase: amylase, lipase

NURSING CONSIDERATIONS

Assess:

- I&O ratio; check for decreasing output; may indicate urinary retention
- Bowel status; constipation is common

⚠ **Withdrawal reactions** in opiate-dependent individuals: PE, vascular occlusion; abscesses, ulcerations, nausea, vomiting, seizures; low potential for dependence

- **CNS changes:** dizziness, drowsiness, hallucinations, euphoria, LOC, pupil reaction
- Allergic reactions: rash, urticaria
- **Respiratory dysfunction: respiratory depression,** character, rate, rhythm; notify prescriber if respirations are <10/min
- **Pain:** type, location, intensity before and 30-60 min after administration; titrate upward with 25%-50% until 50% of pain reduced; need for pain medication by pain sedation scoring, physical dependency

Perform/provide:

- Storage in light-resistant area at room temp

Evaluate:

- Therapeutic response: decrease in pain without respiratory depression

Teach patient/family:

- To report any symptoms of CNS changes, allergic reactions
- That physical dependency may result from long-term use; low potential for dependency
- That withdrawal symptoms may occur: nausea, vomiting, cramps, fever, faintness, anorexia
- To avoid CNS depressants, alcohol
- To avoid driving, operating machinery if drowsiness occurs

TREATMENT OF OVERDOSE:

Naloxone (Narcan) 0.2-0.8 mg IV, O_2, IV fluids, vasopressors

naloxone (Rx)

(nal-oks′one)

Func. class.: Opioid antagonist, antidote

Chem. class.: Thebaine derivative

ACTION: Competes with opioids at opiate receptor sites

USES: Respiratory depression induced by opioids, pentazocine, propoxyphene

Unlabeled uses: IBS, opiate agonist dependence, opiate agonist-induced constipation, pruritus, urinary retention, coma, nausea, vomiting

CONTRAINDICATIONS: Hypersensitivity

Precautions: Pregnancy (C), breastfeeding, children, neonates, CV disease, opioid dependency, seizure disorder, drug dependency

DOSAGE AND ROUTES

Opioid-induced respiratory depression

- **Adult: IV/SUBCUT/IM** 0.4-2 mg, repeat q2-3min if needed, max 10 mg
- **Child <5 yr or ≤20 kg: IV/SUBCUT/IM** 0.01 mg/kg slowly followed by 0.1 mg/kg if needed or as **INF** titrated to response

Postoperative opioid-induced respiratory depression

- **Adult: IV** 0.1-0.2 mg q2-3min prn
- **Child: IV/SUBCUT/IM** 0.005-0.01 mg/kg q2-3min prn

Opioid overdose

- **Adult: IV/SUBCUT/IM** 0.4-2 mg (10 mcg/kg) (not opioid dependent), may repeat q2-3min; 0.1-0.2 mg q2-3min (opioid dependent)

Diagnosis of opiate-agonist dependence (unlabeled)

- **Adult: IM** 0.16 mg; if no withdrawal symptoms after 20-30 min, give 0.24 mg **IV**

Available forms: Inj 0.02, 0.4 mg/ml

Administer:

- Only with resuscitative equipment, O_2 nearby
- Only sol prepared within 24 hr

Direct IV route

- Undiluted with sterile water for inj; give ≤0.4 mg over 15 sec

Continuous IV INF route

- Dilute 2 mg/500 ml 0.9% NaCl or D_5W (4 mcg/ml), titrate to response

Y-site compatibilities: Acyclovir, alfentanil, amikacin, aminocaproic acid, aminophylline, anidulafungin, ascorbic acid, atenolol, atracurium, atropine, azaTHIOprine, aztreonam, benztropine, bivalirudin, bleomycin, bumetanide, buprenorphine, butorphanol, calcium chloride/gluconate, CARBOplatin, caspofungin, cefamandole, ceFAZolin, cefmetazole, cefonicid, cefoperazone, cefotaxime, cefotetan, cefoxitin, ceftazidime, ceftizoxime, cefTRIAXone, cefuroxime, cephalothin, cephapirin, chloramphenicol, chlorproMAZINE, cimetidine, CISplatin, clindamycin, cyanocobalamin, cyclophosphamide, cycloSPORINE, cytarabine, DACTINomycin, DAPTOmycin, dexamethasone, digoxin, diltiazem, diphenhydrAMINE, DOBUTamine, docetaxel, DOPamine, doxacurium, DOXOrubicin, doxycycline, enalaprilat, ePHEDrine, EPINEPHrine, epirubicin, epoetin alfa, eptifibatide, ertapenem, erythromycin, esmolol, etoposide, etoposide phosphate, famotidine, fenoldopam, fentaNYL, fluconazole, fludarabine, fluorouracil, folic acid, furosemide, ganciclovir, gatifloxacin, gemcitabine, gentamicin, glycopyrrolate, granisetron, heparin, hydrocortisone, hydrOXYzine, IDArubicin, ifosfamide, imipenem-cilastatin, inamrinone, indomethacin, insulin (regular), irinotecan, isoproterenol, ketorolac, labetalol, levofloxacin, lidocaine, linezolid, LORazepam, mannitol, mechlorethamine, meperidine, metaraminol, methicillin, methotrexate, methoxamine, methyldopate, methylPREDNISolone, metoclopramide, metoprolol, metroNI-

DAZOLE, mezlocillin, miconazole, midazolam, milrinone, minocycline, mitoxantrone, morphine, moxalactam, multiple vitamins, mycophenolate, nafcillin, nalbuphine, nesiritide, netilmicin, nitroglycerin, nitroprusside, norepinephrine, octreotide, ondansetron, oxacillin, oxaliplatin, oxytocin, paclitaxel, palonosetron, pamidronate, pancuronium, papaverine, pemetrexed, penicillin G potassium/sodium, pentamidine, pentazocine, PENTobarbital, PHENobarbital, phentolamine, phenylephrine, phytonadione, piperacillin, piperacillin-tazobactam, polymyxin B, potassium chloride, procainamide, prochlorperazine, promethazine, propofol, propranolol, protamine, pyridoxine, quiNIDine, quinupristin-dalfopristin, ranitidine, ritodrine, rocuronium, sodium acetate/bicarbonate, succinylcholine, SUFentanil, tacrolimus, teniposide, theophylline, thiamine, ticarcillin, ticarcillin-clavulanate, tigecycline, tirofiban, tobramycin, tolazoline, trimetaphan, urokinase, vancomycin, vasopressin, vecuronium, verapamil, vinCRIStine, vinorelbine, voriconazole, zoledronic acid

SIDE EFFECTS

CNS: Drowsiness, nervousness, **seizures**, tremor

CV: Rapid pulse, increased systolic B/P (high doses), **ventricular tachycardia, fibrillation**, hypo/hypertension, **cardiac arrest, sinus tachycardia**

GI: Nausea, vomiting, **hepatotoxicity**

RESP: Hyperpnea, **pulmonary edema**

PHARMACOKINETICS

Well absorbed IM, SUBCUT; metabolized by liver, crosses placenta; excreted in urine, breast milk; half-life 30-81 min

IM/SUBCUT: Onset 2-5 min, duration 45-60 min

IV: Onset 1 min, duration 45 min

INTERACTIONS

Increase: seizures—tramadol

Decrease: effect of opioid analgesics

Drug/Lab Test

Interference: urine VMA, 5-HIAA, urine glucose

NURSING CONSIDERATIONS

Assess:

- **Withdrawal:** cramping, hypertension, anxiety, vomiting, signs of withdrawal in drug-dependent individuals may occur ≤2 hr after administration
- VS q3-5min
- ABGs including Po_2, Pco_2
- Cardiac status: tachycardia, hypertension; monitor ECG
- **Respiratory dysfunction:** respiratory depression, character, rate, rhythm; if respirations are $<$10/min, administer naloxone; probably due to opioid overdose; monitor LOC
- **Pain:** duration, intensity, location before and after administration; may be used for respiratory depression

Perform/provide:

- Dark storage at room temp

Evaluate:

- Therapeutic response: reversal of respiratory depression; LOC—alert

Teach patient/family:

- When patient is lucid, about reasons for, expected results of product

naltrexone (Rx)

(nal-trex′one)

ReVia, Vivitrol

Func. class.: Opioid antagonist

Chem. class.: Thebaine derivative

ACTION: Competes with opioids at opioid-receptor sites

USES: Blockage of opioid analgesics; used for treatment of opiate addiction, alcoholism

Unlabeled uses: Nicotine withdrawal, opiate-agonist withdrawal, pruritus

CONTRAINDICATIONS: Hypersensitivity, opioid dependence

Black Box Warning: Hepatic failure, hepatitis

Precautions: Pregnancy (C), breastfeeding, children, renal disease, depression, suicidal ideation

Black Box Warning: Hepatic disease

DOSAGE AND ROUTES

Adjunct in opiate-agonist dependence

• **Adult: PO** 25 mg; if no withdrawal symptoms in 1 hr, then 25 mg additionally; if no withdrawal symptoms, then 50-150 mg/day or in divided doses

Adjunct in alcoholism treatment

• **Adult: PO** 50 mg/day with food × 12 wk; **IM** (Vivitrol) 380 mg q4wk

Pruritus (unlabeled)

• **Adult: PO** 50 mg/day × 7 days to 4 wk

Nicotine withdrawal (unlabeled)

• **Adult: PO** 50 mg/day

Ultrarapid opiate detoxification (unlabeled)

• **Adult: PO** 50 mg prior to sedation with midazolam

Available forms: Tabs 25, 50, 100 mg; powder for inj 380 mg/vial kit

Administer:

PO route

• Give with food, antacid to prevent nausea, vomiting

IM route

• IM deep in gluteal, alternate inj sites; use supplied needle to prevent inj site reaction; aspirate before inj

• Only if resuscitative equipment is nearby

SIDE EFFECTS

CNS: *Stimulation, drowsiness,* dizziness, confusion, **seizures**, headache, flushing, hallucinations, nervousness, irritability, **suicidal ideation**, syncope, anxiety

CV: Rapid pulse, **pulmonary edema**, hypertension, DVT

EENT: Tinnitus, hearing loss, blurred vision

GI: *Nausea, vomiting, diarrhea, heartburn,* anorexia, **hepatitis**, constipation, abdominal pain

GU: Delayed ejaculation, decreased potency

INTEG: *Rash,* urticaria, bruising, oily skin, acne, pruritus, inj site reactions

MISC: Increased thirst, chills, fever

MS: Joint and muscle pain

RESP: Wheezing, hyperpnea, nasal congestion, rhinorrhea, sneezing, sore throat, pneumonia

PHARMACOKINETICS

Metabolized by liver, excreted by kidneys; crosses placenta, excreted in breast milk; half-life 4 hr; extensive first-pass metabolism; protein binding 21%-28%

PO: Onset 15-30 min, peak 1-2 hr, duration is dose dependent

IM: Peak 2 hr

INTERACTIONS

Increase: lethargy—phenothiazines

Increase: hepatotoxicity—disulfiram

Increase: bleeding risk—anticoagulants

Decrease: effect of analgesics, antidiarrheals, cough preparations

NURSING CONSIDERATIONS

Assess:

Black Box Warning: Hepatic status: LFTs, jaundice, hepatitis, hepatic failure

• ABGs including Po_2, Pco_2, LFTs, VS q3-5min

• Signs of withdrawal in drug-dependent individuals

• Cardiac status: tachycardia, hypertension

• **Respiratory dysfunction: respiratory depression,** character, rate, rhythm; if respirations <10/min, respiratory stimulant should be administered

• Mental status: depression, suicidal ideation

Perform/provide:

• Storage in tight container

N

Evaluate:
- Therapeutic response: blocking opiate ingestion; successful nicotine, alcohol withdrawal

Teach patient/family:
- That patient must be drug-free to start treatment

⚠ That using opioid while taking this product could prove fatal because high dose is needed to overcome this antagonist; not to self-dose with OTC products unless approved by prescriber
- To carry emergency ID stating product used
- That, if surgery is needed, all involved should be aware of this product
- To use caution while driving or performing other hazardous tasks until effect is known

⚠ That suicidal thoughts/behaviors may occur; to report these immediately

naphazoline nasal agent

See Appendix B

naphazoline ophthalmic

See Appendix B

naproxen (Rx, OTC)

Aleve, Anaprox, Anaprox DS, Apo-Napro-Na ✤, Apo-Naproxen ✤, EC-Naprosyn, Equaline All Day Relief, Gen-Naproxen EC ✤, Good Sense All Day Pain Relief, Leader Naproxen, Midol Extended Relief, Naprelan, Novo-Naprox ✤, Novo-Naprox Sodium ✤, Nu-Naprox ✤, Select Brand Naproxen, Top Care All Day Pain Relief, Wal-Proxen

Func. class.: Nonsteroidal antiinflammatory, nonopioid analgesic

Chem. class.: Propionic acid derivative

Do not confuse:
Naprosyn/Natacyn/Naprelan

ACTION: Completely inhibits COX-1, COX-2 by blocking arachidonate; analgesic, antiinflammatory, antipyretic

USES: Osteoarthritis; rheumatoid, gouty arthritis; primary dysmenorrhea; ankylosing spondylitis, bursitis, tendinitis, myalgia, dental pain

Unlabeled uses: Juvenile rheumatoid arthritis, bone pain, migraine/migraine prophylaxis, heterotropic ossification

CONTRAINDICATIONS: Pregnancy (D) 3rd trimester, hypersensitivity to NSAIDs, salicylates; asthma, severe renal/hepatic disease, ulcer disease

Black Box Warning: Perioperative pain in CABG surgery

Precautions: Pregnancy (C) breastfeeding, children <2 yr, geriatric patients, bleeding disorders, GI disorders, cardiac disorders, hypersensitivity to other antiinflammatory agents, CCr <30 ml/min

Black Box Warning: MI, GI bleeding, stroke

DOSAGE AND ROUTES

200 mg base = 220 mg naproxen sodium

Antiinflammatory/analgesic/antidysmenorrheal

- **Adult: PO** 250-500 mg bid, max 1250 mg/day; **DEL REL** 375-500 mg bid
- **Child ≥2 yr: PO** 5-7 mg/kg q8-12hr

Antigout

- **Adult: PO** 750 mg, then 250 mg q8hr

OTC use

- **Adult: PO** 220 mg q8-12hr or 440 mg then 220 mg q12hr; max 660 mg/24hr taken ≤10 days
- **Geriatric >65 yr: PO** Max 220 mg q12hr

Available forms: Naproxen: tabs 250, 375, 500 mg; del rel tabs (EC-Naprosyn, Naprosyn-E) 250 ♣, 375, 500 mg; oral susp 125 mg/5 ml; ext rel tabs (CR) 375, 500, 750 mg; **naproxen sodium:** tabs 220, 275, 550 mg tab, ext rel 220 mg

Administer:

- With food to decrease GI symptoms; take on empty stomach to facilitate absorption, give with full glass of liquid
- Do not crush, break, or chew ext rel tabs
- OTC for ≤10 days unless approved by prescriber
- **Oral susp:** shake well, use measuring cup provided or other calibrated device

SIDE EFFECTS

CNS: Dizziness, drowsiness, fatigue, tremors, confusion, insomnia, anxiety, depression

CV: Tachycardia, peripheral edema, palpitations, dysrhythmias, **MI, stroke**

EENT: Tinnitus, hearing loss, blurred vision

GI: Nausea, anorexia, vomiting, diarrhea, jaundice, **hepatitis,** constipation, flatulence, cramps, peptic ulcer, **GI ulceration, bleeding, perforation**

GU: **Nephrotoxicity: dysuria, hematuria, oliguria, azotemia**

HEMA: **Blood dyscrasias**

INTEG: Purpura, rash, pruritus, sweating

SYST: **Anaphylaxis**

PHARMACOKINETICS

PO: Peak 2-4 hr, half-life 12-17 hr; metabolized in liver; excreted in urine (metabolites), breast milk; 99% protein binding

INTERACTIONS

Increase: renal impairment—ACE inhibitors

⚠ **Increase: toxicity risk—methotrexate, lithium, antineoplastics, probenecid, radiation treatment**

Increase: bleeding risk—oral anticoagulants, thrombolytic agents, eptifibatide, tirofiban, cefamandole, cefotetan, cefoperazone, clopidogrel, ticlopidine, plicamycin, SSRIs, SNRIs, tricyclics, valproic acid

Increase: GI side effects risk—aspirin, corticosteroids, alcohol, NSAIDs

Decrease: effect of antihypertensives, diuretics

Decreased: absorption of naproxen—antacids, sucralfate, cholestyramine

Drug/Herb

- Bleeding risk: feverfew, garlic, ginger, ginkgo, ginseng *(Panax)*

Drug/Lab Test

Increase: BUN, alk phos

False increase: 5-HIAA, 17KS

NURSING CONSIDERATIONS

Assess:

Black Box Warning: Cardiac status: CV thrombotic events, MI, stroke; may be fatal; not to be used with CABG

Black Box Warning: GI status: ulceration, bleeding, perforation; may be fatal; obtain stool guaiac

- **Pain:** frequency, characteristics, intensity; relief before and 1-2 hr after product
- **Arthritis:** range of motion, pain, swelling before and 1-2 hr after use
- **Fever:** before, 1 hr after use

⚠ **Asthma, aspirin hypersensitivity or nasal polyps, increased risk of hypersensitivity**

• **Renal, hepatic, blood studies:** BUN, creatinine, AST, ALT, Hgb, LDH, blood glucose, Hct, WBC, platelets, CCr before treatment, periodically thereafter during long-term therapy
• Audiometric, ophthalmic exam before, during, after treatment; eye, ear problems: blurred vision, tinnitus (may indicate toxicity)

Perform/provide:
• Storage at room temp

Evaluate:
• Therapeutic response: decreased pain, stiffness, swelling in joints; ability to move more easily

Teach patient/family:
• To use sunscreen to prevent photosensitivity
• To report blurred vision, ringing, roaring in ears (may indicate toxicity)
• To avoid driving, other hazardous activities if dizziness or drowsiness occurs
⚠ To report change in urine pattern, weight increase, edema (face, lower extremities), pain increase in joints, fever, blood in urine (indicates nephrotoxicity); black stools, flulike symptoms
• That therapeutic effects may take up to 1 mo
• To avoid ASA, alcohol, steroids or other OTC medications without prescriber approval
• To report use to all health care providers
• To avoid during pregnancy, breastfeeding

naratriptan (Rx)

(nair′ah-trip-tan)

Amerge

Func. class.: Antimigraine agent, abortive

Chem. class.: 5-HT_1 receptor agonist

ACTION: Binds selectively to the vascular 5-HT_1 B/D receptor subtype, exerts antimigraine effect; causes vasoconstriction in cranial arteries

USES: Acute treatment of migraine with/without aura

CONTRAINDICATIONS: Hypersensitivity, angina pectoris, history of MI, documented silent ischemia, ischemic heart disease, concurrent ergotamine-containing preparations, uncontrolled hypertension, CV syndromes, hemiplegic or basilar migraines, severe renal disease (CCr <15 ml/min); severe hepatic disease (Child-Pugh grade C)

Precautions: Pregnancy (C), breastfeeding, children, geriatric patients, postmenopausal women, men >40 yr, risk factors for CAD, hypercholesterolemia, obesity, diabetes, impaired renal/hepatic function, peripheral vascular disease

DOSAGE AND ROUTES

• **Adult: PO** 1 or 2.5 mg with fluids; if headache returns, repeat 1× after 4 hr; max 5 mg/24 hr

Hepatic/renal dose
• **Adult: PO** CCr 15-39 ml/min, max 2.5 mg/24 hr

Available forms: Tabs 1, 2.5 mg

Administer:
• With fluids as soon as symptoms appear; may take another dose after 4 hr; do not take >5 mg during any 24-hr period

SIDE EFFECTS

CNS: Dizziness, sedation, fatigue
CV: Increased B/P, palpitations, **tachydysrhythmias, PR, QTc prolongation, ST/T wave changes, PVCs, atrial flutter/fibrillation, coronary vasospasm**
EENT: EENT infections, photophobia
GI: *Nausea, vomiting*
MISC: Temperature change sensations; tightness, pressure sensations
MS: *Weakness, neck stiffness,* myalgia

PHARMACOKINETICS

Onset 2-3 hr; peak 2-3 hr; 28%-31% protein binding; half-life 6 hr; metabolized in liver (metabolite); excreted in urine, feces; may be excreted in breast milk

INTERACTIONS

Increase: serotonin syndrome, neuroleptic malignant syndrome—SSRIs (FLUoxetine, fluvoxamine, paroxetine, sertraline), SNRIs, serotonin receptor agonists, sibutramine
Increase: vasospastic effects—ergot, ergot derivatives, other 5-HT_1 agonists
Increase: adverse reactions risk—MAOIs; do not use together
Drug/Herb
• Serotonin syndrome: SAM-e, St. John's wort

NURSING CONSIDERATIONS

Assess:
• **Migraine symptoms:** aura, duration, effect on lifestyle, aggravating/alleviating factors
⚠ **Serotonin syndrome, neuroleptic malignant syndrome:** increased heart rate, shivering sweating, dilated pupils, tremors, high B/P, hyperthermia, headache, confusion; if these occur, stop product, administer serotonin antagonist if needed; at least 2 wk should elapse between discontinuation of serotonergic agents and start of product
⚠ Cardiac status: ECG, increased B/P, dysrhythmias
• Stress level, activity, recreation, coping mechanisms
• Neurologic status: LOC blurred vision, nausea, vomiting, tingling in extremities preceding headache
Perform/provide:
• Quiet, calm environment with decreased stimulation (noise, bright light, excessive talking)
Evaluate:
• Therapeutic response: decrease in frequency, severity of headache
Teach patient/family:
⚠ To report pain, tightness in chest, neck, throat, or jaw; to notify prescriber immediately if sudden, severe abdominal pain occurs
• Not to use if another 5-HT_1 agonist or ergot preparation has been used during past 24 hr; to avoid using >2 days/wk because rebound headache may occur
• To notify prescriber if pregnancy is planned or suspected; to avoid breastfeeding

natalizumab (Rx)

(na-ta-liz′u-mab)

Tysabri

Func. class.: Biologic response modifier, immunoglobulins, monoclonal antibody

ACTION: Biologic-response–modifying properties mediated through specific receptors on cells, may be secondary to blockade of the interaction of inflammatory cells with vascular endothelial cells

USES: Ambulatory patients with relapsing/remitting MS who have not responded to other treatment; those with moderate to severe Crohn's disease

CONTRAINDICATIONS: Hypersensitivity, immunocompromised individuals (HIV, AIDS, leukemia, lymphoma, transplants), PML, murine (mouse) protein allergy

Black Box Warning: Progressive multifocal leukoencephalopathy

Precautions: Pregnancy (C), breastfeeding, geriatric patients, chronic progressive MS, depression, mental disorders, diabetes, TB, active infections, hepatotoxicity

DOSAGE AND ROUTES

• **Adult: IV INF** 300 mg q4wk; give over 1 hr; observe during and for 1 hr after inf
• **Adolescent and child ≥11 yr (unlabeled): IV INF** pediatric Crohn's disease activity index (PCDAI) >30, 3 mg/kg q4wk
Available forms: Single-use vial, 300 mg/100 ml 0.9% NaCl

N

Administer:
- Acetaminophen for fever, headache
- Only after being enrolled in the TOUCH Prescribing Program

Intermittent IV INF route
- Use only clear, colorless solution, without particulates
- Withdraw 15 ml from the vial using aseptic technique: inj conc into 100 ml 0.9% NaCl; do not use other diluents; mix completely; do not shake; inf immediately or refrigerate for ≤8 hr; warm to room temp before using; flush with 0.9% NaCl before, after inf; do not admix or use in same line with other agents
- Withhold product at first sign of PML

SIDE EFFECTS

CNS: *Headache, fatigue,* rigors, syncope, tremors, *depression,* **progressive multifocal leukoencephalopathy (PML), suicidal ideation,** anxiety
CV: Chest discomfort, hypo/hypertension, tachycardia
GI: *Abdominal discomfort,* abnormal LFT, gastroentritis, **severe hepatic injury**
GU: Amenorrhea, *UTI, irregular menses,* vaginitis, urinary frequency
INTEG: *Rash,* dermatitis, pruritus, **skin melanoma,** infusion-related reactions
MS: *Arthralgia,* myalgia
RESP: *Lower respiratory tract infection,* dyspnea
SYST: Anaphylaxis, angioedema

PHARMACOKINETICS

Half-life approximately 11 days

INTERACTIONS

- Do not use with vaccines

Increase: infection—immunosuppressants, antineoplastics, immunomodulators

NURSING CONSIDERATIONS

Assess:

Black Box Warning: Progressive multifocal leukoencephalopathy (weakness, paralysis, vision loss, impaired speech, cognitive deterioration; obtain gadolinium-enhanced MRI scan of the brain, possibly cerebrospinal fluid for JC viral DNA; signs, symptoms of PML (decreased cognition, vision; ataxia, dysphagia)

- Blood, renal, hepatic studies: CBC, differential, platelet counts, BUN, creatinine, ALT, urinalysis, antibody testing
- CNS symptoms: headache, fatigue, depression, rigors, tremors
- GI status: abdominal discomfort, gastroenteritis, severe hepatic injury, abnormal LFTs
- Mental status: depression, depersonalization, suicidal thoughts, insomnia
- **MS symptoms;** product should only be used by patients who have not responded to other treatments

⚠ **Anaphylaxis:** SOB, hives; swelling, tightness in throat, chest pain; usually within 2 hr of inf

Perform/provide:
- Storage of sol in refrigerator; do not freeze or shake; protect from light; use within 8 hr of preparation

Evaluate:
- Therapeutic response: decreased symptoms of MS, Crohn's disease

Teach patient/family:
- Provide patient or family member with written, detailed information about product
- That female patients may experience irregular menses, amenorrhea; to notify prescriber if pregnancy is suspected; to avoid breastfeeding while taking this product

⚠ To notify prescriber of possible infection: sore throat, cough, increased temp, inf site reactions

natamycin ophthalmic

See Appendix B

nebivolol (Rx)

(ne-biv'oh-lol)

Bystolic

Func. class.: Antihypertensive

Chem. class.: β_1-blocker

ACTION: Competitively blocks stimulation of β-adrenergic receptors within vascular smooth muscle; decreases rate of SA node discharge, increases recovery time, slows conduction of AV node, thereby resulting in decreased heart rate (negative chronotropic effect), which decreases O_2 consumption in myocardium due to β_1-receptor antagonism; decreases renin-aldosterone-angiotensin system at high doses, inhibits β_2-receptors in bronchial system at high doses

USES: Hypertension alone or in combination

Unlabeled uses: Heart failure

CONTRAINDICATIONS: Cardiogenic shock, heart failure, severe hepatic disease, severe bradycardia, sick sinus syndrome, AV heart block; hypersensitivity to product, β-blockers

Precautions: Pregnancy (C), breastfeeding, children, major surgery, peripheral vascular disease, diabetes mellitus, thyrotoxicosis disease, COPD, asthma, well-compensated heart failure, renal/hepatic disease, abrupt discontinuation, acute bronchospasm

DOSAGE AND ROUTES

Hypertension

- **Adult: PO** 5 mg/day, may be increased to desired response q2wk; max 40 mg/day
- **Geriatric: PO** max 40 mg/day

Renal/hepatic dose

- **Adult: PO** CCr <30 ml/min, 2.5 mg/day; may increase cautiously; (Child-Pugh class B) 2.5 mg daily, use dose escalation cautiously

Heart failure (unlabeled)

- **Adult: PO** 1.25 mg titrated to max 10 mg/day

Available forms: Tabs 2.5, 5, 10, 20 mg

Administer:

PO route

- Without regard to meals; tab may be crushed or swallowed whole; give with food to prevent GI upset

SIDE EFFECTS

CNS: *Insomnia, fatigue, dizziness, mental changes,* drowsiness, headache

CV: **Bradycardia, MI,** AV heart block, edema

GI: *Nausea, diarrhea,* vomiting, abdominal pain

GU: *Impotence*

HEMA: **Thrombocytopenia**

INTEG: Rash, pruritus, vasculitis, urticaria, psoriasis, **angioedema**

MISC: **Renal failure, pulmonary edema,** hyperuricemia, hypercholesterolemia

RESP: **Bronchospasm,** dyspnea

PHARMACOKINETICS

Peak 1.5-4 hr; half-life 12 hr; metabolized in liver by CYP2D6; 38% excreted in urine, 44% in feces

INTERACTIONS

⚠ Do not give with other β-blockers, mefloquine

Increase: nebivolol action—CYP2D6 inhibitors (amiodarone, buPROPion, chloroquine, chlorpheniramine, chlorproMAZINE, cinacalcet, diphenhydrAMINE, duloxetine, FLUoxetine, haloperidol, imatinib, paroxetine, promethazine, propoxyphene, quiNIDine, quinine, ritonavir, terbinafine, thioridazine), cimetidine, calcium channel blockers (nondihydropyridine)

Decrease: nebivolol action—CYP2D6 inducers (rifampin), sildenafil

Drug/Herb
• May increase nebivolol effect—hawthorn
• May decrease nebivolol effect—ephedra

Drug/Lab Test
Increase: serum lipoprotein levels, BUN, potassium, triglycerides, uric acid, LDH, AST, ALT, blood glucose, alk phos
Positive: ANA titer

NURSING CONSIDERATIONS

Assess:
• **Hypertension:** B/P during beginning treatment, periodically thereafter; apical/radial pulse before administration; notify prescriber of any significant changes (pulse <50 bpm); **signs of CHF** (dyspnea, crackles, weight gain, jugular venous distention)
• Baselines of renal, hepatic function tests before therapy begins and periodically
• Edema in feet, legs daily: monitor I&O
• Skin turgor, dryness of mucous membranes for hydration status, especially among geriatric patients

Perform/provide:
• Storage protected from light, moisture; place in cool environment

Evaluate:
• Therapeutic response: decreased B/P after 1-2 wk; decreased dysrhythmias

Teach patient/family:
⚠ **Not to discontinue product abruptly because severe cardiac reactions may occur, to taper over 2 wk; not to double dose; if dose is missed, to take as soon as remembered up to 4 hr before next dose**
• That product may mask signs of hypoglycemia or alter blood glucose levels
• Not to use OTC products containing α-adrenergic stimulants (nasal decongestants, OTC cold preparations) unless directed by prescriber
• To report low pulse, dizziness, confusion, depression, fever
• To take pulse, B/P at home; advise patient when to notify prescriber
• To comply with weight control, dietary adjustments, modified exercise program
• To carry emergency ID to identify product, allergies
• To avoid hazardous activities if dizziness, drowsiness present
• **To report symptoms of CHF:** difficulty breathing, especially on exertion or when lying down, night cough, swelling of extremities
• To continue with required lifestyle changes (exercise, diet, weight loss, stress reduction)

TREATMENT OF OVERDOSE:
Lavage, IV atropine for bradycardia, IV theophylline for bronchospasm, digoxin, O_2, diuretic for cardiac failure, IV glucose for hypoglycemia, IV diazepam (or phenytoin) for seizures, IV fluids, IV pressors

⚠ HIGH ALERT

nelarabine (Rx)
(nella-ra′ben)
Arranon, Atriance ✱
Func. class.: Antineoplastic
Chem. class.: Purine analog

ACTION: Leukemic blasts allow for incorporation into DNA, thus interfering with cell replication and leading to cell death

USES: T-cell lymphoblastic leukemia, T-cell lymphoblastic lymphoma after relapse or treatment failure with at least 2 chemotherapeutic agents
Unlabeled uses: T-cell leukemia/lymphoma at first relapse or if refractory

CONTRAINDICATIONS: Pregnancy (D), hypersensitivity
Precautions: Breastfeeding, children, geriatric patients, renal/hepatic disease

Black Box Warning: Seizure disorder, IM administration, neurologic disease, peripheral neuropathy

DOSAGE AND ROUTES

- **Adult: IV** 1500 mg/m^2 over 2 hr on days 1, 3, 5, repeated q21days
- **Infant ≥2 mo/child/adolescent: IV** 650 mg/m^2 over 1 hr/day × 5 days, repeated q21days

Available forms: Sol for inj 5 mg/ml (50 ml)

Administer:

Intermittent IV INF route

- Visually inspect for particulate or discoloration whenever possible
- Do not dilute prior to use; transfer needed amount to PVC inf bag or glass container; stable for ≤8 hr in these containers; inf over 2 hr (adult), 1 hr (child)
- IV hydration, allopurinol for risk of hyperuricemia
- Use procedures for proper handling/disposal of anticancer products

SIDE EFFECTS

CNS: Dizziness, *fatigue,* insomnia, rigors, seizures, peripheral neuropathy, **paralysis,** confusion, headache, **Guillain-Barré syndrome,** depression, drowsiness, encephalopathy

CV: Edema

GI: *Nausea, vomiting, anorexia, diarrhea, stomatitis, constipation*

HEMA: **Neutropenia, leukopenia, thrombocytopenia,** anemia

META: Decreased potassium, calcium, magnesium, albumin, bilirubin, AST, ALT, hyperuricemia; increased glucose

MS: Myalgia, arthralgia, back pain, weakness

RESP: **Pleural effusion,** cough, dyspnea, wheezing, epistaxis

SYST: **Tumor lysis syndrome (TLS)**

PHARMACOKINETICS

Metabolized in liver, excreted by kidneys, half-life 30 min-3 hr

INTERACTIONS

- Do not use with live virus vaccinations/toxoids

Increase: bleeding risk—NSAIDs, anticoagulants, platelet inhibitors, salicylates

NURSING CONSIDERATIONS

Assess:

- CBC (RBC, Hct, Hgb), differential, platelet count weekly; withhold product if WBC is <4000/mm^3, platelet count is <75,000/mm^3, or RBC, Hct, Hgb low; notify prescriber of results

⚠ **Tumor lysis syndrome:** hyperkalemia, hyperphosphatemia, hyperuricemia, hypocalcemia

- Renal studies: BUN, serum uric acid, urine CCr, electrolytes before, during therapy
- Monitor temp; fever may indicate beginning infection; no rectal temp
- Hepatic studies before and during therapy: bilirubin, ALT, AST, alk phos as needed or monthly
- **Bleeding:** hematuria, heme-positive stools, bruising or petechiae, mucosa or orifices q8hr

Black Box Warning: Neurotoxicity: somnolence, confusion, seizures, ataxia, paresthesias, hypoesthesia, coma, status epilepticus, craniospinal demyelination; contact prescriber immediately; for those with NCI common toxicity criteria ≥ grade 2, product should be discontinued

- Dyspnea, crackles, unproductive cough, chest pain, tachypnea, fatigue, increased pulse, pallor, lethargy, personality changes
- Buccal cavity for dryness, sores or ulceration, white patches, oral pain, bleeding, dysphagia
- **GI symptoms:** frequency of stools, cramping; if severe diarrhea occurs, fluid, electrolytes may need to be given

Perform/provide:

- Rinsing of mouth tid-qid with water, club soda; brushing of teeth bid-tid with soft brush or cotton-tipped applicators for stomatitis; use unwaxed dental floss
- Storage at room temp

Evaluate:
- Therapeutic response: decreased spread of malignancy

Teach patient/family:
- To avoid foods with citric acid, hot or rough texture if stomatitis present; to avoid OTC products

⚠ **To use contraception while taking this product, pregnancy (D); to avoid breastfeeding**
- To report signs of infection: increased temp, sore throat, flulike symptoms
- To report signs of anemia: fatigue, headache, faintness, SOB, irritability
- To report bleeding; to avoid use of razors, commercial mouthwash
- To report numbness, paresthesias, weakness
- That seizures may occur; not to operate machinery or drive until effects are known
- Not to receive vaccinations while taking this product

nelfinavir (Rx)

(nell-fin′a-ver)

Viracept

Func. class.: Antiretroviral

Chem. class.: Protease inhibitor

ACTION: Inhibits human immunodeficiency virus (HIV-1) protease, which prevents maturation of the infectious virus

Uses: HIV-1 in combination with other antiretrovirals

CONTRAINDICATIONS: Hypersensitivity to protease inhibitors

Precautions: Pregnancy (B), breastfeeding, renal/hepatic disease, hemophilia, PKU, pancreatitis, diabetes, infection

DOSAGE AND ROUTES

HIV infection
- **Adult and child >13 yr: PO** 750 mg tid or 1250 mg bid
- **Child 2-13 yr: PO** 25-35 mg/kg tid, max 2500 mg/day

Prevention of HIV infection after exposure (unlabeled)
- **Adult: PO** 1250 mg bid with 2 other antiretroviral agents × 4 wk

Available forms: Tabs 250, 625 mg; powder, oral 50 mg/g/scoop

Administer:

PO route
- Do not mix with juice or acidic fluids
- **Oral powder:** mixed with fluids if desired; stable mixed for 6 hr, do not mix with water in original bottle
- Tabs may be crushed and dispersed in water or mixed with food; consume immediately

SIDE EFFECTS

CNS: Headache, asthenia, poor concentration, **seizures, suicidal ideation**

CV: Bleeding

ENDO: Hyperglycemia, hyperlipidemia

GI: *Diarrhea,* anorexia, dyspepsia, *nausea, flatulence,* **hepatitis, pancreatitis**

HEMA: **Anemia, leukopenia, thrombocytopenia,** Hgb abnormalities

INTEG: *Rash,* dermatitis, **anaphylaxis**

MS: Pain, arthralgia, myalgia, myopathy

Other: **Hypoglycemia,** redistribution/accumulation of body fat, **immune reconstitution syndrome**

PHARMACOKINETICS

Half-life $3^{1}/_{2}$-5 hr, excreted in feces (87%), peak 2-4 hr, 98% protein binding; metabolized by CYP3A4 enzyme system; potent inhibitor of CYP3A4

INTERACTIONS

Drug/Herb

⚠ **Increase: serious dysrhythmias: amiodarone, ergots, lovastatin, midazolam, pimozide, quiNIDine, simvastatin, triazolam, salmeterol**

Increase: effect of—atorvastatin, azithromycin, rifabutin, indinavir, saquinavir, cycloSPORINE, tacrolimus, sirolimus, sildenafil, alfentanil, alosetron, buprenorphine, busPIRone, bortezomib, calcium channel blockers, cilostazol, disopyramide, dofetilide, docetaxel, donepezil, ethosuximide, fentaNYL, galantamine, gefitinib, levomethadyl, systemic lidocaine, paclitaxel, sibutramine, SUFentanil, vinca alkaloids, ziprasidone, zonisamide, trazadone, tricyclic antidepressants

Increase: nelfinavir levels—ketoconazole, indinavir, ritonavir; delavirdine, other HIV protease inhibitors

Decrease: nelfinavir levels—rifamycins, nevirapine, PHENobarbital, phenytoin, carBAMazepine

Decrease: effect of—didanosine, methadone, oral contraceptives, phenytoin

Drug/Herb

⚠ **Decrease:** antiretroviral effect—St. John's wort; do not use concurrently

Drug/Food

Increase: absorption with food

Drug/Lab Test

Increase: AST, ALT, alk phos, total bilirubin, CPK, LDH

NURSING CONSIDERATIONS

Assess:

- Resistance testing at initiation, with failure of treatment
- Signs of infection, anemia
- Hepatic studies: ALT, AST
- Bowel pattern before, during treatment; if severe abdominal pain with bleeding occurs, product should be discontinued; monitor hydration

⚠ **Immune reconstitution syndrome:** occurs with combination therapy, including MAC, CMV, PCP TB requiring treatment

⚠ **Anaphylaxis, hypersensitivity reaction:** wheezing, flushing; swelling of lips, tongue, throat, skin eruptions, rash, urticaria, itching

- **HIV:** serum lipid profile, plasma HIV RNA, blood glucose, viral load, CD4 cell counts at baseline and throughout treatment

Teach patient/family:

- To avoid taking with other medications unless directed by prescriber
- That product does not cure but does manage symptoms; that product does not prevent transmission of HIV to others
- To use a nonhormonal form of birth control while taking this product
- If dose is missed, to take as soon as remembered up to 1 hr before next dose; not to double dose
- To take with food
- To report symptoms of hyperglycemia, bleeding, abdominal pain; yellowing of skin, eyes

RARELY USED

neomycin (Rx)

(nee-oh-mye′sin)

Neo-Fradin

Func. class.: Antiinfective

USES: Severe systemic infections of CNS, respiratory, GI, urinary tract, eye, bone, skin, soft tissues caused by *Pseudomonas aeruginosa, Escherichia coli, Enterobacter, Klebsiella pneumoniae, Proteus vulgaris;* hepatic coma, preoperatively to sterilize bowel, infectious diarrhea caused by enteropathogenic *E. coli*

CONTRAINDICATIONS: Infants, children, bowel obstruction (oral use), severe renal disease, hypersensitivity, GI disease

Precautions:

Black Box Warning: Dehydration, geriatric patients, hearing impairment, neuromuscular disease, renal disease, respiratory insufficiency

DOSAGE AND ROUTES

Hepatic encephalopathy

- **Adult: PO** 4-12 g/day in divided doses q6hr × 5-6 days
- **Child: PO** 50-100 mg/kg/day in divided doses q6hr × 5-6 days

N

Preoperative intestinal antisepsis
• **Adult: PO** 1 g/hr × 4 hr then 1 g q4hr for remaining 24 hr

neomycin topical

See Appendix B

neostigmine (Rx)

(nee-oh-stig′meen)

Prostigmin

Func. class.: Cholinergic stimulant; anticholinesterase

Chem. class.: Quaternary compound

ACTION:

Inhibits destruction of acetylcholine, which increases concentration at sites where acetylcholine is released; this facilitates transmission of impulses across myoneural junction

USES:

Diagnosis/treatment of myasthenia gravis, nondepolarizing neuromuscular blocker antagonist, postoperative ileus, urinary retention

CONTRAINDICATIONS:

Obstruction of intestine, renal system, bromide sensitivity, peritonitis, urinary tract obstruction, ileus

Precautions: Pregnancy (C), breastfeeding, children, bradycardia, hypotension, seizure disorders, bronchial asthma, coronary occlusion, hyperthyroidism, dysrhythmias, peptic ulcer, megacolon, poor GI motility

DOSAGE AND ROUTES

Myasthenia gravis treatment
• **Adult: PO** 15 mg tid, may increase to 375 mg/day; **IM/IV** 0.5-2.5 mg q1-3hr, max 10 mg/day
• **Child: PO** 0.333 mg/kg q3-4hr; **IM/IV/SUBCUT** 0.01-0.04 mg/kg q2-4hr

Nondepolarizing neuromuscular blocker antagonist
• **Adult: IV** 0.5-2.5 mg slowly, may repeat if needed, max 5 mg (give 0.6-1.2 mg atropine several min before this product)
• **Infant and child: IV** 0.025-0.08 mg/kg/dose (give atropine several min before this product)

Postoperative abdominal distention/ileus
• **Adult: IM/SUBCUT** 0.25-1 mg (1:4000) q4-6hr depending on condition × 2-3 days

Urinary retention treatment
• **Adult: IM/SUBCUT** 0.5-1 mg q3hr × 5 doses after bladder is emptied

Renal dose
• CCr 10-50 ml/min, 50% of dose; CCr <10 ml/min, 25% of dose

Myasthenia gravis diagnosis (unlabeled)
• **Adult: IM** 0.02 mg/kg as single dose
• **Child: IM** 0.04 mg/kg as single dose

Available forms: Tabs 15 mg; inj 0.25, 0.5, 1 mg/ml

Administer:
• Only with atropine sulfate available for cholinergic crisis
• Only after all other cholinergics have been discontinued
• Increased doses, as ordered, if tolerance occurs
• Larger doses after exercise or fatigue, as ordered
• Oral product and injectable version are not equivalent

PO route
• Give with food or milk to minimize gastric upset; for those with difficulty chewing, give 30 min before meals

IM route
• Inject deeply in large muscle, aspirate prior to injecting

SUBCUT route
• Avoid intradermal inj

Direct IV route
• Undiluted, give through Y-tube or 3-way stopcock; give ≤0.5 mg over 1 min

Syringe compatibilities: Glycopyrrolate, heparin, ondansetron, PENTobarbital, thiopental

Y-site compatibilities: Heparin, hydrocortisone, potassium chloride, vit B/C

SIDE EFFECTS

CNS: Dizziness, headache, sweating, weakness, **seizures**, incoordination, **paralysis**, drowsiness, **loss of consciousness**
CV: Tachycardia, dysrhythmias, bradycardia, hypotension, AV block, ECG changes, **cardiac arrest**, syncope
EENT: Miosis, blurred vision, lacrimation, visual changes
GI: *Nausea, diarrhea, vomiting, cramps,* increased peristalsis, salivary and gastric secretions
GU: Urinary frequency, incontinence, urgency
INTEG: Rash, urticaria, flushing
RESP: **Respiratory depression, bronchospasm, constriction, laryngospasm, respiratory arrest**, dyspnea
SYST: **Anaphylaxis**

PHARMACOKINETICS

Metabolized in liver, excreted in urine
PO: Onset 45-75 min, peak 1-2 hr, duration 2½-4 hr
IM/SUBCUT: Onset 20-30 min, duration 2½-4 hr
IV: Onset 1-2 min, duration 2-4 hr

INTERACTIONS

Increase: action of decamethonium, succinylcholine
Increase: bradycardia—β-blockers, calcium channel blockers, digoxin
Decrease: neostigmine action—aminoglycosides, antihistamines, antidepressants, atropine, anticholinergics, local/general anesthetics, corticosteroids, haloperidol, phenothiazines, quiNIDine, disopyramide

NURSING CONSIDERATIONS

Assess:

- **Myasthenia gravis:** before and during treatment; gait, swallowing, respiratory difficulties; chewing, talking, eye muscle weakness
- **Antidote:** use peripheral nerve stimulator to identify reversal of nondepolarizing neuromuscular blocking agents; check for respiratory dysfunction, weakness during recovery
- Pulse, respiratory rate, B/P, neurologic status frequently; ECG IV administration
- **Postoperative urinary retention/abdominal distention:** urinary retention, palpate bladder, I&O ratio; check for incontinence, auscultate bowel sounds, check for distention

⚠ **Bradycardia, hypotension, bronchospasm, headache, dizziness, seizures, respiratory depression; product should be discontinued if toxicity occurs**

Perform/provide:

- Storage at room temp

Evaluate:

- Therapeutic response: increased muscle strength, hand grasp, improved gait, absence of labored breathing (if severe)

Teach patient/family:

- **Myasthenia gravis:** that product is not a cure; it only relieves symptoms; to wear emergency ID specifying myasthenia gravis, products taken; to avoid driving, other hazardous activities until effect is known
- To report respiratory distress, cardiac dysrhythmias

TREATMENT OF OVERDOSE:

Respiratory support, atropine 1-4 mg (IV), aggressive hydration

nepafenac ophthalmic

See Appendix B

N

⚠ HIGH ALERT

nesiritide (Rx)

(neh-seer′ih-tide)

Natrecor

Func. class.: Vasodilator

Chem. class.: Human B-type natriuretic peptide

ACTION: Uses DNA technology; human B-type natriuretic peptide binds to the receptor in vascular smooth muscle and endothelial cells, thereby leading to smooth muscle relaxation

USES: Acutely decompensated CHF

CONTRAINDICATIONS: Hypersensitivity to this product or *Escherichia coli* protein; cardiogenic shock or B/P <90 mm Hg as primary therapy

Precautions: Pregnancy (C); breastfeeding; children; mitral stenosis; significant valvular stenosis, restriction, or obstructive cardiomyopathy, or any condition dependent on venous return; renal disease; constrictive pericarditis

DOSAGE AND ROUTES

- **Adult: IV BOL** 2 mcg/kg then **CONT IV INF** 0.01 mcg/kg/min

Available forms: Powder for inj, 1.5-mg single-use vial

Administer:

IV route

- Do not give through a central catheter containing other products; administer other products through separate catheter or central line heparin-coated catheter because nesiritide binds to heparin
- Reconstitute one 1.5-mg vial/5 ml of diluent from prefilled 250-ml plastic IV bag with diluent of choice (preservative free D_5, 0.9% NaCl, $D_5/^1/_2$ NaCl, D_5/0.2% NaCl); do not shake vial, roll gently; use only clear sol
- Withdraw all contents of reconstituted vial and add to 250-ml plastic IV bag (6 mcg/ml), invert bag several times
- Use within 24 hr of reconstituting
- Prime IV fluid with inf of 5 ml before connecting to patient's vascular access port and before bolus dose or IV inf

Direct IV route

- Prime tubing with 5 ml inf sol; calculate dose based on patient's weight, 0.33 × patient weight (kg) = bolus vol (ml) (6 mcg/ml); withdraw prescribed bolus dose (volume) from prepared inf bag; give over 1 min through IV port

Intermittent IV INF route

- After bolus dose, use inf, give at 0.1 ml/kg/hr (0.01 mcg/kg/min)

Y-site compatibilities: Acyclovir, alfentanil, allopurinol, amifostine, aminocaproic acid, aminophylline, amiodarone, amphotericin B colloidal, amphotericin B lipid complex, amphotericin B liposome, anidulafungin, argatroban, atenolol, atracurium, azithromycin, aztreonam, bivalirudin, bleomycin, buprenorphine, busulfan, butorphanol, calcium acetate/chloride/gluconate, CARBOplatin, carmustine, ceFAZolin, cefotaxime, cefotetan, cefoxitin, ceftazidime, ceftizoxime, cefTRIAXone, cefuroxime, chloramphenicol, cimetidine, ciprofloxacin, cisatracurium, CISplatin, clindamycin, cyclophosphamide, cycloSPORINE, cytarabine, dacarbazine, DACTINomycin, DAUNOrubicin, digoxin, diltiazem, diphenhydrAMINE, docetaxel, dolasetron, doxacurium, DOXOrubicin, doxycycline, droperidol, ePHEDrine, epirubicin, ertapenem, erythromycin, esmolol, etoposide, etoposide phosphate, famotidine, fenoldopam, fentaNYL, filgrastim, fluconazole, fludarabine, fluorouracil, foscarnet, fosphenytoin, ganciclovir, gatifloxacin, gemcitabine, gemtuzumab, glycopyrrolate, granisetron, haloperidol, hydrocortisone, HYDROmorphone, hydrOXYzine, IDArubicin, ifosfamide, imipenem-cilastatin, irinotecan, ketorolac, leucovorin, levofloxacin, lidocaine, linezolid, LORazepam, magnesium sulfate, mannitol, mechlorethamine, melphalan, meropenem, mesna, metaraminol, methohexital, methotrexate, methylPREDNISolone, metoclopramide, metroNIDAZOLE, midazolam, milrinone, minocycline, mitomycin, mitoxantrone, mivacurium, moxifloxacin, mycophenolate, nalbuphine, naloxone, niCARdipine, nitroglycerin, nitroprusside, octreotide, ondansetron, oxaliplatin, oxytocin, paclitaxel, palonosetron, pamidronate, pancuronium, pemetrexed, pentamidine, PENTobarbital, PHENobarbital, phentolamine, phenylephrine, polymyxin B sulfate, potassium chloride/phosphates, prochlorperazine, propranolol, quiNIDine, quinupristin-dalfopristin, ranitidine, remifentanil, rocuronium, sodium acetate/bicarbonate/phosphates, streptozocin, succinylcholine, SUFentanil, tacrolimus, teniposide, theophylline, thiotepa, ticarcillin, tigecycline, tirofiban, tolazoline, topotecan, torsemide, trimethobenzamide, vancomycin, vasopressin, vecuronium, verapamil, vinBLAStine, vinCRIStine, vinorelbine, zidovudine, zoledronic acid

SIDE EFFECTS

CNS: Headache, insomnia, dizziness, anxiety, confusion, paresthesia, tremor
CV: *Hypotension,* tachycardia, dysrhythmias, bradycardia, **ventricular tachycardia, ventricular extrasystoles, atrial fibrillation**
GI: Vomiting, nausea
INTEG: Rash, sweating, pruritus, inj site reaction
MISC: Abdominal pain, back pain
RESP: Increased cough, hemoptysis, **apnea**

PHARMACOKINETICS

Half-life 18 min

INTERACTIONS

Increase: hypotension—ACE inhibitors, antihypertensives, inotropes, IV nitrates

NURSING CONSIDERATIONS

Assess:
- PCWP, RAP, cardiac index, MPAP, B/P, pulse during treatment until stable
- Daily serum creatinine, BUN
- **CHF:** weight gain, dyspnea, crackles, I&O ratios, peripheral edema

Evaluate:
- Therapeutic response: improvement in CHF with improved PCWP, RAP, MPAP

Teach patient/family:
- About purpose of medication, expected results, to report pain at IV site
- To report dizziness, blurred vision, lightheadedness, sweating

nevirapine (Rx)

(ne-veer′a-peen)

Viramune, Viramune XR

Func. class.: Antiretroviral
Chem. class.: Nonnucleoside reverse transcriptase inhibitor (NNRTI)

Do not confuse:
nevirapine/nelfinavir
Viramune/Viracept

ACTION:
Binds directly to reverse transcriptase and blocks RNA, DNA, thus causing a disruption of the enzyme's site

N

USES:
HIV-1 in combination with other highly active antiretroviral therapy (HAART)

CONTRAINDICATIONS:

Black Box Warning: Hypersensitivity, hepatic disease

Precautions: Pregnancy (B), breastfeeding, children, renal disease, Hispanic patients

Black Box Warning: Females, hepatitis

DOSAGE AND ROUTES

Treatment of HIV infection in combination with other antiretrovirals
- **Adult and adolescent: PO** 200 mg/day × 2 wk then 200 mg bid in combination; **EXT REL** tab (adults not currently taking immediate rel nevirapine) 200 mg/day (immediate rel tab) × 14 days with other antiretrovirals; if rash develops

during lead-in periods and persists beyond 14 days, do not use ext rel tab; if no consistent rash present, then give 400 mg/day ext rel tab with other antiretrovirals; if interrupted >7 days, restart 14 day lead-in dosing; for adults switched from immediate rel tab, give 400 mg/day ext rel tab

• **Child/infant/neonate ≥15 days old: PO** 150 mg/m^2/day × 14 days then 150 mg/m^2 bid, max 400 mg/day

Perinatal transmission prophylaxis (unlabeled)

• **Females with no previous antiretroviral therapy: PO** 200 mg as a single dose at onset of labor with zidovudine 2 mg/kg over 1 hr followed by zidovudine 1 mg/kg/hr until delivery

• **Neonate ≥34 wk gestation: PO** Nevirapine 2 mg/kg as single dose at age 48-72 hr and **PO** zidovudine 2 mg/kg q12hr for 6 wk

Hepatic Dose

• **Adult: PO** Do not use with Child-Pugh grade B or C

Available forms: Tabs 200 mg; oral susp 50 mg/5 ml

Administer:

• Do not initiate treatment in females when CD4 counts >250 cells/mm^3 or in males when >400 cells/mm^3 unless benefits outweigh risks

• Without regard to meals

• Oral susp should be shaken prior to giving

SIDE EFFECTS

CNS: *Paresthesia, headache, fever, peripheral neuropathy*

GI: *Diarrhea,* abdominal pain, *nausea, stomatitis,* hepatotoxicity, hepatic failure

HEMA: Neutropenia, anemia, thrombocytopenia

INTEG: *Rash,* toxic epidermal necrolysis

MISC: Stevens-Johnson syndrome, anaphylaxis

MS: Pain, myalgia, rhabdomyolysis

PHARMACOKINETICS

Rapidly absorbed, peak 4 hr, 60% bound to plasma proteins, metabolized by liver; metabolized by hepatic P450 enzyme system, excreted 91% in urine, terminal half-life 25-30 hr, 50% removed by peritoneal dialysis; with hepatic disease and in Hispanics, African Americans, slower rate of clearance

INTERACTIONS

Increase: nevirapine levels—cimetidine, macrolide antiinfectives

Decrease: effects of protease inhibitors, oral contraceptives, ketoconazole, methadone, itraconazole

Decrease: nevirapine levels—rifamycins, anticonvulsants, clonazePAM, diazepam, warfarin

Drug/Herb

Decrease: action of antiretroviral—St. John's wort; do not use concurrently

Drug/Lab Test

Increase: ALT, AST, GGT, bilirubin, Hgb

Decrease: neutrophil count

NURSING CONSIDERATIONS

Assess:

• Resistance testing before therapy and when therapy fails

⚠ Signs of infection, anemia, hepatotoxicity, immune reconstitution syndrome; hepatitis B or C, liver toxicity may occur

• **HIV:** blood studies during treatment: ALT, AST, viral load, CD4, plasma HIV RNA, renal studies; if LFTs elevated significantly, product should be withheld; glucose levels in diabetic patients

⚠ **Rhabdomyolysis:** pain, tenderness, weakness, edema; product should be discontinued

• Bowel pattern before, during treatment; if severe abdominal pain with bleeding occurs, product should be discontinued; monitor hydration

⚠ **Stevens-Johnson syndrome, toxic epidermal necrolysis,** allergies before treatment, reaction to each medication; skin eruptions; rash, urticaria, itching; if rash is severe or systemic symptoms occur, discontinue immediately

Evaluate:

- Therapeutic response: absence of AIDS-defining symptoms, improvement in quality of life; decreased viral load, increase in CD4 count

Teach patient/family:

⚠ To report any right quadrant pain, yellowing of eyes or skin, dark urine, nausea, anorexia, muscle pain or tenderness, rash immediately

- That product may be taken with food, antacids
- To take as prescribed; if dose is missed, to take as soon as remembered up to 1 hr before next dose; not to double dose
- That product is not a cure, does not prevent transmission; controls symptoms of HIV
- To avoid OTC agents unless approved by prescriber
- To use a nonhormonal form of contraception during treatment

niacin (OTC, Rx)

(nye'a-sin)

Equaline Niacin, Niaspan, Ni-Odan ♣, Slo-Niacin

niacinamide (OTC, Rx)

Func. class.: Vit B_3, antihyperlipidemic

Chem. class.: Water-soluble vitamin

ACTION: Needed for conversion of fats, protein, carbohydrates by oxidation reduction; acts directly on vascular smooth muscle, thus causing vasodilation; reduces total cholesterol, LDL, VLDL, triglycerides; increases HDL

USES: Pellagra, hyperlipidemias (types 4, 5), peripheral vascular disease that presents a risk for pancreatitis

CONTRAINDICATIONS: Breastfeeding, hypersensitivity, peptic ulcer, hepatic disease, hemorrhage, severe hypotension

Precautions: Pregnancy (C), breastfeeding, glaucoma, cardiovascular disease, CAD, diabetes mellitus, gout, schizophrenia

DOSAGE AND ROUTES

Niacin deficiency

- **Adult: PO** 100-500 mg/day in divided doses; **IM/SUBCUT** 5-100 mg ≥5×/day; **IV** 25-100 mg bid or tid
- **Child: PO** ≤300 mg/day in divided doses

Adjunct in hyperlipidemia

- **Adult: PO** 250 mg after evening meal; may increase dose at 1-4 wk intervals to 1-2 g tid, max 6 g/day; **EXT REL** 500 mg at bedtime × 4 wk then 1000 mg at bedtime for wk 5-8; do not increase by >500 mg q4wk, max 2000 mg/day

Pellagra

- **Adult: PO** 300-500 mg/day in divided doses; **IM** 50-100 mg 5×/day or **IV** 25-100 mg bid by slow **IV INF**
- **Child: PO** 100-300 mg/day in divided doses; **IV** ≤300 mg/day by slow **IV/INF**

Peripheral vascular disease

- **Adult: PO** 250-800 mg/day in 3-5 divided doses

Available forms: *Niacin:* tabs 50, 100, 250, 500, mg; ext rel caps 250, 500 mg; ext rel tab 250, 500, 750, 1000 mg; *niacinamide:* tab 100, 500 mg

Administer:

- Do not break, crush, or chew ext rel tabs, caps
- With meals for GI symptoms; with 81-325 mg aspirin or NSAIDs 30 min before dose to decrease flushing

SIDE EFFECTS

CNS: Paresthesias, headache, dizziness, anxiety

CV: Postural hypotension, vasovagal attacks, dysrhythmias, vasodilation

EENT: Blurred vision, ptosis

GI: Nausea, vomiting, anorexia, jaundice, hepatotoxicity, diarrhea, peptic ulcer, dyspepsia, hepatitis

GU: Hyperuricemia, glycosuria, hypoalbuminemia
INTEG: Flushing, dry skin, rash, pruritus, itching, tingling

PHARMACOKINETICS

PO: Peak 30-70 min (depends on formulation), half-life 45 min; metabolized in liver; 30% excreted unchanged in urine

INTERACTIONS

Increase: postural hypotension—ganglionic blockers
⚠ **Increase:** myopathy, rhabdomyolysis—HMG-CoA reductase inhibitors
Increase: flushing, pruritus—alcohol, avoid use
Drug/Herb
⚠ **Increase:** myopathy, rhabdomyolysis—red yeast rice
Drug/Lab Test
Increase: bilirubin, alk phos, hepatic enzymes, LDH, uric acid, glucose
Decrease: cholesterol
False increase: urinary catecholamines
False positive: urine glucose

NURSING CONSIDERATIONS

Assess:
- Cardiac status: rate, rhythm, quality; postural hypotension, dysrhythmias
- Nutritional status: liver, yeast, legumes, organ meat, lean poultry; fat in diet

⚠ **Hepatotoxicity:** clay-colored stools, itching, dark urine, jaundice; hepatic studies: AST, ALT, bilirubin, uric acid, alk phos; blood glucose before and during treatment
- CNS symptoms: headache, paresthesias, blurred vision
- **Niacin deficiency:** nausea, vomiting, anemia, poor memory, confusion, dermatitis
- **Hyperlipidemia:** for lipid, triglyceride, cholesterol level; obtain diet history

Evaluate:
- Therapeutic response: decreased lipids, warm extremities, absence of numbness in extremities

Teach patient/family:
- That flushing and increase in feelings of warmth will occur several hr after taking product (PO); after 2 wk of therapy, these side effects diminish
- To remain recumbent if postural hypotension occurs; to rise slowly to prevent orthostatic hypotension
- To abstain from alcohol if product is prescribed for hyperlipidemia
- To avoid sunlight if skin lesions are present

⚠ **Hepatotoxicity:** to report clay-colored stools, anorexia, yellow eyes or skin, dark urine

niCARdipine (Rx)

(nye-card′i-peen)

Cardene IV, Cardene SR

Func. class.: Calcium channel blocker, antianginal, antihypertensive
Chem. class.: Dihydropyridine

Do not confuse:
niCARdipine/NIFEdipine
Cardene/Cardizem
Cardene SR/Cardizem SR

ACTION: Inhibits calcium ion influx across cell membrane during cardiac depolarization; produces relaxation of coronary vascular smooth muscle, peripheral vascular smooth muscle; dilates coronary vascular arteries; increases myocardial oxygen delivery in patients with vasospastic angina

USES: Chronic stable angina pectoris, hypertension

CONTRAINDICATIONS: Sick sinus syndrome, 2nd-/3rd-degree heart block; hypersensitivity to this product or dihydropyridine; advanced aortic stenosis
Precautions: Pregnancy (C), breastfeeding, children, geriatric patients, CHF, hypotension, hepatic injury, renal disease

DOSAGE AND ROUTES

Hypertension

• **Adult: PO** 20 mg tid initially; may increase after 3 days (range 20-40 mg tid) or 30 mg bid **SUS REL**; may increase to 60 mg bid or **IV** 5 mg/hr; may increase by 2.5 mg/hr q15min; max 15 mg/hr

Angina

• **Adult: PO** 20 mg tid; may be adjusted q3days; may use 20-40 mg tid

Renal dose

• **Adult: PO** 20 mg tid or **SUS REL** 30 mg bid

Hepatic dose

• **Adult: PO** 20 mg bid

Available forms: Caps 20, 30 mg; sus rel caps 30, 45, 60 mg; inj 2.5 mg/ml, premixed 20 mg/200 ml, 40 mg/200 ml

Administer:

PO route

• Do not break, crush, chew, or open sus rel cap

• Without regard to meals

IV route

• Dilute each 25 mg/240 ml of compatible sol (0.1 mg/ml), give slowly, titrate to patient response, change IV site q12hr

• Stable at room temp for 24 hr

Solution compatibilities: D_5W, $D_5/0.45\%$ NaCl, $D_5/0.9\%$ NaCl

Y-site compatibilities: Alemtuzumab, amikacin, aminophylline, aztreonam, bivalirudin, butorphanol, calcium gluconate, CARBOplatin, caspofungin, ceFAZolin, ceftizoxime, chloramphenicol, cimetidine, CISplatin, clindamycin, cytarabine, DAPTOmycin, dexmedetomidine, diltiazem, DOBUTamine, docetaxel, DOPamine, DOXOrubicin hydrochloride, enalaprilat, EPINEPHrine, epirubicin, erythromycin, esmolol, famotidine, fenoldopam, fentaNYL, gentamicin, hydrocortisone, HYDROmorphone, labetalol, lidocaine, linezolid, LORazepam, magnesium sulfate, mechlorethamine, methylPREDNISolone, metroNIDAZOLE, midazolam, milrinone, morphine, nafcillin, nesiritide, nitroglycerin, nitroprusside, norepinephrine, octreotide, oxaliplatin, oxytocin, palonosetron, penicillin G potassium, potassium chloride/phosphate, quinupristin/dalfopristin, ranitidine, rocuronium, tacrolimus, tirofiban, tobramycin, trimethoprim/sulfamethoxazole, vancomycin, vasopressin, vecuronium, vinCRIStine, voriconazole, zoledronic acid

SIDE EFFECTS

CNS: *Headache, dizziness,* anxiety, depression, confusion, paresthesia, somnolence, *flushing*

CV: Edema, bradycardia, hypotension, palpitations, **pulmonary edema,** chest pain, tachycardia, increased angina, **arrhythmias, CHF**

GI: Nausea, vomiting, gastric upset, constipation, **hepatitis,** abdominal cramps, dry mouth, sore throat

GU: Nocturia, polyuria

INTEG: Rash, inf site discomfort, **Stevens-Johnson syndrome**

OTHER: Blurred vision, flushing, sweating, SOB, impotence

PHARMACOKINETICS

Metabolized by liver, excreted in urine 60%, feces 35%

PO: Onset 30 min, peak 1-2 hr, duration 8 hr

PO-SR: Onset unknown, peak 2-6 hr, duration 10-12 hr, half-life 2-5 hr

INTERACTIONS

Increase: effects of digoxin, neuromuscular blocking agents, theophylline, other antihypertensives, nitrates, alcohol, quiNIDine

Increase: niCARdipine effects—cimetidine

Increase: toxicity risk—cycloSPORINE, prazosin, carBAMazepine, quiNIDine, propranolol

Decrease: antihypertensive effect—NSAIDs, rifampin

Drug/Herb

Increase: effect—ginkgo, ginseng, hawthorn

Decrease: effect—ephedra, melatonin, St. John's wort, yohimbe

Drug/Food

Increase: hypotensive effect—grapefruit juice

NURSING CONSIDERATIONS

Assess:

⚠ **Cardiac status:** B/P often, pulse, respiration, ECG during long-term treatment

- **Anginal pain:** intensity, location, duration; alleviating, precipitating factors
- Potassium, renal, hepatic studies periodically

⚠ **CHF:** weight gain, crackles, jugular venous distention, dyspnea, I&O

- **Hypertension:** decreasing B/P; assess salt in diet, smoking, exercise, weight

Evaluate:

- Therapeutic response: decreased anginal pain, decreased B/P

Teach patient/family:

- To avoid hazardous activities until stabilized on product, dizziness is no longer a problem
- To limit caffeine consumption; to avoid alcohol products
- To avoid OTC products, grapefruit juice unless directed by prescriber
- **Hypertension:** comply in all areas of medical regimen: diet, exercise, stress reduction, product therapy

⚠ To notify prescriber of irregular heartbeat, SOB, swelling of feet and hands, pronounced dizziness, constipation, nausea, hypotension, change in severity/pattern/incidence of angina

TREATMENT OF OVERDOSE:

Defibrillation, β-agonists, IV calcium, diuretics, atropine for AV block, vasopressor for hypotension

nicotine

(nik′o-teen)

nicotine chewing gum (OTC, Rx)

CVS Nicotine Polacrilex, Equate Nicotine, GNP Nicotine, Good Sense Nicotine, Leader Nicotine Gum, NICOrelief, Nicorette, Publix Stop Smoking Aid, TopCare Nicotine, Walgreens Nicotine

nicotine inhaler (OTC, Rx)

Nicotrol

nicotine lozenge (OTC)

CVS Nicotine Polacrilex, GNP Nicotine Polacrilex, Good Sense Nicotine, Polacrilex Lozenge, TopCare Nicotine Polacrilex, Walgreens Nicotine Polacrilex

nicotine nasal spray (Rx)

Nicotrol NS

nicotine transdermal (OTC, Rx)

CVS Nicotine Transdermal System, Equate Nicotine Transdermal System, Habitrol ✦, Leader Nicotine Transdermal Patch, Nicoderm CQ, Sunmark Nicotine Transdermal System, Walgreens Nicotine Transdermal Patch

Func. class.: Smoking deterrent

Chem. class.: Ganglionic cholinergic agonist

ACTION: Agonist at nicotinic receptors in peripheral, central nervous systems; acts at sympathetic ganglia, on chemoreceptors of aorta, carotid bodies;

also affects adrenalin-releasing catecholamines

USES:
Deter cigarette smoking
Unlabeled uses: Gilles de la Tourette's syndrome, ulcerative colitis

CONTRAINDICATIONS:
Pregnancy (D) (transdermal, inhaler); hypersensitivity, immediate post-MI recovery period, severe angina pectoris
Precautions: Pregnancy (C) (gum); breastfeeding, vasospastic disease, dysrhythmias, diabetes mellitus, hyperthyroidism, pheochromocytoma, esophagitis, peptic ulcer, coronary/renal/hepatic disease; MRI (patch)

DOSAGE AND ROUTES

Nicotine chewing gum
- **Adult:** Chew 1 piece of gum (2 mg nicotine) whenever urge to smoke occurs; dose varies; usually 20 mg/day during first mo, max 30 pieces (60 mg/day), max 3 mo

Nicotine inhaler
- **Adult: INH** 6 cartridges/day for first 3-6 wk, max 16 cartridges/day × 12 wk

Nicotine lozenge
- **Adult:** If cigarette is desired >30 min after awakening, start with 2-mg lozenge; if <30 min after awakening, start with 4-mg lozenge then again q1-2hr, max 20 lozenges/day or 5 lozenges/6 hr × 6 wk, then 1 lozenge q2-4hr × 2 wk, then 1 lozenge q4-8hr × 2 wk, then discontinue

Nicotine nasal spray
- **Adult:** 1 spray in each nostril 1-2×/hr, max 5×/hr or 40×/day, max 3 mo

Nicotine transdermal/inhaler system
- **Habitrol ✱, Nicoderm:** 21 mg/day × 4-8 wk; 14 mg/day × 2-4 wk; 7 mg/day × 2-4 wk
- **Nicotrol:** 15 mg/day × 12 wk; 10 mg/day × 2 wk; 5 mg/day × 2 wk
- **Nicotrol Inhaler:** delivers 30% of nicotine that smoker receives from an actual cigarette

Gilles de la Tourette's syndrome (unlabeled)
- **Adult and child: Chewing gum** 2 mg chewed × 30 min bid for 1-6 mo; **TRANSDERMAL** 7- or 10-mg patch daily × 2 days

Available forms: Transdermal patch (Habitrol ✱, Nicoderm, nicotine transdermal system) delivering 7, 14, 21 mg/day; (Nicoderm) 5, 10, 15 mg/day; **nicotine inhaler** 4 mg delivered; **nasal spray** 0.5 mg nicotine/actuation; gum 2, 4 mg/piece; **lozenge** 2 mg, 4 mg

Administer:
- **Gum:** chew gum slowly for 30 min to promote buccal absorption of product; do not chew >45 min
- Begin product withdrawal after 3 mo of use; do not exceed 6 mo
- **Transdermal patch:** 1×day to nonhairy, clean, dry area of skin on upper body or upper outer arm; rotate sites to prevent skin irritation
- **Inhaler:** puffing on mouthpiece delivers nicotine through mouth

SIDE EFFECTS

CNS: Dizziness, vertigo, insomnia, headache, confusion, seizures, depression, euphoria, numbness, tinnitus, strange dreams
CV: Dysrhythmias, tachycardia, palpitations, edema, flushing, hypertension
EENT: Jaw ache, irritation in buccal cavity
GI: *Nausea, vomiting, anorexia, indigestion,* diarrhea, abdominal pain, constipation, eructation, irritation
RESP: Breathing difficulty, cough, hoarseness, sneezing, wheezing, bronchial spasm

PHARMACOKINETICS

Onset 15-30 min, metabolized in liver, excreted in urine, half-life 2-3 hr, 30-120 hr (terminal)

INTERACTIONS

Increase: vasoconstriction—ergots, bromocriptine, cabergoline

N

Increase: effect of—adenosine
Increase: B/P—buPROPion
Decrease: effect of—α-blockers, insulin
Decrease: nicotine clearance—cimetidine

Drug/Food

• Avoid use of gum with acidic foods (colas, coffee) and for 15 min after

NURSING CONSIDERATIONS

Assess:

• **Smoking:** number of cigarettes smoked, years used; **withdrawal:** headache, cravings, restlessness, irritation, drowsiness, insomnia, sore throat, increased appetite

• Adverse reaction: irritation of buccal cavity, dislike of taste, jaw ache

Evaluate:

• Therapeutic response: decrease in urge to smoke, decreased need for gum after 3-6 mo

Teach patient/family:

• **Gum:** about all aspects of product use; give package insert to patient and explain

• That gum will not stick to dentures, dental appliances

• That gum is as toxic as cigarettes; that it is to be used only to deter smoking

• To avoid use during pregnancy

• **Transdermal patch:** that patch is as toxic as cigarettes; to be used only to deter smoking

• Not to use during pregnancy because birth defects may occur; not to breastfeed

• To keep used and unused system out of reach of children and pets

• To stop smoking immediately when beginning patch treatment

• To apply promptly after removing from protective patch because system may lose strength

• **Nasal spray:** to tilt head back; not to swallow or inhale during administration; after smoking is stopped, to use spray up to 8 wk then discontinue over 6 wk by tapering

• **Lozenges:** to allow to dissolve; to avoid swallowing

• **Inhalation:** to use by inhaler for 20 min

NIFEdipine (Rx)

(nye-fed′i-peen)

Adalat CC, Afedtab CR, Apo-Nifed ✤, Apo-Nifed PA ✤, Nifediac CC, Nifedical XL, Procardia, Procardia XL

Func. class.: Calcium channel blocker, antianginal, antihypertensive

Chem. class.: Dihydropyridine

Do not confuse:
NIFEdipine/niCARdipine/niMODipine

ACTION: Inhibits calcium ion influx across cell membrane during cardiac depolarization; relaxes coronary vascular smooth muscle; dilates coronary arteries; increases myocardial oxygen delivery in patients with vasospastic angina; dilates peripheral arteries

USES: Chronic stable angina pectoris, vasospastic angina, hypertension

Unlabeled uses: Migraines, preterm labor, chronic/acute hypertension (pediatrics), diabetic nephropathy, proteinuria, hiccups

CONTRAINDICATIONS: Hypersensitivity to this product or dihydropyridine; cardiogenic shock

Precautions: Pregnancy (C), breastfeeding, children, CHF, hypotension, sick sinus syndrome, 2nd-/3rd-degree heart block, hypotension <90 mm Hg systolic, hepatic injury, renal disease, acute MI, aortic stenosis, GERD, heart failure

DOSAGE AND ROUTES

• **Adult: PO** Immediate release 10 mg tid, increase in 10-mg increments q7-14days, max 180 mg/24 hr or single dose of 30 mg; **SUS REL** 30-60 mg/day, may increase q7-14days, doses >120 mg not recommended

Hypertension

• **Adult: PO EXT REL** 30-60 mg daily, titrate upward as needed, max 90 mg/day (Adalat CC), 120 mg/day (Procardia XL)

• **Child/adolescent (unlabeled): PO EXT REL** 0.25-0.5 mg/kg/day, max 3 mg/kg/day

Acute hypertensive episodes in pediatric patients (unlabeled)

• **Adolescent/child/infant: PO** 0.2-0.5 mg/kg/dose up to 10 mg (total dose)

Migraine prophylaxis (unlabeled)

• **Adult: PO** 30-180 mg/day

Preterm labor (unlabeled)

• **Pregnant female: PO** Immediate release (Procardia, Adalat) 30-mg loading dose then 10-20 mg q4-6hr; use in monitored settings

Available forms: Caps 5 ♣, 10, 20 mg; ext rel tabs (CC, XL) 10 ♣, 20 ♣, 30, 60, 90 mg; tabs 10 mg ♣

Administer:

• Do not break, crush, or chew ext rel tabs

• Without regard to meals; avoid grapefruit juice

SIDE EFFECTS

CNS: *Headache,* fatigue, drowsiness, *dizziness,* anxiety, depression, weakness, insomnia, light-headedness, paresthesia, tinnitus, blurred vision, nervousness, tremor, *flushing*

CV: Dysrhythmias, edema, hypotension, palpitations, tachycardia

GI: Nausea, vomiting, diarrhea, gastric upset, constipation, increased LFTs, dry mouth, flatulence, gingival hyperplasia

GU: *Nocturia, polyuria*

HEMA: Bruising, bleeding, petechiae

INTEG: Rash, pruritus, flushing, hair loss, **Stevens-Johnson syndrome, toxic epidermal necrolysis, exfoliative dermatitis**

MISC: Sexual difficulties, cough, fever, chills

PHARMACOKINETICS

Metabolized by liver; excreted in urine 60%-80% (metabolites), feces 15%; protein binding 90%-98%

PO: Onset 20 min, peak 0.5-6 hr, duration 6-8 hr, half-life 2-5 hr, well absorbed

PO-ER: Duration 24 hr

INTERACTIONS

⚠ **Contraindicated with strong CYP3A4 inducers**

Increase: level of digoxin, phenytoin, cycloSPORINE, prazosin, carBAMazepine

⚠ **Increase: NIFEdipine, toxicity—cimetidine, ranitidine**

Increase: effects of β-blockers, antihypertensives

Decrease: antihypertensive effect—NSAIDs

Decrease: effects of quiNIDine

Decrease: NIFEdipine level—smoking

Drug/Herb

Increase: effect—ginkgo biloba, ginseng, hawthorn

Decrease: effect—ephedra, melatonin, St. John's wort, yohimbe

Drug/Food

Increase: NIFEdipine level—grapefruit juice

Drug/Lab Test

Increase: CPK, LDH, AST

Positive: ANA, direct Coombs' test

NURSING CONSIDERATIONS

Assess:

• **Anginal pain:** location, intensity, duration, character, alleviating, aggravating factors

• Cardiac status: B/P, pulse, respiration, ECG at baseline and periodically

• Potassium, renal, hepatic studies periodically during treatment

• For bruising, petechiae, bleeding

• **Serious skin disorders: rash that starts suddenly, fever, cutaneous lesions that may have pustules present; discontinue product**

Evaluate:

• Therapeutic response: decreased anginal pain, B/P, activity tolerance

Teach patient/family:

- To avoid hazardous activities until stabilized on product, dizziness is no longer a problem
- To limit caffeine consumption; to avoid alcohol products
- To avoid OTC products unless directed by prescriber
- That ext rel nonabsorbable shell may appear in stools
- **Hypertension:** to comply with all areas of medical regimen: diet, exercise, stress reduction, product therapy
- To change position slowly because orthostatic hypotension is common

⚠ To notify prescriber of dyspnea, edema of extremities, nausea, vomiting, severe ataxia, severe rash; changes in pattern, frequency, severity of angina

- To increase fluid intake to prevent constipation
- To check for gingival hyperplasia and report promptly
- Not to discontinue abruptly; to gradually taper

TREATMENT OF OVERDOSE:
Defibrillation, atropine for AV block, vasopressor for hypotension

nilotinib (Rx)
(nye-loe′ti-nib)

Tasigna

Func. class.: Antineoplastic—miscellaneous

Chem. class.: Protein-tyrosine kinase inhibitor

ACTION:
Inhibits BCR-ABL tyrosine kinase created in patients with chronic myeloid leukemia (CML)

USES:
Chronic phase/accelerated phase Philadelphia-chromosome–positive CML that is resistant or intolerant to imatinib

CONTRAINDICATIONS:
Pregnancy (D), breastfeeding, hypersensitivity

Black Box Warning: Hypokalemia, hypomagnesemia, QT prolongation

Precautions: Children, females, geriatric patients, active infections, anemia, cardiac disease, bone marrow suppression, cholestasis, diabetes, gelatin hypersensitivity, infertility, galactose-free diet, lactase deficiency, neutropenia, pancreatitis, thrombocytopenia

Black Box Warning: Hepatic disease

DOSAGE AND ROUTES

- **Adult: PO** 400 mg q12hr, continue until disease progression or unacceptable toxicity

Escalation regimen for those taking a strong CYP3A4 inducer

- **Adult: PO** Increase dose as required

Adjustment after discontinuation of a strong CYP3A4 inducer

- **Adult: PO** Reduce to 400 mg/bid

For those taking a strong CYP3A4 inhibitor

- **Adult: PO** Reduce dose to 400 mg/day

QT prolongation

- **QTcF >480 msec:** Withhold dose

Myelosuppression

- **ANC 1 × 109/L or platelets <50 × 109/L:** Withhold dose

Hepatic dose

- **Adult: PO** (Child-Pugh A/B/C) newly diagnosed CML 200 mg bid, then escalation to 300 mg bid initially

Available forms: Caps 150, 200 mg

Administer:

- Do not break, crush, or chew caps; if whole capsule cannot be swallowed, disperse capsule contents in 1 tsp. applesauce
- Without regard to meals; separate doses by 12 hr; make-up dose should not be taken if dose is missed

SIDE EFFECTS

CNS: Headache, dizziness, fatigue, fever, flushing, paresthesia

CV: QT prolongation, palpitations, torsades de pointes
GI: *Nausea,* hepatotoxicity, vomiting, dyspepsia, *anorexia, abdominal pain,* constipation, pancreatitis, diarrhea
HEMA: Neutropenia, thrombocytopenia, anemia, pancytopenia
INTEG: *Rash,* alopecia, erythema
META: Hyperamylasemia, hyperbilirubinemia, hyperglycemia, hyperkalemia, hypocalcemia, hyponatremia, hypomagnesemia
MISC: Diaphoresis
MS: Arthralgia, myalgia, back or bone pain, muscle cramps
RESP: Cough, dyspnea
SYST: Bleeding

PHARMACOKINETICS

Protein binding 98%, metabolized by CYP3A4, plasma levels 3 hr, elimination half-life 17 hr

INTERACTIONS

• Product interactions are numerous
• Do not use with phenothiazines, pimozide, ziprasidone
⚠ **Increase:** QT prolongation—class IA/III antidysrhythmics, some phenothiazines, β agonists, local anesthetics, tricyclics, haloperidol, chloroquine, droperidol, pentamidine; CYP3A4 inhibitors (amiodarone, clarithromycin, erythromycin, telithromycin, troleandomycin), arsenic trioxide, levomethadyl; CYP3A4 substrates (methadone, pimozide, QUEtiapine, quiNIDine, risperidone, ziprasidone)
⚠ **Increase:** hepatotoxicity—acetaminophen
Increase: concentrations—ketoconazole, itraconazole, erythromycin, clarithromycin
Increase: plasma concentrations of simvastatin, calcium channel blockers
Increase: plasma concentration of warfarin; avoid use with warfarin, use low-molecular-weight anticoagulants instead
Decrease: concentrations—dexamethasone, phenytoin, carBAMazepine, rifampin, PHENobarbital
Drug/Herb
Decrease: concentration—St. John's wort
Drug/Food
Increase: plasma concentrations—grapefruit juice

NURSING CONSIDERATIONS

Assess:

Black Box Warning: QT prolongation can occur; monitor ECG, left ventricular ejection fraction (LVEF) at baseline periodically; hypertension, assess for chest pain, palpitations, dyspnea

Black Box Warning: Hepatotoxicity: monitor LFTs before treatment and monthly; if liver transaminases $>5 \times$ IULN, withhold until transaminase levels return to $<2.5 \times$ IULN

• **Myelosuppression:** CBC, differential, platelet count; for bleeding: epistaxis, rectal, gingival, upper GI, genital and wound bleeding; tumor-related hemorrhage may occur rapidly
• ANC and platelets; if ANC $<1 \times 10^9$/L and/or platelets $<50 \times 10^9$/L, stop until ANC $>1.5 \times 10^9$/L and platelets $>75 \times 10^9$/L
• **Electrolytes:** calcium, potassium, magnesium, sodium; lipase, phosphate; hypokalemia, hypomagnesemia should be corrected prior to use

Perform/provide:
• Storage at 15° C-30° C (59° F- 86° F)

Evaluate:
• Therapeutic response: decrease in progression of disease

Teach patient/family:
• To report adverse reactions immediately: SOB, bleeding
• About reason for treatment, expected results
• That many adverse reactions may occur
• To avoid persons with known upper respiratory tract infections; immunosuppression is common

• To watch for signs, symptoms of low potassium or magnesium

nilutamide (Rx)

(nye-loo′ta-mide)

Anandron ✱, Nilandron

Func. class.: Antineoplastic-hormone

Chem. class.: Antiandrogen

ACTION: Interferes with testosterone uptake in the nucleus or testosterone activity in target tissues; arrests tumor growth in androgen-sensitive tissue (e.g., prostate gland); prostatic carcinoma is androgen sensitive, so tumor growth is arrested

USES: Metastatic prostatic carcinoma stage D2 in combination with surgical castration (only to be used by men)

CONTRAINDICATIONS: Hypersensitivity, severe hepatic impairment

Black Box Warning: Severe respiratory disease

Precautions: Pregnancy (C), children, alcoholism, Asian patients, breastfeeding, hepatitis, visual disturbances

DOSAGE AND ROUTES

• **Adult: PO** 300 mg/day × 30 days then 150 mg/day

Available forms: Tabs 50, 100 ✱, 150 mg

Administer:

• Without regard to meals

• Start therapy on day of or day after surgery

SIDE EFFECTS

CNS: Hot flashes, drowsiness, insomnia, dizziness, hyperthesia, depression

CV: Heart failure, hypertension

EENT: Delay in adaptation to dark

GI: Diarrhea, nausea, vomiting, increased LFTs, constipation, dyspepsia, hepatotoxicity

GU: Decreased libido, impotence, testicular atrophy, UTI, hematuria, nocturia, gynecomastia

HEMA: Anemia

INTEG: Rash, sweating, alopecia, dry skin

MISC: Edema

RESP: Dyspnea, URI, pneumonia, interstitial pneumonitis

PHARMACOKINETICS

Rapidly and completely absorbed; excreted in urine and feces as metabolites

INTERACTIONS

Increase: toxicity of—vit K, phenytoin, theophylline

NURSING CONSIDERATIONS

Assess:

⚠ **Hepatotoxicity:** AST, ALT, alk phos, which may be elevated; if elevated 3× normal, discontinue product; yellow eyes or skin, dark urine, abdominal pain, clay-colored stools

• For CNS symptoms: insomnia, dizziness

Black Box Warning: Respiratory insufficiency: chest x-rays routinely, baseline pulmonary function studies; dyspnea, cough, which may indicate interstitial pneumonitis; discontinue if this condition is suspected

• PSA, improvement in bone pain

• Hyperglycemia, increased BUN, creatinine, alk phos, leukopenia

Perform/provide:

• Storage at room temp

Evaluate:

• Therapeutic response: decrease in prostatic tumor size, spread of cancer

Teach patient/family:

⚠ To report side effects: decreased libido, impotence, breast enlargement, hot flashes, diarrhea, dyspnea, cough, SOB; if SOB occurs, notify prescriber immediately

⚠ **Hepatotoxicity:** to report dark urine, abdominal pain, clay-colored stools, yellow eyes or skin

- **Visual disturbances:** to wear tinted lenses to alleviate delay in adapting to the dark
- That product is started on day of or day after surgical removal of testes
- To avoid alcohol consumption

TREATMENT OF OVERDOSE:
Induce vomiting, provide supportive care

nisoldipine (Rx)
(nye-sole′dih-peen)

Sular

Func. class.: Calcium channel blocker, antihypertensive

Chem. class.: Dihydropyridine

ACTION: Inhibits calcium ion influx across the cell membrane, thereby resulting in the dilation of peripheral arteries

USES: Essential hypertension, alone or in combination with other antihypertensives

Unlabeled uses: Variant (Prinzmetal's) angina, stable angina pectoris

CONTRAINDICATIONS: Hypersensitivity to this product or dihydropyridines; sick sinus syndrome; 2nd-/3rd-degree heart block; aortic stenosis

Precautions: Pregnancy (C), breastfeeding, children, geriatric patients, CHF, hypotension <90 mm Hg systolic, hepatic injury, renal disease, acute MI, unstable angina, CAD, cardiogenic shock

DOSAGE AND ROUTES
Hypertension

- **Adult: PO** 17 mg/day initially, may increase by 8.5 mg/wk, usual dose 17-34 mg/day, max 34 mg/day
- **Geriatric/hepatic dose: PO** 8.5 mg/day, increase based on patient response

Variant (Prinzmetal's) angina/stable angina pectoris (unlabeled)

- **Adult: PO** 17-34 mg/day, max 34 mg/day

Hepatic dose

- **Adult: PO** 8.5 mg/day

Available forms: Ext rel tabs 8.5, 17, 20, 25.5, 30, 34, 40 mg

Administer:

PO route

- Swallow whole; do not break, crush, or chew
- Once daily as whole tablet; avoid high-fat foods, grapefruit juice

SIDE EFFECTS
CNS: Headache, fatigue, drowsiness, dizziness, anxiety, depression, nervousness, insomnia, lightheadedness, paresthesia, tinnitus, psychosis, somnolence, ataxia, confusion, malaise, migraine, flushing

CV: Dysrhythmia, edema, CHF, hypotension, palpitations, **MI, pulmonary edema,** tachycardia, syncope, AV block, angina, chest pain, ECG abnormalities

GI: Nausea, vomiting, diarrhea, gastric upset, constipation, increased LFTs, dry mouth, dyspepsia, dysphagia, flatulence

GU: Nocturia, hematuria, dysuria

HEMA: **Anemia, leukopenia,** petechiae

INTEG: Rash, pruritus

MISC: Sexual difficulties, cough, nasal congestion, SOB, wheezing, epistaxis, dyspnea, gingival hyperplasia, chills, fever, gout, sweating

PHARMACOKINETICS
Metabolized by liver, excreted in urine, peak 6-12 hr, protein binding 99%, half-life 7-12 hr

INTERACTIONS
Increase: effects of β-blockers, antihypertensives, digoxin

Increase: nisoldipine level—CYP3A4 inhibitors, cimetidine, ranitidine, azole antifungals

Decrease: nisoldipine effect—CYP3A4 inducers, hydantoins

Drug/Herb

Increase: B/P—ephedra, melatonin

Decrease: B/P—hawthorn

Decrease: nisoldipine effect—St. John's wort, ginseng, ginkgo biloba

N

Drug/Food

Increase: nisoldipine level—high-fat foods

Increase: hypotensive effect—grapefruit juice

NURSING CONSIDERATIONS

Assess:

- Cardiac status: B/P, pulse, respiration, ECG before treatment and periodically
- **CHF:** weight gain, jugular venous distention, edema, crackles, I&O ratios

Evaluate:

- Therapeutic response: decreased B/P

Teach patient/family:

- To avoid hazardous activities until stabilized on product, dizziness is no longer a problem
- To report nausea, dizziness, swelling, SOB, palpitations, severe headache
- To avoid OTC products unless directed by prescriber; to avoid grapefruit juice
- About the importance of complying with all areas of the medical regimen: diet, exercise, stress reduction, product therapy
- To rise slowly to prevent orthostatic hypotension
- If dose is missed, to take as soon as remembered; not to double dose
- How to perform B/P monitoring at home

TREATMENT OF OVERDOSE:

Defibrillation, atropine for AV block, vasopressor for hypotension

nitazoxanide (Rx)

(nye-taz-ox′a-nide)

Alinia

Func. class.: Antiprotozoal

ACTION: Interferes with DNA/RNA synthesis in protozoa

USES: Diarrhea caused by *Cryptosporidium parvum* or *Giardia lamblia*

CONTRAINDICATIONS: Hypersensitivity

Precautions: Pregnancy (B), breastfeeding, children <1 yr or >11 yr, renal/hepatic disease, diabetes mellitus (contains sucrose), HIV, immunocompromised patients

DOSAGE AND ROUTES

- **Adult: PO** 500 mg q12hr × 3 days
- **Child 4-11 yr: PO** 10 ml (200 mg) q12hr × 3 days
- **Child 12-47 mo: PO** 5 ml (100 mg) q12hr × 3 days

Available forms: Powder for oral susp 100 mg/5 ml; tab 500 mg

Administer:

PO route

- With food
- Shake oral suspension before giving

SIDE EFFECTS

CNS: *Dizziness, fever, headache*

CV: Hypotension

GI: *Nausea,* anorexia, flatulence, increased appetite, enlarged salivary glands, abdominal pain, diarrhea, vomiting

HEMA: Anemia, leukopenia, neutropenia

INTEG: Pruritus, sweating

MISC: Increased creatinine, pale yellow eye discoloration, rhinitis, discolored urine, infection, malaise

PHARMACOKINETICS

Peak 1-4 hr; excreted in urine, bile, feces; hydrolyzed to active metabolite, which undergoes conjugation; metabolite protein binding >99%

INTERACTIONS

- Competes for binding sites: other highly protein-bound products; phenytoin, salicylates

Drug/Lab Test

Increase: creatinine, GPT

NURSING CONSIDERATIONS

Assess:

- Signs of infection

• Bowel pattern before, during treatment

Evaluate:

• Therapeutic response: C&S negative for organism, decreased diarrhea

Teach patient/family:

• To take with food; shake susp well before each dose, discard susp after 7 days

nitrofurantoin (Rx)

(nye-troe-fyoor'an-toyn)

Apo-Nitrofurantoin ✤, Furadantin, Macrobid, Macrodantin, Novo-Furantoin ✤

Func. class.: Urinary tract antiinfective

Chem. class.: Synthetic nitrofuran derivative

ACTION:
Inhibits bacterial acetyl-CoA inteference with carbohydrate metabolism

USES:
Urinary tract infections caused by *Escherichia coli, Klebsiella, Pseudomonas, Proteus vulgaris, Proteus morganii, Serratia, Citrobacter, Staphylococcus aureus, Staphylococcus epidermidis, Enterococcus, Salmonella, Shigella*

CONTRAINDICATIONS:
Infants <1 mo, hypersensitivity, anuria, severe renal disease CCr <60 ml/min, at term pregnancy (38-42 wk), labor, delivery

Precautions: Pregnancy (B), breastfeeding, geriatric patients, G6PD deficiency, GI disease, diabetes, cholestatic jaundice due to nitrofurantoin therapy

DOSAGE AND ROUTES

Active infections

• **Adult: PO** 50-100 mg qid after meals or 50-100 mg at bedtime for long-term treatment

• **Child: PO** 5-7 mg/kg/day in 4 divided doses; 1-2 mg/kg/day for long-term treatment, max 7 mg/kg/day

Chronic suppression

• **Adult: PO** 50-100 mg q PM

• **Child: PO** 1-2 mg/kg/day in PM or 0.5-1 mg/kg q12hr if dose not well tolerated

Available forms: Caps 25, 50, 100 mg; susp 25 mg/5 ml; macrocrystal caps (Macrodantin) 25, 50, 100 mg; Macrobid cap 100 mg (25 macrocrystals, 75 monohydrate)

Administer:

PO route

• Do not break, crush, chew, or open tabs, caps

• Two daily doses if urine output is high or if patient diabetic

• Use calibrated device to measure liquid product; may mix water, fruit juice; rinse mouth after liquid product; staining of teeth may occur

SIDE EFFECTS

CNS: *Dizziness, headache,* drowsiness, peripheral neuropathy, chills, confusion, vertigo

CV: **Bundle branch block,** chest pain

GI: *Nausea, vomiting, abdominal pain, diarrhea,* **cholestatic jaundice,** loss of appetite, **pseudomembranous colitis, hepatitis, pancreatitis**

HEMA: Anemia, agranulocytosis, hemolytic anemia, leukopenia, thrombocytopenia

INTEG: Pruritus, rash, urticaria, angioedema, alopecia, tooth staining, **exfoliative dermatitis, Stevens-Johnson syndrome**

MS: Arthralgia, myalgia, numbness, peripheral neuropathy

RESP: Cough, dyspnea, pneumonitis, pulmonary fibrosis or infiltrate

SYST: Superinfection, SLE-like syndrome

PHARMACOKINETICS

PO: Half-life 20-60 min; crosses blood-brain barrier, placenta; enters breast milk; excreted as inactive metabolites in liver, unchanged in urine; protein binding 60%-90%

INTERACTIONS

Increase: antagonistic effect—norfloxacin

Increase: levels of nitrofurantoin—probenecid

Decrease: absorption of magnesium trisilicate antacid

Drug/Lab Test

Increase: BUN, alk phos, bilirubin, creatinine, blood glucose

NURSING CONSIDERATIONS

Assess:

- Blood count during chronic therapy, LFTs, pulmonary function tests
- **Urinary tract infection:** burning, pain on urination; fever; cloudy, foul-smelling urine; I&O ratio: C&S before treatment, after completion; serum creatinine, BUN
- CNS symptoms: insomnia, vertigo, headache, drowsiness, seizures

⚠ **Hepatotoxicity:** yellowing of skin or eyes, dark urine, clay-colored stools; monitor AST, ALT

⚠ **Pulmonary fibrosis, pneumonitis:** dyspnea, tachypnea, persistent cough

⚠ **Serious skin disorders:** fever, flushing, rash, urticaria, pruritus

- **Peripheral neuropathy:** paresthesias (more common in diabetes mellitus, electrolyte imbalances, vit B deficiency, debilitated patients)

Evaluate:

- Therapeutic response: decreased dysuria, fever; negative C&S

Teach patient/family:

- To notify prescriber of continued symptoms of UTI, fever, myalgias, arthralgias, numbness or tingling of extremities
- To take with food or milk; to avoid alcohol
- To protect susp from freezing; shake well before taking
- That product may cause drowsiness; to seek aid with walking, other activities; not to drive or operate machinery while taking medication
- That diabetics should monitor blood glucose levels
- That product may turn urine rust-yellow to brown

⚠ **Pseudomembranous colitis:** fever; diarrhea with mucus, pus, or blood

nitrofurazone topical

See Appendix B

nitroglycerin (Rx)

(nye-troe-gli′ser-in)

extended release caps (Rx)

Nitro-Time

topical ointment (Rx)

Nitro-Bid

rectal ointment

Rectiv

SL (Rx)

Nitrostat

translingual spray (Rx)

Nitrolingual

transdermal (Rx)

Minitran, Nitro-Dur

Func. class.: Coronary vasodilator, antianginal

Chem. class.: Nitrate

Do not confuse:
Nitro-Bid/Nicobid

ACTION: Decreases preload and afterload, which are responsible for decreasing left ventricular end-diastolic pressure, systemic vascular resistance; dilates coronary arteries, improves blood flow through coronary vasculature, dilates arterial and venous beds systemically

USES: Chronic stable angina pectoris, prophylaxis of angina pain, CHF, acute MI, controlled hypotension for surgical procedures, anal fissures

⚠ Nurse Alert

Unlabeled uses: Pulmonary hypertension, hemorrhoids, retained placenta

CONTRAINDICATIONS:
Hypersensitivity to this product or nitrites; severe anemia, increased intracranial pressure, cerebral hemorrhage, closed-angle glaucoma, cardiac tamponade, cardiomyopathy, constrictive pericarditis

Precautions: Pregnancy (C), breastfeeding, children, postural hypotension, severe renal/hepatic disease, acute MI, abrupt discontinuation, hyperthyroidism

DOSAGE AND ROUTES

• **Adult: SL** Dissolve tab under tongue when pain begins; may repeat q5min until relief occurs; take ≤3 tabs/15 min; use 1 tab prophylactically 5-10 min before activities; **SUS CAP** q6-12hr on empty stomach; **TOP** 1-2 in q8hr, increase to 4 in q4hr as needed; **IV** 5 mcg/min then increase by 5 mcg/min q3-5min; if no response after 20 mcg/min, increase by 10-20 mcg/min until desired response; **TRANS PATCH** apply a pad daily to a site free of hair; remove patch at bedtime to provide 10-12 hr nitrate-free interval to avoid tolerance

• **Child: IV** Initially 0.25-0.5 mcg/kg/min, titrate to patient response, usual dose 1-3 mcg/kg/min transmucosal

Anal fissures (Rectiv)

• **Adult: Rectal** Apply 1 inch of 0.4% ointment q12hr × 3 wk

Available forms: Translingual aero 0.4 mg/metered spray; sus rel tabs 2.6, 6.5, 9 mg; SL tabs 0.3, 0.4, 0.6 mg; topical oint 2%; trans syst 0.1, 0.2, 0.3, 0.4, 0.6, 0.8 mg/hr; inj sol 25 mg/250 ml, 50 mg/250 ml, 50 mg/500 ml, 100 mg/250 ml, 200 mg/500 ml; rectal ointment 0.4% (Rectiv)

Administer:

• **Topical ointment** should be measured on papers supplied, use paper to spread on nonhairy area of chest, abdomen, thigh skin; thin layer spread over 2-3 inches, do not rub

PO route

• Swallow sus rel products whole; do not break, crush, or chew

• With 8 oz water on empty stomach (oral tablet) 1 hr before or 2 hr after meals

• **SL:** should be dissolved under tongue, not swallowed

• **Aerosol** sprayed under tongue **(nitrolingual),** not inhaled; prime before 1st-time use or if product has not been used in >6 wk; press valve head with forefinger

Transdermal route

• Apply new TD patch daily, remove after 12-14 hr to prevent tolerance

Rectal route

• Cover finger with plastic wrap, disposable glove, or finger cot; lay finger alongside 1-inch dosing line on carton, squeeze tube until equal to 1-inch dosing line; insert covered finger gently into anal canal no further than 1st finger joint and apply to sides; wash hands thoroughly; if too painful, apply directly to outside of anus

Continuous IV INF route

• Diluted in D_5, D_5W, 0.9% NaCl for inf to 200-400 mcg/ml, depending on patient's fluid status; common dilution 50 mg/250 ml, use controlled inf device; use glass inf bottles, non–polyvinyl-chloride inf tubing; titrate to patient response; do not use filters

Y-site compatibilities: Acyclovir, alfentanil, amikacin, aminocaproic acid, aminophylline, amiodarone, amphotericin B cholesteryl, amphotericin B lipid complex, amphotericin B liposome, anidulafungin, argatroban, ascorbic acid, atenolol, atracurium, atropine, azaTHIOprine, aztreonam, benztropine, bivalirudin, bleomycin, bumetanide, buprenorphine, butorphanol, calcium chloride/gluconate, CARBOplatin, caspofungin, cefamandole, ceFAZolin, cefmetazole, cefonicid, cefoperazone, cefotaxime, cefotetan, cefoxitin, ceftazidime, ceftizoxime, cefTRIAXone, cefuroxime, cephalothin, cephapirin, chloramphenicol, chlorproMAZINE, cimetidine, cisatracurium, CISplatin, clindamycin, cloNIDine, cyanocobalamin, cyclophosphamide, cycloSPORINE, cytarabine, DACTINomycin, dexamethasone, digoxin, diltiazem, diphenhydrAMINE, DOBUTamine, docetaxel, DOPamine, doxacurium, DOXOrubicin, doxycycline, drotrecogin alfa, enalaprilat, ePHEDrine, EPINEPHrine, epirubicin, epoetin alfa, eptifibatide, ertapenem, erythromycin, esmolol, etoposide, famotidine, fenoldopam, fentaNYL, fluconazole, fludarabine, fluorouracil, folic acid, ganciclovir, gatifloxacin, gemcitabine, gemtuzumab, gentamicin, glycopyrrolate, granisetron, heparin, hydrocortisone, HYDROmorphone, hydrOXYzine, IDArubicin, ifosfamide, imipenem-cilastatin, indomethacin, insulin (regular), irinotecan, isoproterenol, ketorolac, labetalol, lidocaine, linezolid, LORazepam, magnesium sulfate, mannitol, mechlorethamine, meperidine, metaraminol, methicillin, methotrexate, methoxamine, methyldopate, methylPREDNISolone, metoclopramide, metroNIDAZOLE, mezlocillin, micafungin, miconazole, midazolam, milrinone, minocycline, mitoxantrone, morphine, moxalactam, mycophenolate, nafcillin, nalbuphine, naloxone, nesiritide, netilmicin, niCARdipine, nitroprusside, norepinephrine, octreotide, ondansetron, oxacillin, oxaliplatin, oxytocin, paclitaxel, palonosetron, pamidronate, pancuronium, pantoprazole, papaverine, pemetrexed, penicillin G potassium/sodium, pentamidine, pentazocine, PENTobarbital, PHENobarbital, phentolamine, phenylephrine, phytonadione, piperacillin, piperacillin-tazobactam, polymyxin B, potassium chloride, procainamide, prochlorperazine, promethazine, propofol, propranolol, protamine, pyridoxine, quiNIDine, quinupristin-dalfopristin, ranitidine, remifentanil, ritodrine, rocuronium, sodium bicarbonate, succi-nylcholine, SUFentanil, tacrolimus, teniposide, theophylline, thiamine, thiopental, thiotepa, ticarcillin, ticarcillin-clavulanate, tigecycline, tirofiban, tobramycin, tolazoline, trimetaphan, urokinase, vancomycin, vasopressin, vecuronium, verapamil, vinCRIStine, vinorelbine, voriconazole, warfarin, zoledronic acid

SIDE EFFECTS

CNS: *Headache, flushing, dizziness*
CV: *Postural hypotension,* tachycardia, collapse, syncope, palpitations
GI: Nausea, vomiting
INTEG: Pallor, sweating, rash

PHARMACOKINETICS

Metabolized by liver, excreted in urine, half-life 1-4 min
SUS REL: Onset 20-45 min, duration 3-8 hr
SL: Onset 1-3 min, duration 30 min
TRANSDERMAL: Onset 30 min-1 hr, duration 12-24 hr
AEROSOL: Onset 2 min, duration 30-60 min
TOPICAL OINT: Onset 30-60 min, duration 2-12 hr
IV: Onset 1-2 min, duration 3-5 min

INTERACTIONS

• Severe hypotension, CV collapse: alcohol

Increase: effects of β-blockers, diuretics, antihypertensives, calcium channel blockers
Increase: fatal hypotension—sildenafil, tadalafil, vardenafil; do not use together
Increase: nitrate level—aspirin
Decrease: heparin—IV nitroglycerin

Drug/Lab Test
Increase: urine catecholamine, urine VMA
False increase: cholesterol

NURSING CONSIDERATIONS

Assess:

• **Pain:** duration, time started, activity being performed, character
• Orthostatic B/P, pulse prior to and after administration
• Tolerance if taken over long period

• Headache, lightheadedness, decreased B/P; may indicate a need for decreased dosage

Evaluate:

• Therapeutic response: decrease, prevention of anginal pain

Teach patient/family:

• To place buccal tab between lip and gum above incisors or between cheek and gum

• To keep tabs in original container; to replace q6mo because effectiveness is lost; to keep away from heat, moisture, light

• That if 3 SL tabs in 15 min do not relieve pain, to seek immediate medical attention

• To avoid alcohol

• That product may cause headache; that tolerance usually develops; to use nonopioid analgesic

• That product may be taken before stressful activity: exercise, sexual activity

• That SL may sting when product comes in contact with mucous membranes

• To avoid hazardous activities if dizziness occurs

• To comply with complete medical regimen

• To make position changes slowly to prevent fainting

⚠ **Never to use erectile dysfunction products (sildenafil, tadalafil, vardenafil); may cause severe hypotension, death**

⚠ HIGH ALERT

nitroprusside (Rx)

(nye-troe-pruss′ide)

Nitropress

Func. class.: Antihypertensive, vasodilator

ACTION:
Directly relaxes arteriolar, venous smooth muscle, thereby resulting in reduction in cardiac preload and afterload

USES:
Hypertensive crisis; to decrease bleeding by creating hypotension during surgery; acute CHF

Unlabeled uses: Postoperative hypertension, mitral regurgitation

CONTRAINDICATIONS:
Hypersensitivity, hypertension (compensatory) due to aortic coarctation or AV shunting, acute CHF associated with reduced peripheral vascular resistance, AV shunt, Leber's disease, toxic amblyopia

Black Box Warning: Cyanide toxicity

Precautions: Pregnancy (C), breastfeeding, children, geriatric patients, fluid, electrolyte imbalances, renal/hepatic disease, hypothyroidism

Black Box Warning: Hypotension

DOSAGE AND ROUTES

• **Adult and child: IV INF** 0.25-10 mcg/kg/min; max 10 mcg/kg/min

Renal dose

• **Adult: IV INF** CCr <60 ml/min, maintain doses <3 mcg/kg/min to reduce thiocyanate accumulation

Available forms: Inj 50 mg/2 ml

Administer:

• Antidote is sodium thiosulfate

Continuous IV INF route

• Depending on B/P reading q15min

• Reconstitute 50 mg/2-3 ml of D_5W, further dilute in 250, 500, or 1000 ml of D_5W to 200, 100, 50 mcg/ml, respectively; use inf pump only; wrap bottle with aluminum foil to protect from light; observe for color change in inf; discard if highly discolored (blue, green, dark red); titrate to patient response

Y-site compatibilities: Alfentanil, alprostadil, amikacin, aminocaproic acid, aminophylline, amphotericin B lipid compex, amphotericin B liposome, anidulafungin, argatroban, atenolol, atropine, aztreonam, benztropine, bivalirudin, bleomycin, bumetanide, buprenorphine, butorphanol, calcium chloride/gluconate, CARBOplatin, cefamandole, ceFAZolin, cefmetazole, cefonicid, cefoperazone, cefotaxime, cefotetan, cefoxitin, ceftazidime, ceftizoxime, cefTRIAXone, cefuroxime, cephalothin, chloramphenicol, cimetidine, CISplatin, clindamycin, cyanocobalamin, cyclophosphamide, cycloSPORINE, cytarabine, DACTINomycin, DAPTOmycin, dexamethasone, digoxin, diltiazem, docetaxel, DOPamine, doxacurium, DOXOrubicin, doxycycline, enalaprilat, ePHEDrine, EPINEPHrine, epirubicin, epoetin alfa, eptifibatide, ertapenem, esmolol, etoposide, famotidine, fenoldopam, fentaNYL, fluconazole, fludarabine, fluorouracil, folic acid, furosemide, ganciclovir, gatifloxacin, gemcitabine, gemtuzumab, gentamicin, glycopyrrolate, granisetron, heparin, hydrocortisone, HYDROmorphone, IDArubicin, ifosfamide, inamrinone, indomethacin, insulin (regular), isoproterenol, ketorolac, labetalol, lidocaine, linezolid, LORazepam, magnesium sulfate, mannitol, mechlorethamine, meperidine, metaraminol, methicillin, methoxamine, methyldopate, methylPREDNISolone, metoclopramide, metoprolol, metroNIDAZOLE, mezlocillin, micafungin, miconazole, midazolam, milrinone, minocycline, morphine, moxalactam, multiple vitamins injection, nafcillin, nalbuphine, naloxone, nesiritide, netilmicin, niCARdipine, nitroglycerin, norepinephrine, octreotide, ondansetron, oxacillin, oxaliplatin, oxytocin, paclitaxel, palonosetron, pamidronate, pancuronium, pantoprazole, penicillin G potassium/sodium, pentamidine, PENTobarbital, PHENobarbital, phentolamine, phenylephrine, phytonadione, piperacillin, piperacillin-tazobactam, polymyxin B, potassium chloride/phosphates, procainamide, propofol, propranolol, protamine, pyridoxine, ranitidine, ritodrine, rocuronium, sodium acetate/bicarbonate, succinylcholine, SUFentanil, tacrolimus, teniposide, theophylline, thiamine, ticarcillin, ticarcillin-clavulanate, tigecycline, tirofiban, tobramycin, tolazoline, trimetaphan, urokinase, vancomycin, vasopressin, vecuronium, verapamil, vinCRIStine, zoledronic acid

SIDE EFFECTS

CNS: *Dizziness, headache,* agitation, twitching, decreased reflexes, restlessness

CV: Bradycardia, ECG changes, tachycardia, hypotension

GI: Nausea, vomiting, abdominal pain

INTEG: Pain, irritation at inj site, sweating

MISC: Cyanide, thiocyanate toxicity, flushing, hypothyroidism

PHARMACOKINETICS

IV: Onset 1-2 min, duration 1-10 min, half-life 3 days in patients with abnormal renal function, circulating half-life 2 min; metabolized in liver, excreted in urine

INTERACTIONS

Increase: severe hypotension—ganglionic blockers, volatile liquid anesthetics, halothane, enflurane, circulatory depressants

Drug/Herb

Increase: antihypertensive effect—hawthorn

NURSING CONSIDERATIONS

Assess:

- Electrolytes: K, Na, Cl, CO_2, CBC, serum glucose, serum methemoglobin if pulmonary O_2 levels are decreased; use IV 1-2 mg/kg methylene blue given over several min for methemoglobinemia
- Renal studies: catecholamines, BUN, creatinine
- Hepatic studies: AST, ALT, alk phos
- B/P by direct means if possible; check ECG continuously; pulse, jugular venous distention; PCWP; rebound hypertension may occur after nitroprusside is discontinued
- Weight daily, I&O

⚠ **Thiocyanate, lactate, cyanide toxicity:** obtain levels daily if inf >3 mcg/kg/min; thiocyanate level should be ≤1 mmol/L; thiocyanate toxicity includes

confusion, weakness, seizures, hyperreflexia, psychosis, tinnitus, coma
- Nausea, vomiting, diarrhea
- Edema in feet, legs daily; skin turgor, dryness of mucous membranes for hydration status
- Crackles, dyspnea, orthopnea q30min
- For decrease in bicarbonate, Pco_2 blood pH, acidosis

Evaluate:
- Therapeutic response: decreased B/P, decreasing symptoms of cardiogenic shock or cardiac pump failure

Teach patient/family:
- To report headache, dizziness, loss of hearing, blurred vision, dyspnea, faintness
- About the reason for giving product and expected results

nizatidine (OTC, Rx)

(ni-za′ti-deen)

Apo-Nizatidine ♣, Axid, Axid AR, Gen-Nizatidine ♣, PMS-Nizatidine ♣

Func. class.: H_2-receptor antagonist
Chem. class.: Substituted thiazole

ACTION:
Blocks H_2-receptors, thereby reducing gastric acid output

USES:
Benign gastric and duodenal ulceration, prevention of duodenal ulcer recurrence, symptomatic relief of gastroesophageal reflux, heartburn prevention

CONTRAINDICATIONS:
Hypersensitivity

Precautions: Pregnancy (B), breastfeeding, renal/hepatic impairment (reduce dose in renal impairment)

DOSAGE AND ROUTES

Gastric and duodenal ulcer
- **Adult: PO** 300 mg at night or 150 mg bid for 4-8 wk; maintenance 150 mg at night

Prophylaxis of duodenal ulcer
- **Adult: PO** 150 mg/day at bedtime

Gastroesophageal reflux
- **Adult and child ≥12 yr: PO** 150 mg bid × ≤12 wk, max 300 mg/day

Heartburn prevention
- **Adult: PO** 75 mg before eating bid

Renal dose
- **Adult: PO** CCr 20-50 ml/min, give 150 mg every other day; CCr <20 ml/min, give 150 mg q72hr

Available forms: Caps 150, 300 mg; tabs 75 mg

Administer:
- With meals for prolonged product effect; antacids 1 hr before or 1 hr after product; at bedtime if taken daily

SIDE EFFECTS

CNS: Headache, somnolence, confusion, abnormal dreams, dizziness
CV: **Cardiac dysrhythmias, cardiac arrest**
ENDO: Gynecomastia
GI: Elevated hepatic enzymes, **hepatitis,** jaundice, nausea
HEMA: **Thrombocytopenia, agranulocytosis, aplastic anemia**
INTEG: Pruritus, sweating, urticaria, **exfoliative dermatitis**
METAB: Hyperuricemia
MS: Myalgia
RESP: **Bronchospasm, laryngeal edema, pneumonia**

PHARMACOKINETICS

Partially metabolized by liver, excreted by kidneys, plasma half-life 1-2.8 hr, 70% absorbed orally, small amount (0.1% of plasma concentration) enters breast milk, 35% bound to plasma proteins

INTERACTIONS

Increase: GI obstruction risk—NIFEdipine (ext rel tabs)
Increase: effect of—mefloquine
Decrease: effect of—ketoconazole, itraconazole, atazanavir, cefditoren, cefpodoxime, delavirdine, gefitinib, raltegravir

N

Drug/Lab Test
Increase: ALT, AST, serum creatinine
False negative: allergy skin tests

NURSING CONSIDERATIONS

Assess:

- **GI pain:** epigastric, abdominal, character, alleviating factors, hematemesis, occult blood in stool, heartburn, GERD

⚠ **Agranulocytosis:** CBC with differential if patient receiving long-term therapy

Evaluate:

- Decreased GI pain, heartburn, GERD; resolution of gastric, duodenal ulcers

Teach patient/family:

- That gynecomastia, impotence may occur, are reversible
- To avoid driving or other hazardous activities until stabilized on product; that dizziness may occur
- To avoid black pepper, caffeine, alcohol, harsh spices, extremes in temp of food
- To avoid OTC preparations: aspirin, cough, cold preparations

TREATMENT OF OVERDOSE:

Symptomatic and supportive therapy is recommended; activated charcoal, emesis, or lavage may reduce absorption

⚠ HIGH ALERT

norepinephrine (Rx)

(nor-ep-i-nef′rin)

Levophed

Func. class.: Adrenergic

Chem. class.: Catecholamine

Do not confuse:
norepinephrine/EPINEPHrine

ACTION: Causes increased contractility and heart rate by acting on β-receptors in heart; also acts on α-receptors, thereby causing vasoconstriction in blood vessels; B/P is elevated, coronary blood flow improves, and cardiac output increases

USES: Acute hypotension, shock

CONTRAINDICATIONS: Hypersensitivity to this product or cyclopropane/halothane anesthesia; ventricular fibrillation, tachydysrhythmias, pheochromocytoma, hypotension, hypovolemia

Precautions: Pregnancy (C), breastfeeding, geriatric patients, arterial embolism, peripheral vascular disease, hypertension, hyperthyroidism, cardiac disease

Black Box Warning: Extravasation

DOSAGE AND ROUTES

- **Adult: IV INF** 0.5-1 mcg/min titrated to B/P; maintenance 2-4 mcg/min; max 30 mcg/min
- **Child: IV INF** 0.1-0.2 mcg/kg/min titrated to B/P; max 2 mcg/kg/min

Available forms: Inj 1 mg/ml

Administer:

- Plasma expanders for hypovolemia

Continuous IV INF route

- Dilute with 500-1000 ml D_5W or D_5/0.9% NaCl; average dilution 4 mg/1000 ml diluent (4 mcg base/ml); give as inf 2-3 ml/min; titrate to response

Y-site compatibilities: Alfentanil, amikacin, amiodarone, anidulafungin, argatroban, ascorbic acid, atenolol, atracurium, atropine, aztreonam, benztropine, bivalirudin, bleomycin, bumetanide, buprenorphine, butorphanol, calcium chloride/gluconate, CARBOplatin, caspofungin, cefamandole, ceFAZolin, cefmetazole, cefonicid, cefoperazone, cefotaxime, cefotetan, cefoxitin, ceftazidime, ceftizoxime, ceftobiprole, cefTRIAXone, cefuroxime, cephalothin, chloramphenicol, chlorproMAZINE, cimetidine, cisatracurium, CISplatin, clindamycin, cloNIDine, cyanocobalamin, cyclophosphamide, cycloSPORINE, cytarabine, DAPTOmycin, dexamethasone, digoxin, diltiazem, diphenhydrAMINE, DOBUTamine, docetaxel, DOPamine, doripenem, doxycycline, enalaprilat, ePHEDrine, EPINEPHrine, epirubicin, epoetin alfa, ertapenem, erythromycin, esmolol, etoposide, famotidine, fenoldopam, fentaNYL, fluconazole, fludarabine, gatifloxacin, gemcitabine, gentamicin, glycopyrrolate, granisetron, heparin, hydrocortisone, HYDROmorphone, hydrOXYzine, IDArubicin, ifosfamide, imipenem-cilastatin, irinotecan, isoproterenol, ketorolac, labetalol, lidocaine, linezolid, LORazepam, magnesium sulfate, mannitol, mechlorethamine, meperidine, meropenem, metaraminol, methicillin, methotrexate, methoxamine, methyldopate, methylPREDNISolone, metoclopramide, metoprolol, metroNIDAZOLE, mezlocillin, micafungin, miconazole, midazolam, milrinone, minocycline, mitoxantrone, morphine, moxalactam, multiple vitamins injection, mycophenolate, nafcillin, nalbuphine, naloxone, netilmicin, niCARdipine, nitroglycerin, nitroprusside, octreotide, ondansetron, oxacillin, oxaliplatin, oxytocin, paclitaxel, palonosetron, pamidronate, pancuronium, papaverine, pemetrexed, penicillin G potassium/sodium, pentamidine, pentazocine, phenylephrine, phytonadione, piperacillin, piperacillin-tazobactam, polymyxin B, potassium chloride, procainamide, prochlorperazine, promethazine, propofol, propranolol, protamine, pyridoxine, quiNIDine, ranitidine, remifentanil, ritodrine, succinylcholine, SUFentanil, tacrolimus, teniposide, theophylline, thiamine, thiotepa, ticarcillin, ticarcillin-clavulanate, tigecycline, tirofiban, tobramycin, tolazoline, trimetaphan, urokinase, vancomycin, vasopressin, vecuronium, verapamil, vinCRIStine, vinorelbine, vitamin B complex with C, voriconazole, zoledronic acid

SIDE EFFECTS

CNS: *Headache,* anxiety, dizziness, insomnia, restlessness, tremor, **cerebral hemorrhage**
CV: *Palpitations, tachycardia, hypertension, ectopic beats, angina*
GI: *Nausea, vomiting*
GU: Decreased urine output
INTEG: Necrosis, tissue sloughing with extravasation, **gangrene**
RESP: Dyspnea
SYST: **Anaphylaxis**

PHARMACOKINETICS

IV: Onset 1-2 min; metabolized in liver; excreted in urine (inactive metabolites); crosses placenta

INTERACTIONS

Increase: dysrhythmias—general anesthetics

• Incompatible with alkaline solutions: sodium, bicarbonate

• Severe hypertension: guanethidine

⚠ **Do not use within 2 wk of MAOIs, antihistamines, ergots, methyldopa, oxytocics, tricyclics, guanethidine because hypertensive crisis may result**

Increase: B/P—oxytocics

Increase: pressor effect—tricyclics, MAOIs

Decrease: norepinephrine action—α-blockers

NURSING CONSIDERATIONS

Assess:

• I&O ratio; notify prescriber if output <30 ml/hr

• B/P, pulse q2-3min after parenteral route, ECG during administration continuously; if B/P increases, product is decreased, CVP or PWP during inf if possible

• Paresthesias and coldness of extremities; peripheral blood flow may decrease

Black Box Warning: Extravasation: inj site: tissue sloughing

• Sulfite sensitivity, which may be life-threatening

Perform/provide:

• Storage of reconstituted sol in refrigerator ≤24 hr, protect from light, store unopened product at room temp, do not use discolored sol

Evaluate:

• Therapeutic response: increased B/P with stabilization, adequate tissue perfusion

Teach patient/family:

• About the reason for product administration; to report dyspnea, dizziness, chest pain

TREATMENT OF OVERDOSE:

Administer fluids, electrolyte replacement

norethindrone (Rx)

(nor-eth-in′drone)

Aygestin, Camila, Errin ✦, Heather, Jolivette, Micronor, Nora-BE, Nor-QD, Ortho Micronor

Func. class.: Progestogen

ACTION: Inhibits the secretion of pituitary gonadotropins, which prevents follicular maturation and ovulation; stimulates growth of mammary tissue; antineoplastic action against endometrial cancer

USES: Uterine bleeding (abnormal), amenorrhea, endometriosis, contraception

CONTRAINDICATIONS: Pregnancy (X), breast cancer, hypersensitivity, thromboembolic disorders, reproductive cancer, genital bleeding (abnormal, undiagnosed), liver tumors

Precautions: Breastfeeding, hypertension, asthma, blood dyscrasias, CHF, diabetes mellitus, depression, migraine headache, seizure disorders, bone/gallbladder/renal/hepatic disease, family history of breast or reproductive tract cancer, smoking

DOSAGE AND ROUTES

Amenorrhea, abnormal uterine bleeding (Aygestin)

• **Adult: PO** 2.5-10 mg/day on days 5-25 of menstrual cycle

Endometriosis (Aygestin)

• **Adult: PO** 5 mg/day × 2 wk then increased by 2.5 mg/day × 2 wk up to 15 mg/day, may continue for 6-9 mo

Contraception

• **Adult: PO** 0.35 mg on 1st day of menses then 0.35 mg/day

Available forms: Tabs (Aygestin) 5 mg; tabs 0.35 mg

Administer:

• Titrated dose; use lowest effective dose

• One dose in AM; do not interrupt between pill packs, give at roughly same time of day

• Without regard to meals

SIDE EFFECTS

CNS: Dizziness, headache, migraines, depression, fatigue

CV: Hypotension, **thrombophlebitis,** edema, **thromboembolism, CVA, stroke, PE, MI**

EENT: Diplopia

GI: *Nausea,* vomiting, anorexia, cramps, increased weight, **cholestatic jaundice**

GU: Amenorrhea, cervical erosion, breakthrough bleeding, dysmenorrhea, vaginal candidiasis, breast changes, (gynecomastia, testicular atrophy, impotence), endometriosis, **spontaneous abortion,** breast tenderness

INTEG: Rash, urticaria, acne, hirsutism, alopecia, oily skin, seborrhea, purpura, melasma

META: Hyperglycemia

PHARMACOKINETICS

Duration 24 hr, excreted in urine, feces; metabolized in liver

INTERACTIONS

Decrease: progestin effect—barbiturates, carBAMazepine, fosphenytoin, phenytoin, rifampin

Drug/Herb

Decrease: contraception—St. John's wort

Drug/Food

Increase: caffeine level—caffeine

Drug/Lab Test
Increase: LDL
Decrease: GTT, HDL, alk phos

NURSING CONSIDERATIONS

Assess:
- Weight daily: notify prescriber of weekly weight gain >5 lb
- B/P at beginning of treatment and periodically
- I&O ratio; be alert for decreasing urinary output, increasing edema
- Hepatic studies: ALT, AST, bilirubin periodically during long-term therapy
- Edema, hypertension, cardiac symptoms, jaundice, thromboembolism
- Mental status: affect, mood, behavioral changes, depression
- Hypercalcemia

Perform/provide:
- Storage in dark area

Evaluate:
- Therapeutic response: decreased abnormal uterine bleeding, absence of amenorrhea

Teach patient/family:
- About cushingoid symptoms
- ⚠ To report breast lumps, vaginal bleeding, amenorrhea, edema, jaundice, dark urine, clay-colored stools, dyspnea, headache, blurred vision, abdominal pain, numbness or stiffness in legs, chest pain; impotence or gynecomastia (men)
- To take at same time of day; not to interrupt between pill packs
- To report suspected pregnancy immediately, to wait ≥3 mo after stopping product to become pregnant, (X)
- To avoid smoking; CV reactions may occur
- That product does not protect against HIV, STDs
- That product may mask onset of menopause

norfloxacin ophthalmic

See Appendix B

nortriptyline (Rx)

(nor-trip'ti-leen)

Apo-Nortriptyline ♣, Arentyl ♣, Pamelor

Func. class.: Antidepressant, tricyclic
Chem. class.: Dibenzocycloheptene—secondary amine

Do not confuse:
nortriptyline/amitriptyline

ACTION: Blocks reuptake of norepinephrine and serotonin into nerve endings, thereby increasing action of norepinephrine and serotonin in nerve cells

USES: Major depression
Unlabeled uses: Chronic pain management, PMDD, social phobia, neuropathy, panic disorder, enuresis, migraine prophylaxis

CONTRAINDICATIONS: Pregnancy (D), hypersensitivity to tricyclics, recovery phase of MI, seizure disorders, prostatic hypertrophy
Precautions: Breastfeeding, suicidal patients, severe depression, increased intraocular pressure, closed-angle glaucoma, urinary retention, cardiac/hepatic disease, hyperthyroidism, electroshock therapy, elective surgery

Black Box Warning: Children, suicidal ideation

DOSAGE AND ROUTES

- **Adult: PO** 25 mg tid or qid; may increase to 150 mg/day; may give daily dose at bedtime
- **Adolescent: PO** 1-3 mg/kg/day in 3-4 divided doses or daily at bedtime, max 150 mg/day
- **Child 6-12 yr (unlabeled): PO** 1-3 mg/kg/day in 3-4 divided doses, max 150 mg/day
- **Geriatric: PO** 10-25 mg at bedtime, increase by 10-25 mg at weekly intervals to desired dose; usual maintenance 75 mg/day, max 150 mg/day

Available forms: Caps 10, 25, 50, 75 mg; sol 10 mg/5 ml

Administer:

- Increased fluids, bulk in diet if constipation occurs
- Without regard to meals
- Dosage at bedtime for oversedation during day; may take entire dose at bedtime; geriatric patients may not tolerate once daily dosing
- Gum, hard candy, frequent sips of water for dry mouth
- Oral solution: with fruit juice, water, or milk to disguise taste

SIDE EFFECTS

CNS: *Dizziness, drowsiness,* confusion, headache, anxiety, tremors, stimulation, weakness, insomnia, nightmares, EPS (geriatric patients), increased psychiatric symptoms, seizures

CV: *Orthostatic hypotension, ECG changes, tachycardia,* hypertension, palpitations, dysrhythmias

EENT: *Blurred vision,* tinnitus, mydriasis

GI: *Constipation, dry mouth,* nausea, vomiting, paralytic ileus, increased appetite, cramps, epigastric distress, jaundice, hepatitis, stomatitis

GU: *Urinary retention,* acute renal failure

HEMA: Agranulocytosis, thrombocytopenia, eosinophilia, leukopenia

INTEG: Rash, urticaria, sweating, pruritus, photosensitivity

PHARMACOKINETICS

PO: Steady state 4-19 days; metabolized by liver; excreted by kidneys; crosses placenta; excreted in breast milk; half-life 18-28 hr, protein binding 93%-95%

INTERACTIONS

⚠ **Increase:** QT prolongation—class IA/III antidysrhythmics, some phenothiazines, β agonists, local anesthetics, tricyclics, haloperidol, chloroquine, droperidol, pentamidine; CYP3A4 inhibitors (amiodarone, clarithromycin, erythromycin, telithromycin, troleandomycin), arsenic trioxide, levomethadyl; CYP3A4 substrates (methadone, pimozide, QUEtiapine, quiNIDine, risperidone, ziprasidone)

- Heavy smoking: decreased product effect

⚠ Hyperpyretic crisis, seizures, hypertensive episode: MAOI

Increase: effects of direct-acting sympathomimetics (EPINEPHrine), alcohol, barbiturates, benzodiazepines, CNS depressants, products increasing QT interval, other anticholinergics

⚠ **Increase:** serotonin syndrome, neuroleptic malignant syndrome—SSRIs, SNRIs, serotonin receptor agonists

Decrease: effects of guanethidine, clonidine, indirect-acting sympathomimetics (ePHEDrine)

Drug/Herb

Increase: CNS effect—kava, valerian

Decrease: nortriptyline level—St. John's wort

Drug/Lab Test

Increase: serum bilirubin, blood glucose, alk phos

Decrease: VMA, 5-HIAA

False increase: urinary catecholamines

NURSING CONSIDERATIONS

Assess:

- B/P (lying, standing), pulse q4hr; if systolic B/P drops 20 mm Hg, hold product, notify prescriber; VS q4hr in patients with CV disease
- Blood studies: CBC, leukocytes, differential, cardiac enzymes if patient is receiving long-term therapy
- Hepatic studies: AST, ALT, bilirubin
- Weight weekly; appetite may increase with product

⚠ **PR, QT prolongation:** ECG for flattening of T wave, bundle branch block, AV block, QT prolongation, dysrhythmias in cardiac patients; assess for chest pain, palpitations, dyspnea

- EPS primarily in geriatric patients: rigidity, dystonia, akathisia, preferred tricyclic in geriatric patients
- Mental status changes: mood, sensorium, affect, suicidal tendencies, in-

crease in psychiatric symptoms, depression, panic
• Urinary retention, constipation; constipation is more likely to occur in children
⚠ **Withdrawal symptoms:** headache, nausea, vomiting, muscle pain, weakness; do not usually occur unless product was discontinued abruptly
• Alcohol intake; if alcohol is consumed, hold dose until AM
• **Serotonin syndrome, neuroleptic malignant syndrome:** assess for increased heart rate, shivering, sweating, dilated pupils, tremors, high B/P, hyperthermia, headache, confusion; if these occur, stop product, administer serotonin antagonist if needed (rare)
Perform/provide:
• Storage in tight, light-resistant container at room temp
• Assistance with ambulation during beginning therapy because drowsiness/dizziness occurs; safety measures including side rails, primarily for geriatric patients
Evaluate:
• Therapeutic response: decreased depression
Teach patient/family:
• That therapeutic effects may take 2-3 wk, only small quantities may be dispersed
• To use caution when driving, during other activities requiring alertness because of drowsiness, dizziness, blurred vision
• To avoid alcohol ingestion, other CNS depressants; to avoid MAOIs within 14 days
• Not to discontinue medication quickly after long-term use; may cause nausea, headache, malaise
• To wear sunscreen or large hat because photosensitivity occurs
⚠ To immediately report urinary retention, worsening depression, suicidal thoughts/behaviors

TREATMENT OF OVERDOSE:
ECG monitoring; lavage, activated charcoal; administer anticonvulsant

nystatin (Rx)
(nye-stat′in)
Bio-Statin, Nystat, Nystop, Pedi-Dri, ratio-Nystatin ✦
Func. class.: Antifungal
Chem. class.: Amphoteric polyene

ACTION:
Interferes with fungal DNA replication; binds sterols in fungal cell membrane, which increases permeability, leaking of cell nutrients

USES:
Candida species causing oral, intestinal infections

CONTRAINDICATIONS:
Hypersensitivity
Precautions: Pregnancy (C)

DOSAGE AND ROUTES
Oral infection
• **Adult/adolescent/child: SUSP** 400,000-600,000 units qid, use 1/2 dose in each side of mouth, swish and swallow, use for at least 48 hr after symptoms resolved
• **Infant: SUSP** 200,000 units qid (100,000 units in each side of mouth)
• **Newborn and premature infant: SUSP** 100,000 units qid
• **Adult/child: TROCHES** 200,000-400,000 units qid × ≤2 wk
GI infection
• **Adult: PO** 500,000-1,000,000 units tid
Cutaneous candidiasis
• **Adult/child: Top cream/ointment** apply to affected area bid; **powder** apply to affected area bid-tid
Available forms: Tabs 500,000, 1,000,000 units; powder for oral susp 50 million, 150 million, 500 million; susp 100,000 units per ml; oral caps 500,000, 1,000,000 units, bulk powder
Administer:
• Oral susp dose by placing 1/2 in each cheek, then swallow; do not mix with food

N

• Topical dose after cleansing area; mouth may be swabbed; very moist lesions best treated with topical powder

SIDE EFFECTS/ADVERSE REACTIONS

GI: Nausea, vomiting, anorexia, diarrhea, cramps
INTEG: Rash, urticaria (rare)

PHARMACOKINETICS

PO: Little absorption, excreted in feces

NURSING CONSIDERATIONS

Assess:
• **Allergic reaction:** rash, urticaria, irritated oral mucous membranes; product may have to be discontinued
• Obtain culture, histologic tests to confirm organism
• Predisposing factors: antibiotic therapy, pregnancy, diabetes mellitus, sexual partner infection (vaginal infections)
Perform/provide:
• Storage in refrigerator for oral susp; tabs in tight, light-resistant containers at room temp
Evaluate:
• Therapeutic response: culture negative for *Candida*
Teach patient/family:
• That long-term therapy may be needed to clear infection; to complete entire course of medication
• To avoid commercial mouthwashes for mouth infection
• To shake susp before measuring each dose
• To notify prescriber of irritation; product may have to be discontinued

nystatin topical

See Appendix B

nystatin vaginal antifungal

See Appendix B

octreotide (Rx)

(ok-tree′oh-tide)
Sandostatin, Sandostatin LAR Depot
Func. class.: Growth hormone, antidiarrheal
Chem. class.: Synthetic octapeptide

ACTION: A potent growth hormone similar to somatostatin

USES: **Sandostatin:** acromegaly, improves symptoms of carcinoid tumors, vasoactive intestinal peptide tumors (VIPomas); **LAR Depot:** long-term maintenance of acromegaly, carcinoid tumors, VIPomas

Unlabeled uses: GI fistula, variceal bleeding, diarrheal conditions, pancreatic fistula, irritable bowel syndrome, dumping syndrome, short bowel syndrome, insulinoma, hepatorenal syndrome

CONTRAINDICATIONS: Hypersensitivity

Precautions: Pregnancy (B), breastfeeding, children, geriatric patients, diabetes mellitus, hypothyroidism, renal disease

DOSAGE AND ROUTES

Acromegaly
• **Adult: SUBCUT/IV** (Sandostatin) 50-100 mcg bid-tid, adjust q2wk based on growth hormone levels or **IM** (Sandostatin LAR) 20 mg q4wk × 3 mo, adjust based on growth hormone levels
VIPomas
• **Adult: SUBCUT/IV** (Sandostatin) 200-300 mcg/day in 2-4 doses for 2 wk, max 450 mcg/day or **IM** (Sandostatin LAR) 20 mg q2wk × 2 mo, adjust dose
Flushing/diarrhea in carcinoid tumors
• **Adult: SUBCUT/IV** (Sandostatin) 100-600 mcg/day in 2-4 doses for 2 wk, ti-

trated to patient response or **IM** (Sandostatin LAR) 20 mg q4wk × 2 mo, adjust dose

GI fistula

• **Adult: SUBCUT** (Sandostatin) 50-200 mcg q8hr

Antidiarrheal in AIDS patients (unlabeled)

• **Adult: SUBCUT** (Sandostatin) 50 mcg q8hr prn, increase to 500 mcg q8hr

Irritable bowel syndrome (unlabeled)

• **Adult: SUBCUT** (Sandostatin) 100 mcg in single dose, up to 125 mcg bid

Dumping syndrome (unlabeled)

• **Adult: SUBCUT** (Sandostatin) 50-150 mcg/day

Variceal bleeding (unlabeled)

• **Adult: IV** (Sandostatin) 25-50 mcg/hr **CONT IV INF** for 18 hr-5 days

Available forms: Inj (Sandostatin) 0.05, 0.1, 0.2, 0.5, 1 mg/ml; inj powder for susp (LAR depot) 10, 20, 30 mg/5 ml

Administer:

IM route

• Reconstitute with diluent provided; give in gluteal region

SUBCUT route

• Rotate inj site; use hip, thigh, abdomen

• Avoid using medication that is cold; allow to reach room temp; do not use LAR depot

IV route

• **IV direct:** give over 3 min; during an emergency carcinoid crisis, give rapid bolus

• **Intermittent IV inf:** dilute in 50-200 ml D_5W, 0.9% NaCl; give over 15-30 min

Y-site compatibilities: Acyclovir, alfentanil, allopurinol, amifostine, amikacin, aminocaproic acid, aminophylline, amiodarone, amphotericin B colloidal, amphotericin B lipid complex, amphotericin B liposome, ampicillin, ampicillin-sulbactam, anidulafungin, argatroban, arsenic trioxide, atenolol, atracurium, azithromycin, aztreonam, bivalirudin, bleomycin, bumetanide, buprenorphine, busulfan, butorphanol, calcium chloride/gluconate, capreomycin, CARBOplatin, carmustine, caspofungin, ceFAZolin, cefepime, cefotaxime, cefotetan, cefoxitin, ceftazidime, ceftizoxime, cefTRIAXone, cefuroxime, chloramphenicol, chlorproMAZINE, cimetidine, ciprofloxacin, cisatracurium, CISplatin, clindamycin, cyclophosphamide, cycloSPORINE, cytarabine, dacarbazine, DACTINomycin, DAPTOmycin, DAUNOrubicin, DAUNOrubicin liposome, dexamethasone, digoxin, diltiazem, diphenhydrAMINE, DOBUTamine, docetaxel, dolasetron, DOPamine, DOXOrubicin, DOXOrubicin liposomal, doxycycline, droperidol, enalaprilat, ePHEDrine, EPINEPHrine, epirubicin, eptifibatide, ertapenem, erythromycin, esmolol, etoposide, famotidine, fenoldopam, fentaNYL, fluconazole, fludarabine, fluorouracil, foscarnet, fosphenytoin, furosemide, gallium nitrate, ganciclovir, gatifloxacin, gemcitabine, gentamicin, glycopyrrolate, granisetron, haloperidol, heparin, hydrALAZINE, hydrocortisone, HYDROmorphone, hydrOXYzine, IDArubicin, ifosfamide, imipenem-cilastatin, insulin (regular), irinotecan, isoproterenol, ketorolac, labetalol, lansoprazole, leucovorin, levofloxacin, lidocaine, linezolid, LORazepam, magnesium sulfate, mannitol, mechlorethamine, melphalan, meperidine, meropenem, mesna, methohexital, methotrexate, methyldopate, methylPREDNISolone, metoclopramide, metoprolol, metroNIDAZOLE, midazolam, milrinone, minocycline, mitomycin, mitoxantrone, mivacurium, morphine, moxifloxacin, mycophenolate, nafcillin, nalbuphine, naloxone, nesiritide, niCARdipine, nitroglycerin, nitroprusside, norepinephrine, ondansetron, oxaliplatin, paclitaxel, palonosetron, pamidronate, pancuronium, pemetrexed, pentamidine, pentazocine, PENTobarbital, PHENobarbital, phenylephrine, piperacillin, piperacillin-tazobactam, polymyxin B, potassium acetate/chloride/phosphates, procainamide, prochlorperazine, promethazine, propranolol, quiNIDine, quinupristin-dalfo-

O

pristin, ranitidine, remifentanil, rocuronium, sodium acetate/bicarbonate/phosphates, streptozocin, succinylcholine, SUFentanil, sulfamethoxazole-trimethoprim, tacrolimus, teniposide, thiopental, thiotepa, ticarcillin, ticarcillin-clavulanate, tigecycline, tirofiban, tobramycin, topotecan, vancomycin, vasopressin, vecuronium, verapamil, vinBLAStine, vinCRIStine, vinorelbine, voriconazole, zidovudine, zoledronic acid

SIDE EFFECTS

CNS: *Headache, dizziness, fatigue, weakness,* depression, anxiety, tremors, seizure, paranoia

CV: *Sinus bradycardia, conduction abnormalities,* dysrhythmias, chest pain, SOB, thrombophlebitis, ischemia, CHF, hypertension, palpitations, QT prolongation, ST- or T-wave changes

ENDO: *Hypo/hyperglycemia, ketosis, hypothyroidism,* galactorrhea, diabetes insipidus

GI: *Diarrhea, nausea, abdominal pain, vomiting, flatulence, distention, constipation,* hepatitis, increased LFTs, GI bleeding, pancreatitis, cholelithiasis, ileus

GU: UTI

HEMA: Hematoma of inj site, bruise

INTEG: Rash, urticaria, pain; inflammation at inj site

MS: *Joint and muscle pain*

PHARMACOKINETICS

Absorbed rapidly, completely; peak $^{1}/_{2}$ hr (subcut/IV), 2-3 wk (IM); half-life 1.7 hr, duration 12 hr, excreted unchanged in urine

INTERACTIONS

⚠ **Increase:** QT prolongation—class IA/III antidysrhythmics, some phenothiazines, β agonists, local anesthetics, tricyclics, haloperidol, chloroquine, droperidol, pentamidine; CYP3A4 inhibitors (amiodarone, clarithromycin, erythromycin, telithromycin, troleandomycin), arsenic trioxide, levomethadyl; CYP3A4 substrates (methadone, pimozide, QUEtiapine, quiNIDine, risperidone, ziprasidone)

Decrease: effect of—cycloSPORINE

Drug/Food

Decrease: absorption of dietary fat, vit B_{12} levels

Drug/Lab Test

Decrease: T_4

NURSING CONSIDERATIONS

Assess:

- Growth hormone antibodies, IGF-1 at 1- to 4-hr intervals for 8-12 hr after dose **(acromegaly)**; 5-HIAA, plasma serotonin; blood glucose, serotonin levels **(carcinoid tumors)**, plasma substance P, plasma vasoactive intestinal peptide **(VIP) (VIPoma)**
- Thyroid function tests: T_3, T_4, T_7, TSH to identify hypothyroidism
- Fecal fat, serum carotene
- **Allergic reaction:** rash, itching, fever, nausea, wheezing

⚠ **Cardiac status:** bradycardia, conduction abnormalities, dysrhythmias; monitor ECG for QT prolongation, low voltage, axis shifts, early repolarization, R/S transition, early wave progression

Perform/provide:

- Storage in refrigerator for unopened amps, vials or at room temp for 2 wk; protect from light; do not use discolored or cloudy sol

Evaluate:

- Therapeutic response: relief of diarrhea in patients with AIDS, improves symptoms of carcinoid or VIP tumors; data is insufficient regarding whether products decrease size/rate of tumor growth; decreasing symptoms of acromegaly

Teach patient/family:

- That regular assessments are required, diabetics to monitor blood glucose
- About SUBCUT inj if patient or other persons will be giving inj

⚠ That product may cause dizziness, drowsiness, weakness; to avoid hazardous activities if these occur; to report abdominal pain immediately

ofloxacin (Rx)

(o-flox′a-sin)

Apo-Ofloxacin ✦

Func. class.: Antiinfective

Chem. class.: Fluoroquinolone

ACTION: Interferes with conversion of intermediate DNA fragments into high-molecular-weight DNA in bacteria; inhibits DNA gyrase

USES: Treatment of lower respiratory tract infections (pneumonia, bronchitis), genitourinary infections (prostatitis, UTIs) caused by *Escherichia coli, Klebsiella pneumoniae, Chlamydia trachomatis,* skin and skin-structure infections; gonorrhea, otitis media, PID

Unlabeled uses: Leprosy, anthrax, epididymitis, meningococcal infection, prophylaxis, mycobacterium avium complex (MAC), plague, proctitis, traveler's diarrhea, typhoid fever

CONTRAINDICATIONS: QT prolongation, hypersensitivity to quinolones

Precautions: Pregnancy (C), breastfeeding, children, geriatric patients, renal disease, seizure disorders, excessive sunlight, hypokalemia

Black Box Warning: Tendon pain/rupture, tendinitis, myasthenia gravis

DOSAGE AND ROUTES

Lower respiratory tract infections/ skin and skin-structure infections

- **Adult: PO** 400 mg q12hr × 10 days

Cervicitis, urethritis

- **Adult: PO** 300 mg q12hr × 7 days (non-gonococcal); 400 mg as a single dose (Gonococcal)

Prostatitis from *E. coli*

- **Adult: PO** 300 mg q12hr × 6 wk

Urinary tract infection

- **Adult: PO** 200 mg q12hr × 10 days

Pelvic inflammatory disease

- **Adult: PO** 400 mg q12hr × 10-14 days

Renal dose

- **Adult: PO** CCr 10-50 ml/min, give q24hr; CCr <10 ml/min, give 50% of dose q24hr

Hepatic dose

- **Adult (Child-Pugh class C): PO** max 400 mg/day

Available forms: Tabs 200, 300, 400 mg

Administer:

PO route

- 2 hr before or 2 hr after antacids, calcium, iron, zinc products, without regard to food, maintain hydration
- After clean-catch urine for C&S

SIDE EFFECTS

CNS: *Dizziness, headache, fatigue, somnolence,* depression, insomnia, lethargy, malaise, **seizures,** vertigo

CV: **QT prolongation, dysrhythmias,** chest pain

EENT: Visual disturbances

GI: *Diarrhea, nausea, vomiting,* anorexia, flatulence, heartburn, dry mouth, increased AST, ALT, abdominal pain, constipation, **pseudomembranous colitis,** abnormal taste, xerostomia

HEMA: **Blood dyscrasias**

INTEG: Rash, pruritus, photosensitivity

MS: Tendinitis, **tendon rupture, rhabdomyolysis**

SYST: **Anaphylaxis, Stevens-Johnson syndrome, toxic epidermal necrolysis**

PHARMACOKINETICS

PO: Peak 1-2 hr; half-life 4-8 hr; steady state 2 days; excreted in urine as active product, metabolites; 90%-95% bioavailability

INTERACTIONS

Black Box Warning: Increase: tendon rupture/tendinitis—corticosteroids

- May alter blood glucose levels: antidiabetics

• Possible theophylline toxicity: theophylline

⚠ **Increase:** QT prolongation—class IA/III antidysrhythmics, some phenothiazines, β-agonists, local anesthetics, tricyclics, haloperidol, methadone, chloroquine, clarithromycin, droperidol, erythromycin, pentamidine

Increase: CNS stimulation, seizures—NSAIDs

Increase: anticoagulation—warfarin

Decrease: absorption—antacids with aluminum, magnesium, iron products, sucralfate, zinc products; separate by 2 hr

NURSING CONSIDERATIONS

Assess:

Black Box Warning: Tendon rupture/tendinitis: more common in lung, heart, kidney transplants or geriatric patients; assess for pain or inflammation

• Blood studies: BUN, creatinine, AST, ALT, CBC, blood glucose

• **CNS symptoms:** insomnia, vertigo, headache, agitation, confusion

• **Allergic reactions:** rash, flushing, urticaria, pruritus

Perform/provide:

• Storage at room temp, protect from light

Evaluate:

• Therapeutic response: urine culture, absence of symptoms of infection

Teach patient/family:

• That if dizziness or lightheadedness occurs, to ambulate, perform activities with assistance

• To complete full course of therapy, take with plenty of fluids

• To avoid iron- or mineral-containing supplements within 2 hr before or after dose

• To avoid sun exposure, photosensitivity can occur

ofloxacin ophthalmic

See Appendix B

OLANZapine (Rx)

(oh-lanz′a-peen)

Zyprexa, Zyprexa IntraMuscular, Zyprexa Relprevv, Zyprexia Zydis

Func. class.: Antipsychotic, neuroleptic

Chem. class.: Thienbenzodiazepine

Do not confuse:

OLANZapine/osalazine

Zyprexa/Celexa/Zyrtec

ACTION: May mediate antipsychotic activity by both dopamine and serotonin type 2 (5-HT2) antagonists; may antagonize muscarinic receptors, histaminic (H_1)- and α-adrenergic receptors

USES: Schizophrenia, acute manic episodes with bipolar disorder, acute agitation

Unlabeled uses: Acute psychosis

CONTRAINDICATIONS: Hypersensitivity

Precautions: Pregnancy (C), breastfeeding, geriatric patients, hypertension, cardiac/renal/hepatic disease, diabetes, agranulocytosis, abrupt discontinuation, Asian patients, closed-angle glaucoma, coma, leukopenia, QT prolongation, tardive dyskinesia, torsades de pointes

Black Box Warning: Dementia, postinjection delirium/sedation syndrome

DOSAGE AND ROUTES

Schizophrenia

• **Adult: PO** 5-10 mg/day initially, may increase dosage by 5 mg at ≥1 wk intervals; **ORALLY DISINTEGRATING** tabs: open blister pack, place tab on tongue, let disintegrate, swallow, max 20 mg/day

• **Geriatric: PO** 5 mg, may increase cautiously at 1-wk intervals, max 20 mg/day

• **Adolescent: PO** 2.5 or 5 mg/day, target 10 mg/day

• **Child 6-12 yr (unlabeled): PO** 2.5 mg q day, may increase to 5 mg/day after 4-7 days

Bipolar mania

• **Adult: PO** 10-15 mg/day, may increase dose after >24 hr by 5 mg

• **Adolescent: PO** 2.5 or 5 mg/day, target 10 mg/day

Agitation associated with schizophrenia, bipolar I mania

• **Adult: IM** 10 mg

Severe behavioral disturbances in geriatric patients (unlabeled)

• **Adult: PO** 2.5-5 mg/day; **acute psychosis PO** 5-10 mg every night

Available forms: Tab 2.5, 5, 7.5, 10, 15, 20 mg; **orally disintegrating tabs** 5, 10, 15, 20 mg (Zyprexia Zydis); **powder for inj** 10 mg; **ext rel powder for susp for inj** 210, 300, 405 mg (Zyprexa Relprevv)

Administer:

• Decreased dose in geriatric patients

PO route

• With full glass of water, milk, food to decrease GI upset

• **Orally disintegrating tabs:** open blister pack; place tab on tongue until dissolved; swallow; no water needed

IM route (Zyprexa Intramuscular)

• Dissolve contents of vials with 2.1 ml sterile water for inj (5 mg/ml), use immediately

• Do not use IV or SUBCUT

• Inject slowly, deep into muscle mass

IM route (Zyprexa Relprevv)

Black Box Warning: Available only through restricted distribution program due to postinjection delirium/sedation syndrome, given at a facility with emergency services

• Use deep IM gluteal inj only

• Use only diluent provided in kit; give q2-4wk using 19G, 1.5-inch needle in kit, for obese patients, use 19G, 2-inch or larger needle

SIDE EFFECTS

CNS: EPS: (pseudoparkinsonism, akathisia, dystonia, tardive dyskinesia), **seizures, headache, neuroleptic malignant syndrome (rare)**, agitation, nervousness, hostility, *dizziness,* hypertonia, *tremor,* euphoria, confusion, *drowsiness,* fatigue, *abnormal gait, insomnia, fever*

CV: Hypotension, tachycardia, chest pain, **heart failure, sudden death (geriatric patients, IM)**, orthostatic hypotension

ENDO: Increased prolactin levels, hypoglycemia

GI: *Dry mouth, nausea, vomiting, appetite, dyspepsia,* anorexia, *constipation,* abdominal pain, *weight gain,* jaundice, **hepatitis**

GU: Urinary retention, urinary frequency, enuresis, impotence, amenorrhea, gynecomastia, breast engorgement, premenstrual syndrome

HEMA: **Neutropenia**

INTEG: Rash

MISC: Peripheral edema, accidental injury, hypertonia, hyperlipidemia

MS: *Joint pain,* twitching

RESP: *Cough, pharyngitis;* **fatal pneumonia (geriatric patients, IM)**

PHARMACOKINETICS

Well absorbed (60%), peak 6 hr; metabolized by liver, glucuronidation/oxidation by CYP1A2 and CYP2D6; excreted in urine (57%), feces (30%); 93% bound to plasma proteins; half-life 21-54 hr, extended in geriatric patients; clearance decreased in women, increased in smokers

INTERACTIONS

⚠ **Increase: serotonin syndrome, neuroleptic malignant syndrome—SSRIs, SNRIs**

Increase: sedation—other CNS depressants, alcohol, barbiturate anesthetics, antihistamines, sedatives/hypnotics, antidepressants

Increase: OLANZapine levels—CYP1A2 inhibitors (fluvoxamine)

Increase: hypotension—antihypertensives, alcohol, diazepam

Increase: anticholinergic effects—anticholinergics

Decrease: OLANZapine levels—CYP1A2 inducers: carBAMazepine, omeprazole, rifampin

O

Decrease: antiparkinson activity—levodopa, bromocriptine, other DOPamine agonists

Drug/Lab Test

Increase: LFTs, prolactin, CPK

NURSING CONSIDERATIONS

Assess:

Black Box Warning: Postinjection delirium/sedation syndrome (Zyprexa Relprevv); monitor continuously for ≥3 hr after injection; patient must be accompanied when leaving: sedation, coma, delirium, EPS, slurred speech, altered gait aggression, dizziness, weakness, hypertension, seizures; before leaving, confirm that patient is alert, oriented, and free of any other symptoms

- Mental status: orientation, mood, behavior, presence of hallucinations and type before initial administration, monthly; EPS, including akathisia (inability to sit still, no pattern to movements), tardive dyskinesia (bizarre movements of jaw, mouth, tongue, extremities), pseudoparkinsonism (rigidity, tremors, pill rolling, shuffling gait)
- I&O ratio; palpate bladder if low urinary output occurs, urinary retention may be cause, especially in geriatric patients
- Bilirubin, CBC
- Urinalysis recommended before, during prolonged therapy
- Affect, orientation, LOC, reflexes, gait, coordination, sleep pattern disturbances
- B/P sitting, standing, lying: take pulse, respirations q4hr during initial treatment; establish baseline before starting treatment; report drops of 30 mm Hg; obtain baseline ECG
- Dizziness, faintness, palpitations, tachycardia on rising

⚠ **Geriatric patients for serious reactions:** fatal pneumonia, heart failure, stroke leading to death (IM)

⚠ **Neuroleptic malignant syndrome:** hyperpyrexia, muscle rigidity, increased CPK, altered mental status, for acute dystonia (check chewing, swallowing, eyes, pill rolling)

- Constipation, urinary retention daily; increase bulk, water in diet
- Weight gain, hyperglycemia, metabolic changes in diabetic patients

Perform/provide:

- Supervised ambulation until patient stabilized on medication; do not involve patient in strenuous exercise program because fainting is possible; patient should not stand still for long periods
- Storage in tight, light-resistant container

Evaluate:

- Therapeutic response: decrease in emotional excitement, hallucinations, delusion, paranoia, reorganization of patterns of thought, speech

Teach patient/family:

Black Box Warning: About postinjection delirium/sedation syndrome: teach about all symptoms

- To use good oral hygiene; frequent rinsing of mouth, sugarless gum, candy, ice chips for dry mouth
- To avoid hazardous activities until product response is determined
- That orthostatic hypotension occurs often; to rise from sitting or lying position gradually
- To avoid hot tubs, hot showers, tub baths because hypotension may occur
- To avoid abrupt withdrawal of this product because EPS may result; product should be withdrawn slowly
- To avoid OTC preparations (cough, hay fever, cold) unless approved by prescriber because serious product interactions may occur; to avoid use with alcohol, CNS depressants because increased drowsiness may occur
- That, in hot weather, heat stroke may occur; to take extra precautions to stay cool

TREATMENT OF OVERDOSE:

Lavage if orally ingested; provide airway; do not induce vomiting or use EPINEPHrine

olmesartan (Rx)

(ol-meh-sar′tan)

Benicar

Func. class.: Antihypertensive

Chem. class.: Angiotensin II receptor (type AT_1) antagonist

ACTION: Blocks the vasoconstrictor and aldosterone-secreting effects of angiotensin II; selectively blocks the binding of angiotensin II to the AT_1 receptor found in tissues

USES: Hypertension, alone or in combination with other antihypertensives

CONTRAINDICATIONS: Hypersensitivity, pregnancy 2nd/3rd trimesters (D)

Precautions: Pregnancy (C) 1st trimester, breastfeeding, children, geriatric patients, hepatic disease, CHF

DOSAGE AND ROUTES

- **Adult: PO** Single agent 20 mg/day initially in patients who are not volume depleted, may be increased to 40 mg/day if needed after 2 wk

Available forms: Tabs 5, 20, 40 mg

Administer:

- Without regard to meals, refrigerate susp and store up to 1 mo, shake susp before use

SIDE EFFECTS

CNS: *Dizziness,* fatigue, headache, insomnia

CV: Chest pain, peripheral edema, tachycardia

EENT: Sinusitis, rhinitis, pharyngitis

GI: *Diarrhea,* abdominal pain

MS: Arthralgia, pain

RESP: *Upper respiratory infection,* bronchitis

SYST: Angioedema

PHARMACOKINETICS

Peak 1-2 hr; excreted in urine, feces; half-life 13 hr; protein binding 99%

INTERACTIONS

Increase: antihypertensive effects—other antihypertensives, diuretics

Increase: hyperkalemia—potassium supplements, potassium-sparing diuretics

Increase: effect of lithium, antioxidants

Decrease: antihypertensive effect—NSAIDs

Drug/Herb

Increase: antihypertensive effect—hawthorn

Decrease: antihypertensive effect—ephedra

NURSING CONSIDERATIONS

Assess:

⚠ **Pregnancy;** product can cause fetal death when given during pregnancy (D) 2nd/3rd trimesters

- Response, adverse reactions, especially in renal disease
- **Hypertension:** B/P, pulse q4hr; note rate, rhythm, quality; electrolytes: K, Na, Cl; baselines for renal, hepatic studies before therapy begins
- Skin turgor, dryness of mucous membranes for hydration status; angioedema: facial swelling, dyspnea

Evaluate:

- Therapeutic response: decreased B/P

Teach patient/family:

- To comply with dosage schedule, even if feeling better
- To notify prescriber of mouth sores, fever, swelling of hands or feet, irregular heartbeat, chest pain
- That excessive perspiration, dehydration, vomiting, diarrhea may lead to fall in B/P; to consult prescriber if these occur
- That product may cause dizziness, fainting, lightheadedness
- To rise slowly to sitting or standing position to minimize orthostatic hypotension

O

• To notify prescriber immediately if pregnant; not to use during breastfeeding
• To avoid all OTC medications unless approved by prescriber
• To inform all health care providers of medication use
• To use proper technique for obtaining B/P, acceptable parameters

olopatadine nasal agent

See Appendix B

olopatadine ophthalmic

See Appendix B

olsalazine (Rx)

(ohl-sal′ah-zeen)

Dipentum

Func. class.: Antiinflammatory
Chem. class.: Salicylate derivative

Do not confuse:
olsalazine/OLANZapine

ACTION: Bioconverted to 5-aminosalicylic acid, which decreases inflammation

USES: Maintenance of remission of ulcerative colitis in patients intolerant to sulfasalazine

CONTRAINDICATIONS: Hypersensitivity to this product or salicylates
Precautions: Pregnancy (C), breastfeeding, children <14 yr; impaired renal/hepatic function; severe allergy; bronchial asthma

DOSAGE AND ROUTES

• **Adult: PO** 500 mg bid, max 3 g/day
Available forms: Caps 250 mg
Administer:
• Total daily dose evenly spaced to minimize GI intolerance, give with food

SIDE EFFECTS

CNS: Headache, hallucinations, depression, vertigo, fatigue, dizziness
GI: Nausea, vomiting, abdominal pain, hepatitis, diarrhea, bloating, pancreatitis
HEMA: Leukopenia, neutropenia, thrombocytopenia, agranulocytosis, anemia
INTEG: Rash, dermatitis, urticaria

PHARMACOKINETICS

Partially absorbed, peak 1½ hr, half-life 30-90 min (rectal), 2-15 hr (PO), excreted in urine as 5-aminosalicylic acid and metabolites, crosses placenta

INTERACTIONS

Increase: azaTHIOprine toxicity—azaTHIOprine
Increase: myelosuppression—mercaptopurine, thioguanine
Increase: PT, INR—warfarin
Drug/Lab Test
Increase: AST, ALT

NURSING CONSIDERATIONS

Assess:
• **Colitis:** bowel pattern, number of stools, consistency, frequency, pain, mucus before treatment and periodically
⚠ **Blood dyscrasias:** skin rash, fever, sore throat, bruising, bleeding, fatigue, joint pain (rare); CBC before treatment and periodically
• **Allergic reaction:** rash, dermatitis, urticaria, pruritus, dyspnea, bronchospasm; allergy to salicylates
Perform/provide:
• Storage in tight, light-resistant container at room temp
Evaluate:
• Therapeutic response: absence of fever, mucus in stools, decreased diarrhea, abdominal pain
Teach patient/family:
• To report diarrhea, rash, bleeding, bruising, fever, hallucinations
• That product may cause dizziness; to avoid hazardous activities until reaction is known

• To take even if feeling better; to take as directed; to take missed dose when remembered; but not to double

omalizumab (Rx)

(oh-mah-lye-zoo′mab)

Xolair

Func. class.: Antiasthmatic

Chem. class.: Monoclonal antibody

ACTION: Recombinant DNA-derived humanized IgG murine monoclonal antibody that selectively binds to IgE to limit the release of mediators in the allergic response

USES: Moderate to severe persistent asthma

Unlabeled uses: Seasonal allergic rhinitis, food allergy

CONTRAINDICATIONS: Hypersensitivity to hamster protein

Black Box Warning: Hypersensitivity to this product

Precautions: Pregnancy (B), breastfeeding, children <12 yr, acute attacks of asthma, lymphoma, nephrotic disease, bronchospasm, neoplastic disease, status asthmatics

DOSAGE AND ROUTES

• **Adult/adolescent/child ≥12 yr: SUBCUT** 150-375 mg × 2-4 wk, divide inj into 2 sites if dose >150 mg; dose is adjusted based on IgE levels, significant changes in body weight

Available forms: Powder for inj, lyophilized 202.5 mg (150 mg/1.2 ml after reconstitution)

Administer:

SUBCUT route

• Reconstitute using 1.4 ml sterile water for inj (150 mg/1.2 ml or 125 mg/ml); gently swirl to dissolve; allow vial to stand and q5min gently swirl for 5-10 sec to dissolve, some vials may take ≥20 min, do not use if contents do not dissolve within 40 min, should be clear or slightly opalescent; use large-bore needle to withdraw medication; replace needle with small-bore needle

• Given q2-4wk; product is viscous; if >150 mg is given, divide into 2 sites; inj may take 5-10 sec to administer

SIDE EFFECTS

CV: **Heart failure**, cardiomyopathy, hypotension

HEMA: **Serious systemic eosinophilia**

INTEG: Pruritus, dermatitis, inj site reactions, rash

MISC: Earache, dizziness, fatigue, pain, **malignancies**, viral infections, **anaphylaxis, thrombocytopenia**, headache

MS: Arthralgia, fracture, leg, arm pain

RESP: Sinusitis, upper respiratory infections, pharyngitis, pulmonary hypertension, **bronchospasm**

PHARMACOKINETICS

Slowly absorbed, peak 7-8 days, half-life 26 days, degradation by liver, excretion in bile

INTERACTIONS

• Use cautiously with live virus vaccines

NURSING CONSIDERATIONS

Assess:

• **Asthma:** respiratory rate, rhythm, depth; auscultate lung fields bilaterally; notify prescriber of abnormalities; monitor pulmonary function tests; serum IgE (may increase and continue for 1 year)

• **Inj site reactions:** inflammation, edema, redness, warmth at site; may occur within 60 min of inj, may decrease with repeated dosing

Black Box Warning: Anaphylaxis, allergic reactions: rash, urticaria, inability to breathe, edema of throat; product should be discontinued; have emergency equipment available, observe for 2 hr, reaction can occur ≤24 hr

O

Evaluate:
• Therapeutic response: ability to breathe more easily

Teach patient/family:
• That improvement will not be immediate
• Not to stop taking or decrease current asthma medications unless instructed by prescriber
• To avoid live virus vaccines while taking this product

Black Box Warning: To report signs of allergic reaction

omeprazole (OTC, Rx)
(oh-mep′ray-zole)

Apo-Omeprazole ✱, Good Sense Omeprazole, Losec ✱, Prilosec, Prilosec OTC

Func. class.: Antiulcer, proton pump inhibitor

Chem. class.: Benzimidazole

Do not confuse:
Prilosec/Prinivil/Prozac/predniSONE

ACTION: Suppresses gastric secretion by inhibiting hydrogen/potassium ATPase enzyme system in gastric parietal cells; characterized as gastric acid pump inhibitor because it blocks the final step of acid production

USES: Gastroesophageal reflux disease (GERD), severe erosive esophagitis, poorly responsive systemic GERD, pathologic hypersecretory conditions (Zollinger-Ellison syndrome, systemic mastocytosis, multiple endocrine adenomas); treatment of active duodenal ulcers with/without antiinfectives for *Helicobacter pylori*

Unlabeled uses: NSAID-induced ulcer prophylaxis, stress gastritis prophylaxis

CONTRAINDICATIONS: Hypersensitivity

Precautions: Pregnancy (C), breastfeeding, children

DOSAGE AND ROUTES

Active duodenal ulcers
• **Adult: PO** 20 mg/day × 4-8 wk; associated with *H. pylori* 40 mg q AM and clarithromycin 500 mg tid on days 1-14 then 20 mg/day on days 15-28

Severe erosive esophagitis/poorly responsive GERD
• **Adult: PO** (del rel cap/del rel susp) 20 mg/day × 4-8 wk

Pathologic hypersecretory conditions
• **Adult: PO** 60 mg/day; may increase to 120 mg tid; daily doses >80 mg should be divided

Gastric ulcer
• **Adult: PO** 40 mg/day 4-8 wk
• **Geriatric: PO** ≤20 mg/day

Heartburn (OTC)
• **Adult: PO** 1 del rel tab (20 mg)/day before AM meal with glass of water

Available forms: Del rel caps 10, 20, 40 mg; del rel tabs 20 mg; granules for oral susp 2.5, 10 mg (del rel)

Administer:
• Swallow caps whole; do not crush or chew; caps may be opened and sprinkled over applesauce
• Before eating, usually in the AM, separate with other medications
• **Oral susp powder:** give on empty stomach ≥1 hr before food; if there is NG or enteral feeding tube, do not feed 3 hr before or 1 hr after giving product: contents of packet should be mixed with 1-2 tbls water, add 20 ml water for NG tube; for oral, stir well, drink, add more water, and drink

SIDE EFFECTS

CNS: *Headache, dizziness, asthenia*

CV: Chest pain, angina, tachycardia, bradycardia, palpitations, peripheral edema, **heart failure**

EENT: Tinnitus, taste perversion

GI: *Diarrhea, abdominal pain, vomiting, nausea, constipation, flatulence, acid regurgitation,* abdominal swelling, anorexia, irritable colon, esophageal candidiasis, dry mouth, **hepatic failure**

GU: UTI, urinary frequency, increased creatinine, **proteinuria, hematuria,** testicular pain, glycosuria
HEMA: **Pancytopenia, thrombocytopenia, neutropenia, leukocytosis,** anemia
INTEG: *Rash,* dry skin, urticaria, pruritus, alopecia
META: Hypoglycemia, increased hepatic enzymes, weight gain, hypomagnesemia, hyponatremia, vit B12 deficiency
MISC: *Back pain,* fever, fatigue, malaise
RESP: *Upper respiratory infections, cough,* epistaxis, **pneumonia**
SYST: **Angioedema, exfoliative dermatitis, Stevens-Johnson syndrome, toxic epidermal necrolysis**

PHARMACOKINETICS

Bioavailabity 30%-40%; peak ½-3½ hr; half-life ½-1 hr; protein binding 95%; eliminated in urine as metabolites and in feces; in geriatric patients, elimination rate decreased, bioavailability increased; metabolized by CYP2C19 enzyme system

INTERACTIONS

Increase: bleeding—warfarin
Increase: serum levels of diazepam, phenytoin, flurazepam, triazolam, cycloSPORINE, disulfiram, digoxin
Decrease: effect of iron salts, ketoconazole, cyanocobalamin, calcium carbonate, ampicillin, indinavir, gefitinib
Drug/Lab Test
Increase: alk phos, AST, ALT, bilirubin, gastrin

NURSING CONSIDERATIONS

Assess:
• **GI system:** bowel sounds q8hr, abdomen for pain, swelling, anorexia, blood in stools
• **Electrolyte imbalances:** hyponatremia; hypomagnesemia in patients using product (3 mo-1 yr); if hypomagnesemia occurs, use of magnesium supplements may be sufficient, if severe, discontinue product
• **Hepatic enzymes:** AST, ALT, alk phos during treatment; **blood studies:** CBC, differential during treatment, blood dyscrasias may occur; vit B12 in long-term treatment
• **Serious skin reactions:** toxic epidermal necrolysis, Stevens-Johnson syndrome, angioedema, exfoliative dermatitis; fever, sore throat, fatigue, thin ulcers, lesions in mouth, lips; discontinue product, some serious skin disorders may be fatal

Evaluate:
• Therapeutic response: absence of epigastric pain, swelling, fullness, bleeding: decreased GERD, esophagitis symptoms

Teach patient/family:
• To report severe diarrhea; black, tarry stools; abdominal cramps/pain; or continuing headache; product may have to be discontinued
• That, if diabetic, hypoglycemia may occur
• To avoid hazardous activities because dizziness may occur
• To avoid alcohol, salicylates, NSAIDs; may cause GI irritation
• To take as directed, even if feeling better; to take missed dose as soon as remembered; not to double

ondansetron (Rx)

(on-dan-seh'tron)

Zofran, Zofran ODT, Zuplenz

Func. class.: Antiemetic

Chem. class.: 5-HT_3 receptor antagonist

Do not confuse:
Zofran/Zantac

ACTION: Prevents nausea, vomiting by blocking serotonin peripherally, centrally, and in the small intestine

USES: Prevention of nausea, vomiting associated with cancer chemotherapy, radiotherapy; prevention of postoperative nausea, vomiting
Unlabeled uses: Pruritus (rectal use), alcoholism, hyperemesis gravidarum

CONTRAINDICATIONS:

Hypersensitivity; phenylketonuric hypersensitivity (oral disintegrating tab), torsades de pointes

Precautions: Pregnancy (B), breastfeeding, children, geriatric patients, granisetron hypersensitivity

DOSAGE AND ROUTES

Prevention of nausea/vomiting (cancer chemotherapy)

- **Adult and child 4-18 yr: IV** 0.15 mg/kg infused over 15 min given 30 min before start of cancer chemotherapy; 0.15 mg/kg given 4 hr and 8 hr after 1st dose or 32 mg as single dose; dilute in 50 ml of D_5 or 0.9% NaCl before giving; **RECT** (unlabeled) 16 mg/day 2 hr prior to chemotherapy; **PO** 8 mg ½ hr prior to chemotherapy, repeat 4, 8 hr after 1st dose
- **Child ≥4 yr: PO** 4 mg ½ hr prior to chemotherapy

Prevention of nausea/vomiting (radiotherapy)

- **Adult: PO** 8 mg tid, may repeat q8hr

Prevention of postoperative nausea/vomiting

- **Adult: IV/IM** 4 mg undiluted over >30 sec prior to induction of anesthesia
- **Child 2-12 yr: IV** 0.1 mg/kg (≤40 kg); **IV** 4 mg (≥40 kg), give over ≥30 sec

Hepatic dose

- **Adult: PO/IM/IV** Max dose 8 mg/day

Hyperemesis gravidarum (unlabeled)

- **Adult: PO/IV** 4-8 mg bid-tid

Pruritus (unlabeled)

- **Adult: PO** 4 mg bid

Alcoholism (unlabeled)

- **Adult: PO** 4 mcg/kg bid

Available forms: Inj 2 mg/ml, 32 mg/50 ml (premixed); tabs 4, 8 mg; oral sol 4 mg/5 ml; oral disintegrating tabs 4, 8 mg; oral dissolving film 4, 8 mg

Administer:

PO route

- **Oral disintegrating tab:** do not push through foil; gently remove, immediately place on tongue to dissolve; swallow with saliva
- **Oral dissolving film:** fold pouch along dotted line to expose tear notch; while folded, tear and remove film, place film on tongue until dissolved, swallow after dissolved; to reach desired dose, administer successive films, allowing each to dissolve before using another

Direct IV route

- After diluting single dose in 50 ml NS or D_5W, 0.45% NaCl or NS; give over 15 min

Y-site compatibilities: Aldesleukin, amifostine, amikacin, aztreonam, bleomycin, CARBOplatin, carmustine, ceFAZolin, cefmetazole, cefotaxime, cefoxitin, ceftazidime, ceftizoxime, cefuroxime, chlorproMAZINE, cimetidine, cisatracurium, CISplatin, cladribine, clindamycin, cyclophosphamide, cytarabine, dacarbazine, DACTINomycin, DAUNOrubicin, dexamethasone, diphenhydrAMINE, DOPamine, DOXOrubicin, DOXOrubicin liposome, doxycycline, droperidol, etoposide, famotidine, filgrastim, floxuridine, fluconazole, fludarabine, gallium, gentamicin, haloperidol, heparin, hydrocortisone, HYDROmorphone, hydrOXYzine, ifosfamide, imipenem-cilastatin, magnesium sulfate, mannitol, mechlorethamine, melphalan, meperidine, mesna, methotrexate, metoclopramide, miconazole, mitomycin, mitoxantrone, morphine, paclitaxel, pentostatin, piperacillin/tazobactam, potassium chloride, prochlorperazine, promethazine, ranitidine, remifentanil, streptozocin, teniposide, thiotepa, ticarcillin, ticarcillin-clavulanate, vancomycin, vinBLAStine, vinCRIStine, vinorelbine, zidovudine

SIDE EFFECTS

CNS: *Headache, dizziness, drowsiness, fatigue, EPS*

GI: *Diarrhea, constipation,* abdominal pain, dry mouth

MISC: Rash, bronchospasm (rare), *musculoskeletal pain, wound problems, shivering, fever, hypoxia, urinary retention*

PHARMACOKINETICS

IV: Mean elimination half-life 3.5-4.7 hr, plasma protein binding 70%-76%, extensively metabolized in the liver, excreted 45%-60% in urine

INTERACTIONS

Decrease: ondansetron effect—rifampin, carBAMazepine, phenytoin

NURSING CONSIDERATIONS

Assess:

- Absence of nausea, vomiting during chemotherapy
- Hypersensitivity reaction: rash, bronchospasm (rare)
- **EPS:** shuffling gait, tremors, grimacing, rigidity periodically

Perform/provide:

- Storage at room temp for 48 hr after dilution

Evaluate:

- Therapeutic response: absence of nausea, vomiting during cancer chemotherapy

Teach patient/family:

- To report diarrhea, constipation, rash, changes in respirations, or discomfort at insertion site
- Headache requiring analgesic is common

orlistat (Rx, OTC)

(or'lih-stat)

Alli, Xenical

Func. class.: Weight-control agent

Chem. class.: Lipase inhibitor

ACTION: Inhibits the absorption of dietary fats

USES: Obesity management

CONTRAINDICATIONS: Breastfeeding, hypersensitivity, chronic malabsorption syndrome, cholestasis

Precautions: Pregnancy (B), children, hypothyroidism, other organic causes of obesity, anorexia nervosa, bulimia, nephrolithiasis, GI disease, diabetes, fat-soluble vitamin deficiency

DOSAGE AND ROUTES

- **Adult: PO** (Alli) 60 mg, (Xenical) 120 mg tid with each main meal containing fat, max 360 mg/day

Available forms: Caps (Alli) 60 mg, (Xenical) 120 mg

Administer:

- For obesity only if patient on weight-reduction program that includes dietary changes, exercise; patient should be on a diet with 30% of calories from fat; omit dose of orlistat if meal contains no fat

SIDE EFFECTS

CNS: *Insomnia,* depression, anxiety, dizziness, headache, fatigue

GI: *Oily spotting, flatus with discharge, fecal urgency, fatty/oily stool, oily evacuation, fecal incontinence, frequent defecation,* nausea, vomiting, abdominal pain, infectious diarrhea, rectal pain, tooth disorder, hypovitaminosis, **hepatic failure, hepatitis, pancreatitis**

GU: UTI, vaginitis, menstrual irregularity

INTEG: Dry skin, rash

MS: Back pain, arthritis, myalgia, tendinitis

RESP: Influenza, URI, LRI, EENT symptoms

PHARMACOKINETICS

Minimal absorption, peak 8 hr, 99% protein binding, excretion in feces, half-life 1-2 hr

INTERACTIONS

Increase: lipid-lowering effect—pravastatin

Increase: effects of warfarin

Decrease: absorption—fat-soluble vitamins (A, D, E, K), cycloSPORINE

NURSING CONSIDERATIONS

Assess:

- Weight weekly; diabetic patients may need reduction in oral hypoglycemics

O

• For misuse in certain populations (anorexia nervosa, bulimia)

⚠ **Hepatotoxicity/pancreatitis:** jaundice, weakness, abdominal pain (rare)

Evaluate:

• Therapeutic response: decrease in weight

Teach patient/family:

• That 60-mg cap can be obtained OTC; 60 mg tid is highest OTC dose

• That safety and effectiveness beyond 2 yr have not been determined

• To read patient information sheet; to discuss unpleasant GI side effects

• To take multivitamin containing fat-soluble vitamins 2 hr before or after orlistat; that psyllium taken with each dose or at bedtime may decrease GI symptoms

• To avoid hazardous activities until stabilized on medication; to discuss unpleasant side effects

• To notify prescriber if pregnancy is planned or suspected

⚠ **Hepatotoxicity/pancreatitis:** yellowing of skin, eyes; dark urine; weakness; abdominal pain

oseltamivir (Rx)

(oss-el-tam′ih-veer)

Tamiflu

Func. class.: Antiviral

Chem. class.: Neuramidase inhibitor

ACTION: Inhibits influenza virus neuraminidase with possible alteration of virus particle aggregation and release

USES: Prevention and treatment of influenza type A or B

Unlabeled uses: Avian flu (H5N1), avian influenzae A (H5N1), swine flu (H1N1), encephalitis

CONTRAINDICATIONS: Hypersensitivity

Precautions: Pregnancy (C), neonates, breastfeeding, infants, children, geriatric patients, renal/hepatic/pulmonary/cardiac disease, psychosis, viral infection

DOSAGE AND ROUTES

Treatment of influenza

• **Adult/child >40 kg: PO** 75 mg bid × 5 days, begin treatment within 2 days of onset of symptoms

• **Child 23-40 kg and ≥1 yr: PO** 60 mg bid

• **Child 15-23 kg and ≥1 yr: PO** 45 mg bid

• **Child ≤15 kg and ≥1 yr: PO** 30 mg bid

Prevention of influenza

• **Adult/child ≥13 yr: PO** 75 mg/day × ≥7 days; begin treatment within 2 days of contact, max use 6 wk

Renal dose

• **Adult: PO** CCr 10-30 ml/min, 75 mg/day × 5 days (treatment); 75 mg every other day or 30 mg/day (prophylaxis)

H1N1 influenzae A virus (swine flu) (unlabeled)

• **Adult/adolescent/child >40 kg: PO** 75 mg bid × 5 days

• **Adolescent/child 24-40 kg: PO** 60 mg bid × 5 days

• **Child >1 yr and 15-23 kg: PO** 45 mg bid × 5 days

• **Child >1 yr and ≤15 kg: PO** 30 mg bid × 5 days

Available forms: Caps 30, 45, 75 mg; powder for oral susp 6 mg/ml

Administer:

• Within 2 days of symptoms of influenza; continue for 5 days

• At least 4 hr before bedtime to prevent insomnia

• Without regard to food; give with food for GI upset

• **Oral susp:** 6 mg/ml conc, take care to administer correct dose; loosen powder from side of bottle, add 55 ml, shake well (6 mg/ml), remove child-resistant cap, push bottle adapter into neck of bottle, close tightly with child-resistant cap to ensure sealing, use within 17 days of preparation when refrigerated or within 10 days at room temp, write expiration date on bottle, shake well prior to use, use oral syringe provided but only with markings for 30, 45, 60 mg, confirm that dosing instructions are in same units as syringe provided

SIDE EFFECTS

CNS: *Headache, dizziness,* fatigue, *insomnia,* **seizures,** delirium, **self-injury (children)**
ENDO: Hyperglycemia
GI: *Nausea, vomiting,* diarrhea, abdominal pain
INTEG: **Toxic epidermal necrolysis, Stevens-Johnson syndrome, erythema multiforme**
RESP: Cough

PHARMACOKINETICS

Rapidly absorbed, protein binding 40%-45%, converted to oseltamivir carboxylate (active form), active forms half-life 1-3 hr, metabolite 6-10 hr, excreted in urine (99%), protein binding 3%

INTERACTIONS

- Avoid use with H1N1 virus vaccine, intranasal influenzae vaccine

NURSING CONSIDERATIONS

Assess:
- Bowel pattern before, during treatment
- **Influenza:** fever, fatigue, sore throat, headache, muscle soreness, aches

Perform/provide:
- Storage in tight, dry container

Evaluate:
- Therapeutic response: absence of fever, malaise, cough, dyspnea in infection

Teach patient/family:
- About aspects of product therapy
- To avoid hazardous activities if dizziness occurs
- To take as soon as symptoms appear; to take full course even if feeling better
- To take missed dose as soon as remembered if within 2 hr of next dose

⚠ **To stop immediately; to report to prescriber skin rash, delirium, psychosis, hallucinations (child)**
- That this product should not be substituted for flu shot
- To avoid other products unless approved by prescriber

oxacillin (Rx)

(ox-a-sill'in)
Func. class.: Antiinfective
Chem. class.: Penicillinase-resistant penicillin

ACTION:
Interferes with cell wall replication of susceptible organisms; osmotically unstable cell wall swells, bursts from osmotic pressure

USES:
Effective for gram-positive cocci *(Staphylococcus aureus, Streptococcus pneumoniae),* infections caused by penicillinase-producing *Staphylococcus*

Unlabeled uses: *Corynebacterium diphtheriae,* erysipelothrix rhusiopathiae

CONTRAINDICATIONS:
Hypersensitivity to penicillins or corn

Precautions: Pregnancy (B), breastfeeding, neonates, hypersensitivity to cephalosporins, GI/renal/hepatic disease; hypersensitivity to carbapenem

DOSAGE AND ROUTES

- **Adult/adolescent/child ≥40 kg: IM/IV** 0.25-0.5 g q4-6hr (mild to moderate infections); 1 g q4-6hr (severe infections), max 6 g/day
- **Adolescent <40 kg/child/infant: IM/IV** 50-100 mg/kg/day in divided doses q4-6hr, max 4 g/day

Available forms: Powder for inj 250, 500 mg, 1, 2, 4, 10 g

Administer:
- Product after C&S completed

IM route
- Reconstitute 250, 500 mg, 1, 2, 4 g/1.4, 2.8, 5.7, 11.4, 21.8 ml, respectively, of sterile water for inj, 0.45% NaCl, 0.9% NaCl to 167 mg/ml, shake until clear

• IM inj deep in gluteal muscle

IV route

Direct intermittent IV INJ

• Reconstitute 250 mg/5 ml sterile water for inj, 0.45% NaCl, 0.9% NaCl, (50 mg/ml); 500 mg 1, 2, 4 g/5, 10, 20, 40 ml, respectively; shake until clear; give over 10 min

Intermittent IV INF

• Reconstituted powder may be further diluted to 0.5-40 mg/ml, give over 1 hr

Y-site compatibilities: Acyclovir, cyclophosphamide, diltiazem, famotidine, fluconazole, foscarnet, heparin, hydrocortisone, HYDROmorphone, labetalol, magnesium sulfate, meperidine, methotrexate, morphine, perphenazine, potassium chloride, tacrolimus, vit B/C, zidovudine

SIDE EFFECTS

CNS: Lethargy, hallucinations, anxiety, depression, twitching, coma, seizures

GI: *Nausea, vomiting, diarrhea,* increased AST/ALT, abdominal pain, glossitis, colitis, pseudomembranous colitis, hepatotoxicity

GU: Oliguria, proteinuria, hematuria, *vaginitis, moniliasis,* glomerulonephritis, acute interstitial nephritis

HEMA: Anemia, increased bleeding time, bone marrow depression, granulocytopenia, eosinophilia

INTEG: Exfoliative dermatitis, rash

SYST: Anaphylaxis, serum sickness, Stevens-Johnson syndrome

PHARMACOKINETICS

Metabolized in liver; excreted in urine, bile, breast milk; crosses placenta

IM: Peak 30-60 min, duration 4-6 hr

IV: Peak 5 min, duration 4-6 hr, half-life 30-60 min

INTERACTIONS

• Do not mix or give together with aminoglycosides

Increase: oxacillin concentrations—probenecid

Decrease: oxacillin effect—tetracyclines, rifampin, erythromycins, chloramphenicol, cholestyramine, colestipol, sulfonamides

Drug/Lab Test

False positive: urine glucose, urine protein

NURSING CONSIDERATIONS

Assess:

• I&O ratio; report hematuria, oliguria because penicillin in high doses is nephrotoxic

• **Pseudomembranous colitis:** diarrhea, abdominal pain, fever, fatigue, anorexia; possible anemia, elevated WBC, low serum albumin; stop product; usually either vancomycin or IV metroNIDAZOLE is given

• Hepatic studies: AST, ALT

• Blood studies: WBC, RBC, Hct, Hgb, bleeding time

• Renal studies: BUN, creatinine, urinalysis, protein

• C&S before therapy; product may be given as soon as culture is taken

• Bowel pattern before and during treatment

• Respiratory status: rate, character, wheezing, tightness in chest

• **Anaphylaxis:** wheezing, pruritus, rash, laryngeal edema; discontinue product, notify prescriber, have emergency equipment nearby; skin eruptions after administration of penicillin to 1 wk after discontinuing product

Perform/provide:

• Adrenalin, suction, tracheostomy set, endotracheal intubation equipment

• Scratch test to assess allergy after securing order from prescriber; usually done when penicillin is only product of choice

Evaluate:

• Therapeutic response: absence of fever, draining wounds

Teach patient/family:

• All aspects of product therapy, including need to complete course of medication to ensure organism death (10-14 days); culture may be taken after completed course

- To report sore throat, fever, fatigue **(superinfection)**; persistent diarrhea **(pseudomembranous colitis)**; CNS toxicity
- To wear or carry emergency ID if allergic to penicillins

TREATMENT OF ANAPHYLAXIS: Withdraw product, maintain airway, administer EPINEPHrine, O_2, IV corticosteroids

⚠ HIGH ALERT

oxaliplatin (Rx)

(ox-al-i′plat-in)

Eloxatin

Func. class.: Antineoplastic

Chem. class.: 3rd-generation platinum analog

ACTION:
Forms crosslinks, thereby inhibiting DNA replication and transcription; not specific to cell cycle

USES:
Metastatic carcinoma of the colon or rectum in combination with 5-FU/leucovorin

Unlabeled uses: Relapsed or refractory non-Hodgkin's lymphoma; advanced ovarian cancer; breast, head/neck, testicular, pancreatic, gastric cancer; mesothelioma

CONTRAINDICATIONS:
Pregnancy (D), breastfeeding, radiation therapy or chemotherapy within 1 mo, thrombocytopenia, smallpox vaccination

Black Box Warning: Hypersensitivity to this product or other platinum products

Precautions: Children, geriatric patients, pneumococcus vaccination, renal disease

DOSAGE AND ROUTES

Dosage protocols may vary

Colorectal cancer

- **Adult: IV INF** *Day 1:* oxaliplatin 85 mg/m^2 in 250-500 ml D_5W and leucovorin 200 mg/m^2 in D_5W, give both over 2 hr at the same time in separate bags using a Y-line, followed by 5-FU 400 mg/m^2 **IV BOL** over 2-4 min then 5-FU 600 mg/m^2 **IV INF** in 500 ml D_5W as a 22-hr **CONT INF;** *day 2:* leucovorin 200 mg/m^2 **IV INF** over 2 hr, then 5-FU 400 mg/m^2 **IV BOL** over 2-4 min, then 5-FU 600 mg/m^2 **IV INF** in 500 ml D_5W as a 22-hr **CONT INF;** repeat cycle q2wk

Advanced ovarian cancer (unlabeled)

- **Adult: IV** 130 mg/m^2 q3wk as a single agent in those previously treated

Advanced breast cancer (unlabeled)

- **Adult: IV** 130 mg/m^2 on day 1 plus 5-fluorouracil (1000 mg/m^2 **CONT IV INF** days 1-4) q3wk

Pancreatic cancer (unlabeled)

- **Adult: IV** 100 mg/m^2 on day 2, with gemcitabine 1000 mg/m^2 on day 1, repeat q2wk; 625 mg/m^2 bid throughout treatment or fluorouracil 200 mg/m^2/day throughout treatment

Gastric cancer (unlabeled)

- **Adult: IV** 130 mg/m^2 over 2 hr on day 1 with epirubic 50 mg/m^2 and capecitabine

Available forms: Powder for inj 50, 100-mg single-use vials (5 mg/ml)

Administer:

Intermittent IV INF route

- Premedicate with antiemetics including $5HT_3$ blockers, with or without dexamethasone; prehydration not needed
- Do not reconstitute or dilute with sodium chloride or any chloride-containing sol, do not use aluminum equipment during any preparation or administration, will degrade platinum; do not refrigerate unopened powder or sol; do not freeze; protect from light
- Use cytotoxic handling procedures; prepare in biologic cabinet using gown, gloves, mask; do not allow product to come in contact with skin; use soap and water if contact occurs

• EPINEPHrine, antihistamines, corticosteroids for hypersensitivity reaction
• **Lyophilized powder:** reconstitute vial 50 mg/10 ml or 100 mg/20 ml sterile water for inj or D_5W; after reconstitution, sol may be stored for ≤24 hr in refrigerator; after dilution in 250-500 ml D_5W, may store ≤24 hr in refrigerator or 6 hr at room temp, infuse over 2 hr
• **Aqueous solution:** dilute in 250-500 ml of D_5W; after dilution, may store ≤24 hr refrigerator, 6 hr at room temp, infuse over 2 hr

Y-site compatibilities: Alfentanil, amifostine, amikacin, aminocaproic acid, amiodarone, amphotericin B colloidal, amphotericin B lipid complex, amphotericin B liposome, ampicillin, ampicillin-sulbactam, anidulafungin, atenolol, atracurium, azithromycin, aztreonam, bivalirudin, bleomycin, bumetanide, buprenorphine, butorphanol, calcium chloride/gluconate, CARBOplatin, caspofungin, ceFAZolin, cefotaxime, cefotetan, cefoxitin, ceftazidime, ceftizoxime, cefTRIAXone, cefuroxime, chloramphenicol, chlorproMAZINE, cimetidine, ciprofloxacin, cisatracurium, CISplatin, clindamycin, cyclophosphamide, cycloSPORINE, cytarabine, dacarbazine, DACTINomycin, DAPTOmycin, DAUNOrubicin, dexamethasone, digoxin, diltiazem, diphenhydrAMINE, DOBUTamine, docetaxel, dolasetron, DOPamine, doxacurium, DOXOrubicin, doxycycline, droperidol, enalaprilat, ePHEDrine, EPINEPHrine, epirubicin, ertapenem, erythromycin, esmolol, etoposide, famotidine, fenoldopam, fentaNYL, fluconazole, fludarabine, foscarnet, fosphenytoin, furosemide, gatifloxacin, gemcitabine, gemtuzumab, gentamicin, glycopyrrolate, granisetron, haloperidol, heparin, hydrALAZINE, hydrocortisone, HYDROmorphone, hydrOXYzine, IDArubicin, ifosfamide, imipenem-cilastatin, inamrinone, insulin (regular), irinotecan, isoproterenol, ketorolac, labetalol, leucovorin, levofloxacin, levorphanol, lidocaine, linezolid, LORazepam, magnesium sulfate, mannitol, meperidine, meropenem, mesna, metaraminol, methyldopate, methylPREDNISolone, metoclopramide, metoprolol, metroNIDAZOLE, midazolam, milrinone, minocycline, mitomycin, mitoxantrone, mivacurium, morphine, nafcillin, nalbuphine, naloxone, nesiritide, niCARdipine, nitroglycerin, nitroprusside, norepinephrine, octreotide, ondansetron, paclitaxel, palonosetron, pancuronium, pemetrexed, pentamidine, pentazocine, phenylephrine, piperacillin, polymyxin B, potassium chloride/phosphates, procainamide, prochlorperazine, promethazine, propranolol, quiNIDine, quinupristin-dalfopristin, ranitidine, rocuronium, sodium acetate/phosphates, succinylcholine, SUFentanil, sulfamethoxazole-trimethoprim, tacrolimus, teniposide, theophylline, thiotepa, ticarcillin, ticarcillin-clavulanate, tigecycline, tirofiban, tobramycin, tolazoline, topotecan, trimethobenzamide, vancomycin, vasopressin, vecuronium, verapamil, vinBLAStine, vinCRIStine, vinorelbine, voriconazole, zidovudine, zoledronic acid

SIDE EFFECTS

CNS: Peripheral neuropathy, fatigue, headache, dizziness, insomnia
CV: Cardiac abnormalities, thromboembolism
EENT: *Decreased visual acuity, tinnitus, hearing loss*
GI: *Severe nausea, vomiting, diarrhea, weight loss,* stomatitis, anorexia, gastroesophageal reflux, constipation, dyspepsia, mucositis, flatulence
GU: Hematuria, dysuria, creatinine
HEMA: Thrombocytopenia, leukopenia, pancytopenia, neutropenia, anemia, hemolytic uremic syndrome
INTEG: *Alopecia,* rash, flushing, extravasation, redness, swelling, pain at inj site
META: Hypokalemia
RESP: Fibrosis, dyspnea, cough, rhinitis, URI, pharyngitis
SYST: Anaphylaxis, angioedema

PHARMACOKINETICS

Metabolized in liver, excreted in urine; after administration, 15% of platinum in systemic circulation, 85% either in tissues or being eliminated in urine; half-life 390 hr; protein binding >90%

INTERACTIONS

Increase: bleeding risk—NSAIDs, alcohol, anticoagulants, platelet inhibitors, thrombolytics, salicylates
Increase: oxaliplatin toxicity—tannins
Increase: myelosuppression—myelosuppressive agents, radiation
Increase: nephrotoxicity—aminoglycosides, loop diuretics
Decrease: antibody response—live virus vaccines

Drug/Lab Test
Increase: ALT, AST, bilirubin, creatinine
Decrease: potassium, neutrophils, WBC, platelets

NURSING CONSIDERATIONS

Assess:

⚠ **Bone marrow depression:** CBC, differential, platelet count each cycle; withhold product if WBC is <4000 or platelet count is <100,000; notify prescriber of results

• Renal/hepatic studies: BUN, creatinine, serum uric acid, urine CCr before, electrolytes during therapy; dose should not be given if BUN >19 mg/dl; creatinine <1.5 mg/dl; I&O ratio; report fall in urine output of <30 ml/hr; LFTs

Black Box Warning: Anaphylaxis: wheezing, tachycardia, facial swelling, fainting; discontinue product, report to prescriber; resuscitation equipment should be nearby

⚠ **Pulmonary fibrosis:** cough, crackles, dyspnea, pulmonary infiltrate; discontinue immediately, death may occur

• Monitor temp; may indicate beginning infection

• Hepatic studies before each cycle (bilirubin, AST, ALT, LDH) as needed or monthly

• **Bleeding:** hematuria, guaiac, bruising or petechiae, mucosa or orifices; obtain prescription for viscous lidocaine (Xylocaine)

• Effects of alopecia on body image; discuss feelings about body changes

• Edema in feet, joint pain, stomach pain, shaking

Perform/provide:

• Comprehensive oral hygiene

• All medications PO if possible; avoid IM inj when platelets <100,000/mm^3

• Increase fluid intake to 2-3 L/day to prevent urate deposits, calculi formation; elimination of product

• Blankets, hat, gloves for cold prevention

Evaluate:

• Therapeutic response: decreased tumor size, spread of malignancy

Teach patient/family:

⚠ To report signs of **infection:** increased temp, sore throat, flulike symptoms

• To report signs of **anemia:** fatigue, headache, faintness, SOB, irritability

• To report **bleeding;** to avoid use of razors, commercial mouthwash

• To avoid aspirin, ibuprofen, NSAIDs, alcohol; may cause GI bleeding

⚠ To report any changes in breathing, coughing

• That hair may be lost during treatment; that a wig or hairpiece may make patient feel better; that new hair may be different in color, texture

• To report numbness, tingling in face or extremities, poor hearing or joint pain or swelling

• Not to receive vaccines during treatment

⚠ To use contraception during treatment and for 4 mo after; that product may cause infertility, pregnancy (D)

• **Dysesthesias:** to avoid contact with cold (air, ice, liquid)

oxaprozin (Rx)

(ox-a-proe'zin)

Apo-Oxaprozin ✱, Daypro

Func. class.: Nonsteroidal antiinflammatory, antirheumatic

Chem. class.: Propionic acid derivative

Do not confuse:
Daypro/Diupres
Oxaprozin/Oxazepam

ACTION:
Completely inhibits COX-1, COX-2 by blocking arachidonate; analgesic, antiinflammatory, antipyretic

USES:
Acute and long-term management of osteoarthritis, RA, juvenile RA

CONTRAINDICATIONS:
Pregnancy (D) 3rd trimester, hypersensitivity, asthma, patients in whom aspirin has induced symptoms of allergic reactions or asthma

Black Box Warning: Perioperative pain in CABG surgery

Precautions: Pregnancy (C), breastfeeding, children, geriatric patients, bleeding/GI/cardiac disorders, hypersensitivity to other antiinflammatory agents, severe renal/hepatic disease, CHF

Black Box Warning: GI bleeding, MI, stroke

DOSAGE AND ROUTES

- **Adult: PO** 600-1200 mg/day; max 1800 mg/day or 26 mg/kg, whichever is lower
- **Adult <50 kg: PO** 600 mg/day

Juvenile rheumatoid arthritis

- **Child 6-16 yr: PO** (22-31 kg) 600 mg/day; (32-54 kg) 900 mg/day; (≥55 kg) 1200 mg q day

Available forms: Tabs 600 mg

Administer:

- With food to decrease GI symptoms
- May be given in divided doses; give with a full glass of water

SIDE EFFECTS

CNS: Dizziness, headache, drowsiness, fatigue, tremors, confusion, insomnia, anxiety, depression

CV: Tachycardia, peripheral edema, palpitations, dysrhythmias, MI, stroke

EENT: Tinnitus, hearing loss, blurred vision

GI: Nausea, anorexia, vomiting, diarrhea, jaundice, cholestatic hepatitis, constipation, flatulence, cramps, dry mouth, peptic ulcer, GI bleeding, perforation, ulceration, dyspepsia

GU: Nephrotoxicity: dysuria, hematuria, oliguria, azotemia

HEMA: Increased bleeding time, pancytopenia

INTEG: Purpura, rash, pruritus, sweating, photosensitivity

MISC: Anaphylaxis, angioneurotic edema, toxic epidermal necrolysis, Stevens-Johnson syndrome

PHARMACOKINETICS

PO: Onset 1 wk, peak 1.5-3.5 hr, duration unknown, half-life 40-50 hr; metabolized in liver; excreted in urine/feces (metabolites), breast milk; 99% protein binding

INTERACTIONS

Increase: toxicity—aspirin, cycloSPORINE, methotrexate, probenecid

Increase: bleeding risk—oral anticoagulants, thrombolytics, cefamandole, cefotetan, cefoperazone, clopidogrel, eptifibatide, plicamycin, ticlopidine, tirofiban

Increase: levels of phenytoin, lithium; avoid concomitant use

Increase: GI side effects—aspirin, corticosteroids, NSAIDs, alcohol, potassium supplements

Decrease: effect—antihypertensives, diuretics

Drug/Herb

Increase: bleeding risk—garlic, ginger, ginkgo

Drug/Lab Test

Increase: BUN, alkaline phosphatase

False positive: increased 5-HIAA, benzodiazepine urine assay
False increase: 17-KS

NURSING CONSIDERATIONS

Assess:

- **Pain:** frequency, intensity, characteristics; relief of pain, ROM after med

⚠ Cardiac status: CV thrombotic events, MI, stroke; may be fatal

Black Box Warning: GI status: ulceration, bleeding, perforation; may be fatal

⚠ For Stevens-Johnson syndrome, anaphylaxis, toxic epidermal necrolysis, angioneurotic edema

⚠ Asthma, aspirin hypersensitivity, oronasal polyps; increased hypersensitivity reactions

- Renal, hepatic, blood studies: BUN, creatinine, stool guaiac, AST, ALT, CBC, before treatment, periodically thereafter
- Audiometric, ophthalmic exam before, during, after treatment
- For eye, ear problems: blurred vision, tinnitus; may indicate toxicity

Perform/provide:

- Storage at room temp

Evaluate:

- Therapeutic response: decreased pain, stiffness, swelling in joints; ability to move more easily

Teach patient/family:

⚠ To report blurred vision, ringing, roaring in ears; may indicate toxicity

- To avoid driving, other hazardous activities if dizziness, drowsiness occurs

⚠ To report change in urine pattern, increased weight, edema, increased pain in joints, fever, blood in urine; indicates nephrotoxicity

- That therapeutic effects may take up to 1 mo
- To take with a full glass of water to enhance absorption; to sit upright for 1/2 hr after dose
- To avoid prolonged sun exposure; to use sunscreen, wear protective clothing
- To avoid ASA, alcohol, other OTC medications without prescriber approval
- To inform all health care providers that product is being used

oxazepam (Rx)

(ox-ay′ze-pam)

Apo-Oxazepam ✦

Func. class.: Sedative/hypnotic; antianxiety

Chem. class.: Benzodiazepine, short acting

Controlled Substance Schedule IV

ACTION: Potentiates the actions of GABA, especially in the limbic system and the reticular formation

USES: Anxiety, alcohol withdrawal, insomnia

CONTRAINDICATIONS: Pregnancy (D), breastfeeding, children <12 yr, hypersensitivity to benzodiazepines, closed-angle glaucoma, psychosis

Precautions: Geriatric patients, debilitated, renal/hepatic disease, depression, suicidal ideation, dementia, sleep apnea, seizure disorder

DOSAGE AND ROUTES

Anxiety

- **Adult: PO** 10-30 mg tid-qid, max 120 mg/day
- **Geriatric: PO** 5 mg daily-bid initially, may increase, max 15 mg qid

Alcohol withdrawal

- **Adult: PO** 15-30 mg tid-qid

Available forms: Caps 10, 15, 30 mg

Administer:

- Without regard to food

SIDE EFFECTS

CNS: *Dizziness, drowsiness,* confusion, headache, anxiety, tremors, fatigue, depression, insomnia, hallucinations, paradoxical excitement, transient amnesia

O

CV: *Orthostatic hypotension,* ECG changes, tachycardia, hypotension
EENT: *Blurred vision,* tinnitus, mydriasis
GI: Nausea, vomiting, anorexia
HEMA: Leukopenia
INTEG: Rash, dermatitis, itching
SYST: Dependence

PHARMACOKINETICS

Peak 2-4 hr; metabolized by liver; excreted by kidneys; half-life 5-15 hr; crosses placenta, breast milk; protein binding 97%

INTERACTIONS

Increase: oxazepam effects—CNS depressants, alcohol, disulfiram, oral contraceptives
Decrease: oxazepam effects—oral contraceptives, phenytoin, theophylline, valproic acid
Decrease: effects of levodopa
Drug/Herb
Increase: CNS depression—kava, melatonin, valerian
Drug/Lab Test
Increase: AST, ALT, serum bilirubin
Decrease: RAIU
False increase: 17-OHCS

NURSING CONSIDERATIONS

Assess:

- B/P (lying, standing), pulse; if systolic B/P drops 20 mm Hg, hold product, notify prescriber
- ⚠ Mental status: mood, sensorium, affect, sleeping pattern, drowsiness, dizziness, **suicidal thoughts/behaviors**
- ⚠ **Physical dependency, withdrawal symptoms:** headache, nausea, vomiting, muscle pain, weakness, tremors, seizures (long-term use)

Perform/provide:

- Assistance with ambulation during beginning therapy because drowsiness, dizziness occurs
- Safety measures, including side rails

Evaluate:

- Therapeutic response: decreased anxiety, restlessness, insomnia

Teach patient/family:

- That product may be taken with food
- That medication not to be used for everyday stress or used >4 mo unless directed by prescriber; not to take more than prescribed dose because product may be habit forming
- To avoid OTC preparations (cough, cold, hay fever) unless approved by prescriber
- To avoid driving, activities that require alertness because drowsiness may occur
- To avoid alcohol, other psychotropic products unless directed by prescriber
- Not to discontinue product abruptly after long-term use
- To rise slowly because fainting may occur, especially among geriatric patients
- That drowsiness may worsen at beginning of treatment

OXcarbazepine (Rx)

(ox′kar-baz′uh-peen)

Trileptal

Func. class.: Anticonvulsant
Chem. class.: CarBAMazepine analog

ACTION: May inhibit nerve impulses by limiting influx of sodium ions across cell membrane in motor cortex

USES: Partial seizures
Unlabeled uses: Trigeminal neuralgia, atypical panic disorder, bipolar disorder

CONTRAINDICATIONS: Hypersensitivity
Precautions: Pregnancy (C), breastfeeding, children <4 yr, hypersensitivity to carBAMazepine, renal disease, fluid restriction, hyponatremia, abrupt discontinuation, suicidal ideation

DOSAGE AND ROUTES

Seizures, adjunctive therapy

- **Adult: PO** 300 mg bid, may be increased by 600 mg/day in divided doses bid at weekly intervals; maintenance 1200 mg/day

- **Child 4-16 yr: PO** 8-10 mg/kg/day divided bid; dose determined by weight, increase by 5 mg/kg/day q3days, max doses weight dependent

Conversion to monotherapy for partial seizures

- **Adult: PO** 300 mg bid with reduction in other anticonvulsants; increase OXcarbazepine by 600 mg/day each week over 2-4 wk; withdraw other anticonvulsants over 3-6 wk; max 2400 mg/day

Initiation of monotherapy for partial seizures

- **Adult: PO** 300 mg bid, increase by 300 mg/day q3days to 1200 mg in divided doses bid

Renal dose

- **Adult: PO** CCr <30 ml/min, 150 mg bid, increase slowly

Bipolar disorder/trigeminal neuralgia (unlabeled)

- **Adult: PO** 300 mg bid, may increase by ≤600 mg/day

Available forms: Film-coated tabs 150, 300, 600 mg; oral susp 300 mg/5 ml

Administer:

PO route

- Without regard to meals
- **Oral susp:** shake well, use calibrated oral syringe provided, use or discard within 7 days of opening

SIDE EFFECTS

CNS: *Headache, dizziness, confusion, fatigue,* feeling abnormal, ataxia, abnormal gait, tremors, anxiety, agitation, **worsening of seizures, suicidal thoughts/behaviors**

CV: *Hypotension,* chest pain, edema

EENT: *Blurred vision, diplopia, nystagmus,* rhinitis, sinusitis

GI: *Nausea, constipation, diarrhea,* anorexia, vomiting, abdominal pain, gastritis

INTEG: Purpura, rash, acne

SYST: **Angioedema, anaphylaxis, Stevens-Johnson syndrome, toxic epidermal necrolysis, drug reaction with eosinophilia and systemic symptoms (DRESS)**

PHARMACOKINETICS

PO: Onset unknown; peak 4-6 hr; metabolized by liver to active metabolite; terminal half-life 7-9 hr metabolite; inhibits P450 CYP2C19, induces CYP3A4/5

INTERACTIONS

⚠ **Contraindicated: MAOIs, ranolazine, nisoldipine**

Increase: CNS depression—alcohol

Decrease: effects—felodipine, oral contraceptive, carBAMazepine

Decrease: OXcarbazepine levels—carBAMazepine, PHENobarbital, phenytoin, valproic acid, verapamil

Drug/Herb

Increase: anticonvulsant effect—ginkgo

Decrease: anticonvulsant effect—ginseng, santonica

NURSING CONSIDERATIONS

Assess:

- Description of seizures: frequency, duration, aura
- Hyponatremia: headache, nausea, confusion
- Electrolyte: sodium; T_4; phenytoin (when given together)

⚠ **Serious reactions: angioedema, anaphylaxis, Stevens-Johnson syndrome**

- CNS/mental status: mood, sensorium, affect, behavioral changes, confusion, **suicidal thoughts/behaviors;** if mental status changes, notify prescriber
- Eye problems: need for ophthalmic exams before, during, after treatment (slit lamp, funduscopy, tonometry)

Perform/provide:

- Storage at room temp
- Hard candy, gum, frequent rinsing for dry mouth
- Assistance with ambulation during early part of treatment because dizziness occurs

Evaluate:

- Therapeutic response: decreased seizure activity

Teach patient/family:

- To avoid driving, other activities that require alertness

O

• Not to discontinue medication quickly after long-term use
• To inform prescriber if hypersensitive to carBAMazepine; multisystem hypersensitivity may occur, to report fever, other allergic symptoms
• To avoid use of alcohol while taking product
• To use alternative contraception if using hormonal method

TREATMENT OF OVERDOSE:

Activated charcoal; give 0.9% NaCl (hypotensive state), atropine (bradycardia); use benzodiazepines, barbiturates for seizures

oxybutynin (Rx)

(ox-i-byoo′ti-nin)

Ditropan ✦, Ditropan XL, Gelnique, Oxytrol ✦, Oxytrol Transdermal, Uromax ✦

Func. class.: Anticholinergic

Chem. class.: Synthetic tertiary amine

Do not confuse:
Ditropan/diazepam

ACTION: Relaxes smooth muscles in urinary tract by inhibiting acetylcholine at postganglionic sites

USES: Antispasmodic for neurogenic bladder, overactive bladder

CONTRAINDICATIONS: Hypersensitivity, GI obstruction, urinary retention, glaucoma, severe colitis, myasthenia gravis, unstable CV disease

Precautions: Pregnancy (B), breastfeeding, children <12 yr, geriatric patients, suspected glaucoma, cardiac disease, dementia

DOSAGE AND ROUTES

• **Adult: PO** 5 mg bid-tid, max 5 mg qid; **EXT REL** 5-10 mg/day, may increase by 5 mg, max 30 mg/day; **TD** apply 1 patch to abdomen, hip, buttock 2×/wk (q3-4 days); **GEL** apply contents of 1 packet to abdomen, upper arms, shoulders, thighs daily
• **Geriatric: PO** 2.5-5 mg bid-tid, increase by 2.5 mg q several days
• **Child >6 yr: PO** 5 mg bid, max 5 mg tid; **EXT REL** 5 mg/day, max 20 mg/day
• **Child 1-5 yr: PO** 0.2 mg/kg/dose bid-tid

Available forms: Syr 5 mg/5 ml; tabs 5 mg; ext rel tabs 5, 10, 15 mg; TD 3.9 mg/day; top gel 10% (Gelnique)

Administer:

PO route
• Do not crush, break, or chew ext rel tabs
• Without regard to meals

Topical route
• Wash hands; apply to clean, dry, intact skin on abdomen, upper arms/shoulders, thighs; avoid navel, rotate sites
• Squeeze contents into palm of hand or directly on site, rub gently
• Do not bathe, exercise, swim for 1 hr after application
• Allow to dry before putting on clothing
• Do not be near flame, fire, or smoke until gel has dried
• Delivers 100 mg

Transdermal route
• Apply to clean, dry, intact skin on abdomen, hip, buttock; use firm pressure; not affected by showering/bathing; rotate sites
• Delivers 3.9 mg/day

SIDE EFFECTS

CNS: *Anxiety, restlessness, dizziness, somnolence, insomnia, nervousness,* seizures, headache, *drowsiness,* confusion

CV: *Palpitations, sinus tachycardia,* hypertension, peripheral edema, **QT prolongation**

EENT: *Blurred vision, dry eyes,* increased intraocular tension, *dry mouth,* throat

GI: *Nausea, vomiting, anorexia,* abdominal pain, *constipation, dyspepsia,* diarrhea, taste perversion, GERD

GU: Dysuria, impotence, *urinary retention, hesitancy*
MISC: Hyperthermia, anaphylaxis, angioedema

PHARMACOKINETICS

Onset ½-1 hr, peak 3-6 hr, duration 6-10 hr; metabolized by liver, excreted in urine; terminal half-life 2-3 hr

INTERACTIONS

• Altered pharmacokinetic parameters: CYP3A4 inhibitors
Increase: CNS depression—benzodiazepines, sedatives, hypnotics, opioids
Increase: levels of atenolol, digoxin, nitrofurantoin
Increase: anticholinergic effects—antihistamines, amantidine, other anticholinergics
Increase or decrease: levels of phenothiazines
Decrease: levels of acetaminophen, haloperidol, levodopa
Decrease: effects of oxybutynin—CYP3A4 inducers

NURSING CONSIDERATIONS

Assess:
• **Urinary patterns:** distention, nocturia, frequency, urgency, incontinence, I&O ratios; cystometry to diagnose dysfunction
⚠ **Allergic reactions:** rash, urticaria; if these occur, product should be discontinued; angioedema
⚠ **QT prolongation:** ECG for QT prolongation, ejection fraction; assess for chest pain, palpitations, dyspnea
• CNS effects: confusion, anxiety; anticholinergic effects in geriatric patients
Evaluate:
• Urinary status: dysuria, frequency, nocturia, incontinence
Teach patient/family:
• To avoid hazardous activities because dizziness, blurred vision may occur
• To avoid OTC medications with alcohol, other CNS depressants
• To avoid hot weather, strenuous activity because product decreases perspiration
• About the correct application of each product form

⚠ *HIGH ALERT*

oxyCODONE (Rx)

(ox-i-koe′done)

ETH-Oxydose, Oxecta, Oxy-CONTIN, Roxicodone, Supeudol ✦

oxyCODONE/aspirin (Rx)

Endodan, Percodan

oxyCODONE/acetaminophen (Rx)

Endocet, Magnacet, Percocet, Primalev, Roxicet, Tylox, Xolox

oxyCODONE/ibuprofen (Rx)

Func. class.: Opiate analgesic
Chem. class.: Semisynthetic derivative

O

Controlled Substance Schedule II

Do not confuse:
Percodan/Decadron
Roxicet/Roxanol
Tylox/Xanax/Trimox/Wymox

ACTION: Inhibits ascending pain pathways in CNS, increases pain threshold, alters pain perception

USES: Moderate to severe pain
Unlabeled uses: Postherpetic neuralgic (cont rel)

CONTRAINDICATIONS: Hypersensitivity, addiction (opiate), asthma, ileus
Black Box Warning: Respiratory depression

Precautions: Pregnancy (B), breastfeeding, child <18 yr, addictive personality, increased intracranial pressure, MI (acute), severe heart disease, renal/hepatic disease, bowel impaction

Black Box Warning: Opioid-naive patients, substance abuse

DOSAGE AND ROUTES

• **Adult: PO** 10-30 mg q4hr (5 mg q6hr for concentrated product) **Conc sol is extremely concentrated; do not use interchangeably CONT REL** 10 mg q12hr for opiate-naive patients

Available forms: OxyCODONE: cont rel tabs (OxyContin) 10, 15, 20, 40, 80, 160 mg; immediate rel tabs 5, 15, 30 mg; immediate rel caps 5 mg; oral sol 5 mg/5 ml, 20 mg/ml; **oxyCODONE with acetaminophen:** tabs 2.5 mg/300 mg, 2.5 mg/325 mg, 5 mg/300 mg, 5 mg/325 mg, 7.5 mg/325 mg, 7.5 mg/500 mg, 10 mg/325 mg, 10 mg/400 mg, 10 mg/650 mg; caps 5 mg/500 mg; oral sol 5 mg/325 mg/5 ml; **oxyCODONE with aspirin:** 4.88/325 mg; **oxyCODONE with ibuprofen:** 5 mg/400 mg

Administer:

• Do not break, crush, or chew controlled rel tabs; give q12hr, no more frequently

• 80-, 160-mg cont rel tabs (OxyCONTIN) only to opioid-tolerant patients

• With antiemetic if nausea, vomiting occur

• When pain is beginning to return; determine dosage interval by response

SIDE EFFECTS

CNS: *Drowsiness, dizziness, confusion, headache, sedation, euphoria,* fatigue, abnormal dreams/thoughts, hallucinations

CV: Palpitations, bradycardia, change in B/P

EENT: Tinnitus, blurred vision, miosis, diplopia

GI: *Nausea, vomiting, anorexia, constipation, cramps,* gastritis, dyspepsia, biliary spasms

GU: Increased urinary output, dysuria, urinary retention

INTEG: *Rash,* urticaria, bruising, flushing, diaphoresis, pruritus

RESP: **Respiratory depression**

PHARMACOKINETICS

PO: Onset 15-30 min, peak 1 hr, duration 3-4 hr, metabolized by liver, excreted in urine, crosses placenta, excreted in breast milk, half-life 3-5 hr, protein binding 45%

INTERACTIONS

Increase: effects with other CNS depressants—alcohol, opioids, sedative/hypnotics, antipsychotics, skeletal muscle relaxants

Increase: toxicity—cimetidine, MAOIs

Drug/Herb

Increase: sedative effect—kava, St. John's wort, valerian

Drug/Lab Test

Increase: amylase, lipase

NURSING CONSIDERATIONS

Assess:

• **Pain:** intensity, location, type, characteristics; need for pain medication by pain/sedation scoring; physical dependence

• I&O ratio; check for decreasing output; may indicate urinary retention

• **CNS changes:** dizziness, drowsiness, hallucinations, euphoria, LOC, pupil reaction

• **Allergic reactions:** rash, urticaria

Black Box Warning: Respiratory dysfunction: respiratory depression, character, rate, rhythm; notify prescriber if respirations are <10/min; B/P, pulse

• **Bowel status:** constipation; stimulant laxative may be needed with fluids, fiber

Perform/provide:

• Storage in light-resistant area at room temp

• Assistance with ambulation

• Safety measures: night-light, call bell within easy reach

Evaluate:
- Therapeutic response: decrease in pain without dependence

Teach patient/family:
- To report any symptoms of CNS changes, allergic reactions
- That physical dependency may result from extended use
- That withdrawal symptoms may occur after long-term use: nausea, vomiting, cramps, fever, faintness, anorexia
- To avoid CNS depressants, alcohol
- To avoid driving, operating machinery if drowsiness occurs

TREATMENT OF OVERDOSE:
Naloxone (Narcan) 0.2-0.8 mg IV, O_2, IV fluids, vasopressors

oxymetazoline nasal agent
See Appendix B

oxymetazoline ophthalmic
See Appendix B

⚠ HIGH ALERT

oxymorphone (Rx)
(ox-i-mor′fone)

Opana, Opana ER

Func. class.: Opiate analgesic

Chem. class.: Semisynthetic phenanthrene derivative

Controlled Substance Schedule II

ACTION: Inhibits ascending pain pathways in CNS, increases pain threshold, alters pain perception

USES: Moderate to severe pain

CONTRAINDICATIONS: Hypersensitivity, addiction (opiate), asthma, hepatic disease, ileus, intrathecal use, surgery

Black Box Warning: Respiratory depression

Precautions: Pregnancy (B) (short-term), breastfeeding, children <18 yr, addictive personality, increased intracranial pressure, MI (acute), severe heart disease, respiratory depression, renal/hepatic disease, bowel impaction

Black Box Warning: Alcoholism, opioid-naive patients, substance abuse

DOSAGE AND ROUTES
- **Adult: IM/SUBCUT** 1-1.5 mg q4-6hr prn; **IV** 0.5 mg q4-6hr prn; *opiate naive* **PO** (immediate release only) 5-20 mg q4-6hr prn; *opiate naive* **PO-ER** 5 mg q12hr in those requiring around-the-clock dosing

Labor analgesia
- **Adult: IM** 0.5-1 mg

Available forms: Inj 1, 1.5 mg/ml; ER tab 5, 10, 20, 40 mg; tabs 5, 10 mg

Administer:
- 1 hr before or 2 hr after food (PO)
- With antiemetic for nausea, vomiting
- Do not break, crush, chew ER product
- When pain is beginning to return; determine interval by response

CONTROLLED REL
- **Opiate naive:** start with lowest dose, titrate upward 5-10 mg q12hr q3-7days to therapeutic response
- When converting from immediate rel to ext rel, give ½ daily dose of ext rel product q12hr

SUBCUT route
- Rotate inj sites
- Do not use if respirations are <12/min

IV route
- Give undiluted over 2-3 min

Syringe compatibilities: Glycopyrrolate, hydrOXYzine, ranitidine

SIDE EFFECTS

CNS: *Drowsiness, dizziness, confusion, headache,* hallucinations, increased intracranial pressure, *sedation,* seizures, *euphoria (geriatric patients)*
CV: Palpitations, bradycardia, change in B/P, hypotension
EENT: Tinnitus, blurred vision, miosis, diplopia
GI: *Nausea, vomiting, anorexia, constipation, cramps*
GU: Dysuria, urinary retention
INTEG: *Rash,* urticaria, bruising, flushing, diaphoresis, pruritus
RESP: Respiratory depression

PHARMACOKINETICS

Metabolized by liver, excreted in urine, crosses placenta, half-life 2.5-4 hr
PO: Peak 1 hr (fasting)
SUBCUT/IM: Onset 10-15 min, peak $1^1/_2$ hr, duration 3-6 hr
IV: Onset 5-10 min, peak 15-30 min, duration 3-6 hr

INTERACTIONS

⚠ **Increase:** effects with other CNS depressants—alcohol, opiates, sedative/hypnotics, antipsychotics, skeletal muscle relaxants
⚠ **Increase:** unpredictable effects/reactions—MAOIs

Drug/Herb
Increase: sedative effect—kava, St. John's wort, valerian

Drug/Lab Test
Increase: amylase

NURSING CONSIDERATIONS

Assess:

- **Pain:** location, intensity, type, other characteristics before and 1 hr after (IM) IV 30 min; need for pain medication, physical dependence, give 25%-50% until pain reduction of 50% on pain rating scale, repeat dose may be given at time of peak if previous dose does not control pain and respiratory depression has not occurred; give short-acting opioids for breakthrough pain if patient receiving controlled rel product
- I&O ratio for decreasing output; may indicate urinary retention
- **Bowel status:** constipation; may need stimulative laxative, increased fluids, fiber
- **CNS changes:** dizziness, drowsiness, hallucinations, euphoria, LOC, pupil reaction
- **Allergic reactions:** rash, urticaria

Black Box Warning: Respiratory dysfunction: respiratory depression, character, rate, rhythm; notify prescriber if respirations are <10/min

Perform/provide:

- Storage in light-resistant area at room temp

Evaluate:

- Therapeutic response: decrease in pain

Teach patient/family:

- To report any symptoms of CNS changes, allergic reactions
- That physical dependency may result from extended use
- That withdrawal symptoms may occur: nausea, vomiting, cramps, fever, faintness, anorexia
- Not to drive or operate machinery if drowsiness occurs

⚠ Not to use other CNS depressants, alcohol

- To make position changes slowly to prevent orthostatic hypotension

TREATMENT OF OVERDOSE:

Naloxone (Narcan) 0.2-0.8 mg IV, O_2, IV fluids, vasopressors

⚠ HIGH ALERT

oxytocin (Rx)
(ox-i-toe′sin)
Pitocin
Func. class.: Hormone
Chem. class.: Oxytocic, uterine-active agent

ACTION:
Acts directly on myofibrils, thereby producing uterine contraction; stimulates milk ejection by the breast; vasoactive antidiuretic effect

USES:
Stimulation, induction of labor; missed or incomplete abortion; postpartum bleeding

CONTRAINDICATIONS:
Hypersensitivity, serum toxemia, cephalopelvic disproportion, fetal distress, hypertonic uterus, prolapsed umbilical cord, active genital herpes

Precautions: Cervical/uterine surgery, uterine sepsis, primipara >35 yr, 1st/2nd stage of labor

Black Box Warning: Elective induction of labor

DOSAGE AND ROUTES

Postpartum hemorrhage

• **Adult: IV** 10-40 units in 1000 ml nonhydrating diluent infused at 20-40 mU/min

• **Adult: IM** 3-10 units after delivery of placenta

Contraction stress test (CST)

• **Adult: IV** 0.5 mU/min, increase q20min until 3 contractions within 10 min

Stimulation of labor

• **Adult: IV** 1-2 mU/min, increase by 1-2 mU q15-60min until contractions occur then decrease dose

Incomplete abortion

• **Adult: IV INF** 10 units/500 ml D_5W or 0.9% NaCl at 10-20 mU/min, max 30 units/12 hr

Available forms: Inj 10 units/ml

Administer:

IV route

• Use infusion pump

Labor induction

• After diluting 10 units/1000 ml of 0.9% NS or D_5 NS run at 1-2 mU/min at 15- to 30-min intervals to begin normal labor; dilute 10-40 mU/min; titrate to control postpartum bleeding; dilute 10 units/500 ml sol; run 10 units-20 mU/ml; administer by only 1 route at a time; use inf pump; rotate inf to provide mixing; do not shake

Control of postpartum bleeding

• Dilute 10-40 units/1000 ml of sol; run at 10-20 mU/min; adjust rate as needed

• With crash cart available on unit (magnesium sulfate at bedside)

Incomplete, inevitable, elective abortion

• Dilute 10 units/500 ml compatible IV sol

Y-site compatibilities: Heparin, hydrocortisone, insulin (regular), meperidine, morphine, potassium chloride, vit B/C, warfarin

SIDE EFFECTS

CNS: **Seizures, tetanic contractions**

CV: Hypo/hypertension, dysrhythmias, increased pulse, bradycardia, tachycardia, PVC

FETUS: Dysrhythmias, jaundice, hypoxia, **intracranial hemorrhage**

GI: Anorexia, nausea, vomiting, constipation

GU: **Abruptio placentae, decreased uterine blood flow**

HEMA: Increased hyperbilirubinemia

INTEG: Rash

RESP: **Asphyxia**

SYST: Water intoxication of mother

PHARMACOKINETICS

IM: Onset 3-7 min, duration 1 hr, half-life 12-17 min

IV: Onset 1 min, duration 30 min, half-life 12-17 min

O

INTERACTIONS

- Hypertension: vasopressors

Drug/Herb

- Hypertension: ephedra

NURSING CONSIDERATIONS

Assess:

- I&O ratio
- B/P, pulse; watch for changes that may indicate hemorrhage
- Respiratory rate, rhythm, depth; notify prescriber of abnormalities
- Length, intensity, duration of contraction; notify prescriber of contractions lasting >1 min or absence of contractions; turn patient on her side; discontinue oxytocin
- FHTs, fetal distress; watch for acceleration, deceleration; notify prescriber if problems occur; fetal presentation, pelvic dimensions; turn patient on left side if FHT change in rate, give O_2

⚠ **Water intoxication;** confusion, anuria, drowsiness, headache

Evaluate:

- Therapeutic response: stimulation of labor, control of postpartum bleeding

Teach patient/family:

- To report increased blood loss, abdominal cramps, fever, foul-smelling lochia
- That contractions will be similar to menstrual cramps, gradually increasing in intensity

paclitaxel (Rx)

(pa-kli-tax′el)

Taxol

paclitaxel nanoparticle albumin-bound (Rx)

Abraxane

Func. class.: Antineoplastic—miscellaneous

Chem. class.: Taxane

Do not confuse:

paclitaxel/PARoxetine/Paxil

Taxol/Paxil/Taxotere

ACTION:

Inhibits reorganization of microtubule network needed for interphase and mitotic cellular functions; causes abnormal bundles of microtubules during cell cycle and multiple esters of microtubules during mitosis

USES:

Taxol: metastatic carcinoma of the ovary, breast; AIDS-related Kaposi's sarcoma (2nd-line), non–small-cell lung cancer (1st-line), adjuvant treatment for node-positive breast cancer

Unlabeled uses: Advanced head, neck, small-cell lung cancer; non-Hodgkin's lymphoma, adenocarcinoma of the upper GI tract, hormone-refractory prostate cancer, bladder cancer

CONTRAINDICATIONS:

Pregnancy (D); hypersensitivity to paclitaxel or other products with polyoxyethylated castor oil, albumin

Black Box Warning: Neutropenia of <1500/mm^3

Precautions: Breastfeeding, children, females, geriatric patients, cardiovascular/hepatic/renal disease, CNS disorder, bone marrow suppression, dental disease/work, extravasation, herpes, infection, infertility, jaundice, ocular exposure, radiation therapy, thrombocytopenia, vaccination

Black Box Warning: Taxane hypersensitivity

DOSAGE AND ROUTES

Paclitaxel

Ovarian carcinoma

- **Adult: IV INF** 135 mg/m^2 given over 24 hr q3wk then CISplatin 75 mg/m^2; or 175 mg/m^2 over 3 hr q3wk; or 175 mg/m^2 over 3 hr

Advanced ovarian carcinoma

- **Adult: IV/INF** 175 mg/m^2 with CISplatin 75 mg/m^2 using a 3-hr regimen q3wk

Breast carcinoma

- **Adult: IV INF** 175 mg/m^2 over 3 hr q3wk × 4 courses

AIDS-related Kaposi's sarcoma
- **Adult: IV INF** 135 mg/m² over 3 hr q3wk or 100 mg/m² over 3 hr q2wk

1st-line non–small-cell lung cancer
- **Adult: IV INF** 135 mg/m²/24 hr inf with CISplatin 75 mg/m² × 3 wk

Bladder cancer (unlabeled)
- **Adult: IV** 175 mg/m² over 3 hr with CARBOplatin

Head/neck cancer (unlabeled)
- **Adult: IV** 250 mg/m² over 24 hr or 175-300 mg/m² over 3 hr

Stem cell transplant/bone marrow ablation (unlabeled)
- **Adult: IV** 250-775 mg/m² over 24 hr in combination with other chemotherapy

Paclitaxel protein-bound particles
- **Adult: IV** 260 mg/m² q3wk

Available forms: Inj 30 mg/5-ml vial, 100 mg/16.7-ml vial, 150 mg/24-ml vial, 300 mg/5-ml vial; powder for inj, lyophilized 100 mg in single-use vials (Abraxane)

Administer:

Continuous IV INF route
- After premedicating with dexamethasone 20 mg PO 12 hr and 6 hr before paclitaxel, diphenhydrAMINE 50 mg IV ½-1 hr before paclitaxel and cimetidine 300 mg or ranitidine 50 mg IV ½-1 hr before paclitaxel
- For extravasation if given by regular IV, not port

Paclitaxel
- After diluting in 0.9% NaCl, D_5, D_5 and 0.9% NaCl, D_5LR (0.3-1.2 mg/ml), chemo dispensing pin or similiar devices with spikes should not be used in vials of Taxol; use in-line filter ≤0.22 micron; may be given as 3-hr or 24-hr inf
- Using only glass bottles, polypropylene, polyolefin bags and administration sets; do not use PVC inf bags or sets

Y-site compatibilities: Acyclovir, amikacin, aminophylline, ampicillin/sulbactam, bleomycin, butorphanol, calcium chloride, CARBOplatin, cefepime, cefotetan, ceftazidime, cefTRIAXone, cimetidine, CISplatin, cladribine, cyclophosphamide, cytarabine, dacarbazine, dexamethasone, diphenhydrAMINE, DOXOrubicin, droperidol, etoposide, famotidine, floxuridine, fluconazole, fluorouracil, furosemide, ganciclovir, gentamicin, granisetron, haloperidol, heparin, hydrocortisone, HYDROmorphone, ifosfamide, LORazepam, magnesium sulfate, mannitol, meperidine, mesna, methotrexate, metoclopramide, morphine, nalbuphine, ondansetron, pentostatin, potassium chloride, prochlorperazine, propofol, ranitidine, sodium bicarbonate, thiotepa, vancomycin, vinBLAStine, vinCRIStine, zidovudine

Abraxane

Intermittent IV INF route
- Reconstitute vial by injecting 20 ml of 0.9% NaCl; slowly inject 20 ml of 0.9% NaCl over at least 1 min to direct sol flow on wall of vial; do not inject 0.9% NaCl directly onto lyophilized cake (foaming will occur); allow vial to sit for at least 5 min to ensure proper wetting of lyophilized cake; gently swirl or invert vial slowly for ≥2 min until completely dissolved
- Calculate dose by dosing vol/ml = total dose (mg) ÷ 5 (mg/ml)

SIDE EFFECTS

CNS: *Peripheral neuropathy*
CV: Bradycardia, *hypotension,* abnormal ECG, **supraventricular tachycardia (SVT)**
GI: *Nausea, vomiting, diarrhea, mucositis, stomatitis, increased bilirubin, alk phos, AST*
HEMA: **Neutropenia, leukopenia, thrombocytopenia, anemia, bleeding, infections**
INTEG: *Alopecia,* tissue necrosis, generalized urticaria, *flushing*
MS: *Arthralgia, myalgia*
RESP: **Pulmonary embolism,** dyspnea
SYST: *Hypersensitivity reactions,* **anaphylaxis, Stevens-Johnson syndrome, toxic epidermal necrolysis, angioedema**

PHARMACOKINETICS

89%-98% of product serum protein bound, metabolized in liver, excreted in

P

bile and urine; terminal half-life 5.3-17.4 hr

INTERACTIONS

Increase: myelosuppression—other antineoplastics, radiation

Increase: DOXOrubicin levels—DOXOrubicin

⚠ **Increase:** toxicity, decrease metabolism—ketoconazole; avoid concurrent use

Increase: bleeding risk—NSAIDs, anticoagulants

Decrease: paclitaxel metabolism—verapamil, diazepam, cycloSPORINE, teniposide, etoposide, quiNIDine, dexamethasone, vinCRIStine, testosterone

Decrease: paclitaxel levels—CYP2C8, CYP2C9 inducers

Decrease: immune response—live virus vaccines

NURSING CONSIDERATIONS

Assess:

- CBC, differential, platelet count before treatment and weekly; withhold product if WBC is <1500/mm^3 or platelet count is <100,000/mm^3; notify prescriber
- **Cardiovascular status:** ECG continuously in CV conditions; monitor for hypotension, sinus bradycardia/tachycardia
- **Peripheral neuropathy:** paresthesias, numbness; during inf, use ice packs on extremities to lessen continued neuropathy; may use acupuncture for some relief
- **Arthralgia, myalgia:** may begin 2-3 days after inf and continue for 4-5 days; may use analgesics
- **Nausea, vomiting:** premedicate with antiemetics; nausea and vomiting occur often
- Hepatic studies before, during therapy (bilirubin, AST, ALT, LDH) prn or monthly, check for jaundiced skin and sclera, dark urine, clay-colored stool, itchy skin, abdominal pain, fever, diarrhea
- VS during 1st hr of inf, check IV site for signs of infiltration

⚠ **Hypersensitivity reactions, anaphylaxis:** hypotension, dyspnea, angioedema, generalized urticaria; discontinue inf immediately; keep emergency equipment available, monitor continuously during first 30-60 min then periodically

- **Taxol flush:** for mild to moderate flush, may continue diphenhydrAMINE for ≤48 hr
- Effects of alopecia on body image; discuss feelings about body changes

Perform/provide:

- Confirmation that dexamethasone was given 12 hr and 6 hr before inf begins
- Storage of prepared sol up to 27 hr in refrigerator

Evaluate:

- Therapeutic response: decreased tumor size, spread of malignancy

Teach patient/family:

- To report signs of infection: fever, sore throat, flulike symptoms
- To report signs of anemia: fatigue, headache, faintness, SOB, irritability
- To report bleeding; to avoid use of razors, commercial mouthwash; to use soft-bristle toothbrush; to use viscous xylocaine or compounded formula for stomatitis
- To avoid use of aspirin, ibuprofen
- To avoid crowds, persons with known infections
- That hair may be lost during treatment; that a wig or hairpiece may make patient feel better; that new hair may be different in color, texture
- That pain in muscles and joints 2-5 days after inf is common
- To use nonhormonal contraception
- To avoid receiving vaccinations while taking product

paliperidone (Rx)

(pal-ee-per′i-done)

Invega, Invega Sustenna

Func. class.: Antipsychotic

Chem. class.: Benzisoxazole derivative

Do not confuse:

Invega/Iveegam

paliperidone/risperidone

ACTION:
Mediated through both DOPamine type 2 (D_2) and serotonin type 2 ($5\text{-}HT_2$) antagonism

USES:
Schizophrenia

CONTRAINDICATIONS:
Breastfeeding, geriatric patients, seizure disorders, AV block, QT prolongation, torsades de pointes; hypersensitivity to this product, risperidone

Precautions: Pregnancy (C), children, renal/hepatic disease, obesity, Parkinson's disease

Black Box Warning: Dementia

DOSAGE AND ROUTES

• **Adult: PO** 6 mg/day, max 12 mg/day; **IM** 234 mg on day 1 then 156 mg 1 wk later; after 2nd dose, give 117 mg each mo; range 39-234 mg

• **Child/adolescent ≥12 yr and ≥51 kg: PO** 3 mg daily, may increase if needed by 3 mg/day in intervals of >5 days, up to max 12 mg/day; <51 kg max 6 mg/day

Renal dose

• **Adult: PO** CCr 50-79 ml/min, 3 mg/day, max 6 mg/day; **EXT REL IM** 156 mg on day 1, 117 mg 1 wk later, then 78 mg each mo; CCr 10-49 ml/min, 1.5 mg/day, max 3 mg/day

Available forms: Ext rel tabs 1.5, 3, 6, 9 mg; ext rel susp for inj 39 mg/0.25 ml, 78 mg/0.5 ml, 117 mg/0.75 ml, 156 mg/ml, 234 mg/1.5 ml

Administer:

• Avoid use with CNS depressants

PO route

• Do not break, crush, or chew ext rel tabs

• Without regard for food

• Reduced dose for geriatric patients

IM route

• Use for IM only, do not use IV or subcut; inj kits contain prefilled syringe and 2 safety needles, for single use only, shake for 10 sec; **deltoid inj:** ≥90 kg, use 1.5-inch, 22G needle, <90 kg, use 1-inch, 23G needle, alternate injections between deltoid muscles; **gluteal inj:** use 1.5-inch, 22G needle; while holding syringe upright, twist rubber tip clockwise to remove, peel safety needle pouch halfway open, grasp needle sheath using plastic peel pouch, attach needle to Luer connection in clockwise motion, pull needle sheath away using straight pull, bring syringe with attached needle upright to de-aerate, de-aerate, inject; after inj, use finger, thumb, or flat surface to activate needle protection system until click heard, use deltoid × 2 doses

SIDE EFFECTS

CNS: *EPS, pseudoparkinsonism, akathisia, dystonia, tardive dyskinesia; drowsiness, insomnia, agitation, anxiety, headache,* **seizures, neuroleptic malignant syndrome,** dizziness

CV: Orthostatic hypotension, tachycardia; **heart failure, QT prolongation, heart** block, dysrhythmias

EENT: Blurred vision

ENDO: Hyperinsulinemia

GI: *Nausea,* vomiting, *anorexia, constipation,* weight gain in adolescents, xerostomia

GU: Priapism

HEMA: Agranulocytosis

PHARMACOKINETICS

Peak 24 hr; elimination half-life 23 hr; excreted 80% urine, 11% feces

INTERACTIONS

Increase: sedation—other CNS depressants, alcohol, sedative/hypnotics, opiates

Increase: EPS—other antipsychotics

⚠ **Increase: QT prolongation—class IA, III antidysrhythmics, azole antifungals, tricyclics (high doses), some phenothiazines, β-blockers, chloroquine, pimozide, droperidol, some antipsychotics, abarelix, alfuzosin, amoxapine, apomorphine, dasatinib, dolasetron, flecainide, halogenated anesthetics**

Increase: serotonin syndrome, neuroleptic malignant syndrome—SSRIs, SNRIs

Decrease: effect of paliperidone—carBAMazepine
Decrease: levodopa effect—levodopa
Drug/Lab Test
Increase: prolactin levels

NURSING CONSIDERATIONS

Assess:

Black Box Warning: Mental status: mood, behavior, confusion, orientation, suicidal thoughts/behaviors; dementia, especially in geriatric patients before initial administration

⚠ **QT prolongation:** ECG for QT prolongation, ejection fraction; chest pain, palpitations, dyspnea

- Swallowing of PO medication; check for hoarding, giving of medication to others
- Affect, orientation, LOC, reflexes, gait, coordination, sleep pattern disturbances
- B/P (standing, lying), pulse, respirations; q4hr during initial treatment; establish baseline before starting treatment; report drops of 30 mm Hg; watch for ECG changes
- **Hyperprolactinemia:** sexual dysfunction, decreased menstruation, breast pain
- Dizziness, faintness, palpitations, tachycardia on rising
- **EPS:** akathisia, tardive dyskinesia (bizarre movements of jaw, mouth, tongue, extremities), pseudoparkinsonism (rigidity, tremors, pill rolling, shuffling gait)

⚠ **Serotonin syndrome, neuroleptic malignant syndrome:** hyperthermia, increased CPK, altered mental status, muscle rigidity, fever, seizures, discontinue

- Constipation, urinary retention daily; if these occur, increase bulk and water in diet; monitor for weight gain, especially among adolescents

Perform/provide:

- Supervised ambulation until patient is stabilized on medication; do not involve patient in strenuous exercise program because fainting is possible; patient should not stand still for a long time
- Increased fluids to prevent constipation
- Sips of water, candy, gum for dry mouth
- Storage in tight, light-resistant container

Evaluate:

- Therapeutic response: decrease in emotional excitement, hallucinations, delusions, paranoia; reorganization of patterns of thought, speech

Teach patient/family:

- That orthostatic hypotension may occur; to rise gradually from sitting or lying position
- To avoid hot tubs, hot showers, tub baths because hypotension may occur
- To avoid abrupt withdrawal of this product because EPS may result; that product should be withdrawn slowly
- To avoid OTC preparations (cough, hay fever, cold) unless approved by prescriber because serious product interactions may occur; to avoid alcohol because increased drowsiness may occur
- To avoid hazardous activities if drowsy or dizzy
- About compliance with product regimen; that nonabsorbable tab shell is expelled in stool
- To report impaired vision, tremors, muscle twitching
- That heat stroke may occur in hot weather; to take extra precautions to stay cool
- To use contraception; to inform prescriber if pregnancy is planned or suspected

Black Box Warning: To notify prescriber of suicidal thoughts/behaviors, other changes in behavior

TREATMENT OF OVERDOSE:

Lavage if orally ingested; provide airway; *do not induce vomiting*

palonosetron (Rx)

(pa-lone-o′se-tron)

Aloxi

Func. class.: Antiemetic

Chem. class.: 5-HT_3 receptor antagonist

ACTION: Prevents nausea, vomiting by blocking serotonin peripherally, centrally, and in the small intestine at the 5-HT_3 receptor

USES: Prevention of nausea, vomiting associated with cancer chemotherapy, postoperative nausea/vomiting

CONTRAINDICATIONS: Hypersensitivity

Precautions: Pregnancy (B), breastfeeding, children, geriatric patients, hypokalemia, hypomagnesium, patients taking diuretics

DOSAGE AND ROUTES

- **Adult: PO** 0.5 mg as single dose 1 hr prior to chemotherapy; **IV** 0.25 mg as single dose over 30 sec ½ hr prior to chemotherapy, max 25 mg **IV** over q7days

Postoperative nausea/vomiting prophylaxis for ≤24 hr after surgery

- **Adult: IV** 0.075 mg given over 10 sec immediately before induction

Available forms: Inj 0.25/5 ml; caps 0.5 mg

Administer:

PO route

- Give 1 hr prior to chemotherapy
- May be taken without regard to food

Direct IV route

- **Chemotherapy nausea/vomiting:** give as single dose over 30 sec
- **Postoperative nausea/vomiting:** give over 10 sec immediately prior to anesthesia induction
- Do not mix with other products; flush IV line before and after administration with 0.9% NaCl

Syringe compatibilities: Dexamethasone

Y-site compatibilities: Alemtuzumab, alfentanil, amifostine, amikacin, aminocaproic acid, aminophylline, amiodarone, amphotericin B liposome, ampicillin, ampicillin/sulbactam, atracurium, atropine, azithromycin, aztreonam, bivalirudin, bleomycin, bumetanide, buprenorphine, busulfan, butorphanol, calcium acetate/chloride/gluconate, CARBOplatin, carmustine, caspofungin, ceFAZolin, cefepime, cefotaxime, cefotetan, cefoxitin, ceftazidime, ceftizoxime, cefTRIAXone, cefuroxime, chloramphenicol, chlorproMAZINE, cimetidine, ciprofloxacin, cisatracurium, CISplatin, clindamycin, cyclophosphamide, cycloSPORINE, cytarabine, dacarbazine, DACTINomycin, dantrolene, DAPTOmycin, DAUNOrubicin, dexamethasone, dexmedetomidine, dexrazoxane, digoxin, diltiazem, diphenhydrAMINE, DOBUTamine, docetaxel, DOPamine, doxacurium, DOXOrubicin hydrochloride, droperidol, enalaprilat, ePHEDrine, EPINEPHrine, epirubicin, eptifibatide, erythromycin, esmolol, etoposide, etoposide phosphate, famotidine, fenoldopam, fentaNYL, fluconazole, fludarabine, fluorouracil, foscarnet, fosphenytoin, furosemide, gemcitabine, gentamicin, glycopyrrolate, haloperidol, heparin, hydrALAZINE, hydrocortisone, HYDROmorphone, IDArubicin, ifosfamide, inamrinone, insulin, irinotecan, isoproterenol, ketorolac, labetalol, leucovorin, levofloxacin, lidocaine, linezolid, LORazepam, magnesium sulfate, mannitol, mechlorethamine, melphalan, meperidine, meropenem, mesna, metaraminol, methotrexate, methyldopate, metoclopramide, metoprolol, metroNIDAZOLE, midazolam, milrinone, mitomycin, mitoxantrone, mivacurium, morphine, nalbuphine, naloxone, neostigmine, nesiritide, niCARdipine, nitroglycerin, nitroprusside, norepinephrine, octreotide, oxaliplatin, oxytocin, pacli-

P

taxel, pamidronate, pancuronium, pentazocine, PHENobarbital, phentolamine, phenylephrine, piperacillin/tazobactam, potassium acetate/chloride/phosphates, procainamide, prochlorperazine, promethazine, propranolol, quinupristin/dalfopristin, ranitidine, remifentanil, rocuronium, sodium acetate/bicarbonate/phosphates, streptozocin, succinylcholine, SUFentanil, tacrolimus, teniposide, theophylline, thiotepa, ticarcillin/clavulanate, tigecycline, tirofiban, tobramycin, topotecan, trimethobenzamide, trimethoprim/sulfamethoxazole, vancomycin, vasopressin, vecuronium, verapamil, vinBLAStine, vinCRIStine, vinorelbine, zidovudine

SIDE EFFECTS

CNS: *Headache, dizziness, drowsiness, fatigue, insomnia*
GI: *Diarrhea, constipation,* abdominal pain
MISC: Weakness, hyperkalemia, anxiety, rash, bronchospasm (rare), arthralgia, *fever, urinary retention*

PHARMACOKINETICS

62% protein bound; metabolized by liver; unchanged product and metabolites excreted by kidney; terminal elimination half-life 40 hr

INTERACTIONS

- Possible QT prolongation: class 1A antidysrhythmics (disopyramide, procainamide, quiNIDine), class III antidysrhythmics (amiodarone, dofetilide, ibutilide, sotalol), chloroquine, clarithromycin, droperidol, erythromycin, haloperidol, levomethadyl, methadone, pentamidine, some phenothiazines, diuretics (except potassium sparing)

NURSING CONSIDERATIONS

Assess:
- For agents that cause QT prolongation, even if manufacturer has removed QT prolongation from warnings
- Absence of nausea, vomiting during chemotherapy
- **Hypersensitivity reaction:** rash, bronchospasm (rare)

Perform/provide:
- Storage at room temp

Evaluate:
- Therapeutic response: absence of nausea, vomiting during cancer chemotherapy, postoperatively

Teach patient/family:
- To report diarrhea, constipation, rash, changes in respirations, or discomfort at insertion site
- To avoid alcohol, barbiturates

pamidronate (Rx)

(pam-i-drone′ate)

Aredia

Func. class.: Bone-resorption inhibitor, electrolyte modifier
Chem. class.: Bisphosphonate

Do not confuse:
Aredia/Adriamycin

ACTION:
Inhibits bone resorption, apparently without inhibiting bone formation and mineralization; adsorbs calcium phosphate crystals in bone and may directly block the dissolution of hydroxyapatite crystals of bone

USES:
Moderate to severe Paget's disease, hypercalcemia, osteolytic bone metastases in breast cancer, patients with multiple myeloma

Unlabeled uses: Postmenopausal osteoporosis and prevention, osteoporosis prophylaxis, ankylosing spondylitis, osteogenesis imperfecta, hyperparathyroidism

CONTRAINDICATIONS:
Pregnancy (D), hypersensitivity to bisphosphonates

Precautions: Children, nursing mothers, renal dysfunction, poor dentition

DOSAGE AND ROUTES

Hypercalcemia of malignancy

• **Adult: IV INF** 60-90 mg as single dose for moderate hypercalcemia, 90 mg for severe hypercalcemia over 2-24 hr; dose should be diluted in 1000 ml 0.45% NaCl, 0.9% NaCl, or D_5W; wait 7 days before 2nd course

Osteolytic lesions

• **Adult: IV** 90 mg/500 ml of D_5W, 0.45% NaCl, or 0.9% NaCl given over 4 hr each mo (multiple myeloma) or over 2 hr q3-4wk (breast carcinoma)

Paget's disease

• **Adult: IV INF** 30 mg/day given over 4 hr × 3 days

Severe osteogenesis imperfecta (unlabeled)

• **Child: IV** 1.5-3 mg/kg/cycle, cycle dose is divided in 3, administered via slow IV over 4 hr/day × 3 days

Hypercalcemia (hyperparathyroidism) (unlabeled)

• **Adult: IV** 15-60 mg as a single dose

Corticosteroid-induced osteoporosis (unlabeled)

• **Adult: IV** 30 mg q3mo × 1 yr

Ankylosing spondylitis (unlabeled)

• **Adult: IV INF** 60 mg over 4 hr; 6-hr inf for 1st dose

Osteoporosis prophylaxis in Crohn's disease (unlabeled)

• **Adult: IV INF** 30 mg over 1 hr q3mo × 1 yr

Available forms: Powder for inj 30, 90 mg/vial; inj 3, 6, 9 mg/ml

Administer:

IV route

• After reconstituting by adding 10 ml sterile water for inj to each vial (30 mg/10 ml or 90 mg/10 ml, depending on vial used); add to 1000 ml of sterile 0.45%, 0.9% NaCl, D_5W, run over 2-24 hr **(hypercalcemia);** dilute reconstituted sol in 500 ml of 0.9% NaCl, 0.45% NaCl, or D_5W, give over 4 hr **(multiple myeloma, Paget's disease);** dilute reconstituted sol in 250 ml of 0.9% NaCl, 0.45% NaCl, or D_5W, give over 2 hr **(osteolytic bone metastases of breast cancer)**

• Do not mix with calcium-containing inf sol such as Ringer's sol

Y-site compatibilities: Acyclovir, alfentanil, allopurinol, amifostine, amikacin, aminocaproic acid, aminophylline, amphotericin B lipid complex, amphotericin B liposome, ampicillin, anidulafungin, atenolol, atracurium, azithromycin, aztreonam, bivalirudin, bleomycin, bumetanide, buprenorphine, butorphanol, CARBOplatin, carmustine, ceFAZolin, cefepime, cefoperazone, cefotaxime, cefotetan, cefoxitin, ceftazidime, ceftizoxime, cefTRIAXone, cefuroxime, chloramphenicol, chlorproMAZINE, cimetidine, ciprofloxacin, cisatracurium, CISplatin, clindamycin, cyclophosphamide, cycloSPORINE, cytarabine, dacarbazine, DAPTOmycin, dexamethasone, dexmedetomidine, dexrazoxane, digoxin, diltiazem, diphenhydrAMINE, DOBUTamine, docetaxel, dolasetron, DOPamine, doxacurium, DOXOrubicin, doxycycline, droperidol, enalaprilat, ePHEDrine, EPINEPHrine, epirubicin, ertapenem, erythromycin, esmolol, etoposide, famotidine, fenoldopam, fentaNYL, fluconazole, fludarabine, fluorouracil, foscarnet, fosphenytoin, furosemide, gallium, ganciclovir, gatifloxacin, gemcitabine, gentamicin, glycopyrrolate, granisetron, haloperidol, heparin, hetastarch 6%, hydrALAZINE, hydrocortisone, HYDROmorphone, hydrOXYzine, ifosfamide, imipenem-cilastatin, inamrinone, insulin (regular), isoproterenol, ketorolac, labetalol, levofloxacin, levorphanol, lidocaine, linezolid, LORazepam, magnesium sulfate, mannitol, mechlorethamine, melphalan, meperidine, meropenem, mesna, metaraminol, methotrexate, methyldopate, methylPREDNISolone, metoclopramide, metoprolol, metroNIDAZOLE, midazolam, milrinone, minocycline, mitoxantrone, mivacurium, morphine, mycophenolate, nafcillin, nalbuphine, naloxone, nesiritide, niCARdipine, nitroglycerin, nitroprusside, norepinephrine,

P

octreotide, ondansetron, oxytocin, paclitaxel, palonosetron, pancuronium, pemetrexed, pentamidine, pentazocine, PENTobarbital, PHENobarbital, phenylephrine, piperacillin, polymyxin B, potassium chloride/phosphates, procainamide, prochlorperazine, promethazine, propranolol, quiNIDine, quinupristin-dalfopristin, ranitidine, remifentanil, rocuronium, sodium acetate/bicarbonate/phosphates, succinylcholine, SUFentanil, sulfamethoxazole-trimethoprim, teniposide, theophylline, thiopental, thiotepa, ticarcillin, ticarcillin-clavulanate, tigecycline, tirofiban, tobramycin, tolazoline, topotecan, trimethobenzamide, vancomycin, vasopressin, vecuronium, verapamil, vinBLAStine, vinCRIStine, vinorelbine, voriconazole, zidovudine

SIDE EFFECTS

CNS: Fever, fatigue
CV: Hypertension, **atrial fibrillation**
EENT: Ocular pain, inflammation, vision impairment
GI: Abdominal pain, anorexia, constipation, nausea, vomiting, dyspepsia
GU: **Renal failure**
INTEG: Redness, swelling, induration, pain on palpation at site of catheter insertion
META: Anemia, *hypokalemia, hypomagnesemia, hypophosphatemia, hypocalcemia,* hypothyroidism
MS: Severe bone pain, myalgia, osteonecrosis of the jaw
RESP: Coughing, dyspnea, upper respiratory tract infection
SYST: **Angioedema, anaphylaxis**

PHARMACOKINETICS

Rapidly cleared from circulation and taken up mainly by bones, primarily in areas of high bone turnover; eliminated primarily by kidneys; half-life 21-35 hr, terminal half-life in bone is 300 days

INTERACTIONS

Increase: hypokalemia—loop diuretics
Increase: nephrotoxicity—aminoglycosides, NSAIDs, vancomycin, radiopaque contrast agents, cycloSPORINE, tacrolimus
Increase: effect of entecavir
Decrease: pamidronate effect—calcium, vit D

NURSING CONSIDERATIONS

Assess:

- **Dental health;** cover with antiinfectives for dental extractions
- Atrial fibrillation
- Electrolytes, calcium, magnesium, phosphate
- **Hypocalcemia:** nausea, vomiting, constipation, thirst, dysrhythmias, hypocalcemia, paresthesia, twitching, laryngospasm, Chvostek's sign, Trousseau's sign; **hypercalcemia:** thirst, nausea, vomiting, dysrhythmias
- Bone pain; use analgesics
- I&O, check for fluid overload edema, crackles, increased B/P; BUN, creatinine

Perform/provide:

- Storage of inf sol up to 24 hr at room temp
- Reconstituted sol with sterile water may be refrigerated for ≤24 hr

Evaluate:

- Therapeutic response: decreased calcium levels

Teach patient/family

- To report hypercalcemic relapse: nausea, vomiting, bone pain, thirst; unusual muscle twitching, muscle spasms; severe diarrhea, constipation
- To continue with dietary recommendations, including calcium and vit D
- To obtain analgesic from provider for bone pain
- That, if nausea, vomiting occur, small, frequent meals may help
- To report ocular symptoms to prescriber: blurred vision, edema, inflammation

pancrelipase (Rx)

(pan-kre-li′pase)

Cotazym-65B ✦, Creon, Creon Mini Microspheres; DMH ✦, Dygase, Lipram, Lipram-CR, Lipram-CR5, Lipram-PN, Lipram-PN10, Lipram-UL, Lipram-UL20, Pancrease ✦, Pancreaze, Panrecarb MS, Ultrase, Ultrase MT, Viokase, Zenpep

Func. class.: Digestant

Chem. class.: Pancreatic enzyme—bovine/porcine

ACTION: Pancreatic enzyme needed for the breakdown of substances released from the pancreas

USES: Exocrine pancreatic secretion insufficiency, cystic fibrosis (digestive aid), steatorrhea, pancreatic enzyme deficiency

CONTRAINDICATIONS: Allergy to pork

Precautions: Pregnancy (B), ileus, pancreatitis, Crohn's disease

DOSAGE AND ROUTES

Many products listed above are not interchangeable

• **Adult/adolescent/child ≥4 yr (del rel caps: Creon Caps, Zenpap Caps, Pancreaze Caps): PO** 500 lipase units/kg/meal, titrate based on patient response, max 2500 lipase units/kg/meal

• **Child 1-4 yr: PO** 1000 lipase units/kg/meal, titrate based on patient response, max 2500 lipase units/kg/meal

Available forms: Powder 16,800 units lipase/70,000 units protease and amylase; caps 8000 units lipase/30,000 units protease and amylase; del rel cap 4000 units lipase/12,000 units protease and amylase, 4000 units lipase/25,000 units protease/20,000 units amylase, 5000 units lipase/20,000 units protease and amylase, 10,000 units lipase/30,000 units protease and amylase, 12,000 units lipase/24,000 units protease and amylase, 12,000 units lipase/39,000 units protease and amylase, 16,000 units lipase/48,000 units protease and amylase, 20,000 units lipase/65,000 units protease and amylase, 24,000 units lipase/78,000 units protease and amylase; del rel cap 5000, 15,000 units

Administer:

• Avoid inhaling powder

• After antacid or cimetidine; decreased pH inactivates product

• Powder mixed in prepared fruit juice for infants, children

• Low-fat diet for GI symptoms

• With ≥8 oz water; do not allow to sit in mouth; have patient sit up during administration; give with meals

SIDE EFFECTS

GI: Anorexia, nausea, vomiting, diarrhea, cramping, bloating

GU: Hyperuricuria, hyperuricemia

INTERACTIONS

Decrease: absorption—cimetidine, antacids, oral iron

Decrease: effect of acarbose, miglitol

NURSING CONSIDERATIONS

Assess:

• Appropriate height, weight development prior to and periodically; may be delayed

• I&O ratio; watch for increasing urinary output

• Fecal fat, nitrogen, PT during treatment

• **(Diabetes mellitus)** for polyuria, polydipsia, polyphagia

• Pork sensitivity; cross-sensitivity may occur

Perform/provide:

• Adequate hydration

• Storage in tight container at room temp

Evaluate:

- Therapeutic response: improved digestion of carbohydrates, protein, fat; absence of steatorrhea

Teach patient/family:

- Not to inhale powder; may be very irritating to mucous membranes; some powder may irritate skin
- To notify prescriber of allergic reactions, abdominal pain, cramping, or blood in urine

⚠ HIGH ALERT

pancuronium (Rx)

(pan-kyoo-roe′nee-um)

Func. class.: Neuromuscular blocker (nondepolarizing)

Chem. class.: Synthetic curariform

ACTION: Inhibits transmission of nerve impulses by binding with cholinergic receptor sites, antagonizing action of acetylcholine

USES: Facilitation of endotracheal intubation, skeletal muscle relaxation during mechanical ventilation, surgery, or general anesthesia

CONTRAINDICATIONS: Hypersensitivity to bromide ion

Precautions: Pregnancy (C), breastfeeding, children <2 yr, neuromuscular/cardiac/renal/hepatic disease, electrolyte imbalances, dehydration, previous anaphylactic reactions (other neuromuscular blockers)

Black Box Warning: Respiratory insufficiency

DOSAGE AND ROUTES

- **Adult/child/infant >1 mo: IV** 0.04-0.1 mg/kg initially or 0.05 mg/kg after initial dose of succinylcholine; maintenance 0.01 mg/kg 60-100 min after initial dose then 0.01 mg/kg q25-60min as needed; for obese patients, use ideal body weight
- **Neonate <1 mo: IV** Test dose 0.02 mg/kg then 0.03 mg/kg/dose initially, repeat 2× as needed at 5-10 min intervals; maintenance 0.03-0.09 mg/kg/dose q30min-4 hr as needed

Available forms: Inj 1, 2 mg/ml

Administer:

Direct IV route

- May be given undiluted over 1-2 min (1 mg/ml [10-ml vial], 2 mg/ml [2-, 5-ml vial])

Intermittent IV INF route

- Add 100 mg of product to 250 ml D_5W, NS, LR (0.4 mg/ml)

Additive compatibilities: Verapamil, ciprofloxacin

Y-site compatibilities: Aminophylline, ceFAZolin, cefuroxime, cimetidine, DOBUTamine, DOPamine, EPINEPHrine, esmolol, fenoldopam, fentaNYL, fluconazole, gentamicin, heparin, hydrocortisone, isoproterenol, levofloxacin, LORazepam, midazolam, morphine, nitroglycerin, ranitidine, trimethoprim-sulfamethoxazole, vancomycin

SIDE EFFECTS

CV: Bradycardia; tachycardia; increased, decreased B/P; ventricular extrasystoles, edema, hypertension

EENT: Increased secretions

INTEG: Rash, flushing, pruritus, urticaria, sweating, salivation

MS: Weakness to prolonged skeletal muscle relaxation

RESP: Prolonged apnea, bronchospasm, cyanosis, respiratory depression, dyspnea

SYST: Anaphylaxis

PHARMACOKINETICS

IV: Onset 3-5 min, dose dependent, peak 3-5 min; metabolized (small amounts), excreted in urine (unchanged), crosses placenta

INTERACTIONS

- Dysrhythmias: theophylline

Increase: neuromuscular blockade—aminoglycosides, clindamycin, enflurane, isoflurane, lincomycin, lithium, local anesthetics, opioid analgesics, polymyxin antiinfectives, quiNIDine, thiazides

Drug/Lab Test

Decrease: cholinesterase

NURSING CONSIDERATIONS

Assess:

- **Respiratory recovery:** decreased paralysis of face, diaphragm, leg, arm, rest of body; allow to recover fully before neurologic assessment
- Electrolyte imbalances (K, Mg); may lead to increased action of product
- VS (B/P, pulse, respirations, airway) until fully recovered; rate, depth, pattern of respirations, strength of hand grip
- I&O ratio; check for urinary retention, frequency, hesitancy

Allergic reactions, anaphylaxis: rash, fever, respiratory distress, pruritus; product should be discontinued

Perform/provide:

- Storage in refrigerator; do not store in plastic; use only fresh sol
- Reassurance if communication is difficult during recovery from neuromuscular blockade
- Frequent (q2hr) instillation of artificial tears, covering of eyes to prevent drying of cornea

Evaluate:

- Therapeutic response: paralysis of jaw, eyelid, head, neck, rest of body

TREATMENT OF OVERDOSE:

Neostigmine, atropine, monitor VS; may require mechanical ventilation

panitumumab (Rx)

(pan-i-tue′moo-mab)

Vectibix

Func. class.: Antineoplastic—miscellaneous

Chem. class.: Multikinase inhibitor, signal transduction inhibitor

ACTION: Decreases growth and survival of cancer cells by competitive inhibition of EGF receptor

USES: EGFR expressing metastatic colorectal cancer; not beneficial with KRAS mutations in codon 12 or 13

CONTRAINDICATIONS: Hypersensitivity

Precautions: Pregnancy (C), breastfeeding, children, hepatic disease, acute bronchospasm, diarrhea, hamster protein allergy, hypomagnesemia, hypotension, pulmonary fibrosis, sepsis, KRAS mutations

Black Box Warning: Exfoliative dermatitis, infusion-related reactions

DOSAGE AND ROUTES

- **Adult: IV INF** 6 mg/kg over 60 min every 2 wk; doses >1000 mg over 90 min

Available forms: Sol for inj 20 mg/ml

Administer:

Intermittent IV INF route

- Give in hospital or clinic setting with full resuscitation equipment
- Only as IV inf using controlled IV inf pump; do not give IV push or bolus; use low-protein binding 0.2- or 0.22-micron in-line filter; flush line with 0.9% NaCl before and after administration
- Give over 60 min through a peripheral line or indwelling catheter; infuse doses of >1000 mg over 90 min
- Dilute in 100 ml of 0.9% NaCl; dilute doses >1000 mg in 150 ml of 0.9% NaCl; mix by inverting; do not exceed 10

mg/ml; use within 6 hr if stored at room temp; can be stored between 2° C and 8° C for up to 24 hr

SIDE EFFECTS

CNS: Fatigue
CV: Peripheral edema
EENT: Ocular irritation, ocular toxicity
GI: *Nausea, diarrhea, vomiting,* anorexia, mouth ulceration, abdominal pain, constipation
HEMA: Thrombophlebitis
INTEG: *Rash,* pruritus, exfoliative dermatitis, skin fissure, angioedema, severe/fatal INF reactions
META: Hypocalcemia, hypomagnesemia, antibody formation
RESP: Bronchospasm, cough, dyspnea, hypoxia, pulmonary fibrosis/embolism, pneumonitis, wheezing

PHARMACOKINETICS

Bioavailability 38%-49%; elimination half-life 7.5 days; peak 3 hr; high-fat meal decreases bioavailability; plasma protein binding 99.5%; metabolized in liver; oxidative metabolism by CYP3A4, glucuronidation by UGT1A9; 77% excreted in feces

INTERACTIONS

• Do not use in combination with other antineoplastics

NURSING CONSIDERATIONS

Assess:

Black Box Warning: Serious skin disorders: fever, sore throat, fatigue, then lesions in mouth, lips; withhold product, notify prescriber

• Serum electrolytes periodically (calcium, magnesium)
• **Infection:** increased temp

Black Box Warning: Inf reactions: bronchospasm, fever, chills, hypotension; may require discontinuation, have emergency equipment available

• **Ocular toxicity:** ocular irritation, hyperemia
• **Pulmonary fibrosis:** dyspnea, cough, wheezing; may require discontinuation

Perform/provide:

• Storage of unopened vials in refrigerator; do not shake; protect from direct sunlight; do not freeze

Evaluate:

• Therapeutic response: decrease in colon carcinoma progression

Teach patient/family:

⚠ To report adverse reactions immediately: difficulty breathing, mouth sores, skin rash, ocular toxicity
• About reason for treatment, expected results, adverse reactions
• To use contraception while taking product, for 6 mo after treatment; not to breastfeed for ≥2 mo after stopping treatment
• To avoid the sun, use sunscreen while taking product

pantoprazole (Rx)

(pan-toe-pray′zole)

Panto ✱, Pantoloc ✱, Protonix, Prontonix IV

Func. class.: Proton pump inhibitor
Chem. class.: Benzimidazole

ACTION:
Suppresses gastric secretion by inhibiting hydrogen/potassium ATPase enzyme system in gastric parietal cell; characterized as gastric acid pump inhibitor because it blocks the final step of acid production

USES:
Gastroesophageal reflux disease (GERD), severe erosive esophagitis; maintenance of long-term pathologic hypersecretory conditions, including Zollinger-Ellison syndrome

Unlabeled uses: Duodenal/gastric ulcer, NSAID ulcer prophylaxis, *Helicobacter-pylori*–associated ulcer, dyspepsia

CONTRAINDICATIONS:
Hypersensitivity to this product or benzimidazole

Precautions: Pregnancy (C), breastfeeding, children, proton pump hypersensitivity

DOSAGE AND ROUTES

GERD

• **Adult: PO** 40 mg/day × 8 wk, may repeat course

Erosive esophagitis

• **Adult: IV** 40 mg/day × 7-10 day; **PO** 40 mg/day × 8 wk; may repeat **PO** course

Pathologic hypersecretory conditions

• **Adult: PO** 40 mg bid; **IV** 80 mg q12hr, max 240 mg/day

Duodenal ulcer/gastric ulcer/ NSAID ulcer prophylaxis (unlabeled)

• **Adult: PO** 40 mg/day

***H. pylori*–associated ulcers (unlabeled)**

• **Adult: PO** 40 mg bid; may be used with other products

Available forms: Del rel tabs 20, 40 mg; powder for inj 40 mg/vial; del rel granules for susp 40 mg

Administer:

PO route

• Swallow del rel tabs whole; do not break, crush, or chew; take del rel tabs at same time of day

• May take with/without food

IV route

• Reconstitute each 40-mg vial with 10 ml 0.9% NaCl

Direct IV route

• Give undiluted (4 mg/mL) over ≥2 min

Intermittent IV INF route

• Further dilute with D_5W, 0.9% NaCl, LR (0.4-0.8 mg/ml), give over 15 min (<3 mg/min)

Y-site compatibilities: Acyclovir, allopurinol, amifostine, amikacin, aminocaproic acid, aminophylline, amoxicillin-clavulanate, amphotericin B liposome, ampicillin, ampicillin-sulbactam, anidulafungin, azithromycin, bleomycin, bumetanide, calcium gluconate, CARBOplatin, carmustine, cefazolin, cefoxitin, ceftazidime, ceftizoxime, cefTRIAXone, cefuroxime, clindamycin, cyclophosphamide, cycloSPORINE, cytarabine, dextrose 3.3% in sodium chloride 0.3%, digoxin, dimenhyDRINATE, docetaxel, DOPamine, doripenem, doxycycline, enalaprilat, EPINEPHrine, ertapenem, fluorouracil, foscarnet, fosphenytoin, furosemide, ganciclovir, gentamicin, granisetron, heparin, hydrocortisone HYDROmorphone, imipenem-cilastatin, inamrinone, insulin (regular), irinotecan, isoproterenol, magnesium, mannitol, mesna, methohexital, methyldopate, metoclopramide, nafcillin, nitroglycerin, nitroprusside, ofloxacin, oxytocin, paclitaxel, pentazocine, PENTobarbital, phenylephrine, piperacillin-tazobactam, potassium chloride, procainamide, rifampin, sodium bicarbonate, succinylcholine, SUFentanil, sulfamethoxazole-trimethoprim, teniposide, theophylline, thiopental, ticarcillin, ticarcillin-clavulanate, tigecycline, tirofiban, tobramycin, tramadol, vasopressin, zidovudine

SIDE EFFECTS

CNS: *Headache,* insomnia

GI: *Diarrhea, abdominal pain,* flatulence, **pancreatitis**

INTEG: *Rash*

META: Hyperglycemia, weight gain/loss, hyponatremia, hypomagnesemia

MS: **Rhabdomyolysis**, myalgia

RESP: **Pneumonia**

SYST: **Stevens-Johnson syndrome, toxic epidermal necrolysis, anaphylaxis, angioedema**

PHARMACOKINETICS

Peak 2.4 hr, duration >24 hr, half-life 1.5 hr, protein binding 97%, eliminated in urine as metabolites and in feces; in geriatric patients, elimination rate decreased; some Asian patients (15%-20%) may be poor metabolizers

P

INTERACTIONS

Increase: pantoprazole serum levels—diazepam, phenytoin, flurazepam, triazolam, clarithromycin
Increase: bleeding—warfarin
Decrease: absorption—sucralfate, calcium carbonate, vit B_{12}, ketoconazole, itraconazole, atazanavir, ampicillin, iron salts
Decrease: clopidogrel effect

NURSING CONSIDERATIONS

Assess:

- **GI system:** bowel sounds q8hr; abdomen for pain, swelling; anorexia
- **Hepatic studies:** AST, ALT, alk phos during treatment
- For vit B_{12} deficiency in patients receiving long-term therapy

▲ **Serious skin reactions:** toxic epidermal necrolysis, Stevens-Johnson syndrome, exfoliative dermatitis: fever, sore throat, fatigue, thin ulcers; lesions in the mouth, lips

- **Electrolyte imbalances:** hyponatremia; hypomagnesemia in patients using product 3 mo to 1 year; if hypomagnesemia occurs, use of magnesium supplements may be sufficient; if severe, discontinuation of product may be required

▲ **Rhabdomyolysis, myalgia:** muscle pain, increased CPK; weakness, swelling of affected muscles

Evaluate:

- Therapeutic response: absence of epigastric pain, swelling, fullness

Teach patient/family:

- To report severe diarrhea; black, tarry stools; abdominal pain; product may have to be discontinued
- That hyperglycemia may occur in diabetic patients
- To avoid alcohol, salicylates, NSAIDs; may cause GI irritation
- To notify prescriber if pregnant or planning to become pregnant; not to breastfeed
- To continue taking even if feeling better

paricalcitol (Rx)

(par-ih-cal′sih-tol)

Zemplar

Func. class.: Vit D analog
Chem. class.: Fat-soluble vitamin

ACTION:
Reduces parathyroid hormone (PTH) levels; suppresses PTH levels in patients with chronic renal failure with absence of hypercalcemia/hyperphosphatemia; serum PO_4, calcium, CaXP may increase

USES:
Hyperparathyroidism in chronic renal failure
Unlabeled uses: Renal osteodystrophy

CONTRAINDICATIONS:
Hypersensitivity, hypercalcemia
Precautions: Pregnancy (C), breastfeeding, children, geriatric patients, CV disease, renal calculi

DOSAGE AND ROUTES

- **Adult: IV BOL** 0.04-0.1 mcg/kg (2.8-7 mcg) no more than every other day during dialysis; may increase by 2-4 mcg q2-4wk until target serum intact PTH (1.5−3× nonuremic upper limit of normal) achieved; **PO** 1 mcg/day or 2 mcg 3×/wk (IPTH ≤500 pg/ml); 2 mcg/day or 4 mcg 3×/wk (IPTH >500 pg/ml)

Available forms: Inj 2, 5 mcg/ml; caps 1, 2, 4 mcg

Administer:

PO route

- Daily or 3×/wk; may give without regard to food

IV route

- By IV bolus only

SIDE EFFECTS

CNS: Lightheadedness
CV: Palpitations
GI: Nausea, vomiting, anorexia, dry mouth
OTHER: Pneumonia, edema, chills, fever, flu, sepsis

PHARMACOKINETICS

Crosses placenta, enters breast milk

INTERACTIONS

Decrease: paricalcitol effect—cholestyramine, colestipol, mineral oil, orlistat, corticosteroids, barbiturates, hydantoins, CYP3A4 enzymes (nevirapine, rifampin, bosentan)
Increase: calcium levels—thiazide diuretics, calcium products, vit D supplements
Increase: effect of cardiac glycosides
Altered: paricalcitol effect—CYP3A4 inhibitors (amiodarone, protease inhibitors, systemic azole antifungals, chloramphenicol, clarithromycin, delavirdine, erythromycin)

NURSING CONSIDERATIONS

Assess:

- **Hypocalcemia:** twitching, dysrhythmias, Chvostek's/Trousseu's signs, paresthesia, laryngospasm, prolonged QTc/ST interval
- Serum calcium, serum intact parathyroid hormone concentrations (iPTH), phosphate 2×/wk during initial therapy; after dose is established, take calcium and phosphorus monthly

Evaluate:

- Decreased hypoparathyroidism with chronic renal disease, normal serum calcium, phosphate, iPTH

Teach patient/family:

- To report weakness, lethargy, headache, anorexia, loss of weight
- To report nausea, vomiting, palpitations
- To adhere to dietary regimen of calcium supplementation/phosphorus restriction
- To avoid excessive use of aluminum compounds, antacids
- Not to breastfeed
- Not to take mineral oil, antacids (magnesium) while taking vit D

PARoxetine (Rx)

(par-ox′e-teen)

Paxil, Paxil CR, Pexeva, Sandoz PARoxetine ✤

Func. class.: Antidepressant, SSRI
Chem. class.: Phenylpiperidine derivative

Do not confuse:
PARoxetine/paclitaxel
Paxil/paclitaxel/Taxol

ACTION: Inhibits CNS neuron uptake of serotonin but not of norepinephrine or dopamine

USES: Major depressive disorder, obsessive-compulsive disorder, panic disorder, generalized anxiety disorder, posttraumatic stress disorder, premenstrual disorders, social anxiety disorder
Unlabeled uses: Premature ejaculation, hot flashes, menopause

CONTRAINDICATIONS: Pregnancy (D), hypersensitivity, MAOI use, alcohol use
Precautions: Breastfeeding, geriatric patients, seizure history; patients with history of mania, renal/hepatic disease

Black Box Warning: Children, suicidal ideation

DOSAGE AND ROUTES

Generalized anxiety disorder

- **Adult: PO** 20 mg/day in AM, range 20-50 mg/day

Posttraumatic stress disorder

- **Adult: PO** 20 mg/day, range 20-60 mg/day

Depression

- **Adult: PO** 20 mg/day in AM; after 4 wk, if no clinical improvement is noted, dose may be increased by 10 mg/day each wk to desired response, max 50 mg/day or **CONT REL** 25 mg/day, may increase by 12.5 mg/day/wk up to 62.5 mg/day
- **Geriatric: PO** 10 mg/day, increase by 10 mg to desired dose, max 40 mg/day

Obsessive-compulsive disorder
- **Adult: PO** 40 mg/day in AM, start with 20 mg/day, increase in 10-mg/day increments, max 60 mg/day

Panic disorder
- **Adult: PO** Start with 10 mg/day, increase in 10-mg/day increments to 40 mg/day, max 60 mg/day or **CONT REL** 12.5 mg/day, max 75 mg/day

Premenstrual disorders
- **Adult: CONT REL** 12.5 mg/day in AM

Renal dose
- **Adult: PO** CCr 30-60 ml/min, lower doses may be needed; CCr <30 ml/min, 10 mg/day initially, regular rel, max 40 mg/day; **CONT REL** 12.5 mg/day initially, max 50 mg/day

Hepatic dose
- **Adult: PO** 10 mg/day initially, max 40 mg **regular rel;** 12.5 mg/day initially, max 50 mg/day **(cont rel)**

Menopause symptoms/hot flashes (unlabeled)
- **Adult: PO (CONT REL)** 12.5 mg/day, may increase to 25 mg/day after 1 wk

Premature ejaculation (unlabeled)
- **Adult: PO** 20 mg/day

Available forms: Tabs 10, 20, 30, 40 mg; oral susp 10 mg/5 ml; cont rel tab 12.5, 25, 37.5 mg

Administer:
- Do not substitute Pexeva with Paxil, Paxil CR, or generic PARoxetine
- Increased fluids, bulk in diet for constipation, urinary retention
- With food, milk for GI symptoms
- Crushed if patient is unable to swallow medication whole (regular rel only)
- Gum, hard candy, frequent sips of water for dry mouth
- Avoid use with other CNS depressants
- **Oral susp:** shake, measure with oral syringe or calibrated measuring device
- **Cont rel tab:** do not cut, chew, crush; do not give concurrently with antacids

SIDE EFFECTS

CNS: *Headache,* nervousness, insomnia, *drowsiness, anxiety, tremor, dizziness,* fatigue, *sedation,* abnormal dreams, agitation, apathy, euphoria, hallucinations, delusions, psychosis, **seizures, neuroleptic-malignant-syndrome–like reactions,** restless leg syndrome

CV: Vasodilation, postural hypotension, palpitations

EENT: Visual changes

GI: *Nausea, diarrhea, dry mouth,* anorexia, dyspepsia, *constipation,* cramps, vomiting, taste changes, flatulence, decreased appetite

GU: Dysmenorrhea, decreased libido, urinary frequency, UTI, amenorrhea, cystitis, impotence; decreased sperm quality, decreased fertility, *abnormal ejaculation (male)*

INTEG: *Sweating,* rash

MS: Pain, arthritis, myalgia, myopathy, myosthenia

RESP: Infection, pharyngitis, nasal congestion, sinus headache, sinusitis, cough, dyspnea, yawning

SYST: Asthenia, fever, abrupt withdrawal syndrome

PHARMACOKINETICS

PO: Peak 5.2 hr, ext rel peak 6-10 hr; metabolized in liver by CYP2D6 enzyme system, unchanged products and metabolites excreted in feces and urine; half-life 21 hr (reg rel); 15-20 hr (cont rel); protein binding 95%

INTERACTIONS

⚠ **Increase:** **serotonin syndrome—SSRIs, SNRIs, atypical psychotics, serotonin-receptor agonists, tricyclics, amphetamines, methylphenidate, tramadol**

Decrease: level of digoxin

⚠ **Do not use with MAOIs, pimozide, thioridazine; potentially fatal reactions can occur**

Increase: bleeding—NSAIDs, thrombolytics, salicylates, platelet inhibitors, anticoagulants

Increase: PARoxetine plasma levels—cimetidine

Increase: agitation—L-tryptophan

Increase: side effects—highly protein-bound products

Increase: theophylline levels—theophylline

Increase: toxicity—CYP2D6 inhibitors (aprepitant, delavirdine, imatinib, nefazodone)

Decrease: PARoxetine levels—PHENObarbital and phenytoin

Drug/Herb

- Avoid use with St. John's wort, kava
- Possible serotonin syndrome: St. John's wort
- Hypertensive crisis: ephedra

Drug/Lab Test

Increase: serum bilirubin, blood glucose, alk phos

Decrease: VMA, 5-HIAA

False increase: urinary catecholamines

NURSING CONSIDERATIONS

Assess:

Black Box Warning: Depression/OCD/anxiety/panic attacks: mental status: mood, sensorium, affect, suicidal tendencies (especially in child/young adult), increase in psychiatric symptoms, decreasing obsessive thoughts, compulsive behaviors, restrict amount available

- **Postural hypotension:** B/P (lying/standing), pulse q4hr; if systolic B/P drops 20 mm Hg, hold product, notify prescriber; take vital signs q4hr for patients with CV disease
- Hepatic/renal studies: AST, ALT, bilirubin, creatinine
- Weight weekly; appetite may decrease with product, constipation
- ECG for flattening of T wave, bundle branch or AV block, dysrhythmias in cardiac patients
- EPS, primarily in geriatric patients: rigidity, dystonia, akathisia
- **Renal status:** BUN, creatinine, urinary retention
- **Withdrawal symptoms:** headache, nausea, vomiting, muscle pain, weakness; not usual unless product discontinued abruptly
- Alcohol intake; if alcohol is consumed, hold dose until morning

⚠ **Serotonin, neuroleptic malignant syndrome:** hallucinations, coma, headache, agitation, shivering, sweating, tachycardia, diarrhea, tremor, hypertension, hyperthermia, rigidity, delirium, coma, myoclonus, agitation, nausea, vomiting

Perform/provide:

- Storage at room temp; do not freeze
- Assistance with ambulation during therapy because drowsiness, dizziness occur
- Safety measures, primarily for geriatric patients

Evaluate:

- Therapeutic response: decreased depression

Teach patient/family:

- That therapeutic effect may take 1-4 wk
- To use caution when driving, performing other activities requiring alertness because of drowsiness, dizziness, blurred vision
- Not to discontinue medication quickly after long-term use; may cause nausea, headache, malaise (abrupt withdrawal syndrome)

Black Box Warning: That depression may worsen, suicidal thoughts/behaviors occur; to notify prescriber

- To avoid alcohol ingestion
- To report bleeding, headache, nausea, anxiety, or if depression continues
- To discuss sexual side effects: impotence, possible male infertility while taking product

TREATMENT OF OVERDOSE:

Gastric lavage, airway; for seizures, give diazepam, symptomatic treatment

P

⚠ HIGH ALERT

pegaspargase (Rx)

(peg-as′per-gase)

Oncaspar, PEG-L-asparaginase

Func. class.: Antineoplastic

Chem. class.: Escherichia coli enzyme

ACTION: Indirectly inhibits protein synthesis in tumor cells; without amino acid, DNA, RNA synthesis is halted; asparagine, protein synthesis is halted; G_1 phase; cell-cycle specific; nonvesicant; modified version of L-asparaginase

USES: Acute lymphocytic leukemia in combination with other antineoplastics

CONTRAINDICATIONS: Breastfeeding, infant, hypersensitivity, pancreatitis, acute bronchospasm, bleeding, coagulopathy, coronary thrombosis, DIC, hypotension

Precautions: Pregnancy (C), CNS/renal/hepatic disease, *Escherichia coli* protein hypersensitivity, hemophilia, tumor lysis syndrome, infection

DOSAGE AND ROUTES

In combination

- **Adult and child: IV/IM** 2500 international units/m^2 q14days, run **IV** over 1-2 hr in 100 ml of NaCl or D_5 through a running **IV**; **IM** should be no more than 2 ml in 1 inj site, used in combination with other chemotherapeutics

Available forms: Inj 750 international units/ml in phosphate-buffered saline sol

Administer:

- Use cytotoxic handling procedures
- Allopurinol or sodium bicarbonate to reduce uric acid levels, alkalinization of urine

IM route

- No dilution needed, inject in large muscle; do not give >2 ml in 1 inj site, aspirate; preferred route

Intermittent IV INF route

- Dilute contents of vial/100 ml NS or D_5W, give over 1-2 hr through freely running IV solution; keep refrigerated, do not freeze

SIDE EFFECTS

CNS: Neuritis, dizziness, headache, coma, depression, fatigue, confusion, hallucinations, seizures, intracranial bleeding

CV: Chest pain, hypotension

ENDO: Hyperglycemia

GI: *Nausea, vomiting, anorexia, cramps, stomatitis,* hepatotoxicity, pancreatitis, *diarrhea*

GU: Urinary retention, renal failure, glycosuria, polyuria, azotemia, uric acid neuropathy

HEMA: Thrombocytopenia, leukopenia, myelosuppression, anemia, decreased clotting factors, pancytopenia, DIC

INTEG: *Rash,* urticaria, chills, fever

RESP: Fibrosis, pulmonary infiltrate, severe bronchospasm

SYST: Anaphylaxis, hypersensitivity, angioedema

PHARMACOKINETICS

Half-life $5^1/_2$ days, onset rapid, duration 2 wk, metabolized in reticuloendothelial system

INTERACTIONS

Increase: hypoglycemia—corticosteroids

Increase: bleeding risk—heparin, warfarin, NSAIDs, salicylates, platelet inhibitors, thrombolytics

Decrease: action of methotrexate

Decrease: immune response—live virus vaccines

NURSING CONSIDERATIONS

Assess:

⚠ **Pancreatitis** (nausea, vomiting, severe abdominal pain), **anaphylaxis** (bronchospasm, dyspnea), cyanosis

- Baseline, periodic D-dimer, fibrinogen, serum albumin, thrombin time

• CBC, differential, platelet count weekly; withhold product if WBC count <4000 or platelet count <75,000; notify prescriber of results; RBC, Hct, Hgb; may be decreased
• Pulmonary function tests, chest x-ray studies before, during therapy; chest x-ray film should be obtained q2wk during treatment; watch for severe bronchospasm, fibrosis, pulmonary infiltrate
• Renal studies: BUN, serum uric acid, ammonia, urine CCr, electrolytes before, during therapy
• I&O ratio; report fall in urine output to ≤30 ml/hr, may indicate renal failure
• Temp q4hr (may indicate beginning infection)
• Hepatic studies before and during therapy (bilirubin, AST, ALT, LDH) as needed or monthly, hepatotoxicity can occur; check for jaundiced skin, sclera; dark urine, clay-colored stools, itchy skin, abdominal pain, fever, diarrhea; watch for pancreatitis
• Serum, urine glucose levels; glycosuria can occur
• Bleeding: hematuria, stool guaiac, bruising or petechiae, mucosa or orifices q8hr
• **Serious allergic reaction:** dyspnea, crackles, nonproductive cough, chest pain, tachypnea, fatigue, increased pulse, pallor, lethargy, swelling around eyes or lips; anaphylaxis may occur
• B/P because hypertension can occur
• Local irritation, pain, burning, discoloration at inj site
• Frequency of stools, characteristics; cramping, acidosis; signs of dehydration: rapid respirations, poor skin turgor, decreased urine output, dry skin, restlessness, weakness

Perform/provide:
• Increased fluid intake to 2-3 L/day to prevent urate deposits, calculi formation
• Warm compresses at inj site for inflammation

Evaluate:
• Therapeutic response: decreased exacerbations with acute lymphocytic leukemia

Teach patient/family:
• To report nausea, vomiting, bruising, bleeding, stomatitis, severe diarrhea, jaundice, chest pain, abdominal pain, trouble breathing, rash
• To avoid vaccinations without advice of prescriber
• To avoid OTC medications, alcohol

pegfilgrastim (Rx)

(peg-fill-grass′stim)

Neulasta

Func. class.: Hematopoietic agent
Chem. class.: Granulocyte colony-stimulating factor

ACTION: Stimulates proliferation and differentiation of neutrophils

USES: To decrease infection in patients receiving antineoplastics that are myelosuppressive; to increase WBC count in patients with product-induced neutropenia

CONTRAINDICATIONS: Hypersensitivity to proteins of *Escherichia coli,* filgrastim

Precautions: Pregnancy (C), breastfeeding, children <45 kg, adolescents, myeloid malignancies, sickle cell disease, leukocytosis, splenic rupture, ARDS, allergic-type reactions, peripheral blood stem cell (PBSC) mobilization

DOSAGE AND ROUTES

• **Adult: SUBCUT** 6 mg, give 1× per chemotherapy cycle

Available forms: Sol for inj 6 mg/0.6 ml

Administer:

SUBCUT route
• Using single-use vials; after dose is withdrawn, do not reenter vial
• Do not use 6-mg fixed dose in infants, children, or others <45 kg
• Inspect sol for discoloration, particulates; if present, do not use

P

• Do not administer during the period 14 days before and 24 hr after cytotoxic chemotherapy

SIDE EFFECTS

CNS: Fever, fatigue, headache, dizziness, insomnia, peripheral edema
GI: *Nausea,* vomiting, diarrhea, mucositis, anorexia, constipation, dyspepsia, abdominal pain, stomatitis, **splenic rupture**
HEMA: **Leukocytosis, granulocytopenia, sickle cell crisis, hemoglobin S disease with crisis**
INTEG: Alopecia
MISC: Chest pain, hyperuricemia, **anaphylaxis, influenza-like illness, angioedema, antibody formation**
MS: Skeletal pain
RESP: **Respiratory distress syndrome**

PHARMACOKINETICS

Half-life: 15-80 hr; 20-38 hr (children)

INTERACTIONS

• Do not use product concomitantly, 2 wk before, or 24 hr after administration of cytotoxic chemotherapy
Increase: release of neutrophils—lithium
Drug/Lab Test
Increase: uric acid, LDH, alk phos

NURSING CONSIDERATIONS

Assess:
⚠ **Allergic reactions, anaphylaxis: rash, urticaria; discontinue product, have emergency equipment nearby**
⚠ **ARDS: dyspnea, fever, tachypnea, occasionally confusion; obtain ABGs, chest x-ray; product may need to be discontinued**
• **Bone pain;** give mild analgesics
• Blood studies: CBC with differential, platelet count before treatment, 2× weekly; neutrophil counts may be increased for 2 days after therapy
• B/P, respirations, pulse before and during therapy
Perform/provide:
• Storage in refrigerator; do not freeze; may store at room temp up to 6 hr; avoid shaking, protect from light
Evaluate:
• Therapeutic response: absence of infection
Teach patient/family:
• How to perform the technique for self-administration if product to be given at home: dose, side effects, disposal of containers and needles; provide instruction sheet
• To notify prescriber immediately of allergic reaction, trouble breathing, abdominal pain

peginterferon alfa-2a (Rx)

(peg-in-ter-feer′on)
Pegasys

peginterferon alfa-2b (Rx)

PegIntron, SYLATRON
Func. class.: Immunomodulator

ACTION: Stimulates genes to modulate many biologic effects, including the inhibition of viral replication; inhibits ion cell proliferation, immunomodulation; stimulates effector proteins; decreases leukocyte, platelet counts

USES: Chronic hepatitis C infections in adults with compensated liver disease; chronic hepatitis B in adults who are HBe AG positive, HBe AG negative; HCV patients coinfected with HIV; nonresponders or relapsers with chronic hepatitis C, malignant melanoma
Unlabeled uses: Adenovirus, coronavirus, encephalomyocarditis virus, herpes simplex types 1 and 2, hepatitis D, acute hepatitis C, HIV, HPV, polio virus, rhinovirus, varicella-zoster, variola, vesicular stomatitis

⚠ Nurse Alert

CONTRAINDICATIONS:

Neonates, infants, sepsis; hypersensitivity to interferons, benzyl alcohol, *Escherichia coli* protein

Precautions: Pregnancy (C), breastfeeding, children <18 yr, geriatric patients, thyroid disorders, myelosuppression, renal/hepatic disease, suicidal/homicidal ideation, preexisting ophthalmologic disorders, pancreatitis, hemodialysis

Black Box Warning: Cardiac disease, depression, autoimmune disease, infection, use with ribavirin

DOSAGE AND ROUTES

Pegasys

- **Adult: SUBCUT** 180 mcg q wk × 48 wk; if poorly tolerated, reduce dose to 135 mcg q wk; in some cases, reduction to 90 mcg may be needed

Peg-Intron (chronic hepatitis C with compensated liver disease)

- **Adult >105 kg: SUBCUT** 1.5 mcg/kg/wk plus ribavirin 600 mg in AM and 800 mg in PM plus a HCV NS3/4A protease inhibitor; **86-105 kg:** 150 mcg/0.5 ml (0.5 ml of 150 mcg vial or Redipen) per wk plus ribavirin 1200 mg/day in 2 divided doses plus a HCV NS3/4A protease inhibitor; **81-85 kg:** 120 mcg/0.5 ml (0.5 ml of 120 mcg vial or Redipen) per wk plus ribavirin 1200 mg/day in 2 divided doses plus a HCV NS3/4A protease inhibitor; **76-80 kg:** 120 mcg/0.5 ml (0.5 ml of 120 mcg vial or Redipen) per wk plus ribavirin 400 mg in AM and 600 mg in PM plus a HCV NS3/4A protease inhibitor; **66-75 kg:** 96 mcg/0.4 ml (0.4 ml of 120 mcg vial or Redipen) per wk plus ribavirin 400 mg in AM and 600 mg in PM plus a HCV NS3/4A protease inhibitor; **61-65 kg:** 96 mcg/0.4 ml (0.4 ml of 120 mcg vial or Redipen) per wk plus ribavirin 800 mg/day in 2 divided doses plus a HCV NS3/4A protease inhibitor; **51-60 kg:** 80 mcg/0.5 ml (0.5 ml of 80 mcg vial or Redipen) per wk plus ribavirin 800 mg/day in 2 divided doses plus a HCV NS3/4A protease inhibitor; **40-50 kg:** 64 mcg/0.4 ml (0.4 ml of 80 mcg vial or Redipen) per wk plus ribavirin 800 mg/day in 2 divided doses plus a HCV NS3/4A protease inhibitor; **<40 kg:** 50 mcg/0.5 ml (0.5 ml of 50 mcg vial or Redipen) per wk plus ribavirin 800 mg/day in 2 divided doses plus a HCV NS3/4A protease inhibitor

Malignant Melanoma (SYLATRON only)

- **Adult: SUBCUT** 6 mcg/kg/wk × 8 wk then 3 mcg/kg/wk × ≤5 yr, premedicate with acetaminophen 500-1000 mg 30 min prior to first dose, prn for subsequent doses

Available forms: Pegasys: inj 180 mcg/0.5 ml; Pegintron: 50, 80, 120, 150 mcg/0.5 ml; SYLATRON 296, 444, 888 mcg powder for inj

Administer:

- In evening to reduce discomfort, to allow patient to sleep through some side effects
- Continue pediatric dose in those who turn 18 yr

Interferon alfa-2a

- Use prefilled syringes, store in refrigerator

Interferon alfa-2b

SUBCUT/IM route

- Reconstitute with 1 ml of provided diluent/10-, 18-, or 50-million unit vials, swirl; sol for inj vials do not need reconstitution

SIDE EFFECTS

CNS: *Headache, insomnia, dizziness,* anxiety, hostility, lability, nervousness, depression, fatigue, poor concentration, pyrexia, **suicidal ideation, homicidal ideation,** relapse of drug addiction, emotional lability, mania, psychosis

CV: **Ischemic CV events**

ENDO: Hypothyroidism, diabetes

GI: *Abdominal pain, nausea, diarrhea, anorexia, vomiting,* dry mouth, **fatal colitis, fatal pancreatitis**

HEMA: **Thrombocytopenia,** neutropenia, anemia, lymphopenia

P

INTEG: *Alopecia, pruritus, rash,* dermatitis
MISC: Blurred vision, inj site reaction, rigors
MS: *Back pain,* myalgia, arthralgia
RESP: Cough, dyspnea

PHARMACOKINETICS

Half-life 15-80 hr, large variability in other pharmacokinetics

INTERACTIONS

• Use caution when giving with theophylline, myelosuppressive agents
Drug/Lab Test
Increase: triglycerides, ALT, neutrophils, platelets
Abnormal: thyroid function test

NURSING CONSIDERATIONS

Assess:
• **Neuropsychiatric symptoms:** severe depression with suicidal ideation; monitor q3wk then 8 wk then q6mo
• B/P, blood glucose, ophthalmic exam, pulmonary function
• ALT, HCV viral load; patients who show no reduction in ALT, HCV unlikely to show benefit of treatment after 6 mo
• Platelet counts, heme concentration, ANC, serum creatinine concentration, albumin, bilirubin, TSH, T_4, AFP
⚠ **Myelosuppression:** hold dose if neutrophil count is $<500 \times 10^6$/L or if platelets are $<50 \times 10^9$/L
• **Hypersensitivity:** discontinue immediately if hypersensitivity occurs
• **Infection:** vital signs, increased WBCs, fever; product may need to be discontinued
⚠ **Colitis/pancreatitis:** may be fatal; diarrhea, fever, nausea, vomiting, severe abdominal pain; if these occur, product should be discontinued
Evaluate:
• Therapeutic response: decreased chronic hepatitis C signs, symptoms; undetectable viral load

Teach patient/family:
• Provide patient or family member with written, detailed information about product
• Use 2 forms of effective contraception throughout treatment and for 6 mo after treatment (men and women) (combination therapy with ribavirin)
• To avoid driving, other hazardous activity if dizziness, confusion, fatigue, somnolence occur
• To use puncture-resistant container for disposal of needles/syringes if using at home
⚠ To report suicidal/homicidal ideation, visual changes, bleeding/bruising, pulmonary symptoms

pegloticase (Rx)

(peg-loe′ti-kase)

Krystexxa

Func. class.: Antigout agent
Chem. class.: Pegylated, recombinant, mammalian urate oxidase enzyme

ACTION:
Lowers plasma uric acid concentration by converting uric acid to allantoin, which is readily excreted by the kidneys

USES:
Chronic gout in patients experiencing treatment failure

CONTRAINDICATIONS:
Hypersensitivity, G6PD deficiency
Precautions: Pregnancy (C), breastfeeding, children/infants/neonates, African-American patients, heart failure

Black Box Warning: Requires specialized setting, experienced clinician

DOSAGE AND ROUTES

• **Adult: IV INF** 8 mg over 2 hr q2wk
Available forms: Sol for inj 8 mg/ml

Administer:

Intermittent IV INF route

- ***Reconstitute:*** Visually inspect for particulate matter, discoloration whenever sol/container permits, use aseptic technique, withdraw 8 mg (1 ml) of product/250 ml 0.9% NaCl or 0.45% NaCl, invert several times to mix, do not shake; discard remaining product in vial
- ***Premedicate:*** With antihistamines and corticosteroids in all patients and acetaminophen if deemed necessary to prevent anaphylaxis, inf site reactions
- ***Infusion:*** If refrigerated, allow to come to room temp, do not warm artificially; give over 120 min, do not give IV push or bolus; use inf by gravity feed, syringe-type pump, or inf pump; given in a specialized setting by those who can manage anaphylaxis or inj site reactions; monitor during and for 1 hr after infusion; if reaction occurs, slow or stop infusion, may be restarted at a slower rate; do not admix

SIDE EFFECTS

CNS: Dizziness, fatigue, fever

CV: *Chest pain,* **heart failure,** hypotension

GI: *Nausea,* vomiting, diarrhea, constipation

GU: Nephrolithiasis

HEMA: Anemia

INTEG: Ecchymosis, *erythema, pruritus, urticaria*

MS: Back pain, arthralgia, muscle spasm

SYST: Antibody formation, infection, anaphylaxis, infusion-related reactions

RESP: *Dyspnea,* upper respiratory infection

PHARMACOKINETICS

Remains primarily in intravascular space after administration, elimination half-life 2 wk, mean nadir uric acid concentration 24-72 hr

NURSING CONSIDERATIONS

Assess:

- **Gout:** pain in big toe, feet, knees, redness, swelling, tenderness lasting a few days to weeks; intake of alcohol, purines, if patient is overweight or taking diuretics
- Obtain uric acid levels at baseline, before administration; 2 consecutive uric acid levels of >6 mg/dl may indicate therapy failure; greater chance of anaphylaxis; infection-related reactions

Perform/provide:

- Storage of diluted product in refrigerator or at room temp for up to 4 hr; refrigerator is preferred, protect from light, do not freeze, use within 4 hr of preparation

Evaluate:

- Therapeutic response: decrease uric acid levels; relief of pain, swelling, redness in toes, feet, knees

Teach patient/family:

- About reason for inf, expected results
- To notify prescriber during inf of allergic reactions or redness, swelling, pain at inf site
- That continuing follow-up exams and uric acid levels will be needed

⚠ HIGH ALERT

pemetrexed (Rx)

(pem-ah-trex′ed)

Alimta

Func. class.: Antineoplastic-antimetabolite

Chem. class.: Folic acid antagonist

ACTION: Inhibits multiple enzymes that reduce folic acid, which is needed for cell replication

USES: Malignant pleural mesothelioma in combination with CISplatin; non–small-cell lung cancer as single agent; nonsquamous, non–small-cell lung cancer (1st-line treatment)

Unlabeled uses: Bladder, breast, colorectal, gastric, head/neck, pancreatic, renal cell cancers

CONTRAINDICATIONS:

Pregnancy (D), hypersensitivity, ANC <1500 cells/mm^3, CCr <45 ml/min, thrombocytopenia (<100,000/mm^3), anemia

Precautions: Breastfeeding, children, renal/hepatic disease

DOSAGE AND ROUTES

- **Adult: IV INF** 500-600 mg/m^2 given over 10 min on day 1 of 21-day cycle with CISplatin 75 mg/m^2 infused over 2 hr beginning $^1/_2$ hr after end of pemetrexed inf
- ANC <500/mm^3 and platelets ≥50,000/mm^3, 75% of previous dose

Renal dose

- **Adult: IV INF** CCr <45 ml/min, not recommended

Available forms: Inj, single-use vials, 500 mg

Administer:

- Vit B_{12} and low-dose folic acid as prophylactic measure to treat related hematologic, GI toxicity; ≥5 daily doses of folic acid must be taken during the 7 days preceding 1st dose
- Premedicate with corticosteroid (dexamethasone) given PO bid day before, day of, and day after administration of pemetrexed

Intermittent IV INF route

- Use cytotoxic handling procedures
- Reconstitute 500-mg vial/20 ml 0.9% NaCl inj (preservative free) = 25 mg/ml, swirl until dissolved, further dilute with 100 ml 0.9% NaCl inj (preservative free), give as IV inf over 10 mg
- Use only 0.9% NaCl inj (preservative free) for reconstitution, dilution

Y-site compatibilities: Acyclovir sodium, alfentanil, allopurinol, amifostine, amikacin, aminocaproic acid, aminophylline, amiodarone, amphotericin B lipid complex, amphotericin B liposome, ampicillin, ampicillin-sulbactam, atenolol, atracurium, azithromycin, aztreonam, bivalirudin, bleomycin, bumetanide, buprenorphine, butorphanol, CARBOplatin, carmustine, ceftizoxime, cefTRIAXone, cefuroxime, cimetidine, cisatracurium, CISplatin, clindamycin, cyclophosphamide, cycloSPORINE, cytarabine, DACTINomycin, DAPTOmycin, dexamethasone, digoxin, diltiazem, diphenhydrAMINE, docetaxel, dolasetron, DOPamine, doxacurium, enalaprilat, ePHEDrine, EPINEPHrine, eptifibatide, ertapenem, esmolol, etoposide, famotidine, fenoldopam, fentaNYL, fluconazole, fludarabine, fluorouracil, foscarnet, fosphenytoin, furosemide, ganciclovir, gatifloxacin, glycopyrrolate, granisetron, haloperidol, heparin, hydrocortisone, HYDROmorphone, hydrOXYzine, ifosfamide, imipenem-cilastatin, insulin (regular), isoproterenol, ketorolac, labetalol, leucovorin, levofloxacin, lidocaine, linezolid, LORazepam, magnesium, mannitol, meperidine, meropenem, mesna, methyldopate, methylPREDNISolone, metoclopramide, metoprolol, midazolam, milrinone, mitomycin, mivacurium, morphine, moxifloxacin, nafcillin, naloxone, nesiritide, nitroglycerin, norEPINEPHrine, octreotide, oxaliplatin, paclitaxel, pamidronate, pancuronium, PENTobarbital, PHENObarbital, piperacillin-tazobactam, polymyxin B, potassium chloride/phosphates, procainamide, promethazine, propranolol, ranitidine, remifentanil, rocuronium, sodium acetate/bicarbonate/phosphates, succinylcholine, SUFentanil, sulfamethoxazole-trimethoprim, tacrolimus, theophylline, thiopental, thiotepa, ticarcillin, ticarcillin-clavulanate, tigecycline, tirofiban, trimethobenzamide, vancomycin, vecuronium, verapamil, vinBLAStine, vinCRIStine, vinorelbine, zidovudine, zoledronic acid

SIDE EFFECTS

CNS: *Fatigue, fever, mood alteration, neuropathy*

CV: Thrombosis/embolism, *chest pain*

GI: *Nausea, vomiting, anorexia, diarrhea, ulcerative stomatitis, constipation, dysphagia, dehydration*

GU: Renal failure, creatinine elevation

HEMA: Neutropenia, leukopenia, thrombocytopenia, myelosuppression, anemia

INTEG: *Rash, desquamation*
RESP: *Dyspnea*
SYST: Infection with/without neutropenia, radiation recall reaction

PHARMACOKINETICS

Not metabolized; excreted in urine (unchanged 70%-90%); not known if excreted in breast milk; half-life 3.5 hr, 81% protein binding

INTERACTIONS

Increase: bleeding risk—NSAIDs, anticoagulants, platelet inhibitors, salicylates, thrombolytics
Decrease: clearance of pemetrexed—nephrotoxic products

NURSING CONSIDERATIONS

Assess:

⚠ Previous radiation treatments; radiation recall reactions have occurred (erythema, exfoliative dermatitis, pain, burning)

⚠ **Bone marrow depression**: CBC, differential, platelet count; monitor for nadir, recovery; new cycle should not begin if ANC <1500 cells/mm³, platelets <100,000 cells/mm³, CCr <45 ml/min

- Renal studies: BUN, serum uric acid, urine CCr, electrolytes before, during therapy
- I&O ratio; report fall in urine output to <30 ml/hr
- Monitor temp q4hr; fever may indicate beginning infection; no rectal temp

⚠ **Neurotoxicity:** CTC grade 2: withhold until resolution to at least pretherapy value/condition, reduce CISplatin by 50%; CTC grade 3-4: immediately discontinue product and CISplatin if given in combination

- **Mucositis:** CTC 3-4: withhold until resolution to at least pretherapy value/condition, reduce dose by 50%; if grade 3/4 occurs after 2 dosage reductions, discontinue product and CISplatin
- **Bleeding:** bleeding time, coagulation time during treatment; bleeding: hematuria, guaiac, bruising or petechiae, mucosa or orifices q8hr
- Buccal cavity q8hr for dryness, sores, ulceration, white patches, oral pain, bleeding, dysphagia

⚠ **Severe allergic reaction:** rash, urticaria, itching, flushing

Perform/provide:

- Rinsing of mouth tid-qid with water, club soda; brushing of teeth bid-tid with soft brush or cotton-tipped applicators for stomatitis; use unwaxed dental floss
- Storage at 77° F, excursions permitted at 59° F to 86° F, not light sensitive, discard unused portions

Evaluate:

- Therapeutic response: decreased spread of malignancy

Teach patient/family:

- To report any complaints, side effects to nurse or prescriber: black, tarry stools, chills, fever, sore throat, bleeding, bruising, cough, SOB, dark or bloody urine
- To avoid foods with citric acid, hot or rough texture if stomatitis is present
- To report stomatitis: any bleeding, white spots, ulcerations in mouth to prescriber; to examine mouth daily, to report symptoms to nurse, to use good oral hygiene
- That contraceptive measures recommended during therapy, for ≤8 wk after cessation of therapy; to discontinue breastfeeding because toxicity to infant may occur
- To avoid alcohol, salicylates, live vaccines
- To avoid use of razors, commercial mouthwash
- To eat foods high in folic acid; to take supplements as prescribed

penciclovir topical

See Appendix B

P

PENICILLINS

penicillin G benzathine (Rx)
(pen-i-sill'in)
Bicillin L-A
penicillin G (Rx)
Pfizerpen
penicillin G procaine (Rx)
penicillin V (Rx)
Apo-Pen-VK ♣, Penicillin VK
Func. class.: Broad-spectrum antiinfective
Chem. class.: Natural penicillin

ACTION: Interferes with cell-wall replication of susceptible organisms; lysis is mediated by cell-wall autolytic enzymes, results in cell death

USES: Respiratory infections, scarlet fever, erysipelas, otitis media, pneumonia, skin and soft-tissue infections, gonorrhea; effective for gram-positive cocci *(Staphylococcus, Streptococcus pyogenes, S. viridans, S. faecalis, S. bovis, S. pneumoniae)*, gram-negative cocci *(Neisseria gonorrhoeae)*, gram-positive bacilli *(Actinomyces, Bacillus anthracis, Clostridium perfringens, C. tetani, Corynebacterium diphtheriae, Listeria monocytogenes)*, gram-negative bacilli *(Escherichia coli, Proteus mirabilis, Salmonella, Shigella, Enterobacter, Streptobacillus moniliformis)*, spirochetes *(Treponema pallidum)*

CONTRAINDICATIONS: Hypersensitivity to penicillins, corn

Precautions: Pregnancy (B), breastfeeding; hypersensitivity to cephalosporins, carbapenem, sulfites; severe renal disease, GI disease, asthma

DOSAGE AND ROUTES

Penicillin G benzathine

Early syphilis

- **Adult: IM** 2.4 million units in single dose

Congenital syphilis

- **Child <2 yr: IM** 50,000 units/kg in single dose, max 2.4 million units as single inj

Prophylaxis of rheumatic fever, glomerulonephritis

- **Adult: IM** 1.2 million units in single dose
- **Child >27 kg: IM** 900,000-1.2 million units as single dose
- **Child ≤27 kg: IM** 300,000-600,000 units as single dose

Upper respiratory infections (group A streptococcal)

- **Adult: IM** 1.2 million units as single dose
- **Child >27 kg: IM** 900,000-1.2 million units as single dose
- **Child <27 kg: IM** 300,000-600,000 units as single dose

Available forms: Inj 600,000 units/ml

Penicillin G

Pneumococcal/streptococcal infections (serious)

- **Adult: IM/IV** 5-24 million units in divided doses q4-6hr
- **Child <12 yr: IV** 150,000-300,000 units/kg/day in 4-6 divided doses; max 24 million units/day

Renal dose

- CCr <10 ml/min, give full loading dose then ½ of loading dose q8-10hr

Available forms: Powder for inj 1, 5, 20 million units/vial; inj 1, 2, 3 million units/50 ml

Penicillin G procaine

Moderate to severe pneumococcal infections

- **Adult/child: IM** 600,000-1 million units as single dose or divided bid doses/day for 10 days to 2 wk

Pneumococcal pneumonia

- **Adult/child >12 yr: IM** 600,000-1 million units/day × 7-10 days

Moderately severe group A streptococcal/staphylococcal pneumonia

- **Adult/adolescent/child ≥60 lbs: IM** 600,000-1 million units/day
- **Adolescent/child <60 lbs: IM** 300,000 units/day

Available forms: Inj 600,000, 1,200,000 units/unit dose

Penicillin V

Pneumococcal/staphylococcal infections

- **Adult/adolescents/child >12 yr: PO** 250-500 mg q6hr
- **Child <12 yr: PO** 25-50 mg/kg/day in divided doses q6-8hr; max 2 g/day

Streptococcal infections

- **Adult/adolescent/child ≥12 yr: PO** 125-250 mg q6-8hr × 10 days
- **Child <12 yr and >27 kg: PO** 500 mg q8 or 12 hr × 10 days
- **Child <12 yr and ≤27 kg: PO** 250 mg q8hr or q12hr or 40 mg/kg/day in 3 divided doses × 10 days

Prevention of recurrence of rheumatic fever/chorea

- **Adult: PO** 125-250 mg bid continuously

Vincent's gingivitis/pharyngitis

- **Adult: PO** 250-500 mg q6-8hr

Renal dose

- Dosage reduction indicated with renal impairment (CCr <50 ml/min) based on clinical response, degree of impairment

Available forms: Tabs 250, 500 mg; powder for oral sol 125, 250 mg/5 ml

Administer:

Penicillin G benzathine

- No dilution needed, shake well, deep IM inj in large muscle mass; avoid intravascular inj; aspirate; do not give IV

Penicillin G

- Penicillin G sodium or potassium can be given IM or IV, vials containing 10 or 20 million units not for IM use

Intermittent IV INF route

- Vials/bulk packages: dilute according to manufacturer's directions
- Frozen bags: thaw at room temp, do not force thaw, no reconstitution needed
- Final conc (100,000-500,000 units/ml—adults; 50,000 units/ml—neonate/infant)
- Total daily dose divided q4-6hr and given over 1-2 hr (adult), 15 min (infant/neonate)

Penicillin G potassium

Y-site compatibilities: Acyclovir, amiodarone, cyclophosphamide, diltiazem, enalaprilat, esmolol, fluconazole, foscarnet, heparin, HYDROmorphone, labetalol, magnesium sulfate, meperidine, morphine, perphenazine, potassium chloride, tacrolimus, theophylline, verapamil, vit B/C

Penicillin G procaine

- No dilution needed, give deep IM inj; avoid intravascular inj; aspirate; do not give IV

Penicillin V

- Orally on empty stomach for best absorption
- Oral susp: tap bottle to loosen, add ½ total amount of water, shake, add remaining water, shake; final conc (125 or 250 mg/ml) store in refrigerator after reconstitution, discard after 14 days

SIDE EFFECTS

CNS: Lethargy, hallucinations, anxiety, depression, twitching, **coma, seizures,** hyperreflexia

GI: *Nausea, vomiting, diarrhea,* increased AST, ALT, abdominal pain, glossitis, colitis, **pseudomembranous colitis**

GU: **Oliguria, proteinuria, hematuria,** *vaginitis, moniliasis,* **glomerulonephritis, renal tubular damage**

HEMA: Anemia, increased bleeding time, **bone marrow depression, granulocytopenia, hemolytic anemia**

META: Hypo/hyperkalemia, alkalosis, hypernatremia

MISC: **Anaphylaxis, serum sickness, Stevens-Johnson syndrome,** *local pain,* tenderness and fever with IM inj

P

PHARMACOKINETICS

Penicillin G benzathine:

IM: Very slow absorption; time to peak 12-24 hr; duration 21-28 days; excreted in urine, feces, breast milk; crosses placenta

Penicillin G:

IV: Peak immediate

IM: Peak $^1/_4$-$^1/_2$ hr

PO: Peak 1 hr, duration 6 hr

Excreted in urine unchanged, excreted in breast milk, crosses placenta, half-life 30-60 min

Penicillin G procaine:

IM: Peak 1-4 hr, duration 15 hr, excreted in urine

Penicillin V:

PO: Peak 30-60 min, half-life 30 min, excreted in urine, breast milk

INTERACTIONS

Increase: penicillin effect—aspirin, probenecid

Increase: effect of heparin, methotrexate

Decrease: effect of oral contraceptives, typhoid vaccine

Decrease: antimicrobial effect of penicillin—tetracyclines

Drug/Lab Test

False positive: urine glucose, urine protein

NURSING CONSIDERATIONS

Assess:

- **Infection:** temp; characteristics of sputum; wounds; urine; stools before, during, after treatment; C&S before therapy; product may be given as soon as culture is taken
- I&O ratio; report hematuria, oliguria because penicillin in high doses is nephrotoxic; renal tests: urinalysis, protein, blood

⚠ **Any patient with compromised renal system because product is excreted slowly with poor renal system function; toxicity may occur rapidly**

- Hepatic studies: AST, ALT
- Blood studies: WBC, RBC, Hct, Hgb, bleeding time

⚠ **Pseudomembranous colitis: diarrhea, mucus, pus; bowel pattern before, during treatment**

- Respiratory status: rate, character, wheezing, tightness in chest

⚠ **Allergies before initiation of treatment, reaction of each medication; because of prolonged action, allergic reaction may be prolonged and severe; watch for anaphylaxis: rash, dyspnea, pruritus, laryngeal edema; skin eruptions after administration of penicillin to 1 wk after discontinuing product**

Perform/provide:

- EPINEPHrine, suction, tracheostomy set, endotracheal intubation equipment
- Adequate fluid intake (2 L) during diarrhea episodes
- Scratch test to assess allergy after securing order from prescriber; usually done when penicillin is only product of choice
- Storage in dry, tight container; oral susp refrigerated 2 wk

Evaluate:

- Therapeutic response: resolution of infection

Teach patient/family:

- To report sore throat, fever, fatigue; may indicate superinfection; CNS effects: depression, hallucinations, seizures
- To wear or carry emergency ID if allergic to penicillins
- To report diarrhea, with blood, pus, mucous to prevent dehydration
- To shake susp well before each dose; to store in refrigerator for up to 2 wk
- To use all medication prescribed
- To use additional contraception if using any of these products

TREATMENT OF ANAPHYLAXIS: Withdraw product; maintain airway; administer EPINEPHrine, aminophylline, O_2, IV corticosteroids

pentamidine (Rx)

(pen-tam′i-deen)

Nebupent, Pentam 300

Func. class.: Antiprotozoal

Chem. class.: Aromatic diamide derivative

ACTION: Interferes with DNA/RNA synthesis in protozoa

USES: Treatment/prevention of *Pneumocystis jiroveci* infections

Unlabeled uses: *Leishmania/Trypanosoma* infections

CONTRAINDICATIONS: Hypersensitivity

Precautions: Pregnancy (C), breastfeeding, children, blood dyscrasias, cardiac/renal/hepatic disease, diabetes mellitus, hypocalcemia, hypo/hypertension, anemia

DOSAGE AND ROUTES

- **Adult and child ≥4 mo: IV/IM** 4 mg/kg/day × 2-3 wk; **NEB** 300 mg via specific nebulizer given q4wk for prevention

Available forms: Inj, aerosol 300 mg/vial; sol for aerosol 60 mg/vial ♣

Administer:

Inhalation route

- Through nebulizer, using Raspirgard II jet nebulizer; mix contents in 6 ml of sterile water; do not use low pressure (<20 psi); flow rate should be 5-7 L/min (40-50 psi) air or O_2 source over 30-45 min until chamber is empty

IM route

- 300 mg diluted in 3 ml sterile water; give deep IM by Z-track; if painful by this route, rotate inj site

Intermittent IV INF route

- Reconstitute 300 mg/3-5 ml of sterile water for inj, D_5W, withdraw dose and further dilute in 50-250 ml D_5W, give over 1-2 hr with patient lying down; check B/P often

Y-site compatibilities: Alfentanil, atracurium, atropine, benztropine, buprenorphine, calcium gluconate, CARBOplatin, caspofungin, chlorpromazine, cimetidine, CISplatin, cyclophosphamide, cycloSPORINE, cytarabine, DACTINomycin, diltiazem, gatifloxacin, zidovudine

SIDE EFFECTS

CNS: Disorientation, hallucinations, *dizziness,* confusion, drowsiness

CV: Hypotension, ventricular tachycardia, **QT prolongation, dysrhythmias**

GI: *Nausea, vomiting, anorexia;* increased AST, ALT; **acute pancreatitis,** metallic taste

GU: **Acute renal failure, increased serum creatinine, renal toxicity,** decreased urination

HEMA: Anemia, **leukopenia, thrombocytopenia**

INTEG: Sterile abscess, pain at inj site, pruritus, urticaria, *rash*

META: *Hyperkalemia,* hypocalcemia, hypoglycemia, hypomagnesemia

MISC: Fatigue, fever, chills, night sweats, **anaphylaxis, Stevens-Johnson syndrome**

RESP: Cough, SOB, **bronchospasm** (with aerosol), sore throat

PHARMACOKINETICS

IV: Peak 1 hr

IM: Peak 30 min

Excreted unchanged in urine (66%); half-life 9-12 hr (IM), 6 hr (IV)

INTERACTIONS

- Nephrotoxicity: aminoglycosides, amphotericin B, CISplatin, NSAIDs, vancomycin

⚠ **Fatal dysrhythmias: erythromycin IV**

Increase: QT prolongation—class IA/III antidysrhythmics, some phenothiazines, β agonists, local anesthetics, tricyclics, haloperidol, chloroquine, droperidol, pentamidine; CYP3A4 inhibitors (amiodarone, clarithromycin, erythromycin, telithromycin, troleandomycin, arsenic trioxide, levomethadyl); CYP3A4 substrates (methadone, pimozide, QUEtia-

pine, quiNIDine, risperidone, ziprasidone)
Increase: myelosuppression—antineoplastics, radiation
Drug/Lab Test
Decrease: WBC, platelets, Hbg, Hct
Increase: BUN, creatitine

NURSING CONSIDERATIONS

Assess:

- Blood tests, blood glucose, CBC, platelets, calcium, magnesium
- I&O ratio; report hematuria, oliguria
- ECG for cardiac dysrhythmias; patient should be lying down when receiving product; severe hypotension may develop; monitor B/P during administration and until B/P stable
- Hepatic studies: AST, ALT
- Renal studies: urinalysis, BUN, creatinine; nephrotoxicity may occur; any patient with compromised renal system; product is excreted slowly with poor renal system function; toxicity may occur rapidly
- Signs of infection, anemia
- Bowel pattern before, during treatment
- Sterile abscess, pain at inj site
- Respiratory status: rate, character, wheezing, dyspnea
- Dizziness, confusion, hallucination
- Allergies before treatment, reaction of each medication; place allergies on chart in bright red letters; notify all people giving products
- Diabetic patients, hypoglycemia may occur, then hyperglycemia with prolonged therapy

Perform/provide:

- Storage in refrigerator protected from light

Evaluate:

- Therapeutic response: resolution of AIDS-related PCP

Teach patient/family:

- To report sore throat, fever, fatigue (may indicate superinfection)
- To maintain adequate fluid intake

⚠ HIGH ALERT

pentazocine (Rx)

(pen-taz'oh-seen)

Talwin, Talwin NX

Func. class.: Opiate analgesic, antagonist

Chem. class.: Synthetic benzomorphan

Controlled Substance Schedule IV

ACTION: Inhibits ascending pain pathways in CNS, increases pain threshold, alters pain perception

USES: Moderate to severe pain

CONTRAINDICATIONS: Hypersensitivity to this product or sulfites; addiction (opiate)

Precautions: Pregnancy (C), breastfeeding, children <18 yr, addictive personality, increased intracranial pressure, MI (acute), severe heart disease, respiratory depression, renal/hepatic disease, seizure disorder, head trauma, bowel impaction, geriatric patients

DOSAGE AND ROUTES

- **Adult: PO** 50-100 mg q3-4hr prn, max 600 mg/day; **IV/IM/SUBCUT** 30 mg q3-4hr prn, max 360 mg/day

Labor

- **Adult: IM** 30 mg; **IV** 20 mg q2-3hr when contractions are regular

Renal dose

- CCr 10-50 ml/min, reduce dose by 25%; CCr <10 ml/min, reduce dose by 50%

Available forms: Inj 30 mg/ml; tabs 50 mg

Administer:

- With antiemetic if nausea, vomiting occur

• When pain is beginning to return; determine dosage interval by patient response

PO route

• Without regard to food

• PO tabs intended for PO; lethal reactions have occurred from giving tabs by inj

IM/SUBCUT route

• Give IM deeply into large muscle mass, rotate sites; SUBCUT may cause necrosis with repeated inj

Direct IV route

• Undiluted or diluted in 5 mg/ml of sterile water for inj; give ≤5 mg over 1 min

Syringe compatibilities: Atropine, benzquinamide, butorphanol, chlorproMAZINE, cimetidine, dimenhyDRINATE, diphenhydrAMINE, droperidol, fentaNYL, HYDROmorphone, hydrOXYzine, meperidine, metoclopramide, morphine, perphenazine, prochlorperazine, promazine, promethazine, ranitidine, scopolamine

Y-site compatibilities: Heparin, hydrocortisone, potassium chloride, vit B/C

SIDE EFFECTS

CNS: *Drowsiness, dizziness, confusion, headache, sedation, euphoria,* hallucinations, dreaming, insomnia, lightheadedness

CV: Palpitations, bradycardia, change in B/P, tachycardia, increased B/P (high doses), hypotension, syncope, flushing

EENT: Tinnitus, blurred vision, miosis, diplopia

GI: *Nausea,* vomiting, anorexia, constipation, *cramps,* dry mouth

GU: Increased urinary output, dysuria, urinary retention

HEMA: **Eosinophilia, decreased WBC**

INTEG: *Rash,* urticaria, bruising, flushing, diaphoresis, pruritus, severe irritation at inj sites, **Stevens-Johnson syndrome**

RESP: **Respiratory depression**

PHARMACOKINETICS

Metabolized by liver, excreted by kidneys, crosses placenta, half-life 2-3 hr, extensive first-pass metabolism with <20% entering circulation

IM/SUBCUT: Onset 15-30 min, peak 1-2 hr, duration 2-4 hr

IV: Onset 2-3 min, duration 4-6 hr

INTERACTIONS

⚠ Unpredictable reactions: MAOIs

Increase: effects—CNS depressants; alcohol, sedative/hypnotics, antipsychotics, skeletal muscle relaxants

Decrease: effects—opiates

Drug/Lab Test

Increase: amylase

NURSING CONSIDERATIONS

Assess:

• **Pain:** intensity, duration, location prior to and 1 hr after PO/SUBCUT/IM dose or 30 min after IV dose

• I&O ratio; check for decreasing output; may indicate urinary retention

• Bowel status: constipation; may need stimulant laxatives/stool softeners

• **Withdrawal symptoms** in opiate-dependent patients

• Abscesses, ulcerations, WBC count

• CNS changes: dizziness, drowsiness, hallucinations, euphoria, LOC, pupil reaction

• Allergic reactions: rash, urticaria

• **Respiratory depression:** character, rate, rhythm; notify prescriber if respirations are <10/min

• Need for pain medication, physical dependence

Perform/provide:

• Storage in light-resistant area at room temp

• Assistance with ambulation

• Safety measures: night-light, call bell within easy reach

Evaluate:

• Therapeutic response: decrease in pain

P

Teach patient/family:
• To report any symptoms of CNS changes, allergic reactions
• That physical dependency may result from extended use
• That withdrawal symptoms may occur: nausea, vomiting, cramps, fever, faintness, anorexia
• To avoid CNS depressants, alcohol
• To avoid driving, operating machinery if drowsiness occurs
• To use good oral hygiene, frequent rinsing of mouth to decrease dry mouth; to avoid gum, candy if drowsy

TREATMENT OF OVERDOSE:
Naloxone (Narcan) 0.2-0.8 mg IV, O_2, IV fluids, vasopressors

pentoxifylline (Rx)
(pen-tox′ih-fill-in)
Apo-Pentoxifylline ✤, ratio-Pentoxifylline ✤, Trental
Func. class.: Hemorheologic agent
Chem. class.: Dimethylxanthine derivative

ACTION: Decreases blood viscosity, stimulates prostacyclin formation, increases blood flow by increasing flexibility of RBCs; decreases RBC hyperaggregation; reduces platelet aggregation, decreases fibrinogen concentration

USES: Intermittent claudication related to chronic occlusive vascular disease
Unlabeled uses: Behçet's syndrome, Kawasaki disease to reduce coronary artery lesions, diabetic neuropathies, sickle cell anemia

CONTRAINDICATIONS: Hypersensitivity to this product or xanthines, retinal/cerebral hemorrhage
Precautions: Pregnancy (C), breastfeeding, children, angina pectoris, impaired renal function, recent surgery, peptic ulceration, cardiac disease, bleeding disorders

DOSAGE AND ROUTES
• **Adult: PO** 400 mg tid with meals, may decrease to bid if side effects occur; must be taken for ≥8 wk for maximal effect
Behçet's syndrome (unlabeled)
• **Adult: PO** 300 mg bid × 2 wk then 300 mg/day
Acute claudication in sickle cell disease/diabetic neuropathy (unlabeled)
• **Adult: PO** 400 mg tid
Kawasaki disease (unlabeled)
• **Child: PO** 20 mg/kg/day in 3 divided doses with aspirin and IVIG
Available forms: Cont rel tabs 400 mg; ext rel tabs 400 mg
Administer:
• Do not break, crush, or chew ext rel tabs
• With meals to prevent GI upset

SIDE EFFECTS
CNS: *Headache,* anxiety, *tremors,* confusion, *dizziness*
GI: *Dyspepsia, nausea, vomiting*

PHARMACOKINETICS
PO: Peak 2-4 hr, half-life ½-1 hr, degradation in liver, excreted in urine

INTERACTIONS
Increase: bleeding risk—warfarin, abciximab, eptifibatide, tirofiban, ticlopidine, clopidogrel, thrombin inhibitor
Increase: theophylline level—theophylline
Increase: hypotension—antihypertensives, nitrates
Increase: pentoxifylline—cimetidine, ciprofloxacin

NURSING CONSIDERATIONS
Assess:
• B/P, respirations of patient also taking antihypertensives; intermittent claudication at baseline and throughout

• PT, Hgb, Hct in patients at risk for hemorrhage
• Serum creatinine/BUN

Evaluate:
• Therapeutic response: decreased pain, cramping, increased ambulation

Teach patient/family:
• That therapeutic response may take 2-4 wk, 8-12 wk to reach full benefit
• To observe feet for arterial insufficiency
• To wear cotton socks, well-fitted shoes; not to go barefoot
• To watch for bleeding, bruises, petechiae, epistaxis
• To avoid smoking to prevent blood vessel constriction
• That there are many drug, herb interactions

perindopril (Rx)
(per-in′doe-pril)
Aceon, Coversye ✦
Func. class.: Antihypertensive
Chem. class.: Angiotensin-converting enzyme inhibitor

ACTION:
Selectively suppresses the renin-angiotensin-aldosterone system; inhibits ACE; prevents the conversion of angiotensin I to angiotensin II and the dilation of arterial and venous vessels

USES:
Hypertension, stable coronary artery disease

Unlabeled uses: Heart failure

CONTRAINDICATIONS:
Hypersensitivity, history of angioedema

Black Box Warning: Pregnancy (D)

Precautions: Breastfeeding, renal disease, hyperkalemia, hepatic failure, dehydration, bilateral renal artery stenosis, cough, angioedema, severe CHF

DOSAGE AND ROUTES

Hypertension
• **Adult: PO** 4 mg/day, may increase or decrease to desired response, range 4-8 mg/day; may give in 2 divided doses or as single dose, max 16 mg/day

Patients on diuretics
• **Adult: PO** 2-4 mg/day in 1-2 divided doses, range 4-8 mg/day

Stable CAD
• **Adult: PO** 4 mg/day × 2 wk then increase as tolerated to 8 mg/day

Renal dose
• **Adult: PO** CCr 16-29 ml/min, 2 mg every other day; CCr 30-59 ml/min, 2 mg/day

Available forms: Tabs scored 2, 4, 8 mg

Administer:
• As single dose or in 2 divided doses, without regard to meals

SIDE EFFECTS

CNS: *Insomnia, dizziness,* paresthesias, headache, fatigue, anxiety, depression
CV: *Hypotension,* chest pain, tachycardia, dysrhythmias, syncope
EENT: *Tinnitus;* visual changes; sore throat; double vision; dry, burning eyes
GI: Nausea, vomiting, colitis, cramps, diarrhea, constipation, flatulence, dry mouth, loss of taste
GU: **Proteinuria, renal failure,** increased frequency of polyuria or oliguria
HEMA: **Agranulocytosis, neutropenia**
INTEG: Rash, purpura, alopecia, hyperhidrosis
META: Hyperkalemia
RESP: Dyspnea, *dry cough,* crackles
SYST: **Angioedema**

PHARMACOKINETICS

Bioavailability 75%; peak 1 hr parent product, 3-7 hr prodrug; protein binding 68%; metabolized by liver (active metabolite perindoprilat); half-life 0.8-10 hr; excreted in urine

INTERACTIONS

Increase: effects of neuromuscular blocking agents, antihypertensives, lithium

Increase: antihypertensive effect—diuretics

Increase: hypersensitivity—allopurinol

Increase: severe hypotension—diuretics, other antihypertensives

Increase: hyperkalemia—salt substitutes, potassium-sparing diuretics, potassium supplements

Decrease: effects of NSAIDs

Decrease: antihypertensive effect—NSAIDs, salicylates

Drug/Herb

Increase: antihypertensive effect—hawthorn

Decrease: antihypertensive effect—ephedra

Drug/Lab Test

Interference: glucose/insulin tolerance tests

NURSING CONSIDERATIONS

Assess:

- **Hypertension:** B/P, pulse q4hr; note rate, rhythm, quality
- Electrolytes: K, Na, Cl during 1st 2 wk of therapy
- Baselines of renal, hepatic studies before therapy begins, 1 wk into therapy
- Skin turgor, dryness of mucous membranes for hydration status, dry mouth
- **CHF:** edema, dyspnea, wet crackles
- **Angioedema:** facial swelling, urticaria; product should be discontinued, may be more common in African Americans

Evaluate:

- Therapeutic response: decreased B/P

Teach patient/family:

- Not to use OTC (cough, cold, allergy) products unless directed by prescriber; to avoid salt substitutes
- To avoid sunlight or to wear sunscreen for photosensitivity
- To comply with dosage schedule, even if feeling better
- To notify prescriber of mouth sores, sore throat, fever, swelling of hands or feet, irregular heartbeat, chest pains, signs of angioedema
- That excessive perspiration, dehydration, vomiting, diarrhea may lead to fall in B/P; to consult prescriber if these occur
- That product may cause dizziness, fainting; that lightheadedness may occur during 1st few days of therapy
- That product may cause skin rash or impaired perspiration; that angioedema may occur and to discontinue product if it occurs
- Not to discontinue product abruptly
- To rise slowly to sitting or standing position to minimize orthostatic hypotension

Black Box Warning: To notify prescriber if pregnancy is planned or suspected; pregnancy category (D)

TREATMENT OF OVERDOSE:

Lavage, IV atropine for bradycardia, IV theophylline for bronchospasm, digoxin, O_2, diuretic for cardiac failure

phenazopyridine (Rx, OTC)

(fen-az-oh-peer'i-deen)

Azo-Gesic, Azo-Standard, Baridium, Geridium, Phenazo ✦, Prodium, Pyridiate, Pyridium, Urodine, Urogesic, UTI-Relief

Func. class.: Urinary analgesic

Chem. class.: Azodye

ACTION: Exerts analgesic, anesthetic action on the urinary tract mucosa

USES: Urinary tract irritation, infection; used with a urinary antiinfective

CONTRAINDICATIONS: Hypersensitivity, renal insufficiency, hepatic disease, uremia

Precautions: Pregnancy (B), breastfeeding, children <12 yr, geriatric patients, contact lens

DOSAGE AND ROUTES

• **Adult: PO** 200 mg tid × ≤2 days when used with antibacterial for UTI
• **Child 6-12 yr: PO** 4 mg/kg tid × 2 days

Renal dose
• **Adult: PO** CCr 50-80 ml/min, give dose 8-16 hr; do not use if CCr <50 ml/min

Available forms: Tabs 95, 97.2, 100, 200 mg

Administer:
• Crushed or whole; chewable tablets may be chewed
• With food, milk to decrease gastric symptoms

SIDE EFFECTS

CNS: Headache
GI: *Nausea,* hepatic toxicity
GU: Renal toxicity, *orange-red urine*
HEMA: Methemoglobinemia
INTEG: *Rash,* skin pigmentation, pruritus
SYST: Anaphylaxis

PHARMACOKINETICS

Metabolized by liver, excreted by kidneys, crosses placenta, peak 6 hr, duration 6-8 hr

INTERACTIONS

Drug/Lab Test
Interference: urinalysis

NURSING CONSIDERATIONS

Assess:
• **Urinary status:** burning, pain, itching, urgency, frequency, hematuria before, after treatment completed
• Hepatic studies: AST, ALT, bilirubin if patient receiving long-term therapy
⚠ **Hepatotoxicity:** dark urine, clay-colored stools, jaundiced skin and sclera, itching, abdominal pain, fever, diarrhea if patient receiving long-term therapy
• **Allergic reactions:** rash; product may have to be discontinued

Evaluate:
• Therapeutic response: decrease in urinary pain

Teach patient/family:
• Not to exceed recommended dosage; to take with meals
• To discontinue after pain is relieved but to continue to take concurrent prescribed antiinfective until finished
• That urine may turn red-orange; that product may stain clothing or contact lenses

⚠ HIGH ALERT

PHENobarbital (Rx)

(fee-noe-bar′bi-tal)

Luminal, PMS-PHENobarbital ✤

Func. class.: Anticonvulsant
Chem. class.: Barbiturate

Controlled Substance Schedule IV

Do not confuse:
PHENobarbital/PENTobarbital

ACTION: Decreases impulse transmission; increases seizure threshold at cerebral cortex level

USES: All forms of epilepsy, status epilepticus, febrile seizures in children, sedation, insomnia

Unlabeled uses: Neonatal hyperbilirubinemia, chronic cholestasis, neonatal abstinence syndrome, febrile seizures in children

CONTRAINDICATIONS: Pregnancy (D), breastfeeding, geriatric patients, hypersensitivity to barbiturates, porphyria, hepatic/respiratory disease, nephritis, hyperthyroidism, diabetes mellitus

Precautions: Anemia, renal disease

P

DOSAGE AND ROUTES

Seizures

- **Adult: PO** 1-3 mg/kg/day in divided doses bid-tid or total dose at bedtime
- **Child 5-12 yr: PO** 3-6 mg/kg/day in 1-2 divided doses
- **Child 1-5 yr: PO** 6-8 mg/kg/day in 1-2 divided doses
- **Infant: PO** 5-6 mg/kg/day in 1-2 divided doses
- **Neonate: PO** 3-4 mg/kg/day as single dose

Status epilepticus

- **Adult: IV INF** 10 mg/kg; run no faster than 50 mg/min; may give up to 30 mg/kg
- **Child: IV INF** 5-10 mg/kg; may repeat q10-15min up to 20 mg/kg; run no faster than 50 mg/min

Insomnia

- **Adult: PO/IM/SUBCUT** 100-200 mg
- **Child (unlabeled): PO/IM/SUBCUT** 3-5 mg/kg

Sedation

- **Adult: PO/IM** 30-120 mg/day in 2-3 divided doses
- **Child: PO** 6 mg/kg/day in 3 divided doses

Preoperative sedation

- **Adult: IM** 100-200 mg 1-1½ hr before surgery
- **Child: PO/IM/IV** 1-3 mg/kg 1-1½ hr before surgery

Available forms: Caps 15 mg; elix 20 mg/5 ml; tabs 15, 30, 32, 60, 65, 100 mg; inj 30, 60, 65, 130 mg/ml

Administer:

PO route

- Tabs may be crushed and mixed with food or fluids
- **Oral sol:** use undiluted or mixed with water or other fluids; use calibrated measuring device

IM route

- IM inj deep in large muscle mass to prevent tissue sloughing; use <5 ml at each site

IV route

- Reconstitute powder for IV with ≥3 ml sterile water for inj; slow IV after dilution with ≥10 ml sterile water for inj regardless of dose; give ≤50 mg/min; titrate to patient response

Y-site compatibilities: Doxapram, enalaprilat, fentaNYL, fosphenytoin, levofloxacin, linezolid, meropenem, methadone, morphine, propofol, SUFentanil

SIDE EFFECTS

CNS: Paradoxic excitement (geriatric patients), drowsiness, lethargy, hangover headache, flushing, hallucinations, **coma**

GI: Nausea, vomiting, diarrhea, constipation

HEMA: Agranulocytosis, megaloblastic anemia, thrombocytopenia, thrombophlebitis

INTEG: Rash, urticaria, **Stevens-Johnson syndrome, angioedema,** local pain, swelling, necrosis, scaling eczema

PHARMACOKINETICS

Metabolized by liver; crosses placenta; excreted in urine, breast milk; half-life 53-118 hr

PO: Onset 20-60 min, duration 6-10 hr

IM/SUBCUT: Onset 10-30 min, duration 4-6 hr

IV: Onset 5 min, peak 30 min, duration 4-6 hr

INTERACTIONS

Increase: effects—CNS depressants, alcohol, chloramphenicol, valproic acid, disulfiram, nondepolarizing skeletal muscle relaxants, sulfonamides, MAOIs

Increase: orthostatic hypotension—furosemide

Decrease: effects—theophylline, oral anticoagulants, corticosteroids, metroNIDAZOLE, doxycycline, quiNIDine, estrogens, hormonal contraceptives

Drug/Herb

Increase: CNS depression—chamomile, eucalyptus, hops, kava, valerian

Decrease: barbiturate effect—St. John's wort

NURSING CONSIDERATIONS

Assess:

- Mental status: mood, sensorium, affect, memory (long, short)
- **Blood dyscrasias:** fever, sore throat, bruising, rash, jaundice
- **Seizures:** type, duration, precipitating factors
- Blood studies, LFTs during long-term treatment
- Therapeutic blood level periodically: 15-40 mcg/ml
- Respiratory status: rate, rhythm, depth, respiratory depression; have emergency equipment nearby
- **Dependence:** physical or psychological, monitor amount given to patient; if patient suicidal, may save medication for attempt
- **Pain:** use pain scale if product used for pain; product may increase pain level

Perform/provide:

- Supervision of ambulation because dizziness, drowsiness may occur

Evaluate:

- Therapeutic response: decreased seizures, increased sedation, adequate sleep

Teach patient/family:

- To use exactly as ordered
- To avoid alcohol, other CNS depressants
- To avoid hazardous activities until patient stabilized on product because drowsiness may occur
- Never to withdraw product abruptly because withdrawal symptoms may occur
- That therapeutic effects (PO) may not be seen for 2-3 wk
- To use additional nonhormonal contraception during treatment; to notify prescriber if pregnancy is planned or suspected

phenylephrine (Rx)

(fen-ill-ef′rin)

Neo-Synephrine

Func. class.: Adrenergic, directacting

Chem. class.: Substituted phenylethylamine

ACTION: Powerful and selective (α_1) receptor agonist that causes the contraction of blood vessels

USES: Hypotension, paroxysmal supraventricular tachycardia, shock; maintain B/P for spinal anesthesia

CONTRAINDICATIONS: Hypersensitivity, ventricular fibrillation, tachydysrhythmias, pheochromocytoma, closed-angle glaucoma, severe hypertension

Precautions: Pregnancy (C), breastfeeding, geriatric patients, arterial embolism, peripheral vascular disease, hyperthyroidism, bradycardia, myocardial disease, severe arteriosclerosis, partial heart block

Black Box Warning: Cardiac disease, extravasation

DOSAGE AND ROUTES

Hypotension

- **Adult: SUBCUT/IM** 2-5 mg; may repeat q10-15min if needed; do not exceed initial dose; **IV** 0.1-0.5 mg; may repeat q10-15min if needed; do not exceed initial dose
- **Child: IM/SUBCUT** 0.1 mg/kg/dose q1-2hr prn

Supraventricular tachycardia

- **Adult: IV BOL** max 0.5 mg; max single dose 1 mg

Shock

- **Adult: IV INF** 10 mg/500 ml D_5W given 100-180 mcg/min (if 20 gtt/ml inf device) then maintenance of 40-60 mcg/min; use inf device
- **Child: IV BOL** 5-20 mcg/kg/dose q10-15min; **IV INF** 0.1-0.5 mcg/kg/min

P

Available forms: Inj 1% (10 mg/ml)

Administer:

IV route

- Plasma expanders for hypovolemia
- IV after diluting 1 mg/9 ml sterile water for inj; give dose over ½-1 min; may be diluted 10 mg/500 ml of D_5W or NS; titrate to response (normal B/P); check for extravasation, check site for infiltration, use inf pump

Additive compatibilities: Chloramphenicol, DOBUTamine, lidocaine, potassium chloride, sodium bicarbonate

Y-site compatibilities: Amiodarone, amrinone, cisatracurium, famotidine, haloperidol, remifentanil, zidovudine

SIDE EFFECTS

CNS: *Headache, anxiety, tremor, insomnia, dizziness*

CV: *Palpitations, tachycardia, hypertension, ectopic beats, angina,* reflex bradycardia, dysrhythmias

GI: *Nausea, vomiting*

INTEG: Necrosis, tissue sloughing with extravasation, gangrene

SYST: Anaphylaxis

PHARMACOKINETICS

IM/SUBCUT: Onset 10-15 min, duration 45-60 min

IV: Onset immediate, duration 20-30 min

INTERACTIONS

- Dysrhythmias: general anesthetics, digoxin

⚠ Do not use within 2 wk of MAOIs because hypertensive crisis may result

Increase: in B/P—oxytocics

Increase: pressor effect—tricyclics, β-blockers, H_1 antihistamines

Decrease: phenylephrine action—α-blockers

NURSING CONSIDERATIONS

Assess:

- I&O ratio; notify prescriber if output <30 ml/hr
- ECG during administration continuously; if B/P increases, product is decreased
- B/P and pulse q5min after parenteral route
- CVP or PWP during inf if possible
- Paresthesias and coldness of extremities; peripheral blood flow may decrease

Perform/provide:

- Storage of reconstituted sol if refrigerated for ≤24 hr
- Discard discolored sol

Evaluate:

- Therapeutic response: increased B/P with stabilization

Teach patient/family:

- About the reason for administration
- To report pain at inf site or other adverse reactions immediately

TREATMENT OF OVERDOSE:

Administer α-blocker

phenylephrine nasal agent

See Appendix B

phenylephrine ophthalmic

See Appendix B

phenytoin (Rx)

(fen′i-toh-in)

Dilantin, Phenytek

Func. class.: Anticonvulsant; antidysrhythmic (IB)

Chem. class.: Hydantoin

ACTION: Inhibits spread of seizure activity in motor cortex by altering ion transport; increases AV conduction

USES: Generalized tonic-clonic seizures; status epilepticus; nonepileptic seizures associated with Reye's syndrome or after head trauma; Bell's palsy, complex partial seizures

Unlabeled uses: Migraines, diabetic neuropathy, neuropathic pain, paroxysmal atrial tachycardia, ventricular tachycardia

CONTRAINDICATIONS:

Pregnancy (D), hypersensitivity, psychiatric condition, bradycardia, SA and AV block, Stokes-Adams syndrome, hepatic failure, acute intermittent porphyria

Precautions: Geriatric patients, allergies, renal/hepatic disease, petit mal seizures, hypotension, myocardial insufficiency, Asian patients positive for HLA-B1502

DOSAGE AND ROUTES

Seizures

- **Adult: PO** 15-20 mg/kg (ext rel) in 3-4 divided doses given q2hr or 400 mg then 300 mg q2hr × 2 doses; maintenance 4-7 mg/kg/day; **IV** 15-20 mg/kg, max 25-50 mg/min, then 100 mg q6-8hr
- **Child: PO** 5 mg/kg/day in 2-3 divided doses, maintenance 4-8 mg/kg/day in 2-3 divided doses, max 300 mg/day; **IV** 15-20 mg/kg at 1-3 mg/kg/min

Status epilepticus

- **Adult: IV** 10-15 mg/kg, max 25-50 mg/min, may give 100 mg q6-8hr thereafter
- **Child: IV** 15-20 mg/kg, max in divided doses 1-3 mg/kg/min

Ventricular dysrhythmias

- **Adult: PO** Loading dose 1 g divided over 24 hr then 500 mg/day × 2 days; **IV** 250 mg over 5 min until dysrhythmias subside or until 1 g is given or 100 mg q15min until dysrhythmias subside or until 1 g is given
- **Child: PO** 3-8 mg/kg or 250 mg/m^2/day as single dose or 2 divided doses; **IV** 3-8 mg/kg over several min or 250 mg/m^2/day as single dose or 2 divided doses

Renal dose

- Do not use loading dose if CCr <10 ml/min or hepatic failure

Neuropathic pain/diabetic neuropathy (unlabeled)

- **Adult: PO** 300 mg/day in divided doses

Migraine prophylaxis (unlabeled)

- **Adult: PO** 200-400 mg/day

Available forms: Susp 25 mg/5 ml; chewable tabs 50 mg; inj 50 mg/ml; ext rel caps 100, 200, 300 mg; prompt rel caps 100 mg

Administer:

PO route

- Do not interchange chewable product with caps, not equivalent; only ext rel caps to be used for once-a-day dosing
- **Oral susp:** shake well before each dose given via G tube/NG tube; dilute susp prior to administration; flush tube with 20 ml water after dose
- Allow 7-10 days between dosage changes
- Divided PO doses with or after meals to decrease adverse effects
- 2 hr before or after antacid, enteral feeding

Direct IV route

- Give undiluted at ≤50 mg/min (adult) 1-3 mg/kg/min (neonates)

Intermittent IV INF route

- Dilute dose in NS to ≤6.7 mg/ml, complete inf within 1 hr of preparation, use 0.22 or 0.45 micron in-line particulate final filter between IV catheter and tubing, flush IV line or catheter with NS before and after use, give at ≤50 mg/min (adult), 0.5-1 mg/kg/min (child, infant, neonate)

Additive compatibilities: Do not admix

Y-site compatibilities: CISplatin, foscarnet, temocillin

SIDE EFFECTS

CNS: Drowsiness, dizziness, insomnia, paresthesias, depression, **suicidal tendencies**, aggression, headache, confusion, slurred speech, peripheral neuropathy

CV: Hypotension, **ventricular fibrillation**

EENT: Nystagmus, diplopia, blurred vision

ENDO: Diabetes insipidus

GI: Nausea, vomiting, constipation, anorexia, weight loss, **hepatitis**, jaundice, gingival hyperplasia

GU: Nephritis, urine discoloration
HEMA: Agranulocytosis, leukopenia, aplastic anemia, thrombocytopenia, megaloblastic anemia
INTEG: Rash, lupus erythematosus, Stevens-Johnson syndrome, hirsutism, toxic epidermal necrolysis
SYST: Hypocalcemia, purple glove syndrome (IV)

PHARMACOKINETICS

Metabolized by liver, excreted by kidneys, protein binding 90%-95%, half-life 7-42 hr, dose dependent
PO: Onset 2-24 hr, peak 1½-2½ hr, duration 6-12 hr
PO-ER: Onset 2-24 hr, peak 4-12 hr, duration 12-36 hr
IV: Onset 1-2 hr, duration 12-24 hr

INTERACTIONS

Increase: phenytoin effect—benzodiazepines, cimetidine, tricyclics, salicylates, valproate, cycloSERINE, diazepam, chloramphenicol, disulfiram, alcohol, amiodarone, sulfonamides, FLUoxetine, gabapentin, H_2 antagonists, azole antifungals, estrogens, succinamides, phenothiazines, methylphenidate, felbamate, trazodone
Decrease: phenytoin effects—alcohol (chronic use), antacids, barbiturates, carBAMazepine, rifampin, folic acid

Drug/Food

Enteral tube feeding: may decrease absorption of oral product; do not use enteral feedings 2 hr before or 2 hr after dose

Drug/Lab Test

Increase: glucose, alk phos, GGT
Decrease: dexamethasone, metyrapone test serum, PBI, urinary steroids

NURSING CONSIDERATIONS

Assess:

⚠ **Phenytoin hypersensitivity syndrome** 3-12 wk after start of treatment: rash, temp, lymphadenopathy; may cause hepatotoxicity, renal failure, rhabdomyolysis

⚠ **Serious skin disorders:** for beginning rash that may lead to Stevens-Johnson syndrome or toxic epidermal necrolysis; phenytoin should not be used again; may occur more often among Asian patients with HLA-B 1502

⚠ **Purple glove syndrome** with IV use

- Phenytoin level: toxic level 30-50 mcg/ml, therapeutic level: 7.5-20 mcg/ml; wait ≥1 wk to draw levels
- **Seizures:** duration, type, intensity, precipitating factors; obtain EEG periodically
- Blood studies: CBC, platelets q2wk until stabilized, then monthly × 12, then q3mo; discontinue product if neutrophils $<1600/mm^3$; renal function: albumin conc; folic acid levels

⚠ Mental status: mood, sensorium, affect, memory (long, short), suicidal thoughts/behaviors

- **Respiratory depression:** rate, depth, character
- **Blood dyscrasias:** fever, sore throat, bruising, rash, jaundice

Evaluate:

- Therapeutic response; decrease in severity of seizures, ventricular dysrhythmias

Teach patient/family:

- That, if diabetic, blood glucose should be monitored
- That urine may turn pink
- Not to discontinue product abruptly because seizures may occur
- **Oral hygiene:** about the proper brushing of teeth using a soft toothbrush, flossing to prevent gingival hyperplasia; about the need to see dentist frequently
- To avoid hazardous activities until stabilized on product
- To carry emergency ID stating product use
- That heavy use of alcohol may diminish effect of product; to avoid OTC medications
- Not to change brands or forms once stabilized on therapy because brands may vary

- Not to use antacids within 2 hr of product
- To use nonhormonal contraception; to notify prescriber if pregnancy is planned or suspected, pregnancy (D)
- To notify prescriber of unusual bleeding, bruising, petechiae (bleeding), clay-colored stools, abdominal pain, dark urine, yellowing of skin or eyes (hepatotoxicity); slurred speech, headache, drowsiness

phosphate/biphosphate (OTC)

Fleet Enema, Phospho-Soda

Func. class.: Laxative, saline

ACTION: Increases water absorption in the small intestine by osmotic action; laxative effect occurs by increased peristalsis and water retention

USES: Constipation, bowel or rectal preparation for surgery, exam

CONTRAINDICATIONS: Hypersensitivity, rectal fissures, abdominal pain, nausea, vomiting, appendicitis, acute surgical abdomen, ulcerated hemorrhoids, sodium-restricted diet, renal failure, hyperphosphatemia, hypocalcemia, hypokalemia, hypernatremia, Addison's disease, CHF, ascites, bowel perforation, megacolon, imperforate anus

Black Box Warning: GI obstruction, renal failure

Precautions: Pregnancy (C)

Black Box Warning: Colitis, geriatric hypovolemia, renal disease

DOSAGE AND ROUTES

- **Adult: PO** 20-30 ml (Phospho-Soda)
- **Child: PO** 5-15 ml (Phospho-Soda)
- **Adult and child >12 yr: RECT** 1 enema (118 ml)
- **Child 2-12 yr: RECT** 1/2 enema (59 ml)

Available forms: Enema 7 g phosphate/19 g biphosphate/118 ml; oral sol 18 g phosphate/48 g biphosphate/100 ml

Administer:

- Alone for better absorption; do not take within 1-2 hr of other products

SIDE EFFECTS

CV: **Dysrhythmias, cardiac arrest, hypotension, widening QRS complex**

GI: *Nausea, cramps,* diarrhea

META: Electrolyte, fluid imbalances

PHARMACOKINETICS

Onset 30 min-3 hr, excreted in feces

NURSING CONSIDERATIONS

Assess:

- **Stools:** color, amount, consistency; bowel pattern, bowel sounds, flatulence, distention, fever, dietary patterns, exercise; cramping, rectal bleeding, nausea, vomiting; if these occur, product should be discontinued
- Blood, urine electrolytes if product used often

Evaluate:

- Therapeutic response: decrease in constipation

Teach patient/family:

- Not to use laxatives for long-term therapy because bowel tone will be lost
- That normal bowel movements do not always occur daily
- Not to use in presence of abdominal pain, nausea, vomiting
- To notify prescriber if constipation unrelieved or if symptoms of electrolyte imbalance occur: muscle cramps, pain, weakness, dizziness, excessive thirst
- To maintain fluid consumption

physostigmine ophthalmic

See Appendix B

P

phytonadione (Rx)

(fye-toe-na-dye′one)

Mephyton, Vit K

Func. class.: Vit K_1, fat-soluble vitamin

ACTION: Needed for adequate blood clotting (factors II, VII, IX, X)

USES: Vit K malabsorption, hypoprothrombinemia, prevention of hypoprothrombinemia caused by oral anticoagulants, prevention of hemorrhagic disease of the newborn

CONTRAINDICATIONS: Hypersensitivity, severe hepatic disease, last few weeks of pregnancy

Precautions: Pregnancy (C), neonates, hepatic disease

Black Box Warning: IV use

DOSAGE AND ROUTES

Hypoprothrombinemia caused by vit K malabsorption

- **Adult: PO/IM** 2.5-25 mg, may repeat or increase to 50 mg
- **Child: PO** 2.5-5 mg
- **Infant: PO/IM** 2 mg

Prevention of hemorrhagic disease of the newborn

- **Neonate: IM** 0.5-1 mg within 1 hr after birth, repeat after 2-3 wk if required

Hypoprothrombinemia caused by oral anticoagulants

- **Adult and child: PO/SUBCUT/IM** 1-10 mg, may repeat 12-48 hr after **PO** dose or 6-8 hr after **SUBCUT/IM** dose based on INR

Available forms: Tabs 5 mg; inj 10 mg/ml, 1 mg/0.5 ml

Administer:

Intermittent IV INF route

- After diluting with ≥10 ml D_5NS; give max 1 mg/min

⚠ IV only when other routes not possible (deaths have occurred)

Y-site compatibilities: Alfentanil, amikacin, aminophylline, ascorbic acid, atracurium, atropine, azaTHIOprine, aztreonam, bumetanide, buprenorphine, butorphanol, calcium chloride/gluconate, ceFAZolin, cefonicid, cefoperazone, cefotaxime, cefotetan, cefoxitin, ceftazidime, ceftizoxime, cefTRIAXone, cefuroxime, chloramphenicol, chlorproMAZINE, cimetidine, clindamycin, cyanocobalamin, cycloSPORINE, dexamethasone, digoxin, diphenhydrAMINE, DOPamine, doxycycline, enalaprilat, ePHEDrine, EPINEPHrine, epoetin alfa, erythromycin, esmolol, famotidine, fentaNYL, fluconazole, folic acid, furosemide, ganciclovir, gentamicin, glycopyrrolate, heparin, hydrocortisone, imipenem/cilastatin, indomethacin, insulin, isoproterenol, ketorolac, labetalol, lidocaine, mannitol, meperidine, metaraminol, methoxamine, methyldopate, metoclopramide, metoprolol, metroNIDAZOLE, midazolam, morphine, multivitamins, nafcillin, nalbuphine, naloxone, nitroglycerin, nitroprusside, norepinephrine, ondansetron, oxacillin, oxytocin, papaverine, penicillin G potassium, pentamidine, pentazocine, PENTobarbital, PHENobarbital, phentolamine, phenylephrine, potassium chloride, procainamide, prochlorperazine, propranolol, pyridoxime, ranitidine, sodium bicarbonate, succinylcholine, SUFentanil, theophylline, thiamine, ticarcillin/clavulanate, tobramycin, tolazoline, trimetaphan, urokinase, vancomycin, vasopressin, verapamil, vitamin B with C

SIDE EFFECTS

CNS: Headache, brain damage (large doses)

GI: Nausea, decreased LFTs

HEMA: Hemolytic anemia, hemoglobinuria, hyperbilirubinemia

INTEG: Rash, urticaria

RESP: Bronchospasm, dyspnea, feeling of chest constriction, respiratory arrest

PHARMACOKINETICS

PO/INJ: Metabolized, crosses placenta

INTERACTIONS

Decrease: action of phytonadione—bile acid sequestrants, sucralfate, antiinfectives, salicylates, mineral oil

Decrease: action of warfarin—large dose of product

NURSING CONSIDERATIONS

Assess:

• **Bleeding:** emesis, stools, urine; pressure on all venipuncture sites; avoid all inj if possible

• PT during treatment (2-sec deviation from control time, bleeding time, clotting time); monitor for bleeding, pulse, and B/P

Perform/provide:

• Storage in tight, light-resistant container

Evaluate:

• Therapeutic response: prevention of hemorrhagic disease of the newborn, resolution of hypoprothrombinemia

Teach patient/family:

• Not to take other supplements, OTC products, prescription products unless directed by prescriber

• About the necessary foods for associated diet

• To avoid IM inj; to use soft toothbrush; not to floss, use electric razor until coagulation defect corrected

• To report symptoms of bleeding

• About the importance of frequent lab tests to monitor coagulation factors

• To notify all health care providers of use of this product

• To carry emergency ID describing condition and products used

pilocarpine ophthalmic

See Appendix B

pimecrolimus topical

See Appendix B

pioglitazone (Rx)

(pie-oh-glye′ta-zone)

Actos

Func. class.: Antidiabetic, oral

Chem. class.: Thiazolidinedione

ACTION: Specifically targets insulin resistance; an insulin sensitizer; regulates the transcription of a number of insulin-responsive genes

USES: Type 2 diabetes mellitus

CONTRAINDICATIONS: Breastfeeding, children, hypersensitivity to thiazolidinedione, diabetic ketoacidosis

Black Box Warning: CHF

Precautions: Pregnancy (C), geriatric patients, geriatric patients with CV disease, renal/hepatic/thyroid disease, edema, polycystic ovary syndrome, bladder cancer, osteoporosis, pulmonary disease, secondary malignancy

DOSAGE AND ROUTES

Monotherapy

• **Adult: PO** 15 or 30 mg/day, may increase to 45 mg/day; with strong CYP2C8, max 15 mg/day; with NYHA class I/II heart failure, max 15 mg/day

Combination therapy

• **Adult: PO** 15 or 30 mg/day with a sulfonylurea, metformin, or insulin; decrease sulfonylurea dose if hypoglycemia occurs; decrease insulin dose by 10%-25% if hypoglycemia occurs or if plasma glucose is $<$100 mg/dl, max 45 mg/day

Hepatic dose

• Do not use in active hepatic disease or if ALT $>$2.5 times ULN

Available forms: Tabs 15, 30, 45 mg

Administer:

• Once a day; without regard to meals

• Tabs crushed and mixed with food or fluids for patients with difficulty swallowing

P

SIDE EFFECTS

CNS: *Headache*

CV: MI, heart failure, death (geriatric patients)

ENDO: Hypo/hyperglycemia

MISC: *Sinusitis, upper respiratory tract infection, pharyngitis,* hepatotoxicity, edema, weight gain, anemia, macular edema; risk of bladder cancer (use >1 yr)

MS: Rhabdomyolysis, fractures (females), myalgia

PHARMACOKINETICS

Maximal reduction in FBS after 12 wk; half-life 3-7 hr, terminal 16-24 hr; protein binding >99%

INTERACTIONS

Decrease: effect of oral contraceptives; use alternative contraceptive method

Decrease: pioglitazone effect—CYP2C8 inducers (ketoconazole, fluconazole, itraconazole, miconazole, voriconazole)

Drug/Herb

Increase: hypoglycemia—garlic, green tea, horse chestnut

Drug/Lab Test

Increase: CPK

NURSING CONSIDERATIONS

Assess:

Black Box Warning: For CHF: excessive/rapid weight gain >5 lb, dyspnea, edema; may need to be reduced or discontinued

- **Rhabdomyolysis:** muscle pain, increased CPK, weakness, swelling of affected muscles; if these occur and if confirmed by CPK, product should be discontinued
- **Hypoglycemic reactions:** sweating, weakness, dizziness, anxiety, tremors, hunger; hyperglycemic reactions soon after meals (rare); do not give with NYHA class III/IV heart failure
- Check LFTs periodically: AST, LDH; do not start treatment in active heart disease or if ALT >2.5× upper limit of normal; if treatment has already begun, follow closely with continuing ALT levels; if ALT increases to >3× upper limit of normal, recheck ALT as soon as possible; if ALT remains >3× upper limit of normal, discontinue
- FBS, glycosylated HbA1c, plasma lipids/lipoproteins, B/P, body weight during treatment
- CBC with differential prior to and during therapy; more necessary in those with anemia

Perform/provide:

- Conversion from other oral hypoglycemic agents; change may be made with gradual dosage change; monitor serum glucose during conversion
- Storage in tight container in cool environment

Evaluate:

- Therapeutic response: decrease in polyuria, polydipsia, polyphagia; clear sensorium; absence of dizziness; stable gait; blood glucose A1c improvement

Teach patient/family:

- To self-monitor using a blood glucose meter
- About the symptoms of hypo/hyperglycemia, what to do about each
- That product must be continued on daily basis; about the consequences of discontinuing product abruptly
- To avoid OTC medications or herbal preparations unless approved by prescriber
- That diabetes is a lifelong illness; that product is not a cure, it only controls symptoms
- To notify prescriber if oral contraceptives are used; not to use product if breastfeeding
- To report symptoms of hepatic dysfunction: nausea, vomiting, abdominal pain, fatigue, anorexia, dark urine, jaundice
- To report weight gain, edema

piperacillin/tazobactam (Rx)

(pip′er-ah-sill′in/ta-zoe-bak′tam)

Zosyn

Func. class.: Antiinfective, broad spectrum

Chem. class.: Extended-spectrum penicillin, β-lactamase inhibitor

ACTION: Interferes with cell-wall replication of susceptible organisms; osmotically unstable cell wall swells and bursts from osmotic pressure; tazobactam is a β-lactamase inhibitor that protects piperacillin from enzymatic degradation

USES: Moderate to severe infections: piperacillin-resistant, β-lactamase–producing strains causing infections in respiratory, skin, urinary tract, bone, gonorrhea, pneumonia; effective for resistant *Staphylococcus aureus,* resistant *Escherichia coli, Bacteroides fragilis, Bacteroides ovatus, Bacteroides thetaiotaomicron, Bacteroides vulgatus, Haemophilus influenzae*

CONTRAINDICATIONS: Hypersensitivity to penicillins; neonates; carbapenem allergy

Precautions: Pregnancy (B), breastfeeding, renal insufficiency in children, hypersensitivity to cephalosporins, CHF, seizures, GI disease, electrolyte imbalances

DOSAGE AND ROUTES

Nosocomial pneumonia

- **Adult: IV** 4.5 g q6hr or 3.375 g q4hr with an aminoglycoside or antipseudomonal fluoroquinolone × 1-2 wk; continue aminoglycoside only if *Pseudomonas aeruginosa* is isolated

Other infections

- **Adult: IV INF** 6-12 g/day given 2.25 g q8hr to 3.375 g q6hr over 30 min × 7-10 days

Renal dose

- **Adult: IV** CCr 20-40 ml/min, give 3.375 g q6hr (nosocomial pneumonia); give 2.25 g q6hr (all other indications); CCr <20 ml/min, give 2.25 g q6hr (nosocomial pneumonia), give 2.25 g q8hr (all other indications)

Available forms: Powder for inj 2 g piperacillin/0.25 g tazobactam, 3 g piperacillin/0.375 g tazobactam, 4 g piperacillin/0.5 g tazobactam, 36 g piperacillin/4.5 g tazobactam

Administer:

- Separate aminoglycoside from piperacillin to avoid inactivation
- Product after C&S is complete

Intermittent IV INF route

- Reconstitute each 1 g of product/5 ml 0.9% NaCl for inj or sterile water for inj, dextrose 5%; shake well; further dilute in ≥50 ml compatible IV sol, run as int inf over ≥30 min

Y-site compatibilities: Alfentanil, allopurinol, amifostine, amikacin, aminocaproic acid, aminophylline, amphotericin B lipid complex, amphotericin B liposome, anidulafungin, atenolol, aztreonam, bivalirudin, bleomycin, bumetanide, buprenorphine, busulfan, butorphanol, calcium acetate/chloride/gluconate, CARBOplatin, carmustine, cefepime, chloramphenicol, cimetidine, clindamycin, cyclophosphamide, cycloSPORINE, cytarabine, DACTINomycin, DAPTOmycin, dexamethasone, dexrazoxane, diazepam, digoxin, diphenhydrAMINE, docetaxel, DOPamine, doxacurium, enalaprilat, ePHEDrine, EPINEPHrine, eptifibatide, erythromycin, esmolol, etoposide, fenoldopam, fentaNYL, floxuridine, fluconazole, fludarabine, fluorouracil, foscarnet, fosphenytoin, furosemide, gallium, granisetron, heparin, hydrocortisone, HYDROmorphone, ifosfamide, isoproterenol, ketorolac, lansoprazole, leucovorin, lidocaine, linezolid, LORazepam, magnesium sulfate, mannitol, mechlorethamine, melphalan, meperidine, mesna, metaraminol, methotrexate, methylPREDNISolone, metoclopramide, metoprolol, metroNI-

P

DAZOLE, milrinone, morphine, naloxone, nitroglycerin, nitroprusside, norepinephrine, octreotide, ondansetron, oxytocin, paclitaxel, palonosetron, pamidronate, pancuronium, pantoprazole, pemetrexed, PENTobarbital, PHENObarbital, phenylephrine, plicamycin, potassium chloride/phosphates, procainamide, ranitidine, remifentanil, riTUXimab, sargramostim, sodium acetate/bicarbonate/phosphates, succinylcholine, SUFentanil, sulfamethoxazole-trimethoprim, tacrolimus, teniposide, theophylline, thiotepa, tigecycline, tirofiban, trimethobenzamide, vasopressin, vinBLAStine, vinCRIStine, voriconazole, zidovudine, zoledronic acid

SIDE EFFECTS

CNS: Lethargy, hallucinations, anxiety, depression, twitching, insomnia, headache, fever, dizziness, seizures, vertigo
CV: Cardiac toxicity
GI: *Nausea, vomiting, diarrhea;* increased AST, ALT; abdominal pain, glossitis, pseudomembranous colitis, constipation
GU: Oliguria, proteinuria, hematuria, *vaginitis, moniliasis,* glomerulonephritis, renal failure
HEMA: Anemia, increased bleeding time, bone marrow depression, agranulocytosis, hemolytic anemia
INTEG: Rash, pruritus, exfoliative dermatitis
META: Hypokalemia, hypernatremia
SYST: Serum sickness, anaphylaxis, Stevens-Johnson syndrome

PHARMACOKINETICS

Half-life 0.7-1.2 hr; excreted in urine, bile, breast milk; crosses placenta; 33% bound to plasma proteins
IV: Peak completion of IV

INTERACTIONS

Increase: effect of neuromuscular blockers, oral anticoagulants, methotrexate
Increase: piperacillin concentrations—aspirin, probenecid
Decrease: antimicrobial effect of piperacillin—tetracyclines, aminoglycosides IV
Decrease: effect of oral contraceptives

Drug/Lab Test

Increase: platelet count, eosinophilia, neutropenia, leukopenia, serum creatinine, PTT, AST, ALT, alk phos, bilirubin, BUN, electrolytes
Decrease: Hct, Hgb, electrolytes
False positive: urine glucose, urine protein, Coombs' test

NURSING CONSIDERATIONS

Assess:

- **Infection:** temp, stools, urine, sputum, wounds
- I&O ratio; report hematuria, oliguria because penicillin in high doses is nephrotoxic; maintain hydration unless contraindicated
- Hepatic studies: AST, ALT before treatment and periodically thereafter
- Blood studies: WBC, RBC, Hct, Hgb, bleeding time before treatment and periodically thereafter; serum potassium
- Renal studies: urinalysis, protein, blood, BUN, creatinine before treatment and periodically thereafter
- C&S before product therapy; product may be given as soon as culture is taken
- **Pseudomembranous colitis:** diarrhea, bloody stools, fever, abdominal cramps; may occur ≤2 mo after treatment; bowel pattern before and during treatment
- Skin eruptions after administration of penicillin to 1 wk after discontinuing product
- Respiratory status: rate, character, wheezing, tightness in chest
- **Anaphylaxis:** wheezing, laryngeal edema, rash, itching; discontinue product, have emergency equipment nearby

Perform/provide:

- Adequate intake of fluids (2 L) during diarrhea episodes
- Discard after 24 hr if stored at room temp or after 48 hr if refrigerated; use single-dose vials immediately after re-

constitution; stable in ambulatory IV pump for 12 hr

Evaluate:

- Therapeutic response: absence of fever, purulent drainage, redness, inflammation; culture shows decreased organisms

Teach patient/family:

- That culture may be taken after completed course of medication
- To report sore throat, fever, fatigue (superinfection); CNS effects (anxiety, depression, hallucinations, seizures); **pseudomembranous colitis:** fever, diarrhea with blood, pus, mucous
- To wear or carry emergency ID if allergic to penicillins
- To notify nurse of diarrhea

TREATMENT OF OVERDOSE:

Withdraw product, maintain airway, administer EPINEPHrine, aminophylline, O_2, IV corticosteroids for anaphylaxis

piroxicam (Rx)

(peer-ox′i-kam)

Apo-Piroxicam ♣, Feldene, Gen-Piroxicam ♣

Func. class.: Nonsteroidal antiinflammatory

Chem. class.: Oxicam derivative

ACTION:

Inhibits COX-1 and COX-2 by blocking arachidonate; has analgesic, antiinflammatory, antipyretic properties

USES:

Mild to moderate pain, osteoarthritis, rheumatoid arthritis

CONTRAINDICATIONS:

Pregnancy (D) (3rd trimester), hypersensitivity to this product, NSAIDs, salicylates; asthma

Black Box Warning: Perioperative pain in CABG surgery

Precautions: Pregnancy (C), avoid during late pregnancy, breastfeeding, children, bleeding/GI/cardiac disorders, hypersensitivity to other antiinflammatory agents, CHF

Black Box Warning: GI bleeding, MI, stroke

DOSAGE AND ROUTES

- **Adult: PO** 20 mg/day or 10 mg bid

Available forms: Caps 10, 20 mg

Administer:

PO route

- Do not break, crush, chew caps
- With food to decrease GI symptoms; take product at same time daily, avoid alcohol
- Higher doses not more effective

SIDE EFFECTS

CNS: Dizziness, *drowsiness,* fatigue, tremors, confusion, insomnia, anxiety, depression, *headache*

CV: Tachycardia, peripheral edema, palpitations, dysrhythmias, hypertension, **MI, stroke, CHF**

EENT: Tinnitus, hearing loss, blurred vision

GI: *Nausea, anorexia, vomiting, diarrhea,* jaundice, **cholestatic hepatitis,** constipation, flatulence, cramps, dry mouth, peptic ulcer, **bleeding, ulceration, perforation,** dyspepsia

GU: **Nephrotoxicity: dysuria, hematuria, oliguria, azotemia**

HEMA: **Blood dyscrasias**

INTEG: Purpura, rash, pruritus, sweating, photosensitivity

MISC: Hyperkalemia, hypoglycemia

SYST: **Anaphylaxis**

PHARMACOKINETICS

Peak 3-5 hr; duration 48-72 hr, half-life 50 hr; metabolized in liver; excreted in urine (metabolites), breast milk; 99% protein binding

INTERACTIONS

Increase: hypoglycemia—oral antidiabetics

Increase: toxicity—cycloSPORINE, methotrexate, lithium, alcohol, oral anticoagulants, aspirin, corticosteroids

P

Increase: bleeding risk—anticoagulants, antiplatelets, thrombin inhibitors, NSAIDs, SSRIs, SNRIs
Decrease: effects of antihypertensives, diuretics

Drug/Herb
Increase: bleeding risk—ginger, garlic, ginkgo

Drug/Lab
Increase: AST, ALT, LDH, BUN, creatinine
Decrease: Hgb/Hct, platelets, leukocytes

NURSING CONSIDERATIONS

Assess:

Black Box Warning: Cardiac status: CV thrombotic events, MI, stroke; may be fatal; do not use for perioperative pain with coronary artery bypass graft (CABG) surgery

⚠ GI status: ulceration, bleeding, perforation; may be fatal

- **Pain:** location, duration, type, ROM before, 1-2 hr after administration
- Renal, hepatic, blood studies: BUN, creatinine, AST, ALT, Hgb, before treatment, periodically thereafter
- Audiometric, ophthalmic exam before, during, after treatment
- For eye, ear problems: blurred vision, tinnitus (may indicate toxicity)

⚠ **Anaphylaxis:** wheezing, laryngeal edema; those with aspirin sensitivity, asthma, nasal polyps may develop allergic reactions

Perform/provide:

- Storage at room temp in light-resistant container

Evaluate:

- Therapeutic response: decreased pain, stiffness, swelling in joints; ability to move more easily

Teach patient/family:

- To report blurred vision or ringing, roaring in ears (may indicate toxicity)
- To avoid driving, other hazardous activities if dizzy or drowsy
- That patient should drink at least 6-8 glasses of water/day unless contraindicated
- To report change in urine pattern, weight increase, edema, pain increase in joints, fever, blood in urine (indicates nephrotoxicity)
- That therapeutic effects may take up to 1 mo
- To avoid ASA, other OTC meds, alcohol, herbal supplements unless approved by prescriber
- To report if pregnancy is suspected or planned; to avoid breastfeeding
- To report bruising; bleeding; black, tarry stools
- To avoid prolonged sun exposure; to wear sunscreen, protective clothing
- To inform all health care providers about product use

pitavastatin (Rx)

(pit′a-va-stat′-in)

Livalo

Func. class.: Antilipidemic
Chem. class.: HMG-CoA reductase inhibitor

ACTION: Inhibits HMG-CoA reductase enzyme, which reduces cholesterol synthesis; high doses lead to plaque regression

USES: As an adjunct for primary hypercholesterolemia (types Ia, Ib), dysbetalipoproteinemia, elevated triglyceride levels, prevention of CV disease by reduction of heart risk in those with mildly elevated cholesterol
Unlabeled Uses: Atherosclerosis

CONTRAINDICATIONS: Pregnancy (X), breastfeeding, hypersensitivity, active hepatic disease, cholestasis
Precautions: Past hepatic disease, alcoholism, severe acute infections, trauma, severe metabolic disorders, electrolyte imbalance, seizures, surgery, organ transplant, endocrine disease, females, hypotension, renal disease

DOSAGE AND ROUTES

• **Adult: PO** 2 mg/day, usual range 1-4, max 4 mg/day

Renal dose

• **Adult: PO** CCr 30-<60 ml/min, 1 mg daily, max 2 mg daily; CCr <30 ml/min on hemodialysis, 1 mg daily, max 2 mg daily; CCr <30 ml/min, not recommended

Atherosclerosis (unlabeled)

• **Adult: PO** 4 mg/day

Available forms: Tabs 1, 2, 4 mg

Administer:

• Total daily dose any time of day without regard to meals

SIDE EFFECTS

CNS: Headache

GI: Constipation, diarrhea

INTEG: Rash, pruritus, alopecia

MS: Arthralgia, myalgia, **rhabdomyolysis**

RESP: Pharyngitis

PHARMACOKINETICS

Peak 1 hr; metabolized in liver, excreted in urine, feces; half-life 12 hr; protein binding 99%; concentrations lower in healthy African Americans

INTERACTIONS

Increase: risk for possible rhabdomyolysis—azole antifungals, cycloSPORINE, erythromycin, niacin, gemfibrozil, clofibrate

Increase: levels of pitavastatin—erythromycin, red yeast rice

Increase: effects of warfarin

Drug/Lab Test

Increase: bilirubin, alk phos, ALT, AST

Interference: thyroid function tests

NURSING CONSIDERATIONS

Assess:

• Diet; obtain diet history including fat, cholesterol in diet

• Cholesterol, triglyceride levels periodically during treatment; check lipid panel 6 wk after changing dose

• Hepatic studies at 12 wk after starting treatment, then q6mo; if AST >3× normal, reduce or discontinue; AST, ALT, LFTs may be increased

• Renal studies in patients with compromised renal system: BUN, I&O ratio, creatinine

⚠ **Rhabdomyolysis: muscle pain, tenderness; obtain CPK baseline; if markedly increased, product may need to be discontinued**

Perform/provide:

• Storage in cool environment in tight container protected from light

Evaluate:

• Therapeutic response: decrease in cholesterol to desired level after 6 wk

Teach patient/family:

• That blood work will be necessary during treatment

• To report blurred vision, severe GI symptoms, headache, muscle pain, weakness, tenderness

• That previously prescribed regimen will continue: low-cholesterol diet, exercise program, smoking cessation

• Not to take product if pregnant (X) or if pregnancy is planned or suspected (notify prescriber); to avoid breastfeeding

P

plasma protein fraction (Rx)

Plasmanate

Func. class.: Hematological agent

Chem. class.: Plasma volume expander

ACTION: Exerts similar oncotic pressure as human plasma, expands blood volume

USES: Hypovolemic shock, hypoproteinemia, ARDS, preoperative cardiopulmonary bypass, acute hepatic failure, nephrotic syndrome, cardiogenic shock

CONTRAINDICATIONS:

Hypersensitivity to this product or albumin; CHF, severe anemia, renal insufficiency, hyponatremia, cardiopulmonary bypass

Precautions: Pregnancy (C), decreased salt intake, decreased cardiac reserve, lack of albumin deficiency, hepatic disease

DOSAGE AND ROUTES

Hypovolemia

- **Adult: IV INF** 250-500 ml (12.5-25 g protein), max 10 ml/min
- **Child: IV INF** 10-30 ml/kg at max 5-10 ml/min

Hypoproteinemia

- **Adult: IV INF** 1000-1500 ml/day, max 8 ml/min

Available forms: Inj 5%

Administer:

IV route

- IV access at distant site from infection or trauma; no dilution required; use inf pump, use large-gauge needle (≥20 G); discard unused portion; infuse slowly to prevent hypotension
- Within 4 hr of opening, discard partially used vials
- Do not use sol that has been frozen
- Adjust rate to changes in B/P

Additive compatibilities: Carbohydrate and electrolyte sol, whole blood, packed RBCs, chloramphenicol, tetracycline

SIDE EFFECTS

CNS: Fever, chills, headache, paresthesias, flushing

CV: Fluid overload, hypotension, erratic pulse

GI: Nausea, vomiting, increased salivation

INTEG: Rash, urticaria, cyanosis

RESP: Altered respirations, dyspnea, PE

PHARMACOKINETICS

Metabolized as a protein/energy source

INTERACTIONS

Drug/Lab Test

False increase: alk phos

NURSING CONSIDERATIONS

Assess:

- Blood studies: Hct, Hgb, electrolytes, serum protein; if serum protein declines, dyspnea, hypoxemia can result
- B/P (decreased), pulse (erratic), respiration during inf
- I&O ratio; urinary output may decrease
- Allergy: fever, rash, itching, chills, flushing, urticaria, nausea, vomiting, hypotension requires discontinuation of inf; use new lot if therapy reinstituted; premedicate with diphenhydrAMINE

⚠ Increased CVP reading: distended neck veins indicate circulatory overload; SOB, anxiety, insomnia, expiratory crackles, frothy blood-tinged cough, cyanosis indicate pulmonary overload

Perform/provide:

- Adequate hydration before administration
- Storage at room temp, max 86° F

Evaluate:

- Therapeutic response: increased B/P, decreased edema, increased serum albumin

plerixafor (Rx)

(pler-ix′a-fore)

Mozobil

Func. class.: Biologic modifier

Chem. class.: Colony-stimulating factor

ACTION:

Competitively inhibits the binding of stromal-derived factors, thereby allowing hematopoietic stem cells to mobilize into peripheral blood

USES:

For peripheral blood stem cell (PBSC) mobilization for collection and autologous transplant in patients with non-Hodgkin's lymphoma, multiple myeloma; used with a granulocyte colony-stimulating factor (G-CSF)

CONTRAINDICATIONS:
Hypersensitivity, breastfeeding, pregnancy (D)

Precautions: Children, renal disease, thrombocytopenia

DOSAGE AND ROUTES

- **Adult: SUBCUT** 0.24 mg/kg daily about 11 hr prior to initiation of apheresis, give for up to 4 consecutive days; give filgrastim 10 mcg/kg; **SUBCUT** daily each AM beginning 4 days prior to the 1st evening dose of plerixafor and on each day of apheresis; give filgrastim before procedure

Available forms: Inj 300 mcg/ml, 480 mcg/1.6 ml, 480 mcg/0.8 ml, 3000 mcg/0.5 ml

Administer:

SUBCUT route

- Each single-use vial contains 24 mg of plerixafor (1.2 ml of 20 mg/ml sol); volume calculated by multiplying 0.012 by actual body weight (kg)
- Give 11 hr before apheresis
- Max 40 mg/day or 27 mg/day in patients with renal disease

SIDE EFFECTS

CNS: Syncope, dizziness, fatigue, headache, insomnia, malaise, paresthesias

GI: *Nausea,* vomiting, diarrhea, abdominal pain, constipation

HEMA: Thrombocytopenia, leukocytosis

INTEG: Rash, skin irritation, pruritus, inj site reaction, erythema, urticaria

MS: Musculoskeletal pain

RESP: Dyspnea, hypoxia

PHARMACOKINETICS

SUBCUT: 30-60 min, peak mobilization 6-9 hr, 58% protein binding, 70% excreted via kidneys (parent drug), terminal half-life 3-5 hr

INTERACTIONS

Increase: adverse reactions—do not use this product concomitantly with lithium, may increase leukocytosis

NURSING CONSIDERATIONS

Assess:

- Blood studies: CBC, differential
- B/P, respirations, pulse before and during therapy
- Bone pain; give mild analgesics

Perform/provide:

- Storage at room temp

Evaluate:

- Therapeutic response: collection of stem cells

Teach patient/family:

- About reason for use and expected results

posaconazole (Rx)

(poe′sa-kon′a-zole)

Noxafil, Posanol ♣

Func. class.: Antifungal—systemic

Chem. class.: Triazole derivative

ACTION:
Inhibits a portion of cell-wall synthesis; alters cell membranes and inhibits several fungal enzymes

USES:
Prevention of aspergillus, candida infection, oropharyngeal candidiasis in immunocompromised patients, chemotherapy-induced neutropenia, mucocutaneous, candidiasis

Unlabeled uses: Aspergillosis, cellulitis, coccidioidomycosis, endocarditis, endophthalmitis, esophageal candidiasis, febrile neutropenia, fungal keratitis, fusariosis, histoplasmosis, infectious arthritis, myocarditis, osteomyelitis, pericarditis, sinusitis, tracheobronchitis

CONTRAINDICATIONS:
Hypersensitivity to this product or other systemic antifungals or azoles; fungal meningitis, onchomycosis or dermatomycosis in cardiac dysfunction

Precautions: Pregnancy (C), breastfeeding, children, cardiac/hepatic disease

P

DOSAGE AND ROUTES

• **Adult: PO** 800 mg/day in 2-4 divided doses

• **Child: PO** 100 mg tid

Available forms: Oral susp 200 mg/5 ml

Administer:

PO route

• **Oral susp:** shake well; use calibrated measuring device; take only with full meal or liquid nutritional supplements such as Ensure; rinse measuring device after each use

SIDE EFFECTS

CNS: *Headache, dizziness,* insomnia, fever, rigors, weakness, anxiety

CV: Hypo/hypertension, tachycardia, anemia

GI: *Nausea, vomiting, anorexia, diarrhea,* cramps, abdominal pain, flatulence, GI bleeding, hepatotoxicity

GU: Gynecomastia, impotence, decreased libido

INTEG: *Pruritus,* fever, *rash,* toxic epidermal necrolysis

MISC: *Edema, fatigue,* malaise, hypokalemia, tinnitus, rhabdomyolysis

PHARMACOKINETICS

Well absorbed, enhanced by food, protein binding 98%-99%, peak 4-11 hr, half-life 19-35 hr, metabolized in liver, excreted in feces (77% unchanged)

INTERACTIONS

⚠ **Increase:** QT prolongation—class IA/III antidysrhythmics, some phenothiazines, β agonists, local anesthetics, tricyclics, haloperidol, chloroquine, droperidol, pentamidine; CYP3A4 inhibitors (amiodarone, clarithromycin, erythromycin, telithromycin, troleandomycin), arsenic trioxide, levomethadyl; CYP3A4 substrates (methadone, pimozide, quetiapine, quiNIDine, risperidone, ziprasidone)

Increase: tinnitus, hearing loss—quiNIDine

Increase: hepatotoxicity—other hepatotoxic products

Increase: severe hypoglycemia—oral hypoglycemics

Increase: sedation—triazolam, oral midazolam

Increase: levels, toxicity—busPIRone, busulfan, calcium-channel blockers, clarithromycin, cycloSPORINE, diazepam, digoxin, felodipine, HMG-CoA reductase inhibitors, indinavir, isradipine, midazolam, niCARdipine, niFEDipine, nimodipine, phenytoin, quiNIDine, ritonavir, saquinavir, sirolimus, tacrolimus, vinca alkaloids, warfarin

Decrease: posaconazole level—cimetidine, phenytoin

Decrease: effect of oral contraceptives

Decrease: posaconazole action—antacids, H_2-receptor antagonists, rifamycin, didanosine

Drug/Food

• Food increases absorption

NURSING CONSIDERATIONS

Assess:

⚠ **Infection:** type of, may begin treatment prior to obtaining results; temp, WBC, sputum at baseline and periodically

• I&O ratio, electrolytes; correct electrolyte imbalances before starting treatment

• For allergic reaction: rash, photosensitivity, urticaria, dermatitis

⚠ **Rhabdomyolysis:** muscle pain, increased CPK; weakness, swelling of affected muscles; if these occur and if confirmed by CPK, product should be discontinued

⚠ **Hepatotoxicity:** nausea, vomiting, jaundice, clay-colored stools, fatigue; hepatic studies (ALT, AST, bilirubin) if patient receiving long-term therapy

⚠ **QT prolongation:** ECG for QT prolongation, ejection fraction; assess for chest pain, palpitations, dyspnea

Perform/provide:

• Storage in tight container in refrigerator; do not freeze

Evaluate:

• Therapeutic response: decreased symptoms of fungal infection, negative C&S for infecting organism

Teach patient/family:
- That long-term therapy may be needed to clear infection (1 wk-6 mo, depending on infection)
- To avoid hazardous activities if dizziness occurs
- To take 2 hr before administration of other products that increase gastric pH (antacids, H_2-blockers, omeprazole, sucralfate, anticholinergics); to notify health care provider of all medications taken
- About the importance of compliance with product regimen; to use alternative method of contraception
- To notify prescriber of GI symptoms, signs of hepatic dysfunction (fatigue, nausea, anorexia, vomiting, dark urine, pale stools)

potassium acetate
potassium bicarbonate (OTC, Rx)

K Effervescent, Klor-Con EF, K-Vescent

potassium bicarbonate and potassium chloride (OTC, Rx)

Neo-K ✤

potassium bicarbonate and potassium citrate (OTC, Rx)

potassium chloride (OTC, Rx)

Epiklor, Klor-Con, K-Tab, Micro-K, Odan K-20 ✤

potassium gluconate (OTC, Rx)

Equaline Potassium Gluconate, Walgreens Finest Natural Potassium Gluconate

Func. class.: Electrolyte, mineral replacement
Chem. class.: Potassium

P

ACTION: Needed for the adequate transmission of nerve impulses and cardiac contraction, renal function, intracellular ion maintenance

USES: Prevention and treatment of hypokalemia

CONTRAINDICATIONS: Renal disease (severe), severe hemolytic disease, Addison's disease, hyperkalemia, acute dehydration, extensive tissue breakdown

Precautions: Pregnancy (C), cardiac disease, potassium-sparing diuretic therapy, systemic acidosis

DOSAGE AND ROUTES

Hypokalemia (prevention) (bicarbonate, chloride, gluconate)

• **Adult: PO** 20 mEq/day in 1-2 divided doses

• **Child: PO** 1-2 mEq/kg/day in 1-2 divided doses

Hypokalemia, digoxin toxicity (acetate, chloride)

• **Adult:** serum potassium conc >2.5 mEq/L: **IV** max 10 mEq/1 hr with 24-hr max dose 200 mEq, initial dose of 20-40 mEq has been recommended; **PO** 40-100 mEq/day in 2-4 divided doses

• **Child: IV** 0.25-0.5 mEq/kg/dose at 0.25-0.5 mEq/kg/hr; **PO** 2-5 mEq/day in divided doses

Available forms: Tabs for sol 6.5, 25 mEq; ext rel caps 8, 10 mEq; powder for sol 3.3, 5, 6.7, 10, 13.3 mEq/5 ml; tabs 2, 4, 5, 13.4 mEq; ext rel tabs 6.7, 8, 10 mEq; elix 6.7 mEq/5 ml; oral sol 2.375 mEq/5 ml; inj for prep of IV 1.5, 2, 2.4, 3, 3.2, 4.4, 4.7 mEq/ml

Administer:

PO route

• Do not break, crush, or chew ext rel tabs, caps or enteric products

• With or after meals; dissolve effervescent tabs, powder in 8 oz cold water or juice; do not give IM, SUBCUT

• Caps with full glass of liquid

IV route

• Through large-bore needle to decrease vein inflammation; check for extravasation; in large vein, avoid scalp vein in child (IV)

Potassium acetate

Additive compatibilities: Metoclopramide

Y-site compatibilities: Ciprofloxacin

Potassium chloride

• **Potassium chloride:** must be diluted; concentrated potassium injections fatal

Continuous IV INF route

• Conc max 80 mcg/L for peripheral line, 120 mEq/L for central line

• Dehydrated patients should receive 1 L of potassium-free hydrating solution then infuse 10 mEq/hr; in severe hypokalemia, rate may be 40 mEq/hr

Additive compatibilities: Aminophylline, amiodarone, atracurium, calcium gluconate, cefepime, cephalothin, cephapirin, chloramphenicol, cimetidine, ciprofloxacin, cisatracurium, clindamycin, cloxacillin, corticotropin, cytarabine, dimenhyDRINATE, DOPamine, DOXOrubicin liposome, enalaprilat, erythromycin, floxacillin, fluconazole, fosphenytoin, furosemide, heparin, hydrocortisone, isoproterenol, lidocaine, metaraminol, methicillin, methyldopate, metoclopramide, mitoxantrone, nafcillin, netilmicin, norepinephrine, oxacillin, penicillin G potassium, phenylephrine, piperacillin, ranitidine, sodium bicarbonate, thiopental, vancomycin, verapamil, vit B/C

Y-site compatibilities: Acyclovir, aldesleukin, allopurinol, amifostine, aminophylline, amiodarone, ampicillin, amrinone, atropine, aztreonam, betamethasone, calcium gluconate, cephalothin, cephapirin, chlordiazePOXIDE, chlorproMAZINE, ciprofloxacin, cladribine, cyanocobalamin, dexamethasone, digoxin, diltiazem, diphenhydrAMINE, DOBUTamine, DOPamine, droperidol, edrophonium, enalaprilat, EPINEPHrine, esmolol, estrogens, ethacrynate, famotidine, fentaNYL, filgrastim, fludarabine, fluorouracil, furosemide, gallium, granisetron, heparin, hydrALAZINE, IDArubicin, indomethacin, insulin (regular), isoproterenol, kanamycin, labetalol, lidocaine, LORazepam, magnesium sulfate, melphalan, meperidine, methicillin, methoxamine, methylergonovine, midazolam, minocycline, morphine, neostigmine, norepinephrine, ondansetron, oxacillin, oxytocin, paclitaxel, penicillin G potassium, pentazocine, phytonadione, piperacillin/tazobactam, prednisoLONE, procainamide, prochlorperazine, propofol, propranolol, pyridostigmine, remifentanil, sargramostim, scopolamine, sodium bicarbonate, succinylcholine, tacrolimus, teniposide, theophylline, thiotepa, trimethaphan, trimethoenzamide, vinorelbine, warfarin, zidovudine

SIDE EFFECTS

CNS: Confusion
CV: Bradycardia, cardiac depression, dysrhythmias, arrest; peaking T waves, lowered R, depressed RST, prolonged P-R interval, widened QRS complex
GI: *Nausea, vomiting, cramps,* pain, *diarrhea,* ulceration of small bowel
GU: Oliguria
INTEG: Cold extremities, rash

PHARMACOKINETICS

PO: Excreted by kidneys and in feces; onset of action ≈ 30 min
IV: Immediate onset of action

INTERACTIONS

Increase: hyperkalemia—potassium phosphate IV; products containing calcium or magnesium; potassium-sparing diuretic or other potassium products; ACE inhibitors

NURSING CONSIDERATIONS

Assess:

- **Hyperkalemia:** indicates toxicity; fatigue, muscle weakness, confusion, dyspnea, palpitation; ECG for peaking T waves, lowered R, depressed RST, prolonged P-R interval, widening QRS complex, hyperkalemia; product should be reduced or discontinued, administer sodium bicarbonate (metabolic acidosis)
- Potassium level during treatment (3.5-5 mg/dl is normal level)
- Determine hydration status, I&O ratio; watch for decreased urinary output; notify prescriber immediately
- Cardiac status: rate, rhythm, CVP, PWP, PAWP if being monitored directly

Perform/provide:

- Storage at room temp

Evaluate:

- Therapeutic response: absence of fatigue, muscle weakness; decreased thirst, urinary output; cardiac changes

Teach patient/family:

- To add potassium-rich foods to diet: bananas, orange juice, avocados, whole grains, broccoli, carrots, prunes, cocoa after product is discontinued
- To avoid OTC products: antacids, salt substitutes, analgesics, vitamin preparations unless specifically directed by prescriber; to avoid licorice in large amounts because it may cause hypokalemia, sodium retention
- To report hyperkalemia symptoms (lethargy, confusion, diarrhea, nausea, vomiting, fainting, decreased output) or continued hypokalemia symptoms (fatigue, weakness, polyuria, polydipsia, cardiac changes)
- To dissolve powder or tablet completely in ≥120 ml water or juice
- About the importance of regular follow-up visits
- That potassium levels will need to be monitored periodically

potassium iodide (Rx)

Lugol's, SSKI, Strong Iodine
Func. class.: Thyroid hormone antagonist
Chem. class.: Iodine product

P

ACTION: Inhibits secretion of thyroid hormone, fosters colloid accumulation in thyroid follicles, decreases vascularity of gland

USES: Preparation for thyroidectomy, thyrotoxic crisis, neonatal thyrotoxicosis, radiation protectant, thyroid storm
Unlabeled uses: Erythema multiforme, erythema nodosum leprosum (ENL), sporotrichosis, thyroid involution induction

CONTRAINDICATIONS: Pregnancy (D), pulmonary edema, pulmonary TB, bronchitis, hypersensitivity to iodine
Precautions: Breastfeeding, children

DOSAGE AND ROUTES

Hyperthyroidism/thyrotoxicosis

• **Adult and child: PO** (SSKI) 250 mg tid × 10-14 days preoperatively

Preparation for thyroidectomy

• **Adult and child: PO** 3-5 gtt strong iodine sol tid or 1-5 drops SSKI in water tid after meals for 10 days prior to surgery

Radiation exposure (radioactive iodine)

• **Adult: PO** 130 mg/day (distribution by government/public health officials or OTC purchase)

• **Child ≥3 yr: PO** 65 mg q day

• **Child/infant >1 mo-3 yr: PO** 32 mg/day

• **Neonate: PO** 16 mg/day

Available forms: Oral sol (Lugol's solution) iodine 5%/potassium iodide 10%; oral sol (SSKI) 1 g/ml

Administer:

• Products are not interchangeable

• Strong iodine solution after diluting with water or juice to improve taste

• Through straw to prevent tooth discoloration

• With meals to decrease GI upset

• At same time each day to maintain product level

• At lowest dose that relieves symptoms; discontinue before RAIU

SIDE EFFECTS

CNS: Headache, confusion, paresthesias

EENT: Metallic taste, stomatitis, salivation, periorbital edema, sore teeth and gums, cold symptoms

ENDO: Hypothyroidism, hyperthyroid adenoma

GI: *Nausea, diarrhea, vomiting,* small-bowel lesions, upper gastric pain, metallic taste

INTEG: Rash, urticaria, angioneurotic edema, acne, mucosal hemorrhage, fever

MS: Myalgia, arthralgia, weakness

PHARMACOKINETICS

PO: Onset 24-48 hr, peak 10-15 days after continuous therapy, uptake by thyroid gland or excreted in urine, crosses placenta

INTERACTIONS

• Hypothyroidism: lithium, other antithyroid agents

Increased: hyperkalemia—angiotensin II receptor antagonist, ACE inhibitors, potassium salts, potassium-sparing diuretics

Drug/Lab Test

Interference: urinary 17-OHCS

NURSING CONSIDERATIONS

Assess:

• Pulse, B/P, temp; serum potassium

• I&O ratio; check for edema: puffy hands, feet, periorbit; indicate hypothyroidism

• Weight daily; same clothing, scale, time of day

• T_3, T_4, which is increased; serum TSH, which is decreased; free thyroxine index, which is increased if dosage is too low; discontinue product 3-4 wk before RAIU

⚠ Overdose: peripheral edema, heat intolerance, diaphoresis, palpitations, dysrhythmias, severe tachycardia, fever, delirium, CNS irritability

• Hypersensitivity: rash; enlarged cervical lymph nodes may indicate product should be discontinued

• Hypoprothrombinemia: bleeding, petechiae, ecchymosis

• Clinical response: after 3 wk should include increased weight, pulse; decreased T_4

Perform/provide:

• Fluids to 3-4 L/day unless contraindicated

Evaluate:

• Therapeutic response: weight gain; decreased pulse, T_4, size of thyroid gland

Teach patient/family:

• To abstain from breastfeeding after delivery

• To keep graph of weight, pulse, mood

• To avoid OTC products that contain iodine

• That seafood, other iodine products may be restricted
• Not to discontinue product abruptly; that thyroid crisis may occur as part of stress response
• That response may take several mo if thyroid is large
• To discontinue product, notify prescriber of fever, rash, metallic taste, swelling of throat; burning of mouth, throat; sore gums, teeth; severe GI distress, enlargement of thyroid, cold symptoms

pramipexole (Rx)
(pra-mi-pex′ol)

Mirapex, Mirapex ER

Func. class.: Antiparkinson agent
Chem. class.: DOPamine-receptor agonist, non-ergot

ACTION:
Selective agonist for D_2 receptors (presynaptic/postsynaptic sites); binding at D_3 receptor contributes to antiparkinson effects

USES:
Idiopathic Parkinson's disease, restless leg syndrome

CONTRAINDICATIONS:
Hypersensitivity

Precautions: Pregnancy (C), cardiac/renal disease, MI with dysrhythmias, affective disorders, psychosis, preexisting dyskinesias, history of falling asleep during daily activities

DOSAGE AND ROUTES

Parkinson's disease
• **Adult: PO** 0.125 mg tid; increase gradually by 0.125 mg/dose at 5- to 7-day intervals until total daily dose of 4.5 mg/day reached; ER 0.375 mg daily initially then up to 0.75 mg/day, may increase by 0.75 mg/day no more than q5-7days as needed, max 4.5 mg/day

Restless leg syndrome
• **Adult: PO** 0.125 mg 2-3 hr prior to bedtime, increase gradually, max 0.5 mg/day

Renal dose
• **Adult: PO** CCr 35-59 ml/min, 0.125 mg bid, may increase q5-7days to 1.5 mg bid if required; CCr 15-34 ml/min, 0.125 mg/day, increase q5-7days to 1.5 mg/day

Available forms: Tabs 0.125, 0.25, 0.5, 1, 1.5 mg; ER tab 0.375, 0.75, 1.5, 3.0, 4.5 mg

Administer:
• Adjust dosage to patient response, titrate slowly, taper when discontinuing
• With meals to minimize GI symptoms
• Do not crush, chew, or break ext rel product

SIDE EFFECTS

CNS: *Agitation, insomnia,* psychosis, hallucinations, depression, dizziness, headache, confusion, amnesia, dream disorder, asthenia, dyskinesia, hypersomnolence, **sudden sleep onset,** impulse control disorders
CV: *Orthostatic hypotension,* edema, syncope, tachycardia
EENT: Blurred vision
GI: *Nausea, anorexia,* constipation, dysphagia, dry mouth
GU: Impotence, urinary frequency
HEMA: **Hemolytic anemia, leukopenia, agranulocytosis**

PHARMACOKINETICS

Minimally metabolized, peak 2 hr, half-life 8 hr, 8.5-12 hr in geriatric patients

INTERACTIONS

Increase: pramipexole levels—levodopa, cimetidine, ranitidine, diltiazem, triamterene, verapamil, quiNIDine
Decrease: pramipexole levels—DOPamine antagonists, phenothiazines, metoclopramide, butyrophenones

P

NURSING CONSIDERATIONS

Assess:

- **Parkinson's disease:** involuntary movements: bradykinesia, tremors, staggering gait, muscle rigidity, drooling
- B/P, ECG, respiration during initial treatment; hypo/hypertension should be reported
- Mental status: affect, mood, behavioral changes, depression; complete suicide assessment, worsening of symptoms of restless leg syndrome, impulse control disorders

⚠ **Sleep attacks:** may fall asleep during activities without warning; may need to discontinue medication

Perform/provide:

- Assistance with ambulation during beginning therapy
- Testing for diabetes mellitus, acromegaly if patient receiving long-term therapy

Evaluate:

- Therapeutic response: movement disorder improves

Teach patient/family:

- That therapeutic effects may take several weeks to a few months
- To change positions slowly to prevent orthostatic hypotension
- To use product exactly as prescribed: if product is discontinued abruptly, parkinsonian crisis may occur; to avoid alcohol, OTC sleeping products
- To notify prescriber if pregnancy is planned or suspected

pramlintide (Rx)

(pram′lin-tide)

Symlin

Func. class.: Antidiabetic

Chem. class.: Synthetic human amylin analog

ACTION:
Modulates and slows stomach emptying, prevents postprandial rise in plasma glucagon, decreases appetite, leads to decreased caloric intake and weight loss

USES:
As an adjunct to insulin therapy for uncontrolled type 1 or type 2 diabetes

CONTRAINDICATIONS:
Hypersensitivity to this product or cresol; gastroparesis

Black Box Warning: Hypoglycemia

Precautions: Pregnancy (C), breastfeeding

DOSAGE AND ROUTES

Type 1 diabetes

- **Adult: SUBCUT** before each meal (≥30 g CHO), titrate up in 15-mcg increments to target dose of 60 mcg/dose; each dose titration should occur after no nausea for 3 days

Type 2 diabetes

- **Adult: SUBCUT** 60 mcg prior to each meal (≥30 g CHO), titrate up to 120 mcg **SUBCUT** with each meal after no nausea for 3-7 days

Available forms: Inj 5-ml vials (0.6 mg/ml)

Administer:

- Premeal insulin should be decreased by 50% when starting and adjusted to therapeutic dose to prevent hypoglycemia

SUBCUT route

- Rotate injection sites, allow solution to warm to room temperature before use
- Take immediately before mealtime or if 30 g of carbohydrates will be consumed
- Do not use if a meal is skipped
- Do not use if discolored; do not give in arm; absorption is variable

Syringe compatibilities: Do not mix with insulin; give separately

SIDE EFFECTS

CNS: *Headache,* fatigue, dizziness

GI: *Nausea, vomiting, anorexia,* abdominal pain

INTEG: Inj site reactions

META: Hypoglycemia

MS: Arthralgia

RESP: *Cough,* pharyngitis

SYST: *Systemic allergy*

PHARMACOKINETICS

Bioavailability 30%-40%, not extensively bound to blood cells or albumin, 40% bound in plasma, half-life 48 min, metabolized by kidneys, peak 20 min, duration 3 hr

INTERACTIONS

• Do not use with erythromycin, metoclopramide

Increase: effect of acetaminophen

Increase: pramlintide action—antimuscarinics, α-glucosidase inhibitors, diphenoxylate, loperamide, octreotide, opiate agonist, tricyclics

Increase: hypoglycemia—ACE inhibitors, disopyramide, anabolic steroids, androgens, fibric acid derivatives, alcohol, corticosteroids, insulin

Increase: hyperglycemia—phenothiazines

Decrease: hypoglycemia—niacin, dextrothyroxine, thiazide diuretics, triamterene, estrogens, progestins, oral contraceptives, MAOIs

NURSING CONSIDERATIONS

Assess:

• Fasting blood glucose, 2 hr post-prandiol (80-150 mg/dl, normal fasting level; 70-130 mg/dl, normal 2 hr level); A1c may also be drawn to identify treatment effectiveness; also monitor weight, appetite

• **Hypoglycemic reaction** sweating; weakness; dizziness; chills; confusion; headache; nausea; rapid, weak pulse; fatigue; tachycardia; memory lapses; slurred speech; staggering gait; anxiety; tremors; hunger

• **Hyperglycemia:** acetone breath; polyuria; fatigue; polydipsia; flushed, dry skin; lethargy

Perform/provide:

• Storage at room temp for ≤30 days; keep away from heat and sunlight; refrigerate all other supply

Evaluate:

• Therapeutic response: decrease in polyuria, polydipsia, polyphagia; clear sensorium; absence of dizziness; stable gait; improving blood glucose, A1c

Teach patient/family:

• That product does not cure diabetes but rather controls symptoms

• To carry emergency ID as diabetic

• To recognize hypoglycemia reaction: headache, fatigue, weakness

• About the dosage, route, mixing instructions, diet restrictions, disease process

• To carry a glucose source (candy or lump sugar) to treat hypoglycemia

• About the symptoms of ketoacidosis: nausea; thirst; polyuria; dry mouth; decreased B/P; dry, flushed skin; acetone breath; drowsiness; Kussmaul respirations

• That a plan is necessary for diet, exercise; that all food on diet should be eaten; that exercise routine should not vary

• About blood glucose testing; how to determine glucose level

• To avoid OTC products, alcohol unless directed by prescriber

• Not to operate machinery or drive until effect is known

TREATMENT OF OVERDOSE:

Glucose 25 g IV or 50 ml dextrose 50% sol or 1 mg glucagon SUBCUT

P

pramoxine topical

See Appendix B

prasugrel (Rx)

(pra′soo-grel)

Effient

Func. class.: Platelet aggregation inhibitor

Chem. class.: ADP receptor antagonist

ACTION: Inhibits ADP-induced platelet aggregation

USES:
Reducing the risk of stroke, MI, vascular death, peripheral arterial disease in high-risk patients

CONTRAINDICATIONS:
Hypersensitivity, stroke, TIA

Black Box Warning: Active bleeding

Precautions: Pregnancy (B), breastfeeding, children, geriatric patients, hepatic disease, increased bleeding risk, neutropenia, agranulocytosis, renal disease, surgery, trauma, thrombotic thrombocytopenic purpura, Asian patients, weight <60 kg, CABG, abrupt discontinuation

DOSAGE AND ROUTES

- **Adult/geriatric <75 yr and ≥60 kg: PO** 60-mg loading dose then 10 mg daily with aspirin (75-325 mg/day)
- **Adult/geriatric <75 yr and <60 kg: PO** 60 mg loading dose then 5 mg daily
- **Geriatric >75 yr:** not recommended

Available forms: Tabs 5, 10 mg

Administer:

- With food to decrease gastric symptoms
- Do not break tablets
- Do not discontinue therapy abruptly

SIDE EFFECTS

CNS: Headache, dizziness

CV: Edema, atrial fibrillation, bradycardia, chest pain, hypo/hypertension

GI: Nausea, vomiting, diarrhea

HEMA: Epistaxis, leukopenia, thrombocytopenia, neutropenia, anaphylaxis, angioedema, anemia

INTEG: Rash, hypercholesterolemia

MISC: Fatigue, intracranial hemorrhage, secondary malignancy

MS: Back pain

PHARMACOKINETICS

Rapidly absorbed; peak 30 min; metabolized by liver (CYP3A4; CYP2B6); excreted in urine, feces; half-life 7 hr

INTERACTIONS

Increase: bleeding risk—anticoagulants, aspirin, NSAIDs, abciximab, eptifibatide, tirofiban, thrombolytics, ticlopidine, SSRIs, treprostinil, rifampin

NURSING CONSIDERATIONS

Assess:

⚠ **Thrombotic/thrombocytic purpura:** fever, thrombocytopenia, neurolytic anemia

- Hepatic studies: AST, ALT, bilirubin, creatinine with long-term therapy
- Blood studies: CBC, differential, Hct, Hgb, PT, cholesterol with long-term therapy

Evaluate:

- Therapeutic response: absence of stroke, MI

Teach patient/family:

- That blood work will be necessary during treatment
- To report any unusual bruising, bleeding to prescriber; that it may take longer to stop bleeding
- To take with food or just after eating to minimize GI discomfort
- To report diarrhea, skin rashes, subcutaneous bleeding, chills, fever, sore throat
- To tell all health care providers that prasugrel is being used; that product may be held before surgery

pravastatin (Rx)

(pra'va-sta-tin)

Apo-Pravastatin ✦, CO Pravastatin ✦, Gen-Pravastatin ✦, Novo-Pravastatin ✦, Nu-Pravastatin ✦, PMS-Pravastatin ✦, Pravachol, ratio-Pravastatin ✦, Sandoz Pravastatin ✦

Func. class.: Antilipemic
Chem. class.: HMG-CoA reductase enzyme

Do not confuse:
Pravachol/Prevacid/propranolol

ACTION: Inhibits HMG-CoA reductase enzyme, which reduces cholesterol synthesis

USES: As an adjunct for primary hypercholesterolemia (types IIa, IIb, III, IV), to reduce the risk for recurrent MI, atherosclerosis, primary/secondary CV events, stroke, TIAs

CONTRAINDICATIONS: Pregnancy (X), breastfeeding, hypersensitivity, active hepatic disease

Precautions: Past hepatic disease, alcoholism, severe acute infections, trauma, severe metabolic disorders, electrolyte imbalances

DOSAGE AND ROUTES

- **Adult: PO** 40 mg/day at bedtime (range 10-80 mg/day); start at 10 mg/day if patient also taking immunosuppressants
- **Adolescent 14-18 yr: PO** 40 mg/day
- **Child 8-13 yr: PO** 20 mg/day
- **Geriatric/renal/hepatic disease: PO** 10 mg/day initially

Renal dose

- **Adult: PO** 10-20 mg daily at bedtime, increase at 4-wk intervals

Available forms: Tabs 10, 20, 40, 80 mg

Administer:

- Without regard to meals, at bedtime
- Give 4 hr after bile acid sequestrants

SIDE EFFECTS

CNS: Headache, dizziness, fatigue
CV: Chest pain
EENT: Lens opacities
GI: Nausea, constipation, diarrhea, flatus, abdominal pain, heartburn, **hepatic dysfunction, pancreatitis, hepatitis**
GU: Renal failure (myoglobinuria)
INTEG: Rash, pruritus
MS: Muscle cramps, myalgia, **myositis, rhabdomyolysis**
RESP: Common cold, rhinitis, cough

PHARMACOKINETICS

Peak 1-1½ hr; metabolized by liver; protein binding 50%; excreted in urine 20%, feces 70%, breast milk; crosses placenta; half-life 1.25-2.25 hr

INTERACTIONS

Increase: myopathy risk—erythromycin, niacin, cycloSPORINE, gemfibrozil, clofibrate, clarithromycin, itraconazole, protease inhibitors
Decrease: bioavailability of pravastatin—bile acid sequestrants

Drug/Herb

Increase: adverse reactions—red yeast rice
Increase: hepatotoxicity—eucalyptus
Decrease: effect—St. John's wort

Drug/Lab Test

Increase: CK, LFTs
Altered: thyroid function tests

NURSING CONSIDERATIONS

Assess:

- Fasting lipid profile: LDL, HDL, triglycerides, cholesterol at baseline, q12wk, then q6mo when stable; obtain diet history
- Hepatic studies: baseline, q12wk, then q6mo for remainder of yr; AST, ALT, LFTs may increase

P

• Renal studies of patients with compromised renal systems: BUN, I&O ratio, creatinine

⚠ **Rhabdomyolysis:** muscle tenderness, pain; obtain CPK at baseline and if these occur, therapy should be discontinued

Perform/provide:

• Storage in cool environment in tight container protected from light

Evaluate:

• Therapeutic response: decrease in LDL total cholesterol, triglycerides; increase in HDL

Teach patient/family:

• That blood work will be necessary during treatment

⚠ To report blurred vision, severe GI symptoms, dizziness, headache, muscle pain, weakness, fever

• That regimen will continue: low-cholesterol diet, exercise program

⚠ To report suspected, planned pregnancy; not to use product during pregnancy, pregnancy category (X); not to breastfeed

prazosin (Rx)

(pray′zoe-sin)

Minipress

Func. class.: Antihypertensive

Chem. class.: α_1-Adrenergic blocker, peripheral

ACTION: Blocks α-mediated vasoconstriction of adrenergic receptors, thereby inducing peripheral vasodilation

USES: Hypertension

Unlabeled uses: Benign prostatic hypertrophy to decrease urine outflow obstruction, heart failure, hypertensive urgency, Raynaud's phenomenon, posttraumatic stress disorder (PTSD)

CONTRAINDICATIONS: Hypersensitivity

Precautions: Pregnancy (C), breastfeeding, children, geriatric patients, renal/hepatic disease, prostate cancer, ocular surgery, orthostatic hypotension

DOSAGE AND ROUTES

Hypertension

• **Adult: PO** 1 mg bid or tid increasing to 20 mg/day in divided doses, if required; usual range 6-15 mg/day, max 1 mg initially; max 20-40 mg/day

• **Child: PO** 5 mcg/kg q6hr; max 400 mcg/kg/day or 15 mg/day

Benign prostatic hyperplasia (unlabeled)

• **Adult: PO** 2 mg bid

Raynaud's phenomenon (unlabeled)

• **Adult: PO** 0.5-3 mg bid

CHF (unlabeled)

• **Adult: PO** 1 mg bid-tid, may gradually increase to max 20 mg/day

• **Child: PO** 5 mcg/kg q6hr, may gradually increase to 25 mcg/kg q6hr

Hypertensive urgency (unlabeled)

• **Adult: PO** 10-20 mg, may repeat after 30 min

Available forms: Caps 1, 2, 5 mg

Administer:

• 1st dose at bedtime to avoid fainting

SIDE EFFECTS

CNS: *Dizziness, headache, drowsiness,* anxiety, depression, vertigo, weakness, fatigue

CV: *Palpitations,* orthostatic hypotension, tachycardia, edema, rebound hypertension

EENT: Blurred vision, epistaxis, tinnitus, dry mouth, red sclera

GI: *Nausea,* vomiting, diarrhea, constipation, abdominal pain

GU: Urinary frequency, incontinence, impotence, priapism; water, sodium retention

PHARMACOKINETICS

Onset 2 hr, peak 2-4 hr, duration 6-12 hr, half-life 2-4 hr; metabolized in liver, excreted via bile, feces (>90%), urine (<10%); protein binding 97%

INTERACTIONS

Increase: hypotensive effects—β-blockers, nitroglycerin, alcohol, phosphodiesterase inhibitors (vardenafil, tadalafil, sildenafil); diuretics, other antihypertensives, MAOIs

Decrease: antihypertensive effect—NSAIDs

Increase: antihypertensive effect—hawthorn

Drug/Lab Test

Increase: urinary norepinephrine, VMA

NURSING CONSIDERATIONS

Assess:

• **Hypertension/CHF:** B/P (sitting, standing) during initial treatment, periodically thereafter; pulse, jugular venous distention

• BUN, uric acid if patient receiving long-term therapy

• Weight daily, I&O; edema in feet, legs daily

• **Benign prostatic hypertrophy (unlabeled):** urinary patterns, frequency, stream, dribbling; flow before, during, and after therapy

Perform/provide:

• Storage in tight container in cool environment

Evaluate:

• Therapeutic response: decreased B/P

Teach patient/family:

• That fainting occasionally occurs after 1st dose; to take 1st dose at bedtime; not to drive or operate machinery for 4 hr after 1st dose; that full effect may take 4-6 wk

• To change positions slowly to prevent orthostatic hypotension

• To avoid OTC medications unless approved by prescriber

TREATMENT OF OVERDOSE:

Administer volume expanders or vasopressors, discontinue product, place patient in supine position

prednisoLONE (Rx)

(pred-niss′oh-lone)

Asmal Pred Plus, Millipred, Orapred, Orapred ODT, Prednoral, Prelone, Veripred

Func. class.: Corticosteroid, synthetic

Chem. class.: Glucocorticoid, immediate acting

Do not confuse:

prednisoLONE/predniSONE

ACTION: Decreases inflammation by the suppression of migration of polymorphonuclear leukocytes, fibroblasts; reversal to increase capillary permeability and lysosomal stabilization

USES: Severe inflammation, immunosuppression, neoplasms

CONTRAINDICATIONS: Children <2 yr, psychosis, hypersensitivity, idiopathic thrombocytopenia, acute glomerulonephritis, amebiasis, fungal infections, nonasthmatic bronchial disease, measles, varicella, Cushing's syndrome

Precautions: Pregnancy (C), breastfeeding, children, diabetes mellitus, glaucoma, osteoporosis, seizure disorders, ulcerative colitis, CHF, myasthenia gravis

DOSAGE AND ROUTES

Rheumatic disorders

• **Adult: PO** 5-60 mg/day or in divided doses

Asthma/antiinflammatory

• **Adult: PO** 40-80 mg/day in 1-2 divided doses

• **Child: PO** 1 mg/kg/day in 2 divided doses

Available forms: Tabs 5 mg; syr 5 mg/5 ml, 15 mg/15 ml; oral liquid 5 mg/ml, tabs 1, 2.5, 5, 10, 20, 50 mg, oral sol 5 mg/ml, 5 mg/5 ml, syr 5 mg/5 ml; oral dissolving tab 10, 15, 30 mg

Administer:

• **Oral sol:** use calibrated measuring device

P

• **Orally disintegrating tabs:** place on tongue; allow to dissolve, swallow or swallow whole; do not cut, split

SIDE EFFECTS

CNS: *Depression,* flushing, sweating, headache, mood changes
CV: *Hypertension,* circulatory collapse, thrombophlebitis, embolism, tachycardia
EENT: Fungal infections, increased intraocular pressure, blurred vision
GI: *Diarrhea, nausea, abdominal distention,* GI hemorrhage, increased appetite, pancreatitis
HEMA: Thrombocytopenia
INTEG: Acne, poor wound healing, ecchymosis, petechiae
MS: Fractures, osteoporosis, weakness, arthralgia, myopathy, tendon rupture

PHARMACOKINETICS

PO: Peak 1-2 hr, duration 2 days

INTERACTIONS

Increase: side effects—alcohol, salicylates, indomethacin, amphotericin B, digitalis, cycloSPORINE, diuretics
Increase: prednisoLONE action—salicylates, estrogens, indomethacin, oral contraceptives, ketoconazole, macrolide antibiotics
Decrease: prednisoLONE action—cholestyramine, colestipol, barbiturates, rifampin, ePHEDrine, phenytoin, theophylline
Decrease: effects of anticoagulants, anticonvulsants, antidiabetics, ambenonium, neostigmine, isoniazid, toxoids, vaccines, anticholinesterases, salicylates, somatrem

Drug/Lab Test

Increase: cholesterol, sodium, blood glucose, uric acid, calcium, urine glucose
Decrease: calcium, potassium, T_4, T_3, thyroid ^{131}I uptake test, urine 17-OHCS, 17-KS, PBI
False negative: skin allergy tests

NURSING CONSIDERATIONS

Assess:

• Potassium, blood glucose, urine glucose while patient receiving long-term therapy; hypokalemia, hyperglycemia
• Weight daily; notify prescriber if weekly gain of >5 lb
• B/P q4hr, pulse; notify prescriber if chest pain occurs
• I&O ratio; be alert for decreasing urinary output, increasing edema
• Plasma cortisol levels with long-term therapy; normal level: 138-635 nmol/L SI units when drawn at 8 AM
• **Infection:** increased temp, WBC, even after withdrawal of medication; product masks infection
• **Potassium depletion:** paresthesias, fatigue, nausea, vomiting, depression, polyuria, dysrhythmias, weakness
• Edema, hypertension, cardiac symptoms
• Mental status: affect, mood, behavioral changes, aggression
• **Adrenal insufficiency:** nausea, vomiting, lethargy, restlessness, confusion, weight loss, hypotension before, during treatment; HPA suppression may be precipitated by abrupt withdrawal

Perform/provide:

• Assistance with ambulation for patient with bone-tissue disease to prevent fractures

Evaluate:

• Therapeutic response: ease of respirations, decreased inflammation

Teach patient/family:

• That emergency ID as steroid user should be carried
• To notify prescriber if therapeutic response decreases; that dosage adjustment may be needed
• Not to discontinue abruptly; that adrenal crisis can result; to take product exactly as prescribed
• To avoid OTC products: salicylates, cough products with alcohol, cold preparations unless directed by prescriber
• About cushingoid symptoms

• About the symptoms of adrenal insufficiency: nausea, anorexia, fatigue, dizziness, dyspnea, weakness, joint pain

prednisoLONE ophthalmic (Rx)

See Appendix B

predniSONE (Rx)

(pred′ni-sone)

Apo-Prednisone ♣, Winpred ♣

Func. class.: Corticosteroid

Chem. class.: Intermediate-acting glucocorticoid

Do not confuse:

predniSONE/methylPREDNISolone/predniso LONE/Prilosec

ACTION: Decreases inflammation by increasing capillary permeability, and lysosomal stabilization, minimal mineralocorticoid activity

USES: Severe inflammation, immunosuppression, neoplasms, multiple sclerosis, collagen disorders, dermatologic disorders

Unlabeled uses: Adjunct for refractory seizures, infantile spasms, acute interstitial nephritis, amyloidosis, autoimmune hepatitis, Behçet's syndrome, Bell's palsy, carpal tunnel syndrome, Churg-Strauss syndrome, dermatomyositis, Duchenne muscular dystrophy, endophthalmitis, Lennox-Gastaut syndrome, lupus nephritis, mixed connective-tissue disease, pericarditis, pneumonia, polyarteritis nodosa, polychondritis, polymyositis, pulmonary fibrosis, rheumatic carditis, temporal arteritis, TB, Wegener's granulomatosis

CONTRAINDICATIONS: Child <2 yr, psychosis, hypersensitivity, idiopathic thrombocytopenia, acute glomerulonephritis, amebiasis, fungal infections, nonasthmatic bronchial disease, AIDS, TB, measles

Precautions: Pregnancy (C), diabetes mellitus, glaucoma, osteoporosis, seizure disorders, ulcerative colitis, CHF, myasthenia gravis, renal disease, esophagitis, peptic ulcer, cataracts, coagulopathy

DOSAGE AND ROUTES

• **Adult: PO** 5-60 mg/day or divided bid-qid

• **Child: PO** 0.05-2 mg/kg/day divided 1-4×/day

Nephrosis

• **Child: PO** 2 mg/kg/day in divided doses, max 28 days, then 1-1.5 mg/kg/day every other day × 4 wk

Multiple sclerosis

• **Adult: PO** 200 mg/day × 1 wk then 80 mg every other day × 1 mo

Available forms: Tabs 1, 2.5, 5, 10, 20, 50 mg; oral sol 5 mg/5 ml; syr 5 mg/5 ml

Administer:

• For long-term use, alternate-day therapy recommended to decrease adverse reactions; give in AM to coincide with normal cortisol secretion

• Titrated dose; use lowest effective dose

• With food or milk to decrease GI symptoms

• *Oral sol:* use calibrated measuring device

SIDE EFFECTS

CNS: Depression, flushing, sweating, headache, mood changes

CV: Hypertension, **circulatory collapse, thrombophlebitis, embolism,** tachycardia

EENT: Fungal infections, increased intraocular pressure, blurred vision

GI: Diarrhea, nausea, abdominal distention, **GI hemorrhage,** increased appetite, pancreatitis

HEMA: **Thrombocytopenia**

INTEG: Acne, poor wound healing, ecchymosis, petechiae

META: Hyperglycemia

MS: Fractures, osteoporosis, weakness

P

PHARMACOKINETICS

PO: Well absorbed PO, peak 1-2 hr, duration 1-1½ days, half-life 3½-4 hr, biologic terminal half-life 18-36 hr, crosses placenta, enters breast milk, metabolized by liver after conversion, excreted in urine

INTERACTIONS

Increase: side effects—alcohol, salicylates, indomethacin, amphotericin B, digoxin, cycloSPORINE, diuretics

Increase: predniSONE action—salicylates, estrogens, indomethacin, oral contraceptives, ketoconazole, macrolide antiinfectives

Decrease: predniSONE action—cholestyramine, colestipol, barbiturates, rifampin, ePHEDrine, phenytoin, theophylline

Decrease: effects of anticoagulants, anticonvulsants, antidiabetics, ambenonium, neostigmine, isoniazid, toxoids, vaccines, anticholinesterases, salicylates, somatrem

Drug/Herb

Decrease: predniSONE effect—ephedra (ma huang)

Drug/Lab Test

Increase: cholesterol, sodium, blood glucose, uric acid, calcium, urine glucose

Decrease: calcium, potassium, T_4, T_3, thyroid ^{131}I uptake test, urine 17-OHCS, 17-KS, PBI

False negative: skin allergy tests

NURSING CONSIDERATIONS

Assess:

- **Adrenal insufficiency:** nausea, vomiting, anorexia, confusion, hypotension, weight loss before, during treatment; HPA suppression may be precipitated by abrupt withdrawal
- Potassium, blood glucose, urine glucose while patient receiving long-term therapy; hypokalemia and hyperglycemia; plasma cortisol with long-term therapy, normal: 138-635 nmol/L SI units drawn at 8 AM
- Weight daily; notify prescriber of weekly gain of >5 lb
- B/P q4hr, pulse; notify prescriber of chest pain; monitor for crackles, dyspnea if edema is present; hypertension, cardiac symptoms
- I&O ratio; be alert for decreasing urinary output, increasing edema
- **Infection:** increased temp, WBC, even after withdrawal of medication; product masks infection
- Potassium depletion: paresthesias, fatigue, nausea, vomiting, depression, polyuria, dysrhythmias, weakness
- Mental status: affect, mood, behavioral changes, aggression

Perform/provide:

- Assistance with ambulation for patient with bone-tissue disease to prevent fractures

Evaluate:

- Therapeutic response: ease of respirations, decreased inflammation

Teach patient/family:

- That emergency ID as corticosteroid user should be carried; provide information about product being taken and condition
- To notify prescriber if therapeutic response decreases; that dosage adjustment may be needed
- To avoid vaccinations

⚠ **Not to discontinue abruptly because adrenal crisis can result**

- To avoid OTC products: salicylates, cough products with alcohol, cold preparations unless directed by prescriber
- **Cushingoid symptoms:** moon face, weight gain; symptoms of adrenal insufficiency: nausea, anorexia, fatigue, dizziness, dyspnea, weakness, joint pain
- That product causes immunosuppression; to report any symptoms of infection (fever, sore throat, cough)
- To notify prescriber if pregnancy is planned or suspected; cleft palate, stillbirth, abortion reported

pregabalin (Rx)

(pre-gab'a-lin)

Lyrica

Func. class.: Anticonvulsant

Chem. class.: γ-Aminobutyric acid (GABA) analog

Controlled Substance Schedule V

ACTION:

Binds to high-voltage–gated calcium channels in CNS tissues; this may lead to anticonvulsant action similar to the inhibitory neurotransmitter GABA; anxiolytic, analgesics, and antiepileptic properties

USES:

Neuropathic pain associated with diabetic peripheral neuropathy, partial-onset seizures, postherpetic neuralgia, fibromyalgia

Unlabeled uses: Moderate pain, social anxiety disorder

CONTRAINDICATIONS:

Hypersensitivity, abrupt discontinuation

Precautions: Pregnancy (C), breastfeeding, children <12 yr, geriatric patients, renal disease, PR interval prolongation, creatine kinase elevations, CHF (class III, IV), decreased platelets, substance abuse, dependence, glaucoma, myopathy, angioedema history, suicidal behavior

DOSAGE AND ROUTES

Diabetic peripheral neuropathic pain

• **Adult: PO** 50 mg tid, may increase to 300 mg/day (max) within 1 wk, adjust in patients with renal disease

Partial-onset seizures

• **Adult: PO** 75 mg bid or 50 mg tid; may increase to 600 mg/day (max)

Postherpetic neuralgia

• **Adult: PO** 150 mg/day in 2-3 divided doses, may increase to 300 mg/day in 2-3 divided doses; if higher dose is required after 2-4 wk, may increase to 600 mg/day in 2-3 divided doses

Fibromyalgia

• **Adult: PO** 75 mg bid, may increase to 150 mg bid within 1 wk and 225 mg bid after 1 wk

Renal dose

• **Adult: PO** CCr 30-60 ml/min, 75-300 mg/day in 2-3 divided doses; CCr 15-30 ml/min, 25-150 mg/day in 1-2 divided doses; CCr <15 ml/min, 25-75 mg/day as a single dose

Social phobia (unlabeled)

• **Adult: PO** 150-600 mg/day in 3 divided doses

Available forms: Caps 25, 50, 75, 100, 150, 200, 225, 300 mg

Administer:

• Do not crush or chew caps; caps may be opened and contents put in applesauce or dissolved in juice
• Give without regard to meals
• Gradually withdraw over 7 days; abrupt withdrawal may precipitate seizures

SIDE EFFECTS

CNS: Dizziness, fatigue, confusion, euphoria, incoordination, nervousness, neuropathy, tremor, vertigo, somnolence, ataxia, amnesia, abnormal thinking, **suicidal ideation**

EENT: Dry mouth, blurred vision, nystagmus, amblyopia, sinusitis

GI: Constipation, flatulence, abdominal pain, weight gain

HEMA: Ecchymosis, **thrombocytopenia**

MS: Back pain, **rhabdomyolysis**, myopathy

OTHER: Pruritus, orgasm/erectile dysfunction, peripheral edema, **angioedema**

RESP: Dyspnea

PHARMACOKINETICS

Well absorbed, absorption decreased with food; peak 1.5 hr; 90% recovered in urine unchanged; negligible metabolism; not bound to plasma proteins; half-life 6 hr

INTERACTIONS

Increase: weight gain/fluid retention—thiazolidinedione; avoid use if possible
Increase: CNS depression—anxiolytics, sedatives, hypnotics, barbiturates, general anesthetics, opiate agonists, phenothiazines, sedating H_1 blockers, thiazolidinediones, tricyclics, alcohol

Drug/Lab Test

Increase: creatine kinase
Decrease: platelets

NURSING CONSIDERATIONS

Assess:

- **Seizures:** aura, location, duration, activity at onset
- **Pain:** location, duration, characteristics if using for diabetic neuropathy
- Renal studies: urinalysis, BUN, urine creatinine q3mo, creatine kinase; if markedly increased, discontinue product

⚠ Mental status: mood, sensorium, affect, behavioral changes, suicidal thoughts/behaviors; if mental status changes, notify prescriber

Perform/provide:

- Storage at room temperature away from heat and light
- Hard candy, frequent rinsing of mouth, gum for dry mouth
- Assistance with ambulation during early part of treatment because dizziness occurs
- Seizure precautions: padded side rails; move objects that may harm patient
- Increased fluids, bulk in diet for constipation

Evaluate:

- Therapeutic response: decreased seizure activity; decrease in neuropathic pain

Teach patient/family:

- To carry emergency ID stating patient's name, products taken, condition, prescriber's name and phone number
- To avoid driving, other activities that require alertness because dizziness, drowsiness may occur
- Not to discontinue medication quickly after long-term use, to taper over ≥1 wk; that withdrawal-precipitated seizures may occur; not to double doses if dose is missed, to take if 2 hr or more before next dose
- To notify prescriber if pregnancy planned or suspected; to avoid breastfeeding
- To report muscle pain, tenderness, weakness when accompanied by fever, malaise, suicidal thoughts/behaviors
- To avoid alcohol

TREATMENT OF OVERDOSE:

Lavage, VS, hemodialysis

primaquine (Rx)

(prim'a-kween)

Func. class.: Antimalarial
Chem. class.: Synthetic 8-aminoquinolone

ACTION: Unknown; thought to destroy exoerythrocytic forms by gametocidal action

USES: Malaria caused by *Plasmodium vivax;* in combination with clindamycin for *Pneumocystis jiroveci* pneumonia

CONTRAINDICATIONS: Lupus erythematosus, rheumatoid arthritis; hypersensitivity to this product or idoquinol
Precautions: Pregnancy (C), breastfeeding, methemoglobin reductase deficiency

Black Box Warning: Bone marrow suppression, hemolytic anemia, G6PD deficiency

DOSAGE AND ROUTES

- **Adult: PO** 15-30 mg (base)/day × 2 wk or 45 mg (base)/day × 8 wk; 26.3-mg tab is 15-mg base
- **Child: PO** 0.5 mg/kg (0.3 mg/base/day) daily × 2 wk

Available forms: Tabs 26.3 mg

Administer:

PO route

- Before or after meals at same time each day to maintain product level; take with food to decrease GI upset

SIDE EFFECTS

CNS: Headache, dizziness
CV: Hypertension, dysrhythmias
EENT: *Blurred vision, difficulty focusing*
GI: *Nausea, vomiting, anorexia,* cramps
HEMA: **Agranulocytosis, granulocytopenia, leukopenia, hemolytic anemia, leukocytosis,** mild anemia, **methemoglobinemia**
INTEG: Pruritus, skin eruptions, pallor, weakness

PHARMACOKINETICS

PO: Metabolized by liver (metabolites), half-life 3.7-9.6 hr

INTERACTIONS

- Toxicity: quinacrine

Decrease: effect of carBAMazepine, PHENobarbital, phenytoins, rifamycins, nafcillin

NURSING CONSIDERATIONS

Assess:

- Ophthalmic test if patient receiving long-term treatment or product dosage of >150 mg/day
- Hepatic studies weekly: AST, ALT, bilirubin if patient receiving long-term therapy
- Blood studies: CBC; blood dyscrasias occur
- Allergic reactions: pruritus, rash, urticaria
- Blood dyscrasias: malaise, fever, bruising, bleeding (rare)
- Renal status: dark urine, hematuria, decreased output

⚠ **Hemolytic reaction: chills, fever, chest pain, cyanosis; product should be discontinued immediately**

Evaluate:

- Therapeutic response: decreased symptoms of malaria

Teach patient/family:

- To report visual problems, fever, fatigue, dark urine, bruising, bleeding; may indicate blood dyscrasias
- To complete full course of therapy
- That an eye exam will be needed q4-6mo if using product for an extended period of time

primidone (Rx)

(pri′mi-done)

Apo-Primidone ✱, Mysoline, PMS-Primidone ✱, Sertan ✱

Func. class.: Anticonvulsant

Chem. class.: Barbiturate derivative

ACTION:

Raises seizure threshold by conversion of product to PHENobarbital, decreases neuron firing

USES:

Generalized tonic-clonic (grand mal), complex seizures

Unlabeled uses: Benign familial tremor (essential tremor)

CONTRAINDICATIONS:

Pregnancy (D), breastfeeding, hypersensitivity, porphyria, hepatic encephalopathy

Precautions: Hyperactive children, COPD, renal/hepatic disease, suicidal ideation/behavior

DOSAGE AND ROUTES

- **Adult and child >8 yr: PO** 125-250 mg at bedtime, increase by 125-250 mg/day q3-7days, usual dose 750-1500 mg/day in 3-4 divided doses, max 2 g/day in divided doses
- **Child <8 yr: PO** 50-125 mg at bedtime, increase by 50-125 mg/day q3-7days, usual dose 10-25 mg/kg/day in 3-4 divided doses
- **Neonate: PO** 12-20 mg/kg/day in 2-4 divided doses, start at lower dose and titrate

P

Benign familial tremor/essential tremor (unlabeled)

• **Adult: PO** 50-62.5 mg, increase as tolerated up to 750 mg/day in 3 divided doses

Renal dose

• **Adult: PO** CCr 10-50 ml/min, increase interval between doses to 8-12 hr; CCr <10 ml/min, increase interval to 12-24 hr

Available forms: Tabs 50, 250 mg; susp 250 mg/5 ml ✤; chew tabs 125 mg ✤

Administer:

PO route

• After shaking liquid susp well
• With food for GI upset
• Tablets crushed and mixed with food or fluid for swallowing difficulties
• Avoid use with CNS depressants

SIDE EFFECTS

CNS: *Stimulation, drowsiness,* irritability, psychosis, ataxia, vertigo, fatigue, emotional disturbances, mood changes, paranoia, suicidal ideation

EENT: Diplopia, nystagmus, edema of eyelids

GI: *Nausea, vomiting, anorexia,* hepatitis

GU: Impotence

HEMA: Thrombocytopenia, leukopenia, neutropenia, eosinophilia, megaloblastic anemia, decreased serum folate level, lymphadenopathy

INTEG: *Rash,* edema, alopecia, lupuslike syndrome

PHARMACOKINETICS

PO: Peak 4 hr; metabolized in liver; excreted by kidneys, in breast milk; half-life 10-12 hr (primidone)

INTERACTIONS

• Primidone levels decreased by acetaZOLAMIDE, succinimides
• May decrease effect of oral contraceptives, acebutolol, metoprolol, propranolol, tricyclics, phenothiazines, lamoTRIgine

Increase: primidone levels—alcohol, heparin, CNS depressants, isoniazid, nicotinamide

Increase: toxicity—CYP3A4 inhibitors (aprepitant, antiretroviral protease inhibitors, delavirdine, fluconazole, imatinib, voriconazole)

Decrease: primidone effect—CYP3A4 inducers (barbiturates, carBAMazepine, efavirenz, phenytoins, nevirapine)

Drug/Herb

• Avoid use with kava, St. John's wort, valerian

Increase: effect—ginkgo

Decrease: effect—ginseng, santonica

NURSING CONSIDERATIONS

Assess:

• **Seizures:** location, duration, type; folic acid deficiency; fatigue, weakness, neuropathy, depression
• Product level: therapeutic level 5-15 mcg/ml; CBC, LFTs should be obtained q6mo

⚠ Mental status: mood, sensorium, affect, memory (long, short), suicidal thoughts/behaviors

• Respiratory depression, wheezing
• Blood dyscrasias: fever, sore throat, bruising, rash, jaundice

Evaluate:

• Therapeutic response: decreased seizures

Teach patient/family:

• Not to withdraw product quickly because withdrawal symptoms may occur
• To avoid hazardous activities until stabilized on product because drowsiness, dizziness may occur
• To carry emergency ID with condition, medication listed
• To recognize signs of blood dyscrasias; about when to notify prescriber
• To avoid alcohol

⚠ Nurse Alert

procainamide (Rx)

(proe-kane-ah′mide)

Func. class.: Antidysrhythmic (class IA)

Chem. class.: Procaine HCl amide analog

ACTION: Depresses excitability of cardiac muscle to electrical stimulation and slows conduction velocity in atrium, bundle of His, and ventricle; increases refractory period

USES: Life-threatening ventricular dysrhythmias

Unlabeled uses: Atrial fibrillation, flutter

CONTRAINDICATIONS: Hypersensitivity, severe heart block, torsades de pointes

Black Box Warning: Lupus erythematosus

Precautions: Pregnancy (C), breastfeeding, children, renal/hepatic disease, CHF, respiratory depression, cytopenia, dysrhythmia associated with digoxin toxicity, myasthenia gravis, digoxin toxicity

Black Box Warning: Bone marrow failure, cardiac arrhythmias

DOSAGE AND ROUTES

Ventricular tachycardia during CPR

• **Adult: IV** loading dose 20 mg/min; either ventricular tachycardia resolves or patient becomes hypotensive; QRS complex is widened by 50% of original width or total is 17 mg/kg (1.2 g for a 70-kg patient); may give up to 50 mg/min in urgent situations; maintenance: 1-4 mg/min **CONT IV INF; IM** 50 mg/kg/day in divided doses q3-6hr

• **Child: IV** PALS 15 mg/kg over 30-60 min

Renal dose

• **Adult: IV** CCr 35-59 ml/min, give 70% maintenance dose; CCr 15-34 ml/min, give 40%-60% maintenance dose; CCr <15 ml/min, individualize dose

Available forms: Inj 100, 500 mg/ml

Administer:

IM route

• IM inj in deltoid; aspirate to avoid intravascular administration, use only when unable to use IV

Direct IV route

• Dilute each 100 mg/10 ml of 0.9% NaCl, give at max 50 mg/min

Intermittent IV INF route

• Dilute 0.2-1 g/50-500 ml of D_5W (2-4 mg/ml), give over 30-60 min at max 25-50 mg/min, use inf pump

Y-site compatibilities: Alfentanil, amikacin, aminocaproic acid, aminophylline, amiodarone, amphotericin B lipid complex, amphotericin B liposome, anidulafungin, ascorbic acid, atenolol, atracurium, atropine, aztreonam, benztropine, bivalirudin, bleomycin, bumetanide, buprenorphine, butorphanol, calcium chloride/gluconate, caspofungin, ceFAZolin, cefmetazole, cefonicid, cefoperazone, cefotaxime, cefotetan, cefoxitin, ceftazidime, cefTRIAXone, cefuroxime, cephalothin, chlorproMAZINE, cimetidine, cisatracurium, CISplatin, clindamycin, cyanocobalamin, cyclophosphamide, cycloSPORINE, cytarabine, DACTINomycin, DAPTOmycin, dexamethasone, digoxin, diphenhydrAMINE, DOBUTamine, docetaxel, DOPamine, doxacurium, DOXOrubicin, doxycycline, enalaprilat, ePHEDrine, EPINEPHrine, epirubicin, epoetin alfa, eptifibatide, ertapenem, erythromycin, esmolol, etoposide, etoposide phosphate, famotidine, fenoldopam, fentaNYL, fluconazole, fludarabine, fluorouracil, folic acid, furosemide, gatifloxacin, gemcitabine, gentamicin, glycopyrrolate, granisetron, heparin, hydrocortisone, HYDROmorphone, IDArubicin, ifosfamide, indomethacin, insulin (regular), irinotecan, isoproterenol, ketorolac, labetalol, lidocaine, linezolid, LORazepam, magnesium sulfate, mannitol, mechlorethamine, meperidine, metaraminol, methicillin, methotrexate,

P

methoxamine, methyldopate, methylPREDNISolone, metoclopramide, metoprolol, mezlocillin, miconazole, midazolam, mitoxantrone, morphine, moxalactam, multiple vitamins, mycophenolate, nafcillin, nalbuphine, naloxone, netilmicin, nitroglycerin, nitroprusside, norepinephrine, octreotide, ondansetron, oxacillin, oxaliplatin, oxytocin, paclitaxel, palonosetron, pamidronate, pancuronium, pantoprazole, papaverine, pemetrexed, penicillin G potassium/sodium, pentamidine, pentazocine, PENTobarbital, PHENobarbital, phenylephrine, phytonadione, piperacillin, piperacillin-tazobactam, polymyxin B, potassium chloride, prochlorperazine, promethazine, propranolol, protamine, pyridoxine, quiNIDine, quinupristin-dalfopristin, ranitidine, remifentanil, ritodrine, rocuronium, sodium bicarbonate, succinylcholine, SUFentanil, tacrolimus, teniposide, theophylline, thiamine, thiotepa, ticarcillin, ticarcillin-clavulanate, tigecycline, tirofiban, tobramycin, tolazoline, trimetaphan, urokinase, vancomycin, vasopressin, vecuronium, verapamil, vinCRIStine, vinorelbine, vitamin B complex/C, voriconazole, zoledronic acid

SIDE EFFECTS

CNS: *Headache, dizziness,* confusion, psychosis, restlessness, irritability, weakness, depression
CV: *Hypotension,* **heart block, cardiovascular collapse, arrest, torsades de pointes**
GI: Nausea, vomiting, anorexia, diarrhea, hepatomegaly, pain, bitter taste
HEMA: SLE syndrome, **agranulocytosis, thrombocytopenia, neutropenia, hemolytic anemia**
INTEG: Rash, urticaria, edema, swelling (rare), pruritus, flushing, **angioedema**
SYST: SLE

PHARMACOKINETICS

Metabolized in liver to active metabolites, excreted unchanged by kidneys (60%), protein binding 15%
IM: Peak 10-60 min, half-life 3 hr

INTERACTIONS

Increase: effects of neuromuscular blockers
Increase: procainamide effects—cimetidine, quiNIDine, trimethoprim, β-blockers, ranitidine
Increase: toxicity—other antidysrhythmics, thioridazine, quinolones
Drug/Lab Test
Increase: ALT, AST, alk phos, LDH, bilirubin

NURSING CONSIDERATIONS

Assess:
⚠ **ECG continuously if using IV to determine increased PR or QRS segments; discontinue immediately; watch for increased ventricular ectopic beats, maximum need to rebolus**
• Blood levels, 3-10 mcg/ml or NAPA levels 10-20 mcg/ml
⚠ **CBC q2wk × 3 mo; leukocyte, neutrophil, platelet counts may be decreased, treatment may need to be discontinued**
• I&O ratio; electrolytes (K, Na, Cl), weight weekly, report gain of >2 lb
⚠ **Toxicity: confusion, drowsiness, nausea, vomiting, tachydysrhythmias, oliguria**
• ANA titer; during long-term treatment, watch for lupuslike symptoms
• Cardiac rate, rhythm, character, B/P continuously for fluctuations
• Respiratory status: rate, rhythm, character, lung fields; bilateral crackles may occur in CHF patient; watch for respiratory depression
⚠ **CNS effects: dizziness, confusion, psychosis, paresthesias, seizures; product should be discontinued**
Evaluate:
• Therapeutic response: decreased dysrhythmias
Teach patient/family:
• That wax matrix may appear in stools

• Not to discontinue without health care provider's advice

⚠ **To notify prescriber immediately if lupuslike symptoms appear (joint pain, butterfly rash, fever, chills, dyspnea)**

⚠ **To notify prescriber of leukopenia (sore mouth, gums, throat) or thrombocytopenia (bleeding, bruising)**

• How to take pulse and when to report to prescriber

• To avoid driving, other hazardous activities until product effect is known

TREATMENT OF OVERDOSE:
O_2, artificial ventilation, ECG, administer DOPamine for circulatory depression, diazepam or thiopental for seizures, isoproterenol

procaine (Rx)
(proe'kane)

Novocain

Func. class.: Local anesthetic

Chem. class.: Ester

ACTION: Competes with calcium for sites in nerve membrane that control sodium transport across cell membrane; decreases rise of depolarization phase of action potential

USES: Spinal anesthesia, epidural, peripheral nerve block, perineum, lower extremities, infiltration, dental anesthesia

CONTRAINDICATIONS: Children <12 yr, hypersensitivity, sulfite allergy, myasthenia gravis, severe hepatic disease

Precautions: Pregnancy (C), geriatric patients, severe product allergies

DOSAGE AND ROUTES

Spinal anesthesia
• **Adult:** 50-200 mg

Perineum anesthesia
• **Adult:** 50-100 mg (0.5-1 ml of 10% solution)

Available forms: Inj 1%, 2%, 10%

Administer:
• Only products that are not cloudy, that do not contain precipitate
• Only with crash cart, resuscitative equipment nearby
• Only products without preservatives for epidural or caudal anesthesia

Additive compatibilities: Ascorbic acid, hydrocortisone, penicillin G, penicillin G sodium, vit B/C

Syringe compatibilities: Ampicillin, cloxacillin, glycopyrrolate, hydrOXYzine, gentamicin

SIDE EFFECTS
CNS: Anxiety, restlessness, **seizures, loss of consciousness**, drowsiness, disorientation, tremors, shivering

CV: **Myocardial depression, cardiac arrest,** dysrhythmias, bradycardia, hypotension, hypertension, fetal bradycardia

EENT: Blurred vision, tinnitus, pupil constriction

GI: Nausea, vomiting

INTEG: Rash, urticaria, allergic reactions, edema, burning, skin discoloration at inj site, tissue necrosis

RESP: **Status asthmaticus, respiratory arrest, anaphylaxis**

PHARMACOKINETICS
Onset 2-5 min, duration 1 hr; metabolized by liver, excreted in urine (metabolites)

INTERACTIONS
• Dysrhythmias: EPINEPHrine, halothane, enflurane
• Hypertension: tricyclics, phenothiazines, class IA/III dysrhythmias, other products that prolong QT interval
• Hypotension: MAOIs

Decrease: action of aminosalicylic acid, sulfonamides

Decrease: action of procaine—chloroprocaine

NURSING CONSIDERATIONS

Assess:

- B/P, pulse, respiration during treatment
- Fetal heart tones if product is used during labor
- Allergic reactions: rash, urticaria, itching
- Cardiac status: ECG for dysrhythmias, pulse, B/P during anesthesia

Perform/provide:

- Use of new sol; discard unused portions, protect from light

Evaluate:

- Therapeutic response: anesthesia necessary for procedure

TREATMENT OF OVERDOSE:

Airway, O_2, vasopressor, IV fluids, anticonvulsants for seizures

procarbazine (Rx)

(proe-kar′ba-zeen)

Matulane

Func. class.: Antineoplastic, alkylating agent

Chem. class.: Hydrazine derivative

ACTION: Inhibits DNA, RNA, protein synthesis; has multiple sites of action; nonvesicant

USES: Lymphoma, Hodgkin's disease, cancers resistant to other therapy

Unlabeled uses: Brain, lung malignancies; other lymphomas; multiple myeloma, malignant melanoma, polycythemia vera

CONTRAINDICATIONS: Pregnancy (D), breastfeeding, hypersensitivity, thrombocytopenia

Black Box Warning: Bone marrow depression

Precautions: Cardiac/renal/hepatic disease, radiation therapy, seizure disorder, anemia

DOSAGE AND ROUTES

- **Adult: PO** 2-4 mg/kg/day for 1st wk; maintain dosage of 4-6 mg/kg/day until platelets, WBC fall; after recovery, 1-2 mg/kg/day
- **Child: PO** 50 mg/m^2/day for 7 days then 100 mg/m^2 until desired response, leukopenia, or thrombocytopenia occurs; 50 mg/m^2/day maintenance after bone marrow recovery

Available forms: Caps 50 mg

Administer:

- In divided doses and at bedtime to minimize nausea and vomiting
- Nonphenothiazine antiemetic 30-60 min before product and 4-10 hr after treatment to prevent vomiting

SIDE EFFECTS

CNS: Headache, dizziness, insomnia, hallucinations, confusion, coma, pain, chills, fever, sweating, paresthesias, seizures, peripheral neuropathy

EENT: Retinal hemorrhage, nystagmus, photophobia, diplopia, dry eyes

GI: *Nausea, vomiting,* anorexia, diarrhea, constipation, dry mouth, stomatitis, elevated hepatic enzymes

GU: Azoospermia, cessation of menses

HEMA: Thrombocytopenia, anemia, leukopenia, myelosuppression, bleeding tendencies, purpura, petechiae, epistaxis, hemolysis

INTEG: *Rash,* pruritus, dermatitis, alopecia, herpes, hyperpigmentation

MS: Arthralgias, myalgias

RESP: Cough, pneumonitis

SYST: Secondary malignancy

PHARMACOKINETICS

Half-life 1 hr; concentrates in liver, kidney, skin; metabolized in liver, excreted in urine

INTERACTIONS

⚠ Hypotension: meperidine; do not use together

- Neuroleptic malignant syndrome, seizures, hyperpyrexia: alcohol, MAOIs, tricyclics, sympathomimetic products, SSRIs, SNRIs

- Hypertension: guanethidine, levodopa, methyldopa, reserpine, caffeine

⚠ Life-threatening hypertension: sympathomimetics

Increase: bleeding risk—NSAIDs, anticoagulants, platelet inhibitors, thrombolytics

Increase: CNS depression—barbiturates, antihistamines, opioids, hypotensive agents, phenothiazines

Drug/Food

- Hypertensive crisis: tyramine foods

NURSING CONSIDERATIONS

Assess:

- **Bone marrow suppression:** CBC, differential, platelet count weekly; withhold product if WBC is <4000/mm³ or platelet count is <100,000/mm³; notify prescriber
- Renal studies: BUN; serum uric acid; urine CCr; electrolytes before, during therapy
- I&O ratio, report fall in urine output to <30 ml/hr
- Monitor temp; fever may indicate beginning infection
- Hepatic studies before, during therapy: bilirubin, AST, ALT, alk phos, LDH prn or q mo
- CNS changes: confusion, paresthesias, neuropathies; product should be discontinued

⚠ Tyramine foods in diet; hypertensive crisis can occur

⚠ **Toxicity:** facial flushing, epistaxis, increased PT, thrombocytopenia; product should be discontinued

- **Bleeding:** hematuria, guaiac stools, bruising or petechiae, mucosa or orifices q8hr
- Effects of alopecia on body image; discuss feelings about body changes
- Jaundiced skin, sclera; dark urine, clay-colored stools, itchy skin, abdominal pain, fever, diarrhea
- Buccal cavity for dryness, sores or ulceration, white patches, oral pain, bleeding, dysphagia
- Alkalosis if vomiting is severe
- GI symptoms: frequency of stools, cramping
- **Acidosis, signs of dehydration:** rapid respirations, poor skin turgor, decreased urine output, dry skin, restlessness, weakness

Perform/provide:

- Storage in tight, light-resistant container in cool environment

Evaluate:

- Therapeutic response: decreasing malignancy

Teach patient/family:

- To report any complaints, side effects to nurse or prescriber: CNS changes, diarrhea, cough, SOB, fever, chills, sore throat, bleeding, bruising, vomiting blood; black, tarry stools
- That hair may be lost during treatment and wig or hairpiece may make patient feel better; that new hair may be different in color, texture
- To avoid sunlight or UV exposure; to wear sunscreen or protective clothing
- To avoid foods with citric acid, hot or rough texture
- To report any bleeding, white spots, ulcerations in mouth to prescriber; to examine mouth daily
- To avoid driving, activities requiring alertness because dizziness may occur
- To use effective contraception; to avoid breastfeeding; that product may cause infertility
- To avoid the ingestion of alcohol, caffeine, tyramine-containing foods; that cold, hay fever, and weight-reducing products may cause serious product interactions; to avoid smoking
- To avoid crowds, persons with infections if granulocytes are low
- To avoid vaccines

P

prochlorperazine (Rx)

(proe-klor-pair′a-zeen)

Compro

Func. class.: Antiemetic, antipsychotic

Chem. class.: Phenothiazine, piperazine derivative

Do not confuse:
prochlorperazine/chlorproMAZINE

ACTION: Decreases dopamine neurotransmission by increasing dopamine turnover through the blockade of the D_2 somatodendritic autoreceptor in the mesolimbic system

USES: Nausea, vomiting, psychotic disorders

Unlabeled uses: Migraine

CONTRAINDICATIONS: Hypersensitivity to phenothiazines, coma; infants, neonates, children <2 yr; surgery

Precautions: Pregnancy (C), breastfeeding, geriatric patients, seizure, encephalopathy, glaucoma, hepatic disease, Parkinson's disease, BPH

Black Box Warning: Dementia

DOSAGE AND ROUTES

Postoperative nausea/vomiting

- **Adult: IM** 5-10 mg 1-2 hr before anesthesia; may repeat after 30 min; **IV** 5-10 mg 15-30 min before anesthesia; **IV INF** 20 mg/L D_5W or **NS** 15-30 min before anesthesia, max 40 mg/day

Severe nausea/vomiting

- **Adult: PO** 5-10 mg tid-qid; **SUS REL** 15 mg/day in AM or 10 mg q12hr; **RECT** 25 mg/bid; **IM** 5-10 mg q3-4hr prn, max 40 mg/day
- **Child 18-39 kg: PO** 2.5 mg tid or 5 mg bid; **IM** 0.132 mg/kg q3-4hr prn, max 15 mg/day
- **Child 14-17 kg: PO/RECT** 2.5 mg bid-tid; **IM** 0.132 mg/kg q3-4hr prn, max 10 mg/day
- **Child 9-13 kg: PO/RECT** 2.5 mg/day-bid; **IM** 0.132 mg/kg q3-4hr prn, max 7.5 mg/day

Antipsychotic

- **Adult and child ≥12 yr: PO** 5-10 mg tid-qid; may increase q2-3days, max 150 mg/day; **IM** 10-20 mg q2-4hr up to 4 doses then 10-20 mg q4-6hr, max 200 mg/day; **RECT** 10 mg tid-qid, may increase by 5-10 mg q2-3days as needed
- **Child 2-12 yr: PO** 2.5 mg bid-tid; **IM** 0.132 mg/kg

Antianxiety

- **Adult and child ≥12 yr: PO** 5 mg tid-qid, max 20 mg/day or >12 wk; **IM** 5-10 mg q3-4hr, max 40 mg/day; **IV** 2.5-10 mg; max 40 mg/day
- **Child 2-12 yr: IM** 0.132 mg/kg

Available forms: Syr 5 mg/ml; inj 5 mg/ml; tabs 5, 10, 25 mg; sus rel caps 10, 15 mg; supp 2.5, 5, 25 mg

Administer:

- Avoid other CNS depressants

IM route

- IM inj in large muscle mass; aspirate to avoid IV administration
- Keep patient recumbent for ½ hr

Direct IV route

- IV after diluting 5 mg/9 ml NaCl for inj (0.5 mg/ml); give ≥5 mg/min

Intermittent IV INF route

- May dilute 10-20 mg/L NaCl and give as inf

Syringe compatibilities: Atropine, butorphanol, chlorproMAZINE, cimetidine, diamorphine, diphenhydrAMINE, droperidol, fentaNYL, glycopyrrolate, hydrOXYzine, meperidine, metoclopramide, nalbuphine, pentazocine, perphenazine, promazine, promethazine, ranitidine, scopolamine, SUFentanil

Y-site compatibilities: Amsacrine, calcium gluconate, cisatracurium, CISplatin, cladribine, cyclophosphamide, cytarabine, DOXOrubicin, DOXOrubicin liposome, fluconazole, granisetron, heparin, hydrocortisone, melphalan, methotrexate, ondansetron, paclitaxel, potassium chloride, propofol, remifentanil, sargramostim, SUFentanil, teniposide, thiotepa, vinorelbine, vit B/C

SIDE EFFECTS

CNS: **Neuroleptic malignant syndrome,** *extrapyramidal reactions, tardive dyskinesia, euphoria,* depression, *drowsiness,* restlessness, tremor, dizziness, headache
CV: **Circulatory failure,** tachycardia, hypotension, ECG changes
EENT: Blurred vision
GI: Nausea, vomiting, anorexia, dry mouth, diarrhea, constipation, weight loss, metallic taste, cramps
HEMA: **Agranulocytosis**
MISC: Impotence
RESP: **Respiratory depression**

PHARMACOKINETICS

Metabolized by liver; excreted in urine, breast milk; crosses placenta; 91%-99% protein binding
PO: Onset 30-40 min, duration 3-4 hr
SUS REL: Onset 30-40 min, duration 10-12 hr
RECT: Onset 60 min, duration 3-4 hr
IM: Onset 10-20 min, duration 12 hr

INTERACTIONS

Increase: anticholinergic action—anticholinergics, antiparkinson products, antidepressants
Increase: CNS depression—CNS depressants
Increase: serotonin syndrome, neuroleptic malignant syndrome—SSRIs, SNRIs
Decrease: prochlorperazine effect—barbiturates, antacids
Drug/Herb
Increase: CNS depression—chamomile, hops, kava, St. John's wort, valerian
Increase: EPS—kava
Drug/Lab Test
Increase: LFTs, cardiac enzymes, cholesterol, blood glucose, prolactin, bilirubin, PBI, ^{131}I, alk phos, leukocytes, granulocytes, platelets
Decrease: hormones (blood and urine)
False positive: pregnancy tests, urine bilirubin
False negative: urinary steroids, 17-OHCS, pregnancy tests

NURSING CONSIDERATIONS

Assess:
- **EPS:** abnormal movement, tardive dyskinesia, akathisia
- VS, B/P; check patients with cardiac disease more often

⚠ **Neuroleptic malignant syndrome: seizures, hypo/hypertension, fever, tachycardia, dyspnea, fatigue, muscle stiffness, loss of bladder control; notify prescriber immediately**

⚠ **CBC, LFTs during course of treatment; blood dyscrasias, hepatotoxicity may occur**

- Respiratory status before, during, after administration of emetic; check rate, rhythm, character; respiratory depression can occur rapidly among geriatric or debilitated patients

Evaluate:
- Therapeutic response: absence of nausea, vomiting; reduced anxiety, agitation, excitability

Teach patient/family:
- To avoid hazardous activities, activities requiring alertness because dizziness may occur
- To avoid alcohol
- Not to double or skip doses
- That urine may be pink to reddish brown
- That suppositories may contain coconut/palm oil
- To report dark urine, clay-colored stools, bleeding, bruising, rash, blurred vision
- To avoid sun; wear sunscreen, protective clothing

P

progesterone (Rx)

(proe-jess′ter-one)

Crinone, Endometrin, First-Progesterone, Prochieve, Prometrium

Func. class.: Progestogen

Chem. class.: Progesterone derivative

ACTION:

Inhibits secretion of pituitary gonadotropins, which prevents follicular maturation, ovulation; stimulates growth of mammary tissue; antineoplastic action against endometrial cancer

USES:

Contraception, amenorrhea, premenstrual syndrome, abnormal uterine bleeding, endometrial hyperplasia prevention, assisted reproductive technology (ART) gel

Unlabeled uses: Corpus luteum insufficiency, early pregnancy failure, PMS, preterm delivery prophylaxis

CONTRAINDICATIONS:

Pregnancy (D), ectopic pregnancy; hypersensitivity to this product or peanut oil; thromboembolic disorders, reproductive cancer, genital bleeding (abnormal, undiagnosed), cerebral hemorrhage, PID, STDs

Black Box Warning: Breast cancer

Precautions: Breastfeeding, hypertension, asthma, blood dyscrasias, CHF, diabetes mellitus, bone disease, depression, migraine headache, seizure disorders, gallbladder/renal/hepatic disease, family history of breast/reproductive tract cancer

Black Box Warning: Cardiac disease, dementia

DOSAGE AND ROUTES

Infertility

- **Adult: VAG** 90 mg/day (micronized gel); 100 mg 2-3 times/day starting day after oocyte retrieval and for ≤10 wk total (insert)

Amenorrhea/functional uterine bleeding

- **Adult: IM** 5-10 mg/day × 6-8 doses

Endometrial hyperplasia prevention

- **Adult: PO** 200 mg/day × 12 days

Assisted reproductive therapy

- **Adult: GEL** 90 mg (8%) vaginally daily for supplementation; 90 mg (8%) vaginally bid for replacement; if pregnancy occurs, continue × 10-12 wk

Corpus luteum insufficiency (unlabeled)

- **Adult: VAG INSERT** 100 mg bid-tid starting at oocyte retrieval and continuing up to 10-12 wk gestation

Available forms: Inj 50 mg/ml; vag gel 4%, 8%; caps 100, 200 mg; vag insert 100 mg; vag supp 25, 100, 200, 500 mg; compounding kit 25, 50, 100, 200, 400 mg

Administer:

PO route

- Do not break, crush, or chew caps
- Titrated dose; use lowest effective dose
- In 1 dose in AM
- With food or milk to decrease GI symptoms
- Start progesterone 14 days after estrogen dose if given concomitantly

Vaginal route

- Wait at least 6 hr after any vaginal treatment before using vaginal gel

IM route

- Shake vial, inject deeply into large muscle, aspirate

SIDE EFFECTS

CNS: Dizziness, headache, migraines, depression, fatigue, mood swings, dementia, drowsiness

CV: Hypotension, thrombophlebitis, edema, thromboembolism, stroke, pulmonary embolism, MI

EENT: Diplopia, retinal thrombosis

GI: *Nausea,* vomiting, anorexia, cramps, increased weight, cholestatic jaundice, constipation

GU: Amenorrhea, cervical erosion, breakthrough bleeding, dysmenorrhea, vaginal candidiasis, breast changes, *gy-*

necomastia, testicular atrophy, impotence, endometriosis, spontaneous abortion, breast pain, ectopic pregnancy
INTEG: Rash, urticaria, acne, hirsutism, alopecia, oily skin, seborrhea, purpura, melasma
META: Hyperglycemia
SYST: Angioedema, anaphylaxis

PHARMACOKINETICS

Excreted in urine, feces; metabolized in liver
IM/RECT/VAG: Duration 24 hr

INTERACTIONS

Increase: progesterone effect—CYP3A4 inhibitors (ketoconazole, cimetidine, clarithromycin, danazol, diltiazem, erythromycin, fluconazole, itraconazole, troleandomycin, verapamil, voriconazole)
Decrease: progesterone effect—barbiturates, phenytoin
Drug/Lab Test
Increase: alk phos, nitrogen (urine), pregnanediol, amino acids, factors VII, VIII, IX, X
Decrease: GTT, HDL

NURSING CONSIDERATIONS

Assess:
- **Abnormal uterine bleeding:** vaginal bleeding; obtain pad count, patient menstrual history
- Weight daily; notify prescriber of weekly weight gain of >5 lb
- B/P at beginning of treatment and periodically
- I&O ratio; be alert for decreasing urinary output, increasing edema
- Hepatic studies: ALT, AST, bilirubin periodically during long-term therapy
- Edema, hypertension, cardiac symptoms, jaundice, thromboembolism
- Mental status: affect, mood, behavioral changes, depression
- Hypercalcemia

Perform/provide:
- Storage in dark area

Evaluate:
- Therapeutic response: decreased abnormal uterine bleeding, absence of amenorrhea

Teach patient/family:
- ⚠ To report breast lumps, vaginal bleeding, edema, jaundice, dark urine, clay-colored stools, dyspnea, headache, blurred vision, abdominal pain, numbness or stiffness in legs, chest pain
- To avoid gel with other vaginal products; if to be used together, to separate by ≥6 hr
- To report suspected pregnancy
- To monitor blood glucose if diabetic

promethazine (Rx)

(proe-meth'a-zeen)

Phenadoz, Phenergan, Promethagan

Func. class.: Antihistamine, H_1-receptor antagonist, antiemetic
Chem. class.: Phenothiazine derivative

Do not confuse:
Phenergan/Theragran

ACTION: Acts on blood vessels, GI, respiratory system by competing with histamine for H_1-receptor sites; decreases allergic response by blocking histamine

USES: Motion sickness, rhinitis, allergy symptoms, sedation, nausea, preoperative and postoperative sedation
Unlabeled uses: Allergic rhinitis, acute peripheral vestibular nystagmus, hyperemesis gravidarum

CONTRAINDICATIONS: Hypersensitivity, breastfeeding, agranulocytosis, bone marrow suppression, coma, jaundice, Reye's syndrome

Black Box Warning: Infants, neonates, children, intraarterial/SUBCUT administration, extravasation

Precautions: Pregnancy (C), cardiac/renal/hepatic disease, asthma, seizure

P

disorder, prostatic hypertrophy, bladder obstruction, glaucoma, COPD, GI obstruction, ileus, CNS depression, diabetes, sleep apnea, urinary retention

Black Box Warning: IV use

DOSAGE AND ROUTES

Nausea/vomiting

- **Adult: PO/IM/IV/RECT** 12.5-25 mg; q4-6hr prn
- **Child >2 yr: PO/IM/IV/RECT** 0.25-0.5 mg/kg q4-6hr prn

Motion sickness

- **Adult: PO** 25 mg bid, give ½-1 hr before departure then q8-12hr prn
- **Child ≥2 yr: PO/IM/RECT** 12.5-25 mg bid, give ½-1 hr before departure then q8-12hr prn

Sedation

- **Adult: PO/IM** 25-50 mg at bedtime
- **Child ≥2 yr: PO/IM/RECT** 12.5-25 mg at bedtime

Sedation (preoperative/postoperative)

- **Adult: PO/IM/IV** 25-50 mg
- **Child >2 yr: PO/IM/IV** 0.5-1.1 mg/kg

Allergy/rhinitis (unlabeled)

- **Adult: PO** 12.5 mg qid or 25 mg at bedtime
- **Child ≥2 yr: PO** 6.25-12.5 mg tid or 25 mg at bedtime

Hyperemesis gravidarum (unlabeled)

- **Pregnant females: PO/RECT/IM/IV** 12.5-25 mg q4hr

Nystagmus (unlabeled)

- **Adult: PO** 12.5-25 mg q4-6hr for ≤48 hr

Available forms: Tabs 12.5, 25, 50 mg; supp 12.5, 25, 50 mg; inj 25, 50 mg/ml

Administer:

- Avoid use with other CNS depressants

PO route

- With meals for GI symptoms; absorption may slightly decrease
- When used for motion sickness, 30 min-1 hr before travel

IM route

- IM inj deep in large muscle; rotate site

Direct IV route

Black Box Warning: Check for extravasation: burning, pain, swelling at IV site; can cause tissue necrosis

- Do not use if precipitate is present
- Rapid administration may cause transient decrease in B/P
- After diluting each 25-50 mg/9 ml of NaCl for inj; give ≤25 mg/2 min

Syringe compatibilities: Butorphanol, chlorproMAZINE, cimetidine, dihydroergotamine, diphenhyDRAMINE, droperidol, fentaNYL, glycopyrrolate, HYDROmorphone, hydrOXYzine, meperidine, metoclopramide, midazolam, pentazocine, perphenazine, prochlorperazine, promazine, ranitidine, scopolamine

Y-site compatibilities: Alfentanil, amifostine, amikacin, aminocaproic acid, amsacrine, anidulafungin, ascorbic acid, atenolol, atracurium, atropine, aztreonam, benztropine, bivalirudin, bleomycin, bumetanide, buprenorphine, butorphanol, calcium chloride/gluconate, CARBOplatin, caspofungin, chlorproMAZINE, cimetidine, ciprofloxacin, cisatracurium, CISplatin, cladribine, codeine, cyanocobalamin, cyclophosphamide, cycloSPORINE, cytarabine, DACTINomycin, DAPTOmycin, dexmedetomidine, digoxin, diltiazem, diphenhydrAMINE, DOBUTamine, docetaxel, DOPamine, doxacurium, DOXOrubicin, doxycycline, enalaprilat, ePHEDrine, EPINEPHrine, epirubicin, epoetin, eptifibatide, erythromycin, esmolol, etoposide, famotidine, fenoldopam, fentaNYL, filgrastim, fluconazole, fludarabine, gemcitabine, gentamicin, glycopyrrolate, granisetron, HYDROmorphone, hydrOXYzine, IDArubicin, ifosfamide, insulin (regular), irinotecan, isoproterenol, labetalol, levofloxacin, lidocaine, linezolid, LORazepam, LR, magnesium sulfate, mannitol, mechlorethamine, melphalan, meperidine, metaraminol, methoxamine, methyldopate, metoclopramide, metoprolol, metroNIDAZOLE, miconazole, midazolam, milrinone, mitoxantrone, morphine, mycophenolate, nalbuphine, naloxone, netilmicin, nitroglycerin, norepinephrine, octreotide, ondansetron, oxaliplatin, oxytocin, paclitaxel, palonosetron, pamidronate, pancuronium, pemetrexed, pentamidine, pentazocine, phenylephrine, polymyxin B, procainamide, prochlorperazine, propranolol, protamine, pyridoxine, quiNIDine, quinupristin-dalfopristin, ranitidine, remifentanil, Ringer's, ritodrine, riTUXimab, rocuronium, sargramostim, sodium acetate, succinylcholine, SUFentanil, tacrolimus, teniposide, theophylline, thiamine, thiotepa, tigecycline, tirofiban, TNA, tobramycin, tolazoline, trastuzumab, trimetaphan, vancomycin, vasopressin, vecuronium, verapamil, vinCRIStine, vinorelbine, voriconazole

SIDE EFFECTS

CNS: *Dizziness, drowsiness,* poor coordination, fatigue, anxiety, euphoria, confusion, paresthesia, neuritis, EPS, **neuroleptic malignant syndrome**

CV: Hypo/hypertension, palpitations, tachycardia

EENT: Blurred vision, dilated pupils, tinnitus, nasal stuffiness; dry nose, throat, mouth; photosensitivity

GI: *Constipation,* dry mouth, nausea, vomiting, anorexia, diarrhea

GU: *Urinary retention,* dysuria, frequency

HEMA: **Thrombocytopenia, agranulocytosis, hemolytic anemia**

INTEG: Rash, urticaria, photosensitivity

RESP: Increased thick secretions, wheezing, chest tightness; **apnea in neonates, infants, young children**

PHARMACOKINETICS

Metabolized in liver; excreted by kidneys, GI tract (inactive metabolites)

PO: Onset 20 min, duration 4-12 hr

IV: Onset 3-5 min

INTERACTIONS

Increase: CNS depression—barbiturates, opioids, hypnotics, tricyclics, alcohol

Increase: promethazine effect—MAOIs

Decrease: oral anticoagulants effect—heparin

Drug/Lab Test

False negative: skin allergy test

False positive: urine pregnancy test

Interference: blood grouping (ABO), GTT

NURSING CONSIDERATIONS

Assess:

- **Antiemetic/motion sickness:** nausea, vomiting before, after dose
- I&O ratio; be alert for urinary retention, frequency, dysuria; product should be discontinued

⚠ **CBC with differential, LFTs during long-term therapy; blood dyscrasias, jaundice may occur**

- Respiratory status: rate, rhythm, increase in bronchial secretions, wheezing, chest tightness
- Cardiac status: palpitations, increased pulse, hypo/hypertension, B/P in those receiving IV doses
- **Neuroleptic malignant syndrome:** fever, confusion, diaphoresis, rigid muscles, elevated CPK, encephalopathy; discontinue product, notify prescriber

Perform/provide:

- Hard candy, gum, frequent rinsing of mouth for dryness
- Storage in tight, light-resistant container

Evaluate:

- Therapeutic response: absence of running, congested nose; rashes; absence of motion sickness, nausea; sedation

Teach patient/family:

- That product may cause photosensitivity; to avoid prolonged exposure to sunlight
- To notify prescriber of confusion, sedation, hypotension, jaundice, fever
- To avoid driving, other hazardous activity if drowsy
- To avoid concurrent use of alcohol or other CNS depressants
- That product may reduce sweating; that there is a risk of heat stroke
- How to use frequent sips of water, gum to decrease dry mouth

propafenone (Rx)

(pro-paff′e-nown)

Apo-Propafenone ♣, Gen-Propafenone ♣, Rythmol, Rythmol SR

Func. class.: Antidysrhythmic (class IC)

ACTION:
Slows conduction velocity; reduces membrane responsiveness; inhibits automaticity; increases ratio of effective refractory period to action potential duration; β-blocking activity

USES:
Sustained ventricular tachycardia, atrial fibrillation (single dose), paroxysmal supraventricular tachycardia (PSVT) prophylaxis, supraventricular dysrhythmias

Unlabeled uses: Wolff-Parkinson-White (WPW) syndrome

CONTRAINDICATIONS:
2nd/3rd-degree AV block, right bundle branch block, cardiogenic shock, hypersensitivity, bradycardia, uncontrolled CHF, sick-sinus syndrome, marked hypotension, bronchospastic disorders, electrolyte imbalance

Precautions: Pregnancy (C), breastfeeding, children, geriatric patients, CHF, hypo/hyperkalemia, nonallergic bronchospasm, renal/hepatic disease, hematologic disorders

Black Box Warning: Recent MI, cardiac arrhythmias, QT prolongation, torsades de pointes

DOSAGE AND ROUTES

• **Adult: PO** 150 mg q8hr; allow 3-4 day interval before increasing dose, max 900 mg/day

Atrial fibrillation

• **Adult: PO** 450 or 600 mg as single dose; SR 225 mg q12hr, may increase to 325 q12hr, max 425 mg q12hr

Available forms: Tabs 150, 225, 300 mg; SR cap 225, 325, 425 mg

Administer:

• Do not break, crush, or chew tabs; swallow whole

• To hospitalized patients because heart monitoring is required

• After hypo/hyperkalemia is corrected

• With dosage adjustment q3-4days

• Without regard to meals

SIDE EFFECTS

CNS: Headache, dizziness, abnormal dreams, syncope, confusion, seizures, insomnia, tremor, anxiety, fatigue

CV: Supraventricular dysrhythmia, ventricular dysrhythmia, bradycardia, prodysrhythmia, palpitations, AV block, intraventricular conduction delay, AV dissociation, hypotension, chest pain, asystole

EENT: Blurred vision, altered taste, tinnitus

GI: *Nausea, vomiting,* constipation, dyspepsia, cholestasis, abnormal hepatic studies, dry mouth, diarrhea, anorexia

HEMA: Leukopenia, agranulocytosis, granulocytopenia, thrombocytopenia, anemia, bruising

INTEG: Rash

RESP: Dyspnea

PHARMACOKINETICS

Peak 3-8 hr, half-life 2-10 hr; metabolized in liver; excreted in urine (metabolite)

INTERACTIONS

Increase: propafenone effects—CYP1A2, CYP2D6, CYP3A4 inhibitors (protease inhibitors, quinine, paroxetine, saquinavir, erythromycin, azole antifungals, sertraline, tricyclics)

Increase: QT prolongation—other class IA/IC antidysrhythmics, arsenic trioxide, chloroquine, clarithromycin, droperidol, erythromycin, haloperidol, levomethadyl, methadone, pentamidine, chlorproMAZINE, mesoridazine, thioridazine

Increase: anticoagulation—warfarin

Increase: CNS effects—local anesthetics

Increase: digoxin level—digoxin

Increase: β-blocker effect—propranolol, metoprolol
Increase: cycloSPORINE levels—cycloSPORINE
Decrease: propafenone effect—rifampin, cimetidine, quiNIDine
Drug/Lab Test
Increase: CPK

NURSING CONSIDERATIONS

Assess:

- GI status: bowel pattern, number of stools

⚠ **QT/PR prolongation:** ECG or Holter monitor prior to and during therapy

- **CHF:** dyspnea, jugular venous distention, crackles, edema in extremities, I&O ratio; check for decreasing output; daily weight
- CBC, ANA titer, LFTs
- Chest x-ray, pulmonary function test during treatment
- Lung fields; bilateral crackles, dyspnea, peripheral edema, weight gain; jugular venous distention may occur in patient with CHF

⚠ **Toxicity:** fine tremors, dizziness, hypotension, drowsiness, abnormal heart rate

Evaluate:

- Therapeutic response: absence of ventricular dysrhythmias; decreasing recurrence of PAF, PSVT

Teach patient/family:

- To avoid hazardous activities until response is known
- To report fever, chills, sore throat, bleeding, SOB, chest pain, palpitations, blurred vision
- To take tab with food
- To carry emergency ID identifying medication and prescriber
- To avoid abrupt discontinuation of product; to take as prescribed; not to miss, double doses

TREATMENT OF OVERDOSE:

O_2, artificial ventilation, defibrillation ECG; administer DOPamine for circulatory depression, diazepam or thiopental for seizures, isoproterenol

proparacaine ophthalmic

See Appendix B

⚠ *HIGH ALERT*

propofol (Rx)

(pro′poh-fole)

Diprivan, Fresenius Propoven

Func. class.: General anesthetic

ACTION: Produces dose-dependent CNS depression by activation of GABA receptor

USES: Induction or maintenance of anesthesia as part of balanced anesthetic technique; sedation in mechanically ventilated patients

CONTRAINDICATIONS: Hypersensitivity to this product or soybean oil, egg, benzyl alcohol (some products)

Precautions: Pregnancy (B), breastfeeding, children, geriatric patients, respiratory depression, severe respiratory disorders, cardiac dysrhythmias, labor and delivery, renal disease, hyperlipidemia

DOSAGE AND ROUTES

Anesthesia

- **Adult <55 yr and ASA I/II IV (Diprivan or generic): IV** 40 mg q10sec until induction onset, maintenance 100-200 mcg/kg/min or **IV BOL** 20-50 mg prn, allow 3-5 min between adjustments; Fresenius Propoven 1% **IV** 20-40 q10sec until induction then 3-6 mg/kg/hr
- **Child ≥3 yr or ASA I or II: IV induction:** 2.5-3.5 mg/kg over 20-30 sec when not premedicated or lightly premedicated

P

• **Child 2 mo-16 yr maintenance: IV** 125-300 mcg/kg/min, lower dose for ASA III or **IV**

ICU sedation

• **Adult: IV** 5 mcg/kg/min over 5 min; may increase by 5-10 mcg/kg/min over 5-10 min until desired response (Diprivan or generic): 0.3-4 mg/kg/hr, max 4 mg/kg/hr (Fresenius Propoven)

Available forms: Inj 10 mg/ml in 20-ml ampule, 50-ml and 100-ml vials

Administer:

IV route

• Shake well before use; dilution is not necessary but, if diluted, use only D_5W to ≥2 mg/ml; give over 3-5 min, titrate to needed level of sedation; use only glass containers when mixing, not stable in plastic; use aseptic technique when transferring from original container

• **Fresenius Propoven 1%:** dilution is not necessary but, if diluted, use D_5W or NS to ≥2 mg/ml (max dilution max 1 part Fresenius Propoven/4 parts D_5W or NS); do not admix; lidocaine can be used to reduce pain at site

• May be given by cont inf; give by inf pump

• Only with resuscitative equipment available; only by qualified persons trained in anesthesia

Y-site compatibilities: Acyclovir, alfentanil, aminophylline, ampicillin, aztreonam, bumetanide, buprenorphine, butorphanol, calcium gluconate, CARBOplatin, ceFAZolin, cefoperazone, cefotaxime, cefotetan, cefoxitin, ceftizoxime, cefTRIAXone, cefuroxime, chlorproMAZINE, cimetidine, CISplatin, clindamycin, cyclophosphamide, cycloSPORINE, cytarabine, dexamethasone, diphenhydrAMINE, DOBUTamine, DOPamine, doxycycline, droperidol, enalaprilat, ePHEDrine, EPINEPHrine, esmolol, famotidine, fentaNYL, fluconazole, fluorouracil, furosemide, ganciclovir, glycopyrrolate, granisetron, haloperidol, heparin, hydrocortisone, HYDROmorphone, hydrOXYzine, ifosfamide, imipenem/cilastatin, inamrinone, regular insulin, isoproterenol, ketamine, labetalol, levorphanol, lidocaine, LORazepam, magnesium sulfate, mannitol, meperidine, mezlocillin, miconazole, morphine, nafcillin, nalbuphine, naloxone, nitroglycerin, norepinephrine, ofloxacin, paclitaxel, PENTobarbital, PHENobarbital, piperacillin, potassium chloride, prochlorperazine, propranolol, ranitidine, scopolamine, sodium bicarbonate, sodium nitroprusside, succinylcholine, SUFentanil, thiopental ticarcillin, ticarcillin/clavulanate, vecuronium, verapamil

Solution compatibilities: if given together via Y-site: D_5W, D_5LR, LR, D_5/0.45% NaCl, D_5/0.2% NaCl

SIDE EFFECTS

CNS: Involuntary movement, headache, jerking, fever, dizziness, shivering, tremor, confusion, somnolence, paresthesia, agitation, abnormal dreams, euphoria fatigue, **increased intracranial pressure, impaired cerebral flow, seizures**

CV: *Bradycardia, hypotension,* hypertension, PVC, PAC, tachycardia, abnormal ECG, ST segment depression, **asystole, bradydysrhythmias**

EENT: Blurred vision, tinnitus, eye pain, strange taste, diplopia

GI: *Nausea, vomiting, abdominal cramping,* dry mouth, swallowing, hypersalivation, **pancreatitis**

GU: Urine retention, green urine, cloudy urine, oliguria

INTEG: *Flushing, phlebitis, hives, burning/stinging at inj site,* rash, pain of extremities

MS: Myalgia

RESP: **Apnea**, *cough, hiccups,* dyspnea, hypoventilation, sneezing, wheezing, tachypnea, hypoxia, respiratory acidosis

SYST: **Propofol infusion syndrome**

PHARMACOKINETICS

Onset 15-30 sec, rapid distribution, half-life 1-8 min, terminal half-life 3-12 hr; 70% excreted in urine; metabolized in liver by conjugation to inactive metabolites, 95%-99% protein binding

INTERACTIONS

- Do not use within 10 days of MAOIs

Increase: CNS depression—alcohol, opioids, sedative/hypnotics, antipsychotics, skeletal muscle relaxants, inhalational anesthetics

Drug/Herb

Increase: propofol effect—St. John's wort

NURSING CONSIDERATIONS

Assess:

- Inj site: phlebitis, burning, stinging
- **ECG** for changes: PVC, PAC, ST segment changes; monitor VS
- **Neurologic excitatory symptoms:** movement, tremors, dizziness, LOC, pupil reaction
- Allergic reactions: hives

⚠ **Respiratory dysfunction:** respiratory depression, character, rate, rhythm; notify prescriber if respirations are <10/min

- **Propofol infusion syndrome:** rhabdomyolysis, renal failure, hyperkalemia, metabolic acidosis, cardiac dysrhythmias, heart failure usually between 35 and 93 hr after inf begun at >5 mg/kg/hr for >58 hr

Perform/provide:

- Storage in light-resistant area at room temp, use within 6 hr of opening
- If transferred from original container to another container, complete inf within 12 hr (Dipravan), 6 hr (generic propofol)

Evaluate:

- Therapeutic response: induction of anesthesia

Teach patient/family:

- That product will cause dizziness, drowsiness, sedation

TREATMENT OF OVERDOSE:

Discontinue product; administer vasopressor agents or anticholinergics, artificial ventilation

propranolol (Rx)

(proe-pran′oh-lole)

Apo-Propranolol ✱, Inderal, Inderal LA, InnoPran XL

Func. class.: Antihypertensive, antianginal, antidysrhythmic (class II)

Chem. class.: β-Adrenergic blocker

Do not confuse:

propranolol/Pravachol

Inderal/Toradol/Inderide/Adderall/Imuran

ACTION: Nonselective β-blocker with negative inotropic, chronotropic, dromotropic properties

USES: Chronic stable angina pectoris, hypertension, supraventricular dysrhythmias, migraine prophylaxis, pheochromocytoma, cyanotic spells related to hypertrophic subaortic stenosis

Unlabeled uses: Anxiety, Parkinson's tremor, prevention of variceal bleeding caused by portal hypertension, akathisia induced by antipsychotics, acute MI, portal hypertension, sclerodermal renal crisis, unstable angina, infantile capillary hemangioma, lithium-induced tremor

CONTRAINDICATIONS: Hypersensitivity to this product; cardiogenic shock, AV heart block; bronchospastic disease; sinus bradycardia; bronchospasm; asthma

Precautions: Pregnancy (C), breastfeeding, children, diabetes mellitus, hyperthyroidism, COPD, renal/hepatic disease, myasthenia gravis, peripheral vascular disease, hypotension, cardiac failure, Raynaud's disease, sick sinus syndrome, vasospastic angina, smoking, Wolff-Parkinson-White syndrome

Black Box Warning: Abrupt discontinuation

P

DOSAGE AND ROUTES

Dysrhythmias

• **Adult: PO** 10-30 mg tid-qid; **IV BOL** 1-3 mg give 1 mg/min; may repeat after 2 min, may repeat q4hr thereafter

• **Child: PO** 1 mg/kg/day in 2 divided doses; **IV** 0.01-0.1 mg/kg over 5 min

Hypertension

• **Adult: PO** 40 mg bid or 80 mg/day (ext rel) initially; usual dose 120-240 mg/day bid-tid or 120-160 mg/day (ext rel)

• **Child: PO** 0.5-1 mg/kg/day divided q6-12hr

Angina

• **Adult: PO** 80-320 mg in divided doses bid-qid or 80 mg/day (ext rel); usual dose 160 mg/day (ext rel)

MI prophylaxis

• **Adult: PO** 180-240 mg/day tid-qid starting 5 days to 2 wk after MI

Pheochromocytoma

• **Adult: PO** 60 mg/day × 3 days preoperatively in divided doses or 30 mg/day in divided doses (inoperable tumor)

Migraine

• **Adult: PO** 80 mg/day (ext rel) or in divided doses; may increase to 160-240 mg/day in divided doses

• **Child >35 kg (unlabeled): PO** 20-40 mg tid

Essential tremor

• **Adult: PO** 40 mg bid; usual dose 120 mg/day

Acute MI (unlabeled)

• **Adult: PO** 180-320 mg/day in 3-4 divided doses

Anxiety (unlabeled)

• **Adult: PO** 10-80 mg given 1 hr prior to anxiety-producing event

Scleroderma renal crisis (unlabeled)

• **Adult: PO** 40 mg bid, may increase q3-7days, max 160-480 mg/day

Esophageal varices (portal hypertension) (unlabeled)

• **Adult: PO** 40 mg bid, titrate to heart rate reduction of 25%

Infantile capillary hemangioma (unlabeled)

• **Infant: PO** 2-3 mg/kg/day

Available forms: Ext rel caps 60, 80, 120, 160 mg; tabs 10, 20, 40, 60, 80, 90 mg; inj 1 mg/ml; oral sol 4 mg/ml, 8 mg/ml; conc oral sol 80 mg/ml

Administer:

PO route

• Do not break, crush, chew, or open ext rel cap

• Do not use ext rel cap for essential tremor, MI, cardiac dysrhythmias; do not use InnoPran XL in hypertropic subaortic stenosis, migraine, angina pectoris

• Ext rel caps should be taken daily; InnoPran XL should be taken at bedtime

• May mix oral sol with liquid or semisolid food; rinse container to get entire dose

• With 8 oz water with food; food enhances bioavailability

• Do not give with aluminum-containing antacid; may decrease GI absorption

Direct IV route

• IV undiluted or diluted 10 ml D_5W for inj; give ≤1 mg/min

Intermittent IV INF route

• May be diluted in 50 ml NaCl and run 1 mg over 10-15 min

Y-site compatibilities: Acyclovir, alfentanil, alteplase, amikacin, aminocaproic acid, aminophylline, anidulafungin, ascorbic acid, atracurium, atropine, azaTHIOprine, aztreonam, benztropine, bivalirudin, bleomycin, bumetanide, buprenorphine, butorphanol, calcium chloride/gluconate, CARBOplatin, carmustine, caspofungin, cefamandole, ceFAZolin, cefmetazole, cefonicid, cefoperazone, cefotaxime, cefotetan, cefoxitin, ceftazidime, ceftizoxime, cefTRIAXone, cefuroxime, cephalothin, cephapirin, chloramphenicol, chlorproMAZINE, cimetidine, CISplatin, clindamycin, cyanocobalamin, cyclophosphamide, cycloSPORINE, cytarabine, DACTINomycin, DAPTOmycin, dexamethasone, digoxin, diltiazem, diphenhydrAMINE, DOBUTamine, docetaxel, DOPamine, doxacurium, DOXOrubicin, doxycycline, enalaprilat, ePHEDrine, EPINEPHrine, epirubicin, epoetin alfa, eptifibatide, ertapenem, erythromycin, esmolol, etoposide, etoposide phosphate, famotidine, fenoldopam, fentaNYL, fluconazole, fludarabine, fluorouracil, folic acid, furosemide, ganciclovir, gatifloxacin, gemcitabine, gemtuzumab, gentamicin, glycopyrrolate, granisetron, heparin, hydrocortisone, HYDROmorphone, hydrOXYzine, IDArubicin, ifosfamide, imipenem-cilastatin, inamrinone, irinotecan, isoproterenol, ketorolac, labetalol, levofloxacin, lidocaine, linezolid, LORazepam, magnesium, mannitol, mechlorethamine, meperidine, metaraminol, methicillin, methotrexate, methoxamine, methyldopate, methylPREDNISolone, metoclopramide, metoprolol, metroNIDAZOLE, mezlocillin, miconazole, midazolam, milrinone, minocycline, mitoxantrone, morphine, moxalactam, multiple vitamins, mycophenolate, nafcillin, nalbuphine, naloxone, nesiritide, netilmicin, nitroglycerin, nitroprusside, norepinephrine, octreotide, ondansetron, oxacillin, oxaliplatin, oxytocin, palonosetron, pamidronate, pancuronium, papaverine, pemetrexed, penicillin G potassium/sodium, pentamidine, pentazocine, PENTobarbital, PHENobarbital, phenylephrine, phytonadione, piperacillin, polymyxin B, potassium chloride, procainamide, prochlorperazine, promethazine, propofol, protamine, pyridoxine, quiNIDine, quinupristin-dalfopristin, ranitidine, ritodrine, rocuronium, sodium acetate/bicarbonate, succinylcholine, SUFentanil, tacrolimus, teniposide, theophylline, thiamine, thiotepa, ticarcillin, ticarcillin-clavulanate, tigecycline, tirofiban, tobramycin, tolazoline, trimetaphan, urokinase, vancomycin, vasopressin, vecuronium, verapamil, vinCRIStine, vinorelbine, vitamin B complex/C, voriconazole, zoledronic acid

SIDE EFFECTS

CNS: Depression, hallucinations, dizziness, *fatigue,* lethargy, paresthesias, bizarre dreams, disorientation

CV: Bradycardia, hypotension, **CHF,** palpitations, AV block, peripheral vascular insufficiency, vasodilation, cold extremities, **pulmonary edema, dysrhythmias**

EENT: Sore throat, **laryngospasm,** blurred vision, dry eyes

GI: Nausea, vomiting, diarrhea, colitis, constipation, cramps, dry mouth, hepatomegaly, gastric pain, acute pancreatitis

GU: Impotence, decreased libido, UTIs

HEMA: **Agranulocytosis, thrombocytopenia**

INTEG: Rash, pruritus, fever

META: Hyperglycemia, hypoglycemia

MISC: Facial swelling, weight change, Raynaud's phenomenon

MS: Joint pain, arthralgia, muscle cramps, pain

RESP: Dyspnea, respiratory dysfunction, *bronchospasm,* cough

PHARMACOKINETICS

Metabolized by liver; crosses placenta, blood-brain barrier; excreted in breast milk; protein binding 90%

PO: Onset 30 min, peak 1-1½ hr, duration 12 hr

PO-ER: Peak 6 hr, duration 24 hr, half-life 8-11 hr

IV: Onset 2 min, peak 1 min, duration 5 min

INTERACTIONS

Increase: toxicity—phenothiazines

Increase: propranolol level—propafenone

Increase: effect of calcium channel blockers, neuromuscular blocker

Increase: negative inotropic effects—disopyramide

Increase: β-blocking effect—cimetidine

Increase: hypotension—quiNIDine, haloperidol, prazosin

Decrease: β-blocking effects—barbiturates

Decrease: propranolol levels—smoking

Drug/Herb

- Avoid use with feverfew

Increase: antihypertensive effect—hawthorn

P

Decrease: antihypertensive effect—ma huang

Drug/Lab Test

Increase: serum potassium, serum uric acid, ALT, AST, alk phos, LDH

Decrease: blood glucose

Interference: glaucoma testing

NURSING CONSIDERATIONS

Assess:

Black Box Warning: Abrupt withdrawal: taper over a few weeks, do not discontinue abruptly; dysrhythmias, angina, myocardial ischemia, or MI may occur, taper over 2 wk

- B/P, pulse, respirations during beginning therapy; notify prescriber if pulse <50 bpm or systolic B/P <90 mm Hg

⚠ **ECG** continuously if using as antidysrhythmic IV, PCWP (pulmonary capillary wedge pressure), CVP (central venous pressure)

- Hepatic enzymes: AST, ALT, bilirubin
- Angina pain: duration, time started, activity being performed, character
- Tolerance with long-term use
- Headache, lightheadedness, decreased B/P; may indicate need for decreased dosage; may aggrevate symptoms of arterial insufficiency
- **Fluid overload:** weight daily; report gain of >5 lb

⚠ I&O ratio, CCr if kidney damage is diagnosed; fatigue, weight gain, jugular distention, dyspnea, peripheral edema, crackles

Perform/provide:

- Protection from light

Evaluate:

- Therapeutic response: decreased B/P, dysrhythmias

Teach patient/family:

⚠ Not to discontinue abruptly; may precipitate life-threatening dysrhythmias, exacerbation of angina, MI; to take product at same time each day, either with or without food consistently; to decrease dosage over 2 wk

- To avoid OTC products unless approved by prescriber; to avoid alcohol
- To avoid hazardous activities if dizzy
- About the importance of compliance with complete medical regimen; to monitor blood glucose, may mask symptoms of hypoglycemia
- To make position changes slowly to prevent fainting
- That sensitivity to cold may occur
- How to take pulse, B/P; to withhold product if <50 bpm or systolic B/P <90 mm Hg

propylhexadrine nasal agent

See Appendix B

propylthiouracil (Rx)

(proe-pill-thye-oh-yoor′a-sill)

Propyl-Thyracil ♣

Func. class.: Thyroid hormone antagonist (antithyroid)

Chem. class.: Thioamide

ACTION: Blocks synthesis peripherally of T_3, T_4 (triiodothyronine, thyroxine), inhibits organification of iodine

USES: Preparation for thyroidectomy, thyrotoxic crisis, hyperthyroidism, thyroid storm

CONTRAINDICATIONS: Pregnancy (D), breastfeeding, hypersensitivity, agranulocytosis, hepatitis, jaundice

Precautions: Infants, bone marrow depression, fever

Black Box Warning: Hepatic disease

DOSAGE AND ROUTES

Thyrotoxic crisis

- **Adult and child: PO** 200-400 mg q4hr for 1st 24 hr

Preparation for thyroidectomy

- **Adult: PO** 600-1200 mg/day
- **Child: PO** 10 mg/kg/day in divided doses

Hyperthyroidism

- **Adult: PO** 100 mg tid increasing to 300 mg q8hr if condition is severe; continue to euthyroid state then 100 mg daily-tid
- **Child >6 yr: PO** 50 mg/day divided q8hr, titrate based on TSH/free T_4 levels
- **Neonate (unlabeled): PO** 5-10 mg/kg/day in divided doses q8hr

Available forms: Tabs 50 mg

Administer:

- With meals to decrease GI upset
- At same time each day to maintain product level
- At lowest dose that relieves symptoms

SIDE EFFECTS

CNS: *Drowsiness, headache, vertigo, fever,* paresthesias, neuritis

GI: *Nausea, diarrhea, vomiting,* jaundice, hepatitis, loss of taste, liver failure, death

GU: Nephritis

HEMA: Agranulocytosis, leukopenia, thrombocytopenia, hypothrombinemia, lymphadenopathy, bleeding, vasculitis, periarteritis

INTEG: *Rash, urticaria, pruritus, alopecia, hyperpigmentation,* lupuslike syndrome

MS: Myalgia, arthralgia, nocturnal muscle cramps, osteoporosis

PHARMACOKINETICS

Onset up to 3 wk, peak 6-10 wk, duration 1 wk to 1 mo, half-life 1-2 hr; excreted in urine, bile, breast milk; crosses placenta; concentration in thyroid gland

INTERACTIONS

- Bone marrow suppression: radiation, antineoplastics
- Agranulocytosis: phenothiazines

Increase: effects—potassium/sodium iodide, lithium

Decrease: anticoagulant effect—heparin, oral anticoagulants

Drug/Lab Test

Increase: PT, AST, ALT, alk phos

NURSING CONSIDERATIONS

Assess:

- **Hyperthyroidism:** weight loss, nervousness, insomnia, fever, diaphoresis, tremors; **hypothyroidism:** constipation, dry skin, weakness, headache
- Pulse, B/P, temp
- I&O ratio; check for edema: puffy hands, feet, periorbits; indicates hypothyroidism
- Weight daily; same clothing, scale, time of day
- T_3, T_4, which are increased; serum TSH, which is decreased; free thyroxine index, which is increased if dosage is too low; discontinue product 3-4 wk before RAIU

⚠ **Blood dyscrasias:** CBC with differential; leukopenia, thrombocytopenia, agranulocytosis

⚠ **Overdose:** peripheral edema, heat intolerance, diaphoresis, palpitations, dysrhythmias, severe tachycardia, increased temp, delirium, CNS irritability

⚠ **Hypersensitivity:** rash, enlarged cervical lymph nodes; product may have to be discontinued

- **Hypoprothrombinemia:** bleeding, petechiae, ecchymosis
- Clinical response: after 3 wk should include increased weight, pulse; decreased T_4
- **Bone marrow suppression:** sore throat, fever, fatigue
- **Hepatotoxicity:** LFTs before, during treatment; jaundice, nausea, vomiting, abdominal pain, anorexia, diarrhea, fatigue

Perform/provide:

- Storage in light-resistant container
- Fluids to 3-4 L/day unless contraindicated

Evaluate:

- Therapeutic response: weight gain, decreased pulse, decreased T_4, decreased B/P

Teach patient/family:

- To abstain from breastfeeding after delivery
- To take pulse daily

P

- To report redness, swelling, sore throat, mouth lesions, which indicate blood dyscrasias; to report symptoms of hepatic dysfunction
- To keep graph of weight, pulse, mood
- To avoid OTC products that contain iodine
- That seafood, other iodine products may be restricted
- Not to discontinue product abruptly because thyroid crisis may occur; about stress response
- That response may take several months if thyroid is large
- About the symptoms/signs of overdose: periorbital edema, cold intolerance, mental depression
- About the symptoms of an inadequate dose: tachycardia, diarrhea, fever, irritability
- To take medication as prescribed; not to skip or double dose; that missed doses should be taken when remembered up to 1 hr before next dose
- To carry emergency ID listing condition, medication

protamine (Rx)

(proe'ta-meen)

Func. class.: Heparin antagonist

Chem. class.: Low-molecular-weight protein

ACTION:
Binds heparin, thereby making it ineffective

USES:
Heparin, LMWH toxicity, hemorrhage

CONTRAINDICATIONS:
Hypersensitivity

Precautions: Pregnancy (C), breastfeeding, fish allergy, diabetes, previous exposure to protamine, insulins, heparin rebound or bleeding

DOSAGE AND ROUTES

Heparin overdose

- **Adult and child:** **IV** 1 mg of protamine/100 units heparin given; administer slowly over 1-3 min; max 50 mg/10 min

Enoxaparin overdose

- **Adult:** **IV** 1 mg protamine/1 mg enoxaparin

Dalteparin/tinzaparin overdose

- **Adult:** **IV** 1 mg protamine/100 anti-Xa unit

Available forms: Inj 10 mg/ml

Administer:

Direct IV route

- After reconstituting 50 mg/5 ml sterile bacteriostatic water for inj; shake, give ≤20 mg over 1-3 min

Y-site compatibilities: Alfentanil, amikacin, aminophylline, ascorbic acid, atracurium, atropine, azaTHIOprine, aztreonam, benztropine, bumetanide, buprenorphine, butorphanol, calcium chloride/gluconate, ceftazidime, chlorproMAZINE, cimetidine, clindamycin, cyanocobalamin, cycloSPORINE, digoxin, diphenhydrAMINE, DOBUTamine, DOPamine, doxycycline, enalaprilat, ePHEDrine, EPINEPHrine, epoetin alfa, erythromycin, esmolol, famotidine, fentaNYL, fluconazole, ganciclovir, gentamicin, glycopyrrolate, hydrOXYzine, imipenem-cilastatin, inamrinone, iohexol, iopamidol, iothalamate, isoproterenol, labetalol, lidocaine, magnesium, mannitol, meperidine, metaraminol, methoxamine, methyldopate, metoclopramide, metoprolol, miconazole, midazolam, minocycline, morphine, multiple vitamins, nalbuphine, naloxone, netilmicin, nitroglycerin, nitroprusside, norepinephrine, ondansetron, oxytocin, papaverine, pentazocine, phenylephrine, polymyxin B, potassium chloride, procainamide, prochlorperazine, promethazine, propranolol, pyridoxine, quiNIDine, ranitidine, Ringer's, ritodrine, sodium bicarbonate, succinylcholine, SUFentanil, theophylline, thiamine, tobramycin, tolazoline, trimetaphan, urokinase, vancomycin, vasopressin, verapamil

SIDE EFFECTS

CNS: Lassitude, flushing
CV: Hypotension, bradycardia, circulatory collapse, capillary leak
GI: Nausea, vomiting, anorexia
HEMA: Bleeding
INTEG: *Rash,* dermatitis, urticaria
RESP: Dyspnea, pulmonary edema, severe respiratory distress, bronchospasm
SYST: Anaphylaxis, angioedema

PHARMACOKINETICS

IV: Onset 5 min, duration 2 hr

NURSING CONSIDERATIONS

Assess:

⚠ **Hypersensitivity:** urticaria, cough, wheezing, have emergency equipment nearby; **allergy to fish;** use with caution; men who have had vasectomies may be more prone to hypersensitivity

- Blood studies (Hct, platelets, occult blood in stools) q3mo
- Coagulation tests (aPTT, ACT) 15 min after dose then again after several hours
- VS, B/P, pulse after 30 min then 3 hr after dose
- Skin rash, urticaria, dermatitis

Perform/provide:

- Storage at 36° F-46° F (2° C-8° C)

Evaluate:

- Therapeutic response: reversal of heparin overdose

Teach patient/family:

- Not to take if allergic to fish

pseudoephedrine (OTC, Rx)

(soo-doh-eh-fed′rin)

Contac, Dimetapp Maximum Strength, Elix Sure Cold, Eltor ✱, Equaline Children's Nasal, Equaline Maximum Strength, Equate Suphedrine, Genaphed, Good Sense Nasal, Leader Pseuphedrine, Silfedrine, Sudafed, Sudafed 24 Hour, Sudogest, Top Care Nasal, Walphed

Func. class.: Adrenergic
Chem. class.: Substituted phenylethylamine

ACTION: Primary activity through α-effects on respiratory mucosal membranes reducing congestion hyperemia, edema; minimal bronchodilation secondary to β-effects

USES: Nasal decongestant, adjunct for otitis media; with antihistamines

CONTRAINDICATIONS: Hypersensitivity to sympathomimetics, closed-angle glaucoma

Precautions: Pregnancy (C), breastfeeding, cardiac disorders, hyperthyroidism, diabetes mellitus, prostatic hypertrophy, hypertension

DOSAGE AND ROUTES

- **Adult and child >12 yr: PO** 60 mg q6hr; **EXT REL** 120 mg q12hr or 240 mg q24hr
- **Geriatric: PO** 30-60 mg q6hr prn
- **Child 6-12 yr: PO** 30 mg q6hr, max 120 mg/day
- **Child 2-6 yr: PO** 15 mg q6hr, max 60 mg/day

Available forms: Ext rel caps 120, 240 mg; oral sol 15 mg, 30 mg/5 ml; drops

P

7.5 mg/0.8 ml; tabs 30, 60 mg; caps 60 mg; ext rel tabs 120, 240 mg

Administer:

- Near bedtime; stimulation can occur

SIDE EFFECTS

CNS: *Tremors, anxiety,* stimulation, insomnia, headache, dizziness, hallucinations, **seizures** (geriatric patients)

CV: Palpitations, tachycardia, hypertension, chest pain, **dysrhythmias, CV collapse**

EENT: Dry nose; irritation of nose and throat

GI: *Anorexia, nausea, vomiting,* dry mouth

GU: Dysuria

PHARMACOKINETICS

PO: Onset 15-30 min; duration 4-6 hr, 8-12 hr (ext rel); metabolized in liver; excreted in feces and breast milk; terminal half-life 9-16 hr

INTERACTIONS

⚠ **Do not use with MAOIs or tricyclics; hypertensive crisis may occur**

Increase: effect of this product—urinary alkalizers, adrenergics, β-blockers, phenothiazines, tricyclics

Decrease: effect of this product—urinary acidifiers

NURSING CONSIDERATIONS

Assess:

- Nasal congestion; auscultate lung sounds; check for tenacious bronchial secretions
- B/P, pulse throughout treatment
- CNS side effects in geriatric patients: excitation, seizures, hallucinations

Perform/provide:

- Storage at room temperature

Evaluate:

- Therapeutic response: decreased nasal congestion

Teach patient/family:

- About the reason for product administration
- Not to use continuously or to take more than recommended dose because rebound congestion may occur

⚠ **To notify prescriber immediately of anxiety; slow or fast heart rate; dyspnea; seizures**

- To check with prescriber before using other products because product interactions may occur
- To avoid taking near bedtime because stimulation can occur
- Not to use if stimulation, restlessness, tremors occur
- That use in children may cause excessive agitation

pseudoephedrine nasal agent

See Appendix B

psyllium (OTC, Rx)

(sill′ee-um)

Hydrocil, Leader Fiber Laxative, Metamucil, Natural Fiber, Natural Vegetable Fiber, Reguloid, Wal-Mucil

Func. class.: Bulk laxative

Chem. class.: Psyllium colloid

ACTION: Bulk-forming laxative

USES: Chronic constipation, ulcerative colitis

Unlabeled uses: Diarrhea, diverticulosis, irritable bowel syndrome, hypercholesterolemia

CONTRAINDICATIONS: Hypersensitivity, intestinal obstruction, abdominal pain, nausea, vomiting, fecal impaction

Precautions: Pregnancy (C)

DOSAGE AND ROUTES

• **Adult: PO** 1-2 tsp in 8 oz water bid or tid then 8 oz water or 1 premeasured packet in 8 oz water bid or tid, then 8 oz water
• **Child >6 yr: PO** 1 tsp in 4 oz water at bedtime
Available forms: Chew pieces 1.7, 3.4 g/piece; effervescent powder 3.4, 3.7 g/packet; powder 3.3, 3.4, 3.5, 4.94 g/tsp; wafers 3.4 g/wafer
Administer:
PO route
• Alone for better absorption, separate from other products by 1-2 hr
• In morning or evening (oral dose)
• Immediately after mixing with water or will congeal
• With 8 oz water or juice followed by another 8 oz of fluid

SIDE EFFECTS

GI: *Nausea, vomiting, anorexia, diarrhea,* cramps, intestinal esophageal blockage

PHARMACOKINETICS

Onset 12-72 hr, excreted in feces, not absorbed in GI tract

INTERACTIONS

Decrease: absorption of cardiac glycosides, oral anticoagulants, salicylates
Drug/Herb
Increase: laxative effect—flax, senna

NURSING CONSIDERATIONS

Assess:
• Blood, urine electrolytes if used often
• I&O ratio to identify fluid loss
• **Constipation:** cause of constipation; fluids, bulk, exercise missing; bowel sounds, distention, usual bowel function; color, consistency, amount
• Cramping, rectal bleeding, nausea, vomiting; product should be discontinued

Evaluate:
• Therapeutic response: decrease in constipation, decreased diarrhea with colitis
Teach patient/family:
• To maintain adequate fluid consumption
• That normal bowel movements do not always occur daily
• Not to use in presence of abdominal pain, nausea, vomiting
• To notify prescriber if constipation unrelieved or if symptoms of electrolyte imbalance occur: muscle cramps, pain, weakness, dizziness, excessive thirst

pyrazinamide (Rx)

(peer-a-zin′a-mide)
Tebrazid ♣
Func. class.: Antitubercular agent
Chem. class.: Pyrazinoic acid amine, nicoturimide analog

ACTION:
Bactericidal interference with lipid, nucleic acid biosynthesis

USES:
Tuberculosis; as an adjunct when other products are not feasible

CONTRAINDICATIONS:
Hypersensitivity, severe hepatic damage, acute gout
Precautions: Pregnancy (C), children <13 yr, renal failure, diabetes, porphyria, chronic gout

DOSAGE AND ROUTES

HIV negative
• **Adult and adolescent: PO** 15-30 mg/kg/day max 30 mg/kg/day or 3 g/day; CDC max 50 mg/kg/dose or 4 g max
Renal dose
• **Adult: PO** CCr 10-50 ml/min, give dose q48-72hr; CCr <10 ml/min, give dose q72hr
Available forms: Tabs 500 mg

P

Administer:

- With meals for GI symptoms
- After C&S is completed; monthly to detect resistance

SIDE EFFECTS

CNS: Headache
GI: Hepatotoxicity, abnormal hepatic studies, peptic ulcer, nausea, vomiting, anorexia, cramps, diarrhea
GU: Urinary difficulty, increased uric acid
HEMA: Hemolytic anemia
INTEG: Photosensitivity, urticaria

PHARMACOKINETICS

Peak 2 hr, half-life 9-10 hr; metabolized in liver, excreted in urine (metabolites, unchanged product)

INTERACTIONS

Drug/Lab Test
Interfere: urine ketone tests
Decrease: 17-KS

NURSING CONSIDERATIONS

Assess:

- **TB:** susceptibility tests before and during treatment; sputum cultures
- Signs of anemia: Hct, Hgb, fatigue
- Temp; if >101° F (38° C), product should be reduced
- Renal status before treatment, monthly: BUN, creatinine, output, specific gravity, urinalysis, uric acid
- **Hepatotoxicity:** decreased appetite, jaundice, dark urine, fatigue; hepatic studies weekly: ALT, AST, bilirubin

Evaluate:

- Therapeutic response: decreased symptoms of TB, culture negative

Teach patient/family:

- That compliance with dosage schedule, length is necessary
- To avoid alcohol
- To report fever, loss of appetite, malaise, nausea, vomiting, darkened urine, pale stools

pyridostigmine (Rx)

(peer-id-oh-stig′meen)

Mestinon, Mestinon Timespan, Regonol

Func. class.: Cholinergic; anticholinesterase

Chem. class.: Tertiary amine carbamate

ACTION:

Inhibits destruction of acetylcholine, which increases concentration at sites where acetylcholine is released; this facilitates the transmission of impulses across the myoneural junction

USES:

Nondepolarizing muscle relaxant antagonist, myasthenia gravis, pretreatment for nerve gas exposure (military only)

CONTRAINDICATIONS:

Bradycardia; hypotension; obstruction of intestine, renal system; bromide, benzyl alcohol sensitivity; adrenal insufficiency; cholinesterase inhibitor toxicity

Precautions: Pregnancy (C), seizure disorders, bronchial asthma, coronary occlusion, hyperthyroidism, dysrhythmias, peptic ulcer, megacolon, poor GI motility

DOSAGE AND ROUTES

Myasthenia gravis

- **Adult: PO** 600 mg/day in 5-6 divided doses, max 1.5 g/day; **IM/IV** 2 mg or 1/30 of **PO** dose; **SUS REL** 180-540 mg/day or bid at intervals of ≥6 hr
- **Child: PO** 7 mg/kg/day in 5-6 divided doses; **IM/IV** 0.05-0.15 mg/kg/dose

Nondepolarizing neuromuscular blocker antagonist

- **Adult:** 0.6-1.2 mg **IV** atropine then 0.1-0.25 mg/kg/dose
- **Child: IV** 0.1-0.25 mg/kg/dose

Nerve gas exposure prophylaxis (military)

- **Adult: PO** 30 mg q8hr if threat of exposure to Soman gas is anticipated; start several hours prior to exposure and discontinue upon exposure; after product is discontinued, give antidotes (atropine, pralidoxime)

Available forms: Tabs 60 mg; ext rel tabs 180 mg; syr 60 mg/5 ml; inj 5 mg/ml

Administer:

- Only with atropine sulfate available for cholinergic crisis
- Only after all other cholinergics have been discontinued
- Increased doses for tolerance as ordered
- Larger doses after exercise or fatigue as ordered
- Do not break, crush, or chew sus rel tabs

PO route

- On empty stomach for better absorption

Direct IV route

- Undiluted (5 mg/ml), give through Y-tube or 3-way stopcock, give ≤0.5 mg/min (myasthenia gravis); 5 mg/min (reversal of nondepolarizing neuromuscular blockers)

Syringe compatibilities: Glycopyrrolate

Y-site compatibilities: Heparin, hydrocortisone, potassium chloride, vit B/C

SIDE EFFECTS

CNS: Dizziness, headache, sweating, weakness, **seizures**, incoordination, paralysis, drowsiness, LOC

CV: Tachycardia, dysrhythmias, bradycardia, AV block, hypotension, ECG changes, **cardiac arrest**, syncope

EENT: Miosis, blurred vision, lacrimation, visual changes

GI: *Nausea, diarrhea, vomiting, cramps, increased salivary and gastric secretions, peristalsis*

GU: Urinary frequency, incontinence, urgency

INTEG: Rash, urticaria, flushing

RESP: **Respiratory depression, bronchospasm, constriction, laryngospasm, respiratory arrest**

SYST: **Cholinergic crisis**

PHARMACOKINETICS

Metabolized in liver, excreted in urine (unchanged)

PO: Onset 20-30 min, duration 3-6 hr

PO-EXT REL: Onset 30-60 min, duration 6-12 hr

IM/IV/SUBCUT: Onset 2-15 min, duration $2^1/_2$-4 hr

INTERACTIONS

Increase: action—succinylcholine

Decrease: action—gallamine, metocurine, pancuronium, tubocurarine, atropine

Decrease: pyridostigmine action—aminoglycosides, anesthetics, procainamide, quiNIDine, mecamylamine, polymyxin, magnesium, corticosteroids, antidysrhythmics, quinolones

NURSING CONSIDERATIONS

Assess:

- **Myasthenia gravis:** fatigue, ptosis, diplopia, difficulty swallowing, SOB, hand/gait before, after product; improvement should be seen after 1 hr
- VS, respiration q8hr
- I&O ratio; check for urinary retention or incontinence
- **Toxicity:** bradycardia, hypotension, bronchospasm, headache, dizziness, seizures, respiratory depression; product should be discontinued if toxicity occurs

Perform/provide:

- Storage at room temperature

Evaluate:

- Therapeutic response: increased muscle strength, hand grasp, improved gait, absence of labored breathing (if severe); reversal of nondepolarizing neuromuscular blockers; prevention of nerve gas toxicity

Teach patient/family:

- **Myasthenia gravis:** that product is not a cure, only relieves symptoms
- To wear emergency ID specifying myasthenia gravis, products taken
- To avoid driving, other hazardous activities until effect is known

P

- To report muscle weakness (cholinergic crisis or underdosage), bradycardia
- Not to drink alcohol
- To take with food to decrease gastric side effects

TREATMENT OF OVERDOSE:
Discontinue product, atropine 1-4 mg IV

pyridoxine (vit B_6) (Rx, OTC)
(peer-i-dox'een)

Equaline Vitamin B6, Neuro-K, Walgreens Finest B-6, Walgreens Gold Seal Vitamin B6

Func. class.: Vit B_6, water soluble

ACTION: Needed for fat, protein, carbohydrate metabolism; enhances glycogen release from liver and muscle tissue; needed as coenzyme for metabolic transformations of a variety of amino acids

USES: Vit B_6 deficiency of inborn errors of metabolism, seizures, isoniazid therapy, oral contraceptives, alcoholic polyneuritis

Unlabeled uses: Palmar-plantar erythrodysesthesia syndrome

CONTRAINDICATIONS: Hypersensitivity

Precautions: Pregnancy (A), breastfeeding, children, Parkinson's disease; patients taking levodopa should avoid supplemental vitamins with >5 mg pyridoxine

DOSAGE AND ROUTES

RDA

- **Adult: PO** (male) 1.7-2 mg; (female) 1.4-1.6 mg
- **Child 9-13 yr: PO** 1 mg/day
- **Child 4-8 yr: PO** 0.6 mg/day
- **Child 1-3 yr: PO** 0.5 mg/day
- **Infant 7-12 mo: PO** 0.3 mg/day

Vit B_6 deficiency

- **Adult: PO** 5-25 mg/day × 3 wk
- **Child: PO** 10 mg until desired response

Pyridoxine deficiency neuritis/seizure (not drug induced)

- **Adult: PO** *without neuritis* 2.5-10 mg/day after corrected 2-5 mg/day; *with neuritis* 100-200 mg/day × 3wk then 2-5 mg/day
- **Child: PO** *without neuritis* 5-25 mg/day × 3wk then 1.5-2.5 mg/day in a multivitamin; *with neuritis:* 10-50 mg/day × 3wk then 1-2 mg/day
- **Neonate with seizures: IM/IV** 50-100 mg as single dose

Deficiency caused by isoniazid, cycloSERINE, hydrALAZINE, penicillamine

- **Adult: PO** 100-300 mg/day
- **Child: PO** 10-50 mg/day

Prevention of deficiency caused by isoniazid, cycloSERINE, hydrALAZINE, penicillamine

- **Adult: PO** 25-100 mg/day
- **Child: PO** 1-2 mg/kg/day

Palmar-plantar erythrodysesthesia syndrome (unlabeled)

- **Adult: PO** 50-150 mg/day

Available forms: Tabs 10, 25, 50, 100 mg; ext rel tabs 100 mg; inj 100 mg/ml; ext rel caps 150 mg

Administer:

PO route

- Do not break, crush, or chew ext rel tabs/caps

IM route

- Rotate sites; burning or stinging at site may occur
- Z-track to minimize pain

IV route

- Undiluted or added to most IV sol; give ≤50 mg/1 min if undiluted

Syringe compatibilities: Doxapram

SIDE EFFECTS

CNS: Paresthesia, flushing, warmth, lethargy (rare with normal renal function)
INTEG: Pain at inj site

PHARMACOKINETICS

PO/INJ: Half-life 2-3 wk, metabolized in liver, excreted in urine

INTERACTIONS

Decrease: effects of levodopa
Decrease: effects of pyridoxine—oral contraceptives, isoniazid, cycloSERINE, hydrALAZINE, penicillamine, chloramphenicol, immunosuppressants

NURSING CONSIDERATIONS

Assess:
- **Pyridoxine deficiency:** seizures, irritability, cheilitis, conjunctivitis, anemia, confusion, red tongue, weakness, fatigue prior to and during treatment; monitor pyridoxine levels
- Nutritional status: yeast, liver, legumes, bananas, green vegetables, whole grains
- Blood studies: Hct, Hgb

Perform/provide:
- Storage in tight, light-resistant container

Evaluate:
- Therapeutic response: absence of nausea, vomiting, anorexia, skin lesions, glossitis, stomatitis, edema, seizures, restlessness, paresthesia

Teach patient/family:
- To avoid vitamin supplements unless directed by prescriber
- To increase meat, bananas, potatoes, lima beans, whole grain cereals in diet
- To take as directed; to continue with follow-up exams, blood work

pyrimethamine (Rx)

(peer-i-meth′a-meen)

Daraprim

Func. class.: Antimalarial, antiprotozoal

Chem. class.: Folic acid antagonist

ACTION: Inhibits folic acid metabolism in parasite, prevents transmission by stopping growth of fertilized gametes

USES: Malaria prophylaxis, *Plasmodium vivax, Pneumocystis jiroveci*
Unlabeled uses: Isosporiasis, pneumocystis pneumonia prophylaxis, toxoplasmic encephalitis prophylaxis

CONTRAINDICATIONS: Hypersensitivity, chloroquine-resistant malaria, megaloblastic anemia caused by folate deficiency
Precautions: Pregnancy (C), breastfeeding, geriatric patients, blood dyscrasias, seizure disorder, G6PD disease, renal/hepatic disease

DOSAGE AND ROUTES

Prophylaxis of malaria

Begin 2 wk before entering endemic area, continue for 6-10 wk after return
- **Adult/child >10 yr: PO** 25 mg/wk
- **Child 4-10 yr: PO** 12.5 mg/wk
- **Child <4 yr: PO** 6.25 mg/wk

Malaria treatment
- **Adult/adolescent/child >10 yr: PO** 25 mg q day × 2 days with a sulfonamide
- **Child 4-10 yr: PO** 25 mg/day × 2 days

Toxoplasmosis
- **Adult: PO** 50-75 mg, then reduce by about 50% for 4-5 wk with 1-4 g sulfadoxine × 1-3 wk, then reduce by 50% for 4-5 wk
- **Child: PO** 1 mg/kg/day in 2 divided doses or 2 mg/kg/day × 3 days then 1 mg/kg/day or divided twice daily × 4 wk, max 25 mg/day

Toxoplasmosis in AIDS patients
- **Adult: PO** 100-200 mg/day × 1-2 days, then 50-100 mg/day × 3-6 wk, then 25-50 mg/day for life (given with clindamycin or sulfADIAZINE)

Isosporiasis (unlabeled)
- **Adult: PO** 75 mg/day with leucovorin 10 mg/day × 14 days

Available forms: Tabs 25 mg; combo tabs 500 mg sulfadoxine/25 mg pyrimethamine

P

Administer:

PO route

- Leucovorin IM 3-9 mg/day × 3 days if folic acid deficiency occurs
- Before or after meals at same time each day to maintain product level, decrease GI symptoms
- **Extemporaneous susp:** tabs may be crushed and mixed with 25 ml distilled water, sucrose-containing solution (1 mg/ml); shake well, stable for 5-7 days at room temperature if mixed with sucrose-containing solutions

SIDE EFFECTS

CNS: Stimulation, irritability, seizures, tremors, ataxia, fatigue, fever

CV: Dysrhythmias

GI: *Nausea, vomiting, cramps, anorexia,* diarrhea, atrophic glossitis, gastritis

HEMA: Thrombocytopenia, leukopenia, pancytopenia, megaloblastic anemia, decreased folic acid, agranulocytosis

INTEG: Skin eruptions, photosensitivity, Stevens-Johnson syndrome

RESP: Respiratory failure

PHARMACOKINETICS

PO: Peak 2 hr, half-life 96 hr, half-life accelerated to 23 hr in AIDS patients, metabolized in liver, highly protein bound, excreted in urine (metabolites)

INTERACTIONS

- Synergistic action: folic acid

Increase: Megaloblastic anemia risk, agranulocytosis, thrombocytopenia—zidovudine

Increase: bone marrow suppression—bone marrow depressants, folate antagonists, radiation therapy

NURSING CONSIDERATIONS

Assess:

- Folic acid level; megaloblastic anemia occurs

⚠ **Blood dyscrasias:** blood studies, CBC, platelets; 2×/wk if dosage is increased

⚠ **Toxicity:** vomiting, anorexia, seizure, blood dyscrasia, glossitis; product should be discontinued immediately

- **Serious skin disorders:** Stevens-Johnson syndrome (swelling of face, lips, throat, fever)

Perform/provide:

- Storage in tight, light-resistant container

Evaluate:

- Therapeutic response: decreased symptoms of malaria, toxoplasmosis

Teach patient/family:

- To report visual problems, fever, fatigue, bruising, bleeding, sore throat; may indicate **blood dyscrasias**
- To immediately report skin rash; to discontinue product

TREATMENT OF OVERDOSE:

Gastric lavage, short-acting barbiturate, leucovorin, respiratory support if needed

QUEtiapine (Rx)

(kwe-tie′a-peen)

Seroquel, Seroquel XR

Func. class.: Antipsychotic

Chem. class.: Dibenzodiazepine

ACTION: Functions as an antagonist at multiple neurotransmitter receptors in the brain, including $5HT_{1A}$, $5HT_2$, dopamine D_1, D_2, H_1, and adrenergic α_1, α_2 receptors

USES: Bipolar disorder, bipolar I disorder, depression, mania, schizophrenia

Unlabeled uses: Agitation, dementia, OCD, acute psychosis

CONTRAINDICATIONS: Hypersensitivity, breastfeeding

Precautions: Pregnancy (C), geriatric patients, hepatic/cardiac disease, breast cancer, long-term use, seizures, QT prolongation, brain tumor, hematologic disease, torsades de pointes, cataracts, dehydration

Black Box Warning: Children, suicide, dementia

DOSAGE AND ROUTES

Bipolar I disorder

• **Adult: PO** (monotherapy or adjunct to lithium, divalproex) 50 mg bid on day 1, 100 mg on day 2 in 2 divided doses as tolerated to 400 mg/day on day 4, range 400-800 mg/day

Psychotic disorders

• **Adult: PO** 25 mg bid, titrate upward; (XR) 300 mg/day in PM, range 400-800 mg/day

Depressive disorder (inadequate response to antidepressants alone)

• **Adult: PO EXT REL** 50 mg/day in PM on days 1, 2; on day 3, give 150 mg in PM

• **Geriatric: PO EXT REL** 50 mg, may increase by 50 mg/day based on response

Available forms: Tabs 25, 50, 100, 200, 300, 400 mg; ext rel tab 50, 150, 200, 300, 400 mg

Administer:

• Reduced dose to geriatric patients

• Anticholinergic agent on order from prescriber for EPS

• Avoid use of CNS depressants

• **Immediate release:** without regard to meals

• **Ext rel:** without food or with light meal; swallow whole; do not split, crush, chew, can switch from immediate release to extended release by giving total daily dose q day

SIDE EFFECTS

CNS: EPS, pseudoparkinsonism, akathisia, dystonia, tardive dyskinesia; *drowsiness,* insomnia, agitation, anxiety, *headache,* seizures, neuroleptic malignant syndrome, *dizziness,* dystonia, restless legs

CV: Orthostatic hypotension, tachycardia, QT prolongation, CV disease, Parkinson's disease, cardiomyopathy, myocarditis

ENDO: SIADH, hyperglycemia

GI: *Nausea, anorexia, constipation,* abdominal pain, dry mouth

HEMA: Leukopenia, agranulocytosis

INTEG: Rash

META: Hyponatremia

MISC: Asthenia, back pain, fever, ear pain

MS: Rhabdomyolysis

RESP: Rhinitis

SYST: Stevens-Johnson syndrome, anaphylaxis

PHARMACOKINETICS

Extensively metabolized by liver, half-life ≥6 hr, peak 1½ hr, inhibits P450 CYP3A4 enzyme system, 83% protein binding

INTERACTIONS

⚠ **Increase:** QT prolongation—class IA/III antidysrhythmics, some phenothiazines, β-agonists, local anesthetics, tricyclics, haloperidol, methadone, chloroquine, clarithromycin, droperidol, erythromycin, pentamidine

Increase: CNS depression—alcohol, opioid analgesics, sedative/hypnotics, antihistamines

Increase: hypotension—alcohol, antihypertensives

Increase: QUEtiapine clearance, decrease QUEtiapine effect—phenytoin, thioridazine, barbiturates, glucocorticoids, carBAMazepine, rifampin

Increase: QUEtiapine action—fluconazole, itraconazole, ketoconazole (CYP3A4 inhibitors)

Increase: effects of erythromycin

Decrease: QUEtiapine clearance—cimetidine

Decrease: effects of DOPamine agonists, levodopa, LORazepam

NURSING CONSIDERATIONS

Assess:

⚠ CV status: QT prolongation, tachycardia, orthostatic B/P

Q

Black Box Warning: Mental status before initial administration, AIMS assessment; affect, orientation, LOC, reflexes, gait, coordination, sleep pattern disturbances; suicidal thoughts/behaviors (child/young adult); dementia (geriatric patients)

Suicide: restrict amount of product given; usually suicidal thoughts/behaviors occur early during treatment and among children/adolescents/young adults

- Baseline blood glucose, LFTs, neurologic function, ophthalmologic exam, cholesterol profile, weight
- B/P standing, lying; pulse, respirations; determine q4hr during initial treatment; establish baseline before starting treatment; report drops of 30 mm Hg; watch for ECG changes
- Dizziness, faintness, palpitations, tachycardia on rising
- **EPS:** including akathisia (inability to sit still, no pattern to movements), tardive dyskinesia (bizarre movements of jaw, mouth, tongue, extremities), pseudoparkinsonism (rigidity, tremors, pill rolling, shuffling gait)

Neuroleptic malignant syndrome: hyperthermia, increased CPK, altered mental status, muscle rigidity, seizures, tachycardia, diaphoresis, hypo/hypertension, fatigue; notify prescriber immediately if symptoms occur

- Constipation, urinary retention daily; if these occur, increase bulk, water in diet

Perform/provide:

- Supervised ambulation until patient stabilized on medication; do not involve patient in strenuous exercise program because fainting possible; patient should not stand still for long period of time
- Sips of water, sugarless candy, gum for dry mouth
- Storage in tight, light-resistant container

Evaluate:

- Therapeutic response: decrease in emotional excitement, hallucinations, delusions, paranoia; reorganization of patterns of thought, speech

Teach patient/family:

- Not to become overheated
- Not to use if pregnancy is planned or suspected, not to breastfeed
- To rise slowly to prevent orthostatic hypotension
- To take medication only as prescribed
- That follow up necessary, including LFTs, blood glucose, neurologic/ophthalmic function, cholesterol profile, weight
- If drowsiness occurs, to avoid hazardous activities such as driving
- To avoid use of OTC meds unless directed by prescriber
- To notify prescriber if pregnancy planned, suspected; not to breastfeed
- To notify prescriber immediately of fever, difficulty breathing, fatigue, sore throat, rash, bleeding
- **Suicide:** thoughts/behaviors, primarily among children/adolescents/young adults

quinapril (Rx)

(kwin′a-pril)

Accupril

Func. class.: Antihypertensive

Chem. class.: Angiotensin-converting enzyme (ACE) inhibitor

ACTION: Selectively suppresses renin-angiotensin-aldosterone system; inhibits ACE, prevents conversion of angiotensin I to angiotensin II; results in dilation of arterial, venous vessels

USES: Hypertension, alone or in combination with thiazide diuretics; systolic CHF

CONTRAINDICATIONS: Children, hypersensitivity to ACE inhibitors, angioedema

Black Box Warning: Pregnancy (D) 2nd/3rd trimester

Precautions: Breastfeeding, geriatric patients, impaired renal/hepatic function, dialysis patients, hypovolemia, blood dyscrasias, COPD, bilateral renal stenosis, asthma, cough, pregnancy (C) 1st trimester, hyperkalemia

DOSAGE AND ROUTES

Hypertension

- **Adult: PO** 10-20 mg/day initially then 20-80 mg/day divided bid or daily (monotherapy); start at 5 mg/day (with diuretics)
- **Geriatric: PO** 10 mg/day, titrate to desired response (monotherapy); start at 2.5 mg/day (with diuretics)

Congestive heart failure

- **Adult: PO** 5 mg bid, may increase weekly until 20-40 mg/day in 2 divided doses

Renal dose

- **Adult: PO** CCr 30-60 ml/min, 5 mg/day initially; CCr <30 ml/min, 2.5 mg/day initially

Available forms: Tabs 5, 10, 20, 40 mg

Administer:

- Tabs may be crushed if necessary
- Take 1-2 hr before food or antacids; avoid high-fat foods
- Store in airtight container at room temp

SIDE EFFECTS

CNS: *Headache, dizziness, fatigue,* somnolence, depression, malaise, nervousness, vertigo

CV: *Hypotension,* postural hypotension, syncope, palpitations, angina pectoris, **MI, tachycardia,** vasodilation, chest pain

GI: *Nausea,* diarrhea, constipation, *vomiting,* gastritis, **GI hemorrhage,** dry mouth

GU: Increased BUN, creatinine; decreased libido, impotence

INTEG: **Angioedema,** rash, sweating, photosensitivity, pruritus

META: Hyperkalemia

MISC: Back pain, amblyopia

MS: Myalgia

RESP: *Cough,* pharyngitis, dyspnea

PHARMACOKINETICS

Bioavailability ≥60%, onset <1 hr, peak 1-2 hr, duration 24 hr, protein binding 97%, half-life 2 hr, metabolized by liver (active metabolites quinaprilat), metabolites excreted in urine (60%)/feces (37%)

INTERACTIONS

- Use caution with vasodilators, hydrALAZINE, prazosin, potassium-sparing diuretics, sympathomimetics, potassium supplements, ACE/angiotensin II receptor antagonists

Increase: hypotension—diuretics, other antihypertensives, ganglionic blockers, adrenergic blockers, phenothiazines, nitrates, acute alcohol ingestion

Increase: toxicity of lithium

Decrease: absorption of tetracycline

Decrease: hypotensive effect of quinapril—NSAIDs

Drug/Lab Test

Increase: potassium, creatinine, BUN, LFTs

NURSING CONSIDERATIONS

Assess:

⚠ **Collagen-vascular disease:** **blood studies: neutrophils, decreased platelets; WBC with differential at baseline, periodically, q3mo; if neutrophils <1000/mm³, discontinue treatment**

- **Hypertension:** B/P, orthostatic hypotension, syncope
- Renal studies: protein, BUN, creatinine; watch for increased levels; may indicate nephrotic syndrome
- Baselines of hepatic studies before therapy, periodically; increased LFTs; uric acid, glucose may be increased
- Potassium levels; hyperkalemia rare
- **CHF:** edema in feet, legs daily; weight daily

⚠ **Allergic reactions: rash, fever, pruritus, urticaria, swelling of eyes/face/throat/neck, SOB, difficulty breathing; product should be discontinued**

Black Box Warning: For pregnancy (D), 2nd/3rd trimester, if pregnancy is suspected, discontinue use

Evaluate:
• Therapeutic response: decrease in B/P
Teach patient/family:
• Not to discontinue product abruptly
• Not to use OTC products (cough, cold, allergy); not to use salt substitutes containing potassium unless directed by prescriber, avoid high-fat meal at same time as product
• To comply with dosage schedule, even if feeling better
• To rise slowly to sitting or standing position to minimize orthostatic hypotension
• To notify prescriber of mouth sores, sore throat, fever, swelling of hands/feet, irregular heartbeat, chest pain, persistent dry cough
• To report excessive perspiration, dehydration, vomiting, diarrhea; may lead to fall in B/P
• That product may cause dizziness, fainting, lightheadedness; may occur during first few days of therapy
• That product may cause skin rash, impaired taste perception
• How to take B/P, normal readings for age group

Black Box Warning: Pregnancy: to report if pregnancy planned, suspected; pregnancy category (D) 2nd/3rd trimester, do not breastfeed

TREATMENT OF OVERDOSE:
0.9% NaCl IV inf

quiNIDine gluconate (Rx)
(kwin′i-deen)
quiNIDine sulfate (Rx)
Func. class.: Antidysrhythmic (Class IA)
Chem. class.: Quinine dextroisomer

Do not confuse:
quiNIDine/quiNINE

ACTION: Prolongs duration of action potential and effective refractory period, thus decreasing myocardial excitability; anticholinergic properties

USES: PVCs, atrial fibrillation, PAT, ventricular tachycardia, atrial flutter, malaria/IV quiNIDine gluconate

CONTRAINDICATIONS: Hypersensitivity, idiosyncratic response, digoxin toxicity, blood dyscrasias, myasthenia gravis

Black Box Warning: History of long QT syndrome, product-induced torsades de pointes, severe heart block

Precautions: Pregnancy (C), breastfeeding, children, geriatric patients, potassium imbalance, renal/hepatic disease, CHF, respiratory depression, bradycardia, hypotension, syncope

Black Box Warning: Cardiac arrhythmias, MI

DOSAGE AND ROUTES
QuiNIDine gluconate
• **Adult: PO** (ext rel) 324-648 mg q8-12hr; **IM** 600 mg then 400 mg q2hr; **IV** give 16 mg/min

QuiNIDine sulfate
Atrial fibrillation/flutter
• **Adult: PO** 200 mg q2-3hr × 5-8 doses; may increase daily until sinus rhythm restored; max 4 g/day given only after digitalization; maintenance 200-300 mg tid-qid or **EXT REL** 300-600 mg q8-12hr

Paroxysmal supraventricular tachycardia
• **Adult: PO** 400-600 mg q2-3hr then 200-300 mg q6-8hr or **EXT REL** 300-600 mg q8-12hr

Premature atrial/ventricular contraction
• **Adult: PO** 200-300 mg q6-8hr or **EXT REL** 300-600 mg q8-12hr; max 4 g/day
• **Child: PO** 30 mg/kg/day or 900 mg/m^2/day in 5 divided doses

Available forms: *Gluconate:* ext rel tabs 324, 330 mg; inj gluconate 80 mg/ml; *sulfate:* tabs 200, 300 mg; sus rel tabs 300 mg

Administer:
- AV node blocker (digoxin) before starting quinidine to avoid increased ventricular rate

PO route
- Do not break, crush, chew ext rel products
- With full glass of water on empty stomach; if GI upset occurs, may take with food
- Sus rel forms not interchangeable

IM route
- IM inj in deltoid; aspirate to avoid intravascular administration

Intermittent IV INF route
- After diluting ≥800 mg/50 ml D_5W (16 mg/ml); give max 0.25 mg/kg/min; quiNIDine absorbed by PVC tubing, minimize length; use inf pump

Y-site compatibilities: Alfentanil, amikacin, anidulafungin, ascorbic acid, atenolol, atracurium, atropine, benztropine, bleomycin, bumetanide, buprenorphine, butorphanol, calcium gluconate, caspofungin, chlorproMAZINE, cimetidine, CISplatin, cyanocobalamin, cycloSPORINE, DACTINomycin, digoxin, diltiazem, diphenhydrAMINE, DOBUTamine, docetaxel, DOPamine, doxycycline, enalaprilat, ePHEDrine, EPINEPHrine, epoetin alfa, erythromycin, esmolol, etoposide, famotidine, fenoldopam, fentaNYL, fluconazole, fludarabine, gatifloxacin, gemcitabine, gentamicin, glycopyrrolate, granisetron, HYDROmorphone, IDArubicin, imipenem-cilastatin, irinotecan, isoproterenol, labetalol, lidocaine, linezolid, LORazepam, magnesium sulfate, mannitol, mechlorethamine, meperidine, metaraminol, methoxamine, methyldopate, metoclopramide, metoprolol, metroNIDAZOLE, miconazole, milrinone, mitoxantrone, morphine, multiple vitamins, mycophenolate, nalbuphine, naloxone, nesiritide, netilmicin, nitroglycerin, norepinephrine, octreotide, ondansetron, oxaliplatin, paclitaxel, palonosetron, pamidronate, pancuronium, papaverine, pentamidine, pentazocine, phenylephrine, phytonadione, polymyxin B, potassium chloride, procainamide, prochlorperazine, promethazine, propranolol, protamine, pyridoxine, ranitidine, ritodrine, succinylcholine, SUFentanil, tacrolimus, teniposide, theophylline, thiamine, thiotepa, tirofiban, tobramycin, tolazoline, trimetaphan, urokinase, vancomycin, vasopressin, verapamil, vinorelbine, voriconazole, zoledronic acid

SIDE EFFECTS

CNS: *Headache, dizziness,* involuntary movement, confusion, psychosis, restlessness, irritability, syncope, excitement, depression, ataxia
CV: **Hypotension,** *bradycardia,* PVCs, **heart block, CV collapse, arrest, torsades** de pointes, widening QRS complex, **ventricular tachycardia**
EENT: Cinchonism: tinnitus, blurred vision, hearing loss, mydriasis, disturbed color vision
GI: Nausea, vomiting, anorexia, abdominal pain, *diarrhea,* **hepatotoxicity**
HEMA: **Thrombocytopenia,** hemolytic anemia, **agranulocytosis,** hypoprothrombinemia
INTEG: Rash, urticaria, **angioedema,** swelling, photosensitivity, flushing with severe pruritus
RESP: Dyspnea, **respiratory depression**

PHARMACOKINETICS

PO: Peak 0.5-6 hr, duration 6-8 hr, half-life 6-7 hr, metabolized in liver, excreted unchanged (10%-50%) by kidneys, protein bound (80%-90%)

INTERACTIONS

- Additive vagolytic effect: anticholinergic blockers
- Additive cardiac depression: other antidysrhythmics, phenothiazines, reserpine

Increase: effects of neuromuscular blockers, digoxin, warfarin, tricyclics, propranolol
Increase: quiNIDine effects—cimetidine, sodium bicarbonate, carbonic anhydrase

inhibitors, antacids, hydroxide suspensions, amiodarone, verapamil, NIFEdipine
Decrease: quiNIDine effects—barbiturates, phenytoin, rifampin, sucralfate, cholinergics
Drug/Herb
Increase: quiNIDine effect—hawthorn
Drug/Food
• Delayed absorption, decreased metabolism: grapefruit juice
Drug/Lab Test
Increase: CPK
Interference: triamterene therapy interferes with quiNIDine test levels

NURSING CONSIDERATIONS

Assess:

⚠ **ECG continuously to determine increased PR or QRS segments, QT interval; discontinue product or reduce dose**
• Blood levels (therapeutic level 2-7 mcg/ml), CBC, LFTs
• B/P continuously for fluctuations
⚠ **For cinchonism: tinnitus, headache, nausea, dizziness, fever, vertigo, tremor; may lead to hearing loss**
• Cardiac status: rate, rhythm, character, continuously
• Respiratory status: rate, rhythm, lung fields for crackles; increased respiration, increased pulse; product should be discontinued
• CNS effects: dizziness, confusion, psychosis, paresthesias, seizures; product should be discontinued

Evaluate:
• Therapeutic response: decreased dysrhythmias

Teach patient/family:
• That if dizziness, drowsiness occurs, to avoid driving or hazardous activities
• To use sunglasses; product may cause sensitivity to light
• To carry emergency ID stating disease, medication use
• How to take pulse, when to notify prescriber
• To avoid all products unless approved by prescriber
• To report signs of cinchonism, diarrhea, anorexia, decreased B/P
• To avoid using with grapefruit

quiNINE (Rx)

(kwye′nine)

Apo-QuiNINE ✦, Qualaquin

Func. class.: Antimalarial
Chem. class.: Cinchona tree alkaloid

ACTION: Inhibits parasite replications, transcription of DNA to RNA by forming complexes with DNA of parasite

USES: *Plasmodium falciparum,* malaria

CONTRAINDICATIONS: Hypersensitivity, G6PD deficiency, retinal field changes, myasthenia gravis
Precautions: Pregnancy (C), breastfeeding, blood dyscrasias, severe GI/hepatic disease, neurologic disease, psoriasis, cardiac dysrhythmias, tinnitus, hypoglycemia

Black Box Warning: Nocturnal leg cramps

DOSAGE AND ROUTES

• **Adult: PO** 648 mg q8hr × 3 days or 7 days in SE Asia; given with tetracycline 250 mg q5hr × 7 days, or clindamycin 900 mg q8hr × 7 days, or doxycycline 100 mg q12hr × 7 days
• **Child: PO** 25 mg/kg/day divided q8hr for 3-7 days in conjunction with another agent

Available forms: Tabs 324 mg

Administer:
• Take with food to decrease GI upset; if dose missed, do not double
• Oral caps not approved for prevention of malaria, treatment of severe malaria, treatment/prevention of leg cramps

SIDE EFFECTS

CNS: Headache, stimulation, fatigue, irritability, **seizures**, bad dreams, dizziness, fever, confusion, anxiety
CV: Angina, dysrhythmias, tachycardia, hypotension, **acute circulatory failure**
EENT: *Blurred vision, corneal changes, retinal changes, difficulty focusing,* tinnitus, vertigo, deafness, photophobia, diplopia, night blindness
ENDO: Hypoglycemia
GI: *Nausea, vomiting, anorexia,* diarrhea, epigastric pain
GU: Renal tubular damage, **anuria**
HEMA: **Thrombocytopenia, purpura, hypothrombinemia, hemolysis**
INTEG: Pruritus, pigmentary changes, skin eruptions, lichen-planus–like eruptions, flushing, facial edema, sweating
MISC: **Hemolytic uremic syndrome**
RESP: Dyspnea

PHARMACOKINETICS

Peak 1-3 hr, metabolized in liver (80%), excreted in urine, half-life 8-12 hr, protein binding 70%-90%

INTERACTIONS

Increase: toxicity—sodium bicarbonate, acetaZOLAMIDE
Increase: QT prolongation—quiNIDine
Increase: levels of digoxin, digitoxin, nondepolarizing neuromuscular blockers, anticoagulants; CYP2D6 substrates (amoxapine, atomoxetine, carvedilol, metoprolol, propranolol, timolol, encainide, flecainide, mexiletine, clozapine, codeine, cyclobenzaprine, fenfluramine, darifenacin, dexfenfluramine, dextromethorphan, donepezil, FLUoxetine, galantamine, haloperidol, HYDROcodone, maprotiline, meperidine, methadonic, methamphetamine, oxyCODONE, paroxetine, risperidone, fluphenazine, perphenazine, thioridazine, tramadol, trazodone, tricyclics, venlafaxine, zolpidem)
Increase: quiNINE levels—CYP3A4 inhibitors (clarithromycin, cycloSPORINE, diltiazem, etravirine, azole antifungals, lapatinib, mifepristone, protease inhibitors, ritonavir)
Increase: treatment failure—rifampin
Decrease: absorption—magnesium or aluminum salts (antacids)
Drug/Herb
Decrease: quiNINE—St. John's wort
Drug/Lab Test
Increase: 17-KS
Interference: 17-OHCS

NURSING CONSIDERATIONS

Assess:
- B/P, pulse; watch for hypotension, tachycardia
- Hepatic studies q wk: ALT, AST, bilirubin
- Blood studies, CBC because blood dyscrasias occur
- **Cinchonism:** nausea, blurred vision, tinnitus, headache, difficulty focusing

Perform/provide:
- Storage in tight, light-resistant container

Evaluate:
- Therapeutic response: decreased symptoms of malaria

Teach patient/family:
- Not to breastfeed while taking medication
- To avoid OTC preparations: cold preparations, tonic water

TREATMENT OF OVERDOSE:

Multiple dosages of activated charcoal

R

rabeprazole (Rx)

(rah-bep′rah-zole)

Aciphex, Pariet ♣

Func. class.: Antiulcer, proton pump inhibitor
Chem. class.: Benzimidazole

ACTION:

Suppresses gastric secretion by inhibiting hydrogen/potassium ATPase enzyme system in the gastric parietal cells; characterized as a gastric acid pump inhibitor because it blocks the final step of acid production

USES:
Gastroesophageal reflux disease (GERD), severe erosive esophagitis, poorly responsive systemic GERD, pathologic hypersecretory conditions (Zollinger-Ellison syndrome, systemic mastocytosis, multiple endocrine adenomas); treatment of active duodenal ulcers with/without antiinfectives for *Helicobacter pylori;* daytime, nighttime heartburn

Unlabeled uses: Gastric ulcer, heartburn, *H. pylori* eradication in children

CONTRAINDICATIONS:
Hypersensitivity

Precautions: Pregnancy (C), breastfeeding, children, Asian patients, diarrhea, geriatric patients, gastric cancer, hepatic/GI disease, IBS, osteoporosis, pseudomembranous colitis, ulcerative colitis, vit B_{12} deficiency

DOSAGE AND ROUTES

Healing of duodenal ulcers

- **Adult: PO** 20 mg/day × ≤4 wk; to be taken after breakfast

Healing of erosive esophagitis or ulcerative GERD

- **Adult: PO** 20 mg/day × 4-8 wk
- **Adolescent and child ≥12 yr: PO** 20 mg/day up to 8 wk

Pathologic hypersecretory conditions

- **Adult: PO** 60 mg/day; may increase to 120 mg in 2 divided doses

Gastric ulcer (unlabeled)

- **Adult: PO** 20 mg/day after AM meal × 3-6 wk

Dyspepsia/heartburn (unlabeled)

- **Adult: PO** 20 mg/day × #14 days

Available forms: Del rel tabs 20 mg

Administer:

- **PO:** Do not break, crush, chew del rel tab; after breakfast daily with full glass of water, without regard to food

SIDE EFFECTS

CNS: *Headache, dizziness, asthenia*

CV: Chest pain, angina, tachycardia, bradycardia, palpitations, peripheral edema

EENT: Tinnitus, taste perversion

GI: *Diarrhea, abdominal pain, vomiting, nausea, constipation, flatulence, acid regurgitation,* abdominal swelling, anorexia, irritable colon, esophageal candidiasis, dry mouth

GU: UTI, urinary frequency, increased creatinine, proteinuria, hematuria, testicular pain, glycosuria

HEMA: Pancytopenia, thrombocytopenia, neutropenia, leukocytosis, anemia

INTEG: *Rash,* dry skin, urticaria, pruritus, alopecia

META: Hypoglycemia, increased hepatic enzymes, weight gain

MISC: *Back pain,* fever, fatigue, malaise, Stevens-Johnson syndrome

RESP: *Upper respiratory tract infections, cough,* epistaxis, pneumonia

PHARMACOKINETICS

Eliminated in urine as metabolites and in feces, terminal half-life 1-2 hr, metabolized by CYP2C19 enzyme system, protein binding 96.3%

INTERACTIONS

Increase: bleeding risk—warfarin, clopidogrel

Increase: serum levels of rabeprazole—benzodiazepines, phenytoin, clarithromycin, antacids, other proton pump inhibitors, H_2 blockers

Increase: levels of—digoxin, nelfinavir/omeprazole

Decrease: levels of rabeprazole—sucralfate, calcium carbonate, vit B_{12}

Decrease: levels of ketoconazole, itraconazole, iron salts, atazanavir/ritonavir, ampicillin

Drug/Herb

Decrease: rabeprazole—St. John's wort

NURSING CONSIDERATIONS

Assess:

- GI system: bowel sounds, abdomen for pain, swelling, anorexia, emesis/stool for occult blood

- Hepatic studies: AST, ALT, alk phos during treatment; CBC with differential periodically

⚠ Serious skin reactions: Stevens-Johnson syndrome

- CBC with differential before, periodically during treatment; blood dyscrasias may occur (rare)

Evaluate:

- Therapeutic response: absence of epigastric pain, swelling, fullness; decreased symptoms of GERD after 4-8 wk

Teach patient/family:

- To report severe diarrhea or black, tarry stools; product may have to be discontinued
- That hypoglycemia may occur if patient is diabetic
- To avoid hazardous activities because dizziness, drowsiness may occur
- To avoid alcohol, salicylates, NSAIDs because they may cause GI irritation; to avoid other OTC, herbal products unless approved by prescriber
- To use as directed for length of time prescribed; to take missed dose when remembered; not to double dose
- To notify prescriber if pregnancy planned, suspected

radioactive iodine (sodium iodide) ^{131}I (Rx)

Func. class.: Antithyroid
Chem. class.: Radiopharmaceutical

ACTION: Converted to protein-bound iodine by thyroid gland for use when needed

USES:

High dose: Thyroid cancer, hyperthyroidism
Low dose: Visualization to determine thyroid cancer, diagnostic aid for thyroid function studies

CONTRAINDICATIONS: Pregnancy (X), breastfeeding, age <30 yr, recent MI, large nodular goiter, vomiting/diarrhea, acute hyperthyroidism, use of thyroid products

DOSAGE AND ROUTES

Thyroid cancer

- **Adult: PO** 50-150 mCi; may repeat, depending on clinical status

Hyperthyroidism

- **Adult: PO** 4-10 mCi, depending on serum thyroxine level

Available forms: Caps 1-50, 0.8-100 mCi; oral sol 7.05 mCi/ml, 3.5-150 mCi/vial; concentrated oral solution 1000 mCi/ml

Administer:

- Only after discontinuing all other antithyroid agents × 5-7 days
- After NPO overnight; food delays action
- During or within 10 days of menstruation
- Do not take antithyroid agents except propranolol, which decreases hyperthyroid symptoms, until total effect of taking ^{131}I has occurred (about 6 wk)

SIDE EFFECTS

EENT: Sore throat, cough
ENDO: Hypothyroidism, **hyperthyroid adenoma**, transient thyroiditis, goiter
GI: *Nausea, diarrhea, vomiting*
HEMA: Eosinophilia, lymphedema, leukemia, bone marrow depression, leukopenia, anemia, lymph node swelling
INTEG: Alopecia

PHARMACOKINETICS

PO: Onset 3-6 days; excreted in urine, sweat, feces, breast milk; crosses placenta; excreted in 56 days

INTERACTIONS

- Hypothyroidism: lithium

Decrease: effect of I^{131}—amiodarone
Decrease: uptake—recent intake of stable iodine, thyroid, antithyroid products

NURSING CONSIDERATIONS

Assess:

- Weight daily with same clothing, scale, time of day
- Blood work, including CBC for blood dyscrasias (leukopenia, thrombocytopenia, agranulocytosis)
- **Overdose:** peripheral edema, heat intolerance, diaphoresis, palpitations, dysrhythmias, severe tachycardia, increased temp, delirium, CNS irritability
- **Hypersensitivity:** rash, enlarged cervical lymph nodes; product may have to be discontinued
- **Hypoprothrombinemia:** bleeding, petechiae, ecchymosis
- Clinical response: after 3 wk should include increased weight, pulse; decreased T_4
- **Bone marrow depression:** sore throat, fever, fatigue

Perform/provide:

- Limited contact with patient: ½ hr/day for each person
- Adequate rest after treatment
- Fluids to 3-4 L/day for 48 hr to remove agent from body

Evaluate:

- Therapeutic response: weight gain, decreased pulse, decreased T_4, B/P

Teach patient/family:

- To fast overnight before treatment, consume increased fluids for 48 hr after therapy
- To empty bladder often during treatment; to avoid irradiation of gonads
- To report redness, swelling, sore throat, mouth lesions; may indicate blood dyscrasias
- To avoid extended contact with children, spouse for 1 wk
- That bathroom may be used by entire family; to flush toilet several times
- To avoid coughing, expectorating for 24 hr (saliva and vomitus highly radioactive for 6-8 hr)

raloxifene (Rx)

(ral-ox'ih-feen)

Evista

Func. class.: Bone resorption inhibitor

Chem. class.: Hormone modifier, selective estrogen receptor modulator (SERM)

ACTION: Tissue-selective estrogen agonist/antagonist; agonist activity in bone and on lipid metabolism; antagonist activity on breast and uterus; reduces resorption of bone and decreases bone turnover

USES: Prevention, treatment of osteoporosis in postmenopausal women; breast cancer prophylaxis in postmenopausal women with osteoporosis or in postmenopausal women at high risk for developing the disease

Unlabeled uses: Uterine leiomyomata in postmenopausal women with osteoporosis or in postmenopausal women who are at high risk for developing the disease

CONTRAINDICATIONS: Pregnancy (X), breastfeeding, hypersensitivity

Black Box Warning: Women with active or history of venous thromboembolic events

Precautions: CV/hepatic disease, cervical/uterine cancer, elevated triglycerides, pulmonary embolism

Black Box Warning: Stroke

DOSAGE AND ROUTES

- **Adult: PO** 60 mg/day, max 60 mg/day

Available forms: Tabs 60 mg

Administer:

- PO: without regard to meals, vit D
- Add calcium supplement if inadequate

SIDE EFFECTS

CNS: Insomnia

CV: Hot flashes, peripheral edema, **thromboembolism, stroke**

EENT: Retinal vein occlusion (rare)
GI: *Nausea,* vomiting, diarrhea, dyspepsia
GU: Vaginitis, leukorrhea, cystitis, *hot flashes,* vaginal bleeding
INTEG: Rash, sweating
META: Weight gain, peripheral edema
MS: Arthralgia, myalgia, *leg cramps,* arthritis
RESP: Sinusitis, pharyngitis, increased cough, pneumonia, laryngitis, bronchitis, **pulmonary embolism,** flulike symptoms

PHARMACOKINETICS

Elimination half-life 28-32 hr; excreted in feces, breast milk; highly bound to plasma proteins

INTERACTIONS

• Administer cautiously with other highly protein-bound products, systemic estrogens

Decrease: action of anticoagulants, dessicated thyroid, levothyroxine, liotrix

Decrease: action of raloxifene—ampicillin, cholestyramine

Drug/Food

Decrease: raloxifene—soy

Drug/Lab Test

Increase: apolipoprotein A-1, hormone-binding globulin

Decrease: total cholesterol, LDL, lipoprotein, apolipoprotein B, serum calcium, albumin, total protein

NURSING CONSIDERATIONS

Assess:

Black Box Warning: History of stroke, TIA, thrombosis, atrial fibrillation, hypertension, smoking; venous thrombosis may occur, avoid prolonged sitting; discontinue 3 days before surgery, other immobilization

• Bone density test at baseline, throughout treatment, bone-specific alk phos, osteocalcin

Evaluate:

• Therapeutic response: prevention, treatment of osteoporosis in postmenopausal women; prevention of breast cancer in postmenopausal women with osteoporosis or in those who are at high risk for developing the disease

Teach patient/family:

Black Box Warning: To discontinue product 72 hr before prolonged bedrest; to avoid staying in one position for long periods

• To take calcium supplements, vit D if intake is inadequate
• To increase exercise using weights
• To stop smoking; to decrease alcohol consumption
• That product does not help to control hot flashes

⚠ To report fever, acute migraine, insomnia, emotional distress; urinary tract infection, vaginal burning/itching; swelling, warmth, pain in calves

⚠ To notify prescriber if pregnancy planned, suspected, pregnancy category (X); to avoid breastfeeding

raltegravir (Rx)

(ral-teg′ra-vir)

Isentress

Func. class.: Antiretroviral
Chem. class.: HIV integrase strand transfer inhibitor (ISTIs)

ACTION: Inhibits catalytic activity of HIV integrase, which is an HIV-encoded enzyme needed for replication

USES: HIV in combination with other antiretrovirals

CONTRAINDICATIONS: Breastfeeding, hypersensitivity

Precautions: Pregnancy (C), children, geriatric patients, hepatic disease, immune reconstitution syndrome, hepatitis, antimicrobial resistance, lactase deficiency

DOSAGE AND ROUTES

• **Adult and adolescent ≥16 yr: PO** 400 mg bid; if using with rifampin, give 800 mg bid; max 800 mg/day with/without food

Available forms: Tabs 400 mg

Administer:

- Do not break, crush, chew tabs
- May give without regard to meals, with 8 oz of water

SIDE EFFECTS

CNS: *Fatigue,* fever, *dizziness, headache,* asthenia, suicidal ideation

CV: MI

GI: *Nausea,* vomiting, diarrhea, abdominal pain, asthenia, gastritis, hepatitis

GU: Oliguria, proteinuria, hematuria, glomerulonephritis, acute renal failure, renal tubular necrosis

HEMA: Anemia, neutropenia

INTEG: Rash, urticaria, pruritus, pain or phlebitis at IV site, unusual sweating, alopecia

META: Hyperamylasia, hyperglycemia

MS: Myopathy, rhabdomyolysis

PHARMACOKINETICS

Max absorption 3 hr if taken on an empty stomach; terminal half-life 9 hr; metabolized in the liver by uridine diphosphate glucuronosyltransferase (UGT A1A enzyme system); excreted in feces 51%, urine 32%

INTERACTIONS

Increase: raltegravir effect—proton pump inhibitors, H_2 blockers; UGT1A1 inhibitors (atazanavir)

⚠ **Increase:** rhabdomyolysis, myopathy, elevated CPK—fibric acid derivatives, HMG-CoA reductase inhibitors

Decrease: raltegravir levels—rifampin, efavirenz, tenofovir, tipranavir/ritonavir

Drug/Lab Test

Increase: AST, ALT, GGT, total bilirubin, alk phos, amylase/lipase, CK, serum glucose

Decrease: Hgb, platelets, ANC

NURSING CONSIDERATIONS

Assess:

- **HIV infection:** CD4, T-cell count, plasma HIV RNA, viral load; resistance testing before therapy, at treatment failure

⚠ **Rhabdomyolysis:** Assess for calf pain, increased CPK, product should be discontinued

- Skin eruptions: rash, urticaria, itching
- **Suicidal thoughts/behaviors:** monitor for depression; more common in those with mental illness

Perform/provide:

- Storage at room temp

Evaluate:

- Therapeutic response: improvement in CD4 counts, T-cell counts

Teach patient/family:

- To take as prescribed; if dose missed, to take as soon as remembered up to 1 hr before next dose; not to double dose; not to share with others
- That sexual partners need to be told that patient has HIV; that product does not cure infection, just controls symptoms, does not prevent infecting others

⚠ To report sore throat, fever, fatigue (may indicate superinfection)

- That product must be taken in equal intervals 2×/day to maintain blood levels for duration of therapy

⚠ To notify prescriber immediately of suicidal thoughts/behaviors

- To notify prescriber if pregnancy planned, suspected; to avoid breastfeeding
- To continue with follow-up exams, blood work

ramelteon (Rx)

(rah-mel'tee-on)

Rozerem

Func. class.: Sedative/hypnotic, antianxiety

Chem. class.: Melatonin receptor agonist

ACTION: Binds selectively to melatonin receptors (MT_1, MT_2); thought to be involved in circadian rhythms and in the normal sleep/wake cycle

USES: Insomnia

CONTRAINDICATIONS: Breastfeeding, children, infants, hypersensitiv-

ity, alcohol intoxication, hepatic encephalopathy
Precautions: Pregnancy (C), hepatic disease, alcoholism, COPD, seizure disorder, sleep apnea, suicidal ideation, angioedema, depression, sleep-related behaviors (sleepwalking), schizophrenia, bipolar disorder

DOSAGE AND ROUTES

- **Adult: PO** 8 mg at bedtime

Hepatic dose

- Do not use with severe hepatic disease; use with caution for mild to moderate hepatic disease

Available forms: Tabs 8 mg
Administer:

- Within 30 min of bedtime for sleeplessness; on empty stomach for fast onset

SIDE EFFECTS

CNS: Dizziness, somnolence, fatigue, headache, insomnia, depression, complex sleep-related reactions (sleep driving, sleep eating), **suicidal thoughts/behaviors**
GI: Nausea, diarrhea, dysgeusia, vomiting
MISC: Myalgia, arthralgia, decreased blood cortisol, influenza, upper RI
SYST: **Severe allergic reactions, angioedema**

PHARMACOKINETICS

Absorbed rapidly; peak 0.75 hr; protein binding 82%; rapid first pass metabolism via liver; 84% excreted in urine, 4% in feces; half-life 2-5 hr

INTERACTIONS

⚠ **Possible toxicity: antiretroviral protease inhibitors**
⚠ **Increase: ramelteon effect, toxicity—alcohol; CYP1A2 inhibitors, azole antifungals (ketoconazole, fluconazole), fluvoxamine, anxiolytics, sedatives, hypnotics, barbiturates, ciprofloxacin**
Decrease: effect of ramelteon—rifampin
Drug/Food

- Prolonged absorption, sleep onset reduced: high-fat/heavy meal

NURSING CONSIDERATIONS

Assess:
⚠ **Severe hypersensitive reactions: Assess for angioedema (facial swelling), product should be discontinued**

- Sleep characteristics: type of sleep problem: falling asleep, staying asleep
- Mental status: mood, sensorium, affect, memory (long, short term), suicidal ideation
- LFTs: before treatment, periodically

Perform/provide:

- Storage in tight container in cool environment

Evaluate:

- Therapeutic response: ability to sleep at night, decreased amount of early morning awakening

Teach patient/family:

- To avoid driving, other activities requiring alertness until product stabilized
- To avoid alcohol ingestion, CNS depressants
- About alternative measures to improve sleep: reading, exercise several hr before bedtime, warm bath, warm milk, TV, self-hypnosis, deep breathing
- To take product immediately before going to bed
- Not to ingest a high-fat/heavy meal before taking product

⚠ **To report cessation of menses, galactorrhea (women), decreased libido, infertility, worsening of insomnia, behavioral changes, severe allergic reactions, suicidal thoughts/behaviors**

ramipril (Rx)

(ra-mi′pril)

Altace

Func. class.: Antihypertensive
Chem. class.: Angiotensin-converting enzyme inhibitor (ACE)

Do not confuse:
ramipril/enalapril
Altace/alteplase

ACTION: Selectively suppresses renin-angiotensin-aldosterone system; inhibits ACE, prevents conversion of angiotensin I to angiotensin II; results in dilation of arterial, venous vessels

USES: Hypertension, alone or in combination with thiazide diuretics; CHF (post MI), reduction in risk for MI, stroke, death from CV disorders
Unlabeled uses: Proteinuria due to diabetic nephropathy

CONTRAINDICATIONS: Breastfeeding, children, hypersensitivity to ACE inhibitors, history of ACE-inhibitor–induced angioedema

Black Box Warning: Pregnancy (D) 2nd/3rd trimesters

Precautions: Geriatric patients, impaired renal/hepatic function, dialysis patients, hypovolemia, blood dyscrasias, CHF, COPD, asthma, renal artery stenosis, cough

DOSAGE AND ROUTES

Hypertension
- **Adult: PO** 2.5 mg/day initially then 2.5-20 mg/day divided bid or daily

CHF post-MI
- **Adult: PO** 1.25-2.5 mg bid; may increase to 5 mg bid

Reduction in risk for MI, stroke, death
- **Adult: PO** 2.5 mg/day × 7 days then 5 mg/day × 21 days, then may increase to 10 mg/day

Renal dose
- **Adult: PO** CCr <40 ml/min, reduce by 50%, titrate upward to max 5 mg/day

Proteinuria due to diabetic nephropathy (unlabeled)
- **Adult: PO** 2.5 mg/day up to 20 mg/day

Available forms: Caps 1.25, 2.5, 5, 10 mg

Administer:
- Without regard to meals
- Caps can be opened, added to food

SIDE EFFECTS

CNS: *Headache, dizziness,* anxiety, insomnia, paresthesia, *fatigue,* depression, malaise, vertigo
CV: *Hypotension,* chest pain, palpitations, angina, syncope, dysrhythmia
EENT: Hearing loss
GI: *Nausea,* constipation, vomiting, dyspepsia, dysphagia, anorexia, diarrhea, abdominal pain, **hepatitis, hepatic failure, pancreatitis, hepatic necrosis**
GU: Proteinuria, increased BUN, creatinine, impotence
HEMA: Decreased Hct, Hgb, **eosinophilia, leukopenia, pancytopenia, thrombocytopenia, agranulocytosis (rare)**
INTEG: Rash, sweating, photosensitivity, pruritus
META: *Hyperkalemia*
MISC: **Angioedema, toxic epidermal necrolysis, anaphylaxis, Stevens-Johnson syndrome**
MS: Arthralgia, arthritis, myalgia
RESP: *Cough,* dyspnea

PHARMACOKINETICS

Bioavailability >50%-60%, onset 1-2 hr, peak 3-6 hr, duration 24 hr, protein binding 73%, half-life 1-2 hr, 9-18 hr for active metabolite, metabolized by liver (metabolites excreted in urine, feces)

INTERACTIONS

Increase: hypotension—diuretics, other antihypertensives, ganglionic blockers, adrenergic blockers, nitrates, acute alcohol ingestion
⚠ **Increase: toxicity—vasodilators, hydrALAZINE, prazosin, potassium-sparing diuretics, sympathomimetics, potassium supplements**
Increase: serum levels of lithium
Decrease: absorption—antacids
Decrease: antihypertensive effect—indomethacin, NSAIDs, salicylates

Drug/Herb
Increase: antihypertensive effect—hawthorn
Decrease: antihypertensive effect—ephedra

Drug/Lab Test
False positive: urine acetone, ANA titer

NURSING CONSIDERATIONS

Assess:

⚠ **Collagen-vascular disease (SLE, scleroderma):** neutrophils, decreased platelets; WBC with differential at baseline, periodically; if neutrophils <1000/mm³, discontinue treatment

- **Hypertension:** B/P, orthostatic hypotension, syncope
- Potassium levels; hyperkalemia occurs
- **Renal disease:** protein, BUN, creatinine at baseline, periodically; increased levels may indicate nephrotic syndrome; renal symptoms: polyuria, oliguria, urinary frequency, dysuria
- **CHF:** edema in feet, legs daily; weight daily

⚠ **Serious allergic reactions:** angioedema, Stevens-Johnson syndrome, rash, fever, pruritus, urticaria; product should be discontinued if antihistamines fail to help

Perform/provide:

- Storage in tight container at ≤86° F (30° C)

Evaluate:

- Therapeutic response: decrease in B/P; CHF

Teach patient/family:

- Not to discontinue product abruptly; to comply with dosage schedule, even if feeling better
- Not to use OTC products (cough, cold, allergy) unless directed by prescriber; not to use salt substitutes containing potassium without consulting prescriber
- To rise slowly to sitting or standing position to minimize orthostatic hypotension

⚠ To notify prescriber of mouth sores, sore throat, fever, swelling of hands or feet, irregular heartbeat, chest pain

- To report excessive perspiration, dehydration, vomiting, diarrhea; may lead to fall in B/P
- That product may cause dizziness, fainting, lightheadedness; that these may occur during 1st few days of therapy
- That product may cause skin rash, impaired perspiration
- How to take B/P, normal readings for age group

Black Box Warning: To inform prescriber if pregnancy planned, suspected, pregnancy category (D); not to breastfeed

TREATMENT OF OVERDOSE:

0.9% NaCl IV inf, hemodialysis

ranibizumab (Rx)

(ran-ih-biz′oo-mab)

Lucentis

Func. class.: Ophthalmic
Chem. class.: Selective vascular endothelial growth factor antagonist

ACTION: Binds to receptor-binding site of active forms of vascular endothelial growth factor A (VEGF-A) that causes angiogenesis and cell proliferation

USES: Macular degeneration (neovascular) (wet), macular edema after retinal vein occlusion (RVO)
Unlabeled uses: Diabetic macular edema

CONTRAINDICATIONS: Hypersensitivity, ocular infections
Precautions: Pregnancy (C), breastfeeding, children, retinal detachment, increased intraocular pressure

DOSAGE AND ROUTES

Macular degeneration/macular edema after retinal vein occlusion (RVO)

- **Adult: INTRAVITREAL** 0.5 mg (0.05 ml) monthly

Diabetic macular edema (unlabeled)

- **Adults: INTRAVITREAL** 0.5 mg then prompt (within 1 wk) or deferred (≥24 wk) laser

Available forms: Sol for inj 0.5 mg/0.05 ml

Administer:

- By ophthalmologist via intravitreal injection using adequate anesthesia; use 19-gauge filter

SIDE EFFECTS

CNS: Dizziness, headache

EENT: Blepharitis, cataract, conjunctival hemorrhage/hyperemia, detachment of retinal pigment epithelium, dry/irritation/pain in eye, visual impairment, vitreous floaters, ocular infection

GI: Constipation, nausea

MISC: Hypertension, UTI, thromboembolism, nonocular bleeding

RESP: Bronchitis, cough, sinusitis, URI

PHARMACOKINETICS

Elimination half-life 9 days

INTERACTIONS

Increase: severe inflammation—verteporfin photodynamic therapy (PDT)

NURSING CONSIDERATIONS

Assess:

- **Eye changes:** redness; sensitivity to light, vision change; increased intraocular pressure change; report infection to ophthalmologist immediately

Perform/provide:

- Storage in refrigerator; do not freeze
- Protect from light

Evaluate:

- Therapeutic response: prevention of increasing macular degeneration

Teach patient/family:

- That, if eye becomes red, sensitive to light, painful, or if there is a change in vision, to seek immediate care from ophthalmologist
- About reason for treatment, expected results

ranitidine (Rx, OTC)

(ra-nit′i-deen)

Equaline Heartburn Relief, Nu-Ranit ✱, Top Care Heartburn Relief, Wal-zan, Zantac, Zantac C ✱, Zantac EFFER-dose

ranitidine bismuth citrate

Tritec

Func. class.: H_2-Histamine receptor antagonist

Do not confuse:
ranitidine/amantadine
Zantac/Xanax/Zofran

ACTION: Inhibits histamine at H_2-receptor site in parietal cells, which inhibits gastric acid secretion

USES: Duodenal ulcer, Zollinger-Ellison syndrome, gastric ulcers, hypersecretory conditions, gastroesophageal reflux disease, stress ulcers, erosive esophagitis (maintenance), active duodenal ulcers with *Helicobacter pylori* in combination with clarithromycin, systemic mastocytosis, multiple endocrine adenoma syndrome, heartburn

Unlabeled uses: Prevention of aspiration pneumonitis, stress ulcers (treatment/prophylaxis), upper GI bleeding, angioedema, gastritis, urticaria, NSAID-induced ulcer prophylaxis

CONTRAINDICATIONS: Hypersensitivity

Precautions: Pregnancy (B), breastfeeding, child <12 yr, renal/hepatic disease

DOSAGE AND ROUTES

Ranitidine

Duodenal ulcer

• **Adult: PO** 150 mg bid or 300 mg/day after PM meal or at bedtime; maintenance 150 mg at bedtime

• **Infant and child: PO** 2-4 mg/kg bid, max 300 mg/day

Zollinger-Ellison syndrome

• **Adult: PO** 150 mg bid, may increase if needed

Gastric ulcer

• **Adult: PO** 150 mg bid × 6 wk then 150 mg at bedtime

• **Infant and child: PO** 2-4 mg/kg bid, max 300 mg/day

GERD

• **Adult: PO** 150 mg bid

Erosive esophagitis

• **Adult: PO** 150 mg qid for up to 12 wk

• **Child ≥1 mo: PO** 5-10 mg/kg/day in 2-3 divided doses

Renal dose

• **Adult:** CCr <50 ml/min, give 50% of dose or extend dosing interval

NSAID-induced ulcer prophylaxis (unlabeled)

• **Adult: PO** 150 mg bid

Stress gastritis prophylaxis (unlabeled)

• **Adult: IM/INT IV INF** 50 mg q6-8hr

Severe, acute urticaria/angioedema (unlabeled)

• **Adult: INT IV INF** 50 mg with H_1-blocker

Ranitidine bismuth citrate

• **Adult: PO** 400 mg bid × 4 wk with clarithromycin 500 mg tid × 1st 2 wk

Available forms: *Ranitidine:* tabs 75, 150, 300 mg; sol for inj 25 mg/ml; effervescent tabs 25 mg; caps 150, 300 mg; syr 15 mg/ml; *ranitidine bismuth citrate:* tabs 400 mg

Administer:

PO route

• Antacids 1 hr before or 1 hr after ranitidine

• Without regard to meals; **EFFERdose tab:** dissolve 25 mg/≥5 ml, give after dissolved; swallow whole or dissolve on tongue, do not chew

IM route

• No dilution needed; inject in large muscle mass, aspirate

Direct IV route

• Dilute to max 2.5 mg/ml (50 mg/20 ml) using 0.9% NaCl (nonpreserved) or D_5W, give dose over ≥5 min (max 4 mg/ml)

Intermittent IV INF route

• Dilute to max 0.5 mg/ml with D_5W, NS, give over 15-20 min (5-7 ml/min); premixed ready-to-use bags as 1 mg/ml (50 mg/50 ml), inf over 15-20 min

Continuous 24 hr IV INF route

• dilute 150 mg/250 ml of D**Adult:** ${}_5$W or NS, run over 24 hr (6.25 mg/hr or as directed); use inf device, use within 48 hr; *Zollinger-Ellison Syndrome:* dilute in D_5W, NS; max conc 2.5 mg/ml, use inf device

Y-site: Acyclovir, aldesleukin, alemtuzumab, alfentanil, allopurinol, amifostine, amikacin, aminophylline, amphotericin B liposome, amsacrine, anikinra, anidulafungin, ascorbic acid, atracurium, atropine, aztreonam, bivalirudin, bumetanide, buprenorphine, butorphanol, calcium chloride/gluconate, CARBOplatin, ceFAZolin, cefepime, cefonicid, cefoperazone, cefotaxime, cefotetan, cefoxitin, ceftazidime, ceftizoxime, cefTRIAXone, cefuroxime, chloramphenicol, chlorproMAZINE, cimetidine, ciprofloxacin, cisatracurium, CISplatin, clindamycin, cyanocobalamin, cyclophosphamide, cycloSPORINE, cytarabine, DACTINomycin, DAPTOmycin, dexamethasone, dexmedetomidine, digoxin, diltiazem, DOBUTamine, docetaxel, DOPamine, doripenem, doxacurium, doxapram, DOXOrubicin, DOXOrubicin liposome, doxycycline, enalaprilat, ePHEDrine, EPINEPHrine, epirubicin, epoetin alfa, ertapenem, erythromycin, esmolol, etoposide, etoposide phosphate, famotidine, fenoldopam, fentaNYL, filgrastim, fluconazole, fludarabine, fluorouracil, folic acid, foscarnet,

R

furosemide, ganciclovir, gemcitabine, gentamicin, glycopyrrolate, granisetron, heparin, hydrocortisone, HYDROmorphone, IDArubicin, ifosfamide, imipenem/cilastatin, inamrinone, indomethacin, isoproterenol, ketorolac, labetalol, levofloxacin, lidocaine, linezolid, LORazepam, magnesium sulfate, mannitol, mechlorethamine, melphalan, meperidine, metaraminol, methotrexate, methoxamine, methyldopate, methylPREDNISolone, metoclopramide, metoprolol, metroNIDAZOLE, midazolam, milrinone, mitoxantrone, morphine, multivitamin, nalbuphine, naloxone, nesiritide, niCARdipine, nitroglycerin, nitroprusside, norepinephrine, octreotide, ondansetron, oxacillin, oxaliplatin, oxytocin, paclitaxel, palonosetron, pancuronium, papaverine, pemetrexed, penicillin G, pentamidine, pentazocine, PENTobarbital, PHENobarbital, phentolamine, phenylephrine, phytonadione, piperacillin/tazobactam, potassium chloride, procainamide, prochlorperazine, promethazine, propofol, propranolol, protamine, pyrdoxime, remifentanil, riTUXimab, rocuronium, sargramostim, sodium acetate/bicarbonate, succinylcholine, SUFentanil, tacrolimus, teniposide, theophylline, thiamine, thiopental, thiotepa, ticarcillin/clavulanate, tigecycline, tirofiban, tobramycin, tolazoline, trastuzumab, trimethaphan, urokinase, vancomycin, vecuronium, vinCRIStine, vinorelbine, warfarin, zidovudine, zoledronic acid

SIDE EFFECTS

CNS: Headache, sleeplessness, dizziness, confusion, agitation, depression, hallucination (geriatric patients)
CV: Tachycardia, bradycardia, PVCs
EENT: Blurred vision, increased ocular pressure
GI: Constipation, abdominal pain, diarrhea, nausea, vomiting, hepatotoxicity
GU: Impotence, acute interstitial nephritis (rare)
INTEG: Urticaria, rash, fever
RESP: Pneumonia
SYST: Anaphylaxis (rare)

PHARMACOKINETICS

PO: Peak 2-3 hr; duration 8-12 hr; metabolized by liver; excreted in urine (30% unchanged, PO), breast milk; half-life 2-3 hr; protein binding 15%

INTERACTIONS

Increase: effect of pramipexole, procainamide, trospium, triazolam, calcium channel blockers, memantine, saquinavir, adefovir
⚠ **Increase:** GI obstruction risk—NIFEdipine ext rel products
Increase: toxicity—sulfonylureas, procainamide, benzodiazepines, calcium channel blockers
Decrease: absorption of ranitidine—antacids, anticholinergics
Decrease: effects of cephalosporins, iron salts, ketoconazole, itraconazole
Increase: GI obstruction risk—NIFEdipine ext rel products
Drug/Lab Test
Increase: AST, ALT, alk phos, creatinine, LDH, bilirubin
False positive: urine protein

NURSING CONSIDERATIONS

Assess:
- **GI complaints:** nausea, vomiting, diarrhea, cramps, abdominal discomfort, jaundice; report immediately
- I&O ratio, BUN, creatinine, LFTs, serum, stool guaiac before, periodically during therapy
- Mental status: confusion, dizziness, depression, anxiety, weakness, tremors, psychosis

Perform/provide:
- Storage at room temp

Evaluate:
- Therapeutic response: decreased abdominal pain, heartburn

Teach patient/family:
- To avoid driving, other hazardous activities until stabilized on product

• That product must be continued for prescribed time to be effective
• To notify prescriber if pregnancy planned, suspected; to avoid breastfeeding, excreted in breastmilk
• Not to take maximum OTC daily dose for >2 wk

ranolazine (Rx)

(ruh-no′luh-zeen)

Ranexa

Func. class: Antianginal

ACTION: Antianginal, antiischemic; unknown, may work by inhibiting portal fatty-acid oxidation

USES: Chronic stable angina pectoris; use in patients who have not responded to other treatment options; should be used in combination with other antianginals such as amlodipine, β-blockers, nitrates

CONTRAINDICATIONS: Preexisting QT prolongation, hepatic disease (Child-Pugh class A, B, C), hypersensitivity, hypokalemia, renal failure, torsades de pointes, ventricular dysrhythmia, ventricular tachycardia, hepatic cirrhosis
Precautions: Pregnancy (C), breastfeeding, children, geriatric patients, hypotension, renal disease

DOSAGE AND ROUTES

• **Adult: PO** 500 mg bid, increased to 1000 mg bid based on response; max 1000 mg bid
Available forms: Ext rel tabs 500, 1000 mg
Administer:
• **Ext rel tabs:** do not break, crush, chew tabs; take product as prescribed; do not double or skip dose
• Without regard to meals, bid; limit grapefruit juice

SIDE EFFECTS

CNS: *Headache, dizziness*
CV: Palpitations, QT prolongation
GI: Nausea, vomiting, constipation, dry mouth
MISC: Peripheral edema
RESP: Dyspnea

PHARMACOKINETICS

Absorption varied; peak 2-5 hr; half-life 7 hr; extensively metabolized by the liver (CYP3A and less by CYP2D6); excreted in urine (75%), feces (25%); protein binding 62%

INTERACTIONS

Increase: ranolazine action—diltiazem, ketoconazole, macrolide antibiotics, dofetilide, PARoxetine, protease inhibitors, quiNIDine, sotalol, thioridazine, verapamil, ziprasidone
Increase: action of digoxin, simvastatin
⚠ **Increase: QTc interval—macrolides (clarithromycin, erythromycin, troleandomycin)**
Increase: ranolazine absorption, toxicity—antiretroviral protease inhibitors
⚠ **Increase: QT prolongation and torsades de pointes—class IA/III antidysrythmics, arsenic trioxide, chloroquine, droperidol, haloperidol, levomethadyl, methadone, pentamidine, chlorproMAZINE, mesoridazine, thioridazine, pimozide; CYP3A4 inhibitors (ketoconazole, fluconazole, itraconazole, IV miconazole, voriconazole, diltiazem, verapamil)**
Drug/Food
• Do not use with grapefruit, grapefruit juice

NURSING CONSIDERATIONS

Assess:
• **Angina:** characteristics of pain (intensity, location, duration, alleviating/precipitating factors)
⚠ **QT prolongation: ECG for QT prolongation, ejection fraction; assess for chest pain, palpitations, dyspnea**
• Cardiac status: B/P, pulse, respirations

R

• LFTs, serum creatinine/BUN, magnesium, potassium before treatment, periodically

Evaluate:

• Therapeutic response: decreased anginal pain

Teach patient/family:

• To avoid hazardous activities until stabilized on product, dizziness no longer a problem

⚠ To avoid OTC drugs, grapefruit juice, products prolonging QTc (quiNIDine, dofetilide, sotalol, erythromycin, thioridazine, ziprasidone or protease inhibitors, diltiazem, ketoconazole, macrolide antibiotics, verapamil) unless directed by prescriber; to notify prescriber of palpitations, fainting

• To comply with all areas of medical regimen

• To take as directed; not to skip dose, double doses

• To notify all health care providers of product use

rasagiline (Rx)

(ra-sa′ji-leen)

Azilect

Func. class.: Antiparkinson agent

Chem. class.: MAOI, type B

ACTION: Inhibits MAOI type B at recommended doses; may increase DOPamine levels

USES: Idiopathic Parkinson's disease monotherapy or with levodopa

CONTRAINDICATIONS: Breastfeeding; hypersensitivity to this product, MAOIs; pheochromocytoma

Precautions: Pregnancy (C), children, psychiatric disorders, moderate to severe hepatic disorders

DOSAGE AND ROUTES

Monotherapy

• **Adult: PO** 1 mg/day

Adjunctive therapy

• **Adult: PO** 0.5 mg/day, may increase 1 mg/day; change of levodopa dose for adjunct therapy; reduced levodopa dose may be needed

Hepatic dose

• **Adult: PO** 0.5 mg for mild hepatic disease

Concomitant ciprofloxacin, other CYP1A2 inhibitors

• **Adult: PO** 0.5 mg; plasma concentrations of rasagiline may double

Available forms: Tabs 0.5, 1 mg

Administer:

⚠ With meals to prevent nausea; continuing therapy usually reduces or eliminates nausea; do not give with foods/liquids containing large amounts of tyramine

• Reduced dose of carbidopa/levodopa cautiously

SIDE EFFECTS

CNS: Drowsiness, hallucinations, depression, headache, malaise, paresthesia, vertigo, syncope

CV: Angina, **hypertensive crisis** (ingestion of tyramine products), orthostatic hypotension

GI: *Nausea*, diarrhea, dry mouth, dyspepsia

GU: Impotence, decreased libido

MISC: Conjunctivitis, fever, flu syndrome, neck pain, allergic reaction, alopecia

MS: Arthralgia, arthritis, dyskinesia

RESP: Rhinitis

PHARMACOKINETICS

Onset, peak, duration unknown; well absorbed; protein binding >88%-94%; metabolized by CYP1A2 in liver; excreted by kidneys

INTERACTIONS

⚠ Do not give with meperidine, other analgesics because serious reactions (including coma and death) may occur; do not give with sympathomimetics

Increase: levels of rasagiline up to 2-fold—ciprofloxacin, CYP1A2 inhibitors (atazanavir, mexiletine, taurine)

Increase: severe CNS toxicity with antidepressants (tricyclics, SSRIs, SNRIs, mirtazapine, cyclobenzaprine)

⚠ **Increase:** hypertensive crisis—MAOIs

Drug/Herb

• Do not give with St. John's wort, yohimbe

Drug/Food

• Do not give with foods/liquids that have large amounts of tyramine

NURSING CONSIDERATIONS

Assess:

• **Parkinson's symptoms:** tremor, ataxia, muscle weakness and rigidity at baseline, periodically; increased dyskinesia, postural hypotension if used in combination with levodopa

• Mental status: hallucinations, confusion, notify prescriber

⚠ **Hypertensive crisis:** severe headache, blurred vision, seizures, chest pain, difficulty thinking, nausea, vomiting, signs of stroke; any unexplained severe headache should be considered to be hypertensive crisis

⚠ **Melanomas;** periodic skin exams by a dermatologist

• Cardiac status: B/P, ECG periodically during beginning treatment

⚠ **Tyramine products:** foods, other medications may lead to hypertensive crisis (tachycardia, bradycardia, chest pain, nausea, vomiting, sweating, dilated pupils)

Evaluate:

• Therapeutic response: improved symptoms in patients with Parkinson's disease

Teach patient/family:

• To change positions slowly to prevent orthostatic hypotension

• To avoid hazardous activities until stabilized on product; that dizziness can occur

• To rinse mouth frequently; to use sugarless gum to alleviate dry mouth

• To take as prescribed; not to miss dose or double doses; to take missed dose as soon as remembered if several hours before next dose

⚠ To prevent hypertensive crisis by avoiding high-tyramine foods (>150 mg)

• To report signs of hypertensive crisis

• To avoid CNS depressants, alcohol

• To notify all health care providers of product use; to avoid elective surgery, other procedures involving CNS depressants

rasburicase (Rx)

(rass-burr'i-case)

Elitek, Fasturtec ✦

Func. class.: Enzyme

Chem. class.: Recombinant urate-oxidase enzyme

ACTION: Catalyzes enzymatic oxidation of uric acid into an inactive and soluble metabolite (allantoin)

USES: To reduce uric acid levels in children with leukemia, lymphoma, solid tumor malignancies who are receiving chemotherapy

CONTRAINDICATIONS: Hypersensitivity

Black Box Warning: G6PD deficiency (Mediterranean, African descendants), hemolytic reactions, methemoglobinemia reactions to product

Precautions: Pregnancy (C), breastfeeding, children <2 yr, anemia

Black Box Warning: Acute bronchospasm, angina, angioedema, atony, African-American and Mediterranean patients, hypotension, urticaria

DOSAGE AND ROUTES

• **Adult/adolescent/infant:** **IV INF** 0.2 mg/kg as single daily dose given as **IV INF** over ½ hr × 5 days

Available forms: Powder for inj 1.5, 7.5 mg/vial

Administer:

Intermittent IV INF route

• Reconstitute with diluent provided, add 1 ml of diluent/each vial, swirl, withdraw amount needed, mix with NS to final volume of 50 ml, use within 24 hr, give over 30 min, do not use filter, use different line; if not possible, flush with ≥15 ml of saline before, after use

• Chemotherapy started 4-24 hr after 1st dose

SIDE EFFECTS

CNS: *Headache,* fever

CV: Chest pain, hypotension

GI: *Nausea, vomiting, anorexia, diarrhea, abdominal pain, constipation, dyspepsia, mucositis*

HEMA: Neutropenia with fever, hemolysis, methemoglobinemia

INTEG: *Rash*

MISC: Edema

RESP: Bronchospasm, wheezing, dyspnea

SYST: Anaphylaxis, hemolysis, methemoglobinemia, sepsis

PHARMACOKINETICS

Elimination half-life 16-21 hr

INTERACTIONS

⚠ **Increase:** toxicity—allopurinol

NURSING CONSIDERATIONS

Assess:

• Blood studies: BUN, serum uric acid, urine creatinine clearance, electrolytes, CBC with differential before, during therapy

• Monitor temp; fever may indicate beginning infection; no rectal temps

⚠ **Anaphylaxis:** dyspnea, urticaria, flushing, wheezing, swelling of lips, tongue, throat; have emergency equipment nearby

⚠ **G6PD deficiency, hemolytic reactions, methemoglobinemia;** these patients should not be given this product; screen patients who are at higher risk for these disorders

• GI symptoms: frequency of stools, cramping; if severe diarrhea occurs, fluid, electrolytes may need to be given

Evaluate:

• Therapeutic response: decreased uric acid levels in children when antineoplastics causing high uric acid levels used

Teach patient/family:

• About the reason for therapy, expected results

⚠ To report trouble breathing, jaundice, chest pain

⚠ HIGH ALERT

remifentanil (Rx)

(rem-ih-fin′ta-nill)

Ultiva

Func. class.: Opiate agonist analgesic

Chem. class.: μ-Opioid agonist

Controlled Substance Schedule II

ACTION:
Inhibits ascending pain pathways in limbic system, thalamus, midbrain, hypothalamus

USES:
In combination with other products for general anesthesia to provide analgesia

CONTRAINDICATIONS:
Hypersensitivity

Precautions: Pregnancy (C), breastfeeding, children <12 yr, geriatric patients, increased intracranial pressure, acute MI, severe heart disease, GI/renal/hepatic disease, asthma, respiratory conditions, seizures disorders, bradyarrhythmias

DOSAGE AND ROUTES

• **Adult:** Induction **IV** 0.5-1 mcg/kg/min with hypnotic or volative agent; maintenance with isoflurane (0.4-1.5 MAC) or propofol (100-200 mcg/kg/min); **CONT INF** 0.25-0.4 mcg/kg/min

• **Child 1-12 yr: CONT IV INF** 0.25 mcg/kg/min with isoflurane
• **Full-term neonate and infant up to 2 mo: CONT IV INF** 0.4 mcg/kg/min with nitrous oxide
Available forms: Powder for inj lyophilized 1, 2, 5 mg
Administer:
• Add 1 ml diluent per mg remifentanil
• Interruption of inf results in rapid reversal (no residual opioid effect within 5-10 min)
Direct IV route
• To be used only during maintenance of general anesthesia; inject into tubing close to venous cannula; give to nonintubated patients over 30-60 sec
Continuous IV INF route
• Use inf device, max 16 hr; do not use same tubing as blood, do not admix

Y-site compatibilities: Acyclovir, alfentanil, amikacin, aminophylline, ampicillin, ampicillin/sulbactam, aztreonam, bumetanide, buprenorphine, butorphanol, calcium gluconate, ceFAZolin, cefepine, cefotaxime, cefotetan, cefoxitin, ceftazidime, ceftizoxime, cefTRIAXone, cefuroxime, cimetidine, ciprofloxacin, cisatracurium, CISplatin, clindamycin, DACTINomycin, dexamethasone, digoxin, diltiazem, diphenhydrAMINE, DOBUTamine, docetaxel, DOPamine, doxacurium, doxycycline, droperidol, enalaprilat, EPINEPHrine, esmolol, etoposide, famotidine, fentaNYL, fluconazole, furosemide, ganciclovir, gatiflexacin, gemcitabine, gentamicin, granisetron, haloperidol, heparin, hetastarch, hydrocortisone sodium succinate, HYDROmorphone, hydrOXYzine, imipenem-cilastatin, inamrinone, isoproterenol, ketorolac, levofloxacin, lidocaine, LORazepam, magnesium sulfate, mannitol, meperidine, methylPREDNISolone sodium succinate, metoclopramide, metroNIDAZOLE, midazolam, minocycline, morphine, nalbuphine, netilmicin, nitroglycerin, norepinephrine, ofloxacin, ondansetron, paclitaxel, palonsetron, phenylephrine, piperacillin, potassium chloride, procainamide, prochlorperazine, promethazine, ranitidine, SUFentanil, sulfamethoxazole, teniposide, theophylline, thiopental, thiotepa, ticarcillin, ticarcillin/clavulanale, tobramycin, trimethoprim, vancomycin, voriconazole, zidovudine
Solution compatibilities: D_5, 0.45% NaCl, LR, D_5 LR, 0.9% NaCl

SIDE EFFECTS

CNS: Drowsiness, *dizziness,* confusion, *headache,* sedation, euphoria, delirium, agitation, anxiety
CV: Palpitations, *bradycardia,* change in B/P, facial flushing, syncope, **asystole**
EENT: Tinnitus, blurred vision, miosis, diplopia
GI: *Nausea, vomiting,* anorexia, constipation, cramps, dry mouth
GU: Urinary retention, dysuria
INTEG: Rash, urticaria, bruising, flushing, diaphoresis, pruritus
MS: Rigidity
RESP: **Respiratory depression, apnea**

PHARMACOKINETICS

70% protein binding, terminal half-life 3-10 min

INTERACTIONS

Increase: respiratory depression, hypotension, profound sedation: alcohol, sedatives, hypnotics, other CNS depressants; antihistamines, phenothiazines
Drug/Herb
Increase: CNS depression—kava

NURSING CONSIDERATIONS

Assess:
• I&O ratio; check for decreasing output; may indicate urinary retention, especially in geriatric patients
• CNS changes; dizziness, drowsiness, hallucinations, euphoria, LOC, pupil reaction
• GI status: nausea, vomiting, anorexia, constipation
• Allergic reactions: rash, urticaria

• **Respiratory dysfunction:** respiratory depression, character, rate, rhythm; notify prescriber if respirations <12/min; CV status; bradycardia, syncope
• Use pain scoring to determine pain perception

Perform/provide:
• Storage in light-resistant area at room temp

Evaluate:
• Therapeutic response: maintenance of anesthesia

Teach patient/family:
• To call for assistance when ambulating or smoking; that drowsiness, dizziness may occur
• To make position changes slowly to prevent orthostatic hypotension

repaglinide (Rx)

(re-pag′lih′nide)

Gluconorm ✱, Prandin

Func. class.: Antidiabetic

Chem. class.: Meglitinide

ACTION:
Causes functioning β-cells in pancreas to release insulin, thereby leading to a drop in blood glucose levels; closes ATP-dependent potassium channels in the β-cell membrane; this leads to the opening of calcium channels; increased calcium influx induces insulin secretion

USES:
Type 2 diabetes mellitus

CONTRAINDICATIONS:
Hypersensitivity to meglitinides; diabetic ketoacidosis, type 1 diabetes

Precautions: Pregnancy (C), breastfeeding, children, geriatric patients, thyroid/cardiac disease, severe renal/hepatic disease, severe hypoglycemic reactions

DOSAGE AND ROUTES

• **Adult: PO** 1-2 mg with each meal, max 16 mg/day; adjust at weekly intervals; oral-hypoglycemic–naive patients or patients with A1c <8% should start with 0.5 mg with each meal

Renal/hepatic dose
• **Adult: PO** CCr 20-39 ml/min, 0.5 mg/day; titrate upward cautiously

Available forms: Tabs 0.5, 1, 2 mg

Administer:
• Up to 15-30 min before meals; 2, 3, or 4×/day preprandially
• Skip dose if meal skipped; add dose if meal added

SIDE EFFECTS

CNS: *Headache, weakness,* paresthesia
ENDO: Hypoglycemia
GI: Nausea, vomiting, diarrhea, constipation, dyspepsia
INTEG: Rash, allergic reactions
MISC: Chest pain, UTI, allergy
MS: Back pains, arthralgia
RESP: URI, sinusitis, rhinitis, bronchitis

PHARMACOKINETICS

Completely absorbed by GI route; onset 30 min; peak 1 hr; duration <4 hr; half-life 1 hr; metabolized in liver; excreted in urine, feces (metabolites); crosses placenta; 98% protein bound

INTERACTIONS

⚠ **Do not use with gemfibrozil**
Increase: in both—levonorgestrel/ethinyl estradiol
Increase: repaglinide metabolism—CYP450 inducers: rifampin, barbiturates, carBAMazepine
Increase: repaglinide effect—NSAIDs, salicylates, sulfonamides, chloramphenicol, MAOIs, coumarins, β-blockers, probenecid, gemfibrozil, simvastatin, fenofibrate
Decrease: repaglinide metabolism—CYP450 inhibitors: antifungals (ketoconazole, miconazole), erythromycin, macrolides
Decrease: repaglinide action—calcium channel blockers, corticosteroids, oral contraceptives, thiazide diuretics, thyroid preparations, estrogens, phenothiazines,

phenytoin, rifampin, isoniazid, PHENObarbital, sympathomimetics
Drug/Herb
Increase: antidiabetic effect—garlic, chromium, horse chestnut
Drug/Food
Decrease: repaglinide level; give before meals

NURSING CONSIDERATIONS

Assess:
⚠ **Hypo/hyperglycemic reaction,** which can occur soon after meals: dizziness, weakness, headache, tremor, anxiety, tachycardia, hunger, sweating, abdominal pain, A1c, fasting, postprandial glucose during treatment
Perform/provide:
- Storage in tight container at room temp

Evaluate:
- Therapeutic response: decrease in polyuria, polydipsia, polyphagia; clear sensorium; absence of dizziness; stable gait; blood glucose, A1c improvement

Teach family/patient:
- About technique for blood glucose monitoring; how to use blood glucose meter
- About the symptoms of hypo/hyperglycemia, what to do about each
- That product must be continued on daily basis; about the consequences of discontinuing product abruptly
- To avoid OTC medications unless ordered by prescriber
- That diabetes is a lifelong illness; that product will not cure disease
- That all food included in diet plan must be eaten to prevent hypoglycemia; to have glucagon emergency kit available; to take repaglinide 15-30 min before meals 2, 3, or 4×/day; to carry emergency ID

TREATMENT OF OVERDOSE:

Glucose 25 g IV via dextrose 50% solution, 50 ml or 1 mg glucagon

retapamulin topical

See Appendix B

Rh_o(D) immune globulin standard dose IM (Rx)

BayRho-D, HyperRHO SD, RhoGAM Ultra-Filtered Plus

Rh_o(D) immune globulin microdose IM (Rx)

MICRhoGAM Ultra-Filtered Plus

Rh_o(D) immune globulin IV (Rx)

Rhophylac, WinRho SDF
Func. class.: Immune globulins

ACTION: Suppresses immune response of nonsensitized Rh_o(D or D^u)-negative patients who are exposed to Rh_o(D or D^u)-positive blood

USES: Prevention of isoimmunization in Rh-negative women given Rh-positive blood after abortions, miscarriages, amniocentesis; chronic idiopathic thrombocytopenia purpura (Rhophylac)

CONTRAINDICATIONS: Previous immunization with this product, Rh_o(O)-positive/D^u-positive patient
Precautions: Pregnancy (C)

DOSAGE AND ROUTES

To reduce risk of Rh isoimmunization antepartum/suppression of Rh isoimmunization postpartum following delivery of full-term infant
- **Adult and adolescent ≥16 yr: IM** (BayRho-D [HyperRHO SD] full dose only) 300 mcg (1500 international units) at 28 wk gestation, repeat within 72 hr of delivery of confirmed Rho(D)-positive infant; dose not needed after

R

delivery if delivery within 3 wk of last dose and no fetal maternal hemorrhage of >15 ml of RBC; **IM** (RhoGam only) 300 mcg (1500 international units) at 26-28 wk gestation, repeat within 72 hr even if status of Rho unknown or if 72 hr have passed; **IM/IV** (WinRho SDF only) 300 mcg (1500 international units) at 28 wk gestation; if given earlier during pregnancy, give at 12-wk intervals during pregnancy, 120-mcg (600 international units) dose; IM/IV should be given as soon as possible and preferably within 72 hr of delivery of confirmed Rho(D)-positive infant and even if status unknown; give ≤ 28 days after delivery

Known or suspected massive fetomaternal hemorrhage (>15 ml of fetal RBC or >30 ml of fetal whole blood)

- **Adult and adolescent ≥16 yr: IM** (BayRho-D [HyperRHO SD] full dose only) 300 mcg (1500 international units) per every 15 ml of fetal blood cells or 30 ml of whole blood; multiple syringes may be injected IM at same time in different sites, give within 72 hr of exposure, repeat dose within 72 hr of delivery; **IM** (RhoGAM only) 300 mcg (1500 international units) for every 15 ml of fetal blood cells or 30 ml of whole blood, give total dose within 72 hr of exposure; **IM/IV** (WinRho SDF only) if large fetomaternal hemorrhage suspected, give **IV** 9 mcg (45 international units) or **IM** 12 mcg (60 international units) for every ml of fetal whole blood, give **IV** 600 mcg (3000 international units) q8hr or **IM** 1200 mcg (6000 international units) q12hr until total dose given, total dose should be given within 72 hr of exposure

Threatened abortion at any stage of pregnancy

- **Adult and adolescent ≥16 yr: IM** (BayRho-D [HyperRHO SD] full dose only) 300 mcg (1500 international units) as soon as possible; if given at 13-18 wk gestation, give another 300 mcg (1500 international units) at 26-28 wk gestation; repeat dose within 72 hr of delivery; **IM** (RhoGam only) 300 mcg (1500 international units) as soon as possible and within 72 hr of exposure; **IM/IV** (Rhophylac only) 300 mcg (1500 international units) as soon as possible and within 72 hr; **IM/IV** (WinRho SDF only) 300 mcg (1500 international units) as soon as possible and within 72 hr, repeat dose at 12-wk intervals during pregnancy and give 120 mcg (600 international units) as soon as possible after delivery and within 72 hr

After spontaneous abortion, induced termination of pregnancy, or ectopic pregnancy that occurs at ≤12 wk gestation

- **Adult and adolescent ≥16 yr: IM** (BayRho-D Minidose, HyperRHO Minidose, MICRhoGAM only) 50 mcg (250 international units) as soon as possible, give within 3 hr of spontaneous or surgical removal, if possible within 72 hr

After spontaneous abortion, induced termination of pregnancy, or ruptured tubal pregnancy that occurs at ≥13 wk

- **Adult and adolescent ≥16 yr: IM** (BayRho-D [HyperRHO SD] full dose, RhoGAM only) 300 mcg (1500 international units) as soon as possible and within 72 hr of event

After spontaneous abortion, induced termination of pregnancy, amniocentesis, chorionic villus sampling, abdominal trauma, ruptured tubal pregnancy, or percutaneous umbilical cord sampling at ≤34 wk gestation

- **Adult and adolescent ≥16 yr: IM/IV** (WinRho SDF only) 300 mcg (1500 international units) within 72 hr, repeat at 12-wk intervals during pregnancy, give 120 mcg (600 international units) as soon as possible and preferably within 72 hr of delivery

Available forms: BayRho-D sol for inj 300 mcg/ml (HyperRHO SD sol for inj), MICRhoGAM Ultra Filtered Plus Solution for inj 50 mcg/ml; RhoGam Ultra Filtered Plus Solution for inj 50 mcg; Rhophylac Pre-Filled Syringes Solution for inj 300 mcg/2 ml; WinRho SDF liquid for inj; WinRho powder for inj

Administer:

- BayRho-D being changed to HyperRHO SD
- BayRho-D (HyperRHO SD), MICRhoGAM, RhoGAM given by IM only; do not give IV
- WinRho SDF and Rhophylac can be given IM or IV
- Inspect for particulate matter; do not use if particulate matter present
- Reconstitute/dilution: no reconstitution or dilution needed for BayRho-D (HyperRHO SD); Rhophylac, MICRhoGAM, RhoGAM, or liquid formulation of WinRho SDF
- WinRho SDF powder for IV use: if giving IV, reconstitute 600 international units or 1500 international units immediately before use with 2.5 ml of sterile diluent; reconstitute 5000 international units with 8.5 ml sterile diluent; add diluent to vial slowly down wall of vial; gently swirl until powder dissolved; do not shake
- WinRho SDF powder for IM use: IV giving IM, reconstitute 600 international units or 1500 international units immediately before use with 1.25 ml of sterile diluent; 5000 international units with 8.5 ml of sterile diluent; add diluent to vial slowly down wall of vial; gently swirl until powder dissolved; do not shake

IM route

- Use aseptic technique, observe for 20 min after administration
- Bring Rhophylac to room temp before use
- Inject into deltoid muscle of upper arm or anterolateral portion of upper thigh; do not inject into gluteal muscle
- If dose calculated requires multiple vials or syringes, use different sites at same time

IV route

- Use aseptic technique
- WinRho SDF: remove entire contents of vial to obtain calculated dose; if partial vial required for dosage calculation, withdraw entire vial contents to ensure correct calculation; infuse correct calculated dose over 3-5 min; do not infuse with other fluids, products
- Rhophylac: bring to room temp; infuse by slow IV; observe for 20 min

SIDE EFFECTS

CNS: Lethargy
CV: Hypo/hypertension
INTEG: Irritation at inj site, fever
MISC: Infection, **ARDs, anaphylaxis, pulmonary edema, DIC**
MS: Myalgia, arthralgia

INTERACTIONS

Decrease: antibody response—live virus vaccines (measles, mumps, rubella)

NURSING CONSIDERATIONS

Assess:

⚠ **Allergies, reactions to immunizations; previous immunization with product**

⚠ **Intravascular hemolysis: back pain, chills, hemoglobinuria, renal insufficiency**

- Type, crossmatch mother and newborn's cord blood; if mother Rh_o(D)-negative, D^u-negative and newborn Rh_o(D)-positive, product should be given

Perform/provide:

- Storage in refrigerator

Evaluate:

- Rh_o(D) sensitivity in transfusion error, prevention of erythroblastosis fetalis for normal vision

Teach patient/family:

- How product works; that product must be given after subsequent deliveries if subsequent babies are Rh-positive

⚠ **To report immediately: shaking, fever, chills, dark urine, swelling of hands or feet, back pain, SOB (intravascular hemolysis)**

R

riboflavin (vit B_2) (OTC)

(rye′boh-flay-vin)

Func. class.: Vit B_2, water soluble

ACTION: Needed for respiratory reactions by catalyzing proteins

USES: Vit B_2 deficiency or polyneuritis; cheilosis adjunct with thiamine

Unlabeled uses: Migraine prophylaxis

DOSAGE AND ROUTES

Deficiency

- **Adult: PO** 5-30 mg/day
- **Child ≥12 yr: PO** 3-10 mg/day then 0.6 mg/1000 calories ingested

RDA

- **Adult: PO** (males) 1.3 mg, (females) 1.1 mg

Migraine prophylaxis (unlabeled)

- **Adult: PO** 400 mg/day × 3 mo

Available forms: Tabs 5, 10, 25, 50, 100, 250 mg

Administer:

- With food for better absorption

SIDE EFFECTS

GU: Yellow discoloration of urine

Precautions: Pregnancy (A)

PHARMACOKINETICS

Half-life 65-85 min, 60% protein bound, unused amounts excreted in urine (unchanged)

INTERACTIONS

Increase: riboflavin need—alcohol, probenecid, tricyclics, phenothiazines

Decrease: action of tetracyclines

Drug/Lab Test

- May cause false elevations of urinary catecholamines

NURSING CONSIDERATIONS

Assess:

- Nutritional status: liver, eggs, dairy products, yeast, whole grains, green vegetables

Perform/provide:

- Storage in airtight, light-resistant container

Evaluate:

- Therapeutic response: absence of headache, GI problems, cheilosis, skin lesions, depression; burning, itchy eyes; anemia

Teach patient/family:

- That urine may turn bright yellow
- About the addition of needed foods rich in riboflavin
- To avoid alcohol

rifabutin (Rx)

(riff′a-byoo-ten)

Mycobutin

Func. class.: Antimycobacterial agent

Chem. class.: Rifamycin S derivative

Do not confuse:
rifabutin/rifampin

ACTION: Inhibits DNA-dependent RNA polymerase in susceptible strains of *Escherichia coli* and *Bacillus subtilis;* mechanism of action against *Mycobacterium avium* unknown

USES: Prevention of *M. avium* complex (MAC) in patients with advanced HIV infection

Unlabeled uses: *Helicobacter pylori* that has not responded to other treatment

CONTRAINDICATIONS: Hypersensitivity, active TB, WBC <1000/mm^3 or platelet count <50,000/mm^3

Precautions: Pregnancy (B), breastfeeding, children, hepatic disease, blood dyscrasias

DOSAGE AND ROUTES

- **Adult: PO** 300 mg/day (may take as 150 mg bid); max 600 mg/day

Renal dose

- **Adult: PO** CCr <30 ml/min, reduce by 50%

Available forms: Caps 150 mg
Administer:
- With food if GI upset occurs; better to take on empty stomach 1 hr before or 2 hr after meals; high-fat foods slow absorption; may take in 2 divided doses, may open capsule, mix with applesauce if unable to swallow whole cap
- Antiemetic if vomiting occurs
- After C&S completed; monthly to detect resistance

SIDE EFFECTS

CNS: *Headache,* fatigue, anxiety, confusion, insomnia
GI: *Nausea, vomiting, anorexia, diarrhea,* heartburn, **hepatitis**, discolored saliva, pseudomembranous colitis
GU: *Discolored urine*
HEMA: Hemolytic anemia, eosinophilia, thrombocytopenia, leukopenia
INTEG: *Rash*
MISC: Flulike symptoms, shortness of breath, chest pressure
MS: Asthenia, arthralgia, myalgia

PHARMACOKINETICS

53% absorbed, peak 2-3 hr, duration >24 hr, half-life 45 hr, metabolized in liver (active/inactive metabolites), excreted in urine primarily as metabolites

INTERACTIONS

Increase: levels of rifabutin: ritonavir
Decrease: action of amprenavir, anticoagulants, β-blockers, barbiturates, busPIRone, clofibrate, corticosteroids, cycloSPORINE, dapsone, delavirdine, disopyramide, doxycycline, efavirenz, estrogens, fluconazole, indinavir, ketoconazole, losartan, nelfinavir, nevirapine, oral contraceptives, phenytoin, quiNIDine, saquinavir, sulfonylureas, theophylline, tricyclic antidepressants, zidovudine, zolpidem
Drug/Food
- High-fat diet decreases absorption

Drug/Lab Test
Interference: folate level, vit B_{12}, BSP, gallbladder studies

NURSING CONSIDERATIONS

Assess:

⚠ **Acute TB:** chest x-ray, sputum culture, blood culture, biopsy of lymph nodes, PPD; product should not be given for active TB
- CBC for neutropenia, thrombocytopenia, eosinophilia

⚠ **Pseudomembranous colitis:** diarrhea, abdominal pain/cramping, fever, bloody stools
- Signs of anemia: Hct, Hgb, fatigue
- Hepatic studies weekly: ALT, AST, bilirubin
- Renal status before, each mo: BUN, creatinine, output, specific gravity, urinalysis
- Hepatic status: decreased appetite, jaundice, dark urine, fatigue

Evaluate:
- Therapeutic response: not used for active TB because of risk for development of resistance to rifampin; culture negative

Teach patient/family:

⚠ That patients using oral contraceptives should consider using nonhormonal methods of birth control, may decrease effect; to notify prescriber if pregnancy planned, suspected
- That compliance with dosage schedule, duration necessary
- That scheduled appointments must be kept because relapse may occur
- That urine, feces, saliva, sputum, sweat, tears may be colored red-orange; soft contact lenses may be permanently stained

⚠ To report flulike symptoms: excessive fatigue, anorexia, vomiting, sore throat; unusual bleeding, yellowish discoloration of skin, eyes; myositis: muscle or bone pain; diarrhea, fever, abdominal cramping, bloody stools

R

rifampin (Rx)

(rif′am-pin)

Rifadin, Rofact ♣

Func. class.: Antitubercular

Chem. class.: Rifamycin B derivative

Do not confuse:
rifampin/rifabutin

ACTION: Inhibits DNA-dependent polymerase, decreases tubercle bacilli replication

USES: Pulmonary TB, meningococcal carriers (prevention)
Unlabeled uses: Endocarditis, *Haemophilus influenzae type B prophylaxis,* Hansen's disease, *Mycobacterium avium* complex (MAC), orthopedic-device–related infection, pruritus

CONTRAINDICATIONS: Hypersensitivity to this product, rifamycins; active *Neisseria meningitidis* infection
Precautions: Pregnancy (C), breastfeeding, children <5 yr, hepatic disease, blood dyscrasias

DOSAGE AND ROUTES

Tuberculosis

- **Adult: PO/IV** Max 600 mg/day as single dose 1 hr before meals or 2 hr after meals or 10 mg/kg/day 2-3×/wk
- **Child >5 yr: PO/IV** 10-20 mg/kg/day as single dose 1 hr before meals or 2 hr after meals, max 600 mg/day with other antituberculars
- **6-mo regimen:** 2 mo treatment of isoniazid, rifampin, pyrazinamide, and possibly streptomycin or ethambutol then rifampin and isoniazid 3 4 mo
- **9-mo regimen:** rifampin and isoniazid supplemented with pyrazinamide, streptomycin, or ethambutol

Meningococcal carriers

- **Adult: PO/IV** 600 mg bid × 2 days, max 600 mg/dose
- **Child >5 yr: PO/IV** 10-20 mg/kg × 2 days, max 600 mg/dose
- **Infant 3 mo-1 yr:** 5 mg/kg **PO** bid × 2 days

Prevention of *H. influenzae* type B infection (unlabeled)

- **Adult: PO** 600 mg/day × 4 days
- **Child: PO** 20 mg/kg/day × 4 days

MAC (unlabeled)

- **Adult: PO/IV** 600 mg/day used with ≥3 other active microbials
- **Child: PO/IV** 10-20 mg/kg/day used with ≥3 other active microbials

Endocarditis with prosthetic valves (unlabeled)

- **Adult: PO** 300 mg q8hr with gentamicin and vancomycin
- **Child: PO** 20 mg/kg/day in 2 divided doses with gentamicin and vancomycin, max 900 mg/day

Available forms: Caps 150, 300 mg; powder for inj 600 mg/vial

Administer:

- After C&S completed; monthly to detect resistance
- Do not give IM, SUBCUT

PO route

- On empty stomach, 1 hr before or 2 hr after meals with full glass of water
- Antiemetic if vomiting occurs
- Capsules may be opened, mixed with applesauce or jelly

Intermittent IV INF route

- After diluting each 600 mg/10 ml of sterile water for inj (60 mg/ml), swirl, withdraw dose and dilute in 100 ml or 500 ml of D_5W given as inf over 3 hr; if diluted in 100 ml, give over ½ hr; do not admix with other sol or products

Y-site compatibilities: amiodarone, bumetanide, midazolam, pantoprazole, vancomycin

SIDE EFFECTS

CNS: Headache, fatigue, anxiety, drowsiness, confusion
EENT: Visual disturbances
GI: *Nausea, vomiting, anorexia, diarrhea,* pseudomembranous colitis, *heartburn,* sore mouth and tongue, pancreatitis, increased LFTs

GU: Hematuria, acute renal failure, hemoglobinuria
HEMA: Hemolytic anemia, eosinophilia, thrombocytopenia, leukopenia
INTEG: *Rash, pruritus, urticaria*
MISC: *Flulike symptoms, menstrual disturbances, edema, SOB,* **Stevens-Johnson syndrome, toxic epidermal necrolysis, angioedema, anaphylaxis**
MS: *Ataxia, weakness*

PHARMACOKINETICS

PO: Peak 1-4 hr, duration >24 hr, half-life 3 hr, metabolized in liver (active/inactive metabolites), excreted in urine as free product (30% crosses placenta) and in breast milk

INTERACTIONS

⚠ Do not use with protease inhibitors
Increase: hepatotoxicity—isoniazid
Decrease: action of acetaminophen, alcohol, anticoagulants, antidiabetics, β-blockers, barbiturates, benzodiazepines, chloramphenicol, clofibrate, corticosteroids, cycloSPORINE, dapsone, digoxin, doxycycline, haloperidol, hormones, imidazole antifungals, NIFEdipine, oral contraceptives, phenytoin, protease inhibitors, theophylline, verapamil, zidovudine
Drug/Lab Test
Interference: folate level, vit B_{12}, gallbladder studies, dexamethasone suppression test
False positive: direct Coombs' test

NURSING CONSIDERATIONS

Assess:
- **Infection:** sputum culture, lung sounds, characteristics of sputum
- Signs of anemia: Hct, Hgb, fatigue
- Hepatic studies monthly: ALT, AST, bilirubin
- Renal status before, each mo: BUN, creatinine, output, specific gravity, urinalysis
- Hepatic status: decreased appetite, jaundice, dark urine, fatigue

⚠ **Serious skin reactions:** fever, sore throat, fatigue, ulcers; lesions in mouth, lips, rash; can be fatal
⚠ **Pseudomembranous colitis:** diarrhea, fever, abdominal pain/cramping, bloody stools, product should be discontinued, prescriber notified
Evaluate:
- Therapeutic response: decreased symptoms of TB, culture negative

Teach patient/family:
- That compliance with dosage schedule, duration necessary
- That scheduled appointments must be kept because relapse may occur
- To avoid alcohol because hepatotoxicity may occur
- That urine, feces, saliva, sputum, sweat, tears may be colored red-orange; that soft contact lenses may be permanently stained

⚠ To report flulike symptoms: excessive fatigue, anorexia, vomiting, sore throat; unusual bleeding; yellowish discoloration of skin, eyes; diarrhea with pus, mucous, blood
- To use nonhormonal form of birth control; to notify prescriber if pregnancy planned, suspected; not to breastfeed

rifapentine (Rx)

(riff′ah-pen-teen)
Priftin
Func. class.: Antitubercular
Chem. class.: Rifamycin derivative

ACTION:
Inhibits DNA-dependent polymerase, decreases tubercle bacilli replication

USES:
Pulmonary TB; must be used with at least one other antitubercular agent

CONTRAINDICATIONS:
Hypersensitivity to rifamycins, porphyria
Precautions: Pregnancy (C), breastfeeding, children <12 yr, geriatric pa-

R

tients, hepatic disease, blood dyscrasias, HIV

DOSAGE AND ROUTES

Intensive phase

• **Adult: PO** 600 mg (four 150-mg tabs) 2×/wk with an interval of 72 hr between doses × 2 mo; must be given with at least 1 other antitubercular agent

Continuation phase

• **Adult: PO** 600 mg q wk × 4 mo in combination with isoniazid or other appropriate antitubercular product

Available forms: Tabs 150 mg

Administer:

• May give with food for GI upset
• Antiemetic if vomiting occurs
• After C&S completed; monthly to detect resistance

SIDE EFFECTS

CNS: Headache, fatigue, anxiety, dizziness

EENT: Visual disturbances

GI: *Nausea, vomiting, anorexia, diarrhea,* bilirubinemia, hepatitis, increased ALT, AST, *heartburn,* pancreatitis, pseudomembranous colitis

GU: Hematuria, pyuria, proteinuria, urinary casts, urine discoloration

HEMA: Thrombocytopenia, leukopenia, neutropenia, lymphopenia, anemia, leukocytosis, purpura, hematoma

INTEG: Rash, pruritus, urticaria, acne

MISC: Increased B/P

MS: Gout, arthrosis

PHARMACOKINETICS

Peak 5-6 hr; half-life 13 hr; metabolized in liver (active/inactive metabolites); excreted in urine, feces, breast milk; protein binding 97%; steady state 10 days; CYP450 3A4, 2C8/9 inducer

INTERACTIONS

⚠ Do not use with protease inhibitors

Decrease: action of amitriptyline, anticoagulants, antidiabetics, barbiturates, β-blockers, chloramphenicol, clarithromycin, clofibrate, corticosteroids, cycloSPORINE, dapsone, delavirdine, diazepam, digoxin, diltiazem, disopyramide, doxycycline, fentaNYL, fluconazole, haloperidol, indinavir, itraconazole, ketoconazole, methadone, mexiletine, nelfinavir, NIFEdipine, nortriptyline, oral contraceptives, phenothiazines, phenytoin, progestins, quiNIDine, quiNINE, ritonavir, saquinavir, sildenafil, tacrolimus, theophylline, thyroid preparations, tocainide, verapamil, warfarin, zidovudine

Drug/Food

Increase: absorption with food

Drug/Lab Test

Interference: folate level, vit B_{12}

NURSING CONSIDERATIONS

Assess:

• Baselines of CBC, AST, ALT, bilirubin, platelets
• **Infection:** sputum culture, lung sounds
• Signs of anemia: Hct, Hgb, fatigue
• Hepatic studies monthly: ALT, AST, bilirubin
• Renal status monthly: BUN, creatinine, output, specific gravity, urinalysis
• Hepatic status: decreased appetite, jaundice, dark urine, fatigue

⚠ **Pseudomembranous colitis:** diarrhea, fever, abdominal pain/cramping, bloody diarrhea; discontinue if present, notify prescriber

Evaluate:

• Therapeutic response: decreased symptoms of TB, culture negative

Teach patient/family:

• That compliance with dosage schedule, duration necessary
• That scheduled appointments must be kept because relapse may occur
• That urine, feces, saliva, sputum, sweat, tears may be colored red-orange; that soft contact lenses, dentures may be permanently stained

⚠ To use alternative method of contraception; that oral contraceptive action may be decreased; to notify prescriber if pregnancy planned, suspected; to avoid breastfeeding

⚠ To report flulike symptoms: excessive fatigue, anorexia, vomiting, sore throat; unusual bleeding, yellowish discoloration of skin, eyes; diarrhea with pus, mucous, blood

rifaximin (Rx)

(rif-ax′i-min)

Xifaxan

Func. class.: Antiinfective—miscellaneous

Chem. class.: Analog of rifampin

Do not confuse:
rifaximin/rifampin

ACTION: Binds to bacterial-DNA–dependent RNA polymerase, thereby inhibiting bacterial RNA synthesis

USES: Traveler's diarrhea in those ≥12 yr caused by *E. coli,* hepatic encephalopathy
Unlabeled uses: Crohn's disease, diverticulitis

CONTRAINDICATIONS: Hypersensitivity to product, rifamycins; diarrhea with fever, blood in stool
Precautions: Pregnancy (C), breastfeeding, children, geriatric patients

DOSAGE AND ROUTES

Traveler's diarrhea
- **Adult and child ≥12 yr: PO** 200 mg tid × 3 days without regard to meals

Hepatic encephalopathy
- **Adult: PO** 550 mg bid

Crohn's disease (unlabeled)
- **Adult: PO** 200 mg tid × 16 wk

Diverticulitis (unlabeled)
- **Adult: PO** 400 mg bid with mesalamine 800 mg tid × 7 days then 7 days/mo

Irritable bowel syndrome (unlabeled)
- **Adult: PO** 550 mg tid × 14 day

Available forms: Tabs 200 mg
Administer:
- Without regard to food

SIDE EFFECTS

CNS: Abnormal dreams, dizziness, insomnia
CV: Hypotension, chest pain, peripheral edema
GI: *Abdominal pain, constipation, defecation urgency, flatulence, nausea, rectal tenesmus,* vomiting, ascites, **pseudomembranous colitis**
MISC: *Headache, pyrexia,* motion sickness, tinnitus, rash, photosensitivity, **exfoliative dermatitis**
MS: Arthralgia
RESP: Dyspnea, cough, pharyngitis

PHARMACOKINETICS

Half-life 1.8-4.5 hr, excreted in feces

NURSING CONSIDERATIONS

Assess:
- GI symptoms: amount, character of diarrhea; abdominal pain, nausea, vomiting, blood in stool

⚠ Overgrowth of infection, pseudomembranous colitis

Evaluate:
- Therapeutic response: absence of infection

Teach patient/family:

⚠ To discontinue rifaximin, notify prescriber if diarrhea persists >24-48 hr, if diarrhea worsens, or if blood in stools and fever present
- To avoid hazardous activities if dizziness occurs
- To notify prescriber if pregnancy planned, suspected
- That headache, rash, insomnia, abnormal dreams, tinnitus may occur

rilpivirine

See Appendix A—Selected new drugs

R

riluzole (Rx)

(rill'you-zole)

Rilutek

Func. class.: ALS agent

Chem. class.: Benzathiazole

ACTION: May act by modulating the release of glutamate and inactivating voltage-dependent sodium channels

USES: Amyotropic lateral sclerosis (ALS)

CONTRAINDICATIONS: Hypersensitivity

Precautions: Pregnancy (C), breastfeeding, children, geriatric patients, neutropenia, renal/hepatic disease, cigarette smoking, febrile illness, pneumonia

DOSAGE AND ROUTES

- **Adult: PO** 50 mg q12hr, take 1 hr before or 2 hr after meals

Available forms: Tabs 50 mg

Administer:

- 1 hr before or 2 hr after meals; high-fat meal decreases absorption

SIDE EFFECTS

CNS: Hypertonia, depression, dizziness, insomnia, somnolence, vertigo, paresthesia

CV: Hypertension, tachycardia, phlebitis, palpitation, postural hypertension

GI: Nausea, vomiting, dyspepsia, anorexia, diarrhea, flatulence, stomatitis, dry mouth, increased LFTs, jaundice, abdominal pain

GU: UTI, dysuria

HEMA: Neutropenia

INTEG: Pruritus, eczema, alopecia, exfoliative dermatitis

MS: Arthralgia

RESP: Decreased lung function, rhinitis, increased cough, pneumonia

PHARMACOKINETICS

Well absorbed; extensively metabolized by liver; excretion in urine, feces

INTERACTIONS

Increase: elimination of riluzole—cigarette smoking, rifampin, omeprazole, charcoal-broiled food

Increase: hepatic injury—allopurinol, methyldopa, sulfasalazine, leflunomide, methotrexate, tacrine

Increase: LFTs—barbiturates, carBAMazepine

Decrease: elimination of riluzole—caffeine, theophylline, amitriptyline, quinolones

Drug/Food

Decrease: absorption—high-fat meal

NURSING CONSIDERATIONS

Assess:

- Clinical improvement of neurologic function
- Hepatic studies: AST, ALT, bilirubin, GGT at baseline, monthly × 3 mo, then q3mo; monitor LFTs
- Neutropenia <500/mm

Evaluate:

- Therapeutic response: improvement in neurologic status

Teach patient/family:

- To report febrile illness, signs of infection, cardiac/respiratory changes, which may indicate neutropenia
- About the reason for the product, expected results

rimantadine (Rx)

(ri-man'tah-deen)

Flumadine

Func. class.: Synthetic antiviral

Chem. class.: Tricyclic amine

Do not confuse:
rimantadine/amantadine/ranitidine

ACTION: Prevents uncoating of nucleic acid in viral cell, thereby preventing the penetration of the virus to the host;

causes the release of dopamine from neurons

USES: Prophylaxis or treatment of influenza type A

CONTRAINDICATIONS: Hypersensitivity to this product, amantadine

Precautions: Pregnancy (C), breastfeeding, children <1 yr, seizure disorders, renal/hepatic disease

DOSAGE AND ROUTES

Influenza type A

Prophylaxis

- **Adult and child >10 yr: PO** 100 mg bid
- **Child 1-10 yr: PO** 5 mg/kg/day, max 150 mg

Treatment

- **Adult: PO** 100 mg bid; start treatment at onset of symptoms, continue for ≥1 wk
- **Child ≥10 yr (unlabeled): PO** 200 mg/day either as single dose or in 2 divided doses
- **Child 1-9 yr (unlabeled): PO** 6.6 mg/kg/day in 2 divided doses, max 150 mg/day in 2 divided doses
- **Geriatric: PO** 100 mg/day

Renal/hepatic dose

- **Adult: PO** ≤10 ml/min, 100 mg daily

Available forms: Tabs 100 mg; syr 50 mg/5 ml

Administer:

- Within 48 hr of exposure to influenza; continue for 10 days after contact
- At least 4 hr before bedtime to prevent insomnia
- After meals for better absorption, to decrease GI symptoms
- In divided doses to prevent CNS disturbances: headache, dizziness, fatigue, drowsiness

SIDE EFFECTS

CNS: *Headache, dizziness,* fatigue, depression, hallucinations, tremors, seizures, insomnia, poor concentration, asthenia, gait abnormalities, *anxiety,* confusion

CV: Pallor, palpitations, edema

EENT: Tinnitus, taste abnormality, eye pain

GI: *Nausea, vomiting,* constipation, *dry mouth, anorexia, abdominal pain,* diarrhea, dyspepsia

INTEG: Rash

PHARMACOKINETICS

PO: Peak 6 hr, elimination half-life 13-65 hr, plasma protein binding (40%)

INTERACTIONS

Increase: rimantadine concentration—cimetidine

Decrease: peak concentration of rimantadine—acetaminophen, aspirin; intranasal influenza vaccine (separate by ≥48 hr)

NURSING CONSIDERATIONS

Assess:

⚠ **Seizures;** if seizures occur, product should be discontinued

- Bowel pattern before, during treatment
- CNS effects in geriatric patients, patients with severe renal/hepatic disease
- Skin eruptions, photosensitivity after administration of product
- Respiratory status: rate, character, wheezing, tightness in chest
- Signs of infection

Perform/provide:

- Storage in tight, dry container

Evaluate:

- Therapeutic response: absence of fever, malaise, cough, dyspnea with infection

Teach patient/family:

- About aspects of product therapy: the need to report dyspnea, dizziness, poor concentration, behavioral changes
- To avoid hazardous activities if dizziness occurs

rimexolone ophthalmic

See Appendix B

R

risedronate (Rx)

(rih-sed′roh-nate)

Actonel, Atelvia

Func. class.: Bone resorption inhibitor

Chem. class.: Bisphosphonate

ACTION: Inhibits bone resorption, absorbs calcium phosphate crystal in bone, and may directly block dissolution of hydroxyapatite crystals of bone

USES: Paget's disease; prevention, treatment of osteoporosis in postmenopausal women; glucocorticoid-induced osteoporosis; osteoporosis in men

Unlabeled uses: Osteolytic metastases

CONTRAINDICATIONS: Hypersensitivity to bisphosphonates, inability to stand or sit upright for ≥30 min, esophageal stricture, achalasia, hypocalcemia

Precautions: Pregnancy (C), breastfeeding, children, renal disease, active upper GI disorders, dental disease, hyperparathyroidism, infection, vit D deficiency, coagulopathy, chemotherapy, asthma

DOSAGE AND ROUTES

Paget's disease

- **Adult: PO** 30 mg/day × 2 mo; patients with Paget's disease should receive calcium and vit D if dietary intake lacking; if relapse occurs, retreatment advised

Treatment/prevention of postmenopausal osteoporosis

- **Adult: PO** 5 mg/day or 35 mg/wk or 75 mg/day × 2 consecutive days 2× monthly or 150 mg/mo

Glucocorticoid osteoporosis

- **Adult: PO** 5 mg/day

Osteoporosis in men

- **Adult: PO** 35 mg/wk

Osteolytic metastases (unlabeled)

- **Adult: PO** 30 mg/day × 6 mo

Renal dose

- **Adult: PO** CCr <30 ml/min, avoid use

Available forms: Tabs 5, 30, 35, 150 mg; tab, gastro-resistant, weekly 35 mg; tab, weekly 35 mg

Administer:

- For 2 months to be effective for Paget's disease
- With a full glass of water; patient should be in upright position for ½ hr; swallow whole; do not crush, break, chew
- Supplemental calcium and vit D for Paget's disease if instructed by prescriber
- Give daily ≥30 min before meals or give weekly

SIDE EFFECTS

CNS: Dizziness, headache, depression

CV: *Chest pain,* hypertension, atrial fibrillation

GI: *Abdominal pain, diarrhea, nausea,* constipation, esophagitis

MISC: Rash, UTI, pharyngitis, hypocalcemia, hypophosphatemia, increase PTH

MS: Osteonecrosis of the jaw, severe muscle/joint/bone pain

SYST: Angioedema

PHARMACOKINETICS

Rapidly cleared from circulation, taken up mainly by bones (50%), eliminated primarily through kidneys, absorption decreased by food, terminal half-life 220 hr

INTERACTIONS

Increase: GI irritation—NSAIDs, salicylates

Decrease: absorption of risedronate—aluminum, calcium, iron, magnesium salts, antacids

Drug/Food

Decrease: bioavailability—take ½ hr before food or drinks other than water

Drug/Lab Test

Interference: bone-imaging agents

NURSING CONSIDERATIONS

Assess:

- **Paget's disease:** headache, bone pain, increased head circumference

- **Osteoporosis:** in men or postmenopausal women; bone density study before and periodically during treatment
- Phosphate, alk phos, calcium; creatinine, BUN (renal disease)
- **Hypocalcemia:** paresthesia, twitching, laryngospasm, Chvostek's/Trousseau's signs

⚠ **Serious skin reactions:** angioedema

- **Dental health:** assess dental health, provide antiinfectives for dental extraction; cover with antiinfectives before dental extraction

⚠ For atrial fibrillation

Perform/provide:

- Storage in cool environment, out of direct sunlight

Evaluate:

- Therapeutic response: increased bone mass, absence of fractures

Teach patient/family:

- To sit upright for ½ hr after dose to prevent irritation
- To comply with diet, vitamin/mineral supplements
- To notify prescriber if pregnancy is suspected or if breastfeeding
- To maintain good oral hygiene
- To notify all health care providers of use
- That musculoskeletal pain may occur within a few days/mo after starting but usually resolves; use acetaminophen
- To exercise regularly; to avoid alcohol, tobacco

risperidone (Rx)

(ris-pehr'ih-dohn)

Risperdal, Risperdal Consta, Risperdal M-TAB

Func. class.: Antipsychotic

Chem. class.: Benzisoxazole derivative

Do not confuse:
Risperdal/reserpine

ACTION: Unknown; may be mediated through both dopamine type 2 (D_2) and serotonin type 2 ($5\text{-}HT_2$) antagonism

USES: Irritability associated with autism, bipolar disorder, mania, schizophrenia

Unlabeled uses: Acute psychosis, agitation, ADHD, dementia, psychotic depression, Tourette's syndrome

CONTRAINDICATIONS: Hypersensitivity

Precautions: Pregnancy (C), children, geriatric patients, cardiac/renal/hepatic disease, breast cancer, Parkinson's disease, CNS depression, brain tumor, dehydration, diabetes, hematologic disease, seizure disorders, breastfeeding, abrupt discontinuation

Black Box Warning: Dementia

DOSAGE AND ROUTES

- **Adult: PO** 2 mg/day as single dose or in 2 divided doses, adjust dose at intervals of ≥24 hr and 1-2 mg/day as tolerated to 4-8 mg/day; **IM** establish dosing with **PO** before **IM** 25 mg q2wk, may increase to max 50 mg q2wk
- **Adolescent: PO** 0.5 mg/day in AM or PM, adjust dose at intervals of ≥24 hr and 0.5-1 mg/day as tolerated to 3 mg/day

R

• **Geriatric: PO** 0.5 mg daily-bid, increase by 1 mg/wk; **IM** 25 mg q2wk

Hepatic/renal dose

• **Adult: PO** 0.5 mg bid, increase by 0.5 mg bid, increase to 1.5 mg bid

Available forms: Tabs 0.25, 0.5, 1, 2, 3, 4 mg; oral sol 1 mg/ml; orally disintegrating tabs 0.5, 1, 2, 3, 4 mg; long-acting inj kit (Risperdal Consta) 12.5, 25, 37.5, 50 mg; oral sol 1 mg/ml (30 ml)

Administer:

• Reduced dose in geriatric patients

• Anticholinergic agent on order from prescriber, to be used for EPS

• Avoid use with CNS depressants

• Conventional tabs: give without regard to meals

• **Oral disintegrating tab** (Risperdal M-TAB): do not open blister pack until ready to use; tear 1 of the 4 units apart at perforation; bend corner where indicated; peel back foil; do not push tab through foil; remove from pack and place product on patient's tongue; tab disintegrates in seconds and can be swallowed with/without liquids

• **Oral sol:** dilute 3-4 oz of beverage, measure dose using calibrated pipette; not compatible with coffee, tea

IM route

• Only use diluent and needle provided; do not substitute, 1 needle is for deltoid use, 1 for gluteal, and are not interchangeable; allow to come to room temp, reconstitute powder using 2-ml prefilled syringe, shake vigorously, mixing is complete when susp is uniform, thick, milky colored; do not combine different strengths in single administration; invert vial and withdraw dose, attach supplied label to syringe for ID purpose, unscrew syringe from SmartSite Access Device, discard vial and access device; attach Needle-Pro device as directed, inj deep IM into upper-outer quadrant of gluteal muscle or deltoid, use within 2 min of reconstitution

• Do not give IV

• When switching from oral to inj, give oral dose with 1st inj, continue for 3 wk, then discontinue

SIDE EFFECTS

CNS: *EPS, pseudoparkinsonism, akathisia, dystonia, tardive dyskinesia; drowsiness, insomnia, agitation, anxiety, headache,* **seizures, neuroleptic malignant syndrome,** dizziness, **suicidal ideation,** head titubation (shaking)

CV: Orthostatic hypotension, **tachycardia; heart failure, sudden death (geriatric patients),** AV block

EENT: Blurred vision, tinnitus

GI: *Nausea,* vomiting, *anorexia, constipation,* jaundice, weight gain

GU: Hyperprolactinemia, gynecomastia, dysuria

HEMA: Neutropenia, granulocytopenia

MISC: Renal artery occlusion; weight gain, hyperprolactinemia (child)

MS: Rhabdomyolysis

RESP: Rhinitis; sinusitis, upper respiratory infection, cough

PHARMACOKINETICS

PO: Extensively metabolized by liver to major active metabolite, plasma protein binding 90%, peak 1-2 hr, excreted 90% in urine, terminal half-life 3-24 hr

INTERACTIONS

⚠ **Possible death in dementia-related psychosis: furosemide**

Increase: sedation—other CNS depressants, alcohol

⚠ **Increase: serotonin syndrome, neuroleptic malignant syndrome—CYP2D6 inhibitors (SSRIs, SNRIs)**

Increase: EPS—other antipsychotics

Increase: risperidone excretion—carBAMazepine

⚠ **Increase: QT prolongation—class IA/III antidysrhythmics, some phenothiazines, β-agonists, local anesthetics, tricyclics, haloperidol, methadone, chloroquine, clarithromycin, droperidol, erythromycin, pentamidine**

Decrease: risperidone action—CYP2D6 inducers (carBAMazepine, barbiturates, phenytoins, rifampin)
Decrease: levodopa effect—levodopa
Drug/Herb
Decrease: risperidone effect—echinacea
Drug/Lab Test
Increase: prolactin levels

NURSING CONSIDERATIONS

Assess:

⚠ **Suicidal thoughts/behaviors:** often when depression is lessened; mental status before initial administration

• Swallowing of PO medication; check for hoarding or giving of medication to other patients

• I&O ratio; palpate bladder if urinary output is low

• Bilirubin, CBC, hepatic studies monthly

• Urinalysis before, during prolonged therapy

• Affect, orientation, LOC, reflexes, gait, coordination, sleep pattern disturbances

⚠ **QT prolongation:** B/P standing, lying; pulse, respirations; take these q4hr during initial treatment; establish baseline before starting treatment; report drops of 30 mm Hg; watch for ECG changes

• Dizziness, faintness, palpitations, tachycardia on rising

• **EPS:** akathisia, tardive dyskinesia (bizarre movements of the jaw, mouth, tongue, extremities), pseudoparkinsonism (rigidity, tremors, pill rolling, shuffling gait)

⚠ **Serious reactions in geriatric patient:** fatal pneumonia, heart failure, sudden death, dementia

⚠ **Neuroleptic malignant syndrome:** hyperthermia, increased CPK, altered mental status, muscle rigidity, seizures, change in B/P, fatigue, tachycardia

• Constipation, urinary retention daily; if these occur, increase bulk, water in diet

• Weight gain, hyperglycemia, metabolic changes in diabetes

Perform/provide:

• Decreased stimuli by dimming lights, avoiding loud noises

• Supervised ambulation until patient stabilized on medication; do not involve patient in strenuous exercise program because fainting is possible; patient should not stand still for a long time

• Increased fluids to prevent constipation

• Sips of water, candy, gum for dry mouth

• Storage in tight, light-resistant container (PO); unopened vials in refrigerator, protect from light; do not freeze

Evaluate:

• Therapeutic response: decrease in emotional excitement, hallucinations, delusions, paranoia; reorganization of patterns of thought, speech

Teach patient/family:

• That orthostatic hypotension may occur; to rise from sitting or lying position gradually

• To avoid hot tubs, hot showers, tub baths because hypotension may occur

• To avoid abrupt withdrawal of product because EPS may result; product should be withdrawn slowly

• To avoid OTC preparations (cough, hay fever, cold) unless approved by prescriber; that serious product interactions may occur; to avoid use of alcohol because increased drowsiness may occur

• To avoid hazardous activities if drowsy or dizzy

• To comply with product regimen

• To report impaired vision, tremors, muscle twitching

• That heat stroke may occur in hot weather; to take extra precautions to stay cool

• To use contraception; to inform prescriber if pregnancy is planned or suspected

• To notify provider of suicidal thoughts/behaviors

TREATMENT OF OVERDOSE:

Lavage if orally ingested; provide airway; *do not induce vomiting*

R

ritonavir (Rx)

(ri-toe′na-veer)

Norvir

Func. class.: Antiretroviral

Chem. class.: Protease inhibitor

Do not confuse:
ritonavir/Retrovir

ACTION: Inhibits human immunodeficiency virus (HIV-1) protease and prevents maturation of the infectious virus

USES: HIV-1 in combination with at least 2 other antiretrovirals

CONTRAINDICATIONS: Hypersensitivity

Black Box Warning: Coadministration with other drugs

Precautions: Pregnancy (B), breastfeeding, hepatic disease, pancreatitis, diabetes, hemophilia, AV block, hypercholesterolemia, immune reconstitution syndrome, neonates, cardiomyopathy

DOSAGE AND ROUTES

- **Adult and adolescent >16 yr: PO** 600 mg bid; if nausea occurs, begin at 1/2 dose and gradually increase, max 1200 mg/day
- **Adolescent ≤16 yr and child, infant: PO** 400 mg/m^2 bid up to 1200 mg/day, may start lower and escalate

Available forms: Caps 100 mg; oral sol 80 mg/ml; tab 100 mg

Administer:

Tablet/capsule

- Take with food, swallow whole; do not crush, break, chew
- When switching from cap to tab, more GI symptoms may occur, will lessen over time
- Use dosage titration to minimize side effects
- **Oral sol:** shake well, use calibrated measuring device
- Mix liquid formulation with chocolate milk or liquid nutritional supplement to improve taste

SIDE EFFECTS

CNS: *Paresthesia, headache,* seizures, fever, dizziness, insomnia, asthenia, intracranial bleeding

CV: QT, PR interval prolongation

GI: *Diarrhea,* buccal mucosa ulceration, *abdominal pain, nausea, taste perversion,* dry mouth, *vomiting, anorexia*

INTEG: Rash

MISC: Asthenia, angioedema, anaphylaxis, Stevens-Johnson syndrome, increase lipids, lipodystrophy

MS: Pain, rhabdomyolysis, myalgia

PHARMACOKINETICS

Well absorbed, 98% protein binding, hepatic metabolism, peak 2-4 hr, terminal half-life 3-5 hr

INTERACTIONS

⚠ **Increase:** toxicity—amiodarone, astemizole, azole antifungals, benzodiazepines, buPROPion, CISapride, clozapine, desipramine, dihydroergotamine, encainide, ergotamine, flecainide, HMG-CoA reductase inhibitors, interleukins, meperidine, midazolam, pimozide, piroxicam, propafenone, propoxyphene, quiNIDine, ranolazine, saquinavir, terfenadine, triazolam, zolpidem

⚠ **Increase:** QT prolongation—class 1A/III antidysrhythmics, some phenothiazines, β-agonists, local anesthetics, tricyclics, haloperidol, chloroquine, droperidol, pentamidine, CYP3A4 inhibitors (amiodarone, clarithromycin, erythromycin, telithromycin, troleandomycin), arsenic trioxide, levomethadyl, CYP3A4 substrates (methadone, pimozide, QUEtiapine, quiNIDine, risperidone, ziprasidone)

Increase: ritonavir levels—fluconazole

Increase: level of both products—clarithromycin, ddI

Increase: levels of—bosentan

Decrease: ritonavir levels—rifamycins, nevirapine, barbiturates, phenytoin

Decrease: levels of anticoagulants, atovaquone, divalproex, ethinyl estradiol, lamotrigine, phenytoin, sulfamethoxazole, theophylline, voriconazole, zidovudine

Drug/Herb

Decrease: ritonavir levels—St. John's wort; avoid concurrent use

• Avoid use with red yeast rice

Drug/Lab Test

Increase: AST, ALT, CPK, cholesterol, GGT, triglycerides, uric acid

Decrease: Hct, Hgb, RBC, neutrophils, WBC

NURSING CONSIDERATIONS

Assess:

• **HIV:** viral load, CD4 at baseline, throughout therapy; blood glucose, plasma HIV RNA, serum cholesterol/lipid profile; resistance testing before starting therapy and after treatment failure

• Signs of infection, anemia

• Hepatic studies: ALT, AST

• Bowel pattern before, during treatment; if severe abdominal pain with bleeding occurs, discontinue product; monitor hydration

• Skin eruptions; rash

⚠ **Rhabdomyolysis:** muscle pain, increased CPK, weakness, swelling of affected muscles; if these occur and if confirmed by CPK, product should be discontinued

⚠ **QT prolongation:** ECG for QT prolongation, ejection fraction; assess for chest pain, palpitations, dyspnea

⚠ **Serious skin disorders:** Stevens-Johnson syndrome, angioedema, anaphylaxis

Perform/provide:

• Store caps in refrigerator

Evaluate:

• Therapeutic response: improvement in HIV symptoms; improving viral load, CD4+ T cells

Teach patient/family:

• To take as prescribed; if dose is missed, to take as soon as remembered up to 1 hr before next dose; not to double dose

• That product not a cure for HIV; that opportunistic infections may continue to be acquired

• That redistribution of body fat or accumulation of body fat may occur

• That others may continue to contract HIV from patient

• To avoid OTC, prescription medications, herbs, supplements unless approved by prescriber; not to use St. John's wort because it decreases product's effect

• That regular follow-up exams and blood work will be required

riTUXimab (Rx)

(rih-tuks'ih-mab)

Rituxan

Func. class.: Antineoplastic—miscellaneous; DMARDs

Chem. class.: Murine/human monoclonal antibody

ACTION: Directed against the CD20 antigen that is found on malignant B lymphocytes; CD20 regulates a portion of cell-cycle initiation/differentiation

USES: Non-Hodgkin's lymphoma (CD20 positive, B-cell), bulky disease (tumors >10 cm), rheumatoid arthritis, Wegener's granulomatosis, microscopic polyangitis

Unlabeled uses: Acquired blood factor deficiency, acute lymphocytic leukemia (ALL), Burkitt's lymphoma, chronic lymphocytic leukemia (CLL), hemolytic anemia, human herpesvirus 8, mantle cell lymphoma (MCL), multicentric Castleman's disease, peripheral blood stem cell (PBSC) mobilization, refractory pemphigus vulgaris, relapsing/remitting MS, ITP with dexamethasone

CONTRAINDICATIONS: Hypersensitivity, murine proteins

Precautions: Pregnancy (C), breastfeeding, children, geriatric patients, pulmonary/cardiac/renal conditions

Black Box Warning: Exfoliative dermatitis, infusion-related reactions, progressive multifocal leukoencephalopathy

DOSAGE AND ROUTES

Non-Hodgkin's lymphoma (NHL), chronic lymphocytic leukemia (CLL)

• **Adult: IV INF** 375 mg/m²/wk × 4 doses; give at 50 mg/hr for 1st inf; if hypersensitivity does not occur, increase rate by 50 mg/hr q½hr, max 400 mg/hr; slow/interrupt inf if hypersensitivity occurs; other inf can be given at 100 mg/hr and increased by 100 mg/hr, max 400 mg/hr

Rheumatoid arthritis; relapsing/remitting MS (unlabeled)

• **Adult: IV** 1000 mg on days 1, 15

Available forms: Inj 10 mg/ml

Administer:

Rheumatoid arthritis:

• Give methylPREDNISolone 100 mg or similar product 30 min before inf to decrease reactions

Intermittent IV INF route

• Hold antihypertensives 12 hr before administration

• After diluting to final conc of 1-4 mg/ml; use 0.9% NaCl, D_5W, gently invert bag to mix; do not mix with other products

Y-site compatibilities: Amcyclovir, amifostine, amikacin, aminophylline, ampicillin, ampicillin/sulbactam, aztreonam, bleomycin, bumetanide, buprenorphine, busulfan, butorphanol, calcium gluconate, CARBOplatin, carmustine, ceFAZolin, cefoperazone, cefotaxime, cefotetan, cefoxitin, ceftazidime, ceftizoxime, cefTRIAXone, cefuroxime, chlorproMAZINE, cimetidine, CISplatin, clindamycin, cyclophosphamide, cytarabine, DACTINomycin, DAUNOrubicin hydrochloride, dexamethasone, dexrazoxane, digoxin, diphenhydrAMINE, DOBUTamine, docetaxel, DOPamine, DOXOrubicin liposome, doxycycline, droperidol, enalaprilat, etoposide phosphate, famotidine, fentaNYL, filgrastim, floxuridine, fluconazole, fludarabine, fluorouracil, ganciclovir, gemcitabine, gentamicin, granisetron, haloperidol, heparin, hydrocortisone, HYDROmorphone, IDArubicin, ifosfamide, imipenem/cilastatin, irinotecan, leucovorin, levorphanol, LORazepam, magnesium sulfate, mannitol, meperidine, mesna, methotrexate, methylPREDNISolone, metoclopramide, metroNIDAZOLE, mitomycin, mitoxantrone, morphine, nalbuphine, netilmicin, paclitaxel, pentamidine, piperacillin/tazobactam, plicamycin, potassium chloride, prochlorperazine, promethazine, ranitidine, sargramostim, streptozocin, teniposide, theophylline, thiotepa, ticarcillin/clavulanate, tobramycin, trimethoprim/sulfamethoxazole, trimethobenzamide, vinBLAStine, vincCRIStine, vinorelbine, zidovudine

SIDE EFFECTS

CNS: Life-threatening brain infection (progressive multifocal leukoencephalopathy)

CV: Cardiac dysrhythmias, heart failure, hypertension, MI, supraventricular tachycardia, angina

GI: *Nausea, vomiting, anorexia,* GI obstruction/perforation

GU: Renal failure

HEMA: Leukopenia, neutropenia, thrombocytopenia, anemia

INTEG: *Irritation at site, rash,* fatal mucocutaneous infections (rare)

MISC: *Fever,* chills, asthenia, *headache,* angioedema, hypotension, myalgia, bronchospasm, ARDs

SYST: Toxic epidermal necrolysis, tumor lysis syndrome, Stevens-Johnson syndrome, exfoliative dermatitis

PHARMACOKINETICS

Half-life 60-174 hr, binds to CD20 sites or lymphoma cells

INTERACTIONS

Increase: bleeding—anticoagulants

• Avoid with vaccines, toxoids

NURSING CONSIDERATIONS

Assess:

⚠ **Fatal inf reaction:** hypoxia, pulmonary infiltrates, ARDS, MI, ventricular fibrillation, cardiogenic shock; most fatal reactions occur with 1st inf; potentially fatal

⚠ **Severe mucocutaneous reactions:** Stevens-Johnson syndrome, lichenoid dermatitis, toxic epidermal lysis; occur 1-13 wk after product given

⚠ **Tumor lysis syndrome:** acute renal failure requiring hemodialysis, hyperkalemia, hypocalcemia, hyperuricemia, hyperphosphatemia

⚠ **Multifocal leukoencephalopathy:** confusion, dizziness, lethargy, hemiparesis; monitor periodically

- CBC, differential, platelet count weekly; withhold product if WBC is <3500/mm^3 or platelet count <100,000/mm^3; notify prescriber of results; product should be discontinued
- ECG, serum creatinine/BUN, electrolytes, uric acid
- GI symptoms: frequency of stools
- **Dehydration:** rapid respirations, poor skin turgor, decreased urine output, dry skin, restlessness, weakness

Perform/provide:

- Increase fluid intake to 2-3 L/day for dehydration unless contraindicated
- Storage of vials at 36° F-40° F, protect vials from direct sunlight, inf sol is stable at 36° F-46° F × 24 hr and at room temp for another 12 hr

Evaluate:

- Therapeutic response: prevention of increasing cancer progression

Teach patient/family:

- To avoid use with vaccines, toxoids
- To use contraception during, for up to 12 mo after therapy

⚠ To report to prescriber possible infection (cough, fever, chills, sore throat), renal issues (painful urination, back/side pain), bleeding (gums, stools, urine, bruising, emesis, fatigue)

- To avoid OTC products
- To avoid crowds, those with known infections
- To maintain fluid intake

rivaroxaban

See Appendix A—Selected new drugs

rivastigmine (Rx)

(riv-as-tig′mine)

Exelon, Exelon Patch

Func. class.: Anti-Alzheimer agent

Chem. class.: Cholinesterase inhibitor

ACTION:
Potent, selective inhibitor of brain acetylcholinesterase (AChE) and butyrylcholinesterase (BChE)

USES:
Mild to moderate Alzheimer's dementia, mild to moderate Parkinson's disease dementia (PDD)

Unlabeled uses: Vascular dementia, dementia with Lewy bodies, Pick's disease

CONTRAINDICATIONS:
Hypersensitivity to this product, other carbamates

Precautions: Pregnancy (B), breastfeeding, children, respiratory/cardiac/renal/hepatic disease, seizure disorder, peptic ulcer, urinary obstruction, asthma, increased intracranial pressure, surgery, GI bleeding, jaundice

DOSAGE AND ROUTES

- **Adult: PO** 1.5 mg bid with food; after ≥4 wk, may increase to 3 mg bid; may increase to 4.5 mg bid and thereafter 6 mg bid, max 12 mg/day; **TRANSDERMAL** apply 4.6 mg/24 hr/day, after ≥4 wk may increase to 9.5 mg/24 hr/day

Available forms: Caps 1.5, 3, 4.5, 6 mg; sol 2 mg/ml; transdermal patch 4.6, 9.5 mg/24 hr

R

Administer:

- Oral sol, caps are interchangeable
- With meals; take with morning and evening meal even though absorption may be decreased
- Discontinue treatment for several doses, restart at same or next lower dosage level if adverse reactions cause intolerance
- If treatment is interrupted for more than several days, treatment should be initiated with lowest daily dose and titrated as indicated previously
- **Oral sol:** measure dose with supplied syringe; may be given undiluted or diluted in a small amount of water, fruit juice, or soda; stir diluted sol well, entire amount should be swallowed; stable for 4 hr when mixed

Transdermal route

- Once a day to hairless, clean, dry skin, not in an area that clothing will rub; rotate sites daily, do not apply to same site more than once q14days; remove liner; apply firmly; may be used during bathing, swimming; avoid saunas, excess sunlight or external heat such as saunas; each 5 cm^2 patch contains 9 mg base, rate of 4.6 mg/24 hr, each 10 cm^2 patch 18 mg base, rate of 9.5 mg/24 hr

SIDE EFFECTS

CV: QT prolongation, AV block, cardiac arrest, angina, MI, palpitations

CNS: *Tremors, confusion, insomnia,* psychosis, hallucination, depression, dizziness, headache, anxiety, somnolence, fatigue, syncope, EPS, exacerbation of Parkinson's disease

GI: *Nausea, vomiting, anorexia, abdominal distress, flatulence,* diarrhea, constipation, dyspepsia, colitis, eructation, fecal incontinence, GI bleeding/obstruction, GERD, gastritis, pancreatitis

MISC: Urinary tract infection, asthenia, increased sweating, hypertension, flulike symptoms, weight change

PHARMACOKINETICS

Rapidly and completely absorbed; metabolized to decarbamylated metabolite; half-life 1.5 hr; excreted via kidneys (metabolites); clearance lowered in geriatric patients, hepatic disease and increased with nicotine use; 40% protein binding

INTERACTIONS

Increase: synergistic effect—cholinergic agonists, other cholinesterase inhibitors

Increase: metabolism—nicotine

Increase: GI effects—NSAIDs

Decrease: rivastigmine effect—anticholinergics, sedating H_1 blockers, tricyclics, phenothiazines

NURSING CONSIDERATIONS

Assess:

- Hepatic studies: AST, ALT, alk phos, LDH, bilirubin, CBC
- **Severe GI effects:** nausea, vomiting, anorexia, weight loss, diarrhea
- B/P, heart rate, respiration during initial treatment; hypo/hypertension should be reported
- **Cognitive/mental status:** affect, mood, behavioral changes, depression, insomnia; complete suicide assessment

Perform/provide:

- Assistance with ambulation during beginning therapy; dizziness may occur

Evaluate:

- Therapeutic response: improved mood/cognition

Teach patient/family:

- About the procedure for giving oral sol; use instruction sheet provided; how to apply transdermal product, to fold in half and throw away, not to get in eyes, to wash hands after application; not to use heating pad, sauna, tanning bed
- To notify prescriber of severe GI effects
- That product may cause dizziness, anorexia, weight loss
- That effect may take weeks or months
- To notify prescriber if pregnancy is planned or suspected

rizatriptan (Rx)

(rye-zah-trip′tan)

Maxalt, Maxalt-MLT

Func. class.: Migraine agent

Chem. class.: 5-HT_{1D} receptor agonist, abortive agent-triptan

ACTION: Binds selectively to the vascular 5-$HT_{1B/1D}$ receptor subtype; exerts antimigraine effect; causes vasoconstriction of the cranial arteries

USES: Acute treatment of migraine

CONTRAINDICATIONS: Angina pectoris, history of MI, documented silent ischemia, Prinzmetal's angina, ischemic heart disease, concurrent ergotamine-containing preparations, uncontrolled hypertension, hypersensitivity, basilar or hemiplegic migraine

Precautions: Pregnancy (C), breastfeeding, children, geriatric patients, postmenopausal women, men >40 yr, risk factors for CAD, hypercholesterolemia, obesity, diabetes, impaired renal/hepatic function

DOSAGE AND ROUTES

- **Adult: PO** 5-10 mg single dose, redosing separated by ≥2 hr, max 30 mg/24 hr; use 5 mg for patient receiving propranolol, max 15 mg/24 hr

Available forms: Tabs (Maxalt) 5, 10 mg; orally disintegrating tabs (Maxalt-MLT) 5, 10 mg

Administer:

- **Orally disintegrating tab:** do not open blister until use; peel blister open with dry hands; place tab on patient's tongue, where it will dissolve, and have patient swallow with saliva (contains phenylalanine)

SIDE EFFECTS

CNS: *Dizziness, drowsiness, headache, fatigue,* warm/cold sensations, flushing

CV: **MI, ventricular fibrillation, ventricular tachycardia, coronary artery vasospasm,** palpitations, hypertension

ENDO: Hot flashes, mild increase in growth hormone

GI: *Nausea,* dry mouth, diarrhea, abdominal pain

RESP: Chest tightness, pressure, dyspnea

PHARMACOKINETICS

Onset of pain relief 10 min-2 hr; peak 1-1½ hr; duration 14-16 hr; 14% plasma protein binding; metabolized in liver (metabolite); excreted in urine (82%), feces (12%); half-life 2-3 hr

INTERACTIONS

⚠ Weakness, hyperreflexia, incoordination: SSRIs

Increase: levels of sibutramine

Increase: rizatriptan action—cimetidine, oral contraceptives, MAOIs, nonselective MAOI (type A and B), isocarboxazide, pargyline, phenelzine, propranolol, tranylcypromine

Increase: vasospastic effects—ergot, ergot derivatives, other 5-HT receptor agonists

Drug/Herb

⚠ Serotonin syndrome: St. John's wort

NURSING CONSIDERATIONS

Assess:

- **Migraine symptoms:** visual disturbances, aura, intensity, nausea, vomiting, photophobia
- Stress level, activity, recreation, coping mechanisms
- Neurologic status: LOC, blurring vision, nausea, vomiting, tingling in extremities preceding headache
- **Ingestion of tyramine foods** (pickled products, beer, wine, aged cheese), food additives, preservatives, colorings, artificial sweeteners, chocolate, caffeine, which may precipitate these types of headaches
- Renal status: urine output

R

Perform/provide:
- Quiet, calm environment with decreased stimulation: noise, bright light, excessive talking

Evaluate:
- Therapeutic response: decrease in frequency, severity of headache

Teach patient/family:
- **About use of orally disintegrating tab:** instruct patient not to open blister until use, to peel blister open with dry hands, to place tab on tongue, where it will dissolve, and to swallow with saliva (contains phenylalanine)
- To report any side effects to prescriber
- To use alternative contraception while taking product if oral contraceptives are being used
- That product does not prevent or reduce number of migraines; if 1st dose does not relieve pain, do not use more, notify prescriber

HIGH ALERT

rocuronium (Rx)

(ro-kyur-oh′nium)

Zemuron

Func. class.: Neuromuscular blocker (nondepolarizing)

Chem. class.: Biquaternary ammonium ester

ACTION: Inhibits transmission of nerve impulses by binding with cholinergic receptor sites, antagonizing action of acetylcholine

USES: Facilitation of endotracheal intubation; skeletal muscle relaxation during mechanical ventilation, surgery, or general anesthesia

CONTRAINDICATIONS: Hypersensitivity

Precautions: Pregnancy (C), breastfeeding, children, geriatric patients, electrolyte imbalances, dehydration, respiratory/neuromuscular/cardiac/renal/hepatic disease

DOSAGE AND ROUTES

- **Adult (intubation): IV** 0.6 mg/kg, max blockade within 4 min; median relaxation time 31 min; 0.45 mg/kg provides about 22 min of relaxation
- **Child 1-12 yr: IV** 0.6 mg/kg; onset 1 min; median relaxation time 27 min
- **Child 3 mo-1 yr: IV** 0.6 mg/kg; onset 1 min; median relaxation time 41 min

Rapid-sequence intubation
- **Adult/geriatric: IV** 0.6-1.2 mg/kg

Available forms: Inj 10 mg/ml

Administer:
- Using peripheral nerve stimulator by anesthesiologist to determine neuromuscular blockade; deep tendon reflexes should be monitored during extended use

Direct IV route
- Undiluted direct IV over 2 min (only by qualified person, usually anesthesiologist); do not administer IM
- Maintenance q20-45min after 1st dose; titrate to response

SIDE EFFECTS

CV: Bradycardia, tachycardia, change in B/P, edema

GI: Nausea, vomiting

INTEG: Rash, flushing, pruritus, urticaria

MS: Myopathy

RESP: Prolonged apnea, bronchospasm, cyanosis, respiratory depression, dyspnea, pulmonary vascular resistance

SYST: Tolerance

PHARMACOKINETICS

Terminal half-life 60-70 min, duration $^1/_2$ hr, metabolized in liver

INTERACTIONS

- Theophylline increases risk of dysrhythmias

Increase: neuromuscular blockade caused by amphotericin B, verapamil, aminoglycosides, clindamycin, enflurane, isoflurane, lincomycin, lithium, opiates, local anesthetics, polymyxin, antiinfectives, quiNIDine, thiazides

NURSING CONSIDERATIONS

Assess:

- Electrolyte imbalances (K, Mg), before product is used; may lead to increased action of product
- VS (B/P, pulse, respirations, airway) until fully recovered; rate, depth, pattern of respirations, strength of hand grip; patient should be intubated before use
- **Recovery:** decreased paralysis of face, diaphragm, leg, arm, rest of body; residual weakness, respiratory problems may occur during recovery
- Allergic reactions: rash, fever, respiratory distress, pruritus; product should be discontinued

Perform/provide:

- Storage in light-resistant area, refrigerate; stable for 30 days at room temp
- Reassurance if communication is difficult during recovery from neuromuscular blockade

Evaluate:

- Therapeutic response: paralysis of jaw, eyelid, head, neck, rest of body as evaluated by peripheral nerve stimulator

Teach patient/family:

- About all procedures or treatments; that patient will remain conscious if anesthesia is not also given

TREATMENT OF OVERDOSE:

Edrophonium or neostigmine, atropine, monitor VS; may require mechanical ventilation

roflumilast

See Appendix A—Selected new drugs

romiplostim (Rx)

(roe-mi-ploe′stim)

Nplate

Func. class.: Thrombopoietin receptor agonist

ACTION: Thrombopoietin-like fusion protein produced by DNA recombinant technology

USES: Chronic idiopathic thrombocytopenic purpura in patients who have had an insufficient response to corticosteroids, immunoglobulins, or splenectomy

CONTRAINDICATIONS: Hypersensitivity to this product or mannitol

Precautions: Pregnancy (C), breastfeeding, children, malignancies, bleeding, bone marrow suppression

DOSAGE AND ROUTES

- **Adult: SUBCUT** 1 mcg/kg/wk, increase weekly by 1 mcg/kg until platelets $\geq$50,000/mm^3, max 10 mcg/kg/wk

Available forms: Inj vials 250, 500 mcg

Administer:

SUBCUT route

- Use syringe with 0.01-ml graduations
- Discard any unused portion in vial; do not pool unused portions from vials
- Dilute 250 mcg/0.72 preservative-free sterile water for inj; 500 mcg/1.2 preservative-free sterile water for inj; final conc 500 mcg/ml
- Gently swirl until dissolved; do not shake
- Do not use if discolored or if particulate matter is present
- Inject into outer aspect of upper arm or abdomen except for 2 inches around navel or front aspect of middle thigh; do not use areas that are bruised, scratched, or scarred
- Rotate inj sites

R

SIDE EFFECTS

CNS: *Dizziness, insomnia, headache,* fatigue
GI: Abdominal pain, dyspepsia, diarrhea
HEMA: Thromboembolism, thrombosis, bleeding, myelofibrosis, erythromelalgia
MS: Myalgia
SYST: Secondary malignancy, antibody formation

PHARMACOKINETICS

Peak 7-50 hr, half-life 1-34 days

INTERACTIONS

• Possible bleeding risk: anticoagulants, NSAIDs, platelet inhibitors, thrombolytics, salicylates

NURSING CONSIDERATIONS

Assess:
• Blood studies: CBC during treatment weekly and for 2 wk after discontinuing
Perform/provide:
• Refrigerated storage of vials, do not freeze; protect from light; diluted sol is stable refrigerated or at room temp for 24 hr
Evaluate:
• Therapeutic response: increase in platelet counts, absence of bleeding
Teach patient/family:
• To report bleeding
• About the reason for product and expected results
• To report a missed dose to prescriber due to increased risk of bleeding

ropinirole (Rx)

(roh-pin′ih-role)
Requip, Requip XL
Func. class.: Antiparkinson agent
Chem. class.: DOPamine-receptor agonist, nonergot

ACTION:

Selective agonist for D_2 receptors (presynaptic/postsynaptic sites); binding at D_3 receptor contributes to antiparkinson effects

USES:

Parkinson's disease, restless leg syndrome (RLS)

CONTRAINDICATIONS:

Hypersensitivity
Precautions: Pregnancy (C), dysrhythmias, affective disorder, psychosis, cardiac/renal/hepatic disease

DOSAGE AND ROUTES

• **Adult: PO** 0.25 mg tid, titrate weekly to max 24 mg/day; (XL) 2 mg/day × 1-2 wk, may increase by 2 mg/day each wk
Restless leg syndrome
• **Adult: PO** 0.25 mg 1-3 hr before bedtime; may increase until symptoms resolve
Available forms: Tabs 0.25, 0.5, 1, 2, 3, 4, 5 mg; ext rel tab 2, 4, 8, 12 mg
Administer:
• Product until NPO before surgery
• Adjust dosage to patient response; taper when discontinuing
• With meals to reduce nausea
• *Extended release:* do not chew, crush, or divide

SIDE EFFECTS

CNS: *Agitation, insomnia,* psychosis, hallucination, dystonia, depression, dizziness, somnolence, **sleep attacks**, impulse control disorders
CV: *Orthostatic hypotension,* tachycardia, hypo/hypertension, syncope, palpitations
EENT: Blurred vision
GI: *Nausea, vomiting, anorexia, dry mouth,* constipation, dyspepsia, flatulence
GU: Impotence, urinary frequency
HEMA: Hemolytic anemia, leukopenia, agranulocytosis
INTEG: Rash, sweating
RESP: Pharyngitis, rhinitis, sinusitis, bronchitis, dyspnea

PHARMACOKINETICS

Peak 1-2 hr, half-life 6 hr, extensively metabolized by liver by P450 CYP1A2 enzyme system, protein binding 40%

INTERACTIONS

Increase: ropinirole effect—cimetidine, ciprofloxacin, diltiazem, enoxacin, erythromycin, fluvoxamine, mexiletine, norfloxacin, tacrine, digoxin, theophylline, L-dopa

Decrease: ropinirole effects—butyrophenones, metoclopramide, phenothiazines, thioxanthenes

NURSING CONSIDERATIONS

Assess:

- **Parkinsonism:** akinesia, tremors, staggering gait, muscle rigidity, drooling
- B/P, respirations during initial treatment; hypo/hypertension should be reported

⚠ **Sleep attacks:** drowsiness, falling asleep without warning even during hazardous activities

- Mental status: affect, mood, behavioral changes, depression; complete suicide assessment; worsening of symptoms in restless leg syndrome

Perform/provide:

- Testing for diabetes mellitus, acromegaly if patient receiving long-term therapy

Evaluate:

- Therapeutic response: improvement in movement disorder

Teach patient/family:

- That therapeutic effects may take several weeks to a few months
- To change positions slowly to prevent orthostatic hypotension
- To use product exactly as prescribed; if product is discontinued abruptly, parkinsonian crisis may occur
- That drowsiness, sleep attacks may occur; to avoid driving, other hazardous activities until response known
- To avoid alcohol, CNS depressants cough and cold products

⚠ To notify prescriber if unusual urges occur

ropivacaine (Rx)

(roe-pi′va-kane)

Naropin

Func. class.: Local anesthetic
Chem. class.: Amide

ACTION:

Competes with calcium for sites in nerve membrane that control sodium transport across cell membrane; decreases rise of depolarization phase of action potential

USES:

Peripheral nerve block, caudal anesthesia, central neural block; vaginal, epidural, spinal block

CONTRAINDICATIONS:

Children <12 yr, geriatric patients, hypersensitivity to amide local anesthetics, severe hepatic disease, severe hypotension, complete heart block

Precautions: Pregnancy (B), severe product allergies, hyperthyroidism, neurologic/CV/hepatic disease

DOSAGE AND ROUTES

Lumbar epidural block for cesarean section

- **Adult:** 20-30 ml of 0.5% sol
- **Adult:** 15-20 ml of 0.75% sol

Thoracic epidural

- **Adult:** 5-15 ml of 0.5% to 0.75% sol

Major nerve block

- **Adult:** 35-50 ml of 0.5% sol
- **Adult:** 10-40 ml of 0.75% sol

Labor pain (epidural)

- **Adult:** 10-20 ml 0.2% sol then 6-14 ml/1 hr

Postop (lumbar or thoracic epidural)

- **Adult:** 6-14 ml/hr of 0.2% sol

Infiltration/minor nerve block

- **Adult:** 1-100 ml of 0.2% sol
- **Adult:** 1-40 ml of 0.5% sol

Available forms: Inj 2, 5, 7.5 mg/ml

Administer:

- Only with crash cart, resuscitative equipment nearby

R

• Only products without preservatives for epidural or caudal anesthesia

SIDE EFFECTS

CNS: Anxiety, restlessness, **seizures, loss of consciousness,** drowsiness, disorientation, tremors, shivering, *paresthesia*
CV: **Myocardial depression, cardiac arrest, dysrhythmias,** bradycardia, *hypo/*hypertension, ***fetal bradycardia***
EENT: Blurred vision, tinnitus, pupil constriction
ENDO: Hypokelamia
GI: *Nausea, vomiting*
GU: Urinary retention
INTEG: Rash, urticaria, allergic reactions; edema, burning, skin discoloration at inj site; tissue necrosis
RESP: **Status asthmaticus, respiratory arrest, anaphylaxis**

PHARMACOKINETICS

Onset, duration vary with inj site; metabolized by liver, excreted in urine (metabolites)

INTERACTIONS

• Dysrhythmias: EPINEPHrine, halothane, enflurane
• Hypertension: MAOIs, tricyclics, phenothiazines
Increase: effect—amiodarone, cimetidine, ciprofloxacin, fluvoxamine, azole antifungals, theophylline, imipramine
Decrease: action of ropivacaine—chloroprocaine

NURSING CONSIDERATIONS

Assess:
• B/P, pulse, respirations during treatment
• Fetal heart tones during labor
• Allergic reactions: rash, urticaria, itching
• Cardiac status: ECG for dysrhythmias, pulse, B/P during anesthesia
Perform/provide:
• Use of new sol; discard unused portions
Evaluate:
• Therapeutic response: anesthesia necessary for procedure

TREATMENT OF OVERDOSE:

Airway, O_2, vasopressor, IV fluids, anticonvulsants for seizures

rosiglitazone (Rx)

(ros-ih-glit′ah-zone)
Avandia
Func. class.: Antidiabetic, oral
Chem. class.: Thiazolidinedione

ACTION: Improves insulin resistance by hepatic glucose metabolism, insulin receptor kinase activity, insulin receptor phosphorylation

USES: Type 2 diabetes mellitus, alone or in combination with sulfonylureas, metformin, insulin
Unlabeled uses: Increased ovulation frequency in those with polycystic ovary syndrome; reduced in-stent restenosis in those with diabetes

CONTRAINDICATIONS: Breastfeeding, children, hypersensitivity to thiazolidinediones, diabetic ketoacidosis, jaundice

Black Box Warning: NYHA III, IV acute heart failure, heart failure

Precautions: Pregnancy (C), geriatric patients, thyroid disease, renal/hepatic disease, heart failure, class I, II NYHA

Black Box Warning: MI

DOSAGE AND ROUTES

• **Adult: PO** 4 mg/day or in 2 divided doses, may increase to 8 mg/day or in 2 divided doses after 12 wk; may be added to metformin, sulfonylurea for adult dose
Available forms: Tabs 2, 4, 8 mg
Administer:
• Once or in 2 divided doses, without regard to food

• Tabs crushed and mixed with food or fluids for patients with difficulty swallowing

SIDE EFFECTS

CNS: Fatigue, *headache*
CV: **MI, CHF, death (geriatric patients)**
ENDO: Hypo/hyperglycemia
GI: Weight gain, **hepatotoxicity**, increase total, LDL, HDL cholesterol; decrease free fatty acids, diarrhea
MISC: Accidental injury, URI, sinusitis, anemia, back pain, diarrhea, edema, bone fractures (female)
SYST: **Anaphylaxis, Stevens-Johnson syndrome, lactic acidosis**

PHARMACOKINETICS

Maximal reductions in FBS after 6-12 wk; protein binding 99.8%; excreted in urine, feces; elimination half-life 3-4 hr; may be excreted in breast milk

INTERACTIONS

Increase: hypoglycemia—gemfibrozil
• Avoid concurrent use with insulin, nitrates
• May increase or decrease level: CYP2C5 inducer/inhibitors

Drug/Herb

Increase: antidiabetic effect—garlic, horse chestnut

NURSING CONSIDERATIONS

Assess:

⚠ **CHF: dyspnea, crackles, edema, weight gain ≥5 lb, jugular venous distention; may need to change dose or discontinue product**

⚠ **Lactic acidosis: dyspnea, abdominal pain, muscle pain; notify prescriber**

• Hypoglycemic reactions (sweating, weakness, dizziness, anxiety, tremors, hunger), hyperglycemic reactions soon after meals

⚠ **Systemic reactions: anaphylaxis, Stevens-Johnson syndrome, lactic acidosis**

⚠ **Hepatotoxicity: LFTs periodically AST, ALT (if ALT $>2.5 \times$ ULN, do not use product)**

• Fasting blood sugar, A1c, plasma lipids/lipoproteins, B/P, body weight during treatment

Perform/provide:

• Conversion from other oral hypoglycemic agents if needed; change may be made without gradual dosage change; monitor blood glucose during conversion
• Storage in tight container in cool environment

Evaluate:

• Therapeutic response: decrease in polyuria, polydipsia, polyphagia; clear sensorium; absence of dizziness; stable gait; blood glucose, A1c improvement

Teach patient/family:

• To monitor blood glucose; that periodic liver function tests mandatory; to report edema, weight gain
• About the symptoms of hypo/hyperglycemia, what to do about each
• That product must be continued on daily basis; about the consequences of discontinuing the product abruptly
• To avoid OTC medications, herbal preparations, nitrates, or insulin unless approved by prescriber
• That diabetes is lifelong; that product is not a cure, only controls symptoms
• That all food included in diet plan must be eaten to prevent hypoglycemia
• To carry emergency ID and glucagon emergency kit

⚠ **To report symptoms of hepatic dysfunction (nausea, vomiting, abdominal pain, fatigue, anorexia, dark urine, jaundice)**

• That 2 wk is needed to see reduction in blood glucose level and 2-3 mo needed to see full effect of product
• To notify prescriber if oral contraceptives are used
• Not to use if breastfeeding, may be secreted in breast milk
• That a medication guide should be dispensed with each prescription/refill

R

rosuvastatin (Rx)

(roe-soo′va-sta-tin)

Crestor

Func. class.: Antilipemic

Chem. class.: HMG-CoA reductase inhibitor

ACTION: Inhibits HMG-CoA reductase enzyme, which reduces cholesterol synthesis

USES: As an adjunct for primary hypercholesterolemia (types IIa, IIb) and mixed dyslipidemia, elevated serum triglycerides, homozygous/heterozygous familial hypercholesterolemia (FH), slowing of atherosclerosis, CV disease prophylaxis

Unlabeled uses: MI, stroke prophylaxis (normal LDL)

CONTRAINDICATIONS: Pregnancy (X), breastfeeding, hypersensitivity, active hepatic disease

Precautions: Children, geriatric patients, past hepatic disease, alcoholism, severe acute infections, trauma, hypotension, uncontrolled seizure disorders, severe metabolic disorders, electrolyte imbalances, severe renal impairment, hypothyroidism, Asian patients

DOSAGE AND ROUTES

Hypercholesterolemia

- **Adult: PO** 5-40 mg/day; initial dose 10 mg/day, reanalyze lipid levels at 2-4 wk, adjust dosage accordingly

Homozygous familial hypercholesterolemia

- **Adult: PO** 20 mg/day, max 40 mg

Dose in patients taking cycloSPORINE/gemfibrozil/lopinavir/ritonavir/atazanavir

- **Adult: PO** 5 mg/day, max 10 mg/day

Asian patients/patients with predisposition for myopathy

- **Adult: PO** 5 mg/day

Atherosclerosis slowing

- **Adult: PO** 10 mg/day (for those not taking cycloSPORINE or gemfibrozil)

Heterozygous familial hypercholesterolemia

- **Females ≥1 yr postmenarche and ≥10 yr) and males ≥10 yr: PO** 5-20 mg/day individualized

MI/stroke prophylaxis (unlabeled)

- **Adult: PO** 20 mg daily

Renal/hepatic dose

- **Adult: PO** CCr <30 ml/min, 5 mg/day; max 10 mg/day; avoid use with hepatic disease

Available forms: Tabs 5, 10, 20, 40 mg

Administer:

- May be taken at any time of day, with/without food

SIDE EFFECTS

CNS: *Headache, dizziness,* insomnia, paresthesia

GI: *Nausea, constipation, abdominal pain, flatus, diarrhea, dyspepsia, heartburn,* **kidney failure, liver dysfunction,** vomiting

HEMA: Thrombocytopenia, hemolytic anemia, leukopenia

INTEG: *Rash, pruritus*

MS: *Asthenia, muscle cramps, arthritis, arthralgia, myalgia,* **myositis, rhabdomyolysis;** leg, shoulder, or localized pain

RESP: Rhinitus, sinusitis, *pharyngitis,* increased cough

PHARMACOKINETICS

Peak 3-5 hr, minimal live metabolism (about 10%), 88% protein bound, excreted primarily in feces (90%), crosses placenta, half-life 19 hr, not dialyzable

INTERACTIONS

Increase: hepatotoxicity—alcohol

Increase: rosuvastatin effect—bile acid sequestrants

⚠ **Increase: myalgia, myositis, rhabdomyolysis—cycloSPORINE, gemfibrozil, niacin, clofibrate, azole antifungals, anti-**

retroviral protease inhibitors, fibric acid derivatives
Increase: bleeding risk—warfarin
Drug/Lab Test
Increase: LFTs

NURSING CONSIDERATIONS

Assess:
- Diet; obtain diet history including fat, cholesterol in diet
- Fasting cholesterol, LDL, HDL, triglycerides at baseline and q4-6wk, then periodically
- LFTs at baseline, 12 wk, then q6mo; AST, ALT, LFTs may increase
- Renal function in patients with compromised renal system: BUN, creatinine, I&O ratio

⚠ **Rhabdomyolysis:** muscle pain, tenderness, obtain CPK; if these occur, product may need to be discontinued; for patients with Asian ancestry: increased blood levels, rhabdomyolysis

Perform/provide:
- Storage in cool environment in airtight, light-resistant container

Evaluate:
- Therapeutic response: decreased LDL, cholesterol, triglycerides, increased HDL, slowing CAD

Teach patient/family:

⚠ To report suspected pregnancy; to use contraception while taking product, pregnancy category (X); not to breastfeed

⚠ To report weakness, muscle tenderness, pain, fever
- That blood work and follow-up exams will be necessary during treatment
- To report severe GI symptoms, dizziness, headache, muscle pain, weakness
- That previously prescribed regimen will continue: low-cholesterol diet, exercise program, smoking cessation

rufinamide (Rx)

(roo-fin′a-mide)

Banzel

Func. class.: Anticonvulsant
Chem. class.: Triazole derivative

ACTION: May act through action at sodium channels; exact action is unknown

USES: Lennox-Gastaut syndrome
Unlabeled uses: Partial seizures

CONTRAINDICATIONS: Hypersensitivity, familial short QT syndrome
Precautions: Pregnancy (C), breastfeeding, children <16 yr, geriatric patients, renal/hepatic disease, depression, dialysis, hazardous activities, suicidal ideation

DOSAGE AND ROUTES

- **Adult: PO** 400-800 mg/day divided bid, increase by 400-800 mg/day q2days to 3200 mg/day
- **Child ≥4 yr: PO** 10 mg/kg/day divided equally bid; increase by 10 mg/kg/day every other day to 45 mg/kg/day or 3200 mg/day, whichever is less

Available forms: Tabs 200, 400 mg; oral susp 40 mg/ml
Administer:
- **PO tabs:** give with food; may give whole, crushed, or halved
- **Oral susp:** shake well before use, use provided adapter and calibrated oral dosing syringe, insert adapter firmly in neck of botte before use, keep in place for duration of bottle use; insert dosing syringe into adapter, withdraw dose from inverted bottle; replace cap after each use, use within 90 days of opening, give with food

SIDE EFFECTS

CNS: Dizziness, ataxia, drowsiness, fever, seizures, tremor, fatigue, headache, gait disturbance

R

EENT: Diplopia, blurred vision, nystagmus
GI: Nausea, hepatitis, vomiting
HEMA: Anemia, leukopenia, neutropenia, thrombocytopenia, lymphadenopathy
INTEG: Rash, urticaria
MISC: Edema, hematuria, influenzae, nephrolithiasis

PHARMACOKINETICS

Peak 4-6 hr, half-life 6-10 hr, metabolized by liver, excreted by kidneys, 34% protein binding

INTERACTIONS

Increase: rufinamide effect—valproate
Decrease: effect of hormonal contraceptives
Decrease: effect of rufinamide—carBAMazepine, phenytoin, primidone, PHENobarbital
Drug/Lab Test
Increase: LFTs

NURSING CONSIDERATIONS

Assess:

• **Seizures:** duration, type, intensity precipitating factors

⚠ **Mental status: mood, sensorium, affect, memory (long, short), increased suicidal thoughts/actions**

Evaluate:

• Therapeutic response: decrease in severity of seizures

Teach patient/family:

• Not to discontinue product abruptly because seizures may occur
• To avoid hazardous activities until stabilized on product
• To carry emergency ID stating product use
• To notify prescriber if pregnancy is planned or suspected; to use alternative form of contraception because effect of hormonal contraceptives may be decreased
• To consume adequate fluids

salicylic acid topical

See Appendix B

salmeterol (Rx)

(sal-met′er-ole)

Serevent ♣, Serevent Diskus

Func. class.: β_2-Adrenergic agonist, bronchodilator

ACTION: Causes bronchodilation by action on β_2 (pulmonary) receptors by increasing levels of cAMP, which relaxes smooth muscle with very little effect on heart rate; maintains improvement in FEV from 3 to 12 hr; prevents nocturnal asthma symptoms

USES: Prevention of exercise-induced bronchospasm, COPD, asthma

CONTRAINDICATIONS: Hypersensitivity to sympathomimetics, tachydysrhythmias, severe cardiac disease, monotherapy treatment of asthma
Precautions: Pregnancy (C), breastfeeding, cardiac disorders, hyperthyroidism, diabetes mellitus, hypertension, closed-angle glaucoma, seizures, acute asthma, as a substitute to corticosteroids, QT prolongation

Black Box Warning: Asthma-related death

DOSAGE AND ROUTES

• **Adult/child ≥4 yr: INH** 50 mcg (1 inhalation as dry powder) q12hr; exercise-induced bronchospasm 50 mcg (1 inhalation) ½-1 hr before exercise

Available forms: Inhalation powder 50 mcg/blister

Administer:

• Gum, sips of water for dry mouth

SIDE EFFECTS

CNS: *Tremors, anxiety,* insomnia, headache, dizziness, fever

CV: Palpitations, tachycardia, hypo/hypertension, angina, dysrhythmias
EENT: Dry nose, irritation of nose and throat
GI: Heartburn, nausea, vomiting, abdominal pain
MS: Muscle cramps
RESP: Bronchospasm, cough

PHARMACOKINETICS

INH: Onset 30-50 min; peak 4 hr; duration 12 hr; metabolized in liver; excreted in urine, breast milk; crosses placenta, blood-brain barrier; protein binding 94%-98%; terminal half-life 3-5 hr

INTERACTIONS

Increase: CV effect—CYP3A4 inhibitors (itraconazole, ketoconazole, nelfinavir, nefazodone, saquinavir)
Increase: action of aerosol bronchodilators
Increase: action of salmeterol—tricyclics, MAOIs
Decrease: salmeterol action—other β-blockers

NURSING CONSIDERATIONS

Assess:
- **Respiratory function:** vital capacity, forced expiratory volume, ABGs, lung sounds, heart rate and rhythm

⚠ **Paradoxical bronchospasm:** dyspnea, wheezing, chest tightness

Perform/provide:
- Storage in foil pouch; do not expose to temp >86° F (30° C); discard 6 wk after removal from foil pouch

Evaluate:
- Therapeutic response: absence of dyspnea, wheezing

Teach patient/family:
- Not to use for exercise-induced bronchospasm, never to exhale into diskus, to hold level, keep mouthpiece dry
- Not to use OTC medications because extra stimulation may occur
- Review package insert with patient
- To avoid getting powder in eyes
- To avoid smoking, smoke-filled rooms, persons with respiratory infections
- Not for treatment of acute exacerbation, a fast-acting b-blocker should be used instead

⚠ To immediately report dyspnea after use if ≥1 canister is used in 2 mo time

TREATMENT OF OVERDOSE:

β_2-Adrenergic blocker

salsalate (Rx)

(sal′sah-late)
Func. class.: Nonopioid analgesic, nonsteroidal antiinflammatory
Chem. class.: Salicylate

ACTION: Blocks formation of peripheral prostaglandins, which cause pain and inflammation; antipyretic action results from the inhibition of the hypothalamic heat-regulating center; does not inhibit platelet aggregation

USES: Mild to moderate pain or fever, including arthritis (osteoarthritis, rheumatoid arthritis)

CONTRAINDICATIONS: Children <3 yr; hypersensitivity to salicylates, NSAIDs; GI bleeding, bleeding disorders; vit K deficiency
Precautions: Pregnancy (C) 1st trimester, breastfeeding, geriatric patients, anemia, renal/hepatic disease, Hodgkin's disease

DOSAGE AND ROUTES

- **Adult: PO** 3 g/day in 2-3 divided doses

Available forms: Tabs 500, 750 mg
Administer:
- With food or milk to decrease gastric symptoms

SIDE EFFECTS

CNS: Stimulation, drowsiness, dizziness, confusion, **seizures**, headache, flushing, hallucinations, **coma**
CV: Rapid pulse, **pulmonary edema**
EENT: Tinnitus, hearing loss

ENDO: Hypoglycemia, hyponatremia, hypokalemia, alteration in acid-base balance
GI: *Nausea, vomiting, GI bleeding, diarrhea, heartburn,* anorexia, hepatotoxicity
HEMA: Thrombocytopenia, agranulocytosis, leukopenia, neutropenia, hemolytic anemia, increased PT
INTEG: *Rash,* urticaria, bruising, exfoliative dermatitis, Stevens-Johnson syndrome, toxic epidermal necrolysis, anaphylaxis, laryngeal edema
RESP: Wheezing, hyperpnea

PHARMACOKINETICS

Full benefit 3-4 days, metabolized by liver, excreted by kidneys, half-life 1 hr, highly protein bound, crosses blood-brain barrier and placenta slowly

INTERACTIONS

Increase: bleeding risk—alcohol, heparin, NSAIDs, warfarin, SSRIs, SNRIs
Increase: effects of anticoagulants, insulin, methotrexate, probenecid, penicillins, phenytoin, NSAIDs, thrombolytics, platelet inhibitors
Decrease: effects of spironolactone, sulfinpyrazone, sulfonamides, loop diuretics
Decrease: effects of salsalate—antacids, corticosteroids, urinary alkalizers
Decrease: blood glucose levels—salicylates

Drug/Food

• Foods that cause acidic urine may increase salsalate levels

Drug/Lab Test

Increase: coagulation studies, hepatic studies, serum uric acid, amylase, CO_2, urinary protein
Decrease: serum potassium, cholesterol, blood glucose
Interference: urine catecholamines, pH, pregnancy test

NURSING CONSIDERATIONS

Assess:

• **Pain:** frequency, intensity, characteristics; relief of pain after medication
⚠ Asthma, aspirin hypersensitivity, nasal polyps; may develop hypersensitivity to product
• **Fever:** monitor temp, sweating/chills
• Renal studies: BUN, urine creatinine with long-term therapy
• Blood studies: CBC, Hct, Hgb, PT, stool guaiac, serum salicylate with long-term therapy
• I&O ratio; decreasing output may indicate renal failure with long-term therapy
⚠ **Hepatotoxicity:** dark urine, clay-colored stools; jaundiced skin, sclera; itching, abdominal pain, fever, diarrhea with long-term therapy; hepatic studies: AST, ALT, bilirubin with long-term therapy
⚠ **Serious skin reactions; allergic reactions:** exfoliative dermatitis, Stevens-Johnson syndrome, toxic epidermal necrolysis, anaphylaxis; rash, urticaria; product may have to be discontinued
⚠ **Ototoxicity:** tinnitus, ringing, roaring in ears; audiometric testing needed before, after long-term therapy
• Visual changes
• Edema in feet, ankles, legs
• Product history; many interactions

Evaluate:

• Therapeutic response: decreased pain, fever

Teach patient/family:

⚠ To report any symptoms of hepatotoxicity, renal toxicity, visual changes, ototoxicity, allergic reactions with long-term therapy
• Not to exceed recommended dosage; acute poisoning may result
• That therapeutic response takes 2 wk (arthritis)
• To avoid alcohol ingestion because GI bleeding may occur; to read label on other OTC products; many contain aspirin and should be avoided
• To watch for signs of bleeding: dark stools

TREATMENT OF OVERDOSE:

Lavage, activated charcoal, monitor electrolytes, VS

saquinavir (Rx)

(sa-quen′ah-veer)

Invirase

Func. class.: Antiretroviral

Chem. class.: Protease inhibitor

ACTION:
Inhibits human immunodeficiency virus (HIV-1) protease, which prevents maturation of the infectious virus

USES:
HIV-1 in combination with other antiretrovirals

CONTRAINDICATIONS:
Hypersensitivity

Precautions: Pregnancy (B), breastfeeding, children, hepatic disease, diabetes, pancreatitis, immune reconstitution syndrome, hemophilia, hyperlipidemia

DOSAGE AND ROUTES

- **Adult: PO** 1000 mg bid with 100 mg bid ritonavir

Available forms: Caps 200 mg; tab 500 mg

Administer:

- Within 2 hr of meal

SIDE EFFECTS

CNS: *Paresthesia,* headache, **seizures**

CV: QT/PR prolongation, 2nd/3rd degree AV block, torsades de pointes

GI: *Diarrhea,* buccal mucosa ulceration, *abdominal pain, nausea,* vomiting

INTEG: *Rash*

MISC.: Asthenia, hyperglycemia, **Stevens-Johnson syndrome**

MS: Pain

PHARMACOKINETICS

Absorption increased with food, protein binding 98%, extensive 1st-pass hepatic metabolism, terminal half-life 12 hr

INTERACTIONS

- Avoid use with HMG-CoA reductase inhibitors

Increase: toxicity—ergots, midazolam, triazolam, dapsone, quiNIDine, calcium channel blockers, clindamycin

⚠ **Increase: vasoconstriction—ergots, do not use concurrently**

⚠ **Increase: CNS depression—midazolam, triazolam, do not use concurrently**

⚠ **Increase: QT prolongation—ritonavir with amiodarone, dofetilide, lovastatin, simvastatin**

Increase: saquinavir levels—ketoconazole, indinavir, delaviridine, nelfinavir, ritonavir, clarithromycin

Decrease: saquinavir levels—rifamycins, carBAMazepine, PHENobarbital, phenytoin, nevirapine, dexamethasone

Drug/Herb

- St. John's wort, garlic may decrease saquinavir levels; avoid concurrent use

Drug/Food

Increase: bioavailability after high-fat meal; grapefruit juice increases levels

Drug/Lab Test

- Interference: CPK, glucose

NURSING CONSIDERATIONS

Assess:

- Signs of infection, anemia
- Blood glucose, viral load, CD4+ T-cell count, plasma HIV RNA, serum cholesterol/lipid profile
- Resistance testing at start of therapy and at treatment failure
- Hepatic studies: ALT, AST
- C&S before product therapy; product may be taken as soon as culture is taken; repeat C&S after treatment; determine presence of other sexually transmitted diseases

⚠ **QT/PR prolongation, 2nd/3rd degree AV block, torsades de pointes; monitor ECG for changes**

- Bowel pattern before, during treatment; if severe abdominal pain with bleeding occurs, product should be discontinued; monitor hydration

S

⚠ **Serious skin disorders:** Stevens-Johnson syndrome; skin eruptions, rash, urticaria, itching
• Allergies before treatment, reaction of each medication

Teach patient/family:
• To take as prescribed within 2 hr of full meal; if dose is missed, to take as soon as remembered up to 1 hr before next dose; not to double dose
• That product must be taken in equal intervals to maintain blood levels for duration of therapy; that product is not a cure
• To take precautions to prevent transmission
• That there are significant product interactions

sargramostim (Rx)
(sar-gram′oh-stim)
Leukine, GM-CSF
Func. class.: Biologic modifier
Chem. class.: Granulocyte macrophage colony-stimulating factor (GM-CSF)

Do not confuse:
Leukine/leucovorin/Leukeran

ACTION: Stimulates proliferation and differentiation of hematopoietic progenitor cells (granulocytes, macrophages)

USES: Acceleration of myeloid recovery in patients with non-Hodgkin's lymphoma, acute lymphoblastic leukemia, acute myelogenous leukemia, autologous bone marrow transplantation in Hodgkin's disease; bone marrow transplantation failure or engraftment delay, mobilization and transplant of peripheral blood progenitor cells (PBPCs)
Unlabeled uses: Aplastic anemia, Crohn's disease, HIV, ganciclovir- or zidovudine-induced neutropenia, malignant melanoma

CONTRAINDICATIONS: Neonates; hypersensitivity to GM-CSF, benzyl alcohol, yeast products; excessive leukemic myeloid blast in bone marrow, peripheral blood
Precautions: Pregnancy (C), breastfeeding, children; lung/cardiac/renal/hepatic disease; pleural, pericardial effusions, peripheral edema, leukocytosis, mannitol hypersensitivity, hepatic/renal disease

DOSAGE AND ROUTES

Myeloid reconstitution after autologous bone marrow transplantation
• **Adult: IV** 250 mcg/m^2/day × 3 wk; give over 2 hr, begin 2-4 hr after bone marrow inf, not <24 hr after last dose of antineoplastics and 12 hr after last dose of radiotherapy, bone marrow transplantation failure, or engraftment delay

Acceleration of myeloid recovery
• **Adult: IV** 250 mcg/m^2/day × 14 days; give over 2 hr; may repeat in 7 days, may repeat 500 mcg/m^2/day × 14 days after another 7 days if no improvement

Mobilization of PBPCs
• **Adult: IV/SUBCUT** 250 mcg/m^2/day during collection of PBPCs

After PBPC transplantation
• **Adult: IV/SUBCUT** 250 mcg/m^2/day until ANC >1500 cells/mm^3 × 3 days

Aplastic anemia (unlabeled)
• **Adult: SUBCUT** 250-500 mcg/day or 5 mcg/kg/day × 14-90 days, used with erythropoietin or immunosuppressive therapy

Malignant melanoma (unlabeled)
• **Adult: SUBCUT** 125 mcg/m^2/day × 14 days, alternate with 14 days off

HIV (unlabeled)
• **Adult: SUBCUT** 250 mcg/day 3×/wk for ≤20 mo

Available forms: Powder for inj lyophilized 250 mcg

Administer:

SUBCUT route

• No further dilution of reconstituted sol is needed; take care not to inject intradermally

Intermittent IV INF route

• After reconstituting with 1 ml sterile water for inj without preservative; do not reenter vial; discard unused portion; direct reconstitution sol at side of vial; rotate contents; do not shake

• Dilute in 0.9% NaCl inj to prepare IV inf; if final concentration is <10 mcg/ml, add human albumin to make final conc of 0.1% to NaCl before adding sargramostim to prevent adsorption; for a final conc of 0.1% albumin, add 1 mg human albumin/1 ml 0.9% NaCl inj run over 2 hr **(bone marrow transplant or failure of graft)**; over 4 hr **(chemotherapy for AML)**; over 24 hr as cont inf **(PBPCs)**; give within 6 hr after reconstitution

Y-site compatibilities: Amikacin, aminophylline, aztreonam, bleomycin, butorphanol, calcium gluconate, CARBOplatin, carmustine, ceFAZolin, cefepime, cefotaxime, cefotetan, ceftizoxime, cefTRIAXone, cefuroxime, cimetidine, CISplatin, clindamycin, cyclophosphamide, cycloSPORINE, cytarabine, dacarbazine, DACTINomycin, dexamethasone, diphenhydrAMINE, DOPamine, DOXOrubicin, doxycycline, droperidol, etoposide, famotidine, fentaNYL, floxuridine, fluconazole, fluorouracil, furosemide, gentamicin, granisetron, heparin, IDArubicin, ifosfamide, immune globulin, magnesium sulfate, mannitol, mechlorethamine, meperidine, mesna, methotrexate, metoclopramide, metroNIDAZOLE, minocycline, mitoxantrone, netilmicin, pentostatin, piperacillin/tazobactam, potassium chloride, prochlorperazine, promethazine, ranitidine, teniposide, ticarcillin, ticarcillin-clavulanate, trimethoprim-sulfamethoxazole, vinBLAStine, vinCRIStine, zidovudine

SIDE EFFECTS

CNS: Fever, malaise, CNS disorder, weakness, chills, dizziness, syncope, headache

CV: **Transient supraventricular tachycardia**, peripheral edema, **pericardial effusion**, hypotension, tachycardia

GI: Nausea, vomiting, diarrhea, anorexia, **GI hemorrhage**, stomatitis, **liver damage**, hyperbilirubinemia

GU: Urinary tract disorder, abnormal kidney function

HEMA: **Blood dyscrasias, hemorrhage**

INTEG: Alopecia, rash, peripheral edema

MS: Bone pain, myalgia

RESP: Dyspnea

PHARMACOKINETICS

Half-life elimination: IV 60 min, SUBCUT 2-3 hr; detected within 5 min after administration, peak 2 hr

INTERACTIONS

• Do not use product concomitantly with antineoplastics

Increase: myeloproliferation—lithium, corticosteroids

NURSING CONSIDERATIONS

Assess:

⚠ **Blood studies: CBC, differential count before treatment, 2 × weekly; leukocytosis may occur (WBC >50,000 cells/mm^3, ANC >20,000 cells/mm^3), platelets; if ANC >20,000/mm^3 or 10,000/mm^3 after nadir has occurred or platelets >500,000/mm^3, reduce dose by 1/2 or discontinue; if blast cells occur, discontinue**

• Renal, hepatic studies before treatment: BUN, creatinine, urinalysis; AST, ALT, alk phos; 2 × weekly monitoring is needed in renal/hepatic disease

• **Hypersensitivity,** rashes, local inj site reactions; usually transient

• Body weight, hydration status; increased fluid retention in cardiac disease; pulmonary function

• Myalgia, arthralgia in legs, feet; use analgesics

Perform/provide:

• Storage in refrigerator; do not freeze

S

Evaluate:

• Therapeutic response: WBC and differential recovery

Teach patient/family:

• To report dyspnea to health care provider

saxagliptin (Rx)

(sax-a-glip′tin)

Onglyza

Func. class.: Antidiabetic, oral

Chem. class.: Dipeptidyl-peptidase-4 inhibitor (DPP-4 inhibitor)

ACTION: Slows the inactivation of incretin hormones; improves glucose homeostasis, improves glucose-dependent insulin synthesis, lowers glucagon secretions, and slows gastric emptying time

USES: In adults, type 2 diabetes mellitus as monotherapy or in combination with other antidiabetic agents

CONTRAINDICATIONS: Hypersensitivity, diabetic ketoacidosis (DKA), type 1 diabetes

Precautions: Pregnancy (B), geriatric patients, GI obstruction, surgery, thyroid/renal/hepatic disease, trauma

DOSAGE AND ROUTES

• **Adult: PO** 2.5-5 mg; may use with other antidiabetic agents other than insulin

Renal Dose

• **Adult: PO** CCr ≤50 ml/min, 2.5 mg daily

Available forms: Tabs 2.5, 5 mg

Administer:

• May be taken with/without food

SIDE EFFECTS

CNS: *Headache*

ENDO: Hypoglycemia (renal impairment)

GI: *Nausea, vomiting,* abdominal pain

INTEG: Urticaria, angioedema

MISC: Lymphopenia, peripheral edema

PHARMACOKINETICS

Rapidly absorbed, excreted by the kidneys (unchanged 24%), terminal half-life 2.5 hr, 3.1 hr metabolite, peak 2 hr, duration 24 hr

INTERACTIONS

Increase: sitagliptin level—cimetidine, disopyramide

Increase: levels of digoxin

Increase: hypoglycemia—androgens, insulins, β-blockers, cimetidine, corticosteroids, salicylates, MAOIs, fibric acid derivatives, FLUoxetine

Decrease: antidiabetic effect—thiazide diuretics, ACE inhibitors, protease inhibitors, sympathomimetics, aripiprazole, clozapine, olanzapine, quetiapine, risperidone, ziprasidone, phenytoin, fosphenytoin, phenothiazines, estrogens, progestins, oral contraceptives

Drug/Herb

Increase: antidiabetic effect—garlic, horse chestnut

NURSING CONSIDERATIONS

Assess:

• **Hypoglycemic reactions** (sweating, weakness, dizziness, anxiety, tremors, hunger); **renal studies:** BUN, creatinine during treatment; HbA1c

• Monitor blood glucose as needed

Perform/provide:

• Conversion from other antidiabetic agents; change may be made with gradual dosage change

• Storage in tight container at room temp

Evaluate:

• Therapeutic response: decrease in polyuria, polydipsia, polyphagia; clear sensorium; absence of dizziness; stable gait, blood glucose at normal level

Teach patient/family:

• To perform regular self-monitoring of blood glucose using blood-glucose meter

• About the symptoms of hypo/hyperglycemia, what to do about each
• That product must be continued on daily basis; about consequences of discontinuing product abruptly
• To avoid OTC medications, alcohol, digoxin, exenatide, insulins, nateglinide, repaglinide, and other products that lower blood glucose unless approved by prescriber
• That diabetes is lifelong; that this product is not a cure, only controls symptoms
• That all food included in diet plan must be eaten to prevent hypo/hyperglycemia
• To carry emergency ID

scopolamine (Rx)

(skoe-pol'a-meen)

Maldemar, Scopace, Transderm Scop

Func. class.: Cholinergic blocker
Chem. class.: Belladonna alkaloid

ACTION: Inhibits acetylcholine at receptor sites in autonomic nervous system, which controls secretions, free acids in stomach; blocks central muscarinic receptors, which decreases involuntary movements

USES: Preoperatively to produce amnesia, sedation and to decrease secretions; motion sickness, parkinsonian symptoms

CONTRAINDICATIONS: Hypersensitivity, closed-angle glaucoma, myasthenia gravis, GI/GU obstruction, hypersensitivity to belladonna, barbiturates
Precautions: Pregnancy (C), breastfeeding, children, geriatric patients, prostatic hypertrophy, CHF, hypertension, dysrhythmia, gastric ulcer, renal/hepatic disease, hiatal hernia, GERD, ulcerative colitis, hyperthyroidism

DOSAGE AND ROUTES

Motion sickness
• **Adult: TD** 1 patch 4 hr prior to travel and q3days
Parkinsonian symptoms
• **Adult: PO** 0.4-0.8 mg q8hr
Preoperatively
• **Adult: IM/IV/SUBCUT** 0.32-0.65 mg; **TD** apply 1 patch PM prior to surgery or 1 hr prior to c-section
Nausea and vomiting
• **Adult: SUBCUT** 0.6-1 mg
• **Child: SUBCUT** 0.006 mg/kg; max 0.3 mg/dose

Available forms: Inj 0.4 mg/ml; TD patch 72 hr (1.5 mg)

Administer:
• Parenteral dose with patient recumbent to prevent postural hypotension
• Parenteral dose slowly; keep patient in bed for ≥1 hr after dose
• With or after meals for GI upset; may give with fluids other than water
• At bedtime to avoid daytime drowsiness in patients with parkinsonism
• With analgesic to avoid behavioral changes when given preoperatively

Direct IV route
• Dilute with equal sterile water; give over 2-3 min

Syringe compatibilities: Atropine, benzquinamide, butorphanol, chlorproMAZINE, cimetidine, diamorphine, dimenhyDRINATE, diphenhydrAMINE, droperidol, fentaNYL, glycopyrrolate, HYDROmorphone, hydrOXYzine, meperidine, metoclopramide, midazolam, morphine, nalbuphine, oxyCODONE, pentazocine, PENTobarbital, perphenazine, prochlorperazine, promazine, promethazine, ranitidine, SUFentanil, thiopental

Y-site compatibilities: FentaNYL, heparin, hydrocortisone, HYDROmorphone, methadone, morphine, potassium chloride, propofol, SUFentanil, vit B/C

SIDE EFFECTS

CNS: Confusion, anxiety, restlessness, irritability, delusions, hallucinations, head-

S

ache, sedation, depression, incoherence, dizziness, excitement, delirium, flushing, weakness, fatigue, loss of memory
CV: Palpitations, tachycardia, postural hypotension, paradoxical bradycardia
EENT: Blurred vision, photophobia, dilated pupils, difficulty swallowing, mydriasis, cycloplegia
GI: *Dryness of mouth, constipation,* nausea, vomiting, abdominal distress, paralytic ileus
GU: Urinary hesitancy, retention
INTEG: Urticaria, dry skin
MISC: Suppression of breastfeeding, nasal congestion, decreased sweating

PHARMACOKINETICS

Excreted in urine, bile, feces (unchanged), half-life 8 hr
SUBCUT/IM: Peak 30-60 min, duration 7 hr
IV: Peak 10-15 min, duration 2 hr

INTERACTIONS

Increase: anticholinergic effect—alcohol, opioids, antihistamines, phenothiazines, tricyclics

NURSING CONSIDERATIONS

Assess:

- VS periodically
- I&O ratio; retention commonly causes decreased urinary output
- **Parkinsonism, EPS:** shuffling gait, muscle rigidity, involuntary movements; affect, mood, CNS depression, worsening of mental symptoms during early therapy
- Urinary hesitancy, retention; palpate bladder if retention occurs
- Constipation; increase fluids, bulk, exercise
- Tolerance during long-term therapy; dose may have to be increased or changed

Perform/provide:

- Storage at room temp in light-resistant container
- Hard candy, frequent drinks, sugarless gum to relieve dry mouth

Evaluate:

- Therapeutic response: decreased secretions

Teach patient/family:

- Not to discontinue product abruptly; to taper off over 1 wk
- To avoid driving, other hazardous activities because drowsiness may occur
- To avoid OTC medication: cough, cold preparations with alcohol, antihistamines unless directed by prescriber
- **Transdermal route:** to apply with clean, dry hands; to wash, dry hands before and after applying to surface behind ear; to press patch firmly
- To avoid hazardous activities, activities requiring alertness because dizziness may occur
- To change patch q72hr
- To apply at least 4 hr before traveling
- If blurred vision, severe dizziness, drowsiness occurs, to discontinue use, use another type of antiemetic, or to rotate patch to other ear
- To read label of all OTC medications; if any scopolamine is found in product, avoid use
- To keep out of children's reach

scopolamine ophthalmic

See Appendix B

selegiline (Rx)

(se-le′ji-leen)

Apo-Selegiline ✤, Eldepryl, Emsam, Gen-Selegiline ✤, Zelapar

Func. class.: Antiparkinson agent
Chem. class.: MAOI, type B

Do not confuse:
Eldepryl/enalapril

ACTION: Increased dopaminergic activity by inhibition of MAO type B activity; not fully understood

USES:
Adjunct management of Parkinson's disease for patients being treated with levodopa/carbidopa who had poor response to therapy; depression (transdermal)

Unlabeled uses: Alzheimer's disease, depression

CONTRAINDICATIONS:
Children/adolescents (suicide/hypertensive crisis), hypersensitivity, breastfeeding

Precautions: Pregnancy (C)

DOSAGE AND ROUTES

• **Adult: PO** 10 mg/day given with levodopa/carbidopa in divided doses, 5 mg at breakfast and lunch; after 2-3 days, begin to reduce dose of levodopa/carbidopa 10%-30%; **ORAL DISINTEGRATING** 1.25 mg (1 tab) × 6 wk or more initially then 2.5 mg (2 tabs) dissolved on tongue daily before breakfast; max 2.5 mg/day; **TRANSDERMAL** 6 mg/24 hr initially, increase by 3 mg/24 hr at ≥2 wk, up to 12 mg/24 hr if needed

Alzheimer's disease (unlabeled)

• **Adult: PO** 5 mg bid AM, PM

Available forms: Tabs 5 mg; caps 5 mg; oral disintegrating tabs 1.25 mg; transdermal 6 mg/24 hr (20 mg/20 cm^2), 9 mg/24 hr (30 mg/30 cm^2), 12 mg/24 hr (40 mg/40 cm^2)

Administer:

PO route

⚠ **Do not use in children due to risk for hypertensive crisis**

• Product until NPO before surgery

• Adjust dosage to response

• With meals; limit protein taken with product

• Dosing bid in AM and afternoon; avoid PM or bedtime dosing

• At doses of <10 mg/day because of risks associated with nonselective inhibition of MAO

• **Oral disintegrating tab:** peel back foil; remove tab, do not push through foil; place tab on tongue, allow to dissolve, swallow with saliva

Transdermal route

• Apply to dry, intact skin on upper torso, upper thigh, or outer surface of upper arm q12hr

SIDE EFFECTS

CNS: Increased tremors, chorea, restlessness, blepharospasm, increased bradykinesia, grimacing, tardive dyskinesia, dystonic symptoms, involuntary movements, increased apraxia, hallucinations, *dizziness,* mood changes, nightmares, delusions, lethargy, apathy, overstimulation, sleep disturbances, headache, migraine, numbness, muscle cramps, confusion, anxiety, tiredness, vertigo, personality change, back/leg pain, **suicide in child/adolescent, suicidal ideation in adults**

CV: Orthostatic hypotension, hypo/hypertension, dysrhythmia, palpitations, angina pectoris, **tachycardia**, edema, **sinus bradycardia**, syncope, **hypertensive crisis (children)**

EENT: Diplopia, dry mouth, blurred vision, tinnitus

GI: Nausea, vomiting, constipation, weight loss, anorexia, diarrhea, heartburn, rectal bleeding, poor appetite, dysphagia, xerostomia

GU: Slow urination, nocturia, prostatic hypertrophy, urinary hesitation, retention, frequency, sexual dysfunction

INTEG: Increased sweating, alopecia, hematoma, rash, photosensitivity, facial hair

RESP: Asthma, SOB

S

PHARMACOKINETICS

Absorption (tab) 40-90 min, (oral disintegrating tab) 10-15 min; peak ½-2 hr; rapidly metabolized (active metabolites: *N*-desmethyldeprenyl, amphetamine, methamphetamine); metabolites excreted in urine; half-life 10 hr, orally disintegrating tab 1.3 hr; protein binding up to 85%

INTERACTIONS

⚠ **Fatal interaction: opioids (especially meperidine); do not administer together**

⚠ Serotonin syndrome (confusion, seizures, fever, hypertension, agitation); death—FLUoxetine, PARoxetine, sertraline, fluvoxamine (discontinue 5 wk prior to selegiline treatment); do not use together

⚠ Fatal interaction: do not use with tricyclics

Increase: side effects of levodopa/carbidopa

Increase: unusual behavior, psychosis—dextromethorphan

Increase: hypotension—antihypertensives

Drug/Lab Test

Decrease: VMA

False positive: urine ketones, urine glucose

False negative: urine glucose (glucose oxidase)

False increase: uric acid, urine protein

NURSING CONSIDERATIONS

Assess:

• **Parkinson's symptoms:** decreased rigidity, unsteady gait, weakness, tremors

• Cardiac status: tachycardia/bradycardia; B/P, respiration throughout treatment

• Mental status: affect, mood, behavioral changes, depression; perform suicide assessment on all patients, suicidal ideation may occur

⚠ Opioids; if patient has received, do not administer selegiline, fatal reactions have occurred

Perform/provide:

• Assistance with ambulation during beginning therapy

Evaluate:

• Therapeutic response: decrease in akathisia, improved mood

Teach patient/family:

• To change positions slowly to prevent orthostatic hypotension

• To report side effects: twitching, eye spasms; indicate overdose

• To use product exactly as prescribed; if discontinued abruptly, parkinsonian crisis may occur

• To avoid foods high in tyramine: cheese, pickled products, wine, beer, large amounts of caffeine

⚠ Not to exceed recommended dose of 10 mg (PO) because this might precipitate hypertensive crisis; to report severe headache, other unusual symptoms

TREATMENT OF OVERDOSE:

IV fluids for hypertension, IV dilute pressure agent for B/P titration

selenium topical

See Appendix B

sennosides (OTC)

(sen′na)

Black Draught, Equaline Senna, Ex-Lax, Fletcher's Laxative, Gentlax, Leader Laxative, Perdiem, Senexon, Senna-Gen, Senna-Lax, Senokot, SenokotXTRA, Senolax, Seno Sol, Walgreens Senna

Func. class.: Laxative-stimulant

Chem. class.: Anthraquinone

ACTION: Stimulates peristalsis by action on Auerbach's plexus; softens feces by increasing water, electrolytes in large intestine

USES: Acute constipation, bowel preparation for surgery or examination, prevention of constipation in those taking opiates long term

CONTRAINDICATIONS: Breastfeeding, hypersensitivity, GI bleeding, obstruction, CHF, abdominal pain, nausea/vomiting, appendicitis, acute surgical abdomen

Precautions: Pregnancy (C)

DOSAGE AND ROUTES

- **Adult: PO** (Senokot) 1-8 tabs/day or 1/2 to 4 tsp of granules (1 tsp-4 ml) added to water or juice; **RECT SUPP** 1-2 at bedtime; **SYR** 1-4 tsp at bedtime, 7.5-15 ml (Black Draught) 3/4 oz dissolved in 2.5 oz liquid given between 2-4 PM day before procedure (X-Prep)
- **Child >27 kg: PO** 1/2 adult dose; do not use Black Draught for children
- **Child 1 mo-1 yr: SYR** (Senokot) 1.25-2.5 ml at bedtime

Available forms: Tabs 6, 8.6, 15, 25 mg; syr 8.8 mg/5 ml; liquid 33.3 mg/ml

Administer:

- In morning or evening (oral dose) with full glass of water
- On empty stomach for more rapid results
- Shake oral sol before giving

SIDE EFFECTS

GI: *Nausea, vomiting, anorexia, cramps,* diarrhea, flatulence
GU: Pink, red or brown, black urine
META: Hypocalcemia, enteropathy, alkalosis, hypokalemia, **tetany**

PHARMACOKINETICS

PO: Onset 6-24 hr, metabolized by liver, excreted in feces

INTERACTIONS

- Do not use with disulfiram (Antabuse)

Drug/Herb
Increase: laxative effect—flax, senna

NURSING CONSIDERATIONS

Assess:

- **Stool:** color, consistency, amount, bowel sounds, distension, cause of constipation; fluids, bulk, exercise missing, constipating products; cramping, rectal bleeding, nausea, vomiting; product should be discontinued

Evaluate:

- Therapeutic response: decrease in constipation

Teach patient/family:

- That urine, feces may turn yellow-brown to red
- Not to use laxatives for long-term therapy because bowel tone will be lost
- That normal bowel movements do not always occur daily
- Not to use in presence of abdominal pain, nausea, vomiting
- To notify prescriber if constipation unrelieved or of symptoms of electrolyte imbalance: muscle cramps, pain, weakness, dizziness, excessive thirst
- To use other ways to decrease constipation: water, bulk in diet, exercise

sertraline (Rx)

(ser′tra-leen)

Zoloft

Func. class.: Antidepressant
Chem. class.: SSRI

Do not confuse:
Zoloft/Zocor

ACTION:
Inhibits serotonin reuptake in CNS; increases action of serotonin; does not affect dopamine, norepinephrine

USES:
Major depressive disorder, obsessive-compulsive disorder (OCD), posttraumatic stress disorder (PTSD), panic disorder, social anxiety disorder, premenstrual dysphoric disorder (PMDD)

Unlabeled uses: Premature ejaculation, pruritus with cholestatic liver disease, hot flashes during menopause, breast cancer patients taking tamoxifen; men with prostate cancer secondary to androgen-deprivation therapy

S

CONTRAINDICATIONS:

Hypersensitivity to this product or SSRIs

Precautions: Pregnancy (C), breastfeeding, geriatric patients, renal/hepatic disease, epilepsy, recent MI, latex sensitivity (dropper of oral conc)

Black Box Warning: Children, suicidal ideation

DOSAGE AND ROUTES

Major depression/OCD

- **Adult/geriatric patient/adolescent (unlabeled): PO** 25-50 mg/day; may increase to max of 200 mg/day; do not change dose at intervals of <1 wk; administer daily in AM or PM
- **Child 6-12 yr (unlabeled): PO** 25 mg/day, increase by 25-50 mg/wk

Premenstrual dysphoric disorder

- **Adult: PO** 50-150 mg nightly

Premature ejaculation (unlabeled)

- **Adult: PO** 50 mg/day

Pruritus (unlabeled)

- **Adult: PO** 50-100 mg/day

Hot flashes (unlabeled)

- **Adult: PO** 50 mg/day × 4 wk; men with prostate cancer (androgen deprivation), 50-100 mg/day

Available forms: Tabs 25, 50, 100 mg; oral sol 20 mg/ml

Administer:

- Increased fluids, bulk in diet for constipation, urinary retention
- With food, milk for GI symptoms
- Crushed if patient is unable to swallow medication whole
- Sugarless gum, hard candy, frequent sips of water for dry mouth
- **Oral conc:** dilute prior to use with 4 oz (1/2 cup) of water, orange juice, ginger ale, or lemon/lime soda; do not mix with other liquids
- Avoid use with other CNS depressants

SIDE EFFECTS

CNS: *Insomnia, agitation, somnolence, dizziness, headache, tremor, fatigue,* paresthesia, twitching, confusion, ataxia, gait abnormality (geriatric patients), **seizures, neuroleptic malignant syndrome–like reaction, serotonin syndrome, suicidal ideation**

CV: Palpitations, chest pain

EENT: Vision abnormalities, yawning

ENDO: SIADH (geriatric patients)

GI: *Diarrhea, nausea, constipation, anorexia, dry mouth,* dyspepsia, *vomiting, flatulence,* weight gain/loss

GU: *Male sexual dysfunction,* micturition disorder

INTEG: Increased sweating, rash, hot flashes

MISC: Hyponatremia

PHARMACOKINETICS

PO: Peak 4.5-8.4 hr; steady state 1 wk; plasma protein binding 98%; elimination half-life 26 hr; extensively metabolized; metabolite excreted in urine, bile; weak inhibitor of CYP3A4, moderate inhibitor of CYP2D6

INTERACTIONS

- Altered lithium levels: lithium
- Disulfiram reaction: disulfiram and oral conc due to alcohol content

⚠ **Fatal reactions: MAOIs, pimozide**

Increase: sertraline levels—cimetidine, warfarin, other highly protein-bound products

Increase: effects of antidepressants (tricyclics), diazepam, TOLBUTamide, warfarin, benzodiazepines, sumatriptan, phenytoin, clozapine

Increase: bleeding risk—anticoagulants, NSAIDs, thrombolytic, platelet inhibitors, salicylates

Increase: serotonin syndrome, neuroleptic malignant syndrome—SSRIs, SNRIs, serotonin-receptor agonists, tricyclics, sibutramine, traZODone, busPIRone, linezolid, tramadol

Drug/Herb

Increase: of SSRI, serotonin syndrome—St. John's wort, SAM-e, tryptophan; do not use together

Increase: CNS effect—kava kava, valerian

Drug/Lab Test

Increase: AST, ALT

NURSING CONSIDERATIONS

Assess:

Black Box Warning: Mental status: mood, sensorium, affect, suicidal tendencies (child/young adult), increase in psychiatric symptoms, depression, panic attacks, OCD, PTSD, social anxiety disorder

⚠ **Serotonin syndrome** (hyperthermia, hypertension, rigidity, delirium, coma, myoclonus) or neuroleptic malignant-like syndrome (muscle cramps, fever, unstable B/P, agitation, tremors, mental changes)

⚠ **Bleeding** (platelet serotonin depletion): GI bleeding, ecchymoses, epistaxis, hematomas, petechiae, hemorrhage

- LFTs at baseline and periodically
- B/P (lying/standing), pulse q4hr; if systolic B/P drops 20 mm Hg, hold product, notify prescriber; VS q4hr in patients with CV disease
- Weight q wk; appetite may decrease with product
- Urinary retention, constipation, especially in geriatric patients
- Alcohol consumption; hold dose until morning

Perform/provide:

- Storage at room temp; do not freeze
- Assistance with ambulation during therapy because drowsiness, dizziness occur
- Safety measures, including raised side rails, primarily for geriatric patients

Evaluate:

- Therapeutic response: significant improvement in depression, OCD

Teach patient/family:

- That therapeutic effect may take ≥1 wk
- To use caution when driving, performing other activities requiring alertness because drowsiness, dizziness, blurred vision may occur
- Not to discontinue medication quickly after long-term use; may cause nausea, headache, malaise
- To avoid alcohol
- To notify prescriber if pregnant or if planning to become pregnant or breastfeed

Black Box Warning: That suicidal thoughts/behaviors may occur in children/adolescents

sildenafil (Rx)

(sil-den′a-fill)

Revatio, Viagra

Func. class.: Erectile agent, antihypertensive, peripheral vasodilator
Chem. class.: Phosphodiesterase type-5 inhibitor

ACTION: Enhances the effect of nitric oxide (NO) by inhibiting phosphodiesterase type 5 (PDE5), which is necessary for degrading cGMP in the corpus cavernosum

USES: Treatment of erectile dysfunction, improvement in exercise ability, pulmonary hypertension

Unlabeled uses: Sexual dysfunction (women); lower urinary tract symptoms and erectile dysfunction (with alfuzosin); pediatrics with primary/secondary pulmonary hypertension, altitude sickness, Raynaud's disease

CONTRAINDICATIONS: Hypersensitivity to this product or nitrates

Precautions: Pregnancy (B), anatomical penile deformities, sickle cell anemia, leukemia, multiple myeloma, retinitis pigmentosa, bleeding disorders, active peptic ulceration, CV/renal/hepatic disease, multiproduct antihypertensive regimens, geriatric patients

DOSAGE AND ROUTES

Erectile dysfunction (Viagra only)

- **Adult male <65 yr: PO** 50 mg 1 hr before sexual activity; may be increased to 100 mg or decreased to 25 mg; max 1×/day

S

• **Adult ≥65 yr (male): PO** 25 mg as needed about 1 hr before sexual activity

Renal/hepatic dose

• **Adult: PO** (Child-Pugh A, B) 25 mg, take 1 hr before sexual activity; max 1×/day; CCr <30 ml/min, 25 mg starting dose

Pulmonary hypertension (Revatio only)

• **Adult: PO** 20 mg tid; take 4-6 hr apart; **IV BOL** 10 mg tid

• **Infant/child/adolescent (unlabeled): PO** 0.25-0.5 mg/kg/dose tid qid

Pulmonary hypertension induced by altitude sickness (unlabeled)

• **Adult: PO** 40 mg 6-8 hr after arriving at 14,272 ft, then 40 mg tid × 6 days

Anorgasmy in antidepressant therapy/sexual dysfunction in women (unlabeled)

• **Adult: PO** 50 mg 60-90 min prior to sexual activity

Available forms: Tabs 20, 25, 50, 100 mg; sol for inj 10 mg/12.5 ml

Administer:

• **Erectile dysfunction:** give approximately 1 hr before sexual activity; do not use more than 1×/day, give on empty stomach for better absorption

• **Pulmonary hypertension:** give 3×/day, 4-6 hr apart

SIDE EFFECTS

CNS: *Headache, flushing, dizziness,* transient global amnesia, seizures

CV: MI, sudden death, CV collapse, TIAs, ventricular dysrhythmias, CV hemorrhage

MISC.: *Dyspepsia, nasal congestion, UTI, abnormal vision, diarrhea, rash,* nonarteritic ischemic optic neuropathy, hearing loss, priapism, sickle cell crisis

PHARMACOKINETICS

Rapidly absorbed; bioavailability 40%; metabolized by P45 CYP3A4, 2C9 in the liver (active metabolites); terminal half-life 4 hr; peak 15-30 min; reduced absorption with high-fat meal; excreted in feces, urine

INTERACTIONS

⚠ Do not use with nitrates; fatal fall in B/P

Increase: sildenafil levels—cimetidine, erythromycin, ketoconazole, itraconazole, antiretroviral protease inhibitors, tacrolimus

Decrease: sildenafil levels—CYP-450 inducers, rifampin, barbiturates, bosentan, carBAMazepine, dexamethasone, phenytoin, nevirapine, rifabutin, troglitazone; antacids

Decrease: B/P—α-blockers, alcohol, amlodipine, angiotensin II receptor blockers

Drug/Food

Increase: product effect—grapefruit

Decrease: absorption—high-fat meal

NURSING CONSIDERATIONS

Assess:

• Erectile dysfunction prior to use

⚠ Any severe loss of vision while taking this or any similar products; products should not be used

⚠ Use of organic nitrates that should not be used with this product

• **Sickle cell crisis (vasoocclusive crisis):** when used for pulmonary hypertension, may require hospitalization

• Cardiac status, hemodynamic parameters, exercise tolerance in pulmonary hypertension: B/P, pulse

Evaluate:

• Therapeutic response: decreasing pulmonary hypertension/improved exercise tolerance; ability to perform sexually (male)

Teach patient/family:

• That product does not protect against sexually transmitted diseases, including HIV

• That product absorption is reduced with a high-fat meal

• That product should not be used with nitrates in any form

• That tabs may be split

⚠ To notify prescriber immediately and to stop taking product if vision loss occurs or erection lasts >4 hr

silodosin (Rx)

(si-lo′do-seen)

Rapaflo

Func. class.: Selective α_1-adrenergic blocker

Chem. class.: Sulfamoylphenethylamine derivative

ACTION: Binds preferentially to α_{1A}-adrenoceptor subtype located mainly in the prostate

USES: Symptoms of benign prostatic hyperplasia (BPH)

CONTRAINDICATIONS: Hypersensitivity, renal failure, hepatic disease

Precautions: Pregnancy (B), breastfeeding, children, females, geriatric patients, renal/hepatic disease, hypotension, ocular surgery, orthostatic hypotension, prostate cancer, syncope

DOSAGE AND ROUTES

- **Adult: PO** 8 mg/day with meal; max 8 mg/day

Renal dose

- **Adult: PO** CCr 30-49 ml/min, 4 mg/day; CCr <30 ml/min, not recommended

Available forms: Tabs 8 mg

Administer:

- Give with meal at same time each day

SIDE EFFECTS

CNS: *Dizziness, headache,* asthenia, insomnia, syncope

CV: Orthostatic hypotension

EENT: Nasal congestion, rhinorrhea, sinusitis

GI: Diarrhea, abdominal pain, jaundice

GU: Abnormal ejaculation, priapism, urinary incontinence

HEMA: Purpura

PHARMACOKINETICS

Decreased absorption with high-fat/high-calorie meal, half-life of metabolite 24 hr, metabolized in liver, excreted via urine, extensively protein bound (97%)

INTERACTIONS

Increase: silodosin effect—CYP3A4 inhibitors (clarithromycin, itraconazole, ritonavir, antiretroviral protease inhibitors, aprepitant, chloramphenicol, conivaptan, dalfopristin, danazol, delavirdine, efavirenz, fosaprepitant, fluconazole, fluvoxamine, imatinib, isoniazid, mifepristone, nefazodone, tamoxifen, telithromycin, troleandomycin, voriconazole, zileuton, zafirlukast)

Drug/Food

Increase: silodosin effect—grapefruit juice

Drug Lab/Test

Increase: LFTs

NURSING CONSIDERATIONS

Assess:

- **Prostatic hyperplasia:** change in urinary patterns at baseline and throughout treatment
- CBC with differential and LFTs; B/P and heart rate
- BUN, uric acid, urodynamic studies (urinary flow rates, residual volume)
- I&O ratios, weight daily; edema, report weight gain or edema

Perform/provide:

- Storage at room temp; protect from light and moisture

Evaluate:

- Therapeutic response: decreased symptoms of BPH

Teach patient/family

- Not to drive, operate machinery until effect known
- Not to use with grapefruit juice

silver nitrate 1% ophthalmic

See Appendix B

silver nitrate sulfacetamide sodium ophthalmic

See Appendix B

silver sulfADIAZINE topical

See Appendix B

simethicone (OTC, Rx)

(si-meth'i-kone)

Barriere ✱, Equaline Extra Strength Gas Relief, Gas Relief ✱, Gas-Relief, Gas-X, Good Sense Ultra Strength Gas Relief, Mylanta Gas Relief, Mylanta Gas, Mylicon, Ovol ✱, Phazyme, Top Care Gas Relief Extra Strength, Walgreens Gas Relief

Func. class.: Antiflatulent

Do not confuse:
Mylicon/Mylanta Gas

ACTION: Disperses/prevents mucus gas pockets in GI system, lowers surface tension of gas bubbles

USES: Flatulence
Unlabeled uses: Dyspepsia

CONTRAINDICATIONS: Hypersensitivity, GI obstruction/perforation
Precautions: Pregnancy (C), abdominal pain, fistula, hiatal hernia

DOSAGE AND ROUTES

- **Adult and child >12 yr: PO** 40-125 mg after meals and at bedtime prn, max 500 mg/day
- **Child 2-12 yr: PO** 40-50 mg after meals and at bedtime prn, max 240 mg/day
- **Child <2 yr: PO** 20 mg qid prn

Available forms: Chew tabs 40, 150, 166 mg; tabs 60, 80, 95, 125 mg; drops 20 mg/0.3 ml, 95 mg/1.425 ml; caps 95, 180 mg; soft gel caps 125, 180 mg; oral dissolving film 62.5 mg

Administer:

- After meals, at bedtime; shake susp well before giving; chew tabs should be chewed

SIDE EFFECTS

GI: Belching, rectal flatus, diarrhea

NURSING CONSIDERATIONS

Assess:

- Reason for excess gas production, decreased bowel sounds, recent surgery, other GI conditions

Evaluate:

- Therapeutic response: reduction of abdominal gas, discomfort

Teach patient/family:

- That tablets must be chewed
- To shake susp well before pouring

simvastatin (Rx)

(sim-va-sta'tin)

Zocor

Func. class.: Antilipemic
Chem. class.: HMG-CoA reductase inhibitor

Do not confuse:
Zocor/Cozaar/Zoloft

ACTION: Inhibits HMG-CoA reductase enzyme, which reduces cholesterol synthesis

USES:
As an adjunct for primary hypercholesterolemia (types IIa, IIb), isolated hypertriglyceridemia (Frederickson type IV) and type III hyperlipoproteinemia, CAD, heterozygous familial hypercholesterolemia

CONTRAINDICATIONS:
Pregnancy (X), breastfeeding, hypersensitivity, active hepatic disease

Precautions: Past hepatic disease, alcoholism, severe acute infections, trauma, severe metabolic disorders, electrolyte imbalances, Chinese patients

DOSAGE AND ROUTES

- **Adult: PO** 20-40 mg/day in PM initially; usual range 5-40 mg/day in PM, max 40 mg/day for most patients, max 80 mg/day for patients taking 80 mg/day chronically without myopathy; dosage adjustments may be made in ≥4-wk intervals; those taking verapamil and amiodarone max 20 mg/day; max <80 mg for Chinese patients taking lipid-modifying niacin doses

With diltiazem/verapamil

- **Adult: PO** 5-10 mg in PM, max 10 mg/day with amiodarone/amLODIPine/ranolazine
- **Adult: PO** 5-20 mg in PM, max 20 mg/day
- **Child/adolescent ≥10 yr including girls ≥1 yr postmenarche: PO** 10 mg in PM, range 10-40 mg/day

Heterozygous familial hypercholesterolemia

- **Adolescent 10-17 yr: PO** 10 mg/day, max 40 mg/day

Available forms: Tabs 5, 10, 20, 40, 80 mg

Administer:

- Total daily dose in evening

SIDE EFFECTS

CNS: Headache

GI: Nausea, constipation, diarrhea, dyspepsia, flatus, abdominal pain, **liver dysfunction, pancreatitis**

INTEG: Rash, pruritus

MS: Muscle cramps, myalgia, myositis, **rhabdomyolysis, myopathy**

RESP: Upper respiratory tract infection

PHARMACOKINETICS

Metabolized in liver (active metabolites); >98% protein bound; excreted primarily in bile, feces (60%), kidneys (15%); peak 1-2 hr; half-life 3 hr

INTERACTIONS

⚠ **Do not use with cycloSPORINE, gemfibrozil**

⚠ **Increase: effects of warfarin**

⚠ **Increase: rhabdomyolysis, myalgia; do not use concurrently—niacin, erythromycin, clofibrate, clarithromycin, ketoconazole, itraconazole, protease inhibitors, macrolide antibiotics, danazol, delavirdine, nefazodone, verapamil, diltiazem, amiodarone, azole antifungals, telithromycin**

Increase: serum level of digoxin

Drug/Herb

Decrease: effect—St. John's wort

Drug/Lab Test

Increase: CK, LFTs

NURSING CONSIDERATIONS

Assess:

- Diet history: fat consumption; baseline and lipid profile: LDL, HDL, TG, cholesterol
- Hepatic studies at baseline, after 4-6 wk, periodically thereafter; AST, ALT, LFTs may increase

⚠ **Rhabdomyolysis: muscle tenderness, increased CPK levels (10× above upper normal limit); therapy should be discontinued**

- Renal studies in patients with compromised renal systems: BUN, I&O ratio, creatinine

Perform/provide:

- Storage in cool environment in tight container protected from light

Evaluate:

- Therapeutic response: decrease in LDL, total cholesterol, triglycerides; increase in HDL; slowing CAD

S

Teach patient/family:
- That blood work will be necessary during treatment
- To report severe GI symptoms, headache
- That previously prescribed regimen will continue: low-cholesterol diet, exercise program
- To notify prescriber if pregnancy is suspected or planned; pregnancy (X); not to breastfeed

sipuleucel-T (Rx)

(si′pu-loo′sel-tee)

Provenge

Func. class.: Antineoplastic-biologic response modifiers

Chem class.: Active cellular immunotherapy

ACTION: Stimulates T-cell immunity against prostatic acid phosphatase (PAP), an antigen expressed in prostatic cancer tissue

USES: Asymptomatic or minimally symptomatic metastatic, hormone-refractory prostate cancer

CONTRAINDICATIONS: Hypersensitivity

Precautions: Child/infant/neonate, cardiac disease, chemotherapy, immunosuppression, inf reaction, pulmonary disease

DOSAGE AND ROUTES

- **Adult male: IV INF** give entire contents of bag over 60 min q2wk × 3 doses; premedicate with acetaminophen and diphenhydrAMINE 30 min prior to inf to minimize acute inf reactions

Available forms: Susp for inj

Administer:

Intermittent IV INF route
- **Premedicate:** with acetaminophen and antihistamine 30 min prior to inf
- **Inf:** visually inspect for particulate or discoloration prior to use; remove bag from container and check for leaks; do not use if leak, particulate, or discoloration is present; product is slightly cloudy cream to pink in color, gently mix, check for clumps of clots; must begin inf prior to expiration date and time indicated on cell product disposition form and product label; infuse entire vol over 60 min, do not use a cell filter; reactions may be treated with acetaminophen, H_1/H_2 blockers, low-dose meperidine; if acute reaction occurs, interrupt or slow inf, do not resume if product has been at room temp >3 hr

SIDE EFFECTS

CNS: Asthenia, dizziness, fatigue, fever, flushing, headache, insomnia, paresthesia, stroke, tremor, chills, hot flashes

CV: Hypertension, hypoxia, sinus tachycardia

GI: Anorexia, constipation, diarrhea, weight loss, nausea, vomiting

GU: Hematuria

HEMA: Anemia

MS: Arthralgia, back/bone pain, muscle cramps, myalgia

RESP: Bronchospasm

PHARMACOKINETICS

T-cell stimulation at 8 wk was 8-fold higher than control

INTERACTIONS

- Do not use with antineoplastics, immunosuppressives

NURSING CONSIDERATIONS

Assess:
- **Prostate cancer:** more normal urinary patterns, hematuria, decreased tumor size
- **Bronchospasm, CV adverse reactions:** ability to breathe easily, B/P, pulse, respirations, sinus tachycardia, hypertension

Perform/provide:
- Storage in refrigerator of unopened bags; do not freeze

Evaluate:
- Therapeutic response: decreasing size of tumor, decreasing PSA level

Teach patient/family:
- To notify health care provider of serious adverse reactions: inability to breathe, blood in urine, rapid heartbeat, allergic reactions
- About reasons for product and expected results

sirolimus (Rx)
(seer-oh-lie′mus)

Rapamune

Func. class.: Immunosuppressant
Chem. class.: Macrolide

ACTION: Produces immunosuppression by inhibiting T-lymphocyte activation and proliferation

USES: Organ transplants to prevent rejection; recommended use is with cycloSPORINE and corticosteroids

CONTRAINDICATIONS: Breastfeeding, hypersensitivity to this product, components of product

Precautions: Pregnancy (C), children <13 yr, severe cardiac/renal/hepatic disease; diabetes mellitus, hyperkalemia, hyperuricemia, hypertension, interstitial lung disease, hyperlipidemia

Black Box Warning: Lymphomas, infection, other malignancies

DOSAGE AND ROUTES
- **Adult/adolescent ≥40 kg: PO** 2 mg/day with 6 mg loading dose
- **Child >13 yr weighing <40 kg (88 lb): PO** 1 mg/m^2/day, 3 mg/m^2 loading dose

Hepatic dose
- **Adult/child ≥13 yr/<40 kg: PO** reduce by 33% for maintenance dose (mild to moderate hepatic impairment); reduce by 50% for maintenance dose (severe hepatic impairment)

Available forms: Oral sol 1 mg/ml; tabs 1 mg, 2 mg

Administer:
- Prophylaxis for *Pneumocystis jiroveci* pneumonia for 1 yr after transplantation; prophylaxis for CMV is recommended for 90 days after transplantation in those at increased risk for CMV
- All medications PO if possible, avoid IM inj; bleeding may occur
- For 3 days before transplant surgery; patients should be placed in protective isolation; give at same time of day, give 4 hr after cycloSPORINE oral sol or caps; do not give with grapefruit juice
- Use amber oral dose syringe and withdraw amount of oral sol needed from bottle, empty correct dose into plastic/glass container holding 60 ml of water/orange juice, stir vigorously and have patient drink at once, refill container with additional 120 ml water/orange juice, stir vigorously and have patient drink at once; if using a pouch, squeeze entire contents into container, follow above directions
- Store protected from light, refrigerate; stable for 30 days after opening (sol)
- Do not crush, chew; store tabs at room temp

SIDE EFFECTS
CNS: *Tremors, headache, insomnia, paresthesia,* chills, fever
CV: Hypertension, *atrial fibrillation, CHF, hypotension, palpitation, tachycardia,* peripheral edema, thrombosis
EENT: Blurred vision, photophobia
GI: Nausea, vomiting, diarrhea, constipation, hepatotoxicity
GU: UTIs, albuminuria, hematuria, proteinuria, renal failure, nephrotic syndrome, increased creatinine
HEMA: Anemia, leukopenia, thrombocytopenia, purpura
INTEG: *Rash, acne,* photosensitivity
META: Hyperglycemia, increased creatinine, edema, hypercholesterolemia, *hyperlipemia,* hypophosphatemia, weight gain, hypo/hyperkalemia, hyperuricemia, hypomagnesemia

S

MS: Arthralgia
RESP: Pleural effusion, atelectasis, *dyspnea*
SYST: Lymphoma, exfoliative dermatitis

PHARMACOKINETICS

Rapidly absorbed; peak 1 hr single dose, 2 hr multiple dosing; protein binding 92%; extensively metabolized by CYP3A4 enzyme system

INTERACTIONS

⚠ **Increase:** angioedema—ACE inhibitors, angiotensin-II–receptor antagonists, cephalosporins, iodine-containing radiopaque contrast media, neuromuscular blockers, NSAIDs, penicillins, salicylates, thrombolytics
Increase: blood levels—antifungals, calcium channel blockers, cimetidine, danazol, erythromycin, cycloSPORINE, metoclopramide, bromocriptine, HIV-protease inhibitors
Decrease: blood levels—carBAMazepine, PHENobarbital, phenytoin, rifamycin, rifapentine
Decrease: effect of vaccines
Drug/Herb
• St. John's wort: may decrease the effect of sirolimus
Drug/Food
• Alters bioavailability; use consistently with/without food; do not use with grapefruit juice

NURSING CONSIDERATIONS

Assess:
• Blood levels in patients who may have altered metabolism, trough level ≥15 ng/ml are associated with increased adverse reactions; monitor trough concentrations in all patients
• **Lipid profile:** cholesterol, triglycerides; lipid-lowering agent may be needed
⚠ Infection and development of lymphoma
⚠ **Bone marrow suppression:** Hgb, WBC, platelets during treatment each mo; if leukocytes $<3000/mm^3$ or platelets $<100,000/mm^3$, product should be discontinued or reduced; decreased hemoglobulin level
⚠ **Hepatotoxicity:** alk phos, AST, ALT, amylase, bilirubin, dark urine, jaundice, itching, light-colored stools; product should be discontinued
Evaluate:
• Therapeutic response: absence of graft rejection; immunosuppression with autoimmune disorders
Teach patient/family:
⚠ To report fever, rash, severe diarrhea, chills, sore throat, fatigue; serious infections may occur; clay-colored stools, cramping **(hepatotoxicity)**
• To avoid crowds, persons with known infections to reduce risk for infection
• To use contraception before, during, for 12 wk after product discontinued; to avoid breastfeeding
• To use sunscreen, protective clothing to prevent burns, skin cancer
• Not to use with grapefruit juice
• To avoid vaccines
• That lifelong use will be required to prevent rejection
• That continuing follow-up exams and blood work will be required

sitagliptin (Rx)

(sit-a-glip′tin)

Januvia

Func. class.: Antidiabetic, oral
Chem. class.: Dipeptidyl-peptidase-4 inhibitor (DPP-4 inhibitor)

ACTION: Slows the inactivation of incretin hormones; improves glucose homeostasis, improves glucose-dependent insulin secretion, lowers glucagon secretions, and slows gastric emptying time

USES: Type 2 diabetes mellitus as monotherapy or in combination with other antidiabetic agents

CONTRAINDICATIONS: Hypersensitivity, diabetic ketoacidosis (DKA)

Precautions: Pregnancy (B), geriatric patients, GI obstruction, surgery, thyroid/renal/hepatic disease, trauma, breastfeeding, pancreatitis, hypercortisolism, hyperglycemia, hyperthyroidism, hypogylcemia, ileus, pituitary insufficiency, surgery, type 1 diabetes mellitus

DOSAGE AND ROUTES

- **Adult: PO** 100 mg/day; may use with antidiabetic agents other than insulin

Renal dose

- **Adult: PO** CCr 30-50 ml/min, 50 mg daily; CCr <30 ml/min, 25 mg daily

Available forms: Tabs 25, 50, 100 mg

Administer:

- May be taken with/without food

SIDE EFFECTS

CNS: *Headache*

ENDO: Hypoglycemia

GI: *Nausea, vomiting,* abdominal pain, diarrhea, **pancreatitis**, constipation

MISC: *Peripheral edema*

SYST: Anaphylaxis, Stevens-Johnson syndrome, angioedema

PHARMACOKINETICS

Rapidly absorbed, excreted by the kidneys (unchanged 79%), terminal half-life 12.4 hr, peak 1-4 hr

INTERACTIONS

Increase: sitagliptan level—cimetidine, disopyramide

Increase: levels of digoxin

Increase: hypoglycemia—androgens, insulins, β-blockers, cimetidine, corticosteroids, salicylates, MAOIs, fibric acid derivatives, FLUoxetine, sulfonylureas

Decrease: antidiabetic effect—thiazide diuretics, ACE inhibitors, protease inhibitors, sympathomimetics, aripiprazole, clozapine, olanzapine, quetiapine, risperidone, ziprasidone, phenytoin, fosphenytoin, phenothiazines, estrogens, progestins, oral contraceptives

Drug/Herb

Increase: antidiabetic effect—garlic, green tea, horse chestnut

NURSING CONSIDERATIONS

Assess:

- **Hypoglycemic reactions:** sweating, weakness, dizziness, anxiety, tremors, hunger; hyperglycemic reactions soon after meals
- ⚠ **Serious skin reactions: swelling of face, mouth, lips, dyspnea, wheezing**
- ⚠ **Pancreatitis: severe abdominal pain, nausea, vomiting; discontinue product**
- **Renal studies:** BUN, creatinine during treatment
- Glycosylated hemoglobin A1c; monitor blood glucose (BG) as needed

Perform/provide:

- Conversion from other antidiabetic agents; change may be made with gradual dosage change
- Storage in tight container at room temp

Evaluate:

- Therapeutic response: decrease in polyuria, polydipsia, polyphagia; clear sensorium; absence of dizziness; stable gait, blood glucose, A1c improvement

Teach patient/family:

- To perform regular self-monitoring of blood glucose using blood-glucose meter
- About the symptoms of hypo/hyperglycemia, what to do about each; to carry emergency ID
- To notify prescriber if pregnancy is planned, suspected
- That product must be continued on daily basis; about consequences of discontinuing product abruptly; to continue health regimen (diet, exercise)
- To avoid OTC medications, alcohol, digoxin, exenatide, insulins, nateglinide, repaglinide, and other products that lower blood glucose unless approved by prescriber
- That diabetes is a lifelong illness; that product is not a cure, only controls symptoms

S

• That all food included in diet plan must be eaten to prevent hypo/hyperglycemia
• To immediately notify prescriber of hypersensitivity reactions (rash, swelling of face, trouble breathing)

sodium bicarbonate (Rx, OTC)

Baking soda, Brioschi-Neut, Citrocarbonate, Neut, Sellymin ✦

Func. class.: Alkalinizer
Chem. class.: $NaHCO_3$

ACTION: Orally neutralizes gastric acid, which forms water, NaCl, CO_2; increases plasma bicarbonate, which buffers H^+ ion concentration; reverses acidosis IV

USES: Acidosis (metabolic), cardiac arrest, alkalinization (systemic/urinary) antacid, salicylate poisoning

Unlabeled uses: Contrast media nephrotoxicity prevention

CONTRAINDICATIONS: Metabolic/respiratory alkalosis, hypochloremia, hypocalcemia

Precautions: Pregnancy (C), children, CHF, cirrhosis, toxemia, renal disease, hypertension, hypokalemia, breastfeeding, hypernatremia, Bartter's syndrome, Cushing's syndrome, hyperaldosteronism

DOSAGE AND ROUTES

Acidosis, metabolic (not associated with cardiac arrest)

• **Adult and child: IV INF** 2-5 mEq/kg over 4-8 hr depending on CO_2, pH

Cardiac arrest

• **Adult and child: IV BOL** 1 mEq/kg of 7.5% or 8.4% sol, then 0.5 mEq/kg q10min, then doses based on ABGs
• **Infant: IV** 1 mEq/kg over several min (use only the 0.5 mEq/ml [4.2%] sol for inj)

Alkalinization of urine

• **Adult: PO** 325 mg to 2 g qid or 48 mEq (4 g) then 12-24 mEq q4hr
• **Child: PO** 84-840 mg/kg/day (1-10 mEq/kg) in divided doses q4-6hr

Antacid

• **Adult: PO** 300 mg to 2 g chewed, taken with water daily-qid

Available forms: Tabs 300, 325, 600, 650 mg; inj 4.2%, 5%, 7.5%, 8.4%

Administer:

PO route

• Chew antacid tablets and drink 8 oz water
• Do not take antacid with milk because milk-alkali syndrome may result

Direct IV route

• Use for cardiac emergencies, not used often in cardiac arrest
• Use ampules or prefilled syringes only; give by rapid bolus dose; flush with NS before, after use

Continuous IV INF route

• Diluted in an equal amount of compatible sol given 2-5 mEq/kg over 4-8 hr, max 50 mEq/hr; slower rate in children
• Extravasation with IV administration (tissue sloughing, ulceration, necrosis)

Y-site compatibilities: Acyclovir, amifostine, asparaginase, aztreonam, bivalirudin, bumetanide, ceFAZolin, cefepime, ceftazidime, ceftizoxime, cefTRIAXone, chloramphenicol, cimetidine, cladribine, clindamycin, cyclophosphamide, cycloSPORINE, cytarabine, DAPTOmycin, DAUNOrubicin, dexamethasone sodium phosphated exmedetomidine, digoxin, docetaxel, DOXOrubicin, enalaprilat, ertapenem, erythromycin, esmolol, etoposide, etoposide phosphate, famotidine, fentaNYL, filgrastim, fluconazole, fludarabine, furosemide, gallium nitrate, gemcitabine, gentamicin, granisetron, heparin, hydrocortisone sodium succinate, ifosfamide, indomethacin, insulin, ketorolac, labetalol, levofloxacin, lidocaine, linezolid, LORazepam, magnesium sulfate, melphalan, mesna, meperidine, methylPREDNISolone sodium succinate, metoclopramide, metoprolol, metroNI-

DAZOLE, milrinone, morphine, nafcillin, nitroglycerin, nitroprusside, paclitaxel, palonosetron, pantoprazole, pemetrexed, penicillin G potassium, phenylephrine, phytonadione, piperacillin/tazobactam, potassium chloride, procainamide, propranolol, propofol, protamine, ranitidine, remifentanil, tacrolimus, teniposide, thiotepa, ticarcillin/clavulanate, tirofiban, tobramycin, tolazoline, vasopressin, vit B complex with C, voriconazole

SIDE EFFECTS

CNS: Irritability, headache, confusion, stimulation, tremors, *twitching, hyperreflexia,* tetany, weakness, seizures of alkalosis
CV: Irregular pulse, cardiac arrest, water retention, edema, weight gain
GI: Flatulence, *belching, distention*
META: *Metabolic alkalosis*
MS: Muscular twitching, tetany, irritability

PHARMACOKINETICS

PO: Onset rapid, duration 10 min
IV: Onset 15 min, duration 1-2 hr, excreted in urine

INTERACTIONS

Increase: effects—amphetamines, mecamylamine, quiNINE, quiNIDine, pseudoephedrine, flecainide, anorexiants, sympathomimetics
Increase: sodium and decrease potassium—corticosteroids
Decrease: effects—lithium, chlorproPAMIDE, barbiturates, salicylates, benzodiazepines, ketoconazole, corticosteroids

Drug/Lab Test
Increase: sodium, lactate
Decrease: potassium

NURSING CONSIDERATIONS

Assess:

- Respiratory and pulse rate, rhythm, depth, lung sounds; notify prescriber of abnormalities
- **Fluid balance** (I&O, weight daily, edema); notify prescriber of fluid overload; assess for edema, crackles, shortness of breath
- Electrolytes, blood pH, PO_2, HCO_3-, during treatment; ABGs frequently during emergencies
- Weight daily with initial therapy
- **Alkalosis:** irritability, confusion, twitching, hyperreflexia stimulation, slow respirations, cyanosis, irregular pulse
- **Milk-alkali syndrome:** confusion, headache, nausea, vomiting, anorexia, urinary stones, hypercalcemia
- For GI perforation secondary to carbon dioxide in GI tract; may lead to perforation if ulcer is severe enough

Evaluate:

- Therapeutic response: ABGs, electrolytes, blood pH, HCO_3 WNL

Teach patient/family:

- Not to take antacid with milk because milk-alkali syndrome may result; not to use antacid for >2 wk

⚠ To notify prescriber if indigestion accompanied by chest pain; trouble breathing; diarrhea; dark, tarry stools; vomit that looks like coffee grounds; swelling of feet/ankles

- About sodium-restricted diet; to avoid use of baking soda for indigestion

S

sodium polystyrene sulfonate (Rx)

(po-lee-stye′reen)

Kayexalate, Kionex, SPS

Func. class.: Potassium-removing resin

Chem. class.: Cation exchange resin

ACTION: Removes potassium by exchanging sodium for potassium in body, primarily in large intestine

USES: Hyperkalemia in conjunction with other measures

CONTRAINDICATIONS: Hypersensitivity to saccharin or parabens that may be in some products, GI obstruction, neonate (reduced gut motility)

Precautions: Pregnancy (C), geriatric patients, renal failure, CHF, severe edema, severe hypertension, sodium restriction, constipation, GI bleeding, hypocalcemia

DOSAGE AND ROUTES

- **Adult: PO** 15 g daily-qid; **RECT** enema 30-50 g q1-2hr initially prn then q6hr prn
- **Child (unlabeled): PO** 1 g/kg q6hr prn; **RECT** 1 g/kg q2-6hr prn

Available forms: Powder for susp 453.6 g, 454 g; oral susp 15 g/60 ml

Administer:

PO route

- Oral dose as susp, mixed with water or syr (20-100 ml)
- Mild laxative (not magnesium) as ordered to prevent constipation, fecal impaction

Rectal route

- Retention enema after mixing with warm water; introduce by gravity, continue stirring, flush with 100 ml fluid, clamp, and leave in place
- Retention of enema for at least 1/2-1 hr
- Irrigation of colon after enema with 1-2 qt nonsodium sol, drain

SIDE EFFECTS

GI: Constipation, anorexia, nausea, vomiting, diarrhea (sorbitol), fecal impaction, gastric irritation

META: Hypocalcemia, hypokalemia, hypomagnesemia, sodium retention

INTERACTIONS

Increase: hypokalemia—loop diuretics, cardiac glycosides

Increase: metabolic alkalosis—magnesium/calcium antacids

⚠ **Increase:** colonic necrosis—sorbitol; do not use concurrently

Decrease: effect of—lithium, thyroid hormones

NURSING CONSIDERATIONS

Assess:

- **Hyperkalemia:** confusion, dyspnea, weakness, dysrhythmias; ECG for spiked T waves, depressed ST segments, prolonged QT and widening QRS complex
- Bowel function daily; note consistency of stools, times/day
- **Hypotension:** confusion, irritability, muscular pain, weakness
- **Electrolytes:** serum potassium, calcium, magnesium, sodium; acid-base balance
- I&O ratio, weight daily; crackles, dyspnea, jugular venous distension, edema
- Digoxin toxicity (nausea, vomiting, blurred vision, anorexia, dysrhythmias) in those receiving digoxin

Perform/provide:

- Storage of freshly prepared sol 24 hr at room temp

Evaluate:

- Therapeutic response: potassium level 3.5-5 mg/dl

Teach patient/family:

- About reason for medication and expected results

⚠ Nurse Alert

• To avoid laxatives, antacids, electrolyte-based products unless approved by prescriber

solifenacin (Rx)

(sol-i-fen′a-sin)

VESIcare

Func. class.: Urinary antispasmodic, anticholinergic

Chem. class.: Anti-muscarinic

ACTION: Relaxes smooth muscles in urinary tract by inhibiting acetylcholine at postganglionic sites

USES: Overactive bladder (urinary frequency, urgency, incontinence)

CONTRAINDICATIONS: Hypersensitivity, uncontrolled closed-angle glaucoma, urinary retention, gastric retention

Precautions: Pregnancy (C), breastfeeding, children, geriatric patients, renal/hepatic disease, controlled closed-angle glaucoma, bladder outflow obstruction, GI obstruction, decreased GI motility, history of QT prolongation

DOSAGE AND ROUTES

• **Adult: PO** 5 mg/day, max 10 mg/day

Renal/hepatic dose

• **Adult: PO** (Child-Pugh B) max 5 mg/day; CCr ≤30 ml/min, 5 mg/day

Available forms: Tabs 5, 10 mg

Administer:

• Without regard to meals

• Swallow product whole with water, liquid

SIDE EFFECTS

CNS: Anxiety, paresthesia, fatigue, *dizziness,* headache, confusion

CV: Chest pain, hypertension, QTc prolongation, peripheral edema

EENT: *Vision abnormalities, xerophthalmia,* nasal dryness

GI: *Nausea, vomiting, anorexia,* abdominal pain, *constipation, dry mouth,* dyspepsia

GU: Dysuria, urinary retention, frequency, UTI

INTEG: Rash, pruritus, angioedema

MISC: Hyperthermia

RESP: Bronchitis, cough, pharyngitis, upper respiratory tract infection

PHARMACOKINETICS

90% absorbed; 98% protein bound; extensively metabolized by CYP3A4; excreted in urine 69% (metabolites), feces 22%; terminal half-life 45-68 hr

INTERACTIONS

Increase: CNS depression—sedatives, hypnotics, benzodiazepines, opioids

Increase: effects—CYP3A4 inhibitors (ketoconazole, clarithromycin, diclofenac, doxycycline, erythromycin, isoniazid, nefazodone, propofol, protease inhibitors, verapamil), max dose 5 mg

Decrease: effects—CYP3A4 inducers (carBAMazepine, nevirapine, PHENobarbital, phenytoin)

Drug/Herb

Decrease: effects—St. John's wort

Drug/Food

Increase: effect—grapefruit juice

NURSING CONSIDERATIONS

Assess:

• **Urinary patterns:** distention, nocturia, frequency, urgency, incontinence

• **Allergic reactions:** rash

• **Angioedema:** of the face, lips, tongue, larynx

⚠ Cardiac patients: monitor ECG for QTc prolongation; avoid products that increase QT prolongation

Evaluate:

• Decreasing dysuria, frequency, nocturia, incontinence

Teach patient/family:

• To avoid hazardous activities because dizziness may occur

• That constipation, blurred vision may occur

• To call prescriber if severe abdominal pain or constipation lasts for ≥3 days
• That heat prostration may occur if used in hot environment
• About **anticholinergic effects:** blurred vision, constipation, urinary retention, hyperthermia

somatropin (Rx)

(soe-ma-troe′pin)

Genotropin, Humatrope, Norditropin, Norditropin Flexpro, Nutropin, Nutropin AQ, Omnitrope, Saizen, Serostim, Tev-Tropin, Zorbtive

Func. class.: Pituitary hormone
Chem. class.: Growth hormone

Do not confuse:
somatropin/sumatriptan

ACTION: Stimulates growth; somatropin is similar to natural growth hormone; both preparations were developed with the use of recombinant DNA

USES: Pituitary growth hormone deficiency (hypopituitary dwarfism), children with human growth hormone deficiency/growth failure, AIDS wasting syndrome, cachexia, adults with somatropin deficiency syndrome (SDS), short stature in Noonan syndrome, SHOX deficiency, Turner's syndrome, Prader-Willi syndrome

CONTRAINDICATIONS: Hypersensitivity to benzyl alcohol, creosol; closed epiphyses, intracranial lesions, acute respiratory failure, Prader-Willi syndrome with obesity, trauma

Precautions: Pregnancy (C), breastfeeding, newborn, geriatric patients, diabetes mellitus, hypothyroidism, prolonged treatment in adults, scoliosis, sleep apnea, chemotherapy, respiratory disease, glycerin hypersensitivity (with formulations that contain these products)

DOSAGE AND ROUTES

Genotropin

• **Child: SUBCUT** 0.16-0.24 mg/kg/wk divided into 6 or 7 daily inj, give in abdomen, thigh, buttocks
• **Adult: SUBCUT** 0.04-0.08 mg/kg/wk divided into 6-7 daily doses

Humatrope

• **Adult: IM** 0.006 international units/kg/day, max 0.0125 units/kg/day
• **Child: SUBCUT/IM** 0.18 mg/kg divided into equal doses either on 3 alternate days or 6×/wk, max weekly dose 0.3 mg/kg

Nutropin/Nutropin AQ (growth hormone deficiency)

• **Child: SUBCUT** 0.3 mg/kg/wk

Serostim

• **Adult: SUBCUT** at bedtime >55 kg, 6 mg; 45-55 kg, 5 mg; 35-45 kg, 4 mg

Norditropin

• **Child: SUBCUT** 0.024-0.034 mg/kg 6-7×/wk

Accretropin

• **Child: SUBCUT** 0.18-0.3 mg/kg/wk divided into 6 or 7 equal daily inj

Replacement of GH in GH deficiency

• **Adult: SUBCUT** (Saizen) 0.005 mg/kg/day; may increase after 4 wk to max 0.01 mg/kg/day

Available forms: Powder for inj (lyophilized) 1.5 mg (4 international units/ml), 4 mg (12 international units/vial), 5 mg (13 international units/vial), 5 mg (15 international units/vial) rDNA origin, 5.8 mg (15 international units/ml), 6 mg (18 international units/ml), 8 mg (24 international units/vial), 10 mg (26 international units/vial); inj 10 mg (30 international units/vial), 5 mg/1.5 ml, 10 mg/1.5 ml, 15 mg/1.5 ml

Administer:

IM route

• Rotate inj site
• **Accretropin:** does not require reconstitution
• **Norditropin:** after reconstituting 4 or 8 mg/2 ml diluent
• **Humatrope:** 5 mg/1.5-5 ml diluent; do not shake

• **Nutropin/Nutropin AQ:** reconstitute 5 mg/1-5 ml or 10 mg/1-10 ml bacteriostatic water for inj (benzyl alcohol preserved)
• **Zorbtive:** reconstitute 4, 5, 6 mg with 0.5-1 ml of sterile water for inj; reconstitute each 8.8 mg with 1-2 ml bacteriostatic water for inj

SIDE EFFECTS

CNS: Headache, growth of intracranial tumor, fever, aggressive behavior
ENDO: Hyperglycemia, ketosis, hypothyroidism
GI: Nausea, vomiting
GU: *Hypercalciuria*
INTEG: Rash, urticaria, pain; inflammation at inj site, hematoma
MS: Tissue swelling, joint and muscle pain
SYST: Antibodies to growth hormone

PHARMACOKINETICS

Half-life 15-60 min, duration 7 days, metabolized in liver

INTERACTIONS

Increase: epiphyseal closure—androgens, thyroid hormones
Decrease: growth—glucocorticosteroids
Decrease: insulin, antidiabetic effect—dosage adjustment may be needed

NURSING CONSIDERATIONS

Assess:
• Signs/symptoms of diabetes
• Growth hormone antibodies if patient fails to respond to therapy
• Thyroid function tests: T_3, T_4, T_7, TSH to identify hypothyroidism
• **Allergic reaction:** rash, itching, fever, nausea, wheezing
• **Hypercalciuria:** urinary stones; groin, flank pain; nausea, vomiting, urinary frequency, hematuria, chills
• Growth rate, bone age of child at intervals during treatment

Perform/provide:
• Storage in refrigerator for <1 mo; if reconstituted, <1 wk; do not use discolored or cloudy sol

Evaluate:
• Therapeutic response: growth in children

Teach patient/family:
• That treatment may continue for years; that regular assessments are required
• To maintain a growth record; to report knee/hip pain or limping
• That treatment is very expensive

sorafenib (Rx)

(sore-ah-fen′ib)

Nexavar

Func. class.: Antineoplastic—miscellaneous
Chem. class.: Multikinase inhibitor, signal transduction inhibitor

ACTION:
Multikinase inhibitor that decreases tumor cell proliferation

USES:
Advanced/metastatic murine renal cell carcinoma, unresectable hepatocellular cancer
Unlabeled uses: Metastatic malignant melanoma

CONTRAINDICATIONS:
Pregnancy (D), hypersensitivity
Precautions: Breastfeeding, children, geriatric patients, cardiac/renal/hepatic disease, GI bleeding infection, surgery, dental disease/work

DOSAGE AND ROUTES

• **Adult: PO** 400 mg bid without food, continue until patient no longer benefiting or until unacceptable toxicity occurs
Available forms: Tabs 200 mg
Administer:
• Swallow tab whole; do not break, crush, or chew
• On empty stomach 1 hr before or 2 hr after meal

S

SIDE EFFECTS

CNS: *Fatigue, weight loss, headache*
CV: Hypertension, cardiac ischemia, infarction, hypertensive crisis, cardiotoxicity, MI, thromboembolism
GI: *Nausea, diarrhea, vomiting,* anorexia, pancreatitis, mouth ulceration, *abdominal pain,* constipation, GI perforation
HEMA: Hemorrhage, leukopenia, lymphopenia, anemia, neutropenia, thrombocytopenia, pancytopenia
INTEG: *Rash,* pruritus, *dry skin,* erythema, *hand-foot syndrome,* exfoliative dermatitis, acne, flushing, *alopecia*
META: *Hypophosphatemia*
MS: *Arthralgia, myalgia*
RESP: *Hoarseness*

PHARMACOKINETICS

Bioavailability 38%-49%, elimination half-life 1-2 days, peak 3 hr, high-fat meal decreases bioavailability, plasma protein binding 99.5%, metabolized in liver, oxidative metabolism by CYP3A4, glucuronidation by UGT1A9, 77% excreted in feces

INTERACTIONS

Increase: bleeding risk—NSAIDs, anticoagulants, platelet inhibitors, thrombolytics
Increase: effect of UGT1A1 substrates (irinotecan, DOXOrubicin, morphine, naltrexone, estradiol, buprenorphine)
Decrease: sorafenib effect—CYP3A4 inducers (barbiturates, bosentan, carBAMazepine, efavirenz, phenytoins, nevirapine, rifabutin, rifampin); use cautiously
Decrease: sorafenib levels—phenytoin, rifampin, cimetidine, ranitidine, sodium bicarbonate, carBAMazepine, dexamethasone, PHENobarbital

Drug/Herb

- Avoid use with St. John's wort

Drug/Lab Test

Increase: lipase, amylase, TSH, bilirubin transaminase
Decrease: RBC, WBC, platelets

NURSING CONSIDERATIONS

Assess:

- CBC with differential, LFTs
- **Skin toxicities:** grade 1, continue therapy, topical treatment for relief; grade 2 (1st episode), continue therapy, if no improvement after 7 days, delay treatment until resolved to grade ≤1, resume dose by 1 dose level; grade 2 (2nd or 3rd episode), delay treatment until resolved to grade ≤1, resume dose by 1 dose level; grade 2 (4th episode), discontinue therapy; grade 3 (1st or 2nd episode), delay treatment until resolved to grade ≤1, resume dose by 1 dose level; grade 3 (3rd episode), discontinue therapy
- **Cardiac events:** B/P weekly × 6 wk (hypertension); cardiac ischemia; bleeding, bruising
- **Hand-foot reactions** during first 6 wk of therapy
- PT, INR (bleeding)

Perform/provide:

- Storage at room temp in dry place

Evaluate:

- Therapeutic response: stabilization of renal cell carcinoma progression

Teach patient/family:

⚠ To report adverse reactions immediately
- About reason for treatment, expected results

⚠ To use contraception during treatment, pregnancy (D); that birth defects may occur; to avoid breastfeeding
- To not double dose if dose missed
- To avoid OTC products without approval of prescriber

sotalol (Rx)

(sot'ah-lahl)

Betapace, Betapace AF, Sorine

Func. class.: Antidysrhythmic group III

Chem. class.: Nonselective β-blocker

ACTION: Blockade of β_1- and β_2-receptors leads to antidysrhythmic effect, prolongs action potential in myocardial fibers without affecting conduction, prolongs QT interval, no effect on QRS duration

USES: Life-threatening ventricular dysrhythmias; Betapace AF: to maintain sinus rhythm with symptomatic atrial fibrillation/flutter

Unlabeled uses: Atrial fibrillation prophylaxis, cardiac surgery, PSVT, Wolff-Parkinson-White (WPW) syndrome

CONTRAINDICATIONS: Hypersensitivity to β-blockers, cardiogenic shock, heart block (2nd/3rd degree), sinus bradycardia, CHF, bronchial asthma, CCr <40 ml/min

Black Box Warning: Congenital or acquired long QT syndrome, hypokalemia

Precautions: Pregnancy (B), breastfeeding, major surgery, diabetes mellitus, renal/thyroid disease, COPD, well-compensated heart failure, CAD, nonallergic bronchospasm, electrolyte disturbances, bradycardia, peripheral vascular disease

Black Box Warning: Cardiac dysrhythmias, torsades de pointes, ventricular dysrhythmias, ventricular fibrillation

DOSAGE AND ROUTES

- **Adult: PO** initial 80 mg bid, may increase to 240-320 mg/day
- **Child >2 yr with normal renal function (unlabeled): PO** 30 mg/m^2 tid, adjust dose gradually after ≥36 hr to max 60 mg/m^2 tid

Renal dose

- **Adult: PO** CCr 30-60 ml/min, give q24hr; CCr 10-29 ml/min, give q36-48hr; CCr <10 ml/min, individualize dose

Life-threatening ventricular dysrhythmias

- **Adult (CCr 40-60 ml/min): IV** 75 mg over 5 hr daily, monitor QTc at end of each inf during initiation and titration; 80 mg PO = 75 mg IV; 120 mg PO = 112.5 mg IV; 160 mg PO = 150 mg IV

Betapace AF

- **Adult: PO** initial 80 mg bid, titrate upward to 120 mg bid during initial hospitalization

Renal dose (Betapace AF)

- **Adult: PO** CCr >60 ml/min, give q12hr; CCr 40-60 ml/min, give q24hr; CCr <40 ml/min, do not use

Available forms: Tabs 80, 120, 160, 240 mg; (Betapace AF) 80, 120, 160 mg; inj 150 mg/10 ml (15 mg/ml)

Administer:

PO route

- Before, at bedtime; tablet may be crushed or swallowed whole; give 1 hr before or 2 hr after meals
- Reduced dosage in renal dysfunction
- Betapace and Betapace AF are not interchangeable
- Do not give within 2 hr of antacids

IV route

- Dilute to vol of either 120 ml or 300 ml with D_5W, LR
- **75 mg dose:** withdraw 6 ml sotalol inj (90 mg), add 114 ml dilute to make 120 ml (0.75 mg/ml) or withdraw 6 ml sotalol inj (90 mg), add 294 ml dilute to make 300 ml (0.3 mg/ml)
- **112.5 mg dose:** withdraw 9 ml sotalol inj (135 ml), add 111 ml dilute to make 120 ml (1.125 mg/ml); or withdraw 9 ml sotalol (135 mg), add 291 ml dilute to make 300 ml (0.45 mg/ml)
- **150 mg dose:** withdraw 12 ml of sotalol (180 mg), add 108 ml to make 120 ml (1.5 mg/ml) or withdraw 12 ml so-

S

talol (180 mg), add 288 ml to make 300 ml (0.6 mg/ml)
• Use inf pump and infuse 100 or 250 ml over 5 hr at a constant rate

SIDE EFFECTS

CNS: Dizziness, mental changes, drowsiness, fatigue, headache, catatonia, depression, anxiety, nightmares, paresthesia, lethargy, insomnia, decreased concentration

CV: Prodysrhythmia, prolonged QT, orthostatic hypotension, bradycardia, CHF, chest pain, ventricular dysrhythmias, AV block, peripheral vascular insufficiency, palpitations, torsades de pointes; life-threatening ventricular dysrhythmias (Betapace AF)

EENT: Tinnitus, visual changes, sore throat, double vision; dry, burning eyes

GI: Nausea, vomiting, diarrhea, dry mouth, flatulence, constipation, anorexia, indigestion

GU: Impotence, dysuria, ejaculatory failure, urinary retention

HEMA: Agranulocytosis, thrombocytopenic purpura (rare), thrombocytopenia, leukopenia

INTEG: Rash, alopecia, urticaria, pruritus, fever, diaphoresis

MISC: Facial swelling, decreased exercise tolerance, weight change, Raynaud's disease

MS: Joint pain, arthralgia, muscle cramps, pain

RESP: Bronchospasm, dyspnea, wheezing, nasal stuffiness, pharyngitis

PHARMACOKINETICS

PO: Onset 1-2 hr, peak 2-4 hr, duration 8-12 hr, half-life 12 hr, excreted unchanged in urine, crosses placenta, excreted in breast milk, protein binding 0%

INTERACTIONS

Increase: QT prolongation—class IA/III antidysrhythmics, some phenothiazines, β agonists, local anesthetics, tricyclics, haloperidol, chloroquine, droperidol, pentamidine; CYP3A4 inhibitors (amiodarone, clarithromycin, erythromycin, telithromycin, troleandomycin), arsenic trioxide, levomethadyl; CYP3A4 substrates (methadone, pimozide, QUEtiapine, quiNIDine, risperidone, ziprasidone)

Increase: hypoglycemia effect—insulin

Increase: effects of lidocaine

Increase: hypotension—diuretics, other antihypertensives, nitroglycerin

Decrease: β-blocker effects—sympathomimetics

Decrease: bronchodilating effects of theophylline, β_2-agonists

Decrease: hypoglycemic effects of sulfonylureas

Drug/Lab Test

False increase: urinary catecholamines

Interference: glucose, insulin tolerance tests

NURSING CONSIDERATIONS

Assess:

• I&O, weight daily; edema in feet, legs daily
• B/P, pulse q4hr; note rate, rhythm, quality
• Potassium, magnesium levels

⚠ **QT syndrome:** apical/radial pulse before administration: notify prescriber of any significant changes; monitor ECG continuously (Betapace AF); use QT interval to determine patient eligibility; baseline QT must be ≤450 msec

• Baselines of renal studies before therapy begins
• Skin turgor, dryness of mucous membranes for hydration status

Perform/provide:

• Storage in dry area at room temp; do not freeze

Evaluate:

• Therapeutic response: absence of life-threatening dysrhythmias

Teach patient/family:

• Not to discontinue product abruptly; to taper over 2 wk or may precipitate angina; to take exactly as prescribed
• Not to use antacids or OTC products containing α-adrenergic stimulants (na-

sal decongestants, OTC cold preparations) unless directed by prescriber
- To report bradycardia, dizziness, confusion, depression, fever
- To take pulse at home; advise patient when to notify prescriber
- To avoid alcohol, smoking, sodium intake
- To carry emergency ID to identify product being taken, allergies
- To avoid hazardous activities if dizziness present
- To report symptoms of CHF including difficulty breathing, especially on exertion or when lying down; night cough, swelling of extremities
- To wear support hose to minimize effects of orthostatic hypotension
- To monitor blood glucose if diabetic

TREATMENT OF OVERDOSE:
Lavage, IV atropine for bradycardia, IV theophylline for bronchospasm, digoxin, O_2, diuretic for cardiac failure; hemodialysis is useful for removal; administer vasopressor (norepinephrine) for hypotension, isoproterenol for heart block

spironolactone (Rx)
(speer′on-oh-lak′tone)

Aldactone, Novo-Spiroton ✦

Func. class.: Potassium-sparing diuretic

Chem. class.: Aldosterone antagonist

ACTION: Competes with aldosterone at receptor sites in distal tubule, thereby resulting in the excretion of sodium chloride and water and the retention of potassium and phosphate

USES: Edema of CHF, hypertension, diuretic-induced hypokalemia, primary hyperaldosteronism (diagnosis, short-term treatment, long-term treatment), edema of nephrotic syndrome, cirrhosis of liver with ascites

Unlabeled uses: CHF, hirsutism in women, bronchopulmonary dysplasia (BPD), PMS, polycystic ovary syndrome, acne vulgaris, premenstrual syndrome

CONTRAINDICATIONS: Pregnancy (D), hypersensitivity, anuria, severe renal disease, hyperkalemia

Precautions: Breastfeeding, dehydration, hepatic disease, renal impairment, electrolyte imbalances, metabolic acidosis, gynecomastia

Black Box Warning: Secondary malignancy

DOSAGE AND ROUTES
Edema/hypertension
- **Adult: PO** 25-200 mg/day in 1-2 divided doses

CHF
- **Adult: PO** 12.5-25 mg/day; max 50 mg/day

Edema
- **Child: PO** 1.5-3.3 mg/kg/day as single dose or in divided doses

Hypertension
- **Child (unlabeled): PO** 1.5-3.3 mg/kg/day in divided doses

Hypokalemia
- **Adult: PO** 25-100 mg/day; if **PO**, potassium supplements must not be used

Primary hyperaldosteronism diagnosis
- **Adult: PO** 400 mg/day × 4 days or 4 wk depending on test, then 100-400 mg/day maintenance

Edema (nephrotic syndrome, CHF, hepatic disease)
- **Adult: PO** 100 mg/day given as single dose or in divided doses, titrate to response
- **Child: PO** 1.5-3.3 mg/kg/day or 60 mg/m²/day given daily or in 2-4 divided doses

Renal dose
- **Adult: PO** CCr 10-50 ml/min; give dose q12-24hr; CCr <10 ml/min, avoid use

Polycystic ovary syndrome/hirsutism in women (unlabeled)
- **Adult: PO** 50-200 mg in 1-2 divided doses

S

Acne vulgaris (unlabeled)
- **Adult: PO** 50-200 mg/day

Available forms: Tabs 25, 50, 100 mg
Administer:
- In AM to avoid interference with sleep
- With food; if nausea occurs, absorption may be decreased slightly

SIDE EFFECTS

CNS: *Headache,* confusion, drowsiness, lethargy, ataxia
ELECT: Hyperchloremic metabolic acidosis, hyperkalemia, hyponatremia
ENDO: Impotence, gynecomastia, irregular menses, amenorrhea, postmenopausal bleeding, hirsutism, deepening voice, breast pain
GI: *Diarrhea,* cramps, bleeding, gastritis, *vomiting,* anorexia, nausea, hepatocellular toxicity
HEMA: Agranulocytosis
INTEG: *Rash, pruritus,* urticaria

PHARMACOKINETICS

Onset 24-48 hr, peak 48-72 hr, metabolized in liver, excreted in urine, crosses placenta, protein binding >90%, terminal half-life 10-35 hr

INTERACTIONS

Increase: action of antihypertensives, digoxin, lithium
Increase: hyperchloremic acidosis in cirrhosis—cholestyramine
Increase: hyperkalemia—potassium-sparing diuretics, potassium products, ACE inhibitors, salt substitutes
Decrease: effect of anticoagulants
Decrease: effect of spironolactone—ASA, NSAIDs
Drug/Herb
Increase: severe photosensitivity—St. John's wort
Drug/Lab Test
Interference: 17-OHCS, 17-KS, radioimmunoassay, digoxin assay

NURSING CONSIDERATIONS

Assess:
- **Hypokalemia:** polyuria, polydipsia; dysrhythmias, inluding a U wave on ECG
- **Hyperkalemia:** weakness, fatigue, dyspnea, dysrhythmias, confusion, fatigue
- Electrolytes: sodium, chloride, potassium, BUN, serum creatinine, ABGs, CBC
- Weight, I&O daily to determine fluid loss; effect of product may be decreased if used daily; ECG periodically with long-term therapy
- Signs of metabolic acidosis: drowsiness, restlessness
- Rashes, temp daily
- Confusion, especially in geriatric patients; take safety precautions if needed
- **Hydration:** skin turgor, thirst, dry mucous membranes

Evaluate:
- Therapeutic response: improvement in edema of feet, legs, sacral area daily if medication is being used in CHF

Teach patient/family:
- To avoid foods with high potassium content: oranges, bananas, salt substitutes, dried apricots, dates; to avoid potassium salt substitutes
- That drowsiness, ataxia, mental confusion may occur; to observe caution when driving
- To notify prescriber of cramps, diarrhea, lethargy, thirst, headache, skin rash, menstrual abnormalities, deepening voice, breast enlargement

TREATMENT OF OVERDOSE:

Lavage if taken orally; monitor electrolytes, administer IV fluids, monitor hydration, renal, CV status

stavudine d4t (Rx)

(sta'vyoo-deen)

Zerit

Func. class.: Antiretroviral

Chem. class.: Nucleoside reverse transcriptase inhibitor (NRTI)

ACTION: Prevents replication of HIV by the inhibition of the enzyme reverse transcriptase; causes DNA chain termination

USES: Treatment of HIV-1 in combination with other antiretrovirals

CONTRAINDICATIONS: Hypersensitivity to this product or zidovudine; didanosine, zalcitabine; severe peripheral neuropathy

Black Box Warning: Lactic acidosis

Precautions: Breastfeeding, advanced HIV infection, bone marrow suppression, renal disease, peripheral neuropathy, osteoporosis, obesity

Black Box Warning: Pregnancy (C), hepatic disease, pancreatitis

DOSAGE AND ROUTES

- **Adult >60 kg: PO** 40 mg q12hr
- **Adult <60 kg: PO** 30 mg q12hr
- **Child <30 kg: PO** 1 mg/kg q12hr
- **Child ≥30 kg, ≤60 kg: PO** 30 mg q12hr
- **Child >60 kg: PO** 40 mg q12hr

Renal dose

- **Adult: >60 kg: PO** CCr 26-50 ml/min, 20 mg q12hr; CCr 10-25 ml/min, 20 mg q24hr
- **Adult: <60 kg: PO** CCr 26-50 ml/min, 15 mg q12hr; CCr 10-25 ml/min, 15 mg q24hr

Available forms: Caps 15, 20, 30, 40 mg; powder for oral sol 1 mg/ml

Administer:

- With/without meals; absorption does not appear to be lowered when taken with food
- Every 12 hr around the clock
- Shake suspension well before using

SIDE EFFECTS

CNS: *Peripheral neuropathy,* insomnia, anxiety, depression, dizziness, confusion, *headache,* chills/fever, malaise, neuropathy

CV: Chest pain, vasodilation, hypertension

EENT: Conjunctivitis, abnormal vision

GI: Hepatotoxicity, *diarrhea, nausea, vomiting,* anorexia, dyspepsia, constipation, stomatitis, pancreatitis

HEMA: Bone marrow suppression, leukopenia, macrocytosis

INTEG: *Rash,* sweating, pruritus, benign neoplasms

MISC: Lactic acidosis, asthenia, lipodystrophy

MS: Myalgia, arthralgia

RESP: Dyspnea, pneumonia, asthma

PHARMACOKINETICS

Excreted in urine, breast milk; peak 1 hr; half-life: elimination 1-1.6 hr, intracellular 3-3.5 hr

INTERACTIONS

Increase: myelosuppression—other myelosuppressants

Increase: peripheral neuropathy—lithium, dapsone, chloramphenicol didanosine, ethambutol, hydrALAZINE, phenytoin, vinCRIStine, zalcitabine

Increase: stavudine levels—probenecid

Decrease: stavudine effect—methadone, zidovudine

NURSING CONSIDERATIONS

Assess:

⚠ **Lactic acidosis and severe hepatomegaly with steatosis:** death may result

⚠ **Pancreatitis:** severe upper abdominal pain, nausea, vomiting throughout treatment; discontinue product

- Blood studies: WBC, differential, RBC, Hct, Hgb, platelets, serum amylase, lipase
- Renal tests: urinalysis, protein, blood, serum creatinine

- C&S before product therapy; product may be given as soon as culture taken
- Bowel pattern before, during treatment
- Weakness, tremors, confusion, dizziness; product may have to be decreased, discontinued
- Viral load, CD4 counts, plasma HIV RNA at baseline and throughout treatment
- Peripheral neuropathy: tingling, pain in extremities; discontinue product

Evaluate:

- Therapeutic response: decreased symptoms of HIV

Teach patient/family:

- **About the signs of peripheral neuropathy:** burning, weakness, pain, prickling feeling in extremities
- That product should not be given with antineoplastics
- That product is not a cure for AIDS but will control symptoms
- To call prescriber if sore throat, swollen lymph nodes, malaise, fever occur; that other products may be needed to prevent other infections
- That, even with use of product, patient may pass AIDS virus to others
- That follow-up visits are necessary; that serious toxicity may occur; that blood counts must be done q2wk

⚠ That serious product interactions may occur if other medications are ingested; to see prescriber before taking chloramphenicol, dapsone, CISplatin, didanosine, ethambutol, lithium, antifungals, antineoplastics

- That product may cause fainting or dizziness

streptomycin (Rx)

(strep-toe-mye′sin)

Func. class.: Antiinfective/antitubercular

Chem. class.: Aminoglycoside

ACTION: Interferes with protein synthesis in bacterial cells by binding to ribosomal 30 S, thereby causing inaccurate peptide sequences to form in the protein chain; bactericidal

USES: Sensitive strains of *Mycobacterium tuberculosis;* nontuberculous infections caused by sensitive strains of *Yersinia pestis, Brucella, Haemophilus influenzae, Klebsiella pneumoniae, Escherichia coli, Enterobacter aerogenes, Streptococcus viridans, Francisella tularensis, Proteus*

CONTRAINDICATIONS: Hypersensitivity

Black Box Warning: Pregnancy (D), severe renal disease

Precautions: Breastfeeding, neonates, geriatric patients, mild renal disease, myasthenia gravis, Parkinson's disease, hepatic disease

Black Box Warning: Hearing deficit, neuromuscular disease

DOSAGE AND ROUTES

General dosing

- **Adult: IM** 1-2 g in divided doses q6-12 hr
- **Child: IM** 20-40 mg/kg/day in divided doses q6-12hr, max adult dose

Tuberculosis (HIV negative)

- **Adult: IM** 15 mg/kg/day (max 1 g) × 2-3 mo then 1 g 2-3×/week with other antitubercular products
- **Child: IM** 20-40 mg/kg/day, max 1 g/day

Enterococcal endocarditis

- **Adult: IM/IV** 15 mg/kg/day divided q12hr
- **Child: IM/IV** 20-30 mg/kg/day divided q12hr

Available forms: Inj 500 mg 🍁, 1 g/ml

Administer:

- IM inj in large muscle mass; rotate inj sites
- Product in evenly spaced doses to maintain blood level

SIDE EFFECTS

CNS: Confusion, depression, numbness, tremors, **seizures**, muscle twitching, **neurotoxicity**, dizziness, headache

CV: Hypotension, myocarditis, palpitations

EENT: **Ototoxicity, deafness**, visual disturbances, tinnitus

GI: *Nausea, vomiting, anorexia;* increased ALT, AST, bilirubin; **hepatomegaly, hepatic necrosis, splenomegaly**

GU: **Oliguria, hematuria, renal damage, azotemia, renal failure, nephrotoxicity**

HEMA: **Agranulocytosis, thrombocytopenia, leukopenia, eosinophilia, anemia**

INTEG: *Rash,* burning, urticaria, dermatitis, alopecia

MS: Arthralgia, weakness

PHARMACOKINETICS

IM: Onset rapid, peak 1-2 hr, plasma half-life 2-2$^1/_2$ hr, not metabolized, excreted unchanged in urine, crosses placental barrier, poor penetration into CSF, small amounts enter breast milk

INTERACTIONS

Increase: ototoxicity, neurotoxicity, nephrotoxicity—other aminoglycosides, amphotericin B, polymyxin, vancomycin, ethacrynic acid, furosemide, mannitol, methoxyflurane, CISplatin, cephalosporins, cidofovir, tacrolimus

Increase: streptomycin effects—nondepolarizing muscle relaxants, succinylcholine, warfarin, NSAIDs

Increase: toxicity—lysine (large amounts)

NURSING CONSIDERATIONS

Assess:

- **Infection:** urine, stool, sputum, wound characteristics, fever, monitor WBC for changes
- Weight before treatment; calculation of dosage is usually based on ideal body weight but may be calculated on actual body weight
- I&O ratio, urinalysis daily for proteinuria, cells, casts; report sudden change in urine output
- Serum peak 30-60 min after IM inj, trough level drawn before next dose; acceptable levels—therapeutic peak 15-40 mg/L, therapeutic trough <5 mg/L
- **Severe renal disease:** renal impairment by collecting urine for CCr testing, BUN, serum creatinine; lower dosage should be given with renal impairment (CCr <80 ml/min), monitor electrolytes: K, Na, Cl, Mg
- **Deafness** by audiometric testing; ringing, roaring in ears; vertigo; assess hearing before, during, after treatment
- **Dehydration:** high specific gravity, decreased skin turgor, dry mucous membranes, dark urine
- **Overgrowth of infection:** fever, malaise, redness, pain, swelling, perineal itching, diarrhea, stomatitis; change in cough, sputum
- C&S before starting treatment to identify infecting organism; use only for susceptible bacteria to prevent development of drug-resistant bacteria
- **Vestibular dysfunction:** nausea, vomiting, dizziness, headache; product should be discontinued if severe
- Inj sites for redness, swelling, abscesses; use warm compresses at site

Perform/provide:

- Adequate fluids of 2-3 L/day unless contraindicated to prevent irritation of tubules
- Supervised ambulation, other safety measures with vestibular dysfunction

Evaluate:

- Therapeutic effect: absence of fever, draining wounds, negative C&S after treatment

Teach patient/family:

- To report headache, dizziness, symptoms of overgrowth of infection, renal impairment
- To report loss of hearing; ringing, roaring in ears; fullness in head

S

TREATMENT OF OVERDOSE:
Hemodialysis; monitor serum levels of product

succimer (Rx)
(sux'i-mer)

Chemet

Func. class.: Heavy metal chelator antagonist

Chem. class.: Chelating agent

ACTION: Binds with ions of lead to form a water-soluble complex excreted by kidneys

USES: Lead poisoning in children with lead levels >45 mcg/dl; may be beneficial in mercury, arsenic poisoning

Unlabeled uses: Adults with lead levels >45 mcg/dl

CONTRAINDICATIONS: Hypersensitivity

Precautions: Pregnancy (C), breastfeeding, children <1 yr, renal/hepatic disease

DOSAGE AND ROUTES

- **Adult: PO** 10-30 mg/kg/day × 5 days
- **Child with lead level >45 mcg/dl: PO** 10 mg/kg or 350 mg/m^2 q8hr × 5 days then 10 mg/kg or 350 mg/m^2 q12hr × 2 wk; another course may be required, depending on lead levels; allow 2 wk between courses

Available forms: Caps 100 mg

Administer:

- To children who cannot swallow capsule by opening capsule and sprinkling contents on food or in a spoon followed by a drink; administer immediately after preparation

SIDE EFFECTS

CNS: Drowsiness, dizziness, paresthesia, sensorimotor neuropathy

EENT: Otitis media, watery eyes, film in eyes, plugged ears

GI: *Nausea, vomiting, diarrhea, metallic taste, anorexia*

GU: Proteinuria, decreased urination, voiding difficulties

HEMA: Increased platelets, intermittent eosinophilia, neutropenia

INTEG: Rash, urticaria, pruritus

META: Increased AST, ALT, alk phos, cholesterol

RESP: Sore throat, rhinorrhea, nasal congestion, cough

SYST: Back, stomach, head, rib, flank pain; abdominal cramps, chills, fever, flulike symptoms, head cold, headache

PHARMACOKINETICS

Peak 1-2 hr, 49% excreted (39% in feces, 25% urine, 1% as CO_2 from lungs), terminal half-life 48 hr

INTERACTIONS

- Not recommended concurrently with other chelating agents

NURSING CONSIDERATIONS

Assess:

- Renal, hepatic studies: ALT, AST, alk phos, BUN, creatinine, serum lead level
- I&O
- Lead sources in home, school
- Allergic reactions: rash, pruritus, urticaria; product should be discontinued if antihistamines fail to help

Perform/provide:

- Adequate fluids; check hydration status daily

Evaluate:

- Therapeutic response: decrease in serum lead level

Teach patient/family:

- That therapeutic effect may take 1-3 mo
- To report urticaria, rash, may occur every time product is used
- To increase fluid intake

⚠ HIGH ALERT

succinylcholine (Rx)

(suk-sin-ill-koe′leen)

Anectine, Quelicin

Func. class.: Neuromuscular blocker (depolarizing, ultra short)

ACTION:
Inhibits transmission of nerve impulses by binding with cholinergic receptor sites, thus antagonizing action of acetylcholine; causes release of histamine

USES:
Facilitation of endotracheal intubation, skeletal muscle relaxation during orthopedic manipulations

CONTRAINDICATIONS:
Hypersensitivity, malignant hyperthermia, trauma

Precautions: Pregnancy (C), breastfeeding, geriatric or debilitated patients, cardiac disease, severe burns, fractures (fasciculations may increase damage) electrolyte imbalances, dehydration, neuromuscular/respiratory/cardiac/renal/hepatic disease, collagen diseases, glaucoma, eye surgery

Black Box Warning: Children <2 yr, hyperkalemia, myopathy, rhabdomyolysis

DOSAGE AND ROUTES

- **Adult:** IV 0.3-1.1 mg/kg, max 150 mg, maintenance 0.04-0.07 mg/kg q5-10min as needed; **CONT IV INF** dilute to conc of 1-2 mg/ml in D_5W or NS 10-100 mcg/kg/min
- **Child:** IV initially 1-2 mg/kg; **CONT IV INF** not recommended

Available forms: Inj 20, 50, 100 mg/ml; powder for inj 100, 500 mg/vial, 1 g/vial

Administer:

- Deep IM inj, preferably high in deltoid muscle

IV route

- Using nerve stimulator by anesthesiologist to determine neuromuscular blockade
- Anticholinesterase to reverse neuromuscular blockade
- IV inf: dilute 1-2 mg/ml in D_5, isotonic saline sol; give 0.5-10 mg/min; titrate to response; may be given directly over 1 min

Additive compatibilities: Amikacin, cephapirin, isoproterenol, meperidine, methyldopate, morphine, norepinephrine, scopolamine

Syringe compatibilities: Heparin

Y-site compatibilities: Etomidate, heparin, potassium chloride, propofol, vit B/C

SIDE EFFECTS

CV: Bradycardia, tachycardia; increased, decreased B/P; **sinus arrest, dysrhythmias**, edema

EENT: Increased secretions, intraocular pressure

HEMA: **Myoglobulinemia**

INTEG: Rash, flushing, pruritus, urticaria

MS: Weakness, muscle pain, fasciculations, prolonged relaxation, myalgia, **rhabdomyolysis**

RESP: **Prolonged apnea, bronchospasm, cyanosis, respiratory depression**, wheezing, dyspnea

SYST: **Anaphylaxis, angioedema**

PHARMACOKINETICS

Hydrolyzed in blood, excreted in urine (active/inactive metabolites)

IM: Onset 2-3 min, duration 10-30 min

IV: Onset 1 min, peak 2-3 min, duration 6-10 min

INTERACTIONS

- Dysrhythmias: theophylline

Increase: neuromuscular blockade—aminoglycosides, β-blockers, cardiac glycosides, clindamycin, lincomycin, procainamide, quiNIDine, local anesthetics, polymyxin antibiotics, lithium, opioids, thiazides, enflurane, isoflurane, magnesium salts, oxytocin

S

Drug/Herb
• Blocks succinylcholine: melatonin

NURSING CONSIDERATIONS

Assess:
• Electrolyte imbalances (K, Mg); may lead to increased action of product
• VS (B/P, pulse, respirations, airway) until fully recovered; rate, depth, pattern of respirations, strength of hand grip
• I&O ratio; check for urinary retention, frequency, hesitancy
• **Recovery:** decreased paralysis of face, diaphragm, leg, arm, rest of body
• **Allergic reactions:** rash, fever, respiratory distress, pruritus; product should be discontinued
• **Myopathy, rhabdomyolysis:** in pediatric patients (rare)

Perform/provide:
• Storage in refrigerator, powder at room temp; close tightly
• Reassurance if communication is difficult during recovery from neuromuscular blockade; postoperative stiffness is normal, soon subsides

Evaluate:
• Therapeutic response: paralysis of jaw, eyelid, head, neck, rest of body

TREATMENT OF OVERDOSE:
Neostigmine, atropine, monitor VS; may require mechanical ventilation

sucralfate (Rx)
(soo-kral′fate)

Carafate, Sulcrate ♣

Func. class.: Protectant, antiulcer
Chem. class.: Aluminum hydroxide, sulfated sucrose

Do not confuse:
Carafate/Cafergot

ACTION: Forms a complex that adheres to ulcer site, adsorbs pepsin

USES: Duodenal ulcer, oral mucositis, stomatitis after radiation of head and neck

Unlabeled uses: Gastric/aphthous ulcers, gastroesophageal reflux, NSAID-induced ulcer prophylaxis, proctitis, stomatitis, stress gastritis prophylaxis, *C. difficile*

CONTRAINDICATIONS: Hypersensitivity

Precautions: Pregnancy (B), breastfeeding, children, renal failure; hypoglycemia (diabetics)

DOSAGE AND ROUTES

Duodenal ulcers
• **Adult: PO** 1 g qid 1 hr before meals, at bedtime
• **Child: PO** 40-80 mg/kg/day divided

Aphthous ulcer/stomatitis (unlabeled)
• **Adult: PO** 5-10 ml (500 mg-1 g) swished in mouth for several min; spit or swallow qid

Gastric ulcer/NSAID-induced ulcer prophylaxis/esophagitis/GERD (unlabeled)
• **Adult: PO** 1 g qid, 1 hr before meals and at bedtime

Available forms: Tabs 1 g; oral susp 1 g/10 ml

Administer:

PO route
• Do not crush or chew tabs; tabs may be broken or dissolved in water
• Do not take antacids 30 min before or after sucralfate
• On an empty stomach 1 hr before meals or other medications and at bedtime

SIDE EFFECTS

CNS: Drowsiness, dizziness

GI: *Dry mouth, constipation,* nausea, gastric pain, vomiting, bezoar (for critically ill patients)

INTEG: Urticaria, rash, pruritus

PHARMACOKINETICS

PO: Duration up to 6 hr

INTERACTIONS

Decrease: action of tetracyclines, phenytoin, fat-soluble vitamins, digoxin, ketoconazole, theophylline
Decrease: absorption of fluoroquinolones
Decrease: absorption of sucralfate—antacids, cimetidine, ranitidine

NURSING CONSIDERATIONS

Assess:
- **GI symptoms:** abdominal pain, blood in stools
- **Hypoglycemia:** may occur in patients with diabetes mellitus

Perform/provide:
- Storage at room temp

Evaluate:
- Therapeutic response: absence of pain, GI complaints

Teach patient/family:
- To take on empty stomach
- To take full course of therapy; not to use for >8 wk; to avoid smoking
- To avoid antacids within 1/2 hr of product
- To increase fluids, bulk, exercise to lessen constipation

sulfasalazine (Rx)

(sul-fa-sal′a-zeen)

Azulfidine, Azulfidine EN-tabs, Salazopyrin ✤

Func. class.: GI antiinflammatory, antirheumatic (DMARD)

Chem. class.: Sulfonamide

Do not confuse:
sulfasalazine/sulfiSOXAZOLE

ACTION: Prodrug to deliver sulfapyridine and 5-aminosalicylic acid to colon; antiinflammatory in connective tissue also

USES: Ulcerative colitis; RA; juvenile RA (Azulfidine EN-tabs)
Unlabeled uses: Crohn's disease

CONTRAINDICATIONS: Pregnancy at term, children <2 yr; hypersensitivity to sulfonamides or salicylates; intestinal, urinary obstruction; porphyria
Precautions: Pregnancy (B), breastfeeding, impaired renal/hepatic function, severe allergy, bronchial asthma, megaloblastic anemia

DOSAGE AND ROUTES

Bowel disease
- **Adult: PO** 3-4 g/day in divided doses; maintenance 2 g/day in divided doses q6hr
- **Child ≥6 yr: PO** 40-60 mg/kg/day in 4-6 divided doses then 30 mg/kg/day in 4 doses, max 2 g/day

Rheumatoid arthritis
- **Adult: PO** 0.5-1 g/day then increase daily dose by 500 mg/wk to 2 g/day in 2-3 divided doses

Juvenile rheumatoid arthritis
- **Child ≥6 yr: PO** 30-50 mg/kg/24 hr in 2 divided doses

Renal dose
- **Adult: PO** CCr 10-30 ml/min, give bid; CCr <10 ml/min, give daily

Crohn's disease (unlabeled)
- **Adult: PO** 1 g/15 kg, max 5 g/day

Available forms: Tabs 500 mg; oral susp 250 mg/5 ml; del rel tabs 500 mg

Administer:
- Do not break, crush, chew del rel tabs
- With full glass of water to maintain adequate hydration; increase fluids to 2 L/day to decrease crystallization in kidneys
- Total daily dose in evenly spaced doses and after meals to help minimize GI intolerance

SIDE EFFECTS

CNS: Headache, confusion, insomnia, hallucinations, depression, vertigo, fatigue, anxiety, seizures, product fever, chills

S

CV: Allergic myocarditis
GI: *Nausea, vomiting, abdominal pain,* stomatitis, hepatitis, glossitis, pancreatitis, diarrhea
GU: Renal failure, toxic nephrosis, increased BUN, creatinine, crystalluria
HEMA: Leukopenia, neutropenia, thrombocytopenia, agranulocytosis, hemolytic anemia
INTEG: Rash, dermatitis, urticaria, Stevens-Johnson syndrome, erythema, photosensitivity
SYST: Anaphylaxis

PHARMACOKINETICS

PO: Partially absorbed; peak 1½-6 hr; duration 6-12 hr; half-life 6 hr; excreted in urine as sulfasalazine (15%), sulfapyridine (60%), 5-aminosalicylic acid, metabolites (20%-33%); excreted in breast milk; crosses placenta

INTERACTIONS

Increase: leukopenia risk—thiopurines (azathioprine, mercaptopurine)
Increase: hypoglycemic response—oral hypoglycemics
Increase: anticoagulant effects—oral anticoagulants
Decrease: effect of cycloSPORINE, digoxin, folic acid
Decrease: renal excretion of methotrexate
Drug/Food
Decrease: iron/folic acid absorption
Drug/Lab Test
False positive: urinary glucose test

NURSING CONSIDERATIONS

Assess:

- Renal studies: BUN, creatinine, urinalysis (long-term therapy)

⚠ **Blood dyscrasias:** skin rash, fever, sore throat, bruising, bleeding, fatigue, joint pain; monitor CBC before therapy and q3mo

⚠ **Allergic reaction:** rash, dermatitis, urticaria, pruritus, dyspnea, bronchospasm

- **Ulcerative colitis, proctitis, other inflammatory bowel disease:** character, amount consistency of stools; abdominal pain, cramping, blood, mucous
- **Rheumatoid arthritis:** assess mobility, joint swelling, pain, ability to complete activities of daily living

Perform/provide:

- Storage in tight, light-resistant container at room temp

Evaluate:

- Therapeutic response: absence of fever, mucus in stools, pain in joints

Teach patient/family:

- To take each oral dose with full glass of water to prevent crystalluria
- That contact lenses, urine, skin may be yellow-orange
- To avoid sunlight or use sunscreen to prevent burns
- To notify prescriber of skin rash, sore throat, fever, mouth sores, unusual bruising, bleeding

sulindac (Rx)

(sul-in′dak)

Apo-Sulin ✤, Clinoril

Func. class.: Nonsteroidal antiinflammatory, antirheumatic

Chem. class.: Indene acetic acid derivative

Do not confuse:
Clinoril/Clozaril/Oruvail/Cleocin

ACTION: Metabolite inhibits COX-1, COX-2 by blocking arachidonate; analgesic, antiinflammatory, antipyretic

USES: Osteoarthritis; RA, gouty arthritis; ankylosing spondylitis; bursitis, tendinitis
Unlabeled uses: Arthralgia, bone pain, desmoid tumor, headache, juvenile RA

CONTRAINDICATIONS: Hypersensitivity, asthma, severe renal/hepatic disease, active ulcers, pregnancy (D) 3rd trimester

Black Box Warning: Perioperative pain during CABG

Precautions: Pregnancy (C) 1st trimester, breastfeeding, children, cardiac disorders, hypersensitivity to other antiinflammatory agents, renal disease

Black Box Warning: GI bleeding, MI, stroke

DOSAGE AND ROUTES

Arthritis

- **Adult: PO** 150 mg bid, may increase to 200 mg bid, max 400 mg/day
- **Child (unlabeled): PO** 2-4 mg/kg/day in divided doses; max 6 mg/kg/day or 200 mg bid, whichever is less (safe and effective dose not established)

Bursitis/acute arthritis

- **Adult: PO** 200 mg bid × 1-2 wk then reduce dose

Available forms: Tabs 150, 200 mg

Administer:

- With food to decrease GI symptoms; take on empty stomach to facilitate absorption; tablet may be crushed
- With a full glass of water

SIDE EFFECTS

CNS: Dizziness, drowsiness, fatigue, tremors, confusion, insomnia, anxiety, depression, headache

CV: Tachycardia, peripheral edema, palpitations, dysrhythmias, **MI, stroke, CHF**

EENT: Tinnitus, hearing loss, blurred vision

GI: *Nausea, anorexia, vomiting, diarrhea,* jaundice, **cholestatic hepatitis,** constipation, flatulence, cramps, dry mouth, peptic ulcer, **bleeding, ulceration, perforation,** dyspepsia

GU: **Nephrotoxicity:** **dysuria, hematuria, oliguria, azotemia**

HEMA: **Blood dyscrasias with prolonged** use

INTEG: Purpura, *rash, pruritus,* sweating, photosensitivity

SYST: **Anaphylaxis, Stevens-Johnson syndrome, toxic epidermal necrolysis**

PHARMACOKINETICS

Peak 2-4 hr; half-life 7.8 hr; metabolized in liver; excreted in urine (metabolites), breast milk; 93% protein binding

INTERACTIONS

Increase: GI side effects: aspirin, corticosteroids, other NSAIDs, tobacco

Increase: CNS stimulation, seizures—quinolones (norfloxacin, ofloxacin, levofloxacin)

Increase: bleeding risk—anticoagulants, thrombolytics, tirofiban, eptifibatide, clopidogrel, ticlopidine, SSRIs, SNRIs, valproic acid

Increase: nephrotoxicity—cycloSPORINE

Increase: toxicity—methotrexate, sulfonamides, sulfonylureas, probenecid, aminoglycosides

Decrease: sulindac effect—antacids

Decrease: effect—antihypertensives

Drug/Herb

Increase: bleeding risk—garlic, ginger, ginkgo

Decrease: effect of—feverfew

NURSING CONSIDERATIONS

Assess:

Black Box Warning: Do not use for perioperative pain during CABG

⚠ **Cardiac status: CV thrombotic events, MI, stroke; may be fatal**

⚠ **GI status: ulceration, bleeding, perforation; may be fatal**

- **Pain:** frequency, intensity, characteristics, relief after med

⚠ **Asthma, aspirin hypersensitivity, nasal polyps; increased hypersensitivity; monitor for rash**

- Renal, hepatic studies: BUN, creatinine, AST, ALT, Hgb before treatment, periodically thereafter
- Have B/P checked monthly; product causes sodium retention
- Audiometric, ophthalmic exam before, during, after treatment
- For eye, ear problems: blurred vision, tinnitus may indicate toxicity

S

Perform/provide:
- Storage at room temp

Evaluate:
- Therapeutic response: decreased pain, stiffness, swelling in joints; ability to move more easily

Teach patient/family:
- To report blurred vision or ringing, roaring in ears (may indicate toxicity)
- To avoid driving, other hazardous activities if dizzy or drowsy
- To report change in urine pattern, weight increase, edema, pain increase in joints, fever, blood in urine (indicates nephrotoxicity)
- That therapeutic effects may take ≤1 mo
- To avoid alcohol and aspirin, NSAIDs
- To take with full glass of water
- To use sunscreen
- To report bruising; black, tarry stools
- To inform all health care providers that this product is being used

sumatriptan (Rx)

(soo-ma-trip′tan)

ALSUMA Auto-injector, Imitrex, Sumavel DosePro

Func. class.: Antimigraine agent

Chem. class.: 5-HT_1B/D receptor agonist, abortive agent, triptan

Do not confuse:
sumatriptan/somatropin

ACTION: Binds selectively to the vascular 5-HT_1B/D receptor subtype, exerts antimigraine effect; causes vasoconstriction in cranial arteries

USES: Acute treatment of migraine with/without aura and cluster headache

CONTRAINDICATIONS: Angina pectoris, history of MI, documented silent ischemia, Prinzmetal's angina, ischemic heart disease, IV use, concurrent ergotamine-containing preparations, uncontrolled hypertension, hypersensitivity, basilar or hemiplegic migraine

Precautions: Pregnancy (C), breastfeeding, children <18 yr, geriatric patients, postmenopausal women, men >40 yr, risk factors for CAD, hypercholesterolemia, obesity, diabetes, impaired renal/hepatic function

DOSAGE AND ROUTES

- **Adult: SUBCUT** ≤6 mg; may repeat in 1 hr; max 12 mg/24 hr; **PO** 25 mg with fluids, if no relief in 2 hr, give another dose, max 200 mg/day; **NASAL** single dose of 5, 10, or 20 mg in 1 nostril, may repeat in 2 hr, max 40 mg/24 hr; 1 puff each nostril q2hr

Hepatic dose
- **Adult: PO** 25 mg; if no response after 2 hr, give ≤50 mg

Available forms: Inj 4, 6 mg/0.5 ml; tabs 25, 50, 100 mg; nasal spray 5 mg/100 mcl-U; dose spray device 20 mg/100 mcl-U

Administer:

PO route
- Swallow tabs whole; do not break, crush, or chew
- Take tabs with fluids as soon as symptoms appear; may take a 2nd dose >4 hr; max 200 mg/24 hr

SUBCUT route

SUBCUT only just below the skin; avoid IM or IV administration; use only for actual migraine attack
- Give 1st dose supervised by medical staff to patients with coronary artery disease or those at risk for CAD

Nasal route
- May give as 2 sprays of 5 mg in 1 nostril or 1 spray in each nostril (10 mg)

SIDE EFFECTS

CNS: *Tingling, hot sensation, burning, feeling of pressure, tightness, numb-*

ness, dizziness, sedation, headache, anxiety, fatigue, cold sensation
CV: *Flushing,* **MI**, hypo/hypertension
EENT: Throat, mouth, nasal discomfort; vision changes
GI: Abdominal discomfort
INTEG: Inj site reaction, sweating
MS: *Weakness, neck stiffness,* myalgia
RESP: Chest tightness, pressure

PHARMACOKINETICS

Onset of pain relief 10 min-2 hr, peak 10-20 min; 10%-20% plasma protein binding; metabolized in liver (metabolite); excreted in urine, feces; nasal spray half-life 2 hr

INTERACTIONS

Increase: vasospastic effects: ergot, ergot derivatives
Increase: serotonin syndrome—SSRIs, SNRIs, serotonin-receptor agonists, sibutramine
Increase: sumatriptan effect—MAOIs
Drug/Herb
• Serotonin syndrome: SAM-e, St. John's wort

NURSING CONSIDERATIONS

Assess:
• **Migraine:** type of pain, aura; alleviating, aggravating factors; sensitivity to light, noise
⚠ **Serotonin syndrome:** delirium, coma, agitation, diaphoresis, hypertension, fever, tremors; may resemble neuroleptic malignant syndrome in patients taking SSRIs, SNRIs
• B/P; signs, symptoms of coronary vasospasms, ECG
• Tingling, hot sensation, burning, feeling of pressure, numbness, flushing, inj site reaction
• Stress level, activity, recreation, coping mechanisms
• Neurologic status: LOC, blurring vision, nausea, vomiting, tingling in extremities preceding headache
• Ingestion of tyramine foods (pickled products, beer, wine, aged cheese), food additives, preservatives, colorings, artificial sweeteners, chocolate, caffeine, which may precipitate these types of headaches
• Renal function, urinary output
Perform/provide:
• Quiet, calm environment with decreased stimuli: noise, bright light, excessive talking
Evaluate:
• Therapeutic response: decrease in frequency, severity of migraine
Teach patient/family:
• To report chest pain, tightness; sudden, severe abdominal pain; swelling of eyelids, face, lips; skin rash to prescriber immediately
• To notify prescriber if pregnancy is planned or suspected; to use contraception while taking product
• **Nasal spray:** to use 1 spray in 1 nostril, may repeat if headache returns; not to repeat if pain continues after 1st dose
• To have a dark, quiet environment
• To avoid hazardous activities if dizziness, drowsiness occur
• To avoid alcohol; may increase headache
• To use SUBCUT inj technique, nasal route if prescribed
• That product does not reduce number of migraines; to be used for acute migraine; to use as symptoms occur

sunitinib (Rx)

(soo-nit′-in-ib)
Sutent
Func. class.: Antineoplastic—miscellaneous
Chem. class.: Protein-tyrosine kinase inhibitor

ACTION:
Inhibits multiple receptor tyrosine kinases (RTKs); some are responsible for tumor growth

USES:
Gastrointesitnal stromal tumors (GIST) after disease progression or intol-

S

erance to imatinib; advanced renal carcinoma, pancreatic neuroendocrine tumors (pNET) in patients with unresectable locally advanced/metastatic disease

CONTRAINDICATIONS:

Pregnancy (D), breastfeeding, hypersensitivity

Precautions: Children, geriatric patients, active infections, QT prolongation, torsades de pointes, stroke, heart failure

DOSAGE AND ROUTES

Gastrointestinal stromal tumors (GIST)/renal cell cancer

• **Adult: PO** 50 mg/day × 4 wk then 2 wk off; may increase or decrease dose by 12.5 mg; if administered with CYP3A4 inducers, give 87.5 mg/day; if given with CYP3A4 inhibitors, give 37.5 mg/day

Pancreatic neuroendocrine (pNET)

• **Adult: PO** 37.5 mg daily continuously, increase or decrease by 12.5 mg based on tolerance, avoid potent CYP3A4 inhibitors/inducers; if used with CYP3A4 inhibitors, decrease sunitinib dose to minimum of 25 mg/day; if used with CYP3A4 inducers, increase sunitinib to max 62.5 mg/day

Available forms: Caps 12.5, 25, 50 mg

Administer:

• With meal and large glass of water to decrease GI symptoms

SIDE EFFECTS

CNS: CNS hemorrhage, headache, dizziness, insomnia, seizures, fatigue

CV: Hypertension, left ventricular dysfunction, QT prolongation, cardiotoxicity, torsades de pointes, thrombotic microangiopathy, cardiac arrest, thromboembolism

ENDO: Hypo/hyperthyroidism

GI: *Nausea,* hepatotoxicity, vomiting, dyspepsia, *anorexia, abdominal pain,* altered taste, *constipation,* stomatitis, mucositis, pancreatitis, diarrhea, GI bleeding/perforation

GU: Nephrotic syndrome

HEMA: Neutropenia, thrombocytopenia, hemolytic anemia, leukopenia

INTEG: *Rash, yellow skin discoloration,* depigmentation of hair or skin, alopecia

MS: Pain, arthralgia, myalgia, myopathy, rhabdomyolysis

RESP: Cough, dyspnea, pulmonary embolism

SYST: Bleeding, electrolyte abnormalities, hand-foot syndrome, serious infection

PHARMACOKINETICS

Protein binding 95%; metabolized by CYP3A4; excreted in feces, small amount in urine; peak plasma levels 6-12 hr; terminal half-life 40-60 hr (sunitnib); active metabolite 80-110 hr

INTERACTIONS

⚠ **Increase:** microangiopathic hemolytic anemia—bevacizumab; avoid concurrent use

⚠ **Increase:** QT prolongation—class IA/III antidysrhythmics, some phenothiazines, β agonists, local anesthetics, tricyclics, haloperidol, chloroquine, droperidol, pentamidine; CYP3A4 inhibitors (amiodarone, clarithromycin, erythromycin, telithromycin, troleandomycin), arsenic trioxide, levomethadyl; CYP3A4 substrates (methadone, pimozide, QUEtiapine, quiNIDine, risperidone, ziprasidone)

Increase: hepatotoxicity—acetaminophen

Increase: plasma concentrations of simvastatin, calcium channel blockers; warfarin; avoid use with warfarin, use low-molecular-weight anticoagulants instead

Decrease: sunitinib concentrations—dexamethasone, phenytoin, carBAMazepine, rifampin, PHENobarbital

Drug/Herb

Decrease: sunitinib concentration—St. John's wort

Drug/Food
Increase: plasma concentrations—grapefruit juice

NURSING CONSIDERATIONS

Assess:

⚠ **ANC and platelets; if ANC $<1 \times 10^9$/L and/or platelets $<50 \times 10^9$/L, stop until ANC $>1.5 \times 10^9$/L and platelets $>75 \times 10^9$/L; if ANC $<0.5 \times 10^9$/L and/or platelets $<10 \times 10^9$/L, reduce dosage by 200 mg; if cytopenia continues, reduce dosage by another 100 mg; if cytopenia continues for 4 wk, stop product until ANC $\geq 1 \times 10^9$/L**

⚠ **CV status: hypertension, QT prolongation can occur; monitor left ventricular ejection fraction (LVEF), (MUGA) at baseline, periodically; ECG**

⚠ **Renal toxicity: if bilirubin $>3 \times$ IULN, withhold sunitinib until bilirubin levels return to $<1.5 \times$ IULN; electrolytes**

⚠ **Hepatotoxicity: monitor LFTs before treatment, monthly; if liver transaminases $>5 \times$ IULN, withhold sunitinib until transaminase levels return to $<2.5 \times$ IULN**

- **CHF:** adrenal insufficiency in those experiencing trauma
- Bleeding: epistaxis; rectal, gingival, upper GI, genital, wound bleeding; tumor-related hemorrhage may occur rapidly

Perform/provide:

- Nutritious diet with iron, vitamin supplement, low fiber, few dairy products
- Storage at 25° C (77° F)

Evaluate:

- Therapeutic response: decrease in size of tumor

Teach patient/family:

- To report adverse reactions immediately: SOB, bleeding
- About reason for treatment, expected result
- That many adverse reactions may occur: high B/P, bleeding, mouth swelling, taste change, skin discoloration, depigmentation of hair/skin
- To avoid persons with known upper respiratory infections; that immunosuppression is common
- To avoid grapefruit juice

⚠ **To report if pregnancy is planned or suspected, pregnancy (D)**

suprofen ophthalmic

See Appendix B

tacrolimus (Rx) (PO, IV)

(tak-roe-li′mus)

Prograf

tacrolimus (topical) (Rx)

Protopic

Func. class.: Immunosuppressant
Chem. class.: Macrolide

ACTION: Produces immunosuppression by inhibiting T-lymphocytes

USES: Organ transplants to prevent rejection; **topical:** atopic dermatitis

Unlabeled uses: Severe recalcitrant psoriasis, contact dermatitis, GVHD prophylaxis/disease, pancreas/heart/kidney/liver/lung/small bowel transplant rejection, uveitis, ulcerative colitis, nephrotic syndrome, lichen sclerosus

CONTRAINDICATIONS: Children <2 yr (topical); hypersensitivity to this product or to some kinds of castor oil; long-term use (topical)

Precautions: Pregnancy (C), breastfeeding, severe renal/hepatic disease; diabetes mellitus, hyperkalemia, hyperuricemia, hypertension

Black Box Warning: Children <12, lymphomas, infection, neoplastic disease

DOSAGE AND ROUTES

Kidney transplant rejection prophylaxis

• **Adult: IV** 0.03-0.05 mg/kg/day as **CONT INF**, give no sooner than 6 hr after transplantation

Liver transplant rejection prophylaxis

• **Adult: PO** 0.10-0.15 mg/kg/day in 2 divided doses q12hr, give no sooner than 6 hr after transplantation; **IV** 0.03-0.05 mg/kg/day as **CONT INF**, give no sooner than 6 hr after transplantation

Heart transplant rejection prophylaxis

• **Adult: PO** 0.075 mg/kg/day in 2 divided doses q12hr, give no sooner than 6 hr after transplantation; **IV** 0.01 mg/kg/day as **CONT INF**, give no sooner than 6 hr after transplantation

Atopic dermatitis

• **Adult: TOP** use 0.03% or 0.1% ointment, apply bid × 7 days after clearing of signs

• **Child ≥ 2-15 yr: TOP** 0.03% ointment, apply bid × 7 days after clearing of signs

Graft-versus-host disease (unlabeled)

• **Adult and adolescent: IV** 0.1 mg/kg/day in 2 divided doses given with other immunosuppressants or **PO** 0.3 mg/kg/day in 2 divided doses

• **Child: CONT IV INF** 0.1 mg/kg/day

Graft-versus-host prophylaxis (unlabeled)

• **Adult: CONT IV INF** 0.03 mg/kg/day starting 1-2 days prior to bone marrow transplant; **PO** 0.12 mg/kg/day in 2 divided doses

• **Adolescent and child: PO** 0.12 mg/kg/day in 2 divided doses

Heart transplant rejection (unlabeled)

• **Adult: IV** 0.05 mg/kg/day or **PO** 0.2-0.3 mg/kg/day in 2 divided doses; adjust to maintain whole blood conc 7-15 ng/ml

Lung transplant rejection (unlabeled)

• **Adult: PO** 0.15 mg/kg/day, maintain 12-hr trough, whole blood conc 1-1.5 ng/ml

Small bowel transplant rejection (unlabeled)

• **Adult: IV** 0.1-0.15 mg/kg/day then **PO** 0.3 mg/kg/day in divided doses

Contact dermatitis (unlabeled)

• **Adult: TOP** 0.1% ointment, apply bid × 8 wk

Available forms: Inj 5 mg/ml; caps 0.5, 1, 5 mg; ointment 0.03%, 0.1%

Administer:

PO route

• With meals to reduce GI upset; nausea common

• For several days before transplant surgery, patients should be placed in protective isolation

Topical route

• Do not use occlusive dressings

Continuous IV INF route

• After diluting in 0.9% NaCl or D_5W to 0.004 to 0.02 mg/ml as continuous inf over 24 hr

Y-site compatibilities: Alemtuzumab, alfentanil, amifostine, amikacin, aminophylline, amiodarone, amphotericin B colloidal, amphotericin B liposome, anidulafungin, argatroban, atracurium, aztreonam, benztropine, bivalirudin, bleomycin, bumetanide, buprenorphine, busulfan, butorphanol, calcium acetate/chloride/gluconate, CARBOplatin, carmustine, caspofungin, ceFAZolin, cefoperazone, cefotaxime, cefotetan, cefoxitin, ceftazidime, ceftizoxime, cefTRIAXone, cefuroxime, chloramphenicol, chlorproMAZINE, cimetidine, ciprofloxacin, cisatracurium, CISplatin, clindamycin, cyclophosphamide, cycloSPORINE, cytarabine, DACTINomycin, DAPTOmycin, dexamethasone, dexmedetomidine, dexrazoxane, digoxin, diltiazem, diphenhydrAMINE, DOBUTamine, docetaxel, dolasetron, DOPamine, doripenem, doxacurium, DOXOrubicin hydrochloride, doxycycline, droperidol, enalaprilat, ePHEDrine, EPINEPHrine, epirubicin, ertapenem, erythromycin, esmolol, etoposide, etoposide phosphate, famotidine, fenoldopam, fentaNYL, fluconazole, fludarabine, foscarnet, fosphenytoin, gemcitabine, gentamicin, glycopyrrolate, granisetron, haloperidol, heparin, hydrALAZINE, hydrocortisone, HYDROmorphone, IDArubicin, ifosfamide, imipenem/cilastatin, inamrinone, insulin, isoproterenol, ketorolac, labetalol, leucovorin, levofloxacin, levorphanol, lidocaine, linezolid, LORazepam, magnesium sulfate, mannitol, mechlorethamine, meperidine, meropenem, mesna, metaraminol, methotrexate, methyldopate, methylPREDNISolone, metoclopramide, metoprolol, metroNIDAZOLE, micafungin, midazolam, milrinone, mitomycin, mitoxantrone, mivacurium, morphine, multivitamins, nafcillin, nalbuphine, naloxone, nesiritide, niCARdipine, nitroglycerin, nitroprusside, norepinephrine, octreotide, ondansetron, oxacillin, oxaliplatin, oxytocin, paclitaxel, palonosetron, pancuronium, pemetrexed, penicillin G, pentamidine, pentazocine, perphenazine, phentolamine, phenylephrine, piperacillin/tazobactam, potassium chloride/phosphates, procainamide, prochlorperazine, promethazine, propranolol, quinapristin/dalfopristin, ranitidine, remifentanil, rocuronium, sodium acetate/bicarbonate/phosphates, streptozocin, succinylcholine, SUFentanil, teniposide, theophylline, thiotepa, ticarcillin/clavulanate, tigecycline, tirofiban, tobramycin, tolazoline, trimethobenzamide, vancomycin, vasopressin, vecuronium, verapamil, vinCRIStine, vinorelbine, voriconazole, zidovudine, zoledronic acid

SIDE EFFECTS

CNS: *Tremors, headache,* insomnia, paresthesia, chills, fever, **seizures, posterior reversible encephalopathy syndrome,** BK-virus–associated nephropathy

CV: Hypertension, myocardial hypertrophy, **prolonged QTc**

EENT: Blurred vision, photophobia

GI: Nausea, vomiting, diarrhea, constipation, **GI bleeding**

GU: UTIs, **albuminuria, hematuria, proteinuria, renal failure**

HEMA: **Anemia, leukocytosis, thrombocytopenia, purpura**

INTEG: Rash, flushing, itching, alopecia

META: Hirsutism, hyperglycemia, hyperuricemia, hypo/hyperkalemia, hypomagnesemia

MS: Back pain, muscle spasms

RESP: **Pleural effusion, atelectasis,** dyspnea, **interstitial lung disease**

SYST: **Anaphylaxis**

PHARMACOKINETICS

PO: Extensively metabolized, half-life 10 hr, 75% protein binding

INTERACTIONS

⚠ **Increase: QT prolongation—class IA/III antidysrhythmics, some phenothiazines, β agonists, local anesthetics, tricyclics, haloperidol, chloroquine, droperidol, pentamidine; CYP3A4 inhibitors (amio-darone, clarithromycin, erythromycin, telithromycin, troleandomycin), arsenic trioxide, levomethadyl; CYP3A4 substrates (methadone, pimozide, QUEtiapine, quiNIDine, risperidone, ziprasidone)**

⚠ **Increase: toxicity—aminoglycosides, CISplatin, cycloSPORINE**

Increase: blood levels—antifungals, calcium channel blockers, cimetidine, danazol, mycophenolate, mofetil

Decrease: blood levels—carBAMazepine, PHENobarbital, phenytoin, rifamycin

Decrease: effect of vaccines

Drug/Herb

Decrease: immunosuppression—astragalus, echinacea, melatonin

Decrease: effect—ginseng, St. John's wort

NURSING CONSIDERATIONS

Assess:

• Blood studies: Hgb, WBC, platelets during treatment monthly; if leukocytes <3000/mm³ or platelets <100,000/mm³, product should be discontinued or reduced; decreased hemoglobulin level may indicate bone marrow suppression

• Hepatic studies: alk phos, AST, ALT, amylase, bilirubin; for hepatotoxicity: dark urine, jaundice, itching, light-colored stools; product should be discontinued

• Serum creatinine/BUN, serum electrolytes, lipid profile, serum tacrolimus conc

⚠ **Anaphylaxis:** rash, pruritus, wheezing, laryngeal edema; stop infusion, initiate emergency procedures

• **QT prolongation:** ECG, ejection fraction; assess for chest pain, palpitations, dyspnea

Evaluate:

• Therapeutic response: absence of graft rejection; immunosuppression in patients with autoimmune disorders

Teach patient/family:

PO route

• To report fever, rash, severe diarrhea, chills, sore throat, fatigue; that serious infections may occur; to report clay-colored stools, cramping (hepatotoxicity), nephrotoxicity, signs of diabetes mellitus

• To avoid crowds, persons with known infections to reduce risk for infection; to avoid eating raw shellfish

• To avoid exposure to natural or artificial sunlight

• Not to breastfeed while taking product

• That repeated lab tests will be needed during treatment

• To avoid vaccines

• Not to use with alcohol, grapefruit

• To report if pregnancy is planned or suspected

Black Box Warning: To report symptoms of lymphoma

tadalafil (Rx)

(tah-dal′a-fil)

Adcirca, Cialis

Func. class.: Impotence agent

Chem. class.: Phosphodiesterase type 5 inhibitor

ACTION: Inhibits phosphodiesterase type 5 (PDE5); enhances erectile function by increasing the amount of cGMP, which causes smooth muscle relaxation and increased blood flow into the corpus cavernosum; improves erectile function for up to 36 hr

USES: Treatment of erectile dysfunction; pulmonary arterial hypertension (PAH) (Adcirca only)

Unlabeled uses: Sexual dysfunction in males receiving antidepressants

CONTRAINDICATIONS: Newborns, children, women, hypersensitivity, patients taking organic nitrates either regularly and/or intermittently, patients taking any α-adrenergic antagonist other than 0.4 mg once-daily tamsulosin

Precautions: Pregnancy (B) although not indicated for females, anatomic penile deformities, sickle cell anemia, leukemia, multiple myeloma, CV/renal/hepatic disease, bleeding disorders, active peptic ulcer, prolonged erection

DOSAGE AND ROUTES

Erectile dysfunction

• **Adult: PO** 10 mg taken prior to sexual activity, dose may be reduced to 5 mg or increased to max 20 mg; usual max dosing frequency is 1×/day; once-daily dosing 2.5 mg/day at same time each day

Renal dose

• **Adult: PO** CCr 51-80 ml/min: no adjustment for erectile dysfunction, 20 mg/day initially for pulmonary hypertension; CCr 31-50 ml/min, 5 mg/day, max 10 mg q48hr; CCr <30 ml/min, max 5 mg q72hr

Hepatic dose
- **Adult: PO** (Child-Pugh A, B) max 10 mg/day or 20 mg/day, (pulmonary hypertension) max 40 mg/day; (Child-Pugh C) not recommended

Concomitant medications
- Ketoconazole, itraconazole, ritonavir, max 10 mg q72hr

Pulmonary hypertension
- **Adult: PO (Adcirca only)** 40 mg daily
- **Adult taking ritonavir: PO** 20 mg daily initially then increase to 40 mg daily as tolerated

Male sexual dysfunction (from antidepressants) (unlabeled)
- **Adult: PO** 10-20 mg prior to sexual activity

Available forms: Tabs 2.5, 5, 10, 20 mg; PO tab (Adcirca) 20 mg

Administer:
- Product should not be used with nitrates in any form
- **Sexual dysfunction:** give prior to sexual activity; do not use more than 1×/day
- **Pulmonary hypertension:** give Adcirca with/without meals

SIDE EFFECTS

CNS: *Headache, flushing, dizziness,* **seizures**, transient global amnesia
CV: Hypotension, **QT prolongation**
INTEG: **Stevens-Johnson syndrome, exfoliative dermatitis**, urticaria
MISC: Back pain/myalgia, *dyspepsia, nasal congestion, UTI,* blurred vision, changes in color vision, *diarrhea,* pruritus, priapism, **nonarteritic ischemic optic neuropathy (NAION)**, hearing loss

PHARMACOKINETICS

Rapidly absorbed; metabolized by liver by CYP3A4; terminal half-life 17.5 hr; peak ½-6 hr; excreted primarily as metabolites in feces, urine; excreted 61% in feces, 36% in urine; 94% protein bound; rate and extent of absorption not influenced by food

INTERACTIONS

⚠ **Do not use with nitrates because of unsafe drop in B/P, which could result in MI or stroke**

Increase: tadalafil levels—itraconazole, ketoconazole, ritonavir (although not studied, may also include other HIV protease inhibitors)

Decrease: B/P—alcohol, α-blockers, amlodipine, angiotensin II receptor blockers, enalapril

Decrease: effects of tadalafil—bosentan, antacids

Drug/Food

Increase: tadalafil effect—grapefruit

NURSING CONSIDERATIONS

Assess:
- **Cialis:** erectile dysfunction prior to treatment; use of organic nitrates that should not be used with this product; any severe loss of vision while taking this or any similar products
- **Adcirca:** hemodynamic parameters at baseline and periodically

Evaluate:
- Therapeutic response: ability to engage in sexual intercourse, improvement in exercise ability in pulmonary hypertension

Teach patient/family:
- That product does not protect against sexually transmitted diseases, including HIV
- That product has no effect in the absence of sexual stimulation; to seek medical help if erection lasts >4 hr
- To tell physician about all medicines, vitamins, herbs being taken, especially ritonavir, indinavir, ketoconozole, itraconazole, erythromycin, nitrates, α-blockers; that tadalafil is contraindicated for use with α-blockers except 0.4 mg/day tamsulosin

⚠ **To notify prescriber immediately and to stop taking product if vision, hearing loss occur or if erection lasts >4 hr**

T

tamoxifen (Rx)

(ta-mox'i-fen)

Apo-Tamox ♣, Nolvadex ♣, Tamofen ♣

Func. class.: Antineoplastic

Chem. class.: Antiestrogen hormone

ACTION: Inhibits cell division by binding to cytoplasmic estrogen receptors; resembles normal cell complex but inhibits DNA synthesis and estrogen response of target tissue

USES: Advanced breast carcinoma not responsive to other therapy in estrogen-receptor–positive patients (usually postmenopausal), prevention of breast cancer, after breast surgery/radiation for ductal carcinoma in situ

Unlabeled uses: Mastalgia, to reduce pain/size of gynecomastia, ovulation stimulation, malignant carcinoid tumor, carcinoid syndrome, metastatic melanoma, desmoid tumors, McCune-Albright syndrome (female pediatric patients), osteoporosis, bipolar I disorder, infertility, precocious puberty, gynecomastia, mastalgia

CONTRAINDICATIONS: Pregnancy (D), breastfeeding, hypersensitivity

Black Box Warning: Thromboembolic disease

Precautions: Women of childbearing age, leukopenia, thrombocytopenia, cataracts

Black Box Warning: Endometrial cancer, stroke

DOSAGE AND ROUTES

Breast cancer

- **Adult: PO** 20-40 mg/day for 5 yr; doses >20 mg/day, divide AM/PM

High risk for breast cancer

- **Adult: PO** 20 mg/day × 5 yr

DCIS

- **Adult: PO** 20 mg/day × 5 yr

McCune-Albright syndrome/ precocious puberty (unlabeled)

- **Child 2-10 yr (girls): PO** 20 mg/day for ≤1 yr

Bipolar I disorder (unlabeled)

- **Adult: PO** 40 mg bid

Stimulation of ovulation with infertility (unlabeled)

- **Adult: PO** 20-80 mg/day × 5 days

Mastalgia (unlabeled)

- **Adult (female): PO** 10-20 mg/day × 3-6 mo

Mastalgia/gynecomastia in men with prostate cancer (unlabeled)

- **Adult (male): PO** 20 mg/day for ≤1 yr

Available forms: Tabs 10, 20 mg

Administer:

- Do not break, crush, or chew tabs
- Antacid before oral agent; give product after evening meal, before bedtime; give with food or fluids for GI symptoms
- Antiemetic 30-60 min before product to prevent vomiting

SIDE EFFECTS

CNS: *Hot flashes, headache, lightheadedness,* depression, mood changes

CV: Chest pain, **stroke,** fluid retention, flushing

EENT: Ocular lesions, retinopathy, cataracts, corneal opacity, blurred vision (high doses)

GI: *Nausea, vomiting,* altered taste (anorexia)

GU: Vaginal bleeding, pruritus vulvae, **uterine malignancies,** *altered menses, amenorrhea*

HEMA: **Thrombocytopenia, leukopenia,** DVT

INTEG: *Rash,* alopecia

META: Hypercalcemia

RESP: **Pulmonary embolism**

PHARMACOKINETICS

PO: Peak 4-7 hr, half-life 7 days (1 wk terminal), metabolized in liver, excreted primarily in feces

INTERACTIONS

⚠ **Increase:** risk for death from breast cancer—PARoxetine
Increase: bleeding—anticoagulants
Increase: tamoxifen levels—bromocriptine
Increase: thromboembolic events—cytotoxics
⚠ **Increase:** toxicity—CYP3A4 inhibitors (aprepitant, antiretroviral protease inhibitors, clarithromycin, danazol, delavirdine, diltiazem, erythromycin, fluconazole, FLUoxetine, fluvoxamine, imatinib, ketoconazole, mibefradil, nefazodone, telithromycin, voriconazole)
Decrease: tamoxifen levels—aminoglutethimide, rifamycin
Decrease: letrozole levels—letrozole
Decrease: tamoxifen effect—CYP3A4 inducers (barbiturates, bosentan, carBAMazepine, efavirenz, phenytoins, nevirapine, rifabutin, rifampin)
Decrease: tamoxifen effects—CYP2D6 inhibitors (antidepressants)

Drug/Herb

- Avoid use with St. John's wort, dong qui, black cohosh

Drug/Lab Test

Increase: serum calcium, T_4, AST, ALT, cholesterol, triglycerides

NURSING CONSIDERATIONS

Assess:

- CBC, differential, platelet count weekly; withhold product if WBC count is <3500 or platelet count is <100,000; notify prescriber; breast exam, mammogram, pregnancy test, bone mineral density, LFTs, serum calcium, serum lipid profile

Black Box Warning: Bleeding q8hr: hematuria, guaiac, bruising, petechiae, mucosa or orifices

- Effects of alopecia on body image; discuss feelings about body changes

⚠ **Uterine malignancies, symptoms of stroke, pulmonary embolism** that may occur in women with ductal carcinoma in situ (DCIS) and women at high risk for breast cancer

⚠ **Severe allergic reactions:** rash, pruritus, urticaria, purpuric skin lesions, itching, flushing

- Bone pain; may give analgesics; pain usually transient

Perform/provide:

- Storage in light-resistant container at room temp

Evaluate:

- Therapeutic response: decreased tumor size, spread of malignancy

Teach patient/family:

- To report any complaints, side effects to prescriber; that use may be 5 yr
- To increase fluids to 2 L/day unless contraindicated
- To wear sunscreen, protective clothing, sunglasses
- That vaginal bleeding, pruritus, hot flashes are reversible after discontinuing treatment
- To immediately report decreased visual acuity, which may be irreversible; about need for routine eye exams; that care providers should be told about tamoxifen therapy
- To report vaginal bleeding immediately
- **Tumor flare**—increase in size of tumor, increased bone pain—may occur and will subside rapidly; may take analgesics for pain
- That premenopausal women must use mechanical birth control because ovulation may be induced
- That hair may be lost during treatment; that a wig or hairpiece may make patient feel better; that new hair may be different in color, texture

tamsulosin (Rx)

(tam-sue-lo′sen)

Flomax

Func. class.: Selective α_1-peripheral adrenergic blocker, BPH agent
Chem. class.: Sulfamoylphenethylamine derivative

Do not confuse:
Flomax/Fosamax/Volmax

ACTION:
Binds preferentially to α_{1A}-adrenoceptor subtype, which is located mainly in the prostate

USES:
Symptoms of benign prostatic hyperplasia (BPH)

CONTRAINDICATIONS:
Hypersensitivity

Precautions: Pregnancy (B), breastfeeding, children, hepatic disease, CAD, severe renal disease, prostate cancer; cataract surgery (floppy iris syndrome)

DOSAGE AND ROUTES

- **Adult: PO** 0.4 mg/day increasing to 0.8 mg/day if required after 2-4 wk

Available forms: Caps 0.4 mg

Administer:

- Swallow caps whole; do not break, crush, or chew
- Give ½ hr after same meal each day

SIDE EFFECTS

CNS: *Dizziness, headache,* asthenia, insomnia

CV: Chest pain, orthostatic hypotension

EENT: Amblyopia, floppy iris syndrome

GI: Nausea, diarrhea, dysgeusia

GU: Decreased libido, abnormal ejaculation, priapism

INTEG: Rash, pruritus, urticaria

MS: Back pain

RESP: Rhinitis, pharyngitis, cough

SYST: Angioedema

PHARMACOKINETICS

Peak 4-5 hr, duration 9-15 hr, half-life 9-13 hr, metabolized in liver, excreted via urine, extensively protein bound (98%)

INTERACTIONS

Increase: B/P—prazosin, terazosin, doxazosin, α-blockers, vardenafil

Increase: toxicity—cimetidine

NURSING CONSIDERATIONS

Assess:

- **Prostatic hyperplasia:** change in urinary patterns at baseline and throughout treatment; I&O ratios, weight daily; edema; report weight gain or edema
- **Orthostatic hypotension:** monitor B/P, standing, sitting

Perform/provide:

- Storage in tight container in cool environment

Evaluate:

- Therapeutic response: decreased symptoms of benign prostatic hyperplasia

Teach patient/family:

- Not to drive or operate machinery for 4 hr after 1st dose or after dosage increase
- To continue to take even if feeling better
- To advise providers of all products, herbs taken
- To make position changes slowly because orthostatic hypotension may occur

tapentadol (Rx)

(ta-pen′ta-dol)

Nucynta

Func. class.: Analgesic, misc.

Chem. class.: μ-Opioid receptor agonist

Controlled Substance Schedule II

ACTION:
Centrally acting synthetic analgesic; μ-opioid agonist activity is thought to result in analgesia; inhibits norepinephrine uptake

USES:
Moderate to severe pain

CONTRAINDICATIONS:
Hypersensitivity, asthma, ileus, respiratory depression

Precautions: Pregnancy (C), breastfeeding, children <18 yr, increased intracranial pressure, MI (acute), severe heart disease, respiratory depression, renal/hepatic disease, GI obstruction, ulcerative colitis, sleep apnea, seizure disorder

DOSAGE AND ROUTES

• **Adult: PO** 50-100 mg q4-6hr, may give 2nd dose ≥1 hr after 1st dose, max 700 mg on day 1, max 600 mg/day thereafter

Available forms: Tabs 50, 75, 100 mg

Administer:

• With antiemetic if nausea, vomiting occur

• When pain is beginning to return; determine dosage interval by response

SIDE EFFECTS

CNS: *Drowsiness, dizziness, confusion, headache, euphoria,* hallucinations, restlessness, syncope, anxiety, flushing, psychological dependence, insomnia, lethargy, tremor, **seizures**

CV: Palpitations, bradycardia, hypo/hypertension, orthostatic hypotension, sinus tachycardia

GI: *Nausea, vomiting, anorexia, constipation, cramps,* gastritis, dyspepsia, biliary spasms

GU: Urinary retention/frequency

INTEG: *Rash,* urticaria, diaphoresis, pruritus

RESP: **Respiratory depression,** cough

SYST: **Anaphylaxis,** infection, serotonin syndrome

PHARMACOKINETICS

Bioavailability 32%, extensively metabolized by liver, excreted in urine 99%, terminal half-life 4 hr, protein binding 20%

INTERACTIONS

Increase: effects with other CNS depressants—alcohol, opioids, sedative/hypnotics, antipsychotics, skeletal muscle relaxants

Increase: toxicity—MAOIs

Increase: serotonin syndrome—SSRIs, SNRIs, serotonin-receptor agonists, tricyclics

Drug/Herb

Increase: sedative effect—kava, St. John's wort, valerian

NURSING CONSIDERATIONS

Assess:

• **Pain:** intensity, location, type, characteristics; need for pain medication by pain/sedation scoring; physical dependence

• I&O ratio; check for decreasing output; may indicate urinary retention

• CNS changes: dizziness, drowsiness, hallucinations, euphoria, LOC, pupil reaction

⚠ **Serotonin syndrome: increased heart rate, shivering, sweating, dilated pupils, tremors, high B/P, hyperthermia, headache, confusion; if these occur, stop product, administer serotonin antagonist if needed**

• Allergic reactions: rash, urticaria, anaphylaxis

• **Respiratory dysfunction:** respiratory depression, character, rate, rhythm; notify prescriber if respirations are <10/min; B/P, pulse

Perform/provide:

• Storage in light-resistant area at room temp

• Assistance with ambulation

• Safety measures: night-light, call bell within easy reach

Evaluate:

• Therapeutic response: decrease in pain

Teach patient/family:

• To report any symptoms of CNS changes, allergic reactions, seizures, serotonin syndrome

• That physical dependency may result from extended use

• That withdrawal symptoms may occur: nausea, vomiting, cramps, fever, faintness, anorexia

• To avoid CNS depressants, alcohol

• To avoid driving, operating machinery if drowsiness, dizziness occur

T

• To change positions slowly to decrease orthostatic hypotension
• To notify prescriber if pregnancy planned, suspected or if breastfeeding

telaprevir

See Appendix A—Selected new drugs

telavancin (Rx)

(tel-a-van′sin)

Vibativ

Func. class.: Antiinfective, miscellaneous

Chem. class.: Lipoglycopeptide, a semisynthetic derivative of vancomycin

ACTION: Inhibits bacterial cell wall synthesis, blocks glycopeptides

USES: Skin/skin-structure infections caused by *Enterococcus faecalis, E. faecium, Staphylococcus aureus* (MSRA), *S. aureus* (MSSA), *S. epidermidis, S. haemolyticus, Streptococcus agalactiae* (group B), *S. dysgalactiae, S. pyogenes* (group A β-tremolytic), *S. anginosus, S. intermedius, S. constellates*

Unlabeled uses: Nosocomial pneumonia caused by susceptible gram-positive bacteria

CONTRAINDICATIONS: Hypersensitivity

Precautions: Breastfeeding, children, geriatric patients, renal disease, antimicrobial resistance, diabetes mellitus, diarrhea, GI disease, heart failure, hypertension, pseudomembranous colitis, QT prolongation, vancomycin hypersensitivity

Black Box Warning: Pregnancy (C), females

DOSAGE AND ROUTES

• **Adult: IV INF** 10 mg/kg over 60 min q24hr × 7-14 days

Nosocomial pneumonia (unlabeled)

• **Adult: IV INF** 10 mg/kg q24hr × 7-21 days

Available forms: Powder for inj 250, 750 mg

Administer:

• Use only for susceptible organisms to prevent drug-resistant bacteria
• Antihistamine if red-man syndrome occurs: decreased B/P; flushing of neck, face

Intermittent IV INF route

• After reconstitution with 15 ml D_5W sterile water for inj; 0.9% NaCl (15 mg/ml) 250-mg vial; add 45 ml to 750-mg vial (15 mg/ml) for dose of 150-800 mg; further dilute with 100-250 ml of compatible sol; for dose $<$150 mg or $>$800 mg, further dilute to conc of 0.6-8 mg/ml with compatible sol; give over 60 min

Solution compatibilities: D_5W, LR, NS

SIDE EFFECTS

CNS: Anxiety, chills, flushing, headache, insomnia

CV: QT prolongation, irregular heartbeat

EENT: Hearing loss

GI: Nausea, vomiting, pseudomembranous colitis, abdominal pain, constipation, diarrhea, metallic taste

GU: Nephrotoxicity, *increased BUN, creatinine,* renal failure, foamy urine

HEMA: Leukopenia, eosinophilia, anemia, thrombocytopenia

INTEG: Chills, fever, rash, thrombophlebitis at inj site; urticaria, pruritus, necrosis (red-man syndrome)

SYST: Anaphylaxis, superinfection

PHARMACOKINETICS

Onset rapid, half-life 8-9 hr, excreted in urine (76%)

INTERACTIONS

⚠ **Increase:** otoxicity or nephrotoxicity—aminoglycosides, cephalosporins, colistin, polymyxin, bacitracin, CISplatin, amphotericin B, nondepolarizing muscle relaxants, cidofovir

⚠ **Increase:** QT prolongation—class IA, III antidysrhythmics; some phenothiazines; chloroquine, clarithromycin, droperidol, dronedarone, erythromycin, haloperidol, levomethadye, methadone, pimozide, ziprasidone

NURSING CONSIDERATIONS

Assess:

- **Infection:** WBC, urine, stools, sputum, characteristics of wound throughout treatment
- I&O ratio; report hematuria, oliguria; nephrotoxicity may occur
- C&S
- Auditory function during, after treatment; hearing loss; ringing, roaring in ears; product should be discontinued
- B/P during administration; sudden drop may indicate red-man syndrome
- Skin eruptions
- Respiratory status: rate, character, wheezing, tightness in chest
- Allergies before treatment, reaction to each medication

Perform/provide:

- Storage in refrigerator
- EPINEPHrine, suction, tracheostomy set, endotracheal intubation equipment on unit; anaphylaxis may occur
- Adequate intake of fluids (2 L/day) to prevent nephrotoxicity

Evaluate:

- Therapeutic response: negative culture

Teach patient/family:

- About all aspects of product therapy; that culture may be taken after completed course of medication
- To report sore throat, fever, fatigue; could indicate superinfection

telbivudine (Rx)

(tel-bi′vyoo-deen)

Sebivo ✤, Tyzeka

Func. class.: Antiretroviral

Chem. class.: Nucleoside reverse transcriptase inhibitor (NRTI)

ACTION: Inhibits replication of HBV DNA polymerase, which inhibits HBV replication

USES: Treatment of chronic hepatitis B

CONTRAINDICATIONS: Hypersensitivity, breastfeeding

Precautions: Pregnancy (B), children, severe renal disease, anemia, organ transplant, dialysis, HIV, obesity, alcoholism; Hispanic or African descendents (safety not established)

Black Box Warning: Impaired hepatic function, lactic acidosis

DOSAGE AND ROUTES

- **Adult and adolescent >16 yr: PO** 600 mg/day; max 600 mg/day, monitor HBV DNA after 24 wk; if viral suppression incomplete (≥300 copies/ml), start alternate therapy; monitor HBV DNA q6mo

Renal dose

- **Adult: PO** CCr 30-49 ml/min, 600 mg tab q48hr or 400 mg oral sol daily; CCr <30 ml/min (not requiring dialysis), 600 mg tab q72hr or 200 mg oral sol daily

Available forms: Tabs 600 mg

Administer:

- With/without food with a full glass of water

SIDE EFFECTS

CNS: *Fever, headache, malaise,* weakness, *dizziness, insomnia*

EENT: Taste change, hearing loss, photophobia

T

GI: *Nausea, vomiting, diarrhea, anorexia,* abdominal pain, hepatomegaly
INTEG: *Rash*
MISC: Lactic acidosis
MS: Myalgia, arthralgia, muscle cramps
RESP: Cough

PHARMACOKINETICS

Excreted by kidneys (unchanged), steady state 5-7 days, protein binding 3.3%, terminal half-life 40-49 hr

INTERACTIONS

• Altered telbivudine levels: any agent altering renal function
Increase: myopathy risk—HMG-CoA reductase inhibitors, fibric acid derivatives, penicillamine, zidovudine, ZDV, cycloSPORINE, erythromycin, niacin, azole antifungals, corticosteroids, hydrochloroquine

NURSING CONSIDERATIONS

Assess:

Black Box Warning: LFTs, hepatitis B serology, creatine kinase, periodically, monitor HBV DNA after 24 wk; if viral suppression incomplete (≥300 copies/ml), start alternate therapy; monitor HBV DNA q6mo

Black Box Warning: Lactic acidosis: obtain baseline liver function tests; if elevated, discontinue treatment; discontinue even if liver function tests normal but lactic acidosis, hepatomegaly present, may be fatal

Perform/provide:
• Storage at room temp
Evaluate:
• Therapeutic response: decreasing hepatitis B serology
Teach patient/family:
• That GI complaints and insomnia may resolve after 3-4 wk of treatment
• That product does not cure hepatitis B and does not stop its spread to others
• That follow-up visits must be continued
• That serious product interactions may occur if OTC products are ingested; to check with prescriber before taking
• That product may cause dizziness; to avoid hazardous activities until response is known
• To report symptoms of cough, difficulty sleeping, excessive headache, muscle pain/weakness

telmisartan (Rx)

(tel-mih-sar'tan)
Micardis
Func. class.: Antihypertensive
Chem. class.: Angiotensin II receptor (Type AT_1) antagonist

ACTION: Blocks the vasoconstricting and aldosterone-secreting effects of angiotensin II; selectively blocks the binding of angiotensin II to the AT_1 receptor found in tissues

USES: Hypertension, alone or in combination; stroke, MI prophylaxis (>55 yr) in patients unable to take ACE inhibitors
Unlabeled uses: Heart failure

CONTRAINDICATIONS: Hypersensitivity

Black Box Warning: Pregnancy (D) 2nd/3rd trimesters

Precautions: Pregnancy (C) 1st trimester, breastfeeding, children, geriatric patients; hypersensitivity to ACE inhibitors; renal/hepatic disease, renal artery stenosis, dialysis, CHF, hyperkalemia, hypotension, hypovolemia

DOSAGE AND ROUTES

• **Adult: PO** 40 mg/day; range 20-80 mg/day
Stroke, MI prophylaxis
• **Adult >55 yr: PO** 80 mg/day
Available forms: Tabs 20, 40, 80 mg

Administer:
- Without regard to meals
- Increased dose to African-American patients or consider alternative agent; B/P response may be reduced

SIDE EFFECTS

CNS: Dizziness, insomnia, *anxiety,* headache, fatigue
GI: Diarrhea, dyspepsia, *anorexia, vomiting*
MS: Myalgia, pain
RESP: Cough, *upper respiratory infection,* sinusitis, pharyngitis

PHARMACOKINETICS

Onset of antihypertensive activity 3 hr, peak 0.5-1 hr, extensively metabolized, terminal half-life 24 hr, protein binding 99.5%, excreted in feces >97%, B/P response is less in African-American patients

INTERACTIONS

Increase: digoxin peak/trough concentrations—digoxin
Increase: antihypertensive action—diuretics, other antihypertensives
Increase: hyperkalemia—potassium-sparing diuretics, potassium salt substitutes
Decrease: antihypertensive effect—NSAIDs, salicylates

NURSING CONSIDERATIONS

Assess:
- B/P, pulse standing, lying; note rate, rhythm, quality
- Electrolytes: K, Na, Cl
- Baselines of renal, hepatic studies before therapy begins
- **CHF:** edema in feet, legs daily; jugular venous distention; dyspnea, crackles

Evaluate:
- Therapeutic response: decreased B/P

Teach patient/family:
- To comply with dosage schedule, even if feeling better; to take at same time of day; that therapeutic effect may take 2-4 wk
- To notify prescriber of mouth sores, fever, swelling of hands or feet, irregular heartbeat, chest pain, decreased urine output
- That excessive perspiration, dehydration, vomiting, diarrhea may lead to fall in blood pressure; to consult prescriber if these occur
- That product may cause dizziness, fainting, lightheadedness

Black Box Warning: To notify prescriber if pregnancy is planned or suspected, pregnancy category (D) 2nd/3rd trimester

- To notify prescriber of all prescriptions, OTC products, and supplements taken

temazepam (Rx)

(te-maz′e-pam)

Restoril

Func. class.: Sedative/hypnotic
Chem. class.: Benzodiazepine, short to intermediate acting

Controlled Substance Schedule IV (USA), Schedule F (Canada)

ACTION: Produces CNS depression at limbic, thalamic, hypothalamic levels of the CNS; may be mediated by neurotransmitter γ-aminobutyric acid (GABA); results are sedation, hypnosis, skeletal muscle relaxation, anticonvulsant activity, anxiolytic action

USES: Insomnia

CONTRAINDICATIONS: Pregnancy (X), breastfeeding, hypersensitivity to benzodiazepines, intermittent porphyria

Precautions: Children <15 yr, geriatric patients, anemia, renal/hepatic disease, suicidal individuals, drug abuse, psychosis, acute closed-angle glaucoma, seizure disorders, angioedema, sleep-related behaviors (sleepwalking), pulmonary disease

DOSAGE AND ROUTES

- **Adult: PO** 7.5 to 30 mg at bedtime
- **Geriatric: PO** 7.5 mg at bedtime

Available forms: Caps 7.5, 15, 22.5, 30 mg

Administer:

- After trying conservative measures for insomnia
- ½-1 hr before bedtime for sleeplessness
- On empty stomach for fast onset; may be taken with food if GI symptoms occur
- Avoid use with CNS depressants; serious CNS depression may result

SIDE EFFECTS

CNS: *Lethargy, drowsiness, daytime sedation,* dizziness, confusion, lightheadedness, headache, anxiety, irritability, complex sleep-related reactions (sleep driving, sleep eating), fatigue

CV: Chest pain, pulse changes, hypotension

EENT: Blurred vision

GI: Nausea, vomiting, diarrhea, heartburn, abdominal pain, constipation, anorexia

SYST: Severe allergic reactions

PHARMACOKINETICS

Onset 30-60 min, duration 6-8 hr, half-life 10-20 hr, metabolized by liver, excreted by kidneys, crosses placenta, excreted in breast milk, 98% protein binding

INTERACTIONS

Increase: effects of cimetidine, disulfiram, oral contraceptives

Increase: action of both products—alcohol, CNS depressants

Decrease: effect of antacids, theophylline, rifampin

Drug/Herb

Increase: CNS depression—hops, kava, valerian

Drug/Lab Test

Increase: ALT, AST, serum bilirubin

Decrease: RAI uptake

False increase: urinary 17-OHCS

NURSING CONSIDERATIONS

Assess:

- Mental status: mood, sensorium, affect, memory (long, short)
- Type of sleep problem: falling asleep, staying asleep
- **Dependency:** restrict amount given to patient, assess for physical/psychological dependency; high-level risk for abuse

Perform/provide:

- Assistance with ambulation after receiving dose
- Safety measures: night-light, call bell within easy reach
- Checking to confirm that PO medication has been swallowed
- Storage in tight container in cool environment

Evaluate:

- Therapeutic response: ability to sleep at night, decreased early morning awakening if taking product for insomnia

Teach patient/family:

- To avoid driving, other activities requiring alertness until stabilized
- To avoid alcohol ingestion
- That effects may take 2 nights for benefits to be noticed
- To limit to 7-10 days of continuous use
- About alternative measures to improve sleep: reading, exercise several hours before bedtime, warm bath, warm milk, TV, self-hypnosis, deep breathing
- Not to discontinue abruptly, withdraw gradually
- That complex sleep-related behaviors may occur: sleep driving/eating
- That hangover, memory impairment are common in geriatric patients but less common than with barbiturates

⚠ **To notify prescriber if pregnancy is planned or suspected, pregnancy (X); to use contraception while taking this product**

TREATMENT OF OVERDOSE:

Lavage, activated charcoal; monitor electrolytes, VS

temozolomide (Rx)

(tem-oh-zole′oh-mide)

Temodar

Func. class.: Antineoplastic-alkylating agent

Chem. class.: Imidazotetrazine derivative

ACTION:

Prodrug that undergoes conversion to MTIC; MTIC action prevents DNA transcription

USES:

Anaplastic astrocytoma with relapse, glioblastoma multiforme, malignant glioma

Unlabeled uses: Metastatic melanoma

CONTRAINDICATIONS:

Pregnancy (D), breastfeeding; hypersensitivity to this product, carbazine, or gelatin

Precautions: Geriatric patients, radiation therapy, renal/hepatic disease, bone marrow suppression, infection, myelosuppression

DOSAGE AND ROUTES

Anaplastic astrocytoma

- **Adult: PO** adjust dose based on nadir neutrophil and platelet counts 150 mg/m^2/day × 5 days during a 28-day cycle

Glioblastoma multiforme

- **Adult: PO/IV** 75 mg/m^2/day × 42 days with focal radiotherapy then maintenance of 6 cycles

Malignant glioma

- **Adult: IV** 150 mg/m^2/day over 90 min on days 1-5 q28days, may increase to 200 mg/m^2/day on days 1-5 q28days if hematologic parameters permit

Available forms: Caps 5, 20, 100, 140, 180, 250 mg; powder for inj 100 mg

Administer:

PO route

- Do not break, crush, chew, open caps
- Antiemetic 30-60 min before product to prevent vomiting
- Caps 1 at a time with 8 oz of water at same time of day
- Fluids IV or PO before chemotherapy to hydrate patient
- If caps accidentally damaged, do not allow contact with skin or inhale
- Use proper procedures for handling/disposing of chemotherapy products
- Give on empty stomach at bedtime to prevent nausea/vomiting

IV route

- Bring vial to room temp
- Inject 41 ml sterile water for inj into vial (2.5 mg/ml)
- Gently swirl, do not shake

Intermittent IV INF route

- Withdraw up to 40 ml from each vial to make total dose, transfer to empty 250-ml PVC inf bag, flush before and after inf
- Run over 90 min
- Use reconstituted sol within 14 hr, including inf time

SIDE EFFECTS

CNS: Seizures, *hemiparesis, dizziness, poor coordination, amnesia, insomnia, paresthesia, somnolence, paresis, ataxia, anxiety, dysphagia, depression, confusion*

GI: *Nausea, anorexia, vomiting,* abdominal pain, constipation

GU: Urinary incontinence, UTI, frequency

HEMA: **Thrombocytopenia, leukopenia,** anemia, **myelosuppression, neutropenia**

INTEG: *Rash, pruritus*

MISC: Headache, fatigue, asthenia, fever, edema, back pain, weight increase, diplopia

RESP: URI, pharyngitis, sinusitis, coughing

SYST: **Anaphylaxis, secondary malignancy**

T

PHARMACOKINETICS

Absorption complete, rapid; crosses blood-brain barrier; excreted in urine, feces; half-life 1.8 hr; peak 1 hr

INTERACTIONS

- Do not use within 24 hr of sargramostim, filgrastim, G-CSF

Increase: myelosuppression—radiation, other antineoplastics

Increase: bleeding risk—NSAIDs, anticoagulants, platelet inhibitors, thrombolytics

Decrease: antibody reaction—live virus vaccines, toxoids

Decrease: action of digoxin

NURSING CONSIDERATIONS

Assess:

- Tumor response during treatment
- CBC on day 22 (21 days after 1st dose), CBC weekly until recovery if ANC is <1.5 × 10^9/L and platelets <100 × 10^9/L, do not administer to patients who do not tolerate 100 mg/m^2, myelosuppression usually occurs late during the treatment cycle
- Seizures throughout treatment; mental status
- Monitor temp; may indicate beginning infection
- Hepatic studies before, during therapy (bilirubin, AST, ALT, LDH), as needed or monthly
- Bleeding: hematuria, guaiac, bruising, petechiae, mucosa or orifices

Perform/provide:

- Storage in light-resistant container in a dry area

Evaluate:

- Therapeutic response: decreased tumor size, spread of malignancy

Teach patient/family:

- To report signs of infection: fever, sore throat, flulike symptoms
- To report signs of anemia: fatigue, headache, faintness, SOB, irritability
- To report bleeding; to avoid use of razors, commercial mouthwash
- To notify prescriber if pregnancy is planned or suspected, pregnancy (D); not to breastfeed

temsirolimus (Rx)

(tem-sir-oh'li-mus)

Torisel

Func. class.: Biologic response modifier

Chem. class.: Kinase inhibitor, mTOR antagonist

ACTION: Inhibits mammalian target of rapamycin (mTOR), a protein kinase

USES: Renal cell carcinoma

Unlabeled uses: Mantle cell lymphoma

CONTRAINDICATIONS: Pregnancy (D), breastfeeding; hypersensitivity to this product or to sirolimus; polysorbate 80

Precautions: Children <13 yr, females, severe pulmonary/renal/hepatic disease (bilirubin >1-1.5×ULN or AST >ULN but bilirubin ≤ULN), diabetes mellitus, hyperkalemia, hyperuricemia, hypertension, bone marrow suppression, hypertriglyceridemia/hyperlipidemia, surgery, brain tumors

DOSAGE AND ROUTES

- **Adult:** IV 25 mg over 30-60 min weekly; treat until disease progression or severe toxicity occurs

Hepatic dose

- **Adult:** IV (mild impairment) bilirubin >1-1.5×ULN or AST >ULN but bilirubin ≤ULN
- Reduce to 15 mg/wk; (moderate or severe impairment, do not use)

Available forms: 25 mg/ml sol for inj kit

Administer:

- Using in-line filter ≤5 microns and inf pump
- Premedicate with 25-50 mg diphenhydrAMINE IV 30 min before dose; if re-

action occurs, stop for $^1/_2$-1 hr, may resume at slower rate
• Over 30-60 min, complete inf within 6 hr
• Dilute product with 1.8 ml provided diluent, result is 3 ml (10 mg/ml); invert to mix well; withdraw required amount and inject rapidly into 250 ml of NS; do not use PVC inf bags/sets
• Protect from light during preparation, use only glass

SIDE EFFECTS

CNS: *Headache,* seizures
CV: Hypertension, **thrombophlebitis**
ENDO: Hypertriglyceridemia, hyperlipidemia, hyperglycemia
GI: Nausea, vomiting, diarrhea, constipation, **bowel perforation**
GU: UTIs, **albuminuria, hematuria, proteinuria, renal failure,** mucositis
HEMA: **Anemia, leukopenia, thrombocytopenia**
INTEG: *Rash,* pruritus
META: Metabolic acidosis, hyperglycemia, hyperlipidemia
RESP: **Interstitial lung disease**
SYST: **Lymphoma**

PHARMACOKINETICS

Rapidly absorbed, peak 0.5-2 hr, extensively metabolized via liver by P450 3A4, eliminated via feces

INTERACTIONS

Increase: blood levels—CYP3A4 inhibitors, antifungals, calcium channel blockers, cimetidine, clarithromycin, danazol, erythromycin, cycloSPORINE, metoclopramide, bromocriptine, HIV-protease inhibitors, benzodiazepines, HMG-CoA reductase inhibitors
Increase: toxicity—sunitinib
Decrease: blood levels—CYP3A4 inducers, carBAMazepine, dexamethasone, PHENobarbital, phenytoin, rifamycin, rifapentine
Decrease: effect of vaccines
• Avoid with vaccines

Drug/Herb
• St. John's wort: may decrease effect of sirolimus
Increase: effect—ginseng, maitake, mistletoe
Decrease: immunosuppression—astragalus, echinacea, melatonin
Drug/Food
• Alters bioavailability; use consistently with/without food; do not use with grapefruit juice

NURSING CONSIDERATIONS

Assess:
• Cardiac status: B/P, heart rate
• Interstitial lung disease
• Hypersensitivity reactions: anaphylaxis
• Lipid profile: cholesterol, triglycerides; lipid-lowering agent may be needed; blood glucose
⚠ **Infection and development of lymphoma**
⚠ **Blood studies: Hgb, WBC, platelets during treatment monthly**
• Renal studies: BUN, creatinine, phosphate potassium; proteinuria, hematuria, albuminemia may indicate renal failure
• **Hepatic disease:** monitor liver function tests at baseline and periodically
Evaluate:
• Therapeutic response: decreased time of progression of renal cell carcinoma
Teach patient/family:
• To report fever, rash, severe diarrhea, chills, sore throat, fatigue; that serious infections may occur; to report clay-colored stools, cramping (hepatotoxicity), excessive thirst, urinary frequency, new or worsening breathing problems, blood in stool, abdominal pain
• To avoid crowds, persons with known infections to reduce risk of infection
⚠ **To use contraception before, during, for 12 wk after product discontinued; to avoid breastfeeding; that men should also use reliable contraception during and for 12 wk after cessation of product, pregnancy (D)**

T

⚠ HIGH ALERT

tenecteplase (TNK-tPA) (Rx)

(ten-ek'ta-place)

TNKase

Func. class.: Thrombolytic

Chem. class.: Tissue plasminogen activator

ACTION: Activates conversion of plasminogen to plasmin (fibrinolysin): plasmin breaks down clots (fibrin), fibrinogen, factors V, VII; occlusion of venous access lines

USES: Acute myocardial infarction, coronary artery thrombosis

CONTRAINDICATIONS: Hypersensitivity, arteriovenous malformation, aneurysm, active bleeding, intracranial/intraspinal surgery or trauma within 2 mo, CNS neoplasms, severe hypertension, severe renal/hepatic disease, history of CVA, increased ICP/stroke

Precautions: Pregnancy (C), breastfeeding, children, geriatric patients, arterial emboli from left side of heart, hypocoagulation, subacute bacterial endocarditis, rheumatic valvular disease, cerebral embolism/thrombosis/hemorrhage, intraarterial diagnostic procedure or surgery (10 days), recent major surgery, dysrhythmias, hypertension

DOSAGE AND ROUTES

Total dose, max 50 mg based on patient's weight

- **Adult <60 kg: IV BOL** 30 mg, give over 5 sec
- **Adult ≥60-<70 kg: IV BOL** 35 mg, give over 5 sec
- **Adult ≥70-<80 kg: IV BOL** 40 mg, give over 5 sec
- **Adult ≥80-<90 kg: IV BOL** 45 mg, give over 5 sec
- **Adult ≥90 kg: IV BOL** 50 mg, give over 5 sec, max 50 mg total dose

Available forms: Powder for inj, lyophilized 50 mg

Administer:

Intermittent IV INF route

- As soon as thrombi identified; not useful for thrombi >1 wk old
- Cryoprecipitate or fresh frozen plasma if bleeding occurs
- Heparin after fibrinogen level >100 mg/dl; heparin inf to increase PTT to 1.5-2× baseline for 3-7 days; IV heparin with loading dose is recommended
- Aseptically withdraw 10 ml of sterile water for inj from diluent vial, use red cannula syringe-filling device, inject all contents of syringe into product vial, direct into powder, swirl, withdraw correct dose, discard any unused sol; stand shield with dose vertically on flat surface and passively recap red cannula, remove entire shield assembly by twisting counter-clockwise, give by IV BOL
- IV therapy: use upper-extremity vessel that is accessible to manual compression
- If product not used immediately, refrigerate, use within 8 hr; not compatible with dextrose; flush dextrose-containing lines with saline before and after administration

SIDE EFFECTS

CV: Dysrhythmias, hypotension, pulmonary edema, **PE, cardiogenic shock, cardiac arrest, heart failure, myocardial reinfarction, myocardial rupture, tamponade, pericarditis, pericardial effusion, thrombosis, CVA**

HEMA: Decreased Hct, **bleeding**

INTEG: Rash, urticaria, phlebitis at IV inf site, itching, flushing

SYST: GI, GU, intracranial, retroperitoneal bleeding, surface bleeding, anaphylaxis

PHARMACOKINETICS

IV: Onset immediate, half-life 20-24 min, metabolized by liver

INTERACTIONS

- Bleeding potential: aspirin, indomethacin, phenylbutazone, anticoagulants, antithrombolytics, glycoprotein IIb/IIIa inhibitors, dipyridamole, clopidogrel, ticlopidine, NSAIDs, cefamandole, cefoperazone, cefotetan

Drug/Herb

Increase: risk of bleeding—anise, basil, dong quai, fenugreek, feverfew, garlic, ginger, ginkgo, ginseng, green tea, horse chestnut

Drug/Lab Test

Increase: PT, aPTT, TT

Decrease: plasminogen, fibrinogen

NURSING CONSIDERATIONS

Assess:

- **Allergy:** fever, rash, itching, chills; mild reaction may be treated with antihistamines

⚠ **Bleeding** during 1st hr of treatment; hematuria, hematemesis, bleeding from mucous membranes, epistaxis, ecchymosis; may require tranfusion (rare), continue to assess for bleeding for 24 hr

- Blood studies (Hct, platelets, PTT, PT, TT, aPTT) before starting therapy; PT or aPTT must be $<2\times$ control before starting therapy; PTT or PT q3-4hr during treatment
- Hypersensitive reactions: fever, rash, dyspnea; product should be discontinued
- VS, B/P, pulse, respirations, neurologic signs, temp at least q4hr; temp $>104°$ F ($40°$ C) indicates internal bleeding; systolic pressure increase >25 mm Hg should be reported to prescriber

⚠ Neurologic changes that may indicate intracranial bleeding

⚠ Retroperitoneal bleeding: back pain, leg weakness, diminished pulses

Perform/provide:

- Bed rest during entire course of treatment
- Avoidance of venous or arterial puncture, inj, rectal temp, any invasive treatment
- Treatment of fever with acetaminophen or aspirin
- Pressure for 30 sec to minor bleeding sites; inform prescriber if this does not attain hemostasis; apply pressure dressing

Evaluate:

- Therapeutic response: resolution of MI

Teach patient/family:

- About proper tooth brushing technique to avoid bleeding
- To notify prescriber immediately of sudden, severe headache
- To notify prescriber of bleeding; hypersensitivity; fast, slow, or uneven heart rate; feeling of faintness; blood in urine, stools; nose bleeds

tenofovir (Rx)

(ten-oh-foh′veer)

Viread

Func. class.: Antiretroviral

Chem. class.: Nucleoside reverse transcriptase inhibitor (NRTI)

ACTION: Inhibits replication of HIV virus by competing with the natural substrate and then incorporating into cellular DNA by viral reverse transcriptase, thereby terminating cellular DNA chain

USES: HIV-1 infection with at least 2 other antiretrovirals, hepatitis B

CONTRAINDICATIONS: Hypersensitivity

Black Box Warning: Lactic acidosis

Precautions: Pregnancy (B), breastfeeding, children, geriatric patients, renal disease, CCr <60 ml/min, osteoporosis, immune reconstitution syndrome

Black Box Warning: Hepatic disease, hepatitis

DOSAGE AND ROUTES

- **Adult: PO** 300 mg/day with meal; if used with didanosine, give tenofovir 2 hr before or 1 hr after didanosine

T

- **Adolescent and child ≥12 yr: PO** 300 mg/day

Renal dose

- **Adult: PO** CCr 30-49 ml/min, 300 mg q48hr; CCr 10-29 ml/min, 300 mg q72-96hr; CCr <10 ml/min, not recommended

Available forms: Tabs 300 mg (300 mg of fumarate salt equivalent to 245 mg tenofovir disoproxil)

Administer:

- PO daily with meal
- 2 hr before or 1 hr after didanosine (if used)

SIDE EFFECTS

CNS: *Headache, asthenia*

GI: *Nausea, vomiting, diarrhea,* anorexia, *flatulence, abdominal pain,* pancreatitis

GU: Renal failure, renal tubular acidosis/necrosis, Fanconi syndrome

HEMA: Neutropenia, osteopenia

INTEG: *Rash,* angioedema

META: Lactic acidosis, hypokalemia, hypophosphatemia

MS: Myopathy, rhabdomyolysis

SYST: Lipodystrophy

PHARMACOKINETICS

Rapidly absorbed, distributed to extravascular space, excreted unchanged in urine 70%-80%, terminal half-life 17 hr

INTERACTIONS

Increase: tenofovir level—cidofovir, acyclovir, valacyclovir, ganciclovir, valganciclovir

Increase: level of didanosine when given with tenofovir

Increase: tenofovir level—any product that decreases renal function

NURSING CONSIDERATIONS

Assess:

- Viral load, CD4+ T-cell count, plasma HIV RNA, serum creatinine/BUN/phosphate
- Resistance testing at start of therapy and at treatment failure
- Hepatic studies: AST, ALT, bilirubin; amylase, lipase, triglycerides periodically during treatment
- Bone, renal toxicity: if bone abnormalities are suspected, obtain tests; serum phosphorus, creatinine
- **Lactic acidosis, severe hepatomegaly with steatosis:** obtain baseline liver function tests; if elevated, discontinue treatment; discontinue even if liver function tests normal but lactic acidosis, hepatomegaly present, may be fatal

Perform/provide:

- Storage at 25° C (77° F)

Evaluate:

- Therapeutic response: decrease in signs, symptoms of HIV

Teach patient/family:

- To take without regard to food
- That GI complaints resolve after 3-4 wk of treatment
- Not to breastfeed while taking this product
- That product must be taken daily even if patient feels better
- That follow-up visits must be continued because serious toxicity may occur; that blood counts must be done q2wk
- That product will control symptoms but is not a cure for HIV; that patient is still infectious, may pass HIV virus on to others
- That other products may be necessary to prevent other infections
- That changes in body fat distribution may occur
- To notify prescriber of symptoms of lactic acidosis

terazosin (Rx)

(ter-ay′zoe-sin)

Func. class.: Antihypertensive

Chem. class.: α-Adrenergic blocker

ACTION: Decreases total vascular resistance, which is responsible for a decrease in B/P; this occurs by the blockade of α_1-adrenoreceptors

USES:
Hypertension, as a single agent or in combination with diuretics or β-blockers; BPH

CONTRAINDICATIONS:
Hypersensitivity

Precautions: Pregnancy (C), breastfeeding, children, prostate cancer, renal disease, syncope

DOSAGE AND ROUTES

Hypertension

- **Adult: PO** 1 mg at bedtime, may increase dose slowly to desired response; max 20 mg/day

Benign prostatic hyperplasia

- **Adult: PO** 1 mg at bedtime, gradually increase up to 5-10 mg; max 20 mg

Available forms: Caps 1, 2, 5, 10 mg

Administer

- Give dose at bedtime; patient should not operate machinery because fainting may occur

SIDE EFFECTS

CNS: *Dizziness, headache, drowsiness,* anxiety, depression, vertigo, weakness, fatigue

CV: Palpitations, orthostatic hypotension, tachycardia, edema, rebound hypertension

EENT: Blurred vision, epistaxis, tinnitus, dry mouth, red sclera, nasal congestion, sinusitis

GI: *Nausea,* vomiting, diarrhea, constipation, abdominal pain

GU: Urinary frequency, incontinence, impotence, priapism

RESP: Dyspnea, cough, pharyngitis

PHARMACOKINETICS

Peak 1 hr; half-life 9-12 hr; protein binding 90%-94%; metabolized in liver; excreted in urine, feces

INTERACTIONS

Increase: hypotensive effects—β-blockers, nitroglycerin, verapamil, other antihypertensives, alcohol

Decrease: hypotensive effects—estrogens, NSAIDs, sympathomimetics, salicylates

Drug/Herb

Increase: antihypertensive effect—hawthorn

Decrease: antihypertensive effect—ephedra

NURSING CONSIDERATIONS

Assess:

- **BPH:** urinary patterns (hesitancy, frequency, change in stream, dribbling, dysuria, urgency)
- Hypertension: crackles, dyspnea, orthopnea q30min; orthostatic B/P, pulse, jugular venous distention q4hr; weight daily, I&O
- BUN, uric acid if patient receiving long-term therapy
- Skin turgor, dryness of mucous membranes for hydration status

Perform/provide:

- Cool storage in tight container

Evaluate:

- Therapeutic response: decreased B/P, edema in feet, legs; decreased symptoms of BPH

Teach patient/family:

- That fainting occasionally occurs after 1st dose; not to drive or operate machinery for 4 hr after 1st dose or after an increase in dose; to take 1st dose at bedtime
- To rise slowly from sitting or lying position
- Not to discontinue abruptly
- Hypertension: to continue with regimen including diet, exercise

T

terbinafine (Rx)

(ter-bin′a-feen)

Lamisil

Func. class.: Antifungal

Chem. class.: Synthetic allylamine derivative

ACTION:
Interferes with cell-membrane permeability of fungi such as

Trichophyton rubrum, Trichophyton mentagrophytes, Trichophyton tonsurans, Epidermophyton floccosum, Microsporum canis, Microsporum audouinii, Microsporum gypseum, Candida; broad-spectrum antifungal

USES:
(Oral) onychomycosis of toenail or fingernail due to dermatophytes
Unlabeled uses: Cutaneous candidiasis, tinea versicolor

CONTRAINDICATIONS:
Hypersensitivity/olfactory, chronic/active hepatic disease, renal disease GFR ≤50 ml/min
Precautions: Pregnancy (B), breastfeeding, children, renal disease

DOSAGE AND ROUTES
- **Fingernail: PO** 250 mg/day × 6 wk
- **Toenail: PO** 250 mg/day × 12 wk

Available forms: Tabs 250 mg
Administer:
- **PO:** without regard to food

SIDE EFFECTS
CNS: Depression
GI: Diarrhea, dyspepsia, abdominal pain, nausea, hepatitis
HEMA: Neutropenia
INTEG: Rash, pruritus, urticaria, Stevens-Johnson syndrome
MISC: Headache, hepatic enzyme changes, taste, visual/olfactory disturbance

PHARMACOKINETICS
Peak 1-2 hr, >99% protein binding, half-life 36 hr

INTERACTIONS
Increase: levels of dextromethorphan
Increase: terbinafine clearance—rifampin
Increase: clearance of cycloSPORINE
Decrease: terbinafine clearance—cimetidine

Drug/Herb
- Side effects: cola nut, guarana, yerba maté, tea (black, green), coffee

NURSING CONSIDERATIONS
Assess:
- Hepatic studies (ALT, AST) prior to beginning treatment; do not use in presence of hepatic disease
- CBC in treatment >6 wk
- Continuing infection: increased size, number of lesions

Perform/provide:
- Storage at <25° C (77° F)

Evaluate:
- Therapeutic response: decrease in size, number of lesions

Teach patient/family:
- To notify prescriber of nausea, vomiting, fatigue, jaundice, dark urine, clay-colored stool, RUQ pain; may indicate hepatic dysfunction

terbinafine topical
See Appendix B

terbutaline (Rx)
(ter-byoo′te-leen)
Brethine, Bricanyl ✦
Func. class.: Selective β_2-agonist; bronchodilator
Chem. class.: Catecholamine

ACTION:
Relaxes bronchial smooth muscle by direct action on β_2-adrenergic receptors through the accumulation of cAMP at β-adrenergic receptor sites; bronchodilation, diuresis, CNS, cardiac stimulation occur; relaxes uterine smooth muscle

USES:
Bronchospasm
Unlabeled uses: Premature labor, nonresponsive status asthmaticus in children (IV)

CONTRAINDICATIONS:
Hypersensitivity to sympathomimetics, closed-angle glaucoma, tachydysrhythmias

Precautions: Pregnancy (B), breastfeeding, geriatric patients, cardiac disorders, hyperthyroidism, diabetes mellitus, prostatic hypertension, hypertension, seizure disorder

Black Box Warning: Labor

DOSAGE AND ROUTES

Bronchospasm

- **Adult and child >12 yr: PO** 2.5-5 mg q8hr; **SUBCUT** 0.25 mg q15-30min, max 0.5 mg in 4 hr
- **Adolescent ≤15 yr and child ≥12 yr: PO** 2.5 mg tid, max 7.5 mg/day
- **Child 6-11 yr (unlabeled): PO** 0.05 mg/kg q8hr, may increase slowly

Renal dose

- **Adult: PO** CCr 10-50 ml/min, 50% of dose; CCr <10 ml/min, avoid use

Tocolytic (preterm labor) (unlabeled)

- **Adult: SUBCUT** 0.25 mg q20min to 6 hr, hold if pulse >120 bpm

Available forms: Tabs 2.5, 5 mg; inj 1 mg/ml

Administer:

- With food; may be crushed
- 2 hr before bedtime to avoid sleeplessness

IV route (unlabeled)

- Only used if subcut is ineffective
- IV after diluting each 5 mg/1 L D_5W for inf
- IV, run 5 mcg/min; may increase 5 mcg q10min, titrate to response; after 1/2-1 hr, taper dose by 5 mcg; switch to PO as soon as possible

Y-site compatibilities: Insulin (regular)

SIDE EFFECTS

CNS: Tremors, anxiety, insomnia, headache, dizziness, stimulation

CV: Palpitations, tachycardia, hypertension, dysrhythmias, **cardiac arrest**

GI: Nausea, vomiting

PHARMACOKINETICS

PO: Onset 1/2 hr, peak 1-2 hr, duration 4-8 hr

SUBCUT: Onset 6-15 min, peak 1/2-1 hr, duration 1 1/2-4 hr

INTERACTIONS

- Incompatible with bleomycin
- Hypertensive crisis: MAOIs

Increase: effects of both products—other sympathomimetics

Decrease: action—β-blockers

Drug/Herb

Increase: effect—green tea (large amounts), guarana

NURSING CONSIDERATIONS

Assess:

- Respiratory function: vital capacity, forced expiratory volume, ABGs, B/P, pulse, respiratory pattern, lung sounds, sputum before and after treatment
- Tolerance in patients receiving long-term therapy; dose may have to be changed; monitor for rebound bronchospasm

⚠ **Paradoxical bronchospasm: dyspnea, wheezing; keep emergency equipment nearby**

- **Labor:** maternal heart rate, B/P, contraction, fetal heart rate; can inhibit uterine contractions, labor; monitor for hypoglycemia

Perform/provide:

- Storage at room temp; do not use discolored sol
- Increase in fluids of >2 L/day

Evaluate:

- Therapeutic response: absence of dyspnea, wheezing

Teach patient/family:

- Not to use OTC medications because extra stimulation may occur
- About all aspects of product; to avoid smoking, smoke-filled rooms, persons with respiratory infections
- To increase fluids by >2 L/day; to allow 15 min between inhalation of product and inhaled product containing steroid

• To take on time; if missed, not to make up after 1 hr, to wait until next dose

terconazole vaginal antifungal

See Appendix B

teriparatide (Rx)

(tah-ree-par'ah-tide)

Forteo

Func. class.: Parathyroid hormone (rDNA)

ACTION: Contains human recombinant parathyroid hormone to stimulate new bone growth

USES: Postmenopausal women with osteoporosis, men with primary or hypogonadal osteoporosis who are at high risk for fracture, glucocorticoid-induced osteoporosis

Unlabeled uses: Hypoparathyroidism

CONTRAINDICATIONS: Hypersensitivity, increased baseline risk for osteosarcoma (Paget's disease, open epiphyses; previous bone radiation), bone metastases, history of skeletal malignancies, other metabolic bone diseases, preexisting hypercalcemia

Precautions: Pregnancy (C), breastfeeding, children, urolithiasis, hypotension, use >2 yr, cardiac disease

Black Box Warning: Secondary malignancy

DOSAGE AND ROUTES

• **Adult: SUBCUT** 20 mcg/day up to 2 yr (osteoporosis); long-term/lifetime use is recommended (glucocorticoid-induced osteoporosis)

Available forms: Prefilled pen delivery device (delivers 20 mcg/day)

Administer:

SUBCUT route

• Give by SUBCUT using disposable pen only; inject in thigh or abdomen; lightly pinch fold of skin; insert needle; release skin; inject at 90-degree angle over 5 sec; rotate inj sites

• Have patient sit or lie down; orthostatic hypotension may occur

SIDE EFFECTS

CNS: Dizziness, headache, insomnia, depression, vertigo

CV: Hypertension, angina, syncope

GI: Nausea, diarrhea, dyspepsia, vomiting, constipation

INTEG: Rash, sweating

MISC: Pain, asthenia, hyperuricemia

MS: Arthralgia, leg cramps, back/leg pain, weakness, **osteosarcoma (rare)**

RESP: Rhinitis, cough, pharyngitis, pneumonia, dyspnea

PHARMACOKINETICS

SUBCUT: Extensively and rapidly absorbed, metabolized by liver, excreted by kidneys, terminal half-life 1 hr

INTERACTIONS

Increase: digoxin toxicity: digoxin

Drug/Lab Test

Increase: calcium

NURSING CONSIDERATIONS

Assess:

Black Box Warning: Secondary malignancy: osteosarcoma, dependent on length of treatment; those at higher risk for osteosarcoma should not use this product

• Uric acid, magnesium, creatinine, BUN, urine pH, vit D, phosphate for normal serum levels; serum calcium may be transiently increased after dosing (max at 4-6 hr after dose)

• Bone pain, headache, fatigue, changes in LOC, leg cramps

• **Signs of persistent hypercalcemia:** nausea, vomiting, constipation, lethargy, muscle weakness

• Nutritional status: diet for sources of vit D (milk, some seafood), calcium (dairy products, dark green vegetables), phosphates (dairy products)

Perform/provide:

• Store refrigerated, do not freeze; may be used for 28 days after first inj

Evaluate:

• Therapeutic response: increased bone mineral density

Teach patient/family:

• About the symptoms of hypercalcemia
• About foods rich in calcium, vit D
• How to use delivery device, dispose of needles; not to share pen with others, to use at same time of day
• To sit or lie down if dizziness or fast heartbeat occurs after 1st few doses
• To rotate administration sites
• To store pen in refrigerator

tesamorelin

See Appendix A—Selected new drugs

testosterone cypionate (Rx)

Depo-Testosterone

testosterone enanthate (Rx)

Delatestryl

testosterone gel (Rx)

AndroGel, FORTESTA, Testim

testosterone pellets (Rx)

Testopel

testosterone transdermal (Rx)

Androderm

testosterone buccal (Rx)

Striant

testosterone topical solution

Axiron

Func. class.: Androgenic anabolic steroid

Chem. class.: Halogenated testosterone derivative

Controlled Substance Schedule III

ACTION: Increases weight by building body tissue; increases potassium, phosphorus, chloride, nitrogen levels, bone development

USES: Female breast cancer, hypogonadism, eunuchoidism, male climacteric, oligospermia, impotence, osteoporosis, weight loss in AIDS patients, vulvar dystrophies, low testosterone levels, delayed male puberty (inj)

CONTRAINDICATIONS: Pregnancy (X), breastfeeding, severe cardiac/renal/hepatic disease, hypersensitivity, genital bleeding (rare), male breast/prostate cancer

Precautions: Diabetes mellitus, CV disease, MI, urinary tract disorders, prostate cancer, hypercalcemia

Black Box Warning: Children, accidental exposure

DOSAGE AND ROUTES

Replacement

• **Adult: IM (base or propionate)** 25-50 mg 2-3×/wk or **(enanthate or cypionate)** 50-400 mg q2-4wk; topical sol (Axiron) 60 mg (2 pump actuations), apply each AM

• **Adult (male) and child: SUBCUT (pellets)** 150-450 mg (2-6 pellets) inserted q3-6mo

• **Adult: TRANSDERMAL (Testoderm)** 4-6 mg applied q24hr; **(Androderm)** 5 mg applied q24hr; **GEL (AndroGel)** 1% 5 mg applied q24hr, once daily; 1.62% 40.5 mg (2 pump actuations) q AM; topical sol **(Axiron)** 30 mg/actuation **BUCCAL** 1 buccal system (30 mg) to the gum region q12hr before meals/PM

Breast cancer

• **Adult: IM** 50-100 mg 3×/wk (propionate) or 200-400 mg q2-4wk (cypionate or enanthate)

Delayed male puberty

• **Child >12 yr: IM** ≤100 mg/mo for ≤6 mo

Available forms: Enanthate: inj 200 mg/ml; **cypionate:** inj 100, 200 mg/ml; pellets 75 mg; **transdermal** 2.5, 4, 5, 6 mg/24 hr; **gel** 1%, 1.62%, 10 mg/actuation; **buccal system** 30 mg

Administer:

• Titrated dose; use lowest effective dose

• IM inj deep into upper outer quadrant of gluteal muscle

• Transdermal patches: Testoderm to skin of scrotum; Androderm to skin of back, upper arms, thighs, abdomen; area must be dry shaved; may be reapplied after bathing, swimming

• **Gel:** products not interchangeable, dosage and administration for AndroGel 1% differs from that of AndroGel 1.62%; apply daily to clean, dry area on shoulders, upper arms, or abdomen; women, children should not touch treated skin

Buccal system route

• Do not chew or swallow buccal system

• Rotate sites; place above incisor tooth on either side of mouth

• Open packet; place rounded side of surface against gum and hold firmly in place with finger over lip for 30 sec; if product falls off, replace with new system; discard in trash can away from children or pets

SIDE EFFECTS

CNS: Dizziness, headache, fatigue, tremors, paresthesias, flushing, sweating, anxiety, lability, insomnia, carpal tunnel syndrome

CV: Increased B/P

EENT: Conjunctival edema, nasal congestion

ENDO: Abnormal glucose tolerance test

GI: Nausea, vomiting, constipation, weight gain, **cholestatic jaundice**

GU: Hematuria, amenorrhea, vaginitis, decreased libido, decreased breast size, clitoral hypertrophy, testicular atrophy, gynecomastia

HEMA: Polycythemia

INTEG: Rash, acneiform lesions, oily hair/skin, flushing, sweating, acne vulgaris, alopecia, hirsutism

MS: Cramps, spasms

PHARMACOKINETICS

PO: Metabolized in liver; excreted in urine, breast milk; crosses placenta

INTERACTIONS

• Edema: ACTH, adrenal steroids, buPROPion

Increase: effects of oxyphenbutazone

Increase: PT—anticoagulants

Decrease: glucose levels may alter need for oral antidiabetics, insulin

Drug/Lab Test

Increase: serum cholesterol, blood glucose, urine glucose

Decrease: serum calcium, serum potassium, T_4, T_3, thyroid ^{131}I uptake test, urine 17-OHCS, 17-KS, PBI

NURSING CONSIDERATIONS

Assess:

- Weight daily; notify prescriber if weekly weight gain >5 lb
- B/P q4hr, Hgb/HCT
- I&O ratio; be alert for decreasing urinary output, increasing edema
- Growth rate, bone age in children; growth rate may be uneven (linear/bone growth) with extended use
- Electrolytes: K, Na, Cl, Ca; cholesterol
- Hepatic studies: ALT, AST, bilirubin
- Edema, hypertension, cardiac symptoms, jaundice
- Mental status: affect, mood, behavioral changes, aggression
- **Signs of masculinization in female:** increased libido, deepening of voice, decreased breast tissue, enlarged clitoris, menstrual irregularities; male: gynecomastia, impotence, testicular atrophy
- **Hypercalcemia:** lethargy, polyuria, polydipsia, nausea, vomiting, constipation; product may have to be decreased
- **Hypoglycemia** in diabetic patients; oral antidiabetic action is increased

Perform/provide:

- Diet with increased calories, protein; decrease sodium if edema occurs

Evaluate:

- Therapeutic response: 4-6 wk with osteoporosis

Teach patient/family:

- That product must be combined with complete health plan: diet, rest, exercise
- To notify prescriber if therapeutic response decreases, if edema occurs
- About changes in sex characteristics: priapism, gynecomastia, increased libido
- That women should report menstrual irregularities, voice changes, acne, facial hair growth; if pregnancy is planned or suspected
- That 1-3-mo course is necessary for response with breast cancer
- About the proper application of patches

tetracaine (Rx)

(tet′ra-kane)

Pontocaine

Func. class.: Local anesthetic

Chem. class.: Ester

ACTION: Competes with calcium for binding sites in nerve membrane that control sodium transport across cell membrane; decreases rise of depolarization phase of action potential

USES: Spinal anesthesia, epidural and peripheral nerve block, perineum, lower extremities

CONTRAINDICATIONS: Hypersensitivity, sulfite allergy, severe hepatic disease, heart block, thrombocytopenia

Precautions: Pregnancy (C), breastfeeding, children ≤12 yr, geriatric patients, severe product allergies, cardiac disease

DOSAGE AND ROUTES

Varies with route of anesthesia

Available forms: Inj 0.2%, 0.3%, 1%; powder

Administer:

- Only if not cloudy; does not contain precipitate
- Only with crash cart, resuscitative equipment nearby
- Only without preservatives for epidural or caudal anesthesia

SIDE EFFECTS

CNS: Anxiety, restlessness, **seizures, loss of consciousness**, drowsiness, disorientation, tremors, shivering

CV: Myocardial depression, cardiac arrest, dysrhythmias, bradycardia, hypo/hypertension, fetal bradycardia

EENT: Blurred vision, tinnitus, pupil constriction

GI: Nausea, vomiting
INTEG: Rash, urticaria, allergic reactions, edema, burning, skin discoloration at inj site, tissue necrosis
RESP: Status asthmaticus, respiratory arrest, anaphylaxis

PHARMACOKINETICS

Onset MS 3 min, spinal 3-8 min; duration 1.5-3 hr; metabolized by liver; excreted in urine (metabolites)

INTERACTIONS

- Dysrhythmias: EPINEPHrine, halothane, enflurane
- Hypertension: tricyclics, phenothiazines
- Hypotension: MAOIs

Decrease: action of tetracaine—chloroprocaine
Decrease: action of sulfonamides

NURSING CONSIDERATIONS

Assess:

- B/P, pulse, respirations during treatment
- Fetal heart tones during labor
- Allergic reactions: rash, urticaria, itching
- Cardiac status: ECG for dysrhythmias, pulse, B/P during anesthesia

Perform/provide:

- Use of new sol, discard unused portions; store in refrigerator, avoid freezing

Evaluate:

- Therapeutic response: anesthesia necessary for procedure

TREATMENT OF OVERDOSE:

Maintain adequate airway, O_2, vasopressor, IV fluids, anticonvulsants for seizures

tetracaine ophthalmic

See Appendix B

tetracaine topical

See Appendix B

tetracycline (Rx)

(tet-ra-sye′kleen)

Apo-Tetra ♣, Nu-Tetra ♣

Func. class.: Broad-spectrum antiinfective
Chem. class.: Tetracycline

ACTION:

Inhibits protein synthesis and phosphorylation in microorganisms; bacteriostatic

USES:

Syphilis, *Chlamydia trachomatis,* gonorrhea, lymphogranuloma venereum; uncommon gram-positive, gram-negative organisms; rickettsial infections

CONTRAINDICATIONS:

Pregnancy (D), breastfeeding, children <8 yr, hypersensitivity to tetracyclines
Precautions: Renal/hepatic disease, UV exposure

DOSAGE AND ROUTES

Susceptible gram-positive/gram-negative infections

- **Adult: PO** 250-500 mg q6hr
- **Child >8 yr: PO** 25-50 mg/kg/day in divided doses q6hr

Chlamydia trachomatis

- **Adult: PO** 500 mg qid × 7 days

Syphilis

- **Adult and adolescent: PO** 500 mg qid × 2 wk; if syphilis duration >1 yr, must treat 30 days

Brucellosis

- **Adult: PO** 500 mg q6hr × 3 wk with **IM** 1 g streptomycin bid × 1st wk then daily × 2nd wk

Urethral, endocervical, rectal infections *(C. trachomatis)*

- **Adult: PO** 500 mg qid × 7 days

Acne

- **Adult and adolescent: PO** 250 mg q6hr then 125-500 mg/day or every other day

Renal dose

• **Adult: PO** CCr 51-90 ml/min, give dose q8-12hr; CCr 10-50 ml/min, give dose q12-24hr; CCr <10 ml/min, give dose q24hr

Available forms: Caps 250, 500 mg

Administer:

• After C&S obtained
• 2 hr before or after iron products; 1 hr after antacid products
• Should be given on empty stomach

SIDE EFFECTS

CNS: Fever, headache, paresthesia
CV: Pericarditis
EENT: Dysphagia, glossitis, decreased calcification, discoloration of deciduous teeth, oral candidiasis, oral ulcers
GI: *Nausea,* abdominal pain, *vomiting, diarrhea,* anorexia, enterocolitis, **hepatotoxicity,** flatulence, abdominal cramps, epigastric burning, stomatitis, **hepatitis, pseudomembranous colitis**
GU: *Increased BUN,* **azotemia, acute renal failure**
HEMA: Eosinophilia, neutropenia, thrombocytopenia, leukocytosis, hemolytic anemia
INTEG: *Rash, urticaria, photosensitivity, increased pigmentation,* **exfoliative dermatitis,** pruritus, **angioedema, Stevens-Johnson syndrome**
MISC: Increased intracranial pressure, candidiasis

PHARMACOKINETICS

PO: Peak 2-3 hr; duration 6 hr; half-life 6-12 hr; excreted in urine, breast milk; crosses placenta; 65% protein bound

INTERACTIONS

⚠ **Fatal nephrotoxicity: methoxyflurane**
Increase: effect of warfarin, digoxin
Decrease: effect of tetracycline—antacids, sodium bicarbonate, dairy products, alkali products, iron, cimetidine
Decrease: effect of penicillins, oral contraceptives

Drug/Herb

• Photosensitivity: dong quai

Drug/Lab Test

False increase: urinary catecholamines

NURSING CONSIDERATIONS

Assess:

⚠ **Pseudomembranous colitis: diarrhea, abdominal pain, fever, fatigue, anorexia; possible anemia, elevated WBC count, low serum albumin; stop product; usually either vancomycin or IV metroNIDAZOLE is given**
• Signs of anemia: Hct, Hgb, fatigue
• I&O ratio
• Blood studies: PT, CBC, AST, ALT, BUN, creatinine
• **Allergic reactions:** rash, itching, pruritus
• **Serious skin reactions:** angioedema, Stevens-Johnson syndrome, exfoliative dermatitis; report immediately after stopping product
• Nausea, vomiting, diarrhea; administer antiemetic, antacids as ordered

⚠ **Overgrowth of infection: fever, malaise, redness, pain, swelling, drainage, perineal itching, diarrhea, changes in cough or sputum**

Perform/provide:

• Storage in tight, light-resistant container at room temp

Evaluate:

• Therapeutic response: decreased temp, absence of lesions, negative C&S

Teach patient/family:

• To avoid sun exposure; that sunscreen does not seem to decrease photosensitivity
• That all prescribed medication must be taken to prevent superinfection
• To avoid milk products, antacids or to separate by 2 hr; to take with full glass of water
• That tooth discoloration may occur
• To notify prescriber immediately of diarrhea with pus, mucous, fever, abdominal pain

⚠ **To notify prescriber if pregnancy is planned or suspected, pregnancy (D)**

tetrahydrozoline nasal agent

See Appendix B

tetrahydrozoline ophthalmic

See Appendix B

theophylline (Rx)

(thee-off'i-lin)

Elixophyllin, Theo-24, Theochron, Uniphyl

Func. class.: Bronchodilator

Chem. class.: Methylxanthine

ACTION:

Relaxes smooth muscle of respiratory system by blocking phosphodiesterase, which increases cAMP; exact action unknown

USES:

Bronchial asthma, bronchospasm of COPD, chronic bronchitis, emphysema

CONTRAINDICATIONS:

Hypersensitivity to xanthines, tachydysrhythmias

Precautions: Pregnancy (C), children, geriatric patients, CHF, cor pulmonale, hepatic disease, active peptic ulcer disease, diabetes mellitus, hyperthyroidism, hypertension, seizure disorder, hypothyroidism

DOSAGE AND ROUTES

Acute exacerbations of reversible airway obstruction

- **Adult: IV** 5 mg/kg loading dose over 20-30 min

COPD, chronic bronchitis

- **Adult: IV** 0.4 mg/kg/hr for nonsmokers or 0.7 mg/kg/hr for smokers
- **Adult/child >45 kg maintenance: PO** (regular rel) 10 mg/kg/day in divided doses q6-8hr, max 300 mg/day; after 3 days, increase dose to 400 mg in divided doses q6-8hr; after 3 more days, increase to 600 mg in divided doses q6-8hr, max 800 mg/day

Apnea of prematurity

- **Neonate: IV** 4 mg/kg over 20-30 min then maintenance
- **Neonate ≥24 days: IV/PO** 1.5 mg/kg q12hr

Available forms: Caps, ext rel 100, 200, 300, 400 mg; tab, ext rel 100, 200, 400, 450, 600 mg; elixir 80 mg/15 ml; sol for inj 250 mg/10 ml, 500 mg/20 ml

Administer:

PO route

- Do not break, crush, chew, or dissolve timed-rel products
- PO with 8 oz of water for GI symptoms; avoid food; absorption may be affected; take dose consistently; do not take Theo-24 with meals
- Contents of bead-filled capsule sprinkled over food for children's use
- Check OTC medications, current prescriptions for ePHEDrine, which will increase stimulation

IV route

- Loading dose over 20-30 min, max 20-25 mg/min; do not give by rapid IV, use only cont inf

Y-site compatibilities: Acyclovir, ampicillin, ampicillin/sulbactam, aztreonam, ceFAZolin, cefotetan, ceftazidime, cefTRIAXone, cimetidine, cisatracurium, clindamycin, dexamethasone, diltiazem, DOBUTamine, DOPamine, doxycycline, erythromycin, famotidine, fluconazole, gentamicin, haloperidol, heparin, hydrocortisone, lidocaine, methyldopate, methylPREDNISolone, metroNIDAZOLE, midazolam, nafcillin, nitroglycerin, penicillin G potassium, piperacillin, potassium chloride, ranitidine, remifentanil, sodium nitroprusside, ticarcillin, ticarcillin/clavulanate, tobramycin, vancomycin

SIDE EFFECTS

CNS: *Anxiety, restlessness, insomnia, dizziness,* seizures, headache, lightheadedness, muscle twitching, tremors

CV: *Palpitations, sinus tachycardia,* hypotension, **dysrhythmias**, fluid retention with tachycardia
ENDO: Hyperglycemia
GI: *Nausea, vomiting, anorexia,* diarrhea, bitter taste, dyspepsia, gastric distress
INTEG: Flushing, urticaria
MISC: SIADH, urinary frequency
RESP: Increased rate, tachypnea

PHARMACOKINETICS

Metabolized in liver; excreted in urine, and breast milk; crosses placenta; protein binding 40%; terminal half-life 6.5-10.5 hr
PO: Peak 1-2 hr
SOL: Peak 1 hr

INTERACTIONS

• Cardiotoxicity: β-blockers
Increase: theophylline action—cimetidine, propranolol, erythromycin, oral contraceptives, influenza vaccine, fluoroquinlones, mexiletine, corticosteroids, disulfiram, fluvoxamine, interferons
Increase: effects of anticoagulants
Decrease: theophylline level—phenytoin, phenobarbital, carBAMazepine, rifampin, smoking
Decrease: effect of lithium
Drug/Herb
• Toxicity: ephedra (ma huang), cola nut, guarana, yerba maté, tea (black, green), coffee
Decrease: theophylline levels—St. John's wort

NURSING CONSIDERATIONS

Assess:
⚠ **Theophylline blood levels (therapeutic level is 5-15 mcg/ml); toxicity may occur with small increase >20 mcg/ml**
• Monitor I&O; diuresis occurs; geriatric patients, children may be dehydrated
• Signs of toxicity: irritability, insomnia, restlessness, tremors, nausea, vomiting
• Respiratory rate, rhythm, depth; auscultate lung fields bilaterally; notify prescriber of abnormalities
• Allergic reactions: rash, urticaria; product should be discontinued
Evaluate:
• Therapeutic response: ability to breathe more easily
Teach patient/family:
• To check OTC medications, current prescription medications for ePHEDrine, which will increase stimulation; to avoid alcohol, caffeine
• To avoid hazardous activities because dizziness may occur
• That, if GI upset occurs, to take product with 8 oz water; to avoid food; to take at same time of day; that absorption may be decreased
• To notify prescriber of toxicity: nausea, vomiting, anxiety, insomnia, seizures
• To notify prescriber of change in smoking habits because dosage may have to be changed

thiamine (vit B_1) (PO-OTC; IV, IM-Rx)

Betalin S, Betaxin ♣, Biamine, Revitonus, Thiamilate
Func. class.: Vit B_1
Chem. class.: Water soluble

Do not confuse:
thiamine/Tenormin

ACTION: Needed for pyruvate metabolism, carbohydrate metabolism

USES: Vit B_1 deficiency or polyneuritis, cheilosis adjunct with thiamine beriberi, Wernicke-Korsakoff syndrome, pellagra, metabolic disorders, alcoholism

CONTRAINDICATIONS: Hypersensitivity
Precautions: Pregnancy (A)

DOSAGE AND ROUTES

RDA
• **Adult: PO** (Males) 1.2-1.5 mg; (females) 1.1 mg; (pregnancy) 1.4 mg; (breastfeeding) 1.4 mg

T

- **Child 9-13 yr: PO** 0.9 mg
- **Child 4-8 yr: PO** 0.6 mg
- **Child 1-3 yr: PO** 0.5 mg
- **Infant 7 mo-1 yr: PO** 0.3 mg
- **Neonate and infant ≤6 mo: PO** 0.2 mg

Beriberi

- **Adult: PO** 5-30 mg daily or in 3 divided doses × 1 mo; **IM/IV** 5-30 mg daily or in 3 divided doses then convert to **PO**
- **Infant/child: PO** 10-50 mg daily × 2 wk then 5-10 mg daily × 1 mo; **IV/IM** 10-25 mg/day × 2 wk then 5-10 mg daily × 1 mo

Available forms: Tabs 50, 100, 250, 500 mg; inj 100 mg/ml; enteric-coated tabs 20 mg

Administer:

IM route

- By IM inj; rotate sites if pain and inflammation occur; do not mix with alkaline sol; Z-track to minimize pain

Direct IV route

- Undiluted at 100 mg/ml over 5 min

Continuous IV INF route

- Diluted in compatible IV sol

Y-site compatibilities: Famotidine

SIDE EFFECTS

CNS: Weakness, restlessness
CV: Collapse, pulmonary edema, hypotension
EENT: Tightness of throat
GI: Hemorrhage, *nausea, diarrhea*
INTEG: Angioneurotic edema, cyanosis, sweating, warmth
SYST: Anaphylaxis

PHARMACOKINETICS

PO/INJ: Unused amounts excreted in urine (unchanged)

NURSING CONSIDERATIONS

Assess:

- **Anaphylaxis (IV only):** swelling of face, eyes, lips, throat, wheezing
- **Thiamine deficiency:** anorexia, weakness/pain, depression, confusion, blurred vision, tachycardia
- Nutritional status: yeast, beef, liver, whole or enriched grains, legumes

Perform/provide:

- Storage in tight, light-resistant container
- Application of cold to help decrease pain

Evaluate:

- Therapeutic response: absence of nausea, vomiting, anorexia, insomnia, tachycardia, paresthesias, depression, muscle weakness

Teach patient/family:

- About the necessary foods to be included in diet: yeast, beef, liver, legumes, whole grains

⚠ HIGH ALERT

thiopental (Rx)

(thye-oh-pen′tal)

Pentothal

Func. class.: General anesthetic
Chem. class.: Barbiturate

Controlled Substance Schedule III

ACTION:
Increases membrane ion conduction to chloride, decreases depolarization due to glutamate and increases in GABA

USES:
Short general anesthesia; narcoanalysis, induction anesthesia before other anesthetics, status epilepticus, increased intracranial pressure

Unlabeled uses: Reduction of intracranial pressure with head trauma

CONTRAINDICATIONS:
Hypersensitivity, status asthmaticus, porphyrias

Precautions: Pregnancy (C), severe CV disease, renal/hepatic disease, hypotension, myxedema, myasthenia gravis, asthma, increased intracranial pressure

DOSAGE AND ROUTES

Induction and anesthesia

- **Adult: IV** 25-75 mg test dose, observe for 60 min; initial dose 50-100 mg given at 20 to 40-sec interval; additional 25-50 mg as needed
- **Child 1-12 yr: IV** 5-6 mg/kg over 10-60 min, maintenance 1 mg/kg as needed
- **Infant: IV** 5-8 mg/kg over 10-60 min
- **Neonate: IV** 3-4 mg over 10-60 min

Rapid induction

- **Adult: IV** 210-280 mg or 3-5 mg/kg in 2-4 divided doses
- **Child: IV** 3-5 mg/kg over 20-30 sec then 1 mg/kg as needed

Narcoanalysis

- **Adult: IV** 100 mg/min, max 50 ml/min

Sedation or narcosis

- **Adult: RECT** 30 mg/kg

Reduction of intracranial pressure during neurosurgery

- **Adult: IV BOL** 1.5-3.5 mg/kg

Reduction of intracranial pressure in head trauma, mechanically ventilated patients only (unlableled)

- **Adult and child: IV BOL** loading dose 10-20 mg/kg then **CONT IV INF** 3-5 mg/kg/hr

Available forms: Powder for inj 2%, 2.5% (20 mg/ml, 25 mg/ml)

Administer:

- Only with crash cart, resuscitative equipment nearby

Intermittent IV INF route

- Dilute to 20-50 mg/ml; give by slow inj over 20-30 sec; max 25 mg/min

Continuous IV INF route

- Dilute to 2-4 mg/ml

Additive compatibilities: Chloramphenicol, hydrocortisone sodium succinate, oxytocin, PENTobarbital, PHENobarbital, potassium chloride, sodium bicarbonate

Solution compatibilities: D_5/0.45% NaCl, D_5W, multiple electrolyte sol, 0.45% NaCl, 0.9% NaCl, 1/6 M sodium lactate

Syringe compatibilities: Aminophylline, hyaluronidase, hydrocortisone sodium succinate, neostigmine, PENTobarbital, propofol, scopolamine, tubocurarine

Y-site compatibilities: Doxacurium, fentaNYL, heparin, milrinone, mivacurium, nitroglycerin, ranitidine, remifentanil

SIDE EFFECTS

CNS: Retrograde amnesia, prolonged somnolence

CV: Tachycardia, hypotension, **myocardial depression, dysrhythmias**

EENT: Sneezing, coughing

INTEG: Chills, *shivering,* necrosis, *pain at inj site*

MISC: **Hemolytic anemia (rare)**

MS: Muscle irritability

RESP: **Respiratory depression, bronchospasm**

PHARMACOKINETICS

IV: Onset 30-60 sec, duration 4-15 min, terminal half-life 3-8 hr, crosses placenta

INTERACTIONS

- Do not use with voriconazole

Increase: hypotension—MAOIs

Increase: action—CNS depressants, probenecid

Drug/Herb

Increase: CNS depression—kava, St. John's wort

NURSING CONSIDERATIONS

Assess:

- VS q3-5min during IV administration, after dose, q4hr postoperatively
- Extravasation; if it occurs, apply moist heat and 1% procaine to affected area
- Dysrhythmias or myocardial depression

Evaluate:

- Therapeutic response: maintenance of anesthesia

T

thioridazine (Rx)

(thye-or-rid'a-zeen)

Func. class.: Antipsychotic, neuroleptic

Chem. class.: Phenothiazine piperidine

Do not confuse:
thioridazine/thiothixene

ACTION:
Depresses cerebral cortex, hypothalamus, limbic system, which control activity, aggression; blocks neurotransmission produced by dopamine at synapse; exhibits strong α-adrenergic and anticholinergic blocking action; mechanism for antipsychotic effects is unclear

USES:
Psychotic disorders, schizophrenia, behavioral problems in children, anxiety, major depressive disorders, organic brain syndrome

Unlabeled uses: Behavioral symptoms associated with dementia in geriatric patients

CONTRAINDICATIONS:
Children <2 yr, hypersensitivity, coma, CNS depression

Black Box Warning: QT prolongation, cardiac dysrhythmias

Precautions: Pregnancy (C), breastfeeding, seizure disorders, hypertension, hepatic/pulmonary disease, renal failure, BPH, glaucoma, phenothiazine hypersensitivity, suicidal ideation, smoking, Reye's syndrome, Parkinson's disease

Black Box Warning: Cardiac disease, dementia, AV block, bundle branch block, torsades de pointes

DOSAGE AND ROUTES

Psychosis

- **Adult: PO** 25-100 mg tid, max 800 mg/day; dose gradually increased to desired response then reduced to minimum maintenance

Depression/behavioral problems/organic brain syndrome

- **Adult: PO** 25 mg tid, range from 10 mg bid-qid to 50 mg tid-qid, max 800 mg/day for short period
- **Geriatric: PO** 10-25 mg daily-bid, increase 4-7 days by 10-25 mg to desired dose, max 300 mg/day for short period
- **Child 2-12 yr: PO** 0.5-3 mg/kg/day in divided doses, max 3 mg/kg/day

Available forms: Tabs 10, 15, 25, 50, 100, 150, 200 mg

Administer:

- Antiparkinsonian agent on order from prescriber for EPS
- Avoid use with CNS depressants
- Antacids separated by 2 hr or more

SIDE EFFECTS

CNS: *EPS: pseudoparkinsonism, akathisia, dystonia, tardive dyskinesia,* seizures, *headache,* confusion, neuroleptic malignant syndrome, dizziness, drowsiness

CV: Orthostatic hypotension, cardiac arrest, ECG changes, tachycardia, QT prolongation, torsades de pointes

EENT: Blurred vision, glaucoma, dry eyes

GI: *Dry mouth, nausea, vomiting, anorexia, constipation,* diarrhea, jaundice, weight gain

GU: Urinary retention, urinary frequency, enuresis, impotence, amenorrhea, gynecomastia, ejaculation dysfunction, priapism

HEMA: Anemia, leukopenia, leukocytosis, agranulocytosis

INTEG: *Rash,* photosensitivity, dermatitis

RESP: Laryngospasm, dyspnea, respiratory depression

PHARMACOKINETICS

PO: Onset erratic; peak 2-4 hr; metabolized by liver; excreted in urine, breast milk; crosses placenta; half-life 26-36 hr; 91%-99% protein binding

INTERACTIONS

⚠ **Increase:** QT prolongation—class IA/III antidysrhythmics, some phenothi-

azines, β agonists, local anesthetics, tricyclics, haloperidol, chloroquine, droperidol, pentamidine; CYP3A4 inhibitors (amiodarone, clarithromycin, erythromycin, telithromycin, troleandomycin), arsenic trioxide, levomethadyl; CYP3A4 substrates (methadone, pimozide, QUEtiapine, quiNIDine, risperidone, ziprasidone)
• Oversedation: other CNS depressants, alcohol, barbiturate anesthetics
Increase: anticholinergic effects—anticholinergics
Increase: levels of this product—CYP2D6 inhibitors
Decrease: levels of this product—CYP2D6 inducers
Decrease: antiparkinson's agent effects
Decrease: thioridazine effect—lithium, barbiturates
Decrease: antihypertensive effect—centrally acting antihypertensives
Decrease: absorption—aluminum hydroxide, magnesium hydroxide antacids

Drug/Lab Test
Increase: LFTs, cardiac enzymes, cholesterol, blood glucose, prolactin, bilirubin, PBI, cholinesterase, ^{131}I
Decrease: hormones (blood, urine)
False positive: pregnancy test, PKU
False negative: urinary steroid, pregnancy test

NURSING CONSIDERATIONS

Assess:
• Mental status before 1st dose
• I&O ratio; palpate bladder if low urinary output occurs, urinary retention may be the cause
• Bilirubin, CBC, LFTs monthly
• Urinalysis recommended before and during prolonged therapy
• Affect, orientation, LOC, reflexes, gait, coordination, sleep pattern disturbances
• B/P standing, lying; include pulse and respirations q4hr during initial treatment; establish baseline before starting treatment; report drops of 30 mm Hg
• Dizziness, faintness, palpitations, tachycardia on rising
• **EPS** including akathisia (inability to sit still, no pattern to movements), tardive dyskinesia (bizarre movements of jaw, mouth, tongue, extremities), pseudoparkinsonism (rigidity, tremors, pill rolling, shuffling gait)
⚠ **Neuroleptic malignancy syndrome:** altered mental status, muscle rigidity, increased CPK, hyperthermia, dyspnea, fatigue
⚠ **QT prolongation:** ECG, ejection fraction; assess for chest pain, palpitations, dyspnea
• Constipation, urinary retention daily; increase bulk, water in diet

Perform/provide:
• Supervised ambulation if needed until stabilized on medication; do not involve patient in strenuous exercise program because fainting is possible; patient should not stand still for long periods
• Increased fluids to prevent constipation
• Sips of water, candy, gum for dry mouth
• Storage in tight, light-resistant container; avoid contact with skin

Evaluate:
• Therapeutic response: decrease in emotional excitement, hallucinations, delusions, paranoia; reorganization of patterns of thought, speech

Teach patient/family:
• That orthostatic hypotension occurs frequently; to rise from sitting or lying position gradually; to avoid hazardous activities until stabilized on medication
• To avoid hot tubs, hot showers, tub baths because hypotension may occur
• To avoid abrupt withdrawal of thioridazine because EPS may result; that product should be withdrawn slowly
• To avoid OTC preparations (cough, hay fever, cold) unless approved by prescriber; that serious product interactions may occur; to avoid use with alcohol because increased drowsiness may occur
• To use sunscreen to prevent burns
• About compliance with product regimen

• About the necessity for meticulous oral hygiene because oral candidiasis may occur
• To report sore throat, malaise, fever, bleeding, mouth sores; if these occur, CBC should be drawn and product discontinued; that product may cause vision impairment, should be reported to prescriber
• That, in hot weather, heat stroke may occur; to take extra precautions to stay cool
• That product may cause discoloration of urine

TREATMENT OF OVERDOSE:

Lavage if orally ingested, provide an airway; do not induce vomiting; CV monitoring, continuous ECG

thyroid USP (desiccated) (Rx)

(thye'roid)

Armour Thyroid, Bio-Throid, Nature Thyroid, NP Thyroid

Func. class.: Thyroid hormone
Chem. class.: Active thyroid hormone in natural state and ratio

ACTION: Increases metabolic rates, increases cardiac output, O_2 consumption, body temp, blood volume; growth, development at cellular level

USES: Hypothyroidism, cretinism (juvenile hypothyroidism), myxedema

CONTRAINDICATIONS: Adrenal insufficiency, MI, thyrotoxicosis, porcine protein hypersensitivity

Black Box Warning: Obesity treatment

Precautions: Pregnancy (A), breastfeeding, geriatric patients, angina pectoris, hypertension, ischemia, cardiac disease

DOSAGE AND ROUTES

Hypothyroidism
• **Adult: PO** 60 mg/day, increased by 30 mg/mo until desired response; maintenance dose 60-120 mg/day
• **Geriatric: PO** 7.5-15 mg/day, increase dose q6-8wk until desired response

Cretinism/juvenile hypothyroidism
• **Child: PO** 15 mg/day, then 30 mg/day after 2 wk, then 60 mg/day after another 2 wk; maintenance dose 60-180 mg/day

Myxedema
• **Adult: PO** 15 mg/day, double dose q2wk, maintenance 60-180 mg/day

Available forms: Tabs 16, 32, 60, 65, 98, 130, 195, 260, 325 mg; enteric-coated tabs 32, 65, 130 mg; sugarcoated tabs 32, 65, 130, 195 mg; caps 65, 130, 195, 325 mg

Administer:
• In AM if possible as single dose to decrease sleeplessness; separate iron, calcium products by 4 hr
• At same time each day to maintain product level
• Only for hormone imbalances; not to be used for obesity, male infertility, menstrual disorders, lethargy
• Lowest dose that relieves symptoms

SIDE EFFECTS

CNS: *Insomnia, tremors,* headache, thyroid storm
CV: *Tachycardia, palpitations, angina, dysrhythmias,* hypertension, cardiac arrest
GI: Nausea, diarrhea, increased or decreased appetite, cramps
MISC: Menstrual irregularities, weight loss, sweating, heat intolerance, fever

PHARMACOKINETICS

PO: Peak 12-48 hr, half-life 6-7 days

INTERACTIONS

Increase: effects of anticoagulants, sympathomimetics, tricyclics, catecholamines

Decrease: thyroid absorption—bile acid sequestrants, aluminum, magnesium, calcium
Decrease: thyroid effects—estrogens
Drug/Herb
Decrease: thyroid effect—soy
Drug/Lab Test
Increase: CPK, LDH, AST, PBI, blood glucose
Decrease: thyroid function tests

NURSING CONSIDERATIONS

Assess:

Black Box Warning: Obesity treatment: use can lead to serious or life-threatening toxicity

- B/P, pulse before each dose
- I&O ratio
- Weight daily in same clothing, using same scale, at same time of day
- Height, growth rate of child
- T_3, T_4, which are decreased; radioimmunoassay of TSH, which is increased; radio uptake, which is decreased if dosage is too low
- PT may require decreased anticoagulant; check for bleeding, bruising
- **Hyperthyroidism:** increased nervousness, excitability, irritability; may indicate too high of a dose of medication, usually after 1-3 wk of treatment
- **Hypothyroidism:** lethargy, cold intolerance, weight gain, constipation, muscle cramps; may indicate too low of a dose
- Cardiac status: angina, palpitation, chest pain, change in VS

Perform/provide:

- Removal of medication 4 wk before RAIU test

Evaluate:

- Therapeutic response: absence of depression; increased weight loss, diuresis, pulse, appetite; absence of constipation, peripheral edema, cold intolerance; pale, cool, dry skin; brittle nails, alopecia, coarse hair, menorrhagia, night blindness, paresthesias, syncope, stupor, coma, rosy cheeks

Teach patient/family:

- That hair loss will occur in child, is temporary
- To report excitability, irritability, anxiety; indicates overdose
- Not to switch brands unless directed by prescriber
- That strong odor is normal
- That hypothyroid child will show almost immediate behavior/personality change
- That treatment product is not to be taken to reduce weight
- To avoid OTC preparations with iodine; to read labels
- To separate iron, calcium products by 4 hr
- To avoid iodine food, iodized salt, soybeans, tofu, turnips, some seafood, some bread

tiagabine (Rx)

(tie-ah-ga′been)

Gabitril

Func. class.: Anticonvulsant

ACTION: Inhibits reuptake and metabolism of GABA, may increase seizure threshold; structurally similar to GABA; tiagabine binding sites in neocortex, hippocampus

USES: Adjunct treatment of partial seizures in adults and children ≥12 yr

CONTRAINDICATIONS: Hypersensitivity

Precautions: Pregnancy (C), breastfeeding, children <12 yr, geriatric patients, renal/hepatic disease, suicidal thoughts/behaviors, status epilepticus, mania, bipolar disorder, abrupt discontinuation, depression

DOSAGE AND ROUTES

When not given with a CYP3A4 enzyme, effect of tiagabine is doubled; lower doses are indicated

• **Adult (those receiving an enzyme-inducing antiepileptic product): PO** 4 mg/day in divided doses, may increase by 4-8 mg/wk until desired response, max 56 mg/day
• **Child 12-18 yr: PO** 4 mg/day, may increase by 4 mg at beginning of wk 2; may increase by 4-8 mg/wk until desired response; max 32 mg/day

Available forms: Tabs 2, 4, 12, 16 mg

Administer:
• With food

SIDE EFFECTS

CNS: *Dizziness, anxiety,* somnolence, ataxia, confusion, *asthenia,* unsteady gait, depression, suicidal ideation
CV: Vasodilation
GI: Nausea, vomiting, diarrhea, increased appetite
INTEG: Pruritus, rash, Stevens-Johnson syndrome
RESP: Pharyngitis, coughing

PHARMACOKINETICS

Absorption >95%; peak 45 min; protein binding 96%; metabolized in the liver via CYP3A4; half-life 7-9 hr without enzyme inducers, 2-5 hr with enzyme inducers

INTERACTIONS

• Lower doses may be needed when used with valproate
Increase: CNS depression—CNS depressants
Decrease: tiagabine effect—sevelamer
Decrease: effect—carBAMazepine, PHENobarbital, phenytoin, primidone

Drug/Food
Decrease: rate of absorption—high-fat meal

NURSING CONSIDERATIONS

Assess:
• Renal studies: urinalysis, BUN, urine creatinine q3mo
• Hepatic studies: ALT, AST, bilirubin
• **Seizures:** location, duration, presence of aura
⚠ Mental status: mood, sensorium, affect, behavioral changes, suicidal thoughts/behaviors; if mental status changes, notify prescriber

Perform/provide:
• Storage at room temp, away from heat and light
• Assistance with ambulation during early part of treatment; dizziness occurs
• Seizure precautions: padded side rails; move objects that may harm patient

Evaluate:
• Therapeutic response: decreased seizure activity; document on patient's chart

Teach patient/family:
• To carry emergency ID stating patient's name, products taken, condition, prescriber's name and phone number
• To avoid driving, other activities that require alertness
• Not to discontinue medication quickly after long-term use
• To take with food

TREATMENT OF OVERDOSE:

Lavage, VS

ticagrelor

See Appendix A—Selected new drugs

ticarcillin/clavulanate (Rx)

Timentin

Func. class.: Broad-spectrum antiinfective
Chem. class.: Extended-spectrum penicillin

ACTION:

Interferes with cell-wall replication of susceptible organisms; osmotically unstable cell wall swells, bursts from osmotic pressure; clavulanate inhibits β-lactamase and protects against enzymatic degradation of ticarcillin

USES:
Respiratory, soft-tissue, and urinary tract infections; bacterial septicemia; effective for gram-positive cocci *(Staphylococcus aureus, Streptococcus faecalis, Streptococcus pneumoniae)*, gram-negative cocci *(Neisseria gonorrhoeae)*, gram-positive bacilli *(Clostridium perfringens, Clostridium tetani)*, gram-negative bacilli *(Bacteroides, Fusobacterium nucleatum, Escherichia coli, Proteus mirabilis, Salmonella, Morganella morganii, Proteus rettgeri, Enterobacter, Pseudomonas aeruginosa, Serratia)*; and *Peptococcus, Peptostreptococcus,* and *Eubacterium*

CONTRAINDICATIONS:
Neonates, hypersensitivity to penicillins

Precautions: Pregnancy (B), hypersensitivity to cephalosporins, renal disease

DOSAGE AND ROUTES

Systemic/urinary tract infections, moderate/severe infections

- **Adult ≥60 kg: IV INF** 3.1 g q4-6hr
- **Adult <60 kg: IV INF** 200-300 mg/kg/day q4-6hr
- **Child >60 kg: IV INF** 3.1 g q4-6hr
- **Child <60 kg: IV INF** 300 mg/kg/day q4hr

Mild to moderate infections

- **Child ≥60 kg: IV INF** 3.1 g q6hr
- **Child <60 kg: IV INF** 200 mg/kg/day q6hr

Renal dose

- **Adult: IV INF** loading dose 3.1 g; CCr 60 ml/min, 3.1 g q4hr; CCr 30-60 ml/min, 2 g q4hr; CCr 10-30 ml/min, 2 g q8hr; CCr <10 ml/min, 2 g q12hr; CCr <10 ml/min with hepatic dysfunction, 2 g q24hr

Available forms: Inj 3 g ticarcillin, 0.1 g clavulanate; IV inf 3 g ticarcillin, 0.1 g clavulanate; powder for inj 3 g ticarcillin, 0.1 g clavulanate

Administer:

- Product after C&S

Intermittent IV INF route

- After diluting ≤3.1 g/13 ml of sterile water or NaCl (200 mg/ml), shake; may further dilute in ≥50-100 ml NS, D_5W, or LR sol and run over 1/2 hr

Y-site compatibilities: Allopurinol, amifostine, amikacin, anidulafungin, atropine, aztreonam, bivalirudin, bumetanide, ceFAZolin, cefepime, cefotaxime, cefoxitin, ceftazidime, ceftizoxime, cefTRIAXone, cefuroxime, chloramphenicol, cimetidine, clindamycin, cyclophosphamide, cycloSPORINE, dexamethasone, dexmedetomidine, digoxin, diltiazem, diphenhydrAMINE, docetaxel, DOPamine, DOXOrubicin liposome, doxycycline, enalaprilat, EPINEPHrine, esmolol, etoposide phosphate, famotidine, fenoldopam, filgrastim, fluconazole, furosemide, gemcitabine, gentamicin, granisetron, heparin, hydrocortisone, HYDROmorphone, imipenem/cilastatin, insulin, isoproterenol, labetalol, levofloxacin, lidocaine, linezolid, LORazepam, melphalan, meperidine, methylPREDNISolone, metoclopramide, metoprolol, metroNIDAZOLE, milrinone, morphine, nitroglycerin, nitroprusside, norepinephrine, ondansetron, palonosetron, pantoprazole, pemetrexed, penicillin G potassium, perphenazine, phenylephrine, procainamide, propofol, propranolol, ranitidine, remifentanil, sargramostim, sodium bicarbonate, tacrolimus, teniposide, theophylline, thiotepa, tirofiban, tobramycin, vasopressin, verapamil, vinorelbine, voriconazole

SIDE EFFECTS

CNS: Lethargy, hallucinations, anxiety, depression, twitching, **coma, seizures,** confusion, drowsiness

GI: *Nausea, vomiting, diarrhea;* increased AST, ALT; abdominal pain, glossitis, colitis, **pseudomembranous colitis, hepatotoxicity**

GU: Oliguria, proteinuria, hematuria, *vaginitis, moniliasis,* **glomerulonephritis**

HEMA: Anemia, increased bleeding time, **bone marrow depression, granulocytopenia**

T

INTEG: Rash, urticaria, toxic epidermal necrolysis
META: Hyperkalemia, hypokalemia, alkalosis, hypernatremia
SYST: Anaphylaxis, Stevens-Johnson syndrome

PHARMACOKINETICS

IV: Peak 30-45 min, duration 4 hr, half-life 64-68 min, excreted in urine

INTERACTIONS

⚠ **Increase:** bleeding—anticoagulants
Increase: methotrexate level—methotrexate
Increase: ticarcillin concentrations—probenecid, sulfipyrazone
Decrease: antimicrobial effect of ticarcillin—tetracyclines, aminoglycosides IV, chloramphenicol, macrolides, sulfonamides
Decrease: effect—oral contraceptives, erythromycin
Drug/Lab Test
False positive: urine glucose, urine protein, Coombs' test

NURSING CONSIDERATIONS

Assess:

- I&O ratio; report hematuria, oliguria because penicillin in high doses is nephrotoxic

⚠ **Pseudomembranous colitis:** diarrhea, abdominal pain, fever, fatigue, anorexia; possible anemia, elevated WBC count, low serum albumin; stop product; usually either vancomycin or IV metroNIDAZOLE is given

⚠ **Serious skin reactions:** Stevens-Johnson syndrome, toxic epidermal necrolysis; anaphylaxis: wheezing, rash, laryngeal edema; have emergency equipment nearby

- Hepatic studies: AST, ALT
- Blood studies: WBC, RBC, Hct, Hgb, bleeding time
- Renal studies: urinalysis, protein, blood, BUN, creatinine
- C&S before product therapy; product may be given as soon as culture taken
- Bowel pattern before, during treatment
- Skin eruptions after administration of penicillin to 1 wk after discontinuing product

Perform/provide:

- EPINEPHrine, suction, tracheostomy set, endotracheal intubation equipment
- Scratch test to assess allergy on order from prescriber; usually done when penicillin is only product of choice
- Storage of reconstituted sol 12-24 hr at room temp, or 3-7 days refrigerated

Evaluate:

- Therapeutic response: absence of fever, purulent drainage, redness, inflammation

Teach patient/family:

- To report persistent diarrhea with blood, pus, mucous, or fever
- That culture may be taken after completed course of medication
- To report sore throat, fever, fatigue (may indicate superinfection); CNS effects (anxiety, depression, hallucinations, seizures)
- To wear or carry emergency ID if allergic to penicillins
- To use alternative birth control method instead of hormonal

TREATMENT OF OVERDOSE:

Withdraw product, maintain airway, administer EPINEPHrine, O_2, IV corticosteroids for anaphylaxis

ticlopidine (Rx)

(tye-cloe′pi-deen)
Func. class.: Platelet aggregation inhibitor
Chem. class.: Thienopyridine compound

ACTION: Irreversible inhibition of platelet aggregation through antagonism of ADP

USES: Reducing the risk for stroke in high-risk patients

Unlabeled uses: Intermittent claudication, chronic arterial occlusion, subarachnoid hemorrhage, uremic patients with AV shunts/fistulas, open heart surgery, coronary artery bypass grafts, primary glomerulonephritis, sickle cell disease, diabetic retinopathy

CONTRAINDICATIONS:

Hypersensitivity, severe hepatic disease, active bleeding, coagulopathy

Black Box Warning: Agranulocytosis, neutropenia, thrombocytopenia, thrombotic thrombocytopenic purpura (TTP)

Precautions: Pregnancy (B), breastfeeding, children, geriatric patients, past hepatic disease, renal disease, increased bleeding risk, peptic ulcer disease, surgery

Black Box Warning: Anemia, hematologic disease

DOSAGE AND ROUTES

- **Adult: PO** 250 mg bid with food

Available forms: Tabs 250 mg

Administer:

- With food to decrease gastric symptoms
- Discontinue when absolute neutrophil count falls during treatment to <1200/mm^3 or platelets <80,000/mm^3

SIDE EFFECTS

CNS: Dizziness

GI: Nausea, vomiting, *diarrhea,* GI discomfort, **cholestatic jaundice, hepatitis,** increased cholesterol, LDL, VLDL, triglycerides

HEMA: Bleeding (epistaxis, hematuria, conjunctival hemorrhage, GI bleeding), agranulocytosis, neutropenia, thrombocytopenia, thrombotic thombocytopenic purpura

INTEG: *Rash,* pruritus

PHARMACOKINETICS

Peak 1-3 hr; metabolized by liver; excreted in urine, feces; half-life increases with repeated dosing, initially 12-36 hr; antiplatelet effect 2-5 days; 98% protein binding

INTERACTIONS

Increase: levels of CYP2C19, CYP2DC substrates, phenytoin, fosphenytoin, ambrisentan, theophylline

Increase: bleeding tendencies—anticoagulants, salicylates, thrombolytics, NSAIDs, abciximab, eptifibatide, tirofiban, thrombin inhibitors, SSRIs, aspirin

Increase: effects of ticlopidine—cimetidine

Decrease: plasma levels of ticlopidine—antacids

Decrease: plasma levels of digoxin, cycloSPORINE

Drug/Herb

Increase: bleeding risk—ginger, ginkgo, garlic, feverfew, horse chestnut, green tea

NURSING CONSIDERATIONS

Assess:

- Hepatic studies: AST, ALT, bilirubin, creatinine with long-term therapy
- ⚠ **Blood studies: CBC; CBC q2wk × 3 mo, Hct, Hgb, PT with long-term therapy**
- ⚠ **Bleeding time at baseline and throughout treatment; levels may be 2-5× normal limit**

Evaluate:

- Therapeutic response: absence of stroke

Teach patient/family:

- That blood work will be necessary during treatment
- To report any unusual bleeding to prescriber
- To report side effects such as diarrhea, skin rashes, subcut bleeding, signs of cholestasis (jaundiced skin and sclera, dark urine, light-colored stools)
- That product should be discontinued 10-14 days before surgery; not to double a missed dose
- That there are many product and herbal interactions

tigecycline (Rx)

(tye-ge-sye'kleen)

Tygacil

Func. class.: Broad-spectrum antiinfective

Chem. class.: Glycylcyclines

ACTION: Inhibits protein synthesis and phosphorylation in microorganisms; bacteriostatic structurally similar to the tetracyclines

USES: Complicated skin/skin-structure infections *(Escherichia coli, Enterococcus faecalis* [vancomycin-susceptible only] *Staphylococcus aureus, Streptococcus agalactiae, S. anginosus* group, *S. pyogenes, Bacteroides fragilis;* complicated intraabdominal infections *[Citrobacter freundii] Enterobacter cloacae, E. coli, Klebsiella oxytoca, K. pneumoniae, E. faecalis* [vancomycin-susceptible only], *S. aureus* [methicillin-susceptible only], *S. anginosus* group, *B. fragilis, Bacteroides thetaiotaomicron, B. uniformis, B. vulgatus, Clostridium perfringens, Peptostreptococcus micros);* community-acquired pneumonia

CONTRAINDICATIONS: Pregnancy (D), breastfeeding, children <18 yr, hypersensitivity to tigecycline

Precautions: Renal/hepatic disease, hypersensitivity to tetracyclines, ventilator-associated/hospital-acquired pneumonias

DOSAGE AND ROUTES

- **Adult: IV** 100 mg then 50 mg q12hr, **IV INF** given over 30-60 min q12hr; given for 5-14 days, depending on infection

Hepatic dose

- **Adult: IV** (Child-Pugh C) 100 mg then 25 mg q12hr

Available forms: Powder for inj, lyophilized 50 mg

Administer:

- After C&S obtained

Intermittent IV INF route

- Reconstitute each vial with 5.3 ml of 0.9% NaCl or D_5 (10 mg/ml); swirl to dissolve; immediately withdraw 5 ml of reconstituted sol and add to 100-ml IV bag for inf (1 mg/ml); may be yellow or orange; if not, sol should be discarded; do not give if particulate matter is present

Y-site compatibilities: Acyclovir, alfentanil, allopurinol, amifostine, amikacin, aminocaproic acid, aminophylline, amphotericin B liposome, ampicillin, ampicillin/sulbactam, argatroban, azithromycin, aztreonam, bivalirudin, bumetanide, buprenorphine, butorphanol, calcium chloride/gluconate, CARBOplatin, carmustine, caspofungin, ceFAZolin, cefepime, cefotaxime, cefotetan, cefoxitin, ceftazidime, ceftizoxime, cefTRIAXone, cefuroxime, cimetidine, ciprofloxacin, cisatracurium, CISplatin, clindamycin, cyclophosphamide, cycloSPORINE, cytarabine, dacarbazine, DACTINomycin, DAPTOmycin, DAUNOrubicin hydrochloride, dexamethasone, dexmedetomidine, dexrazoxane, digoxin, diltiazem, diphenhydrAMINE, DOBUTamine, docetaxel, dolasetron, DOPamine, doripenem, DOXOrubicin hydrochloride, DOXOrubicin liposome, droperidol, enalaprilat, EPINEPHrine, eptifibatide, ertapenem, erythromycin, esmolol, etoposide, etoposide phosphate, famotidine, fenoldopam, fentaNYL, fluconazole, fludarabine, fluorouracil, foscarnet, fosphenytoin, furosemide, ganciclovir, gemcitabine, gentamicin, glycopyrrolate, granisetron, haloperidol, heparin, hydrocortisone, HYDROmorphone, ifosfamide, imipenem/cilastatin, insulin, irinotecan, isoproterenol, ketorolac, labetalol, lansoprazole, lepirudin, leucovorin, levofloxacin, lidocaine, linezolid, LORazepam, magnesium sulfate, mannitol, mechlorethamine, melphalan, meperidine, meropenem, mesna, methohexital, methotrexate, methyldopa, metoclopramide, metoprolol, metroNIDAZOLE, midazolam, milrinone, mitomycin, mitoxantrone, morphine, moxifloxacin, mycophenolate, nafcillin, nalbuphine, naloxone, nesiritide, nitroglycerin, nitroprusside, norepinephrine, octreotide, ondansetron, oxaliplatin, oxytocin, paclitaxel, palonosetron, pamidronate, pancuronium, pantoprazole, pemetrexed, pemtamidine, pentazocin, PENTobarbital, PHENobarbital, phenylephrine, piperacillin/tazobactam, potassium acetate/chloride/phosphate, procainamide, prochlorperazine, promethazine, propofol, propranolol, ranitidine, remifentanil, rocuronium, sodium acetate/bicarbonate/phosphate, streptozocin, succinylcholine, SUFentanil, tacrolimus, teniposide, theophylline, thiopental, thiotepa, ticarcillin/clavulanate, tirofiban, tobramycin, topotecan, trimethoprim/sulfamethoxazole, vancomycin, vasopressin, vecuronium, vinBLAStine, vinCRIStine, vinorelbine, zidovudine, zoledronic acid

SIDE EFFECTS

CNS: Headache, dizziness, insomnia
CV: Hypo/hypertension, phlebitis
EENT: Tooth discoloration
GI: *Nausea, vomiting, diarrhea,* anorexia, constipation, dyspepsia, abdominal pain, **hepatotoxicity, hepatic failure, pseudomembranous colitis**
HEMA: **Anemia, leukocytosis, thrombocytopenia**
INTEG: *Rash,* pruritus, sweating, photosensitivity
META: Increased ALT, AST, BUN, lactic acid, alk phos, amylase; hyperglycemia, hypokalemia, hypoproteinemia, bilirubinemia
MISC: Back pain, fever, abnormal healing, abdominal pain, abscess, asthenia, infection, pain, peripheral edema, local reactions
RESP: Cough, dyspnea
SYST: **Anaphylaxis**

PHARMACOKINETICS

Not extensively metabolized, 22% of unchanged product excreted in urine, terminal half-life 42 hr, primarily biliary excreted, protein binding 71%-89%

INTERACTIONS

Increase: effect of warfarin
Decrease: effect of oral contraceptives

NURSING CONSIDERATIONS

Assess:

⚠ **Pseudomembranous colitis:** diarrhea, abdominal pain, fever, fatigue, anorexia; possible anemia, elevated WBC level, low serum albumin; stop product; usually either vancomycin or IV metroNIDAZOLE is given

- Signs of anemia: Hct, Hgb, fatigue
- Blood studies: PT, CBC, AST, ALT, BUN creatinine

⚠ **Allergic reactions:** rash, itching, pruritus, angioedema

- Nausea, vomiting, diarrhea; administer antiemetic, antacids as ordered
- **Overgrowth of infection:** fever, malaise, redness, pain, swelling, drainage, perineal itching, diarrhea, changes in cough or sputum

Perform/provide:

- Storage in tight, light-resistant container at room temp

Evaluate:

- Therapeutic response: decreased temp, absence of lesions, negative C&S

Teach patient/family:

- To avoid sun exposure; sunscreen does not seem to decrease photosensitivity

⚠ To avoid pregnancy while taking this product; fetal harm may occur

- To report infection, increase in temp

T

timolol (Rx)

(tye'moe-lole)

Apo-Timol ✱, Novo-Timol ✱

Func. class.: Antihypertensive

Chem. class.: Nonselective β-blocker

ACTION: Competitively blocks stimulation of β-adrenergic receptor within vascular smooth muscle (decreases rate of SA node discharge, increases recovery time); slows conduction of AV node and decreases heart rate, which decreases O_2 consumption in myocardium; also decreases renin-aldosterone-angiotensin system; at high doses, inhibits β_2-receptors in bronchial system

USES: Mild to moderate hypertension, migraine prophylaxis, to decrease mortality after MI

Unlabeled uses: Tremors, angina pectoris

CONTRAINDICATIONS: Hypersensitivity to β-blockers, cardiogenic shock, heart block (2nd/3rd degree), sinus bradycardia, CHF, cardiac failure, severe COPD, asthma

Precautions: Pregnancy (C), breastfeeding, major surgery, diabetes mellitus, COPD, well-compensated heart failure, CAD, nonallergic bronchospasm, peripheral vascular disease, thyroid/renal/hepatic disease, diabetes mellitus

Black Box Warning: Abrupt discontinuation

DOSAGE AND ROUTES

Hypertension

- **Adult: PO** 10 mg bid or 20 mg/day, may increase by 10 mg q7days, max 60 mg/day

Myocardial infarction

- **Adult: PO** 10 mg bid beginning 1-4 wk after MI

Migraine headache prevention

- **Adult: PO** 10 mg bid or 20 mg/day; may increase to 30 mg/day, 20 mg in AM, 10 mg in PM; discontinue if not effective after 8 wk

Available forms: Tabs 5, 10, 20 mg

Administer:

- PO before or immediately after meals, at bedtime; tab may be crushed or swallowed whole
- Reduced dosage in renal dysfunction

SIDE EFFECTS

CNS: *Insomnia, dizziness,* hallucinations, anxiety, fatigue, depression, headache

CV: Hypotension, bradycardia, CHF, edema, chest pain, claudication, angina, AV block, ventricular dysrhythmias

EENT: *Visual changes;* sore throat; *double vision;* dry, burning eyes

GI: *Nausea,* vomiting, ischemic colitis, diarrhea, *abdominal pain,* mesenteric arterial thrombosis, flatulence, constipation

GU: Impotence, urinary frequency

HEMA: Agranulocytosis, thrombocytopenia, purpura

INTEG: Rash, alopecia, pruritus, fever

META: Hypoglycemia

MUSC: *Joint pain, muscle pain*

RESP: Bronchospasm, *dyspnea,* cough, crackles, nasal stuffiness

PHARMACOKINETICS

Peak 1-2 hr; half-life 4 hr; metabolized by liver; excreted in urine, breast milk; protein binding $<$10%

INTERACTIONS

Increase: hypotension, bradycardia—hydrALAZINE, methyldopa, prazosin, anticholinergics, alcohol, reserpine, nitrates

Increase: effects of β-blockers, calcium channel blockers

Decrease: antihypertensive effects—NSAIDs, sympathomimetics, thyroid, salicylates

Decrease: hypoglycemic effects—insulin, sulfonylureas
Decrease: bronchodilation—theophyllines
Drug/Lab Test
Increase: renal, hepatic studies, uric acid
Interference: glucose, insulin tolerance test

NURSING CONSIDERATIONS

Assess:

Black Box Warning: Abrupt discontinuation: may result in myocardial ischemia, MI, severe hypotension, ventricular dysrhythmias in those with preexisting cardiovascular disease

- **Headaches:** location, severity, duration, frequency at baseline and throughout treatment
- I&O, weight daily
- B/P during initial treatment, periodically thereafter, pulse q4hr; note rate, rhythm, quality
- Apical/radial pulse before administration; notify prescriber of any significant changes
- Baselines of renal, hepatic studies before therapy begins
- Edema in feet, legs daily
- Skin turgor, dryness of mucous membranes for hydration status

Perform/provide:

- Dry storage at room temp; do not freeze

Evaluate:

- Therapeutic response: decreased B/P after 1-2 wk

Teach patient/family:

- To take before or immediately after meals

Black Box Warning: Not to discontinue product abruptly; to taper over 2 wk; may cause precipitate angina

- Not to use OTC products containing α-adrenergic stimulants (nasal decongestants, cold preparations) unless directed by prescriber
- To report bradycardia, dizziness, confusion, depression, fever, sore throat, SOB to prescriber
- To take pulse at home; advise when to notify prescriber
- To avoid alcohol, smoking, sodium intake
- To comply with weight control, dietary adjustments, modified exercise program
- To carry emergency ID to identify product, allergies
- To avoid hazardous activities if dizziness is present
- To report symptoms of CHF: difficulty breathing, especially on exertion or when lying down; night cough; swelling of extremities
- To take medication at bedtime; to wear support hose to minimize effect of orthostatic hypotension

TREATMENT OF OVERDOSE:

Lavage, IV atropine for bradycardia, IV theophylline for bronchospasm, digoxin, O_2, diuretic for cardiac failure, hemodialysis; administer vasopressor (norepinephrine)

timolol ophthalmic

See Appendix B

tinidazole (Rx)

(tye-ni′da-zole)

Tindamax

Func. class.: Antiprotozoal

Chem. class.: Nitroimidazole derivative

T

ACTION: Interferes with DNA/RNA synthesis in protozoa

USES: Amebiasis, giardiasis, trichomoniasis

Unlabeled uses: *Bacteroides* sp., *Clostridium* sp., *Eubacterium* sp., *Fusobacterium* sp., *Peptococcus* sp., *Peptostreptococcus* sp., gingivitis, urethritis, *Veillonella* sp.

CONTRAINDICATIONS:

Pregnancy, breastfeeding; hypersensitivity to this product or nitroimidazole derivative

Precautions: Children, geriatric patients, hepatic disease, CNS depression, blood dyscrasias, candidiasis, seizures, viral infection, alcoholism, pregnancy (C)

Black Box Warning: Secondary malignancy

DOSAGE AND ROUTES

Amebic involvement of the liver

• **Adult: PO** 2 g/day × 3-5 days

• **Child ≥3 yr: PO** 50 mg/kg/day × 3-5 days, max 2 g

Giardiasis

• **Adult: PO** 2 g as a single dose

• **Child ≥3 yr: PO** 50 mg/kg as a single dose, max 2 g

Trichomoniasis

• **Adult: PO** 2 g as a single dose

Bacterial vaginosis

• **Adult (nonpregnant woman): PO** 2 g/day × 2 days with food or 1 g/day × 5 days with food

Prevention of postoperative infections (unlabeled)

• **Adult: PO** 2 g (single dose) 12 hr prior to surgery

Anaerobic infections (unlabeled)

• **Adult: PO** 2 g on day 1 then 1 g daily or 500 mg bid for 5-6 days

Available forms: Tabs 250, 500 mg

Administer:

• Tabs can be crushed and mixed with artificial cherry syrup

• With food to increase plasma concentrations, minimize epigastric distress and other GI effects

SIDE EFFECTS

CNS: *Dizziness, headache,* seizures, *peripheral neuropathy,* malaise, fatigue

GI: *Nausea, vomiting,* anorexia, increased AST/ALT, constipation, abdominal pain, indigestion, altered taste

HEMA: Leukopenia, neutropenia

INTEG: Pruritus, urticaria, *rash,* oral candidiasis

SYST: Angioedema, cramping

PHARMACOKINETICS

Peak 1½ hr; metabolized extensively in liver; excreted unchanged (20%-25%) in urine, (12%) feces; half-life 12-14 hr; crosses blood-brain barrier

INTERACTIONS

• Do not use within 2 wk of disulfiram

Increase: tinidazole action—CYP3A4 inhibitors (cimetidine, ketoconazole): increased action of tinidazole

Increase: action of anticoagulants, cycloSPORINE, tacrolimus, fluorouracil, hydantoins, lithium

Decrease: tinidazole action—CYP3A4 inducers (PHENobarbital, rifampin, phenytoin); cholestyramine, oxytetracycline: decreased action of tinidazole

Drug/Herb

Increase or decrease: tinidazole level—St. John's wort

Drug/Lab Test

Increase: triglycerides, LDH, AST/ALT, glucose

Decrease: WBCs

NURSING CONSIDERATIONS

Assess:

• **Amebic liver abscess:** CBC, ESR, amebic gel diffusion test, ultrasound; also total and differential leukocyte count

Black Box Warning: Secondary malignancy: avoid unnecessary use

• Signs of infection, anemia

• Bowel pattern before, during treatment

Evaluate:

• Therapeutic response: decrease in infection as evidenced by negative culture

Teach patient/family:

• To take with food to increase plasma concentrations, minimize epigastric distress and other GI effects; not to use alcoholic beverages during or for 3 days after treatment

• **Trichomoniasis:** both partners should be treated at the same time

⚠ HIGH ALERT

tinzaparin (Rx)

(tin-zay-par'in)

Innohep

Func. class.: Anticoagulant

Chem. class.: Unfractionated porcine heparin

ACTION: Increases the inhibitory effect of antithrombin factor Xa, thrombin

USES: Treatment of DVT, PE after abdominal, knee, or hip surgery or after knee or hip replacement

Unlabeled uses: Antiphospholipid antibody syndrome, arterial thromboembolism prophylaxis, cerebral thromboembolism, DVT prophylaxis, PE prophylaxis, thrombosis prophylaxis

CONTRAINDICATIONS: Hypersensitivity to this product, heparin, pork or benzyl alcohol, sulfites; hemophilia, leukemia with bleeding, peptic ulcer disease, thrombocytopenic purpura, heparin-induced thrombocytopenia

Precautions: Pregnancy (B), breastfeeding, children, geriatric patients, alcoholism, severe renal/hepatic disease, blood dyscrasias; severe, uncontrolled hypertension; subacute bacterial endocarditis, acute nephritis; geriatric patients >70 yr (renal disease with DVT/PE)

Black Box Warning: Spinal/epidural anesthesia, lumbar puncture

DOSAGE AND ROUTES

Treatment of DVT

- **Adult: SUBCUT** 175 anti-Xa international units/kg/day ≥6 days and until adequate anticoagulation with warfarin (therapeutic INR ≥2 for 2 consecutive days)

Prophylaxis of DVT in orthopedic procedures (unlabeled)

- **Adult:** 75 anti-Xa units/kg/day started 12-24 hr after surgery

Prophylaxis of DVT/thromboembolism/PE (unlabeled)

- **Adult:** 3500 anti-Xa units (50 anti-Xa units/kg) daily beginning 1-2 hr prior to surgery and continued for 5-10 days

Available forms: Inj 20,000 international units/1 ml

Administer:

- Only after screening patient for bleeding disorders
- For 6 days, until warfarin has been given to result in adequate coagulation
- SUBCUT only; do not give IM
- To recumbent patient; give SUBCUT; rotate inj sites (left/right anterolateral, left/right posterolateral abdominal wall)
- Insert whole length of needle into skin fold held with thumb and forefinger

⚠ Only this product when ordered; not interchangeable with heparin (unfractionated) or LMWHs

- At same time each day to maintain steady blood levels
- Do not massage area or aspirate when giving SUBCUT inj
- Do not mix with other products or inf fluids
- Alternate inj sites
- For excessive bruising at inj site, may use ice before subcut inj

SIDE EFFECTS

CNS: Fever, confusion, dizziness, insomnia

CV: Angina, dysrhythmias, peripheral edema, tachycardia, hypo/hypertension

GI: Nausea, constipation, flatulence, dyspepsia, hepatitis

GU: UTI, hematuria, urinary retention, dysuria

HEMA: Hemorrhage, anemia, thrombocytopenia, bleeding

T

INTEG: Ecchymosis, inj site reaction
MISC: Headache, chest/back pain, hypersensitivity
SYST: Stevens-Johnson syndrome

PHARMACOKINETICS

Onset 2-3 hr, max antithrombin activity (3-5 hr), elimination half-life 4.5 hr

INTERACTIONS

Increase: action of tinzaparin—oral anticoagulants, salicylates, thrombolytics, NSAIDs, platelet inhibitors, ticlopidine, clopidogrel

NURSING CONSIDERATIONS

Assess:

Black Box Warning: Spinal/epidermal anesthesia, lumbar puncture: monitor neurological impairment; if impairment occurs, urgent treatment needed

- Blood studies (Hct, platelets, occult blood in stools), anti-Xa; thrombocytopenia may occur
- **Bleeding:** gums, petechiae, ecchymosis, black tarry stools, hematuria, decreased Hct, Hgb
- Hypersensitivity (fever, urticaria, chills); report to prescriber
- Inj site reactions; do not use IM inj

Perform/provide:

- Storage at 77° F (25° C); do not freeze

Evaluate:

- Therapeutic response: resolution of DVT

Teach patient/family:

- To report any signs of bleeding: gums, under skin, urine, stools

TREATMENT OF OVERDOSE:

Protamine 1 mg/100 anti-Xa international units of tinzaparin

tioconazole vaginal antifungal

See Appendix B

tiotropium (Rx)

(ty-oh′tro-pee-um)

Spiriva HandiHaler

Func. class.: Anticholinergic, bronchodilator

Chem. class.: Synthetic quaternary ammonium compound

ACTION:

Inhibits interaction of acetylcholine at receptor sites on the bronchial smooth muscle, thereby resulting in decreased cGMP and bronchodilation

USES:

COPD; for the long-term treatment and once-daily maintenance of bronchospasm associated with COPD, including chronic bronchitis and emphysema

CONTRAINDICATIONS:

Hypersensitivity to this product, atropine or its derivatives

Precautions: Pregnancy (C), breastfeeding, children, geriatric patients, closed-angle glaucoma, prostatic hypertrophy, bladder neck obstruction, renal disease

DOSAGE AND ROUTES

- **Adult: INH** content of 1 cap/day using HandiHaler inhalation device

Available forms: Powder for INH 18 mcg in blister packs containing 6 caps with inhaler; 30 caps with inhaler

Administer:

Inhalation route

- Caps are for INH only; do not swallow
- Immediately before administration, peel back foil until cap is visible and to "stop" line; remove cap from blister cavity; open dust cap of HandiHaler by pulling upward, then open mouthpiece; place cap in center chamber; firmly close mouthpiece until it clicks, leaving dust cap open
- When finished taking dose, remove used capsule and dispose of it; close mouthpiece and dust cap; store
- Rinse mouth after use

SIDE EFFECTS

CNS: Depression, paresthesia
CV: Chest pain, increased heart rate
EENT: Dry mouth, blurred vision, glaucoma
GI: Vomiting, abdominal pain, constipation, dyspepsia
INTEG: Rash, angioedema
MISC: Urinary difficulty, urinary retention
RESP: *Cough, sinusitis, upper respiratory tract infection,* epistaxis, pharyngitis

PHARMACOKINETICS

Half-life 5-6 days in animals, does not cross blood-brain barrier, very little metabolized in the liver, excreted in urine

INTERACTIONS

- Anticholinergics: avoid use with other anticholinergics

NURSING CONSIDERATIONS

Assess:

- **Respiratory status:** dyspnea, rate, breath sounds before and during treatment; pulmonary function tests at baseline and periodically; upper respiratory infections, cough, sinusitis
- Tolerance over long-term therapy; dose may have to be increased or changed
- Patient's ability to use HandiHaler

Evaluate:

- Therapeutic response: ability to breathe easier

Teach patient/family:

- Signs of closed-angle glaucoma
- That product is used for long-term maintenance, not for immediate relief of breathing problems; that effect takes 20 min, lasts 24 hr
- To avoid getting the powder in the eyes; may cause blurred vision and pupil dilation
- To hold HandiHaler with mouthpiece upward; to press button in once, completely, and release; this allows for medication to be released
- To breathe out completely; not to breathe into mouthpiece at any time
- To raise device to mouth and close lips tightly around mouthpiece
- With head upright, to breathe in slowly and deeply, but allow the cap to vibrate; to breathe until the lungs fill; to hold breath and remove mouthpiece; to resume normal breathing
- To rinse mouth after use; to use hard candy or regular oral hygiene to reduce dry mouth

tipranavir (Rx)

(ti-pran′a-veer)

Aptivus

Func. class.: Antiretroviral
Chem. class.: Protease inhibitor

ACTION: Inhibits human immunodeficiency virus (HIV) protease, thereby preventing the maturation of the virus

USES: HIV in combination with other antiretrovirals

CONTRAINDICATIONS: Hypersensitivity

Black Box Warning: Hepatic disease (Child-Pugh B, C)

Precautions: Pregnancy (C), breastfeeding, children, renal disease, history of renal stones, sulfa allergy, hemophilia, diabetes mellitus, pancreatitis, alcoholism, immune reconstitution syndrome, surgery, trauma, infection

Black Box Warning: Intracranial bleeding, hepatitis

DOSAGE AND ROUTES

Reduce dose with mild to moderate hepatic impairment and ketoconazole coadministration

- **Adult: PO** 500 mg coadministered with ritonavir 200 mg bid with food
- **Adolescent and child ≥2 yr: PO** 14 mg/kg given with ritonavir 6 mg/kg bid

T

or 375 mg/m^2 given with ritonavir 150 mg/m^2 bid, max 500 mg with ritonavir 200 mg bid

Available forms: Caps 250 mg; oral sol 100 mg/ml

Administer:

- Swallow cap whole; do not break, crush, chew
- After meals
- In equal intervals around the clock to maintain blood levels
- Give oral sol using calibrated dosing syringe or 5-ml oral syringe provided

SIDE EFFECTS

CNS: *Headache, insomnia,* dizziness, somnolence, fatigue, *fever,* intracranial bleeding

GI: *Diarrhea, abdominal pain, nausea, vomiting,* anorexia, dry mouth, hepatitis B or C, fatalities when given with ritonavir, pancreatitis

GU: Nephrolithiasis

INTEG: *Rash,* urticaria, lipodystrophy, serious rash

MS: Pain

OTHER: Asthenia, insulin-resistant hyperglycemia, *hyperlipidemia,* ketoacidosis

PHARMACOKINETICS

Terminal half-life 6 hr, plasma protein binding 99.9%, steady state 7-10 days, metabolism CYP3A4, 80% fecal excretion

INTERACTIONS

⚠ **Life-threatening dysrhythmias:** amiodarone, astemizole, cisapride, ergots, flecainide, midazolam, pimozide, propafenone, quiNIDine, rifabutin, rifampin, terfenadine, triazolam

Increase: myopathy, rhabdomyolysis—HMG-CoA reductase inhibitors (lovastatin, simvastatin)

Increase: tipranavir levels—ketoconazole, delavirdine, itraconazole

Increase: levels of both products—clarithromycin, zidovudine

Increase: levels of tipranavir—oral contraception

Decrease: tipranavir levels—rifamycins, fluconazole, nevirapine, efavirenz

Drug/Herb

Decrease: tipranavir levels—St. John's wort; avoid concurrent use

Drug/Food

Decrease: tipranavir absorption—grapefruit juice; high-fat, high-protein foods

Drug/Lab Test

Increase: AST/ALT

NURSING CONSIDERATIONS

Assess:

- Complaints of lower back, flank pain; indicates kidney stones
- Signs of infection, anemia; presence of other sexually transmitted diseases

Black Box Warning: Hepatic studies: ALT, AST; total bilirubin, amylase; all may be elevated

- **HIV:** Viral load, CD4, plasma HIV RNA, serum cholesterol profile, serum triglycerides during treatment
- Bowel pattern before, during treatment; if severe abdominal pain with bleeding occurs, product should be discontinued; monitor hydration
- **Serious rash:** if serious rash occurs, product should be discontinued

Perform/provide:

- Storage for caps in refrigerator prior to use; after opening, store at room temp; use within 60 days
- Storage for oral sol at room temp; use within 60 days after opening bottle

Evaluate:

- Therapeutic response: improving CD4 counts, viral load

Teach patient/family:

- To take as prescribed; if dose is missed, to take as soon as remembered up to 1 hr before next dose; not to double dose
- That product must be taken in equal intervals around the clock to maintain blood levels for duration of therapy

⚠ That hyperglycemia may occur; to watch for increased thirst, weight loss, hunger, dry, itchy skin; to notify prescriber

• To increase fluids to prevent kidney stones; if stone formation occurs, treatment may need to be interrupted
• That product does not cure AIDS, only controls symptoms; not to donate blood

⚠ HIGH ALERT

tirofiban (Rx)

(tie-roh-fee′ban)

Aggrastat

Func. class.: Antiplatelet

Chem. class.: Glycoprotein IIb/IIIa inhibitor

ACTION: Antagonist of platelet glycoprotein (GP) IIb/IIIa receptor that prevents binding of fibrinogen and von Willebrand's factor, which inhibits platelet aggregation

USES: Acute coronary syndrome in combination with heparin

CONTRAINDICATIONS: Hypersensitivity, active internal bleeding, stroke, major surgery, severe trauma within 30 days, intracranial neoplasm, aneurysm, hemorrhage, acute pericarditis, platelets <100,000/mm^3, history of thrombocytopenia, coagulopathy, systolic B/P >180 mm Hg or diastolic B/P >110 mm Hg

Precautions: Pregnancy (B), breastfeeding, children, geriatric patients, renal disease, bleeding tendencies, hypertension, platelets <150,000/mm^3

DOSAGE AND ROUTES

• **Adult:** **IV** 0.4 mcg/kg/min × 30 min then 0.1 mcg/kg/min for 12-24 hr after angioplasty or atherectomy

Renal dose

• **Adult:** **IV** CCr <30 ml/min, 0.2 mcg/kg/min × 30 min then 0.05 mcg/kg/min during angiography and for ≤24 hr after angioplasty

Available forms: Inj for sol 250 mcg/ml, inj 50 mcg/ml

Administer:

Intermittent IV INF route

• Dilute inj: withdraw and discard 100 ml from 500-ml bag of sterile 0.9% NaCl or D_5W and replace this vol with 100 ml of tirofiban inj from 2 vials
• Tirofiban inj for sol is premixed in containers of 500-ml 0.9% NaCl (50 mg/ml), infuse over 30 min
• Minimize other arterial/venous punctures; IM inj, catheter use, intubation, to reduce bleeding risk

Y-site compatibilities: Acyclovir, alfentanil, allopurinol, amifostine, amikacin, aminocaproic acid, aminophylline, amiodarone, ampicillin, ampicillin/sulbactam, anidulafungin, argatroban, arsenic trioxide, atracurium, atropine, azithromycin, aztreonam, bivalirudin, bleomycin, bumetanide, buprenorphine, butorphanol, calcium chloride/gluconate, capreomycin, CARBOplatin, carmustine, caspofungin, ceFAZolin, cefepime, cefotaxime, cefotetan, cefoxitin, ceftazidime, ceftizoxime, cefTRIAXone, cefuroxime, chloramphenicol, chlorproMAZINE, cimetidine, ciprofloxacin, cisatracurium, CISplatin, clindamycin, cyclophosphamide, cycloSPORINE, cytarabine, DACTINomycin, DAPTOmycin, dexamethasone, dexmedetomidine, dexrazoxane, digoxin, diltiazem, diphenhydrAMINE, DOBUTamine, docetaxel, dolasetron, DOPamine, doxacurium, DOXOrubicin, DOXOrubicin liposome, doxycycline, droperidol, enalaprilat, ePHEDrine, EPINEPHrine, epirubicin, eptifibatide, ertapenem, erythromycin, esmolol, etoposide, etoposide phosphate, famotidine, fenoldopam, fentaNYL, fluconazole, fludarabine, fluorouracil, foscarnet, fosphenytoin, furosemide, ganciclovir, gemcitabine, gentamicin, glycopyrrolate, granisetron, haloperidol, heparin, hydrALAZINE, hydrocortisone, HYDROmorphone, IDArubicin, ifosfamide, imipenem/cilastatin, insulin, irinotecan, isoproterenol, ketorolac, labetalol, leucovorin, lidocaine, li-

T

nezolid, LORazepam, magnesium sulfate, mannitol, mechlorethamine, melphalan, meperidine, meropenem, mesna, methylhexital, methotrexate, methyldopate, methylPREDNISolone, metoclopramide, metoprolol, metroNIDAZOLE, midazolam, milrinone, mitoxantrone, morphine, mycophenolate, nafcillin, nalbuphine, naloxone, nesiritide, niCARdipine, nitroglycerin, nitroprusside, norepinephrine, octreotide, ondansetron, oxaliplatin, oxytocin, paclitaxel, palonosetron, pamidronate, pancuronium, pantoprazole, pemetrexed, PENTobarbital, PHENobarbital, phentolamine, phenylephrine, piperacillin/tazobactam, potassium acetate, potassium chloride/phosphates, procainamide, prochlorperazine, promethazine, propranolol, quinupristin/dalfopristin, ranitidine, remifentanil, rocuronium, sodium acetate/bicarbonate, streptozocin, succinylcholine, SUFentanil, tacrolimus, teniposide, theophylline, thiopental, thiotepa, ticarcillin/clavulanate, tigecycline, tobramycin, topotecan, vancomycin, vasopressin, vecuronium, verapamil, vinBLAStine, vinCRIStine, vinorelbine, voriconazole, zidovudine, zoledronic acid

SIDE EFFECTS

CNS: Dizziness, headache
CV: Bradycardia, hypotension
GI: Nausea, vomiting
HEMA: Bleeding, thrombocytopenia
INTEG: *Rash*
MISC: Dissection, edema, pain in legs/pelvis, sweating
SYST: Anaphylaxis

PHARMOCOKINETICS

Half-life 2 hr; excretion via urine, feces; plasma clearance 20%-25% lower in geriatric patients with CAD; renal insufficiency decreases plasma clearance

INTERACTIONS

Increase: bleeding—aspirin, heparin, NSAIDs, abciximab, eptifibatide, clopidogrel, ticlopidine, dipyridamole, cefamandole, cefotetan, cefoperazone, valproic acid, heparins, thrombin inhibitors, SSRIs, SNRIs

NURSING CONSIDERATIONS

Assess:

- **Multiple sclerosis, spinal cord injury:** muscle spasms, dizziness, drowsiness, difficulty moving, coordination, balance

⚠ **Bleeding: platelet counts, Hct, Hgb prior to treatment, within 6 hr of loading dose, and at least daily thereafter; watch for bleeding from puncture sites, catheters or in stools, urine; discontinue if platelets <100,000/mm³**

Evaluate:

- Therapeutic response: treatment of acute coronary syndrome

Teach patient/family:

- That it is necessary to quit smoking to prevent excessive vasoconstriction
- About signs, symptoms of bleeding and low platelets
- That there are many product and herbal interactions

tizanidine (Rx)

(ti-za′nih-deen)

Zanaflex

Func. class.: Skeletal muscle relaxant, α_2-adrenergic agonist
Chem. class.: Imidazoline

Do not confuse:
tizanidine/tiagabine

ACTION: Increases presynaptic inhibition of motor neurons and reduces spasticity by α_2-adrenergic agonism

USES: Acute/intermittent management of increased muscle tone associated with spasticity, symptoms of MS
Unlabeled uses: Tension headache, low back pain, trigeminal neuralgia

CONTRAINDICATIONS: Hypersensitivity

Precautions: Pregnancy (C), breastfeeding, children, geriatric patients, hypotension, renal/hepatic disease

DOSAGE AND ROUTES

- **Adult: PO** 8 mg q6-8hr, max 36 mg/24 hr

Renal dose

- **Adult: PO** CCr <25 ml/min, start with lower dose

Available forms: Tabs 2, 4 mg; caps 2, 4, 6 mg

Administer

- Consistently either with/without food; food may affect absorption
- Titrate doses carefully
- Avoid use with other CNS depressants

SIDE EFFECTS

CNS: Somnolence, dizziness, speech disorder, dyskinesia, nervousness, hallucination, psychosis
CV: Hypotension, bradycardia
GI: Dry mouth, vomiting, increased ALT, abnormal LFTs, constipation
OTHER: Blurred vision, urinary frequency, pharyngitis, rhinitis, tremor, rash, muscle weakness

PHARMACOKINETICS

Completely absorbed, widely distributed, peak 1-2 hr, duration 3-6 hr, half-life 2.5 hr, protein binding 30%, metabolized by liver; excreted in urine, feces

INTERACTIONS

Increase: CNS depression—alcohol, other CNS depressants
Increase: tizanidine levels—other CYP1A2 inhibitors (acyclovir, amiodarone, famotidine, mexiletine, enoxacin, norfloxacin, propafenone, tacrine, verapamil, zileuton, oral contraceptives ciprofloxacin), fluvoxamine; avoid concurrent use
Increase: hypotension—antihypertensives
Increase: effect of rasagiline

Drug/Herb
Increase: CNS depression—kava, St. John's wort

Drug/Lab Test
Increase: alk phos, AST, ALT, serum glucose

NURSING CONSIDERATIONS

Assess:

- **Muscle spasticity** at baseline and throughout treatment
- **Hypotension;** gradual dosage increase should lessen hypotensive effects; have patient rise slowly from supine to upright; watch those patients receiving antihypertensives for increased effects
- Increased sedation, dizziness, hallucinations, psychosis; product may need to be discontinued
- Vision by ophthalmic exam; corneal opacities may occur
- Hepatic studies: 1, 3, 6 mo during treatment and periodically thereafter

Evaluate:

- Therapeutic response: decreased muscle spasticity

Teach patient/family:

- To rise slowly from lying or sitting to upright position to prevent orthostatic hypotension
- To ask for assistance if dizziness, sedation occur; to avoid drinking alcohol; to avoid operating machinery, driving until effects known
- To discontinue gradually

tobramycin (Rx)

(toe-bra-mye'sin)

TOBI

Func. class.: Antiinfective
Chem. class.: Aminoglycoside

ACTION: Interferes with protein synthesis in bacterial cell by binding to ribosomal subunits, thereby causing inaccurate peptide sequences to form in protein chain causing bacterial death

USES: Severe systemic infections of CNS, respiratory, GI, urinary tract, bone, skin, soft tissues caused by *Pseudomonas aeruginosa, Escherichia coli, Enterobacter, Providencia, Citrobacter, Staphylococcus, Proteus, Klebsiella, Serratia;* cystic fibrosis (nebulizer) for *Pseudomonas aeruginosa*

CONTRAINDICATIONS: Hypersensitivity to aminoglycosides

Black Box Warning: Pregnancy (D), severe renal disease

Precautions: Breastfeeding, geriatric patients, neonates, mild renal disease, myasthenia gravis, Parkinson's disease

Black Box Warning: Hearing deficits, neuromuscular disease

DOSAGE AND ROUTES

• **Adult: IM/IV** 3 mg/kg/day in divided doses q8hr; may give up to 6 mg/kg/day in divided doses q8-12hr; once-daily dosing (pulse dosing) (unlabeled) **IV** 5-7 mg/kg, dosing intervals determined using nomogram, based on random levels drawn 8-12 hr after 1st dose

• **Child: IM/IV** 6-7.5 mg/kg/day in 3-4 equal divided doses

• **Child ≥6 yr: NEB** 300 mg bid in repeating cycles of 28 days on/28 days off of product; give **INH** over 10-15 min using a handheld PARI LC PLUS reusable nebulizer with DeVilbiss Pulmo-Aid compressor

• **Neonate <1 wk: IM/IV** ≤4 mg/kg/day divided q12hr

Renal dose

• **Adult: IM/IV** 1 mg/kg then dose determined by blood levels, may be removed by dialysis

Available forms: Inj 10, 40 mg/ml; powder for inj 1.2 g; neb sol 300 mg/5 ml

Administer:

• After obtaining specimen for C&S; begin treatment before results

• Product in evenly spaced doses to maintain blood level; separate aminoglycosides and penicillins by ≥1 hr

• Use only on susceptible organisms to prevent development of product-resistant bacteria

IM route

• IM inj in large muscle mass; rotate inj sites

Nebulizer route

• Give as close to q12hr apart as possible; do not use <6 hr apart

• Do not mix with dornase alfa in nebulizer

• Have patient inhale while sitting or standing, breathe normally through mouthpiece; may use noseclips

Intermittent IV INF route

• Diluted in 50-100 ml 0.9% NaCl D_5W ($D_{10}W$, Ringer's, LR), infuse over 30-60 min

• Do not admix

Y-site compatibilities: Acyclovir, aldesleukin, alfentanil, alprostadil, amifostine, aminophylline, amiodarone, amsacrine, anidulafungin, ascorbic acid, atracurium, atropine, aztreonam, bivalirudin, bretylium, bumetanide, buprenorphine, butorphanol, calcium chloride/gluconate, CARBOplatin, caspofungin, chloramphenicol, cimetidine, ciprofloxacin, cisatracurium, CISplatin, clindamycin, cyanocobalamin, cyclophosphamide, cycloSPORINE, cytarabine, DACTINomycin, DAPTOmycin, dexmedetomidine, digoxin, diltiazem, diphenhydrAMINE, DOBUTamine, docetaxel, DOPamine, doripenem, doxacurium, DOXOrubicin hydrochloride, DOXOrubicin liposome, doxycycline, enalaprilat, ePHEDrine, EPINEPHrine, epirubicin, epoetin alfa, ertapenem, esmolol, etoposide, etoposide phosphate, famotidine, fenoldopam, fentaNYL, filgrastim, fluconazole, fludarabine, fluorouracil, foscarnet, furosemide, gemcitabine, gentamicin, glycopyrrolate, granisetron, HYDROmorphone, ifosfamide, imipenem/cilastatin, isoproterenol, ketorolac, labetalol, levofloxacin, lidocaine, linezolid, LORazepam, magnesium sulfate, mannitol, mechlorethamine, melphalan, meperidine, metaraminol, methicillin, methotrexate, methoxamine, methyldopate, methylPREDNISolone, metoclopramide, metoprolol, metroNIDAZOLE, miconazole, midazolam, milrinone, minocycline, mitoxantrone, morphine, moxalactam, multiple vitamins, nafcillin, nalbuphine, naloxone, niCARdipine, nitroglycerin, nitroprusside, norepinephrine, octreotide, ondansetron, oxaliplatin, oxytocin, paclitaxel, palonosetron, pantoprazole, papaverine, penicillin G, pentazocine, perphenazine, PHENobarbital, phentolamine, phenylephrine, phytonadione, potassium chloride, procainamide, prochlorperazine, promethazine, propranolol, protamine, pyridoxime, quinupristin/dalfopristin, ranitidine, remifentanil, riTUXimab, rocuronium, sodium acetate/bicarbonate, succinylcholine, SUFentanil, tacrolimus, teniposide, theophylline, thiamine, thiotepa, ticarcillin/clavulanate, tigecycline, tirofiban, tolazoline, trastuzumab, trimethaphan, urokinase, vancomycin, vasopressin, vecuronium, verapamil, vinCRIStine, vinorelbine, voriconazole, zidovudine

SIDE EFFECTS

CNS: Confusion, depression, numbness, tremors, **seizures**, muscle twitching, **neurotoxicity**, dizziness, vertigo
CV: Hypo/hypertension, palpitation
EENT: **Ototoxicity**, deafness, visual disturbances, tinnitus
GI: *Nausea, vomiting, anorexia;* increased ALT, AST, bilirubin, hepatomegaly, **hepatic necrosis**, splenomegaly
GU: **Oliguria, hematuria, renal damage, azotemia, renal failure, nephrotoxicity**
HEMA: **Agranulocytosis, thrombocytopenia, leukopenia**, eosinophilia, anemia
INTEG: *Rash,* burning, urticaria, dermatitis, alopecia

PHARMACOKINETICS

Plasma half-life 2-3 hr, prolonged in neonates; not metabolized; excreted unchanged in urine; crosses placental barrier; poor penetration into CSF

IM: Onset rapid, peak 1 hr, duration 8 hr
IV: Onset immediate, peak 30 min, duration 8 hr

INTERACTIONS

Increase: ototoxicity, neurotoxicity, nephrotoxicity—other aminoglycosides, amphotericin B, polymyxin, vancomycin, ethacrynic acid, furosemide, mannitol, methoxyflurane, CISplatin, cephalosporins, bacitracin, acyclovir, penicillins, cidofovir

Drug/Lab Test
Increase: eosinophils, BUN, creatinine, AST, ALT, LDH, alk phos
Decrease: potassium, calcium, sodium, magnesium, WBC, granulocytes, platelets

NURSING CONSIDERATIONS

Assess:
- Weight before treatment; dosage is usually based on ideal body weight but may be calculated on actual body weight
- I&O ratio, urinalysis daily for proteinuria, cells, casts; report sudden change in urine output
- VS during inf; watch for hypotension, change in pulse
- IV site for thrombophlebitis, including pain, redness, swelling q30min; change site if needed; apply warm compresses to discontinued site
- Serum aminoglycoside conc; serum peak drawn at 30-60 min after IV inf or 60 min after IM inj, trough drawn just before next dose, peak 4-10 mcg/ml, trough 0.5-2 mcg/ml

Black Box Warning: Renal impairment: CCr, BUN, serum creatinine; lower dosage should be given in renal impairment (CCr $<$80 ml/min); monitor electrolytes: potassium, sodium, chloride, magnesium monthly if patient receiving long-term therapy

Black Box Warning: Deafness by audiometric testing; ringing, roaring in ears; vertigo; assess hearing before, during, after treatment

• **Overgrowth of infection:** fever, malaise, redness, pain, swelling, perineal itching, diarrhea, stomatitis, change in cough, sputum
• **Vestibular dysfunction:** nausea, vomiting, dizziness, headache; product should be discontinued if severe

Perform/provide:

• Adequate fluids of 2-3 L/day unless contraindicated to prevent irritation of tubules
• Flush of IV line with NS or D_5W after inf
• Supervised ambulation, other safety measures with vestibular dysfunction

Evaluate:

• Therapeutic response: absence of fever, draining wounds, negative C&S after treatment

Teach patient/family:

• To report headache, dizziness, symptoms of overgrowth of infection, renal impairment
• To report loss of hearing; ringing, roaring in ears; feeling of fullness in head

Black Box Warning: To notify prescriber if pregnancy is planned or suspected; pregnancy (D)

Nebulizer

• To use other therapies first, then tobramycin

TREATMENT OF OVERDOSE:

Hemodialysis; monitor serum levels of product

tobramycin ophthalmic

See Appendix B

tocilizumab (Rx)

(toe′si-liz′oo-mab)

Actemra

Func. class.: DMARDs (disease-modifying antirheumatoid drugs)/tumor necrosis factor (TNF) modifier

ACTION: Interleukin-6 (IL-6) receptor inhibiting monoclonal antibody

USES: Rheumatoid arthritis, active systemic juvenile idiopathic arthritis

CONTRAINDICATIONS: Serious infections, risk for GI perforation, active hepatic disease, severe neutropenia/thrombocytopenia, demyelinating disorders

Precautions: Breastfeeding, pregnancy (C)

DOSAGE AND ROUTES

• **Adult: IV** 4 mg/kg over 1 hr q4wk, may increase to 8 mg/kg q4wk based on clinical response, max dose 800 mg/inf; do not initiate if ANC >2000, platelets <100,000

Juvenile idiopathic arthritis

• **Child ≥2 yr/adolescent ≥30 kg: IV** 8 mg/kg over 1 hr q2wk
• **Child ≥2 yr/adolescent <30 kg: IV** 12 mg/kg over 1 hr

Available forms: Sol for inj 80 mg/4 ml, 200 mg/10 ml, 400 mg/20 ml

Administer:

Intermittent IV INF route

• Visually inspect for particulate matter, discoloration before administration whenever sol and container permit; colorless to pale yellow liquid
• From 100-ml inf bag or bottle, withdraw vol of 0.9% sodium chloride inj equal to vol of tocilizumab sol required for patient's dose
• Slowly add tocilizumab from each vial into inf bag or bottle; gently invert bag to avoid foaming; fully diluted sols are compatible with polypropylene, polyethylene, polyvinyl chloride inf bags and polypropylene, polyethylene, glass inf bottles
• Fully diluted sol for infusion may be stored refrigerated or at room temp for ≤24 hr and should be protected from light; do not use unused product remaining in vials; no preservatives
• Allow the fully diluted sol to reach room temp before inf
• Give over 60 minutes with inf set; do not administer as IV push or bolus
• Do not infuse concomitantly in same IV line with other drugs

SIDE EFFECTS

CNS: Headache, dizziness
CV: Hypertension
GI: **Perforation**, abdominal pain, gastritis, mouth ulcerations
HEMA: **Neutropenia, thrombocytopenia**
INTEG: Rash, inf reactions
RESP: Upper respiratory infections, nasopharyngitis, bronchitis
SYST: **Serious infections, anaphylaxis,** infusion-related reactions, antitocilizumab antibody formation

INTERACTIONS

- Do not give with live virus vaccines
- Avoid use with TNF modifiers, DMARDs, immunosuppressives due to increased risk of infection

PHARMACOKINETICS

Half-life approx 6 days with single dose, approx 11 days with multiple (steady-state) doses

NURSING CONSIDERATIONS

Assess:
- **Rheumatoid arthritis:** ROM, pain, stiffness at baseline and periodically
- Blood studies: CBC with differential, LFTs, platelet count, serum lipid profile at baseline and periodically
- Infection before treatment and periodically; obtain TB screening before beginning treatment

Evaluate:
- Therapeutic response: ability to move more easily with less pain

Teach patient/family:
- That this treatment must continue unless safety or effectiveness is an issue
- About reason for use and expected results
- To avoid live vaccines
- To report signs, symptoms of infection, including TB and hepatitis B

tolcapone (Rx)

(toll′cah′pone)

Tasmar

Func. class.: Antiparkinson agent
Chem. class.: COMT inhibitor

ACTION:
Inhibits COMT; used as adjunct to levodopa/carbidopa therapy

USES:
Parkinson's disease

CONTRAINDICATIONS:
Hypersensitivity

Precautions: Pregnancy (C), breastfeeding, cardiac/renal disease, hypertension, asthma, history of rhabdomyolysis

Black Box Warning: Hepatic disease

DOSAGE AND ROUTES

- **Adult: PO** 100-200 mg tid with levodopa/carbidopa therapy; max 600 mg/day, discontinue if no benefit after 3 wk

Available forms: Tabs 100, 200 mg

Administer:
- Only to be used if levodopa/carbidopa does not provide satisfactory results

SIDE EFFECTS

CNS: Dystonia, dyskinesia, dreaming, *fatigue, headache, confusion,* psychosis, hallucination, dizziness, sleep disorders
CV: *Orthostatic hypotension,* chest pain, hypotension
EENT: Cataract, eye inflammation
GI: *Nausea, vomiting, anorexia, abdominal distress,* diarrhea, constipation, **fatal hepatic failure,** increased LFTs
GU: UTI, urine discoloration, uterine tumor, micturition disorder, hematuria
HEMA: **Hemolytic anemia, leukopenia, agranulocytosis**
INTEG: Sweating, alopecia
MS: **Rhabdomyolysis**

PHARMACOKINETICS

Rapidly absorbed, peak 2 hr, protein binding 99%, extensively metabolized, half-life 2-3 hr, excreted in urine (60%)/feces (40%)

INTERACTIONS

- May influence pharmacokinetics of α-methyldopa, DOBUTamine, apomorphine, isoproterenol
- Inhibition of normal catecholamine metabolism: MAOIs, MAO-B inhibitor may be used

NURSING CONSIDERATIONS

Assess:

Black Box Warning: Hepatic disease: AST, ALT, alk phos, LDH, bilirubin, CBC; monitor ALT, AST q2wk × 1 yr, then q4wk × 6 mo, then q8wk thereafter; if LFTs elevated, product should not be used

- Involuntary movements of parkinsonism: akinesia, tremors, staggering gait, muscle rigidity, drooling
- B/P, respiration during initial treatment; hypo/hypertension should be reported
- Mental status: affect, mood, behavioral changes

Evaluate:

- Therapeutic response: decrease in akathisia, increased mood

Teach patient/family:

- To change positions slowly to prevent orthostatic hypotension
- That urine, sweat may change color
- That food taken within 1 hr before meals or 2 hr after meals decreases action of product by 20%

Black Box Warning: To report signs of hepatic injury: clay-colored stools, jaundice, fatigue, appetite loss, lethargy

- To report nausea, vomiting, anorexia; that nausea may occur at beginning of treatment

tolnaftate topical

See Appendix B

tolterodine (Rx)

(toll-tehr′oh-deen)

Detrol, Detrol LA

Func. class.: Overactive bladder product

Chem. class.: Muscarinic receptor antagonist

ACTION: Relaxes smooth muscles in urinary tract by inhibiting acetylcholine at postganglionic sites

USES: Overactive bladder (urinary frequency, urgency), urinary incontinence

CONTRAINDICATIONS: Hypersensitivity, uncontrolled closed-angle glaucoma, urinary retention, gastric retention

Precautions: Pregnancy (C), breastfeeding, children, renal/hepatic disease, controlled closed-angle glaucoma, bladder obstruction, QT prolongation, decreased GI motility

DOSAGE AND ROUTES

- **Adult and geriatric: PO** 2 mg bid; may decrease to 1 mg bid; **EXT REL** 4 mg/day, may decrease to 2 mg/day if needed, max 4 mg/day

Hepatic/renal dose

- **Adult: PO** 1 mg bid (50% dose) or **EXT REL** 2 mg/day; CCr ≤30 ml/min, reduce by 50%

Available forms: Tabs 1, 2 mg; ext rel caps 2, 4 mg

Administer:

- Whole; take with liquids; do not crush, chew or break ext rel product; without regard to meals

SIDE EFFECTS

CNS: Anxiety, paresthesia, fatigue, *dizziness, headache;* increasing dementia, memory impairment

CV: Chest pain, hypertension, QT prolongation

EENT: Vision abnormalities, xerophthalmia
GI: *Nausea, vomiting, anorexia,* abdominal pain, constipation, dry mouth, dyspepsia
GU: Dysuria, urinary retention, frequency, UTI
INTEG: Rash, pruritus
RESP: Bronchitis, cough, pharyngitis, upper respiratory tract infection
SYST: **Angioedema, Stevens-Johnson syndrome**

PHARMACOKINETICS

Rapidly absorbed; highly protein bound; extensively metabolized by CYP2D6; a portion of the population may be poor metabolizers; excreted in urine, feces

INTERACTIONS

⚠ **Increase:** **QT prolongation—class IA/III antidysrhythmics, some phenothiazines, β-agonists, local anesthetics, tricyclics, haloperidol, methadone, chloroquine, clarithromycin, droperidol, erythromycin, pentamidine**
Increase: action of tolterodine—antiretroviral protease inhibitors, macrolide antiinfectives, azole antifungals
Increase: anticholinergic effect—antimuscarinics
Increase: urinary frequency—diuretics
Drug/Food
• Food increases bioavailability of tolterodine

NURSING CONSIDERATIONS

Assess:
• **Urinary patterns:** distention, nocturia, frequency, urgency, incontinence
⚠ **Serious skin disorders: angioedema, Stevens-Johnson syndrome; allergic reactions: rash; if this occurs, product should be discontinued**
• LFTs at baseline, periodically
⚠ **QT prolongation: ECG, ejection fraction; assess for chest pain, palpitations, dyspnea**

Evaluate:
• Decreasing dysuria, frequency, nocturia, incontinence
Teach patient/family:
• To avoid hazardous activities; dizziness may occur
• Not to drink liquids before bedtime
• About the importance of bladder maintenance
• Not to breastfeed
• To report signs of infection, skin effects

tolvaptan (Rx)

(tole-vap′tan)

Samsca

Func. class.: Vasopressin receptor antagonist, V2

ACTION:

Arginine vasopressin (AVP) antagonist with affinity for V2 receptors; level of circulating AVP in circulating blood is critical for the regulation of water and the electrolyte balance, and it is usually elevated with euvolemic/hypervolemic hyponatremia

USES:

Hypervolemic/euvolemic hyponatremia with heart failure, cirrhosis, SIADH

CONTRAINDICATIONS:

Hypersensitivity, hypovolemia, anuria
Precautions: Pregnancy (C), breastfeeding, children, dehydration, geriatric, hepatic disease, hyperkalemia
Black Box Warning: Alcoholism, malnutrition

T

DOSAGE AND ROUTES

• **Adult: PO** 15 mg daily; after 24 hr, may increase to 30 mg daily; max 60 mg/day
Available forms: Tab 15, 30 mg
Administer:
• PO with/without food
• Avoid fluid restriction for first 24 hr
• Initiate in hospital setting

SIDE EFFECTS

CNS: Fever
CV: Ventricular fibrillation, DIC, stroke, thrombosis
GI: Nausea, vomiting, constipation, colitis
GU: Polyuria
HEMA: Bleeding
META: Dehydration, hyperglycemia, hyperkalemia, hypernatremia
MS: Rhabdomyolysis
RESP: Respiratory depression, pulmonary embolism

PHARMACOKINETICS

Peak 2-4 hr, protein binding 99%, metabolized by CYP3A4, terminal half-life 12 hr

INTERACTIONS

Increase: plasma concentrations of tolvaptan—CYP3A4 inhibitors (efavirenz, fosamprenavir, quiNINE); P-gp inhibitors (cycloSPORINE, azithromycin, mefloquine, palperidone, propafenone, quiNIDine, testosterone)
Decrease: plasma conc of tolvaptan—CYP3A4 inducers (carBAMazepine, dexamethasone, etravirine, flutamide, griseofulvin, metyrapsone, modafinil, nafacillin, nevirapine, OXcarbazepine, phenytoin, rifampin, rifabutin, rifapendine, topiramate)
Drug/Herb
Decreased: tolvaptan effect: CYP3A4 inducer (St. John's wort)

NURSING CONSIDERATIONS

Assess:
- Renal, hepatic function
- Frequent sodium vol status; overly rapid correction of sodium conc (12 mEq/L per 24 hr), may result in osmotic demyelination syndrome
- CV status: ventricular fibrillation, hypertension; monitor B/P, pulse
- Monitor electrolytes (sodium, potassium)

Evaluate:
- Therapeutic response: correction of serum sodium levels

Teach patient/family:
- To avoid pregnancy, breastfeeding while taking this product
- About administration procedure and expected results

topiramate (Rx)

(toh-pire′ah-mate)

Topamax, Topamax Sprinkle, Topiragen

Func. class.: Anticonvulsant—miscellaneous
Chem. class.: Monosaccharide derivative

ACTION: May prevent seizure spread as opposed to an elevation of seizure threshold, increases GABA activity

USES: Partial seizures in adults and children 2-16 yr old; tonic-clonic seizures; seizures with Lennox-Gastaut syndrome; migraine prophylaxis
Unlabeled uses: Infantile spasms, bipolar disorder, alcohol dependence, absence seizures, neuropathic pain, cluster headaches, mania

CONTRAINDICATIONS: Hypersensitivity, metabolic acidosis, pregnancy (D)
Precautions: Breastfeeding, children, renal/hepatic disease, acute myopia, secondary closed-angle glaucoma, behavioral disorders, COPD, dialysis, encephalopathy, status asthmaticus, status epilepticus, surgery, paresthesias, maculopathy

DOSAGE AND ROUTES

Adjunctive therapy for seizures

• **Adult/adolescent/child ≥10 yr: PO** 25-50 mg/day initially, titrate by 25-50 mg/wk, up to 200-400 mg/day in 2 divided doses

• **Child 2-9 yr: PO** week 1: 25 mg in PM, then 25 mg bid if tolerated (week 2), then increase by 25-50 mg/day each week as tolerated over 5 to 7-wk titration period, maintenance given in 2 divided doses; <11 kg, minimum 150 mg/day, max 250 mg/day; 12-25 kg, minimum 200 mg/day, max 300 mg/day; 23-35 kg, minimum 200 mg/day, max 350 mg/day; 32-38 kg, minimum 250 mg/day, max 350 mg/day; >38 kg, minimum 250 mg/day, max 400 mg/day

Migraine prophylaxis

• **Adult: PO** 25 mg/day initially, increase by 25 mg/day/wk up to 100 mg/day in 2 divided doses

Renal dose

• **Adult: PO** CCr <70 ml/min, give ½ dose

Atonic/atypical absence/myoclonic seizures (unlabeled)

• **Adult/adolescent >16 yr: PO** 50 mg/day, titrate slowly by 50 mg/wk to 100-300 mg tid

• **Child 2-16 yr: PO** 0.5-1 mg/kg, max 25 mg, initially daily × 7 days then increase by 0.5-1 mg/kg/day weekly up to 3-6 mg/kg/day in divided doses

Refractory infantile spasms (unlabeled)

• **Child: PO** 25 mg/day, may increase by 25 mg q2-3days until spasms controlled, max 24 mg/kg/day

Alcoholism (unlabeled)

• **Adult: PO** 25 mg/day, titrated to max 300 mg/day in divided doses

Neuropathic pain (unlabeled)

• **Adult: PO** 12.5-25 mg q day or bid × 4 wk then double dose q4wk to max 100-200 mg/day in divided doses

Bipolar disorder (unlabeled)

• **Adult: PO** 25 mg/day then increase by 25-mg increments to 200 mg/day

Available forms: Tabs 25, 50, 100, 200 mg; sprinkle caps 15, 25 mg

Administer:

• Swallow tabs whole; do not break, crush, or chew tabs; very bitter

• May take without regard to meals

• Sprinkle cap can be given whole or opened and sprinkled on soft food; do not chew

SIDE EFFECTS

CNS: *Dizziness, fatigue*, cognitive disorders, insomnia, *anxiety*, depression, paresthesia, *memory loss, tremor,* motor retardation, **suicidal ideation**

EENT: Diplopia, *vision abnormality*

GI: Diarrhea, *anorexia, nausea, dyspepsia*, abdominal pain, constipation, dry mouth, **pancreatitis**

GU: Breast pain, dysmenorrhea, menstrual disorder

INTEG: Rash

MISC: Weight loss, leukopenia, metabolic acidosis, increased body temperature; **unexplained death (epilepsy)**

RESP: Upper respiratory tract infection, pharyngitis, sinusitis

PHARMACOKINETICS

Well absorbed, peak 2 hr, terminal half-life 19-25 hr, excreted in urine (55%-97% unchanged), crosses placenta, excreted in breast milk, protein binding (9%-17%), steady state 4 days

INTERACTIONS

Increase: renal stones—carbonic anhydrase inhibitors

Increase: effect of amitriptyline

Increase: CNS depression—alcohol, CNS depressants

Increase: topiramate levels—metformin, hydrochlorothiazide, lamotrigine

Decrease: levels of oral contraceptives, estrogen, digoxin, valproic acid, lithium, risperidone

Decrease: topiramate levels—phenytoin, carBAMazepine, valproic acid, probenecid

T

NURSING CONSIDERATIONS

Assess:

- **Seizures:** location, type, duration, aura
- **Bipolar disorder:** mood, behavior
- Renal studies: urinalysis, BUN, urine creatinine q3mo; symptoms of renal colic
- Hepatic studies: ALT, AST, bilirubin if patient receiving long-term treatment
- CBC during long-term therapy (anemia); serum bicarbonate (metabolic acidosis)
- Migraines: pain location, duration; alleviating factors

⚠ Mental status: mood, sensorium, affect, behavioral changes, **suicidal thoughts/behaviors;** if mental status changes, notify prescriber

- Body weight, evidence of cognitive disorder

Perform/provide:

- Storage at room temp away from heat, light
- Assistance with ambulation during early part of treatment; dizziness occurs
- Seizure precautions: padded side rails, move objects that may harm patient

Evaluate:

- Therapeutic response: decreased seizure activity

Teach patient/family:

- To carry emergency ID stating patient's name, products taken, condition, prescriber's name and phone number
- To avoid driving, other activities that require alertness
- Not to discontinue medication quickly after long-term use
- To notify prescriber immediately of blurred vision, periorbital pain
- To maintain adequate fluid intake
- To use nonhormonal contraceptive; that effect of oral contraceptives is decreased, pregnancy (D)

⚠ HIGH ALERT

topotecan (Rx)

(toh-poh-tee′kan)

Hycamtin

Func. class.: Antineoplastic, natural; topoisomerase inhibitor

Chem. class.: Camptothecin analog

ACTION:

Antitumor product with topoisomerase-I–inhibitory activity; topoisomerase I relieves torsional strain in DNA by causing single-strand breaks; also causes double-strand DNA damage

USES:

Metastatic ovarian cancer after failure of traditional chemotherapy; relapsed small-cell lung cancer; cervical cancer

Unlabeled uses: Non–small-cell lung cancer (NSCLC), rhabdomyosarcoma

CONTRAINDICATIONS:

Pregnancy (D), breastfeeding, hypersensitivity, severe bone marrow depression

Black Box Warning: Neutropenia

Precautions: Children, renal disease

DOSAGE AND ROUTES

- **Adult: IV INF** 1.5 mg/m^2 over 30 min daily × 5 days starting on day 1 of 21-day course × 4 courses; may be reduced to 0.25 mg/m^2 for subsequent courses if severe neutropenia occurs; **PO** 2.3 mg/m^2/day on days 1-5 of 21-day course (relapsed small-cell lung cancer in those with prior response)

Renal dose

- **Adult: IV** CCr 20-39 ml/min, 0.75 mg/m^2/day × 5 days starting on day 1 of 21-day course

Available forms: Lyophilized powder for inj 4 mg; caps 0.25, 1 mg

Administer:

PO route

- Do not break, crush, chew, or open caps
- Take without regard to food

IV route
- Give as IV INF

SIDE EFFECTS

CNS: Arthralgia, *asthenia, headache,* myalgia, *pain,* weakness
GI: *Abdominal pain, constipation,* diarrhea, obstruction, *nausea,* stomatitis, *vomiting;* increased ALT, AST; anorexia
HEMA: Neutropenia, leukopenia, thrombocytopenia, anemia, sepsis
INTEG: *Total alopecia*
RESP: Dyspnea, cough, **interstitial lung disease**

PHARMACOKINETICS

Rapidly and completely absorbed, excreted in urine and feces as metabolites, half-life 2.8 hr, 7%-35% bound to plasma proteins

INTERACTIONS

- Avoid use with P-glycoprotein, breast cancer resistance protein inhibitors (amiodarone, clarithromycin, diltiazem, erythromycin, indinavir), quiNIDine, testosterone, verapamil, tamoxifen, itraconazole, mefloquine, RU-486, niCARdipine, vaccines, toxoids

Increase: myelosuppression when used with CISplatin
Increase: bleeding risk—NSAIDs, anticoagulants, thrombolytics, platelet inhibitors

Drug/Food
- Avoid use with grapefruit juice

NURSING CONSIDERATIONS

Assess:
- Hepatic studies: AST, ALT, alk phos, which may be elevated; creatinine, BUN

Black Box Warning: CBC, differential, platelet count weekly; withhold product if WBC is $<3500/mm^3$ or platelet count is $<100,000/mm^3$; notify prescriber of results; product should be discontinued

- Buccal cavity for dryness, sores or ulcerations, white patches, oral pain, bleeding, dysphagia
- GI symptoms: frequency of stools, cramping
- Signs of dehydration: rapid respiration, poor skin turgor, decreased urine output, dry skin, restlessness, weakness

Perform/provide:
- Storage of caps in refrigerator; IV INF unopened at room temp; protect both from light
- Increased fluid intake to 2-3 L/day to prevent dehydration unless contraindicated
- Rinsing of mouth tid-qid with water, club soda; brushing of teeth bid-tid with soft brush or cotton-tipped applicator for stomatitis; use unwaxed dental floss
- Nutritious diet with iron, vit K supplements, low fiber, few dairy products

Evaluate:
- Therapeutic response: decreased tumor size, spread of malignancy

Teach patient/family:
- That total alopecia may occur; that hair grows back but is different in color and texture
- To avoid foods with citric acid or hot or rough texture if stomatitis is present; to drink adequate fluids
- To report stomatitis and any bleeding, white spots, ulcerations in mouth; to examine mouth daily; to report symptoms
- To report signs of anemia: fatigue, headache, faintness, SOB, irritability
- To use effective contraception during treatment and for ≤6 mo after; to avoid breastfeeding
- To avoid OTC products without approval of prescriber
- To avoid driving or other activities requiring alertness
- To avoid vaccines, toxoids

T

toremifene (Rx)

(tor-em′ih-feen)

Fareston

Func. class.: Antineoplastic
Chem. class.: Antiestrogen hormone

ACTION: Inhibits cell division by binding to cytoplasmic estrogen receptors; resembles normal cell complex but inhibits DNA synthesis and estrogen response of target tissue

USES: Advanced breast carcinoma not responsive to other therapy in estrogen-receptor–positive patients (usually postmenopausal)
Unlabeled uses: Prostate cancer prophylaxis

CONTRAINDICATIONS: Pregnancy (D), hypersensitivity, history of thromboembolism

Black Box Warning: QT prolongation
Precautions: Breastfeeding, children, leukopenia, thrombocytopenia, cataracts, hypercalcemia, hepatic disease, endometrial hyperplasia

DOSAGE AND ROUTES

- **Adult: PO** 60 mg/day

Available forms: Tabs 60 mg
Administer:

- Antacid before oral agent; give product after evening meal, before bedtime
- Antiemetic 30-60 min before product to prevent vomiting

SIDE EFFECTS

CNS: *Hot flashes, headache, lightheadedness,* depression
CV: CHF, MI, PE, chest pain, angina
EENT: Ocular lesions, retinopathy, corneal opacity, blurred vision (high doses)
GI: *Nausea, vomiting,* altered taste (anorexia)
GU: Vaginal bleeding, pruritus vulvae
HEMA: Thrombocytopenia, leukopenia, thrombosis
INTEG: Rash, alopecia, *sweating*
META: Hypercalcemia
RESP: Pulmonary embolism

PHARMACOKINETICS

Peak 3 hr, excreted primarily in feces, 99.5% protein binding, terminal half-life 5-6 days, metabolized by liver

INTERACTIONS

- May increase effect of warfarin

⚠ **Increase:** QT prolongation—class IA/III antidysrhythmics, some phenothiazines, β agonists, local anesthetics, tricyclics, haloperidol, chloroquine, droperidol, pentamidine; CYP3A4 inhibitors (amio-darone, clarithromycin, erythromycin, telithromycin, troleandomycin), arsenic trioxide, levomethadyl; CYP3A4 substrates (methadone, pimozide, QUEtiapine, quiNIDine, risperidone, ziprasidone)
⚠ **Increase:** toxicity—CYP3A4 inhibitors (aprepitant, antiretroviral protease inhibitors, clarithromycin, danazol, delavirdine, diltiazem, erythromycin, fluconazole, FLUoxetine, fluvoxamine, imatinib, ketoconazole, mibefradil, nefazodone, telithromycin, voriconazole)
Decrease: toremifene effect—CYP3A4 inducers (barbiturates, bosentan, carBAMazepine, efavirenz, phenytoins, nevirapine, rifabutin, rifampin)
Drug/Herb

- Avoid use with St. John's wort

Drug/Lab Test
Increase: serum calcium

NURSING CONSIDERATIONS

Assess:

- CBC, differential, platelet count weekly; withhold product if WBC is <3500/mm^3 or platelet count is <100,000/mm^3; notify prescriber; LFTs, serum calcium
- **Bleeding:** hematuria, guaiac, bruising, petechiae, mucosa or orifices q8hr
- Effects of alopecia on body image; discuss feelings about body changes

⚠ **Severe allergic reactions:** rash, pruritus, urticaria, purpuric skin lesions, itching, flushing

Black Box Warning: QT prolongation: ECG, ejection fraction; assess for chest pain, palpitations, dyspnea

Perform/provide:

- Increase fluid intake to 2-3 L/day to prevent dehydration
- Nutritious diet with iron, vitamin supplements as ordered; avoid use of herbals
- Storage in light-resistant container at room temp

Evaluate:

- Therapeutic response: decreased tumor size, spread of malignancy

Teach patient/family:

- To report any complaints, side effects to prescriber
- That vaginal bleeding, pruritus, hot flashes are reversible after discontinuing treatment
- To report immediately decreased visual acuity, which may be irreversible; about need for routine eye exams; that health care providers should be told about tamoxifen therapy
- To report vaginal bleeding immediately
- **That tumor flare**—increase in size of tumor, increased bone pain—may occur and will subside rapidly; to take analgesics for pain
- That premenopausal women must use mechanical birth control because ovulation may be induced
- That hair may be lost during treatment; that a wig or hairpiece may make patient feel better; that new hair may be different in color, texture

torsemide (Rx)

(tor'suh-mide)

Demadex

Func. class.: Loop diuretic

Chem. class.: Sulfonamide derivative

ACTION: Acts on loop of Henle by inhibiting absorption of chloride, sodium, water

USES: Treatment of hypertension and edema with CHF, ascites

CONTRAINDICATIONS: Infants, hypersensitivity to sulfonamides, anuria

Precautions: Pregnancy (B), breastfeeding, diabetes mellitus, dehydration, severe renal disease, electrolyte depletion, hypovolemia, syncope, ventricular dysrhythmias

DOSAGE AND ROUTES

CHF

- **Adult: PO/IV** 10-20 mg/day, may increase as needed, max 200 mg/day

Edema in chronic renal failure

- **Adult: PO/IV** 20 mg/day, may increase to 200 mg/day

Hepatic cirrhosis in combination with aldosterone antagonist/ potassium-sparing diuretic

- **Adult: PO/IV** 5-10 mg/day, may increase as needed, max 40 mg/day

Hypertension

- **Adult: PO** 5 mg/day, may increase to 10 mg/day

Available forms: Tabs 5, 10, 20, 100 mg; inj 10 mg/ml

Administer:

- In AM to avoid interference with sleep if using product as diuretic
- Potassium replacement if potassium <3 mg/dl
- With food or milk if nausea occurs; absorption may be decreased slightly

SIDE EFFECTS

CNS: *Headache, dizziness,* asthenia, insomnia, nervousness
CV: Orthostatic hypotension, chest pain, ECG changes, **circulatory collapse,** ventricular tachycardia, edema
EENT: *Loss of hearing,* ear pain, tinnitus, blurred vision
ELECT: *Hypokalemia, hypochloremic alkalosis, hyponatremia,* metabolic alkalosis
ENDO: *Hyperglycemia, hyperuricemia*
GI: *Nausea,* diarrhea, dyspepsia, cramps, constipation
GU: *Polyuria,* **renal failure,** glycosuria
INTEG: *Rash,* photosensitivity, pruritus
MS: Cramps, stiffness
RESP: Rhinitis, cough increase

PHARMACOKINETICS

PO: Rapidly absorbed; duration 6 hr; breast milk; crosses placenta; half-life 3.5 hr; protein binding 97%-99%, cleared through hepatic metabolism

INTERACTIONS

• Incompatible with any product in syringe
Increase: toxicity—lithium, nondepolarizing skeletal muscle relaxants, digoxin
Increase: action of antihypertensives, oral anticoagulants, nitrates
Increase: ototoxicity—aminoglycosides, CISplatin, vancomycin
Decrease: antihypertensive effect of torsemide—indomethacin, carBAMazepine, PHENobarbital, phenytoin, rifampin, NSAIDs
Drug/Herb
• Severe photosensitivity: St. John's wort
Drug/Lab Test
Interference: GTT

NURSING CONSIDERATIONS

Assess:
• Hearing when giving high doses
• Weight, I&O daily to determine fluid loss; effect of product may be decreased if used daily
• Rate, depth, rhythm of respiration; effect of exertion
• B/P lying, standing; postural hypotension may occur
• Electrolytes: potassium, sodium, chlorine; include BUN, blood glucose, CBC, serum creatinine, blood pH, ABGs, uric acid, Ca, Mg
• Glucose in urine of diabetic patients
• **Signs and symptoms of metabolic alkalosis:** drowsiness, restlessness
• **Signs and symptoms of hypokalemia:** postural hypotension, malaise, fatigue, tachycardia, leg cramps, weakness
• Rashes, temp elevation daily
• Confusion, especially in geriatric patients; take safety precautions if needed
Evaluate:
• Therapeutic response: improvement in edema of feet, legs, sacral area daily if medication is being used with CHF
Teach patient/family:
• To rise slowly from lying, sitting position
• To recognize adverse reactions: muscle cramps, weakness, nausea, dizziness, tinnitus
• To take with food or milk for GI symptoms; to limit alcohol use
• To take early during the day to prevent nocturia

TREATMENT OF OVERDOSE:

Lavage if taken orally; monitor electrolytes, administer dextrose in saline; monitor hydration, CV, renal status

trace elements (Rx)

Concentrated Multiple Trace Elements, ConTE-PAK-4, M.T.E.-4, M.T.E.-4 Concentrated, M.T.E.-5, M.T.E.-5 Concentrated, M.T.E.-6, M.T.E.-6 Concentrated, M.T.E.-7, MulTE-PAK-4, MulTE-PAK-5, Multiple Trace Element, Multiple Trace Element Neonatal, Multiple Trace Element Pediatric, Neotrace 4, PedTE-PAK-4, Pedtrace-4, P.T.E.-4, P.T.E.-5

Func. class.: Mineral supplements

ACTION: Needed for adequate absorption and synthesis of amino acids

USES: Prevention of trace element deficiency

Precautions: Pregnancy (C), breastfeeding, biliary/hepatic disease, vomiting, diarrhea

DOSAGE AND ROUTES

Usual dosage may be given in TPN sol

Chromium

- **Adult: IV** 10-15 mcg/day
- **Child: IV** 0.14-0.20 mcg/kg/day

Copper

- **Adult: IV** 0.5-1.5 mg/day
- **Child: IV** 0.05-0.2 mg/kg/day

Iodine

- **Adult: IV** 1 mcg/kg/day

Manganese

- **Adult: IV** 0.15-0.8 mg/day

Selenium

- **Adult: IV** 20-40 mcg/day
- **Child: IV** 3 mcg/kg/day

Zinc

- **Adult: IV** 2-4 mg/day
- **Child: IV** 0.05 mg/kg/day

Available forms: Many forms available; see particular elements

Administer:

- By IV inf, often mixed with TPN solution

SIDE EFFECTS

CHROMIUM: Seizures, coma, nausea, vomiting, ulcers, renal/hepatic toxicity

COPPER: Personality changes, diarrhea, weakness, photophobia, muscle weakness

IODINE: Headache, edema of eyelids, acne, metallic taste, sore mouth, runny nose

MANGANESE: Incoordination, headache, irritability, lability, slurred speech, impotence

SELENIUM: Alopecia, depression, vomiting, GI cramping, nervousness, garlic smell

ZINC: Vomiting, oliguria, hypothermia, vision changes, tachycardia, jaundice, coma

NURSING CONSIDERATIONS

Assess:

- Trace element levels; notify prescriber if low; copper 0.07-0.15 mg/ml, zinc 0.05-0.15 mg/100 ml, manganese 4-20 mcg/100 ml, selenium 0.1-0.19 mcg/ml
- Trace element deficiency of patient receiving TPN for extended period

Evaluate:

- Therapeutic response: absence of element deficiency

tramadol (Rx)

(tram′a-dole)

Rybix, Ryzolt, Ultram, Ultram ER, Zytram ✤

Func. class.: Analgesic—miscellaneous

Do not confuse:
tramadol/Toradol

ACTION: Binds to μ-opioid receptors, inhibits reuptake of norepinephrine, serotonin

USES: Management of moderate to severe pain, chronic pain

Unlabeled uses: Restless leg syndrome (RLS), postoperative shivering, arthralgia/myalgia, bone/dental/neuropathic pain

CONTRAINDICATIONS:
Hypersensitivity, acute intoxication with any CNS depressant, alcohol, asthma, respiratory depression

Precautions: Pregnancy (C), breastfeeding, children, geriatric patients, seizure disorder, renal/hepatic disease, respiratory depression, head trauma, increased intracranial pressure, acute abdominal condition, drug abuse, depression, suicidal ideation

DOSAGE AND ROUTES

Mild to moderate pain

- **Adult: PO** 50-100 mg prn q4-6hr; max 400 mg/day; orally disintegrating tab 50 mg/day, titrate by 50 mg q3day, separate doses to 200 mg/day (50 mg qid)
- **Geriatric >75 years: PO** <300 mg/day in divided doses

Moderate to severe chronic pain

- **Adult: PO-ER** (Ultram ER) 100 mg, titrate upward q5days in 100-mg increments, max 300 mg/day; (Ryzolt) 100 mg, titrate upward q2-3days in 100-mg increments, max 300 mg/day; products are not interchangeable

Renal dose

- **Adult: PO** CCr <30 ml/min, give q12hr, max 200 mg/day; do use ext rel tab

Hepatic dose

- **Adult (Child-Pugh C): PO** 50 mg q12hr, do not use ext rel tab

Restless leg syndrome (RLS) (unlabeled)

- **Adult: PO** 50-150 mg/day × 15-24 mo

Available forms: Tabs 50 mg; ext rel tab 100, 200, 300 mg; orally disintegrating tab 50 mg

Administer:

- *Ext rel products* (Ryzolt/Ultram ER) are not interchangeable
- Do not break, crush, or chew ext rel product
- With antiemetic for nausea, vomiting
- When pain is beginning to return; determine dosage interval by patient response

SIDE EFFECTS

CNS: Dizziness, CNS stimulation, somnolence, headache, anxiety, confusion, euphoria, **seizures,** hallucinations, sedation, **neuroleptic-malignant-syndrome–like reactions**

CV: Vasodilation, orthostatic hypotension, tachycardia, hypertension, abnormal ECG

EENT: Visual disturbances

GI: Nausea, constipation, vomiting, dry mouth, diarrhea, abdominal pain, anorexia, flatulence, *GI bleeding*

GU: Urinary retention/frequency, menopausal symptoms, dysuria, menstrual disorder

INTEG: Pruritus, rash, urticaria, vesicles, flushing

SYST: **Anaphylaxis, Stevens-Johnson syndrome, toxic epidermal necrolysis,** serotonin syndrome

PHARMACOKINETICS

Rapidly and almost completely absorbed, steady state 2 days, peak 1.5 hr, duration 6 hr, terminal half-life 7.9-8.8 hr, may cross blood-brain barrier, extensively metabolized, 30% excreted in urine as unchanged product

INTERACTIONS

- Inhibition of norepinephrine and serotonin reuptake: MAOIs; use together with caution

Increase: CNS depression—alcohol, sedatives, hypnotics, opiates

⚠ **Increase:** serotonin syndrome—**SSRIs, SNRIs, serotonin-receptor agonists**

Increase: tramadol levels—CYP3A4 inhibitors (aprepitant, antiretroviral protease inhibitors, clarithromycin, danazol, delavirdine, diltiazem, erythromycin, fluconazole, FLUoxetine, fluvoxamine, imatinib, ketoconazole, mibefradil, nefazodone, telithromycin, voriconazole)

Decrease: tramadol effects—CYP3A4 inducers (barbiturates, bosentan, carBAM-

azepine, efavirenz, phenytoins, nevirapine, rifabutin, rifampin)
Decrease: levels of tramadol—carBAMazepine
Drug/Herb
• Avoid use with St. John's wort
Increase: CNS depression—chamomile, hops, kava, skullcap, valerian
Drug/Lab Test
Increase: creatinine, hepatic enzymes
Decrease: Hgb

NURSING CONSIDERATIONS

Assess:
• **Pain:** location, type, character, give before pain becomes extreme
• I&O ratio: check for decreasing output; may indicate urinary retention
• Need for product; dependency
• Bowel pattern; for constipation, increase fluids, bulk in diet
• CNS changes: dizziness, drowsiness, hallucinations, euphoria, LOC, pupil reaction
• Allergic reactions: rash, urticaria
• Increased side effects in renal/hepatic disease
⚠ **Serotonin syndrome, neuroleptic malignant syndrome:** increased heart rate, shivering, sweating, dilated pupils, tremors, high B/P, hyperthermia, headache, confusion; if these occur, stop product, administer serotonin antagonist if needed
Perform/provide:
• Storage in cool environment, protected from sunlight
• Assistance with ambulation
• Safety measures: side rails, night-light, call bell within easy reach
Evaluate:
• Therapeutic response: decrease in pain
Teach patient/family:
• To report any symptoms of CNS changes, allergic reactions, serotonin syndrome, seizures
• That drowsiness, dizziness, and confusion may occur; to avoid hazardous activities
• To make position changes slowly because orthostatic hypotension may occur
• To avoid OTC medications, herbs, supplements, CNS depressants and alcohol unless approved by prescriber

trandolapril (Rx)

(tran-doe′la-prill)
Mavik
Func. class.: Antihypertensive
Chem. class.: Angiotension-converting enzyme inhibitor

ACTION: Selectively suppresses renin-angiotensin-aldosterone system; inhibits ACE; prevents conversion of angiotensin I to angiotensin II, dilates arterial and venous vessels, lowers B/P

USES: Hypertension, heart failure, left ventricular dysfunction post MI

CONTRAINDICATIONS: Breastfeeding, hypersensitivity, history of angioedema
Black Box Warning: Pregnancy (D) 2nd/3rd trimester
Precautions: Geriatric patients, hyperkalemia, hepatic disease, bilateral renal stenosis, after kidney transplant, aorta/mitral valve stenosis, cirrhosis, severe renal disease, untreated CHF, autoimmune disease, cough, pregnancy (C) 1st trimester

DOSAGE AND ROUTES

Hypertension
• **Adult: PO** 1 mg/day; 2 mg/day in African-Americans; make dosage adjustment ≥1 wk; max 8 mg/day
Heart failure, left ventricular dysfunction post MI
• **Adult: PO** 1 mg/day, titrate upward to 4 mg/day if tolerated
Renal/hepatic dose
• **Adult: PO** CCr <30 ml/min or hepatic disease, 0.5 mg/day
Available forms: Tabs 1, 2, 4 mg

T

Administer:
- Discontinue diuretic 2-3 days before starting this product; if not possible, decrease initial dose to 0.5 ml
- Make dosage changes ≥1 wk

SIDE EFFECTS

CNS: *Dizziness, syncope,* paresthesias, headache, fatigue, drowsiness, depression, sleep disturbances, anxiety
CV: *Hypotension,* MI, palpitations, angina, TIAs, stroke, *bradycardia,* dysrhythmias
GI: Nausea, vomiting, cramps, diarrhea, constipation, pancreatitis, *dyspepsia*
GU: Proteinuria, renal failure
HEMA: Agranulocytosis, neutropenia, leukopenia, anemia
INTEG: Rash, purpura, pruritus
MISC: Hyperkalemia, hyponatremia, impotence, *myalgia,* angioedema, muscle cramps, *asthenia,* hypocalcemia, gout
RESP: Dyspnea, *cough*

PHARMACOKINETICS

Peak 4-10 hr, duration 24 hr, half-life 6-10 hr, metabolized by liver (active metabolite trandolaprilat), excreted in urine, protein binding 65%-94%

INTERACTIONS

Increase: effects—phenothiazines, diuretics
Increase: severe hypotension—diuretics, other antihypertensives
Increase: potassium levels—salt substitutes, potassium-sparing diuretics, potassium supplements
Increase: effects of ergots, neuromuscular blocking agents, antihypertensives, hypoglycemics, barbiturates, reserpine, levodopa, lithium
Decrease: effects of trandolapril—antacids, NSAIDs, salicylates

NURSING CONSIDERATIONS

Assess:
- B/P, pulse q4hr; note rate, rhythm, quality
- Electrolytes: K, Na, Cl
- Baselines of renal, hepatic studies before therapy begins
- Edema in feet, legs daily
- Skin turgor, dryness of mucous membranes for hydration status
- Symptoms of CHF: edema, dyspnea, wet crackles

Evaluate:
- Therapeutic response: decreased B/P

Teach patient/family:
- Not to use OTC (cough, cold, or allergy) products unless directed by prescriber
- To comply with dosage schedule even if feeling better
- To notify prescriber of mouth sores, sore throat, fever, swelling of hands/feet, irregular heartbeat, chest pain, signs of angioedema
- That excessive perspiration, dehydration, vomiting, diarrhea may lead to fall in B/P; to consult prescriber if these occur
- That product may cause dizziness, fainting; lightheadedness may occur during 1st few days of therapy
- That product may cause skin rash or impaired perspiration
- Not to discontinue product abruptly
- To rise slowly to sitting or standing position to minimize orthostatic hypotension

Black Box Warning: To notify prescriber if pregnancy is planned or suspected; pregnancy (D)

⚠ HIGH ALERT

trastuzumab (Rx)

(tras-tuz′uh-mab)

Herceptin

Func. class.: Antineoplastic—miscellaneous

Chem. class.: Humanized monoclonal antibody

ACTION: DNA-derived monoclonal antibody selectively binds to extracellular portion of human epidermal growth factor receptor 2; it inhibits the proliferation of cancer cells

USES:
Breast cancer; metastatic with overexpression of HER2, early breast cancer (adjuvant, neoadjuvant), gastric cancer

CONTRAINDICATIONS:
Pregnancy (D); hypersensitivity to this product, Chinese hamster ovary cell protein

Precautions: Breastfeeding, children, geriatric patients, pulmonary disease, anemia, leukopenia

Black Box Warning: Cardiac disease, respiratory distress syndrome, respiratory insufficiency, infusion-related reactions

DOSAGE AND ROUTES

Breast cancer

- Several regimens may be used
- **Adult:** IV 4 mg/kg given over 90 min then maintenance 2 mg/kg given over 30 min; do not give as IV push or bol; may be given in combination with other antineoplastics

Gastric cancer

- **Adult:** IV 8 mg/kg over 90 min on day 1 then 6 mg/kg over 30-90 min q21days from day 22, give with CISplatin 80 mg/m^2 on day 1 plus 5-fluorouracil 800 mg/m^2 CONT INF on days 1-5 or capecitabine 1000 mg/m^2 bid on days 1-14, repeat cycle q3wk

Available forms: Lyophilized powder 440 mg

Administer:

- Acetaminophen as ordered to alleviate fever and headache

Intermittent IV INF route

- After reconstituting vial with 20 ml bacteriostatic water for inj, 1.1% benzyl alcohol preserved (supplied) to yield 21 mg/ml, mark date on vial 28 days from reconstitution date; if patient is allergic to benzyl alcohol, reconstitute with sterile water for inj; use immediately, infuse over 90 min; q3wk give 8 mg/kg loading dose over 90 min, subsequent 6 mg/kg dose may be given over 30-60 min
- Do not mix or dilute with other products or dextrose sol

SIDE EFFECTS

CNS: *Dizziness, numbness, paresthesias,* depression, *insomnia,* neuropathy, peripheral neuritis
CV: Tachycardia, CHF
GI: Nausea, vomiting, *anorexia, diarrhea,* abdominal pain, **hepatotoxicity**
HEMA: *Anemia,* leukopenia
INTEG: Rash, acne, herpes simplex
META: Edema, peripheral edema
MISC: *Flulike symptoms; fever, headache, chills*
MS: Arthralgia, *bone pain*
RESP: *Cough, dyspnea, pharyngitis, rhinitis,* sinusitis, **pneumonia, pulmonary edema/fibrosis**
SYST: **Anaphylaxis, angioedema**

PHARMACOKINETICS

Half-life 1-32 days

INTERACTIONS

Increase: bleeding risk—warfarin
Increase: cardiomyopathy—anthracyclines, cyclophosphamide; avoid use
Decrease: immune response—vaccines, toxoids

NURSING CONSIDERATIONS

Assess:

- CBC, HER2 overexpression

Black Box Warning: CHF, other cardiac symptoms: dyspnea, coughing; gallop; obtain full cardiac workup including ECG, echo, MUGA

- Symptoms of infection; may be masked by product
- CNS reaction: LOC, mental status, dizziness, confusion

⚠ **Hypersensitive reactions, anaphylaxis**

Black Box Warning: Inf reactions that may be fatal: fever, chills, nausea, vomiting, pain, headache, dizziness, hypotension; discontinue product

Perform/provide:
- Increased fluid intake to 2-3 L/day

Evaluate:
- Therapeutic response: decrease in size of tumors

Teach patient/family:
- To take acetaminophen for fever
- To avoid hazardous tasks because confusion, dizziness may occur
- To report signs of infection: sore throat, fever, diarrhea, vomiting
- That emotional lability is common; to notify prescriber if severe or incapacitating
- To use contraception while taking this product; pregnancy (D); to avoid breastfeeding

travoprost ophthalmic
See Appendix B

traZODone (Rx)
(tray′zoe-done)

Oleptro

Func. class.: Antidepressant—miscellaneous

Chem. class.: Triazolopyridine

Do not confuse:
traZODone/traMADol

ACTION: Selectively inhibits serotonin uptake by brain; potentiates behavorial changes

USES: Depression

Unlabeled uses: Alcoholism, anxiety, panic disorder, insomnia

CONTRAINDICATIONS: Hypersensitivity to tricyclics, recovery phase of MI, seizure disorders, prostatic hypertrophy

Precautions: Pregnancy (C), suicidal patients, severe depression, increased intraocular pressure, closed-angle glaucoma, urinary retention, cardiac/hepatic disease, hyperthyroidism, electroshock therapy, elective surgery, bleeding, abrupt discontinuation, bipolar disorder, breastfeeding, dehydration, hyponatremic, hypovolemia

Black Box Warning: Suicidal ideation in children/adolescents

DOSAGE AND ROUTES
- **Adult: PO** 150 mg/day in divided doses, may increase by 50 mg/day q3-4days, max 400 mg/day (outpatient), 600 mg/day (inpatients); **EXT REL** 150 mg in PM, may increase gradually by 75 mg/day q3days, max 375 mg/day
- **Child 6-18 yr (unlabeled): PO** 1.5-2 mg/kg/day in divided doses, may increase q3-4days up to 6 mg/kg/day or 400 mg/day, whichever is less
- **Geriatric: PO** 25-50 mg at bedtime, increase by 25-50 mg q3-7days to desired dose, usually 75-150 mg/day

Alcoholism (unlabeled)
- **Adult: PO** 50-100 mg/day

Panic disorder (unlabeled)
- **Adult: PO** 150 mg in divided doses, may increase by 50 mg/day q3-4days

Insomnia (unlabeled)
- **Adult: PO** 50 mg at bedtime

Available forms: Tabs 50, 100, 150, 300 mg; ext rel tabs 150, 300 mg

Administer:
- Increased fluids, bulk in diet if constipation occurs, especially in geriatric patients
- With food, milk for GI symptoms
- Dosage at bedtime for oversedation during day; may take entire dose at bedtime; geriatric patients may not tolerate daily dosing
- Gum, hard candy, frequent sips of water for dry mouth
- Avoid use of CNS depressants
- Do not crush, break, chew ext rel product

SIDE EFFECTS

CNS: *Dizziness, drowsiness,* confusion, headache, anxiety, tremors, stimulation, weakness, insomnia, nightmares, EPS (geriatric patients), increase in psychiatric symptoms, **suicide in children/adolescents**

CV: *Orthostatic hypotension, ECG changes, tachycardia,* **hypertension,** palpitations

EENT: *Blurred vision,* tinnitus, mydriasis

GI: *Diarrhea, dry mouth,* nausea, vomiting, **paralytic ileus,** increased appetite, cramps, epigastric distress, jaundice, **hepatitis,** stomatitis, constipation

GU: *Urinary retention,* **acute renal failure,** priapism

HEMA: **Agranulocytosis, thrombocytopenia, eosinophilia, leukopenia**

INTEG: Rash, urticaria, sweating, pruritus, photosensitivity

PHARMACOKINETICS

Peak 1 hr without food, 2 hr with food; metabolized by liver (CYP3A4); excreted by kidneys, in feces; half-life 4.4-7.5 hr

INTERACTIONS

⚠ **Hyperpyretic crisis, seizures, hypertensive episode: MAOIs; do not use within 14 days of traZODone**

Increase: toxicity, serotonin syndrome—FLUoxetine, nefazodone, other SSRIs, SNRIs

Increase: effects of direct-acting sympathomimetics (EPINEPHrine), alcohol, barbiturates, benzodiazepines, CNS depressants, digoxin, phenytoin, carBAMazepine

Increase: effects of traZODone—CYP3A4, 2D6 inhibitors (phenothiazines, protease inhibitors, azole antifungals)

Increase or decrease: effects of warfarin

Decrease: effects of guanethidine, cloNIDine, indirect-acting sympathomimetics (ePHEDrine)

Drug/Herb

Increase: serotonin syndrome—SAM-e, St. John's wort

Increase: CNS depression—hops, kava, lavender, valerian

Drug/Lab Test

Increase: serum bilirubin, blood glucose, alk phos

Decrease: VMA, 5-HIAA

False increase: urinary catecholamines

NURSING CONSIDERATIONS

Assess:

- **Pain:** location, duration, intensity before, 1-2 hr after medication
- B/P lying, standing; pulse q4hr; if systolic B/P drops 20 mm Hg, hold product, notify prescriber; take vital signs q4hr in patients with CV disease
- Blood studies: CBC, leukocytes, differential, cardiac enzymes if patient is receiving long-term therapy
- Hepatic studies: AST, ALT, bilirubin
- Weight weekly; appetite may increase with product
- ECG for flattening of T wave, bundle branch block, AV block, dysrhythmias in cardiac patients
- EPS, primarily in geriatric patients: rigidity, dystonia, akathisia

Black Box Warning: Mental status changes: mood, sensorium, affect, suicidal tendencies, increase in psychiatric symptoms, depression, panic; observe for suicidal behaviors in children/adolescents

- Urinary retention, constipation; constipation most likely in children
- **Withdrawal symptoms:** headache, nausea, vomiting, muscle pain, weakness; not usual unless product discontinued abruptly
- Alcohol consumption; hold dose until morning

⚠ **Serotonin syndrome, neuroleptic malignant syndrome:** increased heart rate, shivering, sweating, dilated pupils, tremors, high B/P, hyperthermia, headache, confusion; if these occur, stop product, administer serotonin antagonist if needed

Perform/provide:
- Storage in tight, light-resistant container at room temp
- Assistance with ambulation during beginning therapy for drowsiness, dizziness
- Safety measures including side rails, primarily for geriatric patients
- Check to confirm that PO medication swallowed

Evaluate:
- Therapeutic response: decreased depression

Teach patient/family:
- That therapeutic effects may take 2-3 wk; to take product before bedtime
- To use caution when driving, performing other activities requiring alertness because of drowsiness, dizziness, blurred vision
- To avoid alcohol ingestion
- Not to discontinue medication quickly after long-term use; may cause nausea, headache, malaise
- To report urinary retention, priapism >4 hr immediately
- To wear sunscreen or large hat because photosensitivity occurs

Black Box Warning: That suicidal thoughts/behaviors may occur (adolescents/children)

TREATMENT OF OVERDOSE:
ECG monitoring; lavage, activated charcoal; administer anticonvulsant, atropine for bradycardia

treprostinil (Rx)
(treh-prah′stin-ill)

Remodulin, Tyvaso

Func. class.: Antiplatelet agent
Chem. class.: Tricyclic benzidine prostacyclin analog

ACTION:
Direct vasodilation of pulmonary, systemic arterial vascular beds; inhibition of platelet aggregation

USES:
Pulmonary arterial hypertension (PAH) NYHA class II through IV

Unlabeled uses: Pulmonary arterial hypertension in children/adolescents, pediatric patients transitioning from epoprostenol to treprostinil, claudication

CONTRAINDICATIONS:
Hypersensitivity to this product, other prostacyclin analogs

Precautions: Pregnancy (B), breastfeeding, children, geriatric patients, past renal/hepatic disease, thromboembolic disease, abrupt discontinuation, IV administration

DOSAGE AND ROUTES
- **Adult: SUBCUT INF** 1.25 ng/kg/min by **CONT INF**, may reduce to 0.625 ng/kg/min if not tolerated; may increase by 1.25 ng/kg/min q wk for first 4 wk then 2.5 ng/kg/min/wk for remainder of inf; **ORAL INH** 3 breaths via Tyvaso inh system qid

Hepatic dose
- **Adult: SUBCUT INF** 0.625 ng/kg ideal body weight/min; increase cautiously

Available forms: Inj 1, 2.5, 5, 10 mg/ml; neb sol 1.74 mg/2.9 ml

Administer:
- Sudden decreased doses, abrupt withdrawal may worsen pulmonary arterial hypertension symptoms

SUBCUT route
- By continuous inf
- No dilution required

Continuous IV INF route
- By surgically placed CV catheter using ambulatory inf pump
- IV pump, product, patient education can be obtained from Priority Healthcare in United States
- Must be diluted with sterile water for inj or 0.9% NaCl
- Conc should be calculated using this formula: diluted conc = [dose (ng/kg/min) × weight (kg) × 0.00006] / inf rate (ml/hr)]

Oral INH route

- Avoid skin, eyes; do not take orally; use Tyvaso Inhalation System only
- Patient should have backup Optineb-ir device to avoid interruptions
- Follow instructions for use, cleaning
- Do not mix with other medications in Optineb-ir device
- Twist off cap, squeeze total contents into medicine cup; vol is sufficient for 4 treatments

SIDE EFFECTS

CNS: Dizziness, headache
CV: Vasodilation, hypotension, edema
GI: Nausea, *diarrhea*
INTEG: *Rash,* pruritus
OTHER: Jaw pain
SYST: Inf site reactions, pain; increased risk for infection

PHARMACOKINETICS

Metabolized by liver; excreted in urine, feces; terminal half-life 2-4 hr; 90% protein binding

INTERACTIONS

- Excessive hypotension: diuretics, antihypertensives, vasodilators, MAOIs, β-blockers, calcium channel blockers

Increase: bleeding tendencies—anticoagulants, aspirin, NSAIDs, thrombin inhibitors, SSRIs

NURSING CONSIDERATIONS

Assess:

- Hepatic studies: AST, ALT, bilirubin, creatinine with long-term therapy
- ⚠ Blood studies: CBC; CBC q2wk × 3 mo, Hct, Hgb, PT with long-term therapy
- ⚠ Bleeding time at baseline, throughout treatment; levels may be 2-5× normal limit

Evaluate:

- Therapeutic response: decreased pulmonary arterial hypertension (PAH)

Teach patient/family:

- That blood work will be necessary during treatment
- To report side effects such as diarrhea, skin rashes
- That therapy will be needed for prolonged periods of time, sometimes years
- To prevent infection, aseptic technique must be used for preparation, administration of treprostinil
- That there are many product, herbal interactions
- About signs, symptoms of bleeding; blood in urine, stools

tretinoin (vit A acid, retinoic acid) (Rx)

(tret′i-noyn)

Avita, Renova, Retin-A, Retin-A Micro, Stieva-A ✤

Func. class.: Vit A acid, acne product; antineoplastic (miscellaneous)
Chem. class.: Tretinoin derivative

ACTION: (Topical) Decreases cohesiveness of follicular epithelium, decreases microcomedone formation; (PO) induces maturation of acute promyelocytic leukemia, exact action is unknown

USES: (Topical) Acne vulgaris (grades 1-3); (PO) acute promyelocytic leukemia, facial wrinkles, photoaging

Unlabeled uses: Acne rosacea, actinic keratosis, ichthyosis, Kaposi's sarcoma, keloids, keratosis follicularis, melasma

CONTRAINDICATIONS: Hypersensitivity to retinoids or sensitivity to parabens

Black Box Warning: Pregnancy (D) (PO)

Precautions: Pregnancy (C) (topical), breastfeeding, eczema, sunburn, sun exposure

Black Box Warning: Rapid-evolving leukocytosis, respiratory compromise, acute promyelocytic leukemia differentiation syndrome

T

DOSAGE AND ROUTES

• **Adult and child: TOP** cleanse area, apply 0.025%-0.1% cream or 0.05% liquid gel at bedtime, cover lightly

Promyelocytic leukemia

• **Adult: PO** 45 mg/m^2/day given as 2 evenly divided doses until remission, discontinue treatment 30 days after remission or 90 days of treatment, whichever is first

Available forms: Cream 0.01%, 0.02%, 0.025%, 0.05%, 0.1%; gel 0.01%, 0.025%, 0.04%, 0.05%, 0.1%; liquid 0.05%; caps 10 mg

Administer:

Topical route

• Once daily before bedtime; cover area lightly using gauze; use gloves to apply

SIDE EFFECTS

Oral

CNS: *Headache, fever, sweating,* fatigue

CV: Cardiac dysrhythmias, pericardial effusion

GI: *Nausea, vomiting,* hemorrhage, *abdominal pain, diarrhea, constipation, dyspepsia, distention, hepatitis*

Topical

INTEG: Rash, stinging, warmth, redness, erythema, blistering, crusting, peeling, contact dermatitis, hypo/hyperpigmentation, dry skin, pruritus, scaly skin, retinoic acid syndrome (RAS)

META: Hypercholesterolemia, hypertriglyceridemia

RESP: Pneumonia, upper respiratory tract disease

PHARMACOKINETICS

PO: Terminal half-life 0.5-2 hr

TOPICAL: Poor systemic absorption

INTERACTIONS

• Use with caution: medicated, abrasive soaps; cleansers that have a drying effect; products with high conc of alcohol astringents (topical)

Increase: peeling—medication containing agents such as sulfur, benzoyl peroxide, resorcinol, salicylic acid (topical)

Increase: plasma concentrations of tretinoin—ketoconazole (PO)

⚠ **Increase:** ICP, risk of pseudotumor cerebri—tetracyclines; do not use together

Increase: photosensitivity—retinoids, quinolones, phenothiazines, sulfonamides, sulfonylureas, thiazide diuretics

Increase: thrombotic complications—aninocaproic acid, aprotinin, tranexamic acid

Drug/Lab Test

Increase: AST, ALT

NURSING CONSIDERATIONS

Assess:

Topical route

• Area of body involved, what helps or aggravates condition; cysts, dryness, itching; lesions may worsen at beginning of treatment

PO route

• Hepatic function, coagulation, hematologic parameters; also cholesterol, triglycerides

Perform/provide:

Topical route

• Storage at room temp

• Hand washing after application

Evaluate:

• Therapeutic response: decrease in size, number of lesions

Teach patient/family:

Topical route

• To avoid application on normal skin; to avoid getting cream in eyes, nose, other mucous membranes; not to use product on areas with cuts, scrapes

• To use cream/gel by applying a thin layer to affected skin; to rub gently; to use liquid; to apply with fingertip or cotton swab

• To avoid sunlight, sunlamps; to use protective clothing, sunscreen

• That treatment may cause warmth, stinging; that dryness, peeling will occur

• That cosmetics may be used over product; not to use shaving lotions

• That rash may occur during first 1-3 wk of therapy

- That product does not cure condition, only relieves symptoms
- That therapeutic results may be seen in 2-3 wk but may not be optimal until after 6 wk

PO route

Black Box Warning: To notify prescriber if pregnancy is planned or suspected; pregnancy (D) PO

tretinoin topical

See Appendix B

triamcinolone (Rx)

(trye-am-sin′oh-lone)

Aristospan, Kenalog-10, Kenalog-40, Tac-3, Triesence

Func. class.: Corticosteroid, synthetic

Chem. class.: Glucocorticoid, intermediate acting

See ophthalmic in Appendix B

ACTION: Decreases inflammation by suppression of migration of polymorphonuclear leukocytes, fibroblasts; reversal of increased capillary permeability and lysosomal stabilization

USES: Severe inflammation, immunosuppression, neoplasms, asthma (steroid dependent); collagen, respiratory, dermatologic/rheumatic disorders

CONTRAINDICATIONS: Children <2 yr, psychosis, hypersensitivity, idiopathic thrombocytopenia, acute glomerulonephritis, amebiasis, fungal infections, nonasthmatic bronchial disease, AIDS, TB, adrenal insufficiency, acute bronchospasm, neonatal prematurity; epidural/intrathecal administration (Triamcinolone acetonide injections [Kenalog])

Precautions: Pregnancy (C), breastfeeding, diabetes mellitus, glaucoma, osteoporosis, seizure disorders, ulcerative colitis, CHF, myasthenia gravis, renal disease, esophagitis, peptic ulcer, acne, cataracts, coagulopathy, head trauma

DOSAGE AND ROUTES

- **Adult: PO** 4-12 mg/day in divided doses daily-qid; **IM** (acetonide, diacetate) 40 mg/wk; (diacetate, acetonide) 5-48 mg into neoplasms; (diacetate, acetonide) 2-40 mg into joint or soft tissue; (hexacetonide) 0.5 mg/in^2 of affected intralesional skin; (hexacetonide) 2-20 mg into joint or soft tissue
- **Child: PO** 117 mcg/kg/day in divided doses

Asthma

- **Adult: INH** 2 tid-qid, max 16 inh/day
- **Child 6-12 yr: INH** 1-2 tid-qid, max 12 inh/day

Severe/incapacitating allergic conditions such as asthma

- **Adult: IM** (Trivaris) 60 mg, titrate, usual range 40-80 mg
- **Child: IM** (Trivaris) 0.11-1.6 mg/kg/day (3.2-48 mg/m^2/day) in 3-4 divided doses

Available forms: Inj 25, 40 mg/ml diacetate; inj 3, 10, 40 mg/ml acetonide; inj 20, 5 mg/ml hexacetonide; aerosol actuation/100 mcg (acetonide)

Administer:

- After shaking susp (parenteral)
- Titrated dose; use lowest effective dose
- IM inj deep in large muscle mass; rotate sites; avoid deltoid; use 21G needle
- In 1 dose in AM to prevent adrenal suppression; avoid SUBCUT administration, may damage tissue
- Mouth should be rinsed after inhalations

SIDE EFFECTS

CNS: *Depression, flushing, sweating,* headache, mood changes

CV: *Hypertension,* **circulatory collapse, thrombophlebitis, embolism,** tachycardia, edema

EENT: Fungal infections, increased intraocular pressure, blurred vision

T

GI: *Diarrhea, nausea, abdominal distention,* GI hemorrhage, *increased appetite,* pancreatitis
HEMA: Thrombocytopenia
INTEG: Acne, poor wound healing, ecchymosis, petechiae
MS: Fractures, osteoporosis, weakness

PHARMACOKINETICS

PO/IM: Peak 1-2 hr, half-life 2-5 hr

INTERACTIONS

Increase: side effects—alcohol, salicylates, indomethacin, amphotericin B, digoxin, cycloSPORINE, diuretics
Increase: action of triamcinolone—salicylates, estrogens, indomethacin, oral contraceptives, ketoconazole, macrolide antiinfectives
Decrease: action of triamcinolone—cholestyramine, colestipol, barbiturates, rifampin, ePHEDrine, phenytoin, theophylline
Decrease: effects of anticoagulants, anticonvulsants, antidiabetics, ambenonium, neostigmine, isoniazid, toxoids, vaccines, anticholinesterases, salicylates, somatrem

Drug/Herb
- Hypokalemia: aloe, cascara, senna

Drug/Lab Test
Increase: cholesterol, sodium, blood glucose, uric acid, calcium, urine glucose
Decrease: Ca, K, T_4, T_3, thyroid ^{131}I uptake test, urine 17-OHCS, 17-KS, PBI
False negative: skin allergy tests

NURSING CONSIDERATIONS

Assess:
- Potassium, blood glucose, urine glucose while patient receiving long-term therapy; hypokalemia and hyperglycemia
- Weight daily; notify prescriber if weekly gain of >5 lb
- B/P, pulse; notify prescriber if chest pain occurs
- I&O ratio; be alert for decreasing urinary output, increasing edema
- Plasma cortisol levels during long-term therapy (normal level: 138-635 nmol/L SI units when drawn at 8 AM)
- **Infection:** increased temp, WBC even after withdrawal of medication; product masks infection
- Potassium depletion: paresthesias, fatigue, nausea, vomiting, depression, polyuria, dysrhythmias, weakness
- Edema, hypertension, cardiac symptoms
- Mental status: affect, mood, behavioral changes, aggression

Perform/provide:
- Assistance with ambulation for patient with bone-tissue disease to prevent fractures
- Use of spacer device for geriatric patients with inhaler

Evaluate:
- Therapeutic response: ease of respirations, decreased inflammation

Teach patient/family:
- That emergency ID as corticosteroid user should be carried
- To notify prescriber if therapeutic response decreases; that dosage adjustment may be needed
- Not to discontinue abruptly because adrenal crisis can result
- To avoid OTC products: salicylates, alcohol in cough products, cold preparations unless directed by prescriber
- About cushingoid symptoms
- About the symptoms of adrenal insufficiency: nausea, anorexia, fatigue, dizziness, dyspnea, weakness, joint pain

triamcinolone nasal agent

See Appendix B

triamcinolone ophthalmic

See Appendix B

triamcinolone topical

See Appendix B

triamcinolone (topical-oral) (OTC)

(trye-am-sin′oh-lone)

Kenalog in Orabase, Oralone Dental

Func. class.: Topical anesthetic

Chem. class.: Synthetic fluorinated adrenal corticosteroid

ACTION: Binds with steroid receptors, decreases inflammation

USES: Oral pain

CONTRAINDICATIONS: Infants <1 yr, hypersensitivity, application to large areas; presence of fungal, viral, or bacterial infections of mouth or throat

Precautions: Pregnancy (C), children <6 yr, sepsis, denuded skin

DOSAGE AND ROUTES

• **Adult and child: TOP** Press 1/4 inch into affected area until film appears, repeat bid-tid

Available forms: Paste 0.1%

Administer:

• After cleansing oral cavity after meals

SIDE EFFECTS

INTEG: Rash, irritation, sensitization

NURSING CONSIDERATIONS

Assess:

• Allergy: rash, irritation, reddening, swelling

• Infection: if affected area is infected, do not apply

Evaluate:

• Therapeutic response: absence of pain in affected area

Teach patient/family:

• To report rash, irritation, redness, swelling

• How to apply paste

triazolam (Rx)

(trye-ay′zoe-lam)

Apo-Triazo ✦, Halcion

Func. class.: Sedative-hypnotic, antianxiety

Chem. class.: Benzodiazepine, short acting

Controlled Substance Schedule IV (USA), Targeted (CDSA IV) (Canada)

ACTION: Produces CNS depression at limbic, thalamic, hypothalamic levels of CNS; may be mediated by neurotransmitter γ-aminobutyric acid (GABA); results are sedation, hypnosis, skeletal muscle relaxation, anticonvulsant activity, anxiolytic action

USES: Insomnia, sedative/hypnotic

CONTRAINDICATIONS: Pregnancy (X), breastfeeding, hypersensitivity to benzodiazepines, intermittent porphyria

Precautions: Children <15 yr, geriatric patients, anemia, renal/hepatic disease, suicidal individuals, drug abuse, psychosis, acute closed-angle glaucoma, seizure disorders, angioedema, respiratory disease, depression, sleep-related behaviors (sleep walking)

DOSAGE AND ROUTES

• **Adult: PO** 0.125-0.5 mg at bedtime, max 0.5 mg/day

• **Geriatric: PO** 0.0625-0.125 mg at bedtime, max 0.25 mg/day

Available forms: Tabs 0.125, 0.25 mg

T

Administer:

- After trying conservative measures for insomnia
- $^{1}/_{2}$ hr before bedtime for sleeplessness
- On empty stomach for fast onset; may be taken with food if GI symptoms occur
- Avoid use with CNS depressants; serious CNS depression may result

SIDE EFFECTS

CNS: *Headache, lethargy, drowsiness, daytime sedation,* dizziness, confusion, lightheadedness, anxiety, irritability, amnesia, poor coordination, complex sleep-related reactions: sleep driving, sleep eating

CV: Chest pain, pulse changes

GI: Nausea, vomiting, diarrhea, heartburn, abdominal pain, constipation, hepatic injury

HEMA: Leukopenia, granulocytopenia (rare)

SYST: Severe allergic reactions

PHARMACOKINETICS

Onset 30-45 min, duration 6-8 hr, metabolized by liver, excreted by kidneys (inactive metabolites), crosses placenta, excreted in breast milk, half-life 2-3 hr

INTERACTIONS

- Smoking may decrease hypnotic effect

Increase: triazolam levels—CYP3A4 inhibitors, protease inhibitors

⚠ **Increase:** effects of cimetidine, disulfiram, erythromycin, clarithromycin, probenecid, isoniazid, oral contraceptives; do not use concurrently

Increase: action of both products—alcohol, CNS depressants

Decrease: effect of antacids, theophylline, rifampin, smoking

Drug/Herb

Increase: CNS depression—chamomile, hops, kava, lavender, valerian

Drug/Lab Test

Increase: ALT, AST, serum bilirubin

Decrease: RAI uptake

False increase: urinary 17-OHCS

NURSING CONSIDERATIONS

Assess:

- Blood studies: Hct, Hgb, RBC if blood dyscrasias suspected (rare)
- Hepatic studies: AST, ALT, bilirubin if hepatic damage has occurred
- Mental status: mood, sensorium, affect, memory (long, short term), insomnia, withdrawal symptoms, excessive sedation, impaired coordination
- Blood dyscrasias: fever, sore throat, bruising, rash, jaundice, epistaxis (rare)
- Type of sleep problem: falling asleep, staying asleep

Perform/provide:

- Assistance with ambulation after receiving dose
- Safety measures: side rails, night-light, call bell within easy reach
- Check to confirm that PO medication has been swallowed
- Cool storage in tight container

Evaluate:

- Therapeutic response: ability to sleep at night, decreased amount of early morning awakening if taking product for insomnia

Teach patient/family:

- To use reliable contraception; pregnancy category (X)
- That dependence is possible after long-term use
- To avoid driving, other activities requiring alertness until product is stabilized
- To avoid alcohol ingestion
- That effects may take 2 nights for benefits to be noticed; that product is for short-term use only; to use for 7-10 continuous nights
- About alternative measures to improve sleep: reading, exercise several hours before bedtime, warm bath, warm milk, TV, self-hypnosis, deep breathing
- That complex sleep-related behaviors (sleep eating/driving) may occur
- That hangover common in geriatric patients but less common than with barbiturates; that rebound insomnia may occur for 1-2 nights after discontinuing

product; to discontinue by decreasing dose by 50% q2 nights until 0.125 mg for 2 nights, then stop

TREATMENT OF OVERDOSE:
Lavage, activated charcoal; monitor electrolytes, VS

trifluridine ophthalmic
See Appendix B

trimethobenzamide (Rx)
(trye-meth-oh-ben′za-mide)

Tigan

Func. class.: Antiemetic, anticholinergic

Chem. class.: Ethanolamine derivative

ACTION:
Acts centrally by blocking chemoreceptor trigger zone, which in turn acts on vomiting center

USES:
Nausea, vomiting

CONTRAINDICATIONS:
Children (parenterally), hypersensitivity to opioids, shock

Precautions: Pregnancy (C), children, geriatric patients, cardiac dysrhythmias, acute febrile illness, encephalitis, gastroenteritis, dehydration, electrolyte imbalances, Reye's syndrome

DOSAGE AND ROUTES
Nausea/vomiting
- **Adult: IM** 200 mg 3-4×/day; **PO** 300 mg 3-4×/day

Postoperative
- **Adult: IM** 200 mg followed by 2nd dose 1 hr later

Renal dose
- **Adult: IM** CCr 15-30 ml/min, give 50% of dose

Available forms: Caps 300 mg; inj 100 mg/ml

Administer:

PO route
- Capsules may be swallowed whole, chewed, allowed to dissolve

IM route
- Inj in large muscle mass; aspirate to avoid IV administration; inj not to be used in children or infants

Syringe compatibilities: Butorphanol, glycopyrrolate, HYDROmorphone, midazolam, nalbuphine

SIDE EFFECTS
CNS: *Drowsiness,* headache, dizziness, confusion, disorientation, **coma, seizures,** depression, *vertigo,* EPS

CV: Hypo/hypertension, palpitation, **cardiac dysrhythmias**

EENT: Dry mouth, blurred vision, photosensitivity

GI: Nausea, diarrhea, vomiting, difficulty swallowing

INTEG: Rash, urticaria, fever, chills, flushing, hyperpyrexia

PHARMACOKINETICS
Metabolized by liver, excreted by kidneys

PO: Onset 20-40 min, duration 3-4 hr

IM: Onset 15-35 min, duration 2-3 hr

INTERACTIONS
Increase: effect—CNS depressants, alcohol

NURSING CONSIDERATIONS
Assess:
- Nausea, vomiting before, after treatment
- VS, B/P; check patients with cardiac disease more often
- Signs of toxicity of other products or masking of symptoms of disease: brain tumor, intestinal obstruction
- Observe for drowsiness, dizziness

Evaluate:
- Therapeutic response: decreased nausea, vomiting

Teach patient/family:
- To avoid hazardous activities, activities requiring alertness because dizziness

T

may occur; to request assistance with ambulation
- To avoid alcohol, other depressants
- To keep out of children's reach

trimethoprim-sulfamethoxazole (Rx)

(trye-meth'oh-prim–sul-fa-meth-ox'a-zole)

Apo-Sulfatrim ✤, Bacter-Aid DS, Bactrim DS, Novo-Trimel ✤, Nu-Cotrimox ✤, Septra, Septra DS, Sultrex, SMZ/TMP

Func. class.: Antiinfective
Chem. class.: Sulfonamide—miscellaneous

ACTION: Sulfamethoxazole (SMZ) interferes with the bacterial biosynthesis of proteins by competitive antagonism of PABA when adequate levels are maintained; trimethoprim (TMP) blocks the synthesis of tetrahydrofolic acid; the combination blocks 2 consecutive steps in the bacterial synthesis of essential nucleic acids and protein

USES: UTI, otitis media, acute and chronic prostatitis, shigellosis, *Pneumocystis jiroveci* pneumonitis, chronic bronchitis, chancroid, traveler's diarrhea

CONTRAINDICATIONS: Breastfeeding, infants <2 mo; hypersensitivity to trimethoprim or sulfonamides; pregnancy at term, megaloblastic anemia, CCr <15 ml/min, porphyria, hyperkalemia

Precautions: Pregnancy (C), geriatric patients, infants, renal disease, G6PD deficiency, impaired hepatic/renal function, possible folate deficiency, severe allergy, bronchial asthma, UV exposure

DOSAGE AND ROUTES

Based on TMP content

UTI
- **Adult: PO** 160 mg TMP q12hr × 10-14 days
- **Child: PO** 8 mg/kg TMP/day in 2 divided doses q12hr

Otitis media
- **Child: PO** 8 mg/kg TMP/day in 2 divided doses q12hr × 10 days

Chronic bronchitis
- **Adult: PO** 160 mg TMP q12hr × 10-14 days

Pneumocystis jiroveci *pneumonitis*
- **Adult and child: PO** 15-20 mg/kg TMP daily in 4 divided doses q6hr × 14 days; **IV** 15-20 mg/kg/day (based on TMP) in 3-4 divided doses for ≤14 days
- Dosage reduction necessary in moderate to severe renal impairment (CCr <30 ml/min)

Available forms: Tabs 80 mg trimethoprim/400 mg sulfamethoxazole, 160 mg trimethoprim/800 mg sulfamethoxazole; susp 40 mg/200 mg/5 ml; IV 16 mg/80 mg/ml

Administer:

PO route
- Medication after C&S; repeat C&S after full course of medication
- With resuscitative equipment, EPINEPHrine available; severe allergic reactions may occur
- On an empty stomach 1 hr before or 2 hr after meals
- With full glass of water to maintain adequate hydration; increase fluids to 2 L/day to decrease crystallization in kidneys

Intermittent IV INF route
- After diluting 5 ml of product/125 ml D_5W, run over 1-1½ hr

Y-site compatibilities: Acyclovir, aldesleukin, allopurinol, amifostine, amphotericin B cholesteryl, atracurium, aztreonam, cefepime, cyclophosphamide, diltiazem, DOXOrubicin liposome, enalaprilat, esmolol, filgrastim, fludarabine, gallium, granisetron, HYDROmorphone, labetalol, LORazepam, magnesium sulfate, melphalan, meperidine, morphine, pancuronium, perphenazine, piperacillin/tazobactam, remifentanil, sargramostim, tacrolimus, teniposide, thiotepa, vecuronium, zidovudine

SIDE EFFECTS

CNS: Headache, insomnia, hallucinations, depression, vertigo, fatigue, anxiety, **seizures**, product fever, chills, **aseptic meningitis**

CV: **Allergic myocarditis**

EENT: Tinnitus

GI: *Nausea, vomiting, abdominal pain,* stomatitis, **hepatitis**, glossitis, **pancreatitis**, diarrhea, **enterocolitis**, anorexia, **pseudomembranous colitis**

GU: **Renal failure, toxic nephrosis**; increased BUN, creatinine; crystalluria

HEMA: **Leukopenia, neutropenia, thrombocytopenia, agranulocytosis, hemolytic anemia, hypoprothrombinemia, Henoch-Schönlein purpura, methemoglobinemia, eosinophilia I**

INTEG: Rash, dermatitis, urticaria, **Stevens-Johnson syndrome**, erythema, photosensitivity, pain, inflammation at inj site, **toxic epidermal necrolysis, erythema multiforme**

RESP: Cough, SOB

SYST: **Anaphylaxis, SLE**

PHARMACOKINETICS

PO: Rapidly absorbed; peak 1-4 hr; half-life 8-13 hr; excreted in urine (metabolites and unchanged), breast milk; crosses placenta; 68% bound to plasma proteins; TMP achieves high levels in prostatic tissue and fluid

INTERACTIONS

Increase: thrombocytopenia—thiazide diuretics

Increase: potassium levels—potassium-sparing diuretics, potassium supplements

Increase: hypoglycemic response—sulfonylurea agents

Increase: anticoagulant effects—oral anticoagulants

Increase: levels of dofetilide

Increase: crystalluria—methenamine

Increase: bone marrow depressant effects—methotrexate

Decrease: hepatic clearance of phenytoin, CYP2C9, CYP3A4 inducers

Decrease: response—cycloSPORINE

Drug/Lab Test

Increase: alk phos, creatinine, bilirubin, AST, ALT

NURSING CONSIDERATIONS

Assess:

- I&O ratio; note color, character, pH of urine if product administered for UTI; output should be 800 ml less than intake; if urine is highly acidic, alkalization may be needed
- Renal studies: BUN, creatinine, urinalysis with long-term therapy
- Type of infection; obtain C&S before starting therapy
- Blood dyscrasias, skin rash, fever, sore throat, bruising, bleeding, fatigue, joint pain
- **Allergic reaction:** rash, dermatitis, urticaria, pruritus, dyspnea, bronchospasm; product should be discontinued at 1st sign of rash; AIDS patients more susceptible

Perform/provide:

- Storage in tight, light-resistant container at room temp

Evaluate:

- Therapeutic response: absence of pain, fever; C&S negative

Teach patient/family:

- To take each oral dose with full glass of water to prevent crystalluria; to drink 8-10 glasses of water/day; to take product on an empty stomach 1 hr before meals, 2 hr after meals
- To complete full course of treatment to prevent superinfection
- To avoid sunlight; to use sunscreen to prevent burns
- To avoid OTC medications (aspirin, vit C) unless directed by prescriber
- To use alternative contraceptive measures; that decreased effectiveness of oral contraceptives may occur
- To notify prescriber if skin rash, sore throat, fever, mouth sores, unusual bruising, bleeding occur; to notify prescriber of CNS effects: anxiety, depression, hallucinations, seizures

tropicamide ophthalmic

See Appendix B

trospium (Rx)

(trose′pee-um)

Sanctura, Sanctura XR

Func. class.: Anticholinergic

Chem. class.: Muscarinic receptor antagonist

ACTION: Relaxes smooth muscles in bladder by inhibiting acetylcholine effect on muscarinic receptors

USES: Overactive bladder (urinary frequency, urgency)

CONTRAINDICATIONS: Hypersensitivity, uncontrolled closed-angle glaucoma, urinary retention, gastric retention, myasthenia gravis

Precautions: Pregnancy (C), breastfeeding, children, geriatric patients, renal/hepatic disease, controlled closed-angle glaucoma, ulcerative colitis, intestinal atony, bladder outflow obstruction

DOSAGE AND ROUTES

- **Adult <75 yr: PO** 20 mg bid 1 hr before meals or on empty stomach; **ER** 60 mg in AM
- **Geriatric ≥75 yr: PO** titrate down to 20 mg/day based on response and tolerance

Renal dose

- **Adult: PO** CCr <30 ml/min, 20 mg/day at bedtime, ext rel product not recommended

Available forms: Tabs 20 mg; caps ext rel 60 mg

Administer:

- 1 hr before meals or on empty stomach (reg rel); in AM (ext rel) ≥1 hr before meal

SIDE EFFECTS

CNS: Fatigue, dizziness, headache
CV: Tachycardia
EENT: Dry eyes, vision abnormalities
GI: Flatulence, abdominal pain, *constipation, dry mouth,* dyspepsia
GU: Urinary retention, UTI
INTEG: Dry skin, **angioedema**
MISC: Heat stroke, fever

PHARMACOKINETICS

Rapidly absorbed (10%); peak 5-6 hr; protein bound (50%-85%); extensively metabolized; excreted in urine, feces; excreted in urine by active tubular secretion; half-life 20 hr

INTERACTIONS

Increase: drowsiness—CNS depressants, alcohol

Increase or decrease: trospium effect—products excreted by active renal secretion (amiloride, digoxin, morphine), metformin, quiNIDine, procainamide, ranitidine, tenofovir, triamterene, vancomycin

Drug/Food

Decrease: absorption—high-fat meal

NURSING CONSIDERATIONS

Assess:

- **Urinary patterns:** distention, nocturia, frequency, urgency, incontinence

Evaluate:

- Therapeutic response: correction of urinary status: absence of dysuria, frequency, nocturia, incontinence

Teach patient/family:

- To avoid hazardous activities because dizziness may occur
- That alcohol may increase drowsiness
- About anticholinergic effects that may occur
- That overheating may occur with strenuous exercise

undecylenic acid topical

See Appendix B

unoprostone ophthalmic

See Appendix B

⚠ HIGH ALERT

urokinase (Rx)

(yoor-oh-kin′ase)

Kinlytic

Func. class.: Thrombolytic

Chem. class.: β-Hemolytic streptococcus filtrate (purified)

ACTION: Promotes thrombolysis by directly converting plasminogen to plasmin

USES: Pulmonary embolism

Unlabeled uses: Acute MI, arterial thromboembolism, coronary artery thrombosis, DVT, occluded IV catheter, percutaneous coronary intervention, venous thrombosis, arterial embolism

CONTRAINDICATIONS: Hypersensitivity to this product or other thrombolytic enzymes; internal active bleeding, intraspinal surgery, neoplasms of CNS, ulcerative colitis/enteritis, severe uncontrolled hypertension, renal/hepatic disease, hypocoagulation, COPD, subacute bacterial endocarditis, rheumatic valvular disease, cerebral embolism/thrombosis/hemorrhage, intraarterial diagnostic procedure or surgery (10 days), recent major surgery/trauma, aneurysm AV malformation

Precautions: Pregnancy (B), arterial emboli from left side of heart, hepatic disease

DOSAGE AND ROUTES

Lysis of pulmonary emboli

- **Adult: IV** 4400 international units/kg over 10 min (90 ml/hr) then **CONT IV INF** 4400 international units/kg/hr × 12 hr (15 ml/hr); flush line at end of INF

Acute MI

- **Adult: Intracoronary administration: INSTILL** 6000 international units/min into occluded artery for 1-2 hr after giving **IV BOL** of heparin 2500-10,000 units
- May also give as **IV INF** 2 million-3 million units over 45-90 min

Venous catheter occlusion (unlabeled)

- **Adult and child: INSTILL** 5000 international units into line, wait 5 min, then aspirate, repeat aspiration attempts q5min × ½ hr; if occlusion not removed, cap line, wait ½-1 hr, then aspirate; may need 2nd dose if still occluded

Available forms: Powder for inj, lyophilized 250,000 international units/vial; powder for catheter clearance

Administer:

Intermittent IV INF route

- Using programmable inf pump, terminal filter ≤0.45 μm
- Reconstitute only with 5 ml sterile water for inj (not bacteriostatic water)/250,000 international units urokinase (Kinlytic), roll (do not shake) to enhance reconstitution; further dilute with 190 ml; give as intermittent inf or give to clear cannula by using 1 ml diluted product; inject into cannula slowly, clamp 5 min, aspirate clot; avoid excessive pressure when urokinase is injected into catheter; force could rupture catheter or expel clot into circulation
- As soon as thrombi identified; not useful for thrombi >1 wk old
- Cryoprecipitate or fresh frozen plasma if bleeding occurs
- Loading dose at beginning of therapy; may require increased loading doses
- Heparin therapy after thrombolytic therapy is discontinued, TT or APTT <2× control (about 3-4 hr)

U

Y-site compatibilities: Alfentanil, amikacin, aminophylline, ascorbic acid, atracurium, atropine, aztreonam, benztropine, bumetanide, buprenorphine, butorphanol, calcium chloride/gluconate, ceFAZolin, cefoperazone, cefotaxime, cefotetan, cefoxitin, ceftazidime, cefuroxime, chloramphenicol, cimetidine, clindamycin, cyanocobalamin, cycloSPORINE, dexamethasone, digoxin, diphenhydrAMINE, DOBUTamine, DOPamine, doxycycline, enalaprilat, ePHEDrine, EPINEPHrine, epoetin, erythromycin, esmolol, famotidine, fentaNYL, fluconazole, folic acid, furosemide, gentamicin, glycopyrrolate, heparin, hydrocortisone, imipenem-cilastatin, insulin, isoproterenol, ketorolac, labetalol, lidocaine, magnesium sulfate, mannitol, meperidine, metaraminol, methoxamine, methyldopate, metoclopramide, metoprolol, midazolam, morphine, multivitamins, nafcillin, nalbuphine, naloxone, nitroglycerin, nitroprusside, norepinephrine, ondansetron, oxytocin, papaverine, penicillin G, pentamidine, pentazocine, PENTobarbital, PHENobarbital, phenylephrine, phytonadione, potassium chloride, procainamide, propranolol, protamine, pyridoxime, ranitidine, sodium bicarbonate, streptokinase, succinylcholine, SUFentanil, theophylline, thiamine, ticarcillin/clavulanate, tobramycin, tolazoline, trimetaphan, vasopressin, verapamil

SIDE EFFECTS

CNS: *Headache,* fever
CV: Hypotension, dysrhythmias
GI: *Nausea, vomiting*
HEMA: *Decreased Hct,* bleeding
INTEG: *Rash, urticaria,* phlebitis at IV inf site, itching, flushing
MS: Low back pain
RESP: Altered respirations, SOB, bronchospasm, cyanosis
SYST: GI, GU, intracranial, retroperitoneal bleeding, surface bleeding, anaphylaxis (rare)

PHARMACOKINETICS

IV: Half-life 10-20 min; small amounts excreted in urine, cleared by liver

INTERACTIONS

Increase: bleeding potential—aspirin, indomethacin, phenylbutazone, anticoagulants, other NSAIDs, abciximab, eptifibatide, tirofiban, clopidogrel, ticlopidine, some cephalosporins, plicamycin, valproic acid, dipyridamole, glycoprotein IIb, IIIa inhibitors

Drug/Lab Test
Increase: PT, APTT, TT

NURSING CONSIDERATIONS

Assess:

- VS, B/P, pulse, resp, neurologic signs, temp at least q4hr; temp >104° F (40° C) indicates internal bleeding; cardiac rhythm after intracoronary administration
- Neurologic changes that may indicate intracranial bleeding
- **Retroperitoneal bleeding:** back pain, leg weakness, diminished pulses
- Peripheral pulses, lung sounds, respiratory function
- **Hypersensitivity:** fever, rash, itching, chills, facial swelling, dyspnea; mild reaction may be treated with antihistamines; notify prescriber of severe reactions, stop product, keep resuscitative equipment nearby
- **Bleeding** during 1st hr of treatment (hematuria, hematemesis, bleeding from mucous membranes, epistaxis, ecchymosis)
- Blood studies (Hct, platelets, PTT, PT, TT, APTT) before starting therapy; PT or APTT must be <2× control before starting therapy; TT or PT q3-4hr during treatment
- ECG continuously, cardiac enzymes, radionuclide myocardial scanning/coronary angiography

Perform/provide:

- Storage in refrigerator; use immediately after reconstitution

• Bed rest during entire course of treatment; use caution when handling patients
• Avoidance of venous/arterial puncture procedures, inj, rectal temp
• Treatment of fever with acetaminophen or aspirin
• Placement of sign above patient's bed stating urokinase therapy
• Pressure for 30 sec to minor bleeding sites, 30 min to sites of arterial puncture followed by pressure dressing; inform prescriber if hemostasis not attained, apply pressure dressing

Evaluate:
• Therapeutic response: decreased clotting, thrombosis, embolism

Teach patient/family:
• To report immediately any sign of bleeding, easy bruising, urinating less than usual or not at all, weak or shallow breathing
• That bed rest is needed during treatment
• About reasons for treatment and expected results

ursodiol (Rx)
(ur-soh-die′-ohl)

Actigall, Urso

Func. class.: Gallstone solubilizing agent

Chem. class.: Ursodeoxycholic acid

ACTION: Suppresses hepatic synthesis, secretion of cholesterol; inhibits intestinal absorption of cholesterol

USES: Dissolution of radiolucent, noncalcified gallbladder stones (<20 mm in diameter) for which surgery is not indicated; biliary cirrhosis, gallstone prophylaxis

Unlabeled uses: Severe pruritus, cholestasis secondary to cystic fibrosis, intrahepatic cholestasis of pregnancy (ICP), nonalcoholic steatosis-hepatitis (NASH)

CONTRAINDICATIONS: Calcified cholesterol stones, radiopaque stones, radiolucent bile pigment stones, chronic hepatic disease, hypersensitivity, biliary obstruction, pancreatitis compelling for cholecystectomy

Precautions: Pregnancy (B), breastfeeding, children

DOSAGE AND ROUTES
• **Adult: PO** 8-10 mg/kg/day in 2-3 divided doses using gallbladder ultrasound q6mo; determine if stones have dissolved; if so, continue therapy, repeat ultrasound within 1-3 mo

Primary biliary cirrhosis
• **Adult: PO** (Urso tabs) 13-15 mg/kg/day in divided doses 2-4×/day

Gallstone prophylaxis with rapid weight loss
• **Adult: PO** 300 mg bid AM and PM with food

Available forms: Caps 300 mg; tabs 250, 500 mg

Administer:
• Up to 6-24 mo; if no improvement seen, discontinue product; dosing depends on size, composition of stones

SIDE EFFECTS
CNS: Headache, anxiety, depression, insomnia, fatigue

GI: Diarrhea, nausea, vomiting, abdominal pain, constipation, stomatitis, flatulence, dyspepsia, biliary pain

INTEG: Pruritus, rash, urticaria, dry skin, sweating, alopecia

MS: Arthralgia, myalgia, back pain

OTHER: Cough, rhinitis

PHARMACOKINETICS
80% excreted in feces; 20% metabolized, excreted into bile, lost in feces

INTERACTIONS
Increase: risk of stone formation—clofibrate, gemfibrozil, estrogens, oral contraceptives

U

Decrease: action of ursodiol—cholestyramine, colestipol, aluminum-based antacids

NURSING CONSIDERATIONS

Assess:

- **GI status:** diarrhea, abdominal pain, nausea, vomiting; product may have to be discontinued if side effects severe
- Skin for pruritus, rash, urticaria, dry skin; provide soothing lotion to lesions
- Musculoskeletal status: aches or stiffness in joints

Evaluate:

- Therapeutic response: decreasing size of stones on ultrasound

Teach patient/family:

- That anxiety, depression, insomnia are side effects and are reversible after discontinuing product

valacyclovir (Rx)

(val-a-sye′kloh-vir)

Valtrex

Func. class.: Antiviral

Chem. class.: Acyclic purine nucleoside analog

Do not confuse:

valacyclovir/valganciclovir

Valtrex/Valcyte

ACTION: Interferes with DNA synthesis by conversion to acyclovir, thereby causing decreased viral replication, time of lesional healing

USES: Treatment or suppression of herpes zoster (shingles), genital herpes, herpes labialis (cold sores), varicella, varicella-zoster

Unlabeled uses: CMV with advanced HIV, posttransplant patients, Bell's palsy, herpes simplex virus prophylaxis, acute retinal necrosis (ARN), encephalitis

CONTRAINDICATIONS: Hypersensitivity to this product or acyclovir, valganciclovir

Precautions: Pregnancy (B), breastfeeding, geriatric patients, hepatic/renal disease, electrolyte imbalance, dehydration, penciclovir, famciclovir, ganciclovir, hypersensitivity, varicella

DOSAGE AND ROUTES

Herpes zoster

- **Adult: PO** 1 g tid × 1 wk

Genital herpes (suppressive, initial)

- **Adult: PO** 1 g bid × 10 days initially

Genital herpes (recurrent episodes)

- **Adult: PO** 500 mg bid × 3 days

Genital herpes (suppressive therapy)

- **Adult: PO** 1 g/day with normal immune function; 500 mg/day for those with ≤9 recurrences/yr; 500 mg bid for HIV-infected patients with CD4 count ≥100

Reduction of transmission

- **Adult: PO** 500 mg/day for source partner

Herpes labialis

- **Adult: PO** 2 g bid × 1 day at 1st sign of lesions

Varicella (chickenpox) in immunocompetent patients

- **Adolescent and child ≥2 yr: PO** 20 mg/kg/dose tid × 5 days, max 3 g/day; start at 1st sign, preferably within 24 hr of rash

Renal dose

- **Adult: PO** CCr 30-49 ml/min, 1 g q12hr (for regimens 1 g q8hr); 1 g q12hr × 1 day (herpes labialis); CCr 10-29 ml/min, 1 g q24hr (genital herpes/herpes zoster); 500 mg q24hr (recurrent genital herpes); CCr <10 ml/min, 500 mg q24hr (genital herpes/herpes zoster), 500 mg q24hr (recurrent genital herpes)

Available forms: Tabs 500 mg, 1 g

Administer:

- As soon as possible (herpes labialis, genital herpes); within 24 hr of rash (varicella)
- Within 72 hr of outbreak (herpes zoster)
- Without regard to food

• Caps may be made into susp by pharmacy

SIDE EFFECTS

CNS: Tremors, lethargy, *dizziness, headache,* weakness, depression
ENDO: *Dysmenorrhea*
GI: *Nausea,* vomiting, diarrhea, abdominal pain, constipation, *increased AST*
HEMA: Thrombocytopenic purpura, hemolytic uremic syndrome
INTEG: *Rash*

PHARMACOKINETICS

Onset unknown; terminal half-life $2^1/_2$-$3^1/_2$ hr; converted to acyclovir that crosses placenta, enters breast milk; excreted in urine primarily as acyclovir; protein binding 13.5%-17.9%

INTERACTIONS

Increase: blood levels of valacyclovir—cimetidine, probenecid; only significant with renal disease

NURSING CONSIDERATIONS

Assess:
• **Infection;** characteristics of lesions; therapy should be started at 1st sign or symptom of herpes; most effective within 72 hr of outbreak
⚠ **Thrombocytopenic purpura, hemolytic uremic syndrome; may be fatal**
• C&S before product therapy; product may be taken as soon as culture is taken; repeat C&S after treatment; determine presence of other sexually transmitted diseases
• Bowel pattern before, during treatment
• Skin eruptions: rash
• Allergies before treatment, reaction of each medication

Perform/provide:
• Storage at room temp; protect from light, moisture

Evaluate:
• Therapeutic response: absence of itching, painful lesions; crusting and healed lesions

Teach patient/family:
• To take as prescribed; if dose is missed, to take as soon as remembered up to 2 hr before next dose; not to double dose
• That product may be taken orally before infection occurs; that product should be taken when itching or pain occurs, usually before eruptions
• That partners need to be told that patient has herpes because they can become infected; that condoms must be worn to prevent reinfections
• That product does not cure infection, just controls symptoms; that product does not prevent infection of others

valganciclovir (Rx)

(val-gan-sy′kloh-veer)

Valcyte

Func. class.: Antiviral
Chem. class.: Synthetic nucleoside

Do not confuse:
valganciclovir/valacyclovir
Valcyte/Valtrex

ACTION: Metabolized to ganciclovir; inhibits replication of human cytomegalovirus in vivo and in vitro by selective inhibition of viral DNA synthesis

USES: Cytomegalovirus (CMV) retinitis in immunocompromised persons, including those with AIDS, after indirect ophthalmoscopy confirms diagnosis; prevention of CMV with transplantation; prevention of CMV in at-risk patient going through transplant (kidney, heart, pancreas)
Unlabeled uses: Colitis, Epstein-Barr virus, esophagitis, herpes simplex type 1, 2; human herpesvirus 6, 8; multicentric Castleman's disease, varicella-zoster virus

CONTRAINDICATIONS: Breastfeeding, hypersensitivity to ganciclovir, valacyclovir; absolute neutrophil count

<500/mm^3; platelet count <25,000/mm^3; hemodialysis; liver transplantation

Precautions: Pregnancy (C), children, geriatric patients, renal function impairment; hypersensitivity to acyclovir, penciclovir, famciclovir

Black Box Warning: Preexisting cytopenias, secondary malignancy, infertility, anemia

DOSAGE AND ROUTES

Treatment of CMV

• **Adult and adolescent (unlabeled): PO** induction 900 mg bid × 21 days with food; maintenance 900 mg/day with food

Transplant (CMV prophylaxis)

• **Adult/adolescent >16 yr: PO** 900 mg/day with food starting 10 days prior to transplantation until day 100 after transplantation

• **Infant ≥4 mo/child/adolescent ≤16 yr: PO** give within 10 days of heart/kidney transplant; calculate dose as 7 × BSA × CCr, give as single daily dose

Renal dose

• **Adult: PO** CCr ≥60 ml/min, same as above; CCr 40-59 ml/min, 450 mg bid for 21 days then 450 mg/day; CCr 25-39 ml/min, 450 mg/day then 450 mg q2days; CCr 10-24 ml/min, 450 mg q2days then 450 mg 2×/week

Available form: Tabs 450 mg, powder for oral sol 50 mg/ml

Administer:

PO tab

• With food for better absorption; avoid getting product on skin; do not break

Oral sol

• Measure 9 ml purified water in graduated cylinder, shake bottle to loosen powder, add 1/2 liquid, shake well, add remaining water, shake; remove child-resistant cap and push bottle adapter into neck of bottle, close with cap, give using dispenser provided

SIDE EFFECTS

CNS: *Fever,* chills, coma, *confusion,* abnormal thoughts, dizziness, bizarre dreams, *headache, insomnia,* psychosis, tremors, somnolence, *paresthesia, weakness,* seizures

EENT: Retinal detachment with CMV retinitis

GI: Abnormal LFTs, *nausea, vomiting, anorexia, diarrhea, abdominal pain,* hemorrhage

GU: Hematuria, increased creatinine, BUN

HEMA: Granulocytopenia, thrombocytopenia, irreversible neutropenia, anemia, eosinophilia

INTEG: *Rash,* alopecia, *pruritus,* urticaria, pain at site, phlebitis, Stevens-Johnson syndrome

MISC: Local and systemic infections, sepsis

PHARMACOKINETICS

Metabolized to ganciclovir, which has a half-life of 3-4 1/2 hr; excreted by kidneys (unchanged); crosses blood-brain barrier, CSF

INTERACTIONS

• Severe granulocytopenia: zidovudine, antineoplastics, radiation; do not use together

Increase: toxicity—dapsone, pentamidine, flucytosine, vinCRIStine, vinBLAStine, adriamycin, DOXOrubicin, amphotericin B, trimethoprim-sulfamethoxazole combinations or other nucleoside analogs, cycloSPORINE

Increase: seizures—imipenem-cilastatin

Increase: effect of didanosine

Decrease: renal clearance of valganciclovir—probenecid

Drug/Food

Increase: absorption, high-fat meal

NURSING CONSIDERATIONS

Assess:

• CMV retinitis by ophthalmoscopy before beginning treatment, q2wk

• Culture for CMV retinitis

• **Infection:** sore throat, cough, fever, chills, back pain; notify prescriber

Black Box Warning: Leukopenia/neutropenia/thrombocytopenia: WBCs, platelets q2days during 2×/day dosing then q1wk; leukopenia with daily WBC count in patients with prior leukopenia with other nucleoside analogs or for whom leukopenia counts are <1000 cells/mm^3 at start of treatment

- Serum creatinine or CCr ≥q2wk

Evaluate:

- Therapeutic response: decreased symptoms of CMV

Teach patient/family:

- That product does not cure condition; that regular ophthalmologic and blood tests necessary
- That major toxicities may necessitate discontinuing product
- To use contraception during treatment; that infertility may occur; that men should use barrier contraception for 90 days after treatment
- To take with food
- ⚠ **To report infection: fever, chills, sore throat; blood dyscrasias: bruising, bleeding, petechiae**
- To avoid crowds, persons with respiratory infections
- To use sunscreen to prevent burns

valproate (Rx)

(val′proh-ate)

Depacon

valproic acid (Rx)

(val′proh-ik)

Depakene, Stavzor

divalproex sodium (Rx)

(dye-val′proh-ex)

Depakote, Depakote ER, Epival ✦

Func. class.: Anticonvulsant, vascular headache suppressant

Chem. class.: Carboxylic acid derivative

ACTION: Increases levels of γ-aminobutyric acid (GABA) in the brain, which decreases seizure activity

USES: Simple (petit mal), complex (petit mal), absence, mixed, seizures; manic episodes associated with bipolar disorder, prophylaxis of migraine, adjunct for schizophrenia, tardive dyskinesia, aggression in children with ADHD, organic brain syndrome, mania, migraines; tonic-clonic (grand mal), myoclonic seizures

Unlabeled uses: Rectal for seizures (valproic acid)

CONTRAINDICATIONS: Hypersensitivity, urea cycle disorders

Black Box Warning: Pregnancy (D), hepatic disease, pancreatitis

Precautions: Breastfeeding, geriatric patients

Black Box Warning: Children <2 yr

DOSAGE AND ROUTES

Epilepsy

- **Adult and child: PO** 10-15 mg/kg/day in 2-3 divided doses, may increase by 5-10 mg/kg/day weekly, max 60 mg/kg/day in 2-3 divided doses; **IV** ≤20 mg/min over 1 hr

Status epilepticus refractory to diazepam IV (unlabeled)

- **Adult: RECT** 400-600 mg PR as enema or wax-based suppository (not commercially available)
- **Child: RECT** 20 mg/kg/dose

Mania (divalproex sodium)

- **Adult: PO** 750 mg/day in divided doses, max 60 mg/kg/day or 3000 mg/day

Mania (valproic acid: Stavzor)

- **Adult: DEL REL CAP** 750 mg/day in divided doses

Migraine (divalproex sodium)

- **Adult: PO** 250 mg bid, may increase to 1000 mg/day if needed or 500 mg (Depakote ER) daily × 7 days, then 1000 mg/day

Available forms: *Valproate:* inj 100 mg/ml; *valproic acid:* caps 250 mg; syr 250 mg/5 ml; del rel cap (Stavzor) 125 mg; *divalproex:* del rel tabs 125, 250,

V

500 mg; ext rel tabs 250, 500 mg; sprinkle cap 125 mg

Administer:

PO route

- Swallow tabs or caps whole; do not break, crush, or chew ext rel tabs
- Sprinkle cap contents on food
- Elixir alone; do not dilute with carbonated beverage; do not give syrup to patients with sodium restrictions
- Give with food or milk to decrease GI symptoms

SIDE EFFECTS

CNS: *Sedation, drowsiness,* dizziness, headache, incoordination, depression, hallucinations, behavioral changes, tremors, aggression, weakness, **coma, suicidal ideation**

EENT: Visual disturbances, taste perversion

GI: *Nausea, vomiting, constipation, diarrhea, dyspepsia,* anorexia, cramps, **hepatic failure, pancreatitis, toxic hepatitis,** stomatitis, weight gain

GU: Enuresis, irregular menses

HEMA: **Thrombocytopenia, leukopenia, lymphocytosis,** increased PT, bruising, epistaxis

INTEG: *Rash,* alopecia, photosensitivity, dry skin

PHARMACOKINETICS

Metabolized by liver; excreted by kidneys, in breast milk; crosses placenta; half-life 6-16 hr; 90% protein binding

PO: Peak 4 hr (regular rel); 4-17 hr (ext rel)

INTERACTIONS

Increase: valproic acid level—erythromycin, felbamate

Increase: CNS depression—alcohol, opioids, barbiturates, antihistamines, MAOIs, sedative/hypnotics

Increase: toxicity of valproic acid—salicylates

Increase: action of phenytoin, tricyclics, carBAMazepine, ethosuximide, barbiturates, zidovudine, LORazepam, rufinamide

Increase: bleeding—antiplatelets, NSAIDs, tirofiban, eptifibatide, abciximab, cefoperazone, cefotetan, heparin, thrombolytics

Increase: toxicity of carBAMazepine ethosuximide, lamoTRIgine, zidovudine

Decrease: metabolism of valproic acid—cimetidine

Decrease: valproic acid level—rifampin carBAMazepine, lamoTRIgine

Drug/Lab Test

False positive: ketones, urine

Interference: thyroid function tests

NURSING CONSIDERATIONS

Assess:

- Seizure disorder: location, aura, activity, duration; seizure precautions should be in place
- ⚠ **Mental status: bipolar disorder: mood, activity, sleeping/eating, behavior; suicidal thoughts/behaviors**
- Migraines: frequency, intensity, alleviating factors
- Blood studies: Hct, Hgb, RBC, serum folate, PT/PTT, serum ammonia, platelets, vit D if patient receiving long-term therapy

Black Box Warning: Hepatic studies: AST, ALT, bilirubin; hepatic failure has occurred

- Blood levels: therapeutic level 50-100 mcg/ml, during seizures
- Respiratory dysfunction: respiratory depression, character, rate, rhythm; hold product if respirations are <12/min or if pupils are dilated

Black Box Warning: Pancreatitis; may be fatal

Evaluate:

- Therapeutic response: decreased seizures

Teach patient/family:

- That physical dependency may result from extended use
- To avoid driving, other activities that require alertness

• Not to discontinue medication quickly after long-term use because seizures may result
• To report visual disturbances, rash, diarrhea, abdominal pain, light-colored stools, jaundice, protracted vomiting to prescriber
• To use contraception while taking this product; pregnancy category (D)

valsartan (Rx)

(val′sahr-tan)

Diovan

Func. class.: Antihypertensive

Chem. class.: Angiotensin II receptor antagonist (Type AT_1)

ACTION: Blocks the vasoconstrictor and aldosterone-secreting effects of angiotensin II; selectively blocks the binding of angiotensin II to the AT_1 receptor found in tissues

USES: Hypertension, alone or in combination in patients >6 yr, CHF, post MI with left ventricular dysfunction/failure in stable patients

CONTRAINDICATIONS: Hypersensitivity, severe hepatic disease, bilateral renal artery stenosis

Black Box Warning: Pregnancy (D) 2nd/3rd trimester

Precautions: Breastfeeding, children, geriatric patients, hypersensitivity to ACE inhibitors; CHF, hypertrophic cardiomyopathy aortic/mitral valve stenosis, CAD, angioedema, renal/hepatic disease, hyperkalemia, hypovolemia

DOSAGE AND ROUTES

Hypertension

• **Adult: PO** 80 or 160 mg/day alone or in combination with other antihypertensives, may increase to 320 mg
• **Child and adolescent 6-16 yr: PO** 1.3 mg/kg/day, max 40 mg/day

CHF

• **Adult: PO** 40 mg bid, up to 160 mg bid

Post MI

• **Adult: PO** 20 mg bid as early as 12 hr post MI, may be titrated within 7 days to 40 mg bid, then titrate to maintenance of 160 mg bid

Available forms: Tabs 40, 80, 160, 320 mg

Administer:

• Without regard to meals

SIDE EFFECTS

CNS: *Dizziness, insomnia,* drowsiness, vertigo, headache, fatigue

CV: Angina pectoris, 2nd-degree AV block, **cerebrovascular accident**, hypotension, **MI**, *dysrhythmias*

EENT: Conjunctivitis

GI: *Diarrhea,* abdominal pain, nausea, **hepatotoxicity**

GU: Impotence, **nephrotoxicity**

HEMA: *Anemia,* neutropenia

META: Hyperkalemia

MISC: Vasculitis

MS: Cramps, myalgia, pain, stiffness

RESP: *Cough*

PHARMACOKINETICS

Onset up to 2 hr; peak 4-6 hr; duration 24 hr; extensively metabolized; protein binding 95%; half-life 6 hr; excreted in feces, urine, breast milk

INTERACTIONS

Increase: effects of lithium

Increase: hyperkalemia—potassium-sparing diuretics, potassium supplements, ACE inhibitors

Decrease: antihypertensive effects—NSAIDs, salicylates

V

NURSING CONSIDERATIONS

Assess:

• B/P, pulse q4hr lying, sitting, standing; note rate, rhythm, quality periodically
• Blood studies; BUN, creatinine, LFTs, total/direct bilirubin before treatment
• Angioedema: facial swelling; SOB; edema in feet, legs daily

• Skin turgor, dryness of mucous membranes for hydration status; correct volume depletion before initiating therapy

Evaluate:

• Therapeutic response: decreased B/P

Teach patient/family:

• To comply with dosage schedule, even if feeling better; that, if dose is missed, to take it as soon as possible unless it is within 1 hr of next dose

• To notify prescriber of fever, swelling of hands or feet, irregular heartbeat, chest pain, dizziness, persistent cough

• That excessive perspiration, dehydration, diarrhea may lead to fall in blood pressure; to consult prescriber if these occur

• That product may cause dizziness, fainting, lightheadedness; to rise slowly to sitting or standing position to minimize orthostatic hypotension; to take B/P readings

Black Box Warning: Not to take product if pregnant (D) or breastfeeding

vancomycin (Rx)

(van-koe-mye′sin)

Vancocin

Func. class.: Antiinfective—miscellaneous

Chem. class.: Tricyclic glycopeptide

ACTION: Inhibits bacterial cell wall synthesis, blocks glycopeptides

USES: Resistant staphylococcal infections, pseudomembranous colitis, staphylococcal enterocolitis, endocarditis prophylaxis for dental procedures, diphtheroid endocarditis

CONTRAINDICATIONS: Hypersensitivity, previous hearing loss

Precautions: Pregnancy (B), breastfeeding, neonates, geriatric patients, renal disease

DOSAGE AND ROUTES

Serious staphylococcal infections

• **Adult: IV** 500 mg q6-8hr or 1 g q12hr

• **Child: IV** 40-60 mg/kg/day divided q6-8hr

• **Neonate: IV** 15 mg/kg initially, then 10 mg/kg q8-24hr

Pseudomembranous/ staphylococcal enterocolitis

• **Adult: PO** 125 mg qid × 10-14 days

• **Child: PO** 40 mg/kg/day divided q6hr × 7-10 days, max 2 g/day

Endocarditis prophylaxis

• **Adult: IV** 1 g over 1 hr given 1 hr before procedure

• **Child: IV** 20 mg/kg over 1 hr given 1 hr prior to procedure

Renal dose

• **Adult: IV** CCr >70 ml/min, no dosage adjustment; CCr 50-70 ml/min, loading dose of 15 mg/kg, reduce dose to 750 mg-1 g q18-24 hr; CCr <49 ml/min, initial loading dose of 15 mg/kg, with subsequent dosing based on concentration, may be q24-72hr or longer

Available forms: Pulvules 125, 250 mg; powder for inj 500 mg, 1, 5, 10 g

Administer:

• Use only for susceptible organisms to prevent product-resistant bacteria

• Antihistamine if red-man syndrome occurs: decreased B/P, flushing of neck, face

• Dose based on serum concentration

Retention enema

• Dilute 500 mg/1000 ml NS q6hr

IT route

• Use preservative-free 0.9% NaCl (2-5 mg/ml final conc), instill into ventricular cerebrospinal fluid

Intermittent IV INF route

• After reconstitution with 10 ml sterile water for inj (500 mg/10 ml); further dilution is needed for IV, 500 mg/100 ml 0.9% NaCl, D_5W given as intermittent inf over 1 hr; decrease rate of inf if red-man syndrome occurs

Continuous IV INF route

• May infuse 1-2 g in volume to give over 24 hr if intermittent IV route cannot be used

Y-site compatibilities: Acyclovir, allopurinol, amifostine, amiodarone, amsacrine, atracurium, cisatracurium, cyclophosphamide, diltiazem, DOXOrubicin liposome, enalaprilat, esmolol, filgrastim, fluconazole, fludarabine, gallium, granisetron, HYDROmorphone, insulin (regular), labetalol, LORazepam, magnesium sulfate, melphalan, meperidine, meropenem, midazolam, morphine, ondansetron, paclitaxel, pancuronium, perphenazine, propofol, remifentanil, sodium bicarbonate, tacrolimus, teniposide, theophylline, thiotepa, tolazoline, vecuronium, vinorelbine, warfarin, zidovudine

SIDE EFFECTS

CV: Cardiac arrest, vascular collapse (rare), hypotension

EENT: *Ototoxicity, permanent deafness,* tinnitus, nystagmus

GI: Nausea, pseudomembranous colitis

GU: Nephrotoxicity, *increased BUN, creatinine, albumin,* fatal uremia

HEMA: Leukopenia, eosinophilia, neutropenia

INTEG: Chills, fever, rash, thrombophlebitis at inj site, urticaria, pruritus, necrosis (red-man syndrome), skin/subcutaneous tissue disorders

RESP: Wheezing, dyspnea

SYST: Anaphylaxis, superinfection

PHARMACOKINETICS

PO: Absorption poor

IV: Onset rapid, peak 1 hr, half-life 4-8 hr, excreted in urine (active form)

INTERACTIONS

Increase: ototoxicity or nephrotoxicity—aminoglycosides, cephalosporins, colistin, polymyxin, bacitracin, CISplatin, amphotericin B, nondepolarizing muscle relaxants, cidofovir

NURSING CONSIDERATIONS

Assess:

- **Infection:** WBC, urine, stools, sputum, characteristics of wound throughout treatment
- I&O ratio; report hematuria, oliguria; nephrotoxicity may occur
- Serum levels: peak 1 hr after 1-hr inf 25-40 mg/L, trough before next dose 5-10 mg/L
- C&S
- Auditory function during, after treatment
- B/P during administration; sudden drop may indicate red-man syndrome
- Hearing loss, ringing, roaring in ears; product should be discontinued
- Skin eruptions
- Respiratory status: rate, character; wheezing, tightness in chest
- Allergies before treatment, reaction of each medication

Perform/provide:

- Storage at room temp for ≤2 wk after reconstitution
- EPINEPHrine, suction, tracheostomy set, endotracheal intubation equipment on unit; anaphylaxis may occur
- Adequate intake of fluids (2 L/day) to prevent nephrotoxicity

Evaluate:

- Therapeutic response: absence of fever, sore throat; negative culture

Teach patient/family:

- About all aspects of product therapy; about the need to complete entire course of medication to ensure organism death (7-10 days); that culture may be taken after completed course of medication
- To report sore throat, fever, fatigue; could indicate superinfection
- That product must be taken in equal intervals around the clock to maintain blood levels

vardenafil (Rx)

(var-den′a-fil)

Levitra, Staxyn

Func. class.: Erectile dysfunction agent

Chem. class.: Phosphodiesterase type 5 inhibitor

ACTION: Inhibits phosphodiesterase type 5 (PDE5), enhances erectile function by increasing the amount of cGMP, which in turn causes smooth muscle relaxation and increased blood flow into the corpus cavernosum

USES: Treatment of erectile dysfunction

CONTRAINDICATIONS: Hypersensitivity, coadministration of α-blockers or nitrates, renal failure, congenital or acquired QT prolongation

Precautions: Pregnancy (B); not indicated for women, children, or newborns; hepatic impairment, retinitis pigmentosa, anatomical penile deformities, sickle cell anemia, leukemia, multiple myeloma, bleeding disorders, active peptic ulceration, CV/renal disease

DOSAGE AND ROUTES

- **Adult: PO** 10 mg taken 1 hr before sexual activity; dose may be reduced to 5 mg or increased to max 20 mg; max dosing frequency once daily; orally disintegrating tab 10 mg 60 min before sexual activity; do not use with potent CYP3A4 inhibitors
- **Geriatric >65 yr: PO** 5 mg initially, titrated as needed/tolerated

Hepatic dose

- **Adult: PO** (Child-Pugh B) 5 mg, max 10 mg/day

Concomitant medications

- Ritonavir, max 2.5 mg q72hr; for indinavir, ketoconazole 400 mg/day and itraconazole 400 mg/day, max 2.5 mg/day; for ketoconazole 200 mg/day, itraconazole 200 mg/day and erythromycin max 5 mg/day

Available forms: Tabs 2.5, 5, 10, 20 mg; orally disintegrating tab 10 mg

Administer:

- Approximately 1 hr before sexual activity; do not use more than once daily; orally disintegrating tabs are not interchangeable with film-coated tabs
- Without regard to food; avoid taking with high-fat meal

SIDE EFFECTS

CNS: *Headache, flushing, dizziness, insomnia,* seizures, transient global amnesia

CV: Hypertension, MI, CV collapse, chest pain

EENT: Conjunctivitis, tinnitus, photophobia, diminished vision, glaucoma, hearing loss

GU: Abnormal ejaculation, priapism

MISC: Rash, GERD, GGTP increased, NAION (nonarteritic ischemic optic neuropathy), dyspepsia

MS: Myalgia, arthralgia, neck pain

RESP: Rhinitis, sinusitis, dyspnea, pharyngitis, epistaxis

PHARMACOKINETICS

Rapidly absorbed, bioavailability 15%, protein binding 95%, metabolized by liver, terminal half-life 4-5 hr, onset 20 min, peak ½-1½ hr, duration <5 hr, reduced absorption with high-fat meal, primarily excreted in feces (91%-95%)

INTERACTIONS

⚠ Do not use with nitrates because of unsafe decrease in B/P, which could result in MI or stroke

⚠ Serious dysrhythmias: class IA/III antiarrhythmics, clarithromycin, droperidol, procainamide, quiNIDine, quinolones; do not use concurrently

Increase: hypotension—α-blockers, protease inhibitors, metoprolol, NIFEdipine, alcohol, amLODIPine, angiotensin II receptor blockers; do not use concurrently

Increase: vardenafil levels—erythromycin, azole antifungals (ketoconazole, itraconazole), cimetidine, antiretroviral protease inhibitors

Drug/Food

Decrease: absorption—high-fat meal

Drug/Lab Test

Increase: CK

NURSING CONSIDERATIONS

Assess:

- Erectile dysfunction prior to treatment
- ⚠ **Any severe loss of vision while taking this or similar products; products should not be used**
- ⚠ **Use of organic nitrates that should not be used with this product**

Teach patient/family:

- That product does not protect against STDs, including HIV
- That product absorption is reduced with high-fat meal
- That product should not be used with nitrates in any form; to inform physician of all medications being taken
- That product has no effect in the absence of sexual stimulation; that patient should seek immediate medical attention if erections last >4 hr
- ⚠ **To notify prescriber immediately and stop taking product if vision loss occurs**

varenicline (Rx)

(var-e-ni′kleen)

Champix ♣, Chantix

Func. class.: Smoking cessation agent

Chem. class.: Nicotine receptor agonist

ACTION: Partial agonist for nicotine receptors; partially activates receptors to help curb cravings; occupies receptors to prevent nicotine binding

USES: Smoking deterrent

CONTRAINDICATIONS: Hypersensitivity, eating disorders

Precautions: Pregnancy (C), breastfeeding, children <18 yr, geriatric patients, renal disease, recent MI, angioedema

Black Box Warning: Bipolar disorder, depression, schizophrenia, suicidal ideation

DOSAGE AND ROUTES

- **Adult: PO** therapy should begin 1 wk prior to smoking stop date (i.e., take product plus tobacco for 7 days); titrate for 1 wk; days 1 through 3, 0.5 mg/day; days 4 through 7, 0.5 mg bid; day 8 through end of treatment, 1 mg bid; treatment is for 12 wk and may be repeated for another 12 wk

Renal dose

- **Adult: PO** CCr ≤50 ml/min, titrate to max 0.5 mg bid

Available forms: Tabs 0.5, 1 mg; Chantix continuing month PAK; Chantix starting month PAK

Administer:

- Do not break, crush, or chew tabs
- Increased fluids, bulk in diet if constipation occurs
- After eating with a full glass of water
- Sugarless gum, hard candy, or frequent sips of water for dry mouth

SIDE EFFECTS

CNS: Headache, agitation, dizziness, insomnia, abnormal dreams, fatigue, malaise, behavior changes, depression, suicidal ideation, **suicide**, amnesia, hallucinations, hostility, mania, psychosis, tremor

CV: Dysrhythmias, hypo/hypertension, palpitations, tachycardia, angina, **MI**

EENT: *Blurred vision,* tinnitus

GI: *Nausea, vomiting,* anorexia, *dry mouth,* increased/decreased appetite, *constipation,* flatulence, GERD

GU: Erectile dysfunction, urinary frequency, menstrual irregularities

INTEG: Rash, pruritus, **angioedema, Stevens-Johnson syndrome**

V

MISC: Weight loss or gain
RESP: Dyspnea, rhinorrhea

PHARMACOKINETICS

Elimination half-life 24 hr; metabolism minimal; 93% excreted unchanged in urine; steady state 4 days

NURSING CONSIDERATIONS

Assess:

- Renal function in geriatric patients
- Smoking cessation after 12 wk; if progress not made, product may be used for additional 12 wk

Black Box Warning: Neuropsychiatric symptoms: mood, sensorium, affect; behavior changes, agitation, depression, suicidal ideation; suicide has occurred; possible worsening of depression, schizophrenia, bipolar disorder

Evaluate:

- Therapeutic response: smoking cessation

Teach patient/family:

- That treatment for smoking cessation lasts 12 wk and that another 12 wk may be required
- To use caution when driving, performing other activities requiring alertness; blurred vision may occur
- To set a date to quit smoking and to initiate treatment 1 wk prior to that date
- How to titrate product
- Not to use with nicotine patches unless directed by prescriber; may increase B/P
- To notify prescriber if pregnancy planned or suspected
- About common side effects to be expected

vasopressin (Rx)

(vay-soe-press'in)

Pitressin, Pressyn ♣

Func. class.: Pituitary hormone

Chem. class.: Lysine vasopressin

ACTION: Promotes the reabsorption of water via action on the renal tubular epithelium; causes vasoconstriction

USES: Diabetes insipidus (nonnephrogenic/nonpsychogenic), abdominal distention postoperatively, bleeding esophageal varices

CONTRAINDICATIONS: Hypersensitivity, chronic nephritis

Precautions: Pregnancy (C), breastfeeding, CAD, asthma, vascular/renal disease, migraines, seizures

DOSAGE AND ROUTES

Diabetes insipidus

- **Adult: IM/SUBCUT** 5-10 units bid-qid as needed; **CONT IV INF** 0.0005 units/kg/hr (0.05 milliunit/kg/hr), double dose q30min as needed
- **Child: IM/SUBCUT** 2.5-10 units bid-qid as needed; **IM/SUBCUT** 1.25-2.5 units q2-3days (Pitressin Tannate) for chronic therapy

Abdominal distention

- **Adult: IM** 5 units then q3-4hr, increasing to 10 units if needed (aqueous)

Available forms: Inj 20, 5 units/ml (tannate)

SIDE EFFECTS

CNS: Drowsiness, headache, lethargy, flushing, vertigo
CV: Increased B/P, dysrhythmias, **cardiac arrest, shock**, chest pain, **MI**
EENT: Nasal irritation, congestion, rhinitis
GI: Nausea, heartburn, cramps, vomiting, flatus
GU: Vulval pain, uterine cramping

MISC: Tremor, sweating, vertigo, urticaria, bronchial constriction

PHARMACOKINETICS

Nasal: Onset 1 hr; duration 3-8 hr; half-life 15 min; metabolized in liver, kidneys; excreted in urine

INTERACTIONS

Increase: antidiuretic effect—tricyclics, carBAMazepine, chloropromide, fludrocortisone, clofibrate, urea
Decrease: antidiuretic effect—lithium, demeclocycline

NURSING CONSIDERATIONS

Assess:

- Pulse, B/P when giving product IV or IM
- I&O ratio, weight daily; fluid/electrolyte balance; check for edema in extremities; if water retention is severe, diuretic may be prescribed
- **Water intoxication:** lethargy, behavioral changes, disorientation, neuromuscular excitability
- Small doses may precipitate coronary adverse effects; keep emergency equipment nearby

Evaluate:

- Therapeutic response: absence of severe thirst, decreased urine output, osmolality

Teach patient/family:

- To measure and record I&O
- To avoid alcohol, all OTC medications unless approved by prescriber

⚠ HIGH ALERT

vecuronium (Rx)

(vek-yoo-roe′nee-um)
Func. class.: Neuromuscular blocker, nondepolarizing
Chem. class.: Monoquaternary analog of pancuronium

ACTION:
Inhibits transmission of nerve impulses by binding with cholinergic receptor sites and antagonizing action of acetylcholine

USES:
Facilitation of endotracheal intubation, skeletal muscle relaxation during mechanical ventilation, surgery, general anesthesia

CONTRAINDICATIONS:
Hypersensitivity

Precautions: Pregnancy (C), breastfeeding, children <2 yr, electrolyte imbalances, dehydration, hepatic/cardiac/neuromuscular disease

Black Box Warning: Respiratory disease

DOSAGE AND ROUTES

- **Adult and child >1 yr: IV** initially 0.08-0.1 mg/kg or 0.04-0.06 mg/kg if given with succinylcholine, maintenance 0.01-0.015 mg/kg 25-40 min after initial dose then 0.01-0.015 mg/kg q12-15min
- **Infant 7 wk-1 yr: IV** 0.08-0.1 mg/kg, maintenance 0.05-0.1 mg/kg q60min as needed
- **Neonate: IV** 0.1 mg/kg/dose, maintenance 0.03-0.15 mg/kg/dose q1-2hr as needed

Available forms: 10 mg/5-ml vial

Administer:

- With diazepam or morphine when used for therapeutic paralysis; provides no sedation alone
- Using nerve stimulator by anesthesiologist to determine neuromuscular blockade
- Anticholinesterase to reverse neuromuscular blockade

• IV after diluting with diluent provided; give by direct IV over 1 min; may give as continuous inf 10-20 mg/100 ml; titrate to patient response (only by qualified person)

Y-site compatibilities: Aminophylline, ceFAZolin, cefuroxime, cimetidine, diltiazem, DOBUTamine, DOPamine, EPINEPHrine, esmolol, fentanyl, fluconazole, gentamicin, heparin, hydrocortisone, HYDROmorphone, isoproterenol, labetalol, LORazepam, midazolam, milrinone, morphine, niCARdipine, nitroglycerin, norepinephrine, propofol, ranitidine, sodium nitroprusside, trimethoprim-sulfamethoxazole, vancomycin

SIDE EFFECTS

CNS: Skeletal muscle weakness or paralysis (rare)
INTEG: Urticaria, flushing
MISC: Myopathy, hypotension
RESP: **Prolonged apnea, possible respiratory paralysis**, bronchospasm, tachycardia, dyspnea
SYST: **Anaphylaxis**

PHARMACOKINETICS

IV: Onset 2-3 min; peak 3-5 min; duration 15-25 (recovery index) min; half-life 65-75 min; not metabolized; excreted in urine, feces; crosses placenta

INTERACTIONS

• Dysrhythmias: theophylline

Increase: neuromuscular blockade—aminoglycosides, amphotericin B, clindamycin, lincomycin, quiNIDine, local anesthetics, polymyxin antibiotics, lithium, opioid analgesics, phenytoin, piperacillin, thiazides, enflurane, isoflurane, succinylcholine, verapamil

NURSING CONSIDERATIONS

Assess:

Black Box Warning: VS (B/P, pulse, respirations, airway) q15min until fully recovered; rate, depth, pattern of respirations, strength of hand grip

• I&O ratio; check for urinary retention, frequency, hesitancy

• Recovery: decreased paralysis of face, diaphragm, leg, arm, rest of body; allow patient to recover fully before completing neurologic assessment

• Allergic reactions: rash, fever, respiratory distress, pruritus; product should be discontinued

Perform/provide:

• Storage in refrigerator; discard in 24 hr

• Reassurance if communication is difficult during recovery from neuromuscular blockade

Evaluate:

• Therapeutic response: paralysis of jaw, eyelid, head, neck, rest of body

TREATMENT OF OVERDOSE:

Edrophonium or neostigmine, atropine, monitor VS; may require mechanical ventilation

vemurafemib

See Appendix A—Selected new drugs

venlafaxine (Rx)

(ven-la-fax′een)

Effexor ✱, Effexor XR

Func. class.: Antidepressant—SNRI
Chem. class.: SNRI

ACTION: Potent inhibitor of neuronal serotonin and norepinephrine uptake, weak inhibitor of dopamine; no muscarinic, histaminergic, or α-adrenergic receptors in vitro

USES: Prevention/treatment of major depression; depression at the end of life; long-term treatment of general anxiety disorder, panic disorder, social anxiety disorder (Effexor XR only)

Unlabeled uses: Hot flashes, premenstrual dysphoric disorder (PMDD), headache, neuropathic pain, fibromyalgia, diabetic neuropathy

CONTRAINDICATIONS:
Hypersensitivity, bipolar disorder, interstitial lung disease

Precautions: Pregnancy (C), breastfeeding, geriatric patients, mania, hypertension, seizure disorder, recent MI, cardiac/renal/hepatic disease, eosinophilic pneumonia, desvenlafaxine hypersensitivity

Black Box Warning: Children, suicidal ideation

DOSAGE AND ROUTES

Depression

- **Adult: PO** 75 mg/day in 2-3 divided doses; taken with food, may be increased to 150 mg/day; if needed, may be further increased to 225 mg/day; increments of 75 mg/day at intervals of ≥4 days; some hospitalized patients may require up to 375 mg/day in 3 divided doses; **EXT REL** 37.5-75 mg PO daily, max 225 mg/day; give XR daily

Anxiety disorders

- **Adult: PO** 75 mg/day or 37.5 mg/day × 4-7 days initially, max 225 mg/day

Renal dose

- **Adult: PO** CCr 10-70 ml/min, reduce dose by 25%-50%; CCr <10 ml/min, reduce dose by 50%

Hepatic dose

- **Adult: PO** Moderate impairment, 50% of dose

Hot flashes (unlabeled)

- **Adult (male, prostate cancer): PO** 12.5 mg bid × 4 wk; females 37.5-75 mg/day

Neuropathic pain, diabetic neuropathy, headache, fibromyalgia (unlabeled)

- **Adult: PO** 37.5-75 mg/day, max 75 mg bid (regular rel) or 150 mg/day (ext rel)

Premenstrual dysphoric disorder (PMDD) (unlabeled)

- **Adult female: PO** 50-200 mg/day, start at 50 mg/day for 1st cycle, titrate upward

Available forms: Tabs scored 25, 37.5, 50, 75, 100 mg; ext rel cap (Effexor XR) 37.5, 75, 150 mg; ext rel tab 37.5, 75, 150, 225 mg

Administer:

- With food, milk for GI symptoms; do not crush, chew caps; caps can be opened and contents sprinkled on applesauce, given with full glass of water
- Sugarless gum, hard candy, frequent sips of water for dry mouth
- Avoid use with CNS depressants
- In small amounts because of suicide potential, especially at beginning of therapy

SIDE EFFECTS

CNS: Emotional lability, *vertigo, dizziness, weakness,* apathy, ataxia, CNS stimulation, euphoria, hallucinations, hostility, increased libido, hypertonia, hypotonia, psychosis, insomnia, anxiety, **suicidal ideation in children/adolescents, seizures, neuroleptic-malignant-syndrome–like reaction**

CV: *Migraine,* angina pectoris, hypertension, **sustained hypertension, change in QTc interval**, increased pulse, increased cholesterol, extrasystoles, postural hypotension, syncope, thrombophlebitis

EENT: *Abnormal vision,* taste, *ear pain,* cataract, conjunctivitis, corneal lesions, dry eyes, otitis media, photophobia

GI: *Dysphagia, eructation,* nausea, anorexia, dry mouth, colitis, gastritis, gingivitis, **rectal hemorrhage**, stomatitis, stomach and mouth ulceration

GU: *Anorgasmia,* abnormal ejaculation, *dysuria, hematuria, metrorrhagia, vaginitis, impaired urination,* albuminuria, amenorrhea, kidney calculus, cystitis, nocturia, breast and bladder pain, polyuria, **uterine hemorrhage, vaginal hemorrhage**, moniliasis

HEMA: **Agranulocytosis, aplastic anemia, neutropenia, pancytopenia, abnormal bleeding**

INTEG: Ecchymosis, acne, alopecia, brittle nails, dry skin, photosensitivity, sweating, **angioedema (ext rel)**

V

META: *Peripheral edema, weight loss or gain,* diabetes mellitus, edema, glycosuria, hyperlipemia, hypokalemia
MS: Arthritis, bone pain, bursitis, myasthenia, tenosynovitis, arthralgia
RESP: *Bronchitis, dyspnea,* asthma, chest congestion, epistaxis, hyperventilation, laryngitis
SYST: *Malaise, neck pain,* enlarged abdomen, cyst, facial edema, hangover, hernia

PHARMACOKINETICS

Well absorbed; extensively metabolized in liver by CYP2D6 to active metabolite; 87% of product recovered in urine; 27% protein binding; half-life 5, 11 hr (active metabolite), respectively

INTERACTIONS

⚠ **Hyperthermia, rigidity, rapid fluctuations of vital signs, mental status changes, neuroleptic malignant syndrome: MAOIs**
Increase: bleeding risk—salicylates, NSAIDs, platelet inhibitors, anticoagulants
Increase: venlafaxine effect—cimetidine
Increase: CNS depression—alcohol, opioids, antihistamines, sedative/hypnotics
Increase: levels of clozapine, desipramine, haloperidol, warfarin
Increase: serotonin syndrome—sibutramine, sumatriptan, traZODone, traMADol, SSRIs, serotonin receptor agonist
Decrease: effect of indinavir
Decrease: venlafaxine effect—cyproheptadine

Drug/Herb

• Serotonin syndrome: St. John's wort, tryptophan
Increase: CNS depression—kava, valerian

Drug/Lab Test

Increase: alk phos, bilirubin, AST, ALT, BUN, creatinine, serum cholesterol, CPK, LDH

NURSING CONSIDERATIONS

Assess:

Black Box Warning: Mental status: mood, sensorium, affect, increase in psychiatric symptoms; depression, panic; assess for suicidal ideation in children/adolescents

• B/P lying, standing; pulse q4hr; if systolic B/P drops 20 mm Hg, hold product, notify prescriber; take VS q4hr in patients with CV disease
⚠ **Bleeding:** GI, ecchymosis, epistaxis, hematomas, petechiae, hemorrhage
• Blood studies: CBC, differential, leukocytes, cardiac enzymes if patient is receiving long-term therapy
• Hepatic studies: AST, ALT, bilirubin
• Weight weekly; weight loss or gain; appetite may increase; peripheral edema may occur; monitor cholesterol
• **Withdrawal symptoms:** flulike symptoms, headache, nervousness, agitation, nausea, vomiting, muscle pain, weakness; not usual unless product is discontinued abruptly
⚠ **Serotonin syndrome, neuroleptic malignant syndrome:** increased heart rate, shivering, sweating, dilated pupils, tremors, high B/P, hyperthermia, headache, confusion; if these occur, stop product, administer serotonin antagonist if needed

Perform/provide:

• Storage in tight container at room temp; do not freeze
• Assistance with ambulation during beginning therapy because drowsiness, dizziness occur

Evaluate:

• Therapeutic response: decreased depression, anxiety; increased well-being

Teach patient/family:

• To notify prescriber of rash, hives, allergic reactions, bleeding
• To use with caution when driving, performing other activities requiring alertness because of drowsiness, dizziness, blurred vision

Black Box Warning: That worsening of symptoms, suicidal thoughts/behaviors may occur in children/young adults

- To avoid alcohol ingestion
- Not to discontinue medication abruptly after long-term use; may cause nausea, headache, malaise
- To wear sunscreen or large hat because photosensitivity occurs
- To avoid pregnancy or breastfeeding while taking this product
- To monitor B/P with hypertension

TREATMENT OF OVERDOSE:

ECG monitoring; lavage, activated charcoal; administer anticonvulsant; may require whole-bowel irrigation for ext rel product

verapamil (Rx)

(ver-ap′a-mill)

Apo-Verap ♣, Calan, Calan SR, Covera-HS, Isoptin SR, Nu-Verap ♣, Verelan, Verelan PM

Func. class.: Calcium channel blocker; antihypertensive; antianginal, antidysrhythmic (class IV)

Chem. class.: Diphenylalkylamine

ACTION: Inhibits calcium ion influx across cell membrane during cardiac depolarization; produces relaxation of coronary vascular smooth muscle; dilates coronary arteries; decreases SA/AV node conduction; dilates peripheral arteries

USES: Chronic stable, vasospastic, unstable angina; dysrhythmias, hypertension, supraventricular tachycardia, atrial flutter or fibrillation

Unlabeled uses: Prevention of migraine headaches, claudication, mania

CONTRAINDICATIONS: Sick sinus syndrome, 2nd-/3rd-degree heart block, hypotension <90 mm Hg systolic, cardiogenic shock, severe CHF

Precautions: Pregnancy (C), breastfeeding, children, geriatric patients, CHF, hypotension, hepatic injury, renal disease, concomitant β-blocker therapy

DOSAGE AND ROUTES

Angina

- **Adult: PO** 80-120 mg tid, increase weekly, max 480 mg/day

Dysrhythmias

- **Adult: PO** 240-480 mg/day in 3-4 divided doses in digitalized patients
- **Adult: IV BOL** 5-10 mg (0.075-0.15 mg/kg) over 2 min, may repeat 10 mg (0.15 mg/kg) 1/2 hr after 1st dose
- **Child 1-15 yr: IV BOL** 0.1-0.3 mg/kg over ≥2 min, repeat in 30 min, max 5 mg in single dose
- **Child 0-1 yr: IV BOL** 0.1-0.2 mg/kg over ≥2 min, may repeat after 30 min

Hypertension

- **Adult: PO** 80 mg tid, may titrate upward; **EXT REL** 120-240 mg/day as single dose, may increase to 240-480 mg/day

Hepatic disease/geriatric patients/compromised ventricular function

- **Adult: PO** 40 mg tid initially, increase as tolerated

Claudication due to PVD (unlabeled)

- **Adult: PO** 120-480 mg/day in divided doses

Mania (unlabeled)

- **Adult: PO** 160-320 mg/day in divided doses, may be given with lithium

Migraine prophylaxis (unlabeled)

- **Adult: PO** 80 mg tid

Available forms: Tabs 40, 80, 120 mg; ext rel tabs 120, 180, 240 mg; inj 2.5 mg/ml in ampules, syringes, vials; ext rel caps 100, 200, 240, 300 mg

Administer:

PO route

- Do not crush or chew ext rel products; caps may be opened and contents sprinkled on food; do not dissolve chew cap contents
- Before meals, at bedtime; give ext rel product with food

V

Direct IV route

- Undiluted through Y-tube or 3-way stopcock of compatible sol; give over 2 min or 3 min for geriatric patients, discard unused solution

Y-site compatibilities: Alfentanil, amikacin, argatroban, ascorbic acid, atracurium, atropine, aztreonam, bivalirudin, bumetanide, buprenorphine, butorphanol, calcium chloride/gluconate, CARBOplatin, caspofungin, ceFAZolin, cefonicid, cefotaxime, cefotetan, cefoxitin, ceftizoxime, cefTRIAXone, cefuroxime, chlorproMAZINE, cimetidine, ciprofloxacin, clindamycin, cyanocobalamin, cyclophosphamide, cycloSPORINE, cytarabine, DACTINomycin, DAPTOmycin, dexamethasone, dexmedetomidine, digoxin, diltiazem, diphenhydrAMINE, DOBUTamine, docetaxel, DOPamine, doxacurium, DOXOrubicin hydrochloride, doxycycline, enalaprilat, ePHEDrine, EPINEPHrine, epirubicin, epoetin alfa, eptifibatide, erythromycin, esmolol, etoposide, etoposide phosphate, famotidine, fenoldopam, fentaNYL, fluconazole, fludarabine, gemcitabine, gentamicin, glycopyrrolate, granisetron, heparin, hydrALAZINE, hydrocortisone, HYDROmorphone, ifosfamide, imipenem/cilastatin, inamrinone, insulin, isoproterenol, ketorolac, labetalol, levofloxacin, lidocaine, linezolid, LORazepam, magnesium sulfate, mannitol, mechlorethamine, meperidine, metaraminol, methotrexate, methoxamine, methyldopate, methylPREDNISolone, metoclopramide, metoprolol, metroNIDAZOLE, miconazole, midazolam, milrinone, mitoxantrone, morphine, multivitamins, nalbuphine, naloxone, nesiritide, nitroglycerin, nitroprusside, norepinephrine, octreotide, ondansetron, oxaliplatin, oxytocin, paclitaxel, palonosetron, papaverine, pemetrexed, penicillin G, pentamidine, pentazocine, phentolamine, phenylephrine, phytonadione, piperacillin/tazobactam, potassium chloride, procainamide, prochlorperazine, promethazine, propranolol, protamine, pyridoxime, quinupristin/dalfopristin, ranitidine, rocuronium, sodium acetate, succinylcholine, SUFentanil, tacrolimus, teniposide, theophylline, thiamine, ticarcillin/clavulanate, tirofiban, tobramycin, tolazoline, trimethaphan, urokinase, vancomycin, vasopressin, vecuronium, vinCRIStine, vinorelbine, voriconazole

SIDE EFFECTS

CNS: *Headache, drowsiness,* dizziness, anxiety, depression, weakness, insomnia, confusion, lightheadedness, asthenia, fatigue
CV: *Edema,* CHF, bradycardia, hypotension, palpitations, AV block, **dysrhythmias**
GI: *Nausea,* diarrhea, gastric upset, *constipation,* increased LFTs
GU: Impotence, gynecomastia, nocturia, polyuria
HEMA: Bruising, petechiae, bleeding
INTEG: Rash, bruising
MISC: Gingival hyperplasia
SYST: **Stevens-Johnson syndrome**

PHARMACOKINETICS

Metabolized by liver, excreted in urine (70% as metabolites)
PO: Onset variable; peak 3-4 hr; duration 17-24 hr; half-life (biphasic) 4 min, 3-7 hr (terminal)
IV: Onset 3 min, peak 3-5 min, duration 10-20 min

INTERACTIONS

Increase: hypotension—prazosin, quiNIDine, fentanyl, other antihypertensives, nitrates
Increase: effects of verapamil—β-blockers, cimetidine, telithromycin
Increase: levels of digoxin, theophylline, cycloSPORINE, carBAMazepine, nondepolarizing muscle relaxants
Decrease: effects of lithium
Decrease: antihypertensive effects—NSAIDs

Drug/Food

Increase: hypotensive effects—grapefruit juice

Drug/Lab Test
Increase: AST, ALT, alk phos, BUN, creatinine, serum cholesterol

NURSING CONSIDERATIONS

Assess:

- **Cardiac status:** B/P, pulse, respiration, ECG intervals (PR, QRS, QT); notify prescriber if pulse <50 bpm, systolic B/P <90 mm Hg

⚠ **CHF: I&O ratios, weight daily; crackles, weight gain, dyspnea, jugular venous distention**

- Renal, hepatic studies during long-term treatment, serum potassium periodically

Evaluate:

- Therapeutic response: decreased anginal pain, decreased B/P, dysrhythmias

Teach patient/family:

- To increase fluids, fiber to counteract constipation
- How to take pulse, B/P before taking product; to keep record or graph
- To avoid hazardous activities until stabilized on product, dizziness no longer a problem
- To limit caffeine consumption; to avoid alcohol products
- To avoid OTC or grapefruit products unless directed by prescriber
- To comply with all areas of medical regimen: diet, exercise, stress reduction, product therapy
- To change positions slowly to prevent syncope
- Not to discontinue abruptly because chest pain may occur

⚠ **To report chest pain, palpitations, irregular heart beats, swelling of extremities, skin irritation, rash, tremors, weakness**

TREATMENT OF OVERDOSE:

Defibrillation, atropine for AV block, vasopressor for hypotension, IV calcium

vidarabine ophthalmic

See Appendix B

vigabatrin (Rx)

(vye-ga′ba-trin)

Sabril

Func. class.: Anticonvulsant
Chem. class.: GABA transaminase inhibitor

ACTION: May inhibit reuptake and metabolism of GABA, may increase seizure threshold; structurally similar to GABA

USES: Adjunct treatment of partial seizures in adults and children ≥12 yr, infantile spasm

CONTRAINDICATIONS: Hypersensitivity to this product

Precautions: Pregnancy (C), breastfeeding, children <2 yr, geriatric patients, renal/hepatic disease, suicidal thoughts/behaviors, abrupt discontinuation

Black Box Warning: Visual disturbance

DOSAGE AND ROUTES

Partial seizures

- **Adult: PO** 500 mg bid, titrate in 500-mg increments at weekly intervals up to 1.5 g bid

Infantile spasm

- **Infant >1 mo, child ≤2 yr: PO** 50 mg/kg/day in 2 divided doses, titrate in 25 to 50-mg/kg/day increments q3days, max 150 mg/kg/day

Renal dose

- **Adult: PO** CCr 50-80 ml/min, reduce dose by 25%; CCr 30-50 ml/min, reduce dose by 50%; CCr 10-30 ml/min, reduce dose by 75%

Available forms: Powder for sol; tabs 500 mg

Administer:

PO route (tab)

- Give without regard to meals

PO route (oral sol)

- Reconstitute immediately before using
- Empty contents into clean cup

- For each packet, dissolve 10 ml water, conc 50 mg/ml; do not use other liquids
- Stir until dissolved, sol should be clear
- Use calibrated oral syringe to measure correct dosage
- Discard any unused sol

SIDE EFFECTS

CNS: *Dizziness,* irritability, lethargy, malignant hyperthermia, insomnia
CV: Edema
EENT: Visual impairment
GI: Nausea, vomiting, diarrhea, increased appetite, abdominal pain, GI bleeding, hemorrhoids, weight gain, constipation
HEMA: Anemia
INTEG: Pruritus, rash
RESP: Coughing, respiratory depression, pulmonary embolism

PHARMACOKINETICS

Absorption >95%, no protein binding, widely distributed, not metabolized, excretion in urine 80% parent drug, excretion slowed in renal disease, peak 2 hr, half-life 7.5 hr

INTERACTIONS

Increase: CNS depression—CNS depressants

- Serious ophthalmic effects (glaucoma, retinopathy): azaTHIOprine, chloroquine, corticosteroids, deferoxamine, ethambutol, hydroxychloroquine, interferons, loxapine, mecasermin, rh-IGF-1, pentostatin, phenothiazine, phosphodiesterase inhibitors, tamoxifen, thiothixene; avoid concurrent use

NURSING CONSIDERATIONS

Assess:

- Renal studies: urinalysis, BUN, urine creatinine q3mo
- Hepatic studies: ALT, AST, bilirubin
- Description of seizures: location, duration, presence of aura
- Mental status: mood, sensorium, affect, behavioral changes; if mental status changes, notify prescriber

Perform/provide:

- Storage at room temp
- Assistance with ambulation during early part of treatment; dizziness occurs
- Seizure precautions: padded side rails; move objects that may harm patient

Evaluate:

- Therapeutic response: decreased seizure activity; document on patient's chart

Teach patient/family:

- To carry emergency ID stating patient's name, products taken, condition, prescriber's name and phone number
- To avoid driving, other activities that require alertness
- Not to discontinue medication quickly after long-term use

vilazodone (Rx)

(vil-az′oh-done)

Viibryd

Func. class.: Antidepressant, miscellaneous

ACTION: Novel antidepressant unrelated to other antidepressants, enhances serotonergic action by a dual mechanism

USES: Major depression

CONTRAINDICATIONS: Concomitant use of MOA inhibitors or within 14 days after discontinuing MOA inhibitor or within 14 days after discontinuing vilazodone

Precautions: Pregnancy (C), labor, infants, geriatric patients, abrupt discontinuation, bipolar disorder, bleeding, operating machinery, ECT, hepatic disease, hyponatremia, hypovolemia, substance abuse, history of seizures, serotonin syndrome, neuroleptic malignant syndrome; use with serotonin precursors (e.g., tryptophan) or serotonergic drugs; suicidal ideation, worsening depression or behavior

Black Box Warning: Children, suicidal ideation

DOSAGE AND ROUTES

- **Adult: PO** 10 mg × 7 days, then 20 mg × 7 days, then 40 mg/day; if taking potent CYP3A4 inhibitor, max 20 mg/day

Available forms: Tabs 10, 20, 40 mg

Administer:

- With food to increase absorption

SIDE EFFECTS

CNS: Restlessness, dizziness, drowsiness, fatigue, mania, insomnia, migraine, **neuroleptic-malignant–like syndrome**, paresthesias, **seizures, suicidal ideation**, tremor, night sweats, dream disorders

EENT: Cataracts, blurred vision

GI: Nausea, vomiting, flatulence, diarrhea, xerostomia, altered taste, gastroenteritis

GU: Decreased libido, ejaculation disorder, increased frequency of urination, sexual dysfunction

HEMA: Bleeding, decreased platelets

MS: Arthralgia

SYST: Neonatal abstinence syndrome, withdrawal, **serotonin syndrome**

INTERACTIONS

⚠ **Do not use with MAO inhibitors**

⚠ **Increased:** **serotonin syndrome—SSRIs, SNRIs, serotonin receptor agonists, selegiline, busPIRone, dextromethorphan, ergots, fenfluramine, dexfluramine, lithium, meperidine, fentaNYL, methylphenidate, dexmethylphenidate, metoclopramide, mirtazapine, nefazodone, pentazocine, phenothiazines, haloperidol, loxapine, thiothixene, molindone, amphetamines**

Increased: bleeding—anticoagulants, thrombolytics, platelet inhibitors, salicylates

Increased: vilazodone levels—CYP3A4 inhibitors

Drug/Food

- Avoid use with grapefruit juice

Drug/Herb

Increased: serotonin syndrome—St. John's wort

PHARMACOKINETICS

Protein binding 96%-99%, metabolized by liver by CYP3A4 (major) and CYP2C19 and CYP2D (minor) and non-CYP pathways, peak 4-5 hr, half-life 25 hr

NURSING CONSIDERATIONS

Assess:

Black Box Warning: Mental status: orientation, mood behavior initially and periodically; initiate suicide precautions if indicated; history of seizures, mania

- Renal/hepatic status: hyponatremia

Perform/provide:

- Storage at room temp, away from moisture, heat

Evaluate:

- Therapeutic response: remission of depressive symptoms

Teach patient/family:

- To take as directed; not to double dose
- To avoid abrupt discontinuation unless approved by prescriber
- Not to drive or operate machinery until effects are known
- Not to use other products unless approved by prescribed

⚠ **To contact prescriber regarding the following: allergic reactions; personality changes (aggression, anxiety, anger, hostility); extreme sleepiness or drowsiness; feeling confused, nervous, restless or clumsy; numbness, tingling, or burning pain in hands, arms, legs, or feet; tremors; unusual behavior or thoughts about hurting oneself**

V

⚠ HIGH ALERT

vinBLAStine (VLB) (Rx)

(vin-blast′een)

Func. class.: Antineoplastic

Chem. class.: Vinca rosea alkaloid

Do not confuse:
vinBLAStine/vinCRIStine

ACTION: Inhibits mitotic activity, arrests cell cycle at metaphase; inhibits RNA synthesis, blocks cellular use of glutamic acid needed for purine synthesis; vesicant

USES: Breast, testicular cancer, lymphomas, neuroblastoma; Hodgkin's/non-Hodgkin's lymphoma; mycosis fungoides, histiocytosis, Kaposi's sarcoma, Langerhans cell histiocytosis

Unlabeled uses: Lung, bladder, prostate cancer; desmoid tumor, malignant melanoma

CONTRAINDICATIONS: Pregnancy (D), breastfeeding, infants, hypersensitivity, leukopenia, granulocytopenia, bone marrow suppression, infection

Black Box Warning: Intrathecal use

Precautions: Renal/hepatic disease, tumor lysis syndrome

Black Box Warning: Extravasation

DOSAGE AND ROUTES

Breast cancer

- **Adult: IV** 4.5 mg/m^2 on day 1 of every 21 days in combination with DOXOrubicin and thiotepa

Hodgkins disease

- **Adult: IV** 6 mg/m^2 on days 1 and 15 of every 28 days with DOXOrubicin, bleomycin, dacarbazine (ABVD regimen)
- **Child: IV** 2.5-6 mg/m^2/day once q1-2wk × 3-6 wk, max weekly dose 12.5 mg/m^2

Available forms: Inj, powder 10 mg for 10 ml IV; sol for inj 1 mg/ml

Administer:

- Antiemetic 30-60 min before product and prn to prevent vomiting

Black Box Warning: Hyaluronidase 150 units/ml in 1 ml NaCl, warm compress for extravasation for vesicant activity treatment

Black Box Warning: Do not administer intrathecally; fatal

IV inj route

- After diluting 10 mg/10 ml NaCl; give through Y-tube or 3-way stopcock or directly over 1 min

Intermittent IV INF route

- Further dilute in 50-100 ml of NS, infuse over 15-30 min

Additive compatibilities: Bleomycin

Syringe compatibilities: Bleomycin, CISplatin, cyclophosphamide, droperidol, fluorouracil, leucovorin, methotrexate, metoclopramide, mitomycin, vinCRIStine

Y-site compatibilities: Allopurinol, amifostine, amphotericin B cholesteryl, aztreonam, bleomycin, CISplatin, cyclophosphamide, DOXOrubicin, DOXOrubicin liposome, droperidol, filgrastim, fludarabine, fluorouracil, granisetron, heparin, leucovorin, melphalan, methotrexate, metoclopramide, mitomycin, ondansetron, paclitaxel, piperacillin/tazobactam, sargramostim, teniposide, thiotepa, vinCRIStine, vinorelbine

SIDE EFFECTS

CNS: Paresthesias, peripheral neuropathy, depression, headache, seizures, malaise

CV: Tachycardia, orthostatic hypo/hypertension

GI: *Nausea, vomiting,* ileus, *anorexia, stomatitis, constipation,* abdominal pain, GI/rectal bleeding, hepatotoxicity, pharyngitis

GU: Urinary retention, renal failure, hyperuricemia

HEMA: Thrombocytopenia, leukopenia, myelosuppression, agranulocytosis, granulocytosis, aplastic anemia, neutropenia, pancytopenia

INTEG: *Rash, alopecia,* photosensitivity, extravasation, tissue necrosis

META: SIADH

RESP: Fibrosis, pulmonary infiltrate, bronchospasm
SYST: Tumor lysis syndrome (TLS)

PHARMACOKINETICS

Half-life (triphasic) <5 min, 50-155 min, 23-85 hr; metabolized in liver; excreted in urine, feces; crosses blood-brain barrier

INTERACTIONS

- Synergism: bleomycin
- Bronchospasm: mitomycin
- Do not use with radiation

Increase: bleeding risk—NSAIDs, anticoagulants
Increase: toxicity, bone marrow suppression—antineoplastics
Increase: action of methotrexate
Increase: adverse reactions—live virus vaccines
⚠ **Increase:** toxicity—CYP3A4 inhibitors (aprepitant, antiretroviral protease inhibitors, clarithromycin, danazol, delavirdine, diltiazem, erythromycin, fluconazole, FLUoxetine, fluvoxamine, imatinib, ketoconazole, mibefradil, nefazodone, telithromycin, voriconazole)
Decrease: vinBLAStine effect—CYP3A4 inducers (barbiturates, bosentan, carBAMazepine, efavirenz, phenytoins, nevirapine, rifabutin, rifampin)

Drug/Herb

- Avoid use with St. John's wort

NURSING CONSIDERATIONS

Assess:

⚠ CBC, differential, platelet count weekly; withhold product if WBC is <2000/mm³ or platelet count is <75,000/mm³; notify prescriber; RBC, Hct, Hgb may be decreased

- Pulmonary function tests, chest x-ray studies before, during therapy; chest x-ray film should be obtained q2wk during treatment
- Neurologic status: sensory–vibratory evaluation if side effects occur
- Renal studies: BUN, serum uric acid, urine CCr, electrolytes before, during therapy; I&O ratio; report fall in urine output of 30 ml/hr
- Monitor temp; may indicate beginning infection
- Hepatic studies before, during therapy (bilirubin, AST, ALT, LDH) as needed or qmo
- Bleeding: hematuria, guaiac, bruising, petechiae, mucosa or orifices
- Dyspnea, crackles, unproductive cough, chest pain, tachypnea, fatigue, increased pulse, pallor, lethargy
- Effects of alopecia on body image; discuss feelings about body changes
- Sensitivity of feet/hands, which precedes neuropathy
- Jaundiced skin, sclera; dark urine, clay-colored stools, itchy skin, abdominal pain, fever, diarrhea
- Buccal cavity q8hr for dryness, sores, ulcerations, white patches, oral pain, bleeding, dysphagia

Black Box Warning: Local irritation, pain, burning, discoloration at inj site, extravasation

- Symptoms indicating severe allergic reaction: rash, pruritus, urticaria, purpuric skin lesions, itching, flushing
- Frequency of stools and characteristics: cramping; acidosis; signs of dehydration: rapid respirations, poor skin turgor, decreased urine output, dry skin, restlessness, weakness
- Gout, joint pain, swelling, increased uric acid; allopurinol or other treatment may be used

Perform/provide:

- Increased fluid intake to 2-3 L/day to prevent urate deposits, calculi formation
- Brushing of teeth bid-tid with soft brush or cotton-tipped applicator for stomatitis; use unwaxed dental floss

Evaluate:

- Therapeutic response: decreased tumor size, spread of malignancy

Teach patient/family:

- To report any complaints or side effects to nurse or prescriber

- To report any changes in breathing or coughing; to avoid exposure to persons with infection
- That hair may be lost during treatment, that a wig or hairpiece may make patient feel better; that new hair may be different in color, texture
- To report change in gait or numbness in extremities; may indicate neuropathy
- To avoid foods with citric acid, hot or rough texture
- To report any bleeding, white spots, ulcerations in mouth to prescriber; to examine mouth daily
- To wear sunscreen, protective clothing, sunglasses
- To avoid receiving vaccinations

⚠ To use effective contraception, pregnancy (D); to avoid breastfeeding; that product may cause male infertility

⚠ *HIGH ALERT*

vinCRIStine (VCR) (Rx)

(vin-kris′teen)

Vincasar PFS

Func. class.: Antineoplastic—miscellaneous

Chem. class.: Vinca alkaloid

Do not confuse:
vinCRIStine/vinBLAStine

ACTION: Inhibits mitotic activity, arrests cell cycle at metaphase; inhibits RNA synthesis, blocks cellular use of glutamic acid needed for purine synthesis; vesicant

USES: Lymphomas, neuroblastoma, Hodgkin's disease, acute lymphoblastic and other leukemias, rhabdomyosarcoma, Wilms' tumor, non-Hodgkin's lymphoma, malignant glioma, soft-tissue sarcoma

Unlabeled uses: Lung, breast, colorectal, head/neck, osteogenic sarcomas; small-cell lung cancer, trophoblastic disease

CONTRAINDICATIONS: Pregnancy (D), breastfeeding, infants, hypersensitivity, radiation therapy

Black Box Warning: Intrathecal use

Precautions: Renal/hepatic disease, hypertension, neuromuscular disease

Black Box Warning: Extravasation

DOSAGE AND ROUTES

- **Adult:** IV 0.4-1.4 mg/m^2/wk, max 2 mg
- **Child:** IV 1-2 mg/m^2/wk, max 2 mg

Available forms: Inj 1 mg/ml; powder for inj 5 mg/vial

Administer:

- Antiemetic 30-60 min before product and prn
- Antispasmodic for GI symptoms

Black Box Warning: Do not give intrathecally; fatal

IV route

- After diluting with diluent provided or 1 mg/10 ml sterile water or NaCl; give through Y-tube or 3-way stopcock or directly over 1 min

Black Box Warning: Hyaluronidase 150 units/ml in 1 ml NaCl; apply warm compress for extravasation

Additive compatibilities: Bleomycin, cytarabine, fluorouracil, methotrexate

Syringe compatibilities: Bleomycin, CISplatin, cyclophosphamide, doxapram, DOXOrubicin, droperidol, fluorouracil, heparin, leucovorin, methotrexate, metoclopramide, mitomycin, vinBLAStine

Y-site compatibilities: Allopurinol, amifostine, amphotericin B cholesteryl, aztreonam, bleomycin, CISplatin, cladribine, cyclophosphamide, DOXOrubicin, DOXOrubicin liposome, droperidol, filgrastim, fludarabine, fluorouracil, granisetron, heparin, leucovorin, melphalan, methotrexate, metoclopramide, mitomycin, ondansetron, paclitaxel, piperacillin/tazobactam, sargramostim, teniposide, thiotepa, vinBLAStine, vinorelbine

SIDE EFFECTS

CNS: *Decreased reflexes, numbness, weakness, motor difficulties,* CNS depression, cranial nerve paralysis, seizures, peripheral neuropathy
CV: Orthostatic hypotension
EENT: *Diplopia*
GI: *Nausea, vomiting, anorexia, stomatitis, constipation,* paralytic ileus, *abdominal pain,* hepatotoxicity
GU: Renal tubular obstruction
HEMA: Thrombocytopenia, leukopenia, myelosuppression, anemia
INTEG: *Alopecia,* extravasation
SYST: Tumor lysis syndrome (TLS)

PHARMACOKINETICS

Half-life (triphasic) <5 min, 50-155 min, 23-85 hr; metabolized in liver; excreted in bile, feces; crosses placental, blood-brain barrier

INTERACTIONS

- Neurotoxicity: peripheral nervous system products
- Do not use with radiation
- Acute pulmonary reactions: mitomycin-c

⚠ **Increase:** toxicity—CYP3A4 inhibitors (aprepitant, antiretroviral protease inhibitors, clarithromycin, danazol, delavirdine, diltiazem, erythromycin, fluconazole, FLUoxetine, fluvoxamine, imatinib, ketoconazole, mibefradil, nefazodone, telithromycin, voriconazole)
Decrease: immune response—vaccines, toxoids
Decrease: digoxin level—digoxin
Decrease: vinCRIStine effect—CYP3A4 inducers (barbiturates, bosentan, carBAMazepine, efavirenz, phenytoins, nevirapine, rifabutin, rifampin)
Drug/Herb
- Avoid use with St. John's wort

NURSING CONSIDERATIONS

Assess:
- CBC, differential, platelet count before each dose; withhold product if WBC is <4000/mm^3 or platelet count is <75,000/mm^3; notify prescriber; RBC, Hct, Hgb; may be decreased
- Renal studies: BUN, serum uric acid, urine CCr; electrolytes before, during therapy; I&O ratio; report fall in urine output of 30 ml/hr
- Monitor temp q4hr; may indicate beginning infection
- Hepatic studies before, during therapy (bilirubin, AST, ALT, LDH) as needed or monthly
- Deep tendon reflexes; product is neurotoxic
- Sensitivity of feet/hands, which precedes neuropathy
- **Tumor lysis syndrome:** hyperkalemia, hyperphosphatemia, hyperuricemia, hypocalcemia

Black Box Warning: Extravasation: pain, swelling, poor blood return; if extravasation occurs, local inj of hyaluronidase and moderate heat to area may help disperse product

Intrathecal administration
- **Bleeding:** hematuria, guaiac, bruising, petechiae, mucosa or orifices q8hr
- Effects of alopecia on body image; discuss feelings about body changes
- Jaundiced skin, sclera; dark urine, clay-colored stools, itchy skin, abdominal pain, fever, diarrhea
- Buccal cavity q8hr for dryness, sores, ulcerations, white patches, oral pain, bleeding, dysphagia
- Symptoms indicating severe allergic reaction: rash, pruritus, urticaria, purpuric skin lesions, itching, flushing

Perform/provide:
- Brushing of teeth bid-tid with soft brush or cotton-tipped applicator for stomatitis; use unwaxed dental floss

Evaluate:
- Therapeutic response: decreased tumor size, spread of malignancy

Teach patient/family:
- To report change in gait or numbness in extremities; may indicate neuropathy
- To report any complaints or side effects to nurse or prescriber
- To report any bleeding, white spots or

V

ulcerations in mouth to prescriber; to examine mouth daily

- To increase bulk, fluids, exercise to prevent constipation
- To avoid persons with infections
- To avoid vaccinations
- That hair may be lost; that hair will grow back but with different texture, color

⚠ To use effective contraception during and for 2 mo after therapy, pregnancy (D), to avoid breastfeeding

⚠ HIGH ALERT

vinorelbine (Rx)

(vi-nor′el-bine)

Navelbine

Func. class.: Antineoplastic—miscellaneous

Chem. class.: Semisynthetic vinca alkaloid

ACTION: Inhibits mitotic spindle activity, arrests cell cycle at metaphase; inhibits RNA synthesis, blocks cellular use of glutamic acid needed for purine synthesis; vesicant

USES: Unresectable advanced non–small-cell lung cancer (NSCLC) stage IV; may be used alone or in combination with cisplatin for stage III or IV NSCLC

Unlabeled uses: Hodgkin's disease, breast/ovarian/head/neck cancer, desmoid tumor

CONTRAINDICATIONS: Pregnancy (D), breastfeeding, infants, hypersensitivity, granulocyte count <1000 cells/mm^3 pretreatment

Black Box Warning: Severe neutropenia, intrathecal administration

Precautions: Children, geriatric patients, renal/hepatic/pulmonary/neurologic disease, anemia, bone marrow suppression

Black Box Warning: Extravasation

DOSAGE AND ROUTES

- **Adult:** IV 30 mg/m^2/wk
- **ANC 1000-1499:** Give 50% of dose; <1000, hold dose; <1000 × 3 wk, discontinue

Hepatic dose

- **Adult:** IV total bilirubin 2.1-3 mg/dl 15 mg/m^2/wk; total bilirubin ≥3 mg/dl 7.5 mg/m^2/day

Available forms: Inj 10 mg/ml

Administer:

Black Box Warning: Do not give intrathecally; fatal

- Antiemetic 30-60 min before product and prn to prevent vomiting

Intermittent IV INF route

- Dilute to 0.5-2 mg/ml with 0.9% NaCl, 0.45% NaCl, D_5W, D_5/0.45% NaCl, LR, Ringer's sol, give over 6-10 min into Y-site or central line, flush line

Black Box Warning: Hyaluronidase 150 units/ml in 1 ml NaCl, warm compress for extravasation for vesicant activity treatment

Continuous IV INF route

- 40 mg/m^2 q3wk after IV bol of 8 mg/m^2; may be given in combination with DOXOrubicin, fluorouracil, CISplatin

Y-site compatibilities: Amikacin, aztreonam, bleomycin, bumetanide, buprenorphine, butorphanol, calcium gluconate, CARBOplatin, carmustine, cefotaxime, ceftazidime, ceftizoxime, chlorproMAZINE, cimetidine, CISplatin, clindamycin, cyclophosphamide, cytarabine, dacarbazine, DACTINomycin, DAUNOrubicin, dexamethasone, diphenhydrAMINE, DOXOrubicin, DOXOrubicin liposome, doxycycline, droperidol, enalaprilat, etoposide, famotidine, filgrastim, floxuridine, fluconazole, fludarabine, gallium, gentamicin, granisetron, haloperidol, heparin, hydrocortisone, HYDROmorphone, hydrOXYzine, IDArubicin, ifosfamide, imipenem-cilastatin, LORazepam, mannitol, mechlorethamine, melphalan, meperidine, mesna, methotrexate, metoclopramide, metroNIDAZOLE, minocycline, mitoxantrone, morphine, nalbuphine, netilmicin, ondansetron, plicamycin, streptozocin, teniposide, ticarcillin, ticarcillin-clavulanate, tobramycin, vancomycin, vinBLAStine, vinCRIStine, zidovudine

SIDE EFFECTS

CNS: Paresthesias, peripheral neuropathy, depression, headache, seizures, weakness, jaw pain, asthenia
CV: Chest pain
GI: *Nausea, vomiting,* ileus, *anorexia, stomatitis,* constipation, abdominal pain, *diarrhea,* **hepatotoxicity, GI obstruction/perforation**
HEMA: **Neutropenia, anemia, thrombocytopenia, granulocytopenia**
INTEG: *Rash, alopecia,* photosensitivity, inj site reaction, necrosis
META: SIADH
MS: Myalgia
RESP: SOB

PHARMACOKINETICS

Half-life 27-43 hr; peak 1-2 hr; highly bound to platelets, lymphocytes; metabolized in liver; excreted in feces; small amount unchanged in kidneys

INTERACTIONS

Increase: bleeding risk—NSAIDs, anticoagulants
⚠ **Increase: toxicity—CYP3A4 inhibitors (aprepitant, antiretroviral protease inhibitors, clarithromycin, danazol, delavirdine, diltiazem, erythromycin, fluconazole, FLUoxetine, fluvoxamine, imatinib, ketoconazole, mibefradil, nefazodone, telithromycin, voriconazole)**
Decrease: vinorelbine effect—CYP3A4 inducers (barbiturates, bosentan, carBAMazepine, efavirenz, phenytoins, nevirapine, rifabutin, rifampin)
Drug/Herb
- Avoid use with St. John's wort

NURSING CONSIDERATIONS

Assess:
- B/P (baseline, q15min) during administration

Black Box Warning: CBC, differential, platelet count before each dose; withhold product if WBC is <4000/mm^3 or platelet count is <75,000/mm^3; notify prescriber of results; recovery will take 3 wk
- Respiratory status: dyspnea, crackles, unproductive cough, chest pain, tachypnea
- Renal studies: BUN, serum uric acid, urine CCr before, during therapy; I&O ratio; report fall in urine output to <30 ml/hr; decreased hyperuricemia
- **Infection,** cold, fever, sore throat; notify prescriber if these occur; effects of alopecia on body image
- **Bleeding:** hematuria, guaiac, bruising, petechiae, mucosa or orifices, no rectal temps; avoid IM inj; apply pressure to venipuncture sites
- Nutritional status: antiemetic may be needed
- Hepatic function tests: AST, ALT, bilirubin, LDH

⚠ **Severe allergic reactions: rash, pruritus, urticaria, itching, flushing, bronchospasm, hypotension; EPINEPHrine and crash cart should be nearby**
- Neurologic status: numbness, pain, tingling, loss of Achilles reflex, weakness, palsies
- **Gout:** pain, swelling, increased uric acid levels

Perform/provide:
- Brushing of teeth bid-tid with soft brush or cotton-tipped applicator for stomatitis; unwaxed dental floss

Evaluate:
- Therapeutic response: decreased tumor size, spread of malignancy

Teach patient/family:
- To report change in gait or numbness in extremities, continuing constipation; may indicate neurotoxicity
- To report any complaints or side effects to nurse or prescriber
- To examine mouth daily for bleeding, white spots, ulcerations; to notify prescriber
- To avoid crowds, people with infections, vaccinations, OTC products

⚠ To use effective contraception during treatment and for ≥2 mo after product is discontinued, pregnancy (D); to avoid breastfeeding
• That hair may be lost; that hair will grow back but with different texture, color

vitamin A (Rx, OTC)

Aquasol A, Del-Vi-A, Vitamin A
Func. class.: Vitamin, fat soluble
Chem. class.: Retinol

ACTION: Needed for normal bone, tooth development; visual dark adaptation; skin disease; mucosa tissue repair; assists with production of adrenal steroids, cholesterol, RNA

USES: Vit A deficiency

CONTRAINDICATIONS: Pregnancy (X), hypersensitivity to vit A, malabsorption syndrome, hypervitaminosis A, parenteral, IV administration
Precautions: Pregnancy (C) (PO), breastfeeding, impaired renal function, children, hepatic disease, infants, alcoholism, hepatitis

DOSAGE AND ROUTES

• **Adult and child >8 yr: PO** 100,000-500,000 international units/day × 3 days then 50,000/day × 2 wk; dose based on severity of deficiency; maintenance 10,000-20,000 international units for 2 mo
• **Child 1-8 yr: IM** 5000-15,000 international units/day × 10 days
• **Infant <1 yr: IM** 5000-15,000 international units × 10 days
Maintenance
• **Child 4-8 yr: IM** 15,000 international units/day × 2 mo
• **Child <4 yr: IM** 10,000 international units/day × 2 mo
Available forms: Caps 10,000, 25,000, 50,000 international units; drops 5000 international units; inj 50,000 international units/ml; tabs 10,000, 25,000, 50,000 international units
Administer:
PO route
• With food (PO) for better absorption
• Do not administer IV because of risk of anaphylactic shock; IM only
• Oral preparations not indicated for vit A deficiency in those with malabsorption syndrome
IM route
• Give deep in large muscle mass; do not use deltoid muscle for administration of >1 ml

SIDE EFFECTS

CNS: Headache, **increased intracranial pressure, intracranial hypertension,** lethargy, malaise
EENT: Gingivitis, papilledema, exophthalmos, inflammation of tongue and lips
GI: Nausea, vomiting, anorexia, abdominal pain, jaundice
INTEG: Drying of skin, pruritus, increased pigmentation, night sweats, alopecia
META: Hypomenorrhea, hypercalcemia
MS: Arthralgia, retarded growth, hard areas on bone

PHARMACOKINETICS

Stored in liver, kidneys, fat; excreted (metabolites) in urine, feces

INTERACTIONS

Increase: levels of vit A—corticosteroids, oral contraceptives
Decrease: absorption of vit A—mineral oil, cholestyramine, colestipol
Drug/Lab Test
False increase: bilirubin, serum cholesterol

NURSING CONSIDERATIONS

Assess:
• Nutritional status: yellow and dark green vegetables, yellow/orange fruits, vit-A–fortified foods, liver, egg yolks
• Vit A deficiency: decreased growth; night blindness; dry, brittle nails; hair

loss; urinary stones; increased infection; hyperkeratosis of skin; drying of cornea

Perform/provide:

- Storage in tight, light-resistant container

Evaluate:

- Therapeutic response: increased growth rate, weight; absence of dry skin and mucous membranes, night blindness

Teach patient/family:

- That, if dose is missed, it should be omitted
- That ophthalmic exams may be required periodically throughout therapy
- Not to use mineral oil while taking this product
- To notify prescriber of nausea, vomiting, lip cracking, loss of hair, headache
- Not to take more than prescribed amount

TREATMENT OF OVERDOSE:
Discontinue product

vitamin E (OTC)

Amino-Opti-E, Aquasol E, Daltose ✱, E-Complex-600, E-Ferol, E-Vitamin Succinate, E-200 I.U. Softgels, Gordo-Vite E, Tocopherol, Vita-Plus E Softgels, Vitec

Func. class.: Vit E

Chem. class.: Fat soluble

ACTION: Needed for digestion and metabolism of polyunsaturated fats; decreases platelet aggregation, blood clot formation; promotes normal growth and development of muscle tissue, prostaglandin synthesis

USES: Vit E deficiency, impaired fat absorption, hemolytic anemia in premature neonates, prevention of retrolental fibroplasia, sickle cell anemia, supplement for malabsorption syndrome

CONTRAINDICATIONS: IV use in infants

Precautions: Pregnancy (A), anemia, breastfeeding, hypoprothrombinemia

DOSAGE AND ROUTES

Deficiency

- **Adult: PO** 60-75 international units/day
- **Child: PO** 1 international units/kg (malabsorption)

Prevention of deficiency

- **Adult: PO** 30 international units/day; **TOP** apply to affected areas
- **Infant: PO** 5 international units/day

Available forms: Caps 100, 200, 400, 500, 600, 1000 international units; tabs 100, 200, 400 international units; drops 50 mg/ml; chew tabs 400 units; ointment; cream; lotion; oil

Administer:

PO route

- Administer with or after meals
- Chew chewable tabs well
- Sol may be dropped in mouth or mixed with food

Topical route

- To moisturize dry skin

SIDE EFFECTS

CNS: Headache, fatigue
CV: Increased risk for thrombophlebitis
EENT: Blurred vision
GI: Nausea, cramps, diarrhea
GU: Gonadal dysfunction
INTEG: Sterile abscess, contact dermatitis
META: Altered metabolism of hormones (thyroid, pituitary, adrenal), altered immunity
MS: Weakness

V

PHARMACOKINETICS

PO: Metabolized in liver, excreted in bile

INTERACTIONS

Increase: action of oral anticoagulants
Decrease: absorption—cholestyramine, colestipol, mineral oil, sucralfate

NURSING CONSIDERATIONS

Assess:

• Nutritional status: wheat germ; dark green, leafy vegetables; nuts; eggs; liver; vegetable oils; dairy products; cereals

Perform/provide:

• Storage in tight, light-resistant container

Evaluate:

• Therapeutic response: absence of hemolytic anemia, adequate vit E levels, improvement in skin lesions, decreased edema

Teach patient/family:

• About the necessary foods for diet
• To omit dose if missed
• To avoid vitamin supplements unless directed by prescriber

voriconazole (Rx)

(vohr-i-kahn′a-zol)

Vfend

Func. class.: Antifungal, systemic
Chem. class.: Triazole derivative

ACTION: Inhibits fungal CYP 450-mediation demethylation; needed for biosynthesis; causes leakage from cell membrane

USES: Invasive aspergillosis, serious fungal infections (*Candida* sp., *Scedosporium apiospermum, Fusarium* sp., *Monosporium, Apiospermum*)

Unlabeled uses: *Acremonium sp., Blastomyces dermatitidis, Coccidioides immitis, Cryptococcus neoformans,* febrile neutropenia, fungal keratitis, *Histoplasma capsulatum,* oropharyngeal candidiasis, *Rhodotorula sp., Scedosporium sp.,* cutaneous aspergillosis, candidemia (premature neonates), fungal infections in children ≥12 yr

CONTRAINDICATIONS: Pregnancy (D), breastfeeding, children, hypersensitivity, severe bone marrow depression, severe hepatic disease

Precautions: Renal disease (IV); patients of Asian/African descent; cardiomyopathy, cholestasis, chemotherapy, lactase deficiency, visual disturbances, renal failure, pancreatitis, QT prolongation, hypokalemia; ventricular dysrhythmias, torsades de pointes

DOSAGE AND ROUTES

• **Adult/geriatric/child ≥12 yr: PO** give 1 hr before or after meals; ≥40 kg, loading dose 400 mg q12hr on day 1 then 200 mg q12hr; <40 kg, loading dose 200 mg q12hr on day 1 then 100 mg q12hr

• **Adult/geriatric/child ≥12 yr: IV INF** Loading dose 6 mg/kg q12hr × 2 dose then 4 mg/kg q12hr; may switch to oral dosing

CNS blastomycosis/blastomycosis meningitis (unlabeled)

• **Adult: PO** 200-400 mg bid × at least 12 mo and until resolution of CSF abnormalities

Renal dose

• **Adult: PO** CCr <50 ml/min, use orally only

Hepatic dose

• **Adult: PO** 6 mg/kg q12hr × 2 doses then 2 mg/kg q12hr or 100 mg q12hr if >40 kg; 50 mg q12hr if <40 kg

Available forms: Tabs 50, 200 mg; powder for inj, lyophilized 200 mg voriconazole, powder for oral susp 45 g (40 mg/ml after reconstitution)

Administer:

PO route

• Oral susp: tap bottle; add 46 ml of water to bottle; shake well; remove cap; push bottle adaptor into neck of bottle; replace cap; write expiration date (14 days); shake well before each use; administer using only oral dispenser supplied, 1 hr before or after meals; tabs and susp may be interchanged

Intermittent IV INF route

• Product only after C&S confirms organism, product needed to treat condition; make sure product used in life-threatening infections

- Reconstitute powder with 19 ml water for inj to 10 mg/ml, shake until dissolved; infuse over 1-2 hr at conc of ≤5 mg/ml; do not admix with other products, 4.2% sodium bicarbonate inf
- Store at room temp (powder, tabs)

Y-site compatibilities: Acyclovir, alfentanil, allopurinol, amifostine, amikacin, aminocaproic acid, aminophylline, amiodarone, amphotericin B liposome, ampicillin, ampicillin/sulbactam, anidulafungin, azithromycin, aztreonam, bivalirudin, bleomycin, bumetanide, buprenorphine, butorphanol, calcium acetate/chloride/gluconate, CARBOplatin, carmustine, caspofungin, ceFAZolin, cefotaxime, cefotetan, cefoxitin, ceftazidime, ceftizoxime, cefTRIAXone, chloramphenicol, chlorproMAZINE, cimetidine, ciprofloxacin, cisatracurium, CISplatin, clindamycin, cyclophosphamide, cytarabine, dacarbazine, DACTINomycin, DAPTOmycin, DAUNOrubicin, dexamethasone, dexmedetomidine, dexrazoxane, digoxin, diltiazem, diphenhydrAMINE, DOBUTamine, docetaxel, dolasetron, DOPamine, doripenem, doxacurium, doxycycline, droperidol, enalaprilat, ePHEDrine, EPINEPHrine, epirubicin, ertapenem, erythromycin, esmolol, etoposide, etoposide phosphate, famotidine, fenoldopam, fentaNYL, fluconazole, fludarabine, fluorouracil, foscarnet, fosphenytoin, furosemide, ganciclovir, gemcitabine, gentamicin, glycopyrrolate, granisetron, haloperidol, heparin, hydrALAZINE, hydrocortisone, ifosfamide, imipenem/cilastatin, inamrinone, insulin, irinotecan, isoproterenol, ketorolac, labetalol, leucovorin, levofloxacin, lidocaine, linezolid, LORazepam, magnesium sulfate, mannitol, mechlorethamine, melphalan, meperidine, meropenem, mesna, metaraminol, methohexital, methotrexate, methyldopate, methylPREDNISolone, metoclopramide, metoprolol, metroNIDAZOLE, midazolam, milrinone, mitomycin, morphine, nafcillin, nalbuphine, naloxone, niCARdipine, nitroglycerin, norepinephrine, octreotide, ondansetron, oxaliplatin, oxytocin, paclitaxel, pamidronate, pancuronium, pentamidine, pentazocine, PENTobarbital, PHENobarbital, phentolamine, phenylephrine, piperacillin/tazobactam, potassium chloride/phosphates, procainamide, promethazine, propranolol, quinupristin/dalfopristin, remifentanil, rocuronium, sodium acetate/bicarbonate/phosphates, streptozocin, succinylcholine, SUFentanil, tacrolimus, teniposide, theophylline, thiotepa, ticarcillin/clavulanate, tirofiban, tobramycin, topotecan, trimethobenzamide, trimethoprim/sulfamethoxazole, vancomycin, vasopressin, vecuronium, verapamil, vinBLAStine, vinCRIStine, vinorelbine, zidovudine

SIDE EFFECTS

CNS: *Headache,* paresthesias, peripheral neuropathy, hallucinations, psychosis, EPS, depression, Guillain-Barré syndrome, insomnia, suicidal ideation, dizziness

CV: **Tachycardia,** hypo/hypertension, vasodilation, **atrial arrhythmias, atrial fibrillation, AV block, bradycardia, CHF, MI, QT prolongation, torsades de pointes**

EENT: Blurred vision, eye hemorrhage

GI: *Nausea, vomiting, anorexia,* diarrhea, cramps, **hemorrhagic gastroenteritis, acute hepatic failure, hepatitis, intestinal perforation, pancreatitis**

GU: *Hypokalemia,* azotemia, **renal tubular necrosis, permanent renal impairment, anuria, oliguria**

HEMA: Anemia, **eosinophilia,** hypomagnesemia, **thrombocytopenia, leukopenia, pancytopenia**

INTEG: *Burning, irritation,* pain, necrosis at inj site with extravasation, dermatitis, rash, photosensitivity

MISC: Respiratory disorder

SYST: **Stevens-Johnson syndrome, toxic epidermal necrolysis, sepsis;** melanoma (photosensitivity reactions)

PHARMACOKINETICS

By CYP3A4, CYP2C9 enzymes, protein binding 58%; max serum conc 1-2 hr after dosing; eliminated via hepatic metabolism; protein binding 58%; elimination half-life 6 hr (dose dependent)

INTERACTIONS

Increase: effects of benzodiazepines, calcium channel blockers, cycloSPORINE, ergots, HMG-CoA reductase inhibitors, pimozide, quiNIDine, prednisoLONE, sirolimus, sulfonylureas, tacrolimus, vinca alkaloids, warfarin, rifabutin, proton pump inhibitors, NNRTIs, protease inhibitors, phenytoin

Increase: nephrotoxicity—other nephrotoxic antibiotics (aminoglycosides, CISplatin, vancomycin, cycloSPORINE, polymyxin B)

Increase: hypokalemia—corticosteroids, digoxin, skeletal muscle relaxants, thiazides

⚠ **Increase:** QT prolongation—class IA/III antidysrhythmics, some phenothiazines, β agonists, local anesthetics, tricyclics, haloperidol, chloroquine, droperidol, pentamidine; CYP3A4 inhibitors (amiodarone, clarithromycin, erythromycin, telithromycin, troleandomycin), arsenic trioxide, levomethadyl; CYP3A4 substrates (methadone, pimozide, QUEtiapine, quiNIDine, risperidone, ziprasidone)

Drug/Herb

- Do not use with St. John's wort

Drug/Food

- Avoid use with high-fat meals, take 1 hr before or after meal

NURSING CONSIDERATIONS

Assess:

- VS q15-30min during first inf; note changes in pulse, B/P
- I&O ratio; watch for decreasing urinary output, change in specific gravity; discontinue product to prevent permanent damage to renal tubules
- Blood studies: CBC, K, Na, Ca, Mg q2wk; BUN, creatinine weekly
- Weight weekly; if weight increases >2 lb/wk, edema is present; renal damage should be considered

⚠ **Renal toxicity:** increasing BUN, serum creatinine; if BUN is >40 mg/dl or if serum creatinine >3 mg/dl, product may be discontinued or dosage reduced

⚠ **Hepatotoxicity:** increasing AST, ALT, alk phos, bilirubin

- **Allergic reaction:** dermatitis, rash; product should be discontinued, antihistamines (mild reaction) or epinephrine (severe reaction) administered
- **Hypokalemia:** anorexia, drowsiness, weakness, decreased reflexes, dizziness, increased urinary output, increased thirst, paresthesias
- **Ototoxicity:** tinnitus (ringing, roaring in ears), vertigo, loss of hearing (rare); visual disturbance
- **QT prolongation:** ECG, ejection fraction; assess for chest pain, palpitations, dyspnea

Evaluate:

- Therapeutic response: decreased fever, malaise, rash, negative C&S for infecting organism

Teach patient/family:

- That long-term therapy may be needed to clear infection (2 wk-3 mo, depending on type of infection)
- To notify prescriber of bleeding, bruising, soft-tissue swelling, dark urine, persistent nausea or diarrhea, headache, rash, yellow skin/eyes
- Take 1 hr before or after meal
- Do not drive at night because of vision changes
- Avoid strong, direct sunlight
- Women of childbearing age should use effective contraceptive

⚠ HIGH ALERT

warfarin (Rx)

(war'far-in)

Coumadin, Jantoven

Func. class.: Anticoagulant

Chem. class.: Coumarin derivative

Do not confuse:
Coumadin/Cardura/Compazine

ACTION:
Interferes with blood clotting by indirect means; depresses hepatic synthesis of vit-K–dependent coagulation factors (II, VII, IX, X)

USES:
Antiphospholipid antibody syndrome, arterial thromboembolism prophylaxis, DVT, MI prophylaxis, after MI, stroke prophylaxis, thrombosis prophylaxis

Unlabeled uses: Angina, unstable angina

CONTRAINDICATIONS:
Pregnancy (X), breastfeeding, hypersensitivity, hemophilia, leukemia with bleeding, peptic ulcer disease, thrombocytopenic purpura, hepatic disease (severe), malignant hypertension, subacute bacterial endocarditis, acute nephritis, blood dyscrasias, eclampsia, preeclampsia, hemorrhagic tendencies; surgery of CNS, eye; traumatric surgery with large open surface, bleeding tendencies of GI/GU/respiratory tract, stroke, aneurysms, pericardial effusion, spinal puncture, major regional/lumbar block anesthesia

Black Box Warning: Bleeding

Precautions: Geriatric patients, alcoholism, CHF, debilitated patients, trauma, indwelling catheters, severe hypertension, active infections, protein C deficiency, polycythemia vera, vasculitis, severe diabetes, Asian patients (CYP2C9, VKORC1)

DOSAGE AND ROUTES

- **Adult: PO/IV** 2.5-10 mg/day × 2-4 days then titrated to INR/PT
- **Adolescent/child/infant: PO/IV** 0.2 mg/kg/day × 2 days titrated to INR

Available forms: Tabs 1, 2, 2.5, 3, 4, 5, 6, 7.5, 10 mg; inj 5 mg powder for inj

Administer:

- At same time each day to maintain steady blood levels without regard to food; food decreases rate but not extent of absorption; do not change brands
- Tabs whole or crushed
- Avoiding all IM inj that may cause bleeding

Direct IV route

- Reconstitute with 2.7 ml sterile water for inj (2 mg/ml); do not use sol that is discolored or that has particulates
- Give over 1-2 min into peripheral vein

Y-site compatibilities: Amikacin, ascorbic acid, bivalirudin, ceFAZolin, cefTRIAXone, DOPamine, EPINEPHrine, heparin, lidocaine, metaraminol, morphine, nitroglycerin, oxytocin, potassium chloride, ranitidine

SIDE EFFECTS

CNS: *Fever,* dizziness, fatigue, headache, lethargy

CV: Angina, chest pain, edema, hypotension, syncope

GI: *Diarrhea,* nausea, vomiting, anorexia, stomatitis, cramps, **hepatitis,** cholestatic jaundice

GU: **Hematuria**

HEMA: **Hemorrhage, agranulocytosis, leukopenia, eosinophilia,** anemia, **ecchymosis, petechiae**

INTEG: *Rash,* dermatitis, urticaria, alopecia, pruritus

MISC: Epistaxis, hemoptysis, mouth ulcers, taste disturbances, priapism, dyspnea

MS: Bone fractures

SYST: **Anaphylaxis, coma,** cholesterol, **microembolism, exfoliative dermatitis, purple toe syndrome**

W

PHARMACOKINETICS

PO: Onset 12-24 hr, peak $1^{1}/_{2}$-4 days, duration 3-5 days, effective half-life 20-60 hr; metabolized in liver; excreted in urine, feces (active/inactive metabolites); crosses placenta, 99% bound to plasma proteins

INTERACTIONS

Increase: warfarin action—allopurinol, amiodarone, chloral hydrate, chloramphenicol, cimetidine, clofibrate, cotrimoxazole, COX-2 selective inhibitors, dextrothyroxine, diflunisal, disulfiram, erythromycin, ethacrynic acids, furosemide, glucagon, heparin, HMG-CoA reductase inhibitors, indomethacin, isoniazid, mefenamic acid, metroNIDAZOLE, mifepristone, NSAIDs, oxyphenbutazones, penicillins, phenylbutazone, quiNIDine, quinolone antiinfectives, RU-486, salicylates, sulfinpyrazone, sulfonamides, sulindac, SSRIs, steroids, thrombolytics, thyroid, tricyclics

Increase: toxicity—oral sulfonylureas, phenytoin

Decrease: warfarin action—aprepitant, azathioprine, barbiturates, bile acid sequestrants, bosentan, carBAMazepine, dicloxacillin, estrogens, ethchlorvynol, factor IX/VIIa, griseofulvin, nafcillin, oral contraceptives, phenytoin, rifampin, sucralfate, sulfasalazine, thyroid, vit K, vit K foods

Drug/Herb

Increase: risk for bleeding—angelica, anise, basil, chamomile, chondroitin, dong quai, evening primrose, feverfew, garlic, ginger, ginkgo, ginseng, horse chestnut, kava, licorice, melatonin, red yeast rice, saw palmetto

Decrease: anticoagulant effect—coenzyme Q10, St. John's wort

Drug/Lab Test

Increase: T_3 uptake, LFTs

Decrease: uric acid

NURSING CONSIDERATIONS

Assess:

Black Box Warning: Blood studies (Hct, PT, platelets, occult blood in stools) q3mo; INR: in hospital daily after 2nd or 3rd dose; when in therapeutic range for 2 consecutive days, monitor 2-3× wk for 1-2 wk then less frequently, depending on stability of INR results; *Outpatient:* monitor every few days until stable dose then periodically thereafter, depending on stability of INR results

Black Box Warning: Bleeding gums, petechiae, ecchymosis, black tarry stools, hematuria; fatal hemorrhage can occur

⚠ Fever, skin rash, urticaria

Perform/provide:

- Storage in tight container

Evaluate:

- Therapeutic response: decrease in deep venous thrombosis

Teach patient/family:

- To avoid OTC preparations that may cause serious product interactions unless directed by prescriber
- To carry emergency ID identifying product taken
- About the importance of compliance
- To report any signs of bleeding: gums, under skin, urine, stools; to use soft-bristle toothbrush to avoid bleeding gums; to use electric razor
- To avoid hazardous activities (football, hockey, skiing), dangerous work
- About the importance of avoiding unusual changes in vitamin intake, diet, or lifestyle
- To inform all health care providers of anticoagulant intake

TREATMENT OF OVERDOSE:

Administer vit K

xylometazoline nasal agent

See Appendix B

zafirlukast (Rx)

(za-feer′loo-cast)

Accolate

Func. class.: Bronchodilator

Chem. class.: Leukotriene receptor antagonist

ACTION: Antagonizes the contractile action of leukotrienes (LTD_4, LTE_4) in airway smooth muscle; inhibits bronchoconstriction caused by antigens

USES: Prophylaxis and chronic treatment of asthma in adults/children >5 yr

Unlabeled uses: Allergic rhinitis

CONTRAINDICATIONS: Hypersensitivity, hepatic disease, hepatic encephalopathy

Precautions: Pregnancy (B), breastfeeding, children, geriatric patients, hepatic disease, Churg-Strauss syndrome, acute bronchospasm

DOSAGE AND ROUTES

- **Adult and child ≥12 yr: PO** 20 mg bid, take 1 hr before or 2 hr after meals
- **Child 5-11 yr: PO** 10 mg bid

Available forms: Tabs 10, 20 mg

Administer:

- 1 hr before or 2 hr after meals; absorption may be decreased if given with food
- With water if GI upset occurs

SIDE EFFECTS

CNS: Headache, dizziness, **suicidal ideation**, insomnia, fever

GI: Nausea, diarrhea, abdominal pain, vomiting, dyspepsia, **hepatic failure, hepatitis**

HEMA: Agranulocytosis

OTHER: Infections, pain, asthenia, myalgia, fever, increased ALT, urticaria, rash, **angioedema**

PHARMACOKINETICS

Rapidly absorbed, peak 3 hr, 99% protein binding (albumin), extensively metabolized, inhibits CYP2C9 and 3A4 enzyme systems, excreted in feces, clearance reduced in geriatric patients, hepatic impairment, half-life 10 hr

INTERACTIONS

Classifications

Avoid use with: CYP3A4 metabolizers (alfentanil, aripiprazole, busPIRone, buprenorphine, carBAMazepine, many corticosteroids, cyclobenzaprine, cycloSPORINE, darifenacin, disopyramide, calcium channel blockers, eplerenone, ergots, fentaNYL, galantamine, halofantrine, levomethadyl, systemic lidocaine, lovastatin, oxybutynin, paricalcitol, quiNIDine, simvastatin, solifenacin, tadalafil, tolterodine, zonisamide): dosage reduction may be needed

Avoid use with: CYP2C9 metabolizers (some COX-2 inhibitors, chlorpropamide, diclofenac, dronabinol, THC, flurbiprofen, fluvastatin, glimepiride, glipizide, glyburide, ibuprofen, indomethacin, irbesartan, losartan, meloxicam, naproxen, nateglinide, phenytoin, piroxicam, rosiglitazone, TOLBUTamide, valsartan): dosage reduction may be needed

Increase: plasma levels of zafirlukast—aspirin

Increase: PT—warfarin

Decrease: plasma levels of zafirlukast—erythromycin, theophylline

Drug/Herb

Increase: effect—green tea (large amounts), guarana

Drug/Food

Decrease: bioavailability

NURSING CONSIDERATIONS

Assess:

⚠ **Adult patients carefully for symptoms of Churg-Strauss syndrome** (rare), including eosinophilia, vasculitic rash, worsening pulmonary symptoms, cardiac complications, neuropathy

• Respiratory rate, rhythm, depth; auscultate lung fields bilaterally; notify prescriber of abnormalities
• **Hepatic disease:** monitor liver function tests

Evaluate:
• Therapeutic response: ability to breathe more easily

Teach patient/family:
• To check OTC medications, current prescription medications that may increase stimulation
• To avoid hazardous activities because dizziness may occur
• That, if GI upset occurs, to take product with 8 oz water; to avoid taking with food if possible because absorption may be decreased
• To notify prescriber of nausea, vomiting, diarrhea, abdominal pain, fatigue, jaundice, anorexia, flulike symptoms (hepatic dysfunction)
• Not to use for acute asthma episodes
• Not to take if breastfeeding
• To take even if symptom free

zaleplon (Rx)

(zal′eh-plon)

Sonata

Func. class.: Sedative/hypnotic, nonbarbiturate
Chem. class.: Pyrazolopyrimidine

Controlled Substance Schedule IV

ACTION: Binds selectively to omega-1 receptor of the $GABA_A$ receptor complex; results are sedation, hypnosis, skeletal muscle relaxation, anticonvulsant activity, anxiolytic action

USES: Insomnia

CONTRAINDICATIONS: Hypersensitivity, severe hepatic disease
Precautions: Pregnancy (C), breastfeeding, children <15 yr, geriatric patients, respiratory/renal/hepatic disease, psychosis, angioedema, depression, sleep-related behaviors (sleep walking)

DOSAGE AND ROUTES

• **Adult: PO** 10 mg at bedtime; may increase dose to 20 mg at bedtime if needed; 5 mg may be used in low-weight persons
• **Geriatric: PO** 5 mg at bedtime; may increase if needed

Available forms: Caps 5, 10 mg

Administer:
• After removal of cigarettes to prevent fires
• After trying conservative measures for insomnia
• Immediately before bedtime for sleeplessness
• On empty stomach for fast onset
• Avoid use with CNS depressants

SIDE EFFECTS

CNS: *Lethargy, drowsiness, daytime sedation,* dizziness, confusion, anxiety, amnesia, depersonalization, hallucinations, hyperesthesia, paresthesia, somnolence, tremor, vertigo, complex sleep related reactions: sleep driving, sleep eating
EENT: Vision change, ear/eye pain, hyperacusis, parosmia
GI: Nausea, abdominal pain, constipation, anorexia, colitis, dyspepsia, dry mouth
MISC: Asthenia, fever, headache, myalgia, dysmenorrhea
SYST: Severe allergic reactions

PHARMACOKINETICS

Rapid onset, metabolized by liver extensively, excreted by kidneys (inactive metabolites), half-life 1 hr

INTERACTIONS

Increase: effect of zaleplon—cimetidine
Decrease: effect of zaleplon—rifampin
Increase and decrease: zaleplon levels—CYP3A4 inhibitors/inducers

Drug/Herb
Increase: CNS depression—chamomile, hops, kava, valerian
Drug/Food
• Prolonged absorption, sleep onset reduced: high-fat/heavy meal

NURSING CONSIDERATIONS

Assess:
• Mental status: mood, sensorium, affect, memory (long, short term), excessive sedation, impaired coordination
• **Sleep disorder:** type of sleep problem: falling asleep, staying asleep
Perform/provide:
• Assistance with ambulation after receiving dose
• Safety measure: night-light, call bell within easy reach
• Check to see if PO medication has been swallowed
• Storage in tight container in cool environment
Evaluate:
• Therapeutic response: ability to sleep at night, decreased amount of early morning awakening
Teach patient/family:
• To avoid driving or other activities requiring alertness until product is stabilized
• To avoid alcohol ingestion
• About alternative measures to improve sleep: reading, exercise several hours before bedtime, warm bath, warm milk, TV, self-hypnosis, deep breathing
• That product may cause memory problems, dependence (if used for longer periods of time), changes in behavior/thinking, complex sleep-related behaviors (sleep eating/driving)
• That product is for short-term use only
• To take immediately before going to bed
• Not to ingest a high-fat/heavy meal before taking

zanamivir (Rx)

(zan′ah-mih-veer)

Relenza

Func. class.: Antiviral

Chem. class.: Neuramidase inhibitor

ACTION:
Inhibits neuramidase enzyme needed for influenza virus replication

USES:
Treatment of influenza types A and B for patients who have been symptomatic for ≤2 days
Unlabeled uses: Prophylaxis against influenza and biinfections; swine flu (H1N1)

CONTRAINDICATIONS:
Hypersensitivity
Precautions: Pregnancy (C), breastfeeding, children <7 yr, geriatric patients, respiratory disease, angioedema, milk protein hypersensitivity, Reye's syndrome

DOSAGE AND ROUTES

• **Adult/child >7 yr: INH** 2 inhalations (two 5-mg blisters) q12hr × 5 days; on the 1st day, 2 doses should be taken with at least 2 hr between doses
H1N1 (swine flu) (unlabeled)
• **Adult/adolescent/child ≥7 yr: INH** 2 bid × 5 days
Available forms: Blisters of powder for inhalation: 5 mg
Administer:
• Within 2 days of symptoms of influenza; continue for 5 days
• Give patient "Patient's Instructions for Use", review all points before using delivery system
• Do not use as nebulized sol or in mechanical ventilation

SIDE EFFECTS

CNS: *Headache, dizziness,* seizures, fatigue; self-injury, delirium (child)
EENT: Ear, nose, throat infections

GI: *Nausea, vomiting,* diarrhea
RESP: Nasal symptoms, cough, sinusitis, bronchitis, bronchospasm
SYST: Angioedema

PHARMACOKINETICS

Half-life $2^{1}/_{2}$-5 hr, not metabolized, excreted in urine unchanged

INTERACTIONS

- May decrease intranasal influenzae vaccine; separate by ≥48 hr, do not restart antiviral products for ≥2 wk

NURSING CONSIDERATIONS

Assess:
- Bowel pattern before, during treatment
- Skin eruptions, photosensitivity after administration of product
- Respiratory status: rate, character, wheezing, tightness in chest
- Allergies before initiation of treatment, reaction of each medication
- Signs of infection

Perform/provide:
- Storage in tight, dry container

Evaluate:
- Therapeutic response: absence of fever, malaise, cough, dyspnea with infection

Teach patient/family:
- That product does not reduce transmission risk of influenza to others
- That patients with asthma or COPD should carry a fast-acting inhaled bronchodilator because bronchospasm may occur; to use scheduled inhaled bronchodilators before using product
- To avoid hazardous activities if dizziness occurs
- To take product exactly as prescribed

zidovudine (Rx)

(zye-doe′-vue-deen)

Novo-AZT ✱, Retrovir

Func. class.: Antiretroviral
Chem. class.: Nucleoside reverse transcriptase inhibitor (NRTI)

ACTION:
Inhibits replication of HIV-1 virus by incorporating into cellular DNA by viral reverse transcriptase, thereby terminating the cellular DNA chain

USES:
Used in combination with at least 2 other antiretrovirals for HIV-1 infection

Unlabeled uses: Epstein-Barr virus, hepatitis B, human T-lymphotropic virus type I (HTLV-I), thrombocytopenia

CONTRAINDICATIONS:
Hypersensitivity

Precautions: Pregnancy (C), breastfeeding, children, granulocyte count <1000/mm^3 or Hgb <9.5 g/dl, severe renal disease, obesity

Black Box Warning: Impaired hepatic function, anemia, lactic acidosis, myopathy, neutropenia

DOSAGE AND ROUTES

- **Adult: PO** 600 mg/day in divided doses, either 200 mg tid or 300 mg bid in combination with other antiretrovirals; **IV** 1 mg/kg q4hr, initiate **PO** as soon as possible up to 1000 mg
- **Child 6 wk-12 yr: PO** 160 mg/m^2 q8hr (480 mg/m^2/day, max 200 mg q8hr) in combination with other antiretrovirals; **IV** same as adult
- **Neonate: PO** 2-3 mg/kg/dose q6hr; **IV** 1.5 mg/kg infused over 30 min q6hr

Treatment of HIV in combination with other antiretrovirals
- **Adult/adolescent/child ≥30 kg: PO** 300 mg bid or 200 mg tid

• **Child ≥4 wk and weight 4-9 kg/infant: PO** total daily dose 24 mg/kg/day given 12 mg/kg bid or 8 mg/kg tid
• **Neonate (unlabeled): PO** 2 mg/kg q6hr
• **Premature neonate (unlabeled): PO** 2 mg/kg q12hr, increase to 2 mg/kg q8hr at 2 wk for neonates ≥30 wk gestation or at 4 wk for neonates <30 wk gestation

Perinatal transmission prophylaxis
• **Full-term neonate: PO** 2 mg/kg or **IV** 1.5 mg/kg q6h starting 12 hr after birth, continue up to 6 wk of age
• **Preterm neonate: PO** 2 mg/kg or **IV** 1.5 mg/kg q12hr; if >30 wk gestation at birth, advance to q8hr at 2 wk of age; if <30 wk gestation at birth, advance to q8hr at 4 wk of age

Prevention of maternal–fetal HIV transmission
• **Neonatal: PO** 2 mg/kg/dose q6hr × 6 wk beginning 8-12 hr after birth; **IV** 1.5 mg/kg/dose over 30 min q6hr until able to take **PO**
• **Maternal (>14 wk gestation): PO** 100 mg 5×/day until start of labor then during labor/delivery **IV** 2 mg/kg over 1 hr followed by **IV INF** 1 mg/kg/hr until umbilical cord clamped

Symptomatic HIV infection
• **Adult: PO** 100 mg q4hr; **IV** 1-2 mg/kg over 1 hr q4hr
• **Child 3 mo-12 yr: PO** 90-180 mg/m^2 q6hr (max 200 mg q6hr); **IV** 1-2 mg/kg over 1 hr q4hr

Prevention of HIV after needlestick
• **Adult: PO** 200 mg tid plus lamiVUDine 150 mg bid plus a protease inhibitor for high-risk exposure; begin within 2 hr of exposure

Thrombocytopenia associated with HIV infection (unlabeled)
• **Adult: PO** 500 mg qid × 2 wk then 250 mg qid × 6 wk

T-cell leukemia/lymphoma in combination with interferon-alfa in patients infected with T-lymphotropic virus type I (HTLV-I) (unlabeled)
• **Adult: PO** 200 mg q4hr while awake, continue for ≥4 wk after remission, adjust for hematologic toxicity

Available forms: Caps 100; tabs 300 mg; inj 200 mg/20 ml; oral syr 50 mg/5 ml

Administer:
• By mouth; capsules should be swallowed whole
• Bid or tid
• Trimethoprim-sulfamethoxazole, pyrimethamine, or acyclovir as ordered to prevent opportunistic infections; if these products are given, watch for neurotoxicity

Intermittent IV INF route
• After diluting each 1 mg/0.25 ml or more D_5W to ≤4 mg/ml; give over 1 hr

Y-site compatibilities: Acyclovir, allopurinol, amifostine, amikacin, amphotericin B, amphotericin B cholesteryl, aztreonam, cefepime, ceftazidime, cefTRIAXone, cimetidine, cisatracurium, clindamycin, dexamethasone, DOBUTamine, DOPamine, DOXOrubicin liposome, erythromycin, filgrastim, fluconazole, fludarabine, gentamicin, granisetron, heparin, imipenem-cilastatin, LORazepam, melphalan, metoclopramide, morphine, nafcillin, ondansetron, oxacillin, paclitaxel, pentamidine, phenylephrine, piperacillin, piperacillin-tazobactam, potassium chloride, ranitidine, remifentanil, sargramostim, teniposide, thiotepa, tobramycin, trimethoprim-sulfamethoxazole, trimetrexate, vancomycin, vinorelbine

SIDE EFFECTS

CNS: *Fever, headache, malaise,* diaphoresis, *dizziness, insomnia,* paresthesia, somnolence, chills, tremor, twitching, anxiety, confusion, depression, lability, vertigo, loss of mental acuity, **seizures,** malaise

Z

EENT: Taste change, hearing loss, photophobia
GI: *Nausea, vomiting, diarrhea, anorexia,* cramps, *dyspepsia, constipation,* dysphagia, *flatulence,* rectal bleeding, mouth ulcer, abdominal pain, hepatomegaly
GU: Dysuria, polyuria, urinary frequency, hesitancy
HEMA: Granulocytopenia, anemia
INTEG: *Rash,* acne, pruritus, urticaria
MS: Myalgia, arthralgia, muscle spasm
RESP: Dyspnea
SYST: Lactic acidosis

PHARMACOKINETICS

PO: Rapidly absorbed from GI tract, peak $^1/_2$-1$^1/_2$ hr, metabolized in liver (inactive metabolites), excreted by kidneys, protein binding 38%, terminal half-life $^1/_2$-3 hr

INTERACTIONS

- Toxicity: probenecid, fluconazole

Increase: bone marrow depression—antineoplastics, radiation, ganciclovir, valganciclovir, trimethoprim-sulfamethoxazole
Increase: zidovudine level—methadone

NURSING CONSIDERATIONS

Assess:

Black Box Warning: Blood counts q2wk; watch for decreasing granulocytes, Hgb; if low, therapy may have to be discontinued and restarted after hematologic recovery; blood transfusions may be required; viral load, CD4 counts, LFTs, plasma HIV RNA, serum creatinine/BUN at baseline and throughout treatment

Black Box Warning: Lactic acidosis, severe hepatomegaly with steatosis: Obtain baseline liver function tests, if elevated, discontinue treatment; discontinue even if liver function tests are normal but lactic acidosis, hepatomegaly are present; may be fatal

Perform/provide:

- Storage in cool environment; protect from light

Evaluate:

- Blood dyscrasias (anemia, granulocytopenia): bruising, fatigue, bleeding, poor healing

Teach patient/family:

- That GI complaints and insomnia resolve after 3-4 wk of treatment
- That product not cure for AIDS but will control symptoms
- To notify prescriber of sore throat, swollen lymph nodes, malaise, fever because other infections may occur
- That patient is still infective, may pass AIDS virus on to others
- That follow-up visits must be continued because serious toxicity may occur; that blood counts must be done q2wk
- That product must be taken bid or tid
- That serious product interactions may occur if OTC products are ingested; to check with prescriber before taking aspirin, acetaminophen, indomethacin
- That other products may be necessary to prevent other infections
- That product may cause fainting or dizziness

zinc (Rx, otc)

Orazinc, PMS Egozinc ✱, Verazinc, Zinca-Pak, Zincate, Zinc 15, Zinc-220

Func. class.: Trace element; nutritional supplement

ACTION: Needed for adequate healing, bone and joint development (23% zinc)

USES: Prevention of zinc deficiency, adjunct to vit A therapy
Unlabeled uses: Wound healing
Precautions: Pregnancy (C) parenteral; breastfeeding, neonates, hypocupremia, neonatal prematurity, renal disease

DOSAGE AND ROUTES

Dietary supplement (elemental zinc)

- **Adult/adolescent/pregnant female: PO** 11-13 mg/day
- **Adult/lactating female: PO** 12-14 mg/day × 12 mo
- **Adult/adolescent male ≥14 yr: PO** 11 mg/day
- **Adult female ≥19 yr: PO** 8 mg/day
- **Adolescent female ≥14 yr: PO** 9 mg/day
- **Child 9-13 yr: PO** 8 mg/day
- **Child 4-8 yr: PO** 5 mg/day
- **Child 1-3 yr: PO** 3 mg/day
- **Infant 7-12 mo: PO** 3 mg/day
- **Infant birth to 6 mo: PO** 2 mg/day (adequate intake)

Nutritional supplement (IV)

- **Adult: IV** 2.5-4 mg/day; may increase by 2 mg/day if needed
- **Child 1-5 yr: IV** 50 mcg/kg/day

Wound healing

- **Adult: PO** 50 mg tid until healed (elemental zinc)

Available forms: Tabs 66, 110 mg; caps 220 mg; inj 1 mg, 5 mg/ml

Administer:

- With meals to decrease gastric upset; avoid dairy products

SIDE EFFECTS

GI: Nausea, vomiting, cramps, heartburn, ulcer formation

OVERDOSE: Diarrhea, rash, dehydration, restlessness

INTERACTIONS

Decrease: absorption of fluoroquinolones—tetracyclines

NURSING CONSIDERATIONS

Assess:

- Zinc levels during treatment

Evaluate:

- Therapeutic response: absence of zinc deficiency

Teach patient/family:

- That element must be taken for 2-3 mo to be effective
- To immediately report nausea, diarrhea, rash, severe vomiting, restlessness, abdominal pain, tarry stools

ziprasidone (Rx)

(zi-praz′ih-dohn)

Geodon, Zeldox ♣

Func. class.: Antipsychotic/neuroleptic

Chem. class.: Benzisoxazole derivative

ACTION:
Unknown; may be mediated through both dopamine type 2 (D_2) and serotonin type 2 ($5\text{-}HT_2$) antagonism

USES:
Schizophrenia, acute agitation, acute psychosis, bipolar disorder, mania, psychotic depression

Unlabeled uses: Tourette's syndrome

CONTRAINDICATIONS:
Breastfeeding, hypersensitivity, acute MI, heart failure, QT prolongation

Precautions: Pregnancy (C), children, geriatric patients, cardiac/renal/hepatic disease, breast cancer, diabetes, seizure disorders, AV block, CNS depression

Black Box Warning: Dementia

DOSAGE AND ROUTES

Schizophrenia

- **Adult: PO** 20 mg bid with food, adjust dosage every 2 days upward to max of 80 mg bid; **IM** 10-20 mg; may give 10 mg q2hr; doses of 20 mg may be given q4hr; max 40 mg/day

Bipolar disorder

- **Adult: PO** 40 mg bid with food; on day 2 increase to 60 or 80 mg bid, then adjust to response; maintenance as adjunct to lithium/valproate 40-80 mg bid

Tourette's syndrome (unlabeled)
• **Adolescent and child ≥7 yr: PO** 5 mg/day, may increase in divided doses to 20 mg bid

Available forms: Caps 20, 40, 60, 80 mg; inj 20 mg/ml

Administer:

PO route
• Reduced dose in geriatric patients
• Anticholinergic agent on order from prescriber to be used for EPS
• Avoid use with CNS depressants
• With food; increases absorption

IM route
• Add 1.2 ml sterile water for inj to vial; shake vigorously until product is dissolved; do not admix; give only IM

SIDE EFFECTS

CNS: *EPS, pseudoparkinsonism, akathisia, dystonia, tardive dyskinesia; drowsiness, insomnia, agitation, anxiety, headache,* seizures, neuroleptic malignant syndrome, dizziness, tremor, facial droop

CV: Orthostatic hypotension, tachycardia, prolonged QT/QTc, hypertension; sudden death, heart failure (geriatric patients), torsades de pointes

EENT: Blurred vision, diplopia

ENDO: Metabolic changes

GI: *Nausea,* vomiting, *anorexia, constipation,* jaundice, weight gain, diarrhea, dry mouth, abdominal pain

GU: Enuresis, urinary incontinence, gynecomastia, impotence, priapism

RESP: Rhinitis, dyspnea, infection, cough

PHARMACOKINETICS

PO: Extensively metabolized by liver to major active metabolite, plasma protein binding 90%, peak 6-8 hr, terminal half-life 7 hr

INTERACTIONS

⚠ **Increase:** QT prolongation—class IA/III antidysrhythmics, some phenothiazines, β-agonists, local anesthetics, tricyclics, haloperidol, methadone, chloroquine, clarithromycin, droperidol, erythromycin, pentamidine, moxifloxacin

Increase: sedation—other CNS depressants, alcohol

Increase: EPS—other antipsychotics, lithium

Increase: ziprasidone excretion—carBAMazepine

Increase: ziprasidone level—ketoconazole

Increase: hypotension—antihypertensives

Increase: serotonin syndrome, neuroleptic malignant syndrome—SSRIs, SNRIs

Drug/Herb

Increase: CNS depression—chamomile, hops, kava, skullcap, valerian

NURSING CONSIDERATIONS

Assess:
• Mental status before initial administration

Black Box Warning: Geriatric patient with dementia closely; heart failure, sudden death have occurred

• Swallowing of PO medication; check for hoarding or giving of medication to other patients
• I&O ratio; palpate bladder if urinary output is low
• Bilirubin, CBC, LFTs, fasting blood glucose monthly
• Urinalysis before, during prolonged therapy
• Affect, orientation, LOC, reflexes, gait, coordination, sleep-pattern disturbances
• B/P standing and lying; also pulse, respirations; take these q4hr during initial treatment; establish baseline before starting treatment; report drops of 30 mm Hg; watch for ECG changes; QT prolongation may occur
• Dizziness, faintness, palpitations, tachycardia on rising; metabolic changes, weight gain
• **EPS,** including akathisia (inability to sit still, no pattern to movements), tardive dyskinesia (bizarre movements of the jaw, mouth, tongue, extremities),

pseudoparkinsonism (rigidity, tremors, pill rolling, shuffling gait)
Neuroleptic malignant syndrome, serotonin syndrome: hyperthermia, increased CPK, altered mental status, muscle rigidity
- Constipation, urinary retention daily; if these occur, increase bulk and water in diet

Perform/provide:
- Decreased stimulus by dimming lights, avoiding loud noises
- Supervised ambulation until patient is stabilized on medication; do not involve patient in strenuous exercise program because fainting is possible; patient should not stand still for a long time
- Increased fluids to prevent constipation
- Sips of water, candy, gum for dry mouth
- Storage in tight, light-resistant container

Evaluate:
- Therapeutic response: decrease in emotional excitement, hallucinations, delusions, paranoia; reorganization of patterns of thought, speech

Teach patient/family:
- That orthostatic hypotension may occur; to rise from sitting or lying position gradually
- To avoid hot tubs, hot showers, tub baths because hypotension may occur
- To avoid abrupt withdrawal of product because EPS may result; that product should be withdrawn slowly
- To avoid OTC preparations (cough, hay fever, cold) unless approved by prescriber because serious product interactions may occur; to avoid use with alcohol because increased drowsiness may occur
- To avoid hazardous activities if drowsy or dizzy
- About compliance with product regimen
- To report impaired vision, tremors, muscle twitching
- In hot weather, that heat stroke may occur; to take extra precautions to stay cool

TREATMENT OF OVERDOSE:
Lavage if orally ingested; provide airway; *do not induce vomiting*

zoledronic acid (Rx)
(zoh′leh-drah′nick ass′id)

Reclast, Zometa

Func. class.: Bone-resorption inhibitor

Chem. class.: Bisphosphonate

ACTION:
Potent inhibitor of osteoclastic bone resorption; inhibits osteoclastic activity, skeletal calcium release caused by stimulating factors released by tumors; reduction of abnormal bone resorption is responsible for therapeutic effect with hypercalcemia; may directly block dissolution of hydroxyapatite bone crystals

USES:
Moderate to severe hypercalcemia associated with malignancy; multiple myeloma; bone metastases from solid tumors (used with antineoplastics); active Paget's disease; osteoporosis, glucocorticoid-induced osteoporosis, osteoporosis prophylaxis in postmenopausal women

CONTRAINDICATIONS:
Pregnancy (D), breastfeeding; hypersensitivity to this product or bisphosphonates; hypocalcemia

Precautions: Children, geriatric patients, renal dysfunction, aspirin sensitive asthma, asthmatic patients, acute bronchospasm, anemia, chemotherapy, coagulopathy, dehydration, dental disease, diabetes mellitus, renal disease, electrolyte imbalance, hypertension, hypomagnesemia, hypophosphatemia, hypovolemia, infection, multiple myeloma, phosphate hypersensitivity

Z

DOSAGE AND ROUTES

Hypercalcemia of malignancy

• **Adult: IV INF** 4 mg, given as single inf over ≥15 min; may re-treat with 4 mg if serum calcium does not return to normal within 1 wk

Multiple myeloma/metastatic bone lesions

• **Adult: IV INF** 4 mg, give over 15 min q3-4wk

Osteoporosis

• **Adult: IV INF** 5 mg over ≥15 min q12mo

Active Paget's disease

• **Adult: IV INF** 5 mg over ≥15 min

Osteoporosis prophylaxis (Reclast), postmenopausal women

• **Adult: IV INF** 5 mg every other year

Osteoporosis prophylaxis (Reclast) when taking systemic glucocorticoids

• **Adult: IV** 5 mg every yr

Available forms: (Zometa) sol for inj 4 mg/5 ml; (Reclast) inj 5 mg/100 ml

Administer:

• Saline hydration must be performed before administration; urine output should be 2 L/day during treatment; do not overhydrate patient

IV route

Zometa

• Administer after reconstituting by adding 5 ml of sterile water for inj to each vial then add to ≥100 ml of sterile 0.9% NaCl, D_5W; run over ≥15 min

• Administer in separate IV line from all other products

Reclast

• No further dilution required

• Infuse over ≥15 min at constant rate; max 5 mg

SIDE EFFECTS

CNS: Dizziness, headache, anxiety, confusion, insomnia, agitation

CV: Hypotension, leg edema, atrial fibrillation, chest pain

GI: Abdominal pain, anorexia, constipation, nausea, diarrhea, vomiting, taste change

GU: UTI, possible reduced renal function, renal damage

META: Anemia, hypokalemia, hypomagnesemia, hypophosphatemia, hypocalcemia, increased serum creatinine

MISC: *Fever, chills, flulike symptoms*

MS: Severe bone pain, *arthralgias, myalgias,* osteonecrosis of jaw

PHARMACOKINETICS

Rapidly cleared from circulation, taken up mainly by bones, not metabolized, eliminated primarily by kidneys, approximately 50% eliminated in urine within 24 hr of administration, max effect 7 days; terminal half-life 167 hr, protein binding 22%

INTERACTIONS

• Hypomagnesemia, hypokalemia: digoxin

• Do not mix with calcium-containing infusion sol such as lactated Ringer's sol

Increase: nephrotoxicity—aminoglycosides, NSAIDs, radiopaque contrast agents

Decrease: effect of zoledronic acid—calcium, vit D

Decrease: serum calcium, aminoglycosides, loop diuretics

NURSING CONSIDERATIONS

Assess:

• Renal tests, calcium, phosphate, magnesium, potassium; creatinine, BUN; if creatinine elevated, hold treatment

• **Hypocalcemia:** paresthesia, twitching, laryngospasm; Chvostek's/Trousseau's signs

• Dental status; cover with antiinfectives for dental extraction

• Atrial fibrillation

Perform/provide:

• Sol reconstituted with sterile water may be stored under refrigeration for up to 24 hr

• Acetaminophen before and for 72 hr after to decrease pain

Evaluate:
- Therapeutic response: decreased calcium levels, increased bone density

Teach patient/family:
- To report hypercalcemic relapse: nausea, vomiting, bone pain, thirst
- To continue with dietary recommendations, including calcium and vit D; to take a multiple vitamin daily as well as 500 mg of calcium, 400 international units vit D with multiple myeloma
- If nausea or vomiting occurs, to eat small, frequent meals, to use lozenges or chewing gum
- If bone pain occurs, to notify prescriber to obtain analgesics
- To avoid use during pregnancy
- To continue good oral hygiene

zolmitriptan (Rx)
(zole-mih-trip′tan)

Zomig, Zomig-ZMT

Func. class.: Migraine agent, abortive

Chem. class.: 5-HT_{1B}/5HT_{1D} receptor agonist (triptan)

ACTION: Binds selectively to the vascular 5-HT_{1B}/5HT_{1D} receptor subtype, exerts antimigraine effect; causes vasoconstriction in cranial arteries

USES: Acute treatment of migraine with/without aura

CONTRAINDICATIONS: Angina pectoris, history of MI, documented silent ischemia, ischemic heart disease, uncontrolled hypertension, hypersensitivity, basilar or hemiplegic migraine, risk of CV events

Precautions: Pregnancy (C), breastfeeding, children, postmenopausal women, men >40 yr, geriatric patients, risk factors for CAD, hypercholesterolemia, obesity, diabetes, impaired renal/hepatic function

DOSAGE AND ROUTES
- **Adult: PO** start at ≤2.5 mg (tab may be broken), may repeat after 2 hr, max 10 mg/24 hr; **NASAL** 1 spray in 1 nostril at onset of migraine, repeat in 2 hr if no relief

Available forms: Tabs 2.5, 5 mg; orally disintegrating tabs 2.5, 5 mg; nasal spray 5 mg

Administer:
- Take with fluids as soon as symptoms of migraine occur

SIDE EFFECTS
CNS: *Tingling, hot sensation, burning, feeling of pressure, tightness, numbness, dizziness, sedation*

CV: Palpitations, chest pain

GI: Abdominal discomfort, nausea, dry mouth, dyspepsia, dysphagia

MISC: Odd taste (spray)

MS: *Weakness, neck stiffness,* myalgia

RESP: Chest tightness, pressure

PHARMACOKINETICS
Duration 2-3½ hr; 25% plasma protein binding; half-life 3-3½ hr; metabolized in liver (metabolite); excreted in urine (60-80%), feces (20-40%)

INTERACTIONS
⚠ Extended vasospastic effects: ergot, ergot derivatives

⚠ Do not use within 2 wk of MAOIs

⚠ Weakness, hyperreflexia, incoordination: SSRIs (FLUoxetine, fluvoxamine, PARoxetine, sertraline)

Increase: half-life of zolmitriptan—cimetidine, oral contraceptives

Increase: zolimitriptan levels—sibutramine

Drug/Herb
- Serotonin syndrome: SAM-e, St. John's wort

NURSING CONSIDERATIONS
Assess:
- Tingling, hot sensation, burning, feeling of pressure, numbness, flushing

- Stress level, activity, recreation, coping mechanisms
- Neurologic status: LOC, blurring vision, nausea, vomiting, tingling in extremities preceding headache
- Ingestion of tyramine foods (pickled products, beer, wine, aged cheese), food additives, preservatives, colorings, artificial sweeteners, chocolate, caffeine, which may precipitate these types of headaches
- **Serotonin syndrome** if also taking SSRI
- Kidney function, urine output

Perform/provide:
- Quiet, calm environment with decreased stimulation: noise, bright light, excessive talking

Evaluate:
- Therapeutic response: decrease in frequency, severity of headache

Teach patient/family:
- To report any side effects to prescriber
- To use contraception while taking product
- That product does not prevent or reduce number of migraines

zolpidem (Rx)

(zole′pih-dem)

Ambien, Ambien CR, Edluar, Zolpimist

Func. class.: Sedative/hypnotic
Chem. class.: Imidazopyridine

Controlled Substance Schedule IV

ACTION: Produces CNS depression at limbic, thalamic, hypothalamic levels of CNS; may be mediated by neurotransmitter γ-aminobutyric acid (GABA); results are sedation, hypnosis, skeletal muscle relaxation, anticonvulsant activity, anxiolytic action

USES: Insomnia, short-term treatment; insomnia with difficulty of sleep onset/maintenance (ext rel)

CONTRAINDICATIONS: Hypersensitivity to benzodiazepines

Precautions: Pregnancy (C), breastfeeding, children <18 yr, geriatric patients, anemia, renal/hepatic disease, suicidal individuals, drug abuse, psychosis, seizure disorders, angioedema, depression, respiratory disease, sleep apnea, sleep-related behaviors (sleepwalking), myasthenia gravis

DOSAGE AND ROUTES

- **Adult: PO** 10 mg at bedtime × 7-10 days only; total max dose 10 mg; **EXT REL** 12.5 mg immediately before bedtime, may be useful for ≤ 24 wk in people 18-64 yr with primary insomnia; **oral spray** (Zolpimist) 10 mg (2 sprays) immediately before bedtime, max 10 mg/day; **SL** (Edluar) 10 mg just before bedtime
- **Geriatric: PO** 5 mg at bedtime; **EXT REL** 6.25 mg

Available forms: Tabs 5, 10 mg; ext rel tabs 6.25, 12.5 mg; SL: 5, 10 mg; oral spray 5 mg/spray

Administer:

PO route
- Do not break, crush, or chew ext rel
- After trying conservative measures for insomnia, take with full glass of water
- ½-1 hr before bedtime (PO); right before retiring (ext rel)
- On empty stomach for fast onset; may be taken with food if GI symptoms occur
- Avoid use with CNS depressants; serious CNS depression may result

Spray route
- Prime before first use or if pump is not used for ≥ 14 days
- Do not use spray with or after a meal

Sublingual route
- Separate blister pack at perforation, peel paper and push product through, place product under tongue, allow to dissolve before swallowing; do not take with water

SIDE EFFECTS

CNS: Headache, lethargy, drowsiness, daytime sedation, dizziness, confusion, lightheadedness, anxiety, irritability, amnesia, poor coordination, complex sleep-related reactions (sleep driving, sleep eating), depression, somnolence, **suicidal ideation, abnormal thinking/behavioral changes**

CV: Chest pain, palpitations

GI: Nausea, vomiting, diarrhea, heartburn, abdominal pain, constipation

HEMA: **Leukopenia, granulocytopenia** (rare)

MISC: Myalgia

SYST: **Severe allergic reactions**

PHARMACOKINETICS

PO: Onset up to 1.5 hr, metabolized by liver, excreted by kidneys (inactive metabolites), crosses placenta, excreted in breast milk, half-life 2-3 hr

INTERACTIONS

Increase: action of both products—alcohol, CNS depressants

Increase or decrease: zolpidem levels—CYP3A4 inhibitors/inducers

NURSING CONSIDERATIONS

Assess:

⚠ **Mental status: mood, sensorium, affect, memory (long, short term), excessive sedation, impaired coordination, suicidal thoughts/behaviors**

- Blood dyscrasias: fever, sore throat, bruising, rash, jaundice, epistaxis (rare)
- Type of sleep problem: falling asleep, staying asleep

Perform/provide:

- Assistance with ambulation after receiving dose
- Storage in tight container in cool environment

Evaluate:

- Therapeutic response: ability to sleep at night, decreased amount of early morning awakening if taking product for insomnia

Teach patient/family:

- That dependence is possible after long-term use

⚠ **That complex sleep-related behaviors may occur (sleep driving/eating)**

- To avoid driving or other activities requiring alertness until dosage is stabilized
- To avoid alcohol ingestion
- That effects may take 2 nights for benefits to be noticed
- About alternative measures to improve sleep: reading, exercise several hours before bedtime, warm bath, warm milk, TV, self-hypnosis, deep breathing
- Not to use during pregnancy, breastfeeding
- That hangover is common in geriatric patients but less common than with barbiturates; that rebound insomnia may occur for 1-2 nights after discontinuing product; not to discontinue abruptly; to taper

TREATMENT OF OVERDOSE:

Lavage, activated charcoal; monitor electrolytes, VS

zonisamide (Rx)

(zone-is′a-mide)

Zonegran

Func. class.: Anticonvulsant

Chem. class.: Sulfonamides

ACTION: May act through action at sodium and calcium channels, but exact action is unknown; serotonergic action

USES: Epilepsy, adjunctive therapy for partial seizures

Unlabeled uses: Bipolar disorder (mania)

CONTRAINDICATIONS: Hypersensitivity to this product or sulfonamides; psychiatric condition, hepatic failure

Z

Precautions: Pregnancy (C), breastfeeding, children <16 yr, geriatric patients, allergies, renal/hepatic disease

DOSAGE AND ROUTES

• **Adult and child >16 yr:** 100 mg/day, may increase after 2 wk to 200 mg/day, may increase q2wk, max dose 600 mg/day

Mania (unlabeled)

• **Adult: PO** 100-200 mg/day, max 600 mg/day

Available forms: Caps 25, 50, 100 mg

SIDE EFFECTS

CNS: Dizziness, insomnia, paresthesias, depression, fatigue, headache, confusion, somnolence, agitation, irritability, speech disturbance, suicidal ideation

EENT: Diplopia, verbal difficulty, speech abnormalities, taste perversion

GI: Nausea, constipation, anorexia, weight loss, diarrhea, dyspepsia

HEMA: Aplastic anemia, granulocytopenia (rare)

INTEG: Rash

SYST: Stevens-Johnson syndrome, metabolic acidosis

PHARMACOKINETICS

Peak 2-6 hr, half-life in RBCs 105 hr, metabolized by liver, excreted by kidneys, protein binding 40%

INTERACTIONS

Decrease: half-life of zonisamide—carBAMazepine, phenytoin, PHENobarbital

Altered product levels: CYP3A4 inhibitors/inducers

Increase: CNS depression—alcohol

Drug/Herb

Increase: effect of this product—St. John's wort

Drug/Food

• Do not use with grapefruit

NURSING CONSIDERATIONS

Assess:

• **Seizures:** duration, type, intensity, precipitating factors

• Renal function: albumin conc, BUN, creatinine, serum bicarbonate at baseline and periodically

⚠ Mental status: mood, sensorium, affect, memory (long, short term), **suicidal thoughts/behaviors**

• Rash, hypersensitivity reactions

Evaluate:

• Therapeutic response: decrease in severity of seizures

Teach patient/family:

• Not to discontinue product abruptly because seizures may occur

• To avoid hazardous activities until stabilized on product

• To carry emergency ID stating product use

• To notify prescriber of rash immediately; to notify prescriber of back pain, abdominal pain, blood in urine; to increase fluid intake to reduce risk of kidney stones

• To notify prescriber if pregnancy planned, suspected

• To drink adequate fluids; to avoid grapefruit

Appendix A

Selected new drugs

abiraterone
Zytiga
Func. class.: Androgen inhibitor

ACTION: Converted to abiraterone which inhibits CYP17, the enzyme required for androgen biosynthesis; androgen-sensitive prostate cancer responds to treatment that decreases androgens

USES: Metastatic castration-resistant prostate cancer in combination with predniSONE for patients who have received prior chemotherapy containing docetaxel

CONTRAINDICATIONS: Pregnancy (X), women, children
Precautions: Adrenal insufficiency, cardiac disease, MI, heart failure, hepatic disease, hypertension, hypokalemia, infection, surgery, ventricular dysrhythmia

DOSAGE AND ROUTES
• **Adult males: PO** 1000 mg/day with predniSONE 5 mg bid
Hepatic dose
• **Adult males (Child-Pugh B, 7-9): PO** 250 mg/day with predniSONE; (Child-Pugh C, >10) do not use
Available forms:
Tabs 250 mg
Administer:
PO route
• Give whole, on empty stomach two hrs before or 1 hr after meals with full glass of water
⚠ Women who are pregnant or may become pregnant should not touch tabs without gloves

SIDE EFFECTS
CV: Angina, dysrhythmia exacerbation, atrial flutter/fibrillation/tachycardia, AV block, chest pain, edema, heart failure, MI, hypertension, QT prolongation, sinus tachycardia, supraventricular tachycardia, ventricular tachycardia
ENDO: Hot flashes
GI: Diarrhea, dyspepsia
GU: Increased urinary frequency, nocturia, urinary tract infection
META: Adrenocortical insufficiency, hyperbilirubinemia, hypertriglyceridemia, hypokalemia, hypophosphatemia
MS: Arthralgia, myalgia
RESP: Cough, upper respiratory infection
SYST: Infection

PHARMACOKINETICS
99% protein binding, converted to abiraterone (active metabolite), mean terminal half-life 7-17 hr; excreted 88% in feces, 5% in urine; high-fat food increases effect, give on empty stomach; increased effect in hepatic disease

INTERACTIONS
Avoid use with: CYP3A4 inhibitors (clarithromycin, atazanavir, nefazodone, saquinavir, telithromycin, ritonavir, indinavir, nelfinavir, voriconazole, ketoconazole, itraconazole)
Avoid use with: CYP3A4 inducers (carBAMazepine, phenytoin, rifampin, rifabutin, rifapentine, PHENobarbital)
Increase action of CYP2D6 substrate—dextromethorphan, thioridazine; dose of these products should be reduced
Drug/Food
Increase: abiraterone action—must be taken on an empty stomach

NURSING CONSIDERATIONS

Assess:

• **Prostate cancer:** monitor prostate specific antigen (PSA), serum potassium

⚠ **Hepatotoxicity:** monitor liver function tests (AST/ALT) at baseline, every 2 wk for 3 mo, monthly thereafter in patients with no known hepatic disease; interrupt treatment in patients without known hepatic disease at baseline who develop ALT/AST >5 × ULN or total bilirubin >3 × ULN; patients with moderate hepatic disease at baseline, measure ALT, AST, bilirubin before the start of treatment, every wk for 1 month, every 2 wk for the following 2 mo, monthly thereafter; if elevations in ALT and/or AST >5 × ULN or total bilirubin >3 × ULN occur in patients with moderate hepatic impairment at baseline, discontinue and do NOT restart; measure serum total bilirubin, AST/ALT if hepatotoxicity is suspected; elevations of AST, ALT, bilirubin from baseline should prompt more frequent monitoring.

• Musculoskeletal pain, joint swelling, discomfort: arthritis, arthralgia, joint swelling, and joint stiffness, some severe; muscle discomfort that included muscle spasms, musculoskeletal pain, myalgia, musculoskeletal discomfort, and musculoskeletal stiffness may be relieved with analgesics

• Signs, symptoms of adrenocorticoid insufficiency; monthly for hypertension, hypokalemia, fluid retention

⚠ **QT prolongation:** Monitor ECG for QT prolongation, ejection fraction in patients with cardiac disease, small increases in the QTc interval such as <10 ms have occurred; monitor for arrhythmia exacerbation such as sinus tachycardia, atrial fibrillation, supraventricular tachycardia (SVT), atrial tachycardia, ventricular tachycardia, atrial flutter, bradycardia, AV block complete, conduction disorder, bradyarrhythmia

Perform/provide:

• Storage of tabs at room temp

Teach patient/family:

⚠ That women must not come in contact with tabs; wear gloves if product needs to be handled, pregnancy (X)

• To report chest pain, swelling of joints, burning/pain when urinating

aflibercept

EYLEA

Func. class.: Biologic response modifier; signal transduction inhibitor (STIs) (Ophthalmic)

ACTION: A recombinant fusion protein consisting of portions of human VEGF receptors 1 and 2 extracellular domains fused to human IgG1; acts as a soluble decoy receptor that binds vascular endothelial growth factor-A (VEGF-A) and placental growth factor (PIGF); can act as mitogenic, chemotactic, vascular permeability factors for endothelial cells; VEGF-A interacts with VEGFR-1 and VEGFR-2 on the surface of endothelial cells; results in neovascularization and vascular permeability; binding of aflibercept to VEGF-A and PIGF prevents activation of these receptors

USES: For treatment of neovascular (wet) age-related macular degeneration (AMD)

CONTRAINDICATIONS: Hypersensitivity, ocular/periocular infection, active intraocular inflammation

Precautions: Neonates, infants, children, adolescents, pregnancy (C), breastfeeding; history of glaucoma, ocular surgery; driving or operating machinery

DOSAGE AND ROUTES

• **Adult: Intravitreal INJ** 2 mg (0.05 ml) into affected eye(s) q4wk × 12 wk, then 2 mg (0.05 ml) q8wk

Available forms: Solution for injection 2 mg/0.05 ml

Administer:

Intravitreal route

- Visually inspect for particulate matter, discoloration before use; do not use if particulates, cloudiness, discoloration are visible; only for use by physicians trained in administration
- Use controlled aseptic conditions (sterile gloves, sterile drape, sterile eyelid speculum); adequate anesthesia, topical broad-spectrum antiinfective should be given before use
- Use each vial for treatment of single eye only; if other eye is being treated, use new vial and change the sterile field, syringe, gloves, drapes, eyelid speculum, filter, injection needles before administering to the other eye
- Use aseptic technique, withdraw all of vial contents through a 5-micron 19-G filter needle attached to 1-ml syringe supplied by manufacturer; after vial contents are withdrawn, discard filter needle and replace with sterile 30-G × ½ inch needle for intravitreal injection; expel any air bubbles and contents of syringe until plunger tip is aligned with line that marks 0.05 ml
- Immediately after the intravitreal injection, monitor patient for elevation in intraocular pressure (IOP); appropriate monitoring may consist of a check for perfusion of optic nerve head or tonometry; sterile paracentesis needle should be available if required

SIDE EFFECTS

CV: Thromboembolism, nonfatal stroke, nonfatal myocardial infarction, vascular death

EENT: *Ocular hemorrhage, ocular pain, cataracts, vitreous detachment, vitreous floaters,* conjunctival hyperemia, corneal erosion, detachment of retinal pigment epithelium, injection site pain, foreign body sensation, increased lacrimation, blurred vision, retinal pigment epithelium tear, injection site hemorrhage, blepharedema, corneal edema

SYST: Hypersensitivity

PHARMACOKINETICS

Absorbed into systemic circulation; present in its unbound form and stable inactive form bound with endogenous VEGF; elimination by binding to free endogenous VEGF; metabolism by proteolysis; terminal half-life in plasma 5-6 days

NURSING CONSIDERATIONS

Assess:

- **Infection:** monitor for infection during week after injection to permit early treatment of any ocular infection that may develop; proper aseptic injection technique should be used to minimize infection
- **Increased** intraocular pressure: monitor for acute increases in intraocular pressure within 60 min of injection; sustained increases in intraocular pressure have been reported after repeated intravitreal dosing; monitor intraocular pressure and optic nerve head perfusion, a sterile paracentesis needle should be available

Perform/provide:

- Storage: do not freeze, protect from light, refrigerate, store in original package until time of use

Evaluate:

- Prevention of further vision loss

Teach patient/family:

⚠ To seek immediate care if symptoms of endophthalmitis or retinal detachment develop (ocular pain, hyperemia of the conjunctiva, photophobia, blurry vision)

aminophylline (theophylline ethylenediamine) (Rx)

(am-in-off'i-lin)

Phyllocontin ✱, Theochron, Theo-24, Uniphyl

Func. class.: Bronchodilator, spasmolytic

Chem. class.: Methylxanthine

DOSAGE AND ROUTES

Reversible airways obstruction (bronchospasm prophylaxis) associated with asthma or chronic obstructive pulmonary disease (COPD, emphysema, chronic bronchitis)

Calculate initial mg/kg dose based on ideal body weight as theophylline distributes poorly into body fat

Acute exacerbations of the symptoms and reversible airflow obstruction associated with asthma and other chronic lung diseases (COPD) along with inhaled beta-2 selective agonists and systemic corticosteroids

- **Adult <60 yr/adolescent ≥16 yr: IV CONT INF** expressed in theophylline; initially, 0.4 mg/kg/hr; max 900 mg/day (otherwise healthy nonsmokers); patients who smoke may require an increased dose; give 0.2 mg/kg/hr (≥400 mg/day) in CHF, cor pulmonale, liver dysfunction, sepsis with multiorgan failure, shock; reduced doses may be needed in patients receiving other drugs that decrease theophylline clearance; adjust dosage based on serum concentrations
- **Adult ≥60 yr: IV CONT INF** initially, 0.3 mg/kg/hour; give 0.2 mg/kg/hr in CHF, cor pulmonale, liver dysfunction, sepsis with multiorgan failure, shock; reduced doses may be needed in patients receiving other drugs that decrease theophylline clearance; adjust dosage based serum concentrations; max 400 mg/day unless serum concentration and patient condition require a higher dose
- **Child ≥12 yr/adolescent ≥15 yr: IV CONT INF** Initially, 0.5 mg/kg/hr (healthy nonsmokers (up to 900 mg/day); 0.7 mg/kg/hr in smokers; 0.2 mg/kg/hr (up to 400 mg/day) in cardiac decompensation, cor pulmonale, liver dysfunction, sepsis with multiorgan failure, or shock); adjust dosage based on serum concentrations
- **Child 9-11 yr: IV CONT INF** Initially, 0.7 mg/kg/hr; reduced doses may be needed in patients receiving other drugs that decrease theophylline clearance; give 0.2 mg/kg/hr (up to 400 mg/day) in cardiac decompensation, cor pulmonale, liver dysfunction, sepsis with multiorgan failure, or shock; adjust dosage based on serum concentrations
- **Child 1-8 yr: IV CONT INF** Initially, 0.8 mg/kg/hr; reduced doses may be needed in patients receiving other drugs that decrease theophylline clearance; 0.2 mg/kg/hr (up to 400 mg/day) in cardiac decompensation, cor pulmonale, liver dysfunction, sepsis with multiorgan failure, or shock; adjust dosage based on serum concentrations
- **Infant 6-52 wk: IV CONT INF** Calculate initial dosage using the following equation: (0.008 × age in wk) + 0.21 = theophylline dosage in mg/kg/hour IV; reduced doses may be needed in patients with risk factors for reduced theophylline clearance (cimetidine therapy, cardiac or liver dysfunction, renal impairment in infant <3 mo); adjust dosage based on serum concentrations

For maintenance therapy of asthma or COPD

- **Adult/adolescent/child >45 kg: PO** (Expressed in theophylline and reg release products) PO Initially, 300 mg/day in divided doses q6-8hr; after 3 days, if tolerated, increase dose to 400 mg/day in divided doses q6-8hr; after 3 more days, if tolerated, increase dose to 600 mg/day PO in divided doses q6-8hr; adjust dose to maintain therapeutic range; doses of 400-1600 mg/day may be needed, max

400 mg/day in patients with risk factors for decreased theophylline clearance (elderly >60 yr); NIH recommends initial dose for asthma of 10 mg/kg/day (max: 300 mg/day) titrated to serum concentration of 5-15 mcg/ml (usual max: 800 mg/day in ≥12 yr and 16 mg/kg/day in children 1-11 yr)

• **Child/adolescent ≤15 yr old and ≤45 kg: PO** Initially, 12-14 mg/kg (max 300 mg) per day in divided doses q4-6hr; after 3 days, if tolerated, may increase to 16 mg/kg (max 400 mg) per day in divided doses q4-6hr; after 3 more days, if tolerated and if needed, increase dose to 20 mg/kg (max 600 mg) per day in divided doses q4-6hr; adjust dose to maintain therapeutic range (doses of 10-36 mg/kg/day in child 1-9 yr may be needed); max 16 mg/kg (400 mg) per day in patients with risk factors for decreased theophylline clearance or who cannot receive recommended serum concentration monitoring; NIH recommends initial dose for asthma of 10 mg/kg/day (max 300 mg/day) titrated to serum concentration of 5-15 mcg/ml (usual max 800 mg/day in patients ≥12 yr and 16 mg/kg/day in children 1-11 yr)

• **Neonate/infant ≤52 wk: PO** Calculate initial dose using the following equation: [(0.2 × age in wks) + 5] × (kg body weight) = theophylline dosage in mg/day; in infants ≤26 wk, divide dose and administer q8hr and in infant >26 wk, divide dose and give q6hr; adjust dose to maintain a steady-state serum concentration of 5-10 mcg/ml in neonates and 10-15 mcg/ml in infants; NIH recommends initial dose for asthma of 10 mg/kg/day titrated to theophylline serum concentration of 5-15 mcg/ml, max in mg/kg/day = [(0.2 × age in weeks) + 5]

• Extended-release products are to be used only for chronic disease management; do not use in treatment of acute symptoms of asthma and reversible bronchospasm

• **Adult/adolescents/child ≥12 yr and >45 kg: (Theo-24 Cap) PO** Initially, 300-400 mg/day q24hr; evening dosing is not recommended; after 3 days, if tolerated, increase to 400-600 mg/day q24hr; adjust dose to maintain therapeutic range; doses of 400-1600 mg/day may be needed; max 400 mg/day in patients with decreased theophylline clearance, (elderly >60 yr), and in those who cannot receive recommended serum concentration monitoring

• **Child >12 yr/adolescent <16 yr and <45 kg: (Theo-24 Cap) PO** Initially, 12-14 mg/kg (max 300 mg) per day q24hr; evening dosing is not recommended; after 3 days, if tolerated, may increase to 16 mg/kg (max 400 mg) per day; after 3 more days, if tolerated and if needed, increase to 20 mg/kg (max 600 mg) per day; adjust dose to maintain therapeutic range; max 16 mg/kg/day up to 400 mg/day in patients with decreased theophylline clearance

Treatment of methotrexate toxicity (unlabeled)

• **Adult/adolescents/child ≥3 yr: IV** 2.5 mg/kg over 45-60 min

asparaginase *Erwinia chrysanthemi*

Erwinaze

Func. class.: Antineoplastic, natural and semi-synthetic

ACTION: Contains an asparaginase specific enzyme L-asparaginase derived from Erwinia chrysanthemi, which catalyzes of asparagine to aspartic acid and ammonia and causes reduced circulating concentrations of asparagine; efficacy of asparaginase *Erwinia chrysanthemi* may be leukemic cell cytotoxicity from asparagine deficiency

USES: Treatment of acute lymphocytic leukemia (ALL) in combination with other chemotherapeutic agents in patients who have developed hypersensitivity to *E. coli*-derived asparaginase

CONTRAINDICATIONS:
Hypersensitivity, breastfeeding, history of serious pancreatitis, bleeding, or serious thrombosis with prior L-asparaginase therapy

Precautions: pregnancy (C), children <2 yr, hepatic disease, diabetes mellitus

DOSAGE AND ROUTES

• **Adult, adolescent, child ≥2 yr (substitute for pegaspargase): IM** 25,000 IU/m² 3 ×/wk (Monday/Wednesday/Friday) × 6 doses for each planned dose of pegaspargase within a treatment

• **Adult (substitute for L-asparaginase *E. coli*): IM** 25,000 IU/m² for each scheduled dose of native *E. coli* asparaginase within a treatment

Available forms: Powder for inj 10,000 Units

Administer:

• Slowly inject 1 or 2 ml of preservative-free sterile sodium chloride (0.9%) inj against inner vial wall; do not forcefully inject sol directly onto or into powder; if 1 ml of NS is used, conc is 10,000 IU/ml; if 2 ml of NS is used, conc is 5000 IU/ ml; dissolve contents by gentle mixing or swirling; do not shake or invert vial

• Reconstituted sol should be clear and colorless; discard if any visible particles or protein aggregates are present

• Calculate the volume needed to obtain dose; withdraw volume containing calculated dose from vial into polypropylene syringe within 15 min of reconstitution

IM route

Administer dose by IM inj within 4 hr of reconstitution; limit volume to 2 ml per inj site; multiple inj sites may be needed

SIDE EFFECTS

ENDO: Hyperglycemia
GI: Pancreatitis
HEMA: Bleeding, serious thrombosis
INTEG: Local inj site reaction
MISC: Hyperammonemia (seizure, headache), neurotoxicity, elevated hepatic enzymes, hyperbilirubinemia
SYST: Anaphylaxis

PHARMACOKINETICS

Achieved serum trough asparaginase activity concentrations ≥0.1 IU/ml by 72 hr after dose 3

INTERACTIONS

Synergistic or antagonistic action of: methotrexate
Increase: neurotoxicity—vinCRIStine
Increase: pancreatitis risk—cytarabine
Increase: hyperglycemia—corticosteroids
Increase: bleeding risk—NSAIDs, thrombolytics, salicylates, anticoagulants, platelet inhibitors

Drug/Lab Test

Increase: liver function tests, ammonia
Decrease: fibrinogen, protein C activity, protein S activity, anti-thrombin III

NURSING CONSIDERATIONS

Assess:

• **Anaphylaxis:** give only with resuscitation equipment and other agents necessary to treat anaphylaxis; if a serious hypersensitivity reaction occurs, discontinue product

• **Bleeding:** identify if NSAIDs, salicylates, thrombolytics, platelet inhibitors, anticoagulants have been used; grade 1 or 2 bleeding or coagulation abnormalities may occur (serious thrombosis, sagittal sinus thrombosis); discontinue for a thrombotic or hemorrhagic event until symptoms resolve; after resolution, treatment may be resumed; coagulation proteins were decreased in most patients after a 2-wk course: fibrinogen, protein C activity, protein S activity, antithrombin III

⚠ **Pancreatitis:** discontinue for severe or hemorrhagic pancreatitis (abdominal pain >72 hr and amylase elevation ≥2 × upper limit of normal); mild pancreatitis, hold until the signs, symptoms subside and amylase concentrations return to normal, then resume

• **Hyperglycemia:** glucose intolerance that is irreversible in some cases; monitor baseline and periodic glucose concentration; administer insulin therapy as needed

⚠ **Hyperammonemia/neurotoxicity: seizures, headache; asparagine rescue may be used to treat acute CNS toxicity; doses of asparagine used were 1-2 mmol/kg/day continuous IV inf × 5 days**
Monitor liver function tests and for hyperbilirubinemia
Local injection site reaction: no more than 2 ml of the reconstituted product is to be administered at a single injection site

Perform/provide:
• Do not freeze or refrigerate the reconstituted solution; discard any unused portions

Evaluate:
• Decreased spread of malignancy

Teach patient/family:
⚠ **To get immediate medical advice if they experience abdominal pain, nausea, vomiting, diarrhea; pancreatitis may occur**
⚠ **To get immediate medical advice if experiencing anaphylactic reactions**
• To contact provider if patient experiences excessive thirst or any increase in volume or frequency of urination; hyperglycemia may occur

axitinib

Inlyta

Func. class.: Antineoplastics, biologic response modifiers, signal transduction inhibitors (STIs)

Chem. class.: Tyrosine kinase inhibitor

ACTION: Inhibits receptor tyrosine kinases including vascular endothelial growth factor receptors (VEGFR)-1, VEGFR-2, and VEGFR-3; inhibits tumor growth and phosphorylation of VEGFR-2 and VEGF-mediated endothelial cell proliferation

USES: Treatment of advanced renal cell cancer after failure of one prior systemic therapy

CONTRAINDICATIONS: Pregnancy (D), breastfeeding

Precautions Risk for or history of thromboembolic disease, recent bleeding, untreated brain metastasis, recent GI bleeding, GI perforation, fistula, surgery, moderate hepatic disease, uncontrolled hypertension, hyper/hypothyroidism, proteinuria, infertility, end-stage renal disease (CrCl <15 ml/min); not intended for use in adolescents, children, infants, neonates

DOSAGE AND ROUTES

• **Adult:** PO 5 mg bid (at 12 hr intervals), may increase to 7 mg bid and then to 10 mg bid in those not receiving antihypertensives who tolerate the lower dosage for at least 2 consecutive wk with no more than grade 2 adverse reactions. Reduce to 3 mg bid if a dose reduction is needed; if further reduction is necessary, reduce to 2 mg bid
• **Adult receiving a strong CYP 3A4/5 inhibitor:** Reduce dose by 1/2, adjust as needed

Administer:
• Give with or without food; swallow tablet whole with a glass of water
• If patient vomits or misses a dose, an additional dose should not be taken; the next dose should be taken at the usual time

SIDE EFFECTS

CNS: Dizziness, headache, **reversible posterior leukoencephalopathy syndrome (RPLS)**, fatigue
CV: Hypertension, arterial thromboembolic events (ATE), venous thromboembolic events (VTE)
ENDO: Hypothyroidism, hyperthyroidism
GI: lower GI bleeding/perforation/fistula, abdominal pain, constipation, diarrhea, dysgeusia, dyspepsia, dysphonia, hemorrhoids, nausea, mucosal inflammation, stomatitis, vomiting, increased ALT/AST
GU: Proteinuria
HEMA: Bleeding intracranial bleeding, anemia, polycythemia, decreased/in-

creased hemoglobin, lymphopenia thrombocytopenia, neutropenia
INTEG: Palmar-plantar erythrodysesthesia (hand and foot syndrome) rash, dry skin, pruritus, alopecia, erythema
MISC: Weight loss dehydration metabolic and electrolyte laboratory abnormalities included
MS: Asthenia, arthralgia, musculoskeletal pain, myalgia
RESP: Cough, dyspnea

PHARMACODYNAMICS

Absorption: bioavailability 58%; distribution: protein binding >99%; metabolized in liver by CYP3A4/5, CYP1A2, CYP2C19, and UGT1A1; metabolites are carboxylic acid, sulfoxide, and N-glucuronide; excretion 41% in feces and 23% in urine, 12% unchanged; half-life: 2.5-6.1 hr; steady state 2-3 days; onset unknown, peak 2.5-4.1 hr, increased in moderate hepatic disease; duration unknown

INTERACTIONS

Increase: effect of axitinib—CYP3A4/5 inhibitor, strong, moderate (ketoconazole, boceprevir, chloramphenicol, conivaptan, delavirdine, fosamprenavir, imatinib, indinavir, isoniazid itraconazole, dalfopristin, quinupristin, posaconazole, ritonavir, telithromycin, tipranavir (boosted with ritonavir), darunavir (boosted with ritonavir), aldesleukin, IL-2, amiodarone, aprepitant, fosaprepitant atazanavir, bromocriptine, clarithromycin, crizotinib, danazol, diltiazem dronedarone, erythromycin, fluvoxamine, lanreotide, lapatinib, miconazole, mifepristone, nefazodone, nelfinavir, niCARdipine, octreotide pantoprazole, saquinavir, tamoxifen, verapamil, voriconazole, grapefruit juice)
Decrease: effect of axitinib—CYP3A4/5 inducers, strong/moderate (rifampin, carBAMazepine, dexamethasone, phenytoin, PHENobarbital rifabutin, rifapentine, St. John's wort, ethanol, bexarotene, bosentan, efavirenz, etravirine, griseofulvin, metyrapone, modafinil, nafcillin, nevirapine, OXcarbazepine, vemurafenib, pioglitazone, topiramate)
Increase or decrease: effect of axitinib—CYP3A4/5 inhibitor and inducers (quiNINE)

Drug/Lab Test

Increase: creatinine, lipase, amylase, sodium, potassium, glucose
Decrease: bicarbonate, calcium, albumin, glucose, phosphate, sodium
Increase or decrease: sodium, glucose

Drug/Herb

Decrease: effect of axitinib—St. John's wort

NURSING CONSIDERATIONS

Assess:

- **Bleeding:** monitor for GI bleeding or perforation; temporarily discontinue therapy if a patient develops any bleeding that requires treatment
- **Surgery:** discontinue ≥24 hr before surgery, may be resumed after adequate wound healing
- **Hepatic/renal disease:** dosage should be reduced in patients with moderate (Child-Pugh Class B) hepatic disease, monitor liver function tests (ALT, AST, bilirubin) before and periodically during therapy; monitor CCr before and during treatment
- **Hypertension:** B/P should be well controlled before starting treatment; monitor patients for hypertension and administer antihypertensive therapy as needed before and during therapy; dose should be reduced for persistent hypertension; therapy should be discontinued if B/P remains elevated after a dosage reduction or if there is evidence of hypertensive crisis; after discontinuation monitor B/P for hypotension in those receiving antihypertensives
- **Hyper/hypothyroidism:** monitor thyroid function tests before and periodically during therapy; thyroid disease should be treated with rd thyroid medications

• Monitor for proteinuria before and periodically during therapy; product may need to be decreased or discontinued if moderate to severe proteinuria occurs

⚠ **Pregnancy/breastfeeding:** pregnancy category D; determine if the patient is pregnant or breastfeeding before using this product; may also cause infertility

Perform/provide:

• Storage at room temperature

Evaluate:

• Decreased spread of malignancy

Teach patient/family:

⚠ To use contraception during treatment (pregnancy category D) or to avoid use of this product; to notify prescriber if pregnancy is planned to suspected, not to breastfeed

⚠ To notify prescriber of bleeding that is severe or that requires treatment

• That product will be discontinued ≥24 hr before surgery; may be resumed after adequate wound healing

• That laboratory testing will be required before and periodically during product use

• How to monitor B/P and that B/P products should be continued as directed by prescriber

azilsartan

Edarbi

Func. class.: Antihypertensive

Chem. class.: Angiotensin II receptor antagonist

ACTION: Antagonizes angiotensin II at the AT_1 receptor in tissues like vascular smooth muscle and the adrenal gland. Two angiotensin II receptors, AT_1 and AT_2, have been identified; azilsartan exhibits more than 10,000-fold greater affinity for the AT_1 receptor than the AT_2 receptor.

USES: Hypertension, alone or in combination with other antihypertensives

CONTRAINDICATIONS:

Black Box Warning: Pregnancy (D) 2nd/3rd trimesters

Precautions: Pregnancy (C) 1st trimester, breastfeeding, children, geriatric patients, angioedema, African descent, renal disease, renal artery stenosis, heart failure, hypovolemia

DOSAGE AND ROUTES:

• **Adult: PO** 80 mg/day, may give an initial dose of 40 mg/day in patients receiving high-dose diuretic therapy

Available forms: Tabs 40, 80 mg

Administer:

• May administer without regard to food

SIDE EFFECTS

CNS: Dizziness, fatigue, asthenia

CV: Hypotension, orthostatic hypotension

GI: Nausea, diarrhea

HEMA: Anemia

INTEG: Angioedema

MS: Muscle cramps

RESP: Cough

SYST: Secondary malignancy

PHARMACOKINETICS:

Protein binding >99% to serum albumin; metabolized by CYP2C9; elimination half-life 11 hr, steady state within 5 days and no accumulation in plasma occurs with once-daily dosing; elimination 55% in feces, 42% in urine; hydrolyzed to the active metabolite, azilsartan, in GI tract during absorption, rapidly absorbed, peak 1.5-3 hr; absolute bioavailability (60%) not affected by food

INTERACTIONS:

Increase: hypotensive effect—other antihypertensives, other angiotensin receptor antagonists, MAOIs

Increase: hypoglycemia—antidiabetics

⚠ **Increase:** renal failure risk—cyclosporine, diuretics, NSAIDs in those with poor renal function; monitor closely

⚠ **Increase:** lithium toxicity—lithium

⚠ **Increase:** phosphate nephropathy—sodium phosphate monobasic monohydrate; sodium phosphate dibasic anhydrous

Drug/Herb:

Increase: antihypertensive effect—Hawthorn

Decrease: antihypertensive effect—ephedra

NURSING CONSIDERATIONS

Assess:

⚠ **Angioedema:** Assess for facial swelling, difficulty breathing

Black Box Warning: For pregnancy (D) 2nd/3rd trimester, can cause fetal death

- Response and adverse reactions especially in renal disease
- B/P, pulse when beginning therapy and periodically thereafter; note rhythm, rate, quality; obtain electrolytes before beginning therapy

Perform/provide:

- Use original package to protect from light and moisture beat

Evaluate:

- Therapeutic response: decreased B/P

Teach patient/family:

- To comply with dosage schedule even if feeling better

⚠ To notify prescriber of facial swelling; if pregnancy is planned or suspected (category D 2nd/3rd trimester)

- That diarrhea, dehydration, excessive perspiration, vomiting, may lead to fall in B/P; to consult prescriber if these occur
- To rise slowing from lying or sitting to minimize orthostatic hypotension; that product may cause dizziness
- To avoid OTC medications unless approved by prescriber; to inform all health care providers of product use
- To use proper technique for obtaining B/P

belatacept

See page 169

belimumab

See page 171

boceprevir

See page 193

brentuximab

See page 198

crizotinib

See page 337

desvenlafaxine

See page 385

ezogabine

See page 510

fidaxomicin

See page 534

glucarpidase

See page 593

indacaterol

See page 647

ipilimumab

See page 665

linagliptin

See page 717

rilpivirine

Edurant

Func. class.: Antiretroviral

Chem. class.: Non-nucleoside transcriptase inhibitors (NNTIs)

ACTION: Inhibits HIV-1 reverse transcriptase; unlike nucleoside reverse transcriptase inhibitors (NRTIs), it does not compete for binding nor does it require phosphorylation to be active. Binds directly to a site on reverse transcriptase causing disruption of the enzyme's active site thereby blocking RNA-dependent and DNA-dependent DNA polymerase activities

USES: HIV in combination with other antiretrovirals

CONTRAINDICATIONS: Hypersensitivity

Precautions: Pregnancy (category B), breastfeeding, neonates, infants, children, adolescents <18 yr, immune reconstitution syndrome, antimicrobial resistance, pancreatitis, depression, suicidal ideation, QT prolongation, torsades de pointes, hyperlipidemia, hypertriglyceridemia, hypercholesterolemia

DOSAGE AND ROUTES

Antiretroviral treatment-naive adults (HIV) in combination with other antiretroviral agents

- **Adults:** PO 25 mg/day with a meal

Available forms: Tab 25 mg

Administer:

- Give combination with other antiretroviral agents; in antiretroviral treatment–naive adults, rilpivirine is utilized as an alternative to efavirenz in NNRTI-based treatment regimens; potential rilpivirine-based treatment regimens combine rilpivirine with either tenofovir plus emtricitabine or lamiVUDine; or abacavir plus emtricitabine or lamiVUDine; or zidovudine plus emtricitabine or lamiVUDine
- Give with a meal

SIDE EFFECTS

CNS: Depressed mood, dysphoria, major depression, mood alteration, negative thoughts, **suicide attempts**, fatigue, headache, dizziness, drowsiness

GI: Nausea, vomiting, abdominal pain, diarrhea, cholecystitis, cholelithiasis, decreased appetite, elevated hepatic enzymes, hyperbilirubinemia, hypercholesterolemia

GU: Glomerulonephritis membranous/glomerulonephritis mesangioproliferative

PHARMACOKINETICS:

Protein binding (99.7%) to albumin; metabolism via oxidation CYP3A; terminal elimination half-life 50 hr, excretion feces (85%), 25% excreted unchanged; urine (6.1%); peak 4-5 hrs; increased effect 40% (food), decreased effect 50% (high protein drink)

INTERACTIONS:

Increase: rilpivirine effect—CYP3A4 inhibitors (delavirdine, efavirenz, darunavir, tipranavir, atazanavir, fosamprenavir, indinavir, nelfinavir, aldesleukin IL-2, amiodarone aprepitant, basiliximab, boceprevir, bromocriptine, chloramphenicol, clarithromycin, conivaptan danazol, dalfopristin, dasatinib, diltiazem, dronedarone, erythromycin, ethinyl estradiol, fluconazole, FLUoxetine, fluvoxamine, fosaprepitant, imatinib, isoniazid, itraconazole, ketoconazole, lanreotide, lapatinib, miconazole, nefazodone, niCARdipine, octreotide, posaconazole, quiNINE, ranolazine, rifaximin, tamoxifen, telaprevir, telithromycin, troleandomycin, verapamil, voriconazole, zafirlukast)

⚠ **Increase: QT prolongation—class IA/III antidysrhythmics, some phenothiazines, β agonists, local anesthetics, tricyclics, chloroquine, droperidol, haloperidol, pentamidine; CYP3A4 inhibitors (amiodarone, clarithromycin, erythromycin, telithromycin, troleandomycin, arsenic trioxide, levomethadyl); CYP3A4 substrates (methadone, pimozide, QUEtiapine,** quiNIDine, risperidone, ziprasidone, lopinavir, saquinavir, fluconazole, posaconazole, dasatinib, dronedarone, lapatinib, octreotide, ranolazine, citalopram, abarelix, alfuzosin, amoxapine, apomorphine, artemether, lumefantrine, asenapine, ofloxacin, ciprofloxacin, clozapine, cyclobenzaprine, dolasetron, eribulin, flecainide, gatifloxacin, gemifloxacin, halogenated anesthetics, iloperidone, levofloxacin, maprotiline, mefloquine, moxifloxacin, nilotinib, norfloxacin, olanzapine, ondansetron, paliperidone, palonosetron, QUEtiapine)

Increase: rilpivirine adverse reactions, fungal infections—fluconazole, voriconazole

Decrease: rilpivirine effect, treatment failure—CYP3A4 inducers (phenytoin, fosphenytoin, barbiturates, OXcarbazepine, carBAMazepine, rifabutin, rifampin, rifapentine, dexamethasone), efavirenz, nevirapine, ritonavir; aminoglutethimide, bexarotene, bosentan, griseofulvin, metyrapone, modafinil, flutamide, nafcillin, pioglitazone, primidone, topiramate); proton pump inhibitors (PPIs)

Decrease: rilpivirine effect, treatment failure—H2 receptor antagonists (cimetidine, famotidine, nizatidine, ranitidine), give 12 hr before or 4 hr after rilpivirine

Decrease: rilpivirine effect—antacids, use >2 hrs before, or 4 hr after rilpivirine

Drug/Food

Increase: adverse reactions—grapefruit juice

NURSING CONSIDERATIONS

Assess:

- **HIV:** Assess symptoms of HIV including opportunistic infections before and during treatment, some may be life threatening; monitor plasma HIV RNA, CD4+, CD8 + cell counts, serum β-2 microglobulin, serum ICD+24 antigen levels; treatment failures occur more frequently in those with baseline HIV-1 RNA concentrations >100,000 copies/ml than in patients with concentrations <100,000 copies/ml; monitor serum cholesterol, lipid panel
- Antiretroviral drug resistance testing is recommended before initiation of therapy in antiretroviral treatment–naive patients
- For adults and adolescents, initiation of antiretroviral therapy is recommended in any patient with a history of an AIDS-defining infection; with a CD4 ≤500/mm^3; who is pregnant; who has HIV-associated nephropathy; or who is being treated for hepatitis B (HBV) infection.

⚠ **Suicidal thoughts/behaviors:** Assess frequently for suicidal ideation, report any increase in depressive symptoms

- Hepatic disease: monitor for elevated hepatic enzymes (>2.5 × ULN); grade 3 and 4 may be higher in patients co-infected with hepatitis B or C

Perform/Provide:

- Storage at room temperature away from heat and moisture

Teach Patient/family:

- That product is not a cure, but controls symptoms
- That product must be taken in combination with other prescribed products

rivaroxaban

Xarelto

Func. class.: Anticoagulant
Chem. class.: Factor Xa inhibitor

ACTION: A novel, oral anticoagulant that selectively and potently inhibits coagulation factor Xa

USES: For deep venous thrombosis (DVT) prophylaxis, which may lead to pulmonary embolism (PE), in patients undergoing knee or hip replacement surgery; for stroke prophylaxis and systemic embolism prophylaxis in patients with nonvalvular atrial fibrillation

CONTRAINDICATIONS Severe hypersensitivity

Black Box Warning: Active bleeding

Precautions Pregnancy (category C), breastfeeding, neonates, infants, children, adolescents, geriatric patients, moderate or severe hepatic disease (Child-Pugh Class B or C), hepatic disease associated with coagulopathy, creatinine clearance <30 ml/min for use as DVT prophylaxis and <15 ml/min for stroke and systemic embolism prophylaxis in nonvalvular atrial fibrillation, dental procedures, aneurysm, diabetes retinopathy, diverticulitis, endocarditis, GI bleeding, hypertension, obstetric delivery, peptic ulcer disease, stroke, surgery

Black Box Warning: Abrupt discontinuation, epidermal/spinal anesthesia

Patients, especially those with dental disease, should be instructed in proper oral hygiene, including caution in use of regular toothbrushes, dental floss, toothpicks

DOSAGE AND ROUTES

Deep venous thrombosis (DVT) prophylaxis, which may lead to pulmonary embolism (PE) (knee or hip replacement)

- **Adult: PO** 10 mg/day × 12 days after knee replacement surgery or × 35 days after hip replacement; administer the initial dose ≥6-10 hr after surgery once hemostasis has been established

Stroke prophylaxis and systemic embolism prophylaxis (with nonvalvular atrial fibrillation)

- Unless pathological bleeding occurs, do not discontinue rivaroxaban in the absence of alternative
- **Adult: PO** 20 mg/day with evening meal (CrCl >50 ml/min)

Converting from warfarin to rivaroxaban

- Discontinue warfarin and start rivaroxaban when INR is <3

Converting from another anticoagulant other than warfarin to rivaroxaban

- Start rivaroxaban 0-2 hr before the next scheduled evening administration of anticoagulant (omit that dose of anticoagulant); for continuous inf of unfractionated heparin, stop the inf and initiate rivaroxaban simultaneously

Converting from rivaroxaban to another anticoagulant with rapid onset (not warfarin)

- Discontinue rivaroxaban and give the first dose of the other anticoagulant (oral or parenteral) at the time that the next dose of rivaroxaban would have been administered

Available forms: Tabs 10, 20, 50 mg

Administer:

⚠ **For DVT prophylaxis:** give daily without regard to food, give initial dose ≥6-10 hr after surgery when hemostasis has been established

⚠ **For stroke/systemic embolism prophylaxis:** give daily with evening meal

- If dose is not given at correct time, give as soon as possible on the same day

SIDE EFFECTS

GI: Increased hepatic enzymes, hyperbilirubinemia, jaundice, nausea, cholestasis, **cytolytic hepatitis**

HEMA: **Bleeding, intracranial bleeding, epidural hematoma, GI bleeding, retinal hemorrhage, adrenal bleeding, retroperitoneal hemorrhage, cerebral hemorrhage, subdural hematoma, epidural hematoma, hemiparesis, thrombocytopenia**

INTEG: Pruritus, blister, hypersensitivity, **anaphylactic reaction, anaphylactic shock**

SYST: **Stevens-Johnson syndrome**

PHARMACOKINETICS

Bioavailability 80%-100%, protein binding (92%-95%) albumin, excreted in urine 66% (36% unchanged, 30% metabolites), 28% in feces (7% unchanged, 21% metabolites), unchanged drug excreted in urine (via active tubular secretion, glomerular filtration); terminal elimination half-life 5-9 hr, peak 2-4 hr; increased effect in hepatic/renal disease, Japanese patients, increased terminal half-life in geriatric patients

INTERACTIONS

Increase: rivaroxaban effect, possible bleeding—ketoconazole itraconazole, ritonavir, lopinavir/ritonavir; conivaptan, clarithromycin, erythromycin, salicylates, NSAIDs, other anticoagulants, thrombolytics, platelet inhibitors, niCARdipine
Decrease: rivaroxaban effect—carBAMazepine, phenytoin, rifampin
Increase: rivaroxaban effect in renal impairment—telithromycin, darunavir, mifepristone, nelfinavir, pantoprazole, posaconazole, saquinavir, tamoxifen, lapatinib, azithromycin, diltiazem, verapamil, quiNIDine, ranolazine, dronedarone, amiodarone, felodipine
Drug/Herb:
Decrease: rivaroxaban effect—St. John's wort
Drug/Food:
Increase: rivaroxaban effect in renal disease—grapefruit juice
Decrease: rivaroxaban effect—food

NURSING CONSIDERATIONS

Assess:

Black Box Warning: Bleeding: monitor for bleeding, including bleeding during dental procedures (easy bruising, blood in urine, stools, emesis, sputum, epistaxis); there is no specific antidote

Black Box Warning: Abrupt discontinuation: avoid abrupt discontinuation unless an alternative anticoagulant in those with atrial fibrillation; discontinuing puts patients at an increased risk of thrombotic events; if product must be discontinued for reasons other than pathological bleeding, consider administering another anticoagulant

• **Pregnancy/breastfeeding:** pregnancy category C; identify if pregnancy is suspected or planned; pregnancy related hemorrhage may occur and anticoagulation cannot be monitored with standard laboratory testing; breastfeeding should be discontinued before beginning use of this product

Black Box Warning: Epidural/spinal anesthesia: epidural or spinal hematomas that result in long-term or permanent paralysis may occur in patients who have received anticoagulants and are receiving neuraxial anesthesia or undergoing spinal puncture; epidural catheter should not be removed <18 hr after the last dose of rivaroxaban; do not administer the next rivaroxaban dose <6 hr after the catheter removal; delay rivaroxaban administration for 24 hr if traumatic puncture occurs; monitor for neuro changes

• **Hepatic/renal disease:** increase in effect of product in hepatic disease (Child-Pugh Class B or C), hepatic disease with coagulopathy; renal failure/severe renal impairment (creatinine clearance <30 ml/min in DVT prophylaxis and <15 ml/min for stroke or systemic embolism prophylaxis in nonvalvular atrial fibrillation); product should be discontinued in acute renal failure; reduce dose in those with atrial fibrillation and CrCl 15-50 ml/min; monitor renal function periodically (creatinine clearance, BUN)

Perform/provide:

• Storage at room temperature

Evaluate:

• Prevention of DVT, stroke and systemic embolism

Teach patient/family:

• To report if pregnancy is planned or suspected, not to breastfeed

Black Box Warning: To report bleeding (bruising, blood in urine, stools, sputum, emesis, heavy menstrual flow); use soft toothbrush, electric shaver

• To inform all health care providers of use

Black Box Warning: To avoid abrupt discontinuation without another blood thinner

roflumilast

Daliresp

Func. class.: Respiratory anti-inflammatory agent

Chem. class.: Phosphodiesterase-4 (PDE4) inhibitor

ACTION: Roflumilast (and the active metabolite roflumilast N-oxide) selectively inhibit phosphodiesterase-4 (PDE4); not a bronchodilator; inhibition of the PDE4 enzyme blocks the hydrolyses and inactivation of cyclic adenosine monophosphate (cAMP), resulting in intracellular cAMP accumulation; decreases inflammatory activity, PDE4 inhibition may affect migration and actions of pro-inflammatory cells (neutrophils, other leukocytes, T-lymphocytes, monocytes, macrophages, fibroblasts)

USES: For the prevention of COPD exacerbations in patients with severe chronic obstructive pulmonary disease (COPD) associated with chronic bronchitis and a history of exacerbations

CONTRAINDICATIONS: *Moderate to severe hepatic disease* (Child-Pugh B or C)

Precautions: Pregnancy (category C), breastfeeding, neonates, infants, children, adolescents, acute bronchospasm, anxiety, insomnia, depression, suicidal ideation or behavior

DOSAGE AND ROUTES

- **Adult: PO** 500 mcg/day

Available forms: Tabs 500 mcg

Administer:

PO route

- Give without regard to meals

SIDE EFFECTS

CNS: Insomnia, anxiety, depression, headache, dizziness, tremor, suicidal ideation

EENT: Rhinitis, sinusitis

GI: *Weight loss, diarrhea, nausea*, anorexia, abdominal pain, dyspepsia, gastritis, vomiting

GU: Urinary tract infection

MS: Back pain, muscle cramps/spasm

SYST: Infections, influenza

PHARMACOKINETICS

80% absolute bioavailability; protein binding 99% (roflumilast); 97% (N-oxide metabolite); low penetration across the blood–brain barrier; extensively metabolized (liver); metabolism by CYP3A4 and CYP1A2 produces (active metabolite N-oxide); half-life parent drug 17 hr, metabolite 30; steady state 4 days (parent drug), 6 days (metabolite); 70% excreted in urine; parent drug peak 1 hr (range, 0.5 to 2 hr), metabolite peak 8 hr (range, 4 to 13 hr); contraindicated in moderate to severe hepatic impairment; use with caution in patients with mild hepatic

INTERACTIONS

Increase: roflumilast effect—CYP3A4/CYP1A2 inhibitors (enoxacin, cimetidine, delavirdine, indinavir, isoniazid, itraconazole, dalfopristin, quinupristin, tipranavir)

Increase: roflumilast effect—oral contraceptives (gestodene and ethinyl estradiol)

Decrease: roflumilast effect—CYP3A4 inducers (rifampin, barbiturates, carBAMazepine, phenytoin, erythromycin, ketoconazole, fluvoxamine, alcohol, etravirine, ritonavir, bexarotene, rifabutin, OXcarbazepine, nevirapine, modafinil, metyrapone, PHENobarbital, bosentan, dexamethasone)

Altered effect of: fosamprenavir

Drug/Herb

Decrease: roflumilast effect—St. John's wort

NURSING CONSIDERATIONS

Assess:

- Lung sounds and respiratory function baseline and periodically thereafter

⚠ Behavioral changes including mood, depression, suicidal thoughts/behaviors

• Liver function tests baseline and periodically thereafter; if increases in liver function studies occur, product should be discontinued

• Weight; weight loss is common

Perform/provide:

• Storage at room temperature

Evaluate:

• Decreasing exacerbations in COPD

Teach patient/family:

• To take product as directed, not to skip or double doses, to take missed doses as soon as remembered unless almost time for next dose

• Not to use OTC or other products without prescriber approval; not to discontinue other respiratory products unless approved by prescriber

• Not to be used for acute bronchospasm, but may be continued during acute asthma attacks

⚠ **Suicidal thoughts/behaviors:** To notify prescriber of worsening depression or suicidal thoughts/behaviors

telaprevir

Incivek

Func. class.: Antivirals, anti-hepatitis agent

Chem. class.: NS3/4A protease inhibitor

ACTION: Prevents hepatitis C viral (HCV) replication by blocking the proteolytic activity of HCV NS3/4A serine protease; hepatitis C virus NS3/4A serine protease is an enzyme responsible for the conversion of HCV encoded polyproteins to mature/functioning viral proteins. These proteins (NS4A, NS4B, NS5A, NS5B), are needed for viral replication.

USES: Chronic hepatitis C

CONTRAINDICATIONS: Pregnancy (X) in combination, male partners of women who are pregnant

Precautions: Breastfeeding, neonates, infants, children, adolescents <18 years of age, anemia, neutropenia, thrombocytopenia, HIV, hepatitis B, decompensated hepatic disease, liver or other organ transplants, serious rashes

DOSAGE AND ROUTES

Chronic hepatitis C infection (genotype 1) in adults with compensated liver disease without cirrhosis who are previously untreated or have relapsed after treatment with interferon and ribavirin therapy

• **Adults:** PO 750 mg tid (q7-9 hr) with peginterferon alfa and ribavirin; duration is determined by patient's HCV RNA level at treatment wk 4, 12; if the HCV RNA is undetectable at wk 4, 12, give three-drug regimen for 12 wk then give an additional 12 wk of only peginterferon alfa and ribavirin (24 wk total); if the HCV RNA is detectable but #1000 international units/ml at wk 4 or 12, give three-drug regimen × 12 wk then an additional 36 wk of only peginterferon alfa and ribavirin (48 wk total)

Patients without cirrhosis who are previously partial or null responders to interferon and ribavirin therapy/or those with cirrhosis:

• Adults: PO 750 mg tid (q7-9 hr) with peginterferon alfa and ribavirin; give three-drug regimen × 12 wk then another 36 wk (48 wk total) of only peginterferon alfa and ribavirin

Available forms: Tab 375 mg

Administer:

• Only use in combination with peginterferon alfa and ribavirin; never give as monotherapy

⚠ Discontinue in all patients with hepatitis C virus RNA concentrations ≥1000 IU/ml at wk 4 or 12 or a confirmed detectable HCV RNA concentration at wk 24

⚠ Any contraindication to peginterferon alfa or ribavirin also applies to this product; see ribavirin or peginterferon alfa monographs for additional information regarding contraindications and warning associated with these products

- For relief of mild to moderate rashes, give oral antihistamines and/or topical corticosteroids; treatment with systemic steroids is not recommended
- Give with food, not low-fat

SIDE EFFECTS

CNS: Fatigue

GI: Hemorrhoids, anorectal discomfort, pruritus ani, rectal burning, nausea, diarrhea, vomiting, dysgeusia, hyperbilirubinemia

HEMA: **Anemia, decreased Hgb, lymphopenia, leukopenia, neutropenia, thrombocytopenia**

INTEG: **Drug reaction with eosinophilia, and systemic symptoms (DRESS), Stevens-Johnson Syndrome (SJS),** rash, pruritus, severe rashes (bullous rash, vesicular rash, and skin ulcerations)

META: Increased uric acid

PHARMACOKINETICS

59%-76% plasma protein binding, primarily to α 1-acid glycoprotein and albumin; metabolized extensively in liver by hydrolysis, oxidation, reduction by CYP3A4; excreted in feces (82%), exhaled (9%), excreted in urine (1%); elimination half life 4-4.7 hr; steady state half life 9-11 hr, peak 4-5 hr; food increases effect; steady state is reduced by 15% in mild hepatic disease, 46% in moderate hepatic disease (Child-Pugh class B)

INTERACTIONS

⚠ **Increase: life-threatening reactions of each product—alfuzosin, ergots (dihydroergotamine, ergotamine, ergonovine, methylergonovine), cisapride, pimozide, lovastatin, simvastatin, ezetimibe, niacin with simvastatin and boceprevir; triazolam, oral midazolam; sildenafil, tadalafil (pulmonary arterial hypertension); do not use concurrently**

Increase: effect and adverse reactions of each product—phosphodiesterase type 5 (PDE5) inhibitors (for erectile dysfunction), atorvastin, lidocaine, atorvastatin, amiodarone, bepridil, flecainide, propafenone, quinidine, digoxin, ketoconazole, itraconazole, posaconazole, voriconazole, desipramine, traZODone, erythromycin, clarithromycin, telithromycin, rifabutin, dexamethasone, felodipine, niCARdipine, NIFEdipine, budesonide, bosentan, warfarin, astemizole, boceprevir, bupivacaine, busPIRone, cevimeline, chloroquine, cilostazol, cinacalcet, clomipramine, clonazePAM, clopidogrel, clozapine, cyclobenzaprine, dapsone, dextromethorphan, diazepam, diclofenac, disopyramide, disulfiram, dolasetron, donepezil, colchicine, cycloSPORINE, tacrolimus, sirolimus, buprenorphine, salmeterol, vardenafil, alprazolam, citalopram, amLODIPine, diltiazem, nisoldipine, verapamil, systemic corticosteroids, acetaminophen, alfentanil, aliskiren, almotriptan, alosetron, aripiprazole, dutasteride, ebastine, eplerenone, erlotinib, omeprazole, estazolam, eszopiclone, ethosuximide, exemestane, finasteride, flunitrazepam, flurazepam, galantamine, gefitinib, granisetron, halofantrine, haloperidol, HYDROcodone, ifosfamide, imipramine, indiplon, isradipine, ivermectin, ixabepilone, losartan, meloxicam, mirtazapine, montelukast, nateglinide, oxybutynin, oxyCODONE, palonosetron, paricalcitol, prasugrel, praziquantel, quazepam, QUEtiapine, quinacrine, ramelteon, repaglinide, ropivacaine, selegiline, sibutramine, sitaxsentan, solifenacin, SUFentanil, sunitinib, theophylline, aminophylline, tiagabine, tinidazole, tolterodine, traMADol, venlafaxine, amitriptyline, carvedilol, daunorubicin, loratadine, desloratadine, lansoprazole, dexlansoprazole, docetaxel, DOXOrubicin, droperidol, eletriptan, etoposide, fentaNYL, fexofenadine, glyburide, irinotecan, loperamide, maraviroc, mefloquine, mitomycin, morphine, nortriptyline, ondansetron, paclitaxel, plicamycin, risperidone, sertraline, silodosin, teniposide, terfenadine, testosterone, tolvaptan, vinBLAStine, vinCRIStine and others; use cautiously, may need to reduce dose

Increase: hyperkalemia—drospirenone

Decrease: estrogen levels—ethinyl estradiol

Decrease: telaprevir effect—CYP3A4 inhibitors (phenytoin, carBAMazepine, PHENobarbital, rifampin)

Decrease: effect of—methadone

Possible treatment failure: efavirenz, ritonavir, atazanavir, lopinavir with ritonavir

Drug/Herb

⚠ Do not use with St. John's wort

NURSING CONSIDERATIONS

Assess:

⚠ **Pregnancy:** pregnancy (X) combination therapy; obtain a pregnancy test before, monthly during, and for 6 months after treatment is completed; those who are not willing to practice strict contraception should not receive treatment with these products; report any cases of prenatal ribavirin exposure to the Ribavirin Pregnancy registry at (800) 593-2214

⚠ **Anemia:** monitor hemoglobin before, at treatment wk 4, 8, 12, and as needed; if Hgb is <10 g/dL, decrease ribavirin dosage; if Hgb is <8.5 g/dL, discontinuation of therapy is recommended; telaprevir dosage should not be altered based on adverse reactions; anemia may be managed through ribavirin dose modifications; never alter the dose of telaprevir; if anemia persists despite a reduction in ribavirin dose, consider discontinuing telaprevir; if management of anemia requires permanent discontinuation of ribavirin, treatment with telaprevir must also be permanently discontinued; once telaprevir has been discontinued, it must not be restarted; monitor CBC with differential at treatment wk 4, 8, 12, and at other treatment points

⚠ **Stevens-Johnson syndrome:** eosinophilia, fever, mucosal skin erosion, mucosal ulceration, target lesions; if serious skin reaction occurs, immediately discontinue all components of the three-drug regimen and refer the patient for urgent medical care

- Thyroid function tests, LFTs, serum bilirubin/creatinine, BUN, bilirubin, serum electrolytes, serum uric acid, baseline and periodically during treatment

Perform/provide:

- Storage of tablet at room temperature

Evaluate:

- Decreasing hepatitis C viral infection

Teach patient/family:

⚠ To use 2 forms of effective contraception (intrauterine devices and barrier methods) during treatment and for 6 months after treatment (pregnancy category X), not to breastfeed

⚠ That if a serious skin reaction occurs, to seek urgent medical care; all components of the triple-drug regimen must be discontinued immediately

tesamorelin

Egrifta

Func. class.: Pituitary hormone, growth hormone modifiers

ACTION: Binds to growth hormone releasing factor receptors on the pituitary somatotroph cells; binding stimulates the production, release of endogenous growth hormone (GH)

USES: Treatment of excess abdominal fat in HIV-infected patients with lipodystrophy

CONTRAINDICATIONS: Hypersensitivity to this product or mannitol, neoplastic disease, pregnancy X, *disruption of the hypothalamic-pituitary axis* (hypothalamic-pituitary-adrenal (HPA) suppression) due to hypophysectomy, hypopituitarism, pituitary tumor/surgery, radiation therapy of the head or head trauma, IV/IM administration

Precautions: Breastfeeding, CABG, diabetes, diabetic retinopathy, edema, geriatrics, children, infants, adolescents

DOSAGE AND ROUTES

- **Adult:** SUBCUT 2 mg/day

Available forms: Powder for injection 1 mg

Administer:

Subcut route:

- Visually inspect parenteral products for particulate matter and discoloration before use whenever sol and container permit
- To reconstitute, inject 2.1 ml sterile water for inj into the 2-mg vial; use syringe with needle already attached; to avoid foaming, push plunger in slowly with needle on a slight angle so sterile water goes down the inside wall of vial; with needle and syringe attached to vial, keep vial upright and gently roll vial for 30 sec until mixed; do not shake; withdraw 2.1 ml of the reconstituted sol
- To administer, take syringe out of vial, place needle cap on its side against a clean flat surface, do not touch needle, hold syringe and slide needle into cap, push cap all the way or until it snaps shut; do not touch cap until it covers needle completely; remove needle, insert a 0.5 inch 27-G safety injection needle onto syringe; use immediately; throw away any unused product or used sterile water for inj, sol should be clear, do not use if discolored, cloudy, or has particles; slight foaming is acceptable; inject subcut into abdomen; avoid scar tissues, bruises, or navel; rotate inj sites in abdomen; slowly push plunger down until all sol has been injected
- After removing needle from skin, flip back needle shield until it snaps, covering the injection needle completely; keep pressing until you hear a click, that means the injection needle is protected
- Use a piece of sterile gauze to rub the inj site clean; if bleeding, apply pressure to site with gauze for 30 sec; if bleeding continues, apply a bandage to site
- Properly dispose of used syringe, needles, vial, and sterile water for injection bottle in a sharps container

SIDE EFFECTS

CNS: Depression, peripheral neuropathy paresthesias, hypoesthesia, spasms, flushing, night sweats, insomnia, headache

CV: Chest pain, palpitations, hypertension, edema, peripheral edema

GI: Nausea, vomiting, upper abdominal pain, dyspepsia diarrhea

INTEG: Pruritus, urticaria, rash, flushing, injection site reactions

MS: Arthralgia, joint swelling, stiffness, myalgias, carpal tunnel syndrome

RESP: Upper respiratory tract infection

SYST: Secondary malignancy

PHARMACOKINETICS

Half-life 26 min in healthy patients, 38 min and those with HIV infection; peak 0.15 hr

INTERACTIONS

Decrease: effect of—simvastatin, ritonavir, cortisone, prednisone

NURSING CONSIDERATIONS

Assess:

- **Lipodystrophy:** Assess for sunken cheeks, thinning arms and legs, fat accumulation in the abdomen, jaws and back of neck; after treatment these should lessen
- Monitor glycosylated hemoglobin A1c (HbA1c), serum IGF-1 concentrations, ophthalmologic exam

Evaluate:

- Decreasing lipodystrophy in HIV patients

ticagrelor

Brilinta

Func. class.: Platelet inhibitor

Chem. class.: ADP receptor antagonist

ACTION: Reversibly bind to the platelet receptor, preventing platelet activation

USES: Arterial thromboembolism prophylaxis in acute coronary syndrome (ACS) (unstable angina, acute MI), including in patients undergoing percutaneous coronary intervention (PCI)

CONTRAINDICATIONS: Hypersensitivity, severe hepatic disease

Black Box Warning: Bleeding, intracranial bleeding

Precautions: Pregnancy (category C), breastfeeding, infants, neonates, children, GI bleeding, hepatic disease, abrupt discontinuation

Black Box Warning: Coronary artery bypass graft surgery (CABG), surgery

DOSAGE AND ROUTES

- **Adult: PO** loading dose 180 mg with aspirin (usually 325 mg PO); then, give 90 mg bid with aspirin 75-100 mg/day, do not give maintenance doses of aspirin >100 mg/day

Available forms: Tab 90 mg

Administer:

- May be taken without regard to food
- Discontinue 5-7 days before surgery

SIDE EFFECTS

CNS: Headache, dizziness, fatigue

CV: Hypertension, hypotension, chest pain, atrial fibrillation, bradyarrhythmias, syncope, ventricular pauses

GI: Nausea, diarrhea

HEMA: Serious, fatal bleeding

MISC: Back pain, hyperuricemia, gynecomastia

RESP: Dyspnea, cough

PHARMACOKINETICS

Absolute bioavailability 36%, protein binding (>99%), metabolism by CYP3A4, weak P-glycoprotein substrates and inhibitors, elimination for product and metabolite are hepatic and biliary, 84% excreted in feces, 26% in urine, half-life is 7 hr for ticagrelor, 9 hr for metabolite, maximum inhibition of platelet aggregation (IPA) effect 2 hr, maintained ≥8 hrs, peak 1.5 hr product, 2.5 hr metabolite

INTERACTIONS

Increase: bleeding risk—CYP3A4 inhibitors (ketoconazole, itraconazole, voriconazole, clarithromycin, telithromycin, nefazodone, ritonavir, lopinavir, ritonavir, saquinavir, nelfinavir, indinavir, atazanavir, delavirdine, isoniazid, dalfopristin, quinupristin, tipranavir

Decrease: ticagrelor action—CYP3A4 inducers (rifampin, dexamethasone, phenytoin, carBAMazepine, PHENobarbital

Increase: effect of—simvastatin lovastatin

Increase: bleeding risk—NSAIDs, anticoagulants, platelet inhibitors

Increase or decrease: digoxin

Drug/Lab Test

Increase: serum creatinine

NURSING CONSIDERATIONS

Assess:

- **Thromboembolism:** Monitor CBC with differential with platelet count baseline and periodically during treatment

Black Box Warning: Bleeding: Assess for bleeding that may occur when aspirin is combined with this product, some bleeding can be fatal

- **Abrupt discontinuation:** Do not discontinue abruptly, may increase risk for MI, stent thrombosis, death

Perform/provide:

- Storage at room temperature, in original container in dry place

Evaluate:

- Prevention of thromboembolism

Teach patient/family:

- To take only as prescribed, not to skip or double doses; if a dose is missed, to take next dose at scheduled time

Black Box Warning: To notify prescriber of chills, fever, bruising, bleeding

- Not to use any prescription, OTC products, herbs without approval of prescriber; products with aspirin, NSAIDs may cause bleeding

- To notify all health care providers of product use
- That product can be taken without regard to meals
- That it may take longer for bleeding to stop

vemurafenib

Zelboraf

Func. class.: Biologic response modifiers; signal transduction inhibitors (STIs)

ACTION: Inhibitor of some mutated forms of BRAF serine threonine kinase, thereby blocking cellular proliferation in melanoma cells with the mutation; inhibits other kinases including CRAF, ARAF, wild-type BRAF, SRMA, ACK1, MAP4H5, and FGR; potent adenosine triphosphate-competitice inhibitor of RAFs, with a modest preference for mutant BRAF and CRAF as compared with wild-type BRAF

USES: Unresectable or metastatic malignant melanoma with V600E mutation of the BRAF gene

Precautions: Pregnancy (D), breastfeeding, children, infants, neonates, hepatic disease, QT prolongation, secondary malignancy, torsades de pointes, hypokalemia, hypomagnesia, sunlight exposure

DOSAGE AND ROUTES

- **Adult: PO** 960 mg (4 tablets) bid about q12hr

Dose adjustments for toxicity due to symptomatic adverse reactions or QTc prolongation

Grade 1 or tolerable grade 2 adverse events: no dosage change; **intolerable grade 2 or grade 3 adverse events (1st episode):** interrupt treatment until toxicity resolves to grade ≤1, when resuming, reduce dosage to 720 mg (3 tabs) bid; **intolerable grade 2 or grade 3 adverse events (2nd episode):** interrupt treatment until toxicity resolves to grade ≤1, when resuming, reduce dose to 480 mg (2 tabs) bid; **intolerable grade 2 or grade 3 adverse events (3rd episode)** discontinue treatment permanently; **grade 4 adverse events (1st episode):** discontinue permanently or interrupt until toxicity resolves to grade ≤1, when resuming, reduce dose to 480 mg (2 tabs) bid; **grade 4 adverse events (2nd episode):** discontinue permanently

Available forms: Tabs 240 mg

Administer:

- Continue until disease progresses or unacceptable toxicity occurs
- Missed doses can be taken up to 4 hours before the next dose is due, take about 12 hrs apart, take without regard to meals
- Swallow whole with a full glass of water, do not crush or chew

SIDE EFFECTS

CNS: Fatigue, fever, asthenia, headache, dizziness, peripheral neuropathy, muscle paralysis

CV: QT prolongation, atrial fibrillation, peripheral edema, hypotension

EENT: Uveitis, blurred vision, iritis, photophobia

GI: Nausea, diarrhea, vomiting, constipation, dysgeusia, decreased appetite, weight loss

INTEG: Alopecia, pruritus, hyperkeratosis, maculopapular rash, actinic keratosis, xerosis/dry skin, papular rash, palmar-plantar erythrodysesthesia (hand and foot syndrome), photosensitivity

MS: Arthralgia, myalgias, extremity pain, musculoskeletal pain, back pain, arthritis

RESP: Cough

SYST: Secondary malignancy, anaphylaxis

PHARMACOKINETICS

>99% protein binding (albumin and alpha-1 acid glycoprotein) an inhibitor of CYP1A2, 2A6, 2C9, 2C19, 2D6, 3A4/5 CYP1A2 inhibitor, a weak CYP2D6 inhibi-

tor, and a CYP3A4 inducer; elimination 94% in feces, 1% in urine, half-life 57 hr

INTERACTIONS

Increase: vemurafenib effect—CYP3A4/CYP1A2 inhibitors (enoxacin, cimetidine, delavirdine, indinavir, isoniazid, itraconazole, dalfopristin, quinupristin, tipranavir)

⚠ **Increase:** QT prolongation, torsades de pointes—arsenic trioxide, certain phenothiazines (chlorpromazine, mesoridazine, thioridazine), grepafloxacin, levomethadyl, pentamidine, probucol, sparfloxacin, troleandomycin, class IA antiarrhythmics (disopyramide, procainamide, quiNIDine), class III antiarrhythmics (amiodarone, dofetilide, ibutilide, sotalol), clarithromycin, ziprasidone, pimozide, haloperidol, halofantrine, quiNIDine, chloroquine, dronedarone, droperidol, erythromycin, methadone, posaconazole, propafenone, saquinavir, abarelix, amoxapine, apomorphine, asenapine, β-agonists, ofloxacin, eribulin, ezogabine, flecainide, gatifloxacin, gemifloxacin, halogenated anesthetics, iloperidone, levofloxacin, local anesthetics, magnesium sulfate, potassium sulfate, sodium, maprotiline, moxifloxacin, nilotinib, norfloxacin, ciprofloxacin, OLANZapine, paliperidone, some phenothiazines (fluphenazine, perphenazine, prochlorperazine, trifluoperazine), telavancin, tetrabenazine, tricyclic antidepressants, venlafaxine, vorinostat, citalopram, alfuzosin, clozapine, cyclobenzaprine, dolasetron, palonosetron, QUEtiapine, rilpivirine, sunitinib, tacrolimus, tacrolimus, vardenafil, indacaterol, dasatinib, fluconazole, lapatinib, lopinavir/ritonavir, mefloquine, octreotide, ondansetron, ranolazine, risperidone, telithromycin, vemurafenib

Decrease: vemurafenib effect—CYP3A4 inducers (rifampin, barbiturates, carBAMazepine, phenytoin, erythromycin, ketoconazole, fluvoxamine, alcohol, etravirine, ritonavir, bexarotene, rifabutin, OXcarbazepine, nevirapine, modafinil, metyrapone)

Drug/Lab Test:

Increase: serum creatinine, LFTs, alkaline phosphatase, bilirubin

NURSING CONSIDERATIONS

Assess:

- **Hepatic Disease:** Liver function test (LFT) abnormalities, altered bilirubin levels, may occur during treatment; monitor LFTs and bilirubin levels prior to treatment, then monthly; more frequent testing is needed in those presenting with grade 2 or greater toxicities; laboratory alterations should be managed with dose reduction, treatment interruption, or discontinuation

⚠ **QT prolongation**: has been reported with the use of crizotinib; therefore, crizotinib should be avoided in patients with. Monitor ECG and electrolytes in those with congestive heart failure, bradycardia, electrolyte imbalance (hypokalemia, hypomagnesemia), or in those who are taking concomitant medications known to prolong the QT interval; treatment interruption, dosage adjustment, treatment discontinuation may be needed in those who develop QT prolongation

⚠ **Pregnancy/breastfeeding:** Identify if pregnancy is planned or suspected, pregnancy category D, avoid breastfeeding

- Serum electrolytes

Perform/provide:

- Storage at room temperature, in original container

Evaluate:

- Decreased spread of malignancy

Teach patient/family:

- Teach patient missed doses can be taken up to 4 hrs before the next dose is due to maintain the twice daily regimen

⚠ Teach patient to use reliable contraception, both women and men of childbearing age should use adequate contraceptive methods during therapy and for at least 90 days after completing treatment, pregnancy category D

Appendix B

Ophthalmic, otic, nasal, and topical products

OPHTHALMIC PRODUCTS

α-ADRENERGIC BLOCKER

dapiprazole (Rx)
(da-pip′ra-zole)
Rev-Eyes

ANESTHETICS

lidocaine (Rx)
Akten

proparacaine (Rx)
(proe-par′a-kane)
Alcaine, Diocaine ✦, Ophthaine, Ophthetic

tetracaine (Rx)
(tet′ra-kane)
Minims Tetracaine ✦, Pontocaine, Tetracaine

ANTIHISTAMINES

alcaftadine (Rx)
Lastacaft

azelastine (Rx)
(ay-zell′ah-steen)
Optivar

emedastine (Rx)
(ee-med′ah-steen)
Emadine

epinastine (Rx)
(ep-een′as-teen)
Elestat

ketotifen (Rx, OTC)
(kee-toh-tif′en)
Zaditor

levocabastine (Rx)
(lee-voh-cab′ah-steen)
Livostin

olopatadine (Rx)
(oh-loh-pat′ah-deen)
Patanol

ANTIINFECTIVES

azithromycin (Rx)
(ay-zi-thro-my′sin)
AzaSite

besifloxacin (Rx)
(be′si-flox′a-sin)
Besivance

chloramphenicol (Rx)
(klor-am-fen′i-kole)
AK-Chlor, Chloramphenicol, Chloromycetin Ophthalmic, Chloroptic, Chloroptic S.O.P., Fenicol ✦, Isopto Fenicol ✦, Pentamycin ✦

ciprofloxacin (Rx)
(sip-ro-floks′a-sin)
Ciloxan

erythromycin (Rx)
(er-ith-roe-mye′sin)
Erythromycin, Ilotycin

ganciclovir (Rx)
(gan-sye′kloe-vir)
Virgan

gatifloxacin (Rx)
(gat-i-flox′a-sin)
Zymar, Zymaxid

gentamicin (Rx)
(jen-ta-mye′sin)
Garamycin Ophthalmic, Genoptic Ophthalmic, Genoptic S.O.P., Gentacidin, Gentamicin Ophthalmic, Gentak

levofloxacin (Rx)
(lee-voh-floks′a-sin)
Quixin

moxifloxacin (Rx)
(mox-i-flox′a-sin)
Vigamox

natamycin (Rx)
(nat-a-mye′sin)
Natacyn

norfloxacin (Rx)
(nor-floks′a-sin)
Chibroxin

ofloxacin (Rx)
(oh-flox′a-sin)
Ocuflox

silver nitrate 1% (Rx)

silver nitrate

sulfacetamide sodium (Rx)
(sul-fa-seet′a-mide)
AK-Sulf, Bleph-10, Bleph-10 S.O.P., Cetamide, Isopto Cetamide, Ocusulf-10, Sodium Sulamyd, Sodium Sulfacetamide, Storzsulf, Sulf-10, Sulster

tobramycin (Rx)
(toe-bra-mye′sin)
AKTob, Defy, Tobrex

trifluridine (Rx)
(trye-floor′i-deen)
Viroptic

vidarabine (Rx)
(vye-dare′a-been)
Vira-A

β-ADRENERGIC BLOCKERS

betaxolol (Rx)
(beh-tax′oh-lole)
Betoptic, Betoptic S

carteolol (Rx)
(kar-tee′oh-lole)
Carteolol HCl, Ocupress

levobetaxolol (Rx)
(lee-voh-beh-tax′oh-lole)
Betaxon

levobunolol (Rx)
(lee-voe-byoo′no-lole)
AKBeta, Betagen

metipranolol (Rx)
(met-ee-pran′oh-lole)
OptiPranolol

timolol (Rx)
(tye′moe-lole)
Apo-Timop 🍁, Betimol, Timoptic, Timoptic-XE

CARBONIC ANHYDRASE INHIBITORS

brinzolamide (Rx)
(brin-zoh′la-mide)
Azopt

dorzolamide (Rx)
(dor-zol′a-mide)
Trusopt

CHOLINERGICS (Direct-acting)

acetylcholine Rx)
(ah-see-til-koe′leen)
Miochol-E

carbachol (Rx)
(kar′ba-kole)
Carbastat, Carboptic, Isopto Carbachol, Miostat

pilocarpine (Rx)
(pye-loe-kar′peen)
Adsorbocarpine, Akarpine, Isopto Carpine, Ocu-Carpine, Ocusert Pilo-20, Ocusert Pilo-40, Pilagan, Pilocar, pilocarpine, Pilopine HS, Piloptic-1/2, Piloptic-1, Piloptic-2, Piloptic-3, Piloptic-4, Piloptic-6, Pilostat, Pilopto-Carpine

CHOLINESTERASE INHIBITORS

demecarium (Rx)
(dem-e-kare′ee-um)
Humorsol

echothiophate (Rx)
(ek-oh-thye′eh-fate)
Phospholine Iodide

isoflurophate (Rx)
(i-se-flur′e-fate)
Floropryl

physostigmine (Rx)
(fi-zoe-stig′meen)
Eserine Salicylate, Isopto Eserine

CORTICOSTEROIDS

dexamethasone (Rx)
(dex-a-meth′a-sone)
AK-Dex, Decadron Phosphate, Dexamethasone Ophthalmic Suspension, Maxidex, Ozurdex

difluprednate (Rx)
(dye′floo-pred′nate)
Durezol

fluocinolone (Rx)
(floo-oh-sin′oh-lone)
Retisert

fluorometholone (Rx)
(flure-oh-meth′oh-lone)
Flarex, Fluor-Op, FML, FML Forte, FML S.O.P.

loteprednol (Rx)
(loe-tee-pred′nole)
Alrex, Lotemax

medrysone (Rx)
(me′dri-sone)
HMS

prednisoLONE (Rx)
(pred-niss′oh-lone)
Econopred, Econopred Plus, AK-Pred, Inflamase Forte, Inflamase Mild, Pred-Forte

rimexolone (Rx)
(ri-mex′a-lone)
Vexol

triamcinolone (Rx)
(trye-am-sin′oh-lone)
Triesence

MYDRIATICS

atropine (Rx)
(a′troe-peen)
Atropine-1, Atropine Care, Atropine Sulfate Ophthalmic, Atropisol, Isopto Atropine

cyclopentolate (Rx)
(sye-kloe-pen′toe-late)
AK-Pentolate, Cyclogyl, Cyclopentolate HCl

homatropine (Rx)
(home-a′troe-peen)
Homatrine HBr, Isopto Homatropine, Minims Homatropine ✱

phenylephrine (OTC)
(fen-ill-ef′rin)
AK-Dilate, AK-Nefrin, Isopto Frin, Neo-Synephrine 2.5%, Neo-Synephrine 10%, phenylephrine HCl, 2.5% Mydfrin, Phenoptic Relief, Prefrin

scopolamine (Rx)
(skoe-pol′a-meen)
Isopto Hyoscine

tropicamide (Rx)
(troe-pik′a-mide)
Mydriacyl, Opticyl, Tropicacyl, Tropicamide

NONSTEROIDAL ANTIINFLAMMATORIES

bromfenac (Rx)
(brome′fen-ak)
Xibrom

diclofenac (Rx)
(dye-kloe′fen-ak)
Voltaren

flurbiprofen (Rx)
(flure-bih-proh′fen)
Ocufen

ketorolac (Rx)
(kee-toe′role-ak)
Acular, Acurail

nepafenac (Rx)
(ne-pa-fen′ak)
Nevanac

suprofen (Rx)
(soo-proe′fen)
Profenal

SYMPATHOMIMETICS

apraclonidine (Rx)
(a-pra-klon′i-deen)
Iopidine

brimonidine (Rx)
(brih-moh′nih-deen)
Alphagan, Alphagan P

dipivefrin (Rx)
(dye-pi′vef-rin)
Propine, AKPro

EPINEPHrine/ epinephryl borate (Rx)
(ep-i-nef′rin)
Epifrin, Glaucon/Epinal, Eppy 🍁

OPHTHALMIC DECONGESTANTS/ VASOCONSTRICTORS

lodoxamide
(loe-dox′a-mide)
Alomide

naphazoline (OTC, Rx)
(naf-az′oh-leen)
20/20 Eye Drops, Allergy Drops, AK-Con, Albalon, Allerest Eye Drops, Clear Eyes, Clear Eyes ACR, Comfort Eye Drops, Degest 2, Maximum Strength Allergy Drops, Nafazair, naphazoline HCl, Naphcon, Naphcon Forte, Opcon, Vasoclear, Vasocon Regular

oxymetazoline (Rx)
(ox-i-meth′oh-leen)
OcuClear, Visine L.R.

tetrahydrozoline (OTC)
(tet-ra-hye-dro′zoe-leen)
Collyrium Fresh, Eyesine, Geneye, Geneye Extra, Mallazine Eye Drops, Murine Plus, Optigene 3, tetrahydrozoline HCl, Tetrasine, Tetrasine Extra, Visine Moisturizing

MISCELLANEOUS OPHTHALMICS

bimatoprost (Rx)
(bih-mat′o-prost)
Latisse, Lumigan

latanoprost (Rx)
(la-tan′oh-prost)
Xalatan

travoprost (Rx)
(tra′voe-prost)
Travatan

unoprostone (Rx)
(un-oh-proe′stone)
Rescula

β-Adrenergic blockers

ACTION: Reduces production of aqueous humor by unknown mechanism

USES: Ocular hypertension, chronic open-angle glaucoma

Anesthetics

ACTION: Decreases ion permeability by stabilizing neuronal membrane

USES: Cataract extraction, tonometry, gonioscopy, removal of foreign objects, corneal suture removal, glaucoma surgery (ophthalmic); pruritus, sunburn, toothache, sore throat, cold sores, oral pain, rectal pain and irritation, control of gagging (topical)

Antiinfectives

ACTION: Inhibits folic acid synthesis by preventing PABA use, which is necessary for bacterial growth

Uses: Conjunctivitis, superficial eye infections, corneal ulcers, prophylaxis against infection after removal of foreign matter from the eye

Antiinflammatories

ACTION: Decreases inflammation, resulting in decreased pain, photophobia, hyperemia, cellular infiltration

USES: Inflammation of eye, eyelids, conjunctiva, cornea; uveitis, iridocyclitis, allergic conditions, burns, foreign bodies, postoperatively in cataract

Carbonic anhydrase inhibitor

ACTION: Converted to EPINEPHrine, which decreases aqueous production and increases outflow

Uses: Open-angle glaucoma, ocular hypertension

Direct-acting miotic

ACTION: Acts directly on cholinergic receptor sites; induces miosis, spasm of accommodation, fall in intraocular pressure, caused by stimulation of ciliary, pupillary sphincter muscles, which leads to pulling away of iris from filtration angle, resulting in increased outflow of aqueous humor

Uses: Primary glaucoma, early stages of wide-angle glaucoma (less useful in advanced stages), chronic open-angle glaucoma, acute closed-angle glaucoma before emergency surgery; also neutralizes mydriatics used during eye exam; may be used alternately with mydriatics to break adhesions between iris and lens

CONTRAINDICATIONS: Hypersensitivity

Precautions: Pregnancy, breastfeeding, children, aphakia, hypersensitivity to carbonic anhydrase inhibitors, sulfonamides, thiazide diuretics, ocular inhibitors, hepatic/renal insufficiency

SIDE EFFECTS

CNS: Headache

CV: Hypertension, tachycardia, dysrhythmias

EENT: Burning, stinging

GI: Bitter taste

NURSING CONSIDERATIONS

Assess:

- Ophth exams and intraocular pressure readings
- Blood counts; hepatic, renal function tests and serum electrolytes during long-term treatment

Perform/provide:

- Storage at room temperature away from light

Evaluate:

- Positive therapeutic response
- Absence of increased intraocular pressure

Teach patient/family:

- How to instill drops
- That product may cause burning, itching, blurring, dryness of eye area

NASAL AGENTS

NASAL ANTIHISTAMINES

olopatadine (Rx)
(oh-low-pat′uh-deen)
Patanase

NASAL DECONGESTANTS

azelastine (Rx)
(ay-zell′ah-steen)
Astelin, Astepro

desoxyephedrine (OTC)
(des-oxy-e-fed′rin)
Vicks Vapor Inhaler

ePHEDrine (OTC)
(e-fed′rin)
Pretz-D

EPINEPHrine (OTC)
(ep-i-neff′rin)
Adrenalin

naphazoline (OTC)
(naff-a-zoe′leen)
Privine

oxymetazoline (OTC)
(ox-i-met-az′oh-leen)
12-Hour Nasal, Afrin 12-Hour Original, Afrin 12-Hour Original Pump Mist, Afrin Severe Congestion with Menthol, Afrin Sinus with Vapornase, Afrin No-Drip 12-Hour, Afrin No-Drip 12-Hour Extra Moisturizing, Dristan, Duramist Plus, Duration, Genasal, Nafrine ✤, Nasal Relief, Neo-Synephrine 12-Hour, Nostrilla, oxymetazoline HCl, Nasal Decongestant Maximum Strength, Vicks Sinex 12-Hour Long-Acting, Vicks Sinex 12-Hour Ultra Fine Mist for Sinus Relief

phenylephrine (OTC)
(fen-ill-eff′rin)
Alconefrin 12, Children's Nostril, Neo-Synephrine, Sinex

propylhexadrine (OTC)
(proe-pil-hex′a-dreen)
Benzedrex Inhaler

pseudoephedrine (Rx, OTC)
(soo-doe-e-fed′rin)
Cenafed, Decofed, Dimetapp, Genaphed, Sudafed, Triaminic

tetrahydrozoline (OTC)
(tet-ra-hye-dro′zoe-leen)
Tyzine, Tyzine Pediatric

xylometazoline (OTC)
(zye-loh-meh-tazz′oh-leen)
Natru-vent, Otrivin, Otrivin Pediatric Nasal

NASAL CORTICOSTEROIDS

beclomethasone (Rx)
(be-kloe-meth′a-sone)
Beconase AQ Nasal, Beco-nase Inhalation, Vancenase AQ Nasal, Vancenase Pocket Inhaler

budesonide (Rx)
(byoo-des′oh-nide)
Rhinocort, Rhinocort Aqua

flunisolide (Rx)
(floo-niss′oh-lide)
Nasalide, Nasarel

fluticasone (Rx)
(floo-tic′a-son)
Flonase, Veramyst

triamcinolone (Rx)
(trye-am-sin′oh-lone)
Nasacort AQ

NONSTEROIDAL ANTIINFLAMMATORY

Ketorolac (Rx)

(kee'toe-role'ak)

Sprix

ACTION:
Produces vasoconstriction (rapid, long acting) of arterioles, thereby decreasing fluid exudation, mucosal engorgement by stimulation of α-adrenergic receptors in vascular smooth muscle

USES:
Nasal congestion

CONTRAINDICATIONS:
Hypersensitivity to sympathomimetic amines

Precautions: Pregnancy (C), children <6 yr, geriatric, diabetes, CV disease, hypertension, hyperthyroidism, increased intracranial pressure, prostatic hypertrophy, glaucoma

DOSAGE AND ROUTES

Desoxyephedrine

- **Adult and child >6 yr: 1-2 INH** in each nostril q2hr or less

ePHEDrine

- **Adult:** Fill dropper to the level marked, then use in each nostril q4hr or less

EPINEPHrine

- **Adult and child >6 yr:** Apply with swab, drops, spray prn

Naphazoline

- **Adult and child >6 yr:** 1-2 drops/spray q6hr or less

Oxymetazoline

- **Adult and child >6 yr: INSTILL** 2-3 gtt or sprays to each nostril bid
- **Child 2-6 yr: INSTILL** 2-3 gtt or sprays 0.025 sol bid, max 3 days

Phenylephrine

- **Adult and child >12 yr:** 2-3 drops/spray (0.25-0.5) in each nostril q3-4hr or less; or 2-3 drops/spray (1%) in each nostril q4hr or less
- **Child 6-12 yr:** 2-3 drops/spray (0.25%) in each nostril q3-4hr
- **Infant >6 mo:** 1-2 drops (0.16%) in each nostril q3hr

Propylhexadrine

- **Adult and child >6 yr:** 1-2 **INH** in each nostril q2hr or less

Tetrahydrozoline

- **Adult and child >6 yr:** 2-4 drops (0.1%) q3-4hr prn or 3-4 sprays in each nostril q4hr prn
- **Child 2-6 yr:** 2-3 drops (0.05%) in each nostril q4-6hr prn

Xylometazoline

- **Adult and child >12 yr:** 2-3 drops/spray (0.1%) in each nostril q8-10hr
- **Child 2-12 yr:** 2-3 drops (0.05%) in each nostril q8-10hr

Available forms: Nasal sol 0.025%, 0.05%

Administer:

- Having patient tilt head back, squeeze bulb to create a vacuum, and draw correct amount of sol into dropper; insert 2 gtt of sol into nostril; repeat in other nostril
- Store in light-resistant container; do not expose to high temperature or let sol come into contact with aluminum
- For <4 consecutive days
- Environmental humidification to decrease nasal congestion, dryness

SIDE EFFECTS

CNS: Anxiety, restlessness, tremors, weakness, insomnia, dizziness, fever, headache

EENT: Irritation, burning, sneezing, stinging, dryness, rebound congestion

GI: Nausea, vomiting, anorexia

INTEG: Contact dermatitis

NURSING CONSIDERATIONS

Assess:

- For redness, swelling, pain in nasal passages before and during treatment
- For systemic absorption; hypertension, tachycardia; notify prescriber; systemic absorption occurs at high doses or after prolonged use

Evaluate:

- Therapeutic response: decreased nasal congestion

Teach patient/family:

- That stinging may occur for several applications; drying of mucosa may be decreased by environmental humidification
- To notify prescriber if irregular pulse, insomnia, dizziness, or tremors occur
- Proper administration to avoid systemic absorption
- To rinse dropper with very hot water to prevent contamination

TOPICAL GLUCOCORTICOIDS

betamethasone (Rx)
(bay-ta-meth′a-sone)
Alphatrex, Beben ✦, Betacort ✦, Betatrex, Beta-Val, Betnovate ✦, Celestoderm ✦, Diprosone, Ectosone ✦, Luxiq, Maxivate, Metaderm ✦, Psorion, Valisone

betamethasone (augmented) (Rx)
(bay-ta-meth′a-sone)
Diprolene, Diprolene AF

clobetasol (Rx)
(kloe-bay′ta-sol)
Clobex, Cormax, Dermovate ✦, Embeline E 0.05%, Temovate

desonide (Rx)
(dess′oh-nide)
Verdeso Foam

desoximetasone (Rx)
(dess-ox-i-met′a-sone)
Topicort, Topicort LP

dexamethasone (Rx)
(dex-a-meth′a-sone)
Aeroseb-Dex, Decaspray

fluocinolone (Rx)
(floo-oh-sin′oh-lone)
Derma-Smoothe/FSoil, Fluocin, Licon, Lidemol ✦, Lidex, Lyderm ✦, Topsyn ✦, Vasoderm

flurandrenolide (Rx)
(flure-an-dren′oh-lide)
Cordran, Cordran SP, Drenison 1/4 ✦, Drenison Tape ✦

fluticasone (Rx)
(floo-tik′a-sone)
Cutivate

halcinonide (Rx)
(hal-sin′oh-nide)
Halog, Halog-E

hydrocortisone (Rx)
(hye-droe-kor′ti-sone)
Acticort, Aeroseb-HC, Ala-Cort, Allercort, Alphaderm, Anusol HC, Bactine, Barriere-HC ✦, Calde-CORT Anti-Itch, Carmol HC, Cetacort, Cortacet ✦, Cortaid, Cortalo, Cortate ✦, Cort-Dome, Cortef ✦, Corticaine, Corticreme ✦, Cortifair, Corti-zone, Cortoderm ✦, Cortril, Delcort, Dermacort, DemiCort, Dermtex HC, Emo-Cort, Epifoam, FoilleCort, Gly-Cort, Gynecort, Hi-Cor, Hycort, Hyderm ✦, Hydro-Tex, Hytone, Lacti-Care-HC, Lanacort, Lemoderm, Locoid, Locoid Lotion, My Cort, Novohydrocort ✦, Nutracort Pharm, Pharmacort, Pentacort, Rederm, Rhulicort S-T Cort, Synacort, Sarna HC ✦, Texa-Cort, Unicort ✦, Westcort

triamcinolone (Rx)
(trye-am-sin′oh-lone)
Aristocort, Delta-Tritex, Flutex, Kenac, Kenalog, Kenonel, Triaderm, Trianide ✦, Triderm, Trymex

ACTION: Antipruritic, antiinflammatory

USES: Psoriasis, eczema, contact dermatitis, pruritus; usually reserved for severe dermatoses that have not responded to less potent formulation

CONTRAINDICATIONS: Hypersensitivity, viral infections, fungal infections

Precautions: Pregnancy (C)

DOSAGE AND ROUTES

- **Adult and child:** Apply to affected area

Administer:

- Only to affected areas; do not get in eyes
- Leaving site uncovered or lightly covered; occlusive dressing is not recommended—systemic absorption may occur
- Use only on dermatoses; do not use on weeping, denuded, or infected area
- Cleansing before application of product
- Continuing treatment for a few days after area has cleared
- Store at room temperature

SIDE EFFECTS

INTEG: *Acne, atrophy, epidermal thinning, purpura, striae*

NURSING CONSIDERATIONS

Assess:

- Temp; if fever develops, product should be discontinued
- For systemic absorption, increased temp, inflammation, irritation

Evaluate:

- Therapeutic response: absence of severe itching, patches on skin, flaking

Teach patient/family:

- To avoid sunlight on affected area, burns may occur
- To limit treatment to 14 days

TOPICAL ANTIFUNGALS

clotrimazole (OTC)
(kloe-trye′ma-zole)
Canestew ✤, Clotrimaderm ✤, Clotrimazole, Cruex, Desenex, Lotrimin AF, Myclo ✤, Neozol ✤

econazole (OTC)
(ee-kon′a-zole)
Spectazole

ketoconazole (OTC)
(kee-toe-kon′a-zole)
Nizoral, Xolegel

miconazole (OTC)
(mye-kon′a-zole)
Absorbine Antifungal Foot Powder, Breeze Mist Antifungal, Fungoid Tincture, Lotrimin AF, Maximum Strength Desenex Antifungal, Micatin, Monistat-Derm, Ony-clear, Tetterine, Zeasorb-AF

nystatin (OTC)
(nye-stat′in)
Mycostatin, Nadostine ✤, Nilstat, Nyaderm ✤, Nystex

selenium (OTC)
(see-leen′ee-um)
Exsel, Head and Shoulders Intensive Treatment, Selenium Sulfide, Selsun, Selsun Blue

terbinafine (OTC)
(ter-bin′a-feen)
Lamisil

tolnaftate (OTC)
(tole-naf′tate)
Absorbine Athlete's Foot Cream, Aftate for Athlete's Foot, Aftate for Jock Itch, Genaspor, Quinsana Plus, Tinactin, Ting, tolnaftate

undecylenic acid (OTC)
(un-deh-sih-len'ik)
Blis-To-Sol, Breeze Mist, Caldesene, Cruex, Decylenes, Desenex, Desenex Maximum Strength, Pedi-Pro, Phicon F, Protectol

ACTION:
Interferes with fungal cell membrane permeability

USES:
Tinea cruris, tinea pedis, diaper rash, minor skin irritations; amphotericin B is used for candida infections

CONTRAINDICATIONS:
Hypersensitivity

Precautions: Pregnancy (B), breastfeeding, children

DOSAGE AND ROUTES

- Massage into affected area, surrounding area daily or bid, continue for 7-14 days, not to exceed 4 wk

Administer:

Topical route

- To affected area, surrounding area; do not cover with occlusive dressings
- Store below 30° C (86° F)

SIDE EFFECTS

INTEG: Burning, stinging, dryness, itching, local irritation

NURSING CONSIDERATIONS

Assess:

- Skin for fungal infections; peeling, dryness, itching before and throughout treatment
- For continuing infection; increased size, number of lesions

Evaluate:

- Therapeutic response: decrease in size, number of lesions

Teach patient/family:

- To apply with glove to prevent further infection; not to cover with occlusive dressings
- That long-term therapy may be needed to clear infection (2 wk-6 mo depending on organism); compliance is needed even after feeling better
- Proper hygiene; hand-washing technique, nail care, use of concomitant top agents if prescribed
- To avoid use of OTC creams, ointments, lotions unless directed by prescriber
- To use medical asepsis (hand washing) before, after each application; to change socks and shoes once a day during treatment of tinea pedis
- To report to health care prescriber if infection persists or recurs; if blisters, burning, oozing, swelling occur
- To avoid alcohol because nausea, vomiting, hypertension may occur
- To use sunscreen or avoid direct sunlight to prevent photosensitivity
- To notify health care prescriber of sore throat, fever, skin rash, which may indicate overgrowth of organisms

TOPICAL ANTIINFECTIVES

azelaic acid (Rx)
(a-zuh-lay'ic)
Azelex, Finacen

bacitracin (OTC)
(bass-i-tray'sin)
Bacitin ♣, Bacitracin

clindamycin (Rx)
(klin-da-my'sin)
Cleocin T, Clindagel, ClindaMax, Clindets

erythromycin (Rx, OTC)
(er-ith-roe-mye'sin)
A/T/S, Akne-Mycin, Eryderm, Erygel, Erythromycin, Staticin, T-Stat

gentamicin (Rx)
(jen-ta-mye'sin)
Gentamicin

mafenide (Rx)
(ma′fe-nide)
Sulfamylon
metroNIDAZOLE (Rx)
(met-roh-nye′da-zole)
MetroGel, MetroCream, MetroLotion, Noritate
mupirocin (Rx)
(myoo-peer′oh-sin)
Bactroban
neomycin (OTC)
(nee-oh-mye′sin)
Neomycin Sulfate
nitrofurazone (Rx)
(nye-troe-fyoor′a-zone)
Furacin, Nitrofurazone
retapamulin (Rx)
(re-tap′a-mue′lin)
Altabax
salicylic acid (Rx)
(sal′i-sil′ik)
Salitop
silver sulfADIAZINE (Rx)
(sul-fa-dye′a-zeen)
Flamazine ✤, Silvadene, SSD, SSD AF, Thermazene
tretinoin (Rx)
(treh′tih-noyn)
Atralin

ACTION: Interferes with bacterial protein synthesis

USES: Skin infections, minor burns, wounds, skin grafts, primary pyodermas, otitis externa

CONTRAINDICATIONS: Hypersensitivity, large areas, burns, ulcerations
Precautions: Pregnancy (C), breastfeeding, impaired renal function, external ear or perforated eardrum

Administer:
- Enough medication to cover lesions completely
- After cleansing with soap, water before each application; dry well
- To less than 20% of body surface area when patient has impaired renal function

SIDE EFFECTS

INTEG: Rash, urticaria, scaling, redness

NURSING CONSIDERATIONS

Assess:
- Allergic reaction: burning, stinging, swelling, redness
- For signs of nephrotoxicity or ototoxicity

Perform/provide:
- Storage at room temperature in dry place

Evaluate:
- Therapeutic response: decrease in size, number of lesions

TOPICAL ANTIVIRALS

acyclovir (Rx)
(ay-sye′kloe-ver)
Zovirax
penciclovir (Rx)
(pen-sye′kloe-ver)
Denavir

ACTION: Interferes with viral DNA replication

USES: Simple mucocutaneous herpes simplex, in immunocompromised clients with initial herpes genitalis

CONTRAINDICATIONS: Hypersensitivity
Precautions: Pregnancy (C), breastfeeding

Administer:
- Using finger cot or rubber glove to prevent further infection

- Enough medication to cover lesions completely
- After cleansing with soap, water before each application; dry well

SIDE EFFECTS

INTEG: Rash, urticaria, stinging, burning, pruritus, vulvitis

NURSING CONSIDERATIONS

Assess:

- Allergic reaction: burning, stinging, swelling, redness, rash, vulvitis, pruritus

Perform/provide:

- Storage at room temperature in dry place

Evaluate:

- Therapeutic response: decrease in size, number of lesions

Teach patient/family:

- Not to use in eyes or when there is no evidence of infection
- To apply with glove to prevent further infection
- To avoid use of OTC creams, ointments, lotions unless directed by prescriber
- To use medical asepsis (hand washing) before, after each application and avoid contact with eyes
- To adhere strictly to prescribed regimen to maximize successful treatment outcome
- To begin taking product when symptoms arise

TOPICAL ANESTHETICS

benzocaine (OTC)
(ben′zoe-kane)
Americaine Anesthetic, Anbesol Maximum Strength, Baby Anbesol, Biozene, Boil-Ease, Children's Chloraseptic, Dermoplast, Foille, Foille Plus, Hurricaine, Lanacane, Medamint, Orabase, Oracin, Ora-Jel

dibucaine (OTC)
(dye′byoo-kane)
Dibucaine, Nupercainal

lidocaine (Rx, OTC)
(lye′doe-kane)
Anestacon, Burn-O-Jel, Derma Flex, Dentipatch, ELA-Max, Lidoderm, Numby Stuff, Solarcaine Aloe Extra Burn Relief, Xylocaine, Xylocaine 10% oral, Xylocaine Viscous, Zilactin-L

pramoxine (OTC)
(pra-mox′een)
Itch-X, PrameGel, Prax, Tronothane

tetracaine (Rx, OTC)
(tet′ra-cane)
Pontocaine, Viractin

ACTION: Inhibits conduction of nerve impulses from sensory nerves

USES: Oral irritation, sore throat, toothache, cold sore, canker sore, sunburn, minor cuts, insect bites, pain, itching

CONTRAINDICATIONS: Hypersensitivity, infants <1 yr, application to large areas

Precautions: Pregnancy (C), children <6 yr, sepsis, denuded skin

DOSAGE AND ROUTES

• **Adult and child: TOP** apply qid as needed; **RECT** insert tid and after each BM

SIDE EFFECTS

INTEG: Rash, irritation, sensitization

NURSING CONSIDERATIONS

Assess:

• Pain: location, duration, characteristics before and after administration

• For infection: redness, drainage, inflammation; this product should not be used until infection is treated

Perform/provide:

• Storage in tight, light-resistant container; do not freeze, puncture, or incinerate aerosol container

Evaluate:

• Therapeutic response: decreased redness, swelling, pain

Teach patient/family:

• To avoid contact with eyes

• Not to use for prolonged periods: use for <1 wk; if condition remains, prescriber should be contacted

TOPICAL MISCELLANEOUS

docosanol (OTC)

(doe-koe′san-ole)

Abreva

pimecrolimus (Rx)

(pim-eh-croh′lim-us)

Elidel

ACTION: Docosanol unknown; pimecrolimus may bind with macrophilin and inhibit calcium-dependent phosphatase

USES: Docosanol applied to fever blisters to promote more rapid healing; pimecrolimus used to treat mild to moderate atopic dermatitis in nonimmunocompromised patients ≥2 yr who are unresponsive to other treatment

CONTRAINDICATIONS: Hypersensitivity

Precautions: Pregnancy (C), breastfeeding, dermal infections

DOSAGE AND ROUTES

Docosanol

• **Adult: TOP** Rub into blisters 5×/day until healing occurs

Pimecrolimus

• **Adult and child ≥2 yr: TOP** Apply thin layer 2×/day and rub in, use as long as needed

Administer:

• To skin, rub in gently

SIDE EFFECTS

Pimecrolimus

INTEG: Burning

NURSING CONSIDERATIONS

Assess:

• Skin condition (color, pain, inflammation) before and after administration

• For signs and symptoms of skin infections (redness, draining lesions); if present, avoid use of product (pimecrolimus)

Evaluate:

• Therapeutic response: decreased inflammation, redness

Teach patient/family:

• To avoid contact between medication and eyes

• To discontinue use of product when condition clears

VAGINAL ANTIFUNGALS

butoconazole (OTC)
(byoo-toh-kone′ah-zole)
Femstat-3, Gynazol-1, Mycelex-3

clotrimazole (OTC)
(kloe-trye′ma-zole)
Canesten ♣, Clotrimazole, Gyne-Lotrimin 3, Gyne-Lotrimin 7, Mycelex 7, Myclo ♣

miconazole (OTC)
(mye-kon′a-zole)
Femizole-M, Monistat, Monistat 3, Monistat 7, Monistat Dual Pak, M-Zole 7 Dual Pack

nystatin (OTC)
(nye-stat′in)
Nystatin

terconazole (OTC)
(ter-kone′ah-zole)
Terazol 7, Terazol 3

tioconazole (OTC)
(tye-oh-kone′ah-zole)
Gyne-Trosyd ♣, Monistat 1, Vagistat-1

ACTION: Interferes with fungal DNA replication; binds sterols in fungal cell membranes, which increases permeability, leaking of nutrients

USES: Vaginal, vulval, vulvovaginal candidiasis (moniliasis)

CONTRAINDICATIONS: Hypersensitivity
Precautions: Pregnancy, breastfeeding, children <2 yr

DOSAGE AND ROUTES

Butoconazole
- **Adult: VAG** 5 g (1 applicator) at bedtime × 3-6 days

Clotrimazole
- **Adult:** 100 mg (1 vag tab, 100 mg) at bedtime × 1 wk, or 200 mg (2 vag tab, 100 mg) at bedtime × 3 nights, or 500 mg (1 vag tab, 500 mg); or 5 g (1 applicator) at bedtime × 1-2 wk

Miconazole
- **Adult:** 200 mg supp at bedtime × 3 days or 100 mg supp × 1 wk

Nystatin
- **Adult:** 100,000 units daily × 2 wk

Terconazole
- **Adult:** VAG 5 g (1 applicator) at bedtime × 7 days

Tioconazole
- **Adult:** 1 applicator at bedtime × 1 wk

Administer:
Topical route
- One full applicator every night high into the vagina
- Store at room temperature in dry place

SIDE EFFECTS

GU: Vulvovaginal burning, itching, pelvic cramps
INTEG: Rash, urticaria, stinging, burning
MISC: Headache, body pain

NURSING CONSIDERATIONS

Assess:
- For allergic reaction: burning, stinging, itching, discharge, soreness

Evaluate:
- Therapeutic outcome: decrease in itching or white discharge (vaginal)

Teach patient/family:
- About asepsis (hand washing) before, after each application
- To apply with applicator only; to avoid use of any other vaginal product unless directed by prescriber; sanitary napkin may prevent soiling of undergarments
- To abstain from sexual intercourse until treatment is completed; reinfection and irritation may occur
- To notify prescriber if symptoms persist

OTIC ANTIINFECTIVES

boric acid (OTTTC)
(bor'ik as'id)
Auro-Dri, Dri/Ear, Ear Dry

chloramphenicol (Rx)
(klor-am-fen'i-kole)
Chloromycetin Otic

ciprofloxacin (Rx)
Cetraxel

ACTION: Inhibits protein synthesis in susceptible microorganisms

USES: Ear infection (external), short-term use

CONTRAINDICATIONS: Hypersensitivity, perforated eardrum
Precautions: Pregnancy (C)

Administer:
- After removing impacted cerumen by irrigation
- After cleaning stopper with alcohol
- After restraining child if necessary
- After warming sol to body temp

SIDE EFFECTS

EENT: Itching, irritation in ear
INTEG: Rash, urticaria

NURSING CONSIDERATIONS

Assess:
- For redness, swelling, fever, pain in ear, which indicates superinfection

Evaluate:
- Therapeutic response: decreased ear pain

Teach patient/family:
- The correct method of instillation using aseptic technique, including not touching dropper to ear
- That dizziness may occur after instillation

Appendix C Vaccines and toxoids

GENERIC NAME	TRADE NAME	USES	DOSAGE AND ROUTES	CONTRAINDICATIONS
advenovirus vaccine		Prevention of advenovirus types 4/7	Adult ≤50 yr/adolescent ≥17 yr in the military PO 1 tab of each 4/7 or a single dose	Pregnancy
avian influenza A (H5N1) virus vaccine		Prophylaxis	Adult: IM 1 ml (90 mcg) 2 doses, 28 days apart	IV
anthrax vaccine	BioThrax	Pre-/postexposure prophylaxis	**Preexposure** Adult: SUBCUT 0.5 ml at 0, 2, 4 wk, then 0.5 ml at 6, 12, 18 mo **Postexposure** Adult: SUBCUT 0.5 ml 0, 2, 4 wk, with antibiotics	Hypersensitivity
BCG vaccine	TICE BCG	TB exposure	Adult and child >1 mo: 0.2-0.3 ml Child <1 mo: Reduce dose by 50% using 2 ml of sterile water after reconstituting	Hypersensitivity, hypogamma-globulinemia, positive TB test, burns
cholera vaccine	No trade name	Immunization for cholera outside the United States	Adult and child >10 yr: IM/SUBCUT 2× of 0.5 ml, 7-30 days before traveling to cholera areas Booster is used q6mo 0.5 ml prn	Hypersensitivity, acute febrile illness
diphtheria and tetanus toxoids, adsorbed	No trade name	Induces antitoxins to provide immunity to diphtheria and tetanus	Adult and child ≥7 yr: IM (adult strength) 0.5 ml q4-8wk × 2 doses, then 3rd dose 6-12 mo after 2nd dose, booster IM 0.5 ml q10yr Child 1-6 yr: IM (pediatric strength) 0.5 ml q4wk × 2 doses, booster 6-12 mo after 2nd dose Infant 6 wk-1 yr: IM (pediatric strength) 0.5 ml q4wk × 3 doses, booster 6-12 mo after 3rd dose	Hypersensitivity to mercury, thimerosal; immunocompromised patients; radiation; corticosteroids; acute illness
diphtheria and tetanus toxoids and whole-cell pertussis vaccine (DPT, DTP)	DTwP, Tr-Immunol	Prevention of diphtheria, tetanus, pertussis	Doses vary Check product information	Hypersensitivity, active infection, poliomyelitis outbreak, immunosuppression, febrile illness

diphtheria and tetanus toxoids and acellular pertussis vaccine	Adacel, Boostrix, Daptacel, Infranrix, Tripedia			
diphtheria, tetanus, pertussis, haemophilus, polio IPV	Pentacel	Immunity to diphtheria, tetanus, pertussis, haemophilus, polio IPV	Infant >6 wk and child ≤5 yr: IM 0.5 ml at 2, 4, 6, and 15-18 mo	Hypersensitivity, polio outbreak, acute infection, immunosuppression
diphtheria, tetanus, pertussis, polio vaccine IPV	Kinrix	Immunity to diphtheria, tetanus, pertussis, polio vaccine IPV	Child: IM 0.5 ml	Hypersensitivity, polio outbreak, acute infection, immunosuppression
H1N1 influenza A (swine flu) virus vaccine	Influenza A (H1N1)	Immunity to H1N1	Adult <50 yr, adolescent, child ≥2 yr: Intranasal 1 dose (roughly 0.1 ml) into each nostril; child 2-9 repeat dose ≥4 wk later Adult, adolescent, child ≥3 yr: IM 0.5 ml as a single dose; child 3-9 yr repeat dose ≥4 wk later (Sanofi) (CSL); child 4-9 yr repeat dose ≥4 wk later (Novartis); infants ≥6 mo-child <36 mo: IM 0.25 ml, repeat in 4 wk (Sanofi) Adult: IM 0.5 ml as a single dose (GSK)	
haemophilus b conjugate vaccine, diphtheria CRM_{197} protein conjugate (HbOC)	HibTITER	Polysaccharide immunization of children 2-6 yr against *H. influenzae* b, conjugate	**HibTITER (IM only)** Child: IM 0.5 ml Child 2-6 mo: 0.5 ml q2mo × 3 inj	Hypersensitivity, febrile illness, active infection
haemophilus b conjugate vaccine, meningococcal protein conjugate (PRP-OMP)	PedvaxHIB	Immunization of child 2, 4, 6 mo	Child 7-11 mo: Previously unvaccinated 0.5 ml q2mo inj Child 12-14 mo: Previously unvaccinated 0.5 ml × 1 inj **PedvaxHIB (IM only)** Child 2-14 mo: 0.5 ml × 2 inj at 2, 4 mo of age (6 mo dose not needed), then booster at 12-18 mo against invasive disease Child ≥15 mo: Previously unvaccinated 0.5 ml inj	

Continued

Appendix c Vaccines and toxoids—cont'd

GENERIC NAME	TRADE NAME	USES	DOSAGE AND ROUTES	CONTRAINDICATIONS
hepatitis A vaccine, inactivated	Havrix, VAQTA	Active immunization against hepatitis A virus	Adult: IM 1440 EL units (Havrix) or 50 units (VAQTA) as a single dose; booster dose is the same given at 6, 12 mo Child 2-18 yr: IM 720 EL units (Havrix) or 25 units (VAQTA) as a single dose, booster dose is the same given at 6, 12 mo	Hypersensitivity
hepatitis B vaccine, recombinant	Engerix-B, Recombivax HB	Immunization against all subtypes of hepatitis B virus	Varies widely	Hypersensitivity to this vaccine or yeast
herpes zoster virus vaccine	Zostavax	Prevention of herpes zoster	Adult $\geq$60 yr: SUBCUT 0.65 ml	$<$60 yr, child, infant, AIDS, IM/IV, leukemia, lymphoma, pregnancy
human papillomavirus recombinant vaccine, quadrivalent	Gardasil	Prevention of HPV types 6, 11, 16, 18, cervical cancer, genital warts, precancerous dysplasic lesions, anal cancer/anal intraepithelial neoplasia	Adult up to 26 yr and child >9 yr to 26 yr: IM give as 3 separate doses; 1st dose as elected; 2nd dose 2 mo after 1st dose; 3rd dose 6 mo after 1st dose	Child $<$9 yr, pregnancy, breastfeeding, geriatric, active disease, hypersensitivity
influenza virus vaccine	Afluria, FluMist, Fluogen, Flu-Shield, Fluviral*, Fluvirin, Fluzone, influenza virus vaccine, trivalent	Prevention of Russian, Chilean, Philippine influenza	Adult and child $>$12 yr: IM 0.5 ml in 1 dose Adult 18-64 yr: ID 0.1 ml as a single dose Child 3-12 yr: IM 0.5 ml, repeat in 1 mo (split) unless 1978-1985 vaccine was given; also given nasal Child 6 mo to 3 yr: IM 0.25 ml, repeat in 1 mo (split) unless 1978-1985 vaccine was given; also given nasal child $\leq$2 yr	Hypersensitivity, active infection, chicken egg allergy, Guillain-Barré syndrome, active neurologic disorders
Japanese encephalitis virus vaccine, inactivated	JE-VAX	Active immunity against Japanese encephalitis (JE)	Adult and child $\geq$3 yr: SUBCUT 1 ml, days 0, 7, 30; booster SUBCUT 1 ml 2 yr after last dose Child 1-3 yr: SUBCUT 0.5 ml, days 0, 7, 30; booster SUBCUT 0.5 ml 2 yr after last dose	Hypersensitivity to murine, thimerosal; allergic reactions to previous dose

Nurse Alert

Lyme disease vaccine (recombinant OspA)	LYMErix	Immunization against Lyme disease	Adult and adolescent 15-70 yr: IM 30 mcg in deltoid, repeat at 1, 12 mo after first dose	Hypersensitivity, antibiotic refractory Lyme arthritis
measles and rubella virus vaccine, live attenuated	M-R-Vax II	Immunity to measles and rubella by antibody production	Adult and child ≥15 mo: SUBCUT 0.5 ml (1000 units)	Hypersensitivity, immunocompromised patients, active untreated TB, cancer, blood dyscrasias, radiation, corticosteroids, pregnancy; allergic reactions to neomycin, eggs
measles, mumps, and rubella vaccine, live	M-M-R-II	Prevention of measles, mumps, rubella	Adult: SUBCUT 1 vial; 2 vials separated by 1 mo, in person born after 1957 Child >15 mo and adult: SUBCUT 0.5 ml	Hypersensitivity, blood dyscrasias, anemia, active infection, immunosuppression; egg, chicken allergy; pregnancy, febrile illness, neomycin allergy, neoplasms
measles, mumps, rubella, varicella	ProQuad	Immunity to measles, mumps, rubella, varicella	Child: SUBCUT 0.5 ml	Hypersensitivity to eggs, neomycin, cancer, radiation, corticosteroids, blood dyscrasias, active untreated TB
measles virus vaccine, live attenuated	Attenuvax	Immunity to measles by antibody production	Adult and child ≥15 mo: SUBCUT 0.5 ml (1000 units), 1 dose 15 mo, 2nd dose age 4-6 or 11, or 12	Hypersensitivity to eggs, neomycin; cancer, radiation, corticosteroids, pregnancy, immunocompromised patients, blood dyscrasias, active untreated TB
meningococcal diphtheria toxoid conjugate vaccine	Menomune, Menactra, Menveo	Prophylaxis to meningococcal meningitis/diphtheria	All doses are different; check product information	Latex hypersensitivity
meningococcal polysaccharide vaccine	Menomune-A/C/Y/W-135, Menactra	Prophylaxis to meningococcal meningitis	Adult and child >2 yr: SUBCUT 0.5 ml	Hypersensitivity to thimerosal, pregnancy, acute illness
mumps virus vaccine, live	Mumpsvax	Active immunity to mumps	Adult and child ≥1 yr: SUBCUT 0.5 ml (20,000 units)	Hypersensitivity to eggs, neomycin; cancer, radiation, corticosteroids, pregnancy, immunocompromised patients, blood dyscrasias, active untreated TB

*Canada only.

Continued

Appendix c Vaccines and toxoids—cont'd

GENERIC NAME	TRADE NAME	USES	DOSAGE AND ROUTES	CONTRAINDICATIONS
plague vaccine	No trade name	Active immunity to *Yersinia pestis* plague	Adult: IM 1 ml, then 0.2 ml in 4-12 wk, then 0.2 ml 5-6 mo after 2nd dose; booster 0.1-0.2 ml q6mo when in plague area	Hypersensitivity to phenol, sulfites, formaldehyde, beef, soy, casein; pregnancy, coagulation disorders
pneumococcal 7-valent conjugate vaccine	Prevnar	Immunity against *Streptococcus pneumoniae*	Child: IM 0.5 ml × 3 doses (7-11 mo); × 2 doses (12-23 mo); × 1 dose >2-9 yr	Hypersensitivity to diphtheria toxoid or this product
pneumococcal vaccine, polyvalent	Pneumovax 23, Pnu-Imune 23	Pneumococcal immunization	Adult and child >2 yr: IM/SUBCUT 0.5 ml	Hypersensitivity, Hodgkin's disease, ARDS
poliovirus vaccine, live, oral, trivalent (TOPV) poliovirus vaccine (IPV)	Orimune, IPOL	Prevention of polio	Adult and child >2 yr: PO 0.5 ml, given q8wk × 2 doses, then 0.5 ml 1/2-1 yr after dose 2 Infant: PO 0.5 ml at 2, 4, 18 mo; booster at 4-6 yr; may also be given: IPV at 2, 4 mo, then TOPV at 12-18 mo, booster at 4-6 yr	Hypersensitivity, active infection, allergy to neomycin/streptomycin, immunosuppression, vomiting, diarrhea
rabies vaccine, adsorbed	No trade name	Active immunity to rabies	**Preexposure** Adult and child: IM 1 ml day 0, 7, 21, or 28 days (total 3 doses); booster IM 1 ml prn q2-5yr **Postexposure** Adult and child not vaccinated: IM 20 international units/kg of human rabies immune globulin (HRIG), give 5 total doses of 1-ml inj of rabies vaccine on days 0, 3, 7, 14, 28	Severe hypersensitivity to previous inj of vaccine, thimerosol
rabies vaccine, human diploid cell (HDCV)	Imovax Rabies, Imovax Rabies I.D.	Active immunity to rabies	**Preexposure** Adult and child: IM 1 ml day 0, 7, 21, or 28 (total 4 doses) **Postexposure** Adult and child: IM 1 ml on day 0, 3, 7, 14, 28 (total 5 doses)	No contraindications

Nurse Alert

rotovirus	RotaTeq, Rotarix	Prevents rotovirus	Infant: PO 3 doses given between 6 and 32 wk of age; 1st dose between 6-12 wk of age; 2nd and 3rd doses q4-10wk	Hypersensitivity to this product or latex, immunocompromised, blood products given within 6 wk, lymphatic disorders
rubella and mumps virus vaccine, live	Biavax II	Immunity to rubella and mumps by antibody production	Adult and child ≥1 yr: SUBCUT 0.5 ml	Hypersensitivity to eggs, neomycin; cancer, radiation, corticosteroids, pregnancy, immunocompromised patients, blood dyscrasias, active untreated TB
rubella virus vaccine, live attenuated (RA 27/3)	Meruvax II	Immunity to rubella by antibody production	Adult and child ≥1 yr: SUBCUT 0.5 ml (1000 units)	Hypersensitivity to eggs, neomycin; cancer, radiation, corticosteroids
smallpox vaccine	ACAM 2000, Dry Vax	Prevention of smallpox	See package insert	No contraindications
tetanus toxoid, adsorbed/tetanus toxoid	No trade name	Tetanus toxoid: Used for prophylactic treatment of wounds	Adult and child: IM 0.5 ml q4-6wk × 2 doses, then 0.5 ml 1 yr after dose 2 (adsorbed); SUBCUT/IM 0.5 ml q4-8wk × 3 doses, then 0.5 ml $^1/_2$-1 yr after dose 3, booster dose 0.5 ml q10yr	Hypersensitivity, active infection, poliomyelitis outbreak, immunosuppression
typhoid vaccine, parenteral typhoid vaccine, oral	No trade name Vivotif Berna Vaccine	Active immunity to typhoid fever	Adult: PO 1 cap 1 hr before meals × 4 doses, booster q5yr Adult and child >10 yr: SUBCUT 0.5 ml, repeat in 4 wk, booster q3yr Child 6 mo-10 yr: SUBCUT 0.25 ml, repeat in 4 wk, booster q3yr	Parenteral: Systemic or allergic reaction, acute respiratory or other acute infection, intensive physical exercise in high temperatures Oral: Hypersensitivity, acute febrile illness, suppressive or antibiotic products
typhoid Vi polysaccharide vaccine	Typhim Vi	Active immunity to typhoid fever	Adult and child ≥2 yr: IM 0.5 ml as a single dose, reimmunize q2yr 0.5 ml IM, if needed	Hypersensitivity, chronic typhoid carriers
varicella virus vaccine	Varivax	Prevention of varicella-zoster (chickenpox)	Adult and child ≥13 yr: SUBCUT 0.5 ml, 2nd dose SUBCUT 0.5 ml 4-8 wk later	Hypersensitivity to neomycin; blood dyscrasias, immunosuppression, active untreated TB, acute illness, pregnancy, diseases of lymphatic system

Continued

Appendix c Vaccines and toxoids—cont'd

GENERIC NAME	TRADE NAME	USES	DOSAGE AND ROUTES	CONTRAINDICATIONS
yellow fever vaccine	YF-Vax	Active immunity to yellow fever	Adult and child ≥9 mo: SUBCUT 0.5 ml deeply, booster q10yr Child 6-9 mo: same as above if exposed	Hypersensitivity to egg or chicken embryo protein, pregnancy, child <6 mo, immunodeficiency
zoster vaccine, live	Zostavax	Herpes zoster prevention	Reconstitute immediately after removing from freezer; give SUBCUT as a single dose; inject total amount of single-dose vial	Immunosuppression; neomycin, gelatin allergy; children, TB, pregnancy (C)

Index

Entries can be identified as follows: DISEASES/DISORDERS, *DRUG CATEGORIES,* generic names, Trade Names.

Entries can be identified as follows: DISEASES/DISORDERS, *DRUG CATEGORIES,* generic names, Trade Names.

Entries can be identified as follows: DISEASES/DISORDERS, *DRUG CATEGORIES,* generic names, Trade Names.

Entries can be identified as follows: DISEASES/DISORDERS, *DRUG CATEGORIES,* generic names, Trade Names.

Entries can be identified as follows: DISEASES/DISORDERS, *DRUG CATEGORIES*, generic names, Trade Names.

D

Entries can be identified as follows: DISEASES/DISORDERS, *DRUG CATEGORIES,* generic names, Trade Names.

Entries can be identified as follows: DISEASES/DISORDERS, *DRUG CATEGORIES,* generic names, Trade Names.

Entries can be identified as follows: DISEASES/DISORDERS, *DRUG CATEGORIES,* generic names, Trade Names.

Entries can be identified as follows: DISEASES/DISORDERS, *DRUG CATEGORIES*, generic names, Trade Names.

J

Entries can be identified as follows: DISEASES/DISORDERS, *DRUG CATEGORIES,* generic names, Trade Names.

Entries can be identified as follows: DISEASES/DISORDERS, *DRUG CATEGORIES*, generic names, Trade Names.

Entries can be identified as follows: DISEASES/DISORDERS, *DRUG CATEGORIES*, generic names, Trade Names.

Entries can be identified as follows: DISEASES/DISORDERS, *DRUG CATEGORIES,* generic names, Trade Names.

Entries can be identified as follows: DISEASES/DISORDERS, *DRUG CATEGORIES,* generic names, Trade Names.

Entries can be identified as follows: DISEASES/DISORDERS, *DRUG CATEGORIES,* generic names, Trade Names.

Entries can be identified as follows: DISEASES/DISORDERS, *DRUG CATEGORIES,* generic names, Trade Names.

Entries can be identified as follows: DISEASES/DISORDERS, *DRUG CATEGORIES*, generic names, Trade Names.

Entries can be identified as follows: DISEASES/DISORDERS, *DRUG CATEGORIES,* generic names, Trade Names.

Formulas

Surface area rule:

$$\text{Child dose} = \frac{\text{Surface area (m}^2\text{)}}{1.73\ \text{m}^2} \times \text{Adult dose}$$

Calculating strength of a solution:

Solution Strength: *Desired Solution*:

$$\frac{x}{100} = \frac{\text{Amount of drug desired}}{\text{Amount of finished solutio}}$$

Calculating flow rate for IV:

$$\text{Rate of flow} = \frac{\text{Amount of fluid} \times \text{Administration set calibration}}{\text{Running time}}$$

$$\frac{x}{1} = \frac{\text{(ml) (gtt/min)}}{\text{min}}$$

Calculation of medication dosages:

Formula method:

$$\frac{\text{Amount ordered}}{\text{Amount on hand}} \times \text{Vehicle} = \text{Number of tablets, capsules, or amount of liquid}$$

Vehicle is the drug form or amount of liquid containing the dosage. Amounts used in calculation by formula must be in same system.

Ratio–proportion method:

1 tablet:tablet in mg on hand::*x* tablet order in mg

Know or have::Want to know or order

Multiply means and extremes, divide both sides by known amount to get *x*. Amounts used in equation must be in same system.

Dimensional analysis method:

$$\text{Order in mg} \times \frac{\text{1 tablet or capsule}}{\text{What 1 tablet or capsule is in mg}} = \text{Tablets or capsules to be given}$$

If amounts are in different systems:

$$\text{Order in mg} \times \frac{\text{1 tablet or capsule}}{\text{What 1 tablet or capsule is in g}} \times \frac{1}{1000\ \text{mg}} = \text{Tablets or capsules to be given}$$

Temperature conversion:

$F = C \times 9/5 + 32$

$C = 5/9\ (F - 32)$

Nomogram for calculation of body surface area

Place a straight edge from the patient's height in the left column to the patient's weight in the right column. The point of intersection on the body surface area column indicates the body surface area (BSA). (Reproduced in Behrman RE, Kliegman RM, Jenson HB: *Nelson textbook of pediatrics,* ed 18, Philadelphia, 2007, WB Saunders; Nomogram modified from data of E. Boyd by CD West.)

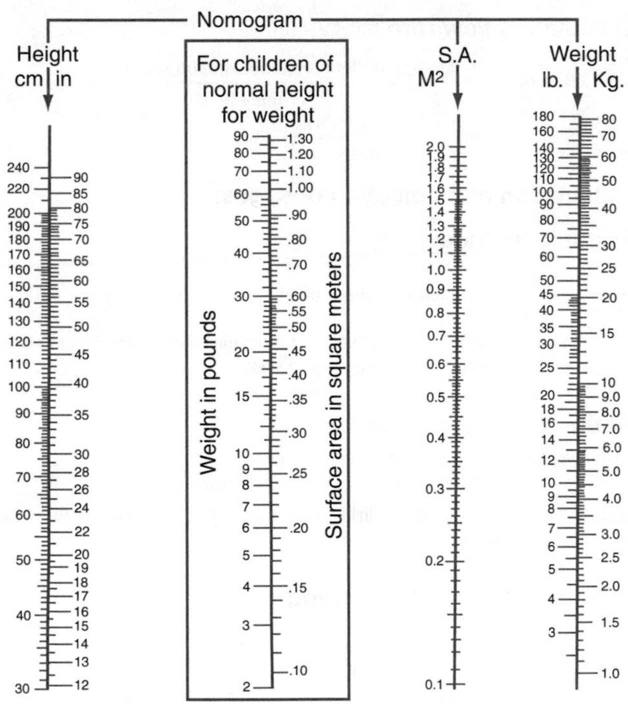

Alternative (Mosteller's formula):

$$\text{Surface area (m}^2\text{)} = \sqrt{\frac{\text{Height (cm)} \times \text{Weight (kg)}}{3600}}$$

Antitoxins and antivenins

GENERIC NAME	TRADE NAME	USES	DOSAGE AND ROUTES	CONTRAINDICATIONS
Black widow spider antivenin *(Lactrodectus mactans)*	No trade name	Black widow spider bite	Adult and child: IM 2.5 ml, 2nd dose may be given if severe; give in anterolateral thigh, obtain test for sensitivity before inj	Hypersensitivity to this product or horse serum
Crotalidae antivenom, polyvalent	No trade name	Rattlesnake bite	Adult and child: IV 20-150 ml depending on seriousness of bite, may give additional doses based on response	Hypersensitivity
Diphtheria antitoxin, equine	No trade name	Diphtheria	Adult and child: IM/slow IV 20,000-120,000 units, may give additional doses after 24 hr	Hypersensitivity
Micrurus fulvius antivenin	No trade name	East/Texas coral snake bite	Adult and child: IV 30-50 ml, give through running IV line of normal saline, give 1st 1-2 ml over 4-5 min, watch for allergic reaction	Hypersensitivity
Scorpion antivenin (centruroides sculpturatus equine)	Anascorp	Scorpion stings	Adult and child: IV 3 vial/50 ml NS given over 10 min, may give other doses 1 vial/50 ml NS over 10 min q30-60min	N/A

Abbreviations

ABG arterial blood gas
ADA American Diabetes Association
ADH antidiuretic hormone
ALT alanine aminotransferase
ANA antinuclear antibody
APLA antiphospholipid antibody syndrome
APTT activated partial thromboplastin time
ASA acetylsalicylic acid, aspirin
AST aspartate aminotransferase (SGOT)
AV atrioventricular
bid twice a day
BPH benign prostatic hypertrophy
BPM beats per minute
BUN blood urea nitrogen
CAD coronary artery disease
CBC complete blood cell count
CCr creatinine clearance
CHF congestive heart failure
CNS central nervous system
CONT continuous
COPD chronic obstructive pulmonary disease
CPAP continuous positive airway pressure
CPK creatine phosphokinase
CPS carbamoyl phosphate synthetase
C&S culture and sensitivity
CSF cerebrospinal fluid
CTCL cutaneous T-cell lymphoma
CV cardiovascular
CVA cerebrovascular accident
CVP central venous pressure
D&C dilatation and curettage
DIC diffuse intravascular coagulation
DIR INF direct infusion
D_5W 5% glucose in distilled water
DVT deep vein thrombosis
ECG electrocardiogram (EKG)
EDTA ethylenediamine tetraacetic acid
EEG electroencephalogram
EPS extrapyramidal symptom
ESR erythrocyte sedimentation rate
EXT REL extended release
FBS fasting blood sugar
FHT fetal heart tones
FSH follicle-stimulating hormone
GABA γ-aminobutyric acid
GPC giant papillary conjunctivitis
gr grain
GT glucose tolerance test
GU genitourinary
GVHD graft-versus-host disease
H_2 histamine$_2$
hCG human chorionic gonadotropin
Hct hematocrit
HDCV human diploid cell rabies vaccine
Hgb hemoglobin
H & H hematocrit and hemoglobin
5-HIAA 5-hydroxyindoleacetic acid
HIV human immunodeficiency virus (AIDS)
HR heart rate
IBD inflammatory bowel disease
IC intracardiac
ICP intracranial pressure
ID intradermal
IgG immunoglobulin G
IM intramuscular
INF infusion
INH inhalation
inj injection
I&O intake and output
INT intermittent
IPPB intermittent positive-pressure breathing
IT intrathecal
ITP idiopathic thrombocytopenic purpura
IUD intrauterine device
IV intravenous
IVP intravenous pyelogram
K potassium
LDH lactic dehydrogenase
LE lupus erythematosus
LFT liver function test
LH luteinizing hormone
LOC level of consciousness
LR lactated Ringer's solution
LT leukotriene
m minim
m^2 square meter
MAC monitored anesthesia care
MAOI monoamine oxidase inhibitor
mcg microgram
mEq milliequivalent
mg milligram
MI myocardial infarction
ml milliliter